FRACTURES AND DISLOCATIONS

This book is dedicated
to the memory of
JACK STEVENS

FRACTURES AND DISLOCATIONS

PRINCIPLES OF MANAGEMENT

———— * ————

EDITED BY

PAUL J. GREGG
MD, FRCS

Professor of Orthopaedic Surgery, School of Medicine
University of Leicester

JACK STEVENS
MA, MD, FRCS, FACS

Emeritus Professor of Orthopaedic Surgery
University of Newcastle upon Tyne

PETER H. WORLOCK
DM, FRCS

Consultant Trauma and Orthopaedic Surgeon,
Trauma Service, John Radcliffe Hospital, Oxford

FOREWORD BY

DAVID L. HAMBLEN

b

Blackwell
Science

DISTRIBUTORS

Marston Book Services Ltd
PO Box 87
Oxford OX2 0DT
(*Orders*: Tel: 01865 791155
        Fax: 01865 791927
        Telex: 837515)

North America
  Blackwell Science, Inc.
  238 Main Street
  Cambridge, MA 02142
  (*Orders*: Tel: 800 215-1000
           617 876-7000
           Fax: 617 492-5263)

Australia
  Blackwell Science Pty Ltd
  54 University Street
  Carlton, Victoria 3053
  (*Orders*: Tel: 03 9347-0300
          Fax: 03 9349-3016)

A catalogue record for this title
is available from the British Library

ISBN 0-632-02303-1

Library of Congress
Cataloging-in-Publication Data

Fractures and dislocations:
principles of management/edited by
  Paul J. Gregg, Jack Stevens,
  Peter H. Worlock: foreword by David L.
  Hamblen.
      p.   cm.
    Includes bibliographical references
    and index.
    ISBN 0-632-02303-1
    1. Fractures.   2. Dislocations.
    I. Gregg, Paul J.   II. Stevens. Jack G.
    III. Worlock, Peter H.
    [DNLM: 1. Fractures — rehabilitation.
  2. Wounds and Injuries — rehabilitation.
  3. Dislocations — rehabilitation.
  WE 175 F79815   1996]
  RD101.F7373   1996
  617.1'5 — dc20
  DNLM/DLC
  for Library of Congress   95-36765
                                        CIP

Contents

List of Contributors, vii

Foreword, xi

Preface, xiii

Part 1: General Principles

1 Biomechanics of Fractures, 3
J.L. Cunningham and J. Kenwright

2 Terminology, Description and Classification, 29
O.O.A. Oni and P.J. Gregg

3 Clinical Features including First Examination
and Detection of Complications, 37
J. Stevens

4 Radiology of Fractures and Dislocations, 43
D.B.L. Finlay

5 The Healing of Injury, 71
Basics of Fracture Healing, 71
A.J. Malcolm
Articular Cartilage, 79
S.B. Trippel and H.J. Mankin
Tendons and Ligaments, 86
G. Hooper

6 Systemic Response to Injury, 91
J.C. Stoddart

7 Early Management, 105
Resuscitation and Multiple Injuries, 105
D.D. Milne
Trauma Scoring, 112
P.H. Worlock
Abdominal Trauma, 114
D.D. Milne

Head Injuries, 126
R.M. Kalbag
Chest Injuries, 139
J.C. Stoddart
Genitourinary Tract Injuries, 149
J.P. Mitchell

8 Definitive Treatment of Fractures and
Dislocations, 167
General Principles, Available Methods and
Methods of Selection, 167
O.O.A. Oni and P.J. Gregg
Anaesthesia, 188
G. Smith
The Tourniquet, 202
L. Klenerman

9 Management of Open Fractures, 207
The Principles of Internal and External
Fixation, 207
R.J. Langstaff, P.H. Worlock and J.K. Webb
Skin Cover, 220
M.J.M. Black

10 Fractures in Children, 237
I.H. Thomas

11 Complications, 249
Classification, 249
P.J. Gregg
Vascular Complications, 250
S.D. Parvin and P.R.F. Bell
Nerve Injuries, 263
I.J. Leslie
Compartment Syndromes, 271
M.J. Allen and M.R. Barnes
Fat Embolism and the Fat Embolism
Syndrome, 283
J.C. Stoddart

Venous Thromboembolism, 286
P.D. Triffitt
Tetanus, 292
J.C. Stoddart
Gas Gangrene, 297
P.J. Gregg
Adult Respiratory Distress Syndrome, 298
J.C. Stoddart
Delayed Union, Non-Union and Infected Non-Union, 302
O.O.A. Oni, P.H. Worlock and P.J. Gregg
Post-Traumatic Reflex Sympathetic Dystrophy, 318
D.P. Conlan
Avascular Necrosis, 322
P.J. Gregg

Part 2: Specific Injuries by Region

12 The Shoulder, 331
Introduction, 331
P.G. Stableforth
Clavicle, 332
H.K. Kalyan and W.A. Wallace
Acromio-clavicular Joint, 353
J.J. Dias and P.J. Gregg
Sternoclavicular Joint, 360
W.A. Wallace
Gleno-humeral Joint, 367
W.A. Wallace and G.H. El-Sobhi
Proximal Humerus, 386
P.G. Stableforth and W.A. Wallace
Rotator Cuff, 396
P.G. Stableforth
Scapula, 397
P.G. Stableforth

13 The Arm, 401
I.H. Thomas

14 The Elbow, 413
R. Hornby

15 The Forearm, 435
A.J. Carr and P.H. Worlock

16 The Wrist, 447
G. Hooper, J.J. Dias and P.J. Gregg

17 The Hand, 495
P.D. Burge

18 The Spine, 551
Cervical Spine, 551
T. McSweeney
Thoracic and Lumbar Spine, 597
D.K. Evans

19 The Pelvis and Acetabulum, 617
P.H. Worlock and M. Tile

20 The Hip Joint, 631
Dislocations and Fracture–Dislocations, 631
D.J. Wood and J. Stevens
Proximal Femoral Fractures, 637
D.J. Wood and J. Stevens
Extracapsular Fractures (Fractures in the Trochanteric Region), 664
R. Hornby

21 The Thigh, 693
A.T. Cross and B.F. Meggitt

22 The Knee, 759
M.L. Harding

23 The Leg, 783
Upper Tibial Metaphyseal Fractures, 783
J.R.W. Hardy
Tibial and Fibular Diaphyseal Fractures, 790
J.K. Webb and J.R.W. Hardy

24 The Ankle, 823
A.H.R.W. Simpson and P.H. Worlock

25 The Foot, 833
Os Calcis, 833
P.D. Triffitt and P.J. Gregg
Talus, Navicular, Metatarsals and Phalanges, 850
H.P.J. Walsh and L. Klenerman

26 Pathological Fractures, 889
C.S.B. Galasko

Index, 909

Colour plate falls between pp. 98 and 99

List of Contributors

MICHAEL J. ALLEN MB BS, FRCS, *Sports Injury Consultant, Department of Sports Medicine, Leicester General Hospital NHS Trust, Gwendolen Road, Leicester LE5 4PW*

MICHAEL R. BARNES Bsc, *Clinical Scientist, Department of Sports Medicine, Leicester General Hospital NHS Trust, Gwendolen Road, Leicester LE5 4PW*

PETER R.F. BELL MD, FRCS, *Professor of Surgery, School of Medicine, University of Leicester, Department of Surgery, Clinical Sciences Building, Leicester Royal Infirmary NHS Trust, PO Box 65, Leicester LE2 7LX*

MICHAEL J.M. BLACK MB BS, FRCS, *Consultant Plastic Surgeon, Royal Victoria Infirmary and Associated Hospitals NHS Trust, Queen Victoria Road, Newcastle upon Tyne NE1 4LP*

PETER D. BURGE FRCS, *Consultant Hand Surgeon, Nuffield Orthopaedic Centre; Clinical Lecturer in Orthopaedic Surgery, University of Oxford; John Radcliffe Hospital and Nuffield Orthopaedic Centre, Headington, Oxford OX3 7LD*

ANDREW J. CARR MA, ChM, FRCS, *Consultant Orthopaedic Surgeon, Shoulder and Elbow Service, Nuffield Orthopaedic Centre; Clinical Lecturer in Orthopaedic Surgery, University of Oxford; Nuffield Orthopaedic Centre, Headington, Oxford OX3 7LD*

DAVID P. CONLAN BSc, FRCS, FRCS(Ed), *Consultant in Trauma and Paediatric Orthopaedics, Addenbrooke's Hospital NHS Trust, Hills Road, Cambridge CB2 2QQ*

ANTHONY T. CROSS MB BS, FRCS, *Consultant Orthopaedic Surgeon, City Hospitals, Sunderland; The Old Vicarage, Tudhoe Village, Spennymoor, Co. Durham DL16 6JY*

JAMES L. CUNNINGHAM BSc, PhD, CEng, MIMechE, MBES, *Senior Lecturer in Biomedical Engineering, Department of Orthopaedic Surgery, University of Bristol, Bristol Royal Infirmary, Bristol BS2 8HW*

JOSEPH J. DIAS MD, FRCS(Ed), *Consultant Orthopaedic Surgeon, The Glenfield Hospital NHS Trust, Groby Road, Leicester LE3 9QP*

GAMAL H. EL-SOBHI MD, *Lecturer in Orthopaedic Surgery and Consultant Orthopaedic Surgeon, Shoubra Hospital, 1 Arab El-Tawaila Street, Ezbet El-Nachl, Cairo, Egypt*

DAVID K. EVANS MB BS, FRCS(Eng), *Emeritus Consultant Orthopaedic Surgeon, Sheffield Area Health Authority; Townhead House, Parwich, Near Ashbourne, Derbyshire DE6 1QF*

DAVID B.L. FINLAY FRCP(Ed), FRCR, *Consultant Radiologist, Leicester Royal Infirmary NHS Trust, Leicester LE1 5WW*

CHARLES S.B. GALASKO MSc, ChM, FRCS(Eng), FRCS(Ed), *Professor of Orthopaedic Surgery, University of Manchester; Department of Orthopaedic Surgery, Clinical Sciences Building, Hope Hospital, Eccles Old Road, Salford, Lancashire M6 8HD*

PAUL J. GREGG MD, FRCS, *Professor of Orthopaedic Surgery, School of Medicine, University of Leicester; University Department of Orthopaedic Surgery, Clinical Sciences, The Glenfield Hospital NHS Trust, Groby Road, Leicester LE3 9QP*

MICHAEL L. HARDING MS, FRCS, *Consultant Orthopaedic Surgeon, Leicester General Hospital NHS Trust, Gwendolen Road, Leicester LE5 4PW*

JOHN R.W. HARDY BSc, MB BS, FRCS(Ed), FRCS(Eng), *Lecturer in Orthopaedic Surgery, School of Medicine, University of Leicester; University Department of Orthopaedic Surgery, Clinical Sciences, The Glenfield Hospital NHS Trust, Groby Road, Leicester LE3 9QP*

DAVID L. HAMBLEN PhD, FRCS, *Head, Department of Orthopaedic Surgery, Western Infirmary, Glasgow G11 6NT*

GEOFFREY HOOPER MB ChB, MMSc, FRCS(Eng), FRCS(Ed)(Orth), *Consultant Orthopaedic Surgeon, Lothian Health Board; Honorary Senior Lecturer in Orthopaedic Surgery, University of Edinburgh; Princess Margaret Rose Orthopaedic Hospital, Fairmilehead, Edinburgh EH10 7ED*

ROGER HORNBY MB ChB, MD, FRCS(C), FRCS(E), *Consultant Orthopaedic Surgeon, Department of Orthopaedic Surgery, Royal Victoria Infirmary and Associated Hospitals NHS Trust, Queen Victoria Road, Newcastle upon Tyne NE1 4LP*

RAMANAND M. KALBAG BSc, MB BS, FRCS, *Emeritus Consultant Neurosurgeon, Newcastle General Hospital; 3 Towers Avenue, Newcastle upon Tyne NE2 3QE*

HEMANT K. KALYAN MB BS, MS(Orth), DOrtho, FCPS, DSports Med(Ed), *Staff Orthopaedic Surgeon and Sports Medicine Consultant, Lakeside Medical Center and Hospital, 33/4 Meanee Avenue (Tank Road), Bangalore 560 042, India*

JOHN KENWRIGHT BM, BCh, MA, MD(Stockholm), FRCS, *Nuffield Professor of Orthopaedic Surgery, Oxford University; Nuffield Orthopaedic Centre, Headington, Oxford OX3 7LD*

LESLIE KLENERMAN ChM, FRCS(Eng), FRCS(Ed), *Professor and Head of Department of Orthopaedic and Accident Surgery, Department of Orthopaedic and Accident Surgery, Royal Liverpool University Hospital, PO Box 147, Liverpool L69 3BX*

RONALD J. LANGSTAFF MA, FRCS(Ed), *Consultant Orthopaedic Surgeon, Hillingdon Hospital, Uxbridge, Middlesex UB8 3NN*

IAN J. LESLIE MCh(Orth), FRCS, *Consultant in Trauma and Orthopaedic Surgery, Bristol Royal Infirmary; Honorary Senior Lecturer in Orthopaedic Surgery, University of Bristol, Bristol Royal Infirmary, Bristol BS2 8HW*

TERENCE McSWEENEY MB BCh, BAO(NUI), MCH, MCh(Orth), FRCS(Eng), FACS, *Emeritus Consultant, Traumatic and Orthopaedic Surgeon, The Robert Jones and Agnes Hunt Orthopaedic Hospital, Oswestry, Shropshire; 127 Crewe Road, Nantwich, Cheshire CW5 6JW*

ARCHIE J. MALCOLM MB ChB, FRCPath, *Reader and Consultant in Pathology, University Department of Pathology, Royal Victoria Infirmary and Associated Hospitals NHS Trust, Queen Victoria Road, Newcastle upon Tyne NE1 4LP*

HENRY J. MANKIN MD, *Edith M. Ashley Professor of Orthopaedic Surgery, Harvard Medical School; Chief of the Orthopaedic Service, Massachusetts General Hospital, Massachusetts General Hospital, 32 Fruit Street, GRB 606, Boston, Massachusetts 02114-2698, USA*

BERNARD F. MEGGITT MA, FRCS, *Consultant Orthopaedic Trauma Surgeon, Addenbrooke's Hospital NHS Trust, Hills Road, Cambridge CB2 2QQ*

DAVID D. MILNE MB ChB, FRCS, *Consultant Trauma Surgeon, Department of Surgery, Newcastle General Hospital, Westgate Road, Newcastle upon Tyne NE1 4LP*

JOHN P. MITCHELL CBE, TD, MS, FRCS(Ed), FRCS, *Honorary Professor of Surgery (Urology), University of Bristol; Emeritus Consultant, United Bristol Hospitals; Abbey Cottage, Parry's Close, Bristol BS9 1AW*

OLUSOLA O.A. ONI Msc, MD, FRCS, FWACS, FMCS, *Consultant Orthopaedic Surgeon, The Glenfield Hospital NHS Trust, Groby Road, Leicester LE3 9QP*

SIMON D. PARVIN MD, FRCS, *Consultant Vascular Surgeon, Royal Bournemouth Hospital, Castle Lane East, Bournemouth, Dorset BH7 7DW*

A.H.R.W. SIMPSON MA(Cantab), BCh, FRCS, DM(Oxon), *Clinical Reader in Orthopaedic Surgery, University of Oxford; Nuffield Department of Orthopaedic Surgery, Nuffield Orthopaedic Centre, Headington, Oxford OX3 7LD*

GRAHAM SMITH BSc, MD, FRCA, *Professor of Anaesthesia and Head of Department, University Department of Anaesthesia, Leicester Royal Infirmary NHS Trust, Leicester LE1 5WW*

PAUL G. STABLEFORTH MB, FRCS, *Consultant Trauma and Orthopaedic Surgeon, Bristol Royal Infirmary, Bristol BS2 8HW*

JACK STEVENS MA, MD, FRCS, FACS, *(Deceased) Emeritus Professor of Orthopaedic Surgery, University of Newcastle upon Tyne; 29 Woolsington Park South, Newcastle upon Tyne NE13 8BJ*

JOSEPH C. STODDART MD, FRCA, FRCP, *Consultant Emeritus in Anaesthesia and Intensive Therapy, Royal Victoria Infirmary and Associated Hospitals NHS Trust, Queen Victoria Road, Newcastle upon Tyne NE1 4LP*

I. HUW THOMAS MD, FRCS(Ed), *Consultant Orthopaedic Surgeon, The Glenfield Hospital NHS Trust, Groby Road, Leicester LE3 9QP*

MARVIN TILE MD, BSc(Med), FRCS(C), *Professor of Surgery, University of Toronto; Surgeon-in-Chief, Sunnybrook Health Science Centre, 2075 Bayview Avenue, Room A333, Toronto, Ontario, Canada M4N 3M5*

PAUL D. TRIFFITT MA, MD, FRCS, *Senior Lecturer in Orthopaedic Surgery, School of Medicine, University of Leicester; Department of Orthopaedic Surgery, Clinical Sciences, The Glenfield Hospital NHS Trust, Groby Road, Leicester LE3 9QP*

STEPHEN B. TRIPPEL MD, *Assistant Professor of Orthopaedic Surgery, Harvard Medical School; Assistant Orthopaedic Surgeon, Massachusetts General Hospital, Department of Orthopaedic Surgery, 32 Fruit Street, GRB 606, Boston, Massachusetts 02114-2698, USA*

W. ANGUS WALLACE MB ChB, FRCS(Ed), FRCS(Ed)(Orth), *Head, The University Department of Orthopaedic and Accident Surgery, University Hospital Queen's Medical Centre, Nottingham NG7 2UH*

HENRY P.J. WALSH MChOrth, FRCS, *Consultant Orthopaedic Surgeon, Alder Hey and Fazakerly Hospitals, Liverpool; Alder Hey Childrens Hospital, Eaton Road, Liverpool L12 2AP*

JOHN K. WEBB FRCS, *Consultant Spine Surgeon, Centre for Spinal Studies and Surgery, Queen's Medical Centre, Nottingham NG13 8BP*

DAVID J. WOOD BSc, MB BS, MS(Lond), FRCS, *Professor of Orthopaedic Surgery, University of Western Australia, Nedlands, Perth, Australia 6009*

PETER H. WORLOCK DM, FRCS, *Consultant Trauma and Orthopaedic Surgeon, Trauma Service, John Radcliffe Hospital, Oxford OX3 9DU*

Foreword

Injuries of the musculo-skeletal system form a major and increasing part of the practice of most orthopaedic surgeons. Despite this, the number of advanced textbooks dealing with these important and common problems are surprisingly few. This may reflect a loss of interest in trauma management, which occurred about ten years ago at the time of major advances in elective orthopaedic surgery, particularly in the field of joint replacement. Fortunately this trend has reversed as a new generation of young orthopaedic surgeons has begun to apply the expanding knowledge from applied basic sciences to the care of the injured. These applications range from an improved understanding of the complex disturbances of physiology and metabolism which occur in the polytraumatized patient, to the use of molecular biology techniques for the development of bone morphogenic proteins to stimulate fracture healing in delayed and non-union.

It is therefore timely for the appearance of a new textbook of orthopaedic trauma care based on scientific principles. In the era of Watson-Jones and Bohler, one man could encompass the range of knowledge and opinions necessary to write such a textbook. The complexity of the subject and the rapid advances in knowledge now demands a team approach, as does the care of the patient with multiple injuries! The Editors have gathered an impressive team of contributors to present a logical and co-ordinated approach to all aspects of the subject. The systematic approach to each tissue, region, and type of injury should make it easy for the readers to find the information they need to diagnose and treat the individual patient and their problem.

The traditional British approach to the care of the injured has been based on the so-called 'conservative' treatment of fractures. In this volume the Editors have been able to combine this philosophy with the best aspects of the more aggressive surgical treatment of skeletal injuries pioneered by the European surgeons and developed to a high level in the North American Trauma Centres. This balanced approach should prove of value to both the surgeon-in-training and the established specialist in selecting the most appropriate method of treatment for each individual patient.

The management of trauma, including the treatment of skeletal injuries and their complications, is now recognized as one of the priority areas in health care worldwide. The cost of inadequate treatment is high in terms of increased morbidity and mortality in this relatively young patient group. I hope that this new book will help to improve the standards of care we can offer these patients and ensure their rapid rehabilitation to full social and economic activity.

DAVID L. HAMBLEN
Glasgow

Preface

There are very few large textbooks on the management of fractures and joint injuries in adults on the market at the present time. Such books which do currently exist are either extensive reference books, are largely written by orthopaedic surgeons outside the United Kingdom or are significantly out of date. The purpose of this new textbook is to present, in one volume, up to date principles of management of bone and joint injuries in adults suitable for those surgeons embarking on higher surgical training in orthopaedic and traumatic surgery. It is not intended that this is a reference book nor that it is completely comprehensive. Rather, it sets out the principles of management of fractures and joint injuries upon which the trainee can build, with increasing experience, by reference to more specialized texts and published scientific papers. It is hoped that this textbook will provide a sound basis of knowledge for those who now have to sit the FRCS Orthopaedic Examination.

The editors have selected contributors who are, for the most part, from the United Kingdom and are currently active and experienced in the management of orthopaedic trauma.

The textbook is divided into two parts. Part one deals with general principles of the management of trauma, including sections on the basic science of biomechanics of fractures; the healing of bone, articular cartilage and tendon; and the systemic response to injury. In addition the principles of diagnosis and management of associated injuries, for example head, chest and abdomen, are considered. In the second part, specific injuries are considered by region.

We do not presume that this new textbook will be perfect and no doubt some will find fault with some sections. However, if we do not try we will never succeed and it is hoped that, with subsequent development and revisions of this first edition, we will establish the standard textbook of orthopaedic trauma upon which our future trainees will learn their principles of management.

P.J. Gregg
J. Stevens
P.H. Worlock

PART 1
GENERAL PRINCIPLES

1: Biomechanics of Fractures

J.L.CUNNINGHAM AND J.KENWRIGHT

Introduction and basic concepts

Biomechanics is the application of the principles of mechanics to biological systems. Mechanics describes the state of rest or motion of bodies under the action of forces and can be subdivided into statics, which studies the action of forces on bodies at rest, and dynamics, which studies the motion of bodies under the action of forces. Stress analysis is a subset of statics and is concerned with determining the internal stresses and strains on a component generated by an applied external loading. A force applied to any component at rest will produce stresses and strains within the material, the magnitudes of which will be proportional to both the applied load and the dimensions of the component. *Stress* is force per unit area and thus is a measure of the intensity of force within a component. *Strain* is a measure of the deformation of a component under load relative to the pre-deformation dimensions of the component. To obtain a more pictorial description of

stress and strain consider a tensile force F applied to a bar of constant cross-sectional area as shown in Fig. 1.1a. This force will cause the bar to extend by a small amount Δl as shown in Fig. 1.1b. If the applied load F is increased in small amounts from zero, and the extension is measured, then a load−extension curve, such as that shown in Fig. 1.2 will be generated. If the material gives a linear load−extension curve, then the gradient of the linear force−extension graph will be

$$K = \frac{F}{\Delta l}$$

where K is termed the *stiffness* of the material.

To investigate the internal stresses produced in the bar, we make an imaginary cut at section Y−Y as shown in Fig. 1.3. The stress σ at section Y−Y is the average force per unit area, hence

$$\sigma = \frac{\text{force}}{\text{area}} = \frac{F}{A}$$

In the above example the stress σ acts at right angles (or normal) to the cross-section and is therefore known as a *normal stress* and has units of $N\,m^{-2}$ (or $N\,mm^{-2}$ or $GN\,m^{-2}$ etc.); tensile stresses (produced by tensile

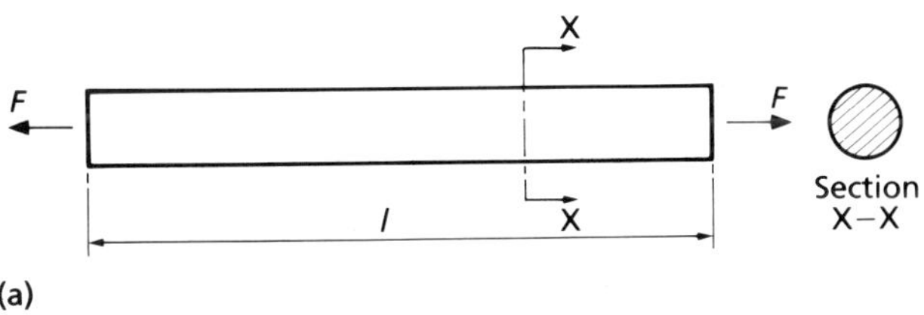

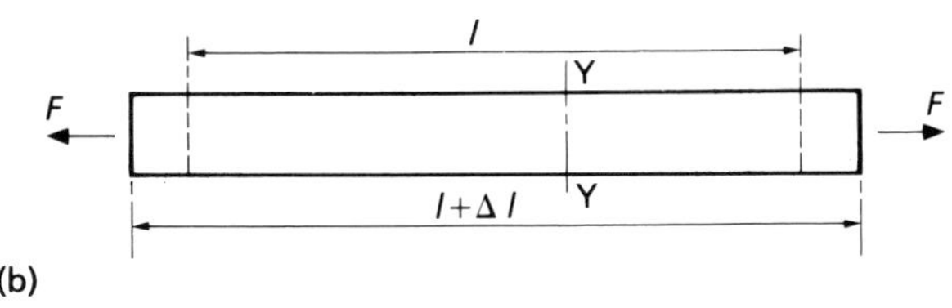

Fig. 1.1 (a) Round bar of initial length l being loaded by a tensile force F. (b) Elongation of bar due to action of tensile force F.

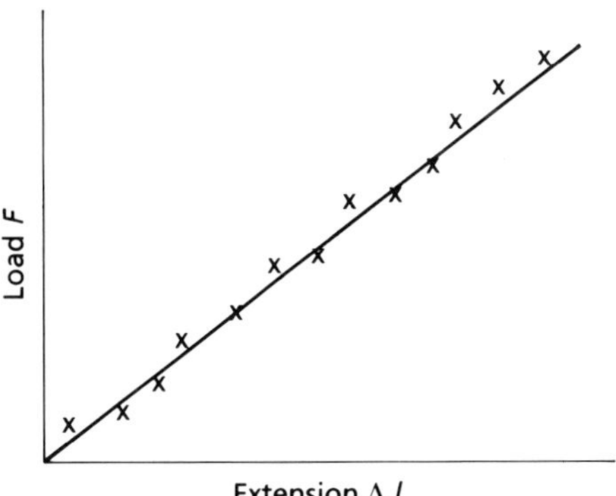

Fig. 1.2 Load−extension graph for a linear elastic material.

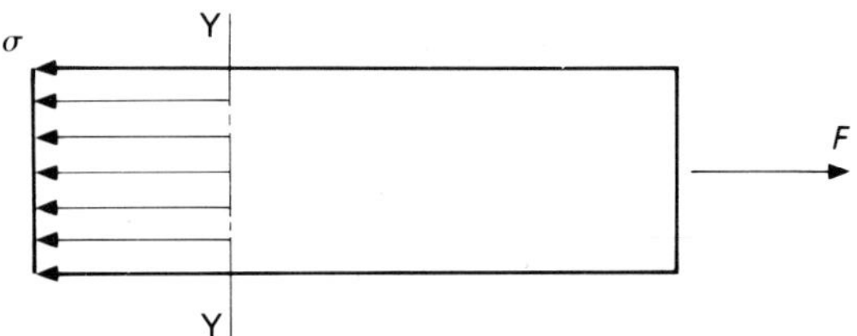

Fig. 1.3 Section through Y–Y of the bar shown in Fig. 1.1 showing internal stress.

forces) are generally considered to be positive while compressive stresses are considered to be negative. Note that $\sigma = F/A$ gives the *average normal stress* which will be constant for most of the length of the bar. However, depending on how the load is applied, the stress distribution may not be uniform and high localized stresses, which are much greater than the average stress, may be generated at the point where the load is applied or at small notches or holes in the structure. Such small discontinuities in a structure are known as stress raisers or stress concentrations.

In the example shown in Figs 1.1a and 1.1b the applied load also produces an extension Δl of the bar and this can be expressed as an elongation per unit length which is termed *strain ε*, i.e.

$$\varepsilon = \frac{\Delta l}{l}$$

Since strain is associated with a normal stress it is termed a normal strain and, also, since strain is a change in length divided by a length it has no dimensions. Strains encountered in practice are generally of the order $10^{-3} - 10^{-6}$ so a convenient method of expressing them is in microstrains (e.g. $10^{-5} = 100$ microstrain).

If the load–extension graph given in Fig. 1.2 is now plotted in terms of stress and strain the graph shown in Fig. 1.4 is obtained. The slope of this graph is called the *modulus of elasticity* (or Young's modulus) of the material and is denoted by E.

$$E = \frac{\sigma}{\varepsilon} = \frac{F/A}{\Delta l/l}$$

Rewriting this equation gives

$$\sigma = E\varepsilon$$

which is known as Hooke's Law and is named after Robert Hooke (1635–1703) who investigated the elastic properties of such diverse materials as metals, wood, bones and sinews. The modulus of elasticity has relatively large values for stiff materials such as structural steel (200 GN m^{-2}) and significantly lower values for less stiff materials such as rubber (0.002 GN m^{-2}). Note that for cortical bone $E = 25$ GN m^{-2}, for a loading direction parallel to the bone axis (Reilly & Burstein 1974).

Most engineering materials, such as steel, give a linear stress–strain curve below the point at which they begin to fail. Biological materials, however, tend to become stiffer the more they are stretched and give a non-linear stress–strain curve such as that shown in Fig. 1.5, which is typical for many soft tissues such as tendon and ligament. The stress–strain behaviour is governed by the constituents of the tissue. At low values of strain the low modulus behaviour typical of elastin predominates, while at higher values of strain the higher modulus collagen fibres take more of the applied load.

Engineering materials, being homogeneous, exhibit the same material properties irrespective of the direction in which they are loaded and are known as *isotropic*. Since many biological materials are fibrous, their properties are very dependent on the orientation of the fibres relative to the applied load and are thus highly *anisotropic*.

The stress–strain characteristics of biological materials are also very dependent on the rate at which

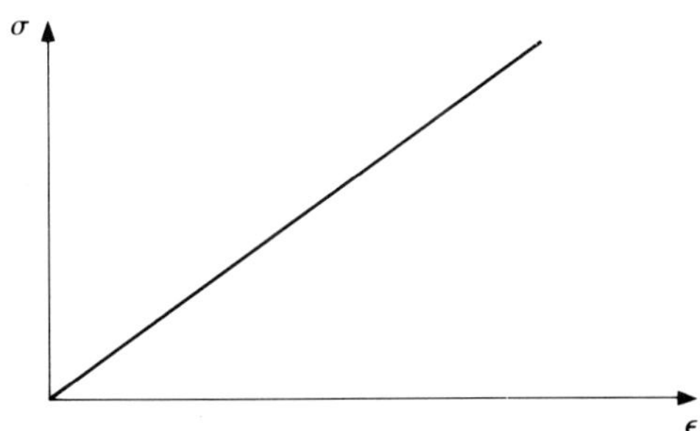

Fig. 1.4 Stress–strain graph for a linear elastic material.

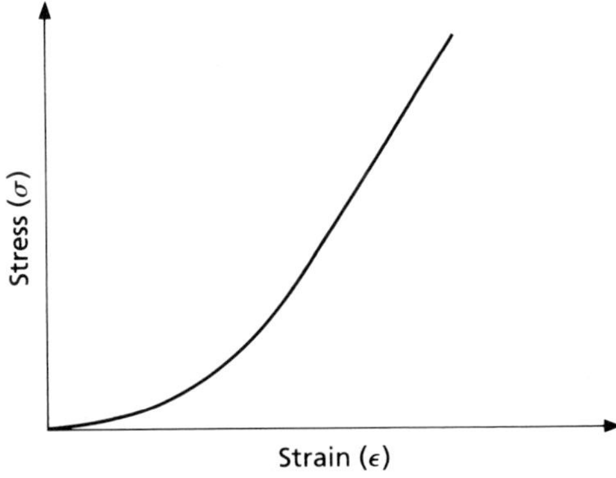

Fig. 1.5 Stress–strain graph for a typical biological material.

they are loaded. For a given applied stress at low loading rates the material undergoes a relatively large amount of strain while at high loading rates the material undergoes a relatively small amount of strain. This rate dependence of material properties is known as *viscoelasticity* and is illustrated in Fig. 1.6.

If, instead of extending or contracting a component, the applied force causes a body to shear (one face of the material slides over an adjacent face) then *shear stresses* are produced in the material. This is illustrated in Fig. 1.7. The shear stress

$$\tau = \frac{\text{shearing force}}{\text{area}} = \frac{V}{A}$$

where the shear stress τ is again an average shear stress. The above is an example of simple or direct shear where the direct action of shearing forces produces shear stress in the material. Direct shear stresses can occur in bolted and adhesive joints. Shear stresses can also be produced by the indirect action of loadings such as torsion and bending.

For a component under a bending load, bending stresses are produced. Consider the beam shown in Fig. 1.8 loaded in bending. Due to the applied bending moment M, surface AB will shorten and thus be in compression while surface CD will lengthen and thus be in tension. Hence there will be a compressive

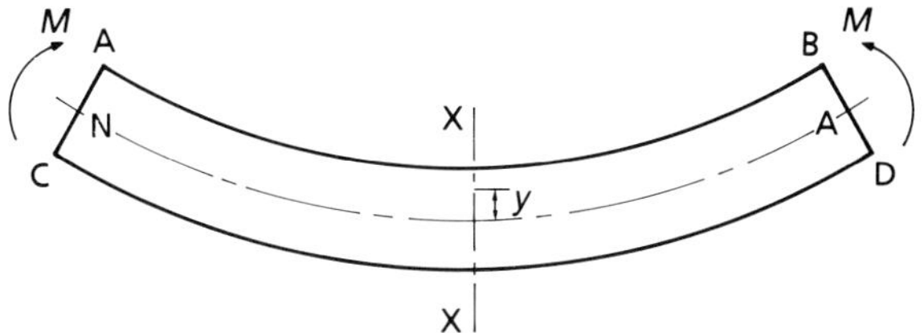

Fig. 1.8 Beam loaded in pure bending by moment M. NA, neutral axis of bending where there is zero stress.

(negative) bending stress on surface AB and a tensile (positive) bending stress on surface CD. The centreline of the beam (NA) will not change in length and hence the stress at the centreline will be zero. The stress in the beam at any distance y from the beam centreline resulting from the action of the bending moment M is given by

$$\sigma = \frac{My}{I}$$

where σ is the bending stress, M is the applied bending moment, I is the second moment of area of the beam and y is the distance from the beam centreline. The second moment of area I is a property of the beam cross-section and for a simple rectangular cross-section, such as that shown in Fig. 1.9

$$I = \frac{bd^3}{12}$$

where b is the width of beam and d is the beam depth.

Note that I increases with the depth of the beam cubed; hence a beam with a large depth has a much higher I value than a beam with a small depth, and is thus able to withstand higher bending loads. A practical demonstration of this is seen if a ruler is bent. With its widest side uppermost the depth of the ruler cross-section is small compared with its width, the I value is therefore relatively low and the ruler bends easily. If the position of the ruler is changed such that its short edge

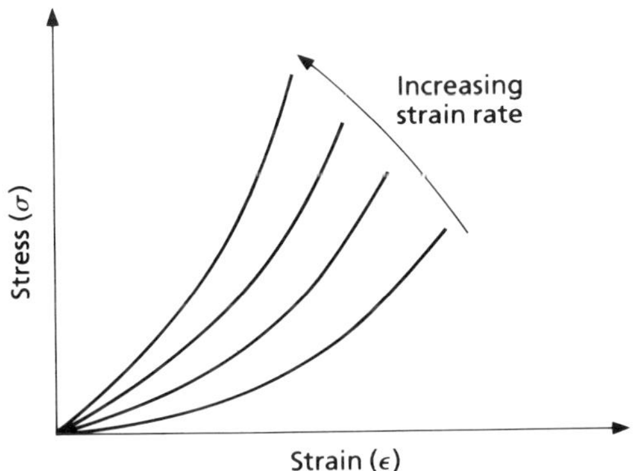

Fig. 1.6 Stress–strain graph for a biological material showing the effect of increasing strain rate.

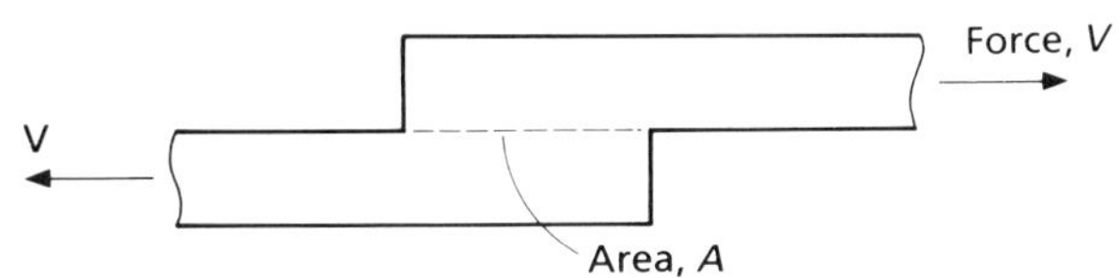

Fig. 1.7 Component loaded so as to produce a shear stress at area A.

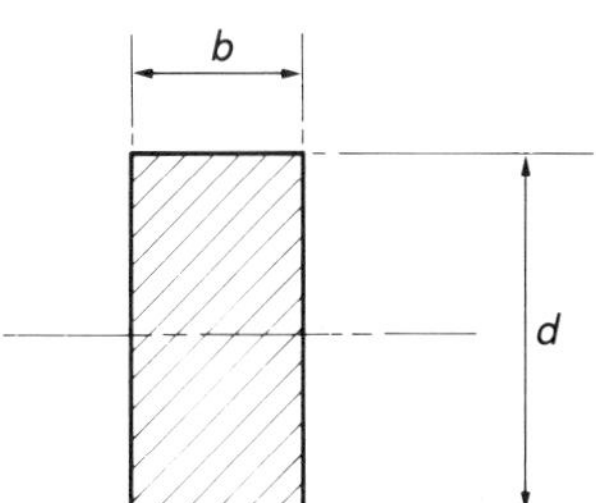

Fig. 1.9 Section X–X of the beam shown in Fig. 1.8.

is now uppermost the depth is large compared with the width, the I value is relatively high, and the ruler is difficult to bend.

Materials fail when the applied loading gives rise to stresses within the material which exceed the failure stress of the material. Materials can fail in either a ductile or a brittle manner; *ductile* materials undergo a large strain before failure while *brittle* materials fail at relatively low values of strain. Typical stress—strain curves of ductile and brittle materials are given in Figs 1.10a and 1.10b. In a ductile material a significant amount of plastic deformation occurs between yield of the material (after which stress and strain are no longer linearly related) and failure, whereas in a brittle material there is none. Examples of ductile materials are mild steel, aluminium, nylon, granular tissue and cartilage while examples of brittle materials include cast iron, concrete, bone cement, cortical bone and glass.

Fractures occur in materials because of microscopic cracks, which are inherent within all materials and will tend to elongate under the action of an applied stress.

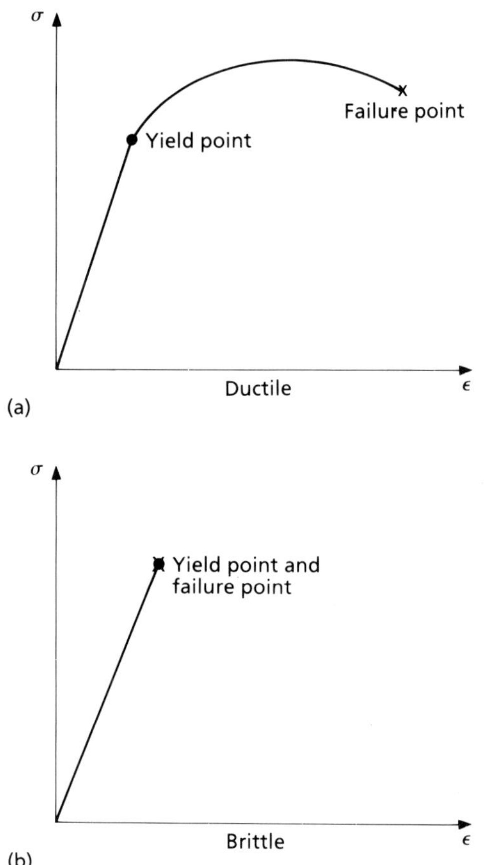

Fig. 1.10 Stress—strain graphs of (a) a ductile material and (b) a brittle material.

The stress required to elongate a crack is dependent in general terms on the length of the crack, the applied stress and the crack resistance or *fracture toughness* of the material. Materials with low fracture toughness (e.g. cortical bone) can only tolerate small cracks before failure while materials with high fracture toughness can tolerate larger cracks without failure for the same applied stress. Cracks may grow progressively in a material under the action of repeated loading until the crack reaches a critical length when one single application of the load will cause complete failure, this failure being known as a *fatigue failure*. On the other hand, the applied load may be so great that even pre-existing cracks in the material will be of a critical length, and failure will occur immediately on one application of the load.

Mechanics of fracture production in bone

Bone is a viscoelastic material and hence its mechanical properties are dependent on the rate of loading (Sammarco *et al.* 1971, Reilly & Burstein 1974, Fischer *et al.* 1986, Currey 1988). Generally, at low loading rates bone exhibits a lower stress to failure than bone loaded at high loading rates, although at very high loading rates the stress to failure begins to decrease (Panjabi *et al.* 1973, Peterson *et al.* 1984). The rate of loading will also affect the energy required to advance a crack and hence the fracture pathway in bone (Pope & Outwater 1972, Behiri & Bonfield 1980, 1984, Bonfield 1987). With low rates of loading, giving conditions for slow or stable crack growth, the fracture will tend to go around the osteons; the resulting crack will be long, the energy required to advance the crack will be relatively large and the microscopic appearance of the fracture will be rough. With a high rate of loading, giving fast and unstable crack growth, the crack will tend to directly cross the osteons; the crack will be short, the energy required to advance the crack will be low and the microscopic appearance of the fracture will be smooth.

The relative density of bone will also affect the fracture stress. As a bone becomes less dense, its susceptibility to fracture increases (Bonfield 1987). However, in immature bone with a relatively low density, incomplete fractures can occur as a result of the increased ability of immature bone to absorb energy and undergo significant plastic deformation (i.e. elongation with minimal increase in stress) before failure (Currey & Butler 1975, Mabrey & Fitch 1989). It has been suggested that this plastic deformation is related to the degree of mineralization and remodelling of immature bone compared to mature bone. Bone with a relatively high density but with poor structural organization, as in osteopetrosis, can fail at low loads and hence give rise to pathological fractures (Bleck & Kleinman 1984).

The direction and nature of the applied loading relative to the bone will determine the type of fracture that occurs (Almo 1961, Harkess *et al.* 1984, Chao & Aro 1989). The applied loading is generally classified as direct, where the force acts directly on the bone to produce the fracture, or indirect, where the force acts at a distance from the fracture. Examples of direct forces are a tapping, crushing or penetrating force, while examples of indirect forces are twisting or torsion, bending and compression or any combination of these. Failure of a material occurs in a macroscopic sense when the applied loading generates an internal stress which is greater than the failure stress of the material. For example, a bending load applied to a long bone produces a tensile stress at one side of the bone and a compressive stress at the other side. Cortical bone, as a semi-brittle solid (Behiri & Bonfield 1984), is generally stronger in compression than in tension (as are most brittle materials) so failure will occur when the tensile stress reaches the tensile failure stress of the material. The bone will thereafter fail progressively across the section and give a transverse fracture, or a transverse fracture with a butterfly fragment if the rate of loading is high (Martens *et al.*, 1986); the butterfly fragment appearing on the side of the fracture that was in compression. A spiral fracture occurs when a bone is loaded in torsion since with this loading the maximum tensile stress is generated within the bone at an angle to the long axis of the bone. A simple demonstration of this type of fracture can be obtained by twisting a piece of chalk. Since chalk, like bone, is also a brittle material, failure will occur when the maximum tensile stress exceeds the tensile failure stress of the material and will give a fracture at 45° to the longitudinal axis. In experimental fracture studies with *in vitro* bone, torsional failure occurs at approximately 30° to the long axis; this results from the anisotropy of the bone and/or the non-uniform cross-section. The principal types of loading modes to cause different types of fracture are shown in Fig. 1.11.

Repetitive loading of bone can enable small inherent flaws within the bone to grow in size, without causing immediate fracture. However, if the rate of crack growth exceeds the rate of repair and remodelling of the bone, then a situation will develop where the crack grows or advances to a sufficient length such that a relatively small load will cause complete propagation of the crack through the bone, thus giving rise to a *stress fracture*.

Comminution of a fracture usually arises as a result of a direct trauma of high energy. Since more energy is absorbed at high rates of loading more energy is there-

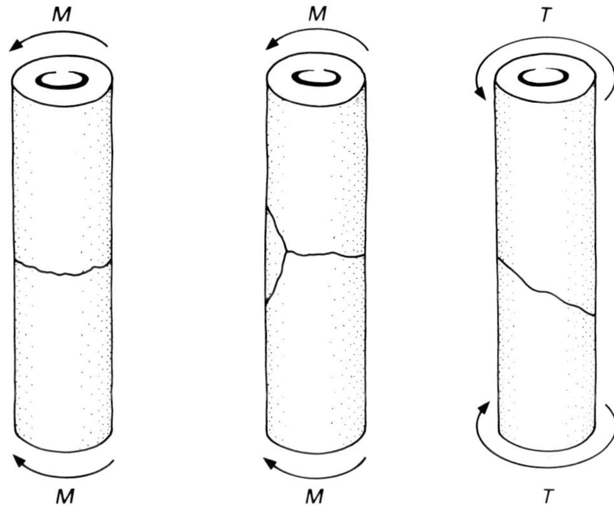

Fig. 1.11 Applied loadings necessary to cause different types of fracture. *M*, bending moment; *T*, torsion. Note that a bending moment can cause a transverse fracture with a butterfly fragment if the rate of loading is high.

fore available once fracture has occurred and this will lead to further fracture with comminution.

Fracture healing

Bone is a remarkable tissue in that following fracture it repairs not with a scar but by reconstitution of the injured tissue in something very like its original form (McKibbin 1978). In this section the biological and mechanical events associated with normal fracture healing will be described. The influence of changes in the mechanical environment at the fracture site upon healing will also be discussed.

Biological process

The process of fracture healing can be described in terms of biochemical events, histological or histochemical observations, radiographs or clinical observations. There have also been many studies of the healing process in cancellous and cortical bone in different animal models and under different conditions. Fracture healing as seen in an experimental model of a diaphyseal fracture can be subdivided into the following steps. A similar sequence probably occurs in humans.

Induction following haematoma formation. Immediately after injury there is bleeding from the damaged bone ends and from the local soft tissues and a haematoma forms. An inflammatory response follows and subsequently there is induction of bone formation. There is still considerable controversy as to whether the osteogenic cells arise from specialized cells that are predetermined to form bone (osteoprogenitor cells) or from 'uncommitted fibroblasts' that are supplied from the surrounding soft tissues.

Callus formation. The granulation tissue is invaded by these osteogenic cells, collagen fibres are laid down and a matrix is formed which is mineralized to make woven bone or provisional callus.

Bridging callus. This forms from the endosteum and periosteum under *secondary* or *indirect bone healing* conditions where there is a significant gap with incomplete reduction of the fracture, giving the potential for interfragmentary movement.

Remodelling. Following bridging of the fracture the remodelling phase is entered. This is a continuation of the replacement and repair process which occurs in a normal bone. The process involves simultaneous bone removal by osteoclasts and replacement by osteoblasts. The woven bone is replaced with lamellar bone over a period of months.

A different pattern of fracture healing may be seen in completely undisplaced fractures in adults (Rahn 1982) and in fractures where there is complete reduction and stable relatively rigid fixation (Perren 1979). Under these conditions *osteonal* or *primary bone healing* may occur (Schenk & Willenegger 1964). Secondary osteons grow directly across the fracture site and haversian remodelling occurs throughout as part of the fracture healing process. Under clinical conditions, even after accurate reduction of a fracture and plate fixation, there are usually distinct gaps. If these are in the region of 1 mm, woven bone is laid down transversely across this small gap; subsequently, secondary osteons can grow directly from one fragment to the other across this woven bone. This is called gap-healing and is a form of osteonal remodelling.

It has been shown that considerable variation can occur in the healing patterns associated with different types of fracture configuration and fixation system; within one fracture different conditions may exist in different zones so that mixtures of the healing patterns just described may be present. Contact healing or primary bone healing and gap-healing can be achieved with or without external callus (Chao & Aro 1989).

Mechanical properties of the healing fracture

Viewed in mechanical terms, fracture healing can be considered as a gradual return of structural integrity. White *et al.* (1977) have identified four distinct stages of fracture repair, according to the mechanical properties of the healing fracture. These vary from low stiffness with rubber-like properties to high stiffness with hard-tissue-like properties. With each increasing stage the stiffness, maximum torque and energy absorbed to failure of the healing fracture increase; the stiffness increases more quickly than both the torque and energy absorbed (Panjabi *et al.* 1977).

The rate of return of structural stiffness to a fracture will be dependent on the rigidity of the healing tissues and on the geometry of the healing fracture. The healing tissues of a fracture experience a 400 000-fold increase in rigidity during healing from a Young's modulus of 0.05 MN m^{-2} for granulation tissue to $20-25$ GN m^{-2} for mature bone (Perren 1979).

For the same material properties of healing tissues a fracture with an external callus gives a stiffer fracture than one with no callus or one with endosteal callus only (Perren 1979, Sarmiento *et al.* 1980). This results from the increased cross-sectional area and second moment of area (see p. 5) occurring with an external callus and is illustrated in Fig. 1.12. Bridging with considerable external callus leads therefore to a marked increase in resistance to axial, bending and shear loading even when the material properties of the callus are relatively low compared with mature bone. Asymmetrical healing will give a greater bending stiffness in the plane of maximum callus formation than in the plane of minimum callus. Asymmetrical healing can also introduce a discontinuity in the healing fracture (Fig. 1.13) which will act as a stress concentration and could lead to refracture if unsupported weight-bearing was permitted. In such circumstances fracture stiffness may be a poor indicator of fracture strength.

The time taken for healing fractures to reach their prefracture stiffness can be considerable. Jernberger (1970) found that in patients the stiffness of a healing tibial fracture did not reach that of the unfractured tibia until at least 1 year after injury. He also found that the majority of increase of stiffness occurred during the first 6 months of healing, and during that time the rate of increase of fracture stiffness was exponential. Several studies of fracture stiffness measurement have attempted to define a value at which unsupported weight-bearing could be permitted (Jorgensen 1972, Hammer *et al.* 1984, Evans *et al.* 1988). This value will be a small percentage, typically $20-25\%$ (Jorgensen 1970), of the

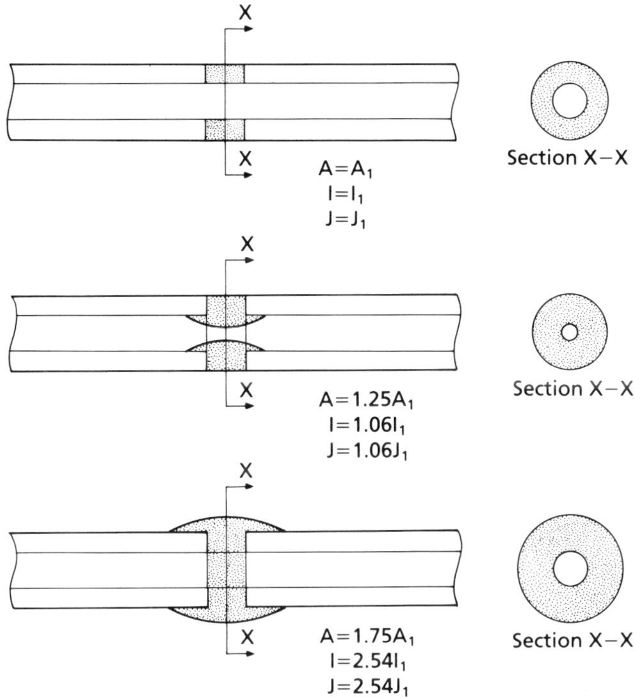

Axial stiffness $= EA; A = \pi/4(d_o - d_i)$
Bending stiffness $= EI; I = \pi/64(d_o^4 - d_i^4)$
Torsional stiffness $= GJ; J = \pi/32(d_o^4 - d_i^4) = 2I$

Fig. 1.12 Influence of callus shape on the axial, bending and torsional stiffness of a healing fracture.

stiffness of the unfractured bone, and will vary according to the predicted loads at different anatomical sites for individuals.

Mechanical influences on fracture healing

Intact bone is a dynamic tissue which is very sensitive to change in mechanical demand. The early observations of Wolff (1986) led to the laws of bone remodelling which incorporate the concepts that both the architecture and the mass of bone tissue are determined by the prevailing forces which act in the bone. Wolff also showed anatomical evidence of remodelling in fractures. In this section evidence will be put forward that the mechanical environment influences the healing of fractures.

Is there any mechanical influence on fracture healing?

Clinical observations certainly suggest that the mechanical conditions at the fracture site have a major influence on healing. The indirect or secondary bone healing pattern described in the previous section is seen in conditions of relative instability when bridging external callus is rapidly produced. This correlation between treatment method and pattern of healing has never been proven by a controlled study in patients, but clinical experience shows obvious major external callus formation when patients are treated for tibial fractures in functional casts (Sarmiento 1974) or by early functional mobility using Perkins treatment for femoral fractures (Buxton 1981). In contrast, if fractures are immobilized with accurate reduction and in such a way as to enforce minimal interfragmentary movement, then direct primary bone healing or gap-healing is observed

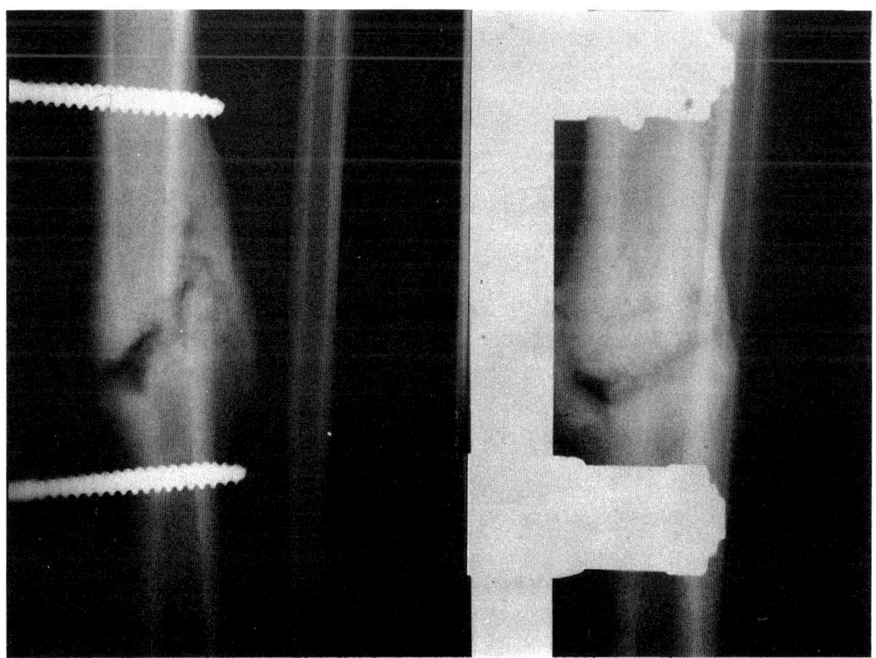

Fig. 1.13 Radiograph of a healing fracture showing asymmetrical callus formation.

(Schenk & Willenegger 1964). Clinically, there is considerable overlap between the types of healing seen but in nearly every instance, after allowing for the severity of injury, the pattern or type of healing appears to correlate with the prevailing mechanical conditions. Studies under the more controlled mechanical conditions of experimental osteotomies have confirmed these observations and a considerable number of experimental investigations have attempted to define the mechanical conditions at the fracture site which would be most appropriate for the advancement of the different stages of fracture healing.

It has been suggested that the *level of strain* prevailing at the fracture site might influence the pattern and rate of tissue differentiation (Yamagishi & Yoshimura 1955, Sarmiento *et al.* 1977, Perren 1979, Wu *et al.* 1984, Goodship & Kenwright 1985, Williams *et al.* 1987). The fracture site strain at any given stage of healing depends on the combined influence of the load applied to the fracture, the size of the fracture gap and the material properties of the tissue in the gap; the rigidity of the method of fracture fixation will influence the loading applied to the fracture. After injury, granulation tissue forms which is easily deformed and which has an ultimate strain of approximately 100%; however, at this stage the functional forces are usually low. As healing proceeds the stiffness of the differentiating tissues increases as does the magnitude of the functional forces acting across the fracture (Meggitt *et al.* 1981, Wardlaw *et al.* 1981, Cunningham *et al.* 1989). Perren (1979) has put forward the hypothesis that there is a relationship between the applied load and tissue stiffness during fracture healing, so that effective differentiation and maturation will not occur unless the appropriate strain acts at each stage of the healing process. Therefore, there should be a balance between the loading (and hence micromovement) of the fracture site and the mechanical characteristics of the healing fracture tissue which will determine the course of all patterns of fracture healing, particularly of secondary fracture healing whilst a bridging callus is being formed.

It should be noted that the strain obtained for a given amount of fracture movement is inversely proportional to the size of the fracture gap (Fig. 1.14). Hence, a very small fracture gap with only very slight interfragmentary motion will give a significant strain to be experienced by the delicate healing tissues. This strain hypothesis has been investigated extensively in experimental studies and most observations support the concept. Many experimental studies have investigated the influence of different overall immobilization regimes on fracture healing using casts, external or internal fixation.

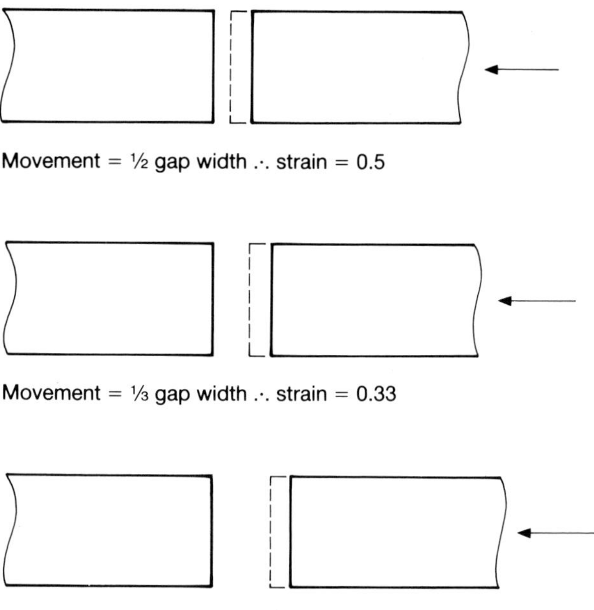

Fig. 1.14 Effect of gap width on fracture site strain for the same amount of movement of one fragment relative to the other.

Such studies suggest that the strain magnitude is of critical importance but that not all micromovement is beneficial. There can be an excess of micromovement as well as too little and both extremes will inhibit indirect fracture healing (Sarmiento & Latta 1981, Kenwright & Goodship 1989).

Similarly, experimental evidence suggests that there are limits to the force of application of any stimulus that is experienced by the healing fracture after which there is inhibition of healing (Goodship 1989). The rate of application of strain also appears important and surprisingly high strain rates, close to the limits of those seen under physiological activities, may stimulate fracture healing more than low strain rates (Goodship & Kenwright 1985). Most clinical observations have shown that early functional loading when using casts or external skeletal fixation is associated with low non-union rates (Sarmiento 1974, De Bastiani *et al.* 1984).

The direction of application of fracture loading may also influence healing. The studies of experimental fracture healing by Yamagishi and Yoshimura (1955) suggested that torsional stress applied across a fracture was disadvantageous. This observation has been generally accepted, but has never been proven clearly, and most fractures must experience considerable torsion during the normal physiological activities of daily life, as has been shown by direct measurement (Lippert & Hirsch 1974).

The effect of loading a fracture also depends upon the stage at which the loading occurs. Most experimental studies suggest that early loading (within the first 6 weeks) is important for fracture healing and this probably also applies to the clinical situation when treating most fractures. The influence of loading on the late remodelling of fractures is not clear, although Wolf *et al.* (1981) demonstrated that it was not until the later stages of fracture healing that cyclical loading was found to enhance fracture stiffness and strength. However, in a more recent study, late dynamic compression of an experimental osteotomy treated with an external fixation frame did not give any increase in new bone formation or fracture stiffness compared to no dynamization of the same frame (Aro *et al.* 1990).

What is the mechanism of mediation of mechanical stimulation of fractures?

This mechanism is, as yet, unknown. It has been noted that deformation of bone cells will lead to immediate changes in biochemistry (Skerry *et al.* 1988). Detailed anatomical connections of the osteocyte show it to be 'ideally' structured to act as a receptor for changes in bone deformation in intact bone so that direct deformation of bone cells may lead to modification of their behaviour. It is also possible that there are piezoelectric effects related to deformation which might mediate the responses leading to osteogenesis.

Have these observations any implications in clinical practice?

Most fractures will heal within wide tolerances of mechanical conditions, for example clavicular fractures. In other fractures the mechanical environment can be very critical, including those with a low potential to heal, for example tibial diaphyseal fractures. There are also circumstances where other treatment aims enforce the use of a potentially unfavourable mechanical environment; this may occur with the use of plates for femoral diaphyseal fractures and external skeletal fixation frames for tibial diaphyseal fractures.

In the next section some applications of our knowledge concerning mechanical influences on fracture healing will be discussed in relation to different treatment methods.

Application of biomechanics to treatment methods

Mechanical and biological considerations have to be co-ordinated for individual fractures. For any fracture one issue usually predominates in order to avoid a particular complication. In intra-articular fractures restoration and maintenance of anatomy may be the predominant issue combined with sufficient internal stability to allow early function of adjacent joints. Restoration of bone length and alignment may predominate in unstable fractures of the tibia and femur; frequently this desire to achieve normal anatomy may make it necessary to increase tissue damage by local dissection. Alternatively, the avoidance of such dissection might be the predominant issue in order to maintain the local blood supply. In each fracture treatment method the influence of the local mechanical environment upon the healing of the fracture also needs to be considered so that inhibition of healing does not result from the treatment.

In the following sections each treatment method will be considered and clinical examples will be used for illustration.

Cast treatment

Most fractures can be, and are, treated in casts and biomechanical principles need to be applied as for other methods of treatment. The biological and mechanical conditions should also be reviewed regularly and, if necessary, adjusted throughout treatment.

Casts are used to meet the following objectives:
1 To relieve pain and allow function of the limb.
2 To maintain anatomy.
3 To lead to appropriate mechanical conditions for fracture healing.
4 To allow soft tissues to heal, without predisposing to permanent disability.

The limitations of cast treatment for maintenance of anatomical position need to be considered for each fracture. Clinical experience, backed up by laboratory studies performed on simulated fractures in postmortem specimens, has shown the positional control which can be obtained with cast treatment of different fracture types (Sarmiento *et al.* 1979, Unsworth & Shannon 1979). Angular deformities can usually be controlled by using the principle of three-point fixation (Charnley 1968), but in order to control rotatory deformity it is nearly always necessary to include the joint above and below the fracture within the cast.

Cast treatment will not usually control length with accuracy in an oblique diaphyseal fracture. This needs to be realized when planning treatment and a small degree of shortening may need to be accepted. It is particularly important to reduce the potential shortening which might develop when treating ipsilateral fractures of the femur and tibia when the accumulated shortening might become excessive. The work of Sarmiento *et al.* (1974) is of great interest in this area. Studies were performed upon fresh fractures of the tibia and fibula when 25 lbf (111 N) of axial loading was applied to the patient's leg, with the patient under general anaesthesia. A longitudinal displacement of 21 mm was measured. A functional brace was applied and the same amount of axial loading then gave a displacement of 2 mm. Pressures were measured from transducers placed within the braces and the pressures recorded from over the gastrosoleus complex were consistently higher than those recorded from the bony prominences. It was concluded from these studies that the cast acts as a rigid shell, restricting the displacement of the soft tissues of the lower leg when the load was applied. This restriction of soft tissue movement in turn restricts the displacement of the bone ends; even if some shortening occurs on loading, the pressures within the soft tissues are sufficient to eliminate this shortening on unloading of the limb. These studies also demonstrated the major importance of the interosseous membrane in resisting deformity. When treating patients with such tibial fractures it is also important to take into account the level and instability of the fracture and the overall shape of the patient's leg since, despite clinical and experimental evidence that angulation and shortening may be well controlled by casts and braces, there are limits of tolerance and significant shortening may yet develop.

Casts will not control reduction accurately if there are disproportionately high unbalanced muscle forces, such as are seen in fractures of the olecranon or in situations where there is an unbalanced force applied to the fractured bone on weight-bearing, as with fractures of the tibia where the fibula is still intact. Despite the application of three-point casts, malunion nearly always occurs in such circumstances.

Cast treatment of fractures which have been displaced requires constant observation to assess whether the cast is providing a suitable mechanical environment for maintaining reduction. The immobilization should be sufficient to enable the leg to weight-bear, and should also be devised so that adjacent joints can be used as soon after injury as possible. This can usually be achieved by the use of knee and ankle hinges.

Cast not too much hope in casts, and know your cast!

Traction

Traction has been used for many centuries for the treatment of fractures and has been found to be very effective under many circumstances. As with cast treatments, it cannot be assumed that the traction will be effective and daily review of its use is needed for individual patients.

Traction will not function to control fracture position unless there is a force acting which is equal in magnitude and opposite in direction to the traction force. In fractures of the shaft of the femur where traction is applied through a tibial pin, the bed must be tipped to a sufficient angle for there to be counter-traction. If fixed traction is supplied through a Thomas splint for femoral fractures, the equal and opposite force will act on the perineum and can cause skin damage.

Traction may not achieve its objective if it leads to insufficient stability. The use of heel wire traction to control fractures of the tibia is frequently advocated to immobilize the fracture and to enhance soft tissue healing. Such immobilization is not usually effective as mobility can still occur at the fracture site despite the traction and such instability often prevents soft tissue healing.

External skeletal fixation

Introduction

There has been a great increase in the use of external fixation over the last 15 years. This has, in part, been due to advances in plastic surgery which enable devastating injuries to be reconstructed; for this surgery to be successful adequate stabilization of the skeleton is essential. There have also been significant biomechanical advances which include the development of more effective and versatile frames, and improved component reliability, resulting in fewer failures. A greater emphasis has also been placed upon sound mechanical principles being applied to the surgical techniques used in the application of frames. Bone screw design and application technique has also advanced so that major screw track infections are much less common.

There is now a vast number of devices available on the market. This is due in part to the increased need for external skeletal fixation, and also to the diverse specifications required for the ideal device, some of which are mutually incompatible. For example, the ideal frame should be strong, versatile, adjustable, user-friendly, light, inexpensive and, ideally, unilateral so as to be unobtrusive.

Types of device

Behrens and Johnson (1989) subdivide external skeletal fixation systems into devices and frames — the latter being configurations of the former. They further divide devices into the following groups: (i) pin devices, which may be simple one-plane unilateral devices such as the Orthofix and Dynabrace, or devices from which more complex two-plane unilateral and bilateral fixators can be constructed, such as the AO and Hoffman; (ii) the ring frame or Ilizarov type device. In these, there is either a circular or semi-circular frame encompassing the limb and thin pre-tensioned wires, which are suspended in the frame, are used for control of the skeleton.

In general, the two main groups show mutually exclusive capabilities and should ideally be used for different clinical indications. Robust pin or screw devices of either unilateral or bilateral type are best used for the treatment of serious fractures to allow rapid stabilization of simple or complex fractures and to permit adequate access for subsequent plastic surgery. Ring fixation systems allow progressive adjustment of fracture position or control of osteotomies, a feature not generally present with the pin devices. Ring frames, however, are complex to apply even with experienced hands, and there is a much higher risk of injury to neurovascular structures; it is usually impossible to insert all the wires through safe corridors (Behrens & Searls 1986, Behrens 1989).

Mechanical characteristics of devices and frame configurations

There is now a considerable amount of literature relating to the mechanical characteristics of each external fixation device in its different configurations. These laboratory studies have enabled measurements of fixator stiffness and fracture gap motion to be obtained on simulated fractures under a variety of loading conditions, in both synthetic materials (Behrens *et al.* 1983, McCoy *et al.* 1983, Finlay *et al.* 1987, Moroz *et al.* 1988) and in *in vitro* bone (Kempson & Campbell 1981, Briggs & Chao 1982). Analytical and finite element models have also been used to enable the stiffness of a given geometry of external fixator to be predicted accurately (Chao *et al.* 1982, Huiskes & Chao 1986). This information should be referred to both when choosing a device for a given hospital and when planning for an individual patient. It is important to know whether the frame will be sufficient for its tasks of both achieving stability and allowing any subsequent adjustment of mechanical characteristics to meet the biological needs of the fracture.

OVERALL FAILURE

All frames will collapse with loss of osteotomy or fracture stability if loaded excessively. Failure of materials or components are rare on modern frames. The most usual site of failure of the device is at the clamp screw connection or at universal joints in the frame, where slippage is common at low loads (Finlay *et al.* 1987, Drijber *et al.* 1990). These potential weaknesses should be borne in mind so that excess loading is avoided.

MECHANICAL CHARACTERISTICS OF DEVICES

The mechanical characteristics of different external fixation devices with different frame configurations are known and can be compared. Of these characteristics it is important to be able to differentiate between overall frame stiffness and the effect of this on fracture site movement.

The overall stiffness of a frame—fracture configuration as measured in the laboratory and calculated from finite element and analytical models depends upon: (i) the components of the fixator; (ii) the geometrical configuration; and (iii) the stability created by the bones at the fracture site.

The components are inherent within any particular device available to the surgeon, although appropriate devices should be chosen for appropriate clinical problems. In practice, if more stability is needed it is better to increase the dimensions of the components rather than add more pins, parts and small pieces. More pins means an increased risk of pin track infections and more components means less access for future surgery.

Predictable increases in overall stiffness can be made by increasing the diameter of the screws or pins or by changing the geometry of the fixator. It should, however, be noted that a given change in fixator configuration will not have an equal effect upon the different fixator stiffnesses. For example, a geometrical change giving a 50% increase in axial stiffness may only give a 20% increase in anteroposterior bending. The most important factors influencing fixator rigidity have been found to be the number of pins or screws used, the screw diameter and the distance from the bone to the support column of the fixator (Chao *et al.* 1982, Huiskes & Chao 1986, Chao & Hein 1988). Screw separation distance and the stiffness of the support column can also influence overall fixator stiffness but by a smaller amount (Kempson & Campbell 1981, Briggs & Chao 1982). Bilateral frames are generally stiffer than unilateral frames, although unilateral frames which use a large diameter bone screw can give comparable values of stiffness to some bilateral frames (Kempson & Campbell 1981, Behrens *et al.* 1983, Behrens & Johnson 1989). Fixation stiffness can also be improved by using two unilateral frames placed at right angles, or by the use of triangulation (Finlay *et al.* 1987, Moroz *et al.* 1988).

Assuming the fixator to be applied to the medial surface of the tibia, most fixators tend to be least rigid in anteroposterior bending and torsion; this applies to both unilateral and bilateral frames (Kempson & Campbell 1981, Kristiansen *et al.* 1987). Significant improvements in fixation stiffness for a given frame geometry can therefore be obtained by placing the screws in the plane of the known major applied bending moment of the limb, e.g. the saggital plane in the tibia (Behrens & Johnson 1989).

Ring or circular frames, such as that of Ilizarov, which use 1.5 or 1.8 mm Kirschner wires tensioned to either 500 or 1300 N within a circular or semi-circular frame can lead to the same or slightly lower rigidity compared with that of the other commonly used frames (McCoy *et al.* 1983, Gasser *et al.* 1990). When loaded in the laboratory the Ilizarov frame demonstrates reasonably high bending stiffness in the anteroposterior and lateral planes with reasonably high torsional stiffness, but in axial loading there is considerable elasticity and a non-linear stiffness behaviour. The possible clinical importance of this in dynamic loading was stressed by Paley *et al.* (1990); weight-bearing when using the Ilizarov system might lead to adequate stability of the fracture and yet allow axial micromovement which could enhance osteogenesis. The stiffness of such circular frames can be enhanced by increasing the tension of the transfixion wires, increasing the separation distance of the rings on either side of the fracture and by decreasing the size of the rings used (McCoy *et al.* 1983, Gasser *et al.* 1990).

INFLUENCE OF FRACTURE STABILITY

Whatever frame configuration is used fixation stiffness will also be altered by the stability of the bony components at the fracture site. For similar fixator configurations and levels of weight-bearing, more movement at the fracture site has been measured in fractures which were longitudinally unstable than in those which were longitudinally stable (Cunningham *et al.* 1989).

SCREWS: PINS AND THE BONE−SCREW CONNECTION

The bone−screw interface is the commonest site for failure when using external skeletal fixation and as such presents a major clinical problem (Seligson *et al.* 1984). A common cause of failure of bone screws is infection associated with poor pin track care, or the clinical necessity to pass pins through extensive layers of soft tissue. However, mechanical influences on screw loosening and subsequent infection and lysis are also important.

The geometry of an external fixator results in large bending loads being carried by the screws and this will result in high stresses in the bone at the points of screw insertion. Unilateral fixators give significantly higher stresses in the proximal cortex than in the distal cortex, while bilateral fixators give similar values of stress in both cortices (Huiskes *et al.* 1985). The maximum stress in the bone can reach a sufficiently high value to cause local bone failure, particularly if the fracture is unstable (Harris *et al.* 1981, Chao & Aro 1989). Cyclical loading of screws *in vivo* has been shown to result in an increased incidence of screw loosening compared with unloaded or statically loaded screws (Pettine *et al.* 1986). Hence, in active or heavy patients particular attention should be paid to loading the bone−screw interface, since the natural rate of bone remodelling may be insufficient to mitigate failure.

If a fixator frame is dynamized, permitting contact of the fracture ends, the stresses in the bone will be reduced during loading of the fixator (Chao & An 1982, Chao & Aro 1989). As healing progresses the fracture callus becomes sufficiently stiff to support an appreciable load and this will result in a marked decrease in loading of the bone−screw interface (Huiskes & Chao 1986). It has also been shown that stress levels at the bone−screw interface can be reduced if the unthreaded shank of the screw perforates the proximal cortex, when screws of a large diameter are used, and if the distance from the bone to the support column of the external fixator is reduced (Klip & Bosma 1978, Harris *et al.* 1981, Behrens 1989). The use of screws of increased diameter will only give a small increase in the risk of fracture through the screw holes provided that the diameter of the screw is less than one-quarter of the minimum width of the bone. Upon fixator removal the screw holes progressively fill with bone and refracture through screw holes is a rare occurrence. The main reason for this low risk is that there is usually considerable remodelling of bone around screw holes and this progresses throughout the time of frame application.

The form of the thread on bone screws can also have an influence on mechanical performance of the screw. Finer screw-thread forms appear to give a higher push-in or pull-out failure load in bone, and the increased surface area of contact of these screws with bone may help to reduce the stresses generated in the bone upon loading of the screws (Wagenknecht *et al.* 1989, Evans *et al.* 1990). Modification of the cutting end of the screw can influence the holding strength, the temperatures generated in the bone and the bone damage which occurs on insertion.

BIOMECHANICAL PRINCIPLES OF APPLICATION

Preplanning of the frame type and configuration is required for individual applications. The site of screw holes should be planned to give appropriate stability and to avoid having to perform repeat placement of screws as this will weaken the bone. The screw sites should be planned to allow screws to pass through the central diameter of the bone.

Pins or screws should be pre-drilled with a low speed drill to prevent thermal necrosis. The screws should be inserted by hand and even then there may be an increase in temperature within the bone which could cause necrosis (Matthews *et al.* 1984). Such details may be very important as frames often have to be left in place for many months. The method of insertion of wires for circular frames is equally important, but in this case the selection of safe corridors for insertion is the predominant problem. Use of these fixators is mainly confined to corrective osteotomies and bone transport where progressive and accurate control of position is needed, so that careful planning, with very accurate insertion of the wires, has to be made (Fig. 1.15). When using circular frames the stability of the system can be adjusted by insertion of the thin wires at as close an angle to 90° as possible, by tensioning the wires, by adding extra rings or by the use of stopwires (olive wires).

At operation, stability can be altered by adjusting the fracture site itself. Anatomical reduction will increase stability; preloading of the fracture by the use of longitudinal axial compression applied via the fixation frame or the use of supplementary lagged internal fixation screws will also increase stability. The use of supplementary internal fixation associated with external fixation, as shown in Fig. 1.16 is, however, controversial. Though such manoeuvres greatly increase stability, they will lead to inhibition of external callus formation. The gap-healing pattern which will follow leads to a prolonged time before protection can be removed without the risk of refracture, and long periods of cast support are normally needed following frame removal.

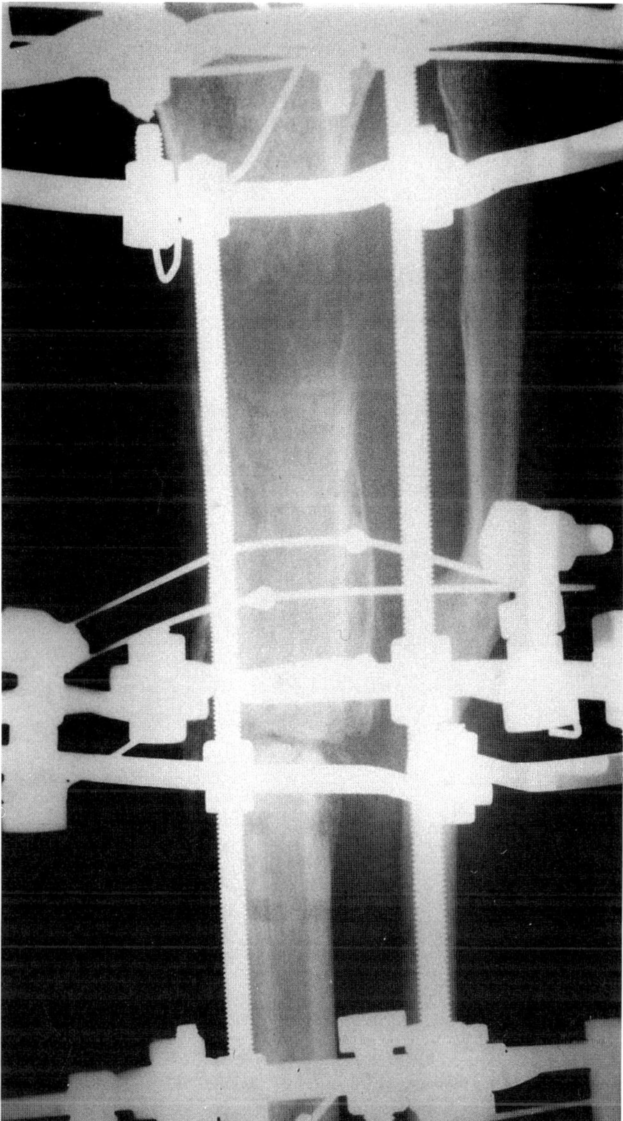

Fig. 1.15 Circular frame used for bone transport. Note the large amount of deformation which has occurred in the olive wires.

SUBSEQUENT TREATMENT, INCLUDING DYNAMIZATION

As described previously, there is probably an appropriate strain for each stage of fracture healing. The appropriate levels are difficult enough to define in experimental models with closely controlled variables, but in human fractures this difficulty is significantly greater.

Passive stimulation can be used within the first week following fracture to stimulate callus formation. Such stimulation does not rely on the patient's ability to weight-bear at this early stage, but provides a known mechanical stimulus to the fracture via a pneumatic

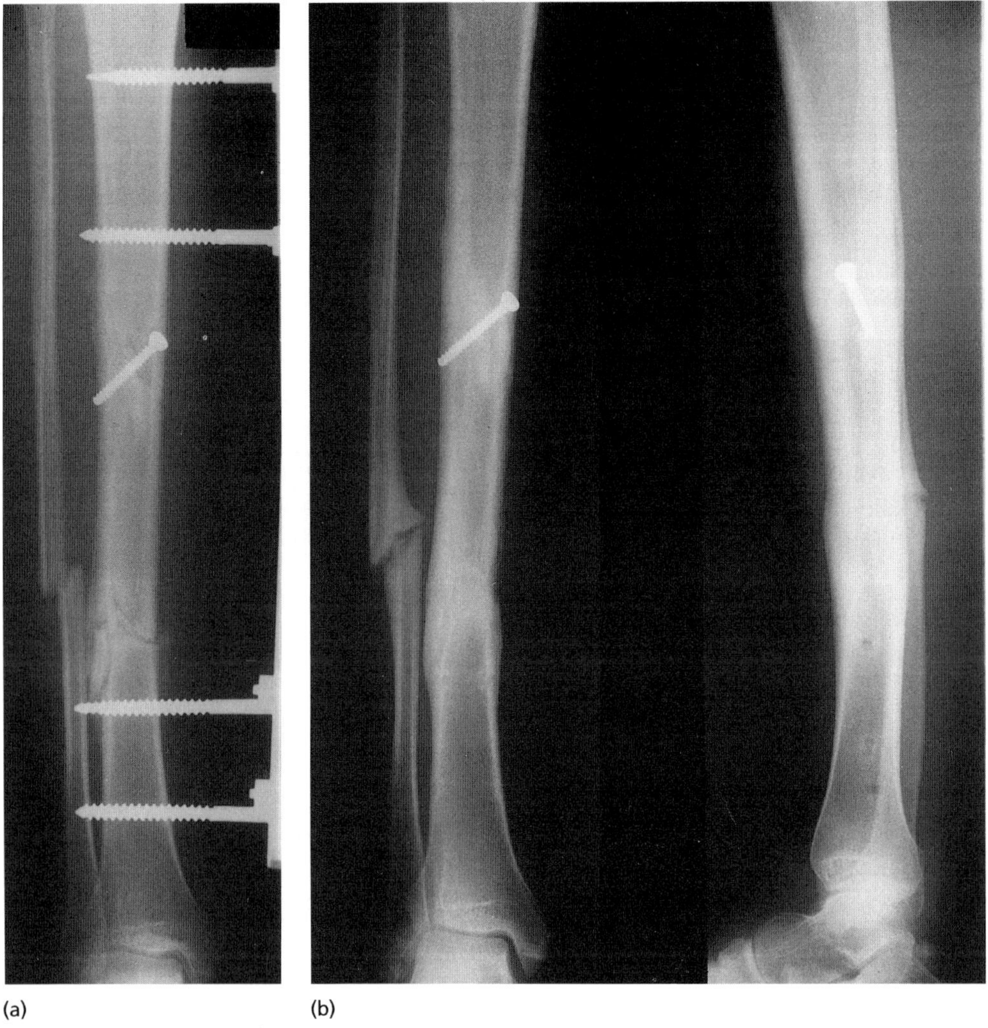

Fig. 1.16 (a) and (b) External fixation supplemented by internal fixation for a segmental tibial fracture. The upper (internally fixed) fracture heals with no callus, while the lower (externally fixed) fracture heals with a callus.

actuator attached to the external fixator (Kenwright & Goodship 1989). Passive stimulation is continued until the patient is able to provide a similar magnitude of stimulus through weight-bearing alone.

Dynamization techniques are considered for loading the fracture once bridging with external callus has occurred; the magnitude of the loading is restricted to less than that which will cause damage to the healing tissues (De Bastiani *et al.* 1984).

Dynamization can be planned in various ways for different devices. Some frames (Orthofix) contain a restraining element which prevents telescoping of the frame, but once bridging with external callus has occurred this element can be removed and dynamization effected during weight-bearing. Other frames (Dynabrace) have a similar system with a spring attached to sliding clamps; pretensioning of the spring

allows a set amount of load to be transferred across the fracture for a certain amount of weight-bearing. Behrens and Johnson (1989) describe dismantling the frame in stages to give a predictable decrease in frame stiffness and to increase the loading of the healing fracture after bridging has occurred. Initially, a triangulated system is converted to a double bar; the double bar is then converted to a single bar configuration and this remaining bar is moved closer to the bone to compensate for the reduction in stiffness obtained by converting from a double to a single bar. This single bar is then progressively placed further from the bone as healing progresses and finally the frame is dismantled. Burny (1979) has used elastic frames in which there is a low amount of frame rigidity to all modes of loading and has shown that it is possible to maintain fracture reduction while permitting significant axial micromovement at the fracture site on functional loading. An interesting concept is that of biocompression proposed by Lazo-Zbikowski *et al.* (1986); a sliding frame is used which allows the patient to dynamize the fracture axially according to the ability to weight-bear. The hypothesis proposes that impulses pass from the leg at each stage in fracture healing to a central neurological mechanism which controls the patient's ability to bear weight according to the amount of healing which has taken place. Hence, through a feedback mechanism the most appropriate load is applied across the fracture at each stage of healing.

Internal fixation

Internal fixation is used very widely in fracture treatment, but it is probably the area of treatment that is most demanding of the surgeon. Its use requires a wide knowledge of the relevant principles of biomechanics and if these are not applied mechanical failure of the implant or non-union may ensue. The relevant biological principles must also be applied, for if excessive surgical dissection is inflicted upon the injured limb in the early days after injury the surrounding vascularity may be impaired and fracture healing inhibited; if infection follows such devascularization this is usually disastrous.

Overall objectives of internal fixation

There are three main objectives related to stabilizing a fracture:

1 Maintaining reduction, which is obviously more important in some fractures than in others.

2 Allowing early function of the limb and particularly of the adjacent joints, muscles and other soft tissues to prevent fracture disease (Danis 1949).

3 Allowing favourable conditions for healing of the fracture.

All these objectives are important but the second is by far the most important as it is loss of joint and soft tissue function which is usually the most disabling permanent problem following any fracture.

Materials for implants

The demands placed upon the materials used for implants are related to the following factors:

1 Materials must be suitable for relatively simple construction into appropriate implants.

2 Corrosion must not occur.

3 The implants must be produced in such a way that there are no defects which would lead to premature failure.

4 The material must undergo some plastic deformation prior to failure to allow contouring of the implant, particularly if it is to be used for plates, and to warn of impending failure of the implant.

5 The material must have the characteristics which enable an implant of low bulk to be formed and which will not fail under the in-service load conditions experienced.

6 Materials should be biologically inert, i.e. no noxious substances must be emitted from them in the short- or long-term.

7 The cost of production of the definitive implant may need to be considered.

8 The relationship between the material properties of the implant and the bone must also be considered; the ideal material will have a high resistance to fatigue and have mechanical properties close to those of bone itself to ensure minimal stress protection and equal sharing of load between the implant and the bone.

Having considered all these aspects, most implants are made from stainless steels, cobalt–chrome–molybdenum alloys (Vitallium, Zimaloy) or titanium–aluminium–vanadium alloys (Tivanium, Tivaloy 12), but certain other materials can be considered for special situations.

Tayton *et al.* (1982) showed that plates made from epoxy-reinforced carbon fibre can have an elasticity which will enhance indirect or secondary fracture healing and reduce osteopenia beneath the plate whilst, at the same time, offering very considerable strength and resistance to fatigue failure. This material, however, does not allow any contouring so that it would be necessary to have available a large number of shapes of plate for different fractures at various levels within any bone.

Polymethylmethacrylate cement is also frequently used for supporting internal fixation, particularly when a destructive metastasis with an associated fracture requires stabilization.

Failure of implants is ultimately due to component failure but this is rarely associated with defects in the construction of implants. Failure is usually due to the implant being inserted in an inappropriate manner, or to damage to the surface of the implant by mishandling during insertion, which can lead to the creation of a stress raiser which will reduce the fatigue life of the plate. Some weakening of implants also occurs due to the plastic deformation produced at the time of contouring of a plate, and this problem is made worse if the surface of the plate has also been damaged.

All metallic implants will corrode to some extent *in vivo* and corrosion is more severe in multicomponent implants such as plates and screws. The host response to such corrosion will depend primarily on the rate of corrosion, but may also depend on a number of other factors such as the local chemical, electrical and mechanical environments (Black 1988). In normal implant use, however, the amount of corrosion occurring should be sufficiently small for it to go unnoticed. If there has been damage to the surface of the implant during insertion the rate of corrosion may increase to an extent where clinical problems manifest themselves. Increased corrosion may also be seen if implants of different alloys are mixed; this is quite a common phenomenon in general hospital practice. Such corrosion can lead to a local inflammatory response with irritation at the implant site. The clinical response to corrosion may be very similar to that of low grade infection but no evidence of sepsis is found when the implant is removed and after removal there is no permanent disability. A comprehensive summary of corrosion and host response as applied to implants is given by Black (1988).

Achievement of stability of fractures

With internal fixation it is necessary to plan and effect operative stabilization so that loads can be applied to the injured limb to allow physiological use of adjacent joints and muscles without risk of disruption at the fracture site. There are several basic principles which should be considered when planning fixation so as to obtain maximum stability. These include the following factors:

1 Reduction of the fracture.
2 The use of interfragmentary compression.
3 The use of an appropriate implant for the predicted loads.
4 Application of the appropriate engineering skills to the insertion of the implant.

The Association for Osteosynthesis (AO) school of fracture treatment has pioneered advances in these concepts and has stressed the importance of considering biological factors such as vascularity of bone as well as the use of sound mechanical principles (Müller *et al.* 1979).

Reduction. Fractures will, of course, heal without perfect reduction, but if the aim is to achieve stability of the fracture then accurate reduction is of prime importance. Accurate reduction increases the area of bony contact and allows the application of interfragmentary compression; in this way there is load sharing between the implant and the bone, and higher levels of bending and

torsional load can be tolerated before there is disruption of the system.

Interfragmentary compression. Experimental work performed on simulated fractures has shown that interfragmentary compression enhances the stability of a fracture to a marked degree, but does not in itself alter the healing pattern when compared with rigid fixation. The interfragmentary compression produced during the application of plates can last for many weeks under experimental conditions (Perren *et al.* 1969) unless there is a high level of movement associated with the compression. Significant necrosis of bone ends does not occur at the levels of compression commonly used in clinical practice. Interfragmentary compression increases stability of the plate–bone complex by ensuring intimate contact of the bone ends and load sharing between the plate and the bone.

Application of biomechanics to implants

Each type of implant will now be considered under the subheadings of mechanical characteristics, biological response and optimal insertion.

SCREW FIXATION

Mechanical characteristics

Figure 1.17 shows the components of a bone screw frequently used for internal fixation. The main aim in screw design for internal fixation in cortical bone is to

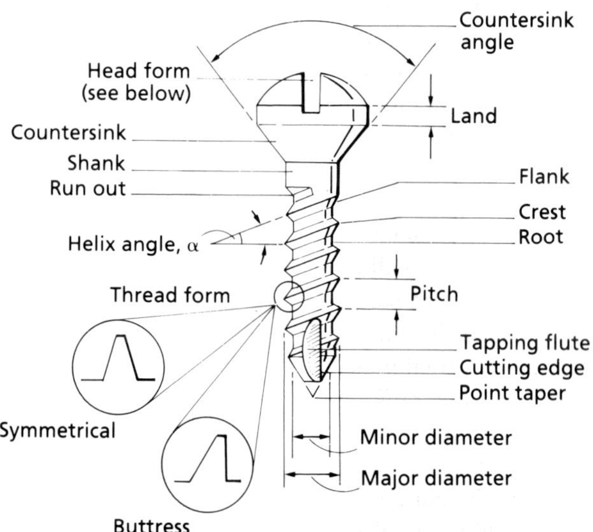

Fig. 1.17 Features of a bone screw used in internal fixation (adapted from Hughes & Jordan 1972).

have a screw which will produce a high level of compression between the bone ends in screw fixation or between the plate and the bone in plate fixation. This compressive stress should be produced with a small tensile stress within the screw and with a reasonably small shear stress in the bone adjacent to the screw; if either of these stresses is too high, fracture of the screw or pull-out failure of the screw will result. An important feature of screw design concerns the core diameter which will have a direct influence on both the tensile and torsional strength of the screw; the material properties of the screw will also affect its failure strength. The thread form will affect both the stripping torque and the pull-out strength of a screw.

The pilot-hole diameter will influence the holding strength of the screw in the bone. If too small a pilot hole is used high levels of torque will be required during screw insertion, and radial cracking in the bone surrounding the screw may occur (Jordan & Hughes 1978). A critical size of pilot hole, above which the holding strength of the screw is reduced, has been defined by Hughes and Jordan (1972) as being between 85 and 90% of the major diameter of the screw. To facilitate easy insertion of screws a large pilot-hole diameter is preferred. However, due to the reduced area of contact between the screw and the bone with a large pilot hole, this may increase the stresses in the bone to an unacceptable level.

The initial fixation of a screw can be improved by the following procedures:

1 *Drilling* a pilot hole greater than the core diameter but less than 85% of the major diameter of the screw.

2 *Tapping*, which allows a more precise introduction with less damage to the bone. Taps allow threads to be cut accurately, and since the tap removes much of the loose bone debris created during tapping, a pre-drilled hole with a diameter close to the screw minor diameter can be used to provide a greater amount of bone to support the screw. Conversely, a self-tapping screw needs a pre-drilled hole of a significantly larger diameter than the minor diameter of the screw to accommodate the debris which will remain.

3 *Lubrication* with saline during pre-drilling can reduce thermal necrosis of the bone, and during screw insertion it can reduce friction at the countersink face.

4 *Cooling during drilling*. Thermal necrosis is commonly created during pre-drilling but can be reduced by using a slow drilling speed (Matthews *et al.* 1984) and by cooling with saline during drilling. The heat produced during drilling can also be reduced by ensuring that the drill used is sharp.

Biological response

Despite the important influences of screw design and method of insertion, the ultimate stability of screw fixation must depend upon the biological response which can change with time.

In experimental studies, the mechanical characteristics of screw fixation have been assessed at defined intervals after insertion. Screws were found to increase their grip up to approximately 6–8 weeks after insertion; after this there was a small decrease, but the level of fixation always remained above the level recorded at the time of insertion (Schatzker *et al.* 1975c).

With time, the woven bone forming around a screw hole is resorbed and is replaced by lamellar bone.

Stability of fixation is essential for the prolonged rigidity of screw fixation. Cortical bone can be subjected to high levels of static compression by screw threads without being resorbed or losing its integrity (Schatzker *et al.* 1975b, Perren 1979). However, relative movement between the screw and the bone causes the migrating cells which fill the microscopic spaces between the screw threads to differentiate into fibroblasts, chondroblasts and osteoclasts. This results in the formation of fibrous and cartilaginous tissue, and existing or newly laid bone is resorbed, thus causing the screw to loosen (Uhthoff 1973, Schatzker *et al.* 1975a, Perren 1979). Conversely, in the absence of relative movement between the screw and the bone, the migrating cells differentiate into osteogenic cells and produce a solid callus which firmly anchors the screw. Uhthoff and Germain (1977) have shown this process to be reversible for a loose screw, i.e. if the relative movement between the screw and the bone is reduced or eliminated, the osteoclastic activity ceases and osteoblastic activity appears, resulting in new bone formation.

Optimal insertion

It can be seen from the above that slow pre-drilling with a pilot-hole diameter greater than the core diameter but not exceeding 85% of the major screw diameter, followed by insertion of a pre-tapped screw of the largest practical core diameter, will lead to the strongest fixation. Screw design should allow high axial forces to be achieved and the instruments available for insertion of screws should not allow forces to be applied which might lead to fracture of the screw or of the bone into which it is to be inserted.

Screws should be inserted to produce interfragmentary compression. For optimal compression the proximal cortical hole should be overdrilled to at least the screw major diameter. Interfragmentary compression, which is vital for close apposition and friction between fragments, cannot be achieved if the cortex is threaded in both fragments. To resist bending, screws should be inserted perpendicular to the axis of the bone, and to resist torsion, screws should be inserted perpendicular to the fracture plane. When fixing a long spiral fracture screws should be inserted at angles between these two optimum values. In these ways sufficient stability can be achieved using only two or three screws for many fractures, although not for long bone diaphyseal fractures.

PLATE FIXATION

Mechanical characteristics

The relative strength of combined implant and bone fixation has been recorded for most types of plate, and the increase in strength and stiffness achieved by changing the characteristics of the plate, either in length, thickness or in number of screws used, has been defined. Manufacturers recommend certain plates for specific clinical indications and these recommendations are best adhered to.

Biological response

The pattern of healing seen with rigid plate fixation with either a gap or no gap has been described in the first section of this chapter, i.e. there is either primary bone healing or gap-healing. If there is callus formation this reflects some instability of fixation, whether this was intentional (as with semi-rigid plates) or not. The late responses to the presence of the plate in relation to bone strength are described on pp. 23–24.

Optimal insertion

Plates are applied for the following mechanical reasons:
1 Having achieved stabilization by interfragmentary compression with the use of screws alone, the resulting fixation may not be sufficient for loading of the implant—bone complex, and a neutralization plate may then be needed to allow for functional loading of the limb. This plate must provide sufficient fixation or early failure will almost certainly result (Fig. 1.18).
2 A similar situation applies when a buttress plate is used to supplement screw fixation in metaphyseal fractures (Fig. 1.19).
3 Plates may also be used for short oblique or for

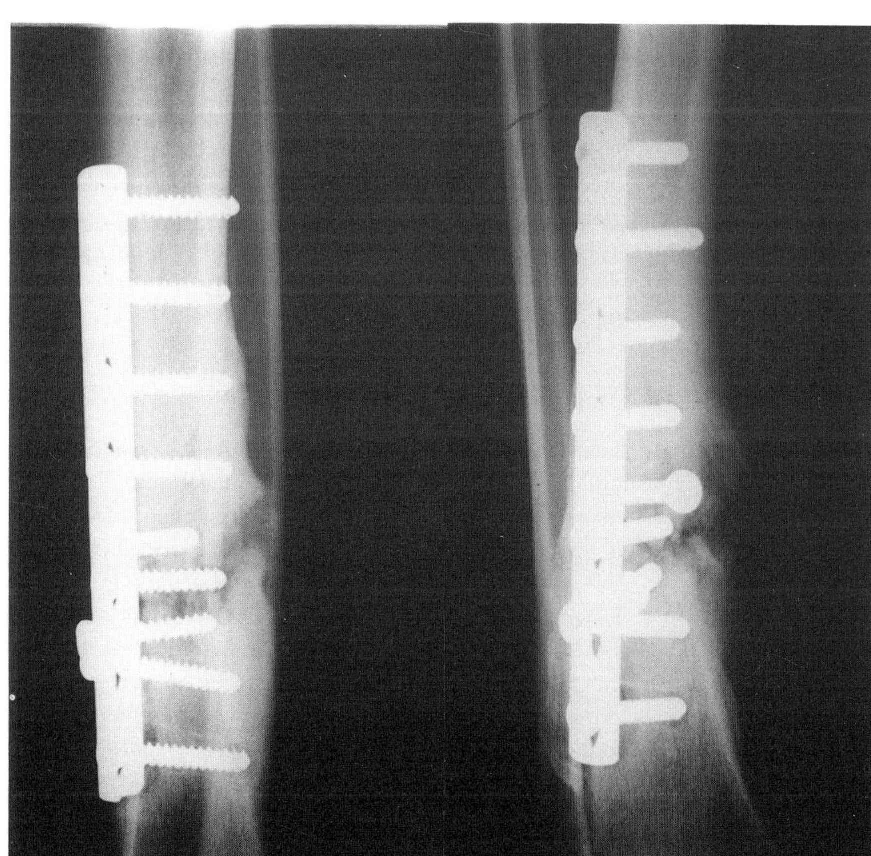

Fig. 1.18 Poor application of a neutralization plate. There are too few screws attached to the distal segment, and one screw is placed through the fracture. Note also that the interfragmentary screw fixation does not cross the fracture site.

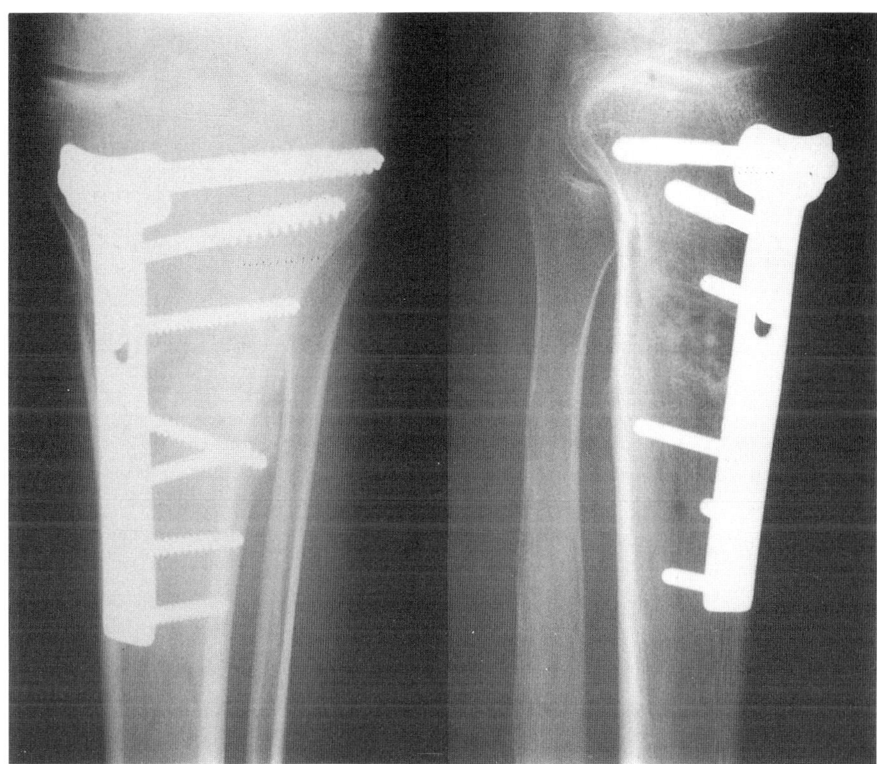

Fig. 1.19 Buttress plate used to supplement screw fixation in metaphyseal fracture. These are needed for intra-articular fractures of the upper tibia after elevation of the fragments.

transverse fractures, with or without compression, for primary fixation. Many experimental studies have been performed with this type of fracture both *in vivo* and *in vitro*, and clinical experience has shown these observations to be relevant to clinical treatment.

As described already, plates should be applied so that on curved long bones they lie on the convex surface of the bone which is the surface normally loaded in tension. On this surface the plate is then loaded in tension and the bone on the opposite surface to the plate is loaded in compression. In these circumstances increases in load through the limb increase the rigidity of fixation; this is improved further by longitudinal compression across the fracture. Placement of the plate on the inappropriate surface of the bone can quickly result in the failure of the fixation (Nunamaker & Perren 1979). Minns *et al.* (1977) have shown by theoretical analysis, for conditions of physiological loading, that the anterolateral surface of the tibia is mainly loaded in tension and is thus more appropriate than the antero-medial surface for application of a plate in order to achieve maximum stiffness of the plate–bone complex.

Slight bending of the plate before insertion leads to enhanced fixation (Nunamaker & Perren 1979). If a straight plate is applied to a bone surface and loading then applied there will be poor bone contact except in the small area adjacent to the plate.

Special precautions need to be taken where the loading axis of the bone is very remote from the axis of the plate. Large bending moments act on the plate in these circumstances, and fatigue failure of plates is very common. Reduced loading of the leg will be necessary until compressive load can be taken by the bone opposite the plate; a bone graft is usually used to enhance this process. This state of affairs is very common in femoral diaphyseal fractures and in unstable femoral trochanteric fractures where large bending moments can occur, and where there is a poor bone on the compression surface (Fig. 1.20). Techniques need to be employed to increase the integrity of the medial bone or relieve the applied bending moment (Fig. 1.21).

INTRAMEDULLARY NAILS

Mechanical characteristics

Many types of intramedullary implant have been devised and they represent the most effective treatment for short oblique diaphyseal fractures in long bones, such as the tibia and femur. Nails of different cross-section with consequent differences in flexibility have been designed. The basic principle of the intramedullary nail is that the nail acts as an internal splint which reduces, but does not eliminate, interfragmentary

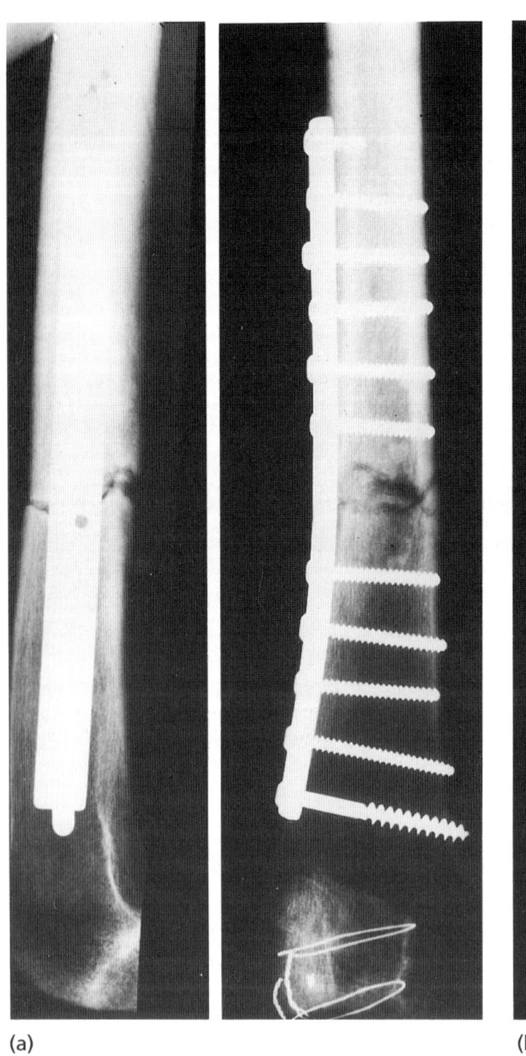
(a)

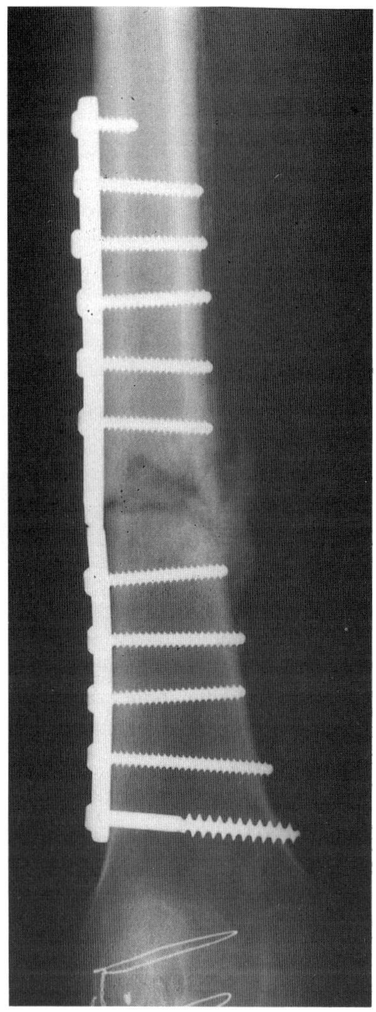
(b)

Fig. 1.20 (a) Femoral plate applied remote from loading axis of bone. (b) Fatigue failure of the plate subsequently occurred since there was no bony support in the cortex opposite the plate. Note that the unfilled screw hole in the plate acts as a stress raiser and provides an initiation site for the fatigue crack.

motion (Perren 1979) so that fracture healing by a secondary means is to be expected. The nail carries predominantly bending and torsional loads from one side of the fracture to the other whilst allowing some axial movement of the fracture ends. By reaming the bone before nail insertion a uniform diameter can be created in the medullary cavity which will provide an optimal fit of the nail.

The fixation of an intramedullary nail, and hence its resistance to deformation, will depend upon the area of contact between the nail and the bone, as well as upon the stiffness characteristics of the nail. Reaming through the isthmus of the bone is usually performed so that the maximum area of contact can be achieved. Four-point fixation of the nail in the medullary canal is sufficient to transmit bending loads large enough to allow early return of function which, in turn, will minimize disuse osteoporosis (Tarr & Wiss 1986). For the nail to effectively transmit torsional loads, however, intimate contact of the nail with the bone over as great an area as possible is required, as is some interlocking of the fracture ends.

The cross-section of the nail will affect its mechanical characteristics. Thin-walled tubular nails with a cloverleaf section are most frequently used as these are flexible across their diameter and thus allow an effective interference fit in the bone. Such nails are weak in torsional loading owing to the open section; indeed, the torsional rigidity of an open section is approximately 1/50 of that of the equivalent closed section (Allen *et al.* 1968). However, these nails resist bending as well as many closed-section nails. The resistance of a nail to bending increases with increasing I (second moment of area; see p. 5) of the nail cross-section which, for a

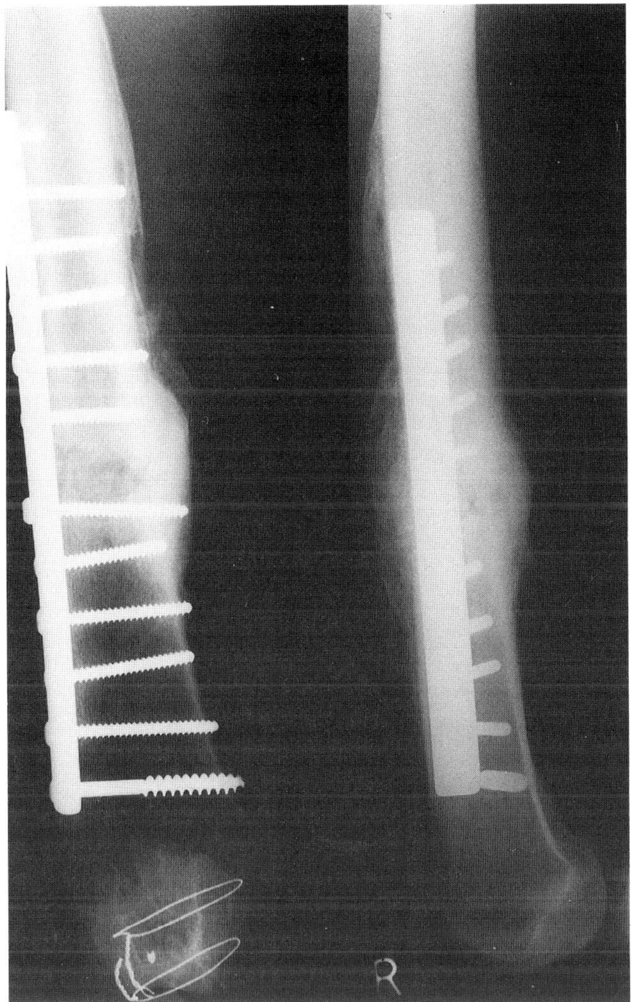

Fig. 1.21 Replating of the fracture shown in Fig. 1.20 has been accompanied by a bone graft to fill the cortical defect.

circular-section nail, is proportional to the fourth power of the diameter of the nail, so that a 15-mm-diameter nail is almost 2.5 times more resistant to bending than a 12-mm-diameter nail.

Biological response

Experimental studies have shown that fractures and simulated fractures fixed with intramedullary nails are markedly less stiff than the equivalent plated fractures (Rand *et al*. 1981, Tencer *et al*. 1984). In experimental studies of fracture healing with intramedullary nails and in clinical practice, indirect healing with external callus formation is nearly always seen.

Intramedullary reaming followed by nail insertion affects the blood supply of the bone throughout its length, including at the fracture site. In experimental conditions a new endosteal blood supply forms rapidly; the normal predominance of the endosteal blood supply of the cortical bone is reversed close to the fracture, so that blood from the periosteal vessels pervades the fracture site. In patients this extraosseous supply might have been damaged at the time of injury, but despite this intramedullary nailing of fractures with severe soft tissue damage does not appear to cause significant bone death at the fracture site.

Optimal insertion

Nails tend to fail by migration, plastic deformation or fatigue failure. Deformation or failure of intramedullary nails as a result of bending or torsional loads is not common in practice. The normal sequence of events is that loss of fracture position occurs by the bone moving on the nail.

A nail of sufficient stiffness for the loads likely to be encountered should be inserted in order to resist plastic deformation of the nail at the fracture site. The medullary shaft of the bone should be reamed at the isthmus to increase the interference fit of the nail, although excessive reaming (to more than 14 mm) can reduce the torsional strength of the bone by over 50% (Pratt *et al*. 1987). In young patients the fixation obtained in the areas of cancellous bone at either end of the bone when using intramedullary nails is strong, but in old people there is little cancellous bone and intramedullary nailing may be associated with a very small area of interference fit. Under these conditions locking of the nail needs to be used or there may be bending at the fracture site or fracture of the nail.

In bones such as the femur the area of fixation for proximal or distal segments is often very different and may be reduced if there is comminution. Longitudinal stability may have to be achieved under these conditions by locking of the nail at each end. Winquist *et al*. (1984) and Brumback *et al*. (1988) have defined the patterns of fracture which require locking nails to be used; however, any degree of comminution leads to a potential instability.

Dynamic loading of the limb can be applied following most forms of intramedullary nailing.

Removal of implants

Implant removal is frequently advised for the following reasons:

1 Plates can act as stress raisers, predisposing to late fracture at the point between the plate and the normal bone. Significant osteoporosis can also occur under a plate due to the effect of stress shielding.

2 Plates and other implants can cause discomfort resulting from friction of the plate with soft tissues or from corrosion responses if low-grade materials are used.
3 The continued presence of an implant might give rise to local infection following haemotological spread.

The risks associated with the removal of plates and intramedullary nails need therefore to be balanced against the gains. The main complication which can follow removal is that of refracture, this being a particular risk following serious diaphyseal fractures where complete revascularization and remodelling of bone at the fracture site may take several years. The risk of refracture is also increased by weakening of the bone beneath the whole of the plate and by the presence of the screw holes. In stable plate fixation, osteonal bone healing leads to a weak fracture in the early months after injury when compared to the strength of similar fractures healing by external callus formation, but it is rarely necessary to consider removal of implants at this early stage. At a later stage, when primary healing is almost complete, remodelling beneath the plate results in bone which is different from that seen in the cortex remote from the plated segment. Uhthoff and Dubuc (1971) have shown that there is cortical thinning at 2, 7, 20 and 24 weeks after compression plating in an experimental model and Tonino *et al.* (1976) showed considerable endosteal resorption and reduced bone mineral mass beneath a rigid plate. Woven bone forms beneath the plate and remodelling does not occur until after plate removal. The bone becomes more porous with widened haversian canals and with decreased density of lamellar bone. There is controversy as to the exact cause of this phenomenon; it may be due to increased vascularity or to decreased loading resulting from stress protection. Such effects undoubtedly exist, and even in experimental osteotomies many weeks may pass before full remodelling has occurred and the bone has regained its former strength.

Added to the problems of bone thinning and porosity beneath the plate is the weakness created around screw holes. If a hole is drilled through a bone, the bone is weaker in both bending and torsion. The hole acts as a stress raiser and Brooks *et al.* (1970) have shown that in the canine femur holes of between 2.8 and 3.6-mm-diameter increase the stress around the hole under torsional loading by a factor of 1.6 compared with normal bone. Fracture was always found to have occurred through the hole.

In the clinical situation further factors need to be considered; there may be relative devitalization of the bone at the fracture site because of the severity of the initial injury, and there may also be small gaps at the fracture site which will act as stress raisers.

The assessment of the above risks is not an exact science and at the present time many factors need to be taken into consideration. As a general rule, however, plate implants used to treat diaphyseal fractures should not be removed until 2 years after injury and significant protection in the form of a lightweight cast or splint is needed for at least 3 months following that time.

Problem areas and conclusions

In all the above sections biomechanical principles have been applied predominantly to normal bone but in clinical practice pathological bone exists and allowance must be made for this when planning the management of a fracture. Common circumstances that require special consideration are:
1 Osteopenia.
2 Cancellous bone in the elderly.
3 Paget's disease.
4 Fractures through the os-calcis and lumbar vertebral bodies.
5 Fracture through metastases.

When planning and carrying out treatment for all fractures the general and local biological and mechanical needs of the injured person must be assessed; in the treatment programme for a particular patient these various needs must be integrated.

References

Allen, W.C., Piotrowski, G., Burstein, A.H. & Frankel, V.H. Biomechanical principles of intramedullary fixation. *Clin Orthop* 1968; **60**: 13−20.

Almo, M. Fracture mechanics. *J Bone Joint Surg* 1961; **43B**: 162−166.

Aro, H.T., Kelly, P.J., Lewallen, D.G. & Chao, E.Y.S. The effects of physiologic dynamic compression on bone healing under external fixation. *Clin Orthop* 1990; **256**: 260−273.

Behiri, J.C. & Bonfield, W. Crack velocity dependence of longitudinal fracture in bone. *J Mater Sci* 1980; **15**: 1841−1849.

Behiri, J.C. & Bonfield, W. Fracture mechanics of bone — the effects of density, specimen thickness and crack velocity on longitudinal fracture. *J Biomech* 1984; **17**: 25−34.

Behrens, F. General theory and principles of external fixation. *Clin Orthop* 1989; **241**: 15−23.

Behrens, F. & Johnson, W. Unilateral external fixation. Methods to increase and reduce frame stiffness. *Clin Orthop* 1989; **241**: 48−56.

Behrens, F. & Searls, K. External fixation of the tibia. Basic concepts and prospective evaluation. *J Bone Joint Surg* 1986; **68B**: 246−254.

Behrens, F., Johnson, W.D., Koch, T.W. & Kovacevic, N. Bending stiffness of unilateral and bilateral fixator frames. *Clin Orthop* 1983; **178**: 103−110.

Black, J. *Orthopaedic Biomechanics in Research and Practice*. Churchill Livingstone: Edinburgh, 1988.

Bleck, E.E. & Kleinman, R.G. Special injuries of the musculo-skeletal system. In: Rockwood, C.A., Wilkins, K.E. & King, R.E. (eds) *Fractures in Children*. Lippincott: Philadelphia, 1984.

Bonfield, W. Advances in the fracture mechanics of cortical bone. *J Biomech* 1987; **20**: 1071–1081.

Briggs, B.T. & Chao, E.Y.S. The mechanical performance of the standard Hoffmann–Vidal external fixation apparatus. *J Bone Joint Surg* 1982; **64A**: 566–573.

Brumback, R.J., Reilly, J.P., Paka, A., Lakatos, R.P., Bathan, G.H. & Burgess, A.R. Intramedullary nailing of femoral shaft fractures. Part 1: Decision making errors with interlocking fixation. *J Bone Joint Surg* 1988; **70A**: 1441–1452.

Brooks, D.B., Burstein, A.H. & Frankel, V.H. The biomechanics of torsional fractures. The stress concentration effect of a drill hole. *J Bone Joint Surg* 1970; **52A**: 507–514.

Burny, F. Elastic external fixation of tibial fractures: study of 1421 cases. In: Brooker, A.F. & Edwards, C.C. (eds) *External Fixation: the Current State of the Art*. Williams & Wilkins: Baltimore, 1979.

Buxton, R.A. The use of Perkins' traction in the treatment of femoral shaft fractures. *J Bone Joint Surg* 1981; **63B**: 362–366.

Chao, E.Y.S. & An, K.N. Biomechanical analysis of external fixation devices for the treatment of open bone fractures. In: Gallagher, R.H., Simon, B.R., Johnson, P.C. & Gross, J.F. (eds) *Finite Elements in Biomechanics*. John Wiley & Sons: New York, 1982.

Chao, E.Y.S. & Aro, H.T. Biomechanics and biology of external fixation. In: Coombs, R., Green, S., & Sarmiento, A. (eds) *External Fixation and Functional Bracing*. Orthotext: London, 1989.

Chao, E.Y.S. & Hein, T.J. Mechanical performance of standard Orthofix external fixator. *Orthopaedics* 1988; **2**: 1057–1069.

Chao, E.Y.S. Kasman, R.A. & An, K.N. Rigidity and stress analysis of external fracture fixation devices — a theoretical approach. *J Biomech* 1982; **15**: 971–983.

Charnley, J. *The Closed Treatment of Common Fractures* 3rd edn. Williams & Wilkins: Baltimore, 1968.

Cunningham, J.L., Evans, M. & Kenwright, J. Measurement of fracture movement in patients treated with external skeletal fixation. *J Biomed Eng* 1989; **11**: 118–122.

Currey, J.D. The evaluation of the mechanical properties of amniote bone. *J Biomech* 1987; **20**: 1035–1044.

Currey, J.D. The effect of porosity and mineral content on the Young's modulus of elasticity of compact bone. *J Biomech* 1988; **21**: 131–139.

Currey, J.D. & Butler, G. The mechanical properties of bone tissue in children. *J Bone Joint Surg* 1975; **57A**: 810–814.

Danis, R. *Theorie et Pratique de l'Osteosynthese*. Masson: Paris, 1949.

De Bastiani, G., Aldegheri, R. & Renzi Brivio, L. The treatment of fractures with a dynamic axial fixator. *J Bone Joint Surg* 1984; **66B**: 538–545.

Drijber, F.L.I., Finlay, J.B., Moroz, T.K. & Rorabeck, C.H. Source of the slippage in the universal joints of the Hoffman external fixator. *Med Biol Eng Comput* 1990; **28**: 8–14.

Evans, M., Kenwright, J. & Cunningham, J.L. Design and performance of a fracture monitoring transducer. *J Biomed Eng* 1988; **10**: 64–69.

Evans, M., Spencer, M., Wang, Q., White, S.H. & Cunningham, J.L. The design and testing of external fixator bone screws. *J Biomed Eng* 1990; **12**: 457–462.

Finlay, J.B., Moroz, T.K., Rorabeck, C.H., Davey, J.R. & Bourne, R.B. Stability of ten configurations of the Hoffmann external fixation frame. *J Bone Joint Surg* 1987; **69A**: 734–744.

Fischer, R.A., Arms, S.W., Pope, M.H. & Seligson, D. Analysis of the effect of using two different strain rates on the acoustic emission in bone. *J Biomech* 1986; **19**: 119–127.

Gasser, B., Bowman, B., Wyder, D. & Schneider, E. Stiffness characteristics of the circular Ilizarov device as opposed to conventional external fixators. *J Biomech Eng* 1990; **112**: 15–21.

Goodship, A.E. Experimental studies of micromotion. In: Coombs, R., Green, S. & Sarmiento, A. (eds) *External Fixation and Functional Bracing*. Orthotext: London, 1989.

Goodship, A.E. & Kenwright, J. The influence of induced micromovement on the healing of experimental tibial fractures. *J Bone Joint Surg* 1985; **67B**: 650–655.

Hammer, R., Edholm., P. & Lindholm, B. Stability of union after tibial shaft fracture. *J Bone Joint Surg* 1984; **66B**: 529–534.

Harkess, J.W., Ramsey, W.C. & Ahmadi, B. Principles of fractures and dislocations. In: Rockwood, C.A. & Green, D.P. (eds) *Fractures in Adults*, Vol. 1, 2nd edn. Lippincott: Philadelphia, 1984.

Harris, J.D., Evans, M. & Kenwright, J. Safe stress levels at the screw interface of an external fixator for long bone fractures. In: Stokes, I.A.F. (ed.) *Mechanical Factors and the Skeleton*. John Libbey: London, 1981.

Hughes, A.N. & Jordan, B.A. The mechanical properties of surgical bone screws and some aspects of insertion practice. *Injury* 1972; **4**: 25–58.

Huiskes, R. & Chao, E.Y.S. Guidelines for external fixation frame rigidity and stresses. *J Orthop Res* 1986; **4**: 68–75.

Huiskes, R., Chao, E.Y.S. & Crippen, T.E. Parametric analysis of pin–bone stresses in external fixation devices. *J Orthop Res* 1985; **3**: 341–349.

Jernberger, A. Measurement of stability of tibial fractures *Acta Orthop Scand Suppl* 1970; **135**.

Jordan, B.A. & Hughes, A.N. A review of the factors affecting the design, specification and material selection of screws for use in orthopaedic surgery. *Eng Med* 1978; **7**: 114–123.

Jorgensen, T.E. Measurements of stability of crural fractures treated with Hoffmann osteotaxis. 2. Measurements on crural fractures. *Acta Orthop Scand* 1972; **43**: 207–218.

Kempson, G.E. & Campbell, D. The comparative stiffness of external fixation frames. *Injury* 1981; **12**: 297–304.

Kenwright, J. & Goodship. A.E. Controlled mechanical stimulation in the treatment of tibial fractures. *Clin Orthop* 1989; **241**: 36–47.

Klip, E.J. & Bosma, R. Investigations into the mechanical behaviour of bone–pin connections. *Eng Med* 1978; **7**: 43–46.

Kristiansen, T., Fleming, B., Neale, G., Reinecke, S. & Pope, M. Comparative study of fracture gap motion in external fixation. *Clin Biomech* 1987; **2**: 191–195.

Lazo-Zbikowski, J., Aguilar, F., Mozo, F., Gonzalez-Buendia, R. & Lazo, J.M. Biocompression external fixation: sliding external osteosynthesis. *Clin Orthop* 1986; **206**: 169–184.

Lippert, F.G. & Hirsch, C. The three-dimensional measurement of tibial fracture movement by photogrammetry. *Clin Orthop* 1974; **105**: 130–143.

Mabrey, J.D. & Fitch, R.D. Plastic deformation in pediatric fractures: mechanism and treatment. *J Pediatr Orthop* 1989; **9**: 310–314.

Martens, M., Van Audekercke, R., de Meester, P. & Mulier, J.C. Mechanical behaviour of femoral bones in bending loading. *J Biomech* 1986; **19**: 443–454.

Matthews, L.S., Green, C.A. & Goldstein, S.A. The thermal effects of skeletal fixation-pin insertion. *J Bone Joint Surg* 1984; **66A**: 1077–1083.

McCoy, M.T., Chao, E.Y.S. & Kasman, R.A. Comparison of mechanical performance in four types of external fixators. *Clin Orthop* 1983; **180**: 23–33.

McKibbin, B. The biology of fracture healing in long bones. *J Bone Joint Surg* 1978; **60B**: 150–162.

Meggitt, B.F., Juett, D.A. & Smith, J.D. Cast bracing for fractures of the femoral shaft. A biomechanical and clinical study. *J Bone Joint Surg* 1981; **63B**: 12–23.

Minns, R.J., Bremble, G.R. & Campbell, J. A biomechanical study of internal fixation of the tibial shaft. *J Biomech* 1977; **10**: 569–579.

Moroz, T.K., Finlay, J.B., Rorabeck, C.H. & Bourne, R.B. Stability of the original Hoffmann and AO tubular external fixation devices. *Med Biol Eng Comput* 1988; **26**: 271–276.

Müller, M.E., Allgower, M., Schneider, R. & Willenegger, H. *Manual of Internal Fixation*. Springer-Verlag: Berlin, 1979.

Nunamaker, D.M. & Perren, S.M. A radiological and histological analysis of fracture healing using prebending of compression plates. *Clin Orthop* 1979; **138**: 167–174.

Paley, D., Fleming, B., Catagni, M., Kristianson, T. & Pope, M. Mechanical evaluation of external fixators used in limb lengthening. *Clin Orthop* 1990; **250**: 50–57.

Panjabi, M.M., White, A.A. & Southwick, W.O. Mechanical properties of bone as a function of rates of deformation. *J Bone Joint Surg* 1973; **55A**: 322–330.

Panjabi, M.M., White, A.A. & Southwick, W.O. Temporal changes in the physical properties of healing fractures in rabbits. *J Biomech* 1977; **10**: 689–699.

Perren, S.M. Physical and biological aspects of fracture healing with special reference to internal fixation. *Clin Orthop* 1979; **136**: 175–196.

Perren, S.M., Haggler, A., Russenberger, M., Allgöwer, M., Mathys, R., Schenk, R., Willenegger, H. & Müller, M.E. The reaction of cortical bone to compression. *Acta Orthop Scand Suppl* 1969; **125**.

Peterson, D.L., Skraba, J.S., Moran, J.M. & Greenwald, A.S. Fracture of long bones: rate effects under singular and combined loading states. *J Orthop Res* 1984; **1**: 244–250.

Pettine, K.A., Kelly, P.J., Chao, E.Y.S. & Huiskes, R. Histologic and biomechanical analysis of external fixator pin–bone interface. *Orthop Trans* 1986; **10**: 337.

Pope, M.H. & Outwater, J.O. The fracture characteristics of bone substance. *J Biomech* 1972; **5**: 457–465.

Pratt, D.J., Papagiannopoulos, G., Rees, P.H. & Quinnell, R. The effects of medullary reaming on the torsional strength of the femur. *Injury* 1987; **18**: 177–179.

Rahn, B.A. Bone healing: histologic and physiologic concepts. In: Sumner-Smith, G. (ed.) *Bone in Clinical Orthopaedics. A Study in Comparative Osteology*. WB Saunders: Philadelphia, 1982.

Rand, J.A., An, K.N., Chao, E.Y.S. & Kelly, P.J. A comparison of the effect of open intramedullary nailing and compression plate fixation on fracture-site blood flow and fracture union.

J Bone Joint Surg 1981; **63A**: 427–442.

Reilly, D.T. & Burstein, A.H. The mechanical properties of cortical bone. *J Bone Joint Surg* 1974; **56A**: 1001–1021.

Sammarco, G.J., Burstein, A.H., Davis, W.L. & Frankel, V.H. The biomechanics of torsional fractures: the effect of loading on ultimate properties. *J Biomech* 1971; **4**: 113–117.

Sarmiento, A. Functional bracing of tibial fractures. *Clin Orthop* 1974; **105**: 202–219.

Sarmiento, A. & Latta, L.L. *Closed Functional Treatment of Fractures*. Springer-Verlag: Berlin, 1981.

Sarmiento, A., Kinman, P.B. & Latta, L.L. Fractures of the proximal tibia and tibial condyles. A clinical and laboratory comparative study. *Clin Orthop* 1979; **145**: 136–145.

Sarmiento, A., Latta, L., Zilioli, A. & Sinclair, W. The role of soft tissues in the stabilization of tibial fractures. *Clin Orthop* 1974; **105**: 116–129.

Sarmiento, A., Mullis, D.L., Latta, L.L., Tarr, R.R. & Alvarez, R.R. A quantitative analysis of fracture healing under the influence of compression plating versus closed weight bearing treatment. *Clin Orthop* 1980; **149**: 232–239.

Sarmiento, A., Schaeffer, J.F., Beckerman, L., Latta, L.L. & Enis, J.E. Fracture healing in rat femora as affected by functional weight bearing. *J Bone Joint Surg* 1977; **59A**: 369–375.

Schatzker, J., Horne, J.G. & Sumner-Smith, G. The effect of movement on the holding power of screws in bone. *Clin Orthop* 1975a; **111**: 257–262.

Schatzker, J., Horne, J.G. & Sumner-Smith, G. The reaction of cortical bone to compression by screw threads. *Clin Orthop* 1975b; **111**: 263–265.

Schatzker, J., Sanderson, R. & Murnaghan, J.P. The holding power of orthopaedic screws *in vivo*. *Clin Orthop* 1975c; **108**: 115–126.

Schenk, R. & Willenegger, H. Zur histologic der primaren Knockenheilung. *Klin Khir* 1964; **308**: 440–452.

Seligson, D., Donald, G.D., Stanwyck, T.S. & Pope, M.H. Consideration of pin diameter and insertion technique for external fixation in diaphyseal bone. *Acta Orthop Belg* 1984; **50**: 441–450.

Skerry, T.M., Bitensky, L., Chayen, J. & Lanyon, L.E. Loading related re-orientation of bone proteoglycan *in vivo*: a strain memory in bone tissue? *J Orthop Res* 1988; **6**: 547–551.

Tarr, R.R. & Wiss, D.A. The mechanics and biology of intramedullary fracture fixation. *Clin Orthop* 1986; **212**: 10–17.

Tayton, K.J.J., Johnson-Nurse, C., McKibbin, B., Bradley, J. & Hastings, G. The use of semi-rigid carbon-fibre-reinforced plastic plates for fixation of human fractures. *J Bone Joint Surg* 1982; **66B**: 105–111.

Tencer, A.F., Johnson, K.D., Johnston, D.W.C. & Gill, K. A biomechanical comparison of various methods of stabilization of subtrochanteric fractures of the femur. *J Orthop Res* 1984; **2**: 297–305.

Tonino, A.J., Davidson, C.L., Klopper, P.J. & Linclau, L.A. Protection from stress in bone and its effects. *J Bone Joint Surg* 1976; **58B**: 107–113.

Uhthoff, H.K. Mechanical factors influencing the holding power of screws in compact bone. *J Bone Joint Surg* 1973; **55B**: 633–639.

Uhthoff, H.K. & Dubuc, F.L. Bone structure changes in the dog under rigid internal fixation. *Clin Orthop* 1971; **81**: 165–170.

Uhthoff, H.K. & Germain, J.-P. The reversal of tissue differentiation around screws. *Clin Orthop* 1977; **123**: 248–252.

Unsworth, A. & Shannon, F.T. A biomechanical study of the treatment of tibial fractures using plaster casts. *Eng Med* 1979; **8**: 4–10.

Wagenknecht, M., Andrianne, Y., Donkerwolcke, M., Zurbuchen, C. & Burny, F. Pin technology. In: Coombs, R., Green, S. & Sarmiento, A. (eds) *External Fixation and Functional Bracing*. Orthotext: London, 1989.

Wardlaw, D., McLauchlan, J., Pratt, D.J. & Bowker, P. A biomechanical study of cast-brace treatment of femoral shaft fractures. *J Bone Joint Surg* 1981; **63B**: 7–11.

White, A.A., Panjabi, M.M. & Southwick, W.O. The four biomechanical stages of fracture repair. *J Bone Joint Surg* 1977; **59A**: 188–192.

Williams, E.A., Rand, J.A., An, K.N., Chao, E.Y.S. & Kelly, P.J. The early healing of tibial osteotomies stabilised with one plane or two plane external fixation. *J Bone Joint Surg* 1987; **69A**: 355–365.

Winquist, R.A., Hansen, S.T. & Clawson, D.K. Closed intramedullary nailing of femoral fractures. *J Bone Joint Surg* 1984; **66A**: 529–539.

Wolf, J.W., White, A.A., Panjabi, M.M. & Southwick, W.O. Comparison of cyclic loading versus constant compression in the treatment of long bone fractures in rabbits. *J Bone Joint Surg* 1981; **63A**: 805–810.

Wolff, J. *The Law of Bone Remodelling*, Maquet, P. & Furlong, R. (trans.). Springer-Verlag: Berlin, 1986.

Wu, J.-J., Shyr, H.S., Chao, E.Y.S. & Kelly, P.J. Comparison of osteotomy healing under external fixation devices with different stiffness characteristics. *J Bone Joint Surg* 1984; **66A**: 1258–1264.

Yamagishi, M. & Yoshimura, Y. The biomechanics of fracture healing. *J Bone Joint Surg* 1955; **37A**: 1035–1068.

2: Terminology, Description and Classification

O.O.A.ONI AND P.J.GREGG

Introduction

There are several reasons for arranging fractures and dislocations into separate groups. First, classification of individual injuries allows surgeons to communicate with each other, regarding fracture management, with some precision. Second, different fractures and dislocations present different sets of problems and have different prognoses. A classification is of practical importance because it may indicate the nature of the clinical problem and the general type of treatment that may be required. Third, a comparison of results of different methods of treatment is impossible unless based on some sort of classification, so that one is sure that the injuries are the same in each treatment group.

General classification of fractures

A fracture is defined as a structural break in the normal continuity of a bone. The break may be either *complete*, or *incomplete*, and a fracture may be classified accordingly in these terms.

Incomplete fractures are rarely observed in adults except in the special circumstances of pathological or fatigue-induced fractures. Incomplete fractures (Fig. 2.1) are common in the more plastic bones of children when they are classified as follows:

Type I — bowing (caused by a bending force; the bone suffers permanent plastic deformation; usually occurs in the ulna or fibula in association with a dislocated radial head or fractured radius or tibia and may prevent accurate closed reduction).

Type II — buckle (torus) fractures (caused by axial compression; the symptoms may be minimal).

Type III — greenstick fractures (caused by a bending force; the cortex breaks on one side and buckles on the other).

Type IV — hairline (crack) fractures (commonly caused

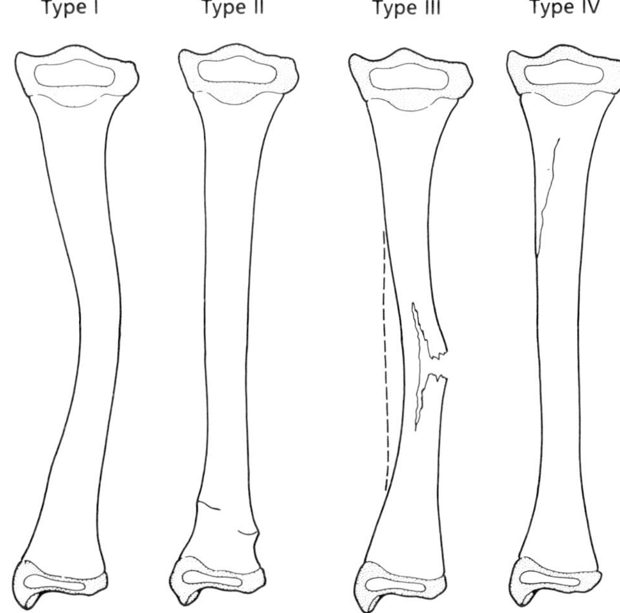

Fig. 2.1 Diagram showing the types of incomplete fractures.

by a twisting force on a loaded bone; the fracture line may be spiral or oblique).

In addition, the classification of fractures is generally based upon the following factors:

1 Anatomical location.
2 Fracture morphology.
3 Mechanism of injury.
4 Severity of fracture.
5 Displacement.
6 Special types.

Anatomical location of fracture

In addition to indicating the actual bone which is fractured, it is customary to indicate the location of the fracture in the bone. This is important since fractures at different regions of a bone pose different problems of management. In addition, healing is different at different locations within a bone. Healing in the hard compact bone of the diaphysis is generally slower than that in the cancellous bone of the metaphysis. In some bones, the blood supply to certain areas is tenuous, for example, the head of the femur and, therefore, easily disrupted by fracture. Fractures through such areas are associated with increased incidence of delayed union, non-union or osteonecrosis.

Fractures of long bones are primarily classified according to their location (Fig. 2.2) as follows:

1 Diaphyseal fractures.

2 Metaphyseal fractures.

3 Epiphyseal fractures.

In diaphyseal fractures, the shaft of long bones is usually divided into equal thirds:

1 Upper (proximal) third fractures.

2 Middle third fractures.

3 Lower (distal) third fractures.

Fractures at the extremities of a long bone may involve the joint in which the bone articulates and this may affect healing or subsequent joint function. There is an infinite variety of these fractures and many have eponyms. However, the following general classification, shown diagramatically in Fig. 2.3, is suitable in most cases:

Type I — extra-articular fractures (the fracture line does not communicate with a joint).

Type II — intra-articular fractures (the fracture line communicates with a joint).

(a) Marginal fractures (fracture line extends from the joint surface into the metaphysis).

(b) T- or Y-fractures (the fracture line extends from the joint surface into the metaphysis which is split to produce two main intra-articular fragments).

(c) Osteochondral fractures (the fracture line runs entirely in the subarticular bone).

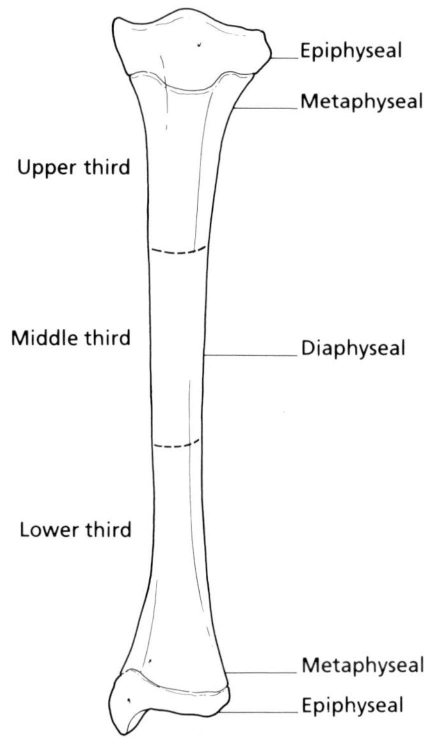

Fig. 2.2 Diagram showing the anatomical regions of a long bone.

Potentially, epiphyseal injuries may result in a disturbance of growth and various attempts have been made to classify these fractures according to the probability of this complication. The most commonly used is the classification (Fig. 2.4) developed by Salter and Harris (1963):

Type I — separation of the epiphysis from the metaphysis.

Type II — epiphyseal separation with a marginal fracture of the metaphysis.

Type III — intra-articular injury consisting of epiphyseal separation and a longitudinal fracture of the epiphysis.

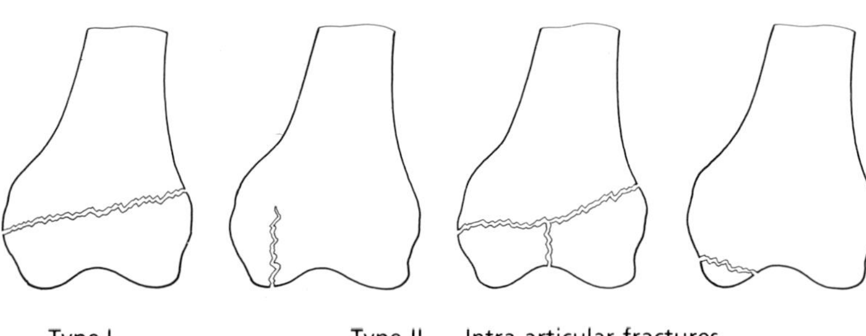

Fig. 2.3 A classification of metaphyseal fractures.

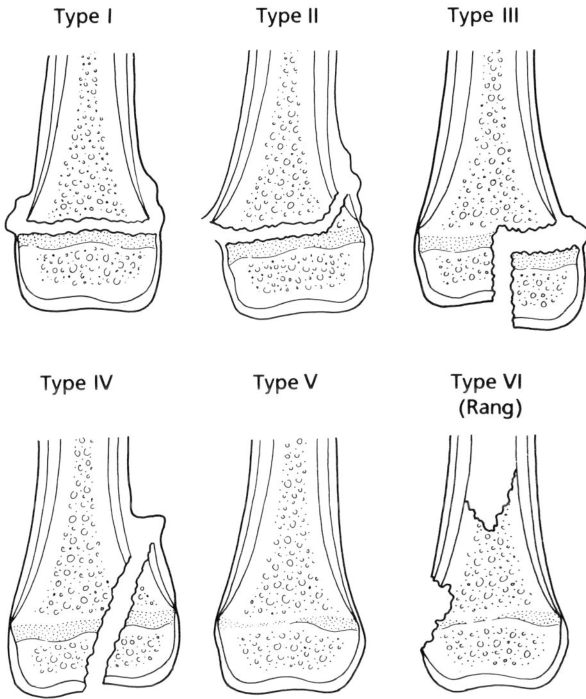

Fig. 2.4 Salter and Harris classification of epiphyseal injuries.

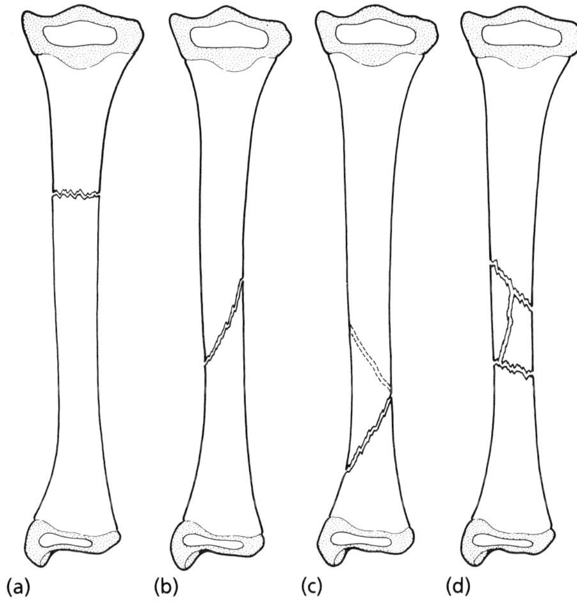

Fig. 2.5 Diagram showing the types of fracture morphology. (a–c) Type I — simple fractures. (d) Type II — comminuted fracture.

Type IV — intra-articular fracture extending across the epiphyseal plate into the metaphysis.

Type V — compression or crush injury of the epiphyseal plate.

Rang (1983) has modified this classification to include a sixth category in which a perichondrial injury has been sustained.

Fracture morphology

The morphology or the orientation of the line of a fracture is determined by the magnitude and direction of the injuring force. The fracture morphology provides information with regards to the potential stability and is one factor of importance in deciding the most suitable treatment method. A correlation has been established by several authors, notably Johner and Wruhs (1983), between fracture morphology and speed of healing. There is also some recent evidence that suggests that different morphological types of fracture sustain different types of associated soft tissue injuries (Oni *et al.* 1988, 1989b).

The shaft of a long bone may break in a variety of ways in response to different types of injuring forces (Fig. 2.5). In addition, the violence of the injury may lead to secondary fractures (Alms 1961) or comminution and this is used to classify fractures into:

Type I — simple (linear) fractures (consist of two fragments).
(a) Transverse (the fracture surface is approximately perpendicular to the longitudinal axis of the shaft; the fracture is stable to compression if end-to-end contact is present).
(b) Oblique (the fracture surface subtends an angle of approximately 45° to the longitudinal axis; the fracture is unstable to compression).
(c) Spiral (the longitudinally oriented fracture line encircles a portion of the shaft; the fracture is unstable to compression unless the fragment spikes are interlocked).
Type II — comminuted fractures (consist of two fragments and one or more intermediate fragments but the primary fracture can still be discerned).
(a) With butterfly fragment.
(b) Segmental fractures (a double fracture isolating a segment of bone or intermediate fragment).
(c) Multiple fragments — not classifiable.

Mechanism of injury

The probable mechanism of injury, which may be deduced from plain radiographs, has been used to classify fractures into those caused by *direct trauma*, or by *indirect trauma*.

Perkins (1958, 1970) has further classified fractures

produced by direct application of a deforming force into:

Type I — tapping fractures (caused by a small force acting over a small area, e.g. a kick on the shin, which results in a transverse fracture line and a localized area of soft tissue damage).

Type II — crush fractures (caused by a large force acting over a large area; transverse or comminuted fracture line and a wide area of soft tissue damage).

Type III — penetrating (missile) fractures (caused by a large force acting over a small area, e.g. gunshot).

(a) Low-velocity (the fracture line may be extensively comminuted but soft tissue damage is minimal).

(b) High-velocity (the bone disintegrates where struck and soft tissue damage is extensive).

Similarly, Alms (1961) further classified fractures produced by indirect application of a deforming force into:

Type I — avulsion (traction) fractures (caused by the forcible contraction of a muscle mass; the failure in tension results in a transverse fracture line, e.g. a fracture of the olecranon or patella (Fig. 2.6)).

Type II — angulation fractures (caused by bending; compression on the concave side and tension on the convex side from where failure propagates into transverse fracture line; soft tissue damage is often significant).

Type III — rotational fractures (caused by twisting; shear stress results in a spiral fracture line — complete rotation around shaft circumference; soft tissue damage may be insignificant).

Type IV — compression fractures (caused by severe violence; the harder shaft driven into cancellous ends gives rise to T- or Y-shaped intra-articular or impacted fractures).

Type V — combination fractures (caused by combinations of compression, bending and/or twisting; most human fractures; oblique fracture lines with varying degrees of comminution).

Severity of fracture

Fractures are frequently classified on the basis of a clinical perception of the severity of the injury measured in terms of the extent of associated soft tissue damage. This is because it has been generally observed that severe damage to the soft tissues impairs fracture healing (Ellis 1958, Bauer *et al.* 1962, Holden 1972).

It is customary to distinguish between *closed* fractures, and *open* (compound) fractures.

The overlying skin is intact in closed fractures but breached in open fractures. Open fractures are deemed to have sustained a more violent injury than closed

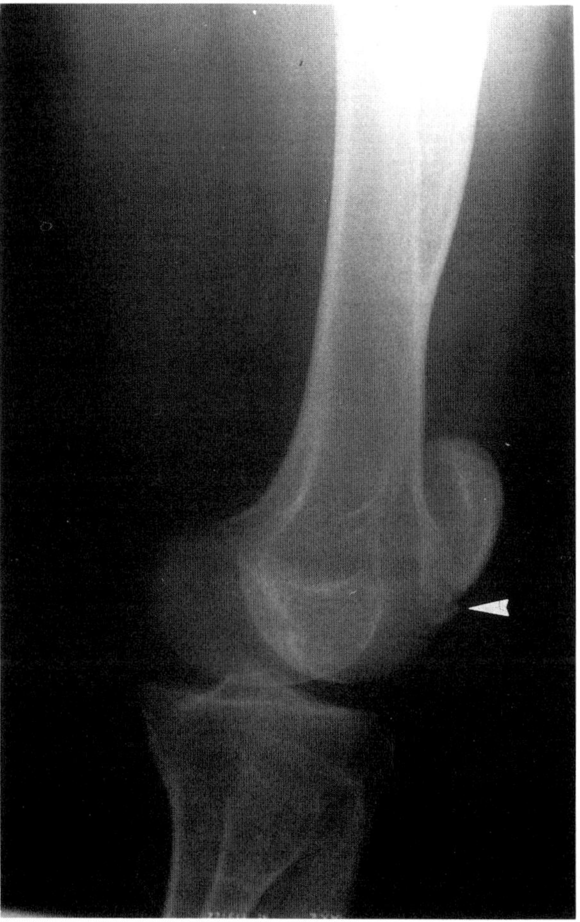

Fig. 2.6 Radiograph showing an avulsion fracture of the patella.

fractures and, hence, have a poorer prognosis. Open fractures have been further classified according to varying degrees of severity.

Some authors distinguish between open fractures which communicate with the external environment and those that do not ('technically compound'). Others differentiate between 'compound from within', where a fracture fragment has penetrated the skin from its deep surface, and 'compound from without', where the object causing the fracture has breached the skin as well (Freedman & Ganes 1958). These distinctions are of little practical use and should not be allowed to alter the recommended surgical treatment for open fractures which is exploration of the wound down to the bone ends and thorough debridement of dead and devitalized tissues in all cases.

A more useful classification of open fractures has been provided by Gustillo and Anderson (1976) which is briefly as follows:

Grade I — open fractures associated with a clean wound less than 1 cm long.

Grade II — open fractures associated with a wound greater than 1 cm in length but not associated with extensive soft tissue damage, tissue/skin flaps or avulsions.

Grade III

(a) open fractures associated with extensive soft tissue damage or traumatic amputations,

(b) severely contaminated wounds or gunshot, farm or vascular injuries.

This classification has been updated and extended by Gustilo *et al.* in 1984.

It is also recognized that closed fractures sustain varying degrees of injuries. Oestern and Tscherne (1984) have provided a classification for these injuries:

Grade 0 — closed fractures with negligible soft tissue damage.

Grade I — closed fractures associated with superficial abrasions or contusions caused from within.

Grade II — closed fractures associated with deeper abrasions and local skin or muscle contusion or with impending compartment syndrome.

Grade III — closed fractures associated with extensive skin and muscle contusion or with decompensated or frank compartment syndrome or with vascular injuries.

This classification is difficult to apply in practice because soft tissue damage cannot be clinically quantified with any degree of accuracy. Recently, Oni *et al.* (1989a) suggested that the serum creatinine phosphokinase (CPK) levels may have a role as an objective measure of soft tissue damage in closed fractures.

Displacement

The deformity which may be present following a fracture, usually referred to as displacement, is described in terms of the position of the fracture fragments in relation to one another. It may be caused by the injuring force, by gravity, by the contraction of the muscles attached to the fragments or during the handling of the patient. The magnitude of the initial displacement may be indicative of the severity of trauma and some authors have used this to predict prognosis in tibial shaft fractures (Weissman *et al.* 1966).

The factors that affect displacement are of considerable importance in relation to treatment; hence, fractures are classified as *displaced*, or *undisplaced*.

Four general types of fracture displacement (Fig. 2.7) are recognized:

Type I — shift (loss of alignment; one fragment is shifted sideways in relation to another in the anterior/posterior and/or medial/lateral directions leading to a loss of continuity of the cortices).

Type II — angulation (loss of normal longitudinal axis of a bone; the axis of one fragment subtends an angle to that of the other in the anterior/posterior and/or medial/lateral directions).

Type III — shortening (loss of length; caused by overlap or impaction).

Type IV — rotation (external and internal; one fragment is twisted about its long axis in relation to that of another).

A fifth category, distraction, which is associated with faulty treatment, particularly excessive traction, may be added.

Angular and rotational deformities are the most important to correct because they may interfere significantly with limb function after the fracture has healed.

Special types of fracture

Most fractures occur as the result of a single application of a force of significant magnitude. In some circumstances the applied force may be repetitive or the bone may be weakened. Fractures under these special circumstances are usually classified separately.

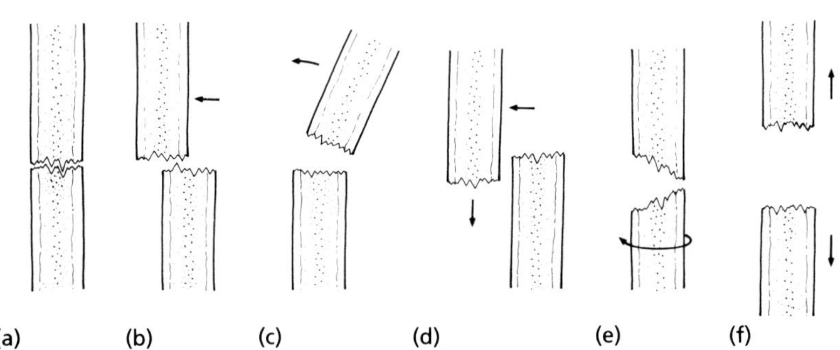

Fig. 2.7 Diagram showing (a) an undisplaced fracture, and the types of fracture displacement: (b) shift, (c) angulation, (d) shortening, (e) rotation, (f) distraction.

Fatigue (stress) fracture

This is caused by stresses generated by excess of a normal activity, e.g. running, or by an unaccustomed activity. Fatigue fractures are usually transverse and undisplaced (Fig. 2.8). Diagnosis, which is suggested by the clinical history and local signs of tenderness, may be difficult (Devas 1961). Plain radiographs may be normal, in which case special tests such as bone scintigraphy (Fig. 2.9) may demonstrate a definite abnormality. There is usually no evidence of a primary bone disease.

Pathological fracture

This is a fracture through abnormal bone, i.e. associated with diseases that weaken or destroy bone (Fig. 2.10). Clinically, these fractures often result, but not always, from a trivial injury or occur spontaneously. Pathological fractures may be further classified into several subgroups according to their cause:

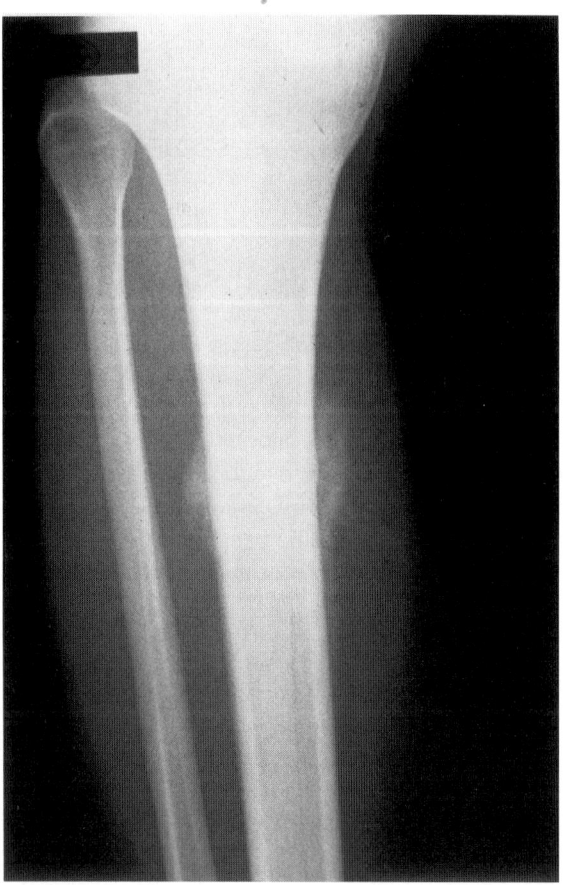

Fig. 2.8 Radiograph showing a fatigue fracture of the proximal tibia. Note the callus response and barely visible 'crack' in the medial cortex.

Type I — congenital abnormalities.
   (a) Localized — pseudarthroses of clavicle and tibia.
   (b) Generalized — in association with multiple enchondromas
Type II — acquired abnormalities.
   (a) Metabolic bone diseases (e.g. rickets, osteoporosis, osteomalacia).
   (b) Inflammatory conditions (e.g. osteomyelitis, rheumatoid arthritis).
   (c) Neuromuscular disorders (e.g. poliomyelitis, muscular dystrophy).
   (d) Avascular necrosis (e.g. caisson disease).
   (e) Neoplasia (primary or secondary).

Birth fracture

This is a fracture that occurs at birth and may be due to an underlying pathological condition of bone, for example osteogenesis imperfecta, or may result purely from the trauma of a difficult delivery.

This fracture is not always easy to diagnose because it is often 'asymptomatic'. A radiological survey of 300 newly born babies revealed a 1.7% incidence of fractures of the clavicle which had not been suspected by routine examination immediately after birth (Ogden 1982). Birth fractures may be incomplete or complete with displacement when they may be confused with congenital pseudarthrosis. Fractures in the upper limb may be associated with brachial plexus injury. Healing of birth fractures is rapid and associated with massive osteoblastic reaction which may be mistaken for osteomyelitis. Birth fractures should not be treated lightly and children sustaining such injuries should be followed closely throughout childhood so that any resulting growth abnormalities may be detected early.

General classification of dislocations

A dislocation is defined as a disruption of a joint such that there is no remaining contact between the articular surfaces. The dislocation may be either *simple*, or *complicated* (when it is associated with a fracture or with damage to other important structures such as nerves or blood vessels).

Dislocations may also be classified as:
Grade I — reducible (by closed manipulation).
Grade II — irreducible (except by open operation).

A subluxation is a partial or incomplete disruption of a joint with some remaining, but abnormal, contact between the articulating surfaces. It may be further classified as:
Type I — ligamentous sprain/rupture.

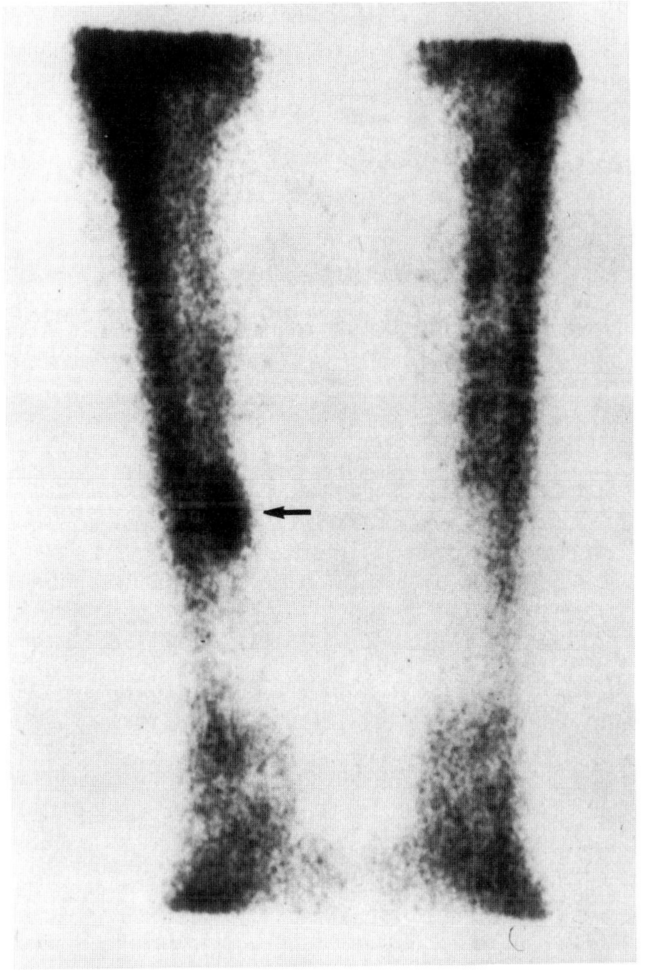
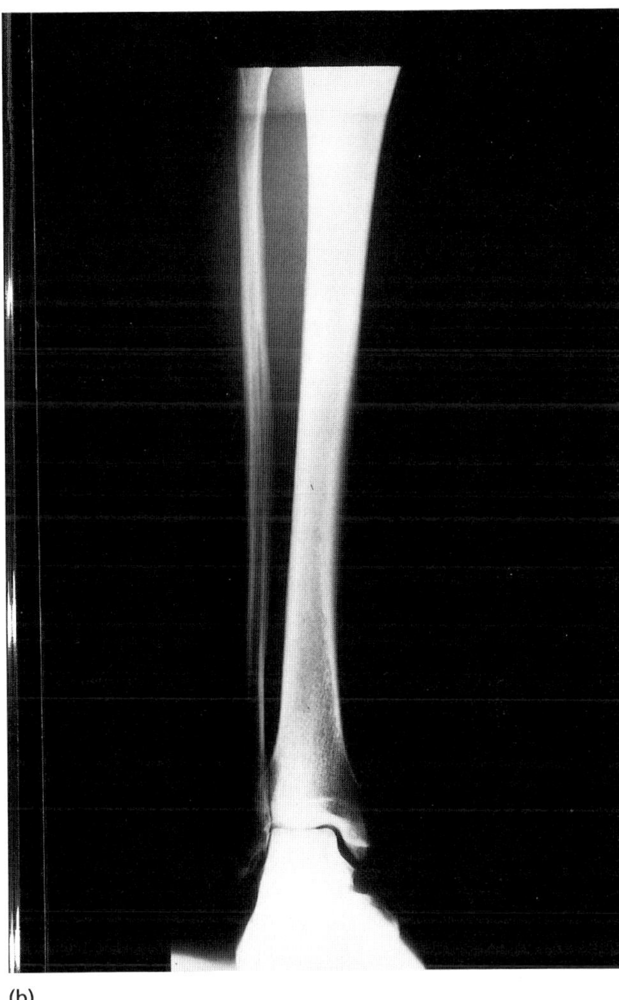

(a)

(b)

Fig. 2.9 Bone scintigraphic appearances of a fatigue fracture. (a) Note localized increase in tracer uptake (arrowed). (b) Note normal radiograph. The patient had recently taken up jogging.

Type II — occult or apparent joint instability (disruption is apparent only when the joint is stressed).

Type III — unstable joint (the joint surfaces lose their normal relationship but retain considerable contact).

The classification of dislocations is not as well developed as that of fractures. Nevertheless, it may be based on the following factors:

1 Onset.
2 Severity of dislocation.
3 Special types.

Onset of dislocation

Cartilage degeneration may occur over a brief period of time following a dislocation and irreversible damage may develop rapidly thereafter. Thus, a temporal classification of dislocations provides an indication of prognosis:

1 Acute (primary) dislocation.
2 Old unreduced dislocation.
3 Recurrent (repetitive) dislocation.

Recurrent dislocations may be further classified as:

Type I — recurrent traumatic dislocation (i.e. caused by a recurrent injury; may be anatomically normal or show minor joint damage).

Type II — recurrent transient dislocation (dislocation by force at the extreme of motion).

Type III — recurrent voluntary dislocation (dislocation under the patient's muscle control — 'party tricks'; usually associated with joint laxity).

(a) Hysterical (poor response to treatment and surgery).

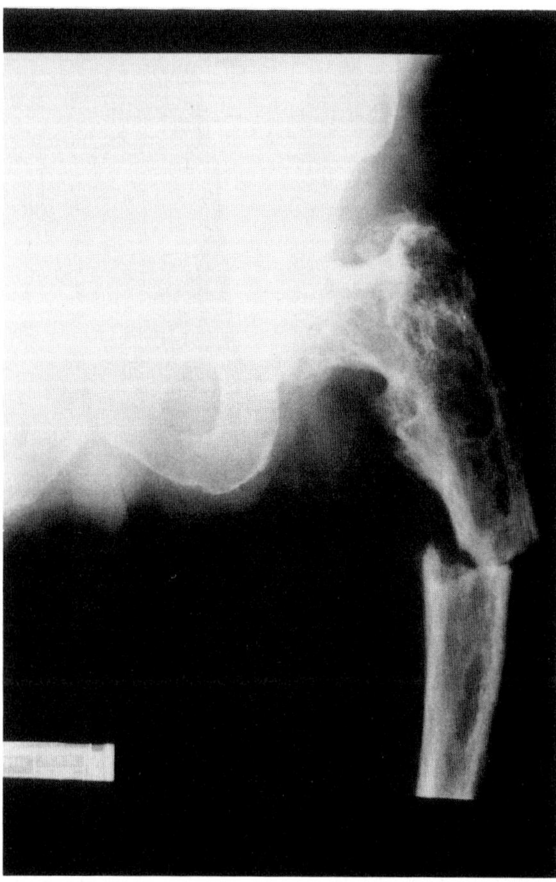

Fig. 2.10 Radiograph showing a pathological fracture through Paget's disease of the left femur.

(b) Non-hysterical (responds to an exercise regime).
Type IV — recurrent involuntary dislocation (multi-directional instability; may be due to a joint abnormality and/or familial joint laxity).

Severity of dislocation

Like fractures, a dislocation may be either *closed*, or *open* (compound), and may be similarly graded.

Special types

Like most fractures, most dislocations are caused by a single application of a significant force. In some circumstances other contributory factors are involved in causing the dislocation.

1 Anatomical abnormality. The dislocation is secondary to underlying anatomical lesions, such as capsular defects or excessive laxity, abnormal bone shapes or muscular paralysis, rupture, contractures or abnormal attachments.

2 Pathological dislocation. The dislocation is associated with disorders of the joint or surrounding tissues such as septic or aseptic joint effusions.

References

Alms, M.A. Fracture mechanics. *J Bone Joint Surg* 1961; **43B**: 162–166.

Bauer, G.C.H., Edwards, P. & Widmark, P.H. Shaft fractures of the tibia. Etiology of poor results in a consecutive series of 173 fractures. *Acta Chir Scand* 1962; **124**: 386–395.

Devas, M.B. Compression stress fractures in man and greyhound. *J Bone Joint Surg* 1961; **43B**: 540–551.

Ellis, H. The speed of healing after fracture of the tibial shaft. *J Bone Joint Surg* 1958; **40B**: 42–66.

Freedman, W.A. & Ganes, A.L. Open tibial shaft fractures — immediate soft tissue closure. *Am J Surg* 1958; **95**: 415–424.

Gustillo, R.B. & Anderson, J.T. Prevention of infection in the treatment of 1025 open fractures of long bones. *J Bone Joint Surg* 1976; **58A**: 453–458.

Gustillo, R.B., Mendoza, R.M. & Williams, D.N. Problems in the management of Type III (severe) open fractures: a new classification of type III open fractures. *J Trauma* 1984; **24**: 742–746.

Holden, C.E.A. The role of blood supply to soft tissues in the healing diaphyseal fractures. *J Bone Joint Surg* 1972; **54A**: 993–1000.

Johner, R. & Wruhs, O. Classification of tibial shaft fractures and correlation with results after rigid internal fixation. *Clin Orthop* 1983; **178**: 7–25.

Ogden, J.A *Skeletal Injury in Childhood*. Lea & Febiger: Philadelphia, 1982.

Oni, O.O.A., Fenton, A., Iqbal, S.J. & Gregg, P.G. Serum creatinine kinase levels as an index of prognosis in tibial shaft fractures. *J Orthop Trauma* 1989a; **3**: 345–347.

Oni, O.O.A., Gregg, P.J., Morrison, C. & Ponter, A.R.S. An investigation of the fracture characteristics of the tibia of mature rabbits. *Injury* 1988; **19**: 172–176.

Oni, O.O.A., Stafford, H. & Gregg, P.G. An experimental study of the patterns of periosteal and endosteal damage in tibial shaft fractures using a rabbit trauma model. *J Orthop Trauma* 1989b; **3**: 142–147.

Oestern, H-J. & Tscherne, H. Pathophysiology and classification of soft tissue injuries. In: Tscherne, H. & Gotzen, L. (eds) *Fractures and Soft Tissue Injuries*. Springer-Verlag: Berlin, 1984.

Perkins, G. *Fractures and Dislocations*. Athlone Press: London, 1958.

Perkins, G. *Ruminations of an Orthopaedic Surgeon*. Butterworth: London, 1970.

Rang, M. *Children's Fractures* 2nd edn. Lippincott: Philadelphia, 1983.

Salter, R.B. & Harris, W.R. Injuries involving the epiphyseal plate. *J Bone Joint Surg* 1963; **45A**: 587–622.

Weissman, S.L., Herold, H.C. & Engelberg, M. Fractures of the middle two-thirds of the tibial shaft. *J Bone Joint Surg* 1966; **48A**: 257–267.

3: Clinical Features Including First Examination and Detection of Complications

J.STEVENS

Introduction

There is no doubt that the diagnosis of a fracture and its associated complications, should any be present, must follow the routine used in medical practice in general, which consists of:

1 History.
2 Physical examination.
3 Differential diagnosis.
4 Special investigations.
5 Final diagnosis.
6 Diagnosis of complications.

If conscientiously followed, with every fracture or potential fracture, then this resumé will give a firm diagnosis in 95 to 99% of cases.

History

In almost every case where a fracture may be present there will be a history of some sort of accidental injury. The exceptions to this rule are of course patients who have non-accidental injury, patients who have stress fractures and some patients who have pathological fractures. It must be remembered that there are patterns of injury associated with different types of accident, for example when one falls from a height and lands on the feet there may be fractures of the os calcis, the spine, the neck of the femur and the upper end of the tibia.

Most patients will be able to give a good history of the site of the pain and the site of the injury which is the cause of that pain, but there are a few cases in which the pain may be referred from the actual site of injury. Classical amongst these is the referral of pain from the hip to the knee and this has, on occasion, caused confusion in the mind of the person carrying out the examination. Similar cases of referred pain, although much less common, are that arising from the upper cervical spine referred to the back of the head, that arising from C5/6 referred down between the shoulder blades and pain from the cervico-thoracic spine referred into the arm. On the left side this may simulate a coronary thrombosis. In the lumbar spine pain may be referred from the L4/5/S1 region to the sacro-iliac joints on either side and may then be referred in a somatic distribution down either or both legs. This pain can be distinguished, as a rule, from that caused by nerve root irritation by the absence of parasthesiae or impulse pain. Pain from the shoulder may be referred to the deltoid insertion and pain from the acromio-clavicular joint into the neck. Pain from the elbow can be referred to the forearm and from the knee it may be referred down the leg.

Doctors who miss the original diagnosis associated with a referred type of pain, for example careful and repeated examination of the knee in a patient in whom the pain is referred from the hip, run the risk of incurring the disbelief of any civilian judge with whom they may ultimately be confronted. We continue to be faced with an increasingly litigious population on the one hand and the need to conserve our resources on the other hand. This therefore raises the question of whether or not to have a radiograph taken. The question of taking 'defensive' radiographs is a very vexed one and where this arises it is believed that if the patient has been seen and examined by a casualty officer, of any status, who decided that no such radiograph is necessary, then confirmation of the decision should be obtained from the consultant in Accident and Emergency Medicine or from an orthopaedic consultant.

It is perhaps worth mentioning at this stage that some bizarre findings may occasionally be encountered. Examples of these are the dislocated shoulder or fractured tibia sustained during football; the team doctor, present at the game, sees the accident and the patient within 5 to 10 minutes, and finds that the patient does not complain at all although there is an obvious deformity. Under these circumstances it is a satisfactory, painless time to carry out an immediate reduction of such a dislocation or to correct the deformity resulting from the fracture. Another, and rather more disconcerting, finding is the absence of total numbness in the sensory distribution of a completely divided nerve. This occurs particularly in the hand after median or ulnar nerve injuries whether or not there is a fracture. Under these circumstances it is appropriate to remember that the specific area supplied by the median nerve is the flexor aspect of the pulp over the distal phalanx of the index finger. The corresponding area of insensibility for the ulnar nerve is the pulp over the flexor aspect of the little finger. However, there may not be any numbness of the fingers at all and indeed so common in this paradox, that a senior hand surgeon has been heard to say that a wound over a nerve is associated with division of that nerve unless it has been *seen* not to be divided.

Non-accidental injuries are fairly typical. They occur in young children or infants and are commonly metaphyseal. Where they are multiple they can be seen radiologically to be of different ages. The first history commonly given, however, is that the baby has fallen out of its cot or the child has fallen downstairs.

Stress fractures are much more common than is generally believed. They occur commonly in the necks of the middle metatarsals in middle-aged people who have recently taken up jogging, around the ankle in ballet dancers, around the upper tibia, femur and neck of the femur in army recruits and it is believed that some spondylolistheses are stress fractures of the pars inter-articularis of the neural arch. These patients are more likely to attend an orthopaedic clinic than at an Accident department. Once a diagnosis of a stress fracture has been made the patient is likely to be referred to the trauma surgeon who should bear in mind that when patients first present with pain (within the first 3 weeks) they may not have any radiological abnormality at all. In these circumstances examination by bone scintigraphy may be useful: a 'hot-spot' is likely to be seen on the scan.

Pathological fractures include such injuries where there is no, or much less than expected, trauma to the part concerned. True pathological fractures (i.e. fractures through abnormal bone) occur in the presence of skeletal metastases. These may just 'give way' and lead to a fracture. The patient will usually, but certainly not always, have a history of previous carcinoma or sarcoma which has known bone-seeking metastatic deposits. For example the breast, the lung, the prostate, the thyroid, the kidney and the gut may produce deposits which can produce pain and lead to an increase in severity of the pain with the occurrence of a fracture. Tumours of the skeletal tissue itself, the marrow and the reticulo-endothelial system, can also produce pathological fractures. Such diseases include multiple myeloma, lymphoma of the various types and disorders of currently unknown nature and cause, such as Paget's disease.

Physical examination

This must be quite thorough. The cardinal signs of a standard fracture are divided into three groups determined by (1) looking at, (2) feeling and (3) moving the part.

Observation

Looking may lead one to see an obvious deformity, an obvious wound, obvious swelling or obvious bruising. However, in stress fractures and some pathological fractures none of these abnormalities may be present. Deformity includes not only an obvious abnormality seen as the patient is resting supine, but may also include a position of deformity that can actually be achieved by gentle manipulation of the part. This can be quite confusing because of the tendency of the various parts of the body to revert to their normal anatomical position after removal of the deforming force. In the conscious patient the anatomy can be seen to be normal, or nearly so, since it is held there by muscle spasm. In this context, ligamentous injury of the knee occurring in association with a fracture of the shaft of the femur, is a well-known entity and may very well be missed unless it is particularly sought by examination under general anaesthetic.

Swelling, which of course is due to oedema and bruising, the result of trauma to the soft tissue more than to the bone, may or may not accompany the fracture. Although it is usually present there are a number of fractures, for example of the neck of the femur, which are not necessarily associated with any visible swelling at all. Of course, the swelling will not always be present within the first hour after a fracture and where the swelling involves a joint, for example the knee, in which the confines of the joint, i.e. the capsule, are disrupted then the swelling will be much less obvious than it would be in the joint whose capsule remained intact. This has some importance in fractures involving joints.

Bruising occurs with fractures which are near the surface of the body when the bruise is due to bleeding from intraosseous vessels and from vessels in the damaged surrounding soft tissues. Of course it is not always possible to tell whether the bleeding has come from a broken bone or whether it has come from damage to the soft tissues. It is often absent with many fractures because of the integrity of the deep fascia within whose compartment the fractured bone will lie and through which the bruise rarely penetrates at an early stage.

Palpation

There are two forms of palpation where bones are concerned. One is the direct palpation of the bone in the position in which it lies, without moving the bone at all. This will give one an opportunity to locate the point of maximum tenderness and probably also the fracture. The second form of palpation is that in which the local joints and the part itself are moved. If this is at all painful then the suspicion of a fracture must be raised. It should be borne in mind that people with spina bifida, for example, may have no pain sensation at all in the legs and can sustain epiphyseal or meta-physeal injuries without the presence of pain or without the typical loss of function. Where accident victims are initially examined in the Accident department a quick routine to detect fractures and dislocations in those with multiple injuries is:

1 Palpation of the skull for any indentations or lacer-ations. Lacerations should be explored with a *sterile* gloved finger.

2 The spine, cervical, dorsal and lumbo-sacral, should not be moved but should be palpated for gaps between the spinous processes, for malalignment of these, or for small amounts of swelling or bruising.

3 The shoulder girdle, upper arm, forearm, wrist and hand can be inspected and their function can be deter-mined by lifting the arm from the resting position into the position of full flexion/abduction. Any painful movement complained of by the patient when this is done will call for the cessation of the test and indicate the need for closer inspection. In the lower limb flexion of the hip with abduction and external rotation (the FABER test) together with flexion of the knee, dorsi-flexion of the ankle and supination of the forefoot, performed as a single comprehensive manoeuvre, will usually give one a firm clue as to any sort of pain, indicating that further examination is required.

Fractures of the thoracic wall can be detected by compressing the chest and similarly fractures of the pelvis can be suspected after the pelvis has been com-pressed from side to side. Where there is any doubt about the presence of fractures, and particularly where the patient is unconscious, then he or she should be turned prone, by careful 'log rolling', so that the spine and the back of the trunk can be properly examined.

Once the patient has been carefully examined the question arises as to which parts of the body should be subjected to radiography. Before this, however, atten-tion must be given to the relief of any pain. For this purpose some sort of splintage of obvious fractured limbs is desirable. Commonly, a pneumatic type of splint is used for the upper limb and a Thomas splint or a pneumatic splint for the lower limb. If the patient has a questionable cervical spine injury, and if unconscious, then it is the duty of the doctor who requests the radiographs to apply a four poster collar and to go to the X-ray department with the patient and remain there to see that a well-intentioned radiographer does not either remove the collar or produce unwanted and unexpected movement of the spinal segment, or both. Whether a patient should be given any analgesia before radio-graphy is still a vexed question. The diminution of pain, once the limb is splinted, will usually keep the patient sufficiently comfortable while radiographs are being made. However, some patients with multiple injuries may warrant the use of morphine or pethidine.

Provisional diagnosis

Whilst the patient is in the X-ray department having films taken, it is common for the doctor to write up a provisional diagnosis. This recording should be done in a sufficient amount of detail, in particular giving the sites of any suspected fractures and whether they are compound or not. A diagram of the skeleton or of the body is very helpful here. Although the films are sub-sequently available to the casualty officer, the vexed question of whether any policy exists for the reporting of films by a radiologist is still not settled in many hospitals. It cannot be expected that every junior staff member in an Accident department will be able to recognize every possible injury shown radiographically. Ideally, the films should be reported upon by someone of at least registrar, but preferably senior registrar or consultant grading in radiology within 48 hours of the patient's attendance at the Accident department. This report should be sent to the consultant in charge of that department if any abnormality is seen on the films.

When the patient has returned from the X-ray depart-ment with the films, then the definitive diagnoses can be made. These should be written down by the casualty officer in the department together with a note of any analgesics given and the time of their administration; a note should be made of the time at which the patient is transferred to the care of the trauma surgeon for de-finitive treatment.

The general principles of the radiology of fractures are discussed in Chapter 4.

Complications of fractures and their detection

The complications of fractures can be described as immediate, early and late.

Immediate complications include:
1 Haemorrhage and shock.
2 Soft tissue injury to arteries, viscera, skin, nerves, ligaments, tendons and muscles in order of decreasing importance.
3 Loss of either soft or hard tissue.

The occurrence of haemorrhage and shock in trauma patients is similar to that occurring in patients with other disorders and apart from mentioning that the neurogenic element of the shock is likely to be greater in someone with an injury, or multiple injuries, than in a postoperative patient, who will be sedated, there is little to add about this. Septic shock, of course, does not come into the clinical picture at first examination.

Arterial injuries

These may be separated into:
1 Those where there is continuity. Such lesions include:
    (a) intramural haematoma,
    (b) intimal rupture.
2 Those where continuity is absent. Such lesions include:
    (a) partial division of the vessel wall (and the distal pulse may still be palpable),
    (b) complete division in which the distal pulse is rarely palpable.

Careful palpation of the known peripheral pulses is important in all injuries. It should be borne in mind that a distal pulse can still be felt in the presence of a compartment compression syndrome — this is a very common cause of the syndrome being missed. The six 'P's' of vascular injuries should be remembered. They are pain, pallor, paralysis, paraesthesiae, pulselessness and 'perishing' cold. These are almost always present when significant ischaemia of the limb has been in existence for some time. However, one would hope to diagnose the ischaemic compromise before there is any question of paraesthesiae or paralysis occurring.

Venous injuries. These are usually regarded as being of little importance. Recently, more interest has been expressed in their occurrence because of the understanding that in a severed limb the venous components as well as the arterial components must be repaired anatomically if a successful replantation is going to be performed.

Of the viscera involved one must consider intrathoracic, intra-abdominal and 'intrapelvic' structures. Care must be taken to check whether these injuries are present since they can rapidly lead to the death of the patient or to very serious complications if they are not treated. For example, a transection of the junction of the arch and the descending parts of the aorta may not immediately be obvious, a rupture of the spleen may be delayed and an extraperitoneal rupture of the bladder or urethra may lead to extravasation of urine with its serious complications. Liver tears or disruptions may not be particularly tender but nowadays they are considered to be repairable by well-trained general surgeons who would be carrying out laporotomy. The possibility of the development and increase of tension pneumothorax in any patient with injuries, particularly to the chest, who is going to be given a general anaesthetic, must be borne in mind.

Skin injuries

Such injuries are not uncommon. They may be from 'without in' when they may be clean lacerations, dirty lacerations or degloving injuries. The presence of an open skin wound in association with a fracture, almost however far apart they may be, renders that fracture open or compound. Wounds from within out occur when a spiral fracture of bone is followed by the pointed fractured bone ends penetrating the skin. The bone may then retract and leave a small laceration over the fracture, possibly some distance away from it, and lead to it being thought not to represent a compound fracture. The occurrence of degloving injury is common after road traffic accidents. Here the skin and superficial tissues are separated from the deep fascia throughout the circumference, or almost the whole circumference, of the limb and the question then arises of how this should be treated. The skin becomes trapped between the tyre of a vehicle and the road and further progression of the wheel causes the skin and subcutaneous tissue to be stripped off since it is fairly elastic. Indeed it is possible to have a circumferential loosening of the skin over a variable distance, but usually just greater than the width of the tyre, without there being any skin break. Needless to say, any fracture deep to this injury would be uncontaminated to start with and may well stay uninfected. However, the almost necessary death of skin will allow the entry of bacteria and lead to secondary infection of the fracture. Other skin lesions can occur from a great variety of causes.

Having mentioned that the fracture is contaminated

by bacteria and possibly also by road dirt, farm dirt, manure and pieces of grass or clothing, the importance of distinguishing between contamination and infection automatically arises. It is generally agreed that the 'golden period' in which a contaminated open fracture can be converted into a clean, closed fracture is the first 6 hours after injury. On occasions this may be extended to 8 or 10 hours and some hand surgeons believe it is a lot longer. However, during the course of this period they cover the wound with a swab soaked in antibiotics. In the hand, where the blood supply is much better than, for example, in the leg, they can expect success whereas in the leg the 6-hour maximum should be observed as rigidly as possible. Where there is delay in treating a patient then the wound ought to be excised and left open for delayed primary or secondary suture at some future date or possibly for skin grafting, either split thickness, or a full thickness, local or free flap.

Nerve injuries

There are four varieties of nerve injury associated with fractures.

1 Neuropraxia, which means that the nerve suffers only a temporary physiological abnormality causing a disturbance of conduction. No anatomical disorder is visible in the nerve and it remains in continuity.

2 Axonotmesis in which the axons in the nerve are ruptured but in which the nerve sheaths (the endoneurium) remain intact. This is easy to conceive if one remembers that the axons are like jelly whereas their sheaths are very much tougher. Therefore a 'karate chop' injury to the nerve will cause disruption of axons but allow the retention of nerve sheaths. Thereafter, there is degeneration back to the nearest node of Ranvier and subsequent regeneration of the nerve along the intact sheath. Given that the distance to be covered by the regenerating nerve is reasonably short (and nothing like as long as the sciatic nerve from the ischium to the foot) then the recovery should be complete or very nearly so.

3 Neurotmesis means division of the two major components of the nerve, the jelly-like axon and the tougher endoneurium. This is usually due to a lacerated injury from without or an injury caused by the broken bone from within. Suture is required.

4 Stretch lesions are a combination of axonotmesis and neurotmesis.

A problem arises when a nerve injury is encountered in combination with a closed fracture. In these circumstances the nerve is usually close to the fractured bone as in the radial nerve within the spiral groove on the back of the humerus, or the common peroneal nerve close to the lateral aspect of the neck of the fibula. Since over 80% of closed nerve injuries are neuropraxias or axonotmeses which do well with no specific treatment at all, then any nerve injury in association with a closed fracture is not explored. Hopefully the nature of the injury will become apparent at a ·later date. If there is no recovery at all within 3 weeks and certainly within 6 weeks, then the nerve lesion has passed out of the realm of a neuropraxia and is almost certain to be a axonotmesis or a neurotmesis. Given a total amount of time for the nerve to recover, up to 9–12 months, then it should be possible to distinguish between axonotmesis and neurotmesis. If there is no recovery at 9–12 months then one is dealing with a neurotmesis and an exploration and nerve suture is appropriate. Where expertise with a microscope is available then this should be used to carry out a fascicular nerve repair, since there is evidence that these do rather better than repair of the nerve as a whole.

A stretch lesion of a nerve represents a serious form of traction injury. Where this has happened, for example in association with posterior dislocation of the hip, and where there is minimal recovery within 9–12 months, then it is generally accepted that the nerve is worth exploring. This, however, is a contentious opinion.

Ligaments and tendons

These structures are among the toughest in the limb and usually hold the distal part to the proximal part for longer than any other structure. The fact that ligaments may be torn is often overlooked, particularly in the instance quoted above where the collateral ligaments of the knee are not examined properly in the presence of a fracture of the shaft of the femur. In the course of examining a joint above a fracture and the joint below a fracture, which should be done routinely, then it ought to be possible to decide about ligamentous damage. However, it must be remembered that an anaesthetic may be required for all but the first examination, because of the awareness and anticipation, on the part of the patient, that pain can ensue. At the same time if the patient is having an anaesthetic for some reason, such as to manipulate a fracture, then the suspected ligament damage can be confirmed or denied under the same anaesthetic, but the operator must be aware of injuries of the ligaments and the methods of testing for these. They will have their own signs of minor or no swelling, minor or no bruising and protection against instability through muscle spasm. Very careful examination is necessary.

Muscle

It is always amazing how much of a muscle or muscle group can be missing and yet still function for the activities of daily living to remain normal. During war-time conditions many servicemen lost large quantities of, for example, calf muscle or thigh muscle and yet were still able to function normally or nearly normally on the small amount that was left behind. It is for this reason that this complication of fractures is regarded as being of least importance.

Complications of fractures are discussed in more detail in Chapter 11.

4: Radiology of Fractures and Dislocations

D.B.L.FINLAY

Introduction

Radiographs are expensive to produce in terms of manpower, equipment and film, and the radiation used in their production is a potential cause of harm to the patient (RCR Working Party, 1993). For these reasons it is important that requests for radiographs be kept to the minimum consistent with good clinical practice. Various authors have produced guidelines as to when radiographs should be obtained, for instance with extremity injuries (Brand *et al.* 1982, De Lacey & Bradbrooke 1979).

Unfortunately, even perfect application of these guidelines may allow fractures to be missed and in practice the guidelines may not be applied perfectly. At present their application depends on local practice in the individual hospital. In some departments radiographs will not be obtained of areas of the body where a specific diagnosis is unlikely to make a difference in management; this occurs in particular for the toes and the sacrum and coccyx. Radiographs should only be obtained after a history and examination of the patient has been undertaken and it is imperative that adequate clinical information be given on the request form. This ensures that the correct area of the body will be radiographed and, if necessary, additional views will be obtained. A knowledge of localizing symptoms and signs has been shown to increase the true positive diagnosis rate by radiologists reading the radiographs (Rickett *et al.* 1992).

There are a number of radiographic techniques used in the diagnosis and management of fractures but plain film radiography still plays the major role for most fractures. Other techniques are used to assess more complicated fractures, particularly preoperatively, com-

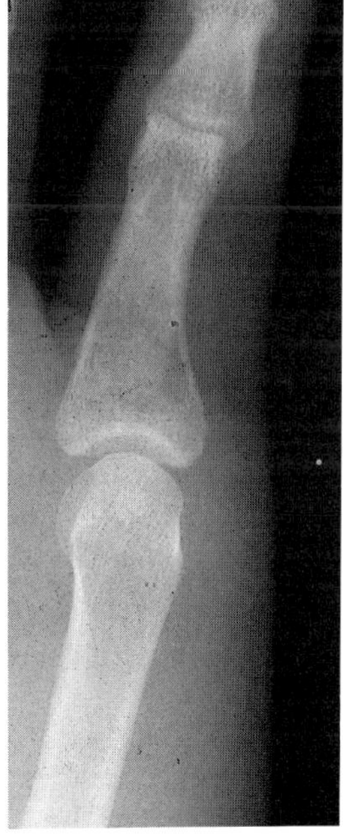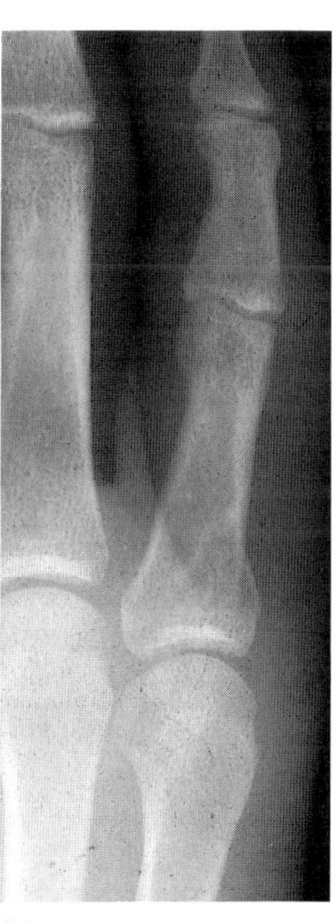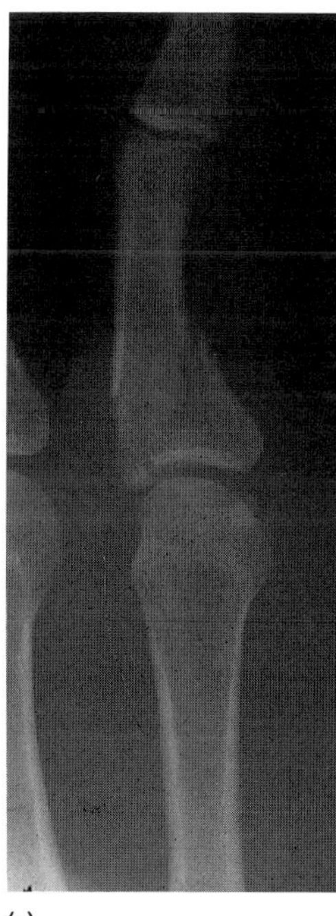

(a) (b) (c)

Fig. 4.1 Fracture of the base of the proximal phalanx of the little finger with intra-articular extension.
(a) Finger posteroanterior — little abnormality seen. (b) Finger postero-anterior oblique — the fracture is not obvious. (c) Finger anteroposterior oblique — at 90° to (b), the fracture is obvious.

plications of fractures in the short- and long-term and to investigate soft tissue injuries. Such techniques include bone scintigraphy, computerized axial tomography (CAT) scanning, magnetic resonance imaging (MRI), arthrography and myelography.

Plain film radiography

A fracture is most commonly seen on a radiograph as a line of lucency (fracture line): the greater the displace-ment of the fragments the wider and more obvious will be the fracture line. The visibility of the line also depends on its alignment with the X-ray beam. If oblique it becomes less visible and there is a degree of obliquity at which each individual fracture line will not be seen (Fig. 4.1). It is, however, unusual for the fracture line not to be visible on a further radiograph obtained at right angles to the first. Dislocation of a joint, although producing abnormal overlapping of bone surfaces or loss of congruity, can easily be missed on a single

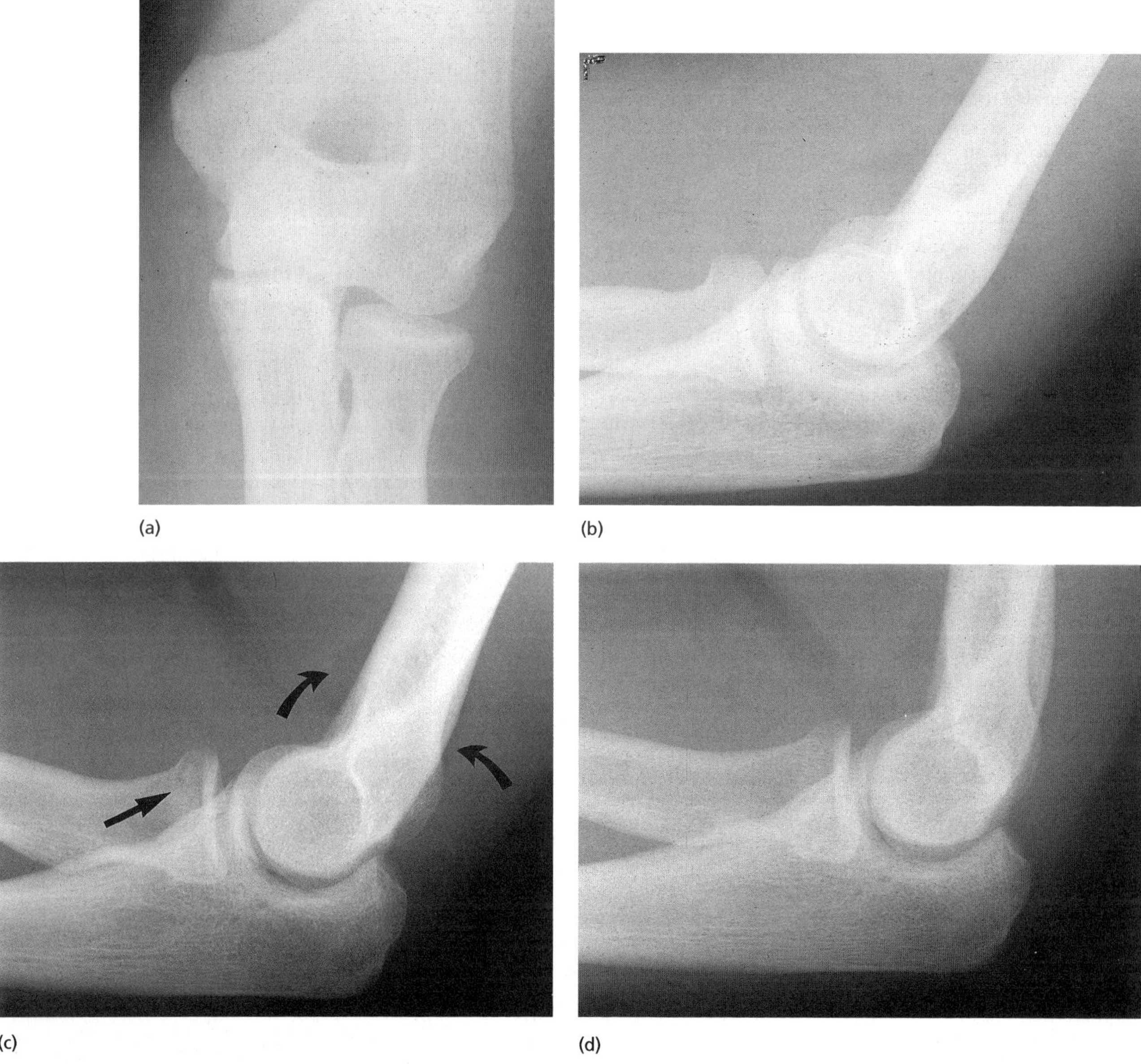

(a)

(b)

(c)

(d)

Fig. 4.2 Fracture of the radial head. (a) Anteroposterior. (b) Lateral with forearm in supination. (c) Lateral with forearm in neutral position. Fracture of the radial head can be seen (arrowed). There is elevation of the anterior and posterior fat pads (curved arrows). (d) Lateral with forearm in pronation.

radiograph (see Fig. 4.4). As a basic principle, therefore, two radiographic views of any injured bone or joint should be obtained, usually at right angles to each other: antero-posterior and lateral. In a small percentage of cases additional radiographs must be obtained to identify the fracture; this is most common in fractures involving the end of a bone within a joint (Fig. 4.2) or the proximal or distal shaft. Diagnosis of scaphoid fractures is particularly difficult. The cortex of the bone should be continous and should not undergo sharp angled variations in its direction. Bone cortex changes direction with smooth curves; straight lines do not occur.

Fractures can also be seen as areas of increased density due to impaction. This is commonly seen in fractures of the femoral neck (Fig. 4.3) and in depressed fractures of the skull vault. In comminuted and other fractures where the alignment of fragments of bone with the X-ray beam is altered, and in dislocated joints where bones overlap, there may be increased density (Fig. 4.4). When a long bone is injured the radiographs should include the joints above and below the site of injury; this is especially important with fractures of the forearm and

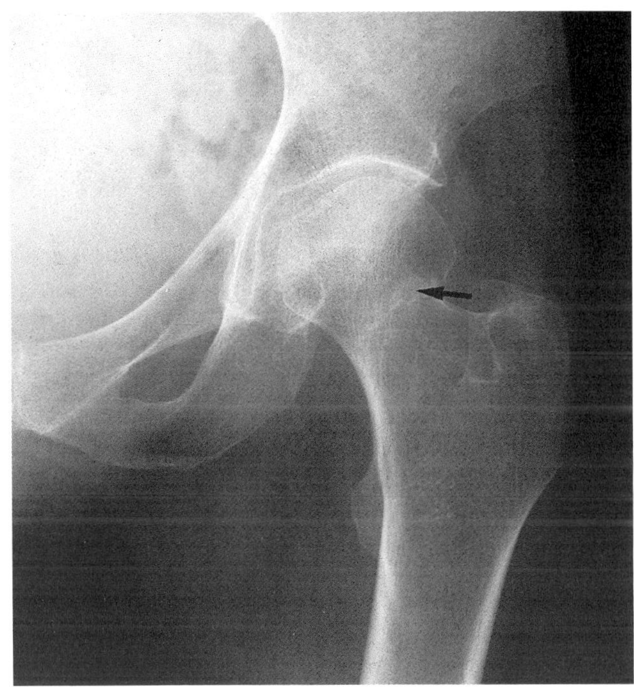

Fig. 4.3 Anteroposterior radiograph of Garden grade I fracture of the femoral neck. Sclerosis is seen in its lateral aspect (arrowed); the head is in valgus.

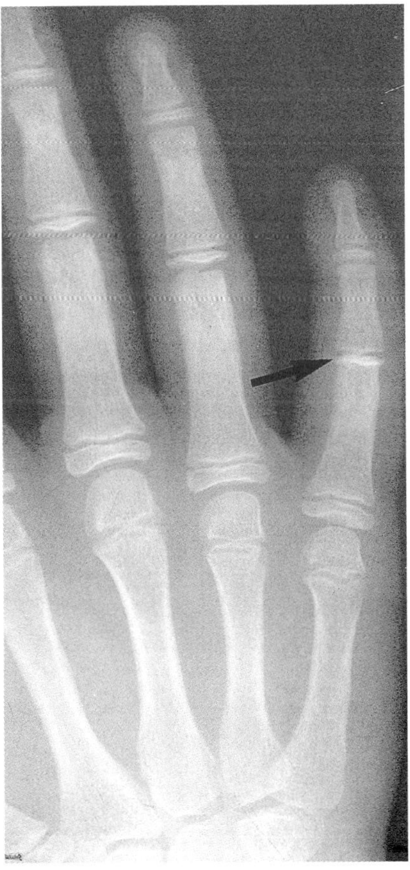

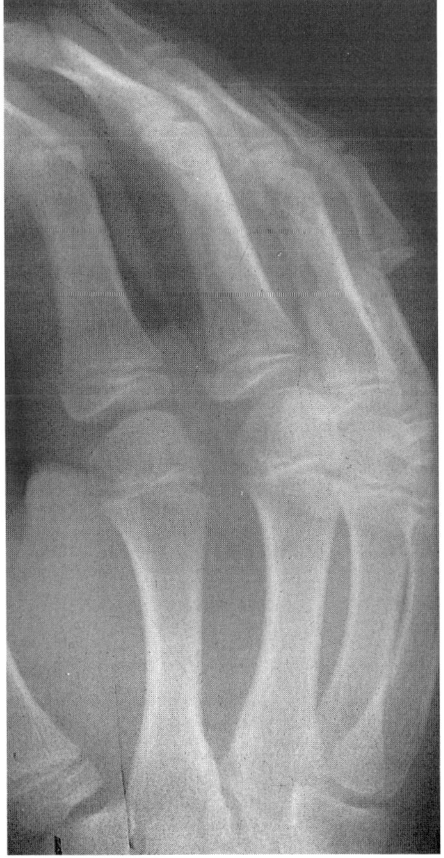

Fig. 4.4 (a) Posteroanterior and (b) oblique radiographs of the hand of a child. The dislocation of the proximal interphalangeal joint of the little finger could easily be missed on the posteroanterior radiograph but it does show an increase in bone density due to overlapping of the fragments (arrowed).

(a)

(b)

femoral shaft. Fractures around joints are particularly easily missed and joint surfaces must be examined for their completeness and congruity.

Soft tissue swelling, for instance around the ankle joint, and obliteration of tissue planes are useful indicators of damage and may be associated with an underlying fracture or ligamentous injury (Fig. 4.5).

By and large, individual fracture types are produced by the same pattern of injury and have the same features, although there are minor variations. A knowledge of the typical radiographic appearance of each fracture type is of great value. Fractures often occur in combination; for example, fractures of the radial head and capitulum may be associated with dislocation of the elbow joint. A fracture of the femoral shaft is sometimes associated with an extracapsular fracture of the femoral neck, especially after high velocity injury.

Classification of fractures by radiological features

Fractures are classified by the direction of the fracture line, the number of component parts and the integrity of the overlying soft tissues.

A complete fracture is one in which both cortices seen on the radiograph are interrupted, resulting in discontinuity between the component parts. In other cases the fracture is incomplete. A transverse fracture is one that is at right angles to the long axis of a bone; such fractures occur as a result of direct trauma and are seen particularly in the ulna and tibia. Fractures in pathological bone are usually transverse. Oblique fractures are the result of angulation and compression forces; a spiral fracture encircles the shaft and is due to torsional forces. Vertical fractures are seen particularly in the tibia or in the proximal phalanx of the thumb and are due to vertical forces. Greenstick fractures occur in children (see Chapter 10). Avulsion fractures occur where fragments of bone are separated by tension forces within the ligaments and tendons at their points of insertion (Fig. 4.6). A comminuted fracture is composed of more than two fragments. A butterfly fragment is an elongated triangular fragment separated from the main proximal and distal components of a long bone fracture. A segmental fracture is where a segment of bone is isolated by proximal and distal fracture lines in the shaft of a bone. Compression fractures may be seen in the vertebral bodies as wedge-shaped deformities or

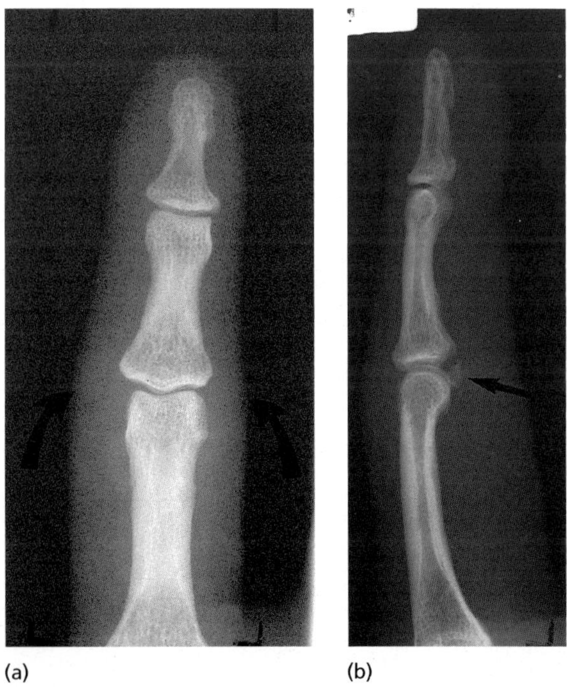

(a)   (b)

Fig. 4.5 Posteroanterior and lateral radiographs of the finger. (a) Posteroanterior radiograph. Soft tissue swelling is present (curved arrows). (b) Avulsion of flexor digitorum superficialis (arrowed), only seen on the lateral radiograph.

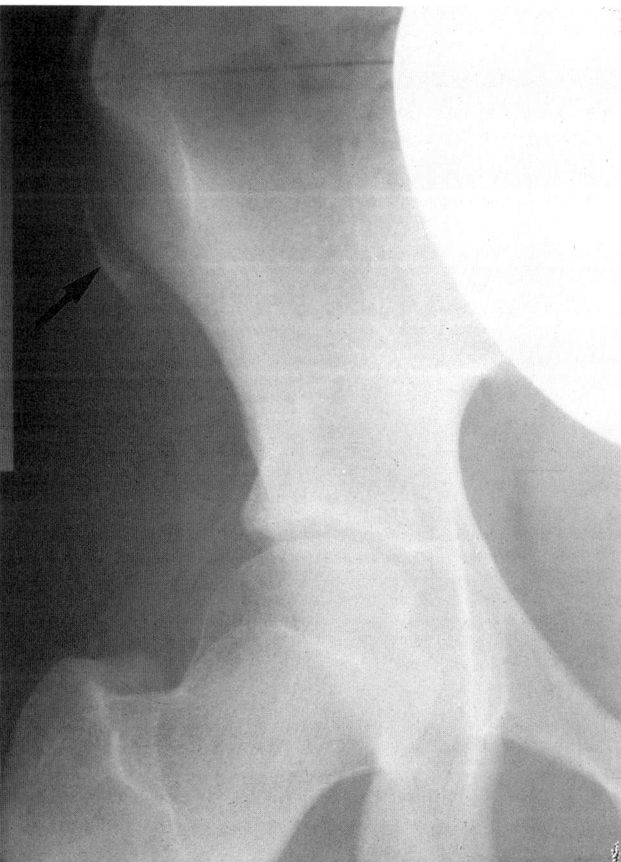

Fig. 4.6 Anteroposterior radiograph of the pelvis. Avulsion of the anterior superior iliac spine (arrowed) by the sartorius.

may occur in association with dislocation of the humeral head, producing a characteristic trough-like depression on the humeral head (Fig. 4.7). Fractures involving the end of a bone often extend into the joint and are known as intra-articular fractures. In childhood, separation and fractures of the epiphyses occur (see Chapter 10).

Dislocation of a joint produces a complete loss of congruity of the joint surfaces. If associated with a fracture the injury is classified as a fracture–dislocation. Impaction forces on the cartilage may produce osteochondral (Fig. 4.8) or chondral fractures; the latter consist entirely of cartilage and will not be visible on a radiograph. Both of these fracture types occur commonly after dislocation of the patella, and in ankle injuries where they involve the dome of the talus. A subluxation is where displacement of the opposing bones of the joint results in partial loss of congruity of the joint surfaces. A diastasis describes displacement of the bone components of a fibrous or cartilaginous joint, for example the symphysis pubis or distal tibio-fibular joint (Fig. 4.9).

Stress fractures can occur in the normal bone of healthy individuals in response to unusual activity. These fractures occur at certain sites, the most common being the distal shafts of the second and third metatarsals, the proximal and distal shafts of the tibia and the pubic rami. Abnormality is demonstrated on the radiograph between 10 days and 3 weeks following the onset of symptoms. The fracture may be visualized as a thin lucent line or may be evident from the presence of periosteal reaction (Fig. 4.10). The fracture may also be seen as a line of sclerosis, particularly in the tibia (Fig. 4.11) and calcaneum. Pathological fractures may occur at any site but are often found in specific sites for which the underlying pathological process has a predilection, for example, the proximal femoral metaphysis in metastatic disease. The injuring force is often of low magnitude or there may be a history of pre-existing pain or the presence of a mass.

Specific injuries

Hand and finger

When a phalanx of the hand is injured it is important to obtain a lateral radiograph. Many of the fractures and dislocations are not visible on the posteroanterior or oblique radiographs usually obtained for the hand. Such injuries include avulsions of the flexor digitorum superficialis, flexor digitorum profundus and extensor tendons from their respective insertions into the phalanges, and phalangeal base fractures. In the case of an avulsion of the flexor digitorum superficialis the fragment from the volar surface of the base of the middle phalanx may be small (Fig. 4.5). Abnormal alignment of one bone with another, even though no fracture is visible, suggests the presence of ligamentous damage and an important clue to this injury is hyperextension of, and soft tissue swelling about, the interphalangeal joint. With an avulsion of the flexor

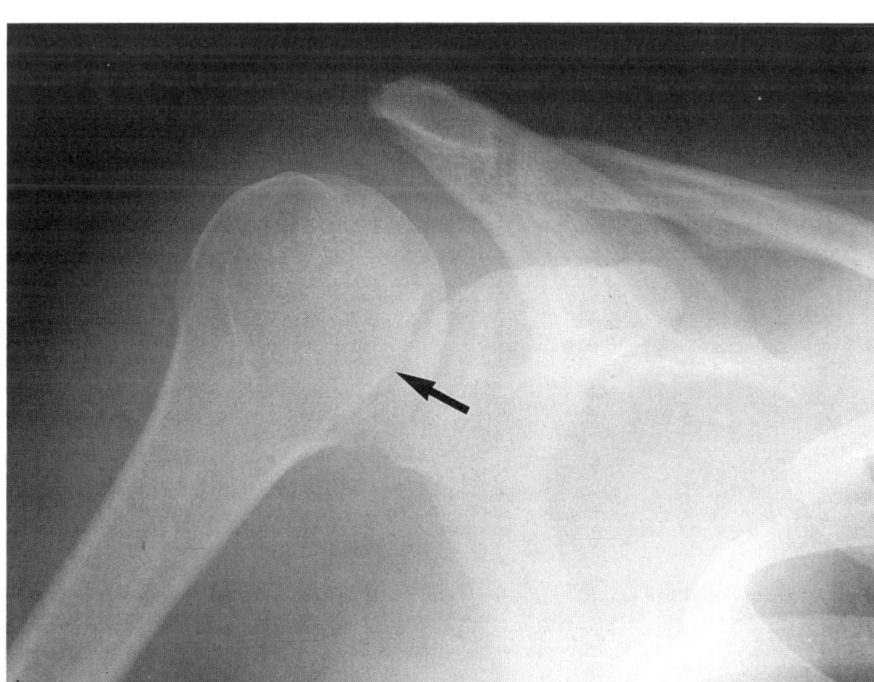

Fig. 4.7 Anteroposterior radiograph of the shoulder. The humeral head is unusually oval in shape. A trough line is present (arrowed).

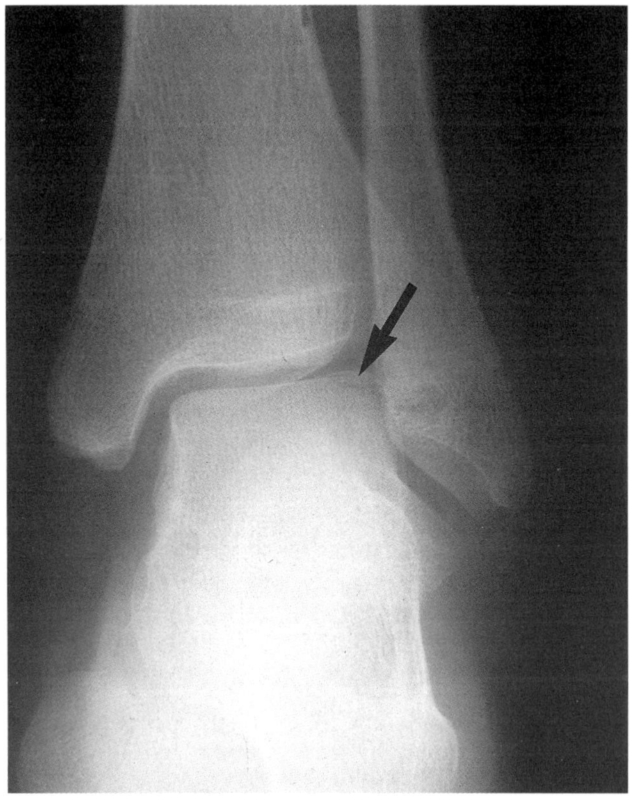 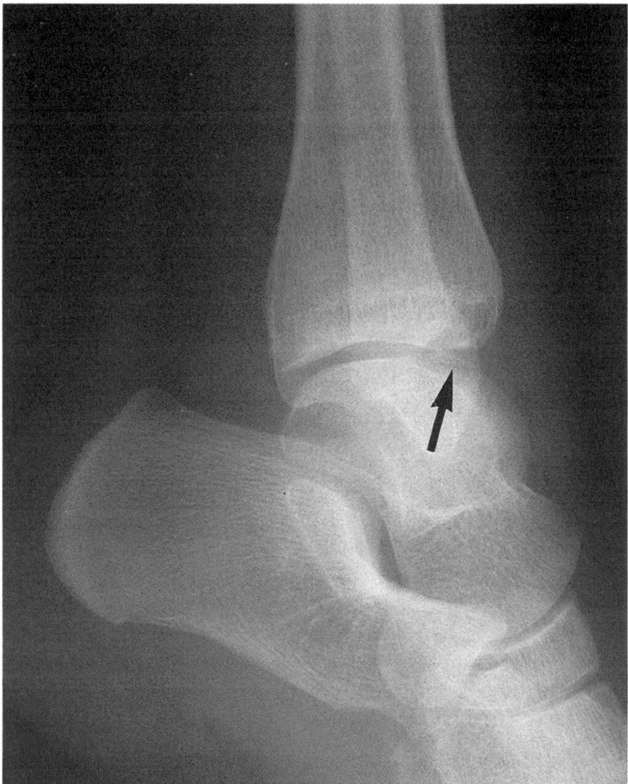

Fig. 4.8 Anteroposterior and lateral radiographs of osteochondral fracture (arrowed) of the lateral dome of the talus.

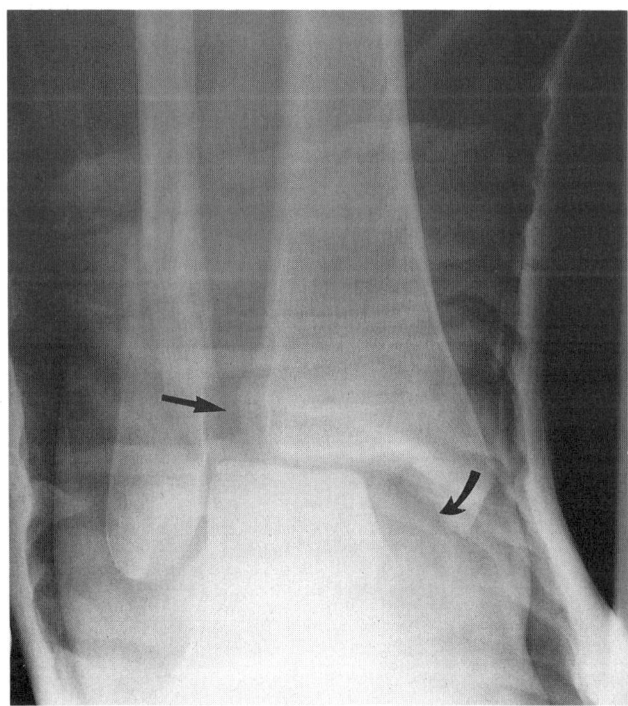 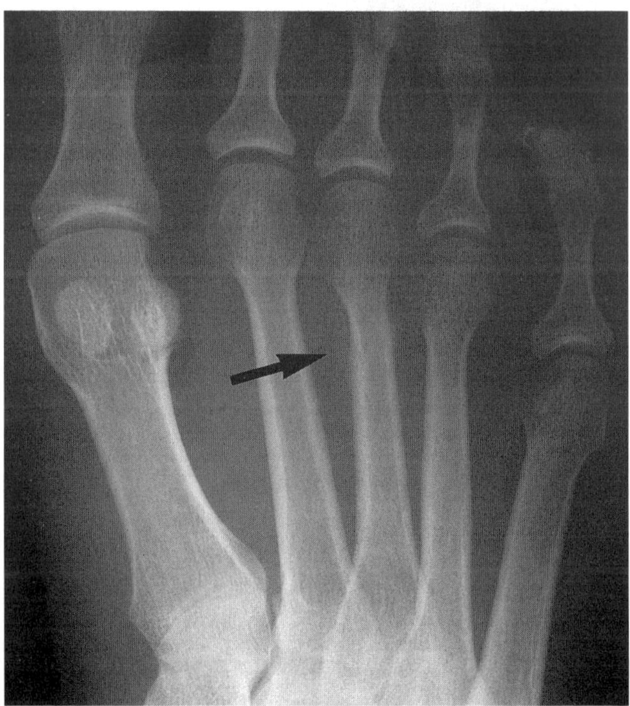

Fig. 4.9 Anteroposterior radiograph of the ankle. There is lateral shift of the talus, widening of the lateral (arrowed) and medial (curved arrow) clear spaces and a fracture of the lateral malleolus.

Fig. 4.10 Anteroposterior radiograph of the foot. March fracture of the neck of the middle metatarsal bone. Periosteal reaction (arrowed) can be seen.

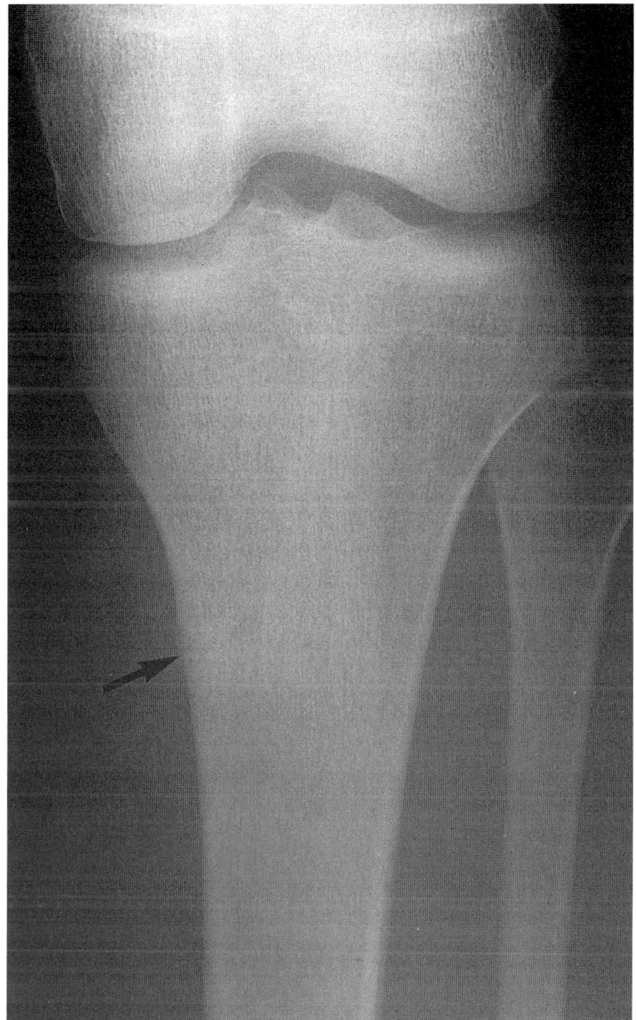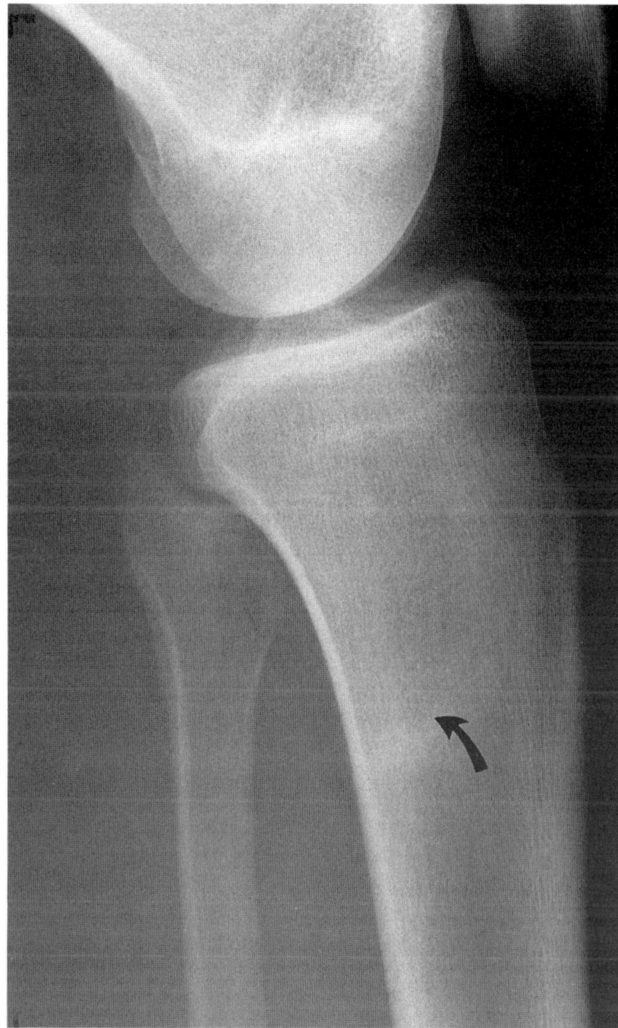

Fig. 4.11 Anteroposterior and lateral radiographs of a stress fracture of the upper tibia which is visualized as periosteal reaction (arrowed) and sclerosis (curved arrow).

digitorum profundus the tendon retracts and a fragment of bone may be seen volar to the proximal interphalangeal joint. This could be mistaken for an avulsion of the volar plate but examination will reveal that the base of the middle phalanx is intact. When an avulsion of the extensor tendon at the base of the distal phalanx occurs there is a variable degree of flexion of the distal interphalangeal joint and an inability to extend the finger — the so-called mallet finger (Fig. 4.12). Commonly no fracture is present. Boutonnière deformity, flexion of the proximal interphalangeal joint associated with extension of the distal interphalangeal joint, occurs when there has been a rupture of the middle slip of the extensor expansion overlying the proximal interphalangeal joint. In some cases there is an associated small avulsion fracture from the base of the middle phalanx. Similarly, dislocations of the phalanges may be easily missed without true lateral films.

In children it is important that an oblique view of the hand is obtained. Fractures of the metacarpals, both at the base and the neck, are often best seen on the oblique views and indeed may only be seen on these.

Rotation of fragments associated with oblique fractures of the metacarpal or phalangeal bones can usually be determined by clinical means but rotation around the long axis of the shaft is signified on the radiograph by a change in width of the cortex or the outside diameter of the fragments.

Wrist

Most scaphoid fractures are undisplaced and many are difficult to see. It is important to examine carefully the cortex, particularly that opposing the capitate (Fig. 4.13). Normally the radiographic views obtained are posteroanterior, lateral, oblique and posteroanterior with ulnar

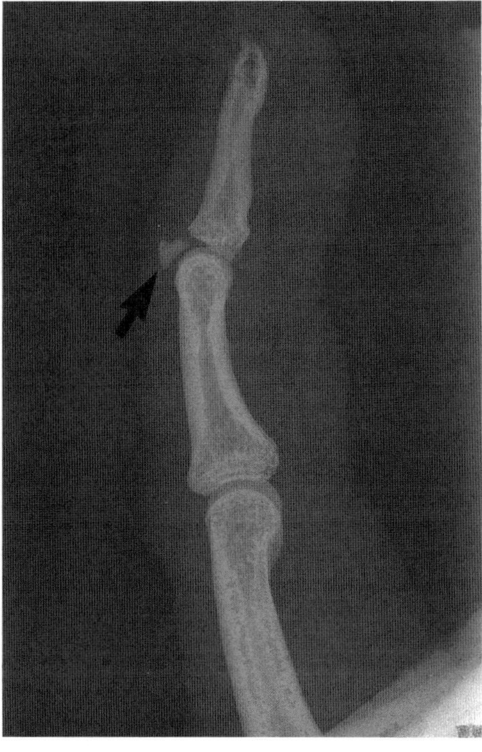

Fig. 4.12 Lateral radiograph of a mallet finger, with an avulsed fragment.

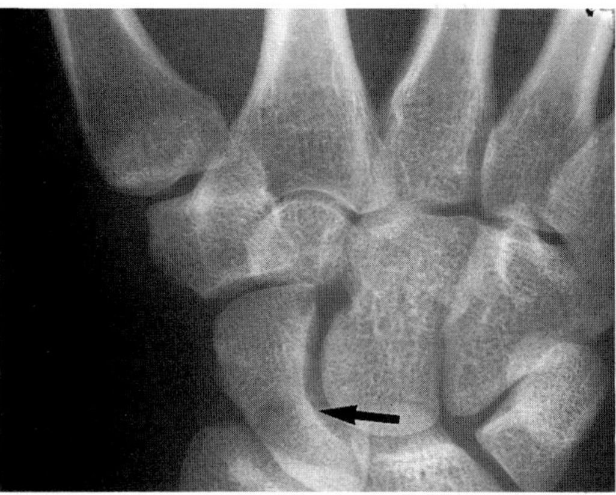

Fig. 4.13 Posteroanterior radiograph of the wrist showing discontinuity of the medial cortex of the scaphoid (arrowed). The fracture was not visible on the other radiographs obtained.

deviation of the hand. Even so, a fracture may not be demonstrated initially (Russe 1960, Leslie & Dickson 1981). Other views, including the so-called Ziter view, can be obtained if indicated (Ziter 1973). The scaphoid fat pad is a line of radiolucency lying parallel to the radial aspect of the scaphoid, seen on the posteroanterior and oblique views. The line is normally concave towards the scaphoid bone, but it may be convex or obliterated

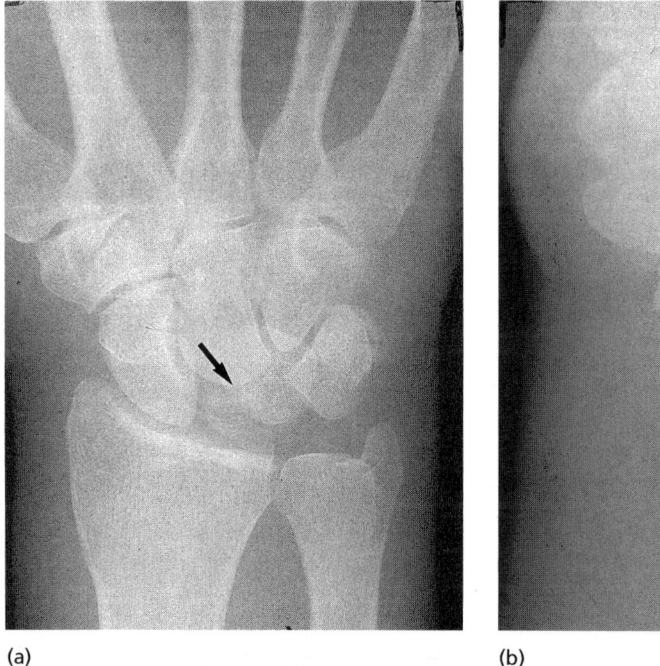

(a)

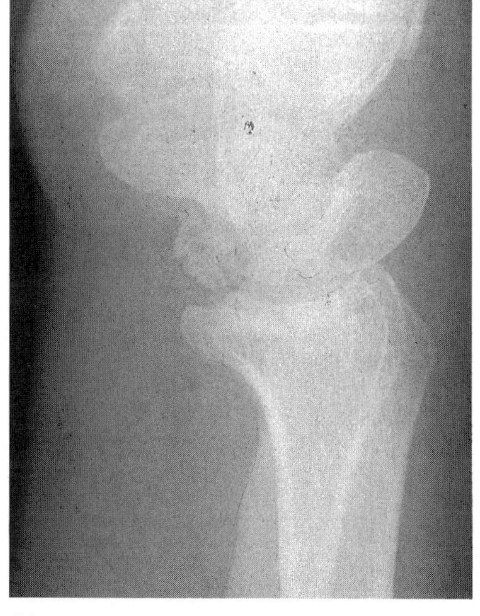

(b)

Fig. 4.14 (a) Posteroanterior radiograph of the wrist does not show the normal relationships of the opposing articular surfaces of the capitate (arrowed) and lunate. (b) Lateral radiograph — fracture dislocation of the lunate. The bulk of the lunate is displaced posteriorly.

with fractures of the scaphoid, radial styloid or base of the thumb metacarpal. The soft tissues on the dorsal aspect of the wrist are normally slightly concave in the region of the carpal bones. In the presence of an injury they may be convex or the fat planes may be obliterated. It must be noted that these signs, like all soft tissue signs of a fracture, are not infallible (Dias *et al.* 1987a). If clinically indicated the case should be treated as a scaphoid fracture and the patient reradiographed after 2–3 weeks when further slight displacement coupled with bone resorption at the fracture site allows visualization of the fracture.

Dislocations around the wrist are easily missed. On the posteroanterior view of the wrist opposing articular surfaces are parallel and do not overlap (Gilula 1979); any loss of this arrangement should suggest the presence of dislocation (Fig. 4.14). On the lateral radiograph the capitate lies between the base of the third metacarpal and the lunate, which overlies the distal radius and ulna. In pure lunate dislocations the lunate is usually displaced forward from between the capitate and the radio-ulnar joint and in distal dislocations the rest of the carpus is displaced on the lunate (MacAusland 1944).

Forearm

When a fracture or dislocation involves either the radius or ulna there is sometimes an injury to the other bone or to its articulations. An example of this is a Monteggia fracture where a fracture of the ulna is associated with dislocation of the head of the radius. On the lateral

projection of the forearm a line along the axis of the radius normally passes through the centre of the capitulum in all degrees of flexion (Storen 1958–1959). If this line is disrupted there is abnormal articulation of the head of the radius and capitulum (Fig. 4.15). When there is a fracture of the shaft of the radius there may be dislocation of the distal radio-ulnar joint seen as an overlapping of the bones on the anterior-posterior radiograph and as a loss of their normal relationship on the lateral radiograph (Galeazzi fracture). When the wrist is truly lateral the capitate and hammate are superimposed, as are the distal radius and ulna.

A fat line, lying volar to the distal radius and ulna and overlying the pronator quadratus, is seen on the lateral radiograph. Alteration, displacement, blurring or obliteration of this fat line (MacEwan 1964) may be due to an underlying fracture of the radius or ulna.

Elbow

In children fractures involving the elbow joint commonly produce an effusion within the joint (Norell 1954). The posterior fat pad behind the distal humerus is not normally visible. If an effusion occurs it is elevated from the bone, as is the anterior fat pad which becomes sail shaped (Fig. 4.2). In adults it is more common to have fractures without an effusion in the joint and it must be remembered that effusion in the joint can occur without a fracture (Quinton *et al.* 1987). Effusion in the joint may also be related to inflammatory conditions (Murphy & Siegel 1977).

In the child a check must be made that the medial

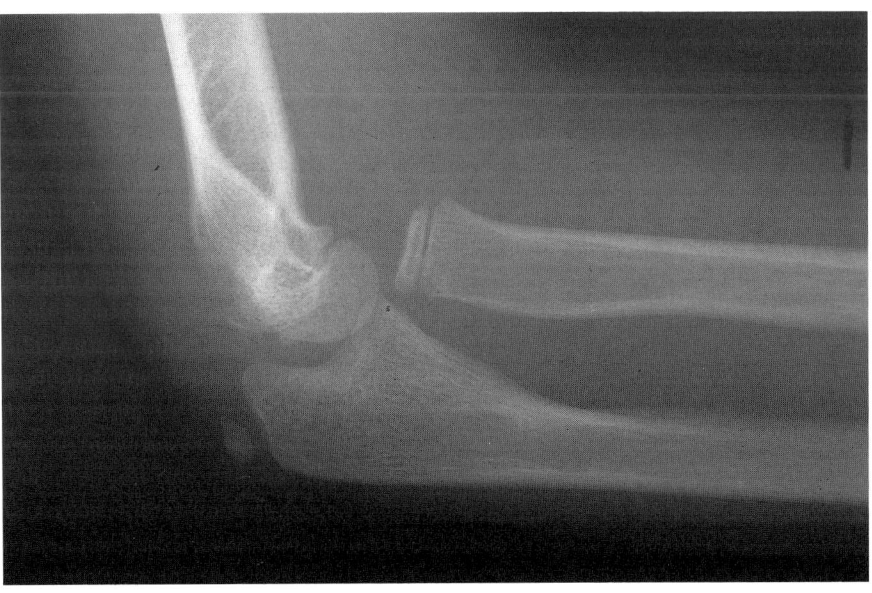

Fig. 4.15 Lateral radiograph of the elbow. Dislocation of the radial head which does not lie in line with the capitulum.

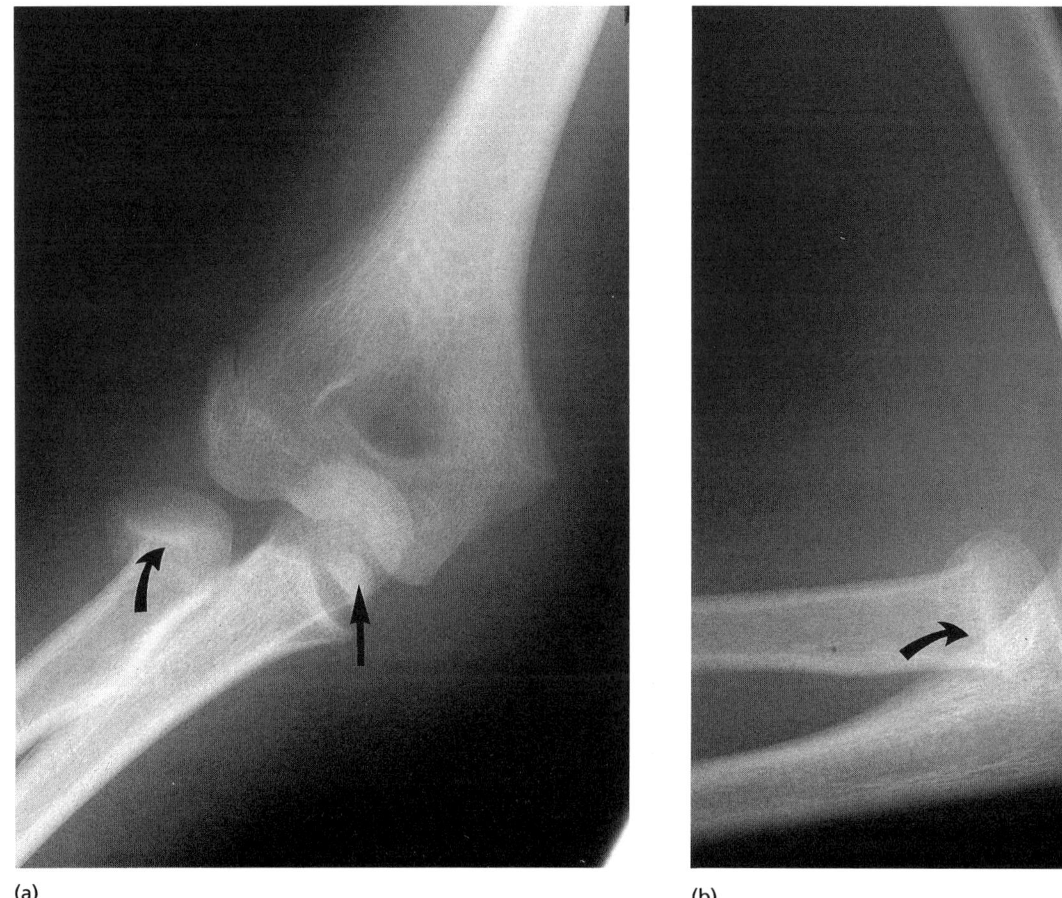

(a)

(b)

Fig. 4.16 (a) Anteroposterior radiograph of the elbow showing absence of the medial epicondyle from its normal position. It is seen in the joint (arrowed). (b) Lateral radiograph showing the medial epicondyle in the joint (arrowed). There is also a fracture of the radial neck which is shown in both illustrations (curved arrow).

epicondyle is situated in its normal position. When the elbow is subject to valgus stress there is opening of the medial side of the elbow joint, following separation of the medial epicondyle which may become trapped within the joint (Fig. 4.16). This may also occur when there has been a complete dislocation of the joint. It is important to remember that the trochlear ossification centre is not seen before that of the medial epicondyle. An apparent trochlear ossification centre on the antero-posterior radiograph with absence of the medial epicondylar epiphysis confirms the diagnosis of dis-placement of the epiphysis which may be in the joint.

In children supracondylar fractures of the humerus may be difficult to see and it is useful to remember that a line drawn down the anterior shaft of the humerus should pass through the middle third of the capitellum (Rogers *et al.* 1978); in children less than 2.5 years old it may pass through the anterior third.

Shoulder

Anterior dislocations of the shoulder joint are usually obvious on both radiographic and clinical examination. Posterior dislocations, however, cause problems. On the anteroposterior radiograph the humeral head is oval in shape (Fig. 4.7) owing to the shoulder being in forced internal rotation (Cisternino *et al.* 1978). Numerous radiological signs have been described which help to make the diagnosis, but they are unreliable and an additional view, showing the head posterior to the glenoid, is necessary. The axillary view is difficult to obtain in a dislocated shoulder but a modified view can be easily obtained (Wallace & Hellier 1983). On the anteroposterior radiograph the humeral head may be displaced lateral to the glenoid rim. The distance between the medial border of the head and the anterior glenoid rim is less than 6 mm in the normal shoulder (Arndt & Sears 1965). On the internally rotated head, a second

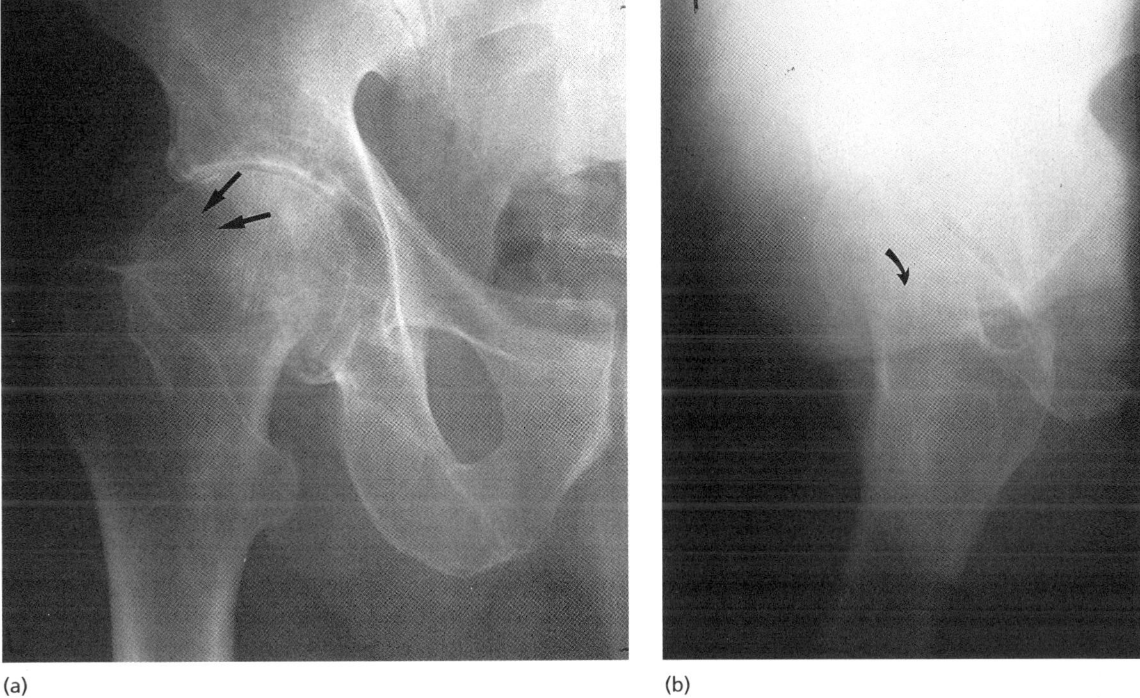

Fig. 4.17 (a) Anteroposterior radiograph of a Garden grade II fracture of the femoral neck. The trabeculae in the femoral neck are interrupted (arrowed). (b) Lateral radiograph of the fracture (curved arrow).

vertical line may be seen lateral to the articular cortex (Fig. 4.7); this is the trough line which shows the margin of an impaction fracture of the head (Cisternino *et al.* 1978).

When a dislocation of the acromio-clavicular joint is suspected, stress views are often required to confirm the injury. Comparative views of both shoulders are obtained with 4.5–6.8 kg weights suspended by loops from the wrists. Although there are normal values for the width of the acromio-clavicular joint and the position of the clavicle with respect to the superior margin of the coracoid process of the scapula, it is safer to consider the difference between the two sides.

Pelvis

Some fractures of the pelvis may not be visualized on the anteroposterior radiograph that is usually obtained. This applies particularly to fractures of the pubic rami, separation of the sacro-iliac joints or fractures in the surrounding bone.

These are commonly better seen on inlet and outlet views of the pelvis (Young *et al.* 1986). It must be remembered that fractures in ring structures commonly occur in pairs.

The obturator internus projects into the pelvis medial to the acetabulum and is normally bilaterally asymmet-

rical. When bulging occurs on one side it is a reliable radiographic sign of underlying bony trauma. Additional views of the acetabulum, such as internal and external oblique views, may give more information (Judet *et al.* 1964) and are sometimes necessary in order to visualize the fracture.

Femoral neck

Intracapsular fractures of the femoral neck may be difficult to visualize when they are undisplaced (Garden grade II). The only abnormality seen on the anteroposterior radiograph may be disruption of the tensile and compressive trabeculae in the femoral neck (Fig. 4.17). It is important that both the anteroposterior and lateral radiographs are carefully examined for breaks in the cortices of the neck. However, a fracture not visualized on the radiographs at presentation is in fact rare (O'Dwyer *et al.* 1992). On the anteroposterior radiograph in a Garden grade I fracture, fracture sclerosis is seen in the lateral part of the neck (Fig. 4.6) and the head is in valgus.

Femoral shaft

When there is a fracture of the femoral shaft adduction of the proximal fragment suggests an associated pos-

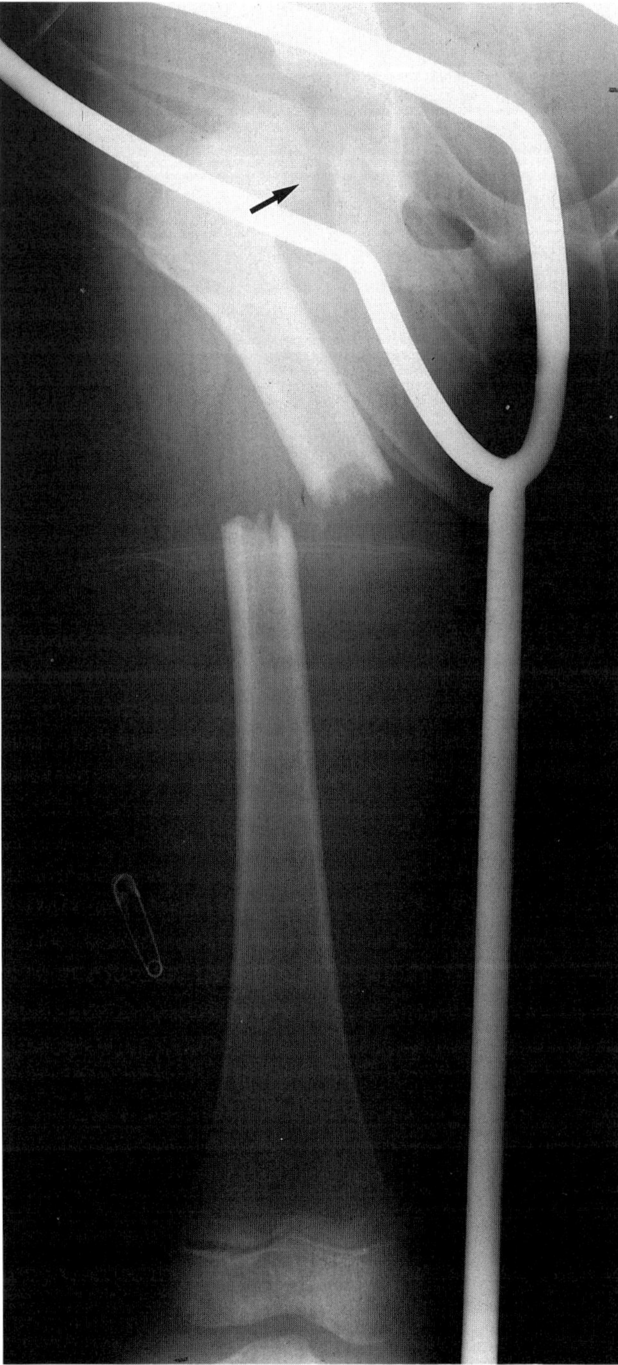

Fig. 4.18 Fracture of the proximal femoral shaft with adduction of the proximal fragment and posterior dislocation of the femoral head (arrowed).

terior dislocation of the hip (Fig. 4.18). By making sure that the joints above and below the fracture of a long bone are present on the radiographs this potential pitfall should be avoided.

Knee

Surprisingly, major fractures of the tibial plateau may not be evident on the anteroposterior and lateral radiographs (Newberg & Greenstein 1978). It is important that when there is clinical suspicion of a fracture oblique radiographs should be obtained. A radiological pointer towards an injury is effusion in the joint (Apple *et al.* 1983); this is seen on the lateral radiograph as a widening of the suprapatellar pouch of the knee joint which separates the fat planes lying anteriorly and posteriorly (Maskell & Finlay 1990). Of greater significance is the presence of a fat fluid level in the knee joint; this is most easily seen on a lateral decubitus film (Fig. 4.19) and signifies a fracture Lee *et al.* (1989). The presence of gas suggests a compound injury (Fig. 4.20). However, gas also occurs in joints which have been distracted but are otherwise normal; this occurs particularly at the shoulder and hip joint in children. It is relatively easy to miss a fragment sheared from a lower femoral condyle in the coronal plane (Fig. 4.21). It is important to be certain that the articular surfaces are congruent. In the elbow likewise an anteriorly displaced fragment from the capitulum is easily missed.

Ankle

Radiology of the ankle joint is complex and commonly the sites of injury are multiple. There may be fractures of the malleoli, either transverse due to ligamentous tensile force or oblique due to impaction by the talus. Ligamentous avulsion from either malleolus may exist with or without an avulsion fracture. The posterior malleolus may be fractured. Important, and not to be missed, is disruption of the tibio-fibular syndesmosis which allows lateral displacement of the talus under the tibia. On the anteroposterior radiograph the lateral clear space (between the medial surface of the fibula and the plain surface of the fibular notch), the tibio-fibular syndesmosis, is well visualized and should be less than 5.5 mm in width (Lauge-Hansen 1954; Fig. 4.22); a measurement greater than this indicates diastasis (Fig. 4.9). The medial clear space between the medial malleolus and talus should measure 3 mm; a width greater than this or a difference greater than 2 mm compared to the normal side suggests rupture of the deltoid ligament (McDade 1975).

If there is widening of the medial clear space, transverse fracture of the medial malleolus, or diastasis of the tibio-fibular syndesmosis or an apparent isolated posterior fracture, there is usually a fracture of the fibula. If this fracture is not visible below the tibial plafond it

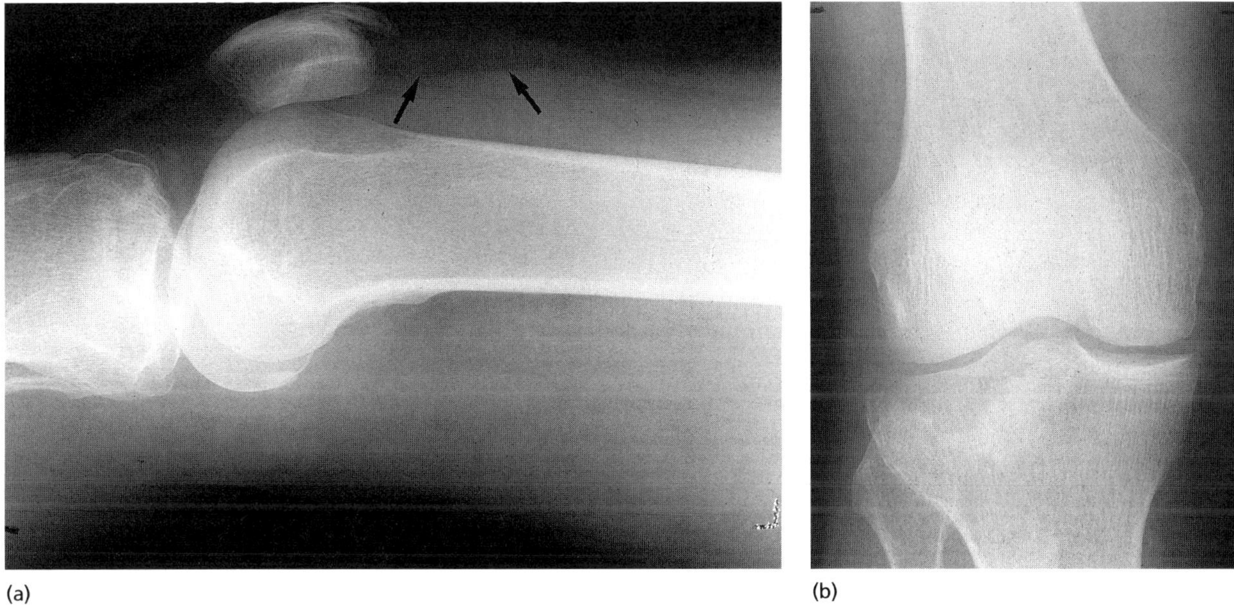

(a) (b)

Fig. 4.19 (a) Horizontal lateral radiograph of the knee joint showing a fat fluid level in the suprapatellar pouch (arrowed). (b) Anteroposterior radiograph showing a depressed fracture of the lateral tibial plateau.

may be above, even in the proximal third of the fibula: the so-called Maisonneuve fracture (Fig. 4.22). A fracture of the fibula above the plafond is almost always associated with diastasis of the tibio-fibular syndesmosis,

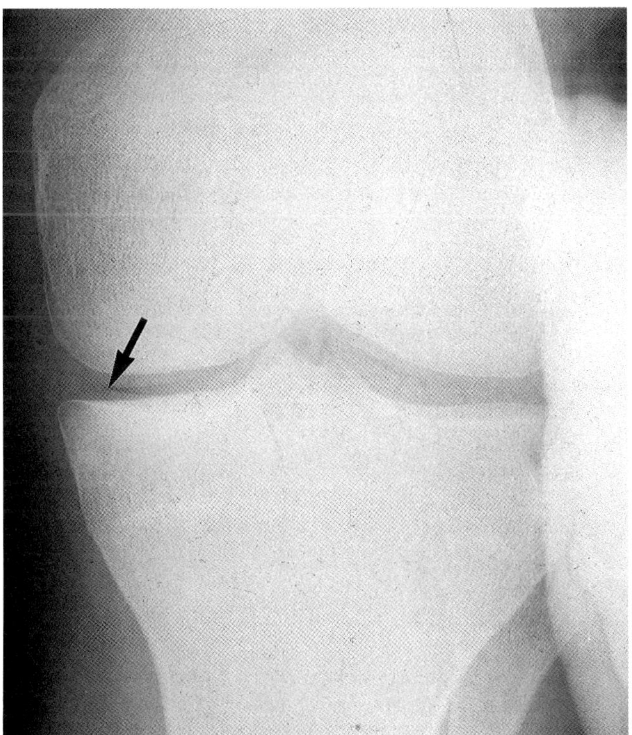

Fig. 4.20 Anteroposterior radiograph of the knee showing gas (arrowed) in the knee joint after a compound injury.

which may be of normal width on the radiograph even though potential diastasis is present.

An additional projection of the ankle joint is the internal oblique view which is obtained with 15−20° of internal rotation of the foot and demonstrates the entire anteroposterior plane of the ankle joint (Goergen *et al.* 1977). This allows assessment of the medial clear space and the talofibular joint which should be approximately the same width; neither should be wider than 4 mm. The significance of increased width of the spaces is the same as for those seen on the anteroposterior radiograph.

Foot

An indicator for compression fractures involving the posterior calcaneal facet is Böhler's angle. This is the angle made by a line drawn from the superior margin of the tuberosity through the superior margin of the posterior facet intersecting a second line from the superior margin of the posterior facet to the superior margin of the anterior process. This angle is normally between 20 and 40°. It must be noted that compression fractures may exist (20%; personal series) without this angle being disturbed.

A tarsometatarsal fracture−dislocation, Lisfranc's fracture−dislocation, is not usually well-demonstrated on the oblique plantar radiograph because there is little evidence of displacement of the metatarsals with respect to the tarsus. Displacement is usually better seen on the

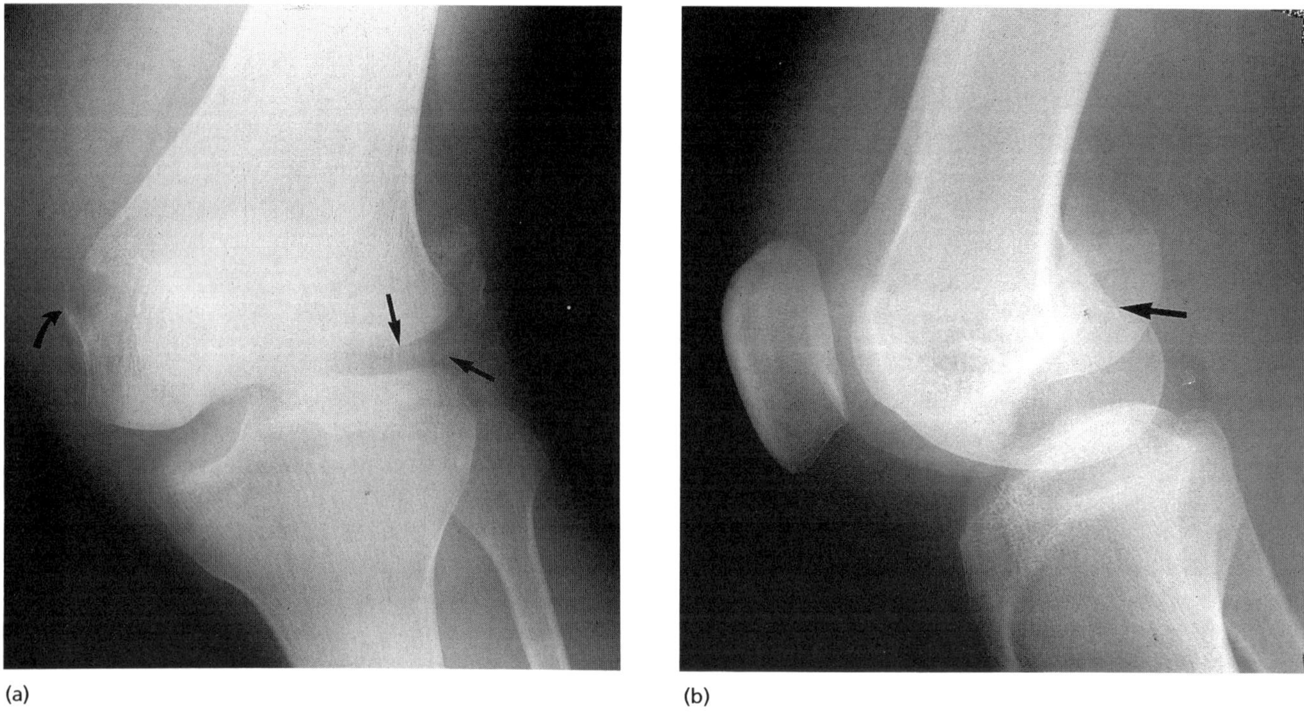

Fig. 4.21 (a) Anteroposterior radiograph of the knee which is in valgus. The lateral joint surfaces are not congruent. The normal femoral condylar articular surface cannot be seen; there appear to be two articular surfaces (arrowed). There has been an avulsion of the medial collateral ligament (curved arrow). (b) Lateral radiograph shows a coronal fracture (arrowed) of the lateral femoral condyle.

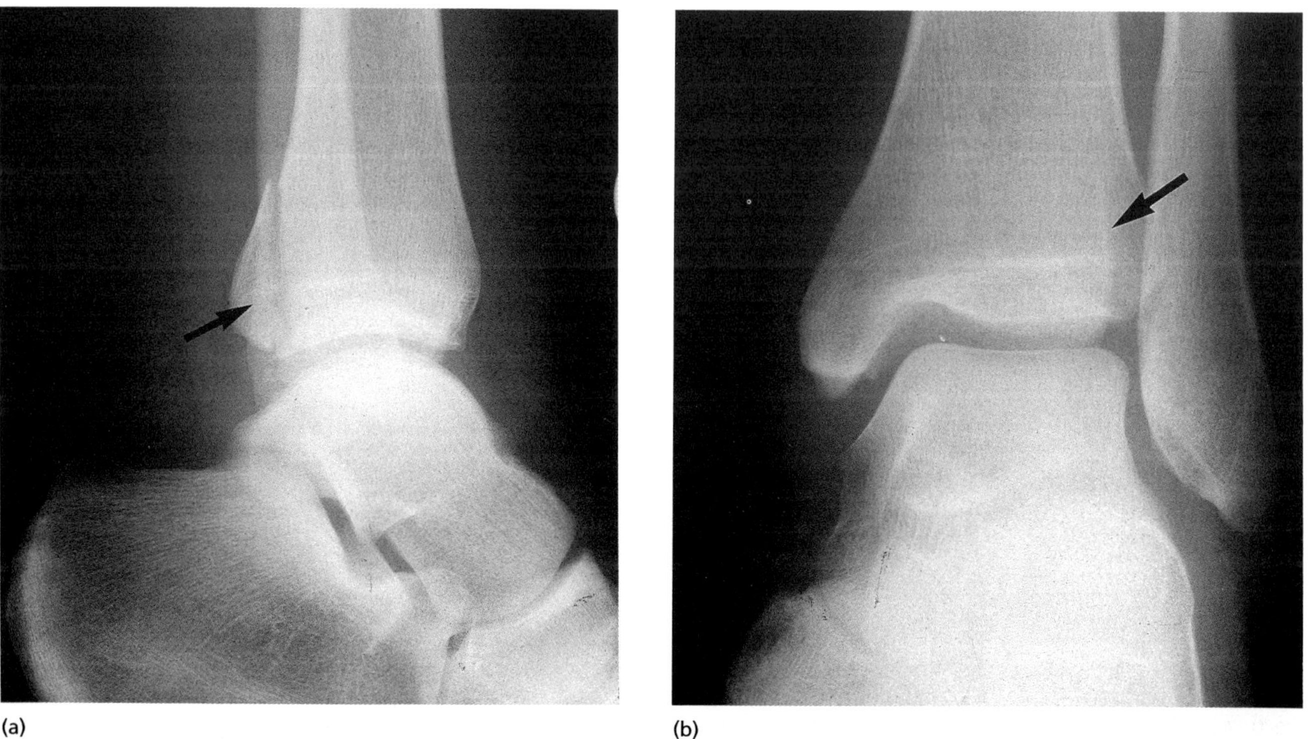

Fig. 4.22 (a) Lateral radiograph of the ankle shows a fracture of the posterior lip of the tibia (arrowed). (b) Mortice view of the ankle demonstrates medial and lateral clear spaces of normal width plain surface of fibular neck (arrowed).

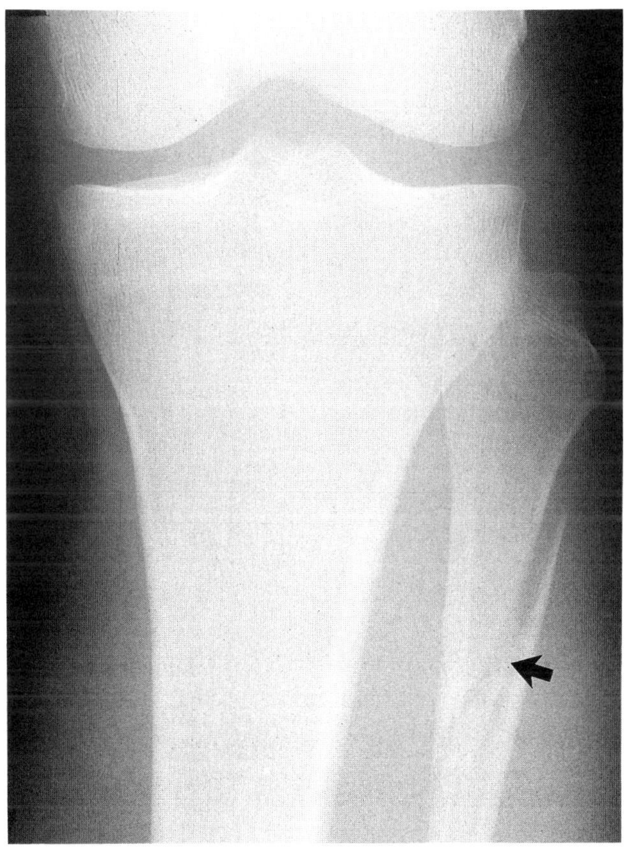

(c)

Fig. 4.22 (*Continued.*) (c) Anteroposterior radiograph of the upper fibula shows a fracture in the proximal third of the fibula (broad arrow).

dorsiplantar radiograph. Radiological pointers for this fracture are that the line which normally joins the medial aspects of the second metatarsal and medial cuneiform is broken (Fig. 4.23) or there are fractures around the bases of the metatarsals.

Spine

In the cervical spine minor fractures are relatively commonly missed (Annis *et al.* 1987), occasionally major ones. Dislocations commonly occur at the lower intervertebral joints and it is important that the lateral radiograph demonstrates the whole cervical spine, including the upper surface of T1. Radiologically, the spine is best thought of as a series of lines connecting similar structures at different levels (Gerlock *et al.* 1978); these lines are along the anterior and posterior edges of the bodies, along the posterior extent of the laminae and along the posterior aspect of the spinous process (Fig. 4.24a). On the anteroposterior radiograph lines can be drawn vertically through the pedicles and the spinous processes, and the gaps between are usually of a similar depth (Fig. 4.24b) (Naidich *et al.* 1977). A fracture or dislocation almost always produces displacement or

angulation of one or more of these lines or interruption by a fragment of bone (Fig. 4.25). Pre-vertebral soft tissue swelling suggests trauma (Miles & Finlay 1988). Fractures at the level of the odontoid process often produce fragments of bone that are superimposed because the odontoid process is displaced anteriorly or posteriorly. An increased density at the base of the odontoid may be seen; these fractures are best seen on a lateral view.

In the thoracic and lumbar spine, of particular importance on anteroposterior radiographs is the line joining the pedicles. Lateral displacement of one or both pedicles indicates that there is a fracture involving the posterior elements (Fig. 4.26). It is important to assess the interspinous gap on the lateral radiograph as widening of this gap similarly indicates instability at this level.

Fractures specific to childhood

In childhood many of the fractures that occur are specific to children and are commonly classed as 'greenstick' fractures. A greenstick fracture is an incomplete fracture where one cortex is fractured and the other is bent or

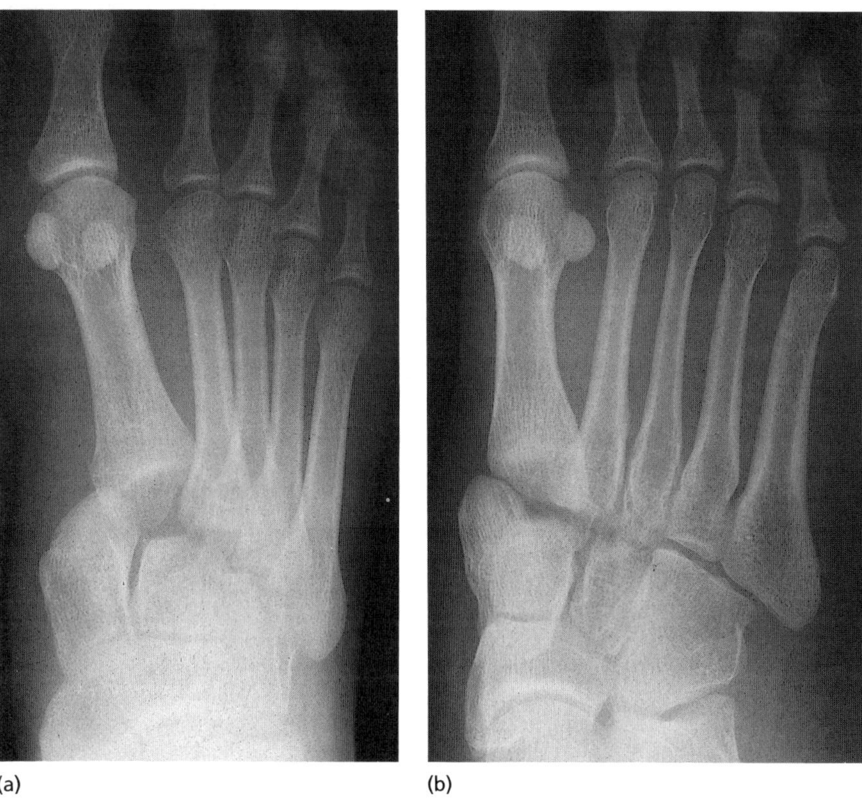

Fig. 4.23 Tarsometatarsal fracture—dislocation. (a) Oblique radiograph shows loss of alignment of the medial aspects of the second metatarsal and the medial aspect of the intermediate cunieform. (b) The dorsiplantar radiograph shows more obvious deformity.

(a)

(b)

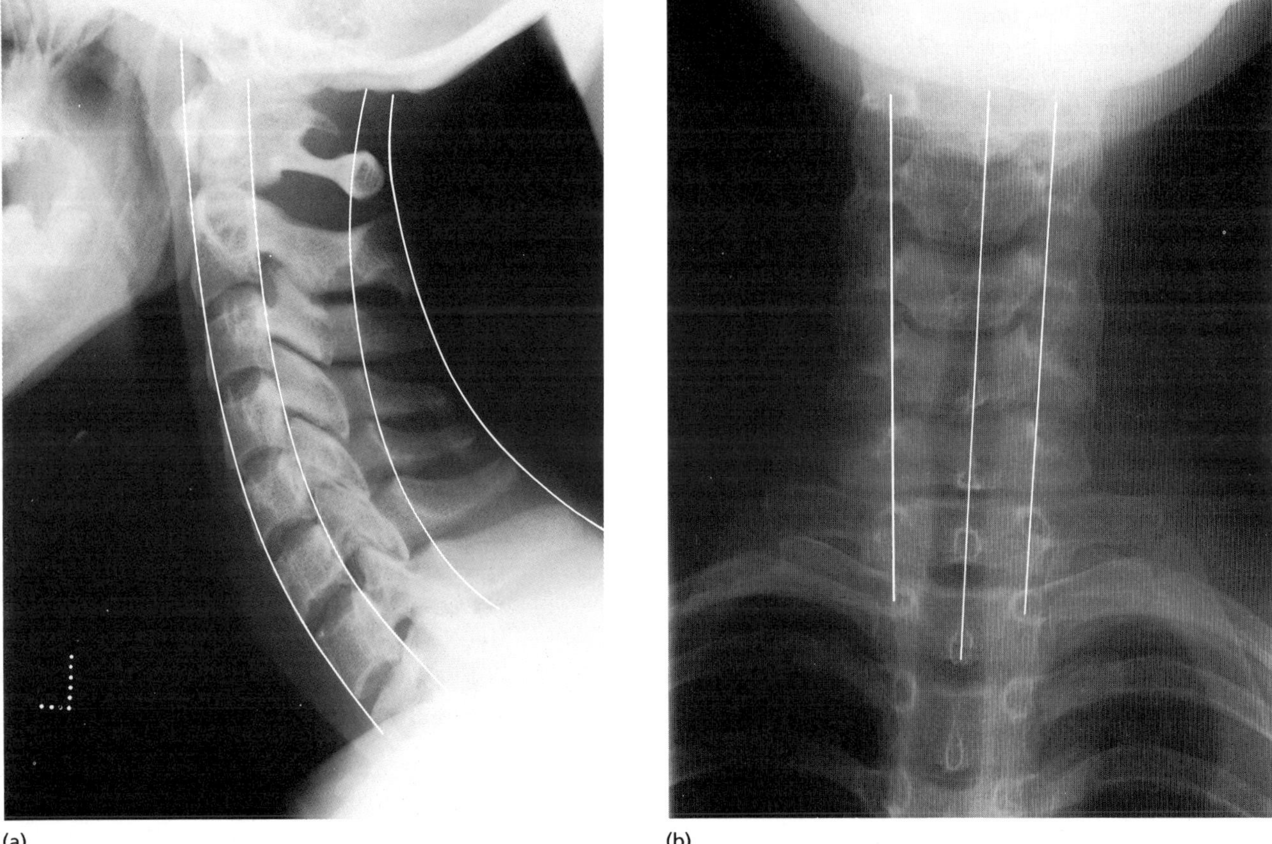

(a)

(b)

Fig. 4.24 (a) Lateral radiograph of the cervical spine with lines. (b) Anteroposterior radiograph of the cervical spine with lines.

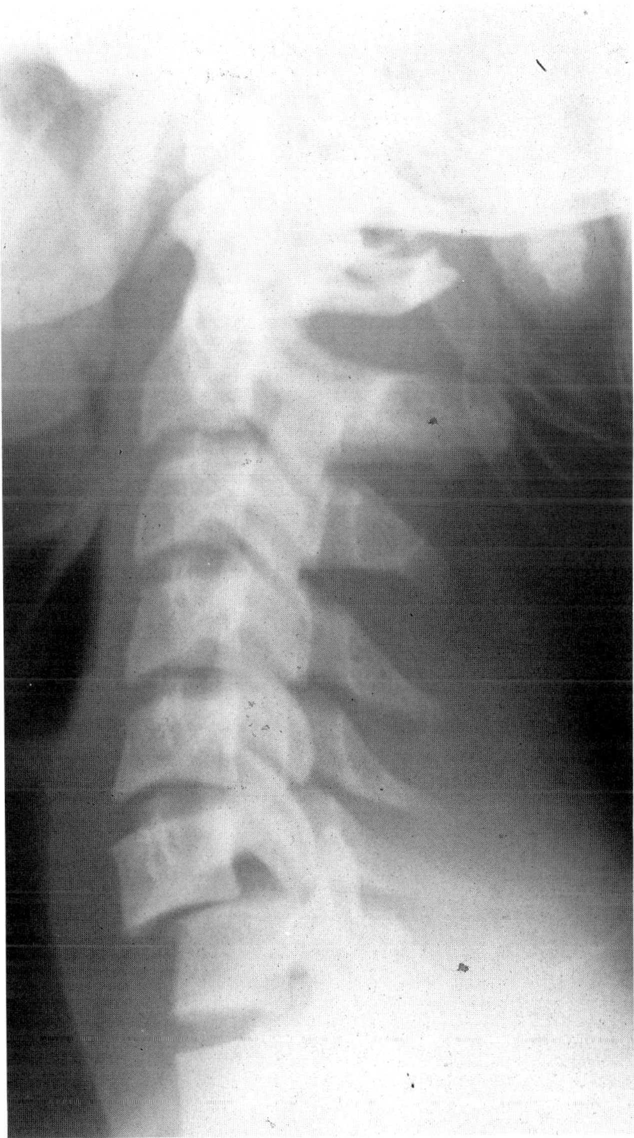

Fig. 4.25 Lateral radiograph of the cervical spine. Bilateral facet dislocation with forward displacement of C6 on C7.

bowed but is otherwise intact. These occur commonly in the mid-shaft of the radius and ulna. Torus fractures occur when there is buckling of the cortex in response to a compressive force; these fractures commonly occur at the end of the long bones, particularly the radius and ulna (Fig. 4.27). These two types of fracture can occur in combination to produce the so-called lead-pipe fracture where one cortex is buckled and the other is fractured. Another type of childhood fracture is a bowing fracture and the resultant deformity usually affects the entire length of a bone, commonly the radius or ulna. Greenstick, torus and lead-pipe fractures are particularly easy to miss and minimal angulation of a cortex, particularly

in the region of a metaphysis, must be sought. The clinical information that a child is unwilling to use a limb is highly indicative of a fracture. A common occurrence in the tibia is a spiral fracture which is not visible on anteroposterior and lateral radiographs; however, it may be seen on oblique radiographs or may be signalled by soft tissue swelling. Alternatively, it may only be demonstrated at a later date by the development of subperiosteal new bone formation. This is the so-called toddler's fracture (Dunbar *et al.* 1964).

A further group of fractures that occur in children are injuries involving the epiphysis (Fig. 4.28). These are classified by the Salter–Harris classification into five types:

I — Separation of the epiphysis without fracture of the metaphysis.

II — A fragment of fractured metaphysis remains attached to the separated epiphysis.

III — Part of the epiphysis is separated with a fracture horizontally through the epiphyseal plate.

IV — There is a vertically orientated line across the epiphysis growth plate and metaphysis separating a fragment.

V — Rarely, there is a crush injury to the epiphyseal growth plate and there are no immediate radiological manifestations.

It is useful to remember that in children epiphyseal separations occur instead of dislocations or ligamentous injury.

Diagnostic problems occasionally arise with respect to normal epiphyses in children. The inclination of the epiphysis of the proximal humerus often produces a double line on the anteroposterior radiograph and this double line may be suspected as a fracture (Fig. 4.29).

Often the normal anatomical position of the epiphysis with respect to the metaphysis suggests trauma. This is seen particularly with the capitular epiphysis (Fig. 4.30). Epiphyses may be multicentred, for example the olecranon or tarsal navicular. Commonly the epiphysis of the proximal phalanx of the big toe is bifid, and the patella may be bi- or tripartite. The multiple epiphyses at the elbow and their different shapes may cause problems and in these cases comparison with the opposite elbow may be of help.

Special consideration must be given to the diagnosis of non-accidental injury. Radiographic evidence consists of multiple injuries in various stages of healing. Fractures of the corners of the metaphysis and marked periosteal new bone formation along the shaft of a long bone are characteristic (Fig. 4.31). Fractures occurring at unusual sites, such as the ribs or the lateral end of the clavicle, and skull fractures are commonly seen.

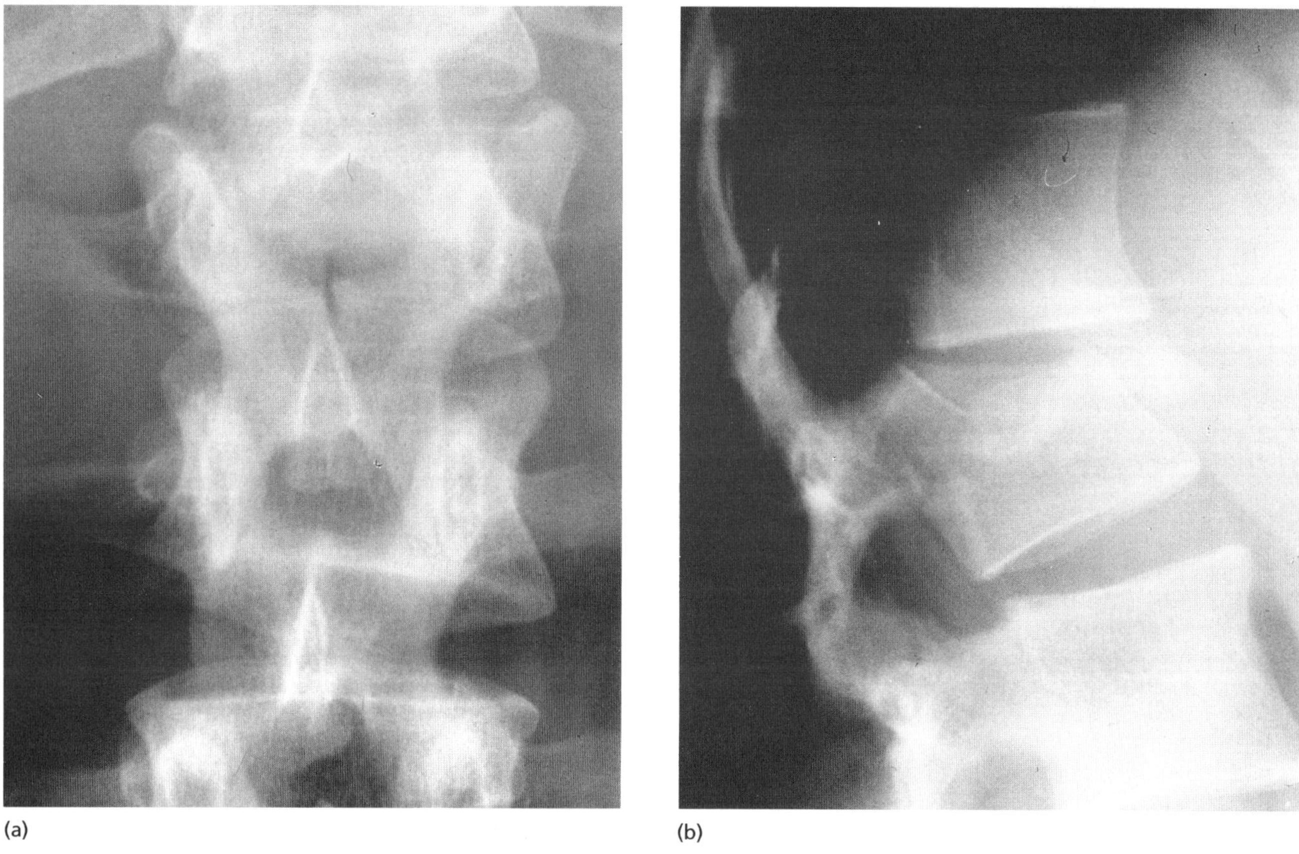

(a)

(b)

Fig. 4.26 (a) Anteroposterior radiograph showing disruption of the lines of the pedicles. (b) Lateral radiograph of a burst fracture.

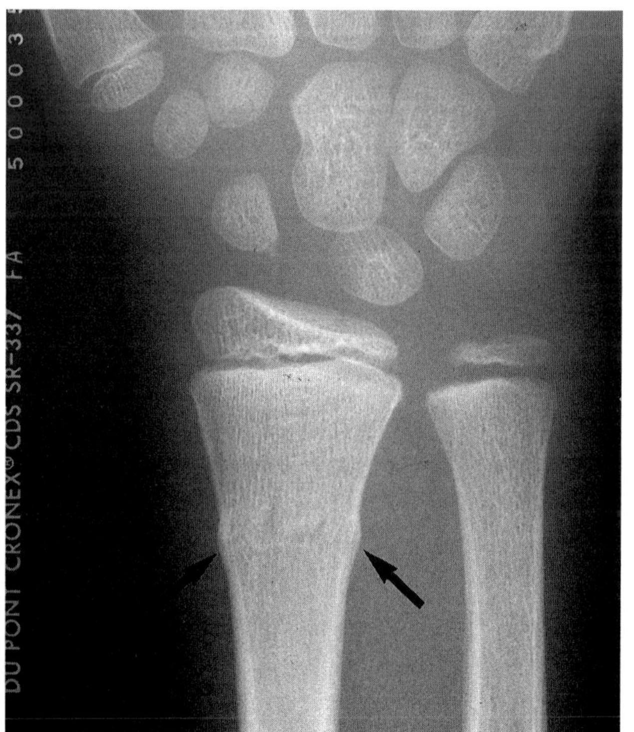

Fig. 4.27 Posteroanterior radiograph of the wrist, in which a torus fracture (arrowed) of the distal radial shaft is seen.

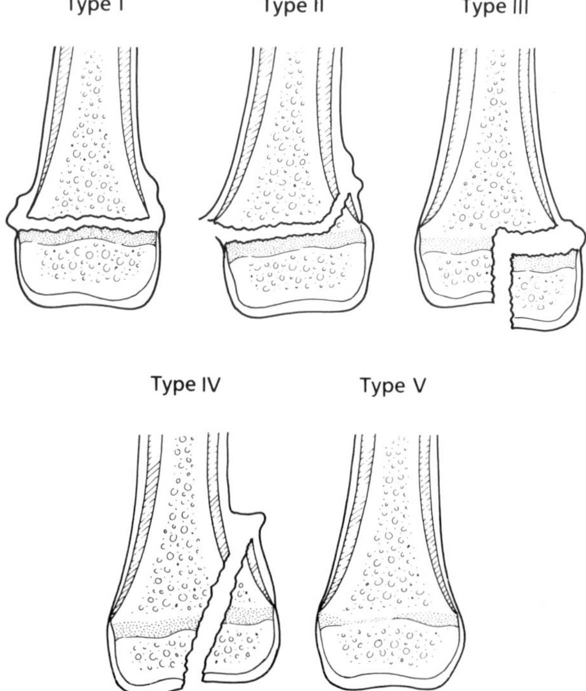

Fig. 4.28 Salter–Harris classification of epiphyseal injuries.

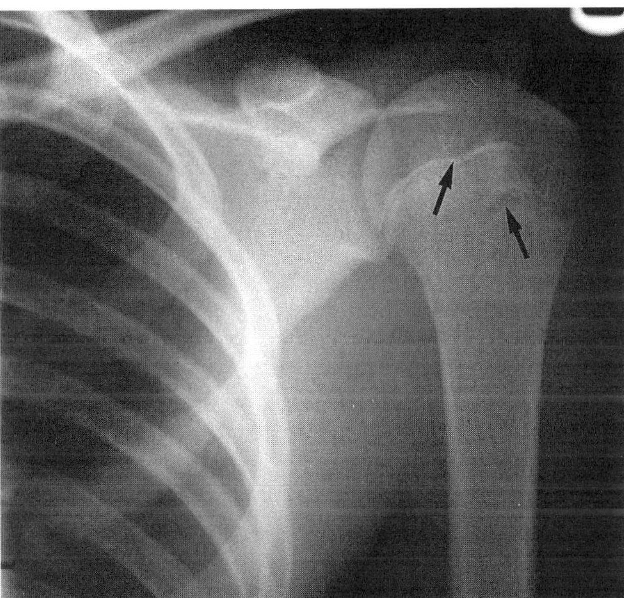

Fig. 4.29 Anteroposterior radiograph of the shoulder showing the normal appearance of the epiphyseal plate (arrowed) of the proximal humerus.

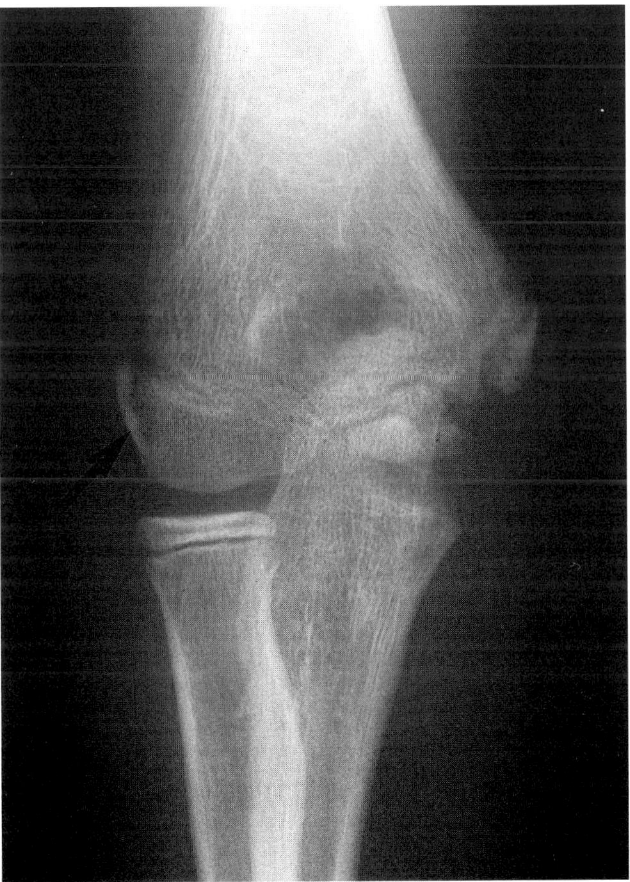

Fig. 4.30 Anteroposterior radiograph of the elbow. A normal but apparently off-set position of the capitellar epiphysis (arrowed); note the different epiphyseal shapes.

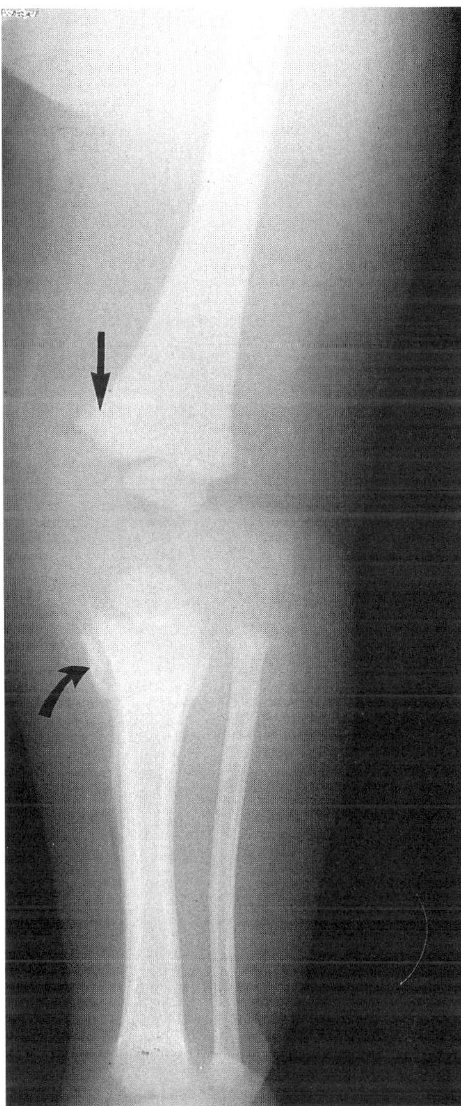

Fig. 4.31 Anteroposterior radiograph of a limb of an infant showing fractures of the corners of the metaphyses (arrowed), and periosteal reaction (curved arrow) characteristic of the battered baby syndrome.

Fracture healing

Within 2 weeks of a fracture, blurring of the opposing margins of the fracture fragment may be seen. Calcified callus eventually appears about the fracture site. Fractures of the long bones develop considerably more callus than those of short bones; in the scaphoid it is minimal. Impacted fractures develop little callus. Callus formation is increased by instability at the fracture site or by infection. Rigid fixation of a fracture reduces the amount of callus, and if much is formed movement at the fracture site or infection should be considered as possible causes.

Bridging across the fracture line by callus is radiographic evidence of union. For confirmation it is necessary to obtain projections at right angles to each other; overlapping of bone can produce the appearance of union when this is not present. It may be necessary to resort to tomography. Whilst this suffices in most cases it may be extremely difficult to tell that bony union has occurred, particularly in the scaphoid (Dias *et al.* 1988).

Non-union may be one of two types; hypertrophic or atrophic. In hypertrophic non-union the fracture is well defined and sclerotic with evidence of callus formation around the end of each fragment. A pseudarthrosis may form at the fracture site; no callus crosses it. In atrophic non-union there is little sclerosis and no evidence of callus formation.

Normal structures mimicking fractures

There are many normal anatomical features in the adult and the child which resemble fractures; these are predictable in their location and appearance (Keats 1984). In the long and short bones vascular foramina sometimes cause a problem. These are sharp, smoothly defined lines which obliquely cross the cortex with their inner limits lying furthest from the fastest growing growth plate. In the femur the nutrient foramen is seen in the posterior cortex with its inner limit lying closest to the knee. In the forearm and fingers the inner limits lie distally (Fig. 4.32). Accessory ossicles occur in characteristic sites and are particularly frequent about the foot (Fig. 4.33) and ankle. In general, they are rounded and have well-defined cortical margins. When two bones overlap, for example the arch of C1 and the odontoid peg, or the lower tibia and fibula, on a lateral radiograph, a line of lucency may be seen parallel to the cortex of one of the two bones. This is an optical illusion (the Mach effect) and produces a simulated fracture (Fig. 4.34). With respect to the chest, lines may be produced across the ribs by soft tissues. Occasionally, fractures may be hidden, particularly by immobilization devices; an example is a Thomas' splint used in the case of a suspected fracture of the femoral neck.

Pathological fractures

Pathological fractures occur characteristically in specific sites. The injury force is usually of low magnitude or there may well have been a history of pre-existing pain or the presence of a mass. Frequently the fracture is seen in an area of bone destruction or expansion. Pathological fractures of the appendicular skeleton are usually

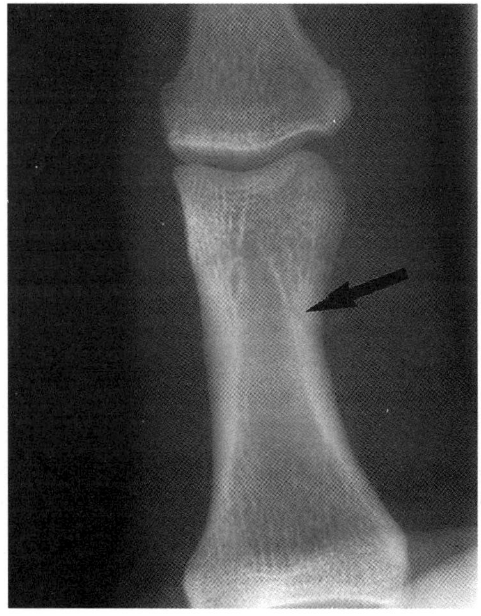

Fig. 4.32 Posteroanterior radiograph of the proximal phalanx of the thumb showing a characteristic vascular foramen (arrowed).

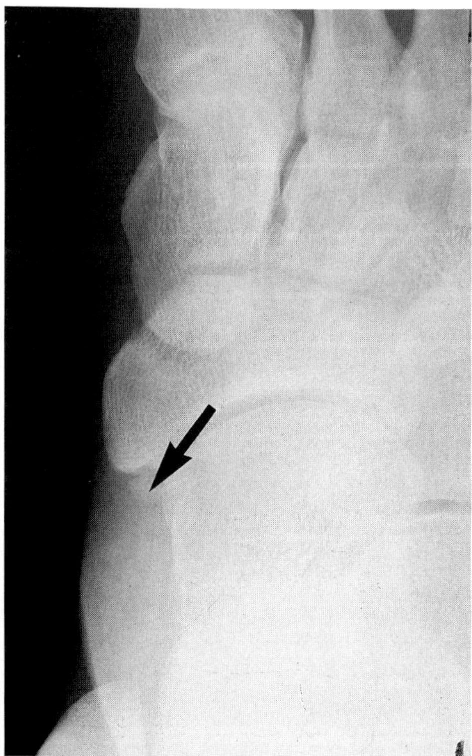

Fig. 4.33 Anteroposterior radiograph of the foot showing os naviculare (arrowed).

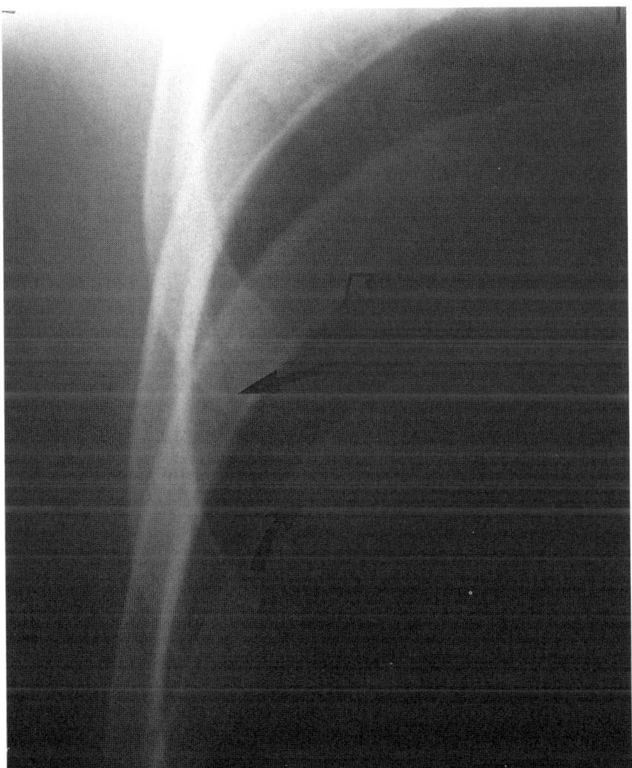

Fig. 4.34 The Mach effect (line arrowed) due to overlap of the lateral border of the scapula (curved arrow) and the posterior aspect of a rib (open arrow).

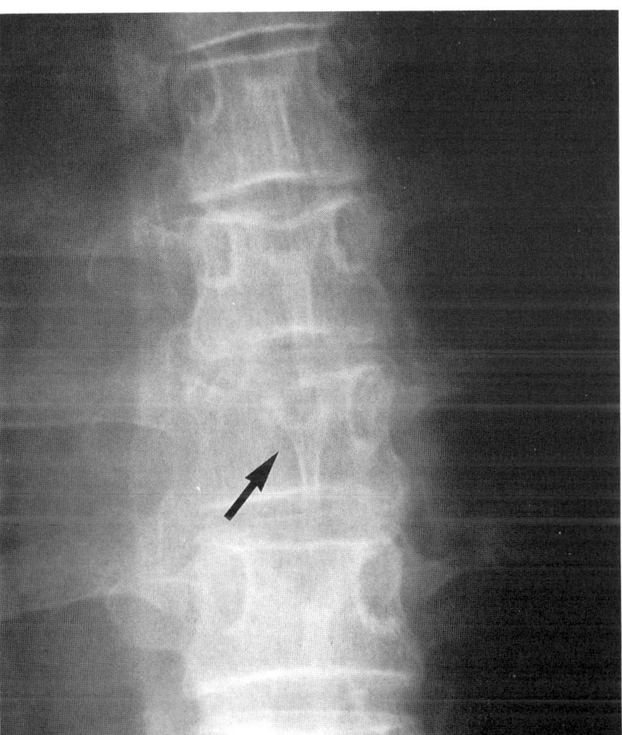

Fig. 4.35 Anteroposterior radiograph of the thoracic spine. The vertebral body (arrowed) only has a right pedicle; the other pedicle has been destroyed.

transverse (uncommon in normal bone). In adults metastases commonly produce extracapsular or sub-trochanteric fractures of the upper femora and less commonly, fractures of the pelvis, humeral neck and tibia. When the spine is involved there is collapse or compression with destruction of the pedicles (Fig. 4.35) Other areas of bone abnormality owing to bone metastases may be identified by plain films or by radio-isotopic study, which is a more sensitive method. Myeloma produces fractures which commonly involve the pelvis or vertebral bodies. Osteomalacia produces fractures which commonly involve the femoral neck. Pathological fractures are uncommon in children and may occur in association with simple bone cysts in the proximal humerus (Fig. 4.36) and femora. Compression fractures of the vertebral bodies are usually associated with leukaemia or histiocytosis. Multiple recurring fractures are seen in osteogenesis imperfecta and non-accidental injury.

Computerized tomography

In skeletal trauma this technique is useful in the assess-ment of complex fractures, particularly if operative

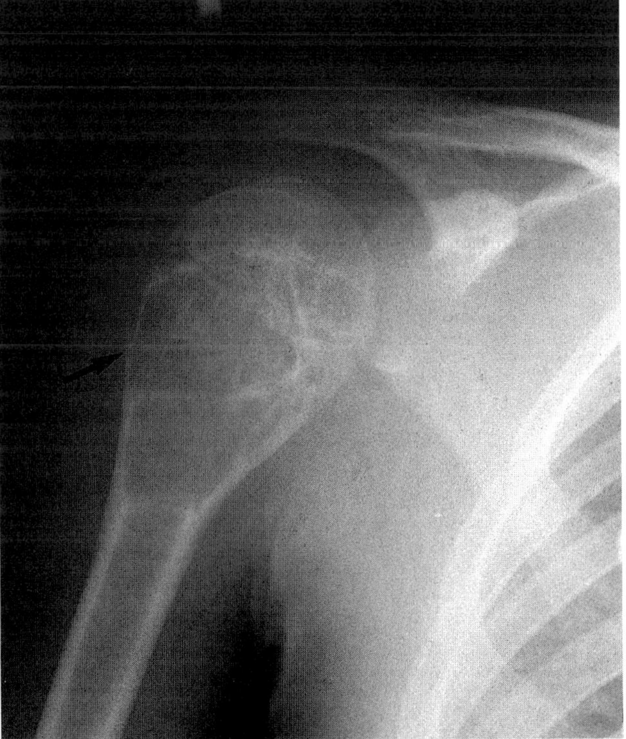

Fig. 4.36 Anteroposterior radiograph of the shoulder. Simple bone cyst in the humeral neck; the fracture can be seen (arrowed).

intervention is considered. It has been used most widely with respect to spinal trauma and here most commonly in the thoracic and lumbar spine. It gives a good assessment of displacement of fragments producing spinal canal narrowing (Fig. 4.37), the degree of which is underestimated by plain film radiography. Fractures involving the neural arch in particular can often be visualized at more than one level when they are not visible on plain films (Lynch *et al.* 1986).

With respect to the pelvis much information can be obtained from plain films (Young *et al.* 1986) but for the hip joint computerized tomography allows an assessment of the position of fragments (Fig. 4.38) and of the direction of fractures, in the transverse plane (Vas *et al.* 1982). Fractures are commonly seen in the sacro-iliac joints; such fractures are not apparent on conventional anteroposterior radiographs (Adam *et al.* 1985). From experimental studies it has been shown that computerized tomography is capable of delineating small (2 mm) loose bodies within the hip joints as accurately as multiplantar tomography (Baird *et al.* 1982).

Plain film tomography has been used to assess the number, size and degree of depression of fragments in fractures of the tibial plateau (Elstrom *et al.* 1976). On plain radiographs the degree of depression is not well seen. This can be overcome to some extent by obtaining anteroposterior radiographs with 15° angulation (Moore & Harvey 1974). Computerized tomography is more accurate (Dias *et al.* 1987b) and has other advantages; in particular, the knee can be examined whilst in plaster.

Computerized tomography has also been used in the assessment of other fractures, including those of the calcaneum (Lowrie *et al.* 1988) and triplane fractures of the lower tibial epiphysis (Cone *et al.* 1984).

Tomography

This is a radiographic technique whereby the structures in a thin horizontal slice of tissue are seen in focus on the radiograph. Shadows above and below are blurred out. The thickness of tissue to be imaged and its plane with respect to the horizontal axis are controlled by pre-set movement of the X-ray source and film. It is used in the diagnosis of fractures of the spine and particularly those of the cervical spine (Maravilla *et al.* 1978). Tomography produced in the lateral plane is often of great value in the diagnosis of odontoid peg fractures.

Isotope bone scanning

The most commonly used radiopharmaceuticals are ^{99m}technetium-labelled compounds, for example meth-

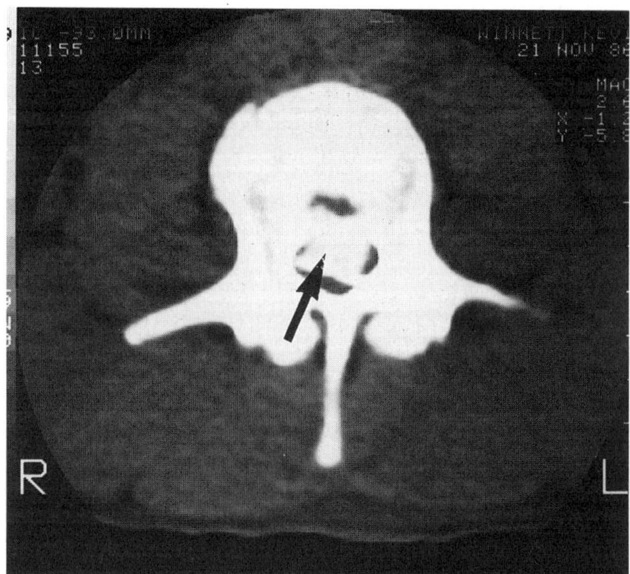

(a)

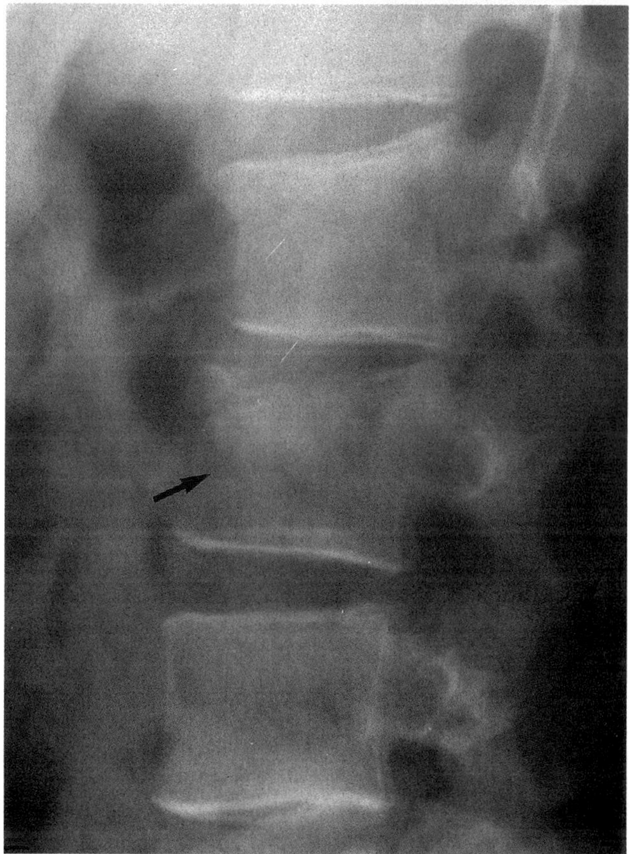

(b)

Fig. 4.37 (a) A transverse computerized tomographic section of a lumbar vertebral body showing almost complete obliteration of the spinal canal by a fragment of bone (arrowed) displaced posteriorly from the body. (b) Lateral radiograph — the corresponding vertebral body is shown (arrowed). There is nothing to suggest the posterior displacement of the large fragment of bone seen in (a).

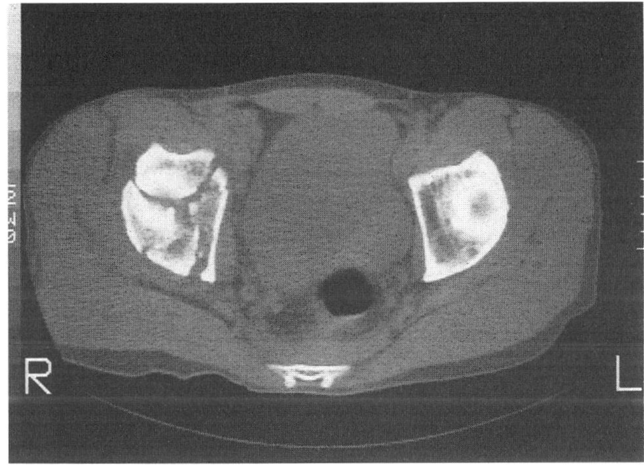

(a)

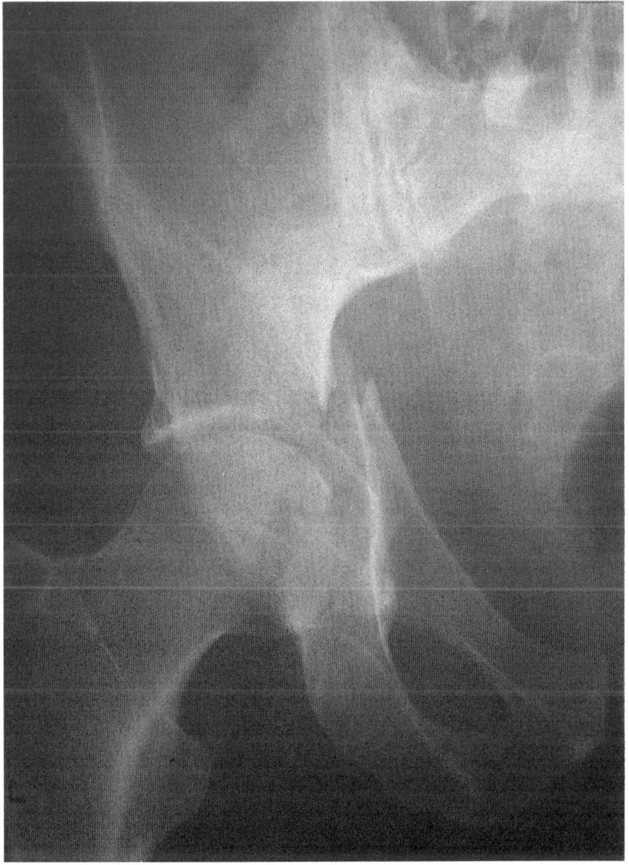

(b)

Fig. 4.38 (a) Computerized tomographic section of the roof of the acetabulum showing displacement of the component parts. (b) Anteroposterior radiograph of the same fracture.

ylene diphosphonate, given by intravenous injection. The patient's skeleton is then imaged by a gamma camera; commonly anterior and posterior views are obtained. The amount of local radioactivity seen on the isotope scan is related to the rate of mineralization of the bone and local blood flow; the predominant finding in pathological processes is increased tracer uptake, so-called 'hot spots'. Occasionally 'cold spots' will be produced when local delivery of the tracer has completely ceased in conditions such as multiple myeloma, aggressive metastatic tumours and absence of blood supply.

In the diagnosis of fractures of the scaphoid, if the examination is performed more than 72 hours after injury, increased activity over the scaphoid (Fig. 4.39) gives a high likelihood that a fracture is present (Rolfe *et al.* 1981). Isotopic examination has also been used to identify fractures in the sacrum, coccyx, ribs, hip (Fairclough *et al.* 1987) and knee and foot (Maurice *et al.* 1987), where fractures are not visible with plain film radiography (Batillas *et al.* 1981). These examinations are highly sensitive but lack specificity. Other conditions, such as a tumour or osteomyelitis, similarly cause increased uptake of radiopharmaceuticals (Kirchner & Simon 1981). Increased uptake also occurs in the articular regions as a result of traumatic synovitis or ligamentous injuries (Rosenthal *et al.* 1976). The increased uptake associated with fractures may still be present in 10% of cases after 2 years (Matin 1979).

Radioisotopic bone scanning has been widely used in the diagnosis of stress fractures, increased uptake being present 2–3 weeks before radiological abnormality is detectable (Geslien *et al.* 1976).

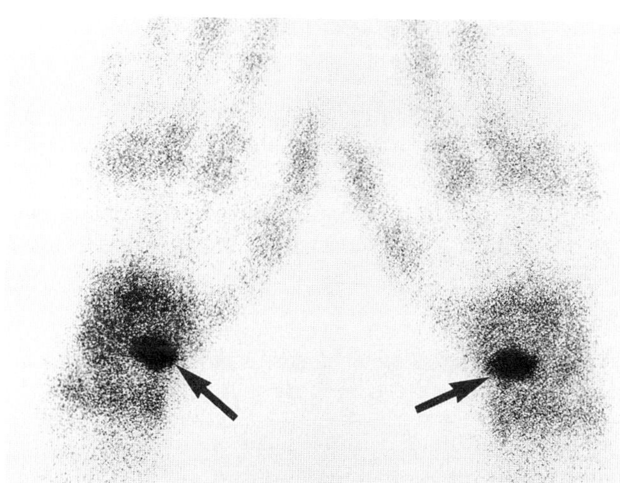

Fig. 4.39 Scaphoid fractures. Images obtained during a bone scan; there is increased uptake (arrowed) related to both scaphoids. There was no abnormality on the radiograph taken at the same time.

Stress views

Stress views are occasionally used and are of particular use with respect to the knee, fingers and thumb. In the knee, for instance, the medial collateral ligament may be injured by a valgus stress, sometimes in association with the anterior cruciate ligament. A stress radiograph obtained in the immediate period after injury will demonstrate opening up of the medial joint space on valgus stressing. Later (after 2 hours), muscle spasm may negate the examination which is better performed under general anaesthetic. In the thumb there may be damage to the ulnar collateral ligament of the metacarpophalangeal joint with or without an avulsion fracture, the so-called gamekeeper's thumb. (Campbell 1955). A valgus stress demonstrates widening of the ulnar margin of the joint and radial subluxation of the proximal phalanx. Stress views may also be used in assessment of the interphalangeal joints of the hand.

Attempts have been made to assess the ligaments of the ankle joint after injury by inversion stress and anterior draw. The results are affected by muscle spasm and have been performed under different conditions, reported in the different series. They are probably only of limited value except when performed under conditions of complete muscle relaxation by general anaesthesia (Staples 1975).

Tenography

This has been used in the assessment of acute rupture of the calcaneo-fibular component of the lateral ligament of the ankle (Blanshard *et al*. 1986). In this technique a needle is introduced directly percutaneously into the tendon sheath immediately behind the ankle and contrast is introduced under image intensification screening. In the acute case examination is performed after peroneal and short saphenous nerve block. When the calcaneofibular ligament is ruptured, contrast passes from the common peroneal tendon sheath into the ankle joint (Fig. 4.40).

Arthrography

This technique, which involves obtaining radiographs after the injection of contrast and air into the joint, gives information about the internal surfaces of the joint. Most of this work is now being taken over by MRI. Where arthrography is available, however, it still of use in the ankle after trauma to the lateral ligament.

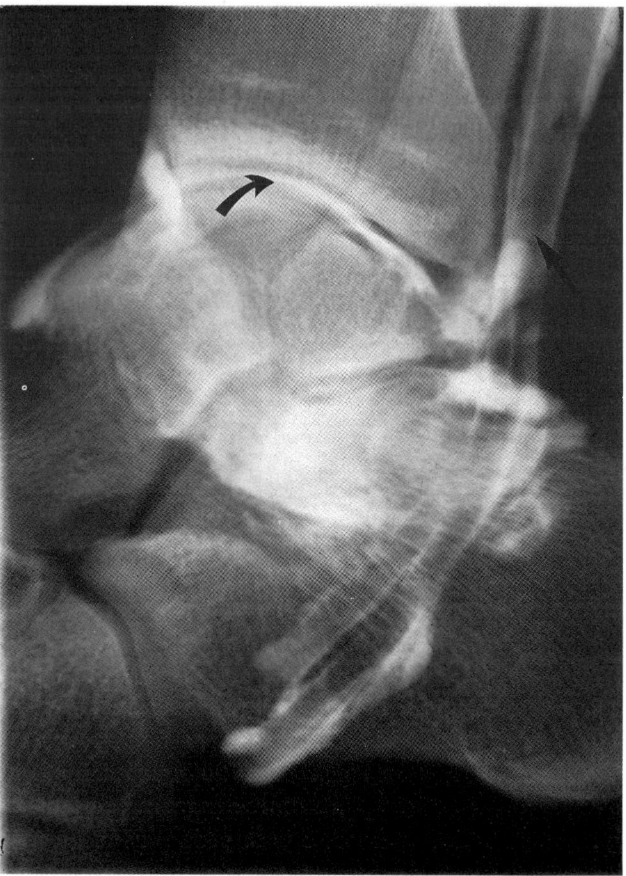

Fig. 4.40 Lateral radiograph obtained after contrast had been introduced into the peroneal tendon sheath (arrowed). Contrast is seen in the ankle joint (curved arrow) signifying communication with the peroneal tendon sheath.

Angiography

Angiography is most commonly used for the assessment of the femoral and popliteal arteries in the presence of a fracture of the lower femoral shaft, dislocations of the knee or displaced fractures around the knee joint. The angiogram can be performed by percutaneous needling or by direct puncture in the operating theatre at the time of exploration. The artery is usually injured at the fracture line and may suffer a complete transection, an intimal tear, thrombosis or compression. Angiography is also used in the assessment of the femoral artery in the adductor canal, of the brachial artery around the elbow and of the subclavian artery in relation to the distal third of the clavicle. It is also used in the assessment of post-fracture bleeding from vessels in the pelvis and their treatment by transcatheter embolization (Ring *et al*. 1974).

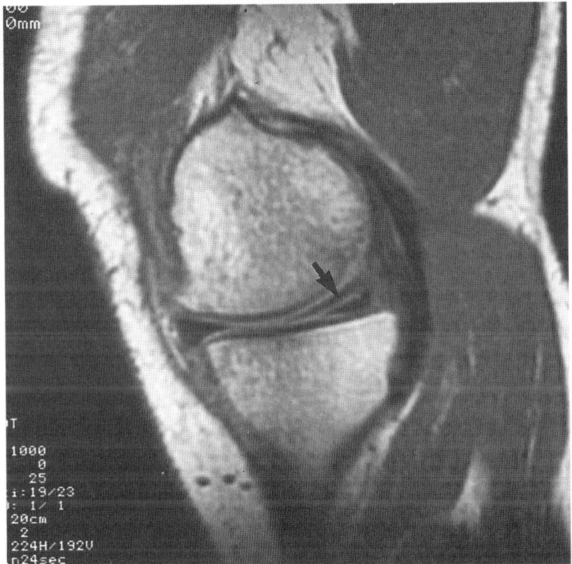

Fig. 4.41 T1 weighted sagittal oblique image of the knee showing an oblique tear (arrowed) of the posterior horn of the medial meniscus.

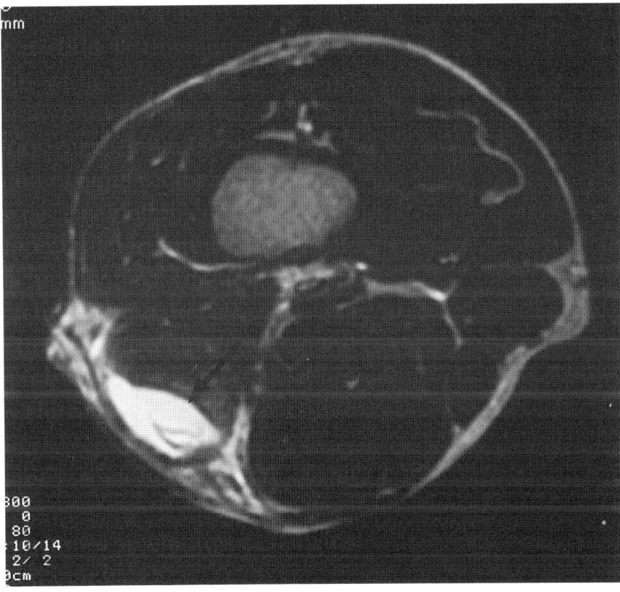

Fig. 4.43 T2 weighted axial image above the knee. Area of well-defined high signal intensity within the biceps femor is arrowed. Haemorrhage due to acute muscle tear.

Magnetic resonance imaging

Where it is available, MRI is now the major investigative technique for the knee, shoulder joint and soft tissues. MRI is highly sensitive to meniscal tears (Fig. 4.41) in the knee, a normal MRI virtually excluding a tear. Unlike arthrography, MRI is also accurate at assessing the anterior (Fig. 4.42) and posterior cruciate ligaments (Spiers *et al.* 1993). In the shoulder, MRI should replace arthrography and computed arthrotomography. MRI is accurate in the diagnosis of both rotator cuff tears and the evaluation of the glenoid labrum. In addition, it is able to diagnose and grade the impingement syndrome (Habibian *et al.* 1989). Injury to the musculotendinous unit can readily be imaged by MRI; typical abnormalities have been shown on MRI in first, second and third degree complete rupture of the musculotendinous unit (Mink & Rosenfeld 1991). In the complete rupture group the damage may lie either in a deep muscles (Fig. 4.43) or in a tendon, most commonly the Achilles (Fig. 4.44). It is quite common for MRI to pick up stress fractures in the tibial condyles (Fig. 4.45) in a patient who has been

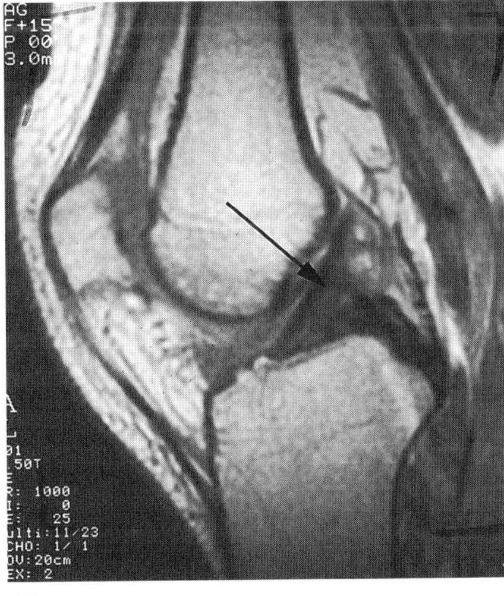

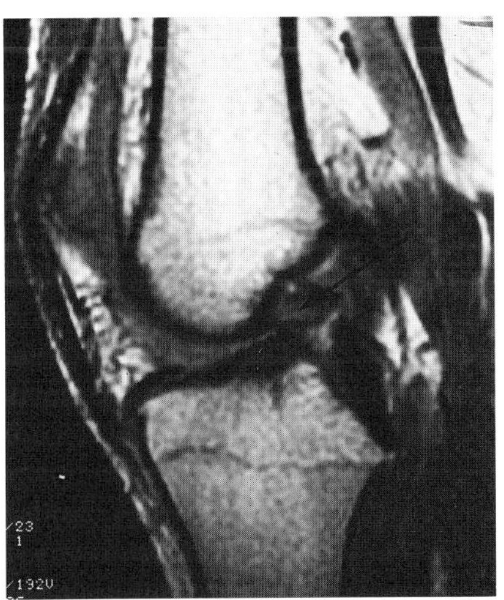

Fig. 4.42 (a) T1 weighted sagittal oblique image of the knee — an intact anterior cruciate ligament (arrowed). (b) T1 weighted sagittal oblique image — a ruptured anterior cruciate (arrowed). The cruciate is no longer straight, is lying in abnormal position and is incomplete superiorly. It has ruptured at its upper end.

(a)

(b)

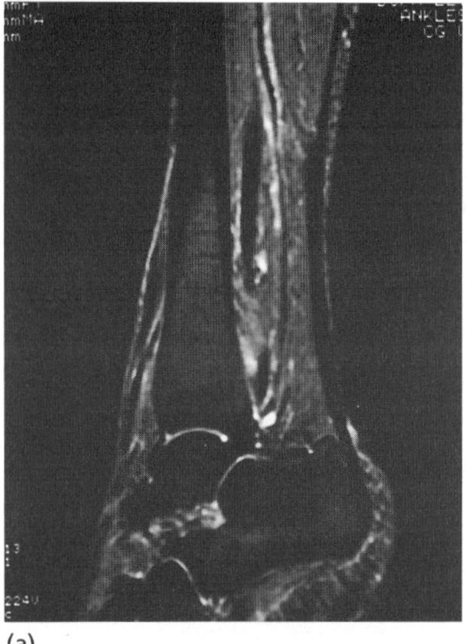

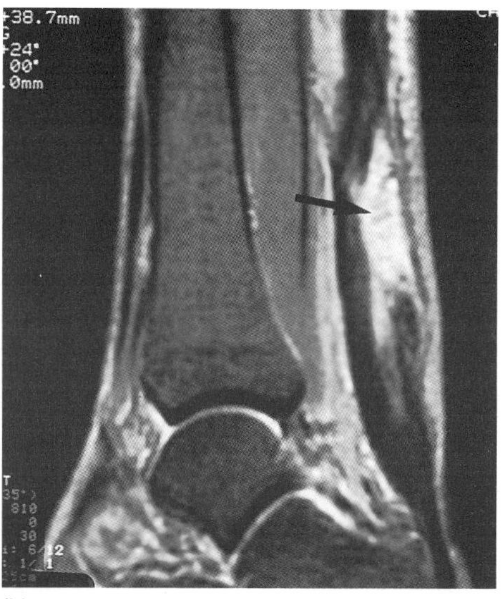

(a)   (b)

Fig. 4.44 (a) T2 weighted sagittal image — normal Achilles tendon. (b) T2 weighted sagittal image — ruptured Achilles tendon. Haemorrhage is seen (arrowed).

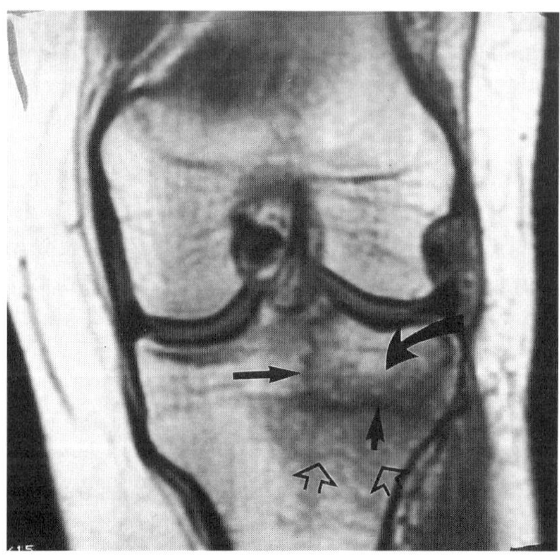

Fig. 4.45 T1 weighted coronal image of the knee showing a fracture of the lateral tibial plateau. Continuous black line (arrowed) is seen around the depressed fragment (curved arrow) and loss of fat signal in adjacent bone (open arrows).

investigated for the clinical diagnosis of a meniscal tear. MRI is of particular value in the investigation of trauma to the cervical spine when no bony injury is visible. Most spinal cord injuries are due to intrinsic lesions, oedema, haemorrhage (Mascalchi 1993), transection as opposed to extrinsic bone fracture, disc or haematoma. MRI does, however, allow assessment of the discs and bony tissues. MRI, where available, has completely replaced the use of myelography in spinal cord assessment.

References

Adam, P., Labbe, J.L., Alberge, Y., Austry, P., Delcroix, P. & Ficat, R.P. The role of computed tomography in the assessment and treatment of acetabular fractures. *Clin Radiol* 1985; **36**: 13−18.

Annis, J.A.D., Finlay, D.B.L., Allen, M.J. & Barnes, M.R. Review of cervical spine radiographs in Casualty patients. *Br J Radiol* 1987; **60**: 1059−1061.

Apple, J.S., Martinez, S., Allen, N.B., Caldwell, D.S. & Rice, J.R. Occult fractures of the knee. Tomographic evaluation. *Radiology* 1983; **148**: 383−387.

Arndt, J.H. & Sears, A.D. Posterior dislocation of the shoulder. *J Bone Joint Surg* 1965; **94A**: 639−645.

Baird, R.A., Schobert, W.E., Pais, M.J., Ahmed, M., Wilson, W.J., Farjalla, G.L. & Imray, T.J. Radiographic identification of loose bodies in the traumatised hip joint. *Radiology* 1982; **145**: 661−665.

Batillas, J., Vasilas, A., Pizzi, W.F. & Gokcebay, T. Bone scanning in the detection of occult fractures. *J Trauma* 1981; **21**: 564−569.

Blanshard, K.S., Finlay, D.B.L., Scott, D.J.A., Ley, C.C., Siggins, D. & Allen, M.J. A radiological analysis of lateral ligament injuries of the ankle. *Clin Radiol* 1986; **37**: 247−251.

Brand, D.A., Frazier, W.H., Kohlhepp, W.C., Shea, K.M., Hoefer, A.M., Ecker, M.D., Kornguth, P.J., Pais, M.J. & Light, T.R. A protocol for selecting patients with injured extremeties who need X-rays. *N Eng J Med* 1982; **306**: 333−339.

Campbell, C.S. Gamekeeper's thumb. *J Bone Joint Surg* 1955; **37B**: 148−149.

Cisternino, S.J., Rogers, L.F., Stufflebam, B.C. & Kruglik, G.D. The trough line; a radiographic sign of posterior shoulder dislocation. *Am J Roentgenol* 1978; **130**: 951−954.

Cone, R.O., Nguyen, V., Flournoy, J.G. & Guerra, J. Tri-plane fracture of the distal tibial epiphysis; radiographic and CT studies. *Radiology* 1984; **153**: 763−767.

De Lacey, G. & Bradbrooke, S. Rationalizing requests for X-ray examination of acute ankle injuries. *Br Med J* 1979; **1**: 1597−1598.

Dias, J.J., Finlay, D.B.L., Brenkel, I.J. & Gregg, P.J. Radiographic assessment of soft tissue signs in clinically suspected scaphoid fractures: the incidence of false negative and false positive results. *J Orthop Trauma* 1987a; **3**: 205−208.

Dias, J.J., Sterling, A.J., Finlay, D.B.L. & Gregg, P.J. Computerised axial tomography for tibial plataeu fractures. *J Bone Joint Surg* 1987b; **69B**: 84−88.

Dias J.J., Taylor, M., Thompson, J., Brenkel, I.J. & Gregg, P.J. Radiographic signs of union of scaphoid fractures. *J Bone Joint Surg* 1988; **70B**: 299−301.

Dunbar, J.S., Owen, H.F., Nogrady, M.B. & McLeese, R. Obscure tibial fractures of infants − the toddler's fracture. *J Assoc Can Radiol* 1964; **15**: 136−144.

Elstrom, J., Pankovich, A.M., Sassoon, H. & Rodriguez, J. The use of tomography in the assessment of fractures of the tibial plateau. *J Bone Joint Surg* 1976; **58A**: 551−555.

Fairclough, J., Colhoun, E., Johnston, D. & Williams, L.A. Bone scanning for suspected hip fractures. A prospective study in elderly patients. *J Bone Joint Surg* 1987; **69B**: 251−253.

Gerlock, A.J., Kirchner, S.G., Heller, R.M. & Kaye, J.J. *The Cervical Spine in Trauma*. WB Saunders: Philadelphia, 1978.

Geslien, G.E., Thrall, H., Espinosa, J.L. & Older, R.A. Early detection of stress fractures using ⁹⁹ᵐTc-polyphosphate. *Radiology* 1976; **121**: 683−687.

Gilula, L.A. Carpal injuries; analytic approach and case exercises. *Am J Roentgenol* 1979; **133**: 503−517.

Goergen, T.G., Danzig, L.A., Resnick, D. & Owen, C.A. Roentgenographic evaluation of the tibiotalar joint. *J Bone Joint Surg* 1977; **59A**: 874−877.

Habibian, A., Stauffer, A., Resnick, D., Reicher, M.A., Rafii, M., Kellerhouse, L., Zlatkin, M.B., Newman, C., Sartoris, D. Comparison of conventional and computed arthrotomography with MR imaging in the evaluation of the shoulder. *J Comput Assist Tomogr* 1989; **13**: 965−975.

Judet, R., Judet, J. & Le Tournel, E. Fractures of the acetabulum; classification and surgical approaches for open reduction. *J Bone Joint Surg* 1964; **46A**: 1615−1675

Keats, T.E. *Atlas of Normal Roentgen Variance*. Year Book Medical Publishers: Chicago, 1984.

Kirchner, P.T. & Simon, M.A. Current concepts review − radioisotopic evaluation of skeletal disease. *J Bone Joint Surg* 1981; **63A**: 673−681.

Lauge-Hansen, N. Fractures of the ankle. III. Genetic roentgenologic diagnosis of fractures of the ankle. *Am J Roentgenol* 1954; **71**: 456−471.

Lee, J.H., Weissman, B.N., Nickpoor, N., Aliabadi, P. & Sosman, L. Lipohemarthosis of the knee: A review of recent experiences. *Radiology* 1989; **173**: 189−191.

Leslie, I.J. & Dickson, R.A. The fractured carpal scaphoid. Natural history and factors influencing outcome. *J Bone Joint Surg* 1981; **63B**: 225−230.

Lowrie, I.G., Finlay, D.B.L., Brenkel, I.J. & Gregg, P.J. Assessment of the subtalar joint in calcaneal fractures. *J Bone Joint Surg* 1988; **70B**: 247−250.

Lynch, D., McManus, F. & Ennis, J.T. Computed tomography in spinal trauma. *Clin Radiol* 1986; **37**: 71−76.

MacAusland, W.R. Peri-lunar dislocation of the carpal bones and dislocation of the lunate bone. *Surg Gynecol Obstet* 1944: **79**: 256−266.

MacEwan, D.W. Changes due to trauma in the fat plane overlying the pronator quadratus muscle − a radiological sign. *Radiology* 1964; **82**: 879−886.

Maravilla, K.R., Cooper, R. & Sklar, F.H. The influence of thin section tomography on the treatment of cervical spine injuries. *Radiology* 1978; **127**: 131−139.

Mascalchi, M., Dal Pozzo, G., Dini, C., Zampa, V., D'Andrea, M., Mizzau, M., Lolli, F., Caramella, D. & Bartolozzi, C. Acute spinal trauma: prognostic value of MRI appearances at 0.5 T. *Clin Radiol* 1993; **48**: 100−108.

Maskell, T.W. & Finlay, D.B.L. The prognostic significance of radiologically detected knee joint affusions in the absence of associated fracture. *Br J Radiol* 1990; **63**: 940−941.

Maurice, H.D., Newman, J.H. & Watt, I. Bone scanning of the foot for unexplained pain. *J Bone Joint Surg* 1987; **69B**: 448−452.

Matin, P. The appearance of bone scans following fractures, including immediate and longterm studies. *J Nucl Med* 1979; **20**: 1227−1231.

McDade, W.C. *Treatment of Ankle Fractures. AAOS Instructional Course Lectures*. CV Mosby: St Louis, 1976.

Miles, K.A. & Finlay, D.B.L. Is pre-vertebral soft tissue swelling a useful sign in injury of the cervical spine. *Injury* 1988; **19**: 177−179.

Mink, J.H. & Rosenfeld, R.T. MR views sports − related bony, muscular injuries. *Diagnostic Imaging* 1991; **13**: 108−114.

Moore, T.M. & Harvey, P. Roentgenographic measurement of tibial-plateau depression due to fracture. *J Bone Joint Surg* 1974; **56A**: 155−160.

Murphy, W.A. & Siegel, M.J. Elbow fat pads with new signs and extended differential diagnosis. *Radiology* 1977; **124**: 659−665.

Naidich, J.B., Naidich, T.P., Garfein, C., Libeskind, A.L. & Hyman, R.A. The widened interspinous distance; a useful sign of anterior cervical dislocation in the supine frontal projection. *Radiology*, 1977; **123**: 113−116.

Newberg, A.H. & Greenstein, R. Radiographic evaluation of tibial plateau fractures. *Radiology* 1978; **126**: 319−323.

Norell, H. Roentgenologic visualisation of extracapsular fat. Its importance in the diagnosis of traumatic injuries of the elbow. *Acta Radiol* 1954; **42**: 205−208.

O'Dwyer, F.G., Harper, W.M., Finlay, D.B.L. Do elderly patients with hip pain following trauma require hospital admission? *Injury* 1992; **23**: 295−296.

Quinton, D.N., Finlay, D.B.L. & Butterworth, R. The elbow fat pad sign. Its clinical and radiological relevance in the diagnosis of an elbow fracture. *J Bone Joint Surg* 1987; **69B**: 844−845.

Rickett, A.D., Finlay, D.B.L. & Jaggar, C. The importance of clinical details when reporting accident and emergency radiographs. *Injury* 1992; **23**: 458−460.

Ring, E.J., Waltman, A.C., Athanasoulis, C., Smith, J.C. & Baum, S. Angiography in pelvic trauma. *Surg Gynecol Obstet* 1974; **139**: 375−380.

Rogers, L.F., Malave, S., White, H. & Tachdjian, M.O. Plastic bowing, torus and greenstick supracondylar fractures of the humerus; radiographic clues to obscure fractures of the elbow in children. *Radiology* 1978; **128**: 145−150.

Rolfe, E.B., Garvaie, N.W., Khan, M.A. & Ackery, D.M. Isotope bone imaging in suspected scaphoid trauma. *Br J Radiol* 1981; **54**: 726−767.

Rosenthal, L., Hill, R.O. & Chuang, S. Observation on the use of ^{99m}Tc-phosphate imaging in peripheral bone trauma. *Radiology* 1976; **119**: 637–641.

RCR Working Party. *Making the Best Use of a Department of Clinical Radiology.* Royal College of Radiologists: London, 1993.

Russe, O. Fracture of the carpal navicular. *J Bone Joint Surg* 1960; **42A**: 759–768.

Spiers, A.S.D., Meagher, T., Ostlere, S.J., Wilson, D.J. & Dodd, C.A.F. Can MRI of the knee affect arthroscopic practice? *J Bone Joint Surg* 1993; **75b**: 49–52.

Staples, O.S. Ruptures of the fibular collateral ligament of the ankle. *J Bone Joint Surg* 1975; **57A**: 101–107.

Storen, G. Traumatic dislocation of the radial head as an isolated lesion in children. *Acta Chir Scan* 1958–1959; **116**: 144–147.

Vas, W.G., Wolverson, M.K., Sundaram, M., Heiberg, E., Pilla, T., Shields, J.B. & Crepps, L. The role of computed tomography in pelvic fractures. *J Comput Assis Tomogr* 1982; **6**: 796–801.

Wallace, W.A. & Hellier, M.H. Improving radiographs of the injured shoulder. *Radiography* 1983; **49**: 229–232.

Young, J.W.R., Burgess, A.R., Brumback, R.J. & Poka, A. Pelvic fractures; value of plain film radiography in early assessment and management. *Radiology* 1986; **160**: 445–451.

Ziter, F.M.H. A modified view of the carpal navicular. *Radiology* 1973; **108**: 706–707.

5: The Healing of Injury

Basics of fracture healing

A.J.MALCOLM

The healing in bones is very similar to the healing in soft tissues. However, primary union of a fracture is exceptional and healing by the proliferation of callus (which is similar to wound healing by second intention) is the rule. Initially there is haemorrhage between the fractured bone ends with the haemorrhage extending into periosteum and soft tissue. This causes a moderate acute inflammatory response. This inflammatory process is followed by a proliferative or reparative phase in which mesenchymal cells, particularly osteogenic cells, play a major role. Continuity between the fractured bone fragments is first established by granulation tissue followed by a mass of new bony trabeculae with some cartilaginous tissue. This mass is called a provisional callus. This callus undergoes slow remodelling with resorption and replacement. In favourable conditions a firm bony union is achieved. Sometimes the uniting and remodelling of a fracture is so good that years later a fracture site cannot be identified. Fracture healing is a continuous process and most of the knowledge of fracture repair is based on animal models although there are some human studies (McKibben 1978, Frost 1989).

Prior to 1965 most authorities considered that osteoblasts were the most important prime movers in the healing of a fracture. It is now known that bone healing requires far more than the stimulation or recruitment of osteoblasts (Brand & Rubin 1987). The healing of bone involves highly specialized physical and biochemical signals being given to cells in the tissues within and around the fracture area. The local and systemic agents that start and ultimately control bone healing do so by acting on the surrounding mesenchymal cells rather than on existing osteoblasts (Urist *et al*. 1983). The formation of granulation tissue, and ultimately callus, requires the activation of local precursor cells and control of the differentiation and function of those cells. Similarly, the remodelling of the fracture callus will depend on recruitment and control of osteoclasts. The exact nature of this local control is poorly understood but the control mechanisms not only control differentiation of cells and their organization within the callus, but also affect the activities of those cells and the amount of matrix those cells will produce. Published histomorphometric data show that if pre-existing osteoblasts only were available to heal a femoral shaft fracture the osteoblasts would require 200–1000 years to make enough callus to allow healing (Frost 1989a). In addition it is known that the osteoblast has a limited life-span which is often less than the length of time the callus is present. Clearly very many new osteoblasts must be recruited both initially and continually during the healing process.

There are very many labile local growth factors and differentiating agents known and it is clear that many of these play a part in the fracture healing process. The epidermal growth factors, various angiogenic growth factors, platelet-derived growth factor, prostaglandins PGE I and II and bone morphogenic protein may all play a part in the stimulation of mesenchymal cells to proliferate in the region of the fracture (Triffit 1987). Tumour necrosis factors and osteoclast-activating factors may play a role in stimulating osteoclasts to remove necrotic bone. In addition to the local factors it is known that growth hormone, thyroid hormone, calcitonin, insulin, vitamins A and D and anabolic steroids may also play a role in fracture healing. Innervation of the region of the fracture must play some role in fracture healing in that patients with denervation show slower fracture healing (Bubenik *et al*. 1981). Fracture healing has been shown to be enhanced in animals and perhaps humans by the application of electrical stimulation (Becker 1978, Lavine & Grodzinski 1987).

There follows a discussion of the stages and phases of

fracture healing but it should be stressed that the events described in one phase often persist into the next phase and that the healing process forms a continuum. This is illustrated in Fig. 5.1(a−e). It is important to note that changes described in the periosteum, the medullary canal and the cortex are taking place simultaneously.

Early stages of fracture healing

Inflammatory phase (0−5 days)

A significant degree of force is normally required to break a bone. The fragments of the fractured bone are often displaced and there is a degree of haemorrhage between the bone ends. In addition, much blood may seep into the tissues from ruptured vessels of the torn periosteum and damaged adjacent soft tissue. This leaked blood rapidly coagulates to form a clot both between the fractured bone ends and in the soft tissues surrounding the fracture. A fibrin network forms within this blood clot. The net result is that the tissues at the fracture site, including the cortex, have their blood supply disrupted which causes further necrosis. The earliest histological change is necrosis of the haemopoietic or fatty marrow cells. The fat released from dead

cells is taken up by macrophages and in addition pools of fat may form which are surrounded by foreign body giant cells (Fig. 5.2). These fat spaces are sometimes referred to as 'fat cysts'. Because of the vascular arrangements within the cortex the cortical bone suffers more extensive necrosis following fracture than does the medullary bone. The exact amount of necrosis depends on the local blood supply to the fractured area. The cortex may undergo necrosis up to 1 cm either side of the fracture and the dead bone is removed by osteoclasis. This is sometimes referred to as 'dying back' of the cortex (Fig. 5.3).

As a result of the necrosis and haemorrhage there is an immediate and intense acute inflammatory response. There is widespread vasodilatation with exudation of plasma resulting in oedema. Acute inflammatory cells, including polymorphonuclear leukocytes, migrate into the margins of the fracture site both within the periosteal area and within the medullary canal. This is soon followed by a migration of macrophages. The polymorphs and macrophages phagocytose the clot and tissue debris. Ingrowth of new blood vessels and fibroblasts enhance the healing process by allowing macrophages access to the necrotic tissue (Fig. 5.4). The larger the mass of clot and tissue between the fractured bone

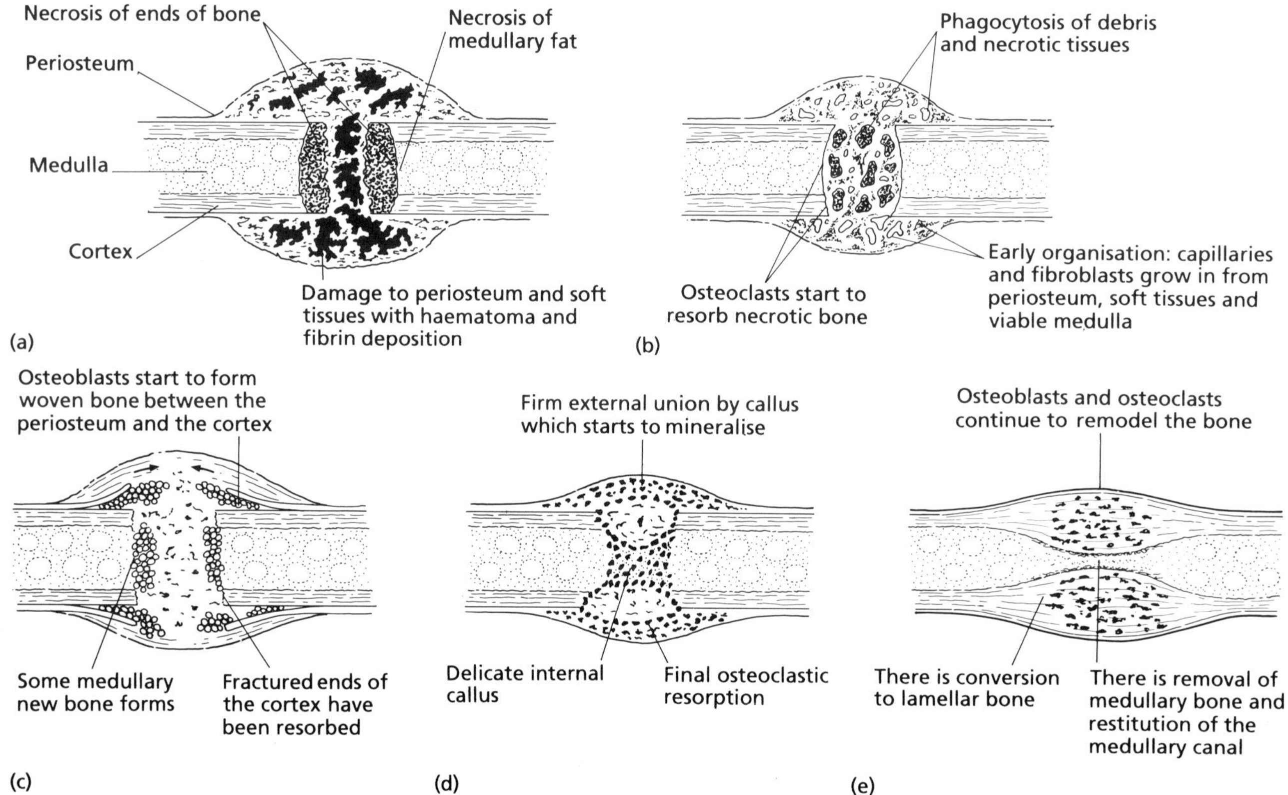

Fig. 5.1 (a−e) A diagrammatic representation of the sequence of events in fracture healing.

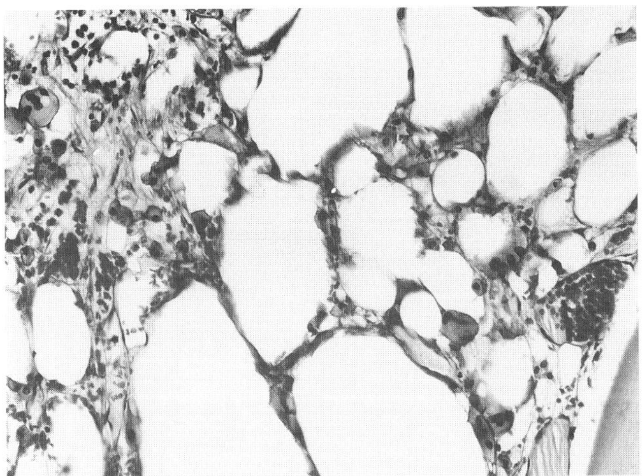

Fig. 5.2 New blood vessels with macrophages and 'fat cysts'. Haematoxylin—eosin ×280.

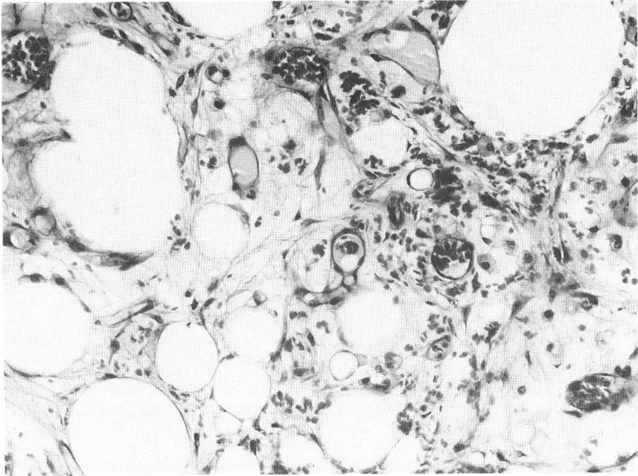

Fig. 5.4 New blood vessels and fibroblasts together with occasional foamy macrophages growing into necrotic fatty marrow. Haematoxylin—eosin ×280.

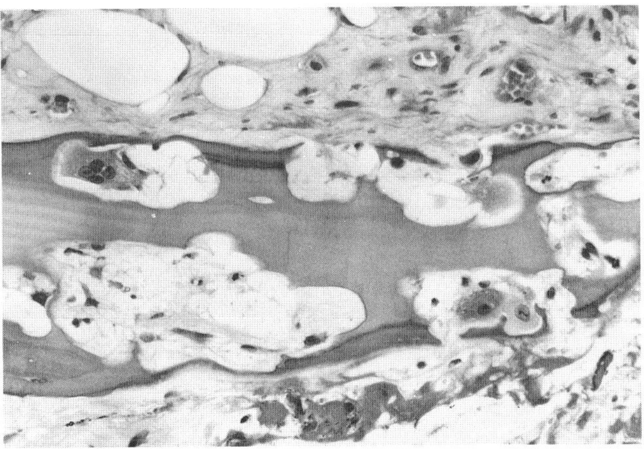

Fig. 5.3 Osteoclastic resorption of dead bone with some adjacent granulation tissue. Haematoxylin—eosin ×470.

ends the longer it may take for the fracture to heal as a result of delay in the removal of necrotic tissue and the delay in ingrowth of granulation tissue.

Reparative phase (5—42 days)

The first step in the reparative phase is the ingrowth of granulation tissue and the organization of the haematoma. The microenvironment about the fracture is acid which may well provide an additional stimulus to local cell behaviour. During the repair process it has been noted that the pH gradually returns to neutral and may even become slightly alkaline (Stirling 1931). Electronegativity is found in the region of a fresh fracture. This electronegativity slowly diminishes until the fracture is united (Friedenberg & Brighton 1966). It has been pos-

tulated that this electrical signal may be one of the stimuli to early osteogenesis and repair.

The periosteal reaction

The cells of the inner layer of the periosteum (the cambium layer) adjacent to the fracture site proliferate in a fairly wide zone overlying the cortex of each fractured bone end. The earliest reaction is the result of proliferation of cells derived from the cambium layer of the periosteum (Tonna & Cronkite 1963) but the majority of cells involved in fracture healing migrate into the fracture site in association with the ingrowth of granulation tissue. It seems likely that the granulation tissue is derived mainly from the periosteal blood supply, the blood supply of the surrounding soft tissues and, to a lesser extent, the medullary canal. There is some evidence to suggest that the periosteum under normal circumstances is the most important but not exclusive source of granulation tissue and osteogenic cells (Rhinelander & Wilson 1982).

The periosteal reaction forms an external provisional callus by proliferation of mesenchymal cells. A cuff of non-calcified tissue is formed around both fractured ends. This consists of fibrous tissue and woven bone trabeculae which are anchored to the cortex with the trabeculae arranged at right angles to the surface (Fig. 5.5). Further woven bone trabeculae form an irregular meshwork and eventually the two cuffs of callus unite so that they form a bridge across the fracture. This mass of tissue helps to immobilize the fractured bone fragments. Admixed with the woven bone being formed there is a variable amount of cartilage. This

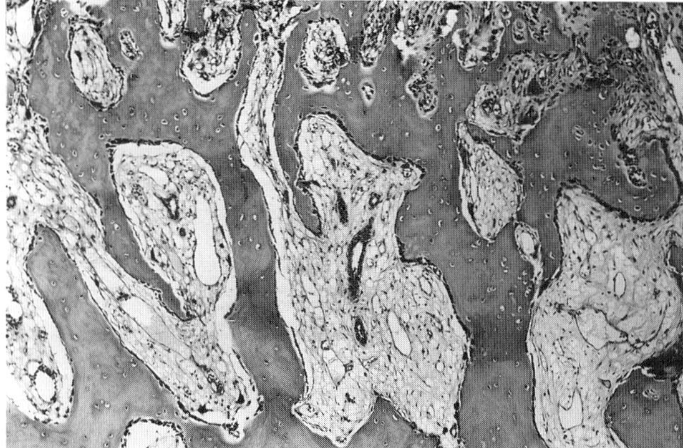

Fig. 5.5 Arcades of reactive subperiosteal new bone. Haematoxylin–eosin ×90.

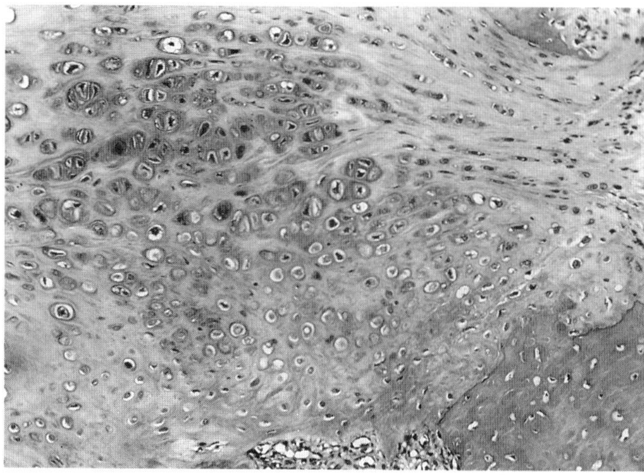

Fig. 5.6 The fracture gap is on the right with reactive new bone in the subperiosteum below. At the fracture gap there is proliferating cartilage. Haematoxylin–eosin ×140.

cartilage is most prominent in the thickest part of the callus and this is usually at the actual line of the fracture (Fig. 5.6).

The amount of cartilage which is formed in a provisional callus varies from species to species. Small mammals such as mice and rats form a predominantly cartilaginous callus while in man the amount, though variable, is much less. The formation of a cartilaginous callus rather than an osseous callus is thought to be the result of either a poor blood supply (Basset 1962) or excess shearing strains and stresses (Albright & Brand 1987) or a combination of both. Any cartilaginous component is eventually replaced by bone as the result of endochrondal ossification. This occurs in a similar fashion to that seen in the epiphyseal cartilage plate except it is less organized.

The two enlarging cuffs of external callus advance towards each other until they unite to bridge the fracture line. This external callus helps to immobilize the bone ends. The amount of bridging external periosteal callus varies depending on the anatomical site of the fracture and on the circumstances in which healing is taking place. The intracapsular part of a bone lacks a periosteal covering and it tends to be separated from surrounding soft tissues and so a fracture at this site often results in poor formation of external callus, the union relying mainly on a medullary reaction. Conversely, poor apposition of the fracture or increased movement at the fracture site are both liable to produce abundant external callus. Good apposition and fixation usually results in union with only a small amount of external callus formation. Indeed bony union with minimal external callus has been reported following compression arthrodesis. This latter situation has been referred to as 'primary union'.

Medullary reaction

At the same time as the periosteal reaction is forming an external callus there is a vigorous response to the fracture within the medullary canal. Granulation tissue with macrophages extends from the viable marrow into the necrotic area. The macrophages phagocytose dead cells and osteoclasts are recruited to resorb the dead bone trabeculae. In addition, osteoclasts start to remove the necrotic endosteal and cortical bone. An 'internal' callus is produced when osteoblasts form new woven bone within the medullary canal at the fracture site. In addition, osteoblasts may form new bone on the surface of some of the dead trabeculae (appositional new bone) (Fig. 5.7). This latter feature may persist for months or even years until this bone is eventually remodelled. Cartilage is very rarely formed within the medullary canal but this may simply reflect the good blood supply within the medullary canal and the relative protection from stress at this site. However, when the external fracture callus reaches the fracture gap a small amount of cartilage may form within the medullary canal.

Cortical reaction

There is striking osteoclastic resorption of the cortical bone at the fracture site with widening of the Haversian canals. This may be seen in the dead cortical bone adjacent to the fracture site and as a result it may cause an initial widening of the fracture gap which may be seen on a radiograph. There may be some resorption of adjacent viable cortical bone causing rarefaction on the radiograph but this is probably related to disuse atrophy

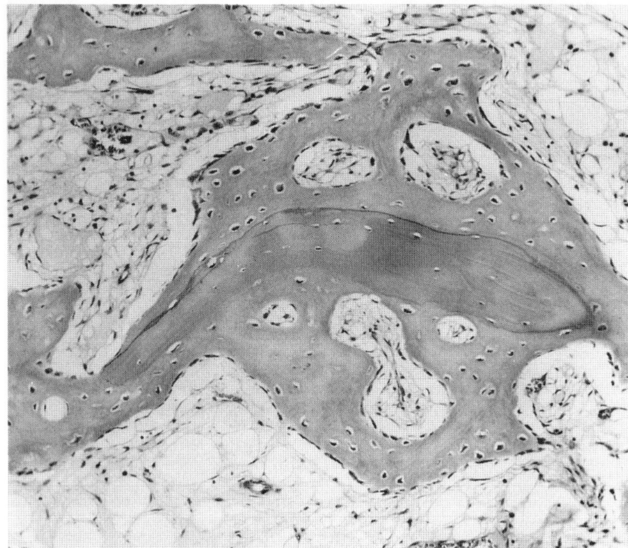

Fig. 5.7 New woven bone formation within the medullary canal, some of which is appositional upon a pre-existing bone trabeculae. Haematoxylin—eosin ×120.

of that part of the cortex. Any osteocytes within cortical or medullary bone that have not undergone ischaemic necrosis play no part in the healing process because these cells are entrapped within their lacunae in calcified bone and are destroyed during resorption (Tonna 1972).

The fracture gap

The periosteal callus joins the two bone fragments externally but does not unite the ends directly. There is a fibrin clot present between the two bone ends which persists for some time. It is eventually replaced by granulation tissue followed by osteogenic and fibroblastic cells. Bone union across the fracture gap can occur in two main ways. Direct ossification is an effective and a more common process of union. This is when bone is formed across the fracture gap resulting in unity of the bone ends. A small amount of cartilage may form at the fracture site but it is rapidly converted to bone by endochondral ossification. An alternative mechanism which is slower is through a fibrous union. This occurs when fibrous tissue grows in from the surrounding tissues or medullary canal and unites the two fracture bone ends. This fibrous tissue often becomes densely collagenized which results in ossification proceeding slowly. Thus, healing may be very slow (delayed union) or may fail completely (non-union). This fibrous union is particularly likely to occur if there is fracture instability, a poor blood supply, extensive disruption of the periosteum, a comminuted fracture or local infection

(Frost 1989b). Delayed or non-union is also more common if the fracture gap is large due to massive tissue necrosis, extensive bone resorption, excess traction or entrapment of soft tissue between the fractured bone ends. In cases of established non-union a dense relatively acellular fibrous tissue forms between the fracture ends which may act as a barrier to vascularization and so to the formation of a calcified callus. When bony union is delayed for a prolonged period fibrocartilaginous tissue may form between the bone ends which may eventually undergo central eosinophilic fibrinoid necrosis. This area of necrotic tissue is inherently weak and movement at the fracture site can cause a transverse split. The split may enlarge into a definite space if movement at the fracture site persists. The tissue either side of the split may become more cartilaginous in nature and some adjacent cells may undergo metaplasia to form a lining indistinguishable from synovium (Fig. 5.8). The bone ends are remodelled to a more smooth outline with some sclerosis. This completes the process of formation of a pseudarthrosis.

Later stages (remodelling) (21—100 days)

The result of the early stages of fracture healing is the presence of a calcified external callus, an internal callus within the medullary canal and bridging of the fracture gap by calcified bone. This will result in restoration of function of the fractured bone and will initiate the remodelling activities of osteoblasts and osteoclasts (Fig. 5.9). The remodelling mechanism does four things.
1 It replaces any mineralized cartilage with woven bone to form a kind of primary spongiosa.
2 It replaces all the woven bone with new lamellar

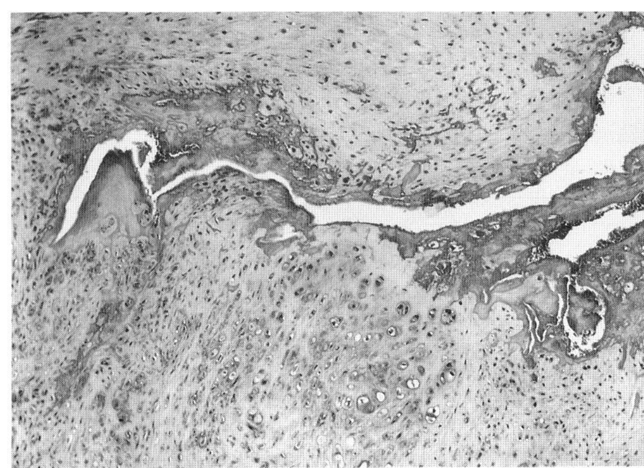

Fig. 5.8 Reactive cartilage above and below with a split containing fibrin and showing the earliest signs of synovial metaplasia. Haematoxylin—eosin ×90.

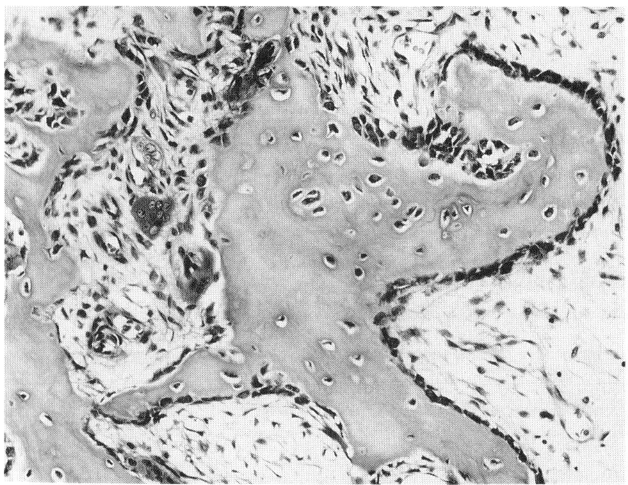

Fig. 5.9 Intense osteoblastic activity particularly on the right with osteoclastic remodelling on the left. Haematoxylin—eosin ×380.

bone. The amount of lamellar bone formed and its distribution appears to reflect the stresses and strains to which the fracture site is subjected. In other words, bone is deposited where the strain is greatest and removed where it serves no useful mechanical function. This is in agreement with the generalization known as Wolff's law (1892) that bone develops a structure that is most suited to resist the forces acting upon it. Thus, if a fracture has united at an angle the remodelled bone persists and is incorporated on the concave side while the callus on the convex side tends to be resorbed.

3 It replaces the bone that has formed between the fractured ends of the cortex with new secondary osteones made of lamellar bone. This new bone is aligned parallel to the lines of stress.

4 It allows removal and remodelling of the callus formed within the medullary canal resulting in reformation of the normal fatty and haemopoietic marrow.

Factors affecting healing

The healing of a fracture is carried out by the proliferation and integration of very many cells. The process can be modified by a large number of endogenous and exogenous factors that have an influence on the metabolic function of the cells. The factors affecting fracture healing can be divided into local and systemic factors.

Local factors

Degree of local trauma

It is recognized that fractures associated with bone

fragmentation, loss of periosteum or extensive trauma to the surrounding soft tissues show retarded healing. This may be the result of severe damage to the tissues causing poor formation of granulation tissue. The larger the haematoma formation the longer it will take to remove the haematoma. This will delay the establishment of a callus. Interposition of soft tissues between the fractured ends will also interfere with normal callus formation. The greater the degree of the local bone necrosis the larger the fracture gap and therefore the healing process will be slower. The repair processes in undisplaced fractures are quicker than in displaced fractures (Rhinelander *et al.* 1968). This is the result of slowing of the rate of callus formation as well as the increased cartilage formation in the displaced fractures. In addition, there tends to be a reduction in the amount of primary bone formation between the fractured ends. Similarly, if large amounts of bone are lost the fracture gap will be much wider and therefore the repair process will be slower.

Type of bone involved

Cortical and cancellous bone react differently to fracture. Cancellous bone unites rapidly but only at the points of direct contact (Uhtoff & Rhan 1981). Where there is no bone contact in a trabecular fracture the gap is filled by the spread of new bone from the remaining points of contact. Repair of cancellous bone is usually rapid because there are often many points of contact and the medullary bone is rich in osteoblastic cells and has a good blood supply. Experimentally, fractures through cancellous bone show a great deal of direct new bone formation and a paucity of cartilage formation. In addition, there is appositional new bone laid down on the surface of the existing necrotic bone trabeculae. This may account for the increase in radiodensity often seen. This contrasts with repair of cortical bone.

Degree of immobilization

Experimentally, repeated manipulation of a fracture site retards fracture healing (Pappas & Radin 1968). This may be the result of disruption of the fibrin formed at the time of initial healing. In addition, cartilaginous rather than bony callus forms which delays healing and this may even prevent healing eventually resulting in a pseudarthrosis. It seems that bone formation is inhibited by significant micromotion.

Infection

If infection is superimposed on the fracture site there will be an exaggerated and persistent acute inflammatory response (Andriole *et al.* 1973). This will interfere with normal healing and reduce or prevent the formation of fracture callus.

Pathological fracture

A pathological fracture is a fracture through a bone already affected by a pathological process. Some pathological fractures may heal normally although many will result in delayed or poor fracture healing. A fracture through a malignant tumour heals poorly because of the presence of the malignant cells at the fracture site. These tumour cells will continue to proliferate at this site and may interfere with the normal healing processes. Indeed, often the malignant tumour can extend out through the fracture site into the surrounding soft tissues and so interpose a cell mass between the fractured bone ends. There is some evidence that Paget's disease and fibrous dysplasia may also interfere with the normal healing process (Nicholas & Killoran 1965). Bone that has been irradiated heals at a much slower rate and there is a risk of non-union. This is partly the result of patchy death of cells within the bone and partly the result of the fibrosis in and around the bone that often results from irradiation.

Avascular necrosis

Fracture healing normally proceeds from both sides of the fracture. The formation of callus is contributed to equally by both fractured ends. If one fracture fragment has been rendered avascular, such as may occur in the femoral head following a fractured neck of femur, the healing process has to depend entirely on ingrowth of capillaries from the living vascularized side. Thus, fractures in these situations may heal but the rate of union is slow and there is a definite risk of non-union. If both fragments are rendered avascular then it is rare for union ever to occur.

Intra-articular fractures

Intra-articular fractures may allow access of synovial fluid to the fracture site. Synovial fluid is rich in fibrinolysins and these may retard the first stage in fracture healing by preventing the formation of fibrin (Lack 1964). Intra-articular fractures do heal but the process may either be delayed or interfered with as a result of the effects of the synovial fluid and poor cartilage healing.

Exercise and local stress

It is recognized that exercise increases the rate of fracture repair (Heikkinen *et al.* 1970). It is likely that bone formation is stimulated by forces acting across the fracture site although the exact mechanism of this is poorly understood. It is also important that appropriate stresses are placed across the fracture if remodelling of the callus is to take place and if lamellar and cortical bone is to reform to prefracture status (Cowin *et al.* 1984).

Denervation

Denervation of the affected tissues may retard fracture healing. The exact mechanism is unknown but it can be seen in patients with peripheral neuropathies and in those with major regional sensory denervations. The slowing of the healing process in these situations may be related to the reduction in the stress across the fracture site as a result of relative immobility, but this is unlikely to be the only mechanism (Frost 1989b). It is interesting to note that patients with head injuries develop exuberant fracture callus in limb fractures with rapid uniting of the fractures.

Electrical stimulation

The application of local electrical current has been demonstrated to stimulate healing in experimental animals (Takahashi *et al.* 1982). The exact mechanism is poorly understood and there is some controversy as to whether this electrical stimulation can promote healing in human subjects (Connolly 1984).

Other local factors

There are some rare conditions that can result in maldifferentiation of the fracture callus or alteration or failure of remodelling of the callus. A fracture in patients with hyperparathyroidism (Frost 1986) or neurofibromatosis (Tachdjian 1972) may result in poor or incomplete callus formation. In addition, children with osteogenesis imperfecta may form a normal callus rapidly but often the callus undergoes incomplete or imperfect remodelling (Sillence 1981). Patients with osteomalacia or rickets may have delayed remodelling of woven bone to calcified lamellar bone.

Systemic factors

Age

It is known that fractures in young people heal much more rapidly than fractures in adults. In addition, the rapid remodelling that accompanies growth seems to allow correction of a greater degree of fracture deformity in young people than would occur in adults. Experimental work has shown that there is a more rapid differentiation of cells from the surrounding mesenchyme in young animals when compared to old animals (Tonna & Cronkite 1963). A good blood supply enhances fracture healing and severe atherosclerosis in the elderly may result in a reduced blood flow and slower fracture healing.

Hormones

In both experimental and clinical situations corticosteroids are powerful inhibitors of the normal fracture healing. They may have an inhibitory effect on the differentiation of osteoblasts from mesenchymal cells and they may also interfere in the formation of the various components of the bone matrix (Cruess & Sakai 1972). Experimental evidence has shown that growth hormone may be a potent stimulator of fracture healing and in the clinical context this may explain in part the better healing of fractures in children (Misol *et al.* 1971). Thyroid hormone, calcitonin, insulin and anabolic steroids have been reported to enhance fracture healing when given to animals. Patients suffering from diabetes mellitus may display poor fracture healing. This is more the result of diabetic angiopathy and neuropathy rather than being a direct effect of deficient insulin.

Nutrition and drugs

Poor nutrition may interfere with fracture healing. This is particularly so if the patient is deficient in either proteins, vitamin A, vitamin C, vitamin D, calcium or essential amino acids. Cytotoxic therapy may also interfere with fracture healing as may local irradiation. It has been suggested that some non-steroidal anti-inflammatory drugs may also have some mild inhibitory effect on fracture healing (Frost 1989b).

References

Albright, J.A. & Brand, R.A. (eds). *The Scientific Basis of Orthopaedics* 2nd edn. Appleton & Lange: Connecticut, 1987.

Andriole, V.T., Nagel, D.A. & Southwick, W.O. A paradigm for human chronic osteomyelitis. *J Bone Joint Surg* 1973; **55A**: 1511–1515.

Basset, C.A.L. Current concepts of bone formation. *J Bone Joint Surg* 1962; **44A**: 1217–1244.

Becker, R.O. Electrical osteogenesis — pro and con. *Calcif Tissue Int* 1978; **26**: 93–97.

Brand, R.A. & Rubin, C.T. Fracture healing. In: Albright, J.A. & Brand, R.A. (eds) *The Scientific Basis of Orthopaedics* 2nd edn. Appleton & Lange: Connecticut, 1987.

Bubenik, G.A., Bubenik, A.B. & Stevens, E.D. The effect of neurogenic stimulation on the development and growth of bony tissues. *J Exp Zool* 1981; **219**: 205–212.

Connolly, J.F. Electrical treatment of non-unions: its use and abuse in 100 consecutive fractures. *Orthop Clin North Am* 1984; **15**: 89–96.

Cowin, S.C., Lanyon, L.E. & Rodan, G. The Kroc Foundation conference on functional adaptation in bone tissue. *Calcif Tissue Int* 1984; **36**: 1–14.

Cruess, R.L. & Sakai, T. Effect of cortisone upon synthesis rates of some components of rat bone matrix. *Clin Orthop* 1972; **86**: 253–259.

Friedenberg, Z.B. & Brighton, C.T. Bioelectric potentials in bone. *J Bone Joint Surg* 1966; **48A**: 915–923.

Frost, H.M. *Intermediary Organisation of the Skeleton.* CRC Press: Florida, 1986.

Frost, H.M. The biology of fracture healing I. *Clin Orthop* 1989a; **248**: 283–293.

Frost, H.M. The biology of fracture healing II. *Clin Orthop* 1989b; **248**: 294–309.

Heikkinen, E., Vihersaari, T. & Penttinen, R. Effect of previous exercise on the development of experimental fracture callus in the mouse. *Scand J Clin Lab Invest* 1970; **25**: 113–132.

Lack, C.H. Proteolytic activity and connective tissue. *Br Med Bull* 1964; **20**: 217–222.

Lavine, L.S. & Grodzinski, A.J. Electrical stimulation of bone. *J Bone Joint Surg* 1987; **69A**: 626–631.

McKibben, B. The biology of fracture healing in long bones. *J Bone Joint Surg* 1978; **60B**: 150–162.

Misol, S., Samaan, N. & Ponseti, I.V. Growth hormone in delayed fracture union. *Clin Orthop* 1971; **74**: 206–208.

Nicholas, J.A. & Killoran, P. Fractures of the femur in patients with Paget's disease. *J Bone Joint Surg* 1965; **47A**: 450–461.

Pappas, A.M. & Radin, E. The effect of delayed manipulation on the rate of fracture healing. *Surg Gynecol Obstet* 1968; **126**: 1287–1297.

Rhinelander, F.W., Phillips, R.S., Steel, W.M. & Beer, J.C. Microangiography and bone healing II. Displaced closed fractures. *J Bone Joint Surg* 1968; **50A**: 643–662.

Rhinelander, F.W. & Wilson, J.W. Blood supply to developing, mature and healing bone. In: Summer-Smith, G. (ed.) *Bone in Clinical Orthopaedics.* WB Saunders: Philadelphia, 1982.

Sillence, D. Osteogenesis imperfecta. An expanding panorama of variants. *Clin Orthop* 1981; **159**: 11–19.

Stirling, R.I. Healing of fractured bones. *Trans R Med Chir Soc Edinb* 1931–32; **46**: 203–228.

Tachdjian, M.O. *Paediatric Orthopaedics.* WB Saunders: Philadelphia, 1972.

Takahashi, H., Watanabe, G., Togawa, Y., Hanzoka, T., Kono, T., Sorto, Y. & Suzuki, H. The effects of various types of electrical current on internal remodelling of bone in dogs. *Orthop Trans* 1982; **2**: 369–377.

Tonna, E.A. An electron microscopic study of osteocyte release during osteoclasis in mice of different ages. *Clin Orthop* 1972; **87**: 311–317.

Tonna, E.A. & Cronkite, E.P. The periosteum; autoradiographic studies on cellular proliferation and transformation utilizing tritiated thymidine. *Clin Orthop* 1963; **30**: 218–233.

Triffit, J.T. Initiation and enhancement of bone formation. *Acta Orthop Scand* 1987; **58**: 673–684.

Uhtoff, H.K. & Rhan, B.A. Healing patterns of metaphyseal fractures. *Clin Orthop* 1981; **760**: 295–303.

Urist, M.R., De Lange, R.J. & Fineman, G.A.M. Bone cell differentiation and growth factors. *Science* 1983, **220**: 680–686.

Wolff, J. Das Gaetz der Transformation. In: *Transformation der Knocken*. Hirschwald: Berlin, 1892.

Articular cartilage

S.B.TRIPPEL AND H.J.MANKIN

Injuries to joint structures are common and may involve either direct or indirect mechanical trauma to the articular cartilage. Although cartilage is considered to be a hardy tissue, it does not heal well and sometimes such injuries result in significant impairment of function and serious sequelae.

In order to understand more fully the effect of such injuries on the cartilage surfaces and the joint, some basic knowledge is required regarding the response of the tissue to trauma. Historically, probably no experiment has been repeated more frequently than surgically injuring the joint (sometimes inadvertently) and observing the manner in which the tissue heals over time. Despite the large amount of data which has accumulated over the years, there remains some confusion as to the nature of the response of articular cartilage to trauma. Some of the controversy is based on the evident fact that cartilage responds to different forms of trauma in different ways (see below); there is also a semantic problem in the definitions of hyaline and fibrocartilages.

Of considerable importance is the current enthusiasm for the management of certain cartilagenous lesions by arthroscopic surgical manoeuvres. One of the more frequent of these ventures is that of 'shaving' the roughened surface of the patella encountered in patients with chondromalacia. The enthusiasm of clinicians for this technique has led them to the opinion that, contrary to prior experimental evidence, such surgery leads to 'healing' of superficial defects, while sceptics consider it possible that there are other aspects of the operative procedure which may improve the symptoms of the patient but, in fact, have no effect on the cartilagenous surface. In any event, there is little question that the

problems of cartilage healing remain relevant to joint biology as well as to our understanding of the basic processes of cartilage metabolism.

Before discussing the response of articular cartilage to mechanical trauma, it is important to consider the 'normal' course of events in the healing of body tissues after trauma and the aberrations seen in articular cartilage based on its avascular state. The general response to injury in vascularized mammalian tissues is a phasic one, so similar for most organs and structures as to be almost stereotypic. The response may be divided into three more or less distinct phases: necrosis, inflammation and repair.

The phase of *necrosis* begins immediately and is characterized by tissue death which varies considerably in extent depending on the type and degree of trauma, the local tissue dependence on its blood supply and the richness of the vascular bed. Injuries of limited extent in a richly vascularized tissue in which the cells are not remarkably susceptible to hypoxia may result in little or no necrosis. In circumstances where the injury is extreme, where the blood supply is marginal and the cells are very susceptible to a decrease in oxygen tension, an extraordinary amount of necrosis may evolve.

The second phase, that of *inflammation*, follows almost immediately after the first and is similar to that seen in infectious or immune challenges of the tissue in that it is almost entirely mediated by the vascular system. Increased blood flow and vascular dilatation occurs and the vessel walls become increasingly permeable and allow their contents to enter the surrounding extracellular spaces. Transudation is followed by exudation and eventually a large mass of cellular and proteinaceous material fills the traumatized area, which, in the presence of fibrin, platelets and the necessary activating factors, becomes a clot. The clot is perhaps significant in part in providing pluripotential cells that yield repair cells and help organize the structure into a fibrous mass.

The third phase of the response of tissues to trauma is that of *repair*. This supervenes when the fibrin clot is invaded by blood vessels and cells, which produce at first a loose vascular granulation tissue, then a fibrous repair matrix and finally a scar which firmly welds the wound edges together and, by subsequently contracting, attempts to close the gap. In certain of the body's connective tissues this final phase is associated with the replacement of the damaged tissue by tissue identical or similar to the original (bone healing with bone, synovium healing with synovium, tendon healing with tendon) rather than the fibrous scar, such as occurs in skin, liver, kidney, etc. In these circumstances, the reparative material undergoes a sometimes prolonged remodelling process to restore or approximate normal anatomy.

In considering the application of this scheme to injuries to hyaline articular cartilage, it is apparent that when subjected to trauma it undergoes the same phase of *necrosis* as any other body tissue. The cells at the site of injury die and matrix disruption occurs consistent with the extent and type of trauma. Since chondrocytes are relatively insensitive to hypoxia, perhaps there is less cell death than one might see in other body tissues. Because there are no blood vessels present, however, the second phase, *inflammation*, which is almost entirely mediated by the vascular system, is absent. No blood escapes from ruptured vessels and no clot can be produced. There are no local blood vessels to undergo vascular dilatation or show increased blood flow and the processes of transudation, exudation and haematoma formation are absent. No fibrin is produced so that the fibrin clot which ordinarily serves as the scaffolding for the repair is absent. If one considers the third phase, *repair*, the absence of an inflammatory or vascular phase to bring in blood vessels and provide reparative cells considerably limits the cells available to respond to the trauma, and the burden for repair falls on the existing chondrocytes. The cells of cartilage are capable of undergoing DNA synthesis and increasing their matrix synthetic activity, but the question arises as to whether the response of only the chondrocytes, sparse in number and presumably limited in their synthetic activities, is sufficient to repair an injury to the articular surface. Without aid from other cellular tissues this burden would seem to be an extraordinary one for a cell with limited potential for metabolic activity and, as will be discussed below, the experimental and clinical circumstances bear out this anticipated limitation for the repair potential for mature articular cartilage in which no vascular system is involved.

It should be clearly noted, however, that if the injury involves the basal layers of the cartilage and, specifically, the damage extends to or through the bony end plate of the underlying subchondral cortex, the previous discussion is inappropriate since in such an injury all three phases of repair are possible. Necrosis (not only of cartilage but of bone as well) is very evidently present, but also since the bone is heavily vascularized, the vascular response of inflammation can and does occur. Furthermore, the underlying bone is a rich source of progenitor cells to generate chondroblasts or fibroblasts and the phase of repair is likely to be very active. Thus, in deeper cartilagenous injuries (those that injure the underlying bone as well) a much more stereotypic response can be anticipated. All three phases of response to injury are demonstrated and the classic form of repair occurs.

Response of articular cartilage to superficial lacerative injuries

As indicated above, the experiment in which a superficial laceration is produced in articular cartilage and the animal is studied for healing at regular intervals is an age-old one and has often been repeated. One of the earliest recorded observations was that of Hunter (1743) who stated, 'from Hippocrates to the present age it is universally allowed that ulcerated cartilage is a troublesome thing and that, once destroyed, it is not repaired'. Since then, numerous studies have demonstrated a disappointing inability of the articular cartilage to produce sufficient tissue to coapt the margins of a lacerative injury or repair an ulcerative defect in the cartilage (Bennett & Bauer 1935, Calandruccio & Gilmer 1962, Campbell 1969, Fuller & Ghadially 1972, Mankin 1975, Ghadially *et al*. 1977). In injuries confined to the substance of the cartilage of adult animals (i.e. not violating the junction of the calcified zone and the underlying bony end plate) the response clearly lacks the *inflammatory* component of the repair process since the avascular tissue has no capillary network. The reaction appears to be independent of extent, depth or orientation of the lesion and is characterized by minimal attempts on the part of the cartilage to add cellular and matrix elements. The repair process observed is almost never effective in healing the defect (Mankin & Boyle 1967, Rosenberg, unpublished data) (Fig. 5.10).

Long-term follow-up of superficial lacerative injuries has demonstrated no further attempt at healing with time but, of some interest, is that there is no evidence of progression to osteoarthritis. In 1963, Meachim described a 'scarification' model in the rabbit, in which multiple superficial slices were made in the articular cartilage (Meachim 1963). It was his contention that the lesions would progress to a disorder resembling chondromalacia. He and other investigators, however, have shown that the lesions remain stable and that only occasionally does one see evidence for early osteoarthritic changes (Thompson 1975). Rosenberg (unpublished data) performed a similar study and using routine histology and safranin-O staining (as a histochemical indicator of proteoglycan concentration) observed the cartilage over time. At the end of 1 year he found the lacerative defects in the cartilage to be essentially unaltered. Not only was there little or no attempt at repair but also there was no indication of

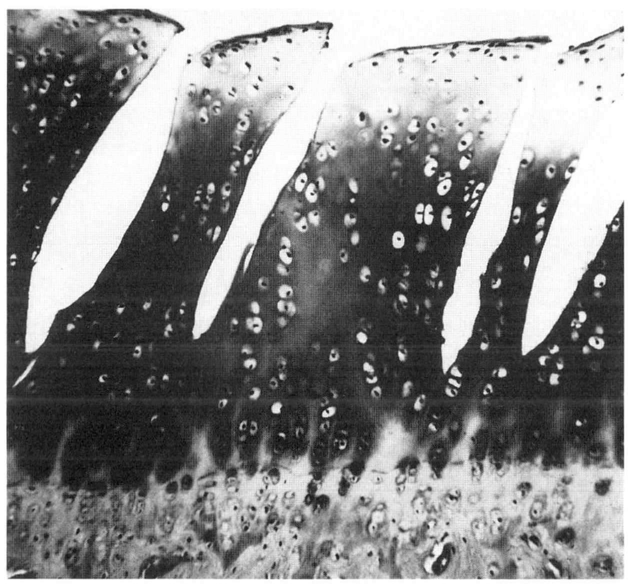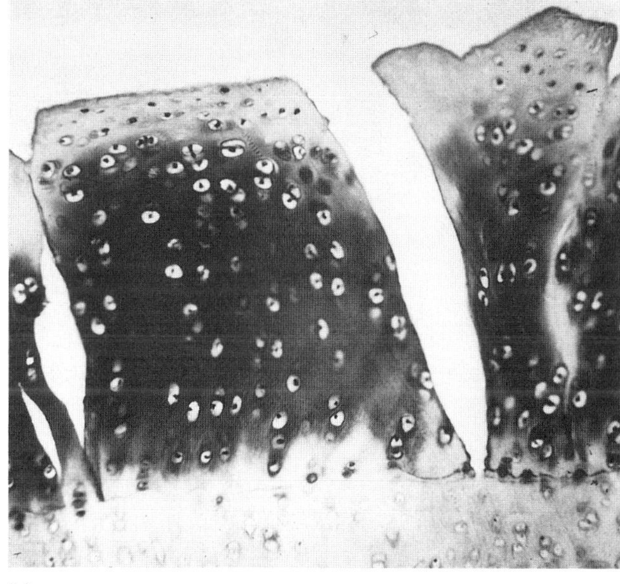

(a)   (b)

Fig. 5.10 Low power photomicrographs of sections of articular cartilage from the distal femur of adult rabbits in which multiple superficial slices have been made. (a) Photomicrograph of the specimen obtained shortly after the surgical procedure; (b) 1 year later. While little healing is evident, one should note the absence of changes consistent with osteoarthritis (see text). Safranin-O−fast green−iron haematoxylin; ×100.

conversion of the lesions to those of chondromalacia or osteoarthritis.

It is apparent from all of these data that lacerative injuries which remain superficial (do not penetrate below the tidemark) generally evoke only a short-lived metabolic and enzymatic response which fails to provide sufficient numbers of new cells or matrix to repair even the minimal defect created by a scalpel blade. Of further interest is the evidence, which has been presented, that these lesions remain as defects for at least a year and do not go on to either chondromalacia or an osteo-arthritic type of degenerative process. The concept has some clinical relevance in that superficial lesions which occur as a result of trauma or surgical procedures may be considered to be of little consequence. Thus, although long-term effects of such injuries are not known, there is reason to speculate on the basis of studies described above that they are generally limited in expression and do not lead to clinical osteoarthritis.

Response of articular cartilage to deep penetrating injuries

Of somewhat greater interest, particularly recently, is the response of the cartilage to the 'deep' lesion, an injury or laceration which crosses the tidemark to violate the vascular underlying bony end plate. As discussed

above and suggested by a number of studies this type of injury, unlike the superficial injury, causes significant interference with the vasculature of the bone and the response is more characteristic of that occurring in other vascularized tissues (Calandruccio & Gilmer 1962, Campbell 1969, Hjertquist & Lemperg 1971, Meachim & Roberts 1971, Mitchell & Shepard 1976, Cheung *et al.* 1980, Rosenberg, unpublished data). The deep defect which passes through the articular cartilage to enter the underlying bone almost immediately fills with blood (Campbell 1969). The haematoma becomes organized into a fibrin clot containing red blood cells, white cells, bone marrow elements and platelets. Undifferentiated cells from the marrow and endothelial lining give rise to fibroblasts (Depalma *et al.* 1966). With the ingrowth of capillaries from the vascular bed in the base of the wound the fibrin clot becomes a vascular fibroblastic tissue (Depalma *et al.* 1966) (Fig. 5.11). With progressive fibrosis of the granulation tissue the defect becomes filled with an initially loose fibrovascular tissue which gradually becomes more fibrous and less vascular (Calandruccio & Gilmer 1962, Campbell 1969). At the base of the lesion, in the region in contact with the injured bone, active new bone formation occurs which extends jointward. For reasons not well understood, however, bone formation generally stops at the margin of the old cartilage−bone junction leaving a vascular

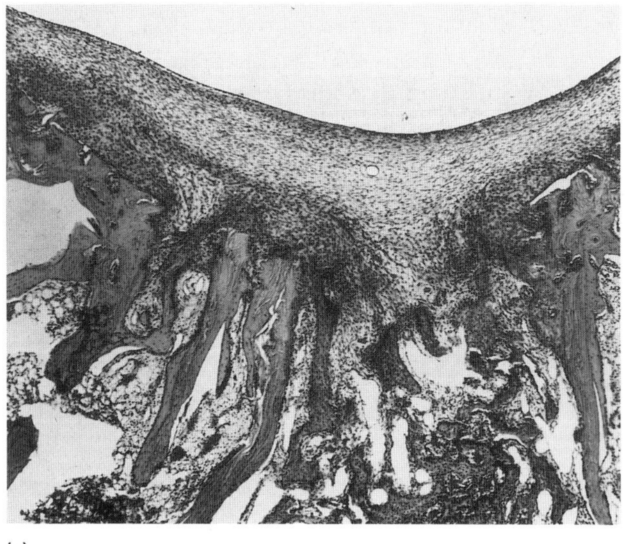

(a)

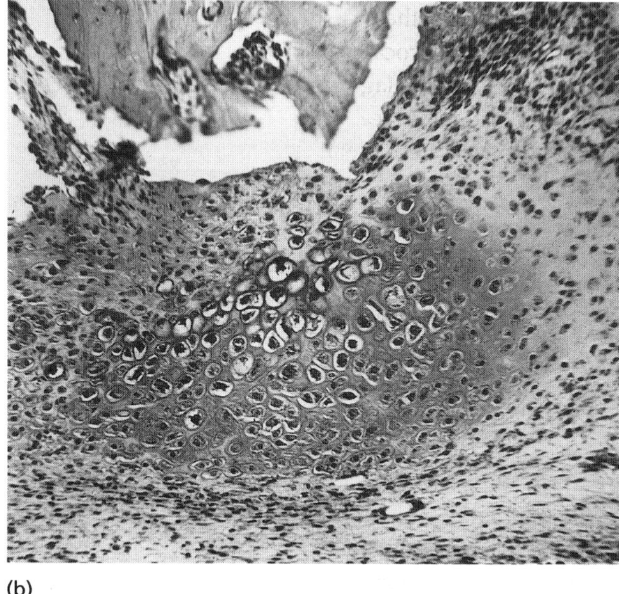

(b)

Fig. 5.11 (a) Low power photomicrograph of deep coring defect in adult rabbit articular cartilage showing the production of exuberant undifferentiated mesenchymal tissue several weeks after injury. The tissue is mostly fibrous and limited in vascularity at this point. (b) A short time later foci of chondrification appear. Haematoxylin—eosin; (a) ×100; (b) ×450.

fibrous tissue to unite the cartilage wound edges. The tissue undergoes progressive hyalinization and subsequently becomes 'chondrified' to produce a fibrocartilagenous mass which, at this point, firmly welds the wound edges together and remains fused to the underlying new bone in the base (Calandruccio & Gilmer 1962, Depalma *et al*. 1966, Rosenberg, unpublished data) (Fig. 5.12).

The biochemical character of the repair tissue has been investigated by Furukawa *et al.* (1980). These authors showed that repair tissue filling deep (bone-penetrating) defects in rabbit knee articular cartilage initially consisted of type I collagen, the major collagen of fibrous tissue, tendon, skin and bone. By 6—8 weeks following injury, type II collagen, the major collagen of cartilage, had become predominant. Even so, the repair cartilage at 1 year continued to contain significant quantities of type I collagen indicating that it never fully achieved the characteristic structure of normal articular cartilage. These data reveal that while full-thickness articular cartilage injuries may heal with a cartilagenous material, this repair tissue does not duplicate normal articular cartilage and retains some of the characteristics of fibrocartilage.

The ultimate fate of the newly formed fibrocartilage tissue is of considerable interest. In a rabbit model of deep cartilage injury, Mitchell and Shepard (1976) demonstrated that early in the course of repair the primary fibrous repair tissue is converted to a hyaline-like chondroid tissue showing evidence of active mitotic

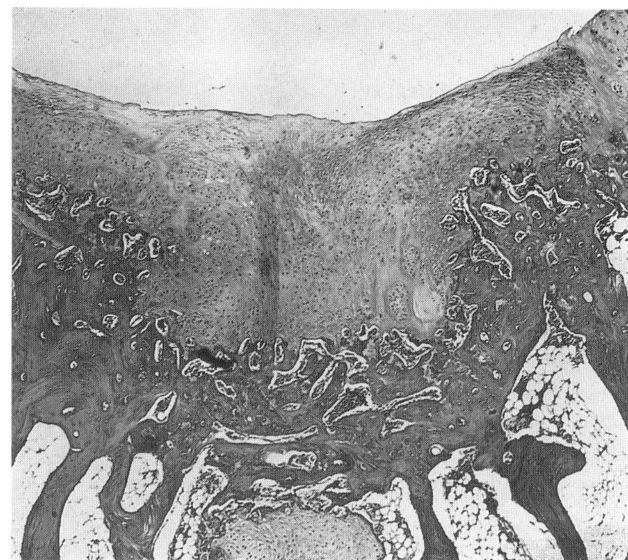

Fig. 5.12 As the coring defect heals, at 6 months chondroid tissue fills the defect and the articular surface is reconstituted. The surface is 'dimpled' but the cartilage present appears hyaline and well-organized. Haematoxylin—eosin; ×100. (Reproduced with permission from Mankin, H.J. The reaction of articular cartilage to injury and osteoarthritis. *N Engl J Med* 1974; **291**: 1285.)

activity and histochemical staining consistent with a high concentration of proteoglycan. By 12 months post injury, however, the cartilagenous nature of the material became less obvious and its appearance more fibrous.

At this later stage, the surface layers and the cells were more typical of fibrocartilage than of hyaline cartilage and the tangential collagen orientation (the 'skin') failed to appear. The surface became fibrillated while the subjacent matrix remained filled with a cartilage-like material (Fig. 5.13). Similar evidence that newly formed cartilage shows signs of degeneration after 6–12 months has been obtained by other investigators as well (Hjertquist & Lemperg 1971). This experience parallels the observation that the site of an old 'deep' laceration or defect may be clearly visible years after injuries as a slightly discoloured, roughened pit or linear groove on the otherwise smooth and quite normal surface of the adjacent hyaline cartilage (Campbell 1969, Stockwell & Meachim 1973) (Plate 5.1, facing p. 98).

Application of this experience to the treatment of articular cartilage injury in the clinical setting has been described (Dandy 1986, Johnson 1986) and abrasion arthroplasty is now a relatively common arthroscopic procedure. Controlled trials of its effects on cartilage repair are, however, not yet available. Reported efforts to produce healing of damaged patello-femoral articular cartilage in the clinical setting have been somewhat discouraging (Milgrem 1985).

Another interesting facet of the problem of cartilage healing is the effect of continuous passive motion (CPM), as reported by Salter *et al.* (1980). Coring defects through the underlying bone were made in the distal femora of rabbits and the animals treated in three ways: by plaster immobilization, cage ambulation (obviously limiting) and by CPM (achieved by placing the rabbits in an assembly in which the firmly held extremities were passively flexed and extended at a slow rate). After 4 weeks, the animals were killed and the cartilage defects studied. In the animals subjected to CPM, the tissue appeared on histological and histochemical staining to more closely approximate hyaline cartilage than fibrocartilage. These data suggest that CPM materially enhances the healing of cartilage defects. Palmoski *et al.* (1980) have shown that motion of the limb without weight-bearing produces an alteration in the chemical structure of normal rabbit articular cartilage, characterized by depletion of proteoglycan, increased water content and diminished synthetic activity. These data would seem inconsistent with Salter's theory, but it is possible that the injured and uninjured surfaces behave differently in their response to passive motion.

The application of CPM to the management of orthopaedic patients has, curiously, achieved its greatest popularity in joint replacement surgery, a setting in which articular cartilage is no longer an issue. Although cases of good clinical results following the use of CPM

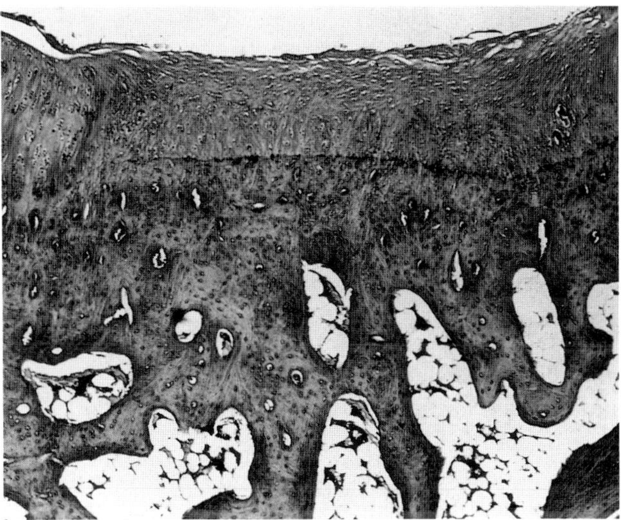

Fig. 5.13 With time, good restoration is noted in the subchondral bone, calcified cartilage and basilar layers. At 1 year, however, in some of the specimens fraying and degeneration of the surface is noted. Haematoxylin–eosin; ×100. (Reproduced with permission from Mankin, H.J. The articular cartilages, cartilage healing, and osteoarthritis. In: Cruess, R.L. & Rennie, W.A.J. (eds) *Adult Orthopaedics*. Churchill Livingstone: New York, 1984.)

for a variety of injuries have been reported (Salter *et al.* 1984) the influence of this treatment on cartilage in these cases is not known. The long-term effect of CPM on articular cartilage in human joint pathology remains to be established.

Response of articular cartilage to blunt impact

There are relatively few studies which have attempted to analyse the results of either single or multiple impacts on articular cartilage. Repo and Finlay (1977) analysed human tissues impacted by a 'drop tower' technique by radioisotopic tracer studies, histology and scanning electron microscopy. All specimens impacted at 10% strain survived without apparent injury to the chondrocytes. All specimens impacted to strains of 40% or more showed some evidence of chondrocyte death. Fissures on the surface were noted on visual inspection in some of the specimens which correlated well with failures of the collagen network as seen on scanning electron microscopy.

On the basis of these studies, and prior studies by a number of investigators, on the effect of compression and repetitive impact loading (Radin *et al.* 1970), it is apparent that there is a threshold for single or multiple impacts which the cartilage can sustain without undergoing significant injury. If the threshold is exceeded, however, cartilage damage ensues which, for the most part, rapidly progresses to an osteoarthritic-like lesion.

It is thus apparent that mechanical injury to articular cartilage has considerable variation in effect depending on the nature of the injury (deep, superficial or impactive) and the extent of the lesion created. Lacerative injuries which do not violate the underlying bone for the most part remain stationary, neither healing nor progressing to osteoarthritis. If the lesion is sufficiently severe, as perhaps occurs in chondromalacia, osteoarthritis may supervene over long observation but, at least in the experimental animal, simple laceration of the cartilagenous surface over at least a year does progress to the classic changes of osteoarthritis.

Deep lacerations, those that violate the underlying bone, produce an exuberant healing response from the underlying bone which ultimately becomes a form of hyaline (with some fibrocartilagenous elements) cartilage. The material initially appears to be reasonably competent cartilage which fills the defect in an appropriate fashion but in many circumstances it undergoes degeneration and leads to a localized focus of osteoarthritis. The focus which develops may remain stationary, however, particularly if the defect is small.

Loading or impactive injuries on the cartilagenous surface, whether single or repetitive and if they exceed a certain threshold, cause injury not only to the chondrocyte but also to the underlying bone and, at least in experimental studies, progress rapidly to an osteoarthritic lesion. Optimistically, evidence from Radin *et al.* (1978) suggests that the lesion may be reversible, particularly if the injury is mild.

New directions

A novel approach to cartilage healing is the biochemical manipulation of chondrocyte metabolic activity. Several low molecular weight peptide growth factors, identified over the last several years, have been found to be highly anabolic for cartilage. These include the somatomedins, or insulin-like growth factors (IGFs), fibroblast growth factor (FGF), epidermal growth factor (EGF), platelet-derived growth factor (PDGF) and insulin.

Osborn *et al.* (1989) found that insulin-like growth factor-I (IGF-I), insulin, FGF and EGF all stimulated sulphate incorporation, an index of matrix synthesis, by adult bovine cartilage in explant culture. Tritiated thymidine incorporation, an index of DNA synthesis, was stimulated by FGF but not by the other individual growth factors. Importantly, however, certain of these factors were found to interact with each other to produce

additive or synergistic effects. Insulin and EGF are two such factors. Acting individually neither was stimulatory for articular cartilage synthesis. Acting together, they generated a 20-fold stimulation of DNA synthesis.

Similarly, Prins *et al.* (1982a,b) and Kato *et al.* (1983) have shown growth factor stimulation of articular chondrocytes in monolayer culture, and at least two studies (Wellmitz *et al.* 1980, Cuevas *et al.* 1988) suggest that peptide growth factors may be effective in healing articular cartilage *in vivo*. The potential roles of such anabolic peptides in the normal homeostasis of articular cartilage and in the repair of damaged cartilage are not yet known.

Normal articular cartilage undergoes constant turnover, a process requiring both synthetic and degradative activity. In progressive cartilage damage, the catabolic side of this equation becomes dominant. Among the presumed major contributors to cartilage degradation is interleukin-1 (IL-1). This peptide acts directly or indirectly on articular chondrocytes, stimulating them to enzymatically digest their surrounding matrix (Dingle *et al.* 1979). IL-1 and its mediators have been shown to be produced both by synovium and by articular chondrocytes themselves (Wood *et al.* 1985, Ollivierre *et al.* 1986) and to contribute with other catabolic factors to cartilage injury in a variety of joint disorders. The specific contribution of such catabolic factors to the articular cartilage damage of acute trauma remains unknown, but in developing methods to improve articular cartilage healing in these injuries, the inhibition or moderation of cartilage catabolic activity will likely play an important role.

Summary

The clinical implications of these observations should be quite apparent. A single lacerative injury to the articular surface should cause little concern. Although the lesion is unlikely to heal, the likelihood of a progression to osteoarthritis is small. Multiple lacerative injuries or even chondromalacia-like lesions which do not violate the underlying bone can be treated by 'shaving' of the articular surfaces but unless the underlying bone is violated in the process of shaving, there is little likelihood that one will obtain 'repair' of the articular cartilage or that new cartilage will grow at the local site. A tangential slice of articular cartilage which is removed, whether by trauma or by the surgeon's knife, will remain a defective area in the cartilagenous surface with little evidence of a repair phenomenon.

If cartilage defects are 'drilled' so that there is violation of the underlying bone, one can anticipate exuberant cartilage formation which, in a very short period of time, should produce a hyaline and fibrocartilagenous mass to replace the damaged cartilage surface or ulcer. The difficulty with this system is that the type of cartilage produced is not 'normal' and this tissue may undergo degeneration over time. There is reason, however, on the basis of Salter's experiments to suggest that early movement of the part following the drilling will lead to improved cartilage formation and perhaps to longer preservation of the hyaline cartilage characteristics necessary for good joint function. Although quite preliminary from a clinical perspective, data on the application of cell-regulatory factors to the problem of cartilage healing are encouraging. With improved understanding of the pathophysiology of cartilage response to injury, it may eventually be possible to influence cartilage healing at the cellular level.

References

Bennett, G.A. & Bauer, W. Further studies concerning the repair of articular cartilage in dog joints. *J Bone Joint Surg* 1935; **17**: 141–150.

Calandruccio, R.A. & Gilmer, W.S. Jr. Proliferation, regeneration and repair of articular cartilage of immature animals. *J Bone Joint Surg* 1962; **44A**: 431–455.

Campbell, C.J. The healing of cartilage defects. *Clin Orthop* 1969; **64**: 45–63.

Cheung, H.S., Lynch, K.L., Johnson, R.P. & Brewer, B.J. *In vitro* synthesis tissue specific type II collagen by healing cartilage. I. Short term repair of cartilage by mature rabbits. *Arthritis Rheum* 1980; **23**: 211–219.

Cuevas, P., Burgos, J. & Baird, A. Basic fibroblast growth factor (FGF) promotes cartilage repair *in vivo*. *Biochem Biophys Res Commun* 1988; **156**: 611–618.

Dandy, J. Abrasion chondroplasty. *Arthroscopy* 1986; **2**: 51–53.

Depalma, A.F., McKeever, C.D. & Subin, S.K. Process of repair in articular cartilage demonstrated by histology and autoradiography with tritiated thymidime. *Clin Orthop* 1966; **48**: 229–242.

Dingle, J.T., Saklatvala, J., Hembry, R., Tyler, J., Fell, H.B. & Jubb, R. A cartilage catabolic factor from synovium. *Biochem J* 1979; **184**: 177–180.

Fuller, J.A. & Ghadially, F.N. Ultrastructural observations on surgically produced partial-thickness defects in articular cartilage. *Clin Orthop* 1972; **86**: 193–205.

Furukawa, T., Eyre, D.R., Koide, S. & Glimcher, M.J. Biochemical studies on repair cartilage resurfacing experimental defects in the rabbit knee. *J Bone Joint Surg* 1980; **62A**: 79–89.

Ghadially, F.N., Thomas, I., Oryshak, A.F. & LaRonde, J.M. Long term results of superficial defects in articular cartilage; a scanning electron microscope study. *Virchows Archiv Cell Pathol* 1977; **25**: 125–136.

Hjertquist, S.O. & Lemperg, R. Histological, autoradiographic and microchemical studies of spontaneously healing osteochondral articular defects in adult rabbits. *Calcif Tissue Res* 1971; **8**: 54–72.

Hunter, W. Of the structure and diseases of articulating cartilage. *Philos Trans R Soc Lond* 1743; **42**: 514–521.

Johnson, L.L. Arthroscopic abrasion arthroplasty historical and pathologic perspectives: present status. *Arthroscopy* 1986; **2**: 54–69.

Kato, Y., Hiraki, Y., Inoue, H., Konoshita, M., Yutani, Y. & Suzuki, F. Differential and synergistic actions of somatomedin-like growth factors, fibroblast growth factor and epidermal growth factor in rabbit costal chondrocytes. *Eur J Biochem* 1983; **192**: 885–890.

Mankin, H.J. The metabolism of articular cartilage in health and disease. In: Burleigh, P.M.C. & Poole, A.R. (eds) *Dynamics of Connective Tissue Macromolecules*. Elsevier: New York, 1975.

Mankin, H.J. & Boyle, C.J. The acute effects of lacerative injury on DNA and protein synthesis in articular cartilage. In: Bassett, C.A.L. (ed.) *Cartilage Degradation and Repair*. National Academy of Sciences, National Research Council: Washington DC, 1967.

Meachim, G. The effect of scarification on articular cartilage in the rabbit. *J Bone Joint Surg* 1963; **45B**: 150–161.

Meachim, G. & Roberts, C. Repair of the joint surface from subarticular tissue in the rabbit knee. *J Anat* 1971; **109**: 317–327.

Milgrem, J.W. Injury to articular cartilage joint surfaces. I. Chondral injury produced by patellar shaving: a histopathologic study of human tissue specimens. *Clin Orthop* 1985; **192**: 168–173.

Mitchell, N. & Shepard, N. The resurfacing of adult rabbit articular cartilage by multiple perforations through the subchondral bone. *J Bone Joint Surg* 1976; **58A**: 230–233.

Ollivierre, F., Gubler, U., Towle, C.A., Laurencin, C. & Treadwell, B.V. Expression of IL-I genes in human and bovine chondrocytes: a mechanism for autocrine control of cartilage matrix degradation. *Biochem Biophys Res Commun* 1986; **141**: 904–911.

Osborn, K.D., Trippel, S.B. & Mankin, H.J. Growth factor stimulation of adult articular cartilage. *J Orthop Res* 1989; **7**: 35–42.

Palmoski, M.J., Colyer, R.A. & Brandt, K.D. Joint motion in the absence of normal loading does not maintain normal articular cartilage. *Arthritis Rheum* 1980; **23**: 325–334.

Prins, A.P.A., Lipman, J.M., McDevitt, C.A. & Sokoloff, L. Effect of purified growth factors on rabbit articular chondrocytes in monolayer culture. II. Sulfated proteoglycan synthesis. *Arthritis Rheum* 1982a; **25**: 1228–1238.

Prins, A.P.A., Lipman, J.M. & Sokoloff, L. Effect of purified growth factors on rabbit articular chondrocytes in monolayer culture. I. DNA synthesis. *Arthritis Rheum* 1982b; **25**: 1217–1227.

Radin, E.L., Ehrlich, M.G., Chernak, B.J., Abernathy, P., Paul, I.L. & Rose, R.M. Effect of repetitive impulsive loading on the knee joint of rabbits. *Clin Orthop* 1978; **131**: 288–293.

Radin, E.L., Paul, I.L. & Lowy, M. A comparison of the dynamic force transmitting properties of subchondral bone and articular cartilage. *J Bone Joint Surg* 1970; **52A**: 444–456.

Repo, R.U. & Finlay, J.B. Survival of articular cartilage after controlled impact. *J Bone Joint Surg* 1977; **59A**: 1068–1076.

Salter, R.B., Hamilton, H.W., Wedge, J.H., Tile, M., Torode, I.P., O'Driscoll, S.W., Murnaghan, J.J. & Saringer, J.H. Clinical application of basic research on continuous passive motion for disorders and injuries of synovial joints. A preliminary report of a feasibility study. *J Orthop Res* 1984; **1**: 325–342.

Salter, R.B., Simmonds, D.F., Malcolm, B.W., Rumble, E.J., McMichael, D., & Clemente, N.D. The biological effect of continuous passive motion on the healing of full thickness defects in articular cartilage. *J Bone Joint Surg* 1980; **62A**: 1232–1251.

Stockwell, R.A. & Meachim, G. The chondrocytes. In: Freeman, M.A.R. (ed.) *Adult Articular Cartilage.* Grune & Stratton: New York, 1973.

Thompson, R.C. Jr. An experimental study of surface injury to articular cartilage and enzyme responses within the joint. *Clin Orthop* 1975; **107**: 239–248.

Wellmitz, G., Petzold, E., Jentzsch, K.D., Heder, G. & Buntrock, P. The effect of brain fraction with fibroblast growth activity on regeneration and differentiation of articular cartilage. *Exp Pathol* 1980; **18**: 282–287.

Wood, D.D., Ihrie, E.J. & Homerman, D. Release of interleukin-I from human synovial tissue *in vitro. Arthritis Rheum* 1985; **28**: 853–862.

Tendons and ligaments

G.HOOPER

Structure and function

Tendons

Tendons transmit the actions of muscles to bones or cartilages. The action of one muscle belly can be transmitted to one bone or to several, depending on the number of tendons associated with that muscle and the arrangement of the tendon insertions. Alternatively the actions of several muscles can be brought to bear on one insertion as is seen in the quadriceps. The direction of muscle pull can be altered by pulleys, fibrous sheaths and retinacula that are associated with tendons; when this happens friction is diminished by surrounding synovial sheaths or sesamoid bones within the tendons.

Tendons consist of fascicles of type I collagen fibrils which are arranged longitudinally and embedded in a proteoglycan–water matrix (Elliott 1965). The fascicles are bound together by endotenon, a delicate connective tissue meshwork containing blood vessels, lymphatics and nerves and which condenses on the surface of tendons to form the epitenon. The sparse cellular elements of tendons may be divided into flattened cells called tenocytes, which are indistinguishable from fibrocytes, and rounder, plumper cells called tenoblasts which correspond to fibroblasts; the latter cells contain more active organelles within the cytoplasm and are probably involved in collagen production.

The attachments of tendons to bone are usually more complex than the classical concept of tendon fibres passing directly into bone as 'Sharpey's perforating fibres'. Cooper and Misol (1970) have described four zones at the insertion of some tendons and ligaments. These are:

Zone I: tendon (or ligament) made up of longitudinal collagen fibres.

Zone II: fibrocartilage.

Zone III: mineralized fibrocartilage which is sharply separated from zone II by a darkly staining 'tidemark' that runs perpendicular to the collagen fibres.

Zone IV: bone.

This arrangement is known as a chondroapophysial attachment. The other arrangement, where tendon collagen becomes continuous with the collagen of bone and periosteum, is called a diaphysoperiosteal attachment (Canoso 1981).

Tendons are surrounded by loose areolar tissue (paratenon) or more specialized synovial tendon sheaths. The latter are found where tendons change direction, particularly around the wrist and the ankle and on the flexor aspect of the digits. At these sites the tendons lie in fibrous tunnels lined with synovium. The arrangement of the synovial membrane around the tendon within a sheath is analogous to that of the peritoneum within the abdomen: the synovial membrane covers the tendon and the inner surface of the sheath, the two layers being reflected to form a mesotenon that carries blood vessels to the tendon (Fig. 5.14). The mesotenon is usually incomplete and this is well seen in the fingers where it is represented by the vincula.

Tendons are relatively avascular structures and the blood flow to tendons is very small. In some areas, notably the volar aspect of the flexor tendons in the hand, no blood vessels can be identified (Lundborg *et al.* 1980). It has been shown that molecules can reach tendons by diffusion across the synovial space as well as via the vascular system (Hooper *et al.* 1984). It is probable that the route of exchange varies in different parts of tendons and varies with metabolic requirements. The metabolic activity of tendons is normally very low but increases during the process of repair (Birdsell *et al.* 1966).

In vitro studies of muscle–tendon–bone preparations have shown that the muscle will tear or the tendon will be avulsed from bone (often with a small fragment of bone) before the tendon itself will rupture, provided that the tendon is normal. A weak area can be created within a tendon by partially dividing it or producing an area of local ischaemic damage (McMaster 1933, Welsh *et al.* 1971).

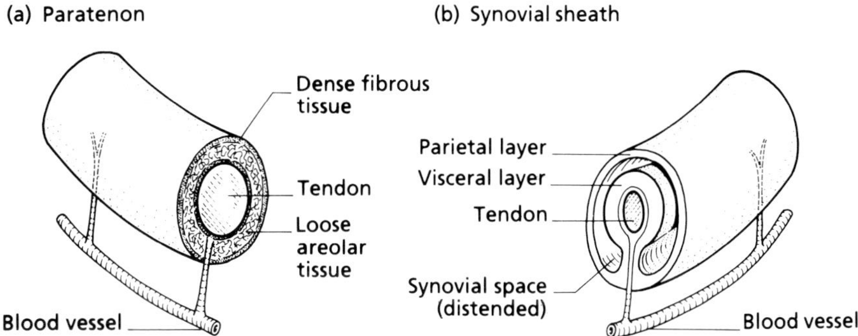

Fig. 5.14 Tendons are surrounded by (a) paratenon or by (b) synovial sheaths. (After Lamb *et al.* 1988.)

Ligaments

Ligaments are fibrous tissue bands that link bones. They maintain the stability of joints and prevent excessive movements. In addition, they play a role in the control of posture. For example, in resting one leg when standing the knee locks into extension and the pelvis is supported by the ipsilateral iliotibial tract which acts as a ligament. This stable position is maintained by ligaments without muscle activity (Evans 1979).

Various types of ligaments are recognized:

Capsular ligaments are thickenings of the joint capsule e.g. the medial collateral ligament of the knee.

Accessory ligaments are separate from the fibrous joint capsule. They may be extracapsular (e.g. the fibular collateral ligament of the knee) or intracapsular (e.g. the cruciate ligaments in the knee).

Vertebral ligaments connect the bony points of the vertebrae and may run the whole length of the vertebral column, being attached to each vertebra.

Other ligaments are not so easily classified. For example, the plantar ligament of the foot is a true ligament inasmuch as it acts as a tie between the calcaneum and the proximal phalanges of the toes, but it is also valid to call it the plantar fascia (since it is a condensation of the deep fascia) or the plantar aponeurosis (since it covers muscles and provides attachments for them). Similar difficulties are encountered when considering the iliotibial tract.

In structure ligaments are similar to tendons, being composed of type I collagen fibrils which are orientated in a longitudinal fashion. Specialized elastic ligaments are found, particularly in the spine; their main component is the microfibrillar protein elastin in a 4:1 ratio with collagen (Serafini-Fracassini *et al.* 1976). The biomechanical properties of elastic ligaments are different from collagenous ligaments and are responsible for the fact that the ligamentum flavum between vertebral laminae can shorten between full flexion and extension of the spine without buckling or pressing on the dura.

The site at which a ligament will rupture when an excessive load is applied to it is probably dependent upon the rate of loading. A rapidly applied strain tends to cause failure within the substance of the ligament whereas a slowly applied strain results in failure at the bony attachment (Noyes *et al.* 1974, Kennedy *et al.* 1976).

Healing

Tendons

Attempts to repair cut flexor tendons in the fibrous flexor sheaths in the hand are notoriously liable to give poor functional results because the tendons become bound down with scar tissue at the site of repair. The functional results of repair of tendons surrounded by paratenon are usually much better. Many experimental studies of repair of flexor tendons have been made, but the repair process in other tendons has been less intensively investigated.

A central problem in the process of healing of flexor tendons is the origin of the cells involved. Do tendons have an intrinsic capacity for healing or is the process dependent upon cells derived from extrinsic tissues?

Peacock (1967) has proposed the 'one wound, one scar' concept in which the tendon is seen as one type of tissue in a single wound that contains several injured tissues. The single wound heals as a single scar and the various tissues within it undergo later remodelling. Reorientation of collagen fibrils within the tendon will allow some movement in relation to surrounding tissues, but implicit in this concept is the inevitability of local tissue adhesions causing some loss of mobility.

Potenza (1962) designed a series of experiments to study the process of healing in cut flexor tendons, using the profundus tendons in the paws of mongrel dogs, where the anatomical arrangement is similar to the human hand. The profundus tendon was repaired with stainless steel wire using a Bunnell-type criss-cross suture. The sublimus tendon was left undisturbed and the tendon sheath was repaired. The technique used ensured that the tendon could not move at the site of repair. Care was taken not to handle the tendon with forceps and other instruments.

Initially there was a proliferation of granulation tissue at the site of suture and this appeared to derive from the synovial layer of the tendon sheath. By 7 days new collagen fibres were evident and by 21 days fibroblasts and collagen fibres were orientated in the longitudinal axis of the tendon. Subsequently, the collagen became organized in bundles. The appearance of the tendon was eventually restored to near-normal by about 112 days after injury although some filmy adhesions remained around the tendons. At no time was there evidence of proliferation of tenocytes within the tendon, or production of collagen by intrinsic cells. Attempts to prevent ingrowth of granulation tissue by isolating the repair with a polyethylene tube resulted in a delay in healing until granulation tissue gained the repair site (Potenza 1963). Potenza also showed that when repaired tendons were further damaged by puncturing or crushing them with forceps, adhesions formed at the site of damage and the quantity of adhesions was proportional to the degree of injury. Adhesions were also increased by excising the sublimus tendon or the fibrous flexor sheath at the time of repair.

Lindsay and Birch (1964) studied the origin of cells involved in the healing process of flexor tendons, using a model similar to Potenza's. Labelled thymidine, which is taken up by dividing fibroblasts, was injected at various times before sacrifice and the distribution of the label was shown by autoradiography. Their experiments (Fig. 5.15) clearly showed that fibroblasts migrated into the tendon during healing.

It would seem clear that tendon healing is an extrinsic process in the experimental model used by Potenza, which closely mimicked the techniques of tendon repair then in common use. His careful studies also identified other factors, such as rough handling and excision of adjacent tissues, that would be likely to affect results adversely.

It must be remembered that in Potenza's model the tendons were repaired with a Bunnell pull-out suture and movement of the tendon was blocked. Matthews and Richards (1974) developed an ingenious experimental model to study healing in partly divided flexor tendons in the rabbit in which the tendon was not sutured or immobilized (Fig. 5.16). They found that when a tendon was partially divided without damaging the fibrous flexor sheath it would heal without adhesions and they believed that the tendons had healed by an

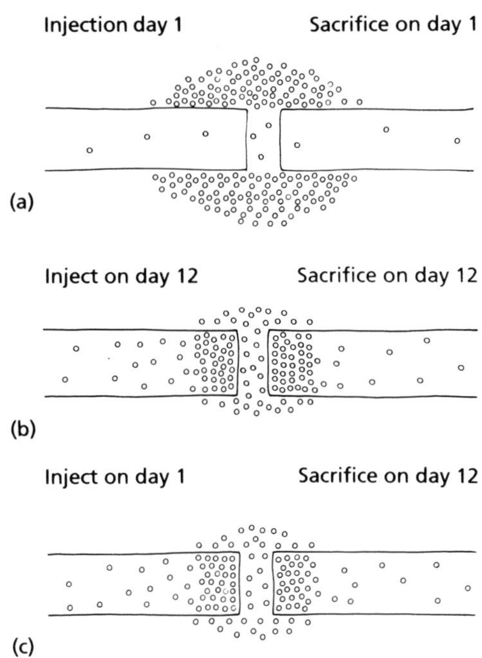

Fig. 5.15 The migration of fibroblasts during tendon healing. Dividing cells take up labelled thymidine. (a) The activity is around the tendon on day 1 after injury and (b) within the tendon on day 12. (c) The cells migrate into the tendon between day 1 and 12. (After Lindsay & Birch 1964.)

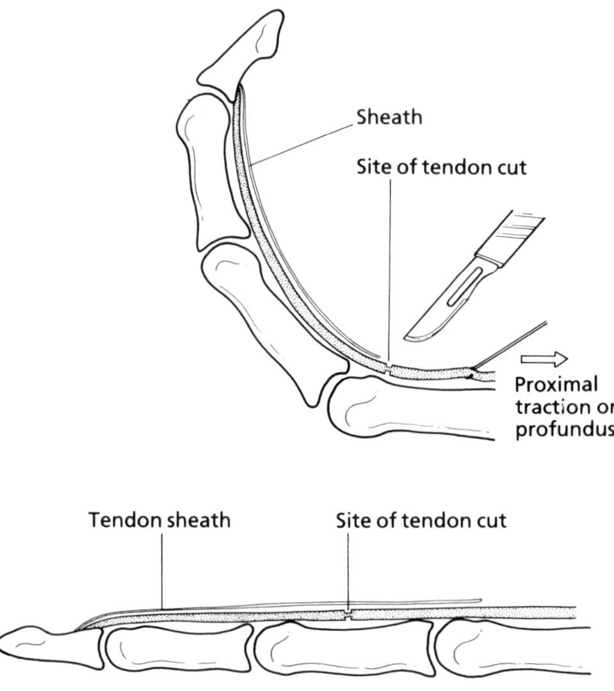

Fig. 5.16 Method of producing a partial division of a tendon without damaging the fibrous flexor sheath. (After Matthews & Richards 1976.)

intrinsic repair process. Similar findings have been reported in dogs (McDowell & Snyder 1977). However, this model did not exclude the possibility that the cells involved in the healing process had seeded on to the tendon from the synovial sheath; it is known that such a process is important in the recellularization of freeze-dried tendon grafts (Potenza & Melone 1978).

Matthews and Richards (1976) studied the effects of various factors, namely splintage, suture and excision of the flexor sheath, alone and in combination, on the formation of adhesions around rabbit flexor tendons that had been partially divided. Individually none of the factors caused adhesions and the tendons appeared to heal by intrinsic activity. When two factors were present there was mild to moderate adhesion formation, but when all factors were present dense, restrictive, persistent adhesions formed (Table 5.1). These important studies indicated that none of the factors commonly present in the clinical situation, i.e. postoperative immobilization, the presence of suture material or damage to the fibrous sheath, is alone responsible for adhesions. However, the authors recognized that in practice it would be impossible to maintain tendon apposition during healing without one or more of these factors being present.

The process of intrinsic healing has been studied by Lundborg (1976) who placed sutured segments of tendons in the rabbit knee joint. Apparent healing took place without the formation of adhesions. Was this true intrinsic healing or had the cells involved seeded on to the surface of the tendons from the synovial fluid? Lundborg clearly recognized this latter possibility but was unable to exclude it completely because he was unsuccessful in isolating tendons within a membrane that was permeable to synovial fluid but not cells (Lundborg & Rank 1980). However, his experiment has been repeated, using irradiated (Potenza & Herte 1982) and freeze-dried tendons (Chow *et al.* 1983) that contained no living cells, with similar results: the tendon remained floating freely and was covered with a thick layer of cells that must have been deposited from synovial fluid.

It may therefore be concluded that, even though no adhesions form, extrinsically derived cells are involved in the healing of tendons in a synovial environment, just as they are when a tendon heals with the formation of adhesions. Nevertheless, *in vitro* studies have shown that there is an intrinsic cellular and biochemical response when tendons are injured (Becker *et al.* 1981, Manske *et al.* 1984, Manske & Lesker 1984). Whether this is relevant in the clinical situation is doubtful and with present knowledge one must conclude that flexor tendon repair is always associated with some adhesion formation (Ketchum 1977). These adhesions may be diminished by minimal handling of the tendon, careful suture technique using inert material and avoidance of further damage to the flexor tendon sheath. The tethering effect of adhesions may also be lessened by early passive mobilization after repair. In the technique popularized by Kleinert (Lister *et al.* 1977) an elastic band attached to the fingernail pulls the finger into flexion when it is not being actively extended. This allows movement of the flexor tendon but diminishes stress at the repair site since the flexor muscles do not undergo active contraction.

It is extremely important to protect the repair from stress in the early stages as tensile strength actually diminishes for a few days because the ends of the tendon soften. Thereafter, there is a steady increase in tensile strength, especially if movement is allowed (Mason & Allen 1941) but the tendon is still subject to rupture for a few weeks after repair.

Table 5.1 The effect of iatrogenic factors on adhesion formation around partly divided tendons. (From Matthews & Richards 1976)

Adverse factors	Adhesions
Nil	−
Immobilization alone	−
Suture alone	−
Excision of sheath alone	−
Immobilization + suture	+
Suture + sheath excision	+
Immobilization + sheath excision	+
Immobilization + suture + sheath excision	+++

Ligaments

In contrast to flexor tendons, the process of repair in ligaments has been little studied, despite the obvious clinical importance of ligamentous injuries.

Most workers have studied the effects of injuries of the various ligaments in the knee joint, using a variety of experimental animals (Miltner *et al.* 1937, Jack 1950, Clayton & Weir 1959, O'Donoghue *et al.* 1961, Clayton *et al.* 1968). When some fibres are torn, or the ligament is repaired, healing takes place in an orderly sequence. During the first week there is an inflammatory cell response; in the second to third weeks there is an invasion of fibroblasts and thereafter collagen is laid down and becomes orientated in the line of the ligament. This process is much slower if the ligament is completely torn and the end result is a diffuse, poorly organized scar tissue with little tensile strength. Intrasynovial ligaments such as the anterior cruciate may completely fail to heal if the stumps are not held in contact by surgical repair (O'Donoghue *et al.* 1964).

The tensile strength of ligaments continues to increase for several weeks after repair but then declines somewhat and is never as great as in the uninjured ligament.

References

Becker, H., Graham, M.F., Cohen, I.K. & Diegelmann, R.F. Intrinsic tendon cell proliferation in tissue culture. *J Hand Surg* 1981; **6**: 616–619.

Birdsell, D.C., Tustanoff, E.R. & Lindsay, W.K. Collagen production in regenerating tendon. *Plast Reconstr Surg* 1966; **37**: 504–511.

Canoso, J.J. Bursae, tendons and ligaments. *Clin Rheum Dis* 1981; **7(1)**: 189–221.

Chow, S.P., Hooper, G. & Chan, C.W. The healing of freeze-dried rabbit flexor tendon in a synovial fluid environment. *Hand* 1983; **15**: 136–142.

Clayton, M.L. & Weir, G.J. Experimental investigations of ligamentous healing. *Am J Surg* 1959; **98**: 373–378.

Clayton, M.L., Miles, J.S. & Abdulla, M. Experimental investigations of ligamentous healing. *Clin Orthop* 1968; **61**: 146–152.

Cooper, R.R. & Misol, S. Tendon and ligament insertion. *J Bone Joint Surg* 1970; **52A**: 1–20.

Elliott, D.H. Structure and function of mammalian tendon. *Biol Rev* 1965; **40**: 392–421.

Evans, P. The postural function of the iliotibial tract. *Ann R Coll Surg Engl* 1979; **61**: 271–280.

Hooper, G., Davies, R. & Tothill, P. Blood flow and clearance in tendons. *J Bone Joint Surg* 1984; **66B**: 441–443.

Jack, E.A. Experimental rupture of the medial collateral ligament of the knee. *J Bone Joint Surg* 1950; **32B**: 396–402.

Kennedy, J.C., Hawkins, R.J., Willis, R.B. & Danylchuk, K.D. Tension studies of human knee ligaments. Yield point, ultimate failure and disruption of the cruciate and tibial collateral ligaments. *J Bone Joint Surg* 1976; **58A**: 350–355.

Ketchum, L.D. Primary tendon healing. A review. *J Hand Surg* 1977; **2**: 428–435.

Lamb, D.W., Kuczynski, K. & Hooper, G. (eds) *The Practice of Hand Surgery* 2nd edn. Blackwell Scientific Publications: Oxford, 1988.

Lindsay, W.K. & Birch, J.R. The fibroblast in flexor tendon healing. *Plast Reconstr Surg* 1964; **34**: 223–232.

Lister, G.D., Kleinert, H.E., Kutz, J.E. & Atasoy, E. Primary flexor tendon repair followed by immediate controlled mobilization. *J Hand Surg* 1977; **2**: 441–451.

Lundborg, G. Experimental flexor tendon healing without adhesion formation — a new concept of tendon nutrition and intrinsic healing mechanism. *Hand* 1976; **8**: 235–238.

Lundborg, G. & Rank, F. Experimental studies on cellular mechanisms in healing tendons. *Hand* 1980; **12**: 3–11.

Lundborg, G., Holm, S. & Myrhage, R. The role of the synovial fluid and tendon sheath for flexor tendon nutrition. *Scand J Plast Reconstr Surg* 1980; **14**: 99–107.

Manske, P.R. & Lesker, P.A. Biochemical evidence of flexor tendon participating in the repair process. An *in vitro* study. *J Hand Surg* 1984; **9B**: 117–120.

Manske, P.R., Gelberman, R.H., Vande Bergh, J.S. & Lesker, P.A. Intrinsic flexor tendon repair. A morphologic study *in vitro*. *J Bone Joint Surg* 1984; **66A**: 385–396.

Mason, M.L. & Allen, H. The rate of healing of tendons; an experimental study of tensile strength. *Ann Surg* 1941; **113**: 424–459.

Matthews, P. & Richards, H. The repair potential of digital flexor tendons. *J Bone Joint Surg* 1974; **56B**: 618–625.

Matthews, P. & Richards, H. Factors in the adherence of flexor tendon after repair. *J Bone Joint Surg* 1976; **58B**: 230–236.

McDowell, G.L. & Snyder, D.M. Tendon healing: an experimental model in the dog. *J Hand Surg* 1977; **2**: 122–126.

McMaster, P.E. Tendon and muscle ruptures. *J Bone Joint Surg* 1933; **15**: 705–722.

Miltner, L.J., Hu, C.H. & Fang, H.C. Experimental joint strain. Pathologic study. *Arch Surg* 1937; **35**: 234–240.

Noyes, F.R., De Lucas, J.L. & Torvik, P.J. Biomechanics of anterior cruciate ligament failure: an analysis of strain rate sensitivity and mechanics of failure in primates. *J Bone Joint Surg* 1974; **56A**: 236–253.

O'Donoghue, D.H., Rockwood, C.A., Frank, G.R., Jack, S.C. & Kenyon, R. A study of repair of the knee ligaments in dogs. Part II. The anterior cruciate ligament. *J Bone Joint Surg* 1964; **46A**: 1362.

O'Donoghue, D.H., Rockwood, C.A., Zaricznyj, B. & Kenyon, R. Repair of knee ligaments in dogs. I. The lateral collateral ligament. *J Bone Joint Surg* 1961; **43A**: 1167–1178.

Peacock, E.E. Biology of tendon repair. *N Engl J Med* 1967; **276**: 680–683.

Potenza, A.D. Tendon healing within the flexor digital sheath in the dog. *J Bone Joint Surg* 1962; **44A**: 49–64.

Potenza, A.D. Critical evaluation of flexor-tendon healing and adhesion formation within artificial digital sheaths. *J Bone Joint Surg* 1963; **45A**: 1217–1233.

Potenza, A.D. & Herte, M.C. The synovial cavity as a "tissue culture *in situ*" — science or nonsense? *J Hand Surg* 1982; **7**: 196–199.

Potenza, A.D. & Melone, C. Evaluation of freeze-dried flexor tendon grafts in the dog. *J Hand Surg* 1978; **3**: 157–162.

Serafini-Fracassini, A., Field, J.M., Smith, J.W. & Stephens, W.G.S. The ultrastructure and mechanics of elastic ligaments. *Adv Exp Med Biol* 1976; **79**: 97–103.

Welsh, R.P., Macnab, I. & Riley, V. Biomechanical studies of rabbit tendon. *Clin Orthop* 1971; **81**: 171–177.

6: Systemic Response to Injury

J.C.STODDART

Acute cardiocirculatory failure

Shock is the term commonly used to describe a state of acute cardiocirculatory failure. It is a complex phenomenon and can only be described in outline here. More comprehensive reviews are referred to at the end of this chapter (Cowley & Trump 1982, Shires 1985, Barrett & Nyhus 1986, Ledingham & Ramsay 1986). It is usual to define three types of shock:
1 Haemorrhagic.
2 Septicaemic.
3 Cardiogenic.

In a previously fit patient the signs and symptoms of haemorrhagic shock usually do not appear until approximately 25% of the circulating blood volume has been abruptly lost. In less fit individuals the effects of a smaller blood loss may be recognizable.

Septicaemic shock is a much more subtle condition and will be described in some detail since it is all too common. It results either from an overwhelming infection, or from failure of the body's defence system to deal with a less obvious microbial invasion.

Cardiogenic shock follows infarction of a mass of left (rarely right) ventricular muscle after coronary thrombosis. It will not be considered further here.

The effects of shock are failure to meet the metabolic needs of organs and tissues. These needs include:
1 The delivery of oxygen, nutrients and other substances (hormones, vasoactive materials, etc.).
2 The removal of organic and inorganic waste products (CO_2, H^+, urea, etc.).
The results of supply failure are tissue starvation and auto-intoxication.

Patients with shock due to haemorrhage or myocardial infarction frequently have a reduced cardiac output initially; patients with shock due to sepsis have a normal or raised cardiac output until the terminal stages of the disorder.

Although the final result of haemorrhagic and septicaemic shock may be similar, haemorrhagic shock is a condition which usually has an identifiable initiation point, the treatment of which follows well-established lines and usually has a favourable outcome. Septicaemic shock is often less obvious in its onset and its management is much less satisfactory, as demonstrated by a mortality rate of approximately 70% (McCabe 1974, Hardaway 1981, Cowan *et al*. 1982, Cowley 1982, Cowan *et al*. 1984).

Cardiac output determinants

The main determinants of cardiac output are the venous return and the rate and force of cardiac contraction. The blood pressure (BP) is maintained by the cardiac output ($\dot{Q}$), the total peripheral resistance (TPR) and a viscosity factor k, i.e.

$$BP = \dot{Q} \times TPR\ (k).$$

A change in any one of the factors in this equation can be compensated by alteration of the others but this may lead to secondary harmful effects, as described later.

Haemorrhagic shock

Haemorrhagic shock has two phases. The first, which gives rise to the clinical signs of the condition, is associated with activation of the baroreceptor system by a fall in cardiac output. This is readily reversed by treatment but if it is not treated the patient may progress to the second phase of organ and tissue damage, which has long-term consequences. Baroreceptor activation is accompanied by the metabolic changes described later.

The baroreceptor system

The baroreceptor system (Fig. 6.1) has evolved to enable the cardiac output and blood pressure to change rapidly in response to changing demands, such as those which

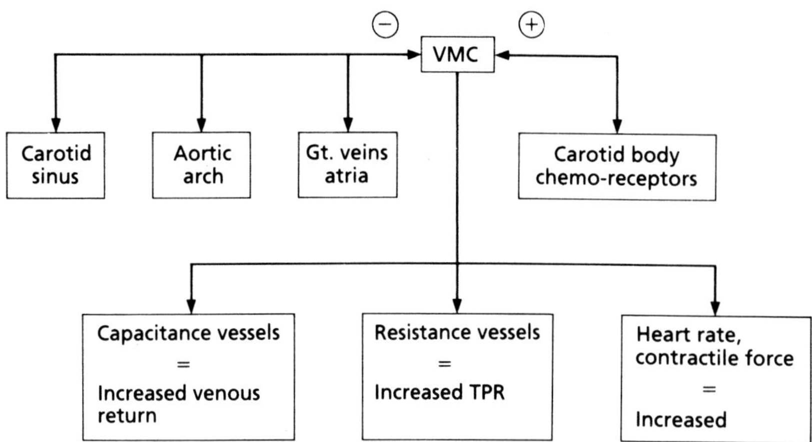

Fig. 6.1 The baroreceptor system. VMC, medullary vasomotor centre; TPR, total peripheral resistance.

follow change of posture or of physical activity. Under these circumstances it works well but it is not intended to cope with a sustained demand, when its responses may be less beneficial for the patient.

The components of the system are:
1 The medullary vasomotor centre (VMC).
2 Baroreceptors in the aortic arch, carotid sinus, great veins and atria.
3 The hypothalamus and autonomic nervous system.

The reactions of this system are reinforced by the renal juxta-glomerular apparatus, the hypothalamic—pituitary axis, the suprarenal glands, the pancreatic islets and other structures, some of which are mentioned below.

Under resting conditions the VMC is in a state of tonic inhibition and its output to the receptor sites (indicated in Fig. 6.1) is minimal. If for any reason the cardiac output or blood pressure falls (postural changes, haemorrhage, myocardial infarction, etc.) inhibition of the VMC is reduced and its output increases. This is shown by increased sympatho-adrenal activity, which is the cause of the early clinical features of shock which inlcude:
Apprehension, alertness.
Pallor.
Cold moist skin.
Tachycardia.
Increased force of cardiac contraction.
Increased TPR.
Contraction of capacitance vessels.
Selective diversion of blood flow.
Oliguria.

Activation of these mechanisms may initially maintain (or even increase) the blood pressure and cardiac output. Selective vasoconstriction ensures that the flow of blood to the brain, heart, lungs and muscles is preserved. This is at the expense of the skin and some other

viscera: in particular the renal blood flow is reduced causing renal ischaemia and oliguria.

The resistance vessels (Fig. 6.1) are the small arteries and arterioles; the capacitance vessels are the larger arteries and veins. Normally, two-thirds of the blood volume is contained within the capacitance vessels. Their contraction temporarily increases venous return; this is augmented by complete emptying of the ventricles with each systolic contraction.

The stress response to injury

Many of the less obvious or less immediate effects of trauma are collectively known as the stress response (Hinshaw 1971, Cuthbertson 1980a,b, Buckingham 1985, Knepel *et al.* 1985, Le Quesne *et al.* 1985, Shires 1985). This is mediated via the hypothalamic—pituitary system which is activated by the secretion of corticotrophin releasing factor (CRF) and other intermediary agents in response to a number of afferent stimuli which include:
Pain.
Fear.
Hypoxia.
Hypercapnia.
Hypoglycaemia.
Acidaemia.
Pyrexia/hypothermia.
Histamine.
Serotonin (5-hydroxytryptamine).
Antidiuretic hormone (ADH)—vasopressin.

Other mediators include some products of tissue injury. Amongst these are:
Bradykinin.
Kalikrein.
Thromboxane.
Prostaglandin $F_{1\alpha}$.
Bacterial toxins may have a similar effect.

The most obvious consequences of stress in the traumatized patient are catecholamine activity and increased corticotrophin release, followed by increased secretion of cortisol. Among other activities, cortisol augments the effects of adrenaline and noradrenaline on the contractility of myocardial and vascular smooth muscle. Gluconeogenesis from amino acids in the liver makes energy substrate available. Protein breakdown may be as great as 250 g in 24 hours. At the very high levels reached in the shocked patient, cortisol causes the renal tubules to retain sodium and water and excrete potassium.

Aldosterone secretion is controlled by three mechanisms: stimulation of the intrathoracic baroreceptors by hypovolaemia; reduced sodium intake; and the renin angiotensin system. When renal blood flow or pressure falls the renal juxta-glomerular body releases renin. Renin converts angiotensinogen to angiotensin I, which is converted to angiotensin II in the lung. In addition to its effects on aldosterone secretion, angiotensin is an effective vasoconstrictor.

Aldosterone causes sodium and water retention in exchange for potassium.

ADH—VASOPRESSIN

ADH—vasopressin is released from the posterior lobe of the pituitary and from the hypothalamus. Its secretion is influenced by factors which include:
Pain, fear.
Circulating catecholamines.
Intrathoracic baroreceptor stimulation.
Changes in plasma osmolality.
The effects of ADH vasopressin are:
1 To increase water reabsorption by the distal renal tubules.
2 To cause vasoconstriction (particularly in the renal cortex).
3 To increase the secretion of corticotrophin.

The baroreceptor and stress responses sustain the blood flow through vital organs and maintain the circulating blood volume and its osmolality. Prompt and effective resuscitation reverses all of the features of haemorrhagic shock; delayed or inadequate resuscitation inevitably permits organ and tissue damage.

OTHER HORMONAL EFFECTS

Shock increases the production of growth hormone, thyroxine and glucagon and inhibits insulin secretion. The consequences include hyperglycaemia and hyperlipidaemia; the benefits or otherwise of these effects are uncertain. Atrial natriuretic peptide (ANP) is produced by the right atrium in response to an increase in venous return. It is possible that a reduction in venous return may inhibit ANP secretion and help to maintain the circulating blood volume (Needleman *et al.* 1985).

The initial metabolic response to trauma or other injury causes a transient fall in metabolic rate (the 'ebb' phase). After 3—12 hours this is succeeded by a 'flow' (or hypercatabolic) phase which is associated with a greatly increased oxygen consumption, and which may last many hours or days (Cuthbertson 1980a,b).

The Starling diagram

Figure 6.2 (the Starling diagram) is a representation of the balance between the intravascular (hydrostatic) pressure and the plasma oncotic pressure across the capillary network. Under normal circumstances the excess hydrostatic pressure at the arteriolar end of the capillary forces fluid outwards; at the venular end the plasma oncotic pressure draws it back into the circulation. When the blood pressure falls, the hydrostatic pressure may be lower than the oncotic pressure and fluid may be drawn into the circulation throughout the length of the capillary. This increases the blood volume but, at the same time, it limits the transport of nutrients to the tissues. The diagram emphasizes the importance of the oncotic pressure, most of which is generated by the serum albumin.

The vascular unit

The distribution of blood to the tissues and organs is through vascular units; their number and reactivity depends upon the tissue supplied. For example, the viscera and muscle are more vascular than fat or skin. Figure 6.3 represents a vascular unit at four stages after activation of the VMC. In the diagram each unit consists of an arteriole which supplies three capillaries which are drained by a venule. In some tissues the capillary network can be short-circuited by an arteriovenous anastomosis. Pre- and post-capillary sphincters are shown; although only the former has been demonstrated histologically, indirect evidence suggests that there is also a post-capillary sphincter.

The flow through the capillary bed is controlled by the hydrostatic pressure, the oncotic pressure and sphincter tone. The latter is influenced by catecholamines and substances produced locally, which include carbon dioxide and hydrogen ions, accumulation of which causes the sphincters to relax. Tissue hypoxia has the same effect.

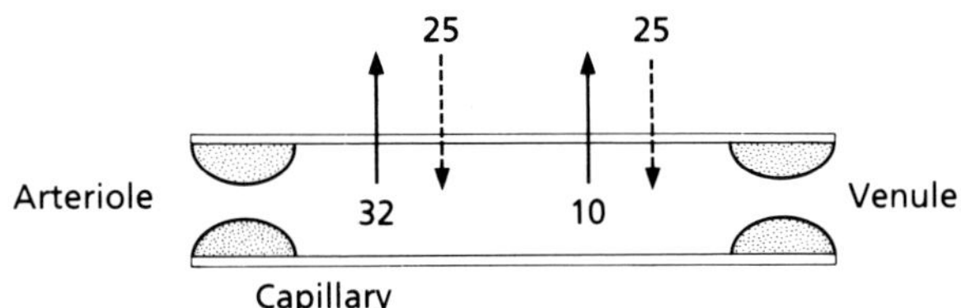

Fig. 6.2 The Starling diagram.

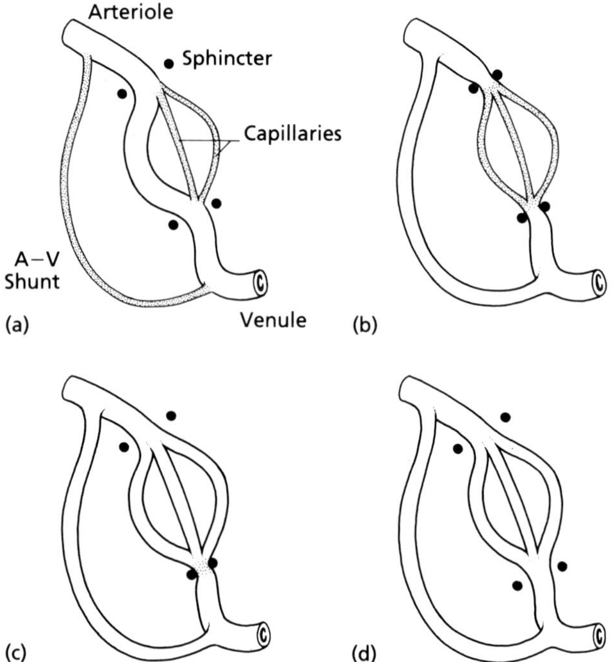

Fig. 6.3 The vascular unit. (a) Normal. (b) Vasoconstriction. (c) Stagnation. (d) Reflow.

The vasomotor response

The four stages of the vasomotor response are indicated in Fig. 6.3. The resting pattern is shown in Fig. 6.3a, with the arteriovenous shunt closed and only one of the capillaries open. Figure 6.3b shows the first stage of the response to activation of the vasomotor centre. Vasoconstriction, which causes a rise in TPR, is accompanied by cessation of capillary blood flow. The blood which flows through the arteriovenous shunt bypasses the tissues which become hypoxic and begin to suffer from auto-intoxication. Prompt resuscitation will reverse these changes completely, but if it is delayed, the pre-capillary sphincter opens while the post-capillary sphincter remains closed (Fig. 6.3c). Blood enters the capillaries and stagnates. The hydrostatic pressure forces fluid and albumin out of the capillaries. The stagnant blood becomes hypoxic and its carbon dioxide tension

and acidity rise; other substances (bradykinin, prostaglandin $F_{2\alpha}$, etc.) accumulate. The plasma lactate may be raised because of tissue ischaemia (Counts *et al.* 1979, Cowan *et al.* 1982, Hillman 1986). Disseminated intravascular coagulation (DIC) may be initiated. In Fig. 6.3d the post-capillary sphincter has finally relaxed, allowing the stagnant blood to re-enter the circulation, carrying with it metabolic waste products. By this time vulnerable organs, particularly the kidneys and liver, will have been damaged. This is the second stage of shock.

Shock and the heart

The work done by the heart depends upon its rate and force of contraction and the TPR. These are increased in the shocked patient. Coronary artery perfusion occurs principally during diastole and is reduced by tachycardia. Young patients with good cardiac reserve should come to no harm, but the elderly or arteriopathic patient may quickly demonstrate clinical, biochemical and electrocardiographic signs of myocardial ischaemia.

There is laboratory evidence which suggests that venous blood from ischaemic tissues contains vasodepressor materials which further reduce cardiac output (Lefer 1978).

Thus, shock both increases the demands upon the heart and reduces its efficiency.

Shock and the lung

This is discussed in detail later (see pp. 298–307).

Shock and the kidneys

Under normal circumstances the kidneys receive approximately 20% of the total cardiac output, with 90% of this being distributed to the renal cortex. When the cardiac output or blood pressure falls, renal blood flow is reduced and the urine output is diminished. Catecholamine secretion causes renal vasoconstriction and oliguria, which is accentuated by the secretion of cortisol, aldosterone and ADH–vasopressin. These processes are reversed by adequate fluid replacement, but if they are allowed to persist, renal failure may develop (prerenal failure) (Kerr & Elliott 1974, Kraman *et al.* 1979, Stoddart 1982, Brenner & Lazarus 1983, Lefer 1983).

If the patient has suffered burns or extensive crush injuries hypotensive vasoconstriction may be aggravated by myoglobinuria. Muscle damage and myoglobin can cause renal failure in the absence of prolonged hypotension and vasoconstriction (Kerr & Elliott 1974, Kraman *et al.* 1979, Brenner & Lazarus 1983).

Shock may cause either acute tubular necrosis (ATN, acute 'reversible' renal failure) or acute cortical necrosis (ACN, acute 'irreversible' renal failure). The distinction may sometimes be made only when the patient either regains or fails to regain renal function. Renal biopsy may be helpful if the condition persists.

DIC (consumption coagulopathy) may cause cortical necrosis. DIC occasionally follows uncomplicated trauma and prolonged intravascular stasis, but more frequently it is associated with systemic sepsis; it may also follow an incompatible blood transfusion (Kerr & Elliott 1974).

RECOGNITION OF ACUTE RENAL FAILURE

A patient is in renal failure when failing to excrete enough urine to maintain fluid balance and to keep the plasma electrolyte, urea and creatinine levels within normal limits. The volume of urine which is needed to achieve homeostasis is not constant: a patient who is normothermic and at rest needs to pass a smaller volume than one who is pyrexial or has recently undergone major surgery or multiple injuries. A figure of 0.5 ml kg^{-1} h^{-1} is usually said to be adequate, but even twice this volume may be insufficient.

The patient's renal function should be assessed daily during the acute phase of any major physical disturbance. No single test is conclusive, and it is usual for a battery of tests to be performed (Table 6.1). For the creatinine clearance to be measured, a 24-hour urine collection must be sent to the laboratory. The other tests can be performed on spot samples of blood and urine. The patient with pre-renal failure usually passes urine which has a high osmolality (more than 350 mosmol l^{-1}), whereas the patient with intrinsic renal failure almost always passes urine with an osmolality of less than 350 mosmol l^{-1}.

PROGNOSIS OF ACUTE RENAL FAILURE

After an episode of ATN most patients who are less than 30 years of age should regain normal renal function, but the older the patient the less complete the degree of recovery. However, for many reasons (including the fact that the patient with acute renal failure frequently had dysfunction of other organs, such as the lung) the overall survival rate is still unsatisfactory. Only a very small minority of patients of any age who develop ACN can expect to regain adequate renal function.

Table 6.1 Renal function tests

Urine volume	At least 0.5 ml kg^{-1} h^{-1}
$\dfrac{\text{Urine osmolality}}{\text{Blood osmolality}}$	At least $\dfrac{1.2}{1}$
$\dfrac{\text{Urine urea}}{\text{Blood urea}}$	Greater than $\dfrac{13}{1}$
Creatinine clearance	Greater than 30 l/24 h

Shock and the liver

The effects of shock upon hepatic function are less immediately apparent than those upon the kidney, but they may carry an even worse prognosis (Mela *et al.* 1971).

The liver obtains only 30% of its oxygen supply from the hepatic artery, the remainder being provided by the portal vein. It is easily damaged by arterial hypotension and by splanchnic vasoconstriction and stagnation. Splanchnic vasostagnation also encourages the absorption of bacterial endotoxin from the gut, which may aggravate liver damage. Endotoxin from the gut is normally destroyed by the hepatic reticuloendothelial system, but this is easily damaged by ischaemia and hypoxia.

Evidence of hepatocellular damage may be obtained from the coagulation screen and liver function tests. Unless these are carried out routinely jaundice may be the first sign of liver damage. This may be due to haemolysis of transfused blood or absorption of haematoma but jaundice which is due to shock or septicaemia has a very bad prognosis.

Stress peptic ulceration

Stress peptic ulceration of the gastric or duodenal mucosa occurs in many patients who have suffered major trauma or sepsis (Lucas *et al.* 1971, Le Gall *et al.* 1976, Priebe *et al.* 1980). This may manifest itself either as haematemesis or melaena, or by a progressive fall in the patient's haemoglobin level, together with occult blood in the stool or gastric aspirate. The causes include increased gastric acidity due to stress and an increased plasma cortisol level, although reduced mucosal blood flow may be important. There is also an increased secretion of gastrins. Inability to take food by mouth reduces the neutralizing effect of foodstuffs against gastric acid. Although emotional stress may play a part, patients who are deeply sedated or unconscious may develop stress ulceration. Every patient who has suffered a major physical insult should routinely be given an H_2-receptor blocker or regular antacids until they are able to eat and drink normally.

Monitoring of haemorrhagic shock

Cardiocirculatory monitoring

The objectives of monitoring are to recognize and record the changes in organ and tissue perfusion as they occur. Many techniques are available, some of which can be used in unsophisticated establishments whilst others are applicable in only a few of the most highly specialized research and treatment centres.

ESSENTIAL INVESTIGATIONS

Cardiocirculatory monitoring requires the recording of pulse rate and rhythm, the electrocardiogram (ECG) pattern and systemic blood pressure. Intra-arterial monitoring is the most reliable method, but indirect ultrasonic or oscillotonometric methods are satisfactory.

Other fundamental investigations must be carried out. These include:

1 Core−skin temperature measurement.
2 Urine output per hour and its osmolality.
3 Central venous pressure (CVP) in response to a fluid challenge.
4 Blood gases, hydrogen ion status and alveolar/arterial (Aa) oxygen tension gradient.
5 Chest radiograph.
6 Blood sugar.
7 Plasma lactate.
8 Cardiac enzymes.
9 Serum amylase.
10 Coagulation screen.

Core−skin temperature measurement

This gradient gives a good indication of the cardiac output (Joly & Weil 1969). The core temperature is recorded with a thermistor probe inserted into the external auditory canal or into the oesophagus at 24 cm from the teeth (in the adult). Probes should be inserted with care since damage to the eardrum or oesophagus is possible. The skin temperature is measured on the dorsum of the hand or foot. The difference should not exceed 3°C unless the patient has been exposed to a low environmental temperature. If the gap is greater than 3°C, the cardiac output and peripheral perfusion are probably reduced and it should narrow in response to infusion. If, in spite of apparently adequate fluid re-

placement, the gap is greater than 3°C and the CVP is high or rising, alpha-blocking drugs may be required (see p. 98). Patients who are suffering from septicaemic shock do not usually have a wide core−skin temperature difference until the preterminal phase of the illness.

CVP monitoring

The CVP level is a guide to right ventricular function, but only when measured in response to the fluid challenge. By itself it does not indicate the state of the circulating blood volume and the practice of 'filling up the CVP' to some predetermined level should be abandoned. If the other indices of organ function are satisfactory (the pulse rate and blood pressure, the core−skin temperature difference and the urine output), the CVP is usually acceptable. It is very easy to overtransfuse patients during the acute stage of resuscitation. The signs of overtransfusion include a triple rhythm audible at the apex of the heart and basal pulmonary crepitations.

The fluid challenge is performed as follows: 200 ml of a suitable fluid (plasma protein fraction (PPF), gelatin, solution, dextran) are infused over 15 minutes; if the CVP rises and does not return to its previous level after a further 15 minutes the infusion rate should be reduced. If the CVP rises but falls again to its previous level after 15 minutes, the central circulation can probably accept further fluid.

Other investigations

The other tests listed are performed for the reasons which have been suggested. Deterioration in respiratory function must be identified as soon as it develops, since this may be due to adult respiratory distress syndrome (ARDS). The blood sugar level should be maintained at the upper limit of normal throughout this critical period to provide a readily available source of calories.

In all but the most complex cases of haemorrhagic shock the monitoring methods described above will provide all the information which is necessary for treatment to be applied. Less essential information may be provided by pulmonary wedge pressure measurement and by cardiac output determination.

Pulmonary wedge pressure measurement

With flow-directed balloon catheters the pulmonary wedge pressure can be measured (Swan *et al.* 1970, Gilbertson 1974). It provides information about the function of the left ventricle and should be taken together with CVP measurement, urine output and core–skin temperature measurement. These data indicate when further transfusion is needed, or when inotropic agents such as dopamine and dobutamine should be used. The normal wedge pressure range is less than 10 mmHg and if it rises above this level during resuscitation, the patient may be fluid overloaded. If pulmonary oedema occurs at a pressure lower than 15 mmHg, ARDS or hypoalbuminaemia are the likely causes (see pp. 298–307).

When multifunction balloon catheters are used, the cardiac output can be calculated by the thermal dilution method and mixed venous blood can be obtained so that tissue oxygen extraction can be calculated. This is of particular value in septicaemic shock, when the arteriovenous oxygen content difference is often less than would be expected from the cardiac output. The risks from pulmonary wedge pressure monitoring are higher than those which accompany CVP monitoring. When the balloon is inflated up to 15% of the blood supply of one lung is occluded and the balloon should be deflated immediately after each measurement has been made. Complications include local and systemic infection, pulmonary infarction, haemorrhage, knotting of the catheter leading to difficulty with withdrawal, cardiac rupture, tamponade and many dysrhythmias (Robin 1985).

Aortovelography

Cardiac output may be measured by the reflection of ultrasound from blood flowing through the aortic arch or pulmonary artery, with the aid of an external sensor system, or with one which is placed in the oesophagus. At the present time this method is only available in centres which are financially well endowed.

Treatment of haemorrhagic shock

Volume replacement

The treatment of haemorrhagic shock is based upon fluid replacement. Until recently it was taught that blood should be replaced as it was lost so as to maintain both the circulating blood volume and its haemoglobin content. However, there is evidence which suggests that there are benefits to be obtained by deliberate haemodilution, although the optimum haematocrit is not known with certainty (Crowell & Smith 1967, Fan *et al.* 1980). Patients whose cardiac output is limited by diseases such as constrictive pericarditis or valvular disease, or those for whom a tachycardia would en-

danger myocardial oxygenation, may require a higher haematocrit. For most other patients it is generally agreed that a haemoglobin level of around 10 g or a haematocrit of around 35% is quite adequate (Shoemaker 1976, Smith & Norman 1982). The filtration of stored blood is probably unnecessary (Derrington 1985).

The choice of blood volume expander

If the patient has suffered a major blood loss of more than 25% of the blood volume, some of this should be replaced in the form of whole blood. Some of the colloid blood substitutes which are available are shown in Table 6.2.

If it were freely available PPF would be the blood volume expander of choice. The gelatin derivatives have a mean molecular weight of around 30 000. Because of this they are quickly cleared from the circulation by the kidneys. Dextran 70 (mean molecular weight 70 000) remains in the circulation for approximately 6 hours. Allergic reactions to gelatin and dextrans occur with similar low frequencies (Ring & Messmer 1977). Hydroxyethyl starch (HES, Hetastarch) has been available for a relatively short time. Its molecular weight ranges between 30 000 and 150 000. A significant proportion of HES stays in the circulation for 24 hours or more and its ultimate fate is not known.

The argument as to whether colloidal fluids (e.g. PPF, gelatin, etc.) are better than crystalloids for resuscitation is not yet resolved (Smith & Norman 1982, Hillman 1986). At present, the evidence suggests that if the patient has normal renal function it may be less dangerous to overtransfuse with crystalloid than with colloid, since the latter seems more likely to cause persistent overload and pulmonary oedema. However, provided that overload is avoided, colloid solutions have other advantages which are discussed in the later section on septicaemic shock (Shoemaker 1976).

Blood conservation (autotransfusion)

Whole blood is scarce and homologous blood transfusion carries many risks, including acquired immune deficiency syndrome (AIDS). There is therefore an increasing tendency to attempt to conserve the patient's blood during surgery and re-infuse it. A number of relatively simple and safe techniques are available. These are principally used during intrathoracic and transplant surgery. They must never be used if there is any chance of bacterial contamination of the blood (Orr 1982, Davies & Cronin 1984).

Table 6.2 Commonly used infusion fluids

	Blood	PPF	Dextran 40	Dextran 70	Gelatine products	HES
Availability	Variable	Variable	Good	Good	Good	Variable
Cost	High	High	Modest	Modest	Modest	High
Hepatitis risk	Present	Absent	—	—	—	—
Allergenicity	Present	Rare	+	++	+	?
Microembolism risk	Present	—	—	—	—	—
Oxygen carriage	Yes, but varies	No	No	No	No	No
Albumin content	30 g l^{-1}	30 g l^{-1}	—	—	—	—
Duration of action as blood volume expander	24 h	12 h	2 h	4 h	2 h	24 h +
Sodium	140 mmol l^{-1}	140 mmol l^{-1}	Available in normal saline or dextrose			140 mmol l^{-1}
Potassium	$3-4$ mmol l^{-1} up to 20 mmol l^{-1}	$2.2-2.4$ mmol l^{-1}	—	—	—	—
Calcium	$0.5-1.5$ mmol l^{-1}	—	—	$3-4$ mmol l^{-1}	—	
Special problems	Microaggregates 2,3-DPG, etc.	May cause renal damage	Cross-match problems	Immiscible with blood	Cross-match problems	

2,3-DPG, 2,3-diphosphoglycerate.

The use of pharmacological agents in haemorrhagic shock

In most cases restoration of the circulating blood volume is all that is required. However, it may be necessary to use drugs to assist cardiac output and regional blood flow.

DOPAMINE

Dopamine stimulates both alpha- and beta-adreno-receptors, but it is usually given because of its vaso-dilatory effects upon the renal dopaminergic receptors. It is a very safe drug and should be used early rather than late; in many centres a dopamine infusion is begun prophylactically in any patient at risk of renal failure. When given at the rate of $2-5$ µg kg^{-1} min^{-1} it has minimal effects upon pulse rate and rhythm or upon blood pressure, but it improves renal blood flow and often causes a diuresis (Henderson *et al.* 1980, Foex 1983).

Dopamine should be given by syringe pump or by a similar device and it should always be infused through a central line because if it extravasates it can cause extensive tissue necrosis (Barrett & Nyhus 1986).

DOBUTAMINE

Dobutamine is primarily a beta-1 agonist which improves cardiac output by increasing the force of cardiac contraction. In the normal therapeutic dose it has little effect upon heart rate and rhythm and, because its alpha stimulant effects are trivial, it can safely be given through a peripheral vein if necessary. The recommended dose ranges from 2.5 to 10 µg kg^{-1} min^{-1} (Foex 1983). It has no specific effects on renal blood flow but may cause a diuresis by increasing the cardiac output. It may be given together with dopamine in the early stages of treatment of septicaemic shock.

ISOPRENALINE

Isoprenaline is a beta-1 agonist which also has beta-2 effects. It is an effective vasodilator but it has largely been superseded by dobutamine except for patients in refractory asystole. It usually causes a tachycardia and may cause other tachydysrhythmias. In addition to its vasodilatory effects on the peripheral circulation it reduces pulmonary arteriolar pressure. It is given by infusion at a rate of 0.05 µg kg^{-1} min^{-1}.

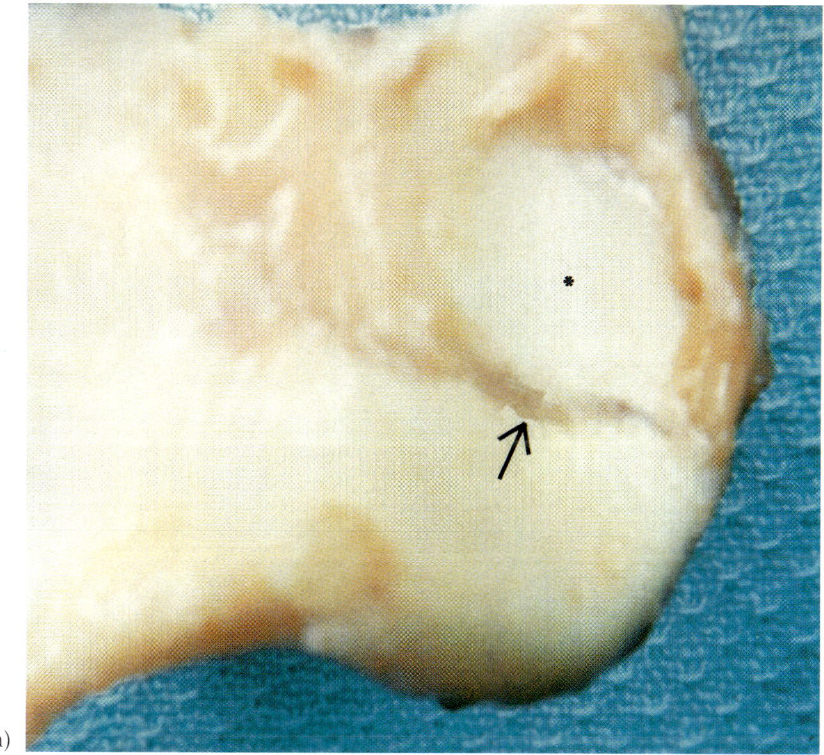

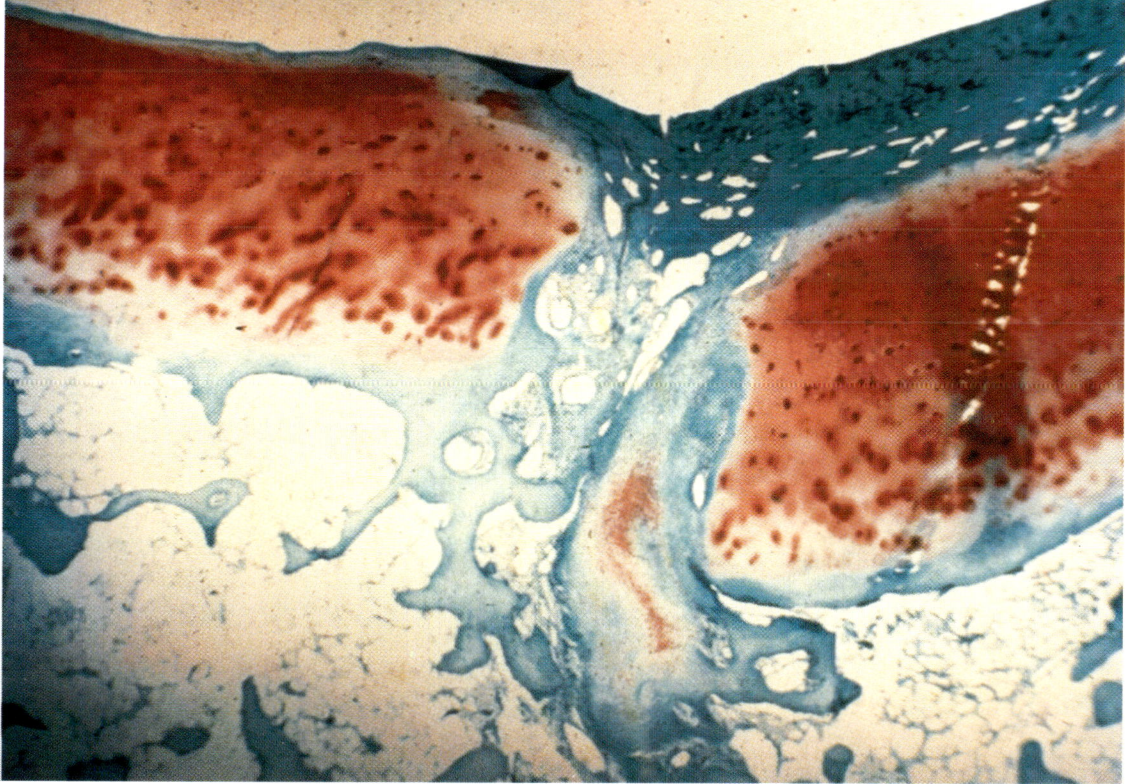

Plate 5.1 Old olecranon fracture treated by revision surgery. (a) Surgical specimen showing normal olecranon articular cartilage (*) and the fracture defect filled by repair tissue (arrow). (b) Low power photomicrograph of the fracture site demonstrating superficial fibrous tissue and deeper fibrocartilage filling the defect. Although the defect is of the deep penetrating type, the articular cartilage repair within the defect is incomplete and the articular step-off has been 'corrected' entirely with fibrous tissue. Proteoglycan-containing cartilage is stained red. Safranin-o-fast green-iron haematoxylin.

[*facing page 98*]

The use of diuretics

Diuretics such as frusemide are not therapeutic agents; they do not cure acute renal failure and there is no firm evidence that they protect the patient against impending renal damage (Kerr & Elliott 1974, Brenner & Lazarus 1983).

Mannitol is an effective osmotic diuretic which is often used prophylactically during operations upon arteriopathic patients, and in hepato-renal failure. It is also a blood volume expander and should not be given to a patient who is volume-overloaded since it may precipitate heart failure.

Alpha-adrenergic blockade

The best peripheral vasodilator is an adequate circulating blood volume, but a patient who has been in peripheral circulatory failure for more than 1 or 2 hours may not respond immediately to simple blood volume replacement. The patient's extremities may remain cold and blue in spite of a rising CVP. These may be indications for the use of alpha-adrenergic blocking agents (Henderson *et al.* 1980, Foex 1983). Phenoxybenzamine is the best known member of this group of drugs (Hardaway 1980). It is usually given by infusion at the rate of 10 mg kg^{-1} h^{-1} after an initial loading dose of 0.5 mg kg^{-1}. It has a duration of action of 6–8 hours and its action cannot easily be reversed.

Chlorpromazine is an effective and safe vasodilator in the dose range 5–25 mg given intravenously.

Chlorpromazine or specific alpha-adrenergic blockers must not be given until the patient has been adequately transfused, as demonstrated by the fluid balance chart and generous allowance should be given for occult losses. The CVP and/or pulmonary wedge pressure must be high.

Alpha-stimulant drugs (methoxamine, noradrenaline, metaraminol, methyl amphetamine, etc.) and corticosteroids are no longer used in the treatment of either haemorrhagic or septicaemic shock.

Other aids to treatment of haemorrhagic shock

THE SPACE BLANKET

This is a lightweight aluminized sheet which is widely used by campers and climbers as a substitute for conventional bedding. In hospital it is used to wrap patients who are hypothermic as a result of trauma (with or without exposure) or surgical procedures. It has become standard practice to wrap a 'space blanket' around any patient who shows signs of peripheral or central cooling. If the patient's core temperature rises and the skin temperature remains static, the space blanket should be removed since the core temperature may overshoot.

THE 'G' SUIT

This is an inflatable double-layered plastic bag which is wrapped around the patient in order to apply external counterpressure. Several sizes are available and it should envelop the patient from the nipple line to the ankles. It is inflated to 30 cm water pressure and is used to arrest retroperitoneal or intramuscular bleeding such as may occur from pelvic, lumbar or closed lower limb injuries. It is most frequently used for the pre- and postoperative care of patients with leaking abdominal aortic aneurysms and it can be effectively used to aid the safe transport of injured patients. It has no place in the treatment of intra-abdominal, as distinct from retroperitoneal, bleeding. It may be applied for periods in excess of 24 hours, and although when it is properly used it does not interfere with spontaneous ventilation, most patients who require this form of treatment can benefit from controlled ventilation.

The 'G' suit can cause skin necrosis and it must be carefully applied, with particular attention being paid to contact points between the knees and ankles, which should be separated by sponge pads.

The medical anti shock trousers (MAST) suit is a similar device which may have some advantages. The lower part of the suit is divided into two which allows it to be used as a splint during transport of a patient.

Trauma and sepsis

A patient who has suffered an injury is at risk from sepsis from two sources:
1 The injury itself.
2 Treatment of the injury (McCabe 1974, Cowley & Trump 1982).

Major trauma reduces the body's resistance to infection by impairing the production of antibacterial antibody and complement and by reducing leukocyte mobility and phagocytosis. These effects are sustained by the high level of cortisol secretion. There is evidence that burned tissue produces a specific toxin which interferes with defence against infection.

The injury itself may increase the risk of infection. If the wound is grossly contaminated, or if the integrity of the gastrointestinal or genitourinary tracts is interrupted, an obvious source of systemic infection is created. Patients who have been immersed in polluted water are exposed to a similar hazard.

Surgical operations and the treatment of many injuries involves the use of invasive techniques or the insertion of foreign materials into tissues. Many of the procedures which are performed for resuscitative, monitoring or therapeutic purposes are potential sources of infection. Intravenous therapy, intravascular monitoring, prolonged endotracheal intubation, tracheostomy, chest drainage and the use of urinary catheters increase the hazard of local and systemic infection.

Septic shock

Septic shock is cardiocirculatory failure due either to an overwhelming bacterial infection or to a less severe bacteriological assault on a patient with reduced resistance. The term 'endotoxic shock' is less satisfactory since shock due to organisms which do not produce an endotoxin (e.g. *Staphylococcus aureus* and *Streptococcus pneumoniae*) is not materially different from that due to *Escherichia coli*.

A fundamental distinction between septic and haemorrhagic shock is that in septicaemia the disturbance begins at the cellular level and all of the tissues and organs are affected simultaneously, though not necessarily to the same degree, by the agents which cause the syndrome. Although the baroreceptors and other components described earlier may be activated in septic shock, many additional factors are involved. Endotoxin is a lipopolysaccharide which originates in the outer membranes of Gram-negative bacteria such as *E. coli* and *Pseudomonas aeruginosa*. *Staph. aureus* produces an alpha-haemolysin which may cause circulatory collapse. No comparable material has yet been identified from organisms such as *Strep. pneumoniae* or the meningococcus.

Other substances may be of secondary importance, arising directly or indirectly from damaged tissues, but they may help to perpetuate or complicate the disturbance. They include lysosomal breakdown products, vasodepressor material (VDM), bradykinin and other tissue kinins, thromboxane, proteinases and prostaglandins (Cowley & Trump 1982, Lefer 1983). Serotonin and histamine released from damaged platelets undoubtedly play a part. Some of these substances are also released in the second phase of haemorrhagic shock.

Other mediators of septic shock

In addition to those mentioned above, a number of other mediators have been found to be involved in the production of the signs and symptoms which typify septic shock. These particularly include the increased cellular permeability which leads to pulmonary and systemic oedema, and the failure of the cardiovascular system to respond to the circulating and fixed catecholamines, i.e. resistant vasodilatation and hypotension.

Tumour necrosis factor (TNF, cachectin) is a cytokine which is secreted by macrophages which have been activated by lipopolysaccharide (LPS, endotoxin), other bacterial products, and also during haemorrhagic shock. In experiments, it has been shown to produce all of the typical features of sepsis, including 'third spaces losses' and the pulmonary changes of the adult respiratory distress syndrome (see pp. 298–307). TNF also facilitates the secretion of prostaglandins, leucotrienes, platelet activating factor and complement C5a and initiates the coagulation cascade. All of these are identifiable during the stages of septic shock (Tracey *et al.* 1986, Rothstein & Schreiber 1988). Monoclonal antibodies to TNF have been raised, and it was hoped that these would be useful in treatment, but they were found to increase mortality overall and were withdrawn from use.

Interleukin 1 is a cytokine which is also produced by macrophages in the presence of LPS. It may be responsible for some of the other features of sepsis, including negative nitrogen balance, pyrexia and neutrophil leucocytosis (Dinarello 1984).

Nitric oxide is generated in damaged cells by TNF and by some cytokines. This substance is also produced during normal cellular activity and plays a part in physiological regulation of vascular smooth muscle tone. However, there is good evidence that in sepsis it is an important cause of the resistant vasodilatation and hypotension referred to earlier, i.e. that it is the endothelium-derived relaxant factor identified by many researchers (Palmer *et al.* 1987; Ochoa *et al.* 1991).

Mode of presentation of septic shock

It usually has an insidious onset, although occasionally it may present as sudden collapse during the course of urinary catheterization, bouginage, cytoscopy or similar procedures. The orthopaedic patient with multiple injuries or with an infected prosthesis is particularly at risk.

Hypotension, tachycardia and pyrexia are prominent features in most cases ('warm shock'); the degree of diastolic hypotension is disproportionate (e.g. BP 80/20) and in many cases the second Korotkof sound cannot be heard. This is a manifestation of peripheral vasodilatation and at this stage the cardiac output is usually elevated. Other signs include mental clouding, confusion, coma and occasionally, grand mal fits. In most cases oliguria is noted and other signs of renal impairment can usually be identified in those patients who are not oliguric. The relationship of shock, sepsis and jaundice has already been referred to.

In the early stages of septic shock the patient has a respiratory alkalaemia with hypocapnia and hypoxia, with an increased Aa oxygen tension gradient. The causes of respiratory impairment in sepsis are discussed later. The arteriovenous oxygen content difference is reduced, which indicates that the cardiac output is increased and that tissue oxygen extraction is subnormal. If the condition does not respond to treatment the patient usually develops a non-respiratory acidaemia, with an elevated blood lactate, together with hypoxaemia which is resistant to all forms of oxygen therapy. Other signs of multiple organ failure are also identifiable. Leukopenia, thrombocytopenia and DIC are common at this stage and are bad prognostic signs (McCabe 1974, Hardaway 1981).

The small proportion of patients who die during the acute phase of septic shock pass from the stage of 'warm shock' to that of acute peripheral circulatory failure ('cold shock') which is resistant to treatment with blood volume expanders and pharmacological agents.

The 'capillary leak' syndrome

Within 1–3 days of its onset, most patients with septic shock show some evidence of the 'capillary leak' syndrome (Ellman 1984). This can be recognized by the appearance of oedema of the face, limbs and flanks, and from radiographic evidence of interstitial pulmonary oedema, accompanied by hypoxaemia. This syndrome is presumed to be caused by the toxic substances listed earlier, which increase capillary permeability by an effect upon either the intercellular cement or the cell wall itself.

Endotoxin is too large a molecule to enter undamaged cells but it probably activates intermediary agents. It also increases the severity of post-capillary venospasm, thus increasing the hydrostatic factor of the Starling equation and aggravating the loss of fluid and albumin from the intravascular compartment. Other studies have demonstrated that patients with septicaemia may lose up to 20% of their serum albumin in each 24 hours. This is partly due to diminished food intake and hypercatabolism, but liver damage and loss of albumin into the interstitial tissues, particularly the lungs, are equally important (Ellman 1984).

Other factors which are involved in the generation of oedema during the acute phase of resuscitation include fluid overload due to an attempt to provoke a diuresis in the oliguric patient. If the patient is receiving intermittent positive pressure ventilation from a ventilator, this may cause periorbital and conjunctival oedema.

With the treatment, described below, most patients with shock due to sepsis should survive the acute phase but up to 70% die days or weeks later from the combination of respiratory, renal and hepatic failure, together with chronic sepsis ('multiple organ failure') (Stoddart 1982, 1988).

Treatment of septicaemic shock

The principles that govern the treatment of this condition are:
1 Maintenance of the circulating blood volume.
2 Support of organ function.
3 Control of the underlying infection.

Volume replacement

Many patients are already hypovolaemic before they develop the signs of septicaemic shock and this must be corrected; others may appear to require large volume transfusions without having lost much fluid externally. This is the main feature of the 'capillary leak' syndrome and indicates that great caution should be observed when planning further infusions (Ellman 1984). The monitoring which was described earlier is also necessary for the septicaemic patient but, in addition, the haematocrit must be measured every 3–6 hours during resuscitation as a guide to plasma losses. If the haematocrit rises inappropriately during resuscitation it indicates that capillary leakage with plasma loss has begun, or that fluid is being lost into closed compartments such as the pleural or peritoneal cavity. Systemic and pulmonary oedema are prominent features of septicaemia.

Choice of volume expander

PPF is the first-choice plasma volume expander for the septicaemic patient, although whole blood may also be required. Even when supplements are given the albumin level may fall below 30 g l^{-1}. The use of albumin solutions in the septicaemic patient has been criticized on the basis that they may aggravate rather than prevent or reduce interstitial pulmonary oedema. This is a difficult problem, but at present it appears to be more logical to use oncotically active agents (colloids) rather than crystalloids in this situation (Hillman 1986).

Use of digoxin and other agents

Both experimental and clinical evidence indicate that every patient with septicaemia and a tachycardia should be digitalized. Because of the high incidence of renal impairment the plasma digoxin level should be monitored after 2 days of treatment with this drug.

The use of dopamine in the shocked patient was described earlier. The indications for its use in septicaemia are similar to those already given, particularly with regard to the prophylaxis and treatment of renal impairment; it may also be used in a higher dose (up to 10 µg kg^{-1} min^{-1}) to support the systemic circulation. When the patient's condition has stabilized the dopamine infusion should be discontinued gradually.

Occasionally a patient is found to have a low ionized calcium level (when corrected for the serum albumin). Although this is of doubtful significance, calcium chloride injections may bring about an improvement in cardiocirculatory function.

Controlled ventilation in septicaemic shock

Of all forms of treatment of septicaemic shock, none has so much improved the prognosis of what is still a lethal condition as the early institution of oxygen therapy and recognition of the need for controlled ventilation. Septicaemia is always associated with a widening of the Aa oxygen tension gradient and if it progresses severe hypoxia is inevitable, leading to irreversible damage to the kidneys, liver and other organs (Stoddart 1988). Every patient with septicaemia should be admitted to the Intensive Therapy Unit because they may have to be intubated and ventilated with oxygen-enriched air (see pp. 298–307). The indications for this treatment include radiographic evidence of pulmonary infiltration with an arterial oxygen tension of less than 7 kPa, when the patient is breathing room air. The causes of respiratory failure in septicaemic patients are listed in Table 6.3.

Control of the underlying infection

This is the most difficult part of the treatment of septicaemia. The factors which are associated with septicaemia are set out in Table 6.4. Although these include the primary cause, including the surgical procedure, many of them are inseparable from septicaemia treatment, including the use of intravenous and intra-arterial lines, endotracheal intubation, intermittent positive pressure ventilation (IPPV) and urinary catheterization. Every form of invasive treatment or monitoring must be balanced against its possible side-effects and dis-

Table 6.3 Reasons for respiratory failure in the septicaemic patient

Fluid overload
Atelectasis
Bronchopneumonia
Hypoproteinaemia
Pulmonary microembolism/microthrombosis/ARDS
Interstitial oedema
Increased metabolic rate/oxygen consumption
Reduced efficiency of the respiratory muscles
Ventilation/perfusion imbalance
Increased alveolar dead space
Intra-abdominal sepsis and diaphragmatic splinting

ARDS, acute respiratory distress syndrome.

Table 6.4 Factors involved in the development of septic shock

Pre-existing factors: diabetes, leukaemia, malignant disease
Extremes of age
Severity of injury, including burns, surgery, compound fractures
Abdominal or genitourinary tract involvement
Invasive monitoring
Intravenous therapy, including intravenous nutrition
Bladder catheterization, endotracheal intubation, tracheostomy, IPPV
Inappropriate antibiotic therapy
Immunosuppressive and corticosteroid drugs

IPPV, intermittent positive pressure ventilation.

continued as soon as possible. Intravenous catheters, such as those used for CVP measurements or parenteral nutrition, should be removed, even if only for 24 hours, until an adequate blood antibiotic level is achieved. They can be reinserted at a different site. Intravenous catheters should not be used for drug injection since this probably increases the risk of secondary infection. Arterial lines should be inspected daily and removed as soon as possible.

RE-EXPLORATION

In many cases the source of the infection may be suspected (e.g. wound infection, infected prosthesis or other localized collection). Many surgeons are unwilling to re-operate upon patients with septicaemia through fear of anaesthetic complications. These are very rare in experienced hands.

Choice of antibiotics

In many cases this is dictated by microbiological evidence obtained before the patient became acutely ill; for example, *Staphylococcus* sp., *E. coli* or *Klebsiella* sp. may have been identified in specimens taken at the operation, or grown from subsequent sputum, wound drainage or urine samples. Many hospitals have an antibiotic policy which is designed to deal with all eventualities and which is partly dependent upon known hospital organisms. A balanced broad-spectrum combination is the first-choice ('best guess') treatment, which may be modified as a result of laboratory identification of organisms from pus, blood cultures or elsewhere. Skin commensals such as *Staph. aureus* and *Staph. albus* are commonly incriminated and the choice should include an effective anti-staphylococcal drug. Metronidazole and an aminoglycoside are often added. The dose of each should be maximal.

The blood antibiotic levels must be monitored daily to reduce the risk of toxicity, particularly if the patient's renal function is impaired, and a special regimen of treatment must be drawn up for the anuric patient.

Before the first dose of antibiotics is given, specimens must be taken from every conceivable source, which includes blood cultures, in an attempt to identify the cause of the illness.

Antibiotic regimens should not be changed until treatment has been given for at least 5 days, unless bacteriological evidence suggests that the 'best guess' regimen is wrong. No course of antibiotics should be continued for more than 7 days unless the patient has a source of infection which cannot be found or relieved. It cannot be overemphasized that the essential part of treatment is to discover the source of the infection, drain it or remove it.

References

Barrett, J. & Nyhus, L.M. *Treatment of Shock* 2nd edn. Lea & Febiger: Philadelphia, 1986.

Brenner, B.M. & Lazarus, M.G. *Acute Renal Failure*. WB Saunders: Philadelphia, 1983.

Buckingham, J.C. Hypothalamo-pituitary responses to trauma. *Br Med Bull* 1985; **41**: 203–209.

Counts, R.B., Haisch, C., Simon, T.L., Maxwell, D.M., Heinbach, D.M. & Carrico, C.J. Hemostasis in massively transfused trauma patients. *Ann Surg* 1979; **190(1)**: 91–99.

Cowan, B.N., Burns, H.J.G., Boyle, P. & Ledingham, I.McA. The relative prognostic value of lactate and haemodynamic measurements in early shock. *Anaesthesia* 1984; **39(8)**: 750–755.

Cowan, B.N., Burns, H.J.G., Cunningham, K. & Ledingham, I.McA. Lactate — haemodynamic changes in early shock. *Br J Anaesth* 1982; **54**: 716–792.

Cowley, R.A. & Trump, B.F. *Pathophysiology of Shock, Anoxia and Ischaemia*. Williams & Wilkins: Baltimore and London, 1982.

Crowell, J.N. & Smith, E.C. Determination of optimal hematocrit. *J Appl Physiol* 1967; **22**: 501–504.

Cuthbertson, D.P. Alterations in metabolism following injury. Part I. *Injury* 1980; **11(4)**: 175–189.

Cuthbertson, D.P. Alterations in metabolism following injury. Part II. *Injury* 1980; **11(4)**: 286–303.

Davies, M.J. & Cronin, K.D. Blood conservation in elective surgery. *Anaesth Intensive Care* 1984; **12**: 229–235.

Derrington, M.C. The present status of blood filtration. *Anaesthesia* 1985; **40**: 334–347.

Dinarello, C.A. Interleukin 1 and the pathogenesis of the acute phase response. *N Engl J Med* 1984; **311**: 1413–1415.

Ellman, H. Capillary permeability in septic patients. *Crit Care Med* 1984; **12**: 629–633.

Fan, F., Chen, R.Y.Z., Schmessler, G.B. & Chien, S. Effects of hematocrit variations on regional hemodynamics and oxygen transport in the dog. *Am J Physiol* 1980; **238(7)**: 545–549.

Foex, P. Inotropic and vasodilator agents. In: Ledingham, I.McA. (ed.) *Recent Advances in Critical Care Medicine*, Vol. 2. Churchill Livingstone: Edinburgh, 1983.

Gilbertson, A.A. Pulmonary artery catheterisation and wedge pressure measurement in the general I.T.U. *Br J Anaesth* 1974; **46**: 97–104.

Hardaway, R. Treatment of severe shock with phenoxybenzamine. *Surg Gynecol Obstet* 1980; **151**: 725–734.

Hardaway, R.M. Prediction of survival or death of patients in a state of severe shock. *Surg Gynecol Obstet* 1981; **152(2)**: 200–206.

Henderson, I.A., Beattie, T.J. & Kennedy, A.C. Dopamine hydrochloride in oliguric states. *Lancet* 1980; **2**: 1329–1334.

Hillman, K. Colloid versus crystalloid fluid therapy in the critically ill. *Intensive Crit Care Digest* 1986; **5(1)**: 7–10.

Hinshaw, L.B. Autoregulation in normal and pathological states including shock and ischaemia. *Circ Res* 1971; **28**: 46–53.

Joly, H.R. & Weil, M.H. Temperature of the great toe as an indication of the severity of shock. *Circulation* 1969; **39**: 131–135.

Kerr, D.N.S. & Elliott, R.W. The pathogenesis of acute renal failure. In: Flynn, C.T. (ed.) *Acute Renal Failure*. Medical & Technical Publishing Co.: Lancaster, 1974.

Knepel, W., Przewlocki, R., Nutto, D. & Herz, A. Foot-shock, stress-induced release of vasopressin. *Endocrinology* 1985; **117(1)**: 292–299.

Kraman, S., Khan, F., Patel, S. & Seriff, N. Renal failure in the intensive care unit. *Crit Care Med* 1979; **7**: 263–266.

Ledingham, I.McA. & Ramsay, G. Hypovolaemic shock. *Br J Anaesth* 1986; **58**: 169–189.

Lefer, A.M. Properties of a cardio-inhibiting factor produced in shock. *Fed Proc* 1978; **37**: 2734–2780.

Lefer, A.M. Role of prostaglandins and thromboxanes in shock states. In: Altura, B.M., Lefer, A.M. & Schumaker, P.T. (eds) *Handbook of Shock and Trauma*, Vol. I *Basic Sciences*. Raven

Press: New York, 1983.

Le Gall, J.R., Mignon, F.C., Rapin, M., Redjemi, M., Harari, A., Bader, J.P. & Soussy, C.J. Acute gastroduodenal lesions related to severe sepsis. *Surg Gynecol Obstet* 1976; **142(3)**: 377−380.

Le Quesne, L.P., Cochrane, J.P.S. & Fieldman, N.R. Fluid and electrolyte changes after trauma: the role of adrenocortical and pituitary hormones. *Br Med Bull* 1985; **41(3)**: 212−217.

Lucas, C.E., Sugawa, C., Riddle, J., Rector, F., Rosenberg, B. & Walt, A.J. Natural history and surgical dilemma of 'stress' gastric bleeding. *Arch Surg* 1971; **102**: 266−273.

McCabe, W.R. Gram negative bacteremia. *Adv Intern Med* 1974; **19**: 135−158.

Mela, L., Bacalzo, L.V. & Miller, L.D. Defective oxidative metabolism of rat liver mitochondria in hemorrhagic and endotoxin shock. *Am J Physiol* 1971; **220**: 571−574.

Needleman, P., Adams, S.P., Cole, B.R., Currie, M.G., Geller, D.M., Michener, M.L., Saper, C.B., Schwartz, D. & Standaert, D.G. Atriopeptins as cardiac hormones. *Hypertension* 1985; **7**: 469−482.

Ochoa, J.B., Udekwu, A.O., Billiar, T.R., Curran, R.D., Cerra, F.B., Simmons, R.L. & Peitzman, A.B. Nitrogen oxide levels in patients after trauma and during sepsis. *Ann Surg* 1991; **213**: 621−625.

Orr M.D. Autotransfusion: intraoperative scavenging. *Int Anesthesiol Clin* 1982; **20**: 97−119.

Palmer, R.M.J., Ferrige, A.C. & Moncada, S. Nitric oxide release accounts for the biological activity of endothelium derived relaxant factor. *Nature* 1987; 357−359.

Priebe, H.J., Skillmann, J.J., Bishnell, L.S., Long, P.C. & Silen, W. Antacid versus cimetidine in preventing acute gastrointestinal bleeding. A randomised trial in 71 critically ill patients. *N Engl J Med* 1980; **302**: 426−430.

Ring, J. & Messmer, K. Incidence and severity of anaphylactic reactions to colloid substitutes. *Lancet* 1977; **1**: 466−469.

Robin, E.G. The cult of the Swan Ganz catheter. *Ann Intern Med* 1985; **102(3)**: 445−449.

Rothstein, J.L. & Schreiber, H. Synergy between tumour necrosis factor and bacterial products causes hemorrhagic necrosis and lethal shock in normal mice. *Proc Nat Sci USA* 1988; **85**: 607−611.

Shires, G.T. *Principles of Trauma Care*. McGraw Hill: New York, 1985.

Shoemaker, W.C. Comparison of the relative effectiveness of whole blood transfusions and various types of fluid therapy in resuscitation. *Crit Care Med* 1976; **4**: 71−76.

Smith, J.A.R. & Norman, J.N. The fluid choice for resuscitation of severe shock. *Brit J Surg* 1982; **69**: 702−705.

Steff, J.S. & Clive, D.M. Role of prostaglandins and thromboxane in acute renal failure. In: Brenner, B.M. & Lazarus, M.G. (eds) *Acute Renal Failure*. W.B. Saunders: Philadelphia, 1983.

Stoddart, J.C. Hospital acquired infection. In: Tinker, J. & Rapin, M. (eds) *Care of the Critically Ill Patient*. Springer-Verlag: Berlin, Heidelberg, New York, 1982.

Stoddart, J.C. Multiorgan failure and its management in the ITU. *Brit Med Bull* 1988; **44(2)**: 475−498.

Swan, H.J.C., Ganz, N., Forrester, J., Marcus, H., Diamond, G. & Chonette, D. Catheterisation of the heart in man with use of flow directed balloon tipped catheter. *New Eng J Med* 1970; **283**: 447−481.

Tracey, K.J., Beutler, B., Lowry, S.F., Merryweather, J., Wolpe, S., Milsark, I.W., Hariri, R.J., Fahey, T.J., Zentella, A., Albert, J.D., Shires, G.T. & Cerami, A. Shock and tissue injury induced by recombinant human cachectin. *Science* 1986; **234**: 470−474.

7: Early Management

Resuscitation and multiple injuries

D.D.MILNE

The management of a patient suffering from multiple injuries should ensure that the examination and treatment proceed simultaneously. Conditions which are life-threatening should be dealt with immediately. Thereafter, by means of a thorough physical examination, an accurate estimate of injuries can be made so that a baseline may be established from which changes in the patient's condition can be measured. If possible a history should be obtained from the patient, any witnesses, Police or Ambulance crews. It may be important in the management to ascertain any previous history of diseases of the cardiovascular, pulmonary or endocrine systems and also information regarding current medication. If any immediate surgery is contemplated it is helpful to the anaesthetist to ascertain when the patient last ate or drank.

The essential measures which may be life-saving include the maintenance of an airway, the control of haemorrhage, the maintenance of cardiac output by external chest compression if necessary and the establishment of intravenous access whereby rapid infusions may be given if the patient is found to be hypovolaemic. The most common cause of the sudden cessation of respiration is obstruction in the pharynx, caused either by the tongue having fallen backwards with relaxation of the jaw or by tracheal obstruction from exudate or aspirated vomitus or blood. A more insidious form of respiratory embarrassment occurs due to a reduction in pulmonary volume caused by traumatic or spontaneous tension pneumothorax or by filling of the pleural space by haemothorax.

It is usually a simple manoeuvre to correct the position of the tongue but in patients who have sustained severe facial injury, with comminuted jaw fractures and possibly tongue lacerations, it may be difficult to maintain patency of the upper airway. In these situations a laryngoscope is necessary as well as a good suction device to clear the pharynx of any blood or secretions and one should attempt to visualize the vocal cords and try to ascertain whether there is any cause for obstruction at a more distal level. If the patient is deeply unconscious an endotracheal tube may be passed at this stage. If the patient will not tolerate an endotracheal tube between the cords, it may be possible as a temporary measure to use an oropharyngeal airway. It is most unusual to have to revert to tracheotomy at an early stage in the initial management but if there is gross facial mutilation it may be the only method of obtaining and maintaining a safe and adequate airway; in addition, the tracheotomy may be welcomed by the faciomaxillary surgeons who will embark on facial reconstruction at a later stage.

Emergency tracheotomy can be carried out without anaesthesia in the unconscious patient. When the patient is conscious all layers should be infiltrated with local anaesthetic solution. For urgent tracheotomy a vertical skin incision should be used although the cosmetic appearance of the resultant scar is not pleasing. Nevertheless, access to the trachea is rapid and blood vessels less troublesome than when a transverse incision is used. A cuffed tracheotomy tube should be inserted and a suction catheter used through the tracheotomy tube to clear the lower respiratory passages of any blood, vomitus or secretions. If, at this stage, adequate spontaneous respiration cannot be maintained, respiration should be assisted or taken over completely by a mechanical respirator. Before a mechanical respirator is used it is essential to exclude pneumothorax. If there is a breach of the visceral pleura with air leakage into the intrapleural space, the positive pressure of the ventilator will very rapidly build up a tension pneumothorax, causing further respiratory embarrassment. The position of the trachea should be checked to see whether it is central or whether it is deviated. Pneumothorax causes

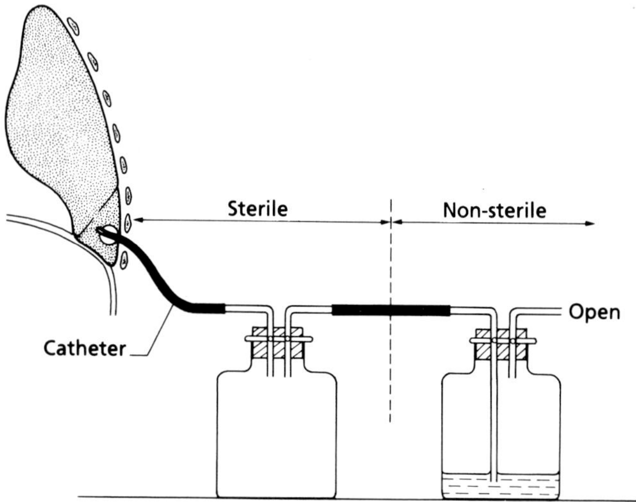

Fig. 7.1 Water-seal drain.

deviation of the trachea away from the affected side. The chest wall should be inspected and palpated for rib fractures and surgical emphysema since pneumothorax is frequently associated with these lesions. Auscultation will fail to reveal any breath sounds on the affected side and on percussion there is a resonant note over the air-filled pleural space. If tension pneumothorax is suspected on clinical examination, intercostal drainage should be instituted immediately using either a wide-bore needle or an intercostal drainage tube connected to an underwater seal bottle (Fig. 7.1). Tension pneumo-thorax can progress rapidly and fatally and one should not wait for time-consuming radiographic confirmation.

Intercostal drains should be inserted with the utmost care; this applies especially to the modern plastic chest drainage tube which uses a long trocar which passes through the bore of the plastic catheter. The author has repaired damage to lung, diaphragm, liver and spleen caused by the hasty insertion of these devices. At all times the drainage bottle should be kept well below the level of the patient's body. If the bottle is raised to a high level there is a danger that its contents may siphon back into the pleural space. It is not an unusual occur-rence to see drainage bottles picked up and placed on the trolley or bed whilst the patient is moved to the X-ray department or to a ward. If this is to be done the tube should be double clamped or other suitable pre-cautions taken.

Control of haemorrhage

External haemorrhage does not usually prove to be a great challenge in the emergency situation. First-aid measures of a simple nature, such as elevation and application of direct pressure by absorbant dressings, generally deal with most bleeding sources. Arterial bleeding following trauma is rarely a major cause for concern. The trauma to the vessel causes contraction and retraction of the vessel — even of large vessels like the femoral artery when a limb is traumatically ampu-tated. The usual source of bleeding is from veins and is often aggravated by the application of tight circum-ferential bandages which act as 'venous tourniquets'. Tourniquets are very rarely necessary, but when used they should be removed as soon as possible and the bleeding controlled by some other means. For stab wounds the most effective method of control is to pack the wound deeply and apply direct digital pressure which must be maintained into the operating theatre and until the vessels can be surgically exposed and either repaired or ligated. There is no place for groping blindly in the depths of a wound with a pair of artery forceps. Frequently, both ends of a divided vessel may be bleeding and irreparable damage may be caused to the vessels or to adjacent nerves, making what might have been an easy repair impossible.

Internal haemorrhage may, at times, be slowly pro-gressive and constitute a major problem in diagnosis. Patients, who are unconscious and possibly have an obvious scalp wound, are frequently seen; it is very tempting to assume that the unconsciousness is due to head injury. Many cases have been seen, diagnosed in this way and transferred, perhaps many miles, by ambu-lance, to a Neurosurgical centre only to arrive moribund or even worse — the true diagnosis is then made at autopsy. Sadly, these unfortunate patients may have passed several hospitals on their journey by ambulance where they could have been capably treated for control of concealed internal haemorrhage. It is a common mistake in the trauma situation to assume that all un-consciousness must be due to head injury.

The major sites of concealed haemorrhage are the serous cavities, pleural, peritoneal and pericardial, but one must not forget that fractures of the pelvis and major long bones result in significant bleeding into the surrounding tissues, and if the injuries are multiple the volume of blood lost from the circulation becomes con-siderable and may be life-threatening.

Bleeding into the pleural space usually comes from a torn intercostal artery which has been damaged as it lies closely bound in the subcostal groove. The other major source of bleeding is the lung parenchyma which may have been lacerated by bone spicules from rib fractures. The pulmonary blood pressure is considerably lower than systemic; therefore, it is unusual to have severe bleeding from this source. Blunt chest trauma, especially if of a crushing nature, has a tendency to cause tears of the pulmonary ligaments at the root of the lung and in this site venous bleeding may be considerable and necessitate thoracotomy and surgical control.

Haemothorax should be suspected when there are classic signs and symptoms of hypovolaemia together with a history, symptoms or signs of trauma to the thorax, e.g. rib fractures, surgical emphysema, stab wounds and increasing respiratory embarrassment. Confirmation is most readily made by a chest radiograph taken in the erect position. If haemothorax is suspected, it is imperative that one does not rely on a film made in the supine position, since a considerable volume of blood can be in the posterior sulcus of a hemithorax without producing any significant radiographic change. It may not be easy to obtain an erect film with an uncooperative or unconscious patient, but by placing a board, or even a long, broad splint, behind the patient's spine it is possible to elevate the head and trunk at least into a semi-erect position and thus obtain a more meaningful radiograph. Any fluid in the pleural space falls by gravity to obliterate the costophrenic angle and causes a fluid level to become readily visible. Any signficant collection should be removed by intercostal drainage placed low in the mid-axillary line of the chest wall, taking great care to avoid perforation of the diaphragm. Controlled suction should be applied to the drainage bottle to facilitate emptying of the chest cavity and to allow the lung to expand into contact with the chest wall (Fig. 7.2). Having established drainage, the majority of cases will settle without further intervention, but should drainage be copious and show no sign of ceasing spontaneously, thoracotomy will be necessary in order to control the bleeding vessel and to evacuate the haematoma.

A haemothorax should never be left in the hope that it will resolve spontaneously. If left untapped the blood will clot and a dense fibrinous layer will develop around the lung. In a short time the layer becomes tough and adherent and after a relatively short period, perhaps only 7 days, it can only be removed by dissection and decortication of the lung. If neglected, the fibrin organizes and forms a dense fibrous tissue which will contract, causing a marked diminution in capacity of the enclosed lung.

Haemopericardium is fortunately not commonly seen in the course of the treatment of trauma. Prior to the introduction of compulsory wearing of seat belts in vehicles the condition was seen following a crush injury of the heart by the vehicle's steering wheel. Many of these injuries were severe with rupture of the heart and, therefore, did not survive the journey to hospital. The condition is now usually seen following stab wounds of the chest with puncture of the ventricular wall. The pericardium having been breached, there is leakage into the pleural space which, to a large extent, alleviates the cardiac tamponade. Nevertheless, a blood clot accumulates in the pericardium and impairs the filling of the chambers of the heart. Clinically, there is distension of the neck veins and decreased pulse pressure. It rapidly becomes obvious that cardiac decompensation is taking place. The patient becomes anxious and breathlessness develops owing to a combination of tamponade and haemothorax causing hypovolaemia. Conservative measures are of no avail in this situation. Immediate thoracotomy and surgical repair are vital.

Intra-abdominal bleeding is a common source of hypovolaemia in the patient suffering from multiple injuries. In the unconscious patient the diagnosis may not be easy. The history and an accurate description of

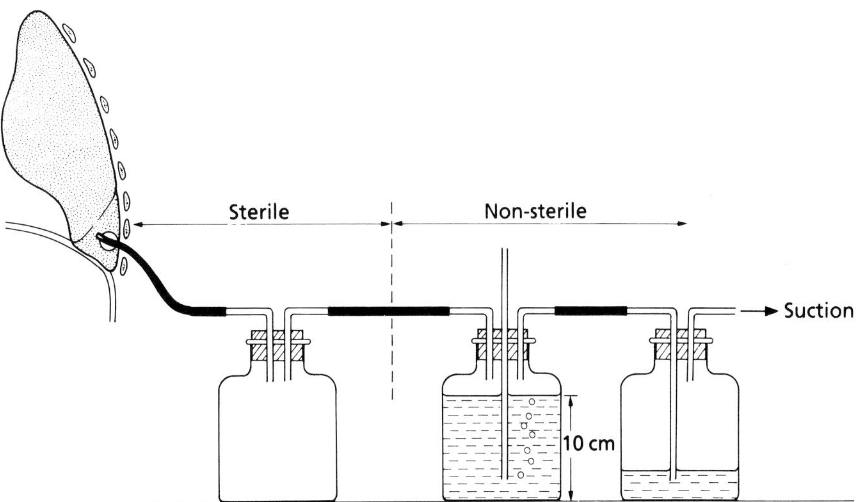

Fig. 7.2 Chest suction. The second bottle is introduced to limit negative pressure, depending on the level of fluid, e.g. 10 cm of water.

the causative mechanism of injury may give a helpful indication of intra-abdominal mischief. Even if the patient is conscious, a complaint of abdominal pain does not confirm or refute the true diagnosis. A history of referred shoulder tip pain may suggest that there is diaphragmatic irritation due to blood in that region. A meticulous examination is the only safe method of making a reasoned diagnosis. A careful search should be made for signs of local trauma to the lower chest with particular note of any bruising or marks of clothing imprint. Careful palpation for evidence of rib fractures should be made — over the liver and spleen laterally and the kidneys posteriorly. The presence of any stab or penetrating wounds should be sought. The anterior abdominal wall should be inspected for abnormal swelling which might indicate a contusion even though there is no discoloration normally associated with bruising. This may take hours to develop. The integrity of the pelvis should be tested by palpation of the pubic rami and by attempting to 'spring' the ala of the pelvis. Any gap at the symphysis should be noted since this would indicate disruption of the pelvic ring. The buttocks and perineum should be inspected for penetrating wounds and a rectal examination carried out. It may be possible to palpate a boggy swelling in the recto-vesical pouch indicating a pelvic haematoma, and blood in the rectum would reveal any lower bowel tear. The femoral pulses should be palpated to ascertain the presence or inequality of the pulses; these may be affected by aortic damage.

Intra-abdominal bleeding usually produces guarding in the muscles of the abdominal wall, even in the unconscious patient, and this is probably the most reliable, easily elicited physical sign of intraperitoneal bleeding. The guarding never progresses to the board-like rigidity of a perforated ulcer, but by repeated examination by the same observer the extent and degree of muscle guarding can be assessed.

A plain radiograph of the abdomen, although not confirmatory of intra-abdominal bleeding, may give useful information and indicate possible likely sources. Fractures of the lower ribs laterally may point to bleeding from the liver or spleen — the two most common sources of severe bleeding. On the left side, medial displacement of the stomach shadow may suggest a perisplenic haematoma. Obliteration of the psoas shadows suggests the presence of blood in the posterior vertebral recesses. A collection of air around the duodenum from rupture may be seen and if the air leak is extensive it may outline the right kidney as a 'renogram'. Similar gas leaks may be seen around the retroperitoneal areas of the colon if there has been visceral rupture,

e.g. seat-belt injury. The absence of free gas under the diaphragm does not exclude bowel damage since a fairly large volume is required and will only be seen on an erect film. The presence of pelvic fractures or separation of the sacro-iliac joint with diastasis of the symphysis pubis will be readily identified on a plain film.

In centres where ultrasound scanning is available, intra-abdominal haematomas may be demonstrated by this means. The method is non-invasive, does not expose the patient to ionizing radiation, and the equipment is transportable, allowing it to be taken to the patient if necessary. Computerized axial tomography (CAT) scanning may be used to demonstrate haematomas, but, although useful, it tends to be time-consuming and, of course, is not portable. It is not always convenient or even advisable to transport a severely injured patient to a scanner for a lengthy radiographic procedure. Formerly, four quadrant needle tap was popular but this tended to produce many false negative and false positive results. The procedure has now been replaced by peritoneal lavage. After emptying the bladder a peritoneal catheter is inserted 2–3 cm below the umbilicus and 500 ml of warm isotonic saline are instilled. If possible, the patient is gently rolled from side-to-side and also a 'head-down' tilt is used to allow the fluid to penetrate to the subdiaphragmatic areas. After 10 minutes the fluid is allowed to return by siphon action. The colour of the fluid is noted and can be sent for red cell count, microscopy and estimation of amylase content. If a significant amount of blood is present the laboratory examination is unnecessary.

Shock (See also Chapter 6)

The clinical condition of 'shock' has been described for centuries but it is only since the beginning of the present century that any attempt has been made to think of the condition in scientific terms. The word 'shock' has been used to describe many conditions ranging from vasovagal syncope, due to psychological trauma, to gross physical injuries sustained on battlefields throughout the ages. It is not surprising that studies have gained impetus during periods of war — in more recent years with the two World Wars, then Vietnam, Northern Ireland and, recently, in the Falkland Islands conflict. Looking back through historical records it is obvious that military surgeons made attempts to control haemorrhage: Ambroise Pare used ligatures in the 16th century (Pare 1948) and Esmarch introduced field dressings in the Franco-Prussian War (Guthrie 1945). However, there did not appear to be any great recognition of the fact that excessive blood loss was a major contributory factor in the overall condition of 'shock'. Blood-letting had been used for many centuries and is well documented. Attempts to give blood did occur but were made for rather esoteric reasons, such as rejuvenation or as an elixir of life. Blood groups and sepsis had not been recognized; therefore, it is doubtful whether any benefit would have been derived from these ventures!

The first recorded intravenous injections appear to have been given by Sir Christopher Wren (1632–1723) and Robert Boyle (1527–1691); they were given to dogs as wine, ale and opium (Oldenburgh 1665). Intravenous saline was first given by Thomas Latta of Leith in 1828 for the treatment of cholera (Latta 1831–1832). It was recorded by Sir William Macewan that Lister had transfused a patient with blood in 1869. Following the work of Landsteiner on blood groups and the Rhesus (Rh) factor, blood transfusion became a reality and was established as a regular therapy after World War I.

The work of Crile (1899) was an extensive study devoted to shock. He noted that if warm saline was administered there was an increase in venous pressure which, in turn, produced a more rigorous heartbeat and output. He believed that shock was produced by exhaustion of the vasomotor centre of the brain, causing pooling of blood in the large veins and, thus, a failure of venous return to the heart. During World War I, an international team, led by Cannon and Bayliss, collected data from battle casualties and also performed animal experiments. Their findings, published in 1923, showed that casualties who were trapped with their legs crushed were stable until they were released, whereupon cardiovascular collapse and, frequently, death occurred. Animal experiments using tourniquets confirmed that a 'toxin' was derived from the ischaemic limb after release of the tourniquet and that this could produce 'shock' in a second animal. Histamine and other substances such as amines from proteolytic action were identified and thought to be the 'toxic substance' responsible for shock. It was also noted that there was considerable fluid loss into the injured part. Vasodilatation of the small vessels due to a 'neurogenic factor' occurred, but it was not appreciated that spinal anaesthesia caused paralysis of the sympathetic control of the small blood vessels.

The development of biochemistry as a study opened up a completely new approach to the understanding of shock and in 1929 Sir David Cuthbertson produced a now classic publication (Cuthbertson 1929). The work of Krebs on cellular metabolism has also led to a better understanding of the pathophysiology of shock.

It is now recognized that shock is the condition which results from failure of the cardiovascular system to fulfil its normal functions, i.e. to supply oxygen and nutrients to the tissue cells and to transport and effect excretion of waste products. This simplistic view has, of course, many interconnected ramifications which encompass several systems of the body. Different causative lesions may interrupt the network at different sites, but the end result does not differ. There is cardiovascular collapse with hypotension affecting many organs, some preferentially in the beginning, but eventually there is generalized hypoxia with organ failures.

Fluid replacement

The effect of blood loss depends on both the rate and volume of loss. Loss of small volumes spread over a prolonged period of time, for example several days, will have a much less dramatic effect than the rapid loss of a large volume. This is brought about by the rate at which various homeostatic mechanisms can react. When there has been a loss of 25–30% of the blood volume, blood transfusion should be used to make up the deficit, at least in part.

Safe blood transfusion became possible after the discovery of blood groups by Landsteiner in 1900; he later identified the Rh factor in 1940. The infusion of a body tissue is not without hazard. The strict criteria of matching specific blood groups requires a disciplined approach to the labelling of specimens during what may be a long process between collection from the donor to infusion into the recipient. Considering the large volumes which may be required quickly and under stressful conditions, great caution must be observed to prevent human error in the handling and distribution. When homologous blood is used there is always the possibility of the transmission of diseases from donor to recipient. Formerly, the main conditions at risk were malaria, syphilis and hepatitis, but in recent years the virus of acquired immune deficiency syndrome (AIDS) may be passed. It is now customary to test all samples of donated blood for these diseases. This is labour-intensive, time-consuming and, therefore, expensive and can only be carried out in countries where well-organized and well-funded blood transfusion facilities exist.

Donated blood is collected and coagulation prevented by the addition of anticoagulant substances. Acid–citrate–dextrose (ACD), citrate–phosphate–dextrose (CPD) or diphosphate–glyceric–dextrose (DPG) are the commonly used anticoagulants. In Europe, since 1965, adenine has been added to prolong the storage life to 5 weeks – 2 weeks longer than with addition of ACD alone. In the United Kingdom there is concern that adenine may cause toxicity, but it would appear that large volumes of blood would have to be used before problems arose.

Stored blood contains high levels of potassium and citrate. When infused, the citrate is metabolized to bicarbonate, but if given in large volumes, and especially if given quickly, steps must be taken to counteract the 'citrate toxicity'. Calcium is a natural antagonist of potassium and neutralizes the toxic effect of citrate. Normally, calcium ions can be quickly mobilized from body tissues but with massive infusions the mobilization of calcium will not be sufficiently rapid. Calcium chloride, 5 ml of a 10% solution should be given for every 3−4 l of blood infused, but it should not be given directly into central lines since this may precipitate bradycardia and asystole by direct effect on the myocardium.

Since blood is stored at 4°C it is not prudent to use large volumes rapidly without taking precautions to prevent cardiac cooling, which may lead to arrhythmias and possibly to cardiac arrest. Blood-warming devices are either of the water-bath type or of the dry-block, electrically heated and thermostically controlled, variety.

Stored blood is found to contain particulate matter made up of aggregates of platelets, red blood cells and granulocytes. These particles can pass through the normal 170-µm filter of an infusion set and may lodge in the pulmonary capillaries where the degradation products of the granulocytes and platelets exert a deleterious effect, as in adult respiratory distress syndrome (ARDS). If more than one or two units of blood are to be given, an additional 70-µm filter should be used to remove the leukocyte aggregates. This means that up to 36% of platelets will be removed (Seibel *et al.* 1985).

Efforts have been made to reduce the demand and expense of homologous transfusion and also to avoid some of the inevitable risks. Certain religious beliefs must be observed when homologous transfusion is refused; autotransfusion may be a useful solution in certain selected cases. In the emergency situation the only possible measure has been to attempt to recover blood from the serous cavities. In general, this has not met with much success. Blood which has been shed into a serous cavity rapidly loses its coagulation factors. Special sterile collecting and filtering equipment is required and quite often the prepared equipment is not used at operation and, thus, is wasted. Frequently, the volume collected is not sufficient to justify the time, effort and expense of collection, and bank blood is freely available.

Over the last decade there has been a move by the National Blood Transfusion Service to supply only limited quantities of whole blood for infusion. Over 80% of blood issued for transfusion is now in the form of packed cells or plasma-reduced blood. Blood plasma is used to manufacture its component factors for the treatment of specific conditions, e.g. haemophilia. Following the recent AIDS epidemic the import of blood products has been strictly curtailed. From every six units of whole blood it is possible to obtain six units of red cell concentrate, six platelet concentrates, six packs of cryoprecipitate, two vials of factor 1X, two 400-ml bottles of plasma protein fraction and seven vials of immunoglobulin.

Packed cells or plasma-reduced blood has a high haemoglobin content and viscosity and will not readily flow through microfilters. In the treatment of hypovolaemia where considerable replacement is necessary the missing plasma can be supplied as colloid or cystalloid solution. The American experience in the Vietnam war, where battle casualties were promptly evacuated from the front-line and taken to well-equipped hospital facilities with good laboratory back-up, allowed an excellent opportunity to study the treatment of trauma and hypovolaemia. The casualties were a highly selected group — all young and previously fit servicemen. This fact alone may make their findings impracticable when applied to peacetime trauma where patients are of a wide age-span and where many are afflicted by pre-existing conditions, such as diabetes, obesity and cardiac and pulmonary conditions.

Plasma expanders and blood substitutes

Electrolyte solutions. Isotonic saline and Ringer's lactate solution have been used for intravenous infusion for many years, but are of little value in replacement of massive blood loss. Their action in the circulation is short-lived. Their main action is to replace extracellular fluid which may have moved into the vascular space, and their value would be confined to the treatment of haemorrhage amounting to no more than 500−1000 ml, where the osmotic pressure will not have been greatly affected by slight haemodilution by a small volume of crystalloid fluid.

Dextran. This is a high molecular weight polysaccharide which has been manufactured in a variety of molecular sizes. Dextran 70 (mol.wt 65 000−70 000) has been made to simulate albumen (mol.wt 65 000). This substance is usually dispensed in saline or glucose as a hypertonic fluid which will absorb its own volume of water. Dextran is largely excreted by the kidneys, but a small amount is metabolized and a further fraction is stored in the liver and reticuloendothelial system prior to being excreted. The haemodilution effect of dextran is frequently used to prevent thromboembolism in postoperative patients. A dosage of 500 ml of dextran 70 is given over a 48-hour period. Dextran 110 (mol.wt 110 000) has also found favour in the treatment of thrombosis. The larger molecule has the advantage of being retained in the circulation for longer periods. Antigen reactions to dextran have been reported, but are infrequent. These are treated by stopping the infusion and administering antihistamines and steroids.

Gelatin. This is produced from skin, tendon and bone and there is therefore a possibility of sensitization and allergic reactions, as one would expect from animal protein derivatives. In practice, the occurrence of reactions is rare. The gelatins used clinically are slightly modified and three groups are currently marketed. The urea-linked preparation (Haemacel) has been available for many years but occasionally produces a histamine-like reaction if given rapidly. Succinylated gelatin (modified fluid gelatin), marketed as Gelofusin or Physiogel, appears to have the lowest incidence of reaction. All gelatin preparations have lower molecular weights (30 000−50 000) than dextrans and absorb more water than their own volume. They are effective volume expanders and their effect lasts 3−4 hours. Thereafter, they are rapidly excreted by the kidneys. Only a small amount is metabolized before excretion. In addition to volume expansion, they cause haemodilution and a lowering of blood viscosity. Gelatin has no effect on blood coagulation factors.

Hydroxyethyl starch (HES). Starch contains 98% amylopectin, which is chemically modified by exposure to ethylene oxide using an alkaline catalyst to form hydroxyethyl starch. By chemical manipulation the chain length can be altered, affecting the time taken for the substance to be hydrolysed in the body. The metabolic fate of the starch products has not been fully explained and at present there is reluctance to make widespread use of the material. In experimental animals large doses cause an increase in weight of internal organs, in particular the adrenals, and also vacuolization of the renal tubular epithelium (Horsey 1980).

Plasma protein fraction (PPF). This is a solution of 4.5% human albumen together with a small proportion of globulins. In addition to its volume expanding effect, the albumen exerts an osmotic effect. Since the albumen is metabolized to produce amino acids it is a very effective form of therapy, although more expensive than whole blood.

Frozen red cells. These can be stored at low temperatures for many years using glycerol as a cryoprotective. Temperatures of −130 to −190°C can be obtained using liquid nitrogen. Although this may appear to be an attractive technique the main disadvantages are the cost and the time (at least 2 hours) taken to thaw the cells and remove the glycerol by washing.

Stroma-free haemoglobin (SFH). Pure haemoglobin in solution retains the capacity for oxygen transport. The solution passes into all the body tissues and is excreted by the kidneys. Its disadvantage is that only a small proportion remains within the circulation and for a relatively short time. Experimentally, SFH has been incorporated into lecithin capsules (0.02−5.0 μm) which are suspended in albumen as a 'synthetic plasma'. Should this technique result in an 'artificial blood' at a realistic price, this would be an ideal solution to the problem of emergency transfusion.

Perfluorochemicals (PFC). These substances have been found to have the ability to transport oxygen in solution, and not in combination as with haemoglobin. Oxygen solubility is greater in PFC than in plasma and is increased with increased inspired oxygen pressures. PFC is not metabolized and is totally excreted in 48 hours. The incidence of side-effects is high and it is doubtful whether a clinical use will be found for them.

Summary

Blood donors regularly lose 1 unit of blood and walk home afterwards! The average healthy patient can withstand the loss of 1 l of blood without any need for blood transfusion. When blood loss is excessive the imminent danger is of hypovolaemia. In the initial period resuscitation can proceed with the rapid infusion of crystalloids up to a volume of perhaps 2 l; thereafter, there is a risk of pulmonary oedema. This can be followed with a further litre of colloid in the form of dextran, gelatin of PPF. After this time, fully cross-matched packed cells or blood should be available.

References

Crile, G.W. *An Experimental Research into Surgical Shock.* Lippincott; Philadelphia, 1899.
Cuthbertson, D.P. The influence of prolonged muscular rest on

metabolism. *Biochem J* 1929; **23**: 1328–1345.

Guthrie, D.A. *History of Medicine*. Thomas Nelson & Son: London, 1945.

Horsey, P.J. Blood transfusion. *Recent Advances in Anaesthesia and Analgesia*. 1980.

Latta, T. Malignant cholera. *Lancet* 1831–1832; **ii**: 274–277.

Oldenburgh, H. *Philos Trans R Soc Lond* 1665; **7**: 119.

Paré, A. *The Collected Works of Ambroise Paré*. Translated from the Latin by T. Johnston, Milford House: Pound Ridge, N.Y. 1948.

Seibel, R., La Duca, J., Hassett, J.M., Babikian, G., Mills, B., Border, D.O. & Border, J.R. Blunt multiple trauma (ISS 36), femur traction, and the pulmonary-failure-septic state. *Ann Surg* 1985; **202**: 3.

Trauma scoring

P.H.WORLOCK

In order to evaluate the delivery of care to the injured it is essential to be able to classify accurately injuries and their physiological sequelae. There are two main categories of assessment:

1 Categorization of specific anatomical injuries.
2 Evaluation of physiological disturbance.

Anatomical scoring systems

In an attempt to establish a uniform assessment of the anatomical effect of injury, the abbreviated injury score (AIS) was introduced in 1971 and has since been developed and revised. AIS describes specific injuries in an individual patient. For scoring, the body is divided into seven separate regions: external, head/face, neck, thorax, abdomen and pelvic contents, spine and extremities.

Within each body region injuries are graded according to severity on a score of 1–6 (Table 7.1). Although AIS is valuable in categorizing individual injuries, it has limitations when applied to multiple injuries. To overcome this, the injury severity score (ISS) was developed by Baker *et al.* in 1974. Using AIS they found that mortality increased in line with the AIS grade of the most serious injury. This relationship was not linear, but mortality increased regularly when plotted against the square of the AIS. They also noted that injuries affecting up to three body regions increased the mortality, while including injuries in more areas did not produce a better correlation.

ISS is defined as the sum of the squares of the highest AIS grade in each of the three most severely injured areas. The body regions used for ISS scoring differ slightly from those initially described for AIS and are: head/neck, face, chest, abdomen and pelvic contents,

Table 7.1 Abbreviated injury scale (AIS)

AIS code	Definition
1	Minor
2	Moderate
3	Serious (not life-threatening)
4	Severe (life-threatening, survival probable)
5	Critical (survival uncertain)
6	Unsurvivable (with current treatment)

extremities/pelvic girdle and external. The maximum ISS is 75. Any patient with an injury coded AIS 6 in any one region automatically scores an ISS of 75 (see Table 7.2).

ISS is now recognized as the best method currently available for the *anatomical* assessment of injury severity. Major trauma is defined as patients with an ISS of 16 or greater. A useful adjunct to ISS is the concept of the LD50 (Bull 1975). The LD50 is defined as the severity of injury that is a 'lethal dose' for 50% of patients injured and is age related: the LD50 is an ISS of 40 for patients between 15 and 44 years of age, 29 for patients between 45 and 64 years of age and 20 for patients over the age of 65 years.

Physiological scoring systems

The first of the commonly used physiological scores to be developed was the Glasgow coma scale (GCS), described by Teasdale and Jennett in 1974 (Table 7.3). This has proved a reliable tool in the assessment of conscious level.

Of the physiological scoring system is use today, the most widely used are the trauma score (TS) and the revised trauma score (RTS). TS was described by

Table 7.2 Example of injury severity score (ISS) scoring

Injury	AIS	ISS region
Minor head injury Unconscious for 3 minutes, GCS 15 and no neurological signs	2*	Head/neck
Right pneumothorax	3*	Chest
Fracture of right acetabulum	3	Extremities/pelvic girdle
Open fracture of right femur	3*	Extremities/pelvic girdle

ISS = $(3^2 + 3^2 + 2^2) = (9 + 9 + 4) = 22$

GCS, Glasgow coma scale.

Table 7.3 Glasgow 'coma' scale

Response	Score
Eye opening	
Spontaneous	4
To speech	3
To pain	2
None	1
Verbal response	
Orientated	5
Confused	4
Inappropriate words	3
Incomprehensible sounds	2
None	1
Best motor response	
Obeys	6
Localizes	5
Flexion/withdrawal	4
Spastic flexion	3
Extension	2
None	1
Maximum	15

Table 7.4 Trauma score (TS)

		TS value
Respiratory rate/min	10−24	4
	25−35	3
	>35	2
	1−9	1
	0	0
Respiratory expansion	Normal	1
	Shallow	0
	Retractive	0
Systolic blood pressure (mmHg)	>90	4
	70−89	3
	50−69	2
	<50	1
	0	0
Capillary refill	Normal	2
	Delayed	1
	None	0
GCS	14−15	5
	11−13	4
	8−10	3
	5−7	2
	3−4	1
Total TS		1−16

GCS, Glasgow coma scale.

Champion *et al.* in 1981 (Table 7.4). As injury severity increases, the physiological disturbance becomes worse and the TS falls. The probability of survival (PS) has been calculated for TS (Table 7.5). TS has been most widely used in pre-hospital care as a triage tool and as a way of assessing the effectiveness of therapeutic intervention in the field. A TS of 13 or less indicates a risk of death of at least 10% and this can be used as a criterion to select the most appropriate hospital for an individual patient. TS is used with ISS in the Major Trauma Out come Study (MTOS), which is described below. Analysis of patients in the North American MTOS database led to the development of the RTS. This system weights elements, such as the GCS, so that the importance of isolated severe head injury is recognized (Table 7.6). TS and RTS are the physiological scoring systems that are most commonly used and most reliable. However, up to 20% of patients with significant injuries may not be detected, either because physiological compensation has already occurred or because assessment has been performed quickly, before physiological changes have developed.

MTOS

It is possible to combine the anatomical and physiological scoring systems already described and create a more refined assessment system. The combination of TS and

Table 7.5 Probability of survival (PS) with trauma score (TS)

TS	PS (%)
16	99
15	98
14	95
13	91
12	83
11	71
10	55
9	37
8	22
7	12
6	7
5	4
4	2
3	1
2	0
1	0

ISS is known as TRISS (Boyd *et al.* 1987). In this system TS and ISS are assessed together with age. With this technique the probability of survival for individual patients can be calculated.

The MTOS is an audit programme run in both North America and the United Kingdom. TRISS data (TS on

Table 7.6 Revised trauma score (RTS)

GCS	Systolic BP (mmHg)	Respiratory rate/min	RTS
13–15	>90	10–29	4
9–12	76–89	>30	3
6–8	50–75	6–9	2
4–5	<50	1–5	1
3	0	0	0

Each component is scored separately and the three scores are added together to give the RTS.
GCS, Glasgow coma scale; BP, blood pressure.

arrival in hospital, ISS on death or discharge, and age) are recorded and individual units can audit their performance on their patients compared with a national/international database. Data are analysed separately for blunt and penetrating trauma. There are details on over 130 000 patients in the North American database and over 15 000 patients in the United Kingdom database.

Data from participating units are confidential and can be used to evaluate overall performance as well as to identify unexpected survivors and unexpected deaths. Such patients are then subject to clinical audit in a continuous attempt to improve the quality of care in an individual unit.

Summary

The scoring systems described (AIS, ISS, GCS, TS, RTS and TRISS) are now part of the modern language of trauma care. Familiarity with the basic systems is essential for all those involved in care of the injured.

References

Baker, S.P., O'Neill, B., Haddon, W. & Long, W.B. The injury severity score. *J Trauma* 1974; **14**: 144–150.
Boyd, C.R., Tolson, M.A. & Copes, W.S. Evaluating trauma care: The TRISS method. *J Trauma* 1987; **27**: 370–378.
Bull, J.P. Measures of severity of injury. *Injury* 1975; **9**: 184–187.
Champion, H.R., Sacco, W.J., Carnazzo, A.J., Copes, W. & Forty, W.J. Trauma score. *Crit Care Med* 1981; **9**: 672–676.
Teasdale, G. & Jennett, B. Assessment of coma and impaired consciousness. A practical scale. *Lancet* 1974; **2**: 81–83.

Abdominal trauma

D.D.MILNE

Abdominal trauma occurs fairly frequently in military practice but in civilian trauma it occurs in approximately 1% of hospital admissions. In warfare, there are many penetrating injuries with the possibility of retained metallic fragments whereas in civilian urban trauma the majority of abdominal injuries are due to road traffic accidents and result from blunt trauma. Review of the literature shows distinct geographical variation in the aetiology of abdominal trauma. In America there is a preponderance of bullet and gunshot wounds and also stabbings, whilst in South Africa the majority are due to stab wounds.

When seat belts in vehicles were made compulsory in the United Kingdom in 1982, the pattern of multiple injuries changed and the seat belt brought its own specific pattern of injuries. There was a marked reduction in severe facial and head injuries and a reduction in severe chest injuries, but the device itself produced 'typical' injuries which include clavicle fractures, sternal and rib fractures, and also compression injuries to the abdominal viscera. The belt traps abdominal viscera against the 'anvil' of the vertebral bodies and applies shearing stresses to the mesenteries, causing tears and avulsion of the more fixed parts of the gut, e.g. colonic flexures and duodeno-jejunal flexure. Fortunately, the majority of these injuries are amenable to repair and there is a good chance of survival, whereas previously the gross cerebral laceration had no hope of therapy or survival.

In civilian practice, as a consequence of the rising frequency of violent crime, there is at times difficulty in diagnosis because of associated drug or alcohol intoxication and there is also often multisystem injuries with head injury and unconsciousness. Penetrating injuries are usually obvious and are frequently confined to one or two stab wounds, the effects of which are localized. This permits early and easy diagnosis. Treatment is usually uncomplicated and the mortality is low.

Conversely, blunt abdominal trauma is frequently associated with multiple injuries, some of which are obvious, e.g. compound limb fractures with deformity or severe head injury. In these cases diagnosis may not be easy and the abdominal injury is often overlooked and only found by a process of exclusion when the reason for profound shock and collapse is investigated.

Diagnosis

History

Attempts should always be made to obtain a history. If the patient is unconscious or inebriated no useful facts may be obtained from the patient; some form of history can always be obtained from Ambulance crews, Police officers or relatives. The circumstances and location of the incident will give some clue as to the mechanism of the injury and the degree of violence applied, and thus one may be directed to certain areas to expect, or at least suspect, a certain type of lesion. It may be possible to ascertain whether the patient had been previously healthy and to obtain details of any current medication and when the patient last ate or drank and the quantities consumed. Witnesses can also give valuable information regarding the state of the patient immediately after the injury and whether the condition has changed with the passage of time. This may be of particular importance if there has been a head injury or if there has been occult internal bleeding. The patient may have lapsed into unconsciousness during transit to hospital, indicating ongoing bleeding in the cranium or in one of the serous cavities.

The conscious patient may be able accurately to describe the circumstances of the incident and will direct the examiner's attention to the relevant injured areas. By careful questioning one may elicit a description of the type of pain experienced, its character, location and whether there is any radiation to the shoulder tip, indicating diaphragmatic irritation. The patient will be able to indicate whether it is aggravated by breathing or by movement.

Clinical examination

Even if one expects that abdominal injury is the only area of concern, it is essential to carry out a thorough examination. The scalp should be inspected for wounds or signs of trauma and the eyes checked for pupillary reflexes. The patient may well require general anaesthesia for treatment of the abdominal condition, and it would be difficult to diagnose an expanding intracranial haematoma in an anaesthetized patient. The neck should be examined for signs of cervical fracture since endotracheal intubation may be required for anaesthesia and this necessitates manipulation of the cervical spine during placement of the tube. Examination of the chest will reveal any sign of surgical emphysema, rib fractures or 'flail segment' and routine clinical examination may suggest pneumo- or haemothorax. These conditions require urgent treatment by intercostal drainage, before embarking on abdominal surgery. The bladder should be emptied by catheterization; this will reveal any haematuria and, as time progresses, the state of urinary output. The pelvis should be examined for evidence of fractures or subluxation of the sacro-iliac joints or symphysis. Careful inspection of the abdominal wall will reveal the presence of any clothing imprints, bruising or wounds. One should remember that the abdomen is accessible to trauma via the lower thorax, the flanks and also from behind. Similarly, the pelvic part of the abdominal cavity can be injured via the buttocks and perineum. The wings of the iliac bones are composed of rather thin plates of bone which can readily be transfixed by penetrating objects, and posteriorly the sciatic notches afford further access. Rectal examination should not be omitted. The presence of blood will indicate internal mischief and palpation may reveal dislocation of the prostate or urethral damage. Sigmoidoscopy at an early stage is indicated if rectal bleeding is noted. Inspection of the external urethral meatus may reveal blood which indicates that further investigation of its source is required. Measurement of abdominal girth is often described but in the author's experience is not a helpful investigation. Frequently, an agitated patient, especially a child, will swallow considerable amounts of air causing gastric distension which increases girth and abdominal discomfort. This makes examination and assessment much more difficult. The passage of a nasogastric tube releases the air, relieves the distension, makes the patient more comfortable and may reveal blood in the gastric aspirate.

Unless a confident diagnosis and a decision regarding the need for urgent laparotomy can be made immediately it will be essential that abdominal examination be repeated at regular intervals of 15–30 minutes. It is preferable that the examinations be made by the same observer, who can decide whether the tenderness or muscle guarding has increased or the area of involvement has extended.

Investigation

It is routine, when intravenous access is being established, to take blood specimens for blood grouping, haemoglobin and electrolyte estimation, level of serum amylase and white cell count. Apart from the preliminary to blood transfusion, these results will give a useful baseline against which any further estimations may be compared. When there is associated chest or head injury it may be informative to know the level of blood gases, since early respiratory assistance may be beneficial in the resuscitation phase of treatment.

Plain radiographs of the abdomen are of surprisingly little value in the assessment of abdominal trauma. Rib fractures may suggest the possibility of liver or spleen damage and fractures of the pelvis may provide an explanation of lower abdominal pain and possible hypovolaemia due to their associated extraperitoneal haematomas which may be considerable. Occasionally, a perisplenic haematoma may displace the air-filled stomach, or herniated viscera may be seen in the chest with diaphragmatic rupture. Obliteration of the psoas shadows is frequently described as a sign of intraperitoneal blood but this is difficult to interpret and is not a convincing and diagnostic radiographic sign. Kester *et al.* (1986), who analysed the value of plain radiographs in the investigation of abdominal stab wounds, found that only 8.5% of films were reported as 'abnormal' and of these 12.5% at exploration had no peritoneal penetration. 'Normal' films were reported in 91.5% of cases and of these 49% had positive findings at laparotomy.

More sophisticated radiology, with contrast studies or angiography, is probably more helpful, but is time-consuming, invasive and not readily available in other than specialized centres. A CAT scan is a useful method of investigation but is not practicable in the profoundly shocked patient, since the patient must be moved to the scanner to traverse the 'doughnut' arrangement of X-ray beams. This is not easy to achieve if the patient has several intravenous lines and/or respiratory assistance from a mechanical respirator.

Ultrasound scanning is at present the most convenient, quickest and most helpful method of assessment of the 'traumatic' abdomen. This non-invasive technique will show the presence of free fluid and the outlines of the solid abdominal viscera. The presence of collections of blood or other fluids within these organs can readily be seen owing to the presence of non-anatomical sonic boundaries.

Laparoscopy is an invasive technique that has been gaining recommendation for use in the assessment of abdominal trauma (Berci *et al.* 1983). The technique appears to be useful in that direct observation may be made — reassuring to the clinician who decides on a conservative policy in the treatment of intra-abdominal bleeding. The distinction between intraperitoneal bleeding and the extraperitoneal haematoma surrounding pelvic fractures can be made. Uwadia (1986) describes the possibility of gas embolism from the pneumoperitoneum. This may occur when the pressure is raised and venous channels have been opened by trauma.

Peritoneal lavage

This technique has now superseded the previously used four quadrant tap. The procedure was first introduced in 1974 (Thal 1977) for the assessment of abdominal stab wounds; it has now become an accepted method of diagnosis and management, including for blunt abdominal trauma. The procedure is helpful in the management of semi- and unconscious patients, where hypovolaemia cannot be readily explained, or where prolonged anaesthesia may be necessary for the treatment of other conditions, making abdominal assessment virtually impossible.

METHOD

The urinary bladder is emptied by a urethral catheter to prevent inadvertent puncture by the lavage cannula. Under local anaesthesia a small mid-line infra-umbilical incision is made and the peritoneum is approached by a cut-down technique. A peritoneal dialysis catheter is carefully inserted. At this stage, frank blood may be found on aspiration; if more than 10 ml is apirated the lavage is considered as 'positive'. If no blood is aspirated 1 l of warm isotonic saline is instilled and the patient is placed in a 'head-down' tilt for 10 minutes. If other injuries do not preclude, the patient should be gently rolled from side-to-side to disperse the lavage fluid. The fluid is allowed to drain from the peritoneal cavity and specimens are taken for red cell count, white cell count, amylase and bilirubin estimations and Gram's stain of a centrifuged deposit. The lavage is considered 'positive' if more than 100 000 red blood cells (rbcs) or more than 500 white blood cells (wbcs) per cubic millimetre are found. Amylase levels greater than 100 units ml^{-1} and bilirubin levels higher than the serum level are highly suggestive of pancreatic, duodenal or biliary damage. Microscopy of the stained deposit may reveal coliform bacilli or faecal residue indicating intestinal perforation.

A 'positive' lavage is usually accepted as one of the criteria for laparotomy. Although various levels of rbc dilution have been suggested, i.e. 1000–100 000, as an indication for surgical exploration, the lower levels appear to make an 'over sensitive' test and lead to an unacceptably high number of negative laparotomies. Even using 100 000 rbcs mm^{-3} as an indication for surgery, exploration may show that the bleeding has stopped and no therapeutic procedure is required. Ryan *et al.* (1986) found a 97% accuracy using peritoneal lavage. In this series, only 73% of 'positive' lavage cases required any surgical procedure. It could be argued that diagnostic laparotomy carries a very low morbidity.

Since trauma patients are usually followed for only a short time after discharge from hospital, complications such as adhesive intestinal obstruction or wound hernia may not be seen as 'complications' as they develop many years later.

The result of peritoneal lavage should not be used as the sole criterion for laparotomy, but should be taken in association with a full clinical assessment. The patient with a 'positive' lavage may be haemodynamically stable and may have responded well to resuscitative measures. Much, of course, will depend on the hospital facilities which are available for close observation — ideally an Intensive Care facility — and also on the immediate availability of a surgical team should there be any sudden deterioration. Such facilities would not be expected in front-line military service, where laparotomy should be undertaken promptly to ensure control of bleeding and make the patient fit for onward transit.

Laparotomy

In a minority of cases laparotomy must be undertaken to control bleeding as part of the resuscitation therapy. Apart from these desperate situations, laparotomy should be performed as early as possible once the decision has been made that there may be persistent bleeding or intestinal perforation. Early intervention will guard against profound shock and ensure that peritonitis due to intestinal leakage is minimal.

General anaesthesia is necessary for exploration of abdominal trauma. This can provide a challenge to the anaesthetist who may find a collapsed patient, who has recently eaten and may be suffering from various pre-existing ailments. By using general anaesthesia and with a cuffed endotracheal tube, a high concentration of oxygen can be ensured. It is necessary to have maximal muscle relaxation in order to ease the task of the operator in making extensive exploration of the abdominal cavity.

Laparotomy should not be commenced until there is a supply of cross-matched blood in the operating room. Apart from any hypotension due to the initial injury, there will be a further fall in blood pressure with the administration of muscle relaxants, which release the 'tamponade' effect of the muscles of the abdominal wall. A further, and often dramatic, fall in blood pressure occurs when the peritoneum is opened. It is prudent to be in readiness for these episodes and to speed up the rate of blood infusion, by pressure, if necessary.

Unless the intention is to explore a specific site, a mid-line incision is the most useful, since it can be extended vertically, circumventing the umbilicus, and, if necessary, lateral extensions can be made — into the flanks or across the costal margin as a combined thoraco-abdominal incision. This incision would be necessary for exploration of the hepatic veins or suprahepatic vena cava.

The first priority is to control bleeding. If there is a massive haemoperitoneum it may be difficult to ascertain the source of bleeding. A preliminary search by palpation of the dome and under-surface of the liver and of the surface of the spleen will identify major tears. If found, these can be occluded with large packs as a temporary measure. The peritoneum should be evacuated of blood and clots as quickly as possible by scooping with the hands and by using a wide-bore suction apparatus. In the young adult it may be possible to slow any massive bleeding by occluding the aorta with digital pressure, and haemorrhage from the liver can be diminished by cross-clamping the portal triad in the free edge of the lesser omentum, using a light clamp. Similarly, bleeding from the spleen can be controlled by digital compression of the splenic pedicle. It is usually possible by these temporary measures to control massive bleeding to allow the anaesthetist to infuse sufficient blood to maintain an adequate blood pressure, since profound hypotension with the abdomen open quickly leads to cardiac arrest. When the blood pressure is above the critical level and the haemoperitoneum evacuated, the site of bleeding usually becomes apparent and steps may be taken to stop the blood loss and to repair any damage.

At the initial exploration, punctures or tears of the hollow viscera may be found with leakage of their contents. The large bowel, and especially the left side, contains a high content of varied faecal bacteria. Further spillage can be prevented by covering the defect with a gauze swab, over which light bowel clamps are placed to temporarily occlude the gut, until full exploration can be performed.

The 'trauma' abdomen should be explored thoroughly since injuries are frequently multiple. The diaphragm should be inspected for tears and this inspection can conveniently be continued downward to search for any wounds of the anterior abdominal wall or peritoneum of the flanks. Stab wounds, for example, should be repaired on their peritoneal aspect in addition to the other layers. The abdominal oesophagus and anterior wall of the stomach and duodenum can readily be seen. Any leakage around the duodenum or upper border of the pancreas should be sought. The gall bladder and bile ducts should be inspected. The transverse colon should now be exteriorized to allow inspection of its mesentery and also the posterior aspect of the stomach. At the same time, the body of the pancreas can be inspected as well as the duodeno-jejunal flexure. It is convenient at this point to follow the small bowel caudally, inspecting for perforations and looking on both side of the mesentery for any tears. When the ileo-caecal valve has been reached it is then possible to follow round the caecum and right side of the colon. Finally, the left colon should be examined down to the peritoneal reflection of the rectum. In the pelvis the pubic rami and symphysis should be palpated for any irregularity which might suggest fracture. In the female the broad ligament should be inspected for haematoma, and in the male inspection and palpation of the bladder and prostate will reveal any damage.

The retroperitoneal areas should be inspected for haematoma and the kidneys palpated for any tears which may be present. Retroperitoneal haematomas tend to be extensive and track for considerable distances. The bleeding may, therefore, have origin from the kidneys, great vessels or from pelvic veins in association with pelvic fractures.

Treatment of specific injuries

Diaphragm

Injury to the diaphragm is estimated to occur in about 4.5% of cases of multiple trauma admitted to hospital. Considerable violence is required to cause diaphragmatic injury, and, in virtually every series reported, the aetiology is the road traffic accident. The majority have been vehicle drivers who have not been wearing seat belts. The mechanism of the injury appears to be a violent anteroposterior compression force applied to the abdomen and which raises the intra-abdominal pressure. This, in association with a Valsalva manoeuvre, results in tearing of the diaphragm and prolapse of the viscera into the thorax. The majority of tears involve the left half of the diaphragm, since the right half is in contact with the large, smooth dome of the superior surface of the liver. Although the incidence of left-sided tears is classically described as 90–98%,

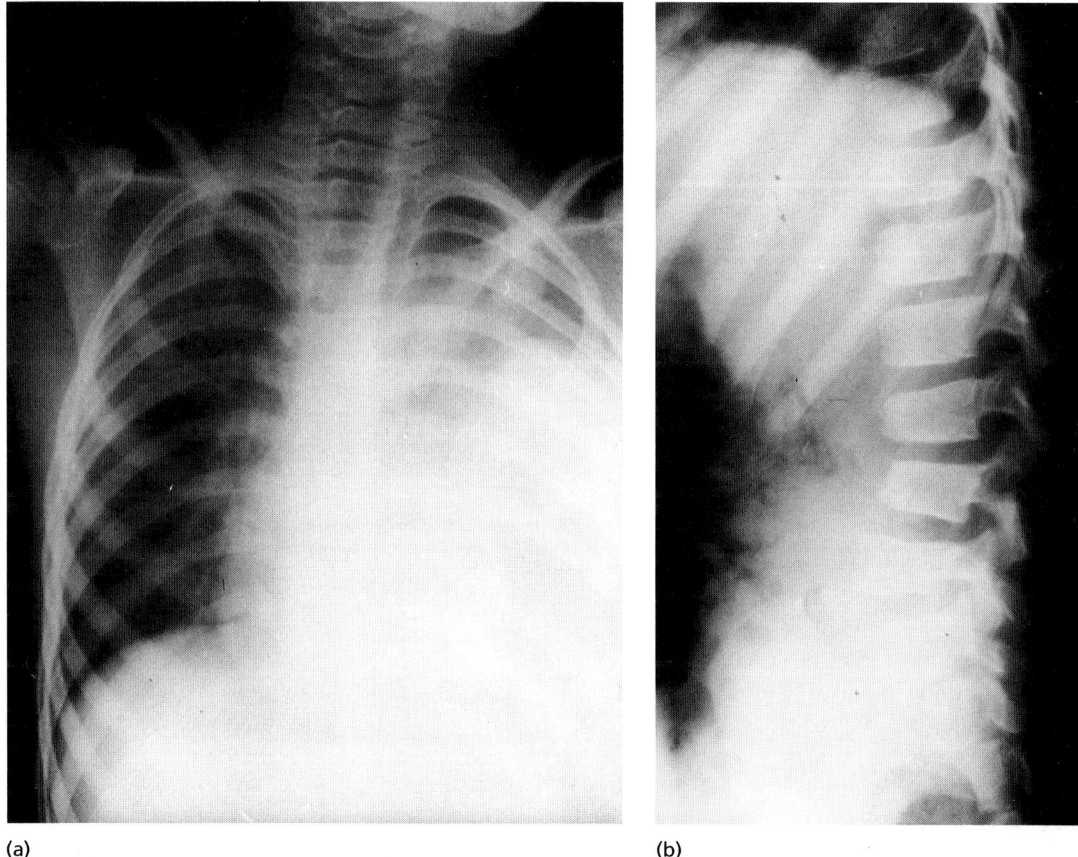

(a)   (b)

Fig. 7.3 (a) Ruptured diaphragm. Left hemithorax contained stomach, spleen and splenic flexure of colon. (b) Associated spinal fractures in the same patient.

Flancbaum *et al.* (1981) describe right-sided tears in 20–45% of cases. Rupture of the central tendon has been reported with prolapse of the transverse colon into the pericardium.

The usual method of diagnosis is the chest radiograph (Fig. 7.3), although a 'normal' radiograph does not preclude a diaphragmatic tear. If there is any suspicion or doubt, passage of a nasogastric tube and instillation of Gastrografin (aqueous radiopaque contrast medium) into the stomach, or induction of a pneumoperitoneum, may reveal the presence of a tear. A CAT or ultrasound scan may resolve a doubtful radiographic appearance. The use of laparoscopy has also been recommended (Adamthwaite 1984).

Associated intra-abdominal injuries are found in virtually 100% of cases and, hence, a mid-line epigastric incision is the access of choice for exploration and repair. The incision can be extended either by sternotomy or by thoraco-abdominal extension to provide more adequate access. Usually, adequate access to the right hemidiaphragm can be obtained by dividing the coronary ligaments and also by detaching the falciform ligament, which can then be used as a 'liver retractor'. If there has been peritoneal soiling due to associated bowel injury, one should hesitate to open the thorax or mediastinum. A diaphragmatic tear can usually be readily repaired using non-absorbable, interrupted sutures. The associated pneumothorax should be drained with an intercostal drain.

Spleen

The spleen is the most commonly injured intra-abdominal viscus following abdominal trauma. For many years the spleen was considered to have no useful function and, accordingly, splenectomy was the only form of surgical treatment for splenic injury. In 1952, King and Schumaker described the increased incidence of infection following splenectomy. Since that time, considerable research into splenic function has taken place and it has been realized that splenectomy may lead to serious complications, especially in certain groups of patients.

The spleen contains about 25% of the body's lymphoid tissue in the adult and plays a major role in humoral and cell-mediated immunity. The organ is responsible for antigen filtration and production of immunoglobulin M (IgM) and, in addition, produces opsonins, tuftsin and properdin, which are all necessary for phagocytosis of bacteria. The spleen has no haemopoetic function in the adult, but is responsible for removal of abnormal and effete red blood cells. Following splenectomy there is an increased number of target cells and cells showing Howell–Jolly bodies. Platelet count increases markedly in the first few weeks after splenectomy and it has been suggested that aspirin or dipyridamole should be given since there may be an increased risk of thromboembolism.

Review of the literature suggests that the risks of postsplenectomy sepsis are greater when the splenectomy has been performed for reasons other than trauma or in very young children. The presence of splenic tissue can be ascertained by a radioisotope scan and following splenectomy areas of functional splenic tissue are seen in 35–40% of cases (personal series). This regeneration of splenic tissue may arise from hypertrophy of splenunculi or from seedlings of splenic tissue which were disseminated at the time of injury.

Splenectomy in children has been estimated to increase the incidence of overwhelming sepsis by a factor of 50–60 when compared with the general population. The patient is most vulnerable to sepsis in the first 2 years after splenectomy, although life-threatening sepsis has been reported 20 years after operation. Efforts to prevent sepsis by recommending long-term antibiotics have failed because of a lack of patient compliance, and the use of polyvalent vaccines has not been entirely satisfactory since they do not cover the entire range of infecting organisms.

In children, there has been considerable success with conservative treatment of splenic injury, if there is haemodynamic stability following resuscitation. The injury is confirmed and followed by CAT, ultrasound or isotope scans. There appears to be success with this mode of therapy in children because the splenic capsule is thicker and there is more smooth muscle and elastic tissue around the blood vessels in the splenic pulp. In the child the ribs are more pliable, so that fractures do not readily occur, resulting in a different type of injury to the underlying spleen. Non-operative treatment must be pursued in an Intensive Care facility with ready access to a surgical team and there must be clear indication that there is no damage to any other intra-abdominal viscus. If there is clinical deterioration, laparotomy should be performed and an attempt made to control the bleeding and to conserve the spleen.

Splenic conservation

Superficial lacerations may be repaired and the bleeding controlled by the application of haemostatic agents such as Surgicel, Gelfoam, Spongistan or thrombin derivatives. Sutures may be required to hold the haemostatic fabric in position. Deeper parenchymal lacerations should be approximated with catgut sutures. Where part of the organ has been avulsed, and provided that there has not been gross damage to the hilum, it may be possible to perform partial splenectomy. If bleeding is found to be difficult to control it is acceptable practice to ligate the splenic artery within the pedicle. Multiple small lacerations can be dealt with by enclosing the spleen with a net made of polyglycolic material (Dexon).

The vast majority of splenic injuries occur as the result of road traffic accidents; there are usually other associated injuries and the incidence of concurrent intra-abdominal injuries has been estimated as being 25–60%. There is, therefore, a considerable risk of over-looking other lesions if a conservative policy is pursued.

In the adult, since the incidence of post-splenectomy sepsis is quite low and since spontaneous haemostasis does not occur so readily as in the child, it is not reasonable to follow a conservative policy. If there are clinical signs of intra-abdominal bleeding laparotomy should be performed. The spleen can be observed directly and steps taken to ensure control of bleeding, or if the damage is considerable and splenography impossible, then splenectomy should be performed. If there is peritoneal soiling due to intestinal perforation, no attempt should be made to preserve the spleen. All haematomas should be evacuated from the peritoneum, thus reducing the possibility of subphrenic abscess. The splenic bed should be drained with a low-vacuum, closed drainage system.

Autotransplantation

If total splenectomy is inevitable, attempts to preserve some splenic function should be made by implanting part of the spleen into an omental pouch. Since any implant has to derive its nourishment from the omentum, the implant should be in the form of small particles or thin slices, to assist in diffusion of nutrients and gases. It has been found in experimental animals (Pabst & Kamran 1986) that the mass or weight of tissue implanted appears to bear no relationship to the eventual mass which will regenerate after a period of necrosis — hence, the optimum amount to implant has not yet been determined. The efficacy of splenic tissue function depends on the total volume of blood subjected to 'splenic filtration'. Unfortunately, to date, the return from implants has not been great, so it is doubtful whether transplant confers any great benefit in protection against post-splenectomy sepsis.

Splenectomy

The stomach should be emptied and decompressed by nasogastric suction prior to surgery. This will ensure better access and prevent aspiration of the gastric contents during manipulation of the stomach. Bleeding from the spleen is readily apparent on exploration. To make a full assessment of the extent of injury to the spleen it is necessary to completely mobilize the organ and to deliver it into the wound where it can be clearly inspected. Prior to mobilization, if bleeding is profuse and hypovolaemia is causing concern, the splenic pedicle can be compressed by digital pressure whilst blood transfusion is accelerated. Mobilization is achieved by division of the lieno-renal ligament, which is usually separated by digital dissection; only a few strands require division with scissors. Frequently, at the lower pole there may be strands of omentum which will require careful separation. Adherent strands of omentum or lieno-renal ligament should be carefully separated, since it is easy to strip the splenic capsule and cause troublesome haemorrhage.

The spleen can be elevated from its bed and brought out from under the costal margin, bringing with its pedicle the tail of the pancreas and the greater curvature of the stomach. A large pack should now be placed in the splenic bed. The splenic artery should first be isolated and divided between clamps; the vessel should be doubly ligated, the distal ligature being a trans-fixation ligature of some non-absorbable material. The veins are then ligated as well as a few branches of the short gastric vessels. Great care should be taken whilst placing the artery forceps. Frequently, the splenic pedicle is very short and the tail of the pancreas and the greater curvature of the stomach lie in close proximity to the splenic hilum. These structures should be clearly identified and protected, since leakage from the pancreatic tail or from a lateral opening in the stomach will prove a difficult complication. Following removal of the spleen, the pack in the splenic bed is removed and any residual bleeding from the lieno-renal ligament or diaphragm is controlled with diathermy. The splenic bed should be drained with a closed vacuum system.

Complications of splenectomy include the following:
1 Haemorrhage.
2 Subphrenic abscess.
3 Basal atelectasis.
4 Pancreatic fistula.
5 Gastric damage.
6 Thromboembolism.
7 Post-splenectomy sepsis.

Liver

The liver may be damaged by either penetrating or blunt trauma. Penetrating injuries are caused by pointed instruments like knives or by missiles. In American reported series penetrating injuries predominate, but in Europe most liver trauma is caused by road traffic accidents.

Blunt liver trauma carries a much higher incidence of mortality, and in approximately 50% of cases, there are associated intra-abdominal injuries. The right lobe of the liver is most commonly injured on the dome and in the form of a stellate 'fracture'. Multiple linear splits may occur, but at times the capsule may remain intact although the underlying parenchyma is lacerated; this gives rise to a subcapsular haematoma, where the laceration is not apparent. An uncommon type of injury is the central rupture, which gives rise to an internal haematoma which, in turn, may produce haemobilia, at times, several weeks after injury. Massive trauma may cause extensive liver lacerations with avulsion of large fragments. The liver may be completely transected, with laceration running backwards to involve the hepatic veins and the vena cava. As one would expect, this type of injury has a very high mortality.

The diagnosis of hepatic trauma is made by an assessment of the history and site of abdominal trauma and the findings on peritoneal lavage. Plain radiography may reveal rib fractures overlying the liver, but otherwise has little to offer. Ultrasound and CAT scans are useful, especially if augmented by visualization of the gastrointestinal tract by water-soluble contrast agents. Contrast enhancement may also be assisted by a bolus intravenous injection of ioxothalamate, 1−2 ml per kilogram of body weight. A CAT scan has better resolution than an ultrasound scan owing to the ability to manipulate the images by computer; it is also useful to visualize intraperitoneal free air or blood, since the relative 'X-ray densities' may be compared and contrasted with the surrounding tissues. Radioisotope scans are time-consuming and of very poor resolution.

Frequently, the diagnosis is made at laparotomy, which may have been performed as a resuscitative procedure in the treatment of profound hypovolaemia which could not otherwise be controlled. Although it is accepted that many smaller lacerations will spontaneously cease to bleed it is prudent to explore any bleeding from liver trauma in the adult since the incidence of associated injuries is very high and would be catastrophic if neglected.

In children, there has been a recent move towards conservative treatment, as with their splenic injuries. In children there is a surprisingly low incidence of associated visceral damage. In evaluating these children, the determination of levels of liver enzymes has shown a remarkable accuracy in the diagnosis of liver trauma (Oldham *et al.* 1984). Within minutes of liver injury there is elevation of both serum glutamic oxaloacetic transaminase (SGOT) and serum glutamic pyruvic transaminase (SGPT). In the reported series all children with liver injuries had SGOT >200 iu and SGPT >100 iu. Children with other intra-abdominal injuries had levels below 130 iu. Provided that the child is haemodynamically stable, he/she may be observed. It has been reported (Cywes *et al.* 1985) that bleeding ceases spontaneously in 70% of cases. Progress is followed by serial CAT or ultrasound scans. The lesion may appear to increase in size in the first 14 days post-injury, but this is thought to be due to coalescence of the lacerations rather than to continued bleeding. Healing gradually takes place over 3−6 months.

Control of haemorrhage

If liver injury is suspected the abdomen should be opened through an upper mid-line or right paramedian incision which can be readily extended. If the incision has to be converted into a thoraco-abdominal incision, the thoracic part should be as high as the sixth or seventh rib to allow access, after opening the diaphragm, to the posterior parts of the liver, the hepatic veins and the vena cava.

The liver has a large blood flow, in excess of $2 \, l \, min^{-1}$. The portal vein carries 70% and the hepatic artery 30%, although the oxygen supply is approximately 50% each. Selective ligation of the branches or main trunk of the hepatic artery may be used in the control of haemorrhage. Bleeding from the edges of lacerations can be temporarily controlled by direct digital pressure on the cut edges and bleeding from the hepatic veins can be controlled by gauze packs. Attempts have been successfully made to allow 'dry-field' repair by forming a by-pass between the right atrium and the inferior vena cava below the liver, by inserting a tube, either from the tube atrium or via the saphenofemoral region, and encircling ligatures, above and below the liver. With the additional use of Pringle's manoeuvre the circulation is effectively occluded. This technique of vascular occlusion is difficult and is a major undertaking in a shocked patient; it should be reserved for those cases in which no other method will control bleeding.

Minor bleeding from superficial lacerations may be controlled by the application of haemostatic agents such as oxidized cellulose or thrombin derivatives. More major lacerations are best treated by isolation of bleeding vessels with 3/o silk or application of metal clips. Thereafter, the edges are approximated with catgut sutures. Individual vessel ligation may be supplemented by the insertion of mattress sutures, placed parallel to the wound edges. The sutures are passed using special liver needles which have blunt points and round edges. It is necessary to tie the sutures sufficiently tight to control bleeding. This requires great care lest the suture cuts through the liver tissue. Historically, several methods of preventing this have been used. Plates made from magnesium, bone and stainless steel have been used and, more recently, various inert plastic plates have been devised to prevent the suture cutting into the liver (Fig. 7.4).

Massive splits in a liver lobe may require amputation of the lobe to effect control of bleeding. Mattress sutures of heavy 2/o catgut are placed 1−2 cm from the edges to control the bleeding and the cut edge should be covered with omentum or detached falciform ligament.

There is still great controversy regarding the advisability of drainage of the common bile duct following repair of massive liver trauma. It appears reasonable to decompress the biliary system to prevent leakage from the damaged radicles. Following repair, all blood, bile and necrotic tissue should be removed from the peritoneum and closed suction drainage instituted.

In the past there has been much discussion on the use of antibiotics following liver trauma. Effective peritoneal drainage and chest physiotherapy are essential in the management, since basal atelectasis is a frequent complication of liver surgery and antibiotics probably have a place in the prophylaxis and treatment of associated respiratory infection.

Haemobilia is an uncommon sequel to liver trauma, presenting as gastrointestinal haemorrhage some time after injury. The condition is best confirmed by endoscopy. A CAT or ultrasound scan usually reveals a cavity within the liver substance containing fluid. The condition may be treated by operative means by opening into the cyst and ligating the bleeding vessels. Selective angiography and embolization have also been used successfully.

Liver regeneration

The liver is unique amongst solid organs of the body in that it has remarkable powers of regeneration. In animal experiments 80% of the liver can be safely removed, and similarly in humans there has been survival after extensive resections. Initially, there are signs of hepatic insufficiency but within a month recovery takes place.

Histologically, components of the lobule bud repeatedly and enlargement takes place by hyperplasia and not by hypertrophy.

Porta hepatis

Injuries of the porta hepatis constitute one of the most difficult problems in abdominal surgery. These injuries are usually associated with multiple intra-abdominal lesions of the liver, pancreas, aorta or vena cava. Vascular injury associated with biliary tract trauma has a mortality of 50−75% for the portal vein, 40−60% for the vena cava and 40−80% for the hepatic artery (Sheldon *et al.* 1985).

Control of bleeding is effected by the application of soft clamps to the free edge of the lesser omentum to occlude the vessels and bile duct. Extensive dissection of the various structures is necessary in order to make an accurate assessment of the damage. To explore the portal vein fully it may be necessary to divide the neck of the pancreas and excise the tail.

If the common bile duct is completely transected, direct repair over a T-tube stent leads to stricture in 90% of cases. In the emergency situation the duct should be repaired over a T-tube, with the intention of a staged procedure at a later date when a ductal-enteric anastomosis can be fashioned. Injuries to the hepatic ducts may require extensive dissection into the liver tissue at the porta in order to identify the structures. Thereafter, a hepatico-jejunostomy must be performed.

The hepatic artery should be repaired if possible, but if it is extensively damaged then it should be ligated. Hepatic necrosis is an unusual sequel to ligation. It may be possible to repair a tear in the portal vein by direct suture. Grafts are not indicated in the emergency situation. The vein should be ligated. Should portal hypertension develop, a porto-systemic shunt can be established when the patient is in a more robust state of health. In recent years there have been moves away from massive resectional therapy since the mortality is excessive. Alternative procedures such as selective arterial ligation and suture techniques should be pursued if possible. The majority of these patients have sustained multiple lesions and may be subject to complications such as disseminated intravascular coagulation and ARDS, in addition to any complications of their specific lesions.

Pancreas

The pancreas, by virtue of its anatomical position, lying transversely in the retroperitoneal tissue of the posterior

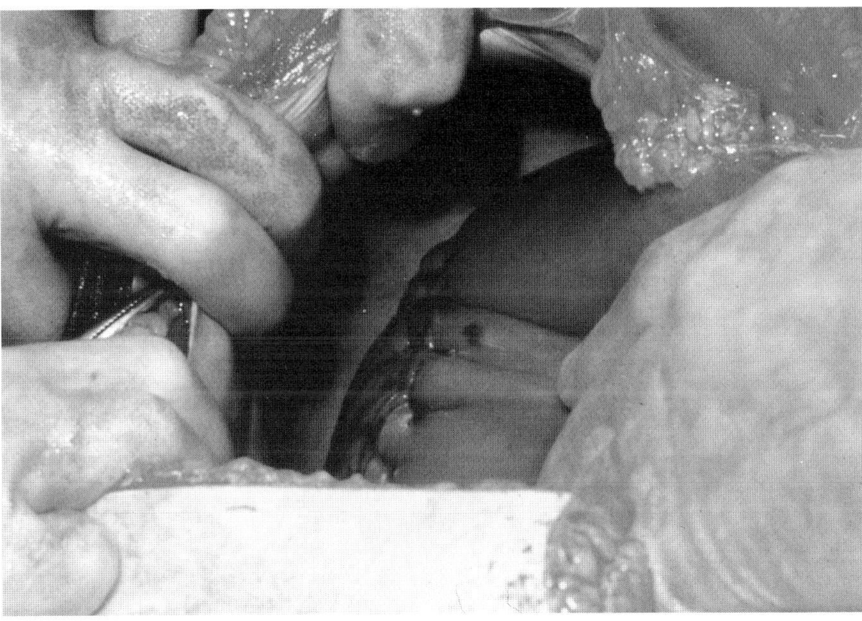

Fig. 7.4 Suture of a liver tear.

abdominal wall, is relatively inaccessible to trauma, except where it lies across the vertebral bodies where it is exposed to crushing injuries. This type of injury is seen as a result of badly positioned seat belts which crush the abdominal viscera against the rigid spine in deceleration accidents. Frequently, pancreatic injury is overlooked and it should be routine practice to consider pancreatic injury in all cases of abdominal trauma and to look specifically for injury in every exploratory laparotomy for trauma.

Diagnosis

Diagnosis may be made by the finding of amylase in peritoneal lavage fluid or by the elevation of serum amylase. Serum amylase is elevated immediately after blunt trauma in 60% of patients and possibly in 90% after a few days. A CAT scan is probably the most helpful diagnostic tool, although ultrasound can visualize fluid collections which may be suspicious around the pancreas. Frequently, the condition is only found at laparotomy and may be one of many intra-abdominal lesions. In American series, where pancreatic injury is most commonly due to penetrating or missile injury, there is often considerable adjacent damage to the duodenum, vena cava or portal vein. These cases carry a high mortality and morbidity.

Treatment

If there is a clinical indication of pancreatic trauma, or if the injury is found at exploratory laparotomy, a thorough examination of the pancreas should be made by opening the gastrohepatic omentum or, to obtain wider access, the gastrocolic omentum. Evidence of pancreatic injury may include blood-stained fluid, oedema, retroperitoneal fat necrosis and bruising or transection of the pancreas.

Essentially, the surgical treatment depends on whether there has been damage to the pancreatic duct system. Any injury which has no duct transection should be treated conservatively with drainage. Ideally, integrity of the duct system should be ascertained by endoscopy and retrograde choledocho-pancreatography. If there is leakage of the contrast agent the lesion should be explored without delay. Transections to the left of the mid-line are most easily treated by resection of the distal pancreas, if possible without injury to the splenic vessels or spleen. Lesions on the right of the mid-line constitute a more difficult problem. Direct repair of the duct should not be attempted. A Roux-Y loop should be fashioned and the damaged duct ends implanted, or the loop opened to cover the site of the damage in the pancreas. Gross injuries to the head of the pancreas will necessitate pancreatico-duodenectomy. This is a formidable procedure (Whipple's operation) in a shocked patient.

Stomach

Injury to the stomach is most frequently caused by penetrating violence, since a considerable area of the organ lies vulnerable across the anterior wall. The fundus of the stomach is at times penetrated through the lower left costal region. Injury due to blunt trauma is not frequent, but may take the form of splits or tears and even complete transection. These are usually seen if violence has occurred soon after a meal has been ingested.

Since the stomach has a thick vascular mucosal layer, there is usually haemorrhage into the peritoneum and also into the lumen of the viscus. This is revealed by haematemesis or aspiration of blood via the nasogastric tube. On exploration, the whole extent of the viscus should be examined, including the posterior aspect, since generating wounds may involve both anterior and posterior walls and even structures behind the stomach. The lesser sac should be opened via the gastrohepatic omentum to allow adequate exploration and, if necessary, repair.

Wounds of the stomach should be treated by excision of any devitalized tissue and ligation of isolated vessels, if they are bleeding profusely. It is usually possible to convert any wound into a linear shape which is readily closed with an inner layer of continuous (haemostatic) catgut suture through all layers of the stomach, followed by an outer layer of interrupted non-absorbable sutures to the seromuscular coats. If the stomach is extensively damaged, e.g. as by gunshot wounds, considerable areas of tissue may be devitalized and require resection. Re-establishment of continuity may necessitate partial gastrectomy and reconstruction as Bilroth or Polya gastrectomy, whichever is more appropriate. Following repair the stomach should be kept empty by nasogastric decompression until peristalsis recommences.

Duodenum

Injury to the duodenum is most frequently encountered during exploration for trauma to other upper abdominal organs. Since the structure is retroperitoneal, unless a careful search is made it is possible to miss areas of doubtful viability which may break down at a later date. Retroperitoneal tears present as discoloured, blackish-green haematomas surrounding the duodenum secondary to leakage of duodenal contents. The duodenum has to be carefully mobilized to allow inspection of the posterior aspect. This may not be an easy dissection, the tissue planes being distorted by haematomas and possibly by trauma to neighbouring structures. The head of the pancreas, extrahepatic bile ducts and duodenal-jejunal junction should be meticulously inspected, paying particular attention to the integrity of the duct system.

The complexity of repair of duodenal injuries will depend on the extent of trauma. In general, minor tears or lacerations can be treated by excision of devitalised areas, meticulous haemostasis and control of bleeding vessels. Thereafter, lacerations, and even complete transection, may be closed transversely, in a two-layer fashion. If the trauma is extensive, especially if there is transection or avulsion of the bile or pancreatic duct systems, then a more extensive procedure will be necessary to restore enteric continuity and duct drainage.

If the upper duodenum has extensive tissue loss, gastric exclusion with partial gastrectomy or gastroenterostomy may be necessary, and if the duct system is still intact duodenal 'diverticulization' may be used. If there is extensive damage to the head of the pancreas, resection may be necessary and drainage established via a Roux-Y loop.

In the emergency situation it is prudent to avoid, if possible, the extensive and complicated procedures since these add considerably to the morbidity and mortality. More extensive injuries are usually associated with multiorgan damage.

Following repair the area should be adequately drained, since there is a high incidence of complications which include bleeding, fistula formation, pancreatitis and subphrenic abscess.

Small bowel and mesentery

Injury to the small bowel and its mesentery is fairly common following both blunt and penetrating trauma. Direct blunt force to the anterior abdominal wall may crush the bowel against the vertebral bodies and cause laceration with perforation or tears of the mesentery. Trauma does not usually involve large areas, but is often multiple.

Trauma from seat belts frequently causes traction injuries affecting the fixed areas of the bowel, i.e. the ligament of Treitz and the ileo-caecal junction. In addition, there may be crushing of the bowel and tears of the mesentery. Since the small bowel has a relatively thick and vascular mucosal layer, blunt trauma may produce intramural bleeding which gives rise to haematoma formation. These may appear to be innocent lesions at primary laparotomy, but some lead to delayed perforation.

Diagnosis

The diagnosis of small bowel injury or perforation may not be easy and may be delayed. Trauma to the bowel results in a localized segment of 'paralytic ileus'. There is not usually a large volume of leakage of the small bowel content. Unlike gastric content, which is acid and highly irritant, small bowel content is of a higher pH and evokes less peritoneal reaction and pain. The volume of gas released through a laceration is not usually sufficient to be seen on radiographic examination of the abdomen.

Treatment

Small, localized wounds or tears are treated by simple suture closure in two layers, aligning the repair transversely to the long axis of the bowel in order to prevent stricture. If multiple perforations or tears are in close proximity to each other it may be simpler and safer to resect the area and perform end-to-end anastomosis.

Injuries to the mesentery are at times troublesome. At laparotomy a large haematoma is found. This should be explored and the bleeding vessel ligated. The associated segment of bowel should be closely examined for viability and, if found to be ischaemic, should be resected.

Major injuries to the superior mesenteric vessels are infrequent, but if the vessel has been transected it must be repaired. Repair of the artery may necessitate the insertion of a graft from the aorta to the damaged vessel.

Colon

World War I brought a dramatic reduction in mortality from colonic injuries; prior to that time there was virtually 100% mortality. It was realized that prompt evacuation, resuscitation and early surgical treatment were vital for survival. During World War II the use of antibiotics was instituted and exteriorization of the damaged bowel was the recommended practice. The mortality fell to 30%. During the Vietnam conflict, with further improvements in speed of evacuation, resuscitation techniques and antibiotic therapy, the mortality fell to 15% (Ziperman 1956).

The colon is commonly injured by penetrating stab wounds or by crush injuries. Anatomically, the colon is large, thin-walled, and apart from the transverse and sigmoid parts, is fixed and retroperitoneal. The colonic contents are of a large volume and have a high content of infective organisms including anaerobes.

Treatment

Since parts of the colon are retroperitoneal a careful search should be made for damaged areas. Haematomas in the paracolic gutters or around the mesenteric aspects of the colon should arouse suspicion. The peritoneum of the paracolic gutter should be opened and any suspect area examined. Frequently, the attention of the operator is attracted by the faecial smell of escaped colonic gas and contents.

Traditionally, there have been three modes of treatment:

1 Military field surgery, where time and facilities are limited, insists that an injured segment of colon should either be exteriorized or functionally excluded by a proximal colostomy (Kirby 1983). In civilian practice, where more time is available for repair, attempts are made to avoid the inconvenience of a colostomy and a second operation to restore bowel continuity.

2 Primary repair, with return of the damaged bowel to the peritoneal cavity, undoubtedly carries a risk of leakage and sepsis.

3 As a compromise it was suggested that primary repair should be made and the damaged area then exteriorized, with a view to returning the segment to the peritoneal cavity after about 10 days. This method carried a high complication rate. The incidence of leakage at the repair site was high and frequently broke down or had to be converted to a colostomy. This method has now been abandoned.

The bacterial count of intestinal flora rises progressively from the right to the left side of the colon and has led to the suggestion that all left-sided colonic injuries must be treated by colostomy. Recently, there have been a number of series which have shown insignificant differences in complication rates when comparing the two sides. (Demetriades *et al.* 1985). There is no doubt that the most important factors in the treatment are the amount of peritoneal soiling found at the time of exploration and the extent of the trauma. If contamination is gross, no attempt should be made to perform primary repair and abdominal closure. On the right side, if the damage is extensive, hemicolectomy may be necessary in order to remove all devitalized tissue. Depending on the circumstances, the bowel ends may be brought our separately as ileostomy and colostomy, or ileo-transverse-colostomy may be used to restore continuity. The transverse colon and left colon are readily mobilized and the damaged segments may be exteriorized and used as a colostomy. The distal colon and rectum should be thoroughly cleansed by lavage and enema.

If the damage to the colon is localized, and there has

not been extensive soiling of the peritoneum, it is probably safe to carry out primary repair, if one can be sure that the distal colon and rectum have been cleared so that there is no build-up of pressure at the site of repair. Antibiotics should include agents specific for anaerobic organisms, e.g. metronidazole.

Rectum

Wounds of the rectum have a high morbidity and mortality since the rectum is in close proximity to the bladder, urethra, pelvic vessels and nerves. The gluteal muscles may be lacerated and contaminated by bowel contents and may form a nidus for anaerobic infection.

Digital rectal examination may reveal bleeding which should be further investigated by proctoscopy and sigmoidoscopy. Any laceration of the rectum must be treated by thorough cleansing of the bowel by irrigation, excision of all devitalized tissue with good haemostasis, and repair by suture. A defunctioning colostomy must be fashioned. The damaged area must be freely drained. If injury has occurred high in the rectum, the repair will have necessitated abdominal operation with incision of the peritoneum of the pelvic floor. Drains should be sited in the recto-vesical pouch. The lower rectum should be drained by a pararectal, perineal incision.

Anal injuries

These are usually obvious and although on first inspection they may not appear to be serious, they should be thoroughly examined to assess the integrity of the anal sphincters. If the sphincter musculature has been completely divided, urgent defunctioning colostomy and distal bowel wash-out are imperative. Any attempted repair without colostomy has little chance of success. The sphincter muscles can be identified with an electric stimulator, provided that muscle relaxants have not been given by the anaesthetist. Meticulous haemostasis and repair of all layers will usually give a good functional result if operation is early.

References

Adamthwaite, D.N. Traumatic diaphragmatic hernia: a new indication for laparoscopy. *Br J Surg* 1984; **71**: 314–316.

Berci, G., Dunkelman, D., Michel, S.L., Sanders, G., Wahlstrom, E. & Morgenstern, L. Emergency minilaparoscopy in abdominal trauma. *Am J Surg* 1983; **146**: 261–265.

Cywes, S., Rode, H. & Millar, A.J.W. Blunt liver trauma in children: Non-operative management. *J Pediatr Surg* 1985; **20(1)**: 14–19.

Demetriades, D., Rabinowitz, B., Sofianos, C. & Prumm, E. The management of colon injuries by primary repair or colostomy. *Br J Surg* 1985; **72**: 881–882.

Flanckbaum, A. Injuries to the diaphragm. In: *Chest Trauma.* Springer-Verlag: New York, 1981.

Glinz, W. Injuries to the diaphragm. *Chest Trauma.* Springer-Verlag: New York, 1981.

Kester, D.E., Andrescy, R.J. & Aust, J.B. Value and cost effectiveness of abdominal roentgenograms in the evaluation of stab wounds of the abdomen. *Surg Gynecol Obstet* 1986; **162**: 337–340.

King, B. & Schumaker, C. Splenic studies — susceptibility to infection after splenectomy performed in infancy. *Ann Surg* 1952; **135**: 239–242.

Kirby, N.G. *Field Surgery.* HMSO; London, 1983.

Oldham, K.T., Gince, K.S., Kaufman, R.A. & Martin, L.W. Blunt hepatic injury and elevated hepatic enzymes. *J Pediatr Surg* 1984; **19**: 457–462.

Pabst, R. & Karman, D. Autotransplantation of splenic tissue. *J Pediatr Surg,* 1986; **21(2)**: 121–125.

Ryan, J.J., Kyes, F.N., Horner, W.R., Young, J.C. & Diamond, D.L. Critical analysis of open peritoneal lavage in blunt abdominal trauma. *Am J Trauma* 1986; **151**: 221–223.

Sheldon, G.F., Lim, R.C., Yee, E.S. & Petersen, S.R. Management of injuries to the porta hepatis. *Ann Surg* 1985; **202(5)**: 539–543.

Thal, E.R. Evaluation of peritoneal lavage and local exploration in abdominal stab wounds. *J Trauma* 1977; **17**: 642–648.

Udwadia, T.E. Peritoneoscopy for surgeons. *Ann R Coll Surg Engl* 1986; **68**: 125–130.

Ziperman, H.H. The management of large bowel injuries in the Korean campaign. *US Armed Med Serv J* 1956; **7**: 85–99.

Head injuries

R.M.KALBAG

About 120 000 head injuries are admitted each year to hospitals in England and Wales. In these days it seems paradoxical that only 5% of these admissions ever come under the care of those best qualified to care for them; the neurosurgeons. The organization varies in different parts of the country; the proportion of patients seen in neurosurgical departments ranges from 1% in some areas to 30% in others. The reasons for this are mainly logistic. Head injuries account for about 10% of all new attenders in Accident and Emergency departments and for 15% of those attending after recent trauma, while about a fifth of these are admitted to hospital (Jennett & MacMillan 1981). Most of those admitted will be ready for discharge in a day or two and few will need the clinical expertise or diagnostic facilities only available, as a rule, in neurosurgical units. The very size of the client population necessitates shared care between specialties. The Hospital Inpatient Enquiry estimates for 1982 showed nearly a third of all head injuries in

England and Wales as having been admitted under orthopaedic surgeons.

Difficulties in organization, posed by the sheer number of patients, are compounded by the times at which most head injuries arrive in Accident and Emergency departments: after normal working hours and at weekends when important decisions, about whom to admit from those with apparently mild head injury and about priorities in the management of unconscious patients, often have to be taken by inexperienced junior doctors. These are decisions for which neither their undergraduate teaching nor their postgraduate experience has equipped them. As a result, a mere sense of inadequacy in the young doctor faced with a frightened toddler may well escalate to panic when confronted with a deeply unconscious patient. The risk of any confidence being shattered is heightened by the fact that a third of all patients who die after reaching a hospital do so before admission to a ward (Field 1976).

The interests of both patient and primary physician demand that the neurosurgeon who cannot deal with all head injury patients has at least an obligation to set down responsible advice in management as simply as possible. This advice should be based on a general consideration of the mechanisms and pathology of head injury.

The primary head injury

The principal concern in head injury is its effect on the brain, but evidence of damage to the scalp or the skull may be important indicators of the complications most likely to develop. What happens to the brain is influenced by:

1 The surface area of the object the head comes into contact with.
2 The velocity of the impact.
3 Whether the head is unsupported and therefore able to move freely or not.

The most common injury seen in peacetime is the *blunt acceleration–deceleration injury* in which the unsupported head is struck by a moving object or the moving head is abruptly brought to a halt when it strikes a blunt or flat surface such as the road. A pedestrian hit by a fast-moving vehicle, for instance, sustains both an acceleration and a deceleration injury. The brain is easily deformed by rotational forces to which it is subjected by the impact, and shearing occurs between structures of differing density, notably the cortex and the white matter. Widespread stretching, sometimes even rupture, of the axons and diffuse neuronal disturbance is responsible for the most characteristic feature of

such injury — *loss of consciousness*. If, at the same time, there is a compound skull fracture, the injury is *open* and carries the additional risk of *infection*. If there is no fracture, it is a closed head injury.

Crushing of the fixed head between two surfaces produces a *compression injury* without loss of consciousness but which may be associated with a compound fracture of the skull base, presenting as cerebrospinal fluid (csf) otorrhoea or rhinorrhoea and lower cranial nerve palsies. Such injury is rare.

A *penetrating injury* is obviously open and carries the risk of infection. The effect on the brain itself depends on the speed at which the head is struck. If the velocity is low the damage is localized to the skull and perhaps the underlying dura and even the brain, but consciousness is retained. The point of entry may be small and it is an injury particularly likely to be missed in children if an adequate history is not obtained, the wound not inspected properly or the surrounding hair not shaved. Any track in the brain may be scarcely wider than the missile.

The damage, however, increases with the speed of the missile: the energy transmitted to the brain is directly related to the square of the missile velocity. Modern rifles with a muzzle velocity more than twice the speed of sound release up to 10 times as much energy as a hand gun. While the latter may produce little generalized damage, the former create an explosive radial force at the point of entry into the cranium, temporary cavitation and a massive increase in intracranial pressure. The rapid deterioration and death seen in such injuries is due to extensive disruption of brain tissue with secondary haemorrhage and oedema. When a high-velocity bullet has passed clean through the skull the exit wound is always larger than the entry wound.

Whatever the mechanism, the primary injury is itself not amenable to treatment and management concentrates on the additional factors that could damage any prospects of recovery. These threats to the brain are, in order of chronological importance, (i) anoxia, (ii) cerebral compression and (iii) infection; they should be borne in mind when assessing any unconscious patient. If the patient is conscious only the likelihood of cerebral compression and infection need be considered, except in cases of multiple or severe extracranial injury.

Anoxia

Every medical undergraduate knows the danger to the brain from anoxia. Yet, after graduation, the same individual faced with an unconscious patient may ignore basic principles familiar to every layman with an elementary knowledge of first aid. One cannot help wondering whether the emphasis placed by neurosurgeons in their ivory towers on early computerized tomography (CT) scanning has not engendered a feeling of frightening impotence in the inexperienced young doctors who actually first see the patient and forget that resuscitation comes first.

Gentleman and Jennett (1981) studied over a 12-month period 150 consecutive patients in coma after head injury who were transferred from other hospitals to a neurosurgical unit; they excluded those who were dead on arrival. Major extracranial injuries, i.e. justifying hospital admission in their own right, were present in 45% of these patients and were more common in victims of road accidents. Hypoxaemia was found in 23% and hypotension in 11%. Most of those with hypotension had one or more inadequately managed major extracranial injuries, mainly fractures of long bones; some of these had not even been recognized in the referring hospitals. In fact, in nearly a third of those with such injuries the initial management was deemed to have been inadequate. Airways obstruction by inhaled vomit, blood or secretions was seen in 27% while 44% of 108 patients transferred without an endotracheal tube were in the supine position and would have been better off in the hands of a Red Cross volunteer than in those of a doctor. That panic was probably at the root of the problem is suggested by the finding that these 'second accidents' were more common in patients referred within the first 6 hours than in those referred later. That, at the same time, 93% of those patients had already had skull radiography before transfer is testimony to the defects in our undergraduate education, a point also alluded to in the Report of the Working Party on Head Injuries to the Royal College of Surgeons of England in June 1986.

The adverse influence of these systemic insults, namely hypoxia with or without hypotension, was particularly striking in the very patients who needed neurosurgery: 76% of patients with a haematoma died and only 4% made a good recovery among those who had suffered a systemic insult as against 47% dead and 16% good recovery in those who had been properly handled in the first hospital. The survey was also of interest in that it confirmed what neurosurgeons have long noted with dismay: in equivalent depths of coma, the patient fortunate enough not to harbour an intracranial clot has a far better outcome than the one who has a clot, no matter how energetic and skilful the management. In patients without a haematoma only 17% died while 47% made a good recovery.

Anoxia may be of the anoxic, stagnant or anaemic type. In its simplest form anoxic anoxia can be prevented by placing the victim in the semi-prone position. However, in the presence of severe facial fractures, endotracheal intubation may be required while a 'flail' chest calls for assisted ventilation. Head and chest injury are frequently associated and the ready availability of an anaesthetist is so important that any Accident department that does not have such anaesthetic cover should be closed down.

Shock produces stagnant anoxia and is always a sign of major extracranial injury. There are three exceptions to this axiom: the infant with an intracranial haematoma; the patient with massive blood loss from a scalp laceration; and the brain-dead victim with a failing circulation. In most circumstances the head injury in an unconscious patient declares itself, not so the others. Thus, of the severe head injuries admitted to a regional Head Injury unit (Miller & Jones 1985) 32% had injuries to limbs, 6% had injuries to the spine and 28% had injury to the thorax and abdomen. All these were of sufficient severity to warrant the intervention of another surgical service. Some of these may be missed unless actively sought. While shock from a limb fracture may call for no more than immediate restoration of blood volume, that from a splenic rupture requires surgical intervention at the same time.

The importance of restoring the blood pressure expeditiously cannot be overstressed. An injured brain rendered ischaemic by the added insult of profound hypotension loses its capacity for autoregulation and swells as the blood pressure is restored, with intracranial pressure passively following the rise in systemic arterial pressure. The resulting clinical picture resembles the neurological deterioration classically associated with an intracranial haematoma but usually with a fatal outcome. Gentleman and Jennett (1981) recorded 75% mortality in patients with hypotension on arrival at the neurosurgical units, while all five of the patients who were hypoxic and in shock died.

In trauma, shock is usually from massive blood loss and the hypoxia therefore of the mixed stagnant and anaemic type. Subtler forms of anoxic anoxia may be seen in some very severe head injuries and in multiple trauma with shock when, due to terminal airway closure, the perfusion of blood through the walls of unaerated alveoli produces a functional pulmonary shunt.

Cerebral compression

Hard on the heels of anoxia as a potential threat to recovery in an injured brain comes the possibility of cerebral compression. Such compression may be due to brain swelling or intracranial haematoma, often both, in patients who have been unconscious from the time of injury. Pathological evidence of raised intracranial pressure was found in 83% of fatal head injuries studied at the Southern General Hospital in Glasgow (Jennett & Teasdale 1981); 68% of these were associated with haematomas. Brain swelling is usually localized in relation to contusions or areas of ischaemic and hypoxic brain damage. Occasionally the swelling may be massive without surface contusion or other obvious focal lesions.

It is customary to divide intracranial haematomas into extradural, subdural and intracerebral, but more than one type of haematoma may be present in the same patient.

Extradural haematoma

Of all the complications of head injury that an undergraduate memory carries over to later years, the extradural haematoma is probably the one that stands out, together with the importance of a lucid interval in the diagnosis. The condition is sometimes also referred to, wrongly, as 'middle meningeal artery haemorrhage': the haematoma is not always in the middle meningeal territory nor necessarily of arterial origin. Even more erroneous is the concept one has heard people, who ought to know better, expound; namely, that a fracture line on the skull radiograph crossing the groove made by the middle meningeal 'artery' is of particular value in the diagnosis of an extradural haematoma. In fact, as any standard anatomy text book will confirm, the groove is occupied by the middle meningeal vein, whilst the artery lies deeper and outside the groove. Veins are thin-walled and easily damaged, and this explains why an extradural haematoma can occur after minor head injury and why in many cases at operation no frank arterial bleeding is seen. Nearly a third of the patients in one of the largest published series of extradural haematomas had had such a trivial head injury that they would not have sought medical attention if the complication had not arisen (Gallagher & Browder 1968). Nevertheless, a lucid interval is not invariable and the absence of one should not be considered to rule out the possibility of a clot.

Any extradural haematoma is directly under the point of impact. Where the urgency of the situation or the absence of a CT scanner makes the evacuation of, or search for, an extradural clot imperative, the external evidence of injury, whether bogginess, bruising or laceration of the scalp, is a more reliable pointer to where the lesion is than any other clinical feature. Even a skull radiograph may be superfluous in certain circumstances. While there is a high degree of correlation between skull fracture and haematoma, and much has been made of this, fatal mistakes, as well as expensive ones in medico-legal terms, have been made from failure to appreciate that there are frequent exceptions, especially among children in whom the dura is less adherent to the inner table of the skull and is more readily separated from it by seemingly mild knocks. In a study of over 4000 consecutive head injuries admitted to the Hospital for Sick Children in Toronto there were just as many extradural haematomas without skull fracture as there were with (Harwood–Nash *et al.* 1971).

Subdural haemorrhage

Subdural haematomas have been conventionally divided into acute, subacute and chronic, according to the interval between injury and recognition by whatever means. In the light of modern practice with emphasis on early CT scanning this classification loses any significance it ever had, and that is debatable. It is probably more realistic and of greater practical value to distinguish between *acute* and *chronic haematomas* with different connotations in terms of pathology, management and prognosis.

The *acute subdural haematoma* is hardly ever a purely subdural collection of blood. In acceleration–deceleration injury as the brain 'swirls' around within the cranium its cortical surface may be damaged by contact with structures projecting into the cranial cavity, in particular the lesser wings of the sphenoid, which accounts for acute 'subdural' haematomas being almost invariably low in the anterior temporal region. Though the clot is seen on opening the dura, it is, in fact, a mixture of subdural and intracerebral blood with pulped, swollen brain and therefore is more accurately designated an *intradural haematoma*. Because the clot is solid, its evacuation demands a craniotomy while the prognosis, despite intensive and early treatment, depends on the severity of the primary impact. The best clinical indicator of the latter is the highest level of responsiveness after injury: a patient who has no response at all to pain has a much worse outlook than one who, though not obeying commands, is able to localize pain.

The *chronic subdural haematoma*, on the other hand, is purely subdural, usually fluid and requires rarely more than burr-hole evacuation. The prognosis is good. In at least half the patients there may be no history of head injury. If there is, it is often trivial with an interval of a fortnight or longer between injury and presentation, and the condition is predominantly an affliction of the middle-aged and elderly.

Pure intracerebral haematomas are rare in older literature but are being recognized more frequently since CT scanning after head injury has become more or less routine in many modern neurosurgical centres. They are mostly in the frontal lobes but their aetiology is not known.

Traditionally, the recognition of life-threatening haematomas after head injury has relied on observed deterioration in the neurological state, especially the level of consciousness. In fact, the principal reason for the admission of hordes of mildly injured persons to hospital is just such observation, though only a few of these will actually prove to need any intracranial surgery. Miller and Jones (1985) found only 12 haematomas in 1616 consecutive admissions after mild head injury.

A frequent cause of concern among neurosurgeons is delay in diagnosis and referral with a consequent increase in mortality and morbidity. Galbraith (1976), in a study of over 300 patients with haematomas arriving at a neurosurgical unit, found, in about a third of them, evidence of deterioration recorded in the notes for more than 12 hours before the patients were referred.

There are many causes of misdiagnosis or delay. Altered consciousness may be attributed to alcohol rather than head injury. The absence of any agreed method of assessing changes in the level of consciousness can lead to a breakdown in communication when there is a change of ward staff. Many of the patients arrive in the observation ward at night when nurse staffing levels are often inadequate, and there is a natural tendency for the staff to concentrate on those who are obviously ill rather than on the minor injuries, few of whom will actually develop any serious complications. In the rare circumstances when there are enough nurses, an understandable reluctance on the part of a nurse to wake up a 'sleeping' patient at regular intervals to record the level of rousability may result in deterioration not being appreciated until one or both pupils have dilated widely and lost their reaction to light.

If a patient is obtunded when first seen, the traditional stress on waiting for deterioration or for lateralizing features, such as inequality of pupils or other focal neurological deficits, for the diagnosis of a haematoma, may mean delay and death.

The advent of CT scanning, with its safety and simplicity in comparison with earlier invasive procedures like carotid angiography, has shown that:

1 A patient who does not obey commands or utter recognizable words when first seen has an even chance of harbouring an intracranial haematoma.

2 Most haematomas are present from the time of injury and will be demonstrated by CT scanning before clinical deterioration occurs.

3 Early evacuation of a haematoma improves the prognosis.

The principal reservation one has about total reliance on CT scanning that this evidence would seem to justify is that not all haematomas seen are necessarily biologically relevant. Carotid angiography in the pre-scan era used to reveal haematomas and contusions that were not suspected clinically and which could often be treated conservatively without prejudice to the patient's welfare. Teasdale *et al.* (1980), in a trial of conservative management, found that less than half the patients with haematomas demonstrated on routine CT scanning eventually needed evacuation of the clot.

As CT scanning becomes increasingly available in District General hospitals, the possibility of screening patients with head injury to avoid unnecessary transfer to a distant neurosurgical department is attractive. This would be particularly true of:

1 A patient with multiple trauma in whom an extracranial injury demands urgent action but who has a head injury.

2 A patient who is confused and has a skull fracture.

3 A patient who remains confused for more than 12 hours in the absence of a skull fracture.

4 A patient who has had fits after injury.

The acute lesions commonly seen on a CT scan after head injury may be:

1 Extracerebral collections of blood.

(a) The acute subdural haematoma (Fig. 7.5) is a concavoconvex enhancing mass covering an extensive area of the cerebral convexity and displacing the midline structures to the opposite side occasionally. The blood may be of the same density as the underlying brain, and the lesion may then be wrongly diagnosed as swollen brain.

(b) The acute extradural haematoma (Fig. 7.6), on the other hand, is a biconvex and more localized enhancing lesion.

2 Lesions within the brain substance.

(a) Cerebral contusions (Fig. 7.7) show a speckled appearance with a mixture of low and high density lesions. Such contusions are particularly liable to become oedematous and produce clinical deterioration. The patient therefore needs to be observed carefully, though in most cases the depression in consciousness in the first instance would be sufficient on its own to warrant consultation with a neurosurgeon.

(b) Intracerebral haematomas (Fig. 7.8) are less frequent and such patients are, again, most likely to be

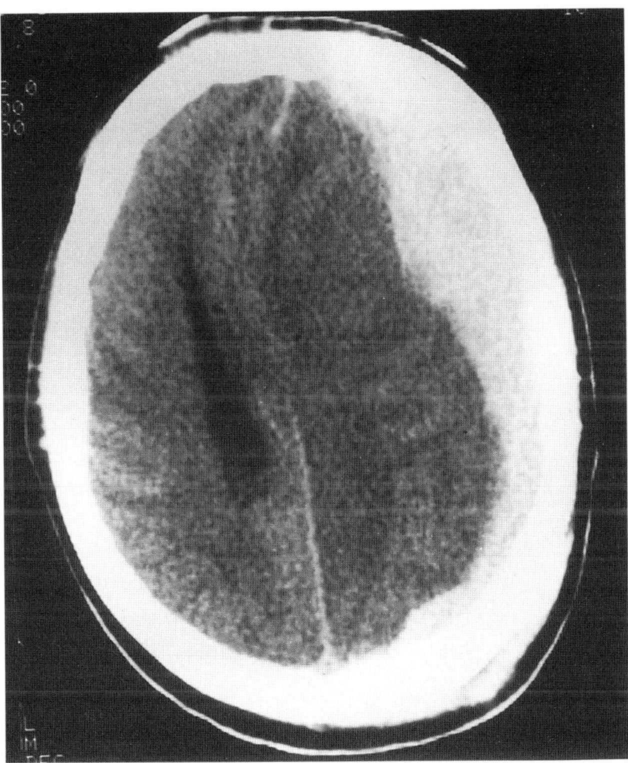

Fig. 7.5 Acute subdural haematoma.

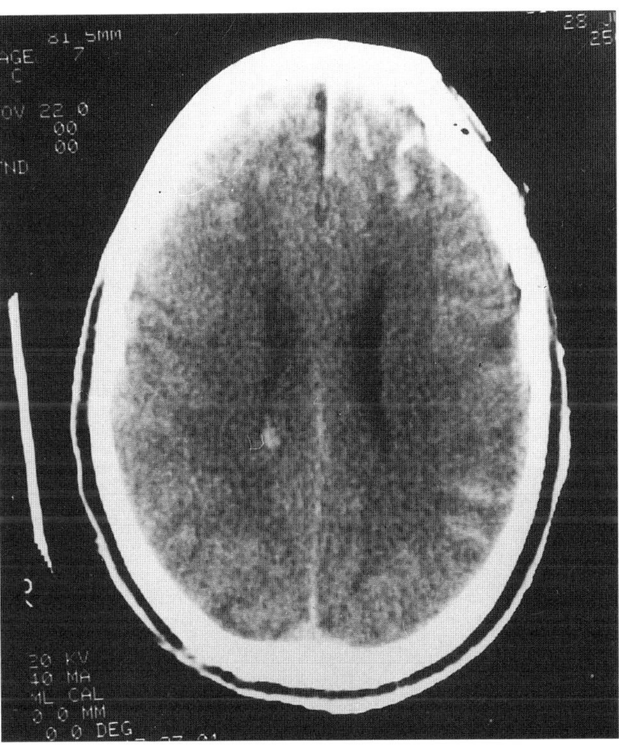

Fig. 7.7 Bilateral frontal contusions.

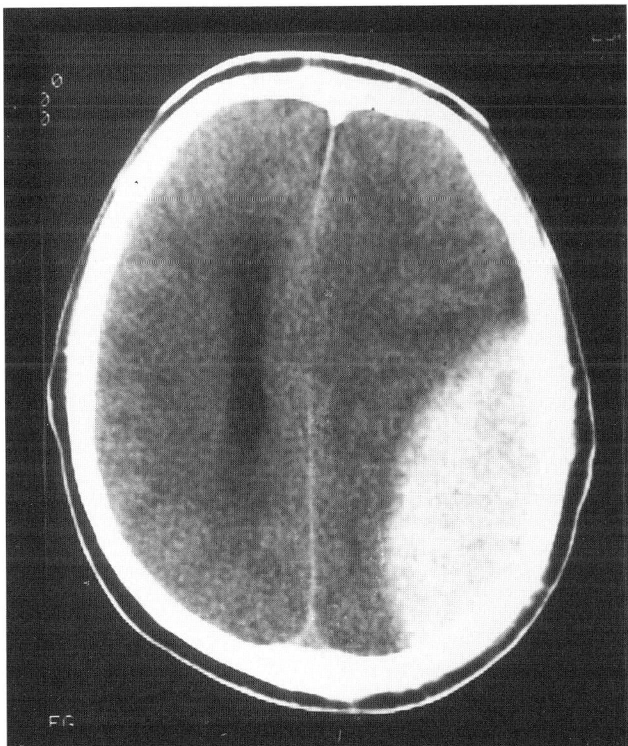

Fig. 7.6 Acute extradural haematoma.

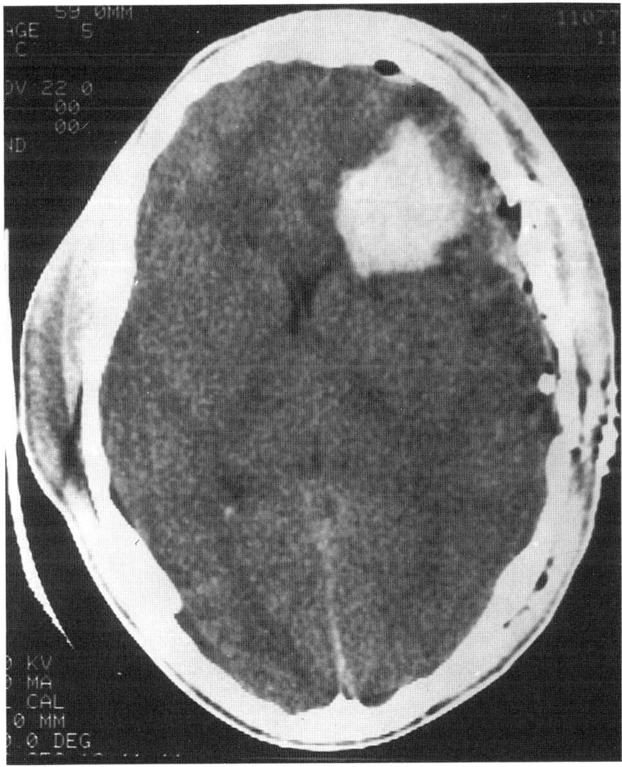

Fig. 7.8 Traumatic intracerebral haematoma.

ill enough anyway for referral to a neurosurgeon.

The value of such preliminary screening is shown by the finding that of patients in deep coma (MacPherson *et al.* 1990) almost a fifth had a normal scan.

In practice, only a few of the many head injuries seen in a large General hospital will justify scanning and the interpretation of radiological findings by non-specialist staff could lead to misdiagnosis. It is now possible to have scanner data transmitted by telephone lines to a neurosurgical unit where the images could be seen by a neurosurgeon who could, at the same time, discuss the patient's clinical condition before giving advice on action.

THE CASE FOR CLINICAL DIAGNOSIS

One of the recommendations of the Working Party on Head Injuries of the Royal College of Surgeons of England in 1986 was that every District General hospital with an Accident department should have a CT scanner. This is improbable in the foreseeable future. Even in hospitals with CT scanners already installed, difficulties in staffing have meant that the service is rarely available when most head injuries are admitted, i.e. outside office hours. Clinical assessment and plain radiographs of the skull will, for all practical purposes, continue to be the cornerstone of head injury management with selective early referral of the high-risk patients to a neurosurgical unit and serial observation in the primary hospital of the 'minor' head injuries for neurological deterioration. Even in neurosurgical departments there are occasions when a patient's life depends on expeditious action based on simple criteria without recourse to plain radiographs, let alone a CT scan. This point tends to be overlooked in a system heavily reliant on sophisticated technology.

The findings of Andrews *et al.* (1986) provide support for a view that is unfashionable in many neurosurgical circles today. One hundred patients arriving at the San Francisco General Hospital within 1 hour of injury and with clinical signs of tentorial herniation or upper brain stem dysfunction had emergency burr-hole exploration after resuscitation and after radiographs of the chest and lateral views of the cervical spine had been taken to rule out major neck injury. Of this group 56 had surface haematomas. In patients with negative exploration a CT scan was carried out postoperatively. Six haematomas were missed but in none of these had a complete bilateral exploration been carried out. The patients in this study were in a category in which prognosis is poor anyway, but there are, and will continue to be, circumstances in which a patient, who is deteriorating rapidly,

will not survive a journey to a distant neurosurgical unit and the only hope is prompt action by the first surgeon, orthopaedic or otherwise, who sees the patient. The diagnostic tool most readily available to a surgeon is the brace and burr.

Where exploration on clinical grounds alone is indicated, three burr holes at most are all that are generally needed: (i) a burr hole over the point of impact on the scalp, as indicated by a bruise, bogginess or contused scalp laceration, will expose an extradural clot if there is one (Fig. 7.9); and (ii) a burr hole low in either temple will reveal any acute intradural haematoma (Fig. 7.9).

When haematomas are missed it is either because further exploration is omitted, if the first drill hole has shown a haematoma, or, as is still recommended in some circles, exploration is carried out at three standard sites: namely, low temporal and the other two just in front of the lambdoid and coronal sutures, respectively, along a parasagittal line passing through the pupil. While acute subdural clots will be revealed by the temporal burr hole, the parasagittal burr holes will only strike 'oil' in a chronic subdural haematoma which does not present with the same dramatic urgency (Fig. 7.10).

What to do when a clot is found will depend on the individual surgeon's experience.

If an extradural clot is found the temptation to suck the clot out through the burr hole must be resisted: this may produced troublesome bleeding before there is enough access to the torn vessel. If the surgeon lacks the confidence or the facilities to do any more, leaving the wound unsutured, covered over with loosely applied generous dressings and a slow intravenous infusion

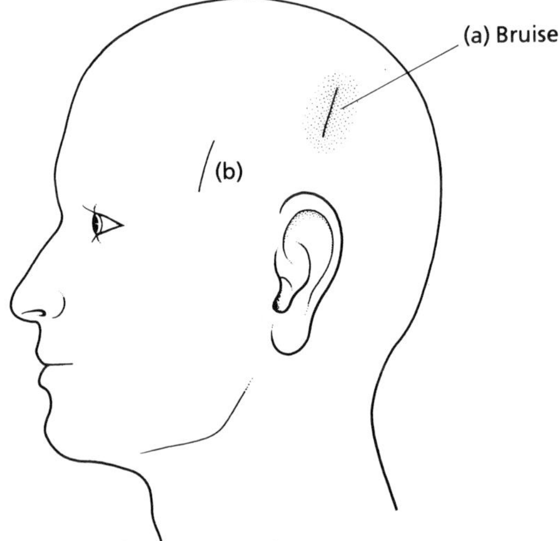

Fig. 7.9 Recommended sites for burrhole exploration. (a) Over bruise for an extradural clot. (b) Low anterior temporal for an acute subdural clot.

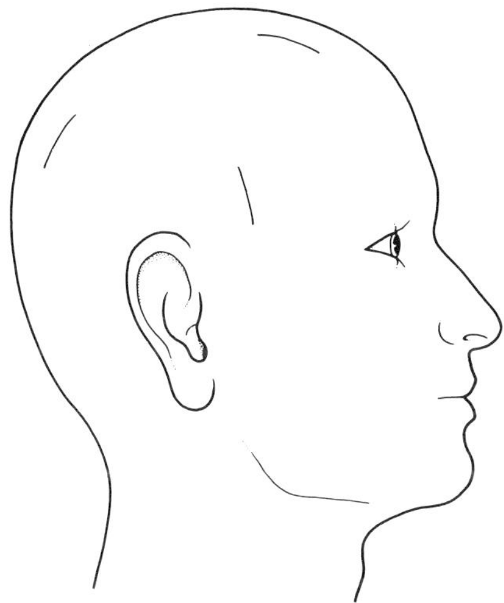

Fig. 7.10 Three conventional sites for burrhole exploration which may miss acute haematomas.

will permit safe transfer to a neurosurgical unit. The pulsating brain will extrude sufficient clot into the dressings to decompress itself.

The surgeon who wishes to perform the whole procedure personally could extend the scalp incision and enlarge the burr hole to uncover as much of the haematoma as possible before removing it; this will provide sufficient access for control of any bleeding with diathermy. Such a 'creeping craniectomy' is safer and quicker than a craniotomy in inexperienced hands. The resulting skull defect can be easily repaired by a neurosurgeon at a later date.

An acute intradural clot of any biological significance will require a formal craniotomy and this is outside the scope of those who have not spent at least a few months in a neurosurgical unit during their training. Many surgical training schemes rotate through neurosurgery and should provide the necessary familiarity. The surgeon who feels diffident can find consolation in the knowledge that the prognosis is poor in the person with a very acute subdural haematoma and who has been deeply unconscious since the moment of injury. While advocating the clinical approach in an extreme situation, one ought to emphasize that in most Western countries it should be exceptional to have to carry out cranial surgery at any hospital less than an hour's journey from a neurosurgical unit.

Brain swelling may be an important contributor to intracranial hypertension with or without haematoma and cannot be distinguished clinically from the latter with any certainty. It should only be diagnosed after exclusion of a haematoma by CT scanning or, exceptionally, after burr-hole exploration.

The level of consciousness is the most sensitive index of brain function and the management of all cerebral disorders, and not just head trauma, depends on the examiner's ability to recognize changes in consciousness. A progressive deterioration in consciousness is the one constant clinical feature of life-threatening haematomas. The assessment of altered consciousness therefore merits separate consideration.

Stupor and coma have no generally accepted definitions and mean different things to different people. The two terms are, strictly speaking, synonymous and are respectively the Latin and Greek terms for sleep. Unconscious means unaware: on its own it conveys nothing unless qualified by indicating what the individual is unaware of. In cerebral disorders consciousness is best described simply in terms of how the patient responds to speech and, failing this, to the more powerful stimulus of pain. The traditional approach has always favoured a description of the patient's responses, or individual departments have instituted their own systems. The absence of a structured approach creates ambiguities in assessment and communication when decisions about the transfer of ill patients to a specialist centre have to be made over the telephone. The Glasgow 'coma' scale (GCS), introduced by Teasdale and Jennett (1974), is now widely accepted and used in most major neurological centres in the Western world. Three features — *eye opening, verbal performance* and *motor response* — are assessed separately (Table 7.3).

Eye opening can be noted in passing when testing verbal and motor responses. One of the more common errors in Accident and Emergency departments is to label a person who gives rational answers as conscious, forgetting that the essential components of full consciousness are orientation in time and space. The lower levels of verbal response are self-explanatory.

The highest motor response is obeying commands; if the patient cannot do this the reaction to pain is observed. Painful stimulation is best applied by firm supraorbital pressure with the pulps of the fingers on either side of the bridge of the nose. If the hand moves above the chin towards the eyebrow, the response is a localizing one, or what used to be traditionally called a purposeful response to pain. Abnormal responses, indicating progressively lower levels of consciousness, are:

1 Flexion withdrawal, where the flexing hand does not move above the chin.

2 Spastic flexion or abnormal flexion, representing what used to be called a decorticate response.

3 Extension at the elbow, corresponding to the conventional decerebrate state.

4 No response at all.

Where there is an asymmetrical response, the better one represents the level of consciousness and the other is due to focal cerebral injury. The Glasgow scale lends itself to being recorded as a score; the lowest response in each feature is 1 and every step up the scale justifies an additional mark. Full consciousness merits a score of 15 while the deepest level in which there is no eye opening, no verbal response and no response even to pain has a score of 3. 'Coma' on the Glasgow scale is defined as *not opening the eyes, not uttering recognizable words* and *not obeying commands*, and has a score of 8 or less.

The lower levels of response are rarely seen outside neurological units, and those who are unfamiliar with them may not readily differentiate between flexion/withdrawal and spastic flexion; therefore, most bedside observation charts in general use allow space for only 'flexion' to be recorded. Many retrospective studies use these charts, and if scores are to be used, then coma on these charts scores 7 or less and full consciousness 14.

A severe injury is defined as one which produces 'coma' lasting for 6 hours or longer. However, this definition has suffered the ravages of early aggressive treatment which often demands tracheal intubation and sedation to allow controlled ventilation so that, in effect, severity is nowadays defined by the level of consciousness soon after resuscitation: a score of 7 or less on the 14-point scale constitutes severe injury, 8—12 signifies a moderate injury and a score above 12 a minor injury. The principal drawback of such a classification is that in comparing the results of varying management patients in 'coma', many of whom, in the author's experience, recover spontaneously in 1—2 hours, may be included in regimens involving ventilation with an inevitable skewing of the outcome figures in favour of ventilation.

On observation wards most patients who do not obey commands resent interference and will push the examiner's hand away if attempts are made, say, to open the eyelids to look at the pupils. Such patients will obviously localize pain, and it is suggested that before applying a painful stimulus the examiner should see whether the person resents interference, the absence of which in modern assessment one notes with dismay. However, this move may spare the infliction of pain on the patient as well as avoiding unpleasant repercussions when dealing with an inebriate head injury.

Infection

Infection is chronologically the last, but not the least, of the major threats to the injured brain and skull. Broadly, the principles are the same as in compound wounds in any other region of the body, but the timing and scope of surgical intervention depend on whether the wound is over the vault or in the base of the skull.

Compound fracture of skull vault

A fracture under a scalp laceration is technically compound but becomes particularly significant if the dura deep to it is also injured by depressed bone fragments with the additional risk of meningitis or brain abscess.

Recognition of a compound depressed fracture depends on getting a proper account of how the laceration was caused and careful inspection of the wound under a good light. The latter means shaving the scalp for at least 5 cm around the laceration. If there is bruising and swelling adjacent to the laceration radiographs of the skull are indicated, as they are also after any laceration, however neat, produced by a pointed object, especially in children.

As with compound fractures elsewhere in the body management consists of exploration of the wound to clean it of all contaminated non-viable tissue and foreign bodies, followed by primary closure. Treatment can, if necessary for any reason, be delayed for up to 24 hours without increasing morbidity, while keeping the patient on prophylactic antibiotics. Penicillin and sulphadimidine are the most commonly used drugs in the United Kingdom. Exploration is preferably carried out by a neurosurgeon, as is conventionally taught, to remove bone fragments where the inner table is depressed more than the thickness of the skull, and to look for any dural tear underneath, which should be repaired using either pericranium from the adjacent intact skull or fascia lata for larger defects. It is doubtful, however, whether such exploration, where the outer table fragments are impacted firmly and without loose pieces of bone, is superior to just cleaning out the wound thoroughly and suturing the scalp without tension. Where the dura has been exposed it is better to replace cleaned fragments of bone, rather than to discard them and leave a skull defect whch will require secondary repair, as long as the surgery is within 24 hours of injury.

Even in high-speed missile wounds (Crockard 1974) it is advisable to defer surgery till the intracranial pressure, invariably high in such patients, has been controlled with mechanical ventilation. Death is inevitable, despite vigorous treatment, in those who do not respond to pain when first seen; it also claims 11% of those who reach hospital conscious and alert. At operation, the necrotic brain contains all the fragments of bone that were driven in and can be safely removed without damaging more brain, but pieces of metal which penetrate more deeply are not actively sought.

Compound fracture of the skull base

The amount of force needed to fracture the heavily buttressed skull base will usually have been enough to render the victim unconscious but the compound fracture may not be recognized unless actively sought. A compound fracture of the anterior cranial fossa should be considered in patients with a frontal impact who also have either fractures of the middle third of the face or periorbital haematoma with discoloration of the eyelids and a clean cut edge at the bony aperture of the orbit (the so-called racoon sign, though this is perhaps better described as the 'eye-shadow' sign) as well as bleeding from the nostrils. An anterior fossa fracture with a dural tear will declare itself in patients with an obvious csf rhinorrhoea, which may be delayed and develop only after the blood clot in the fracture line has resolved and brain swelling subsided.

Routine skull radiographs taken immediately after injury may not reveal a basal fracture unless the latter extends into the skull vault, but it should be diagnosed if the radiographs show air in the cranium, and suspected if there is a fluid level or opacity in the paranasal sinuses, particularly the sphenoid.

Csf otorrhoea, as evidence of a dural tear in the floor of the middle fossa, is usually present soon after injury, but a compound fracture here should be suspected if there is blood in the external auditory canal and bruising over the mastoid process just behind the ear. Rarely, with an intact eardrum, csf from a middle fossa dural defect may run forwards through the Eustachian canal and be seen as rhinorrhoea.

Finally, the first sign of a traumatic basal dural defect may be meningitis.

Controversy surrounds both the management of suspect dural tears and the indications for exploration. The balance of evidence favours the prophylactic use of penicillin and sulphadimidine in every patient with a clinical suspicion of a compound basal fracture, whether there is an obvious csf leak or not (Jennett & Teasdale 1981). If there is no evidence of such a fistula or of air in the cranium, then the antibiotics can be discontinued after 1 week. If a csf leak is present the prophylaxis is continued for a fortnight after the leak has stopped or for a week after surgical repair. Such a policy will reduce the risk of meningitis but not remove it altogether. There is no place whatsoever for broad-spectrum antibiotics in this situation.

Repair of any proven dural tear or exploration to look for one is not an emergency. It is best postponed for a couple of weeks or even longer to allow the patient to recover from the acute phase of the head injury and also to see whether the csf discharge stops of its own accord.

Csf otorrhoea may be profuse soon after injury but it usually stops within a few days and it is exceptional to have to carry out any exploratory operation. A rare but well-recognized cause of persistent, or even copious, leakage of csf from the ear is the presence of a subacute extradural haematoma; the fistula compensates for the increasing pressure from an intracranial haematoma by pouring out csf from the cranium. Such a patient's level of consciousness will therefore remain high until the clot expands to block the dural defect which had allowed the csf to escape; after this, the level of consciousness may decline dramatically.

Surgical repair is obviously called for if a csf leak persists for more than 1 week. Even where there is a transient rhinorrhoea surgery may be advisable if: (i) the fracture is wider than a hairline; or (ii) there is bilateral anosmia and no skull fracture. In wide fracture lines the cessation of rhinorrhoea is due to brain plugging the dural defect. Dural repair also has to be considered when there is: (iii) a persisting aerocoele; or (iv) meningitis (after recovery from the infection). It is best to postpone exploration in all cases until any facial fractures have been reduced; this often succeeds in stopping persistent csf rhinorrhoea. Because such operations are only carried out as planned procedures, appropriate radiography to delineate possible defects in the skull base can be deferred until the patient is awake and able to co-operate.

Early management

The overwhelming majority of patients seen in an Accident department after head injury are talking on arrival and may even have walked in. Apart from the obvious need for treatment of scalp lacerations, it is important to identify those who need admission either because they are at particular risk of harbouring a haematoma or because they have a compound fracture of the skull.

There is also a very small second group who are clearly candidates for admission because they have been brought in with a depressed level of consciousness. In these cases, while the highest priorities are resuscitation and the search for major extracranial injury that might need immediate intervention, decisions have to be made about possible urgent transfer to, or at least consultation with, a neurosurgeon.

Stimulated by studies showing the variability in the

patterns of care in different parts of the United Kingdom and in the incidence of avoidable mortality and morbidity a group of surgeons (Briggs *et al.* 1984), meeting at intervals informally over a period of 3 years, agreed on guidelines in the hope of rationalizing head injury care and helping inexperienced doctors and non-specialists with responsibility for the primary, and often continuing, care of the bulk of head injuries.

Clinical judgement should not be sacrificed to the guidelines, which are not mandatory and are offered as only a guide. It also needs to be stressed that they apply mainly to *adult head injuries* and that they were not endorsed by the Society of British Neurological Surgeons when presented to it at a meeting of its members.

Radiographic examination of the skull after recent head injury

Radiography of the skull is recommended in the following situations:

1 History of loss of consciousness or amnesia at any time.
2 Neurological symptoms or signs, e.g. persistent severe headache, vomiting or fits.
3 Csf or blood flow from the nose or ear.
4 Suspected penetrating injury (a history is important here).
5 Scalp bruising or swelling whether or not in association with a laceration.

A clean laceration of the scalp without bruising of its edges probably does not need radiographic examination and it is also questionable as to whether anything is to be gained by radiography of all cases where the clinical picture alone already calls for admission. This applies especially to confused and restless patients, for whom radiographs of any diagnostic quality may not be practicable, especially in an understaffed District General hospital in the middle of the night. In high-speed accidents and with multiple injury radiographs of the chest and cervical spine may be more important; the skull may also be examined at the same time. On the other hand, radiographs may be all important in asymptomatic patients in whom the demonstration of a skull fracture would dictate admission.

Admission to a District General hospital

The criteria for admission from the accident room to an observation ward are:

1 Confusion or any depression of consciousness at the time of initial examination.
2 Neurological symptoms or signs.

3 Presence of a skull fracture.
4 Difficulty in assessing the patient, e.g. as a result of alcohol, epilepsy or other medical conditions, and children.
5 Lack of a responsible adult to supervise the patient at home, or other social problems.

Historically, in the United Kingdom one of the indications for admission for observation has been amnesia for the injury. In fact, this constitutes the bulk of patients who are admitted for observation and discharged the following day. However, surveys have demonstrated that such patients, if asymptomatic, orientated and without skull fracture, are unlikely to develop complications and need not be admitted (Weston 1981).

Orientation cannot be assessed in infants and young children and, therefore, in the United Kingdom neurosurgeons have often advised that all children brought to the Accident department should be admitted. Paediatricians, on the other hand, are concerned about the long-term psychological trauma produced in children by the mere fact of having been admitted into an unfamiliar environment, even for a single night. A happy compromise is to obtain radiographs of the skulls of all children brought to an Accident department and, even if there is no skull fracture, detain parent and child in the waiting room for a couple of hours. In a busy Accident department at weekends and in the evening this may be the length of waiting time for apparently well patients before radiographs are available anyway. Most children who may be harbouring an extradural haematoma will have developed symptoms of raised intracranial pressure, such as headache and vomiting, within this time. The author knows personally of at least two children without skull fracture for whom this advice proved life-saving.

All patients, young and old, seen in Accident departments and deemed not to warrant admission should only be allowed home with verbal and written instructions to a relative or friend about changes to look for which will require the urgent return of the patient to hospital. These are virtually the same as for patients admitted for observation — altered consciousness, increasing headache, vomiting and fits.

Consultation with a neurosurgeon

Neurosurgeons cannot accept all head injuries into their care, but they are, or should be, prepared to give advice over the telephone or discuss management of any patient that the non-specialist doctor is concerned about. It is recommended that a neurosurgeon is contacted for advice in the following circumstances:

1 'Coma', i.e. not uttering comprehensible words, not opening eyes and not obeying commands *after* resuscitation.

2 Fractured skull with

  (a) confusion or worse impairment of consciousness.

  (b) focal neurological signs.

  (c) epileptic fits.

3 Deterioration in the level of consciousness.

4 Confusion or other neurological disturbances persisting for more than 12 hours, even if there is no fracture.

5 A depressed fracture of the skull vault — simple or compound.

6 A suspect compound fracture of the skull base.

Many neurosurgeons would prefer to have all such patients under their care in neurosurgical departments, at least for assessment, rather than be merely consulted.

Patients in categories 1−3 should be referred urgently *after resuscitation* and after confirming that extracranial injuries that need immediate treatment have not been missed. Precautions should be taken to reduce risks during transfer and the patient should be accompanied by a trained doctor or nurse with all the notes and radiographs. If the patient appears to be deteriorating and if this deterioration appears to be due to raised intracranial pressure, and not to unrecognized extracranial, particularly thoracic, complications, the safest way of transporting such patients to a neurosurgical centre is with controlled mechanical ventilation and an infusion of 20% mannitol $0.5-1$ g kg^{-1} given over $10-15$ minutes. To reduce the effects of hypervolaemia from the use of a hyperosmolar agent 40 mg frusemide is preferably given at the start of the mannitol infusion.

Such extraordinary measures should normally only be instituted after consulting the neurosurgeon and the level of consciousness should be recorded before starting them. Unless dictated by the needs of extracranial problems or by deterioration from rising intracranial pressure, which may prevent the patient from reaching a neurosurgical unit with any prospect of survival, a patient who needs sedation to allow intubation probably does not require this treatment. A factitious argument put forward in support of sedation of such patients is that their intracranial pressure rises to dangerous levels when they cough or are restless. Proponents of this argument ignore the fact that it is not raised intracranial pressure but reduced cerebral perfusion pressure that is dangerous and that patients with a good cough reflex have also retained their capacity for autoregulation of cerebral blood flow.

Minor and moderate head injuries

Only a fraction of the head injuries seen in an Accident department will qualify for immediate transfer or consultation with a neurosurgeon. The rest will be looked after in the primary surgical ward and such patients are usually apparently fit for discharge in a day or two. The problems of management, unless the patient deteriorates while under observation, are of little interest to the average surgeon but they may, nevertheless, be of importance to the nursing and junior medical staff and, not least of all, to the patient.

Intravenous infusion

The average head-injured patient who is not shocked from another injury does not need an intravenous infusion even if oral nutrition is not taken for 12 hours or longer. Most head-injured patients are healthy at the time of injury and are unlikely to come to any harm from such deprivation, though it is no longer considered necessary to dehydrate head injuries deliberately.

Restlessness

Many patients may be restless from alcohol, headache or pain from other injured organs. When close observation of levels of consciousness is the mainstay in management it is important *not to give any sedative drugs*: increasing restlessness is a rare but well-recognized feature of an extradural haematoma. Codeine phosphate is very effective for headache while the pain from limb fractures is best treated by proper immobilization after reduction. Many neurosurgeons used to advise against any treatment under general anesthesia for extracranial injuries, but most adverse effects have been instances of bad anaesthesia rather than of anaesthesia itself. Any anaesthesia in a head injury should be with controlled ventilation. Restless patients can be difficult to nurse and head-injured patients are best looked after in a separate observation ward attached to the Accident department.

Anosmia

This can result from relatively trivial injury as can blindness from *optic nerve damage*. In the latter there is invariably a tell-tale sign of a blow around or above the ipsilateral eyebrow. In the past surgeons have recommended exploration and decompression of the optic nerve in the canal, especially if a depressed spicule of bone is seen protruding into the optic foramen. This is of no value; any partial recovery in due course is part of the natural history where the nerve has not been completely severed. In the unconscious patient the absent light reflex in a relatively large pupil can raise doubts about an intracranial clot, unless the consensual reflex is tested.

Postural vertigo

This can occur even after minor injury and is often associated with headaches. Unless the test for postural vertigo is carried out, and positional nystagmus seen with reproduction of the patient's symptom, it may not be recognized for what it is. The dizziness is a true vertigo, is brought on by a sudden change of position and usually improves spontaneously after a variable length of time. From quite early on the trend to such recovery becomes obvious. If dizziness gets worse, it may be part of an accident or compensation neurosis. But in some victims the feeling of physical insecurity caused by the dizziness can produce a reactive depression, probably resulting from a failure of the patient or doctor to appreciate that symptoms can develop after a trivial head injury.

Post-traumatic syndrome

Dizziness is part of a more complex post-traumatic syndrome, the existence and aetiology of which has been disputed, especially as the severity and duration are out of proportion to the causative injury. Headache, memory impairment and poor concentration are the principal symptoms, in addition to dizziness. The frequent association with a compensation claim (which may be the only time these patients are examined by a specialist) has naturally led to the conclusion that conscious or subconscious motivation towards financial gain perpetuates the symptoms. This is true in most cases in which the disability is so complete as to prevent the individual leading anything resembling a normal personal life, let alone work, and where the symptoms progressively deteriorate with the passage of time. Nevertheless, such symptoms do occur after minor head injury and where there is no question of compensation.

Rimel *et al.* (1981) evaluated 424 minor head injuries in a prospective study. Minor head injury was defined as one with a history of unconsciousness of 20 minutes or less, a GCS of 13–15 and hospitalization not longer than 48 hours. At 3 months 79% had persistent headache, 59% complained of problems of memory and only 16% were symptom-free. Only in six of these patients was there any question of litigation: three had returned

to work before the claim was settled, two were unemployed at the time of the injury and only one had not returned to work. Return to work correlated well with socioeconomic status and occupation of the individual; this may perhaps be explained by greater motivation in patients from a higher social background, though it may just as well be because they generally have more resources to buffer the effects of their injury after return to work. There is evidence in the survey that this morbidity is more likely to be an emotional response to the stress produced by the persistent symptoms from the *injury* than from organic brain damage.

Reassurance at routine follow-up about the self-limiting nature of these symptoms is probably the best way to manage post-traumatic syndrome. After a night or two in an observation ward peremptory discharge without explanation or review is undesirable, but who should provide, or is able to find time for, this is another matter. Most surgeons who have the responsibility for initial care are temperamentally unsuited to such aftercare. The trend towards the appointment in Accident and Emergency departments of consultants without major surgical commitments and often from general medical disciplines should provide an opportunity to remedy a major deficiency in aftercare; the help of a full-time neuropsychologist attached to the department and a social worker would complete the team.

Though by profession committed to the provision of appropriate care once an injury has occurred, it would be short-sighted of the medical profession to ignore the importance of preventing injury, particularly to an organ like the brain which has obvious limitations as an object of therapeutic endeavour.

References

Andrews, B.T., Pitts, L.H., Lovely, M.P. & Bartowski, H. Is computed tomographic scanning necessary in patients with tentorial herniation? Results of immediate surgical exploration without computed tomography in 100 patients. *Neurosurgery* 1986; **19**: 408–414.

Briggs, M., Clark, P., Crockard, A. *et al.* Guidelines for initial management of head injury in adults. *Br Med J* 1984; **288**: 983–985.

Crockard, H.A. Bullet injuries of the brain. *Ann R Coll Surg Engl* 1974; **55**: 111–123.

Field, J.H. *Epidemiology of Head Injuries in England and Wales.* HMSO: London, 1976.

Galbraith, S. Misdiagnosis and delayed diagnosis in traumatic intracranial haematoma. *Br Med J* 1976; **i**: 1438–1439.

Gallagher, J.P. & Browder, E.J. Extradural haematoma. Experience with 167 patients. *J. Neurosurg* 1968; **19**: 1–12.

Gentleman, D. & Jennett, B. Hazards of inter-hospital transfer of comatose head injured patients. *Lancet* 1981; **ii**: 853–855.

Harwood-Nash, D.C., Hendrick, E.B. & Becker, D.P. The significance of skull fracture in children. A study of 1187 patients. *Paediatr Radiol* 1971; **101**: 151–155.

Jennett, B. & MacMillan, R. Epidemiology of head injury. *Br Med J* 1981; **282**: 101–104.

Jennett, B. & Teasdale, G. *The Management of Head Injuries.* FA Davis: Philadelphia, 1981.

MacPherson, P., Jennett, B. & Anderson, E. CT scanning and surgical treatment of 1551 patients admitted to a regional neurosurgical unit. *Clin Radiol* 1990; **42**: 85–87.

Miller, J.D. & Jones, P.A. The work of a regional head injury service. *Lancet* 1985; **i**: 1141–1144.

Rimel, R.W., Giordano, B., Barth, J.T., Boll, T.J. & Jane, J.A. Disability caused by minor head injury. *Neurosurgery* 1981; **9**: 221–228.

Teasdale, G. & Jennett, B. Assessment of coma and impaired consciousness. *Lancet* 1974; **ii**: 81–84.

Teasdale, G., Galbraith, S. & Jennett, B. Operate or observe? ICP and the management of the 'silent' intracranial haematoma. In: Shulman, K., Marmarou, A., Miller, J.D., Becker, D.P., Hochwald, A.M., Brock, M. (eds) *Intracranial Pressure IV.* Springer-Verlag: Berlin, 1980.

Weston, P.A.M. Admission policy for patients following head injury. *Br J Surg* 1981; **68**: 663–664.

Chest injuries

J.C.STODDART

Most major chest injuries result from road traffic accidents, with a small number being caused by other types of trauma. In hospital, an occasional patient may be seen whose chest injuries have been produced by closed chest cardiac massage. Patients who have undergone extensive thoracic or thoraco-abdominal surgery may present a similar problem. In all of these situations the initial management is the same. This is based upon the immediate effects of the injury and concentrates upon (i) cardiocirculatory resuscitation, (ii) pain relief and (iii) gas exchange.

Cardiocirculatory resuscitation

A patient who has sustained a major chest injury may exsanguinate with no external evidence of blood loss. One half of the thoracic cavity can easily accommodate the entire blood volume. Fractured ribs often tear intercostal or internal mammary arteries, and the lungs are very vascular and frequently bleed profusely. More dramatic bleeding may result from damage to the aorta, the vena cava or the heart.

Many patients with chest injuries also have injuries elsewhere which result in significant blood loss and for which the optimum treatment includes large volume fluid replacement. The need to give blood or another blood volume expander, while at the same time protecting the lungs from the danger of overtransfusion, creates a conflict in the treatment of patients with multiple injuries. This explains in part why patients with chest injuries who also have other injuries require more prolonged supportive treatment than those whose injuries are localized to the thorax and its contents.

Pain relief

Even the most trivial chest wall injury is painful and the patient may be in pain from other injuries. Pain restricts respiratory movements and interferes with the efficiency of coughing and of expectoration. The patient who will not, or cannot, cough is in danger of atelectasis, and the ability to expectorate is one of the most useful guides to the severity of the injury. Pain also greatly increases tissue oxygen consumption. The patient must therefore be given effective pain relief as soon as possible, but whichever method is used its side-effects must constantly be borne in mind. Relief of pain may enable the patient to breathe more deeply and to cough and expectorate; on the other hand, it may also cause respiratory depression and encourage the retention of secretions.

Problems of gas exchange

Paradoxical ventilation

Chest wall instability restricts respiratory movements and may cause paradoxical ventilation such that the movement of a part of the thoracic cage is in the opposite direction to the phase of ventilation. It is caused either by fractures in two places in one or more ribs or by the combination of rib fractures with costochondral fracture–dislocation. If the sternum is fractured a further cause for instability is created.

Paradoxical ventilation may be of a minor degree, affecting only one segment of the chest wall, or it may be so extensive that no effective alveolar ventilation or gas exchange can take place. If one side of the chest is totally unstable it is theoretically possible for the respiratory movements to move gas from one lung to the other — the so-called pendelluft (pendulum breathing) — without any external gas exchange taking place. Unless this is treated rapidly it is incompatible with life.

In recent years the effects of small areas of paradoxical ventilation have been shown to be of little significance, although major chest wall instability always causes hypoxia and hypercapnia. On the other hand, if the patient is given effective pain relief adequate ventilation may be possible in the presence of quite extensive bone injury, with or without paradox.

Penetrating injuries

Penetrating injuries and direct pulmonary trauma create problems which may demand urgent treatment such as the insertion of a chest drain or the use of an occlusive pack, together with cardiocirculatory resuscitation. Pneumothorax, with or without haemothorax, usually requires the use of an intercostal drain. Penetrating wounds of the pericardium or heart, with or without tamponade, require urgent surgical treatment. The treatment of tamponade caused by closed trauma is described later. The aorta or vena cava may also be injured directly or indirectly (p. 145). The lungs and bronchi may be damaged; lobectomy or, rarely, pneumonectomy may be required.

Pulmonary contusions

Although the bony injuries may be more obvious, the underlying pulmonary contusion may be more significant. Contused alveoli cannot take part in gas exchange, leading inevitably to hypoxia with a widened alveolar/arterial (Aa) oxygen tension gradient (p. 144).

Classification of the severity of chest injuries

This is based upon the patient's pre-incident physical status, the extent of chest trauma and any associated injuries (Lloyd *et al.* 1965).

The extent and result of the pulmonary injury

The initial assessment of the severity of the injury must include chest radiography and blood gas analysis, although it may be obvious without the aid of these investigations that the patient requires oxygen therapy or ventilatory assistance. If the extent of the injury is not immediately apparent the patient must be kept under constant skilled observation and re-examined at intervals which are dictated by the overall physical status.

If an injured patient becomes confused or begins to behave in a bizarre fashion, hypoxia is the most likely cause and the appropriate steps must be taken to identify and treat it. Brain damage and fat embolism must also be included in the differential diagnosis. Sepsis is a common cause of post-traumatic confusion, but this is a later development. Confusion is not a diagnosis but a symptom and confused patients must never be given sedative, narcotic or similar drugs until the cause of the symptom has been determined.

Blood gas analysis

Blood gas analysis may need to be repeated hourly until a firm decision can be made as to the extent of the injuries and the course of treatment required. Blood gas analysis must always be performed after the patient has been given the first effective dose of an analgesic drug, particularly if the patient is somnolent or asleep, to exclude the possibility of respiratory depression.

The results must be clearly charted since they are the only reliable indication of the progression of the lesion. During the first 48 hours after injury, hypoxia without hypercapnia is usually due to pulmonary contusion, pneumothorax or pulmonary oedema. Hypercapnia means that the patient is underventilating because of either the injury(s) or its treatment. The causes of underventilation include pain, the use of narcotic analgesics and previously undiagnosed head injury. Ventilatory depression due to natural or synthetic narcotics can be reversed with naloxone.

Chest radiography

Chest radiography will reveal the extent of bone damage and underlying pulmonary contusions or other intrathoracic injury; if only portable films can be taken, injuries to the sternum and anterior ribs may not be demonstrated and the shape and size of the heart cannot be determined accurately. It is quite common for previously unrecognized rib fractures to be identified days later during the course of treatment. Pulmonary contusions may not be apparent radiographically until up to 24 hours after the incident.

Whenever possible, the films should be taken with the patient in the erect position. Erect films allow the size of the apical veins to be more accurately assessed and facilitate the recognition and quantification of pleural fluid; the position of the diaphragm and the presence of subphrenic gas may also be more readily determined.

Good quality lateral chest radiographs cannot be obtained after the patient is admitted to the Intensive Therapy unit or ward and, if possible, they should be taken in the X-ray department before admission.

Radiographs may need to be taken daily or more frequently. Complications which may arise during the course of treatment include pneumothorax or the appearance of delayed signs of aortic, pericardial or pleural bleeding. Evidence of bronchopneumonia or pulmonary oedema may also emerge.

Pre-existing health status

A patient who is suffering from an intercurrent disease at the time of injury is at greater risk than a previously healthy person. Such diseases include cardiorespiratory disturbances such as hypertension, myocardial ischaemia and chronic obstructive airways disease, but musculoskeletal disorders, such as rheumatoid arthritis, may also adversely influence the outcome of chest trauma. One of the more common conditions which may have a profound bearing upon the prognosis is obesity, since this influences not only the consequences of the respiratory injury but also the ease with which medical, surgical and nursing procedures can be carried out.

The effects of age

Major chest wall injuries are uncommon in small children both because of their epidemiology and because the infant or child has a thoracic cage which is almost infinitely malleable. Pulmonary contusions are also usually less severe and secondary infection a relatively minor problem. At the other extreme, elderly patients have very brittle bones which fracture readily, do not heal quickly and often pierce underlying structures. They are also more likely to suffer from intercurrent disease and have poor defence against traumatic insults and infection. Therefore, their prognosis is proportionally worse than that of a younger person with injuries of the same extent.

Co-existing injury

Patients who suffer chest injuries following industrial or road traffic accidents frequently sustain extrathoracic injuries. Those which increase the morbidity of the chest injury include faciomaxillary, intra-abdominal and intracranial injuries.

Faciomaxillary injuries

Faciomaxillary injuries may cause airway obstruction and interfere with swallowing, expectoration and oral nutrition. If a patient requires faciomaxillary surgery, including interdental banding, the risk of major respiratory difficulties is greatly increased. This type of injury is also frequently associated with post-concussional confusion.

Intra-abdominal and pelvic injuries

If the patient has sustained intra-abdominal injuries which necessitate an abdominal exploratory laparotomy, the resultant pain and paralytic ileus may interfere with respiratory movements and prevent the patient from breathing deeply, coughing and expectorating. A perforated viscus or bowel resection presents an important potential source of infection and the combination of intra-abdominal sepsis with thoracic trauma has a high mortality rate. Injuries which involve the lumbar vertebrae or pelvis cause extensive retroperitoneal bleeding which may have a similar effect.

These conditions may make enteral feeding impossible for a variable period. For the traumatized patient the maintenance of adequate nutrition is vital: parenteral feeding methods may have to be adopted, with the small but measurable increase in morbidity which inevitably follows.

Injuries which restrict the patient's ability to move in bed, either because of pain or because of extensive orthopaedic treatment, increase the risk of atelectasis, bronchopneumonia and pulmonary embolism. All patients with bone injuries (and rarely, those with soft tissue injuries) are at risk of fat embolism.

Level of consciousness

Any patient whose level of consciousness is impaired — because of direct brain damage, fat embolism or drugs — is in danger of pulmonary complications, either through an inability to co-operate with the nurses and physiotherapists or because of respiratory depression and reduced airway protection.

Diaphragmatic rupture

This injury is relatively rare and is usually caused by trauma to the anterior abdominal wall, although the association between acetabular fractures and diaphragmatic rupture has been recognized for many years; the force of impact is transmitted from the hip joint through the abdominal viscera so that part or all of the stomach, small or large bowel and, occasionally, the spleen herniate into the thoracic cavity. Although injuries to the left hemidiaphragm are more frequently recognized, autopsy examination indicates that the right hemidiaphragm may also be injured, although it retains its normal outline because of the position of the liver.

The diagnosis of diaphragmatic rupture may be suggested by the clinical presentation of dyspnoea and unequal chest movement. Radiologically, the left hemidiaphragm may be distorted and a visceral gas shadow may be visible in the left thoracic cavity. The diagnosis can sometimes be confirmed by passing a radio-opaque nasogastric tube; if the stomach has herniated the position of the tube will make this obvious. If barium is injected down the nasogastric tube, the stomach or other hollow viscus may be seen to be above the diaphragm.

The injury may be symptomless but may cause dyspnoea. Definitive treatment should be delayed until the patient has recovered from other injuries.

Tracheal and bronchial injuries

Injury to the cervical part of the trachea usually causes stridor and asphyxial symptoms. The lower trachea and major bronchi are well protected from the effects of external chest trauma, and the type of injury which is violent enough to cause damage to these structures often causes death very quickly because of damage to other structures (Mills *et al.* 1982, Amanchi *et al.* 1983).

Patients who survive are usually shocked, hypoxic, dyspnoeic and produce blood-stained sputum. They may have surgical emphysema which is localized to the supraclavicular region and to the base of the neck and they may have blood bubbles issuing from the mouth and nose. Chest radiography usually shows complete atelectasis of the affected lung together with mediastinal emphysema, but the cause can be confirmed only by bronchoscopy. The bronchus is usually found to be torn approximately 2 cm from the carina, causing complete obstruction of the distal segment. This condition must be treated surgically and the results are usually good. As with many of the injuries described in this chapter, the diagnosis may occasionally be unrecognized until many months later (Hix 1984).

Treatment of chest injuries

After taking the above factors into consideration the severity of chest injuries can be tabulated as shown in Table 7.7. This demonstrates the cumulative deleterious effects of factors which include increasing age, coma and intra-abdominal injuries. Although it is not intended to be fully comprehensive or to be applied rigidly, the classification is the principal guide to the regimen of treatment which the patient requires.

Patients who have sustained grade 1 injuries require:
1 Titrated analgesia.
2 Physiotherapy.
3 Mobilization.
Patients with grade 2 injuries require:

Table 7.7 A guide to the assessment of the severity of chest injuries

Grade 1	Grade 2	Grade 3
Young patient, multiple rib fractures, nil else	Grade 1 *plus* ileus, hypoxia	Grade 2 plus obtunded
Middle-aged patient, fit, few rib fractures	Middle-aged patient, bronchitic, few rib fractures, hypoxia	Grade 2 *plus* ileus
	Elderly patient, few rib fractures, frail	Grade 2 *plus* hypoxia

1 Titrated analgesia.
2 Physiotherapy.
3 Tracheostomy.
4 Spontaneous ventilation with oxygen enrichment.
Patients with grade 3 injuries require:
1 Titrated analgesia.
2 Physiotherapy.
3 Tracheostomy.
4 Controlled ventilation with oxygen enrichment.

This assessment must be repeated at frequent short intervals until the patient's condition stabilizes, since unexpected deterioration may occur. This implies that the patient should be observed in an Intensive Therapy unit.

Patients with extensive pulmonary contusions and a wide Aa gradient require positive pressure ventilation. However, provided that the contused lung does not become grossly infected and that overtransfusion is avoided, most patients with grade 3 injuries should be able to breathe spontaneously through a tracheostomy after 5–7 days of controlled ventilation. Occasionally this period has to be extended to 2–3 weeks. The mortality rate from chest injuries after the first 72 hours is largely dictated by the presence or absence of intra-abdominal and pulmonary infection.

The patient who has suffered extensive pulmonary contusions and is hypoxic should be given frusemide 40 mg intravenously 12-hourly. This regimen should be continued for up to 3 days or until the blood urea starts to rise. If no sustained improvement in the radiographic appearance or blood gas exchange has been achieved at the end of this period, the frusemide should be discontinued but fluid overload should be avoided at all costs. If the patient is oliguric or in frank renal failure from the time of admission, early haemodialysis must be considered.

The analgesia problem

The importance of pain relief was emphasized at the beginning of this chapter. If the patient has suffered grade 1 injuries almost any analgesic drug can be used as long as its effects are monitored.

For many years tight adhesive strapping was applied over rib fractures to reduce respiratory movement and thus relieve pain. Unfortunately, although this undoubtedly gives some pain relief, it also increases the likelihood of atelectasis in the underlying area of the lung, and this form of treatment has a very limited place.

Epidural analgesia

For patients with grade 2 injuries the ideal form of pain relief is achieved with continuous thoracic epidural analgesia, and for many patients effective analgesia obviates the need for tracheostomy. Although 0.5% bupivacaine is the standard analgesic, epidural analgesics (morphine, fentanyl, etc.) have been used.

Occasionally epidural analgesia may not be entirely satisfactory. It is inadvisable to extend the block above T4 because the patient may become hypotensive. A patchy block may be corrected by withdrawing the catheter slightly, but it may have to be supplemented with systemic analgesics such as buprenorphine. If the patient has suffered very extensive chest injuries, which cannot be adequately treated by epidural analgesia, controlled ventilation is probably required.

When the duration of action of the local anaesthetic agent has been determined, analgesia should be maintained with a syringe pump. In the uncomplicated case it is usually possible to dispense with epidural analgesia after 4–5 days. Patients who have persistent severe chest pain upon coughing or while receiving physiotherapy can be given extra pain relief with entonox or with small doses of systemic narcotics.

Intercostal blockade

Pain relief may also be obtained by intercostal blockade; this usually needs to be repeated at 4- to 6-hour intervals. It carries the risk of pneumothorax, and if more than four intercostal spaces need to be injected the toxic dose of the drug used must be considered.

Recently, continuous intercostal blockade has been successfully used. A catheter is inserted in the inter-costal space at the angle of the rib and after the initial injection has established the position, an infusion can be set up.

Endotracheal intubation and tracheostomy care

In addition to adequate pain relief, patients with grade 2 or grade 3 injuries often require a tracheostomy. Its functions are:
1 To permit the efficient aspiration of secretions and blood.
2 To facilitate the more efficient application of oxygen therapy and humidification.
3 To allow the nurse to measure and record the patient's tidal volume and minute volume.
4 To allow controlled ventilation to be applied if necessary.

Occasionally it may be possible to postpone or avoid the need for a tracheostomy by passing an endotracheal tube, particularly if the clinical presentation suggests that the incident will be short-lived. Patients who have sustained relatively minor chest injuries but have undergone abdominal surgery may be in this category. For intubation the nasotracheal route is preferred because:
1 The tube is more easily secured in position.
2 It is less likely to kink and cannot be chewed by the patient.
3 It causes less salivation and oral sepsis.
4 It is more comfortable and, therefore, more readily tolerated by the patient.

PROBLEMS AFTER INTUBATION
(INCLUDING TRACHEOSTOMY)

Intubation reduces the efficiency of coughing and necessitates regular tracheobronchial suction which must be performed gently and aseptically. It probably also increases the risk of systemic sepsis. Any procedure which breaks mucosal or mucocutaneous continuity, particularly in the immunologically compromised patient, is a likely source of systemic sepsis.

The major problems associated with tracheal intubation and controlled ventilation are technical: namely, ventilator failure, disconnection and obstruction. The inexperienced doctor or nurse naturally assumes that tracheal intubation automatically guarantees a patent airway but this is not the case. Endotracheal tubes and tracheostomy tubes readily become obstructed, kinked, displaced or disconnected from the ventilator or oxygen line. Endotracheal tubes may be too long and enter the right bronchus unless they are measured and inserted correctly.

Patients who require intubation or tracheostomy, with or without controlled ventilation, must be carefully monitored in an Intensive Therapy unit.

The ventilatory treatment of grade 3 injuries

The reasons for applying positive pressure ventilation are:
1 To permit the effective use of systemic analgesics.
2 To achieve satisfactory gas exchange.
3 To apply internal pneumatic fixation.
4 As an aid to the treatment of non-thoracic injuries.

Chest-wall and lung injuries cause hypoventilation (hypercapnia) and ventilation/perfusion ($\dot{V}/\dot{Q}$) imbalance with hypoxia. More extensive lung injuries which involve a whole lobe or lung produce a true shunt. Controlled ventilation in one form or another is the most effective and least traumatic treatment for injuries of this type, although its efficiency is limited by their extent. If blood and oxygen cannot be brought into apposition, the effects of controlled ventilation are limited. It is usually not difficult to correct hypercapnia but hypoxia may be an intractable problem.

Arterial oxygen desaturation due to $\dot{V}/\dot{Q}$ disturbance can usually be corrected by increasing the inspired oxygen concentration (Pio_2), although the Aa oxygen tension gradient may be wide. However, if a true shunt exists, that is, if a significant proportion of the circulating blood volume perfuses lung tissue which is not ventilated, the arterial blood will inevitably be desaturated. This cannot be corrected by increasing the Pio_2 in the perfused and ventilated alveoli. Both $\dot{V}/\dot{Q}$ imbalance and true shunt are found in contused and lacerated lung tissue.

The Aa oxygen gradient

The difference between the partial pressure of oxygen in the alveolar gas (PAo_2) and that in arterial blood (Pao_2) provides a valuable, though indirect, indication of the true shunt; this is known as the Aa gradient and it should be measured and recorded at frequent intervals during the course of treatment since it gives a good guide to the progress of the lung lesion, whether it is caused by trauma, infection or other factors. The alveolar oxygen tension is calculated from the simplified alveolar air equation:

$$PAo_2 = Pio_2 - \frac{Paco_2}{R},$$

where PAo_2 is the partial pressure of oxygen in alveolar gas, Pio_2 is the partial pressure of oxygen in the inspired gas, $Paco_2$ is the partial pressure of carbon dioxide in arterial blood (all gas tensions are in kilopascals) and R is the respiratory exchange ratio which is usually assumed to be 0.8.

The relationship between $\dot{V}E$ and $Paco_2$

Figure 7.11 shows the relationship between the arterial carbon dioxide tension ($Paco_2$) and the minute volume ($\dot{V}E$): when the $\dot{V}E$ is doubled, the $Paco_2$ is halved and vice versa. It also demonstrates that increasing the physiological dead space reduces the efficiency of ventilation.

Pneumothorax and haemothorax

When the lungs are inflated against fractured ribs there is a risk of pneumothorax and haemothorax. This is most likely to occur during the first 3–4 days after instituting controlled ventilation, although it can occur at any time. Physiotherapy may also increase this hazard. If, while undergoing controlled ventilation, a patient's colour deteriorates the attendant must first ascertain that the ventilator is still functioning and that the airway is clear; an erect chest radiograph must be taken as soon as possible (within 15 minutes). However, the medical attendant must be prepared to insert a chest drain without waiting for radiographic confirmation of the diagnosis.

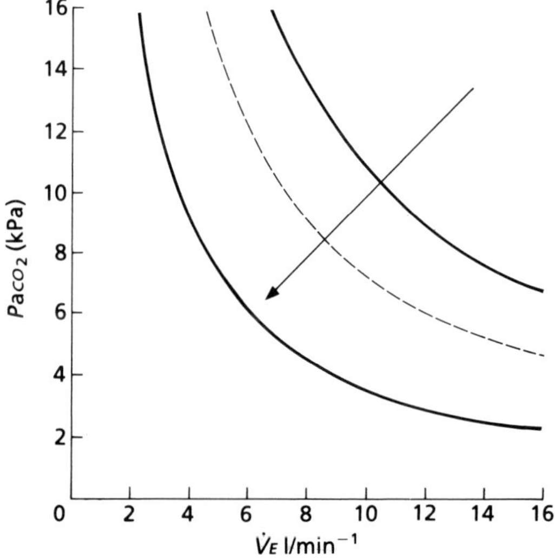

Fig. 7.11 The relationship between $\dot{V}E$ and $Paco_2$.

Indications for discontinuing controlled ventilation

These are:
1 Radiographic resolution of the signs of pulmonary contusion.
2 Narrowing of the Aa oxygen tension gradient.
3 Diminution or safe control of pain.
4 Improvement of the other injuries.

Freedom from pain is particularly important. In other cases once the underlying pulmonary pathology has cleared the bony injuries can be expected to resolve. If these are very extensive and include unstable injuries to the sternum, controlled ventilation may need to be continued for 2–3 weeks. This period is influenced by the extent and significance of other factors, including the patient's pre-incident physical status and the presence of extrathoracic injury. In some centres intermittent mandatory ventilation (IMV) is used as an aid to the weaning process.

Pharmacological aids to controlled ventilation

When controlled ventilation is instituted the patient will require sedation and analgesia to reduce anxiety and to provide relief from pain. Narcotics are used because in addition they depress the respiratory centre and simplify the application of intermittent positive pressure ventilation (IPPV). In the author's department adult patients with grade 3 injuries are given morphine 1–4 mg hourly by continuous infusion and this is reinforced with propofol intravenously 6-hourly. This regimen is usually required for 3–5 days, at the end of which the patients can be given progressively less morphine as they become pain-free and accustomed to the ventilator.

THE USE OF MUSCLE RELAXANTS

Muscle relaxants must never be used in the absence of adequate sedation, but not infrequently a patient who is pain-free and has acceptable blood gases and hydrogen ion status continues to make respiratory efforts. These can usually be overcome by temporarily increasing the alveolar ventilation and thereby causing hypocapnia. When spontaneous ventilatory efforts cease the alveolar ventilation can be reduced gradually without causing the patient to breathe against the ventilator. An alternative method is to insert an extra dead space into the ventilator circuit and then increase the patient's tidal volume by the volume of the dead space, usually 200–250 ml. The resulting increase in chest distension

frequently inhibits voluntary movements and has no effect upon P_{aCO_2}.

If neither of these methods is successful and the patient is still breathing against the machine a muscle relaxant should be used for 24–48 hours. Vicuronium 6–10 mg hourly by infusion is usually given, but only after the patient has been told what is about to happen so that if, by mischance, the analgesia or sedation wears off the patient will understand why he or she cannot move.

When heavy sedation, with or without relaxants, is prescribed the medical attendant must be able to place absolute reliance on the nursing staff and on the ventilator circuitry.

The problem of occult injuries

Intra-abdominal injuries

Patients who have suffered major chest trauma may also have suffered intra-abdominal injuries. The diagnosis of delayed visceral rupture or of splenic or hepatic injury may be very difficult when the patient is sedated and/or paralysed. If there is any question of such an injury being present, a surgeon must be found who is willing to try to exclude it before long-term ventilation is begun. Laparotomy should be performed if there is any direct or indirect evidence which suggests that such an injury may be present. Peritoneal lavage is a valuable technique but it may not establish the presence of ischaemic but intact bowel (Gomez *et al*. 1987).

It was stated earlier that the combination of serious chest injuries with abdominal sepsis carries a high mortality; this can only be increased if the diagnosis is delayed.

Aortic arch rupture

The aortic arch ruptures where its mobile and fixed segments meet, on one or other side of the vertebral column. This is one of the most lethal complications of chest-wall trauma, but provided that the patient reaches hospital alive it can be treated surgically. If the patient is more than 50 years of age the injury is usually immediately fatal because of the rigidity of the aorta, but younger patients may survive with partial rupture for hours, days or even longer.

Clinical features

Aortic arch rupture is usually due to violent forward

flexion of the upper thorax and is often associated with fractures of posterior segments of the second or third rib and wedge fractures of upper thoracic vertebrae. Aortography is potentially lethal in this condition and, if it is available, digital vascular imaging (DVI) provides a less dangerous technique to identify aortic arch rupture.

The diagnosis is suggested if the blood pressure in the right arm is more than 20 mmHg greater than in the left. This examination should be routinely performed on every patient with chest trauma. If the rupture is beyond the left subclavian artery no blood pressure discrepancy is noted in the arms but the femoral pulses may be diminished or absent.

Classically, the chest radiograph shows widening of the superior mediastinum and pleural fluid may be noted, but these signs are not always present.

Treatment

Treatment may involve the use of cardiopulmonary bypass, although a left ventricle-to-descending aorta cannula has been designed to eliminate the need for full bypass. A recent review suggested that the results of 'clamp and sew' treatment are better than those obtained after formal resection (Schmidt and Jacobson 1984). If the diagnosis is made in time the results are quite good, although paraplegia is a recognized complication. Occasionally a false aneurysm forms which is recognized only long after the event (Tengler, 1985).

Pericardial tamponade

This is caused by the accumulation of fluid (usually blood) in the pericardial sac, preventing ventricular filling and leading to a rapidly progressive fall in cardiac output. It may be caused by a penetrating injury, but it most frequently follows the so-called steering column injury. The bleeding originates from either pericardial or epicardial vessels and, rarely, from small cardiac tears. Although the presenting evidence is clinical, the diagnosis may be suggested by radiographic evidence of cardiac enlargement. If there is time it can be confirmed by echocardiography.

Clinical signs

The clinical signs of pericardial tamponade are:
1 Dyspnoea or tachypnoea.
2 A fall in cardiac output.
3 Engorgement of the head, neck and upper limb veins.
4 Pulsus paradoxus.

The conscious patient usually complains of breathlessness, an oppressive central chest discomfort and a feeling of impending death.

Recognition and treatment

A 12- or 14-gauge cannula, such as a Medicut or Abbocath, fitted to a 20-ml syringe via a three-way tap is inserted through the left fifth intercostal space 1 cm from the sternal edge and advanced slowly, aspirating all the way. With an average-sized adult, at a depth of 1.5–2.0 cm blood can be aspirated freely, and when the syringe and inner cannula are removed blood is ejected in a pulsatile manner. If the cannula moves very vigorously with pulsation the right ventricle may have been transfixed, but this is usually accompanied by runs of ectopic beats.

A few millilitres of the aspirated blood should be placed in a glass tube and watched for 4 minutes to see if it clots; pericardial blood is usually defibrinated and does not clot. Most patients with tamponade improve rapidly after 100–300 ml blood are removed but aspiration should continue until the sac is dry. Alternatively, a soft intravascular catheter can be introduced into the pericardial sac via the cannula and allowed to drain spontaneously. If the bleeding persists and only temporary relief is obtained it may be necessary to perform a pericardiectomy or open drainage procedure.

Myocardial contusion

Myocardial contusions, which can give rise to delayed problems, may occur more frequently than is appreciated. These may be suggested by the echocardiogram signs which include ST segment and T wave abnormalities suggestive of myocardial ischaemia. Tachydysrhythmias are common.

If any of these signs is noted, an echocardiogram should be performed since pericardial tamponade is a constant hazard. The measurement of cardiac enzymes is not of great diagnostic value in the traumatized patient, but proof of the existence of myocardial contusions may be obtained only at thoracotomy or at autopsy. If the evidence is suggestive, the patient should be given lignocaine by infusion since ventricular tachycardia and ventricular fibrillation commonly occur (Editorial 1986, Muwanga *et al.* 1986).

Pneumothorax and haemothorax

Probably as many as 20% of all patients with chest injuries show evidence of a pneumothorax on admission to hospital, and a significant number develop this complication after admission — either spontaneously or as a result of treatment. It is often accompanied by haemothorax.

If the patient is breathing spontaneously and is not hypoxic, and the pneumothorax occupies less than one-fifth (estimated) of the thoracic cavity, it may be felt that the risks of inserting a chest tube outweigh its advantages, particularly if the patient is pain-free, breathing and coughing freely. If the patient requires surgical treatment under general anaesthesia, a tube should first be inserted because the pneumothorax may enlarge or become valvular whilst the patient is anaesthetized. If the patient with a pneumothorax is receiving controlled ventilation a chest tube should always be inserted.

Clinical signs

The clinical signs of pneumothorax may be obvious, although patients with low pressure pneumothorax frequently have few diagnostic signs. These are often difficult to elicit because of the pain, dyspnoea and ventilatory limitation caused by the injury. If the patient is receiving IPPV the diagnosis may be even more difficult.

If the patient is breathing spontaneously, examination may reveal:
1 Cyanosis.
2 Dyspnoea and tachypnoea.
3 Tracheal deviation towards the injured side.
4 Reduced chest movement.
5 Increased resonance to percussion.
6 Diminished vocal resonance.
7 Diminished air entry.
Occasionally the patient may cough up blood-stained sputum.

Tension pneumothorax

If the pneumothorax is under tension the respiratory and cardiocirculatory signs are more marked. Acute dyspnoea, cyanosis and greatly reduced cardiac output are accompanied by tracheal deviation away from the injured side together with the other signs listed above. In either case the patient may, if able, complain of a sharp chest pain on the appropriate side.

If the patient is receiving controlled ventilation the position of the trachea may be influenced by the tracheal tube and breath sounds may be transmitted across the mid-line from the other side, making the diagnosis more difficult.

The radiographic signs of tension pneumothorax include displacement of the mediastinum away from the affected collapsed lung and downward displacement of the diaphragm on the same side. Very occasionally, if the patient is receiving controlled ventilation, the diaphragm may actually be inverted.

A high index of suspicion is necessary at all times and, in an emergency, it may be necessary to act on the physical signs alone. Wherever possible a chest radiograph should first be taken since patients with extensive chest injuries frequently present very misleading physical signs. Not infrequently, patients develop bilateral pneumothorax after chest injuries and recognition is extremely difficult without a chest radiograph.

Chest drainage

The optimum site for insertion of chest drains is the mid-axillary line in the fifth, sixth or seventh intercostal space. The traditional anterior 'medical' site is useless for the drainage of fluid, and if the tube is inserted behind the posterior axillary line it readily becomes kinked. The patient's position in bed and ability to move about are also restricted.

The type of tube used is a matter of personal preference, but it should be of an adequate size; a very generous amount of local anaesthetic solution must be infiltrated since it is a painful procedure. The costal periosteum appears to be particularly sensitive and an attempt should always be made to infiltrate the local anaesthetic very close to it.

COMPLICATIONS OF CHEST DRAINAGE

The problems associated with chest drainage include:
1 Unnecessary insertion.
2 Haemorrhage.
3 Sepsis.
4 Fistula formation.
5 Subphrenic insertion.
The first of these may occasionally be unavoidable if the clinician feels impelled to insert a drain without first obtaining a chest radiograph. It may cause pneumothorax, sometimes accompanied by bleeding. Haemorrhage from the insertion of a chest drain in the mid-axillary line is rarely severe, whereas the anterior approach may be associated with heavy bleeding from the internal mammary artery. Exceptionally, an intercostal vessel is damaged but this rarely causes significant bleeding. Sepsis can be avoided only by paying strict attention to aseptic insertion and maintenance, and the tube should be removed as soon as it has fulfilled its function.

Bronchopleural fistula

If the patient is receiving controlled ventilation the tear in the lung may be slow to heal, and much of the tidal volume may be lost through the chest drain so that gas exchange may be inadequate. If it does not show rapid signs of resolution, a thoracotomy and repair are necessary.

Subphrenic insertion

It is surprisingly easy to insert a chest drain below the diaphragm, particularly if the procedure is performed with the patient supine and without the aid of a chest radiograph. If there is any doubt as to the diaphragm's position, and particularly if the patient's abdomen is distended, the drain should be inserted through a higher intercostal space. It is a good practice to first enter the pleural cavity with the needle through which the local anaesthetic is being injected. If air or blood can be aspirated freely, it is usually safe to insert a drainage tube through the same site. However, if the needle is inserted below the diaphragm and the peritoneal cavity contains blood this test is not reliable.

REMOVAL OF CHEST DRAINS

After the lung has been fully expanded for 24 hours, bubbles have ceased to emerge from the underwater drain and any drainage of blood has stopped, a clamp should be placed across the tube. After a further 8 hours an erect chest radiograph should be taken to determine whether or not the pneumothorax has recurred. If it has not, the tube may be removed.

Fractured clavicle

This is usually of little functional importance but if it occurs in association with anterior rib fractures it will increase the degree of chest wall instability and disability. the clavicle may also be fractured following direct injury to the supraclavicular region, which may involve the brachial plexus. The phrenic nerve may be damaged, leading to diaphragmatic paralysis. On its own this should not cause severe incapacity unless the patient has a pre-existing respiratory problem.

Surgical treatment of chest injuries

Chest-wall injuries are still treated surgically in some centres. The treatment ranges from the application of traction to the unstable chest wall, to the open reduction of multiple rib fractures with fixation by wires, plates or a wide variety of clamps. In the author's experience the place for such manoeuvres is strictly limited.

If the patient requires surgical treatment of open chest-wall injuries or because of intrathoracic damage, it is logical to attempt to stabilize the chest wall afterwards. The surgical approach to chest-wall injuries involves the patient in very extensive skin mobilization and prolonged traumatic surgery, with the risks of haemorrhage and infection and a painful postoperative course. If the patient has extensive pulmonary contusions or lacerations controlled ventilation with added oxygen will still be required for a variable period, and the main objective of surgery, which is to avoid such ministrations, will be lost.

Prevention of permanent deformity

If the patient is young and has very extensive chest-wall fractures with deformities which do not respond quickly to controlled ventilation, surgical treatment may be considered. However, in the author's experience, only the elderly are left with much chest-wall deformity and the surgical treatment of chest-wall injuries in patients over the age of 70 years is a hazardous procedure.

References

Amanchi, W., Birolini, D., Bianco, P.O. & de Oliveria, M.R. Injuries to the tracheobronchial tree in closed trauma. *Thorax* 1983; **38**: 923–928.

Editorial. Blunt trauma to the heart. *Lancet* 1986; **ii**: 724.

Gomez, G.A., Alvarez, R., Placencia, G., Echemique, M., Vopal, J.J., Byers, P., Dorte, D.B. & Kreis, D.J. Diagnostic peritoneal lavage in the management of blunt abdominal trauma: a reassessment. *J Trauma* 1987; **27(1)**: 1–5.

Hix, W.R. Residue of thoracic trauma. *Surg Gynecol Obstet* 1984; **158**: 295–301.

Lloyd, J.W., Crampton Smith, A. & O'Connor, B.T. Classification of chest injuries as an aid to treatment. *Br Med J* 1965; **1**: 1518–1521.

Mills, S.A., Johnston, F.R., Hudspeth, A.S., Breyer, R.H., Myers, R.T. & Cordell, A.R. Clinical spectrum of blunt tracheobronchial disruption. *J Thorac Cardiovasc Surg* 1982; **84**: 49–54.

Muwanga, C.L., Cole, R.P., Sloan, J.P. *et al.* Cardiac contusion in patients wearing seat belts. *Injury* 1986; **17**: 37–39.

Schmidt, C.A. & Jacobson, J.C. Thoracic aortic injury: a ten year experience. *Arch Surg* 1984; **119**: 1244–1246.

Tengler, M.L. The spectrum of myocardial trauma. *J Trauma* 1985; **25**: 620–627.

Williams, W.G. & Smith, R.E. *Trauma of the Chest*. John Wright & Son: Bristol, 1977.

Genitourinary tract injuries

J.P.MITCHELL

Injuries to the kidney

In European countries blunt trauma accounts for more than 90% of all renal injuries amongst the civilian population. In contrast, penetrating injuries to the kidney are significantly more common in the United States than in Europe (Hai *et al.* 1977, Mitchell 1984). Considering the relative size of the kidneys it is surprising how uncommon renal gunshot wounds are amongst all abdominal injuries. In Northern Ireland less than 2% of gunshot wounds that reached hospital alive involved one or other kidney (Archbold *et al.* 1981). However, stab wounds of the kidney are more common, presumably because the assailant so often stabs from the back.

Spontaneous rupture of the kidney or renal pelvis is uncommon. Nevertheless, most urologists will have seen at least two or three cases during a lifetime of urological practice.

Mode of injury in closed renal trauma

In the same way as injuries of the spleen can show a split in the line of the rib, so injuries of the kidney will more commonly be seen across the waist or lower pole of the kidney, where the 12th rib makes its impact, compressing the kidney medially against the lumbar spine. Apart from road traffic accidents the types of injury may be a kick in the loin at rugby football or a horse-riding fall across the top bar of a jump.

Occasionally the kidney may be damaged by a blow in the abdomen anteriorly, just below the rib cage, particularly in road traffic accidents, such as when the driver of the vehicle is thrown violently onto the steering wheel (Fig. 7.12).

Closed injury may result from deceleration, particularly falling from a height and landing on the buttocks, when the momentum of the kidney forces it downwards within the perirenal (Gerota's) fascia. The traction force on the renal pedicle can tear the renal artery or one of its major branches. Rupture of a renal vessel may not be lethal as avulsion of a vessel can cause recoil of the intima and endothelial lining, which can be sufficient to occlude the lumen of the vessel in the presence of hypotension from shock. Hence, occasionally, a patient with complete avulsion of the renal pedicle can reach hospital alive.

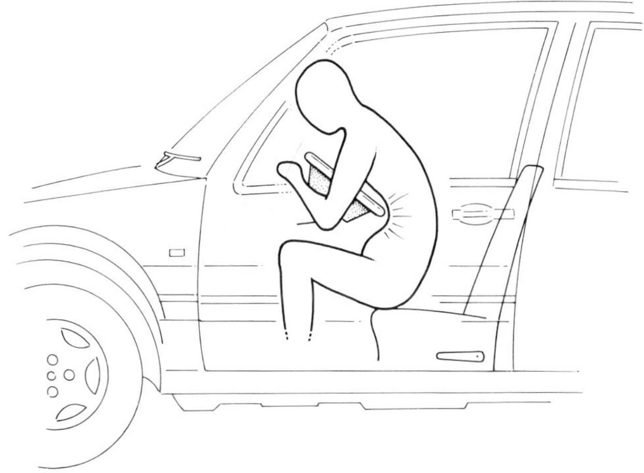

Fig. 7.12 Road traffic accident in which the victim is thrown forwards onto the steering column.

Extent of damage in closed injuries

If the capsular tear does not communicate with the calyces then there will be no immediate haematuria, though delayed bleeding can appear 2–4 days after injury, when blood eventually seeps down the tubules. If no other intra-abdominal structures are injured it is likely that many of these patients will never report to their doctors as it is usually only the haematuria that causes the patient sufficient anxiety to seek medical advice. Therefore, it is probable that many minor renal injuries pass undiagnosed.

Haematuria with the first act of micturition after the accident will indicate that the tear in the cortex of the kidney is deep enough to communicate with a calyx. At the same time some degree of perirenal haematoma always develops. Urine probably will not leak from the renal pelvis into the perirenal tissues if the tear is only a fine split (Fig. 7.13), but if the tear of the renal substance allows some separation then the urine will leak into the perirenal haematoma. If a kidney is split in two, both fragments may still be viable (Fig. 7.14).

Injuries in which the kidney has been fragmented or shattered, or in which the renal pelvis has been avulsed, are of such severity that the patient may be dead before reaching hospital, either from excessive blood loss or from other multiple major injuries. Of the patients with renal injury that reach hospital alive less than 2% are in the category of critical, that is to say they have shattered kidneys or avulsed pedicles (Fig. 7.15).

If the overlying peritoneum is also torn then blood and urine will leak into the peritoneal cavity. This complication is seen more often in children due to their very limited amount of perirenal fat.

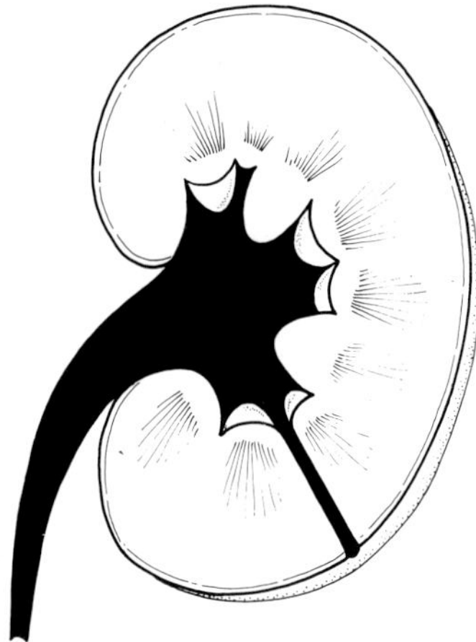

Fig. 7.13 If the tear is only a fine split, urine will probably not leak into the perirenal tissues.

Thrombosis of the main renal artery means death to that kidney unless surgery is attempted without delay. Smaller branches of the renal artery can recanalize with complete restoration of function. Sadly, the inevitable delay in reaching the diagnosis of renal artery thrombosis is nearly always beyond the warm ischaemic time for a viable kidney. Damage to the renal artery may be limited to the intimal layer as a result of acute angulation of the vessel or due to stretching from deceleration.

Blunt injury of the kidney is often associated with fractures of the ribs and lumbar transverse processes. In addition, there may be a pneumothorax and a haemothorax, while below the diaphragm the liver or spleen may be lacerated in as many as 30% of renal injuries.

Associated pathology

The possible presence of some underlying pathology of the kidney should be suspected when haematuria occurs after what appears to be only trivial trauma to the loin and the patient is comparatively fit. Hydronephrosis is the most common renal pathology to be found in association with kidney trauma. Underlying and pre-existing disorders of the kidney may be discovered on investigation of renal injury in children (in as many as 10−15% of cases) and even occasionally in the contralateral kidney.

Spontaneous rupture of the kidney is rare and is nearly always associated with pathology such as a tumour, hypertension, tuberculosis or renal vein thrombosis. Spontaneous leak of urine from the hilum of the kidney at the margin of the renal pelvis can occur when a calculus is impacted in the ureter.

Clinical presentation

The distinction between major and minor injuries of the kidney is virtually academic, as any patient

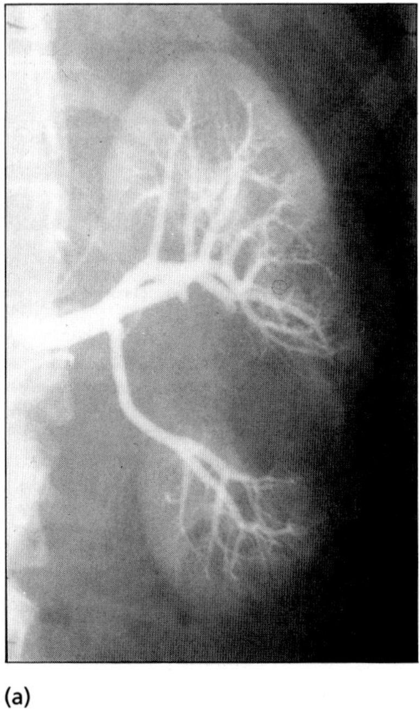

(a)

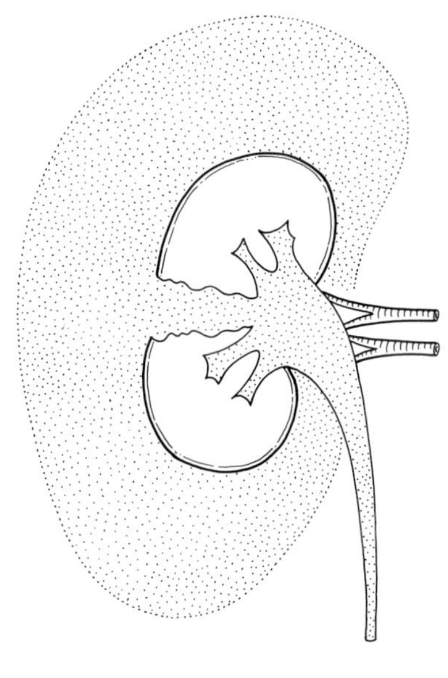

(b)

Fig. 7.14 (a) Angiogram showing complete separation of the lower pole of the kidney which still has a satisfactory blood supply. After the haematoma between the two segments subsided, an intravenous pyelogram eventually showed a normal kidney. (b) Diagrammatic representation of Fig. 7.14 (a).

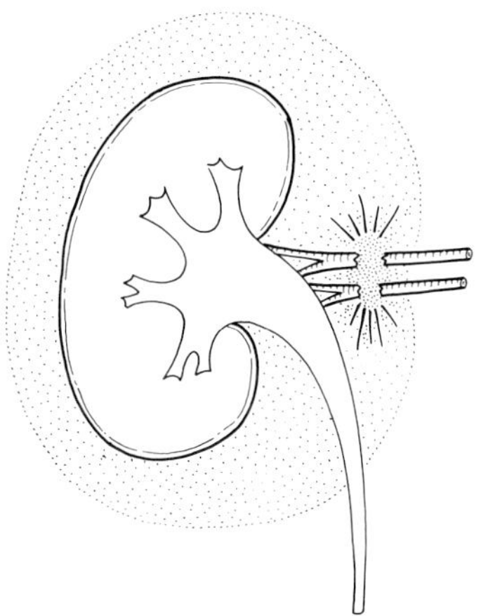

Fig. 7.15 Avulsed pedicle.

presenting with a history of injury in the flank followed by haematuria should be treated as though severe until the haematuria has subsided and investigation has confirmed no urinary leak and no progression of the perirenal haematoma. Furthermore, it is often impossible to determine the severity of the lesion in the early stages.

In sporting injuries the patient may continue to play until the end of the match and it is only when blood-stained urine is passed that the incident of a severe blow in the flank is recalled. In contrast, when the patient has been carried off the field there are, in many instances, either associated injuries such as a ruptured spleen or liver, or fractures of a rib with possible intra-thoracic problems; the symptoms and signs of these associated injuries may obscure the diagnosis of renal trauma.

Not infrequently the possibility of kidney damage may only be suspected after the abdomen has been opened for other abdominal trauma and a retroperi-toneal haematoma is discovered on the posterior abdominal wall. An intravenous urogram obtained on the operating table may be helpful but the usual procedure is to observe the size and extent of the haematoma accurately before and after all other intra-abdominal damage has been repaired, and then to estimate, during that time interval, whether the haematoma has increased in size, indicating the need to explore that area. If it has not increased then it is reasonably safe to be managed conservatively; exploration of a perirenal haematoma is so often tantamount to nephrectomy.

Following a fall from a height there may be no clinical symptoms or signs pointing to renal injury. The fact that the patient has reached hospital alive does not exclude a torn renal vessel. Any suggestion of loin pain or tenderness following a vertical deceleration injury should alert the clinician to the possibility of renal trauma. These injuries are unlikely to produce any haematuria.

Delay in the appearance of blood in the urine suggests that the injury is not severe. Renal colic may be caused by a small clot passing down the ureter. A perinephric haematoma may not be obvious clinically in the early stages as it will be obscured by guarding and rigidity of the abdominal wall. In fact, it is probably unwise, if such an injury is suspected, to risk palpating the loin sufficiently firmly to feel the kidney, for fear of stimulating further bleeding. It may not be until the following morning, when the discomfort is beginning to ease, that examination of the loin will be possible and the outline of the haematoma can be felt.

The inexperienced junior doctor must be aware of the patient complaining of haematuria with a story of a blow in the loin; such a patient may be a drug addict hoping for a 'jab' of powerful analgesic.

Management

The most important and most urgent investigation is an excretory urogram, not only to assess the injured kidney but also to ensure that the opposite kidney is normal. A further reason for some urgency is that delay will allow the development of meteorism to the extent that the intestinal gas can obscure the contrast medium within the calyces or any trace of leakage from the calyces. In addition to the damage to the renal parenchyma or any underlying pathology this radiograph will show other features such as loss of the psoas shadow and renal outline due to the perirenal haematoma, scoliosis of the lumbar spine with the concavity towards the side of the injury due to muscle spasm (Fig. 7.16) and damage to other structures including ribs, transverse processes, herniation through a ruptured diaphragm, a pneumo-thorax or haemothorax or possible escape of intestinal gas into the peritoneal cavity.

Retrograde pyelography is mentioned only to be condemned as it carries a risk of introducing infection into the damaged kidney and perirenal haematoma and is unlikely to provide any useful additional information not obtainable from other, less dangerous invest-igations. Condemning retrograde pyelography may, in part, have contributed during the last 30 years to the marked reduction in post-traumatic pyonephrosis and perinephric abscess resulting in nephrectomy at 10–14 days after injury.

Angiography may be advisable when the injured kidney or part of it fails to opacify, when haematuria

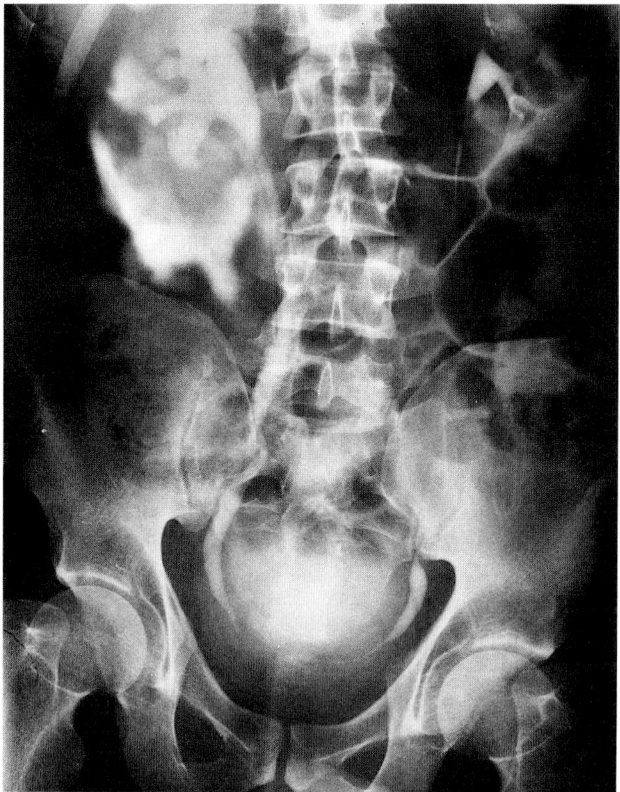

Fig. 7.16 Scoliosis with the concavity to the right, where there has been a rupture of the right kidney with perirenal extravasation.

persists unabated for a week after injury, if hypertension develops some weeks after injury or if an arteriovenous fistula is suspected from an audible bruit over the loin. At the time of admission to hospital, angiography is unlikely to provide any helpful information soon enough to embark on conservative surgery before the warm ischaemic time of that kidney has expired. Ultrasound can give an assessment of the perirenal haematoma and can monitor its progress, whilst CT scanning, if available under the emergency conditions, will give the most accurate information about the tear in the kidney parenchyma and the haematoma. Nuclear magnetic resonance (magnetic resonance imaging — MRI) has the potential to distinguish a leak of urine and blood from a simple haematoma uncontaminated by urine.

The majority of renal injuries can be treated conservatively but this requires careful clinical monitoring. All penetrating injuries, with the exception of shallow stab wounds, should be explored to repair, where necessary, to remove foreign bodies such as pieces of clothing, to debride the track and to inspect the abdomen for possible damage to other structures. The conservative management must be bed rest, monitoring of pulse and blood pressure every 15 minutes and, if there is any deterioration, monitoring with a central venous pressure line. Every specimen of urine must be saved and clearly labelled with the time it was passed, so that at the end of 24 hours the specimens can be compared. Any change from bright red to brown indicates control of the bleeding and usually precedes any diminution in the intensity of the discoloration. Bleeding recurring at about 10–14 days suggests that infection has occurred; this is an ominous sign as it may be followed by a severe secondary haemorrhage requiring emergency exploration.

The serious consequences of any infection of the damaged renal tissue or the perirenal haematoma justifies the use of prophylactic antibiotics. The age group so frequently affected may demand the use of sedatives simply to keep them quiet and in bed as any unnecessary activity can aggravate the bleeding and, thereby, the haematoma. The amount of blood lost in these injuries should be assessed on the patient's clinical condition as a haematoma that may appear small on an ultrasound or CT scan may actually contain as much as a pint or more of blood.

There are three prime indications for surgical intervention in renal trauma: (i) penetrating injuries deep enough to have involved the kidney; (ii) deterioration of the patient as monitored by the central venous pressure, despite all measures to combat shock; and (iii) those patients who, at laparotomy for other abdominal injuries, are found to have a large retroperitoneal haematoma. Exploration for renal vascular injuries in the acute phase must be a matter for personal surgical judgement, but the surgeon should be aware of the increased risk to the life of that kidney that any surgical intervention can cause.

Post-traumatic hypertension may be due to vascular damage or to imprisonment of the kidney in a fibrous sac resulting from the resolving haematoma. Following renal injury occasional checks on the blood pressure should be carried out even though the incidence of hypertension appears to be less than 1%. Otherwise, the post-traumatic complications may be some deformity of the renal outline and calyceal pattern (Fig. 7.17) which may contribute to infection, cyst formation or calculus in less than 5% of all renal injuries.

Injuries to the ureter

As a result of its anatomical position and its free mobility the ureter is rarely involved in blunt trauma. In children, injury is still rare but the few scattered reports in the literature deal principally with patients

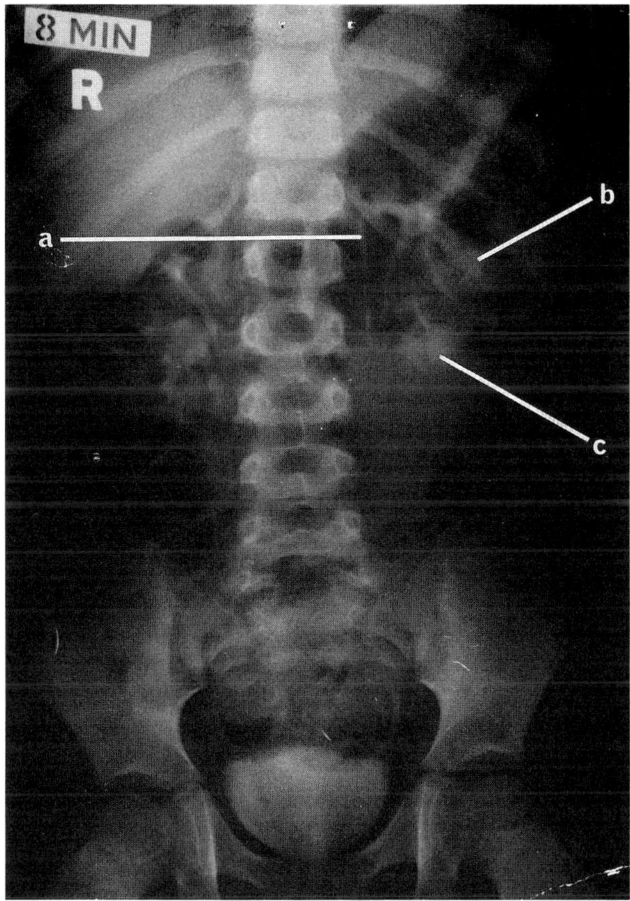

Fig. 7.17 Severe disruption of the left kidney. (a) Extracapsular contrast medium alongside the psoas muscle. (b) Contrast medium filling a split in the kidney. (c) Subcapsular pooling of contrast medium.

around the age of 20. The mode of injury appears to be avulsion at or below the pelvi-ureteric junction or nipping of the ureter between fragments of a spinal fracture. A tear of one of the calyces may occur in association with renal trauma causing a leak of urine

into the perirenal haematoma. Owing to the extreme rarity of this injury and the fact that other intra-abdominal damage is also present in most instances a diagnosis of ruptured ureter is unlikely to be considered before the abdomen has been opened. Ultrasonography may detect a collection of urine (a urinoma).

Gunshot wounds of the ureter have been reported but are far less common than renal trauma in proportion to the size of the two organs. On occasions the first intimation that the ureter has been involved is the development of a fistula following laparotomy for other intraperitoneal damage.

Spontaneous rupture of the ureter usually occurs in association with other pathology, in particular an impacted calculus, and the leak will be either at the junction of the calyces and the renal parenchyma or by necrosis of the wall of the ureter at the site of impaction. The patient will usually present with symptoms and signs of an acute abdomen and often with a recent history of ureteric colic. There will be guarding and ileus will develop at an early stage from the retroperitoneal collection of extravasated urine.

By far the majority of ureteric injuries are iatrogenic, consequent upon pelvic surgery, particularly when the ureter is enclosed in fibrous tissue or distorted from its normal anatomical site by other pathology. The ureter may be clamped, tied, cut or transected (Fig. 7.18).

Investigation of ureteric injury

It is necessary to differentiate between a fistula from one ureter, two ureters, the bladder or any combination. The excretory urogram will usually identify which ureter is affected by some increased fullness of the renal pelvis and ureter on that side (Fig. 7.19). On the other hand, if there is obstruction then there may be delayed function. It may also be possible to visualize the leak radiologically, outlining its track and revealing a faint filling of the

Fig. 7.18 The ureter may be (a) clamped, (b) tied, (c) cut or (d) transected.

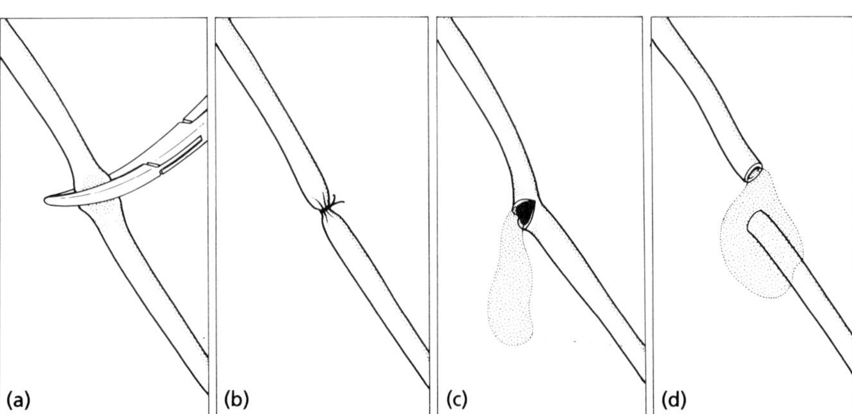

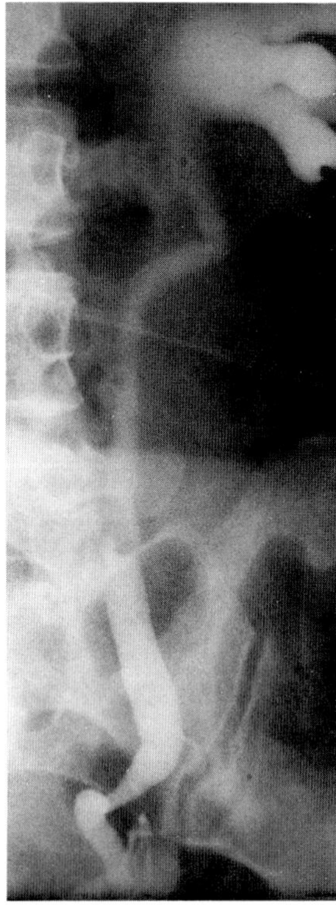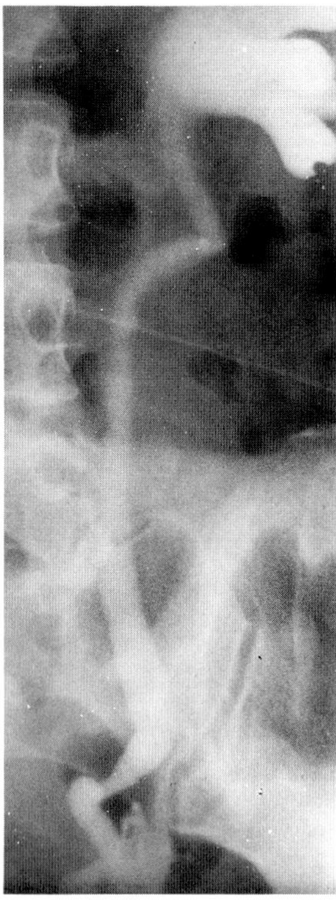

Fig. 7.19 Intravenous pyelogram showing a ureter acutely angulated by a suture high in the pelvis following hysterectomy. The ureter above is dilated and the kidney is hydronephrotic.

vault of the vagina. The distortion of the ureter may be quite surprising even without any leak or obstruction, but this is usually only a temporary deformity and the ureter gradually returns to its normal position.

Ultrasonography can be valuable in monitoring any hydronephrosis or hydroureter, and changes in the size or extent of a urinoma can be seen clearly. A functionless kidney can be outlined by antegrade pyelography after the cannula and catheter have been introduced into the renal pelvis under ultrasonic control. Perhaps the most valuable investigation is endoscopy, which will demonstrate any hole in the bladder and identify both ureteric orifices. After intravenous injection of indigo carmine, the dye will appear in the efflux from the intact ureter, while the leaking ureter will discolour a pack placed in the vault of the vagina. There may, however, be some oedema over the base of the bladder consequent upon recent surgery and this swelling can obscure the ureteric orifices. Finally, having identified the orifices, these should be catheterized to test for occlusion of the lumen and its distance along the ureter.

Repair of the damaged ureter

As with other parts of the urinary track all penetrating injuries will require exploration. Urinomas, if increasing in size, will have to be drained.

Damage to a ureter recognized at the time of surgery should be repaired or drained immediately. Fishtailing the two ends in order to create an oblique suture line will reduce the risk of stricture formation (Fig. 7.20). If the two ends cannot be brought together without tension or if the lower end cannot be identified, then the upper proximal ureter should be drained with a single pigtail-ended catheter to retain the tip inside the renal pelvis. If no pigtail catheter is available, then a length of silicone tubing, about 12 or 14 Charrière, should be tied in the ureter and brought out onto the surface to drain into a bag. A ureter divided in its lower segment can be difficult, if not impossible, to reanastomose in the depths of the pelvis and it is usually simpler and safer to anastomose the proximal cut ureter to the bladder.

If the leak or other ureteric damage is recognized within 2–3 days of injury, then immediate repair can be considered. With a longer time interval the site will probably be infected and the tissues macerated so that they do not hold sutures and it is wise to delay further surgery for 10–12 weeks.

Damage to a ureter in its lower segment will leave

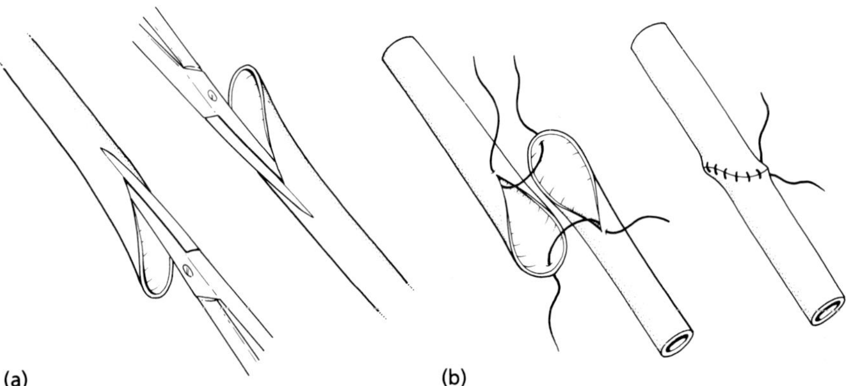

(a)   (b)

Fig. 7.20 (a) A longitudinal cut to fishtail the cut ends of the ureter. (b) Suturing the margins of the ureter in eversion.

enough length of the proximal part to construct a comfortable anastomosis to the side wall of the bladder without tension. There will also be enough to construct an anti-reflux type of anastomosis by laying the terminal 2 cm of ureter in a submucosal tunnel, thus creating a flutter valve.

If the level of ureteric trauma is just below the brim of the pelvis, then reanastomosis should be considered. If, after mobilization, the two ends can be brought together to create a fishtail union without tension over an indwelling catheter, this is probably the method of choice. However, at a second-stage repair it is rarely possible to bring the two ends together without so much mobilization that their viability is endangered. If a rigid urethral dilator is passed to tent up the highest point of the bladder (Fig. 7.21) it is possible to create an end-to-side anastomosis and abandon an anti-reflux technique. In order to avoid tension on the sutures when the bladder contracts, the highest point of the bladder wall should be stitched securely to the fascia and muscles (the psoas) on the posterolateral wall of the pelvis (Turner-Warwick & Worth 1969).

Damage above the pelvic brim should be repaired by reanastomosis wherever possible but, alternatively, the cut end can be transposed and joined to the side of the opposite ureter (uretero-ureterostomy; Fig. 7.22). Turning up a flap of bladder wall (Boari technique; Fig. 7.23) is often recommended but, in practice, a transverse opening in the bladder wall can be sutured vertically with just as much elevation of the bladder vault as in the Boari procedure.

Locating the lower end of the ureter can be aided with a catheter or light guide passed upwards from the ureteric orifice. Identification of the upper ureter will often necessitate locating it in the posterior abdominal wall, where it is still lying in its normal anatomical position, and then tracing it downwards.

Other techniques have been described; these include small gut replacement of the ureter, uretero-calycostomy and autotransplantation of the kidney into the pelvis so that only a short length of ureter is required. These techniques are for the urological specialist.

Whichever method of anastomosis is used the ureter must be drained and the most convenient catheter is the pigtail which coils into the renal pelvis and is therefore self-retaining. Its lower end can be drawn out through the urethra.

Injury to the bladder and posterior urethra

Bladder and posterior urethral injuries should be considered together for three reasons: (i) the differential

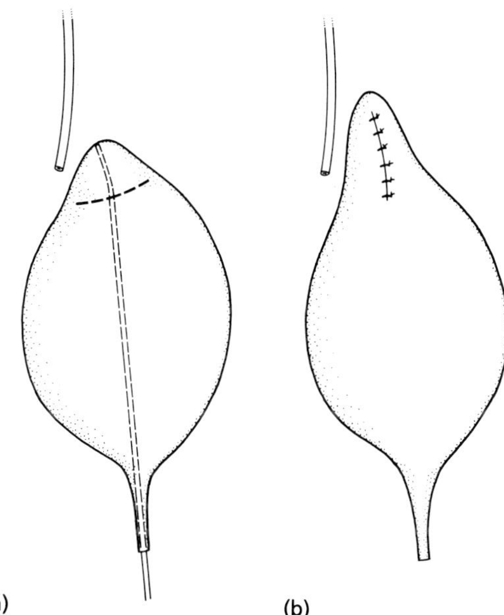

Fig. 7.21 (a) A transverse incision across the bladder at right angles to the instrument tenting the bladder upwards. This incision should be about 4 cm below the highest point of the bladder. (b) The transverse incision is sutured vertically to give extension in the height of the bladder.

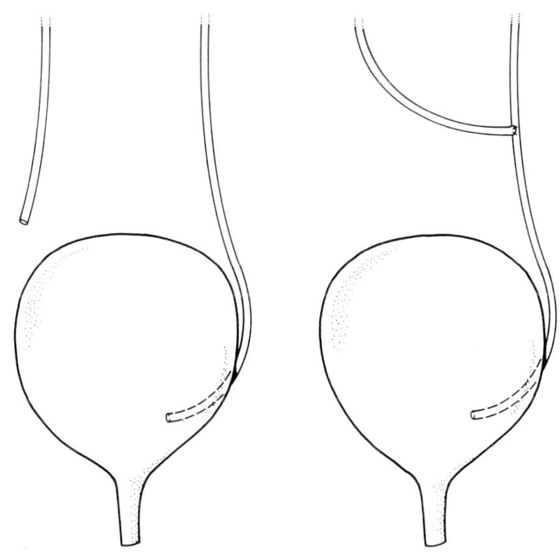

Fig. 7.22 Transuretero-ureterostomy.

diagnosis may not be easy; (ii) both may be associated with a fracture of the pelvis; and (iii) because 20–25% of all bladder injuries also involve the posterior urethra or, to quote the figure in terms of rupture of the posterior urethra then 10–12% will involve the bladder as well. This applies to closed injuries. In the case of penetrating injuries, such as gunshot wounds or stab wounds,

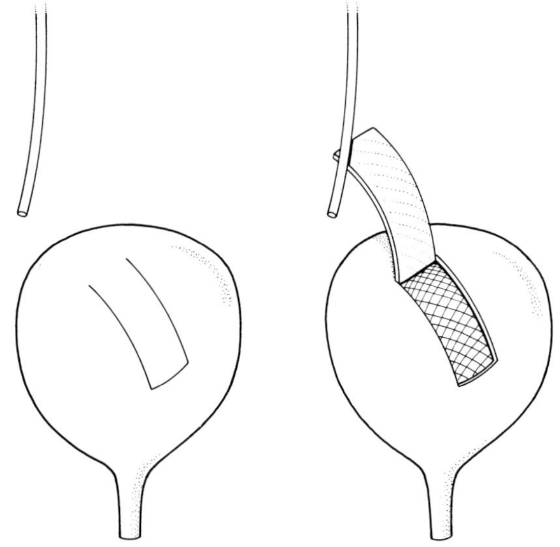

Fig. 7.23 Diagrammatic representation of the construction of a Boari flap to make a tube of bladder wall reaching to a point above the brim of the pelvis.

or falling onto, or astride, stakes or spikes, both the bladder and the posterior urethra may be damaged, though the object usually misses the posterior urethra and passes beside it before penetrating the bladder.

Damage to other intra-abdominal viscera or even vascular injury may add to the difficulty of diagnosis, particularly in penetrating injuries or following a blow to the lower abdomen. In fact, intraperitoneal rupture of the bladder may not be suspected before laparotomy as its presentation in the early stages may be only that of a ruptured hollow viscus leaking into the peritoneal cavity.

Mode of injury of the bladder

Rupture of the bladder can only occur if, at the time of injury, the bladder was full or nearly so. This applies to both intraperitoneal and extraperitoneal ruptures.

Intraperitoneal rupture of the bladder is localized to the vault of that viscus, where it is covered by peritoneum. In its lower part, the bladder wall is supported by the pelvic floor and the bony pelvis, but the vault, being the only part of the bladder that is unsupported, can tear as a result of a sudden increase in intravesical pressure; this can happen when an unanticipated severe blow to the lower abdomen compresses the wall of a full bladder. This produces a bursting type of injury and the tear in the bladder wall will be large; in fact, the rent may be such that the bladder is virtually bivalved. Consequently, very little urine will be retained in this

bladder, as most of the urine will have escaped into the peritoneal cavity.

Extraperitoneal rupture results from the penetration of the bladder wall by a small sharp spicule of bone. Hence, it usually occurs in association with a fracture of the pelvis and the site of penetration is on the anterior wall (Fig. 7.24). In contrast with intraperitoneal rupture the hole may be only a small puncture wound and, consequently, some urine may still be retained in the bladder. As much as 300 ml of only slightly blood-stained urine has been found in a bladder with an extraperitoneal rupture.

Although wide separation of the symphysis pubis may, in some pelvic injuries, be associated with a rupture of the bladder, it is not the fracture that has caused the bladder damage but rather a blow to the lower abdomen, or thereabouts, which has been responsible for both the ruptured viscus and the bony displacement. In these cases the bladder damage is, in fact, usually an intraperitoneal burst.

Mode of injury of the posterior urethra

Almost any variety of disruption of the bony pelvic ring can result in damage to the posterior urethra, but the classical type is the 'stove in' fracture of the anterior central segment in which all four rami have been broken with backward displacement of the symphysis pubis (Fig. 7.25). The prostate lying immediately behind the symphysis is driven backwards and upwards so that the membranous urethra is stretched and torn. The upward displacement of the prostate is further aggravated by the haematoma, the extravasated fluid and the

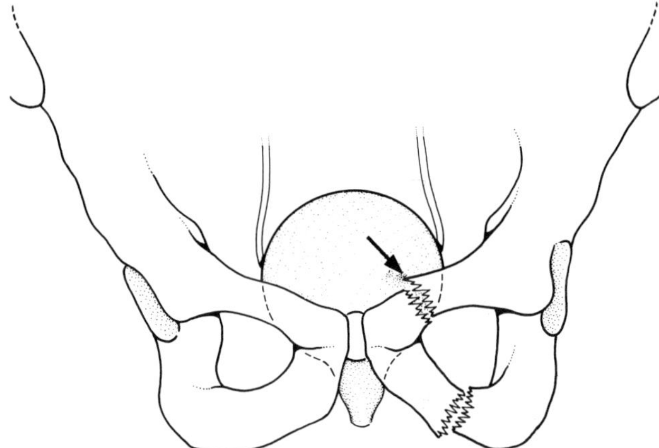

Fig. 7.24 Diagrammatic representation of the type of fracture which could result in extraperitoneal rupture of the bladder by a spicule of bone.

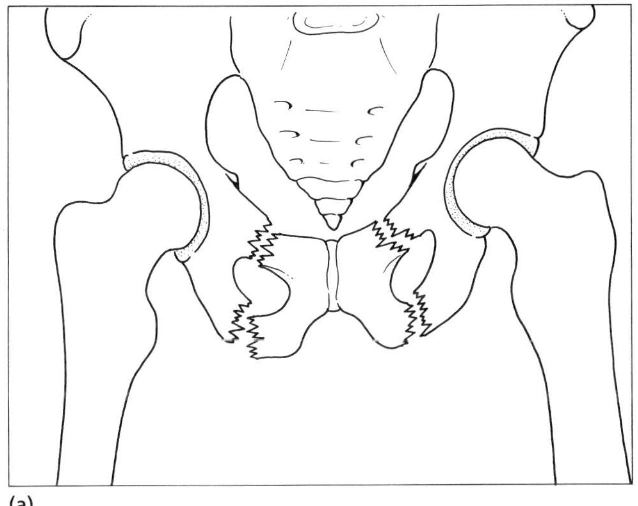

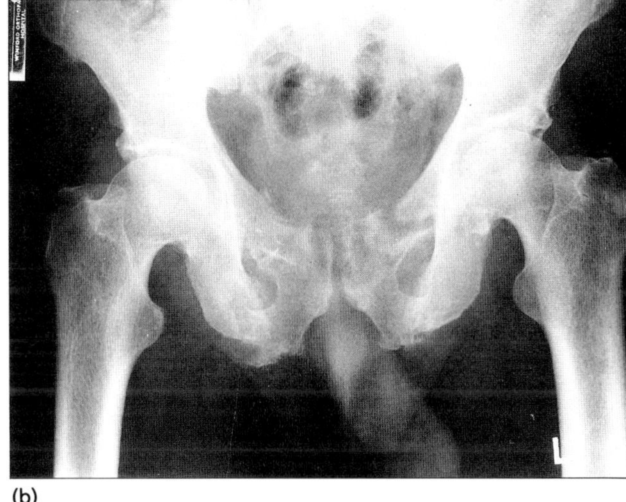

Fig. 7.25 (a) Sketch and (b) radiograph of a 'stove in' fracture of the pelvis with all four rami fractured. This fracture is stable but liable to produce injury of the lower urinary tract.

subsequent oedema. It is for this reason that realignment of the bony ring is an important factor in reconstruction of the ruptured urethra, as otherwise the prostate cannot return to its normal position, even when the haematoma, oedema and extravasated fluid around the bladder have been cleared or resolved.

Rupture of the posterior urethra may occur at any level in the membranous part. Only in penetrating injuries may the prostatic part of the urethra be damaged. The tear in the posterior urethra is frequently only partial and total transection is found in less than 20% of all urethral injuries. As the membranous urethra is stretched by the prostate and is forced backwards and upwards the wall may tear or split anteriorly or posteriorly, though rarely on either side.

Occasionally the urethra may be penetrated by a sharp bony fragment. In the same way a bony fragment may penetrate the rectum also, thus complicating the urethral injury which is thereby converted into an 'open' wound with regard to the risk of infection and subsequent management. In the female, urethral damage associated with fracture of the pelvis is usually due to penetration by a bony fragment. In the absence of the prostate gland no stretching force can be exerted in the length of the urethra and, therefore, rupture of the female urethra is much less common than rupture of the male posterior urethra.

In the young boy, before puberty and before the prostate has fully developed, the site of injury may be at a higher level just below the bladder neck. Theoretically, this could result in subsequent scarring of the ejaculatory ducts and consequent infertility as these ducts are not supported by the prostate gland at that age.

A bivalve type of fracture of the pelvis can be associated with rupture of the posterior urethra, but this appears to be a shearing effect as in all other types of pelvic fracture and not, as has been suggested, a distraction of the urethra from the pull of the two puboprostatic ligaments in opposite directions. This would be expected to result in a longitudinal tear of the urethra, which has not been reported.

Comparative incidence of partial tears and complete transections

Injuries to the lower urinary tract are seen in approximately 5% of all fractures of the pelvis. The incidence of total transection of the posterior urethra is relatively small, being somewhere in the region of 10–15% of all urethral ruptures. The remainder will be partial ruptures retaining some continuity, even though the residual strand between the proximal and distal parts of the tear may only be small. This residual strand may not be viable; nevertheless, it is sufficient to retain some approximation of the two ends. There is now evidence to suggest that in previous years the immediate repair of a ruptured posterior urethra often resulted in damage or destruction of this bridge of tissue during the surgical manipulation to achieve exposure and haemostasis at the site of the urethral tear; consequently, nearly all these injuries were reported erroneously as total transections. It is therefore important that the surgeon managing these cases is aware of the possible presence of this strand of tissue and does not aggravate the damage in the approach to the injury site.

The term 'partial tear' indicates that there has been a breach of the full thickness of the wall and that there is a hole from lumen to periurethral tissues. This is in contrast to 'incomplete tear' or 'contusion', terms which should be reserved for splits of the mucosal lining without penetration through the full thickness of the muscle wall (Fig. 7.26). Even though a contusion injury may be limited to the mucosal layer it can still occasionally produce persistent bleeding from the external urinary meatus.

Mode of injury of the urethra at the junction of posterior and anterior segments

The manner in which this type of injury occurs differs from that of the more proximal part of the urethra in that it is peculiar to a blow to the perineum and is more akin to anterior urethral ruptures caused by falling astride some object. A kick or some other form of violent blow delivered from behind the victim can crush the urethra, at the lowest level of its membranous part, against the posterior aspect of the symphysis pubis. These injuries are often associated with damage to the anus (Mathieson & Mann 1965) and the force of the injury may be sufficient to chip the lower margin of the bone. This particular type of urethral rupture is more frequently a total transection and presents the added problem that the proximal torn end recedes upwards into the pelvis whilst the lower end retracts downwards into the perineal haematoma. Although these urethral injuries are not associated with a fracture of the pelvic ring they should be considered with the posterior urethral injuries as the proximal torn end is no longer accessible via the perineum. These injuries usually develop an extensive area of ecchymosis in the perineum similar to the haematoma that occurs in anterior urethral tears. Having said that, it must be admitted that the extent of perineal ecchymosis can vary in posterior urethral injuries from no discoloration to deeply suffused skin over the whole perineum and scrotum, and it bears little relation to the severity of the lower urinary tract injury.

Management

Most road traffic accidents involve some other injury in addition to the fractured pelvis. This may be abdominal trauma, possibly with a major vessel bleeding. The patient may be unconscious due to a head injury so that voluntary co-operation is impossible; furthermore, some form of urinary drainage may be required to

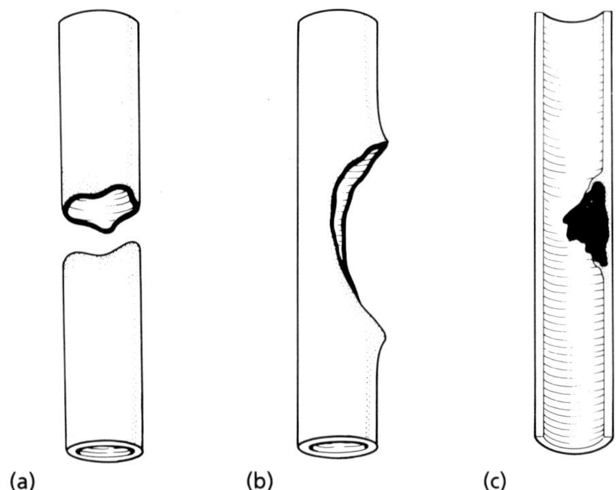

Fig. 7.26 Definition of the extent of injury: (a) complete (transection); (b) partial; (c) contusion.

monitor fluid output. Any of these factors can modify the plan of management.

Although injuries to the lower urinary tract may be severe, they do not need to take priority over other major injuries. Nearly all patients with a fractured pelvis will have sterile urine and extravasated sterile urine is in no way harmful to the patient for 24 hours. In the past, surgery of this condition has been guided by the fear of spreading gangrenous cellulitis of the skin in the suprapubic and perineal areas, but these cases occurred when infected urine extravasated, probably following urethral instrumentation for severe chronic urethral strictures. If the urine is sterile then only chemical irritation can give rise to symptoms within the first few hours. There are, however, parts of the world where underlying pathology, such as bilharzial infestation, may account for secondary bacterial infection and where this is anticipated, then urinary extravasation must be relieved without delay.

Double injuries of the bladder and urethra are common (20% of all bladder ruptures) (Wilkinson 1961, Mitchell 1963, 1968) but these are rarely diagnosed prior to definitive surgery and sometimes not until even later. Persistent haematuria may hint at the possibility of concomitant upper tract damage so that all patients with any injury to the urinary tract at any level should have an excretory urogram performed.

Clinical diagnosis

In many instances the diagnosis of a ruptured bladder is obscure and will only be made when there is a high degree of suspicion. *Intraperitoneal* rupture is rarely obvious when the patient is first admitted to hospital as the low toxicity of the urine results in a delay in the full development of signs of peritoneal irritation. The signs may be masked by other more dramatic trauma.

In the early stages the clinical signs of an *extraperitoneal* rupture may be indistinguishable from those of a posterior urethral injury. A ruptured bladder should be suspected if the patient fails to pass urine within 24 hours and if no distended bladder can be felt suprapubically whilst, at the same time, the patient's condition has deteriorated slowly following injuries such as a blow to the lower abdomen or a fracture of the pelvis.

The classical triad of symptoms and signs of posterior urethral trauma are blood at the external urinary meatus, an inability to pass urine and, after a reasonable time, the patient develops a distended bladder.

Blood at the external urinary meatus may not have been noticed in the Casualty department or may have been wiped away by an enthusiastic nursing attendant in efforts to prepare the patient before transfer to the ward. Although this sign is present in nearly all posterior urethral ruptures, a very high lesion at or above the level of the external sphincter may not show any blood at the meatus if the sphincter is still closed and competent.

The inability to pass urine is due to reflex spasm of the bladder neck and external sphincter mechanisms. There can be no harm in requesting the patient to attempt to pass urine because if the smallest amount of urine leaks through a small tear, it will immediately cause discomfort and the patient will arrest micturition instantly. If the urethra is only contused or if the rupture is only a small puncture wound, the patient may pass some urine, though this will be blood-stained and should indicate the probable diagnosis.

The distended bladder developing within a few hours of injury may not be a reliable sign. Quite apart from the injury to the urethra itself, the patient may develop urinary retention simply from reflex sphincter spasm due to the painful pelvic trauma, comparable to the retention that may occur postoperatively after any pelvic or lower abdominal surgery. Furthermore, the bladder may not fill because the patient had not been drinking any fluid prior to the injury, the patient may be in anuria from shock or a period of hypotension or there may be a concomitant rupture of the bladder wall.

The passage of a diagnostic catheter is mentioned only to be condemned as inconclusive and meddlesome. The successful passage of a catheter and withdrawal of urine does not exclude either a ruptured bladder or a partial rupture of the urethra. Many instances have been reported in the literature where surgeons have

been lulled into a false sense of security after having passed a catheter and drawn urine (Barry 1941, Mitchell 1963, 1968), only to discover subsequently that they have missed either a ruptured bladder or urethra. Failure to withdraw urine can be equally fallacious because the bladder may be empty as the patient has produced no urine or the catheter has simply been obstructed at the neck of the bladder, which is in spasm as a result of the pelvic injury alone. Furthermore, the catheter, acting as a foreign body, can introduce infection into an area of blood clot, extravasated urine, broken bones and damaged tissues which can form a perfect nidus in which organisms can multiply. There is also evidence to suggest that attempts at passing a diagnostic catheter may have aggravated the degree of injury by converting a simple contusion of the mucosa into a partial rupture or even a total transection.

RECTAL EXAMINATION

The clinical value of a rectal examination in cases of fractured pelvis is primarily to note any damage to the rectal wall, which will be revealed by blood on the examining finger or by feeling the sharp projection of a spicule of bone protruding into the lumen of the rectum. If the prostate is palpable then it has not been dislocated upwards and any rupture of the urethra cannot be more than a partial tear, but an inability to feel the prostate certainly does not prove the converse as the outline of the gland can be completely masked by surrounding blood clot and oedema.

EXCRETORY UROGRAPHY

Intraperitoneal rupture of the bladder, in which the leak of urine is gross, can be readily visualized by excretory urography, but in extraperitoneal rupture with only a small puncture hole in the anterior bladder wall excretory urography is unreliable. Contrast medium that has leaked into the peritoneal cavity will outline the loops of the bowel, while perivesical leakage will show contrast medium mixing with the perivesical haematoma.

CYSTOURETHROGRAPHY

Although urethrography can be very helpful in confirming a rupture of the urethra, this investigation is unlikely to demonstrate a leak from an extraperitoneal bladder hole. It is essential that this investigation is performed under screen control, because the first few drops of contrast to extravasate will indicate exactly where the tear has occurred. If the full urethral instillation is given before the picture is taken, then the bolus of extravasated contrast will obscure the exact site of the lesion.

What is described as the 'tear drop bladder', riding high in the pelvis, is a radiological sign of fluid accumulation in the pelvis around the base of the bladder and in the perivesical tissues. This sign does not confirm a rupture of the posterior urethra.

ENDOSCOPY

In the hands of a skilled endoscopist direct visualization of the length of the urethra is probably the most accurate means of confirming the diagnosis. However, there are some instances where the bleeding is so severe and so extensive that an adequate view cannot be obtained. It is suggested that immediate endoscopy is reserved for the patient whose condition requires diagnostic confirmation immediately prior to major surgery for some other feature of multiple injuries. Then, any irrigation fluid that may have extravasated can be aspirated with a sucker when the abdomen is open. Otherwise, endoscopy can be postponed until definitive surgery for the ruptured urethra is planned.

When any urethral injury has been excluded the endoscopist can then proceed to inspect the bladder (Mitchell 1984). An intraperitoneal rupture is easily recognized as the hole is usually large and the diagnosis will be confirmed by the appearance of the small bowel floating in the view. The small puncture wound of an extraperitoneal rupture may not be recognized easily and may be difficult to distinguish from a simple contusion of the bladder wall. Provided that the endoscopist knows exactly where and what to look for, namely an area of hyperaemia, perhaps even a trickle of blood oozing from a point within the hyperaemic oedematous anterior wall of the bladder 3–4 cm from the bladder neck, he or she will concentrate on this point and see if it is possible to demonstrate any flow of the blood through a suspected hole.

If no experienced endoscopist is available, then this investigation is best not attempted as there is a distinct risk of aggravating the damage to the already traumatized urethral wall.

ULTRASOUND AND CT SCANS

As neither an ultrasound nor a CT scan is capable of distinguishing extravasated urine from a blood clot or oedema fluid, these investigations are unlikely to provide any further information which is not already evid-

ent from excretory urography. It remains to be seen whether MRI will recognize extravasated urine.

Treatment

As soon as the clinical diagnosis has been confirmed by investigation, urinary drainage via some form of diversion, such as a suprapubic cystotomy, should be established without further delay, provided that the patient's general condition has been stabilized. The optimum time for definitive surgery is still a matter of very diverse opinion. Those who advocate immediate repair of the ruptured urethra have the satisfaction of knowing, after the procedure, that they have achieved correct alignment of the two ends, but they must be aware that in approaching a ruptured urethra in the depths of the pelvis there is a significant risk of aggravating the damage during the surgical exposure of the site of rupture. In the simple manoeuvres of extracting the blood clots and retracting the tissues to obtain an adequate view it is only too easy to extend the urethral tear and convert a partial rupture into a complete transection. Those who advocate later intervention, but still within the first week, will have the advantage of a surgical field in the pelvis free from oozing blood, but by this stage the tissues may have become macerated and friable in the area of the haematoma. On the other hand, the longer surgery can be withheld to allow the haematoma and other fluid to resorb and the oedema to settle the more complete will be the replacement of the prostate gland into its correct anatomical site.

Intraperitoneal rupture of the bladder will require laparotomy and suture of the full length of the rent, which is often several centimetres long. The mucosa, the muscle layer and the peritoneal covering should each be sutured separately. Assuming there is no urethral damage a catheter can be passed via the urethra and the bladder tested for a watertight closure, after which the catheter is connected for continuous drainage.

An extraperitoneal bladder rupture should be explored after endoscopy in order to drain the retropubic space of extravasated urine and blood. If, as is often the case, the hole is little more than a small puncture wound, then formal suture of the bladder wall is unnecessary and simply the insertion of a catheter drain will suffice. If there is evidence of urethral trauma in addition to the bladder rupture the catheter should be left in as a suprapubic drain but if urethral injury has been excluded, then the catheter can be passed via the urethra.

In all these patients there should be the closest possible co-operation with the orthopaedic surgeons so as to achieve an accurate reconstruction of the bony pelvic ring and, thereby, realignment of the prostate. Most important of all is replacement of the 'stove in' type of pelvic fracture as this gives maximal prostatic displacement, but this type of fracture may be accepted as a stable pelvis and the orthopaedic surgeon may be reluctant to interfere.

Any patient who has had urethral bleeding following an injury should have a suprapubic catheter drain, because the bleeding indicates damage to the urethral mucosa and even if this is due only to a contusion, then a diversion will avoid the risk of extravasation of urine into the wall of the urethra and probable stricture at a later date. The same applies after endoscopic inspection when a mucosal contusion or simple tear, without complete penetration of the urethral wall, has been seen; temporary diversion of the urine will reduce the risk of stricture formation. A temporary suprapubic catheter is a relatively insignificant inconvenience compared with a possible subsequent stricture.

It should be remembered, when suturing any part of the urinary tract, that closure with plain catgut or polyglycolic acid suture material will avoid the risk of phosphatic encrustation which can occur on any foreign body.

The track of all penetrating wounds must be fully explored. Debridement of all dead tissue and foreign material, such as clothing, driven into the wound must be removed and closure with good drainage must be carried out as for other bladder and urethral injuries. If there is a loss of tissue it may be difficult or even impossible to suture wounds of the bladder base satisfactorily and more harm than good will result from attempts to draw the bladder base together under tension.

In these types of injury the rectum is often involved as well, in which case a colostomy will have to be established. Provided that there is free catheter drainage of the bladder and the colostomy is efficient, a proportion of these double injuries to the bladder and rectum will heal spontaneously without fistula formation.

DEFINITIVE SURGERY OF THE URETHRA

If, at the time of performing the suprapubic cystotomy, the bladder and prostate are found to be floating high in the abdomen, having been completely detached from the pelvic tissues, then a complete transection of the posterior urethra must have occurred. Nothing can then be gained from delaying definitive surgery and an immediate realignment should be achieved. A Foley catheter (16 Charrière) is passed via the urethra until it presents in the depths of the pelvis. Another latex Foley catheter (24 Charrière) is passed from the lumen of the bladder down the urethra to present beside the first catheter. The tip of the larger (24 Charrière) catheter is amputated, exposing its lumen, into which the tip of the smaller catheter is firmly tucked (Fig. 7.27) and, if necessary, the two are stitched together. The proximal larger catheter is well lubricated and then withdrawn gently and slowly back into the bladder, carrying the smaller catheter with it. Care must be taken to ensure that the margins of the proximal torn end of the urethra do not invaginate with the catheter as it is withdrawn. The balloon of the smaller catheter is then distended with 15–20 ml of water and the tip is extracted from the end of the larger catheter. Light traction may be applied to the urethral catheter, or larger sutures through the base of the prostate may be passed downwards to present in the perineum, but even without these manoeuvres the prostate and bladder base will return to their normal positions as soon as the oedema and haematoma have absorbed, provided that the bony pelvic ring has been restored accurately.

If the urethral tear is partial and the initial treatment has been simply a suprapubic cystostomy, then subsequent definitive surgery should be preceded by endoscopy. On inspection some stenosis will usually be seen at the site of the tear, and the lumen is visible and can be traced with the beak of the endoscope. Sometimes, however, the track of the normal urethra is not obvious as the mucosal walls of the urethra have adhered together. If, under these circumstances, a flexible endoscope is passed from the suprapubic cystostomy into the bladder and then down the proximal urethra as far as the face of the rupture (Fig. 7.28), the terminal light of the proximal flexible endoscope will be clearly visible via the rigid distal endoscope, which can then be replaced by a viewing urethrotome and a short cut made directly towards the transmitted light. This technique should only be attempted by those skilled in endoscopy. An 18 Charrière catheter can then be passed and left *in situ* as a stent for 2–3 weeks. Alternatively, a length of silicone tubing can be passed into the bladder via the urethrotome sheath and brought out of the suprapubic cystotomy by means of another endoscope equipped with grasping forceps. So effective is this method that it is rarely necessary to explore the rupture site by open surgery. However, if this has to be performed, then the technique is exactly as described for realignment of a total transection.

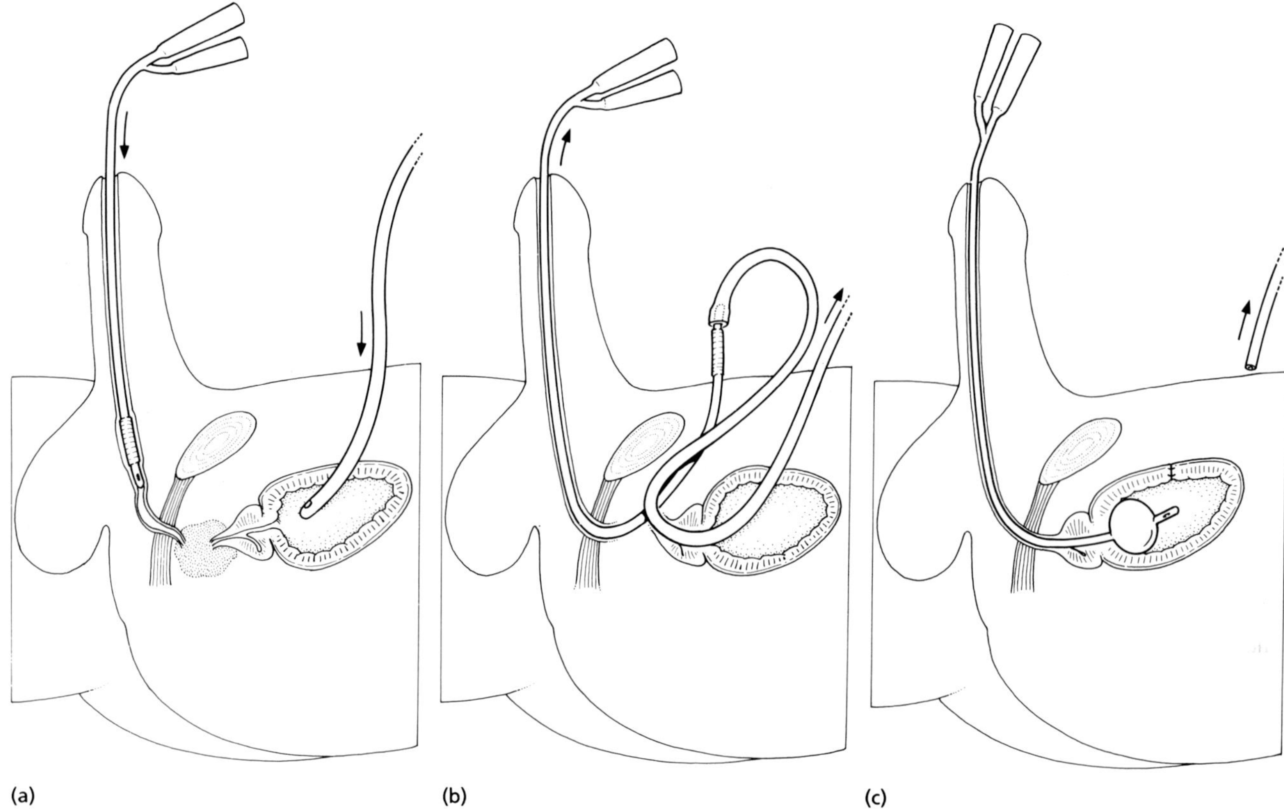

(a)   (b)   (c)

Fig. 7.27 (a) A Foley catheter (16 Charrière) is passed via the urethra to present in the depths of the wound. A similar Foley catheter (24 Charrière) is passed from the bladder via the internal meatus to present in the wound and (b) the two catheters are joined together after amputating the tip of the larger catheter. (c) The larger catheter is withdrawn into the bladder, leaving the smaller catheter as a stent. (In the last diagram, to avoid a complicated picture, the suprapubic catheter is not shown.)

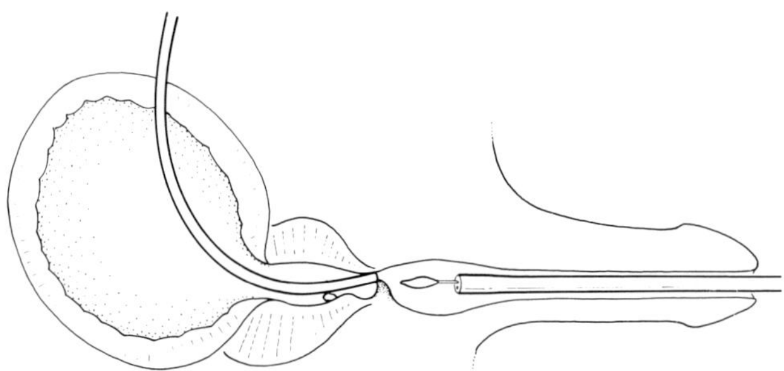

Fig. 7.28 Flexible endoscope passed suprapubically and the rigid urethrotome passed via the urethra.

Complications of bladder and posterior urethral injuries

Except for loss of tissue reducing the capacity of the bladder, the only early complication of any importance is infection and, unless there is any obstruction to the outflow or other underlying pathology, this infection should clear with appropriate antibiotic therapy. Later complications of posterior urethral rupture are stricture formation, incontinence and disabilities in sexual function.

Infection

During the first 4 weeks after injury to the posterior urethra, infection can be a complication with sinister implications. The pelvis contains blood, extravasated urine, broken bone ends and damaged tissue, of which some may not be viable. This is a perfect nidus in which organisms can multiply, resulting in a pelvic cellulitis; when the patient recovers from such a severe infection, then the healing process will inevitably result in dense and distorting fibrosis. This can make realignment at a later stage an extremely difficult problem; therefore, every effort must be made to control and, if possible, avoid infection.

Stricture

Whether a stricture develops depends on how much of the circumference of the urethral wall has been torn and on the state of the blood supply to the apparently intact part and, secondly, whether infection and subsequent fibrosis has occurred. The treatment of a stricture is either by endoscopic urethrotomy or, if that fails, then some form of urethroplasty will be necessary.

Incontinence

Although incontinence carries with it no risk to life it can be an extremely demoralizing and embarrassing disability. Following trauma, incontinence can be due to direct involvement of the urethra and sphincter mechanism, or to neurological impairment from damage to S2/3 outflow at the sacral foramina or within the pelvic cavity. In high posterior urethral ruptures the external sphincter and the lower margin of the prostate may be involved in the original urethral tear, or may subsequently be encased in periurethral scar tissue, resulting from extravasation or infection of a haematoma. In the same way, incontinence can result from rupture of the female urethra but with two additional factors. First, there is the possibility of the tear extending upwards to involve the bladder neck and secondly, the split may extend even higher to tear the bladder wall. The temporary management of incontinence is relatively easy in the male by use of a dribbling bag appliance, but the female has to rely on perineal pads as no satisfactory incontinence appliance has yet been designed for the female. Operations for incontinence following trauma are aimed at restoring the normal anatomy in those patients with sphincter damage, but neurological incontinence will tax the ingenuity of the urologist. Unfortunately, the site of the urethral injury and subsequent fibrosis will, in many cases, preclude the use of any urethral compression implants.

Disabilities of sexual function

The disabilities in sexual function attributable to lower urinary tract injury are impotence, loss of ejaculation and infertility. Defining impotence as an inability to produce an erection adequate for sexual intercourse, at least one-third of all patients with rupture of the posterior urethra will be victims, but here there appears to be a significant difference between the results of delayed and immediate definitive surgery, in that the latter has double the number of patients affected (Morehouse *et al.* 1972). Mobilization of the prostate and the bladder neck appears to be the factor responsible. Following injury within the pelvis, impotence may be due to various causes, including thrombosis of the vessels supplying the corpora cavernosa, involvement of the nervi erigentes either at their outflow from the cord or in their passage across the pelvic floor, or simply the psychological effect of severe trauma. Normal tactile sensation over the penis and scrotum may impair the sexual response. In younger patients potency should improve with the passage of time, particularly when their compensation has been settled.

As with impotence, so a loss of ejaculation can occur when there has been damage in the region of the lower posterior part of the prostate and bladder neck and, again, it is found more commonly in those patients in whom immediate definitive repair was carried out. The cause is often due to failure of the bladder neck to close, resulting in retrograde ejaculation into the bladder. It can also be the result of failure of the seminal vesicles to contract after neurological interference, or the result of a tight stricture of the urethra below the level of the ejaculatory ducts so that semen passes upwards to the bladder more readily than downwards.

Impotence and failure to ejaculate will both contribute to infertility but, in addition, damage to the seminal vesicles, the vas deferens or the ejaculatory ducts, with subsequent scarring, can obstruct the flow of the seminal fluid. In most adults rupture of the posterior urethra occurs below the level of the prostate, but in small boys the rupture appears to occur, in many instances, at a higher level and nearer to the neck of the bladder. It is impossible to assess damage to the vesicles or ducts until adolescence.

Injuries to the anterior urethra and penis

The incidence of rupture of the anterior urethra is one-third of the frequency of posterior urethral trauma. In the majority of cases the injury is due to falling astride some object such as a wall or fence, slipping with one leg on either side of the rung of a ladder or the anecdotal manhole cover (Dudley 1977). The signs of rupture are blood from the external meatus and the rapid development of severe ecchymosis in the perineum owing to haematoma formation. The anterior urethra may be involved in lacerations of the scrotum and perineum or even, occasionally, in gunshot wounds. The extent of the urethral damage may be difficult to assess, even at open operation, because of the intense discoloration of the tissues.

Regeneration of the anterior urethra cannot occur; therefore, when this has been claimed (Mitchell 1984) undoubtedly the surgeon failed to identify a viable length of urethra amongst the grossly blood-stained tissues and haematoma.

The mode of injury in 'falling astride' accidents is

sudden forceful compression of the urethra against the undersurface of the symphysis pubis. As with ruptures of the posterior urethra, the majority of these tears are partial and only a small proportion are total transections. There are various other types of injury of the anterior urethra and penis which may have some sexual association such as fracture of the penis, constricting rings of string or metal, or insertion of the penis into mechanical orifices, of which the most extraordinary and dangerous is the Hoover. Industrial accidents, when clothing may be caught in machinery, can result in degloving of the penis, though fortunately the urethra and corpora cavernosa are usually spared.

Sporting accidents account for occasional anterior urethral injuries. Perhaps the best-known from the literature are the bulbar ruptures resulting from go-kart crashes (Heddle & Robb 1974) in which the driver slides forward onto the steering column. Winter sports accidents have been reported from the downhill slalom when the skier straddles one of the gates at speed.

A iatrogenic injury to the urethra has been reported on the orthopaedic table used for hip and femoral neck surgery when the perineal pillar is made the point of counter-traction. This pillar should have a recess grooved into the cephalic surface to accommodate the anterior urethra and avoid any compression necrosis.

Cardiac surgery has come under particular scrutiny as the cause of postoperative stricture following cardiac bypass surgery; this type of stricture reached almost epidemic proportions (Ruutu 1982). However, the co-incidental use of a particularly toxic catheter was found to be the causative factor.

Management of anterior urethral rupture

In all cases where there is blood oozing from the external urinary meatus and an extensive haematoma of the scrotum and perineum, diversion of the urine must be performed so as to reduce the risk of stricture formation even though the patient may successfully pass urine. There is no need to discourage patients from attempting to pass urine as a trial; if the lesion is minor they will succeed, but if the tear is of any considerable size the pain in attempting to pass water will stop the flow immediately.

If urethral bleeding is not excessive, then the services of a skilled endoscopist will confirm the diagnosis and provide an accurate assessment of the extent of the tear. This investigation should not be attempted by anyone unskilled in the technique, as the risk of aggravating the injury outweighs the benefit of the inspection. If endoscopy reveals anything more than a small longit-udinal split, then the urine should be diverted for at least 2 weeks and the site of rupture should be explored and sutured.

Although the usual indications for exploring a ruptured urethra are a total transection or a severe partial rupture, occasionally a haematoma may be so tense that the viability of the overlying skin is endangered.

Complications

Stricture is the commonest problem following trauma to the anterior urethra and penis, though occasionally there may be post-traumatic distortion of the corpora due to intercavernous fibrosis (Peyronie's disease).

The problems of incontinence, impotence and retrograde ejaculation do not occur with anterior urethral ruptures, but lacerations of the perineum and penile degloving accidents can cause loss of cutaneous sensation.

Injuries to the urethra in children and females

Although damage to the urethra in the female is far less common than rupture of the posterior urethra in the male, the proportional incidence of urethral damage in association with a fracture of the pelvis is very similar in both sexes because fracture of the pelvis is a far less common injury in the female than in the male.

The level at which injury is seen in both children and females can vary considerably throughout the length of the urethra. A kick or other type of blow from behind can damage the lower third of the urethra, whilst a spicule of bone from the posterior aspect of the symphysis pubis can penetrate the most proximal part of the urethra. This is the same site as in young males before the prostate has developed to protect this most proximal part of the posterior urethra.

Most urethral injuries in the female also involve the anterior wall of the vagina; thus, they cannot be regarded as closed injuries. Straddle injuries in the female may cause bruising and laceration of the vulva and clitoris, though occasionally the external urinary meatus or the distal end of the urethra may be damaged. Small foreign bodies introduced into the urethra or larger foreign bodies introduced into the vagina may cause damage to the female urethra. Personal assault seems very rarely to give rise to any urinary tract damage beyond bruising of the vulva.

The high level of injury in the upper part of the posterior urethra in young males not only incurs the risk of involvement of the seminal vesicles and ejaculatory ducts but will often impair the action of the bladder neck sphincter mechanism so that even after realignment of the urethra and an adequate period of recovery there may be considerable difficulty in initiating micturition. Patience on the part of the surgeon and reassurance of the young patient will usually result in successful emptying of the bladder. A too hasty conclusion that the bladder neck should be resected to reduce the outflow resistance can result in infertility due to retrograde ejaculation and may even produce urinary incontinence.

Parental advice, counselling and concern

As soon as the child has recovered from the immediate severe trauma, it is important to have a frank and, at the same time, sympathetic discussion about the possible complications and the child's future. It is no use painting an absurdly rosy picture of the prognosis in young males with posterior urethral ruptures as, sadly, the parents have to be told about the possible risk of impotence and infertility. Comfort can, however, be given as 70–80% develop at puberty into sexually adequate males, but failure to mention these risks means failure to take account of these possibilities in the assessment of compensation after road traffic accidents.

References

Archbold, J.A.A., Barros D'Sa, A.A.B. & Morrison, E. Genito-urinary injuries of civil hostilities. *Br J Surg* 1981; **68**: 625–631.

Barry, H.C. Discussion on rupture of the urethra and its treatment. *Proc R Soc Med* 1941; **35**: 292–293.

Dudley, H.A.F. (ed.) *Hamilton Bailey's Emergency Surgery* 10th edn. Wright: Bristol, 1977.

Hai, M.A., Pontes, E. & Pierce, J.M. Surgical management of major renal trauma: a review of 102 cases treated by conservative surgery. *J Urol* 1977; **118**: 7.

Heddle, R.M. & Robb, W.A. Go-kart injuries of the urethra. *J R Coll Surg Edinb* 1974; **19**: 310–312.

Mathieson, A.J.M. & Mann, T.S. Rupture of the posterior urethra and avulsion of the rectum and anus as a complication of fracture of the pelvis. *Br J Surg* 1965; **52**: 309–310.

McDougal, W.S. & Persky, L. *International Perspectives in Urology*, Vol. 1, *Traumatic Injuries to the Genito-urinary System: Anterior Urethral Injuries*. Williams & Wilkins: Baltimore, 1981.

Mitchell, J.P. Injuries to the lower urinary tract. *Proc R Soc Med* 1963; **56**: 1046–1050.

Mitchell, J.P. Injuries to the urethra. *Br J Urol* 1968; **40**: 649–669.

Mitchell, J.P. *Urinary Tract Trauma*. Wright: Bristol, 1984.

Morehouse, D.D., Belitsky, P. & Mackinnon, K. Rupture of the posterior urethra. *J Urol* 1972; **107**: 255–258.

Ruutu, M. 'Epidemic' of urethral strictures after open heart surgery. *Lancet* 1982; **i**: 218.

Turner-Warwick, R. & Worth, P.H. The psoas bladder hitch procedure for replacement of the lower third of the ureter. *Br J Urol* 1969; **41**: 701–709.

Wilkinson, F.O.W. Rupture of posterior urethra. *Lancet* 1961; **i**: 1125–1129.

8: Definitive Treatment of Fractures and Dislocations

General principles, available methods and methods of selection

O.O.A.ONI AND P.J.GREGG

The management of a patient with a fracture or dislocation begins with making the correct diagnosis. This involves the taking of a thorough history, performing a thorough clinical examination and requesting appropriate investigations which will always include radiographic examination. The fracture or dislocation is then described and classified. These aspects of fracture management have already been described. In addition, potential complications must be sought and, if present, dealt with promptly. Complications and their management are discussed in general in Chapter 11. It is only after these aspects of the injury have been dealt with satisfactorily that attention is focussed on the specific treatment of the fracture or dislocation.

The objectives of fracture management are:
1 To allow a fracture to heal as quickly as possible with restoration of normal or acceptable anatomy and without any complications.
2 To obtain normal fracture union (prevention of malunion and non-union).

The hope is that unimpaired function and a return to normal activities will be achieved in the shortest possible time with the least expense.

One of the principal roles of treatment of fractures is to prevent deformity because the deformity of a long bone may impose abnormal stresses on adjacent joints and subsequently lead to degenerative joint disease. Residual deformity (irregularity) of articular surfaces must also be prevented, if at all possible, because this inevitably leads to the development of secondary degenerative osteoarthrosis.

Fracture reduction

If the ends of a fractured bone are displaced, the question needs to be asked as to whether the degree of displacement is acceptable. What can or cannot be accepted depends upon a number of factors which include the type and site of fracture and the age of the patient. This will be dealt with in greater detail in the sections dealing with specific fractures. Fracture reduction refers to the restoration of normal or acceptable anatomy (alignment) and it may be achieved by closed or open methods:
1 Closed
  (a) Gravity — collar-and-cuff, hanging cast.
  (b) Manipulation.
  (c) Continuous traction — fixed or sliding; skin or skeletal.
2 Open — surgical operation.
3 Semi-open — external fixator.

Fracture stabilization

If a fracture is undisplaced or minimally displaced, the question needs to be asked as to whether the fracture has the potential to displace, i.e. is unstable. If the fracture is unstable, it needs to be stabilized to prevent malunion. Fractures requiring reduction should, by and large, always be regarded as unstable and, therefore, should be stabilized to prevent recurrence of deformity after reduction. Stabilization may be achieved by closed or open methods:
1 Closed methods
  (a) Plaster casts, splints.
  (b) Gravity — collar-and-cuff, hanging casts.
  (c) Continuous traction.
2 Open methods
  (a) Wires, screws.
  (b) Plates, nails, etc.
3 External fixation.

Closed treatment of fractures

Most fractures can be treated adequately without operation. Therefore, it is incumbent on every fracture surgeon to be familiar with closed methods. Yet, while there are many centres offering courses on operative treatment of fractures, there are none in the United Kingdom today offering courses on closed methods.

The closed method consists of closed reduction and application of casts, splints or traction to maintain the reduction until union has occurred. It includes the following:

1 Fracture reduction
   (a) Gravity — via devices such as collar-and-cuff, hanging casts.
   (b) Manipulation
      (i)   Reversal of mechanism of injury.
      (ii) Realignment of fragments.
      (iii) Periosteal hinge technique.
      (iv) Disimpaction–traction technique.
   (c) Traction — sliding.
2 Immobilization
   (a) Gravity — hanging casts etc.
   (b) Plaster casts and splints.
   (c) Traction
      (i) Skin traction — fixed or sliding.
      (ii) Skeletal traction — fixed or sliding.

Fracture reduction

The reduction of fractures is not by ritual movements of the injured limb but by a careful assessment of the influence of various mechanical factors on the fracture fragments and the use of such knowledge to achieve anatomical alignment. The principal components of closed fracture reduction depend upon the type of displacement, whether the fracture is associated with a periosteal hinge and upon the location of the fracture in the shaft.

Gravity

Gravity may be used to give positive help in the reduction of some fractures. The weight of a limb, or part thereof, may be used to overcome muscle contraction which produces overlap or shortening of fracture fragments. The effect of gravity may be harnessed through devices such as the collar-and-cuff sling and hanging casts. This method is used most commonly for fractures of the humeral shaft and proximal humerus. In other instances the elimination of gravity may be used, for example, in reducing displaced trimalleolar fractures (Charnley 1971).

Manipulation

To reduce the fracture anatomically, preliminary manual traction, to overcome shortening and disimpact the fracture fragments, is followed by a reduction manoeuvre. Most commonly, an attempt is made to reverse the mechanism of injury.

Displaced subtrochanteric fractures and fractures of the forearm or leg bones pose a difficult problem. One fracture fragment is usually easily controlled while the other is not. Reduction requires that the 'controllable' fragments, usually the distal, be lined up with the less 'controllable' fragments, usually the proximal.

The reduction manoeuvres for a long bone fracture with a 'periosteal hinge' have been described by Charnley (1971). They consist essentially of: increasing the angulation of the fracture to achieve soft tissue relaxation on the concave side of the deformity and disimpaction of the fragments; the broken edges of the bone are brought into contact by manual traction and by manipulation; the fragments are guided into their anatomical positions and realigned as shown diagrammatically in Fig. 8.1. This tightens up the 'periosteal hinge' and prevents slippage, and rotational deformity is visually corrected.

Impacted metaphyseal fractures, such as those of the distal radius, may be reduced by the method described in Fig. 8.2. The fracture is first disengaged by a combination of traction and manipulation; then, with traction still maintained, one fragment is guided onto the other; and finally, the fracture fragments are 'locked' into place (Charnley 1971).

Reduction is more easily achieved soon after injury because haemorrhage and interstitial oedema, which develop within hours of injury, render the soft tissues inelastic. If gross swelling has already developed it is reasonable to wait until it subsides and this may be assisted by elevation of the part and/or application of ice packs. Before embarking on manipulative reduction, adequate radiographs must be available as these are used to decide beforehand what is indicated and what is achievable (Perkins 1970). Radiographs show the displacement which has to be corrected and make it possible to work out the mechanism of injury which has to be reversed.

Manipulative reduction can be carried out under local or general anaesthesia. Check radiographs must be carried out before discontinuing the anaesthetic to

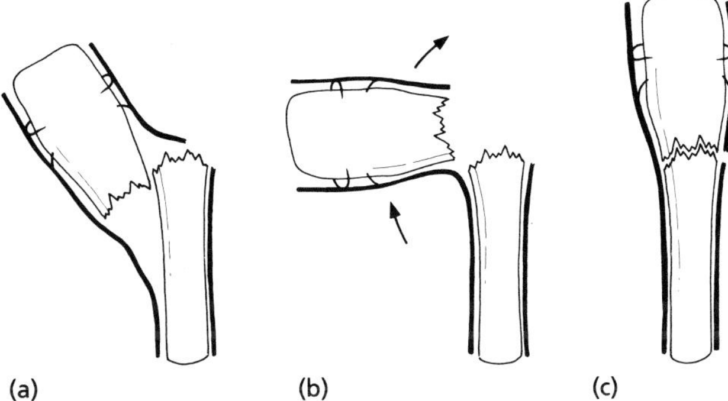

Fig. 8.1 The periosteal hinge reduction technique of Charnley. (a) The periosteum is intact on the concave side of the angulatory fracture deformity but is torn on the convex side. (b) The fracture deformity is first increased to relax the soft tissues, after which the distal fragment is guided into the anatomical position and the fracture is corrected. (c) The intact periosteal hinge helps to prevent overcorrection of the deformity and helps to maintain reduction of the fracture.

determine whether reduction has been adequate and what, if any, other treatment may be necessary. When there is a likelihood that manipulative reduction may fail or there may be other problems, reduction should be attempted under general anaesthesia in an operating theatre so that the surgeon can proceed to internal or external fixation, if necessary, under the same anaesthetic.

Traction

Traction results in the stretching and elongation of the soft tissues and, as a consequence, overcomes the pull of muscles, which produces overlap of fracture fragments and shortening, and disimpacts the fracture fragments. A displaced long bone fracture may be reduced by manual traction or by one device or another as will be discussed later.

Only sliding traction, by definition, may be used to reduce a displaced fracture. A large fracture haematoma or buttonholing of the fracture fragments through the periosteal/soft tissue sleeve may make traction ineffective (Charnley 1971). Furthermore, excessive traction may fail or may rupture the periosteal sleeve and thereby result in delayed union or non-union (Charnley 1971).

Immobilization

After a satisfactory reduction has been achieved, immobilization may be provided by a variety of methods, including plaster of Paris and other casts, splints or continuous traction.

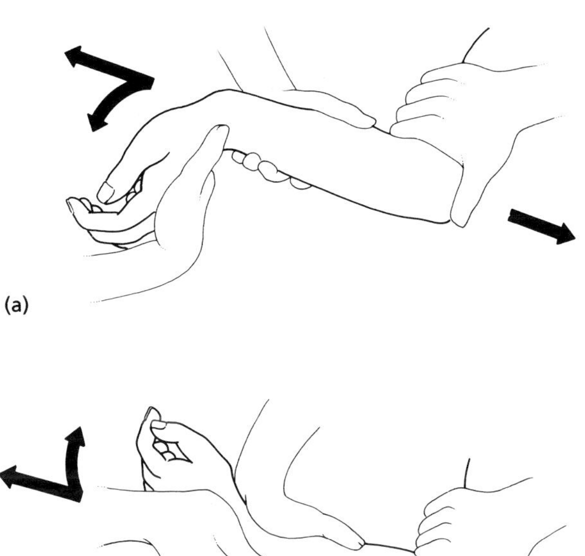

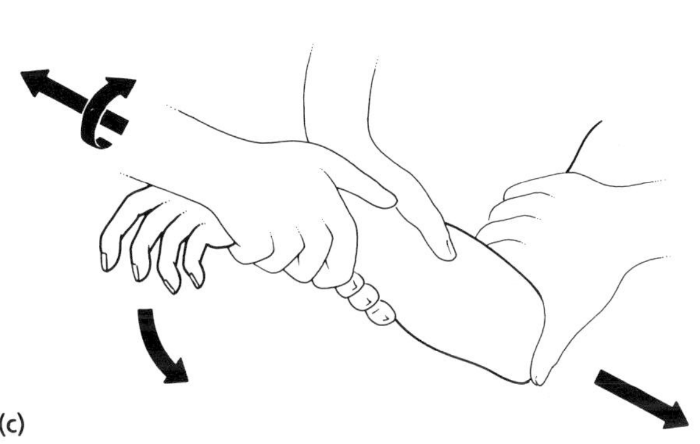

Fig. 8.2 A method of reducing impacted Colles' fracture. (a) Disimpaction by traction and manipulation. (b) Reduction by guiding the distal fragment into the anatomical position. (c) Locking the reduction by pronation.

Gravity

Fractures reduced by gravity may be maintained in their reduced positions by gravity using a variety of devices such as the collar-and-cuff sling. However, such fractures may need splintage to control or prevent angular deformity. A plaster cast may be used in such circumstances to act as a mould.

Plaster of Paris and other casts and splints

Casts and splints are used in fracture treatment to support the injured limb, control movement of the fragments in order to prevent malunion and delayed union and to rest the injured soft tissues. The modern plaster of Paris bandage was developed from a dressing used for battlefield injuries by Mathysen (1854). It consists of a roll of muslin stiffened with starch and impregnated with partially hydrated calcium sulphate. The bandage hardens in an exothermic reaction with water; the reaction may be accelerated by increasing the temperature of the water or by adding alum.

In the treatment of fractures the plaster is wrapped around, or a slab of it is bandaged onto, the limb and held there while it hardens. The safest method of applying the cast is over a stockinet bandage and/or generous padding. A stockinet bandage should not be used if swelling is anticipated. On the other hand, too much padding makes the cast loose-fitting and thereby reduces its efficacy.

After manipulation the plaster cast is applied quickly and dexterously by an assistant, while the reduction is maintained by the surgeon; this is followed by moulding for three-point fixation according to Charnley (1971) 'to overcorrect the original angulation'. In this technique, pressure is exerted at certain precisely determined points on the skeleton on either side of the fracture (Fig. 8.3). According to Charnley (1971), reduction is held because the soft tissues are kept under tension.

In the correct application of the full cast, the first 5 cm or so of the bandage is unrolled. One end of the roll is held in each hand, and the bandage is immersed in water until all the air bubbles have escaped. Then the roll is taken out of the water and squeezed gently. Next, the plaster bandage is rolled onto the limb in the same direction as the padding; each turn slightly overlaps the preceding turn and each turn is smoothed over using the palm of the hand. When the plaster has been completely rolled on, the cast is rubbed and moulded with the palms of the wet hands to assume the desired contour and taking care not to indent it while setting.

A cast should always be made too long and then trimmed to size; it is less satisfactory to increase the length of a short one. After application of a cast to a recently reduced fracture, the limb should be elevated for 2–3 days to minimize swelling. If significant swelling is anticipated the cast should be split. Residual deformities may be corrected by wedging after the cast is dried but this only corrects angulation and not shift or rotation. A plaster cast may be windowed for dressing of wounds, etc., but rectangular shapes should be avoided because they weaken the cast. Windows should never be left open because they allow soft tissues to herniate through.

The plaster of Paris bandage is easy to apply and mould. It is inexpensive and is porous to blood, pus and odour. Nevertheless, there are now casting materials

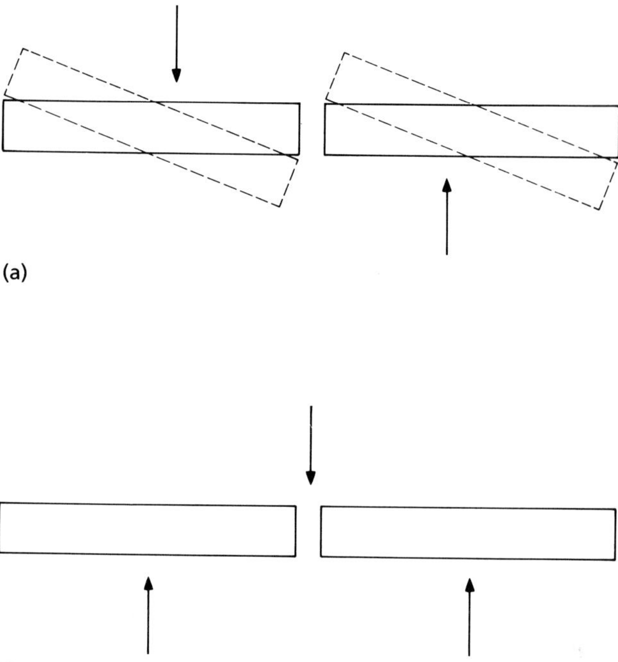

Fig. 8.3 The principles of three-point fixation. (a) Two-point fixation introduces 'coupling' and displacement. (b) Three-point fixation prevents 'coupling' and displacement.

such as fibreglass (e.g. Scotchcast and Baycast) which are lighter, harder wearing, waterproof and more radiolucent. They are particularly suitable for the elderly and for open wounds requiring regular dressings. However, they are less easy to apply and mould satisfactorily.

COMPLICATIONS OF CAST TREATMENT OF FRACTURES

Treatment by plaster casts requires a lot of care and vigilance to prevent serious complications such as circulatory impairment, plaster sores and malunion.

Circulatory impairment

This is the most serious complication. A limb with a fractured bone swells within hours of injury and such a limb encased in a rigid cast may suffer a reduction in the blood supply to muscles and nerves. This can result in ischaemic necrosis of muscles with subsequent fibrotic contractures, and in impaired cutaneous sensibility. The impairment in circulation may occur in the presence of distal peripheral pulses but is usually associated with significant and persistent pain. There may be swelling of the fingers or toes, poor capillary circulation in the nail-beds and/or pain on passively extending the fingers or toes as appropriate. If there is any doubt about the circulation, the plaster should be split from end-to-end and down to the skin. The skin must be exposed by pulling apart the cut edges of the cast.

Plaster sores

These usually occur over bony prominences or beneath areas of indentations in the cast or close to sharp edges. They may also be due to the presence of foreign bodies, such as coins, between the cast and the skin (Fig. 8.4). The mechanism is one of pressure necrosis. The patient usually complains of a burning pain or discomfort. The cast may have a circumscribed area of increased warmth or odour. If the presence of a pressure sore is suspected, the plaster should be windowed immediately to examine the underlying skin. It must be emphasized that a 'wait and see' policy must not be adopted because the pain will pass off when the skin finally becomes necrotic. The pain should not be treated only with analgesics.

Loss of position

This is probably the most common complication of cast treatment of fractures. A plaster cast limits deformity to a minimum by a hydraulic effect and is aided by the splinting effect of the soft tissues as they organize around the fragments, but this does not render a fracture totally stable (Hicks 1960). Encasing joints above and below the fracture does not promote stability; the three-point fixation of the fracture is more important (Charnley 1971). It is advisable to obtain regular radiographs of the fracture in the first few weeks of treatment when remanipulation or wedging may still be possible or the method of treatment revised.

Plaster wedging. Angulation at the fracture site may be corrected by the technique of wedging. There are two methods: opening wedge and closing wedge. In the *opening wedge* method the plaster cast is cut transversely around 50−75% of its circumference on the concave side of the deformity, the edges are spread apart and the cut is strutted open with a predetermined length of cork (Fig. 8.5). In the *closing wedge* method a wide wedge is excised from the convex side of the deformity and closed. It is necessary to remove a wide wedge so that it cannot be completely closed and thereby pinch the soft tissues. The plaster cast is reconstituted by repairing the defect with further plaster bandages after checking the fracture alignment by radiographs.

The wedging of a plaster cast requires as much care and detailed attention as the application of the cast. It

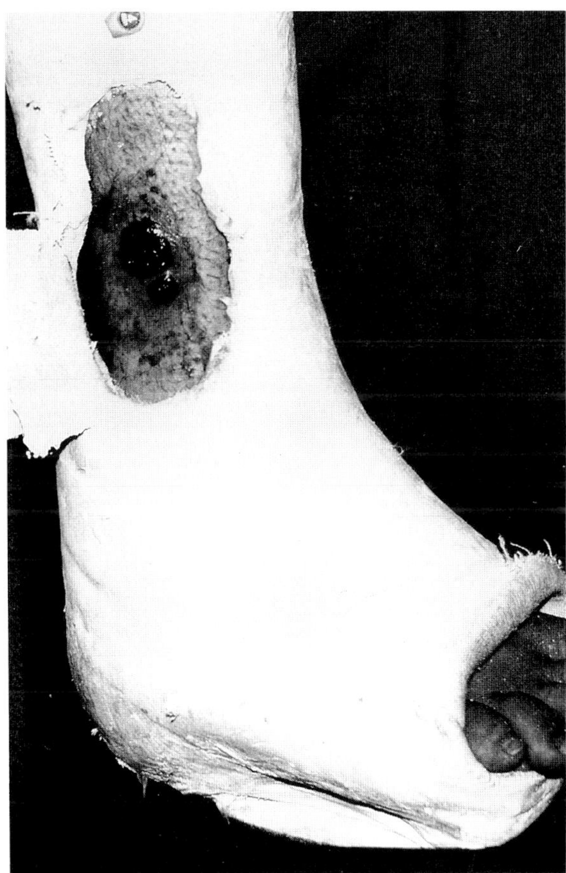

Fig. 8.4 Plaster sore.

should be carried out within a week of the reduction and application of the cast, when the tissues have not yet consolidated around the fracture.

The amount of wedging required is determined from the radiographs:

1 The width of the plaster cast at the fracture site is first measured and noted,

2 The longitudinal axis of both major fracture fragments is then drawn on the anteroposterior or lateral projections as the case may be.

3 A length equal to the width of the plaster cast is measured and marked on each line from the point of intersection of the two lines.

4 The distance between the two marks is equal to the size of wedge required to correct the angulation.

Traction

Traction may be used to overcome deformity and the tendency to shortening produced by muscle contraction. It relieves pain by overcoming muscle spasm and controls movement of the fracture fragments by creating

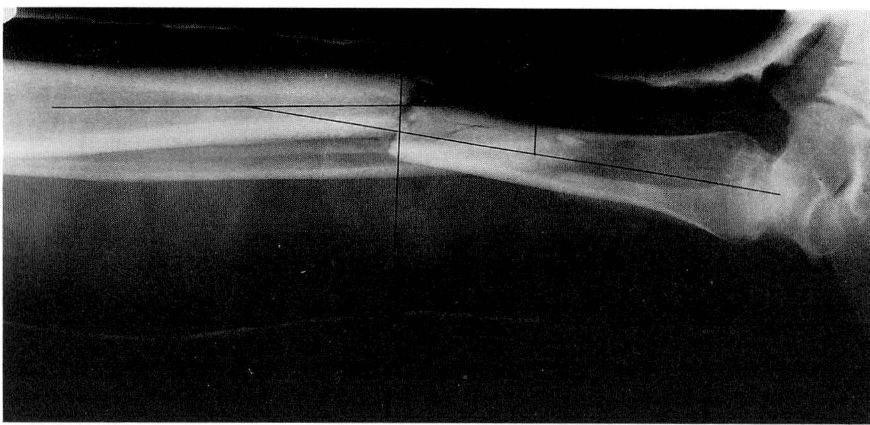

(a)

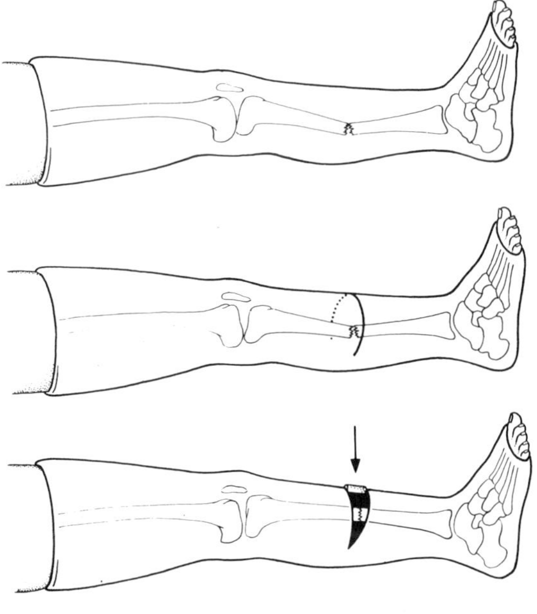

(b)

Fig. 8.5 A method of wedging a plaster cast to correct angulation. (a) A radiograph showing pre-planning. (b) A linear cut is opened to a wedge and held by a cork block (arrow). After confirming the position on a radiograph, the gap is repaired with plaster.

tension in the muscles. Traction may also be used to rest the injured limb in the best functional position.

It is a useful technique for managing fractures too unstable for cast immobilization or too comminuted for prudent surgical intervention, although the latter indication has, to some extent, been overcome by locking nails. It is also a useful method for treating certain fractures in children.

Traction entails obtaining a satisfactory grip on a part of the body to allow the application of a pulling force. In limb fractures the traction force is applied either through the skin or through the skeleton and is supplemented, as required, with pads, slings or pushers to overcome angulation and shift of fragments. It is often used in lower limb fractures, especially femoral shaft fractures, but can also be used in upper limb fractures, for example, fractures of the humeral shaft in a patient with a head injury and who has to be nursed flat, or supracondylar fractures of the elbow in children.

SKIN TRACTION

This is usually applied via commercially available adhesive or non-adhesive tapes. For comfort and efficacy, the traction force is applied over a large skin area and distal to the fracture site. Bony prominences are protected from pressure necrosis by padding proximal to them and the traction tapes are applied evenly without wrinkles or creases — oblique cuts may be made at the edges to make the traction tape conform to the shape of the limb. An elastic bandage is wrapped around the limb over the traction tape (Fig. 8.6). The traction cord(s) is attached to a metal hook or to a block inserted into the loop at the free end. Weights may then be attached to the cord(s), which is passed over a pulley. Alternatively, the cord(s) may be attached to the ends of a splint such as the Thomas' splint (see below).

The force exerted on the skin is dissipated to the soft tissues and this pulls the fracture fragments apart. However, skin tolerates shear forces poorly and, therefore, the maximum weight should not exceed 4.5 kg (10 lb), because otherwise the superficial layers of the skin are peeled off. Rotation of the limb is difficult to control with skin traction and, therefore, this method is unsuitable for most adult fractures other than as a temporary measure to keep the patient comfortable while awaiting more definitive treatment.

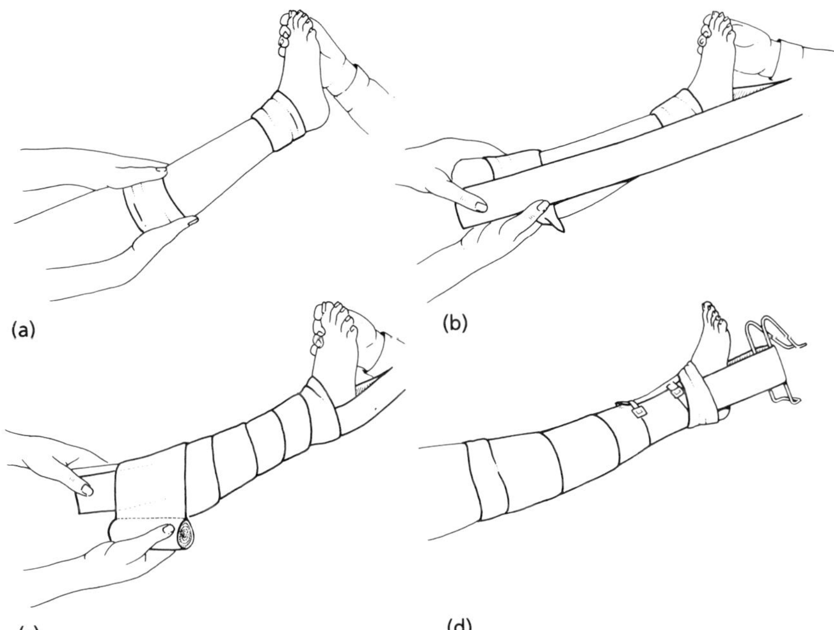

Fig. 8.6 The application of skin traction tapes. (a) Padding felt is applied over the ankle and head of the fibula. (b) The traction tape is applied. (c) The tape is held in place by an elastic wrapping. (d) Skin traction is applied.

Complications of skin traction

Skin traction can be responsible for the development of serious complications including pressure sores over bony prominences, nerve palsies and damage to skin from allergic reactions or slipping of the adhesive tapes. Shaving and the use of adhesives such as tincture of benzoin should be discouraged as they cause irritation and discomfort. The most serious complication of all is limb ischaemia which may result from the application of skin traction in the form of the gallows traction (see below) to children older than 3 years of age or whose weight exceeds 20 kg or 40 lb (Irani *et al.* 1976).

SKELETAL TRACTION

The advantages of skeletal traction over skin traction are that a greater force can be applied and rotation and angulation can be more easily corrected. The traction may be applied via a variety of pins or wires driven through a bone. The Steinman's pin is a 4- to 6-mm-thick rigid stainless steel pin of varying lengths. A modification of this, the Denham pin (Fig. 8.7d), which is especially suitable for cancellous and osteoporotic bones, has a short raised threaded length to engage the bony cortex and prevent sliding of the pin in the bone. The Kirschner (K) wire, which is of smaller diameter and is usually used with a tensioner, has the advantage that it causes less tissue damage.

Under aseptic conditions, and using local or general anaesthesia, the pin is inserted at the appropriate site (Fig. 8.7a−c) as an assistant steadies the limb. The site of insertion on the lateral side of the limb is identified and the skin is incised along Langher's lines with the point of a No. 11 blade. The pin, mounted on an introducer, is driven through the stab wound into the bone from the lateral to the medial with a gentle twisting motion of the wrist. When the point of the pin is felt underneath the skin on the other side, that skin is then incised and the pin is driven through. Betadine-soaked dressings are applied to the wounds around the pin.

The traction pin is attached through a Böhler stirrup (Böhler 1929), Simonis low friction swivel (Fig. 8.8) or other device to the traction cord. Alternatively, the traction pin may be incorporated in a light plaster of Paris cast as practised by Charnley (1971) for femoral shaft fractures (Fig. 8.9). The 'traction unit', as it is called, should be considered whenever a smooth traction pin is used to minimize the potential of the pin to loosen.

Complications of skeletal traction

Skeletal traction is subject to similar complications as skin traction. In addition, it may introduce infection into the bone. Therefore, daily skin-care around the pin sites is mandatory. To prevent infection from skin irritation by the protruding pin, it is advisable to incise the entry and exit wounds. The insertion of a traction pin close to a joint or growth plate may damage these structures. Incorrect placement of the traction pin may result in the failure of the traction system or may make

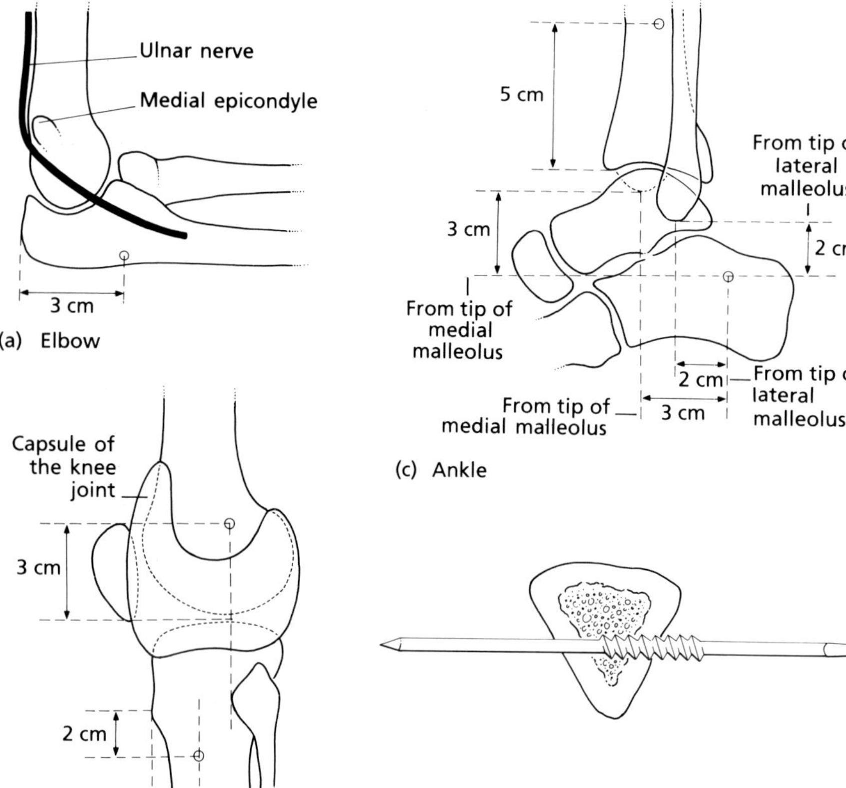

Fig. 8.7 Common pin sites used for skeletal traction.

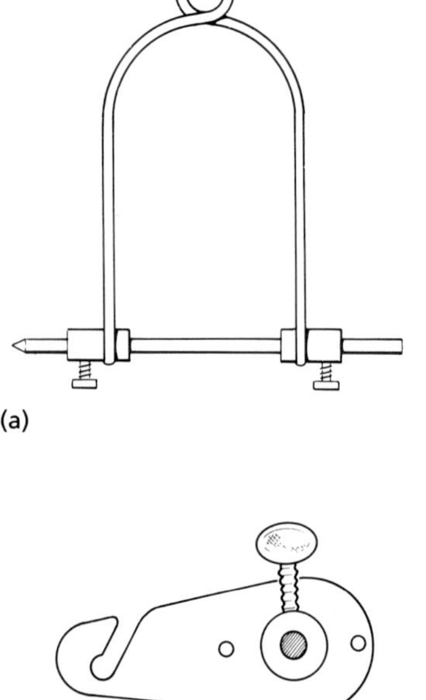

Fig. 8.8 (a) The Böhler stirrup with Steinman's pin and (b) Simonis swivel.

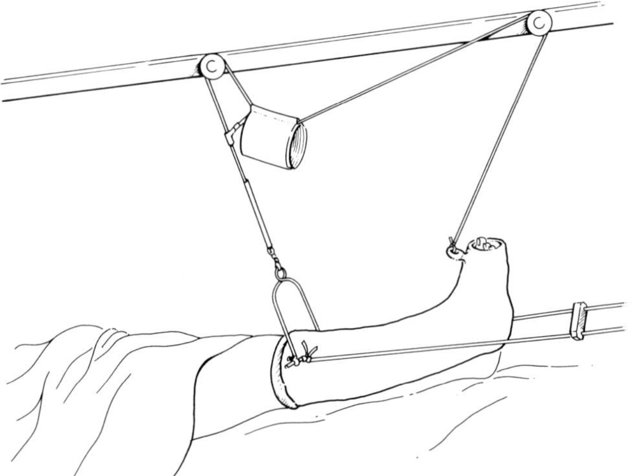

Fig. 8.9 The Charnley traction unit — traction pin incorporated in a plaster cast.

the application of splints difficult. Overdistraction at the fracture site may lead to delayed union.

APPLICATION OF TRACTION FORCE

The effectiveness of a traction system, whether skin or skeletal, depends upon a force (counter-traction) acting in the opposite direction. Counter-traction may be obtained by applying the traction force against a fixed point on the body, proximal to the attachments of the muscles in spasm (fixed traction) or, alternatively, against the weight of the patient's body (sliding traction). A splint is usally required to apply a fixed traction and may be used in sliding traction when it functions merely to support the injured limb.

In *fixed traction* the traction cord is attached to the end of a splint or modified bedframe. Different types of splints are used in the treatment of fractures (Fig. 8.10):
1 The Thomas' splint (Thomas 1876) is a padded oval metal ring attached to the ends of a U-shaped metal loop.
2 The Fisk splint (Fisk 1944) is a modification of the Thomas' splint in which the side bars terminate in small rings distal to the knee joint and a knee-flexion piece is attached just proximal to these rings.
3 The Tulloch Brown splint is a U-shaped metal loop with pre-drilled holes for tibial traction and a hook for attachment of the traction cord.
4 In Bryant's or gallows traction (Bryant 1876) both lower limbs are suspended from an overhead beam.

Details of the application of these splints are beyond the scope of this book and readers are advised to read more authoritative texts on the subject (Brooker & Schmeisser 1980, Stewart & Hallett 1983).

In *sliding traction* a system of pulleys is employed and the traction cord is attached to weights (Fig. 8.11). Lower limb fractures may be treated using Buck's traction which consists of straight skin traction with the injured limb supported on a soft pillow (Buck 1861); when skeletal traction is used in this way it is called Perkins traction (Perkins 1970). The pull on the limb may be increased by the Hamilton Russell (Russel 1921) technique or by the Tulloch Brown U-loop, or the 90/90 traction variations of the technique. These techniques use multiple pulleys to increase the mechanical advantage of the system. Sliding traction may also be provided with a Thomas' splint, to which a knee-flexion piece has been added, or through a Fisk splint or a Braun frame.

Upper limb fractures may be treated by the Dunlop traction system (Dunlop 1939) which consists of vertical skin traction to the forearm and counter-traction provided by a weighted sling around the arm (Fig. 8.12).

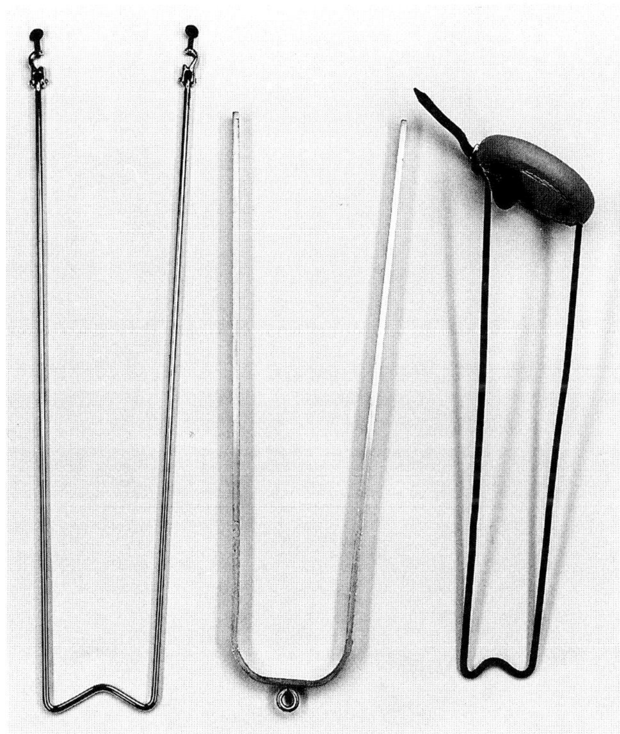

Fig. 8.10 Different types of splint used in fracture treatment. From left to right, Pearson knee flexion piece; Tulloch Brown splint; Thomas' splint.

Alternatively, skeletal traction through an olecranon pin or screw eye may be used. Difficult forearm fractures may be managed with traction through K-wires inserted into the metacarpal bones.

In the sliding traction system the weight needed to reduce the fracture in the early stages is greater than that required to maintain the reduction. The exact weight required is determined by trial and frequent check radiographs are required in the early period following fracture. This is to ensure adequate correction of length on the one hand and avoidance of overdistraction on the other hand.

Traction by casts

Both fixed and dynamic traction may be applied by means of plaster of Paris casts. Humeral shaft fractures are frequently treated by the hanging cast technique (Fig. 8.13). Traction is provided by the combined weight of the cast and the limb under the effect of gravity; anteroposterior angulation may be corrected by varying the length of the collar-and-cuff and lateral angulation may be corrected by varying the location of the cuff from the wrist.

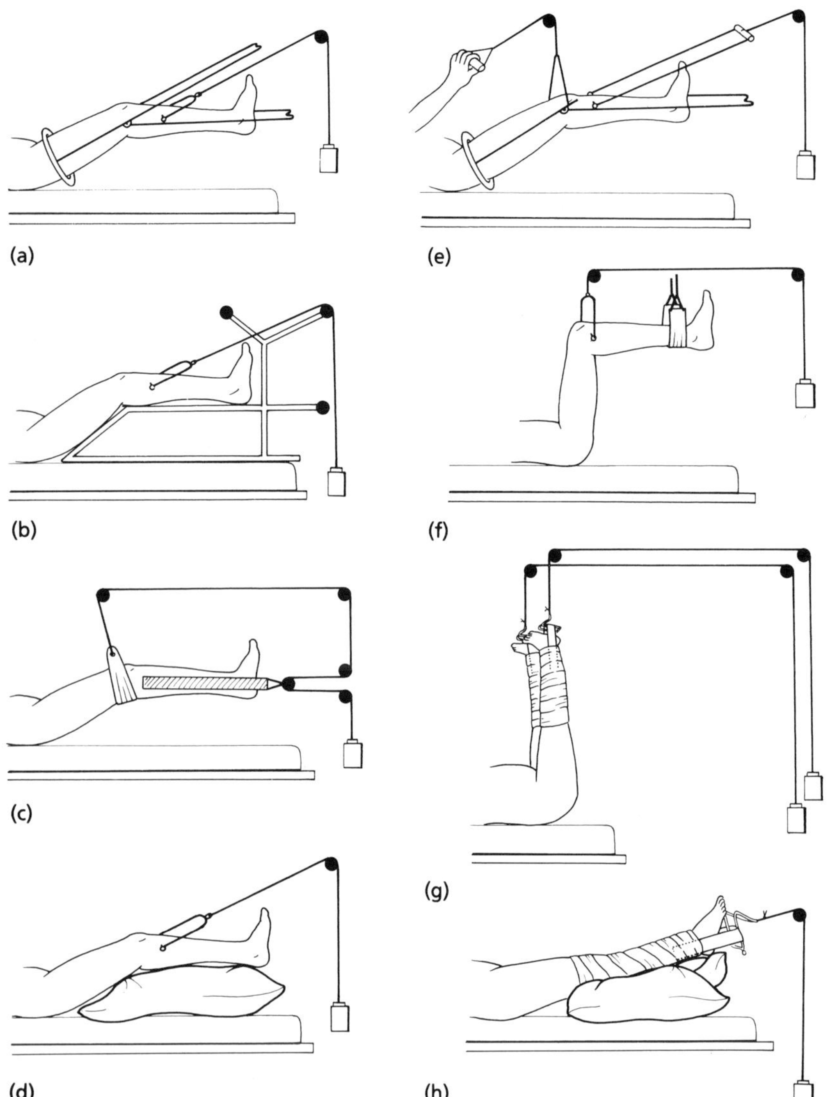

Fig. 8.11 Different types of sliding traction. (a) Thomas' splint and Pearson knee-flexion piece. (b) Braun frame. (c) Hamilton Russell traction. (d) Perkins traction. (e) Fisk traction. (f) 90/90 traction. (g) Gallows traction. (h) Buck's traction.

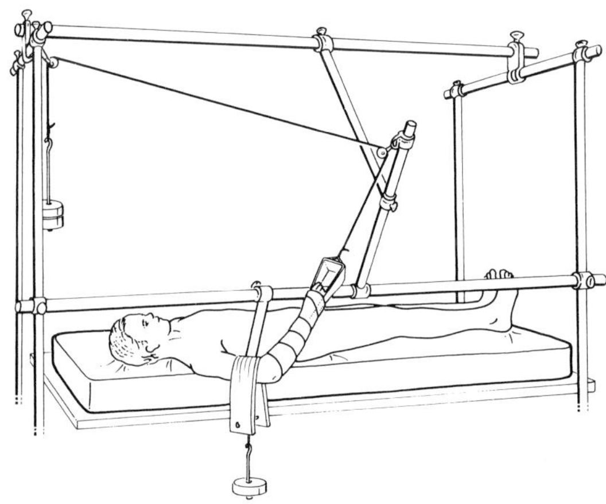

Fig. 8.12 The Dunlop skin traction.

Very unstable fractures have been treated by incorporating pins inserted above and below the fracture in a plaster cast. By this means continuous traction is applied to the fracture. This technique is very demanding and is prone to complications such as pin track infection, slow healing and pin breakage, in addition to overdistraction. It has now largely been replaced by external fixation.

Internal fixation of fractures

Except for fractures of subcutaneous bones, such as the patella and olecranon, open fracture management began as a supplementary measure adopted when conservative treatment had failed. Until the beginning of this century internal fixation was confined to bone suture with wires

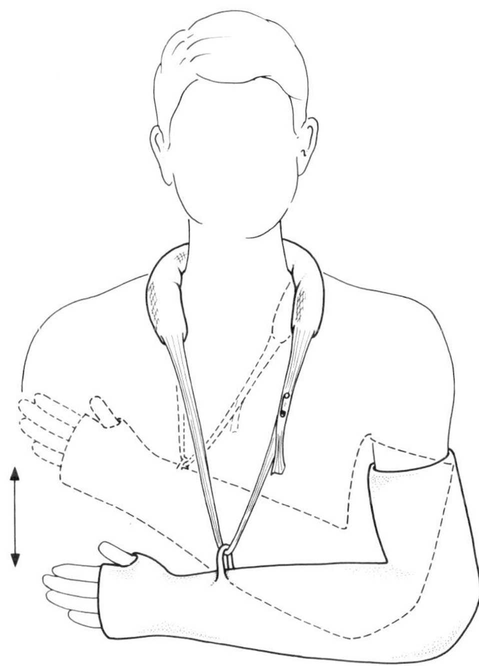

Fig. 8.13 The hanging cast technique. To correct anterior angulation of the distal fragment the sling is lengthened. To correct posterior angulation the sling is shortened. To correct rotation the sling is attached ventrally or dorsally as required.

and screws. Koenig (1931) attempted to improve stability by adding ivory pegs and bone inserts as struts. Lambotte (1913) improved the technique of screw fixation and also experimented with plate and external fixation.

The intramedullary nail was being developed by, amongst others, Hey Groves (*1916*) and Kuntscher (1967). Danis (1949) introduced the concept of 'primary bone healing' (soudure autogene) and helped to perfect devices for internal fixation of fractures (Müller *et al.* 1965); this resulted in the formation in Switzerland in 1956 of the Association for Osteosynthesis/Association for the Study of Problems of Internal Fixation (AO/ASIF) group.

With operative treatment the aim is to anatomically reduce the fracture (although this may not always be achieved!) and this is usually followed by stabilization by means of a metal device implanted on the surface of the bone or within the medullary cavity. Such devices include the following:

1 Screws
  (a) Cortical screws — machine screws, AO cortical screws.
  (b) Cancellous screws — wood screws, AO cancellous screws.

2 Plates
  (a) Non-rigid plates.
  (b) Rigid plates.
  (c) Compression plates.
3 Intramedullary nails
  (a) Rigid nails.
  (b) Solid nails.
  (c) Flexible nails.
  (d) Interlocking nails.
4 Wires
  (a) K-wire.
  (b) Cerclage wire.

The objectives of internal fixation are to eliminate 'fracture disease', such as pain, swelling and joint stiffness, and to stimulate 'primary bone healing'. By providing stable fixation, external splintage is unnecessary and active exercise of muscles and joints can begin immediately.

A detailed description of the whole range of metal implants available, their mode of insertion and specific indications for their use are outwith the scope of this chapter. For more detailed description the reader is referred to various internal fixation manuals (e.g. Heim & Pfeiffer 1974, Müller *et al.* 1991).

Screws (Fig. 8.14)

Fracture fragments, particularly in oblique and long spiral fractures, may be held together by means of one or more screws. *Machine screws*, which are the most commonly used in orthopaedic surgery, have a blunt end and are threaded from head to tip. They are inserted into pre-drilled and pre-tapped holes; a flute-tipped variety is self-tapping. The AO *cortical screw* has a wider thread diameter and its head has a deep hexagonal recess which mates accurately with the screwdriver. *Wood screws*, which are tapered into a sharp end and have an unthreaded neck portion, are designed to be used without pre-drilling. They are suitable only for cancellous bone. True *cancellous screws* have wider threads and are similar to *malleolar screws* which have a sharper point. The AO screw has no specific biomechanical superiority over other similar screws but it is part of a complete and well-engineered internal fixation system.

Intrafragmentary screw fixation

To achieve a lag effect or interfragmentary compression (Fig. 8.15), the fracture is anatomically reduced and held with clamps. The near (gliding) hole is overdrilled, a guide is inserted into this hole until it abuts on the far

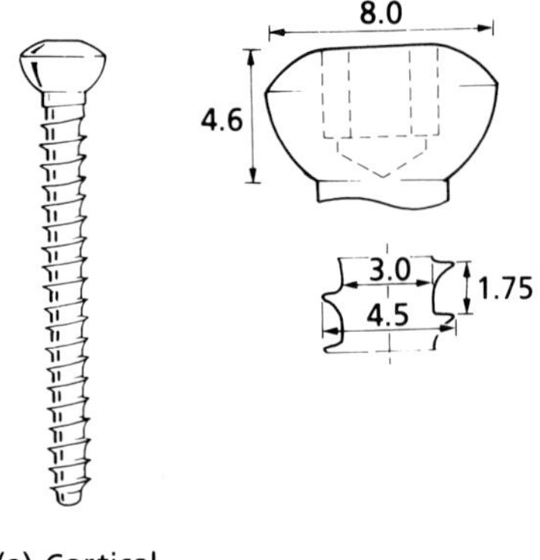

(a) Cortical

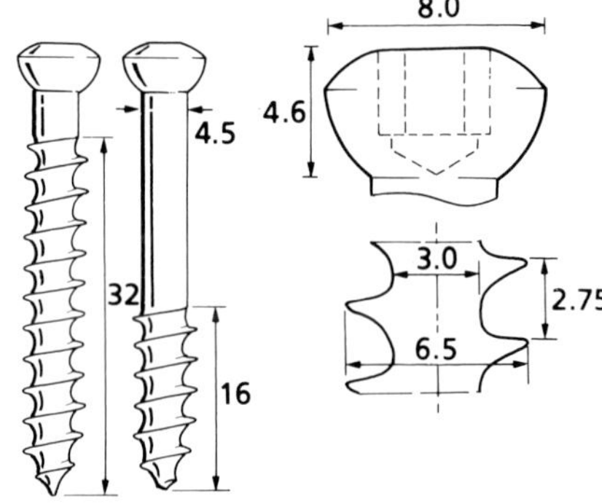

(b) Cancellous

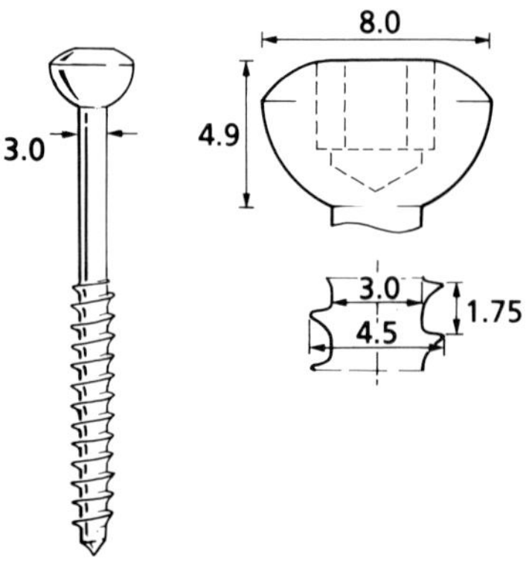

(c) Malleolar

Fig. 8.14 Types of AO bone screw.

cortex and then the screw or thread hole is drilled into it. A recess for the screw head is cut using the countersink cutter. The screw length is measured with a depth gauge prior to tapping and then the screw is inserted.

The most commonly recommended technique of inserting screws at right angles to the fracture line provides the least secure fixation. Screws should be inserted midway between a line perpendicular to the shaft and another perpendicular to the fracture line. The

protection of a plate (neutralization plate) is probably advisable in most cases after interfragmentary screw fixation. Cancellous screws should not be tapped all the way. The smooth portion should cross, and the threaded portion should lie beyond, the fracture line.

Plates (Fig. 8.16)

Plates may be used to provide static or dynamic compression, neutralization (to protect intrafragmentary screws) and a buttress (to protect a cortex from collapsing). The most secure fixation is obtained with strong and heavy plates. Traditional plates such as the Eggers' plate and the self-compressing semi-tubular plates are *non-rigid* and should be used only as 'bone sutures' or when the fracture can be guaranteed to unite quickly. *Rigid plates* such as the AO plates may be too bulky to allow skin closure over subcutaneous bones such as the tibia. *Dynamic compression plates* (DCP) provide axial compression without the use of a compression device because their oval-shaped screw holes allow fracture fragments to be brought together under compression.

Compression plating

In compression plating using the DCP plate (Fig. 8.17) the fracture is anatomically reduced including all small fragments and held with clamps. If there are any gaps cancellous grafts should be inserted. A plate is selected which provides at least three screw holes (i.e. six cortices) above and below the fracture. A malleable template is laid alongside the bone at the fracture site to conform to the contour of the bone. The selected plate is then bent to the shape of the template using a plate-bending press and/or tongs. Next, the plate is applied to the shaft and screws are introduced into the two holes immediately adjacent to the fracture using the eccentric drill guides. Tightening up of the eccentrically placed screws produces motion of the plate and the fracture surfaces are compressed together. The rest of the screws are inserted in turn, one at a time, on either side of the fracture using the neutral drill guide. If more compression is required, subsequent screws may be introduced eccentrically but the tension must be released in previously inserted screws. Each screw is inserted until 'resistance' is felt; they are not fully tightened until the last screw has been inserted to provide uniform tension on the screws.

The technique of inserting the screw is different from that used in interfragmentary fixation. A single hole (pilot hole) is drilled through both cortices, the length of

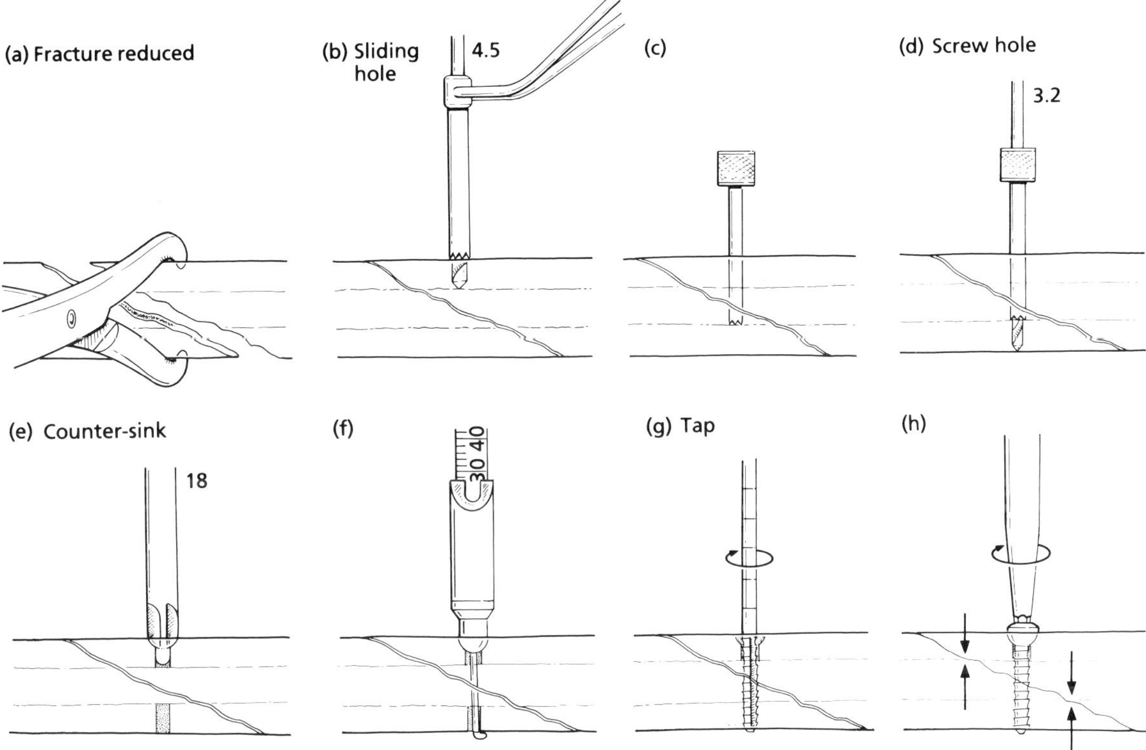

Fig. 8.15 Steps in intrafragmentary screw fixation.

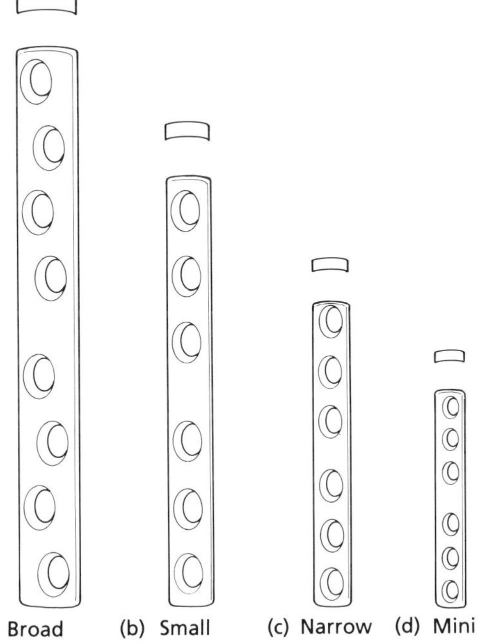

Fig. 8.16 Types of plate.

the screw is measured prior to tapping and the screw is then inserted.

Intramedullary nails

Hey Groves inserted the first intramedullary nail at the beginning of this century and Kuntscher (1967) refined and popularized its use. There are now several varieties of nail on the market, each portending one or other advantage over the others.

Rigid nails (Fig. 8.18) are hollow metal tubes which act by filling the medullary cavity. They are firmly held by the bone for some distance proximal and distal to the fracture. They have great resistance to bending moments but carry very little compression load. The greater the diameter of the nail, the greater the strength; bending rigidity is proportional to the cube of the nail diameter. Consequently, the medullary cavity should be reamed to as large a diameter as possible; this also produces the greatest length of tight fit between nail and bone which, in turn, produces increased resistance to rotational deformity. However, less than 4 mm, or less than half of the original thickness of the cortex, should be removed by reaming, particularly since marrow debris may embolize in the cortex and give rise to extensive

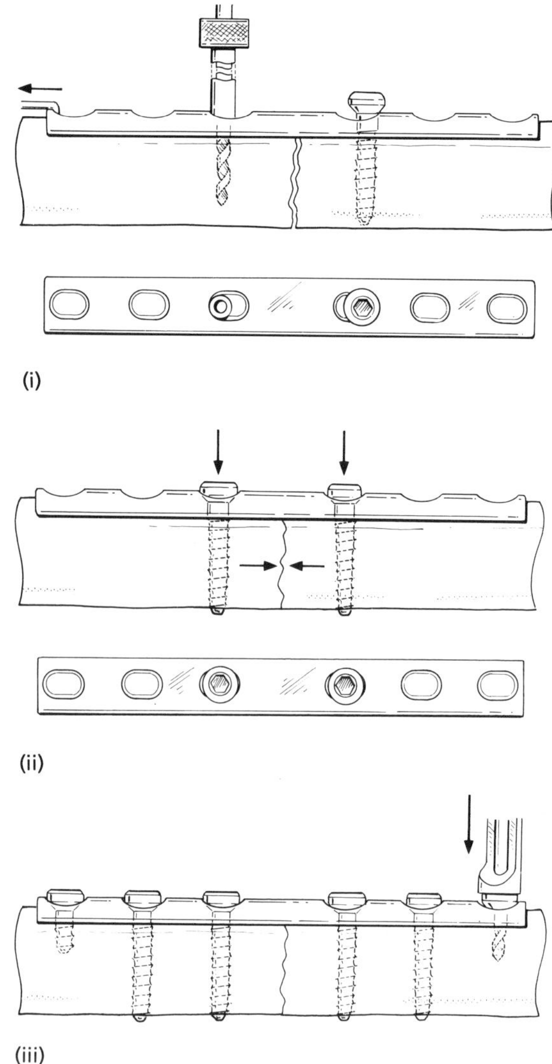

(i)

(ii)

(iii)

Fig. 8.17 Steps in dynamic compression plating.

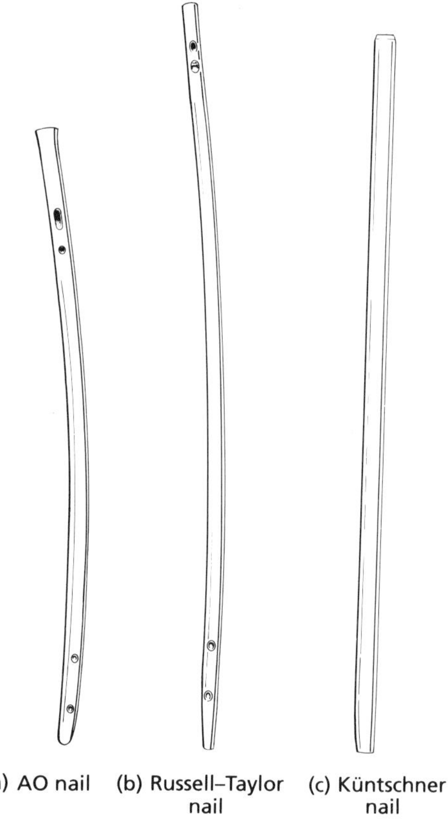

Fig. 8.18 Rigid intramedullary nails.

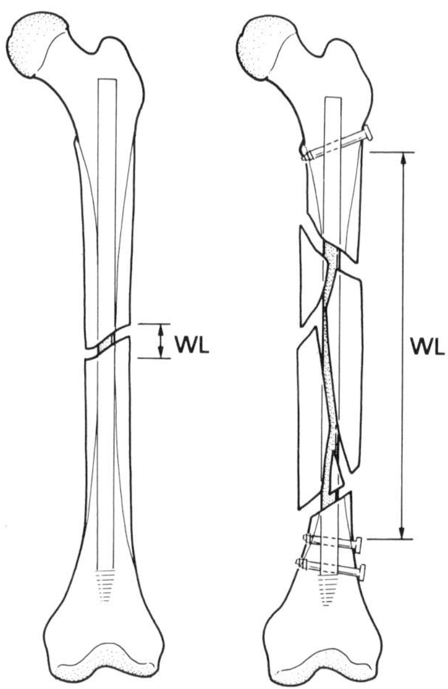

Fig. 8.19 The concept of working length of an intramedullary nail. WL = the length between the two main points where the bone has purchase on the rod.

cortical infarction (Dankwardt-Lilliestrom 1969). These nails prevent medullary callus formation so that the fracture heals entirely by periosteal callus; hence, the ideal method of insertion is the closed technique which preserves the periosteum.

The torsional forces transmitted to a rigid nail depend upon the grip between the nail and bone; this area of contact is enhanced by reaming. The working length which determines the efficacy of rigid nails is defined as the length of nail not protected by intact bone, i.e. the length between the two points where the bone has no purchase on the nail. This ranges from a few millimetres in transverse fractures to several centimetres in comminuted fractures (Fig. 8.19).

There are many varieties of rigid nails but Kuntscher ('K') and AO nails are the most popular in the United

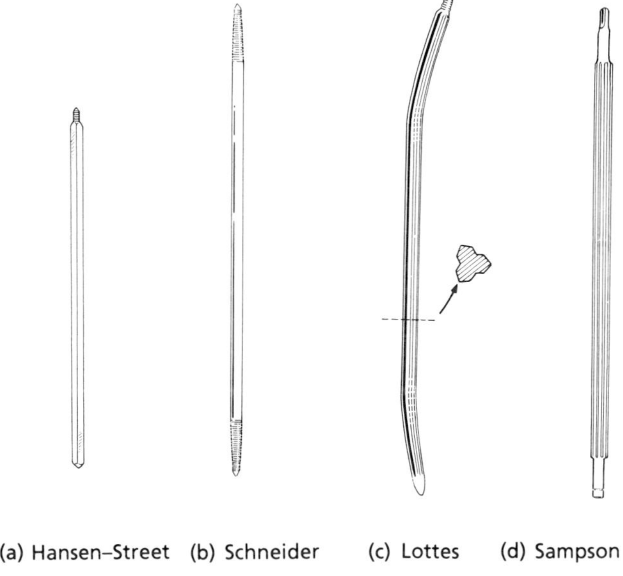

Fig. 8.20 Solid intramedullary nails.

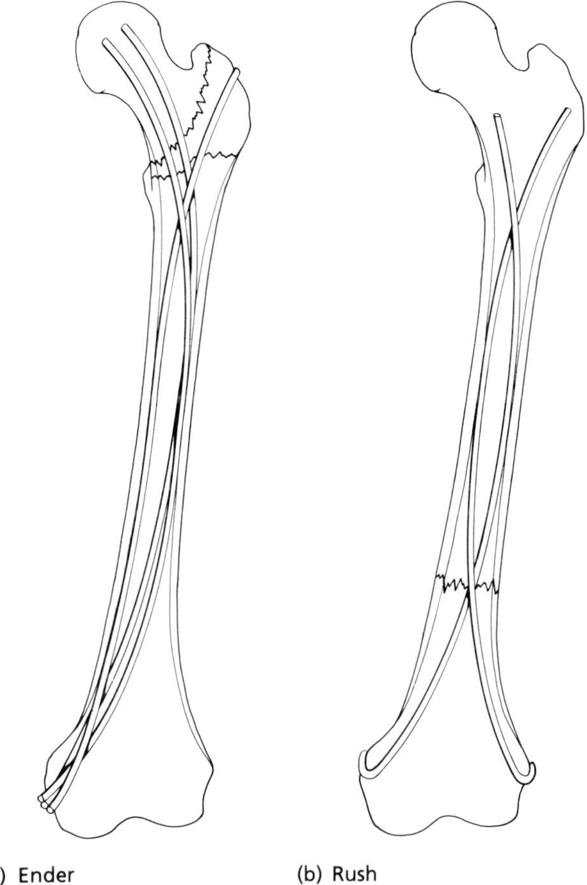

Fig. 8.21 Flexible intramedullary nails.

Kingdom. Both are cloverleaf-shaped in cross-section and have an open section along their lengths. They are designed to be introduced into the medullary cavity over a guide wire after preliminary reaming. The nails are inserted through the greater trochanter or the anterior tibial eminence which makes removal easier. The open section of these nails allows compression and snug (interference) fit at the isthmus of the medullary canal; this prevents loosening and controls rotation (Müller *et al*. 1991). It also permits revascularization of the medullary cavity whilst the nail is *in situ* (Kuntscher 1967).

Solid nails such as the Hansen–Street and Huckstep nails are solid metal rods without a lumen (Fig. 8.20). They do not have the inherent elasticity of the rigid nails. These devices are said to have some particular advantage in terms of rigidity of fixation and biomechanics (Huckstep 1972). However, the general principles of their use are similar to those of the rigid nails.

Flexible nails (Fig. 8.21) are solid metal rods of smaller diameter and in general, because they are curved, they act like tension rods. They are inserted in such a way as to neutralize deforming forces within the fractured bone by three-point fixation. Flexible nails are particularly useful in the treatment of pathological fractures and osteoporotic fractures of the distal femur and humerus.

The most commonly used flexible nails are the Rush pin (Rush 1968) and the Ender nail (Ender 1970). The Rush pin is a curved solid rod with a hook at one end and a bevel at the other. They are usually inserted in

pairs through opposite holes in the condyles and this allows them to exert opposing forces. They may also be used singly in the treatment of metacarpal fractures or fractures of the forearm bones. The Ender nail is similarly curved but it has an eyelet at one end instead of a hook. As many as are acceptable may be introduced into the unreamed medullary cavity as a bundle through a cortical window.

Interlocking nails (Fig. 8.22) have provided the most dramatic innovation in intramedullary nailing and have extended the indications for the procedure. They are rigid nails with prefabricated holes at either end. Inserting screws into these holes proximal and/or distal to a fracture provides rotational stability and prevents shortening. They can be used for dynamic or static fixation. In dynamic fixation screws are only inserted through the nail in the shorter fracture fragment. Stability of the other fragment is achieved by interference fit between nail and bone. In static fixation the nail is fixed to both proximal and distal fragments, thereby providing continuous traction which keeps the fracture out to length.

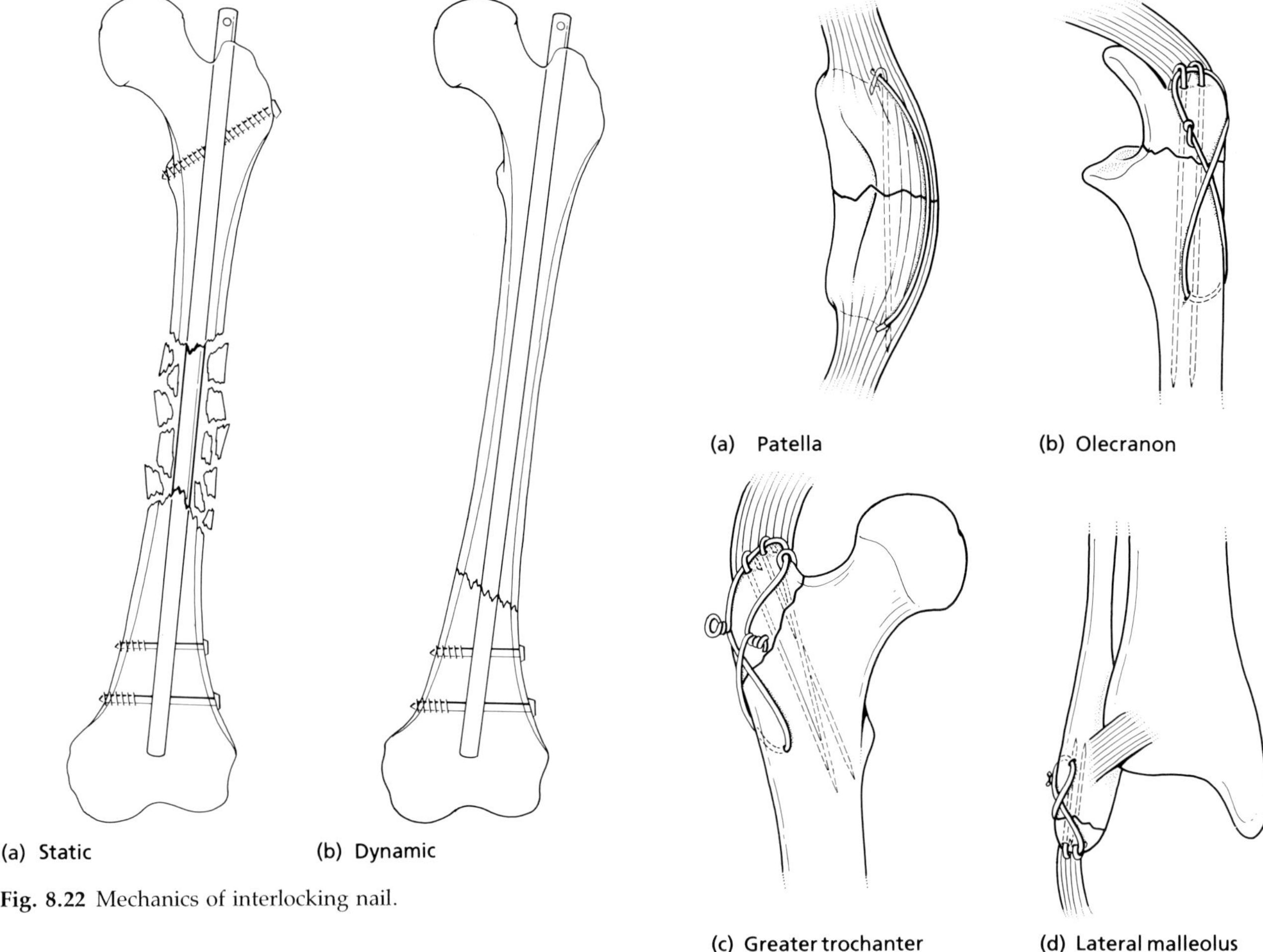

Fig. 8.22 Mechanics of interlocking nail.

Fig. 8.23 The tension-band principle.

Wires

K-wires are extremely useful in providing temporary fixation of complicated fractures prior to applying more rigid devices, but they may also be used in their own right to treat fractures. The fixation is not secure and, therefore, should be supplemented by some form of external immobilization because movement of the fracture fragments will allow the wire to fail or back-out. K-wire fixation may also be supplemented by wire cerclage as in *tension-band* and *compression-band* wiring (Fig. 8.23). Tension-band wiring is useful in fractures of the patella, malleoli and olecranon while compression-band wiring is useful in phalangeal fractures. Details of the principles of these techniques may be found in various internal fixation manuals (e.g. Müller *et al*. 1991).

Cerclage wire fixation (Fig. 8.24) was one of the earliest means of internal fixation of fractures. Its reputation for damaging periosteal blood supply is unfounded (Brookes & Heatley 1984). It can provide a successful means of dealing with complex fractures and is particu-

larly useful in holding in place 'floating' cortical fragments in intramedullary nailing or even in plate fixation.

Complications of internal fixation of fractures

Infection is the most disastrous complication of internal fixation. It is avoided by strict adherence to aseptic techniques, use of clean-air theatres and antibiotics, firm fixation of fracture fragments and by a few days of enforced rest and elevation of the injured parts after operation. If a fracture becomes infected free drainage must be ensured, but provided that the implant continues to fix the fracture firmly it should be left in place until union is complete. If the implant is to be removed because of loosening, debridement of infected bone should be carried out at the same time. The fracture should then be immobilized with an external fixator and the gap left by bone debridement should be filled with autogenous cancellous graft.

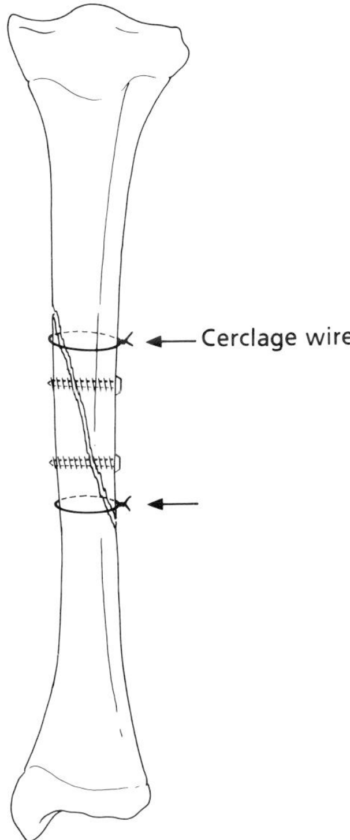

Fig. 8.24 Cerclage wire fixation (arrows).

Operative treatment of fractures may lead to *delayed union* or *non-union* because of rigid fixation (Schenk & Willenegger 1967) and/or indiscriminate periosteal stripping. This tendency to slow healing may be responsible for the increased risk of refracture. Hence, it is advised that the implants, particularly after rigid fixation, be left in place for up to 18 months before removal in adults. Plates and nails may hold the fracture fragments apart and an ill-fitting nail which leads to motion at the fracture site may also result in delayed union, usually of the hypertrophic type. A loose or failed fixation device may be replaced.

External fixation of fractures

External fixation is a method of immobilizing fractures using percutaneous intraosseous pins attached to an external metal frame. The increasing frequency of severe musculoskeletal injuries associated with travel by high-speed vehicles and the use of heavy machinery has stimulated interest in such devices. Early attempts employed a claw-like device for treating patellar fractures (Malgaigne 1859) but the present design is derived from the invention of Lambotte (1913). External fixation of fractures has become popular mainly as a result of the work of Anderson (1934) and Hoffman (1938) (Mears 1979).

The components of the modern fixator include fixing pins, longitudinal supporting rods, connecting elements such as joints (articulations) and ring frames. The transfixing pins may be threaded pins of 4–6 mm diameter or K-wires of 1.5–2 mm diameter. Transfixing pins protrude through the skin on either side of the bone while half pins only penetrate the skin on one side. The threaded portions are designed to engage both cortices. The K-wires are tensioned to 500–1300 N to convert these flexible wires into relatively stiff pins.

Types of fixators

External fixators include the following:
1 Simple fixators.
2 Modular fixators.
3 Ring fixators.
4 Improvised fixators.

Simple linear fixators (Fig. 8.25) such as the Denham and the Roger Anderson fixators have independent articulations which connect each pin to the supporting rod. They are versatile because each pin can be placed at the desired angle, but the fracture must be reduced before applying the fixator.

In *modular fixators* (Fig. 8.26), such as the Hoffman and Shearer fixators, the pins of each principal fragment are held in a clamp device which is then connected to the supporting rod. These fixators permit reduction of displaced fragments by external manoeuvres ('osteotaxis'), compression and neutralization of unstable fractures as well as by distraction to give normal limb length whenever there is loss of bony substance. However, because the size and shape of the clamps determine where the transfixing pins are inserted into the fractured bone, the numbers and locations of the supporting rods that may be used (i.e. the configuration of the fixator) are limited. In addition, the surgeon cannot insert transfixing screws at all the desired locations in the bone. Furthermore, with some fixators, a loose or infected pin cannot be safely exchanged without loss of reduction and the articulations are often weak.

The *ring fixators* (Fig. 8.27) such as the Ilizarov fixators are more popular in Eastern Europe. Pins passed through each principal fragment are held in a ring device which is then connected to rods. The fixator permits graduated adjustments for length and angulation after the application of the frame. The application is time-consuming and hazardous to neurovascular structures.

Improvised fixators consist of systems of fracture management where transfixing pins are connected by bone cement, epoxy-filled tubes (Lundeen *et al.* 1980) and other home-made devices.

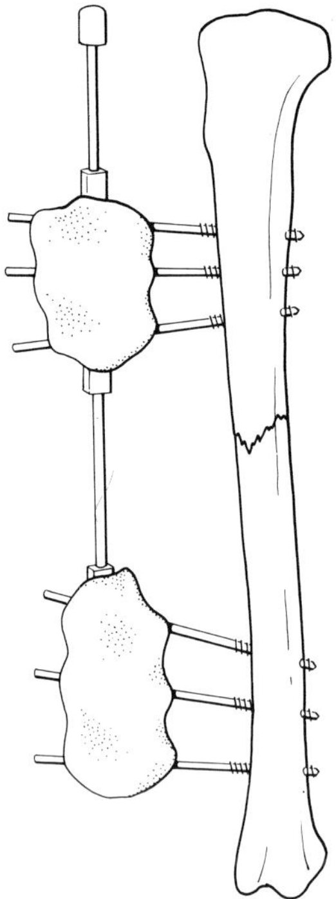

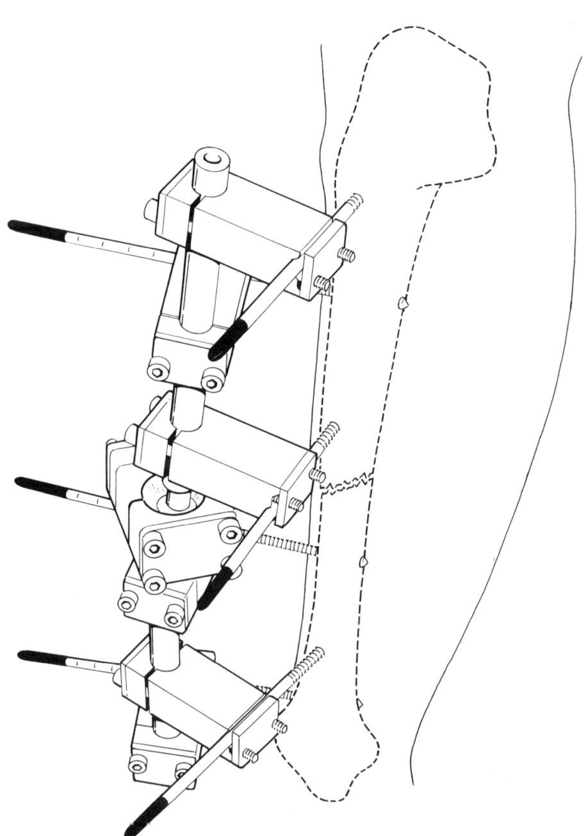

Fig. 8.25 A simple (linear) external fixator.

Fig. 8.26 A modular external fixator.

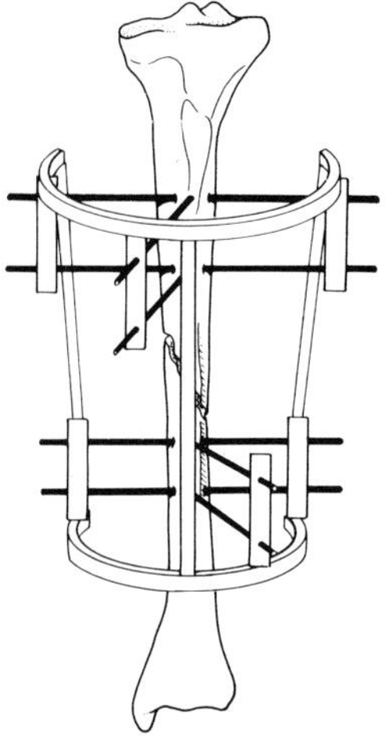

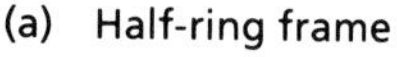

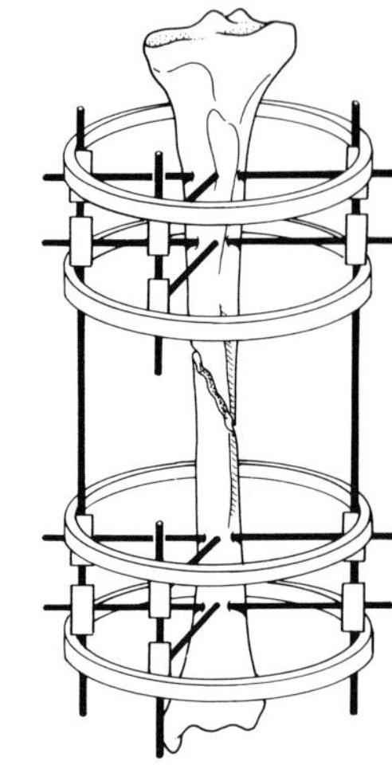

(a) Half-ring frame   (b) Full-ring frame

Fig. 8.27 Ring fixators.

Frame configuration (Fig. 8.28)

The frame configuration determines access to the injured part and the mechanical characteristics. The simplest configuration is a *unilateral frame* such as the Hoffman fixator, which consists of a longitudinal supporting rod connected to half pins. A *bilateral frame* such as the Roger Anderson fixator employs two rods, one on either side of the limb.

These frame configurations may be applied singly (*uniplanar*) or in pairs (*biplanar*) to improve stability.

Ring fixators may utilize *half* or *full* rings.

The application of fixators

The external fixator comes into its own in the treatment of open and infected fractures for it allows easy access to the area of injury. It is possible to graft the bone or skin and dress wounds as required. Because of its stability, it permits suspension and active mobilization while the patient is in bed.

There are, at present, no clear guidelines for the use of external fixators. The situation is further complicated by the multitude of devices and configurations and by the lack of information regarding the ideal mechanical environment for healing (Goodship & Kenwright 1985, Kenwright *et al.* 1987). The potential indications are:

1 Open and complicated fractures.
2 Non-union associated with infection.
3 Major pelvic disruptions.
4 Complex metaphyseal intra-articular fractures.
5 Limb realignment procedures.
6 Arthrodesis.

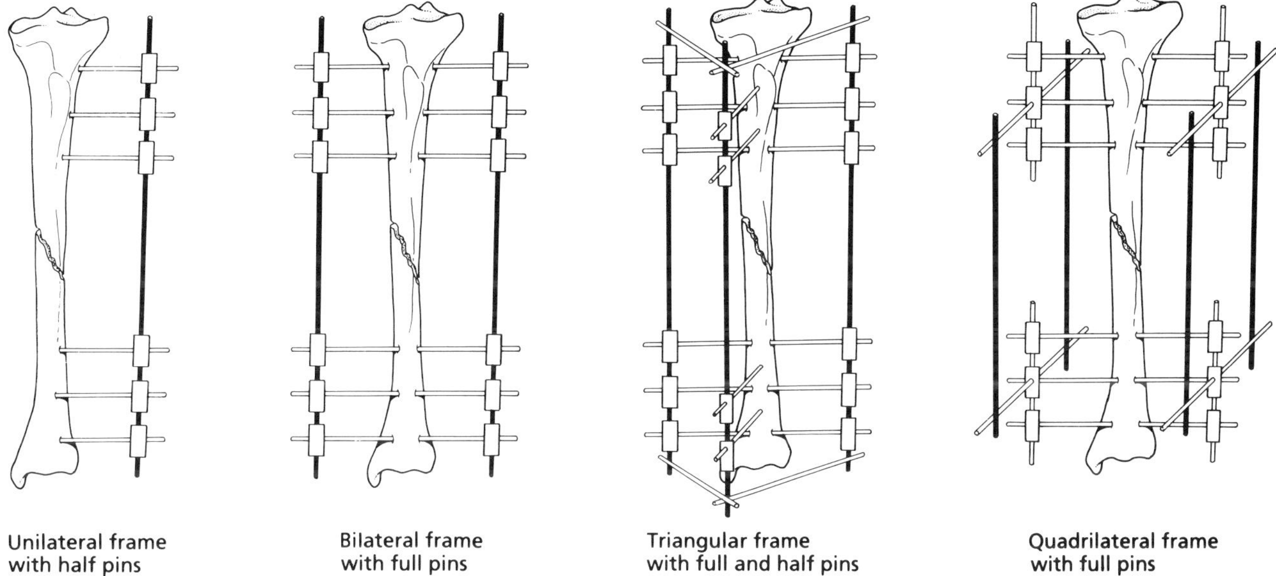

Fig. 8.28 Frame configurations for a simple (linear) fixator.

Preplanning is essential to determine (i) whether external fixation is the best method of treating the patient's injuries, (ii) what type of frame configuration is required and for how long, and (iii) what additional procedure might be required. Severe traumatic limb injuries are best managed with a simple unilateral frame while ring fixators are best suited to correct bone defects and complex malalignments.

The external fixator is applied under a general anaesthetic, sterile conditions and radiographic control. Ideally, a plastic surgeon should review the wound before pin placement so as not to jeopardize future flaps, etc. The fracture fragments should first be reduced by traction and should be held in the reduced position by clamps or interfragmentary screw(s) if the fracture is open. Bone grafting may be carried out for bone defects. The pins are inserted via stab wounds avoiding the danger zones. Holes may be pre-drilled but the pins should be inserted by hand to avoid thermal burns.

With a typical simple (Fig. 8.25) or modular (Fig. 8.26) frame, three pins are inserted in each main fragment in such a way that both sets are in the same plane with the fracture reduced. The connecting elements are attached to the pins and a rod of appropriate length is selected and inserted into these. Fracture reduction is checked, if the fragments had been held in clamps these are removed, and the joints of the connecting elements are tightened; a further radiological check is carried out to determine whether any further adjustments are necessary.

The adjacent joints are splinted in the position of function until active exercise can begin. This is particularly important in the case of the ankle, in tibial shaft fractures, which must be splinted in the neutral position. Meticulous daily care of the pin sites, including cleansing, must be carried out. Pin-site inflammation or discharge is promptly treated with antibiotics, rest and local skin-care, including incision of tight skin. The injured limb is regularly examined and preparation is made early for further soft tissue or bone grafting and for secondary treatment such as cast bracing or internal fixation.

Complications of external fixation of fractures

Pin-site infection may be classified as follows (Gie & MacEachern 1986):

Grade I — settles with improved pin care.

Grade II — antibiotics also required.

Grade III — pin removal also required.

Grade IV — persistent infection and sequestrum formation.

Such infection, which may lead to the serious complication of pin-hole osteomyelitis, is the principal drawback to the use of external fixation. The incidence ranges from 10–50% in reported series (Burny 1979, Green 1981) and relative motion between the pin and adjacent tissues is responsible. Hence, pins incorporated in plaster casts cause a much lower infection rate than pins of external fixators because the cast stabilizes the pins

(Green 1983). The pin-site infection rate may be reduced by protected weight-bearing, sterile techniques, skin incision before placement of pins and a daily pin-care routine.

Transcutaneous pins have the potential to *impale* or *damage major nerves* and *blood vessels*, although reports of serious neurovascular injuries are rare. It would appear from the experimental work of Dwyer (1973) that the pin pushes vessels to one side as it penetrates through the soft tissues. On the other hand, compartment syndromes have been described in association with external fixation of fractures by a mechanism which has not been fully explained. It is incumbent on the practitioner to know the danger zones in each limb and to select pin positions that avoid damage to important structures. Some authors recommend that larger skin incisions be made in order to visualize major neurovascular structures in the vicinity when pins are inserted into certain locations in the body.

Transfixing pins may *restrict joint mobility* by impaling muscles and tendons or by spanning joints. Pain due to pin-site sepsis or other causes may also inhibit joint movement. However, muscle impalement is often unavoidable in external fixation of fractures. This results in a tendency to equinus deformity at the ankle. Therefore, the foot must be maintained in the dorsiflexed position for the first few weeks after operation or until the patient can actively exercise the ankle without pain. It is also advisable to dorsiflex the foot during pin insertion. In the upper limb, although posterior insertion through the triceps is the safest, it may result in significant restriction of elbow motion. This may be prevented by inserting the pins with the elbow flexed to at least 90° followed by manipulation of the joint through a full range of motion.

External fixation has a reputation for causing *slow healing*, although there are no controlled prospective studies to compare union rates with other methods of treatment. Furthermore, in most centres, only very difficult fractures are treated with external fixation. Nevertheless, many workers have now adopted certain measures, such as early removal of the fixator, bone grafting and 'dynamization', which are believed to prevent slow healing (De Bastiani *et al.* 1984).

Choosing a method of treatment

There is no unanimity of opinion about the treatment of most fractures. Even where there is a consensus, for example, fixation of intracapsular fracture of the femoral neck, there is no agreement with regard to the most appropriate device. The AO system of anatomical reduction and rigid internal fixation often appears to be in conflict with the functional fracture bracing system. Yet, in practice, the desired goals of normal union and unimpaired function may be achieved using either system.

In fracture management the specific method chosen should be tailored to the individual fracture and individual patient. The location of a fracture is important; an undisplaced intracapsular fracture of the femoral neck requires internal fixation while a comparable fracture of the humerus requires protection only. In general, stable and undisplaced fractures require much simpler methods of treatment than unstable or displaced fractures. The potential of a fracture to develop complications such as avascular necrosis may need to be considered. On the other hand, a method of treatment is contraindicated if it is inappropriate, superfluous or is likely to make matters worse.

Very simply, fracture treatment can be broken down into five groups

Protection alone. Some undisplaced or relatively stable fractures, particularly of the ribs, clavicle, phalanges, metatarsals and metacarpals, require little more than protection from further injury. This may be accomplished by means of strapping or of a sling in the upper limb and use of crutches to avoid weight-bearing in the lower limb. In either case bandaging may be used to control swelling. Other fractures, such as those of the pubic rami alone, the neck of the humerus, radial head and some fractures of the spine, require only pain relief for a brief period before active mobilization.

Immobilization alone. Undisplaced but potentially unstable fractures require immobilization; reduction is not necessary. This can usually be achieved by the application of a cast or splint but these still require to be moulded to prevent displacement. Regular radiographs may be required to check that the position remains satisfactory and to confirm union.

Closed reduction and immobilization. Many displaced fractures can be adequately reduced by closed methods, and the plaster cast is the commonest method of maintaining this reduction. The only indication for fracture reduction is to reduce a significant displacement which is likely to produce cosmetic or functional disability.

Having decided that the fracture requires reduction, surgeons have to decide when to carry this out. Open fractures, to prevent infection, and diaphyseal fractures, to prevent swelling and compartment syndromes, should be dealt with within 4–6 hours of injury. However, in closed fractures, once significant swelling has developed, it is wise to allow this to subside. If there is any question of a compartment syndrome being present, its treatment, by fasciotomy, takes precedence. Before embarking on the manipulation, surgeons should decide on which method of anaesthesia is appropriate, appraise themselves of the likely mechanism of injury and select the method of immobilization. They should give clear instructions on how the patient is to be managed in the cast. A plaster cast should be checked within 2 days of application to ensure that it is not causing discomfort or neurovascular compromise. Regular radiographs are necessary to follow the progress of the fracture to union.

Open reduction with or without internal or external fixation. All open fractures must be treated surgically to debride wounds, etc., and, usually, to carry out open reduction at the same time. The fracture may then be stabilized by internal fixation, external fixation or cast immobilization.

The place of internal fixation in the management of closed fractures has often been exaggerated by proponents and this has lead to some confusion with regard to the appropriate indications. The indications employed by the authors are as follows:

1 Open fractures.
2 Irreducible or unstable fractures.
3 Pathological fractures.
4 To aid management of soft tissue or neurovascular complications.
5 A patient with significant head injury.
6 Multiple fractures.

Open reduction should be undertaken only for definite and justifiable reasons; for example, when closed reduction is impossible (e.g. small fragments) or has failed, or a reduction cannot be maintained by closed methods. Fractures complicated by nerve and/or vascular injuries, some fractures in patients unable to comply with the rigours of closed methods, and pathological fractures are relative indications.

Operative treatment may result in serious complications or inhibit osteogenesis and this should never be forgotten. The pros and cons should be assessed for each fracture in each individual patient and, in some cases, the final decision as to which treatment is most appropriate, should be taken only after full consultation with the patient.

Replacement of fracture fragments. Where results of internal fixation are relatively unsatisfactory, such as intracapsular fractures of the femoral neck, the articular fragment may be excised and replaced with an appropriate prosthesis.

References

Anderson, R. An automatic method of treatment for fractures of the tibia and the fibula. *Surg Gynecol Obstet* 1934; **58**: 637.

Böhler, L. In: Steinberg, M.E. (trans.) *The Treatment of Fractures.* Maudrich: Vienna, 1929.

Brooker, A.F. & Schmeisser, G. *Orthopaedic Traction Manual.* Williams & Wilkins: Baltimore, 1980.

Brookes, M. & Heatley, F.W. Nylon cerclage: the bone circulation in experimental osteotomy. In: Arlet, J., Ficat, R.P. & Hungerford, D.S. (eds) *Bone Circulation.* Williams & Wilkins: Baltimore, 1984.

Bryant, T. *The Practice of Surgery.* Churchill: London, 1876.

Buck, G. An improved method of treating fractures of the thigh illustrated by cases and drawing. *Trans N York Acad Sci* 1861; **2**: 232.

Burny, F. Elastic external fixation of tibial fractures, study of 1421 cases. In: Brooker, A.F. & Edwards, C.C. (eds) *External Fixation. The Current State of the Art.* Williams & Wilkins: Baltimore, 1979.

Charnley, J. *The Closed Treatment of Fractures.* Churchill Livingstone: Edinburgh, 1971.

Danis, R. *Theorie et Practique de l'Osteosynthese.* Masson: Paris, 1949.

Dankwardt-Lilliestrom, G. Reaming of medullary cavity and its effect on diaphyseal bone: fluorochromic, microangiographic and histologic study on the rabbit tibia and dog femur. *Acta Orthop Scand Suppl* 1969; **50**: 128.

De Bastiani, G., Aldegheri, R. & Brivio, L.R. The treatment of fractures with a dynamic axial fixator. *J Bone Joint Surg* 1984; **66B**: 538.

Dunlop, J. Transcondylar fractures of the humerus in children. *J Bone Joint Surg* 1939; **21**: 59.

Dwyer, N. Preliminary report upon a new fixation device for fractures of long bones. *Injury* 1973; **5**: 141.

Ender, J. Probleme beim frischen per und subtrochanteren Oberschenkelbruch. *H Unfallkeilk* 1970; **106**: 2.

Fisk, G.R. The fractured femoral shaft: new approach to the problem. *Lancet* 1944; **i**: 659.

Gie, G.A. & MacEachern, G.A. Experience with the Orthofix. In: *Recent advances in external fixation.* Riva del Garda: Italy, 1986.

Goodship, A. & Kenwright, J. The influence of induced micromovement upon the healing of experimental tibial fractures. *J Bone Joint Surg* 1985; **67B**: 650.

Green, G.A. *Complications of External Skeletal Fixation.* Charles C. Thomas: Springfield, 1981.

Green, S.A. Complications of external skeletal fixation. *Clin Orthop* 1983; **180**: 109.

Heim, V. & Pfeiffer, K.M. *Small Fragment Set Manual.* Springer-Verlag: Berlin, 1974.

Hey Groves, E.W. *On Modern Methods of Treating Fractures.* Wright: Bristol, 1916.

Hicks, J.H. External splintage as a cause of movement in fractures. *Lancet* 1960; **i**: 667.

Hoffman, R. Rotules à os pour la reduction dirigée, non saglante des fractures (osteotaxis). *Helv Med Acta* 1938; **5**: 844.

Huckstep, R.L. Rigid intramedullary fixation of femoral shaft fractures with compression. *J Bone Joint Surg* 1972; **54B**: 204.

Irani, R.N., Nicholson, J.T. & Chong, S.M.K. Long-term results in the treatment of femoral-shaft fractures in young children by immediate spica immobilisation. *J Bone Joint Surg* 1976; **58A**: 945.

Kenwright, J., Goodship, A.E., Newman, J.H., Harris, J.D., Richardson, J.B., Evans, M., Spriggins, A.J.M., Burrough, S.J. & Rowley, D.I. Effect of controlled axial micromovement on healing of tibial fractures. *Lancet* 1987; **ii**: 1185.

Koenig, F. *Operative Chirurgie der Knochenbruche. 1. Bd.: Operationen am frischen und verschleppten Knochenbruch.* Springer-Verlag: Berlin, 1931.

Kuntscher, G. *The Callus Problem.* W.H .Green: St Louis, 1967.

Lambotte, A. *Chirurgie Operatoire des Fractures.* Masson: Paris, 1913.

Lundeen, M., Jones, R., Mooney, V. & Murray, W. Complex open tibia fractures treated by external fixation. A comparison study using the Roger Anderson device and the Murray external fixation system. *Orthop Trans* 1980; **4**: 348.

Malgaigne, J.F. *Treatise on Fractures.* Lippincott: Philadelphia, 1859.

Mathysen, A. *Plaster-of-Paris in the Treatment of Fractures.* Grandmont-Doners: Liege, 1854.

Mears, D.C. History of external fixation. In: Brooker, A.F. & Edwards, C.C. (eds) *External Fixation. The Current State of the Art.* Williams & Wilkins: Baltimore, 1979.

Müller, M.E., Allgower, M., Schneider, R. & Willenegger, H. *Manual of Internal Fixation of Fractures.* Springer-Verlag: Berlin, 1991.

Müller, M.E., Allgower, M. & Willenegger, H. *Techniques of Internal Fixation of Fractures.* Springer-Verlag: Berlin, 1965.

Perkins, G. *The Ruminations of an Orthopaedic Surgeon.* Butterworth: London, 1970.

Rush, L.V. Dynamic intramedullary fracture-fixation of the femur. Reflections on the use of the round rod after thirty years. *Clin Orthop* 1968; **60**: 21.

Russell, R. Theory and method in extension of the thigh. *Br Med J* 1921; **2**: 637.

Schenk, R.K. & Willenegger, H. Morphological findings in primary fracture healing. *Symp Biol Hung* 1967; **7**: 75.

Stewart, J.D.M. & Hallett, J.P. *Traction and Orthopaedic Appliances.* Churchill Livingstone: Edinburgh, 1983.

Thomas, H.O. *Diseases of the Hip, Knee and Ankle Joints, with Their Deformities, Treated by a New and Efficient Method.* Dobb: Liverpool, 1876.

Anaesthesia

G.SMITH

Patients undergoing elective surgery are usually in optimum physical condition with a definitive surgical diagnosis and with concomitant medical disease under adequate control. In contrast, the patient with a fracture may have additional overt or latent injuries and uncontrolled concomitant medical illness. Thus, the most important principle in the anaesthetic management of a patient with a fracture is that of careful preparation for all potential complications, in particular the problems associated with hypovolaemia and haemorrhage, vomiting and regurgitation and abnormal reactions to drugs in the presence of electrolyte disturbance and renal impairment.

Preoperative assessment

Several of the large-scale epidemiological studies of anaesthetic mortality have indicated that inadequate preoperative preparation of the patient is a major contributory factor to perioperative mortality (Derrington and Smith 1987). It is essential to ascertain the likely surgical diagnosis, the magnitude of the proposed surgery and how urgently the surgery is indicated, as these dictate the extent of preoperative preparation and the method of anaesthesia.

The history and physical examination of the patient should be obtained in the usual way. The systems of greatest relevance to the anaesthetist are the cardiovascular and respiratory systems. Direct questions should be asked about the following items of particular anaesthetic relevance:

1 The family history of hereditary conditions associated with anaesthetic problems, e.g. porphyria, malignant hyperpyrexia, hypercholesterolaemia, haemophilia, cholinesterase abnormalities and dystrophia myotonica.

2 Diseases of the cardiovascular and respiratory systems involve direct questions regarding exertional dyspnoea, paroxysmal nocturnal dyspnoea, orthopnoea, angina of effort, etc.

3 If relevant, it is important to determine if pregnancy is present. In the early stages of pregnancy anaesthetics are theoretically teratogenic and there is also a risk of inducing spontaneous abortion. In late pregnancy the patient presents risks of regurgitation and acid aspiration syndrome. If feasible, a regional anaesthetic technique may be preferable to general anaesthesia for the pregnant patient with a fracture.

4 A history of previous anaesthesia should be sought and specific questions asked regarding allergy. The current recommendation of the Committee of Safety of Medicines is that halothane anaesthesia should not be repeated within 6 months of a previous halothane anaesthetic because of the increased risk of postoperative hepatic dysfunction.

5 A history of allergies to other drugs should be sought.

6 A history of human immunodeficiency virus (HIV) infection or jaundice has important implications as staff need to take additional precautions to prevent the transmission of infection.

7 It is essential that a complete history is obtained regarding concurrent medication. Many drugs interact with agents employed by the anaesthetist. In general, administration of most drugs should be continued up to the time of surgery. Important exceptions to this rule include insulin and mono-amine oxidase inhibitors. With regard to the oral contraceptive pill, it has been recommended that therapy should be discontinued at least two cycles before elective surgery because of the increased risk of deep venous thrombosis (DVT). This policy is under review, however, and some authorities believe that the risk of pregnancy after discontinuing the pill is greater than the risk of DVT; thus, low-dose heparin therapy has been advised with maintenance of oral contraceptive therapy. For emergency surgery, the use of low-dose subcutaneous heparin should certainly be considered; the risk of DVT has to be balanced against the risk of haemorrhage from the fracture site.

Special investigations

It is generally accepted that the clinical history and physical examination represent the best method of screening for the presence of disease. Routine laboratory tests should be obtained only if the results have an impact on the anaesthetic management of the patient.

In order to reduce the volume of routine investigations the following suggestions are made (Fee and McCaughey 1994):

1 Urinalysis should be performed on every patient as it may occasionally reveal an undiagnosed diabetic or urinary tract infection.

2 Haemoglobin concentration should be measured in every patient with a fracture.

3 Urea and electrolyte concentrations are not required routinely but should be obtained if there is a history of diarrhoea or vomiting, metabolic disease, renal or hepatic disease or diabetes and in patients receiving medication with diuretics, digoxin, antihypertensives, steroids or hypoglycaemic agents.

4 Liver function tests are required only in patients with hepatic disease, metabolic disease or where there is a history of a large intake of alcohol.

5 Chest radiography is not required routinely in patients below 60 years of age but should be obtained in the following cases.

(a) In the event of thoracic trauma.

(b) If there is a history of, or physical signs of, cardiac or respiratory disease.

(c) If there may be metastases from carcinoma, e.g. if there is a possibility that a fracture may be meta-static rather than traumatic.

(d) In recent immigrants from countries where tuberculosis is endemic.

6 A 12-lead electrocardiogram (ECG) should be obtained if there is a history of, or physical signs of, cardiac disease, in hypertensive patients and in all patients over the age of 55 years.

7 Blood sugar estimation is required in patients receiving corticosteroid drugs and in those with diabetes.

8 Sickle cell status should be assessed if there is an ethnic origin or family history suggestive of a haemoglobinopathy. Black patients of African origin scheduled for emergency surgery should have a sickle-dex test performed; if this is positive, haemoglobin electrophoresis should be obtained as soon as possible but should not delay emergency surgery.

9 Pulmonary function tests (peak expiratory flow rate and forced vital capacity) should be measured in all patients with severe dyspnoea on mild to moderate exercise. More sophisticated pulmonary function tests do not provide better prognostic criteria of the necessity for postoperative elective ventilation and should not be required by the anaesthetist.

10 Blood gas analysis should be performed in all patients with dyspnoea at rest or in patients with severe thoracic trauma.

11 Coagulation tests should be performed in patients who give a history of bleeding disorders.

Assessment of volaemic status

Assessment of the extent of the intravascular volume is essential in all patients with fractures, as underestimated or unrecognized hypovolaemia may lead to circulatory collapse during induction of anaesthesia. The extent of blood loss may be assessed from the history and the extent of fractures. In the patient with trauma it is important to make repeated assessments to include the possibility of latent intra-abdominal injury, particularly in the presence of head injury where physical signs may be masked.

Clinical evaluation of blood loss relies particularly on heart rate, arterial pressure, state of the peripheral circulation, central venous pressure (CVP) and urinary output. Table 8.1 describes approximate correlations between these indices and the extent of haemorrhage; it should be stressed that these refer to the ideal patient. In young healthy adults, heart rate and arterial pressure may be unreliable guides to volume status. In elderly patients with widespread arterial disease, signs of severe hypovolaemia may become evident when blood volume has been reduced by as little as 15–20%.

In general, hypovolaemia does not become apparent clinically until the blood volume has been reduced by at least 1 l (20% of blood volume). A reduction by more

Table 8.1 Clinical indices of extent of blood loss (Turner 1985)

Grade of hypovolaemia	1 (minimal)	2 (mild)	3 (moderate)	4 (severe)
Blood volume lost (%)	10	20	30	Over 40
Volume lost (ml)	500	1000	1500	Over 2000
Heart rate (beats min^{-1})	Normal	100–120	120–140	Over 140
Arterial pressure (mmHg)	Normal	Orthostatic hypotension	Systolic below 100	Systolic below 80
Urinary output (ml h^{-1})	Normal (1 ml kg^{-1} h^{-1})	20–30	10–20	Nil
Sensorium	Normal	Normal	Restless	Impaired consciousness
State of peripheral circulation	Normal	Cool and pale	Cold and pale; slow capillary	Cold and clammy; peripheral cyanosis
CVP (cmH$_2$O)	Normal	−3	−5	−8

CVP, central venous pressure.

than 30% occurs before the classical shock syndrome is produced; notably, hypotension, tachycardia, oliguria and cold clammy extremities. Haemorrhage in excess of 40% of the blood volume may be associated with loss of compensatory mechanisms maintaining cerebral and coronary blood flow and this should be suspected if a patient becomes restless and agitated and eventually comatose.

In patients with major trauma it is valuable to compare the clinical assessment of the extent of haemorrhage with a measured or assumed loss. A marked disparity between these two estimates leads not infrequently to a diagnosis of a further concealed source of haemorrhage.

The full stomach

Of all the hazards of emergency anaesthesia, vomiting or regurgitation of gastric contents followed by aspiration is one of the most common. The resultant asphyxia, due to obstruction of the airway, or aspiration pneumonitis represent the most common causes of death produced primarily by anaesthesia. Vomiting is an active process occurring in the lighter planes of anaesthesia during induction or recovery from anaesthesia. In contrast, regurgitation is a passive phenomenon and occurs frequently in the presence of deep anaesthesia or at the onset of action of muscle relaxant drugs.

In elective surgery, patients are usually starved of food and drink overnight or for at least 4–6 hours.

However, in emergency surgery, it may be necessary to induce anaesthesia urgently before an adequate period of starvation occurs.

Vomiting and regurgitation are encountered most frequently in anaesthetic practice during induction of general anaesthesia in patients with an acute abdomen or trauma. All patients with even minor trauma (fractures and dislocations) must be assumed to have a full stomach, as gastric emptying virtually ceases at the time of significant trauma as a result of the combined effects of fear, pain, shock and treatment with opioid analgesics. In all trauma patients, the time interval between ingestion of food and the accident is a more reliable index of the degree of gastric emptying than is the period of fasting. It is not uncommon to encounter vomiting occurring up to 24 hours after ingestion of food when trauma has occurred very shortly after the meal. Thus, the 4- to 6-hour rule is quite unreliable.

Head injury

Many patients with trauma have associated head injury, varying from minor trauma to a variable period of loss of consciousness. The most extreme example would be coma prolonged to the time at which surgery becomes essential. All patients with head injury have some oedema of the brain with damage to its blood vessels and some degree of loss of autoregulation of the cerebral circulation. Anaesthesia with volatile agents and spontaneous ventilation causes a severe increase in intracranial pressure (ICP) for two reasons: first, hypercapnia increases the ICP as carbon dioxide is the most potent cerebral vasodilator, and spontaneous ventilation with volatile anaesthetic agents leads invariably to some degree of hypercapnia; secondly, all the volatile anaesthetic agents are cerebral vasodilators and increase cerebral blood flow and intracranial pressure. For these reasons, spontaneous ventilation techniques are contraindicated and, wherever possible, a regional or local anaesthetic technique is to be preferred. Where general anaesthesia is mandatory, it is essential to utilize a technique of intermittent positive pressure ventilation (IPPV) using muscle relaxants, and to avoid the use of volatile anaesthetic agents. The use of IPPV is beneficial as hypocapnia may be produced with resultant cerebral vasoconstriction.

Clinical assessment of the patient with head injury is aided by the use of the Glasgow coma scale (see Table 7.1, p. 112). Investigations may be required, including computerized axial tomography (CAT) scans and arterial blood/gas analysis. Mannitol should not be used routinely but may help to prevent deterioration during patient transfer or to postpone coning when a patient appears to be deteriorating rapidly. Immediate surgery may be required in those patients in whom there is a rapid decline in conscious level or the sudden development of unilateral neurological signs.

It may be seen that the assessment of head injury utilizing the Glasgow coma scale is rendered impossible in the presence of general anaesthesia. For this reason it is preferable to postpone surgery of a concomitant fracture for as long as possible.

Control of raised ICP

Many patients with severe head injury develop an elevation of ICP, resulting from a subdural or extradural haematoma or in the absence of a mass lesion. In the first 24 hours following head injury, the cerebral vasculature in damaged areas of brain dilates and results in an increased cerebral blood volume. Later, both extracellular and intracellular oedema develop, increasing the volume of fluid inside the skull.

Control of raised ICP involves:

1 Position — the patient should be nursed with the head and shoulders elevated at 15° to the horizontal.

2 Oxygenation — hypoxaemia leads to further cerebral vasodilatation and therefore the arterial Po_2 should be maintained above 13 kPa.

3 Controlled ventilation — elective controlled ventilation is used widely in patients whose head injury

results in persistent intracranial hypertension. It is also indicated in hyper- or hypoventilating patients and in the presence of hypoxia (e.g. where $Paco_2$ is less than 3 kPa or Pao_2 is less than 10 kPa with an inspired oxygen concentration of 40%, which is commonly achieved with standard disposable facemasks). When controlled ventilation is instituted, it is necessary to maintain good oxygenation and moderate hypocapnia ($Paco_2$ 3.5–4 kPa) with minimal airway pressure. When elective ventilation is required continuous ICP monitoring must be instituted.

Assessment of the risks of anaesthesia

The Confidential Enquiry into Perioperative Deaths (CEPOD study) indicated that over a broad range of elective and emergency surgery and patient age, the overall mortality rate from surgery is of the order of 0.6%, whereas the overall mortality rate attributable directly to anaesthesia is in the order of 1 in 10000. Anaesthesia is partially responsible for a mortality rate of 1 in 3000. In many of the large-scale studies common factors which have emerged as contributing to anaesthetic mortality include inadequate assessment of patients in the preoperative period, inadequate supervision and monitoring in the intraoperative period and inadequate postoperative supervision and management (Buck, Devlin & Lunn 1987; Campling *et al.* 1993).

It is difficult to quantitate the risk of anaesthesia in an individual patient. Whilst some accuracy is possible for populations of patients, precision does not extend to an accurate prediction of the risk for an individual patient. One of the simplest methods of assessment is the grading system suggested by the American Society of Anesthesiologists (ASA physical status score; Table 8.2) which does correlate, albeit poorly, with the risk of anaesthesia and surgery (Table 8.3).

The greatest interest in risk prediction has centred on cardiovascular risks and a large number of studies have shown that the risk of cardiac death is related closely to the presence of a preoperative myocardial infarction, in particular to the time interval between the first myocardial infarction and surgery. A number of risk factors have been described and Goldman and colleagues have produced a risk index (Table 8.4) for the development of life-threatening cardiovascular complications in the postoperative period (Goldman 1988).

The elderly are subject to increased risks from anaesthesia and surgery, largely because of the association between many diseases of the cardiovascular or respiratory systems and age, and also because routine clinical evaluation often fails to detect cardiorespiratory dys-

Table 8.2 The ASA physical status scale

Class	Description
I	A normally healthy individual
II	A patient with severe systemic disease
III	A patient with severe systemic disease that is not incapacitating
IV	A patient with incapacitating systemic disease that is a constant threat to life
V	A moribund patient who is not expected to survive 24 hours with or without operation
E	Added as a suffix for emergency operation

Table 8.3 Mortality rates after anaesthesia and surgery for each ASA physical status — emergency and elective cases

ASA rating	Mortality rate (%)
I	0.1
II	0.2
III	1.8
IV	7.8
V	9.4

ASA, American Society of Anesthesiologists.

Table 8.4 Goldman's index of cardiac risk in non-cardiac procedures

Risk factor	Points*
Third heart sound or jugular venous distension	11
Myocardial infarction in preceding 6 months	10
Rhythm other than sinus or premature atrial contractions	7
Abdominal, thoracic or aortic operation	3
Age > 70 years	5
Important aortic stenosis	3
Emergency operation	4
Poor conditions as defined by any one of: $Pao_2 < 8$ kPa $Paco_2 > 6.5$ kPa $K^+ < 3.0$ mmol l^{-1} $HCO_3 < 20$ mmol l^{-1} Creatinine > 260 mmol l^{-1} SGOT[†] abnormal Chronic liver disease	3

* 5 points or less indicates a risk of cardiac mortality of 0.2%; 6–25 points indicates a risk of 2%; and >25 points indicates a risk of 56%.

† SGOT, serum glutamic oxaloacetic transaminase.

function in geriatric patients (Krechel 1994).

Factors which are of the greatest importance in predicting the development of postoperative morbidity and mortality include, in decreasing order of importance:

1 Clinical assessment — ASA rating greater than 3.

2 Cardiac failure.

3 Cardiac risk index — as assessed by the score obtained using the Goldman index (see Table 8.4).

4 Pulmonary disease.

5 Pulmonary abnormalities confirmed by chest radiography.

6 ECG abnormalities.

Timing of surgery for fractures

From the orthopaedic viewpoint, it seems sensible to proceed to surgery as soon as possible after the definitive diagnosis of a fracture has been made. However, the anaesthetist may wish to delay anaesthesia for as long as possible and to institute appropriate assessment and preparation it may be permissible to delay surgery of closed fractures for 24–48 hours; there is usually no conflict between the surgeon and anaesthetist in this instance. However, with open fractures, many surgeons insist that surgery should be undertaken as soon as possible in order to minimize the risk of infection. Under these circumstances a compromise has to be reached, based upon the balance of risks of proceeding to early anaesthesia as opposed to the risk of infection of bone and its sequelae.

The anaesthetist's opinion on the optimum time for surgery is governed by three important considerations:

1 *Adequate resuscitation*. It is vital to reiterate that failure to resuscitate a patient adequately may result in profound circulatory shock, and even death, following induction of general anaesthesia because all agents are vasodilators and myocardial depressants. Thus, it is particularly important to assess the patient carefully for concomitant injury which may be clinically latent. If there is any doubt, a central venous catheter should be inserted for monitoring of volaemic status. This important principle may be breached *only* if haemorrhage is extensive and continuous.

2 *Recent ingestion of food*. Wherever possible, induction of general anaesthesia should be postponed for at least 6 hours before proceeding to any form of surgery, either elective or emergency, even though this does not guarantee the presence of an empty stomach in traumatized patients.

3 *Head injury*. Because clinical observation of the response to commands and the conscious level is such an important determinant of the presence or progression of intracerebral pathology, and because general anaesthesia removes the ability to assess these variables, it is important to delay anaesthesia for as long as possible in the patient who has suffered a head injury. As the likelihood of clinically important cerebral pathology diminishes rapidly after the moment of head trauma, it follows that it is useful to delay surgery for as long as possible, even if this involves a period of only 24 hours.

The recently conducted NCEPOD study emphasized many points that are particularly important in considering emergency anaesthesia and surgery. It drew attention to the excessive amount of surgery conducted outside the normal working day; it emphasized the failure of junior anaesthetic and surgical staff to obtain senior advice and assistance; and it confirmed the findings of many previous studies with regard to inadequate assessment and preoperative preparation (Campling *et al.* 1993).

Many fractures fall into these categories. For example, fractures of the proximal femur are dealt with in some hospitals by junior anaesthetists and surgeons operating in the middle of the night on elderly frail patients. Such patients are invariably dehydrated upon admission and require rehydration with fluids. In addition, elderly patients frequently have concomitant medical disease which requires assessment and therapy. To reduce the duration of surgery to a minimum it is also desirable that these patients are treated on an elective operating theatre list by senior anaesthetic and surgical staff.

Choice of anaesthetic technique for fractures

Anaesthetic techniques suitable for patients with a fracture may be classified into general techniques and regional (local) techniques. On occasions, an anaesthetist may give a regional anaesthetic technique to a patient under general anaesthesia in order to reduce the dosage of central nervous system (CNS) and myocardial depressant drugs. The techniques available are:
1 General anaesthesia.
2 Regional (local) anaesthetic techniques
  (a) *Peripheral blocks*
    Field block.
    Peripheral nerve block.
    Plexus block.
    Intravenous regional analgesic (IVRA; Bier's block).
  (b) *Central blocks*
    Subarachnoid (spinal) block.
    Epidural (extradural) block.
3 General anaesthesia and regional block.

The choice of whether to utilize general anaesthesia or local anaesthesia is dependent upon a variety of considerations:
1 Concomitant medical disease
  (a) Cardiovascular disease.
  (b) Respiratory disease.
  (c) Disease of the nervous system.
  (d) Obesity.
  (e) Diabetes.
2 Infection.
3 Bleeding disorders.
4 Sickle cell disease.
5 Concomitant drug therapy.
6 Full stomach.
7 Hypovolaemia.
8 Fracture site.
9 Duration of surgery.

Concomitant medical disease

There is a widespread feeling, particularly amongst surgeons and junior anaesthetists, that regional anaesthesia is safer than general anaesthesia in patients with severe systemic disease. Whilst this may be true for peripheral blocks, it does not apply to central regional blocks (spinal or epidural blocks).

The presence of cardiovascular disease, for example, valvular cardiac disease or ischaemic heart disease, may be an indication for peripheral nerve blocks but central blocks may be avoided in favour of general anaesthesia as it is easier to ensure cardiovascular stability during general anaesthesia.

Respiratory disease is frequently cited as an excellent indication for regional nerve blocks and this is true particularly of peripheral nerve bocks or low spinal or epidural anaesthesia. High spinal and epidural anaesthesia, which interfere with the intercostal muscles, should be avoided.

Pre-existing disease of the nervous system is frequently cited as a contraindication to regional anaesthesia on the grounds that worsening of the patient's neurological condition after a regional anaesthetic is blamed upon the block itself.

Obesity makes the technical performance of regional anaesthesia difficult.

In diabetic patients peripheral nerve blocks may be useful as they cause minimal disruption of the patient's carbohydrate and insulin regimen.

Infection

Infection at, or close to, the site of injection is an absolute contraindication to the use of all local anaesthetic techniques. Insertion of a needle may spread the infection but, in addition, local anaesthetic agents tend to be ineffective because the low pH of inflamed tissue inhibits the dissociation of the local anaesthetic drug.

Bleeding disorders

These are an absolute contraindication to spinal and epidural anaesthesia, and possibly also to regional nerve blocks where it may be difficult to exert local pressure to control bleeding.

Sickle cell disease

Regional anaesthetic techniques are the method of choice in sickle cell disease. Obviously this condition is an absolute contraindication to the use of a tourniquet.

Concomitant drug therapy

Drug interactions are extremely rare with local anaesthetic agents but are relatively common with general anaesthetic agents.

The full stomach

It is frequently assumed, although erroneously, that regional anaesthesia totally avoids the hazards of general anaesthesia.

Patients receiving regional anaesthetic techniques frequently require benzodiazepines to provide sedation. It is difficult to judge the dosage of these drugs and overdosage is common with loss of pharyngeal and laryngeal reflexes. It is feasible, therefore, for patients who are well sedated with benzodiazepines to aspirate regurgitated material. Furthermore, regional anaesthetic techniques are not 100% effective and under some circumstances, where a block is deemed inadequate, it is essential to induce general anaesthesia immediately to avoid suffering.

Toxicity of local anaesthetic agents may be manifested by convulsions; this greatly increases the possibility of regurgitation and poses a very difficult clinical situation to manage.

For all these reasons, therefore, it is essential that patients scheduled to undergo regional anaesthesia are starved for 4−6 hours, i.e. for the same period that would normally be employed for general anaesthesia.

Hypovolaemia

Hypovolaemia is exaggerated and severe hypotension

produced by general anaesthetic agents and by central nerve blocks. Both are therefore contraindicated if this condition is suspected.

Site of fracture

Regional anaesthetic techniques are particularly appropriate for fractures of the upper and lower limbs, as peripheral blocks may be used. Central blocks for fractures involving the pelvis are invariably more dangerous than general anaesthesia and should be avoided. Fractured ribs may be managed by intercostal nerve blocks provided that the technique is confined to one side. Bilateral intercostal nerve blocks are contraindicated because of the small risk of pneumothorax.

Duration of surgery

Regional anaesthetic techniques are only appropriate if the duration of analgesia exceeds the likely duration of surgery (see below). Regional anaesthesia may be prolonged by the use of catheter techniques (catheters placed close to the site of the nerve requiring blockade). Whilst catheter techniques are commonly employed in North America for a variety of peripheral nerve blocks, in the United Kingdom they tend to be used predominantly only for extradural nerve blocks.

General anaesthesia

General anaesthetic techniques, in which the patient breathes spontaneously via a facemask or laryngeal mask, can only be used if there is no doubt that the patient has an empty stomach and the risk of regurgitation is minimal. If these conditions do not apply, it is customary to intubate the trachea by 'a rapid sequence induction'. This comprises preoxygenation of the patient's lungs, rapid intravenous injection of thiopentone followed by suxamethonium, the application of cricoid pressure by an assistant to prevent aspiration, and intubation of the trachea with a cuffed tube.

Following tracheal intubation the patient may either breathe spontaneously a mixture of nitrous oxide and volatile anaesthetic agents in oxygen or, alternatively, muscle relaxation is maintained by a long-acting muscle relaxant drug and the patient's lungs are ventilated artificially for the duration of anaesthesia. The practical conduct of general anaesthesia does not fall within the scope of this book, but there are some important points which the orthopaedic surgeon should note:

1 Hypotension may occur on induction of anaesthesia, particularly if there is any element of hypovolaemia.

2 Vomiting or regurgitation with aspiration is a hazard not only at induction of anaesthesia but also on recovery from anaesthesia. Assistance may therefore be required to place the patient on the side in a head-down position before the trachea is extubated.

3 IPPV carries an extremely small risk of pneumothorax in the patient with healthy lungs because of the increase in alveolar pressure. However, in patients with fractured ribs there is a high risk of producing pneumothorax and tension pneumothorax. In the presence of bilateral fractured ribs following multiple trauma, the author would recommend insertion of bilateral chest drains if IPPV is instituted, even if the pre-anaesthetic chest radiograph fails to demonstrate pneumothorax.

4 The duration of action and efficacy of anaesthetic agents and opioids are prolonged in the presence of shock, metabolic acidosis, debilitated state, etc.

5 Induction of general anaesthesia immediately removes the ability to assess the patient's neurological status.

6 Awareness during relaxant anaesthesia — there is a possibility that the patient may be aware during light anaesthesia employing paralysis with muscle relaxant drugs. This is usually avoided successfully by the addition of a small concentration of a volatile anaesthetic agent. In emergency anaesthesia for multiple trauma the dosage of volatile agent used may be reduced to a minimum because of its profound hypotensive action and awareness is more likely to occur than in other types of anaesthesia. This problem may also be avoided by good resuscitation of the patient, thereby enabling adequate concentrations of volatile agents to be used without undue cardiovascular depression.

Regional anaesthetic techniques

Central regional blocks

Subarachnoid (spinal) and extradural (epidural) anaesthetic techniques are collectively termed central regional blocks. These blocks produce profound physiological changes and must *never* be used unless the operator is skilled in the performance of tracheal intubation and cardiopulmonary resuscitation. Table 8.5 shows a comparison of these two blocks.

The height of a spinal block may be controlled quite

Table 8.5 Comparison of subarachnoid and extradural blocks

	Subarachnoid	Extradural
Doses of drug used	Small	Large systemic absorption occurs with possible CNS effect (drowsiness) and cardiovascular effects (myocardial depression and peripheral dilatation)
Rate of onset of block	Fast (2—8 minutes)	Slow (20—40 minutes)
Success rate	100% if lumbar puncture successful	Missed segments and total failure not uncommon
Intensity of block	May be complete	Rarely complete block of all modalities of sensation
Segmental block	No	Yes
Extent of block	May be widespread — depends on positioning	Depends on total dose of drug injected
Precision in predicting height of block	Good if clinician experienced	Very imprecise, even in experienced hands
Postspinal headache	1—2% with 25 gauge needle; 10% with 22 gauge needle	Absent
Infections — local or systemic	Absolute contraindication	Absolute contraindication
Bleeding disorder	Contraindication	Contraindication

precisely by the skilled operator, but this is not true for epidural blocks. It is therefore possible to maintain a spinal block below the level of L1 and thereby cause minimal peripheral vasodilatation and hypotension. For this reason subarachnoid anaesthesia may be an excellent technique for use in patients with fractures of the lower limb.

As spinal and epidural blocks are normally performed only by specialist anaesthetists, this subject is not considered further. (See Greiff and Cousins 1994 for further information)

Peripheral regional nerve blocks

FACILITIES

It is essential that all forms of local anaesthetic technique are undertaken in an area which is appropriately equipped with intravenous fluids, a tipping trolley, oxygen supply and full resuscitation equipment and drugs, including ECG, defibrillator, laryngoscopes, means of artificial ventilation of the lungs, etc. Where large volumes of local anaesthetic are used for blockade of, for example, brachial plexus, it is essential that a venous cannula be inserted into a suitable vein before institution of the block. Amongst the drugs which should be available immediately are thiopentone, diazepam, suxamethonium, ephedrine, atropine and adrenaline.

PREPARATION OF THE PATIENT

Patients for major nerve blocks should be treated in the same way as patients receiving general anaesthesia and should undergo a similar period of starvation. They should empty the bladder preoperatively.

An adequate explanation of what the patient will experience should be given and specific mention should be made of paraesthesiae if they are to be elicited. If a patient is to remain conscious during the block it is important that a warning is given that some sensation may be preserved and that movement and warmth or cold are likely to be felt — this is important as without such a warning the patient may interpret any sensation as pain.

It is invariably desirable to sedate the patient during major nerve blocks. Premedication may be required using benzodiazepines, e.g. 2.5–10 mg oral diazepam 2 hours before surgery or 10 mg oral temazepam 1 hour before surgery. These drugs may be omitted if the patient has a painful fracture which has received preliminary treatment in the form of opioids.

LOCAL ANAESTHETIC DRUGS

There are three drugs used commonly in the United Kingdom for regional nerve block.

Lignocaine. This is the standard against which all other local anaesthetics are compared. It has been used safely for all types of local anaesthesia and is a standard antiarrhythmic agent. It is available in concentrations of 0.5, 1% and 2% plain and also in solutions containing adrenaline.

The rate of onset of action of lignocaine depends upon the nerve which has been blocked; large fibres taking longer than small fibres to be anaesthetized. However, the onset of action may be expected within 15–30 minutes and the duration of action of the plain solution is 1–2 hours. Addition of adrenaline to the solution almost doubles the length of action.

Prilocaine. This drug is equipotent with lignocaine and, unlike the latter drug, does not cause vasodilatation. The safe dose of the agent is twice that of lignocaine and it has a slightly longer duration of action. It is the drug of choice when the risk of local anaesthetic toxicity is high. Methaemoglobinaemia may be produced when the dosage of the drug exceeds approximately 600 mg; this is considerably greater than the dose used for a single administration.

Bupivacaine. This is a long-acting agent with a toxicity similar to that of lignocaine. It has a slower onset of action than lignocaine (it may take up to 45 minutes for an axillary brachial plexus block) and a considerably longer duration of action. For peripheral nerve blocks the duration may vary between 4 and 11 hours. Bupivacaine is available as a 0.25% or 0.5% solution, with or without adrenaline. The addition of adrenaline has little effect on the duration of action of bupivacaine but it helps to reduce the risk of toxicity by reducing the rate of systemic absorption of the drug.

Dosage of local anaesthetic agents

The concentration and volume of solutions required to produce nerve block vary considerably. Although maximum recommended doses are shown in Table 8.6, it is important to note that the toxicity is dependent upon the peak plasma concentration of local anaesthetic produced and, therefore, the site of administration is almost as important as the dose of drug administered. Absorption from the tracheobronchial tree is almost as fast as that following slow intravenous injection; infiltration

Table 8.6 Maximum recommended doses of local anaesthetic agents

Agent	Dose (mg)	Volume of solution (ml)			
		0.25%	0.5%	1%	2%
Prilocaine					
Without adrenaline	400	160	80	40	20
With adrenaline	600	240	120	60	30
Lignocaine					
Without adrenaline	200	80	40	20	10
With adrenaline	500	200	100	50	25
Bupivacaine					
Without adrenaline	150	60	30	Not available	
With adrenaline	150	60	30	Not available	

Notes: (a) These doses are only approximate recommendations and are dependent on the site of injection and the rate of absorption.
(b) These doses apply to a 70 kg healthy adult male. The dose should be reduced *pro rata* for children and be reduced in the presence of severe systemic disease, liver disease and general debility.
(c) Toxicity of a combination of different local anaesthetics is additive.

into the face or perineal region is also associated with very fast absorption. In contrast, following injection into the brachial plexus sheath, maximum plasma concentrations are not attained within 10 minutes. A well-tolerated single dose of a local anaesthetic may be repeated after a couple of hours (Covino and Wildsmith 1994).

Maintenance of analgesia

It is important when using local anaesthetic techniques to ensure that systemic analgesic agents have been administered to the patient before the local anaesthetic block wears off, otherwise the patient may experience a rapid transition from total analgesia to severe pain within a very short period of time.

DIGITAL NERVE BLOCK

Each digit is supplied by four nerve branches, two dorsal and two palmar, which run forward along the edge of the digit. These nerves are blocked easily at the base of the digit using a total of 2–4 ml of 1 or 2% lignocaine, or a similar volume of 1 or 2% prilocaine. Vasoconstrictors must *not* be used.

Digital nerve blocks are appropriate for injuries of the distal or middle phalanges, but for more extensive injuries it is advisable to choose a more proximal site for the block, e.g. wrist block, block at the elbow or brachial plexus block.

INTRAVENOUS REGIONAL ANAESTHESIA (IVRA) OR BIER'S BLOCK

IVRA is one of the easiest blocks for the inexperienced clinician to perform. However, there are several case reports of inexperienced clinicians using IVRA without understanding the technique or the drugs used and without being able to cope with complications. As a result, fatalities have occurred, usually with bupivacaine and this drug should be avoided for this technique.

The technique produces satisfactory analgesia and muscle relaxation of the hand and forearm in up to 98% of cases and is suitable for open or closed procedures below the elbow if they can be completed within 1 hour. Bier's block is not commonly used for the lower limb, largely because of the volume of local anaesthetic required; this necessitates placing the tourniquet at mid-calf level.

Practical performance of Bier's block

1 The patient should be starved for 4–6 hours.
2 The recommended drug to be used for this block is prilocaine plain (Citanest) which is available as a 0.5% solution. Only the 0.5% solution must be used. The recommended dosage for regional analgesia is 3–4 mg kg^{-1}; Table 8.7 shows the dosage injection volumes for a range of patient weights.
3 Take the patient's blood pressure.
4 Apply a *reliable* tourniquet cuff, over padding, to the upper arm but do not inflate yet. The automatic tourni-

Table 8.7 Injection volume of 0.5% solution of prilocaine for various patient weights

Weight (kg)	Prilocaine dose (mg)	Final injection volume (ml)
70	250	50
60	225	45
50	200	40
40	150	30

quet should have been checked for volume of gas, etc.

5 Insert a small (23 or 25 gauge) indwelling cannula into a suitable vein, preferably on the dorsum of the hand, and secure it. The needle *must* be inserted into a vein as distal as possible and *not* in the antecubital fossa.

6 Insert a small cannula into a vein on the opposite arm and flush to ensure patency.

7 Exsanguinate the limb, either by simple elevation for 2 minutes or by use of an Esmarch elastic bandage.

8 Now inflate the tourniquet cuff to a pressure 100 mmHg higher than the recorded systolic arterial pressure. Maintain the cuff at this pressure for the duration of the procedure. Leakage from the cuff, resulting from a possible fault in the automatic inflating device, should be prevented by the application of a clamp to the rubber connection between machine and tourniquet.

9 Inject the required dose of 0.5% plain prilocaine slowly through the indwelling needle. Check for drowsiness after injecting 10–15 ml. Gently massage the limb to facilitate the spread of the solution. The patient will experience a feeling of warmth and/or paraesthesiae.

10 Wait for analgesia to develop (usually complete within 4–6 minutes). Loss of cutaneous sensation to pinprick is a useful guide. As muscle relaxation occurs the limb should feel 'heavy' to the patient. If analgesia is patchy or inadequate, a further 5–10 ml of the 0.5% prilocaine solution may be given.

11 *After 20 minutes, or on completion of the operation,* whichever is the longer, deflate the cuff in a *stepwise* manner and remove the indwelling needle. Sensation will usually return within several minutes. Allow the patient to recover under supervision.

Precautions and adverse effects of IVRA

As with all local anaesthetic procedures, facilities for resuscitation should be close at hand. Pain from pressure of the tourniquet is an occasional problem, but provided that there is adequate padding beneath the cuff and the

operating time is limited to about 40 minutes, opioid analgesics are rarely required for cuff pain.

Tourniquet pain may be obviated by the use of a double-cuff, which may be available in some hospitals. With this cuff, the block is performed as described above apart from the fact that a special double-cuff tourniquet is used. After exsanguination the *upper* cuff is inflated to a pressure 100 mmHg greater than the systolic arterial pressure. Ten minutes after administration of prilocaine i.v. the *lower* cuff is then inflated and the *upper* cuff is *subsequently deflated*. In this way, the lower cuff is applied to an area of the arm which is anaesthetized. The double-cuff technique carries the risk of accidental early intravascular injection of local anaesthetic, as a result of a simple error in the order of cuff inflation and release and, in practice, it is of no great advantage for surgery of short duration.

Contraindications

These include the presence of severe neurological or vascular disease in the limb, where use of a tourniquet may worsen the condition, or the presence of haemolytic disease, especially sickle cell anaemia.

BRACHIAL PLEXUS ANAESTHESIA

There are three common approaches to local anaesthesia of the brachial plexus — the supraclavicular, the interscalene and the axillary (Chambers & Wildsmith 1994). The interscalene blocks the humerus, shoulder, elbow and lateral aspect of the forearm and hand but misses the medial aspects of the upper arm and therefore is not really appropriate for fractures of the humerus. Fractures of the forearm and hand may be managed satisfactorily using a supraclavicular approach which generally provides block below the elbow in more than 90% of cases. The axillary block occasionally misses the radial nerve and not infrequently misses the musculocutaneous nerve.

Supraclavicular block (Fig. 8.29)

This block is performed at the site where the plexus crosses the first rib.

Method. The patient lies with the head turned away from the site of injection. A point is located 1 cm above and immediately lateral to the mid-point of the clavicle. A fine needle, 5 cm in length, is inserted at this point, inclined at 80° to the skin and directed backwards, inwards and downwards. Paraesthesia indicates contact with the plexus. In the absence of paraesthesia the needle is 'walked' along the rib. It is possible to explore all three main divisions of the plexus, producing paraesthesia in the upper and lower arm and in both sides of the hand. A volume of 8–10 ml of 1.5% lignocaine or prilocaine with adrenaline (1:200 000) is injected into each division.

The limitations of this technique are as follows:

1 The point of injection often does not lie over the first rib.

2 The incidence of pneumothorax is 0.5–6.0%.

3 The subclavian perivascular space is deep and very narrow in its anteroposterior dimension. Thus, the needle is directed across the space at its narrowest diameter, with reduced chance of successful block.

4 The trunks of the plexus tend to lie one on top of the other and not one behind each other in a horizontal plane. Consequently, large volumes of solution may be deposited outside the sheath causing block of phrenic, vagus, recurrent laryngeal and sympathetic nerves — the latter gives rise to Horner's syndrome.

Interscalene block (Fig. 8.30)

The roots of the brachial and cervical plexuses travel between the scalene muscles in the interscalene space. The major part of this space is above the subclavian artery and is ideally suited for plexus blockade.

Method. The patient lies with the head turned away from the side of injection. A line is taken from the level of the cricoid cartilage (C6 level) laterally to the interscalene groove which is identified just lateral to the sternomastoid. At this point a 1.5 in. 22-gauge needle is introduced at right angles to all planes of the skin. The direction of the needle is slightly caudal, posterior and medial. Advancement produces paraesthesia or the needle comes up against the transverse process of the cervical vertebrae.

In the adult, 20 ml of solution injected at this level produces anaesthesia of the cervical and brachial plexuses. Ulnar nerve block may be delayed or absent with this volume, but not if the volume is increased to 40 ml. However, a small volume may be combined with ulnar nerve block at the elbow if a minimal dose of drug is required.

The advantages of this technique are:

1 In the obese patient the block is easier to perform than other approaches to the brachial plexus.

2 It is ideal for shoulder manipulations where high block and good muscle relaxation are produced with a small dose.

3 Pneumothorax is obviated.

The disadvantages include:

1 Slow onset or absence of ulnar nerve block.

2 Subarachnoid and extradural injection may occur.

3 Vertebral artery injection may occur; in this case, the drug is taken straight to the brain. Fatalities have occurred with small volumes of local analgesia solution injected here.

4 Bilateral blockade must be avoided because of frequent phrenic nerve block.

Axillary brachial plexus block (Fig. 8.31)

This is the easiest block of the brachial plexus to perform

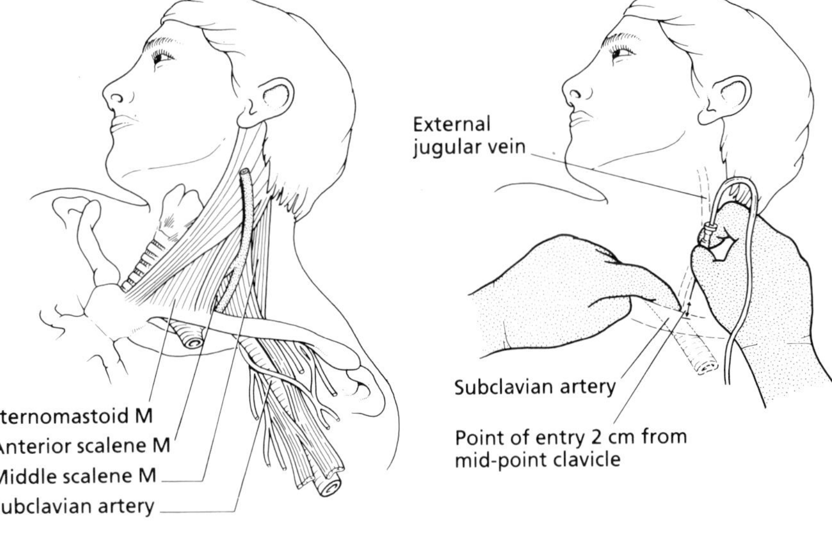

Fig. 8.29 Supraclavicular brachial plexus block. If the artery is palpable the operator's index finger palpates the artery and a needle is inserted backwards, inwards and downwards; paraesthesiae are usually elicited within 1–2 cm of insertion. If paraesthesiae are not evinced, the needle may contact the rib and 'walk' along the rib.

and it is devoid of the serious complication of pneumothorax. Despite the use of large volumes of local anaesthetic solution, the circumflex humeral and musculocutaneous nerves are commonly missed.

Technique. With the patient supine, and the arm abducted to 90° the axillary artery is located and traced until it passes behind the anterior wall of the axilla. With the operator's index finger on the artery, a single injection is made just above the vessel with the needle inclined cephalad. A volume of 30–40 ml of 1% lignocaine or 1.5% prilocaine (with adrenaline) should be injected.

The disadvantages of the axillary approach are that it cannot be used if a patient cannot abduct the arm; intravascular injection is possible and the technique may be difficult in obese patients. However, it obviates the possibility of pneumothorax or block of the phrenic, vagus or recurrent laryngeal nerves or the stellate ganglion; these are complications of all supraclavicular routes.

OTHER PERIPHERAL NERVE BLOCKS FOR THE UPPER LIMB

Nerves may be blocked either at the elbow or at the wrist. Because these involve multiple injections, they are rarely as satisfactory as a good brachial plexus block. Rather, they tend to be used to supplement plexus anaesthesia or to provide analgesia during short procedures on the hand or fingers.

LOWER LIMB BLOCKS

Spinal and epidural anaesthetic techniques are the methods of choice for surgery on the hip and knee and for operations involving the femoral shaft. Nerves to the lower limb may be blocked singly or in combination and by a variety of routes which are discussed in standard textbooks of local anaesthesia.

COMPLICATIONS OF REGIONAL BLOCKS

Inadequate block

The rate of onset of a block may be relatively slow. Peripheral nerve blocks with long-acting agents may take up to 45 minutes to develop, but where a block is only partially developed it may be possible to perform peripheral supplementation.

If a block is persistently inadequate it may be possible to provide satisfactory analgesia by giving the patient small quantities of intravenous opioids. Care should be taken to avoid excessive dosage, otherwise respiratory obstruction and depression or regurgitation and aspiration may occur. The easiest way to deal with an inadequate block may be to induce general anaesthesia. This represents the most valid reason for routine starvation of all patients prior to regional anaesthetic techniques.

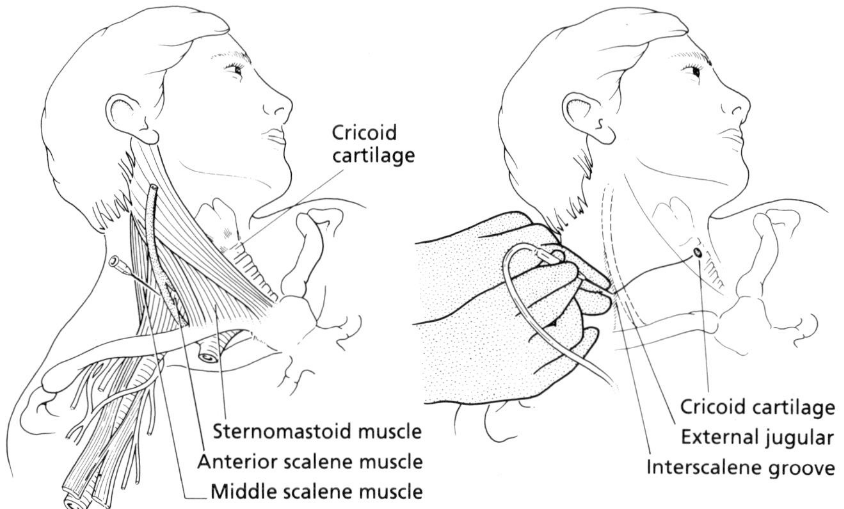

Fig. 8.30 The interscalene block. The posterior border of the sternomastoid is palpated and the interscalene groove is palpated posterior to this with the index finger. At the level of the cricoid cartilage a needle is inserted perpendicular to the skin (i.e. inwards, 45° caudad and slightly backwards. Paraesthesiae are elicited, usually within 2.5 cm of insertion.

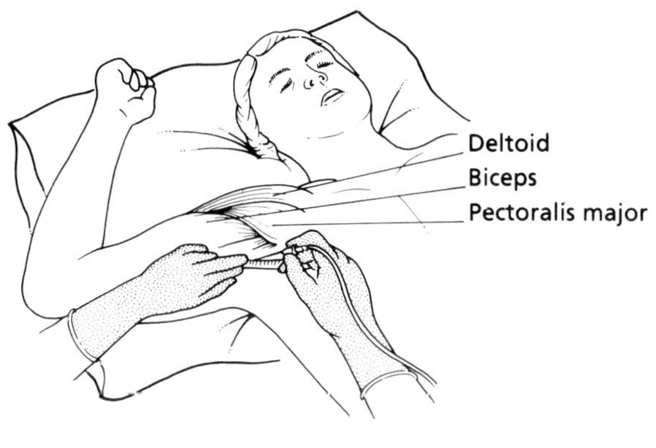

(a) Approach

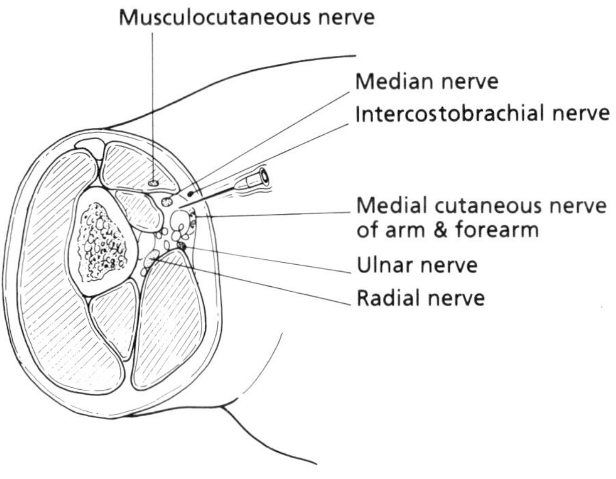

(b) Anatomy

Fig. 8.31 Axillary approach to brachial plexus. With the finger palpating the axillary artery as high as possible, a needle is inserted to enter the axillary sheath just above the artery. Penetration of the axillary sheath is usually felt by the operator. Because of fibrous bands within the sheath, some authorities recommend a second injection just below the artery. A few millilitres of solution are deposited in the subcutaneous tissue upon withdrawal in order to block the intercostobrachial nerve and its communications with the medial cutaneous nerve of the arm.

Central nervous system toxicity

The frequency of CNS toxic reactions to local anaesthetic drugs is extremely low if the techniques are applied carefully. However, reactions do occur and do account for morbidity and mortality unless immediate resuscitative measures are applied.

CNS toxicity may be manifest by twitches, followed by convulsions with cessation of respiration and development of hypoxia, hypercapnia and metabolic acidosis. It should be noted that the toxic effects of a mixture of two local anaesthetics are additive.

Signs of impending neurotoxicity include light-headedness, nausea, sleepiness and disorientation. Early signs include dysarthria, sweating, vomiting, aggressiveness, loquaciousness and drowsiness.

The commonest causes of toxic reactions are: an inadvertent intravenous injection, extra-vascular administration of an excessive dose or injection of a lower dose to a highly vascular area. It is therefore important to aspirate before injection of local anaesthetic solution.

If CNS toxicity does occur, it is essential to:
1 Maintain a clear airway.
2 Institute ventilation of the lungs with oxygen using an Ambu bag and mask.
3 Control the convulsions by administration of thiopentone or diazepam. Administration of these drugs will invariably be subsequently accompanied by profound respiratory depression and it will be essential to ventilate the lungs with oxygen. Alternatively, suxamethonium may be administered and the trachea intubated.

Cardiovascular toxicity of local anaesthetics

Mild overdosage leads to stimulation of the cardiovascular system which is followed, in higher dosage, by severe cardiovascular depression. In the event of profound cardiac depression, treatment of the situation may be similar to that for cardiac arrest, including external cardiac massage.

Allergic reaction to local anaesthetic drugs

Allergic reactions to local anaesthetic drugs are very uncommon. If allergy is suspected, the patient should be referred to the Immunology department for full investigation. Cross-sensitivity occurs between some local anaesthetic agents and advice should be sought before alternative local anaesthetic agents are selected.

Systemic complications of adrenaline

The maximum dosage of adrenaline used in any local block should not exceed 200 µg (i.e. 40 ml of a 1:200 000 solution). Intravenous injection of such a dose may lead to ventricular fibrillation. Because of the dangers of adrenaline overdosage, other vasoconstrictors without sympathomimetic properties, e.g. Felypressin, may be used, although these are not as effective as adrenaline.

In the event of adrenaline overdosage giving rise to tachycardia, hypertension, etc., oxygen should be administered to control tachycardia and glyceryl trinitrate should be given sublingually if the patient experiences angina.

Hypotension

The commonest cause of hypotension with regional anaesthetic techniques is sympathetic blockade produced by high spinal or epidural anaesthesia.

Neurological sequelae

These may be produced by intraneural injection, faulty positioning, incorrect use of a tourniquet and damage caused when eliciting paraesthesiae.

Nerve damage does not occur following extraneural injection of local anaesthetics, but intraneural injection may give rise to prolonged or permanent neural blockade. The risk of complication is increased if adrenaline is present. Common causes of nerve damage include surgical trauma, compression, stretch and ischaemic injury to the nerves.

Miscellaneous complications

Needles may break, particularly where the shaft joins the hub, in the tissue. This is prevented by a good technique. Infection is an uncommon complication of regional anaesthesia and haematoma rarely causes problems.

References

Buck, N., Devlin, H.B. & Lunn, J.N. *Confidential Enquiry into Perioperative Deaths*. 1987.

Campling, E.A., Devlin, H.B., Hoile, R.W. & Lunn, J.N. *Report of the National Enquiry in Perioperative Deaths*, 1991/2. National Confidential Enquiry in Perioperative Deaths: London, 1993.

Chambers, W.A. & Wildsmith, J.A.W. Upper limb. In: Nimmo, W.S., Rowbotham, D.J. & Smith, G. (eds) *Anaesthesia* 2nd edn. Blackwell Scientific Publications: Oxford, 1994.

Covino, B.G. & Wildsmith, J.A.W. General considerations, toxicity and complications of local anaesthesia. In: Nimmo, W.S., Rowbotham, D.J. & Smith, G. (eds) *Anaesthesia* 2nd edn. Blackwell Scientific Publications: Oxford, 1994.

Derrington, M.C. & Smith, G. A review of study of anaesthetic risk, morbidity and mortality. *Br J Anaesth* 1987; **59**: 815–834.

Fee, J.P.H. & McCaughey, W. Preoperative preparation, premedication and concurrent drug therapy. In: Nimmo, W.S., Rowbotham, D.J. & Smith, G. (eds) *Anaesthesia* 2nd edn. Blackwell Scientific Publications: Oxford, 1994.

Goldman, L. Assessment of the patient with known or suspected ischaemic heart disease for non-cardiac surgery. *Br J Anaesth* 1988; **61**: 38–43.

Greiff, J.M.C. & Cousins, M.J. Subarachnoid and extradural anaesthesia. In: Nimmo, W.S., Rowbotham, D.J. & Smith, G. (eds) *Anaesthesia* 2nd edn. Blackwell Scientific Publications: Oxford, 1994.

Krechel, S.W. Anaesthesia and the elderly patient. In: Nimmo, W.S., Rowbotham, D.J. & Smith, G. (eds) *Anaesthesia* 2nd edn. Blackwell Scientific Publications: Oxford, 1994.

Turner, D.A.B. Emergency anaesthesia. In Smith, G. & Aitkenhead, A.R. (eds) *Textbook of Anaesthesia*. Churchill Livingstone: Edinburgh, 1985.

The Tourniquet

L.KLENERMAN

The need for a tourniquet in the surgical management of an injured limb must always be carefully considered. One must remember that it is possible to superimpose a vascular insult on an already damaged limb. It may be possible to avoid the use of a tourniquet altogether in operations on a subcutaneous bone, such as the tibia. A tourniquet should only be applied to a limb that has a normal blood supply and no evidence of ischaemic disease. If there is any doubt, the pressure index should be measured using a Doppler probe, i.e. the ratio of ankle to brachial systolic blood pressure (the normal is ± 1). Extra care and vigilance in the use of a tourniquet is needed where patients have suffered acute haemorrhage or hypoxia, as experimental evidence indicates that the tolerance for increased tissue pressure may be reduced in these subjects (Matsen *et al.* 1981). Where fractures and joint injuries have occurred, tissue pressure is also likely to have been raised as a result of bleeding from the damaged structures.

Types of pneumatic tourniquet

There are two distinct types of pneumatic tourniquet; those which are inflated by direct hand pumping and those which are 'automatic', allowing the cuff to be inflated by the movement of a switch which controls an air/gas supply. There is no place in present-day practice for the use of an Esmarch bandage as a tourniquet, because there is no accurate method of controlling the pressure applied to the limb.

Whatever type of tourniquet is used, it is essential that regular checks, not less frequent than once a month, are made of the accuracy of pressure gauges against a mercury manometer. This is of particular importance with manually operated units, as an accidental drop on the floor or a knock against an operation table can easily damage the aneroid gauge.

Before the application of a tourniquet, it is necessary to exsanguinate the limb to obtain the maximum benefit of a bloodless field. Three methods are available:

1 Simple elevation of the limb to a vertical position.

The maximum decrease in volume occurs within 15–20 seconds (Di Stefano *et al.* 1974). Hinman (1945) has suggested that compensatory vasodilatation occurs after 3 minutes. Elevation is the method of choice where there is infection, in the presence of a neoplasm and in a lower limb immobilized for a week or more, because of the danger of producing pulmonary emboli (Austin 1963, Hoffmann & Wyatt 1985).

2 The use of an Esmarch bandage applied firmly from the distal end of the limb to the level of the tourniquet is common practice. Its disadvantages are that it requires two people, one to hold the limb and the other to apply the bandage. It is difficult to use where there is a fracture and it is possible that, if applied with excessive tension, it could be responsible for nerve damage.

3 The Rhys-Davies exsanguinator has become available during the past few years (Rhys-Davies & Stotter 1985). This is an inflated elastic cylinder which is rolled on to the limb to produce exsanguination (Fig. 8.34). It can be applied single-handed. The degree of inflation may be affected by stretching of the elastomer with time, and can be checked by measurement of the external circumference. Reflation and measurement of the inflation pressure are carried out via a needle through a valve in the wall of the exsanguinator with a connection to a sphygmomanometer. From the surgeon's viewpoint, the degree of exsanguination is the same as that produced by an Esmarch bandage.

The tourniquet cuff should always be applied to the proximal part of the limb, so that there is the maximum bulk of soft tissue for the protection of the major peripheral nerves. One should be aware of the scraggy limb of a patient with rheumatoid arthritis or the thin arm of a child. Padding, in the form of plaster wool, is a useful precaution. The duration of tourniquet ischaemia is always emphasized but the pressure used is equally important. The rule should be to always use the lowest effective pressure. In clinical practice, the cuffs in common use are somewhat narrower than the ideal blood pressure cuff, in order to allow ready access to the surgically draped limb. The wider the cuff, the more diffuse (and safe) is the pressure transmitted to the underlying structures. An unusually wide tourniquet cuff, 12.5 cm as compared with 9 cm, has recently become available (Stelle-Werner U.K., Woking, Surrey), and it has been shown that it can reliably control arterial inflow at an inflation pressure significantly lower than that needed in a narrower cuff (Newman & Muirhead 1986). Until the wider cuff becomes more generally adopted, one should add 50 mmHg pressure to the resting blood pressure of the patient for tourniquet application to the upper limb and simply double the systolic pressure for the cuff applied to the lower limb, provided that the patient is normotensive and not unduly obese (Klenerman & Hulands 1979). The duration of application of the tourniquet and the pressure used should be recorded in the operation note.

Three hours is the upper limit of time for which it is safe to leave a tourniquet in place, and it should be possible to complete the majority of procedures well within this period (Klenerman *et al.* 1980). Release of the tourniquet for 5 minutes after application for 1½ hours has been advocated by Sapega *et al.* (1985) if the tourniquet is likely to be needed for 3 hours. It is suggested from this study in dogs, in the absence of peripheral vascular disease and traumatized soft tissues, that this breathing period reduces the chances of irreversible damage to muscle.

Complications

Swelling

The main effect of the prolonged application of a tourniquet is the production of swelling of the limb. This results from a combination of oedema, produced as a result of anoxia of capillary endothelium, and bleeding. Because of this, the limb feels stiff and the muscles are weak (Patterson *et al.* 1981). Release of the tourniquet to secure haemostasis before closure of the wound, and closing of the skin only, not fascia, is to be re-

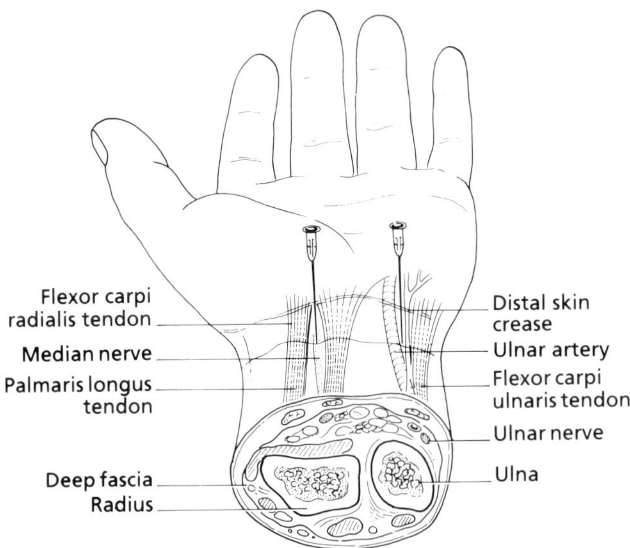

Fig. 8.32 Performance of a wrist block. The median and ulnar nerves may be blocked at the wrist by deposition of small volumes of local anaesthetic. In addition, the radial nerve requires blockade by infiltration into the 'anatomical snuff box' using 2–3 ml of solution in the whole 'snuff box'.

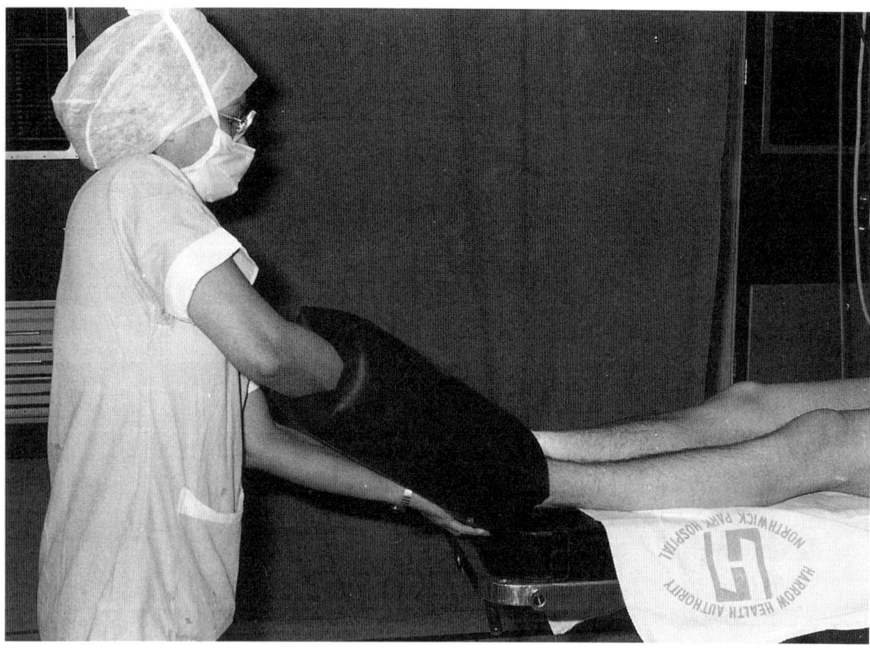

Fig. 8.33 To show the Rhys-Davies exsanguinator and its application by passing it from the arm of the operator on to the limb of the subject.

commended. Adequate allowance for postoperative swelling must be made by the application of well-padded dressings, and by never immobilizing the limb in a complete plaster cast after an operation under a tourniquet; a plaster back-slab or a split plaster is mandatory. Failure to allow for postoperative swelling and increased intracompartmental pressure after prolonged use of a tourniquet may result in a compartment syndrome and, if untreated, lead to a Volkmann's ischaemic contracture. It should be remembered that it may take 12, or even 24, hours for the maximum changes to occur.

Nerve damage

The incidence of damage to peripheral nerves from the use of a tourniquet has been estimated to be 1:8000, with a somewhat higher figure of 1:5000 for the upper limb compared with 1:13000 for the lower limb (Middleton & Varian 1974). All the lower limb palsies were due to the use of an Esmarch bandage as a tourniquet. The arm palsies fell into two groups: one where all three nerves (median, ulnar and radial) were involved below the tourniquet, and a second with isolated radial nerve lesions.

Although upper limb palsies are most common, the lower limb can also be affected, as noted above, even with the use of pneumatic tourniquets. Rorabeck and Kennedy (1980) record five patients with sciatic nerve palsy after operations for knee ligament repair. The significant point about this report was that the tourni-

quet pressure used in all cases was 500 mmHg, which is a higher pressure than is optimal for the average thigh. The cause of nerve damage is abnormally high cuff pressure and, when a pneumatic cuff is used, the usual cause is a faulty gauge (Bruner 1951, Hamilton & Sokoll 1967, Prevoznick 1970, Fry 1972). This may occur both with the aneroid gauges of hand-operated tourniquets or Bourdon gauges of the pneumatic type. The effect is a localized nerve conduction block produced by deformation of nerve fibres (Fowler *et al.* 1972, Ochoa *et al.* 1972). Large myelinated fibres only are affected. This explains the relative sparing of sensation (Gilliatt 1975). The level of tourniquet pressure is more important in the cause of tourniquet paralysis than is the length of time for which the tourniquet has been in place. Fortunately, most tourniquet paralyses recover in about 6 months, and permanent damage is exceptional, (Spiegel & Lewin 1945).

Vascular damage

Damage from pressure on an underlying artery is rare (Giannestras *et al.* 1977), as is an undetected arterial injury from operative dissection (Scott 1955, Webb-Jones 1955). Routine deflation of the tourniquet before the wound is closed should enable one to identify any undue bleeding as a result of a cut vessel. One must be aware of the occasional presence of calcified vessels in the thigh which may be incompressible by a tourniquet cuff inflated to the maximum pressure. This is only likely to occur in the elderly, and the presence of calcified vessels on radiographs should be a warning (Klenerman & Lewis 1976, Jeyaseelan *et al.* 1981, Irvine & Chan 1986).

It is often thought that there is a danger in applying a tourniquet to the limb of a patient with sickle cell disease and thus producing a crisis. Bloodless surgery in the presence of sickle cell disease should be preceded by careful exsanguination of the limb before inflation of the tourniquet. The safety of this recommendation has not been documented in the literature, but the author has been informed by experienced surgeons working in areas where sickle cell disease is common that no problems have arisen by following this technique. Sickle cell trait alone does not itself add any risk.

For surgeons working in Accident departments, it should be remembered, when carrying out an intravenous regional block, that despite the fact that a tourniquet cuff is inflated above systolic pressure, drug leakage can occur. Areas of low pressure exist under tourniquet cuffs and, with a rapid injection, venous pressure rises during injection of the local anaesthetic. When an area of low surface pressure is aligned with a superficial vein, leakage of an injected drug may occur. For this reason, all injections for this procedure should be at the distal end of the limb (Sayegh & Gough 1984).

Digital tourniquets

Numerous techniques have been described for the application of a digital tourniquet, which is an indispensable adjunct in surgery of the hand. Excessive pressure may damage the digital vessels (Dove & Clifford 1982) or traumatize the nerves. Studies using a pressure transducer (Hixson *et al.* 1986) have shown that, using a rubber band (or soft rubber catheter) or a Penrose drain, the pressures produced were often in excess of 500 mmHg. By applying the appropriate finger cut from a rubber glove with its tip removed, it was possible to have a thin rubber cylinder which is rolled from distal to proximal on the injured finger, producing exsanguination. Then, rolled up at the base of the digit, it acts as a tourniquet. The use of a glove, equal to the subject's hand size, uniformly generated pressures under 500 mmHg. However, many variables can influence the pressures that are generated with a rolled surgical glove. First, there is the problem of defining the appropriate glove size for the patient. Secondly, gloves differ in thickness and the material properties could vary from manufacturer to manufacturer. Thirdly, the number of rolls depends on the length of the digit and the amount of glove fingertip removed. The overlapping folds of the rolled glove finger can create high pressures

(Shaw *et al.* 1985). In view of these observations, it is recommended that the safest digital tourniquet is a 0.5 in. Penrose drain stretched to no more than 50% strain.

A miniature pneumatic tourniquet cuff inflated by a syringe has been developed. The air in the syringe can be compressed to a known pressure and held by a spring housing (Tountas 1986). Clearly, this is the safest possible technique and it is hoped that it will become commercially available.

References

Austin, M. The Esmarch bandage and pulmonary embolism. *J Bone Joint Surg* 1963; **45B**: 384−385.

Bruner, J.W. Safety factors in the use of the pneumatic tourniquet for haemostasis in surgery of the hand. *J Bone Joint Surg* 1951; **33A**: 221−224.

Di Stefano, V., Nixon, J.E. & Stone, R.H. Bio-electrical impedance plethysomography as an investigative tool in orthopaedic surgery. *Clin Orthop* 1974; **99**: 203−206.

Dove, A.F. & Clifford, R.P. Ischaemia after use of finger tourniquet. *Br Med J* 1982; **284**: 1162−1163.

Fowler, T.J., Danta, G. & Gilliatt, R.W. Recovery of nerve conduction after a pneumatic tourniquet: observations on the hind limbs of baboons. *J Neurol Neurosurg Psych* 1972; **35**: 638−647.

Fry, D. Inaccurate tourniquet gauges. *Br Med J* 1972; **1**: 151.

Giannestras, N.J., Crawley, J.J. & Lentz, M. Occlusion of the tibial artery after a foot operation under tourniquet. *J Bone Joint Surg* 1977; **59A**: 682−683.

Gilliatt, R.W. Peripheral nerve compression and entrapment. In: Lant, A.J. (ed.) *Proceedings of a Conference held at the Royal College of Physicians of London.* Pitman: London, 1975.

Hamilton, W.K. & Sokoll, M.D. Tourniquet paralysis. *J Am Med Assoc* 1967; **199**: 37.

Hinman, F. The rational use of tourniquets. *Surg Gynecol Obstet* 1945; **81**: 357−366.

Hixson, F.P., Shafiroff, B.B., Werner, F.W. & Palmer, A.K. Digital tourniquets: a pressure study with clinical relevance. *J Hand Surg* 1986; **11A**: 600−601.

Hoffmann, A.A. & Wyatt, R.W.B. Fatal pulmonary embolism following tourniquet inflation. *J Bone Joint Surg* 1985; **67A**: 633−634.

Irvine, G.B. & Chan, R.N.W. Arterial calcification and tourniquets. *Lancet* 1986; **ii**: 127.

Jeyaseelan, S., Stevenson, T.M. & Pfitzner, J. Tourniquet failure and arterial calcification. *Anaesthesia* 1981; **36**: 48−50.

Klenerman, L. & Hulands, G.H. Tourniquet pressures for the lower limb. *J Bone Joint Surg* 1979; **61B**: 124.

Klenerman, L. & Lewis, J. Incompressible vessels. *Lancet* 1976; **i**: 811.

Klenerman, L., Biswas, M., Rhodes, A. & Hulands, G.H. Systemic and local effects of the application of a tourniquet. *J Bone Joint Surg* 1980; **62B**: 385−388.

Matsen, F.A., Wyss, C.R., King, R.V., Barnes, D. & Simmons, C.W. Factors affecting the tolerance of muscle circulation and function for increased tissue pressure. *Clin Orthop* 1981; **155**: 224−230.

Middleton, R.W.D. & Varian, J.P.W. Tourniquet paralysis. *Aust N Z J Surg* 1974; **44**: 124−128.

Newman, R.J. & Muirhead, A. A safe and effective low-pressure tourniquet. A prospective evaluation. *J Bone Joint Surg* 1986; **68B**: 625−628.

Ochoa, J., Fowler, T.J. & Gilliatt, R.W. Anatomical changes in peripheral nerves compressed by a pneumatic tourniquet. *J Anat* 1972; **113**: 433−455.

Patterson, S., Klenerman, L., Biswas, M. & Rhodes, A. The effect of pneumatic tourniquets on skeletal muscle physiology. *Acta Orthop Scand* 1981; **52**: 171−175.

Prevoznik, S.J. Injury from use of pneumatic tourniquets. *Anaesthesiology* 1970; **32**: 177.

Rhys-Davies, N.L. & Stotter, A.T. A safe and effective low pressure tourniquet. *Ann R Coll Surg Engl* 1985; **67**: 193−195.

Rorabeck, C.H. & Kennedy, J.C. Tourniquet-induced nerve ischaemia complicating knee ligament surgery. *Am J Sports Med* 1980; **8**: 98−102.

Sapega, A.A., Heppenstall, R.B., Chance, B., Park, Y.S. & Sokolow, D. Optimizing tourniquet application and release times in extremity surgery. *J Bone Joint Surg* 1985; **67A**: 303−314.

Sayegh, A. & Gough, S.G. *Evaluation of Automatic Cuffs.* University of Salford, Department of Orthopaedic Mechanics 1984, SEV/54/01/1.

Scott, J.H.S. Traumatic aneurysm of the peroneal artery. *J Bone Joint Surg* 1955; **37B**: 439.

Shaw, J.A., De Muth, W.W. & Gillespy, A.W. Guidelines for the use of digital tourniquets based on physiological measurements. *J Bone Joint Surg* 1985; **67A**: 1086−1090.

Spiegel, I.J. & Lewin, P. Tourniquet paralysis. *J Am Med Assoc* 1945; **129**: 432−435.

Tountas, C.P. A disposable pneumatic digital tourniquet. *J Hand Surg* 1986; **11A**: 600−601.

Webb-Jones, A. Aneurysm after foot stabilisation. *J Bone Joint Surg* 1955; **37B**: 440.

9: Management of Open Fractures

The principles of internal and external fixation

R.J.LANGSTAFF, P.H.WORLOCK
AND J.K.WEBB

I can say from experience, that even the best visceral operation never gave me as much satisfaction as the successful treatment of a difficult fracture [Billroth 1866].

Introduction

In the management of the open fracture the surgeon and the patient should have a clear understanding of the objectives of treatment. In simple terms the aim is the restoration of function, not only of the injured part but also of the individual in society. It is no longer good enough to consider outcome in terms of the 'inevitable minimal acceptable deformity'. In today's increasingly litigious age it is, however, imperative that realistic expectations exist on both sides and that patient and surgeon understand the limitations, the risks and the likely course of any management proposed. An open fracture still constitutes a major cause of morbidity, often in the most economically active members of society.

The management of such fractures demands the highest degree of skill, knowledge and commitment on the part of the surgeon if the best possible outcome is to be achieved and iatrogenic complications avoided. Ignorance of modern methods of fracture care too often results in stiff joints, wasted muscles, mal- or non-union and a disabled patient. Surgeons who are incapable of understanding and applying the full range of therapeutic manoeuvres in these most difficult cases should arrange early transfer of the injured to those who are capable of such care.

The general principles of open fracture management are simple:

1 Classification of the injury.
2 Initial management of the soft tissue wound to prevent infection and further damage.
3 Selection of an appropriate method of skeletal stabilization to give stable fixation.
4 Achieve early soft tissue cover.
5 Early movement and rehabilitation of the limb.

Classification of injuries

A number of attempts have been made to classify open fractures and their soft tissue injuries (Allgower 1971, Gustilo & Anderson 1976, Gustilo *et al.* 1984, Tscherne 1984). Whichever system is chosen, it should be logical in that it should be predictive of the likely outcome, and indicative in that it should aid the surgeon in the decision-making process, helping in selection of the most appropriate form of treatment. It should be repeatable with minimal inter- and intra-observer variation and it should be comprehensive without being too complex. The system devised by Gustilo is probably in most common use (Tables 9.1 & 9.2). This grading can only be done at the surgical debridement.

Wound infection rates and eventual outcome have been shown to correlate well with these classification systems, ranging from 2% in type I fractures to 50% in type IIIB and with an amputation rate in IIIC fractures of 50–70% (Gustilo *et al.* 1987, Dellinger *et al.* 1988).

Classification systems should not be blindly applied. Thought must be given to the energy of the injury and to the situation of the fracture. Consideration of the soft tissue envelope surrounding a fracture and the *possible* degree of damage done to it in association with the fracture is less likely to result in misclassification than simply considering the size of the wound. With this in mind the Association for Osteosynthesis (AO) group have recently introduced a classification of open fractures (see Table 9.3). This grading is carried out at surgery and accurately identifies the severity of damage to the skin, musculotendonous units and neurovascular

Table 9.1 Classification of open fractures (after Gustilo & Anderson 1976)

Type I
Clean puncture wound <1 cm
Minimal muscle contusion
No crushing injury
Simple fracture without contamination

Type II
Laceration >1 cm without extensive soft tissue damage, flaps
 or avulsions
Minimal to moderate crushing injury
Simple fracture without comminution

Type III
Extensive soft tissue damage including skin, muscle and
 neurovascular structures
High-energy injury with severe crush
Comminuted fracture component (includes *all* segmental
 fractures, *all* fractures with bone loss, gunshot wounds,
 traumatic amputations and farm injuries with soil
 contamination)

Table 9.2 Classification of type III open fractures (after Gustilo *et al.* 1984)

Type	Definition	Infection rate (%)	Amputation rate (%)
IIIA	Adequate soft tissue coverage of bone despite extensive soft tissue laceration or flaps	4	0
IIIB	Extensive soft tissue injury with periosteal stripping and bone exposure; major wound contamination	52	16
IIIC	Any open fracture associated with an arterial injury requiring repair	42	42

Table 9.3 AO classification of open fractures (after Muller *et al.* 1991)

Skin lesions; integument open (IO)
IO 1   Skin breakage from inside out
IO 2   Skin breakage from outside in (<5 cm), contused
          edges
IO 3   Skin breakage >5 cm, increased contusion,
          devitalized edges
IO 4   Full-thickness contusion/abrasion *or* extensive open
          degloving *or* skin loss

Muscle/tendon injury (MT)
MT 1   No muscle injury
MT 2   Circumscribed muscle injury, one compartment only
MT 3   Considerable muscle injury, two compartments
MT 4   Muscle defect/tendon laceration/extensive muscle
          contusion
MT 5   Compartment syndrome/crush syndrome with wide
          injury zone

Neurovascular injury (NV)
NV 1   No neurovascular injury
NV 2   Isolated nerve injury
NV 3   Localized vascular injury
NV 4   Extensive, segmental vascular injury
NV 5   Combined neurovascular injury, including subtotal
          or total amputation

Initial wound management

The open fracture is an emergency, not in the immediate achievement of skeletal stability, but in the initial management of the soft tissues. The goal is the prevention of further wound contamination and further ischaemic damage. The aim is the conversion as rapidly as possible of the contaminated, contused wound into a clean wound. Current thinking has been well summarized by Tscherne (1984) and more recently by Worlock (1989). In the short term the objective is the avoidance of soft tissue and bone infection. In the long term the ideal is bony union and the restoration of normal soft tissue cover with minimal scarring.

Development of infection in a wound is dependent on a number of factors: the presence and degree of bacterial contamination, the virulence of the contaminating organisms, the presence of dead or dying tissue, the delay between injury and wound excision, the adequacy of wound excision and debridement, and finally the presence or absence of skeletal stability.

Bacterial contamination and virulence

Bacterial contamination of open fractures cannot be prevented. Swabs taken on arrival in hospital show that some 60–70% of all wounds have organisms present before the start of treatment (Patzakis & Ivler 1977). Once the patient has reached hospital further contam-

structures. It should be remembered that the deformity seen on admission to hospital is the residual deformity and may not represent the maximum deformity of the bony skeleton at the time of injury. A fractured long bone may protrude through the skin, contaminate the ends of the bone and then spontaneously reduce. Failure to appreciate the degree of contamination and carry out adequate wound excision and debridement may result in disaster. Indeed, the final grading of the open fracture can *only* be determined at surgery.

Tissue damage is proportional to the amount of energy absorbed by the limb at the time of injury. It is this concept which is fundamental to the philosophy of modern fracture management, and application of it will avoid undertreatment owing to failure to appreciate the severity of the initial injury. The essential consideration is in distinguishing between high- and low-energy injuries.

ination is preventable. Bacteriology swabs should be taken from the wound in the Accident department. The injury is then photographed with a Polaroid camera and the wound covered with a sterile dressing soaked in iodine (Fig. 9.1). This dressing should not be disturbed until the patient reaches the operating theatre. Any organisms grown subsequently may guide treatment if infection should develop. Tscherne *et al.* (1983) reported a reduction in wound infection rates from 19.2 to 4.3% using this technique.

The importance of quantitative bacterial contamination is harder to assess but the critical figure for the development of sepsis has been placed at 10^5 organisms per gram of tissue (Cooney *et al.* 1982). The presence of necrotic tissue and foreign bodies has been reported by Mader and Cierny (1984) to reduce this 'critical inoculum'. Logically, the more heavily contaminated a wound is the more rapidly the critical inoculum will be reached and contamination becomes infection. Contaminated wounds can accumulate 10^5 organisms per gram within 6 hours (Robson *et al.* 1973). In the

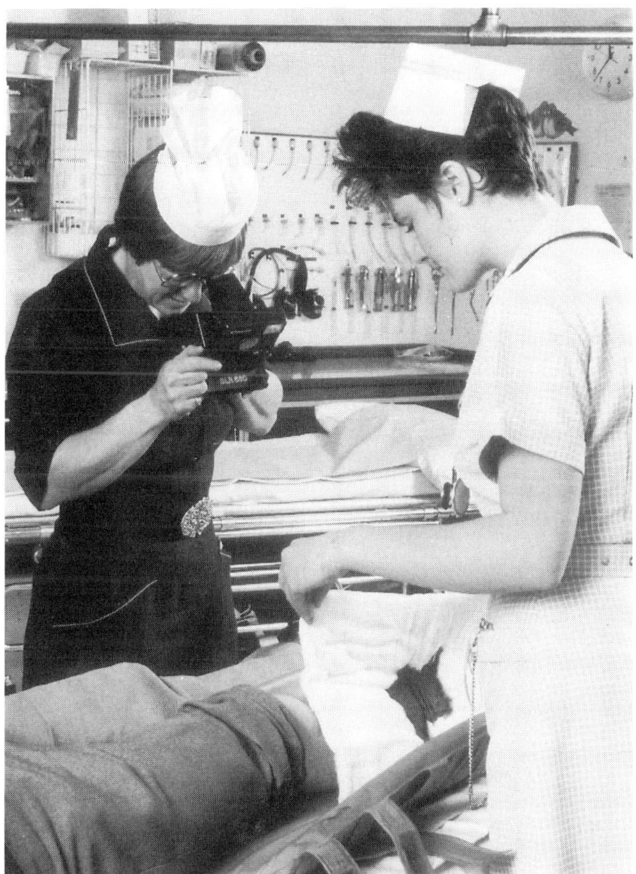

Fig. 9.1 On arrival in the Accident Unit, the wound is photographed with a Polaroid camera and then covered with a sterile dressing. (Reproduced with permission from Worlock 1989.)

clinical situation increased wound infection rates have been demonstrated with a delay in treatment.

Antibiotic policy

Experimental studies have shown that to achieve maximum effect, antibiotics should be present in the tissues at the time of injury (Burke 1961). This is obviously not achievable *in vivo*. Experimentally, Worlock *et al.* (1988) have shown that antibiotics administered post injury do have an effect up to 4 hours after the initial contamination. In clinical trials, Patzakis *et al.* (1974) showed that high-dose cephalosporins were effective in reducing infection after open fracture.

Staphylococcus aureus is still the main contaminating organism, but attention should be paid to the circumstances of the injury. A first- or second-generation cephalosporin is recommended for types I and II injuries, and either a third-generation cephalosporin or a first- or second-generation cephalosporin plus an aminoglycoside for type III injuries (which have an increased incidence of Gram-negative infections) (Gustilo *et al.* 1984). Metronidazole should be added if significant anaerobic contamination is suspected. Treatment should be for no longer than 3 days and in many units is only for 24 hours. There is no evidence that prolonging the treatment course results in lower infection rates (Patzakis *et al.* 1983).

Wound surgery

The objective of wound surgery has been stated to be the conversion of a contaminated wound to a clean surgical wound by the excision of all dead or dying tissue and the removal of all foreign material. This is the process of wound excision. The term debridement is widely and incorrectly used to describe this process. Debridement originates from the French 'debrider', meaning 'to unbridle'; this more properly refers to the process of fasciotomy, a secondary, but equally important, phase of wound care. Wound surgery should always be considered in two phases; wound excision and fasciotomy.

Wound excision

The sterile dressing is removed in the operating theatre and the wound thoroughly irrigated using Hartman's or Ringer's solution. A simple gravity feed via an intravenous giving set works well (Fig. 9.2). Between 4 and 10 litres is recommended, depending on the degree of contamination. The limb may be scrubbed; indeed, this is mandatory where skin surrounding wounds has

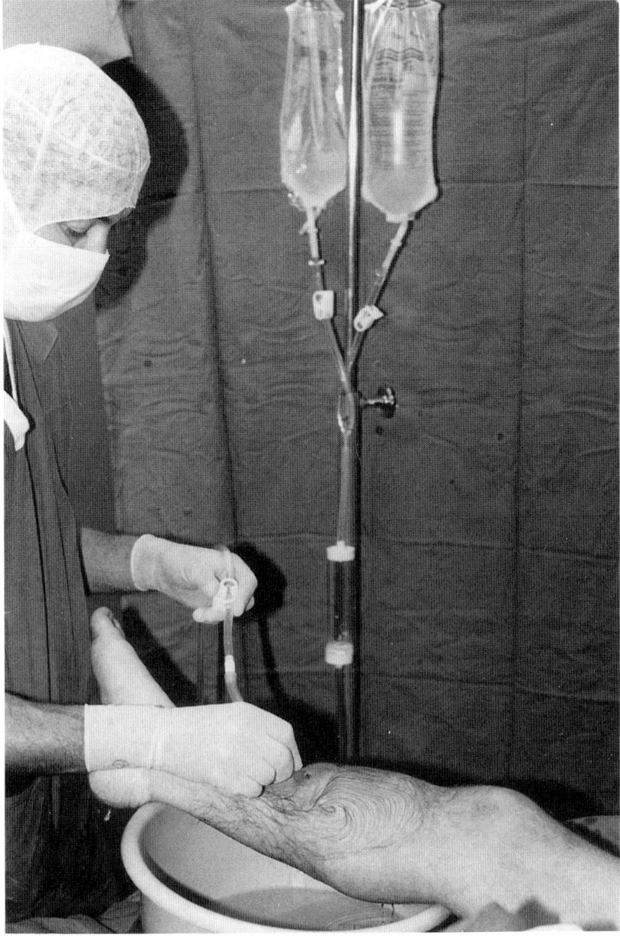

Fig. 9.2 After removal of the sterile dressing in the operating theatre, the wound is irrigated with Hartmann's solution. The sterile end of the intravenous giving set is used to probe the depths of the wound, washing out debris. (Reproduced with permission from Worlock 1989.)

been subjected to road burns and impregnated with dirt. Failure to carry out this procedure will result in the most unsightly tattooing of the skin. Having cleaned the wound in this fashion the operative area is then prepared and draped in the usual fashion.

The operation is performed without a tourniquet as bleeding is a sign of viable tissue. However, it is helpful to have a tourniquet in place as this can be used to control any torrential haemorrhage. All dead tissue must be ruthlessly excised.

SOFT TISSUES

Skin

Skin survives trauma well and most wound edges need only marginal excision.

Fat

Fat survives much less well and should be widely excised.

Muscle

Similar considerations apply to muscle as to fat. Viability of muscle may be assessed by the four 'C's: *colour* — ischaemic muscle has an unhealthy purple sheen; *contractility* — viable muscle contracts when pinched with forceps; *consistency* — dead muscle loses its normal turgor and retains the imprint of the pinching forceps on its surface, with the consistency of a rather coarse paté; and *capillary bleeding* — when cut, viable muscle bleeds from the cut ends.

BONE

Detached bone fragments denuded of their soft tissue attachments should be discarded. Large articular fragments may have to be retained and replaced to rescue the joint. Wounds should be carefully explored for foreign material; a gloved finger is a gentle and highly sensitive instrument in such explorations. If possible, the opening up of previously undisturbed tissue planes and new dissection should be avoided.

Fasciotomy

With the primary process of wound excision completed the necessity of performing a fasciotomy should be considered. The aim is the avoidance of a compartment syndrome, which is a not uncommon complication (Blick *et al*. 1986). The belief that open fractures have performed an autodecompression is a false one. The decision to perform a fasciotomy must be based on a knowledge of the mechanism of injury. A crushing or blast injury is more likely to produce a compartment syndrome than is a low-energy injury producing a type I open fracture. The key is clinical suspicion (Gustilo *et al*. 1990) and it is for this reason that the surgeon is encouraged to consider debridement as a distinct process from that of wound excision. Remembering to 'unbridle' the tissues may help avoid what is still all too common a complication. If fasciotomy is performed it must be over the full length of the compartment and of an open type. There is no place in the management of trauma for the percutaneous fasciotomy.

Finally, the wound should be dressed, not packed, using fluffed-up gauze swabs (crani-swabs are ideal) which will absorb any exudate. The patient is returned to theatre 24–48 hours later for 'second-look surgery' when, under a further general anaesthetic, the dressings are removed and the process of wound excision is repeated. This process continues until the wound is clean and ready for obtaining soft tissue cover. The aim is to establish skin cover at an early stage, ideally by 5–7 days at the latest.

In general, no attempt should be made to close any contaminated wound immediately. Some authorities suggest that type I wounds may be excised and closed primarily if it is possible to do so *without tension*. If there is any doubt wounds should be left open, and although some workers have advocated primary closure of contaminated high-energy wounds after excision (Broome *et al.* 1989), the results are too frequently disastrous to be acceptable.

The principles of wound care outlined above are not new, but need frequent restating. They are basic, surgical tenets and should be familiar to all surgeons. Experience suggests they are not.

Skeletal stabilization

How the surgeon chooses to gain skeletal stability must be based on personal experience and familiarity with the techniques available. There is no room for the occasional operator in modern fracture surgery. Unfamiliarity with the increasingly complex equipment is liable to lead to disaster.

Skeletal stabilization that is rigid enough to permit early mobilization gives the patient the best opportunity for full functional recovery. Skeletal stabilization also reduces the risks of infection (Worlock *et al.* 1994), but absolute rigidity may not be the optimum environment for rapid bony union. Micromovement has a role to play in achieving bony union (Goodship & Kenwright 1985). Skeletal traction is not suitable for definitive management of open fractures and the methods considered here for obtaining skeletal stability are external stabilization with plaster, pins through plaster, external skeletal fixation, and internal fixation with plates, screws and intramedullary nails.

Plaster

Prolonged periods of immobilization in plaster for open fractures promote joint stiffness and prevent adequate wound care. Some workers feel that its use with open fractures is to be discouraged (Schatzker & Tile 1987), except in the simplest of circumstances. Sarmiento *et al.* (1989) have reported on a large, but selected, series of tibial shaft fractures, including open fractures, treated by cast bracing, early mobilization and weight bearing. They reported excellent results but conclude that of type III fractures 'very few are suitable for bracing'. The paper states that the type I and II fractures were initially treated with either an external fixator or a long leg cylinder but it does not make clear the numbers or percentages in each group. A significant proportion (17%) of the total number of patients was lost to follow-up, making difficult the drawing of conclusions from this particular study.

Pins through plaster

Pins in plaster as a method of treatment has in the past been widely used. This combination of fixation is a crude form of external fixation, offering all the disadvantages of plaster in terms of wound access, but none of the advantages of the more modern types of external fixation. We would not advocate it where alternatives are available.

External fixation

Use of the external fixator in Europe was described by Malgaigne in the early part of the nineteenth century. In the last 30 years the principles of, indications for and techniques used in external fixation have become better understood and their use more widespread. Behrens and Searls (1986) have lucidly summarized the terminology and biomechanics in this field and divide fixators into two major types; ring fixators and pin fixators, which have overlapping, but differing, indications for use.

In the West, for trauma care most surgeons use pin fixators. Ring fixators are used more frequently in the correction of deformity rather than in the primary care of the injured limb. External fixation may significantly reduce additional soft tissue trauma while stabilizing the fracture.

Types of external fixators

RING FIXATORS

The principal advantage over other types of fixation device is that multiplanar adjustment of the fracture fragments is possible after application of the device. Application is difficult and time consuming, and there is a higher incidence of complications associated with its use than with the half pin type of fixator. These devices may also be used for segmental bone transport to replace bone loss in open fractures.

PIN FIXATORS

Pin fixators can be divided into two groups on the basis of their adjustability; the simple type, in which each pin is connected directly to the rod (Fig. 9.3), and clamp fixators, in which pins are first connected to a clamp that is then connected to a rod (Fig. 9.4).

Biomechanics of external fixation

The theoretical background to external fixation has been comprehensively covered by Seligson and Pope (1982). Broadly speaking, fracture and fixator behaviour is dependent on fixator rigidity and the stability at the pin−bone interface.

FIXATOR RIGIDITY

In general terms, fixator rigidity is increased by increasing the number and diameter of pins, decreasing pin separation within pin groups and increasing the separation of those groups, increasing the number of bars and decreasing their separation, decreasing the distance from the bars to the skin, and by using bilateral devices with full pins rather than unilateral devices (Fig. 9.5).

PIN−BONE INTERFACE STABILITY

Chao and Pope (1982) listed a number of factors which influence pin−bone interface behaviour. These include:

(i) stresses arising at the pin−bone interface; (ii) pin geometry and thread design; and (iii) pin insertion techniques.

Pin−bone stress

Pin−bone stress is influenced to a major degree by fracture stability. Early weight-bearing should be avoided in unstable fractures. Attempts should be made to increase stability by maximizing cortical contact at the time of application of the fixator. A pair of reduction forceps applied across the fracture, if it is not grossly comminuted, will allow an accurate reduction to be held while the fixator is applied. The wound can be extended to allow accurate reduction.

Pin geometry and thread design

Pin geometry and thread design also affect pin−bone interface stability. Increasing the pin diameter increases pin stiffness, which is a function of the fourth power of the pin diameter. Full-pin, rather than half-pin, frame designs are more stable but suffer from the added complications, associated with full pins, of an increased incidence of damage to neurovascular structures and decreased joint mobility consequent on muscle group transfixion.

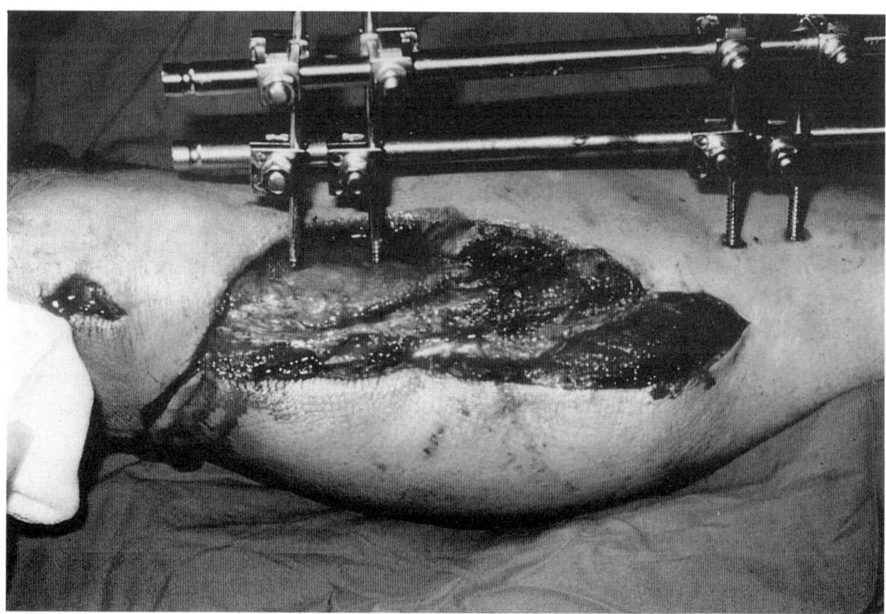

Fig. 9.3 With the AO tubular external fixator, each pin is connected directly to the rod(s).

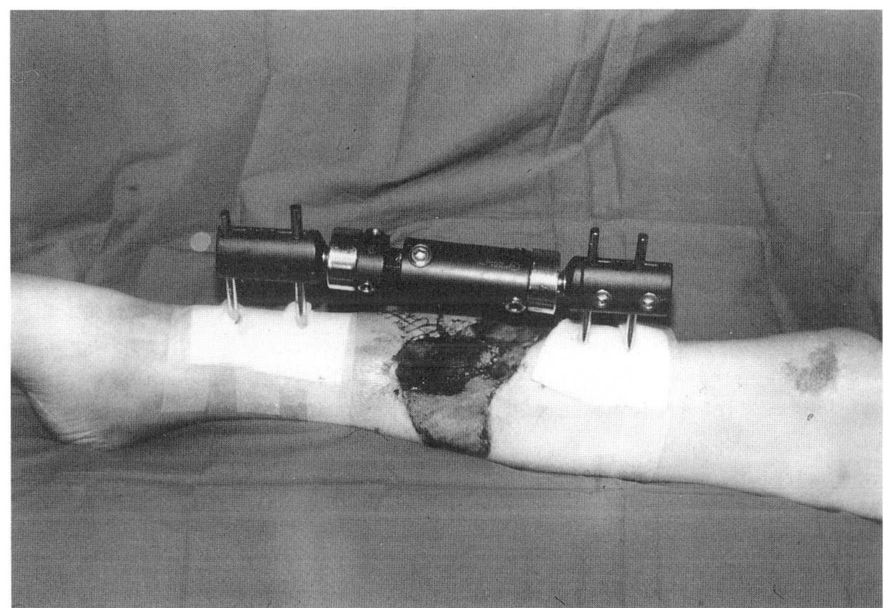

Fig. 9.4 An Orthofix external fixator. The pins are connected in a clamp, which is attached to the body of the external fixator by a lockable universal joint. (Produced with permission from Worlock 1989.)

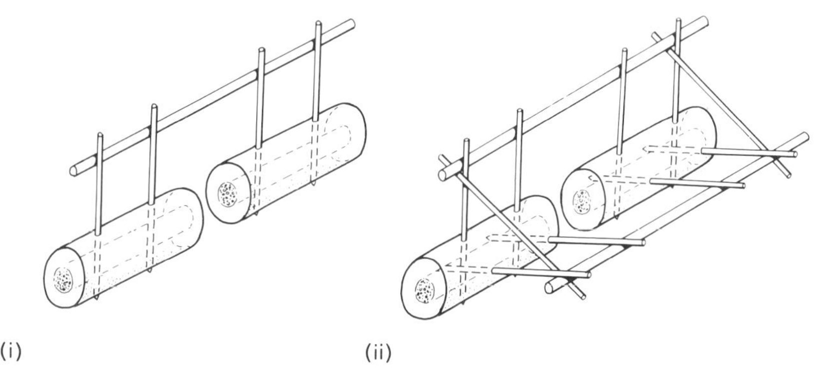

(i)   (ii)

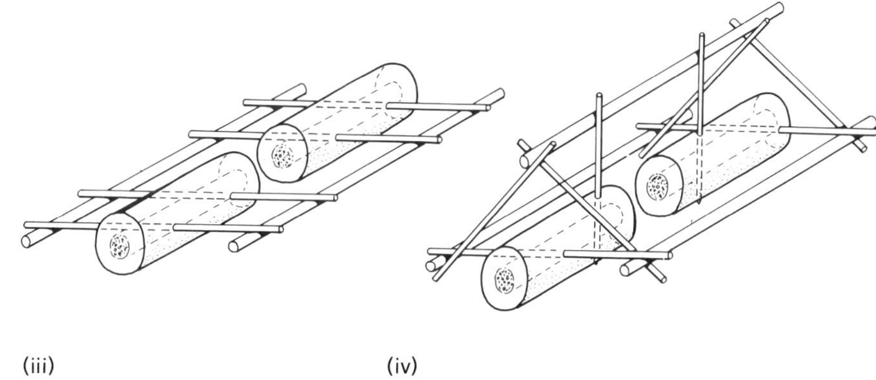

Fig. 9.5 The four basic types of external fixation frames: (I) unilateral half-frame (one plane); (II) unilateral V-frame (two planes); (III) bilateral frame (one plane); (IV) bilateral delta frame (two planes). The stability of the external fixator increases from type I to type IV.

(iii)   (iv)

Pin insertion techniques

The aim of pin insertion techniques is to avoid thermal necrosis of bone, and hence pin–bone interface loosening. The cortex should be pre-drilled and the drill irri- gated to cool it. The pin should be inserted by hand. Half pins should be advanced into the proximal cortex to avoid soft tissue irritation by the threads and to decrease pin–bone interface movement.

Indications for external fixation

The indications for use of the external fixator are not absolute. In general terms, the external fixator is an alternative to internal fixation for long bone diaphyseal fractures when internal fixation is inapplicable, usually because of severe soft tissue injuries.

The advantages of external fixation are a fixation that is rigid enough to give fracture stability but avoids the further soft tissue damage required to provide access for internal fixation. There is good access to the soft tissues for further wound care. There is the stability that is adequate for early joint and patient motion. The best accepted indication for external fixation is in the type III open diaphyseal tibial fracture. Use of external fixators in intra-articular fractures is limited because of their inability to achieve an anatomical reduction of the joint surface, unless combined with limited internal fixation of the articular surface. Several series (Karlstrom & Olerud 1983, Clifford *et al.* 1987, Court-Brown *et al.* 1990b) of open tibial fractures treated using external fixation have been reported and produced good results. However, it is difficult to compare results from different series because of the mix of case and fracture types.

Outcomes and complications of external fixation

Use of the external fixator is not free of complications. The major problems are pin track infection, pin loosening with loss of reduction, delayed union, malunion and a significant incidence of non-union.

Pin track infection rates vary considerably and depend to a certain extent upon how 'infection' is defined (Burny 1979, Green 1983). Pin track infections can be reduced by use of the insertion techniques already described and avoiding soft tissue tension around pins by using adequate relieving incisions. Muscle trans-fixing pins and full pins are associated with a particularly high incidence of pin-site infection (Clifford *et al.* 1987). In circumstances where a bone has a bulky surrounding soft tissue envelope with no subcutaneous border, then consideration should be given to an alternative method of achieving skeletal stability.

Delayed and non-union is not uncommon with external fixation (Karlstrom and Olerud (1983) reported a rate of 18%) and appears to be related to the extreme rigidity of some fixator systems. In the absence of absolute anatomical reduction and in the presence of marked comminution (two situations that occur frequently in fractures treated with external fixation) fracture healing takes place by the formation of callus. Extreme rigidity reduces callus formation. Reducing the stability of the fixator or dynamization of the fixator is necessary to increase stress at the fracture site and to promote micro-movement to encourage callus formation. At what stage dynamization should begin is a matter for speculation. The question of when to remove a fixator has been studied in an experimental model (Terjesen 1984) and it has been suggested that to avoid the effects of stress protection 6 weeks is the optimum time to wait before removal.

Malunion may be due either to a failure to achieve adequate reduction at the time of surgery or to a loss of position secondary to factors causing pin loosening and loss of fixator rigidity (Court-Brown *et al.* 1990b).

Reported rates of non-union in external fixation vary between 5 and 30% and, as might be expected, vary with fracture type; the rate of non-union increases as fracture severity increases (Gustilo *et al.* 1990).

Other complications include damage to surrounding neurovascular structures (more common with full pin fixators) and limited access to wounds because of poorly sited fixators (Seligson & Pope 1982).

External fixation is, almost by definition, used with difficult fractures prone to complications. Careful management and follow-up with early soft tissue cover, bone grafting and avoidance of stress protection is necessary if iatrogenic delay in bony union is to be avoided. Conversely, early fixator removal, if not accompanied by some other form of adequate fracture stabilization, is often associated with a loss of position (Court-Brown & Hughes 1985).

After fixator removal, further management may consist of definitive internal fixation or cast bracing. The frequency of pin track infection with external fixation, particularly for femoral fractures, means that the decision to externally fix a fracture may limit future management options. In particular, the surgeon may be ruling out the later option of secondary internal fixation. The presence of active pin track infection is considered by some to be an absolute contraindication to secondary internal fixation because of an unacceptable rate of infection (Maurer *et al.* 1989). Others report successful internal fixation at varying time intervals following external fixator removal (Biachut *et al.* 1990). It would appear that pin-site colonization and the increased duration of external fixation are both associated with an increased risk of infection when external is succeeded by internal fixation.

Internal fixation

In a text on general principles, there is no room for the technical details of individual fracture fixation. It must be said, however, that familiarity with anatomy, surgical techniques and increasingly complex equipment is a necessity and that departure by the inexperienced from basic principles usually results in disaster.

The use of internal fixation in the management of open fractures is still regarded by some as controversial. Plaster casts or skeletal traction undoubtedly avoid the risks associated with internal fixation, but in complex fractures they do not give sufficient skeletal stability to allow early mobilization. They will fail to hold accurate reduction of the fracture and allow considerable movement at the fracture site. The role of rigidity in preventing infection has already been discussed. Increasing rigidity at the fracture site has also been suggested to increase local tissue oxygenation; O'Sullivan *et al.* (1989) have suggested that this may be important in the promotion of bone, rather than cartilage, production in the process of fracture healing.

For joint surface damage in intra-articular fractures, Salter *et al.* (1980) have demonstrated the value of early continuous movement in the regeneration of articular cartilage in an experimental model. These desirable conditions of fracture stability and accurate reduction to allow early movement are best achieved by means other than plaster or skeletal traction. The indications for internal fixation in open fractures have been summarized by Webb (1983) and more recently by Schatzker and Tile (1987). The choice was considered to be between internal fixation using plates and screws or external fixation. Medullary nailing was not recommended in the acute management of open fractures (Smith 1964, Schatzker & Tile 1987). This view has been challenged and there are an increasing number of reports of acute intramedullary nailing in open fractures of both the femur and the tibia (Christie *et al.* 1988, Lhowe & Hansen 1988, Brumback *et al.* 1989, Court-Brown *et al.* 1990a, Wiss *et al.* 1991).

Plates and screws

Rigid plating according to the principles of the AO group is said to result in primary bone union (Danis 1947). It is probably true to say that the desirability of primary bone union is under question as more is learnt about the mechanisms which control fracture healing. Absolute rigidity is unphysiological. It is the stability of the fracture, allowing early mobilization of the limb, rather than absolute rigidity at the fracture site which is attractive. In a comminuted fracture, extensive soft tissue stripping to position multiple interfragmentary screws results in devitalization of bony fragments and is not to be encouraged. Stable fixation above and

below the area of comminution is preferable, with the preservation of soft tissue attachments of, and hence the blood supply to, the multiple small fragments. Under these circumstances healing takes place by the formation of callus in the presence of micromovement between the fragments. This is the concept of 'biological fixation'. The fixation must, however, still be stable enough to permit early mobilization (Fig. 9.6). Callus is no longer necessarily considered to be a sign of inadequate fracture fixation.

There are no absolute indications for plating open fractures but the commonest indication is probably the type I or II metaphyseal fracture with or without an intra-articular component. Type I or II diaphyseal fractures that can be reduced and fixed without further major soft tissue dissection may also be considered for internal fixation. The surgical approach may either incorporate the wound to provide access or a separate incision may be used if an adequate (at least 5 cm) soft tissue bridge can be left between the two incisions. Clifford *et al.* (1988) reported a series of open tibial fractures treated with internal fixation with excellent results, which in terms of infection compared well with more conservative methods of management, but in terms of functional outcome gave much better results. Similar excellent results for open forearm fractures have recently been reported (Chapman *et al.* 1989). Comparative studies are sparse and for the treatment of open fractures there are no prospective randomized trials of internal fixation versus external splintage, or traction, to be found in the scientific press.

If the decision is made to internally fix an open fracture with plates and screws, then meticulous preoperative planning is called for. This will minimize operative time and demonstrate the feasibility, or otherwise, of the proposed method of fixation. Impossibility is better demonstrated on paper than on the patient. Holdsworth (1989) has recently eloquently summarized the techniques of fracture planning.

Infection rates rise with the severity of the initial soft tissue injury, as might be expected. Even if infection does supervene, then as long as fracture stability with no implant loosening is maintained, there is no indication for implant removal. A stable fracture will heal in the presence of soft tissue infection. Removal of implants simply converts an infected but stable fracture to an infected unstable fracture, which is a much less satisfactory situation. The instinctive reaction to remove metalwork in the presence of infection must be avoided unless the implant shows signs of loosening. Continued stability will allow management of the soft tissues and control of any sepsis.

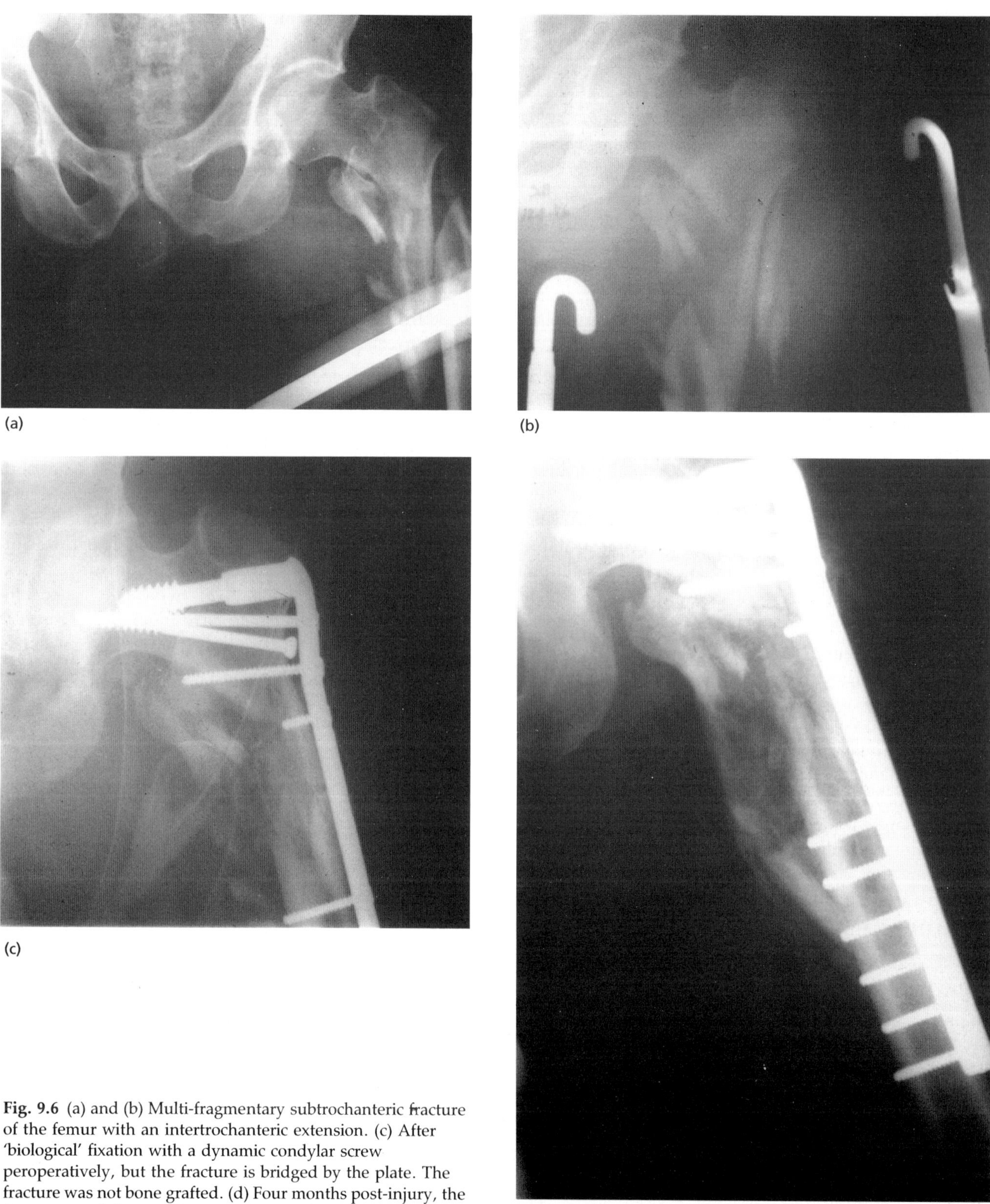

Fig. 9.6 (a) and (b) Multi-fragmentary subtrochanteric fracture of the femur with an intertrochanteric extension. (c) After 'biological' fixation with a dynamic condylar screw peroperatively, but the fracture is bridged by the plate. The fracture was not bone grafted. (d) Four months post-injury, the fracture is solidly united.

Intramedullary nailing

Hey-Groves described intramedullary nailing in the UK during the early part of the twentieth century (1912). Major advances were made by Küntscher in Germany during the Second World War. With the introduction of proximal and distal locking in the latter half of the twentieth century, the application of intramedullary nailing can span virtually the entire length of the long bones. Intramedullary nails act as load-sharing rather than load-bearing devices and are less rigid than plates. Rand *et al.* (1981) compared nailing with plating and showed increased periosteal new bone formation with nailing. Nails may be either reamed or unreamed. Reaming undoubtedly disrupts the endosteal circulation, producing local bone ischaemia (Smith *et al.* 1987), which together with an open wound and the lack of absolute rigidity may theoretically predispose the patient to infection. In a large series of nailings Winquist *et al.* (1984) reported three infections in 86 open fractures nailed at varying time intervals after injury. The immediate nailing of open fractures remains highly controversial, principally because of the fear of overwhelming sepsis. Schatzker and Tile (1987) have stated that primary intramedullary nailing is not indicated and that this should be performed as a delayed procedure 5–14 days later, depending on the state of the soft tissues. Other authors disagree, and more recently several reports have appeared suggesting that the use of immediate nailing in the open fracture is safe and not accompanied by any increased frequency of overwhelming sepsis, or an undue incidence of other complications. The advantages of immediate nailing in open fractures are the same as for closed fractures, namely control of angulation, rotation and length plus all the benefits of early mobilization already described (Fig. 9.7).

Lhowe and Hansen (1988) reported a series of 67 patients with open femoral fractures treated by intramedullary nailing. They concluded that their technique showed no increase in complication rates and produced results comparable with those in closed fractures. Christie *et al.* (1988) have reported no increase in infection rates with immediate nailing in a group of 20 open fractures of the femur, including eight type III injuries. Brumback *et al.* (1989) described 86 open femoral fractures, 56 of which were nailed immediately. They concluded that the key to avoiding infection was early wound excision and debridement; this allowed immediate nailing of type I and II fractures with no increased risk of sepsis. Interestingly, their results also called into question the idea that delayed nailing reduces the sepsis rate, and they suggest that there is no advantage to be gained by delay if adequate wound toilet can be carried

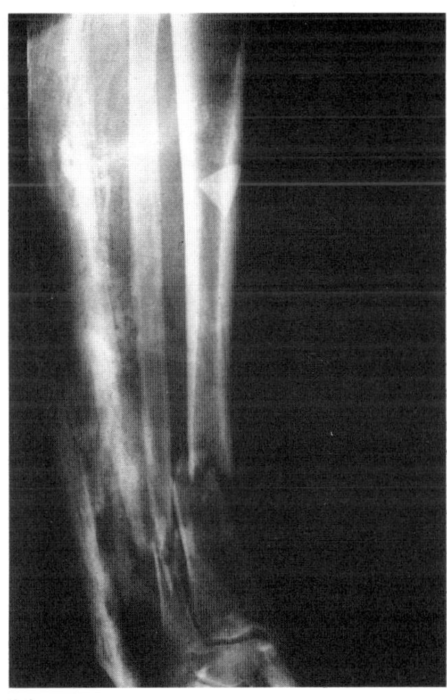 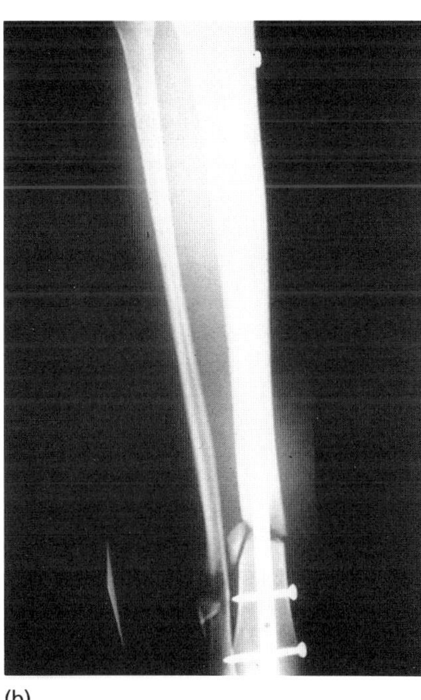 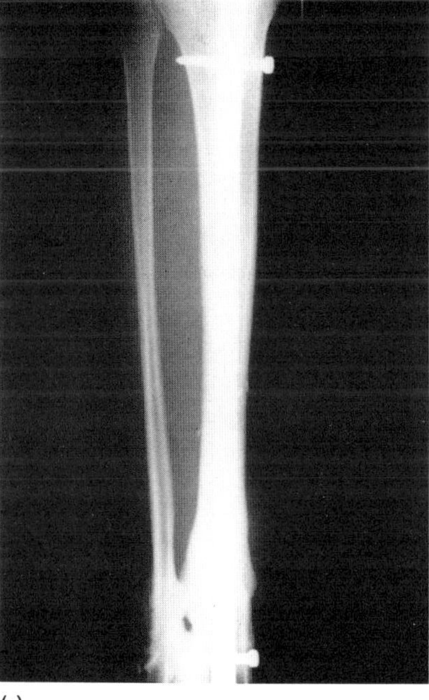

(a)   (b)   (c)

Fig. 9.7 (a) A type III B open fracture of the distal tibia. (b) After debridement, the fracture was stabilized with an unreamed tibial nail. Four days post-injury the wound was closed with a latissimus dorsi free flap. (c) Although there was uneventful wound healing, fracture union was only achieved after exchange nailing, three months post-injury.

out within 8 hours. The final outcome in patients who did develop infection was still good. Treatment of sepsis involved either removal of the nail, overreaming and renailing or repeated debridements and antibiotics. Despite the theoretical disadvantages with disruption of the blood supply, these fractures do unite following intramedullary nailing and there is a low incidence of non-union and infection.

In the tibia, the situation is less clear. These fractures are notoriously prone to non-union and the lack of a good soft tissue envelope combined with the eccentric placement of the bone may theoretically increase the risks of infection and non-union where attempts are made at reamed nailing in open fractures. Court-Brown *et al.* (1990a, 1991) have shown, however, in spite of these theoretical disadvantages, that reamed tibial nailing is an acceptable method of treating type I open fractures; there is a low complication rate that compares well with other methods of treatment. Unreamed nailing of the tibia has theoretical attractions such as less interference with the endosteal blood supply.

Wiss (1986) and Velazco *et al.* (1983) have reported on unreamed tibial nails in types I and II open tibial fractures. The outcomes were satisfactory with infection rates of 3–7%. A recent prospective, randomized study by Holbrook *et al.* (1989) suggested that unreamed nailing may have advantages over external fixation, or is at least as good as external fixation, for type I or II open fractures; there were lower rates of delayed union in comparison with the externally fixed group. Unreamed nailing is not recommended for type III open injuries or for the mechanically unstable Winquist type IV injuries because of the lack of control over shortening and rotation.

Intramedullary nailing as a primary procedure should not be contemplated for open fractures unless early and adequate wound surgery has been carried out, and there is considerable familiarity with the technique.

Having achieved skeletal stability, by whatever method, the key to successful management of the open fracture is the achievement of early soft tissue cover (see next Section). Delay in reaching this is associated with increased rates of infection, which remains the most potent cause of disaster and is a common cause of eventual amputation.

Conclusion

Every fracture is unique. Familiarity must not breed contempt. Management must be active, with careful and constant reassessment and prompt intervention when required. Treatment must be based on an assess-ment of the 'personality' of the fracture, as suggested by its causative mechanism, soft tissue damage, bony configuration and mechanical stability. There must be a clear plan of treatment with specific aims and objectives and the patient should be kept informed. The selection of a particular treatment modality must also be based on a consideration of the patient's needs and expectations and, finally, the ability and experience of the surgeon.

References

Allgower, M. Weichteilprobleme und Infektionsrisiko der Osteosynthese. *Arch F Klin Chir* 1971; **329**: 1128.

Behrens, F. & Searls, K. External fixation of the tibia. Basic concepts and prospective evaluation. *J Bone Joint Surg* 1986; **68B**: 246–254.

Biachut, P.A., Meek, R.N. & O'Brien, P.J. External fixation and delayed intramedullary nailing of open fractures of the tibial shaft. A sequential protocol. *J Bone Joint Surg* 1990; **72A**: 729–735.

Blick, S., Brumback, R.J., Poka, A., Burgess, A.R. & Ebraheim, N.A. Compartment syndrome in open tibial fractures. *J Bone Joint Surg* 1986; **68A**: 1348–1353.

Broome, G., Butler-Manuel, A., Broo, J., Carter, P.G. & Warlow, T.A. The Hungerford shooting incident. *Injury* 1988; **19**: 313–317.

Brumback, R.J., Ellison, P.S., Poka, A., Lakatos, R., Bathon, G.H. & Burgess, A.R. Intramedullary nailing of open femoral fractures. *J Bone Joint Surg* 1989; **71A**: 1324–1330.

Burke, J.F. The effective period of preventive antibiotic action in experimental incisions and dermal incisions. *Surgery* 1961; **50**: 161–168.

Burny, F. Elastic external fixation of tibial fractures. Study of 1421 cases. In: Brooker, A.F. & Edwards, C.L. (eds) *External Fixation: The Current State of the Art.* Williams & Wilkins: Baltimore, 1979.

Chao, E.Y.S. & Pope, M.H. The mechanical basis of external fixation. In: Seligson, D. & Pope, M. (eds) *Concepts in External Fixation.* Grune & Stratton: New York, 1982.

Chapman, M.W., Gordon, E. & Zissimos, A.G. Compression-plate fixation of acute fractures of the diaphysis of the radius and ulna. *J Bone Joint Surg* 1989; **71A**: 159–169.

Christie, J., Court-Brown, C.M., Kinninmouth, A.W.G. & Howie, C.R. Intramedullary locking nails in the management of femoral fractures. *J Bone Joint Surg* 1988; **70B**: 206–210.

Clifford, R.P., Lyons, T.J. & Webb, J.K. Complications of external fixation of compound tibial fractures. *Injury* 1987; **18**: 174–176.

Clifford, R.P., Webb, J.K., Beauchamp, C.G., Kellan, J.F. & Tile, M. Plate fixation of open fractures of the tibia. *J Bone Joint Surg* 1988; **70B**: 644–648.

Cooney, W.P., Fitzgerald, R.H., Dobyns, J.H. & Washington, J.A. Quantitative wound cultures in upper extremity trauma. *J Trauma* 1982; **22**: 112–117.

Court-Brown, C.M. & Hughes, S.P.F. Hughes external fixator in the treatment of tibial fractures. *J R Soc Med* 1985; **78**: 830–837.

Court-Brown, C.M., Christie, J. & McQueen, MM. Closed intramedullary tibial nailing; its use in closed and type I open fractures. *J Bone Joint Surg* 1990a; **72B**: 605−611.

Court-Brown, C.M., Wheelwright, E.F., Christie, J. & McQueen, M.M. External tibial fixation for type III open fractures. *J Bone Joint Surg* 1990b; **72B**: 801−804.

Court-Brown, C.M., McQueen, M.M., Quabra, A. & Christie, J. Locked intramedullary nailing of open tibial fractures. *J Bone Joint Surg* 1991; **73B**: 959−964.

Danis, R. *Theorie et Practique de l'Osteosynthese*. Masson: Paris, 1947.

Dellinger, E.P., Miller, S.D., Wertz, M.J., Grypma, M. Droppert, B. & Anderson, P.A. Risk of infection after open fracture of the arm or leg. *Arch Surg* 1988; **123**: 1320−1327.

Goodship, A.E. & Kenwright, J. The influence of induced micromovement upon the healing of experimental tibial fractures. *J Bone Joint Surg* 1985; **67B**: 650−655.

Green, S.A. Complications of external skeletal fixation. *Clin Orthop* 1983; **180**: 109−116.

Gustilo, R.B. & Anderson, J.T. Prevention of infection in the treatment of one thousand and twenty-five fractures of long bones. *J Bone Joint Surg* 1976; **58A**: 453−458.

Gustilo, R.B., Gruninger, R.P. & Davis, T. Classification of type III (severe) open fractures relative to treatment and results. *Orthopaedics* 1987; **10**: 1781−1788.

Gustilo, R.B., Mendoza, R.M. & Williams, D.N. Problems in the management of type III (severe) open fractures; a new classification of type III open fractures. *J Trauma* 1984; **24**: 742−746.

Gustilo, R.B., Merkow, R.L. & Templeman, D. The management of open fractures. *J Bone Joint Surg* 1990; **72A**: 299−304.

Hey-Groves, E.W. Some clinical and experimental observations on the operative treatment of fractures, with especial reference to the use of intramedullary pegs. *Br Med J* 1912; **2**: 1102−1105.

Holbrook, J.L., Swiontkowski, M.F. & Saunders, R. Treatment of open fractures of the tibial shaft: Ender nailing versus external fixation. *J Bone Joint Surg* 1989; **71A**: 1231−1238.

Holdsworth, B.J. Planning in fracture surgery. In: Bunker, T.D., Colton, C.L. & Webb, J.K. (eds) *Frontiers in Fracture Management*. Martin Dunitz: London, 1989.

Karlstrom, G. & Olerud, S. External fixation of severe open tibial fractures with the Hoffman frame. *Clin Orthop* 1983; **180**: 63−67.

Lhowe, D.W. & Hansen, S.T. Immediate nailing of open fractures of the femoral shaft. *J Bone Joint Surg* 1988; **70A**: 812−820.

Mader, J.T. & Cierny, G. The principles of the use of preventative antibiotics. *Clin Orthop* 1984; **190**: 75−82.

Maurer, D.J., Merkow, R.L. & Gustilo, R.B. Infection after intramedullary nailing of severe open tibial fractures initially treated with external fixation. *J Bone Joint Surg* 1989; **71A**: 835−838.

Muller, M., Allgower, M., Schneider, R. & Willemegger, H. (eds) *Manual of Internal Fixation*, 3rd edn. Springer-Verlag: 1991.

O'Sullivan, M.E., Chao, E.Y.S. & Kelly, P.J. The effects of fixation on fracture healing. *J Bone Joint Surg* 1989; **71A**: 306−309.

Patzakis, M.J. & Ivler, D. Antibiotic and bacteriologic considerations in open fractures. *South Med J* 1977; **70**: 46−80.

Patzakis, M.J., Harvey, J.P. & Ivler, D. The role of antibiotics in the management of open fractures. *J Bone Joint Surg* 1974; **56A**: 532−541.

Patzakis, M.J., Willkins, J. & Moore, T.M. Considerations in reducing the infection rate in open tibial fractures. *Clin Orthop* 1983; **178**: 36−41.

Rand, J.A., Rand, J.A., An, K.N., Chao, E.Y.S. & Kelly, P.J. A comparison of open intramedullary nailing and compression plate fixation on fracture site blood flow and fracture union. *J Bone Joint Surg* 1981; **63A**: 427−442.

Robson, M.C., Duke, W.F. & Krizek, T.J. Rapid bacterial screening in civilian wounds. *J Surg Res* 1973; **14**: 426−433.

Salter, R.B., Summonds, D.F., Malcolm, B.N., Rumble, E.J., McMichael, D. & Clements, N.D. The biological effects of continuous passive motion on full thickness defects in articular cartilage. An experimental investigation in the rabbit. *J Bone Joint Surg* 1980; **62A**: 1232−1251.

Sarmiento, A., Gersten, L.M., Sobol, P.A., Shankwiler, J.A. & Vangsness, C.T. Tibial shaft fractures treated with functional braces. *J Bone Joint Surg* 1989; **71B**: 602−609.

Schatzker, J. & Tile, M. *The Rationale of Operative Fracture Care*. Springer-Verlag: Berlin, 1987.

Seligson, D. & Pope, M. (eds) *Concepts in External Fixation*. Grune & Stratton: New York, 1982.

Smith, J.E.M. The results of early and delayed internal fixation of fractures of the shaft of the femur. *J Bone Joint Surg* 1964; **46B**: 28−31.

Smith, S.R., Bronk, J.T. & Kelly, P.J. Effects of fixation on fracture blood flow. *Orthop Trans* 1987; **11**: 295−295.

Terjesen, T. Healing of rabbit tibial fractures using external fixators. Effects of removal of the fixation device. *Acta Orthop Scand* 1984; **55**: 192−196.

Tscherne, H. The management of open fractures. In: Tscherne, H. & Gotzen, L. (eds) *Fractures with Soft Tissue Injuries*. Springer-Verlag: Berlin, 1984.

Tscherne, H., Oesterne, H.J. & Sturm, J. Osteosynthesis of major fractures in poly-trauma. *World J Surg* 1983; **7**: 80−87.

Velazco, A., Whitesides, T.E. Jr. & Fleming, L. Open fractures of the tibia treated with the Lottes nail. *J Bone Joint Surg* 1983; **65A**: 879−885.

Webb, J.K. The indications for internal fixation. In: Ackroyd, C.E., O'Connor, B.T. & De Bryn, P.F. (eds) *The Severely Injured Limb*. Churchill Livingstone: Edinburgh, 1983.

Winquist, R.A., Hansen, S.T. & Clawson, D.K. Closed intramedullary nailing of femoral fractures. A report of five hundred and twenty cases. *J Bone Joint Surg* 1984; **66A**: 529−539.

Wiss, D.A. Flexible medullary nailing of acute tibial shaft fractures. *Clin Orthop* 1986; **212**: 122−132.

Wiss, D.A., Brien, W.W. & Becker, V. Interlocking nailing for the treatment of femoral fractures due to gunshot wounds. *J Bone Joint Surg* 1991; **73A**: 588−606.

Worlock, P.H. The prevention of infection in open fractures. In: Bunker, T.D., Colton, C.L. & Webb, J.K. (eds) *Frontiers in Fracture Management*. Martin Dunitz: London, 1989.

Worlock, P.H., Slack, R.C.B., Harvey, L. & Mawhinney, R.R. The prevention of infection in open fractures: An experimental study of the effects of antibiotic therapy. *J Bone Joint Surg* 1988; **70A**: 1341−1347.

Worlock, P.H., Slack, R.C.B., Harvey, L. & Mawhinney, R.R. The prevention of infection in open fractures: an experimental study of the effect of fracture stability. *Injury* 1994; **25**: 31−38.

Skin cover

M.J.M.BLACK

General principles

In recent years the methods available for the management of open fractures have improved dramatically. Perhaps the most important advance has been an enhanced understanding of the principles of wound care. Prompt and adequate debridement makes it possible to proceed to successful wound closure at an early stage, and reduce dramatically the time to recovery and the incidence of complications.

The development of modern external fixation devices has been another major contribution to fracture management and wound care. However, such methods must be applied with considerable thought, care and early collaboration, so that the isolated needs of fracture management are not allowed to compromise the possibilities for early wound closure. Bone pins may be inadvertently inserted through the middle of the best muscle or myocutaneous flap donor site, or the external device positioned in such a way as to impede access to vessels required for microvascular anastomosis. They may also damage the arterial blood supply to a limb, with associated arteriovenous fistula or false aneurysm formation (Fig. 9.8a & b).

Also of importance has been a greater, and still increasing, understanding of the blood supply to the skin. This has led to the development of far more reliable and effective methods for the provision of skin cover, with consequent reduction of sepsis, non-union and bone loss. Especially important has been the con-

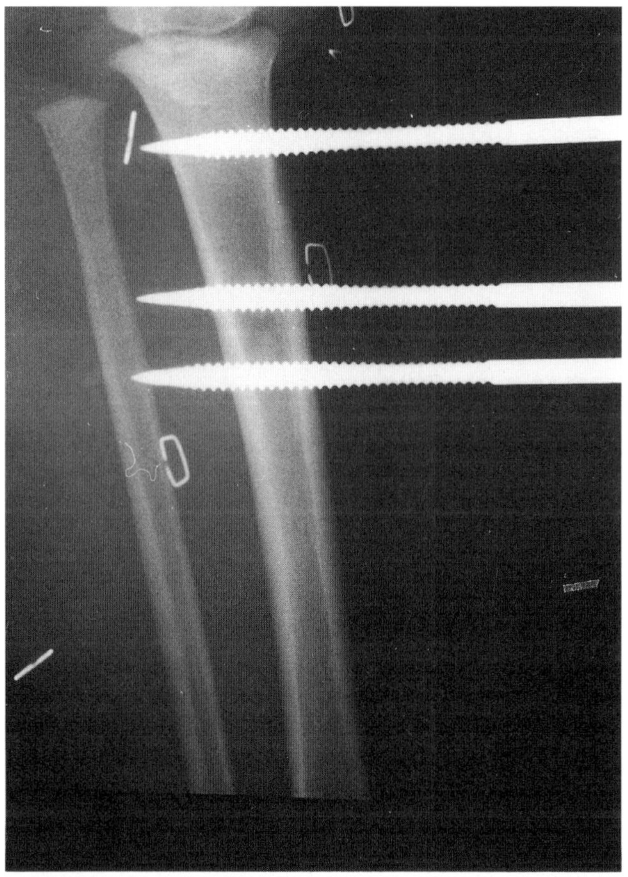

(a)

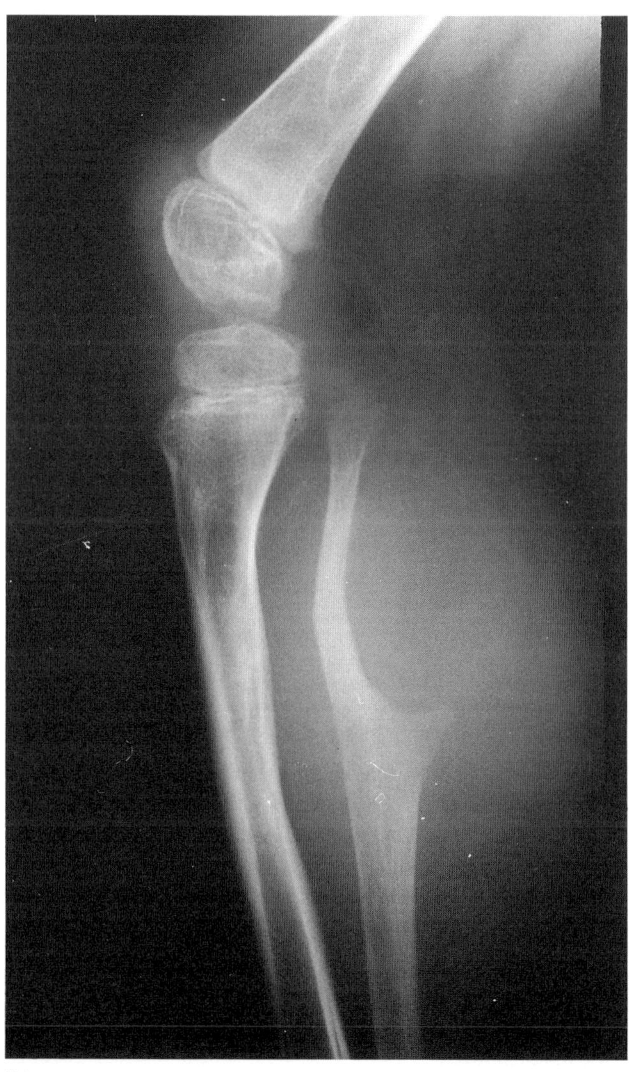

(b)

Fig. 9.8 (a) Fixation of a severe knee injury. The tip of the centre pin is at the site of the peroneal artery. (b) Fibula deformity as a result of a large false aneurysm of the peroneal artery.

tribution of microvascular free tissue transfer, especially free muscle transfer.

It has been stressed that the proper approach should be to achieve well-vascularized soft tissue cover as soon as possible (Maxwell & Hoopes 1979). Exposed bone can only come to harm if left uncovered. This concept demands aggressive initial debridement. Placing muscle or skin flaps onto necrotic tissue, or even worse, using such non-viable tissues for closure, can only result in sepsis and failure. The traditional secondary closure method of management of severe compound fractures is well known to lead to a high incidence of complications, including sepsis, delayed union, non-union and limb loss.

The successful aggressive approach to wound management has been well described (Byrd *et al.* 1981, 1985, Godina 1985, Yaremchuk *et al.* 1987). In summary, the best results with flap closure are seen in the 'acute' closure group, closure being achieved after thorough debridement. Closure in the 'subacute' phase is associated with sepsis and further tissue loss, including a higher incidence of flap loss. If the subacute phase is reached without achieving closure, then conservative wound management is indicated until the chronic phase is reached. At this stage flap closure has again a higher success rate.

The classification of open fractures according to severity has its value in understanding the damage to the blood supply of the bone (Table 9.4). From the point of view of wound closure the indication of the extent of

Table 9.4 Classification of open tibial fractures (Byrd *et al.* 1985)

Type 1
Low-energy forces causing a spiral or oblique fracture pattern with skin lacerations less than 2 cm and a relatively clean wound

Type 2
Moderate-energy forces causing a comminuted or displaced fracture pattern with skin lacerations greater than 2 cm and moderate adjacent skin and muscle contusion but *without* devitalized muscle

Type 3
High-energy forces causing a significantly displaced fracture pattern with severe comminution, segmental fracture, or bone defect with extensive associated skin loss and devitalized muscle

Type 4
Fracture pattern as in type 3 but with extreme-energy forces as in high-velocity gunshot or shotgun wounds, a history of crush or degloving, or associated vascular injury requiring repair

---

soft tissue damage is of equal importance. Not only is an indication of the required extent of debridement given, but the feasibility, or otherwise, of using local tissues for repair will also be indicated. In the more severe injuries many of the local muscle and skin flaps are doomed to failure because they themselves are damaged and not able to tolerate the extra surgical insult. Also, both the periosteal and endosteal blood supply to the bone will have been lost. Healing will then be dependent upon ingrowth of blood supply from the surrounding soft tissues. The sooner well-vascularized soft tissue cover is provided, the greater the chance of survival of the bone and subsequent healing.

Types 1 and 2 may not necessarily present a particular problem so far as wound closure is concerned. It is the more severe type 2, and types 3 and 4 that require special attention. Although the above classification applies to tibial fractures, the principles are the same for all severe open fractures.

Note that the first indication of the likely extent of soft tissue damage comes from the history, followed by the preoperative clinical and radiological examination. But it is at operation that one sees the full extent of the damage, although already it may have been made clear that local muscle flaps, for example, could and should not be relied upon.

We may now consider the principles of management based upon the concept of early soft tissue cover. Note the expression 'soft tissue cover', not necessarily 'skin' cover. So far as bone is concerned, muscle provides the best environment, not skin. If the bone is covered by muscle, actual skin closure can easily be achieved by simple skin grafting. Another major advantage of muscle flaps is their ability to fill the full extent of an irregular wound, thus closing all dead space and therefore reducing the risk of haematoma and sepsis.

The first step after evaluation is thorough debridement within 6 to 8 hours of injury. Good advice is that this should be repeated at 48 hours and again after a further 48 hours if there was no assurance that all necrotic tissue had finally been removed. This is to cope with doubt about viability of tissue and the possibility of progressive necrosis. Godina (1985), however, has advocated an even more radical approach, resulting in closure of wounds either immediately or after 72 hours at the latest. The key to this approach is thorough primary debridement. Godina stated that the reason for the 72-hour delay in his experience was usually organizational, rather than as a result of doubt about the adequacy of debridement, meaning that the resources required for microvascular free tissue transfer were not immediately available. Occasionally, the general condition of the patient precluded the immediate reconstruction. Godina's approach to debridement was somewhat different from the usual. He advocated meticulous debridement under tourniquet control, stating that otherwise, as a result of bleeding, with the consequent tissue staining and obscuring of the operative field, adequate excision was impossible, as it was not possible to identify clearly the tissue that had to be excised. A further advantage of the use of the tourniquet was that the often severe blood loss associated with this surgery was avoided. For many trauma teams this would be a revolutionary approach. Most would not be able to offer an immediate on-site microvascular free tissue repair service, but at least the crucial radical debridement could be completed in one stage, and arrangements made for reconstruction within 72 hours. Even that would test the resources of many centres. The reward would be the dramatic reduction in failures and complications as reported by Godina. A further advantage of very early closure of wounds is that primary repairs of vessels, nerves and tendons demand such cover to be successful. Godina divided the phases for wound closure into three: phase one — up to 72 hours; phase two — 72 hours to 3 months; and phase three — later than 3 months. The flap failure rate in each phase was 0.75, 12 and 9.5%, respectively. Infection occurred in 1.5, 17.5 and 6% of cases. Bone healing took 6.8, 12.5 and 29 months, respectively, and the hospital stay was for 27, 130 and 256 days. The average number of operations required was 1.3, 4.1 and 7.8. It can be seen that by far the best results were in the early aggressively managed group. If that opportunity is missed then reconstruction should probably best be further delayed until the wound is again in a more favourable phase.

Although degloving injuries are not necessarily associated with fracture, it is perhaps appropriate to mention this clinical problem here. The classical cause of such injuries is the pneumatic tyre. A shearing force separates the skin of the limb from the underlying deep fascia and from its blood supply. Actual tears in the skin are common but not universal, and usually do not indicate the full extent of the injury (Fig. 9.9a & b). Much of the non-viable skin may not be directly injured,

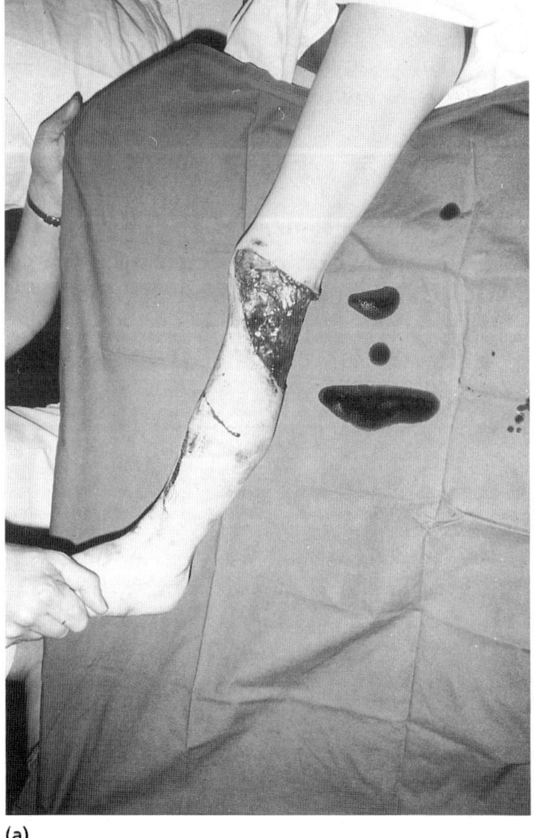

(a)

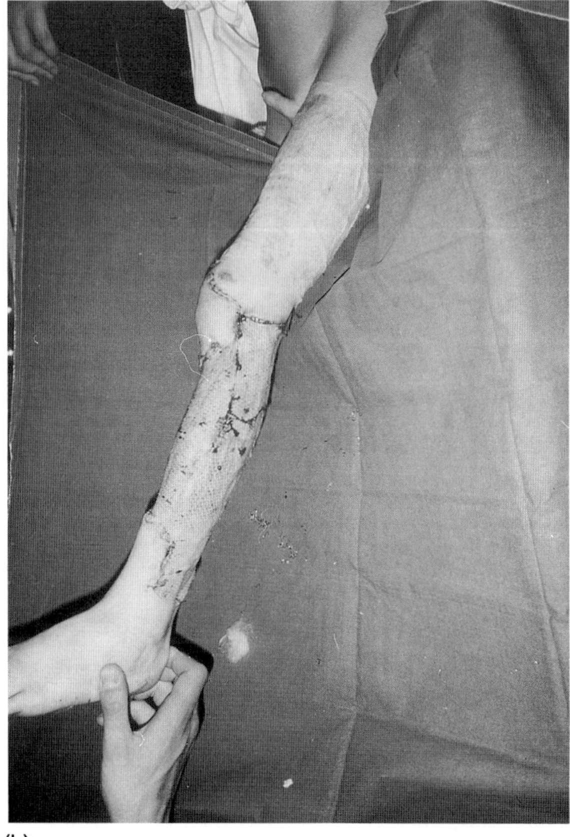

(b)

Fig. 9.9 (a) Pneumatic tyre degloving injury. (b) The eventual extent of skin grafting required. Note the use of a local skin flap to cover the knee.

so even Godina's criteria for excision would provide no guide. The use of intravenous fluorescein may be of assistance in assessing skin viability (McCraw *et al.* 1977). It is because much of the skin is not itself damaged that such attempts have been made to revascularize by microvascular anastomosis. However, the pathological anatomy is such that attempts are hardly ever practical. The problem therefore comes down to an exercise in deciding what will die through lack of blood supply and what will not. Usually, a wait-and-see policy with repeated visits to the operating theatre at 48-hour intervals is best, so long as this does not become a situation of neglect; skin cover should be provided at the earliest opportunity.

Fasciotomy should be undertaken as indicated. If damaged tissues are allowed to swell within closed fascial compartments, their blood supply and viability will be compromised. Fasciotomy wounds should be closed early with split-thickness skin grafts to reduce the risk of sepsis, and maintain the momentum towards recovery.

An external fixation device should be applied with due consideration of the points made above with regard to access to the wound, to potential repair tissue donor sites and to major limb vessels which may be required for microvascular free tissue transfer. The clinical situations are of course legion, and each case is unique. Perhaps the collaborative approach, as advocated by Godina, is the ideal to avoid errors. In my experience the commonest problem is the external fixation frame that obscures access to the posterior tibial vessels. Such devices have, on occasion, had to be moved at the time of free tissue transfer.

The wound should be covered with a moist dressing that will prevent desiccation of exposed structures, and this applies especially to periosteum. A wide choice is available, ranging from saline-soaked gauze to lyophilized porcine skin. The performance of the most expensive does not necessarily justify the cost. A non-adherent layer against the wound is helpful. Modern hydrocolloid materials are useful, but simple saline will do, so long as the dressing is not allowed to dry out.

Prophylactic antibiotic therapy is given.

These comments apply to the management of the acute referral.

Byrd *et al.* (1985) also described three phases of the open fracture wound; acute, subacute and chronic (Table 9.5).

As already stated, it has usually been considered to be less than ideal to attempt to close a subacute wound. Unfortunately, a large number of wounds referred for closure fall into this category, as it has been seen that

Table 9.5 Biological phases of the open fracture wound (Byrd *et al.* 1985)

Category	Clinical features	Time since injury
Acute	Contaminated but not infected Haemorrhagic and oedematous Presence of ischaemic and devitalized soft tissue and bone Serosanguineous drainage	1–5 days
Subacute	Colonized and infected wound Seropurulent drainage Erythema, increased swelling, cellulitis Exudative wound surfaces	1–6 weeks

Chronic	Infection limited to scar and
	   sequestrae in fracture
	Granulating, contracting wound
	Soft tissues 'stuck' to healthy bone
	   outside of fracture
		>6 weeks

this is the least favourable as measured by most parameters other than time to recovery. This should be recognized and preferably time should be spent in preparation by local wound care and antibiotic therapy. Formal surgical debridement may be required. Local wound care consists of the removal of necrotic material as a ward procedure, and frequent dressing changes. Highly absorbent modern dressing materials, such as the alginates, have much to offer. When combined with proper wound cleansing they can result in significant reduction in sepsis, even without antibiotic therapy. Split-thickness skin grafting of exposed soft tissues, including infected granulation tissue, can be a very helpful interim procedure at this stage. By such means the overall burden of sepsis is reduced, and the evolution from the dangerous subacute to the more favourable chronic phase hastened. Mesh grafting, as later described, is usually the most successful in this situation.

Yaremchuk *et al.* (1987) and others, however, have shown that closure during this period can succeed. It becomes a matter for careful judgement in each case. It is the more severe high-energy wounds that tend to fall into this delayed group because several debridements may have been undertaken before one becomes convinced that all non-viable tissue has been removed. These authors stress that it is important to remove devascularized bone fragments as well as soft tissues. They stress also the universal value of muscle flaps in this situation. In the more severe injuries these will have to be free muscle transfers. Another point of interest is the timing and method of bone defect reconstruction. Muscle flap healing is achieved before bone grafting.

Primary cancellous and free osteocutaneous flap repair are associated with a high failure rate. Osteocutaneous free flaps in particular, because of their rather rigid configuration, cannot fill the confines of an irregular contaminated wound in the way that muscle can, thus leaving dead space and leading to sepsis. It is becoming accepted that the approach to bone defects should be first to heal the wound with muscle flaps and skin graft, and then to bone graft at 4 to 6 weeks from successful healing. For tibial defects less than 8 cm long, cancellous bone grafting has proved to be adequate. For defects over 8 cm long, a microvascular free fibular transfer is considered to be the most suitable (Yaremchuk *et al.* 1987). In other situations there will, of course, be other choices.

Reconstructive methods

Skin grafts

Skin grafts may be either full thickness or partial (split) thickness. Split-thickness grafts are tangentially cut to include all the epidermis but only a proportion of the underlying dermis, leaving behind the deeper dermis with many epithelial cells in sectioned hair follicles, sweat glands and sebaceous glands, from which healing will occur. The grafts may be thin (Thiersch), intermediate (medium) or thick, depending upon the amount of dermis included (Fig. 9.10). The great advantage of split-thickness grafts is that the donor site will heal within a few days. Thin grafts offer the advantage of more reliable take and very rapidly healing donor sites. They lack, however, durability and they contract excessively. Thick-graft donor sites may be subject to delayed healing, or even failure to heal, especially in the elderly, or to the formation of hypertrophic scar. It is therefore intermediate-thickness grafts that are most useful, as they provide the best compromise between the reconstructive requirements and donor site morbidity, and that is a central theme in reconstructive surgery.

For grafts to be successful they must be placed in immobile contact with a viable recipient site. In the first few days the grafts survive by diffusion from the recipient site, until vascular connections have been established; this is really why they have to be thin, the diffusion process cannot cope with anything more.

Split-thickness skin grafts are valuable for two purposes. First, for the provision of skin cover of those parts of wounds that are suitable for that method, and

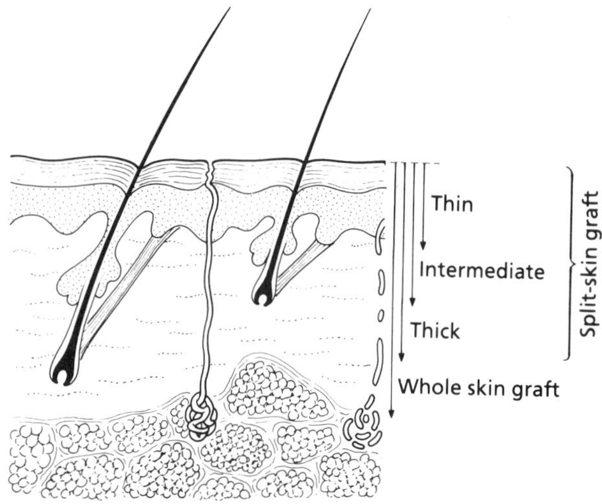

Fig. 9.10 Skin graft thicknesses, showing the level of cut.

that do not require cover by skin or muscle flaps. This allows the size of any skin flap that is required to be kept to the essential minimum, as there are usually donor site morbidity considerations. It is the bone that needs to be covered by flap, as it cannot support a graft; surrounding muscle, for example, will readily accept split-thickness skin grafts. Second, for the cover of local or free muscle flaps. The use of muscle flaps with split-thickness skin grafts has become one of the most valuable methods for soft tissue cover of compound fractures. Grafts are also very useful in the subacute wound as a means of helping to bring infection under control, as described above.

Meshing (MacMillan 1970), with or without expansion, has enormously enhanced the success rate of split-thickness skin grafting (Fig. 9.11). Such grafts may be applied with confidence to surfaces that would be problematic for sheet grafts. Exudate, whether septic, serous or haemorrhagic, will escape through the slits rather than lift the graft from its bed and thus prevent take. Another advantage is that meshed grafts will more readily conform to the irregular surfaces that are common in these situations. Various meshing machines are commercially available (Fig. 9.12a & b). The use of a powered dermatome is recommended because the resultant strips of graft fit the meshing machine more satisfactorily than grafts cut with a hand knife, and the donor sites heal better than those resulting from the use of hand knives, being more even in depth and with less jagged edges; however, such a machine is not indispensable (Fig. 9.13). Probably many surgical units will not have access to a powered dermatome. There are

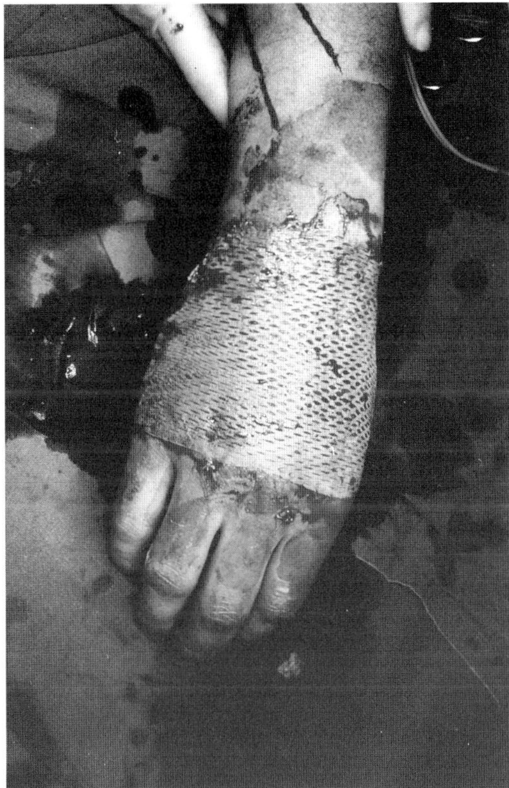

Fig. 9.11 Meshed skin graft applied to the dorsum of a hand.

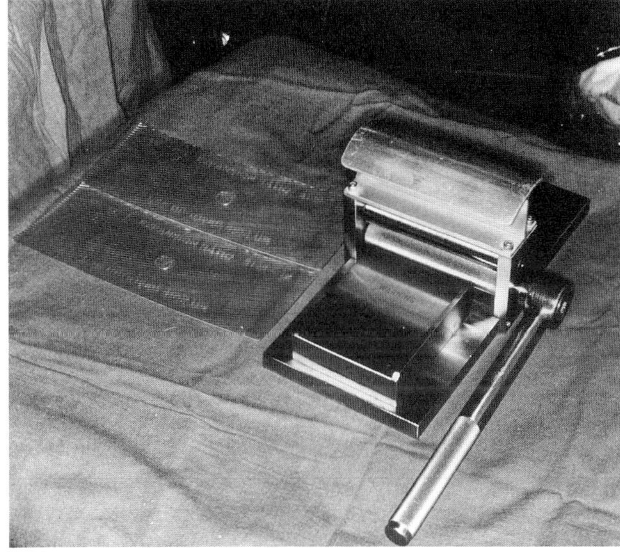

(a)

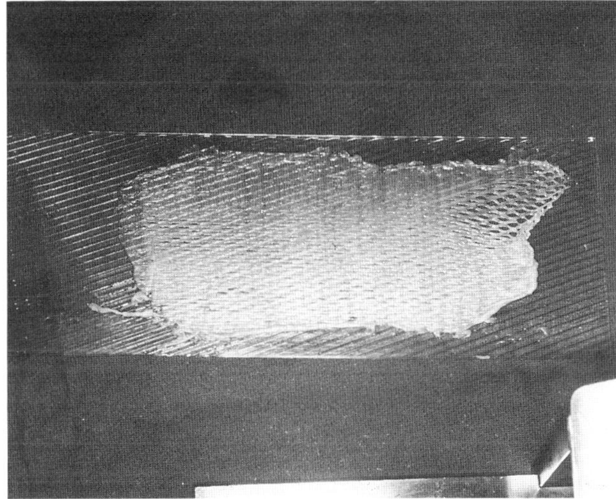

(b)

Fig. 9.12 (a) A skin meshing machine. (b) Meshed skin on the carrier board after passage through the machine.

many designs of skin graft knives. The author prefers the Watson pattern as it is sturdy and reliable (Fig. 9.14). The choice of donor sites is more limited if one is having to use a hand knife, for purely technical reasons. A site that can be flattened, held under moderate tension and accessed with a hand knife is required. The most useful donor site is the thigh. Although the bar or roller at the leading edge of most knives flattens the skin in advance of the blade, it is useful for the lubricated edge of a board to be pressed on the skin ahead of the knife. This helps to tension as well as flatten the donor site.

The available expansion ratio of meshed skin depends upon either the machine used, or the choice of carrier board chosen for those machines that use such boards. In the relevant situation a carrier giving a ratio of 1:1.5 will be appropriate, although hardly any expansion may actually be used. To a limited extent, the advantages of meshing can be achieved by cutting multiple slits in the graft with a scalpel, when no machine is available.

The dressing of donor sites is a subject of much variance in practice. Much work has been done in recent times in studying the best conditions for wound healing, and that has included examination of many old and new wound-dressing techniques. The best environ-ment is moist and sterile. Semi-permeable adhesive films are excellent where a good area around the actual donor site is available for seal. Exudate collection can be a problem. It has recently been shown that the use of alginate sheet (Kaltostat) dressings results in more rapid healing, and can be used under semi-permeable film. Where film is not suitable, a more conventional dressing of absorbent layers of cotton gauze will be satisfactory. Healing takes 7 to 14 days, depending upon the depth. The dressing should be allowed to separate spon-taneously, or the delicate freshly healed epithelium will be ripped off.

There are two absolute requirements for successful

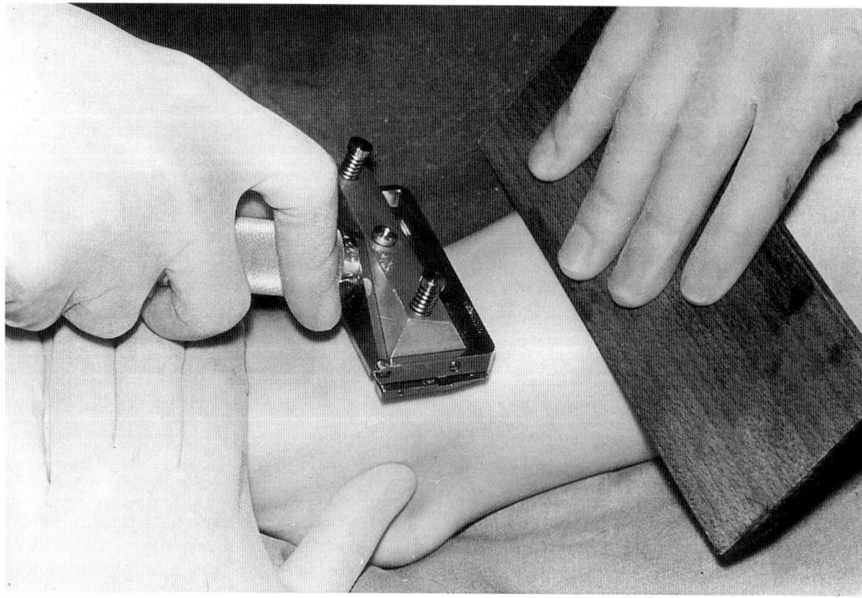

Fig. 9.13 Electric-powered dermatome.

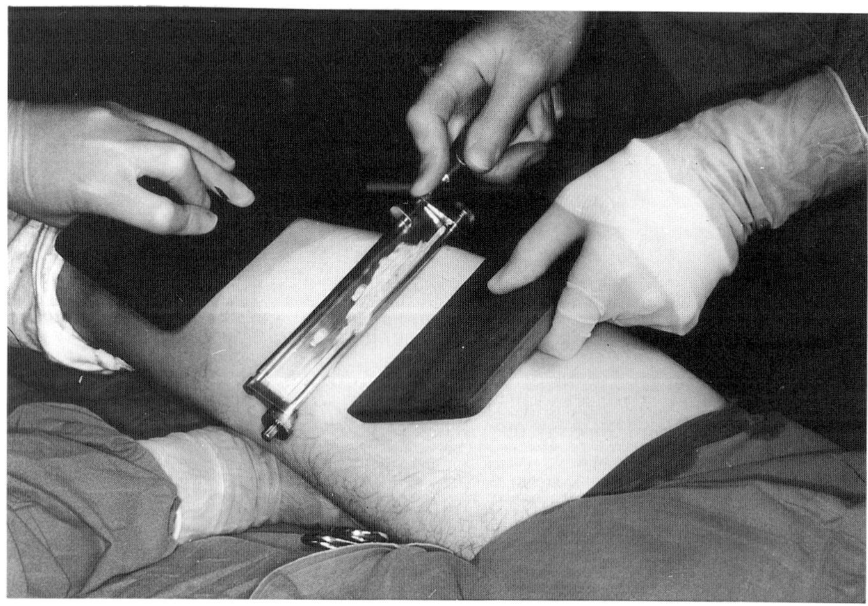

Fig. 9.14 Hand skin graft knife (Watson pattern).

graft take; immobility on, and contact with, the recipient site. Poor haemostasis, leading to haematoma under the graft, is a common cause of graft failure. Both requirements may be met by, or frustrated by, dressings. These, therefore, need to be thought out and applied with care. It is often helpful to suture grafts into place, although staples may be quicker to use and cause less bleeding. Sometimes the best dressing is no dressing! At other times a carefully applied dressing will enhance graft take, provide greater security and reduce nursing requirements. A non-adherent layer, such as Vaseline gauze, absorbent padding and compressing bandages are usually applicable.

One organism that is fatal to skin grafts is the beta haemolytic streptococcus, Lancefield group A. This organism should be eradicated before grafting. Some other organisms reduce graft take, e.g. *Pseudomonas*, but as discussed above skin grafting can be a useful method of bringing such infection under control. It can be a hopeless task trying to sterilize wounds unless one heals them!

Grafts may be stored at 4°C in a fridge, wrapped in

saline-soaked gauze, in a sterile container. The graft will remain usable for several days but its viability will gradually decline. It is essential to label the container with the patient's name and to avoid even accidental allografting, as this practice has been known to transmit human immunodeficiency virus (HIV).

Grafts take time to consolidate. Grafts on the leg require prolonged compression support if they are not to blister and separate as the limb becomes dependent once again.

Flaps

Flaps, by definition, bring their own blood supply with them and are therefore independent of the recipient site for their nutrition. In fact, and often crucially, they bring blood supply to the defect, thus directly aiding the healing process.

Flaps may be:

1 Skin.
2 Muscle.
3 Myocutaneous.

Depending upon the pattern of the blood supply, skin flaps may be:

1 Random pattern.
2 Axial pattern.
3 Fasciocutaneous.
4 Septocutaneous.

Cormack and Lamberty (1986) have provided a detailed, up-to-date description of the blood supply of skin flaps. The classification given above is probably not definitive, as the topic is the subject of considerable current debate.

In the case of random pattern flaps, the blood supply enters the base, or pedicle, through small vertically aligned musculocutaneous perforating vessels, each of which supplies a limited area of skin. The size of such flaps is therefore necessarily limited.

Axial pattern flaps contain a horizontal vessel, called a direct cutaneous vessel, of some size within the subcutaneous tissue. Because the head of pressure is carried well into the vascular territory of such a flap, it may be larger and longer than a random pattern flap, as well as more reliable. In addition, the pedicle may be narrowed down to even the single artery and vein, thus allowing greater ease of transposition. The final step is that such a pedicle may lend itself to division followed by microvascular anastomosis at the recipient site, thereby allowing immediate distant transfer. One of the first-described axial pattern flaps, the groin flap supplied by the superficial circumflex iliac artery, is still popular as a pedicled flap for hand cover (Fig. 9.15), and sometimes still as a free flap (Fig. 9.16a & b).

Flaps may also be: (i) local or (ii) distant. Local flaps are found adjacent to the defect to be repaired and are transposed directly in one way or another to that defect, without severance of the pedicle. Distant flaps are found at sites away from the defect. They may be: (i) direct or (ii) indirect.

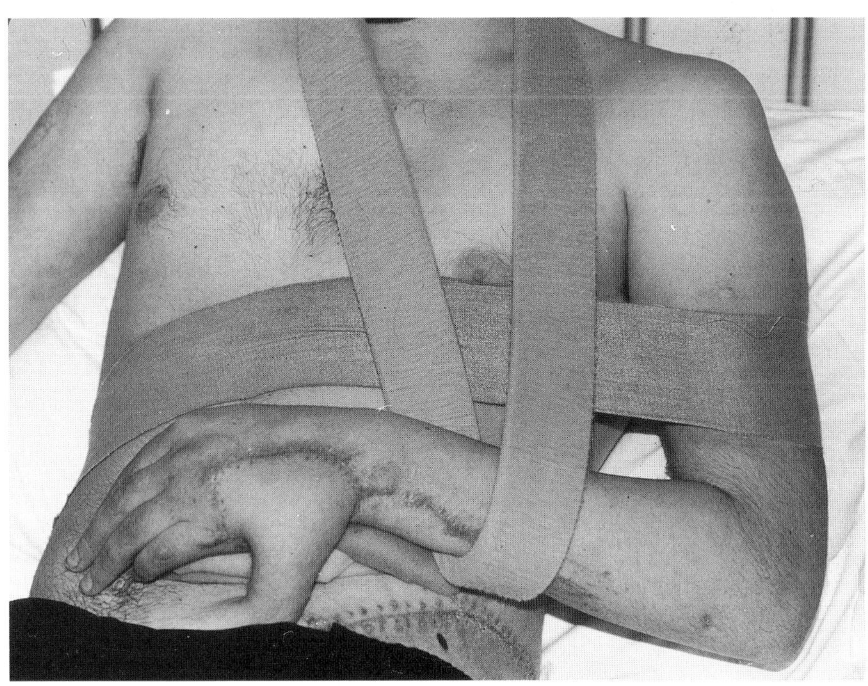

Fig. 9.15 Pedicled groin axial pattern flap to a hand.

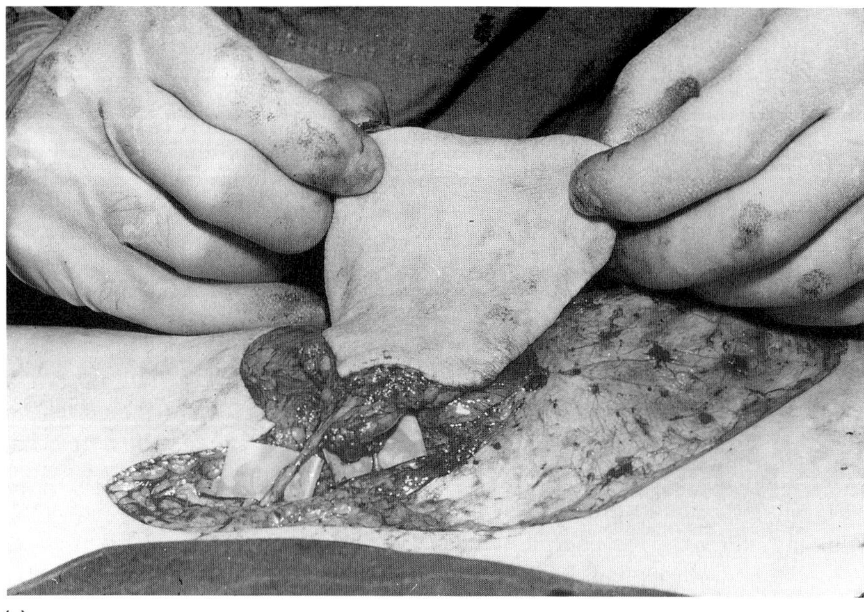

(a)

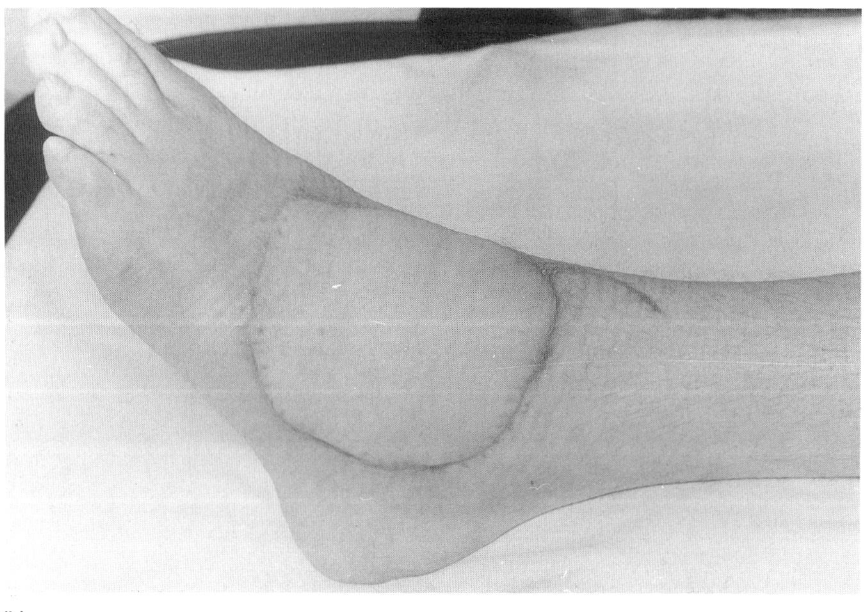

(b)

Fig. 9.16 (a) A groin flap raised as an island ready for microvascular free transfer. (b) The free groin flap healed onto a foot.

A distant direct flap is brought 'directly' to the recipient site by approximation of donor and recipient sites, e.g. a cross leg flap, where the two legs can be suitably positioned together (Fig. 9.17). Indirect flaps can only reach their intended site by means of temporary attachment to a carrier such as a wrist, or by means of the traditional waltzing and caterpillaring techniques that were used for tube pedicles. These are now rarely used. Both these classes of more traditional distant flaps suffer from what may be a disadvantage in that the blood supply brought by the flap will be lost at final pedicle division. The flap then relies for permanent nutrition upon the recipient site, or at least those parts of it that are capable of such provision, usually the edges.

A special class of distant direct flap is the microvascular free flap which is brought from a distance to the recipient site in one stage, as described above. Any flap that depends for its blood circulation upon an artery and vein that can be anastomosed by microsurgical means is a possible free flap (Figs 9.18 & 9.19). These flaps tend to have an enhanced blood circulation over the often more precarious pedicled flaps. Axial pattern skin flaps, some septocutaneous skin flaps,

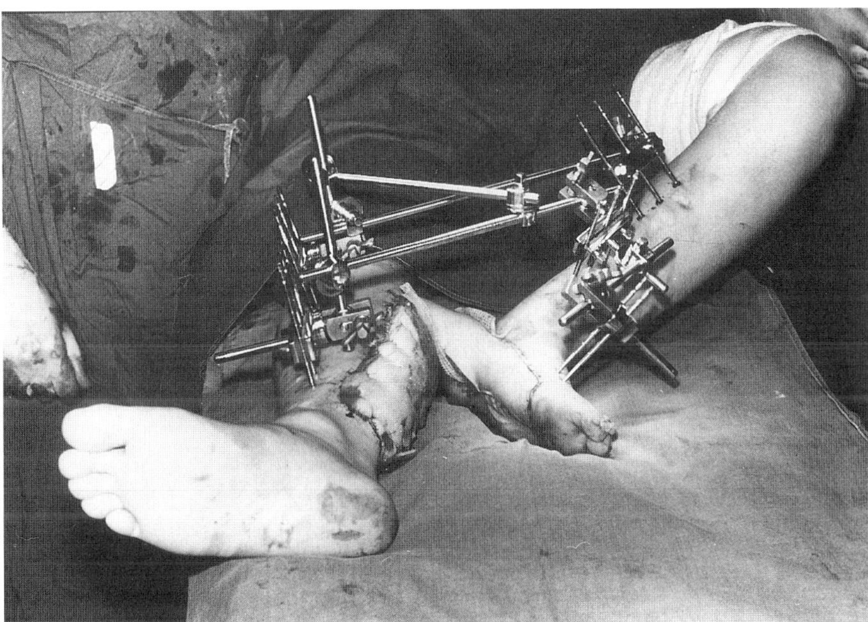

Fig. 9.17 A cross leg myocutaneous flap. The external fixation device offers ease of adjustment, better access and greater comfort compared with the traditional plaster technique.

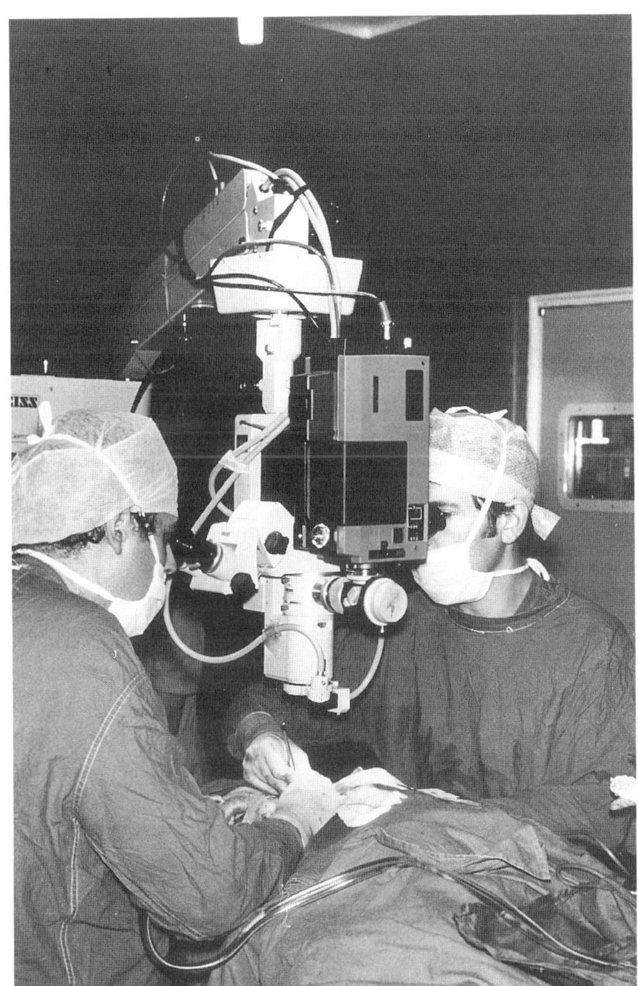

Fig. 9.18 A modern operating microscope.

muscle and myocutaneous flaps are all candidates for free flap transfer.

Most muscle flaps are equivalent to axial pattern skin flaps, although the details of the anatomy of the blood supply of individual muscles is a massive and important subject in its own right. The principle of the myocutaneous flap is that the muscle acts as an axial flap carrying overlying skin, supplied via the usual small musculocutaneous perforating vessels. Such skin would otherwise be subject to all the limitations of the random pattern blood supply. The discovery and development of such flaps has been an advance of equal importance to reconstructive surgery as microvascular free flap surgery.

Muscle flaps — local

The principle that muscle flaps may be used to cover defects not suitable for simple skin grafting was expounded by Ger (1970, 1972, 1975) and elaborated by others (Mathes *et al.* 1974, Pers & Medgyesi 1975, Vasconez *et al.* 1974, 1977, Vasconez & McGraw 1976).

A prerequisite for their use is that the proposed donor muscle should be viable enough to withstand such use. This is often not possible in the more severe injuries. The muscle must, of course, be functionally expendable. Finally, it is of course essential to know the anatomy of the chosen muscle and especially of its blood supply.

Mathes and Nahai have provided an excellent reference source of the donor sites and potential applications

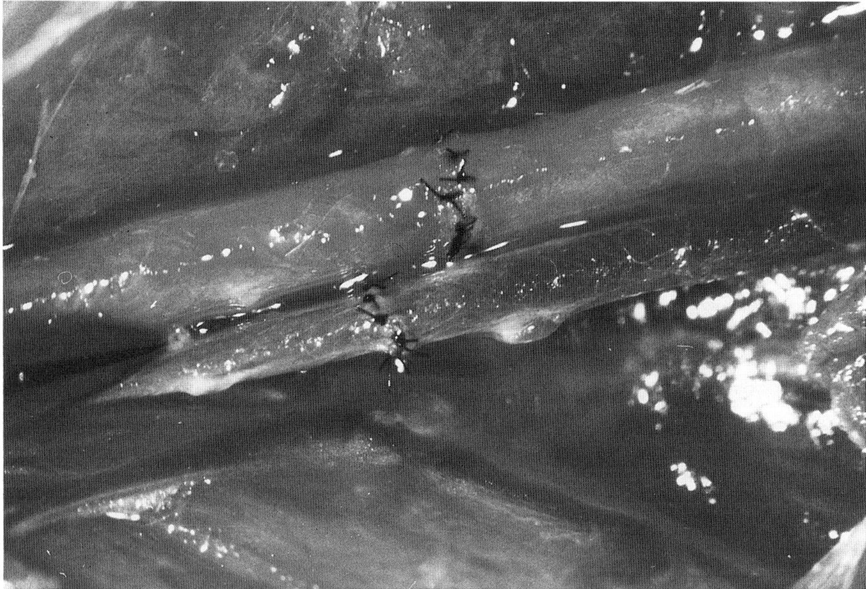

Fig. 9.19 Anastomosed artery of 1.0-mm diameter and vein of 0.5 mm.

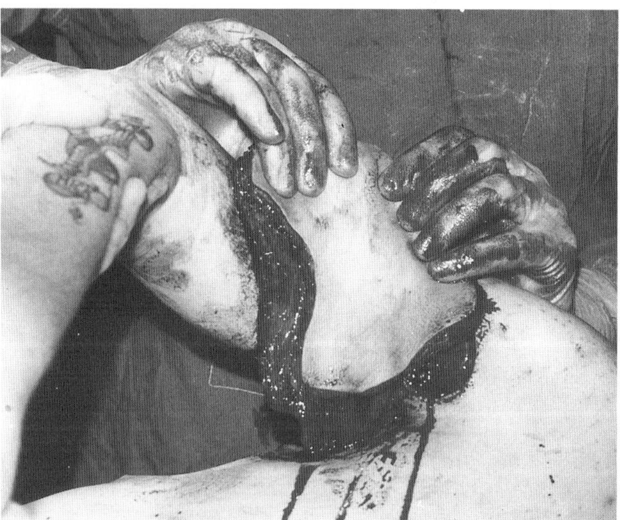

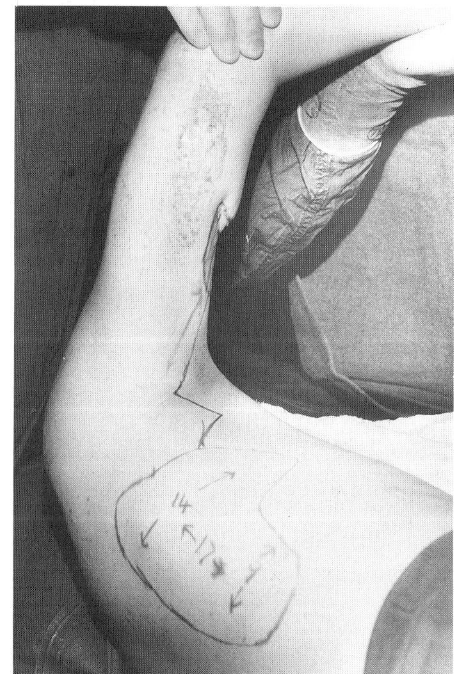

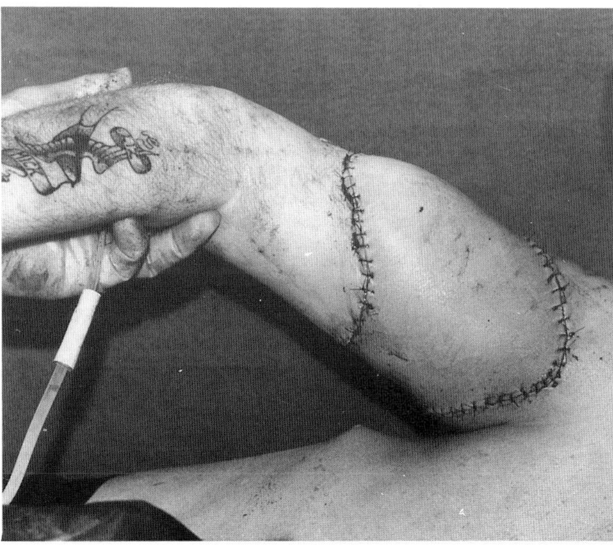

Fig. 9.20 (*Above*.) Planning for transfer of a latissimus dorsi myocutaneous flap to an arm defect. (*Top left*.) The flap raised upon the axillary pedicle as a skin island. (*Lower left*.) The flap in place.

of each recognized donor site (Mathes & Nahai 1979). This is highly recommended.

Much of the discussion in this chapter has concerned tibial injuries. This is because such injuries present us with the majority of severe fracture cover problems. The muscles available to cover the upper third of the tibia are the medial and lateral heads of gastrocnemius. Soleus can be mobilized to cover much of the middle third, augmented by flexor digitorum longus. The latter also contributes to lower-third cover. Other muscles of more limited application are flexor hallucis longus, tibialis anterior, extensor digitorum longus and extensor hallucis longus. Around the foot and ankle, the use of abductor hallucis, flexor digitorum brevis, abductor digiti minimi and extensor digitorum brevis has been described.

One of the most important muscles for reconstructive purposes is latissimus dorsi. It is used as either a muscle or myocutaneous flap, either pedicled at the axilla to reach the shoulder and arm (Fig. 9.20a–c), or as a free flap to any site that requires its size (Fig. 9.21a–c). The rectus abdominis is gaining popularity, especially as a free flap upon the inferior epigastric vessels.

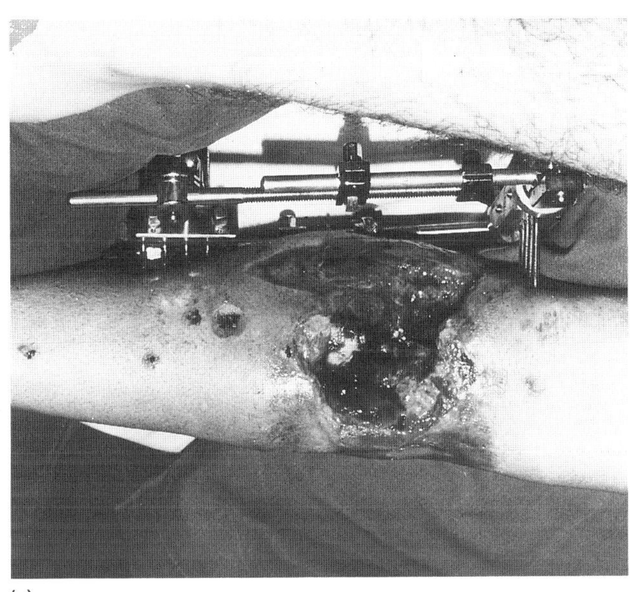

(a)

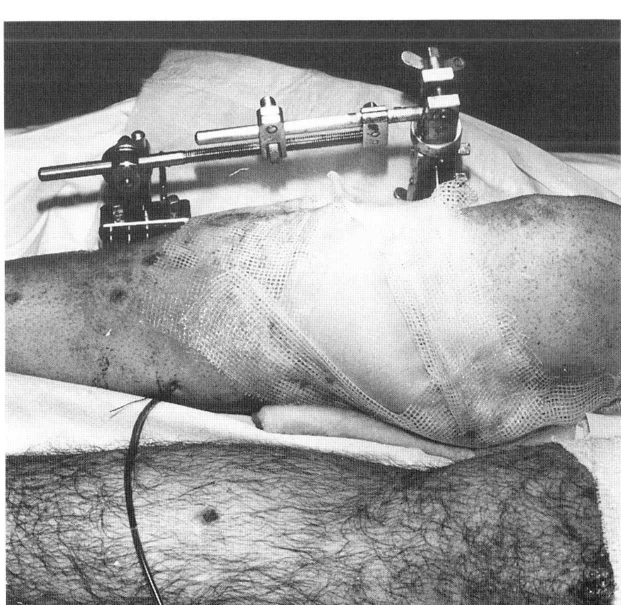

(c)

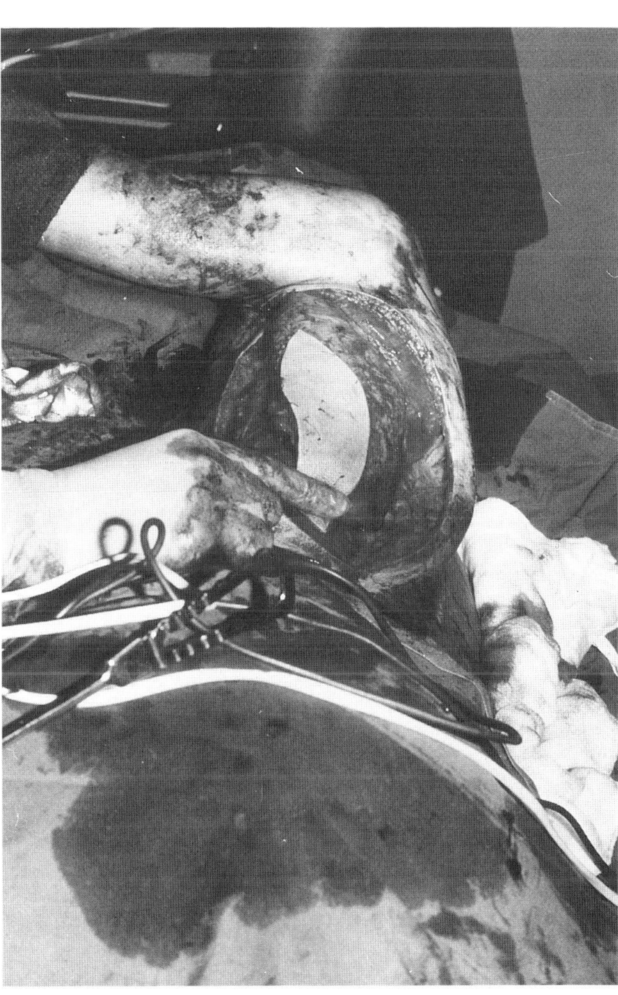

(b)

Fig. 9.21 (a) Compound tibial fracture requiring free flap repair. (b) Latissimus dorsi myocutaneous flap being raised for free transfer. (c) The flap after transfer.

Myocutaneous flaps

As already stated, many muscles provide nutrition for an area of overlying skin through musculocutaneous perforating vessels. This area of skin may be transferred as an island with the muscle, even though the skin alone could not survive as such an extensive flap. By this means good-quality skin repair may be obtained and a useful clinical indicator of flap viability provided by direct observation of the skin circulation. A disadvantage is the possibly increased donor site morbidity and cosmetic damage where skin grafting of the donor site might be necessary. The latissimus dorsi has already been referred to, but there are many more examples. One of the earliest to be used was the medial gastrocnemius myocutaneous flap, which has greater reach than the muscle flap alone. The cutaneous territories of supply of all those body muscles that contribute such supply has been mapped in recent years.

Fasciocutaneous and septocutaneous flaps

These flaps are a relatively recent discovery and indeed not yet fully understood. New donor sites are regularly being described. Perhaps the first such description was the 'super flap' originally presented as an alternative to the medial gastrocnemius myocutaneous flap (Ponten 1981) (Fig. 9.22). It was demonstrated that this area of skin could survive upon blood supply from fasciocutaneous vessels rather than the myocutaneous perforators that had been thought to be essential. The

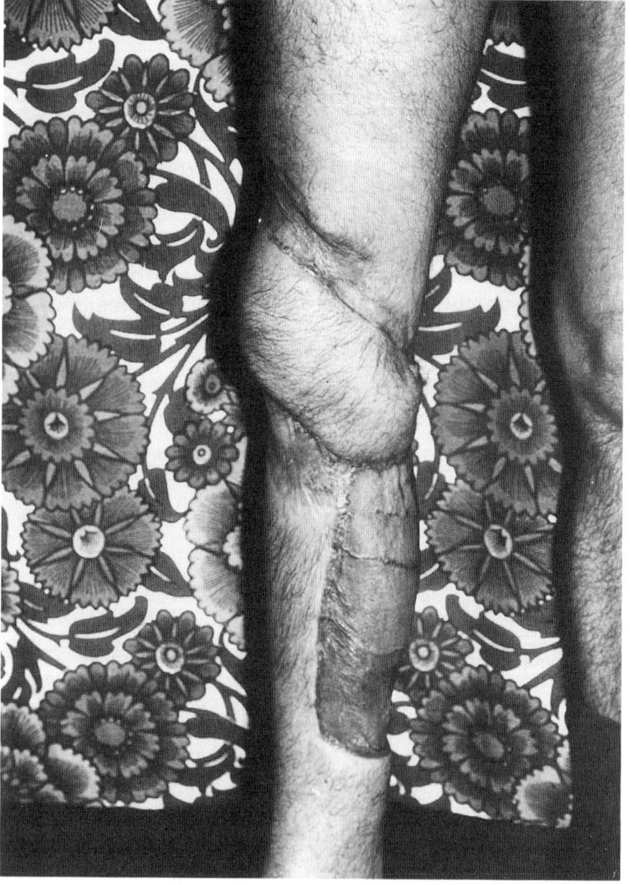

Fig. 9.22 A long fasciocutaneous flap, based proximally for coverage of the patella. Note the split-thickness skin grafts applied to the flap donor site.

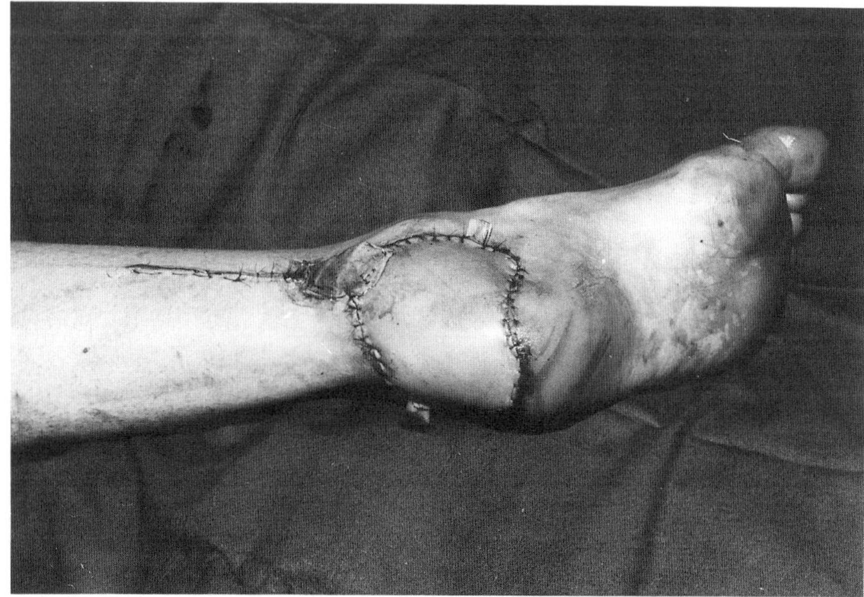

Fig. 9.23 A microvascular free radial forearm flap for heel coverage.

fasciocutaneous vessels run horizontally in relation to the deep fascia, which must be included in the flap, hence the terminology. They are not of the same dimension as most direct cutaneous vessels, but do allow the flap to be designed and used similarly to an axial pattern flap. In the case of septocutaneous flaps, the vessels come to the surface through intermuscular septa rather than through muscle. Once there, they spread out over a large area, initially within the deep fascia, which has to be included. To this extent they are, therefore, also fasciocutaneous. One can see why there is still debate about the terminology of flaps. The radial forearm flap is one of the most widely used septocutaneous flaps, both locally pedicled but especially as a free flap (Souter *et al*. 1983). This flap is particularly useful on the distal parts of both upper and lower limbs because it is thin (Fig. 9.23). In the case of the hand, the pedicle may be distal, so long as the flow across the palmar arch is

adequate to sustain backflow up the radial artery, and so long as the radial artery can otherwise be dispensed with, thus obviating the need for microvascular anastomosis (Fig. 9.24a−c). Other advantages are that the vascular pedicle may be long and the vessels are of large diameter; both features facilitate free transfer.

Microvascular free flaps

Such a flap may be any of the flap types described above, so long as it can be raised as an island on a supplying artery and a draining vein, and that these are suitable for microvascular anastomosis to vessels at the recipient site, e.g. muscle, myocutaneous, axial pattern skin, or even more complex compound transfers containing bone or other tissues required for repair. The possible donor sites have proliferated in the last few years and a wide choice is now available. Each site has

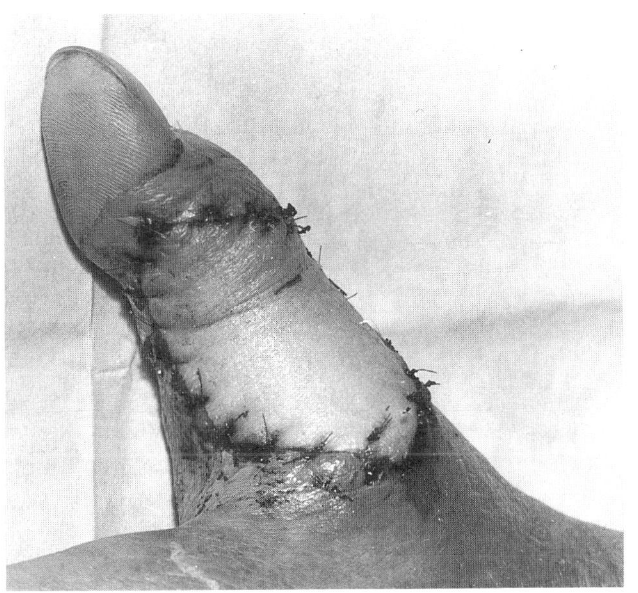

(a)

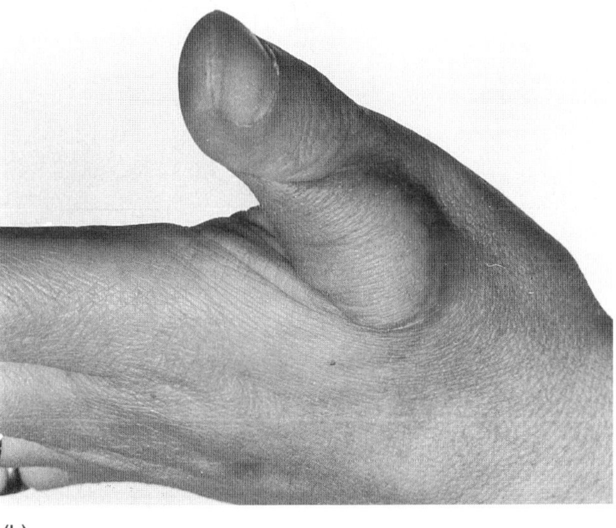

(b)

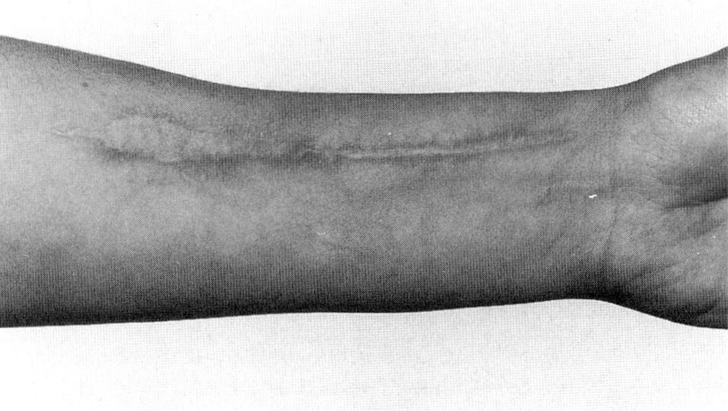

(c)

Fig. 9.24 (a) A distally pedicled radial forearm flap to a thumb defect. (b) The later result. (c) The donor site.

its advantages and disadvantages, as well as suitabilities for any particular reconstructive problem.

For fracture coverage purposes, free muscle flaps are often the best choice when local flaps are not available. They bring in highly vascular tissue to aid healing. They are economical at the donor site, as the skin is spared. They conform very well to the irregularities of complex recipient sites, and they accept skin grafts readily.

Potentially the two most useful donor sites for major fracture coverage are the latissimus dorsi and rectus abdominis muscles. Both are reasonably expendable and have comparatively long and large vascular pedicles; they are thus safe and dependable. Latissimus dorsi offers a huge area and mass of tissue, although the size of the flap can, within limits, be tailored to the requirements (Fig. 9.25a–d). The rectus abdominis has been used to a lesser extent to date, but has the advan-

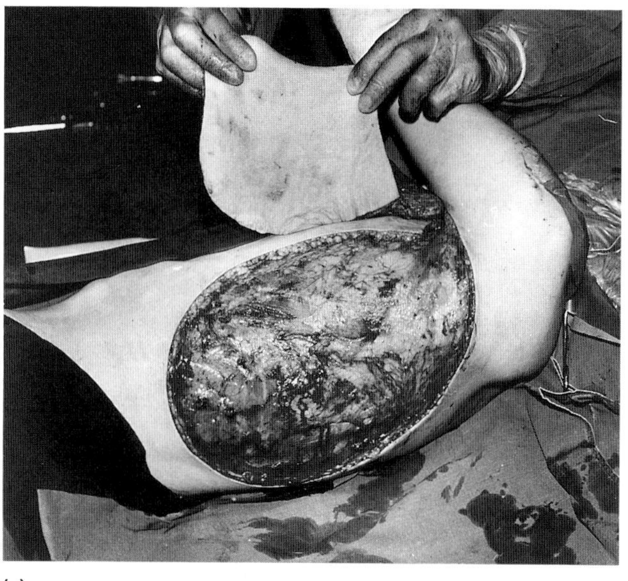

(a)

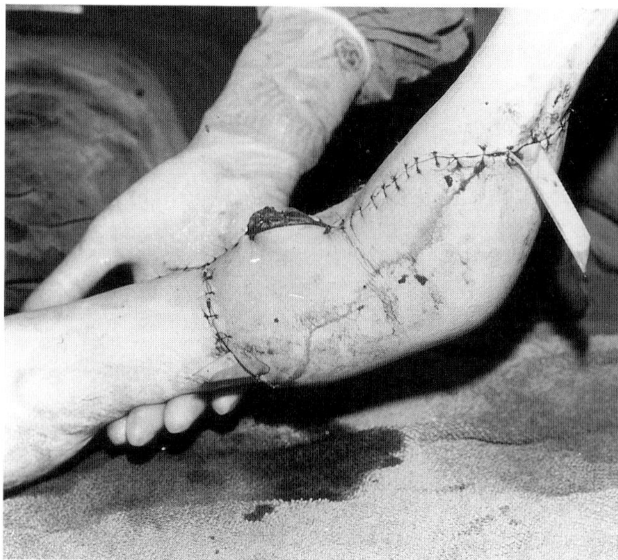

(b)

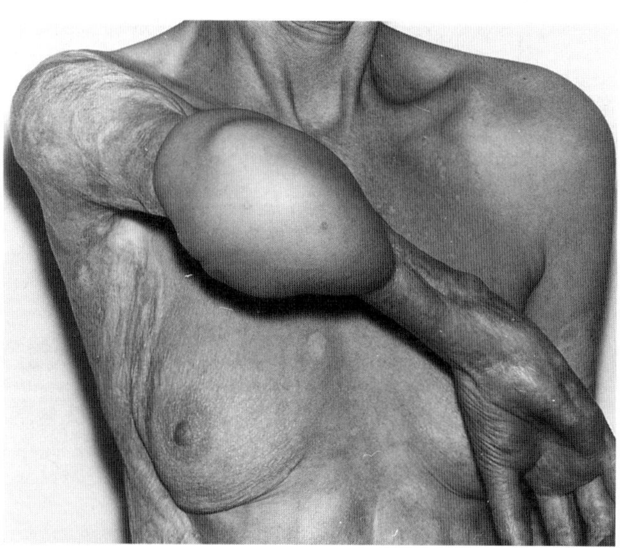

(c)

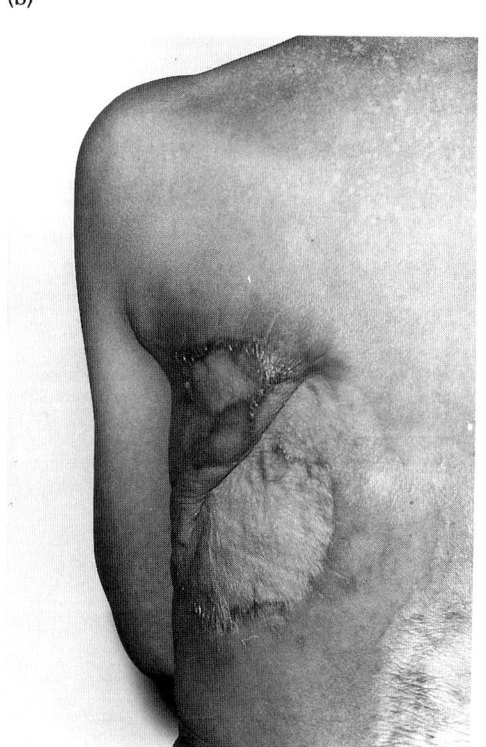

(d)

Fig. 9.25 (a) A very large latissimus dorsi myocutaneous flap being raised for free transfer to an exposed elbow joint. (b) The flap in place. (c) The later result. (d) The skin-grafted donor site. Nowadays, one would probably use muscle alone, covered with skin grafts, to minimize donor site morbidity.

tage that the patient may remain supine (this is only an advantage if, in such a position, the recipient site is accessible!). Both may be myocutaneous flaps if required, to provide total skin repair, or partial with the assistance of skin grafts, although it must be remembered that such flaps are more bulky than muscle flaps with skin grafts. This is especially evident on the distal parts of the limbs.

Although this is not a treatise on microvascular technique, it is worth restating here that the use of end-to-side anastomosis has greatly contributed to the success rate of free flap transfer, especially to the leg. The reasons for this are that the spasm associated with complete severance of a leg vessel is avoided, and the blood flow past an end-to-side anastomosis is faster, thus reducing the incidence of thrombosis. The preservation of the distal blood flow down the main artery is also an important consideration. It is essential to site the anastomoses where the recipient vessels are not damaged, as suturing damaged vessels is a potent cause of thrombosis. The advantage of long free flap pedicles will now be appreciated: they can reach well away from the site of actual trauma. It is common practice, for example, to anastomose free flap vessels onto the posterior tibial artery and adjacent vein, distally at the ankle, even when the site of trauma is more proximal. The vessels are certainly more accessible at that site. Sometimes it will be more appropriate with proximal tibial injuries to anastomose well up onto the popliteal artery to get away from the area of local tissue damage.

Conclusion

It will be apparent from this discussion that the modern management of severe open fractures should be an early collaborative effort between those who can provide the necessary expertise. The application of such modern understanding and techniques provides the potential for the more rapid rehabilitation of patients, and the reduction of the incidence of complications.

References

Byrd, S.H., Cierney, G. & Tebbetts, J.B. The management of open tibial fractures with associated soft-tissue loss: external pin fixation with early flap coverage. *Plast Reconstr Surg* 1981; **68**: 73–79.

Byrd, S.H., Spicer, T.E. & Cierney, G. Management of open tibial fractures. *Plast Reconstr Surg* 1985; **76**: 719–730.

Cormack, G.C. & Lamberty, B.G.H. *The Arterial Anatomy of Skin Flaps.* Churchill Livingstone: Edinburgh, 1986.

Ger, R. New operative approach in the treatment of chronic osteomyelitis of the tibial diaphysis. *Clin Orthop* 1970; **70**: 165.

Ger, R. Surgical treatment of ulcerative lesions of the leg. *Curr Probl Surg* 1972; **9**: 1–52.

Ger, R. The surgical management of ulcers of the heel. *Surg Gynecol Obstet* 1975; **140**: 909–911.

Godina, M. Early reconstruction of complex trauma of the extremities. *Plast Reconstr Surg* 1985; **78**: 285–292.

MacMillan, B.G. The use of mesh skin grafting in treating burns. *Surg Clin North Am* 1970; **50**: 1347–1359.

Mathes, S.J. & Nahai, F. *Clinical Atlas of Muscle and Musculocutaneous Flaps.* CV Mosby: St Louis, 1979.

Mathes, S.J., McCraw, J.B. & Vasconez, L.O. Muscle transposition flaps for coverage of lower extremity defects: anatomic considerations. *Surg Clin North Am* 1974; **54**: 1337–1354.

Maxwell, G.P. & Hoopes, J.E. Management of compound injuries of the lower extremity. *Plast Reconstr Surg* 1979; **63**: 176–185.

McCraw, J.B., Myers, B. & Shanklin, K.D. The value of fluorescein in predicting the viability of arterialized flaps. *Plast Reconstr Surg* 1977; **60**: 710–719.

Pers, M. & Medgyesi, S. Pedicle muscle flaps and their applications in the surgery of repair. *Br J Plast Surg* 1975; **26**: 313–321.

Ponten, B. The fascio-cutaneous flap: its use in soft tissue defects of the lower leg. *Br J Plast Surg* 1981; **34**: 215–220.

Souter, D.S., Scheker, L.R., Tanner, N.S.B. & McGregor, I.A. The radial forearm flap: a versatile method for intra-oral reconstruction. *Br J Plast Surg* 1983; **36**: 1–8.

Vasconez, L.O. & McCraw, J.B. The use of muscle in plastic and reconstructive surgery. In: Krizec, T.L. & Hoopes, J.E. (eds) *Symposium on Basic Science: Applications to Plastic Surgery.* CV Mosby: St. Louis, 1976.

Vasconez, L.O., Bostwick, J. & McCraw, J.B. Coverage of exposed bone by muscle transposition and skin grafting. *Plast Reconstr Surg* 1974; **53**: 526–530.

Vasconez, L.O., Schneider, W.B. & Jurkiewicz, M.J. The treatment of 'pressure sores'. *Curr Probl Surg* 1977; **14**: 1–62.

Yaremchuk, M.J., Brumback, R.J., Manson, P.N., Burgess, A.R., Poka, A. & Weiland, A.J. Acute and definitive management of traumatic osteocutaneous defects of the lower extremity. *Plast Reconstr Surg* 1987; **80**: 1–12.

10: Fractures in Children

I.H.THOMAS

Introduction

Children's bones differ from those of adults in several ways. This is due to differences in structure, growth and faster rates of healing. As the developing skeleton grows and matures from infancy to adulthood it becomes susceptible to different patterns of failure which influence the approach to treatment. Particular problems arise in the diagnosis of some fractures of the growth plate and in suspected non-accidental injury. The importance of a thorough examination of the injured child and the development of a satisfactory working relationship not only with the patient but also with the parents cannot be overemphasized.

Structure and behaviour under stress of growing bone

The diaphysis. Growing bone is extremely vascular and therefore more porous when compared with a cross-section of mature bone. In the neonate the diaphysis consists of woven bone which is subsequently transformed into lamellar bone by the development of Haversian systems and apposition of bone by the periosteum. With increasing age there is an increase in the stiffness, strength and resistance to a bending (tension) stress. This is due to the increase in bone mass and the longitudinal orientation of the osteons and collagen fibres. In children the endosteal bone is stronger than the subperiosteal bone. This explains why, in an adult, a tension stress sufficient to produce a diaphyseal fracture may result, in a young child, in plastic deformation and a bent bone, without a visible fracture on the radiograph and, in the older child, in a greenstick fracture.

The metaphysis. Compared with that in the adult the cortex of the metaphyseal region is thinner and perforated by more foramina. Because bones increase in length from the ends there is considerable metabolic activity in the metaphyseal region with new bone formation and remodelling. This accounts for the increased uptake demonstrated by a radionuclide bone scan. Metaphyseal cancellous bone does not develop secondary Haversian systems until the late stages of maturation. This probably accounts for the susceptibility of metaphyseal bone to fail under compression whereas adult cancellous bone fails more readily under tension.

The epiphysis. With the exception of the distal femur all the epiphyses at birth consist only of cartilage. The secondary centres of ossification form at a time characteristic for each epiphysis. Those around the elbow, for example, appear in the following order: capitulum, 5 years; medial epicondyle, 7 years; trochlear, 9 years and the lateral epicondyle at 11 years (Hensinger 1986). As the secondary centres of ossification increase in size they become stiffer than the more resilient epiphyseal cartilage. This has a bearing on the age at which certain epiphyseal fractures tend to occur. The superficial layers of epiphyseal cartilage develop into adult-type hyaline cartilage and lose the ability to become transformed into bone. For this reason unreduced rotated epiphyseal fractures fail to unite.

The growth plate (physis). Being responsible for longitudinal growth this is the most important part of the skeleton. The growth plates in long bones are discoid and initially planar but with growth they become contoured and develop interdigitations (the mammillary processes). These increase the intrinsic stability of the growth plate to shearing stress. The germinal layer of cells is attached to the epiphysis and receives its blood supply from the epiphyseal vessels (Fig. 10.1). This may be jeopardized in total separation of those epiphyses entirely covered with cartilage, the capital femoral epiphysis and head of radius, with the possible result of avascular necrosis and cessation of growth. In those

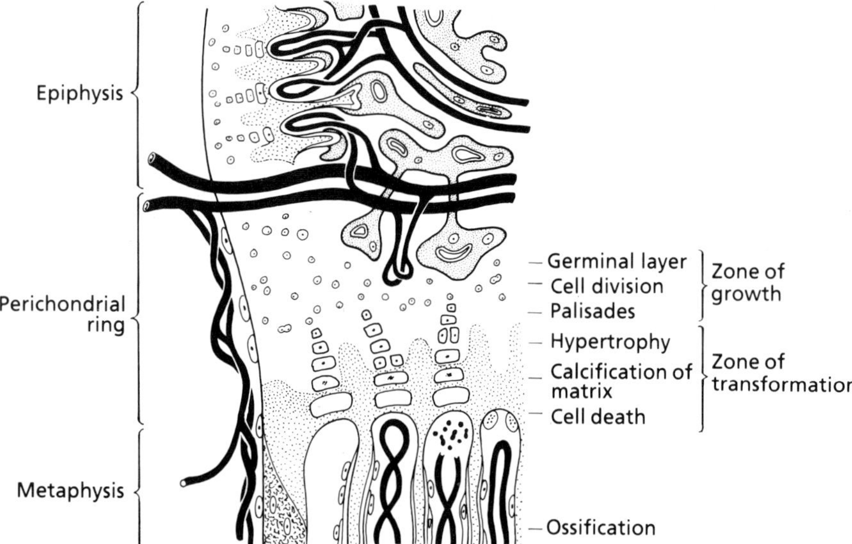

Fig. 10.1 The epiphysis, growth plate (physis) and perichondrial ring.

epiphyses which receive their blood supply through soft tissue attachments, a soft tissue hinge remains attached after separation and preserves the circulation. The viscoelastic nature of cartilage allows the epiphyseal cartilage and the growth plate to withstand large forces when applied rapidly. In decreasing order the growth plate is most resistant to pure axial tension, bending and torsion. Interstitial cracks can appear in the growth plate with half the stress necessary to produce total separation (Bright *et al.* 1974). When separation does occur it usually does so through the zone of cartilage transformation between the uncalcified and calcified cartilage layers (lower hypertrophic zone). However, with increasing age separation may occur through part of the germinal layer and result in asymmetrical longitudinal growth.

The periosteum. In children this is thicker and stronger than in adults. It is relatively loosely attached to the diaphysis and is easily elevated at operation. In the metaphyseal region it is more densely attached and blends into the perichondrial ring and perichondrium. The perichondrial ring (Fig. 10.1) completely encircles the growth plate and is considered to play an important role in increasing the width of the growth plate. Peripherally, it consists of fibrocartilage and receives its blood supply from branches of metaphyseal periosteal vessels. Muscles are attached to the periosteum, and tendons and ligaments into the fibrous and fibrocartilaginous regions of the metaphysis, perichondrial ring and epiphysis. All these soft tissue attachments contribute significantly to the stability of the epiphysis. Experimentally, four times the force is required to disrupt a growth plate if all the soft tissue connections remain. Because of the nature of the soft tissue attachments and the fact that the growth plate is the weakest of these tissues, sprains and dislocations are therefore uncommon in childhood.

Classification

Fractures are the most common type of skeletal injury in childhood and are usually the result of low energy trauma. Many fractures seen in adults, for example, fractures and dislocations of the hand, and fractures of the spine, hip and foot and open fractures, are uncommon in children. Fractures of the clavicle and supracondylar region of the humerus are common in children and growth plate injuries are obviously confined to the growing child. Fractures of the upper limb predominate.

Buckle fracture (Fig. 10.2)

This is most commonly seen in the metaphysis of the distal forearm and tibia. It is the result of an axial compression force. Buckle fractures occur in young children and appear as a kink in the cortex with minimal displacement.

Bend of bone

This is an uncommon injury and occurs mainly in the ulna and fibula in association with a complete fracture of the radius and tibia without obvious angular deformity; it is due to plastic deformation of the bone. In the very young a bend in the ulna may be associated

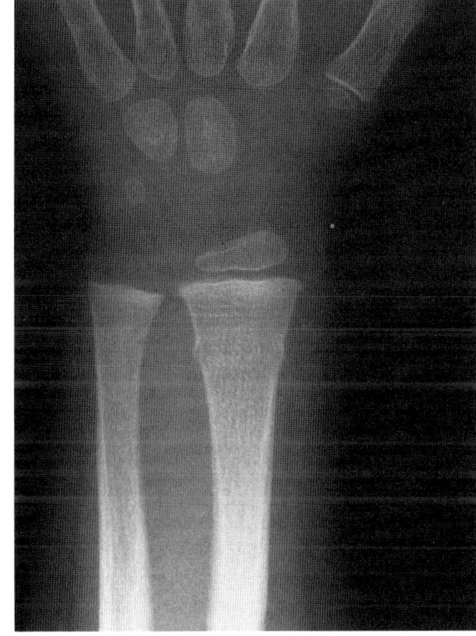

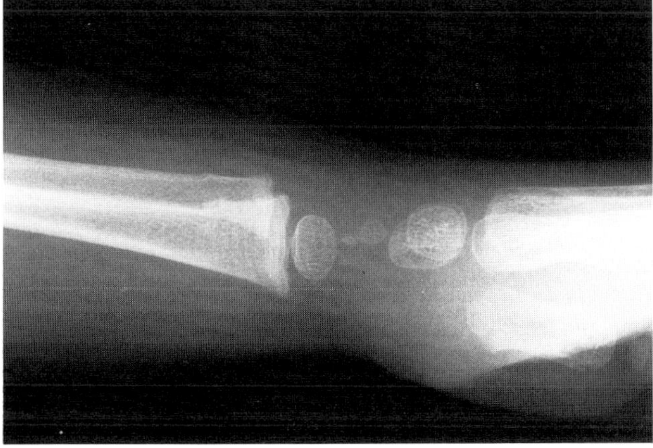

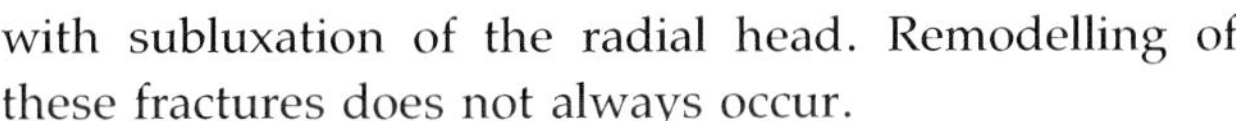

Fig. 10.2 (a) Anteroposterior and (b) lateral radiograph of a 'buckle' fracture of the distal radius and ulna.

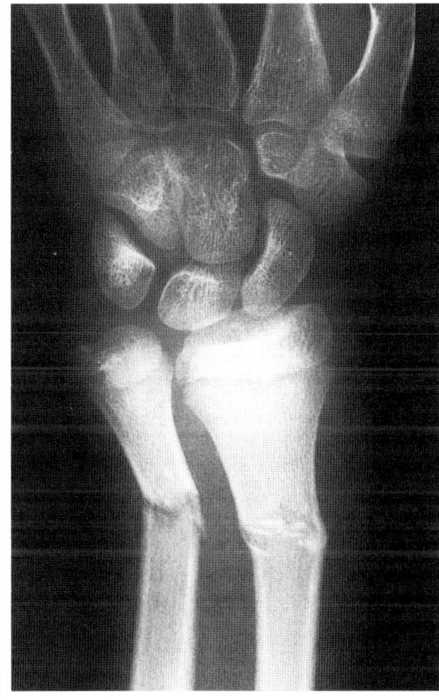

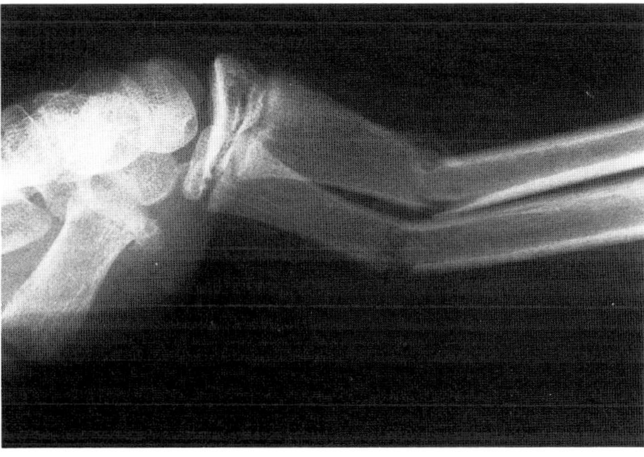

Fig. 10.3 (a) Anteroposterior and (b) lateral radiograph of 'greenstick' fractures of the distal radius and ulna.

with subluxation of the radial head. Remodelling of these fractures does not always occur.

Greenstick fractures (Fig. 10.3)

These commonly occur in the metaphysis. Mid-diaphyseal forearm and tibial greenstick fractures occur in neonates and infants but are rare in older children. They arise when an angulatory force, sufficient to disrupt the periosteum and cortex under tension, is applied. A compression fracture occurs in the opposite cortex.

Complete fracture (Fig. 10.4)

This is an injury of older children. The majority of these fractures are diaphyseal; displacement is common but comminution is rare.

Epiphyseal and growth plate injuries

Of all fractures 20% occur through the growth plate or epiphysis (Peterson & Peterson 1972). They are twice as common in boys. The peak incidence in girls is between 11 and 12 years of age and in boys it occurs 2

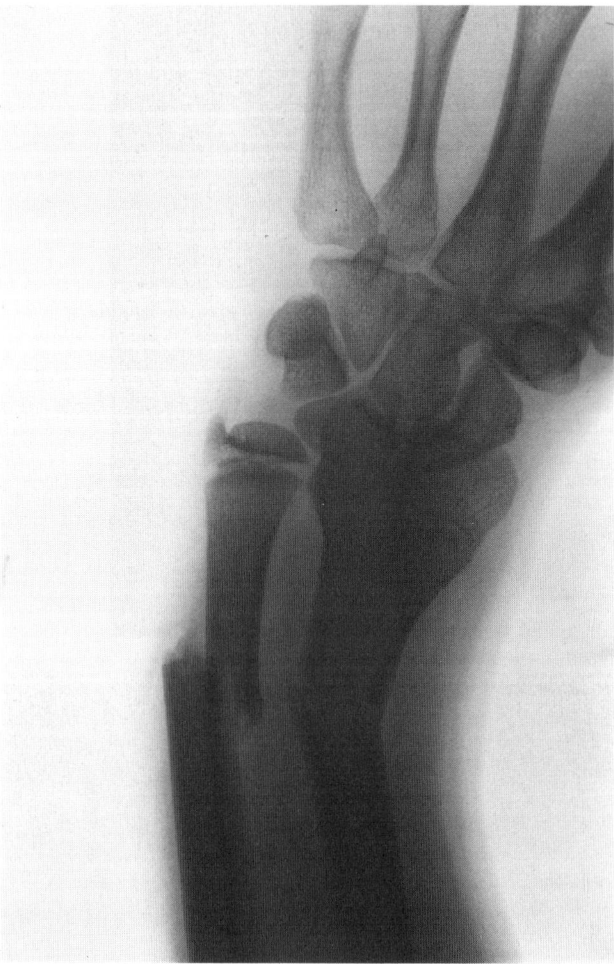

(a)

(b)

Fig. 10.4 (a) Anteroposterior and (b) lateral radiograph of complete fracture of diaphysis of radius and ulna.

years later. The most frequently affected sites are the distal radius and tibia and together these make up half of the fractures.

Epiphyseal fractures (Rang 1983a)

These usually involve the growth plate, with three exceptions:

1 Avulsion by a ligament. The radiograph may only show small osseous fragments but there is always a substantially larger fragment of epiphyseal cartilage. Common sites include the avulsion of the anterior tibial spine by the anterior cruciate ligament, the ulna styloid by the collateral ligament and the bases of the phalanges by collateral ligaments. Displaced fragments may block joint movement and cause symptoms of instability. If unreduced there is a significant risk of non-union.

2 Osteochondral fractures. Traumatic dislocation of the patella is not uncommonly associated with an osteochondral fracture of the lateral femoral condyle or medial facet of the patella. This should be suspected in all patella dislocations because the bony elements may be small and therefore not readily visible on the radiographs.

3 Compression fractures. These are rare and tend to occur in osteoporotic epiphyses secondary to either disuse or paralytic conditions.

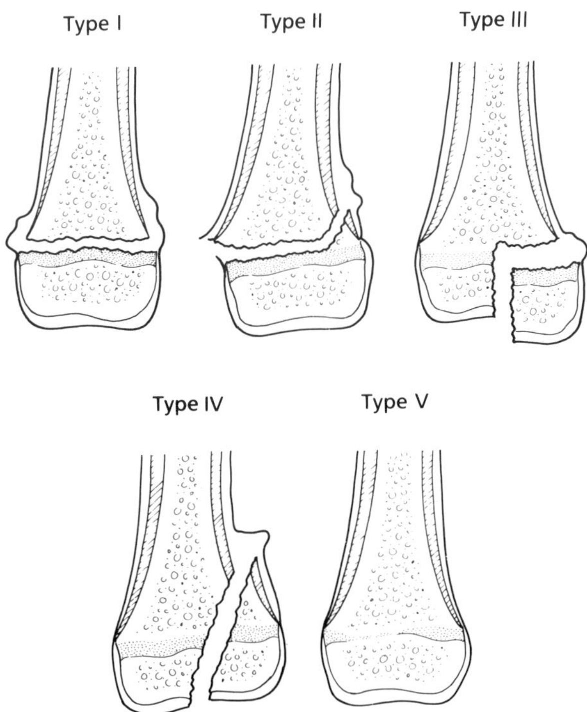

Fig. 10.5 Salter and Harris classification of growth plate fractures.

Growth plate fractures

Several classifications of these injuries (Salter & Harris 1963, Poland 1965, Weber 1980, Ogden 1982), whose major complication is the development of significant deformity, have been described to help the clinician distinguish those injuries which have a good prognosis from those which do not and hence, to guide the management. The classification by Salter and Harris (1963) is the most practical and is used worldwide (Fig. 10.5). However, because the classification is based on radiographic appearances the prognostic value of the classification is not as accurate as initially proposed. This is because fractures with the same radiological appearance may not have the same outcome due to differences in the precise mechanism of the injury.

Type I (6%) (Rogers 1970) (Fig. 10.6). In this type of injury the epiphysis separates from the metaphysis without extension through either the epiphysis itself or the metaphysis. This is usually seen as a birth injury in infants, young children or occasionally as a pathological fracture secondary to scurvy, rickets or osteomyelitis. There is tenderness at the level of the growth plate in undisplaced fractures which are often diagnosed as 'sprains'. Rarely displaced fractures may be associated with damage to the central portion of the growth plate as the displaced epiphysis is compressed by the trailing edge of the metaphysis.

Type II (75%) (Fig. 10.7). This is the most common type overall and is particularly prevalent in children over the age of 10. The fracture plane extends from a tear in the periosteum, through the growth plate and out through a variable portion of the metaphysis. The triangle of metaphyseal bone with its attached hinge of periosteum can be used to stabilize the reduction in displaced fractures. In about 20% of cases reduction in longitudinal growth may occur with most effect if it occurs in the distal femur. It is perhaps fortunate that this injury tends to occur in the older child.

Type III (8%) (Fig. 10.8). This takes the form of an intra-articular fracture of the epiphysis communicating with a horizontal cleavage of the growth plate. The fracture may arise and propagate from either end. It is most common in the distal tibia of the adolescent, when part of the plate has closed and growth disturbance is not therefore a significant clinical problem. Some type III fractures, especially of the medial malleolus, may displace late in a cast because of disruption of the soft tissue attachments.

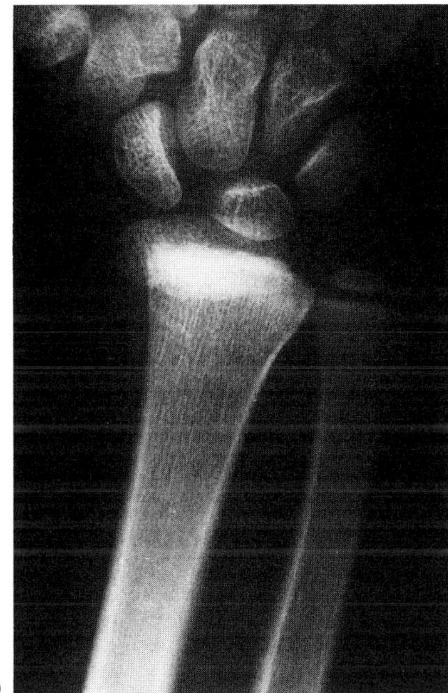
(a)

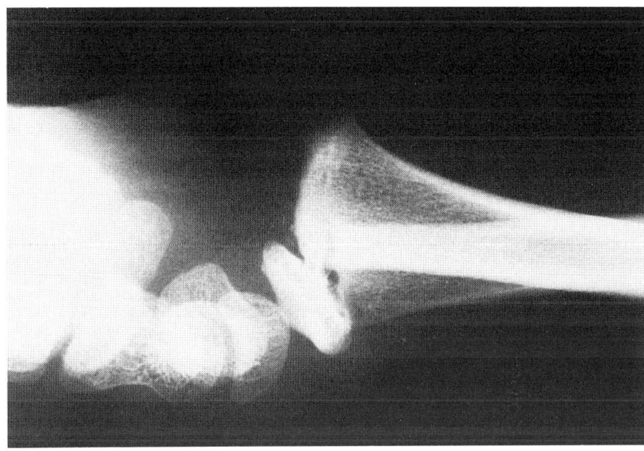
(b)

Fig. 10.6 Salter and Harris type I fracture of the distal radius.

Type IV (10%) (Fig. 10.9). The fracture starts at the joint surface, splits the epiphysis, crosses the growth plate, exits through the metaphysis and usually displaces towards the diaphysis. If initially undisplaced, displacement often occurs in the cast. If displacement is allowed to persist cross-union occurs between the displaced epiphysis and the remaining undisplaced metaphysis. Not all type IV injuries are the same, for example, if the fracture passes through the cartilaginous part of an epiphysis (Fig. 10.9) bridging is unlikely and a stepped fracture line may be stable after closed reduction.

Type V (1%) (Fig. 10.10). This occurs as a result of an axial compression force crushing part or all of the growth plate. The extent of the damage depends on the precise

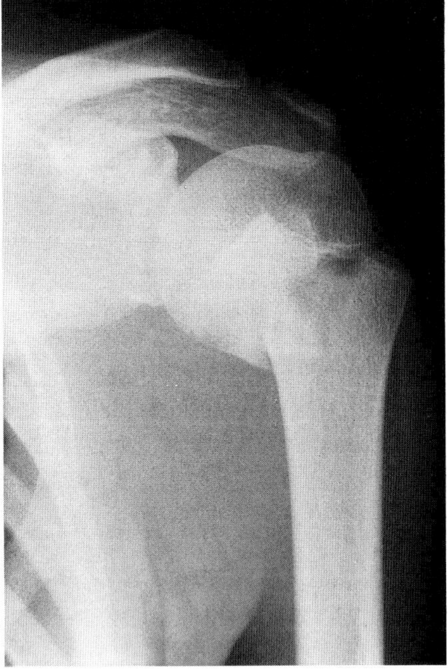

Fig. 10.7 Salter and Harris type II fracture of the proximal humerus.

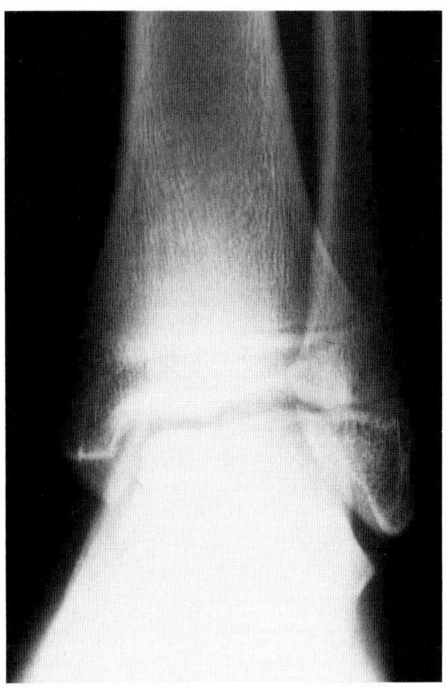

Fig. 10.8 Salter and Harris type III fracture of the distal tibia.

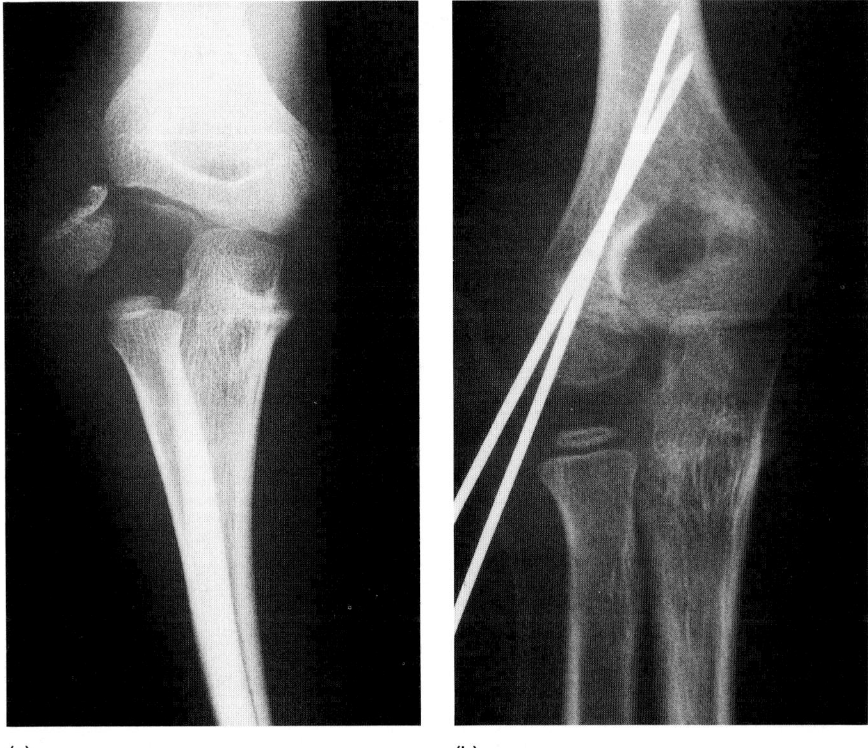

(a)   (b)

Fig. 10.9 (a) Salter and Harris type IV fracture of the capitulum. (b) Post open reduction and Kirschner wire stabilization.

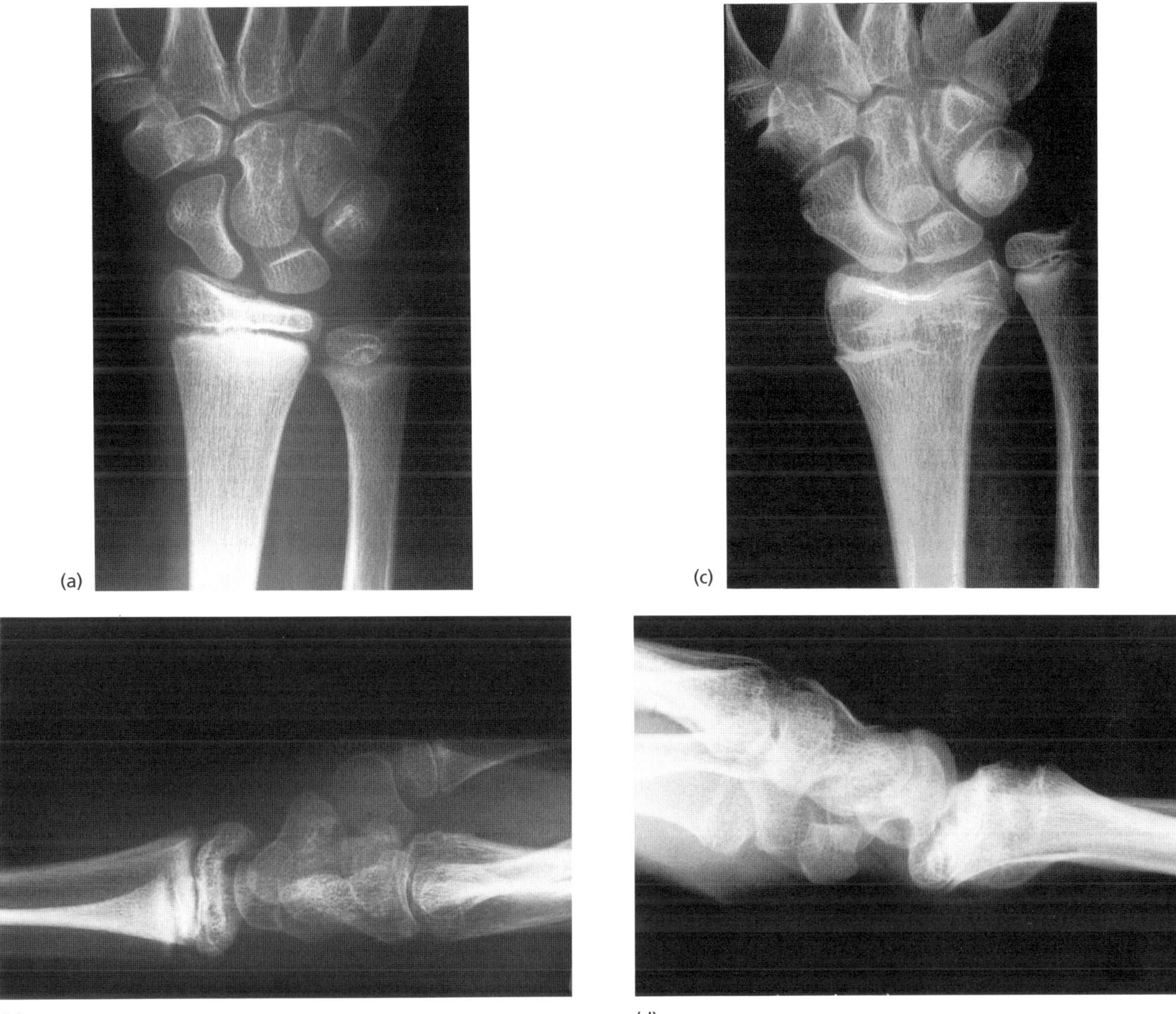

Fig. 10.10 Salter and Harris type III/V fracture of the distal radius. (a) Anteroposterior and (b) lateral radiograph of the initial injury to the distal radius; (c) anteroposterior and (d) lateral radiograph 22 months later showing asymmetrical growth arrest with shortening and dorsal tilt of the epiphysis.

magnitude and vector of the force. This injury is impossible to diagnose initially and may occur in association with type I, II and III (Fig. 10.10) fractures. Metaphyseal osteomyelitis may similarly leave permanent damage to the growth plate. The end result is either partial or complete arrest of growth with shortening and/or angulation.

Type VI. Rang (1983b) described growth disturbance following damage to the perichondrial ring. This is not a true injury of the growth plate, more a disruption of the perichondrial soft tissues. The injury may occur as a closed injury with local haematoma formation or as the result of a burn or degloving injury involving loss of part of the perichondrial ring. This leads to either the formation of a bony bar and rapidly developing angular deformity or an osteochondroma.

Pathological fractures

These do occur and they may be the first indication of an underlying disease. Treatment is determined by the nature of the lesion. The fractures are almost invariably the result of a trivial injury and occur through either a lytic lesion, such as a simple bone cyst, fibrous cortical defect, fibrous dysplasia or aneurysmal bone cyst, or in bone weakened by osteoporosis secondary to paralytic disorders and osteogenesis imperfecta.

Healing

Fractures in children heal rapidly, many in half the time it takes for an adult fracture to unite. This is very apparent in the young and non-union seldom occurs.

Remodelling

With further growth the potential to remodel a fracture is greater than that in the adult, in whom only a 'round-ing off' occurs. In children the growth plate may realign by differential growth until it is perpendicular to the axis of the joint movement (Ryoppy & Karaharju 1974). To a much greater extent, remodelling takes place by appositional growth and resorption but this is not true realignment. The potential for remodelling is greater the younger the child is, with displacement in the plane of the axis of movement in the neighbouring joint and in metaphyseal fractures (Fig. 10.11). In the latter this is most evident at the ends of those bones which con-

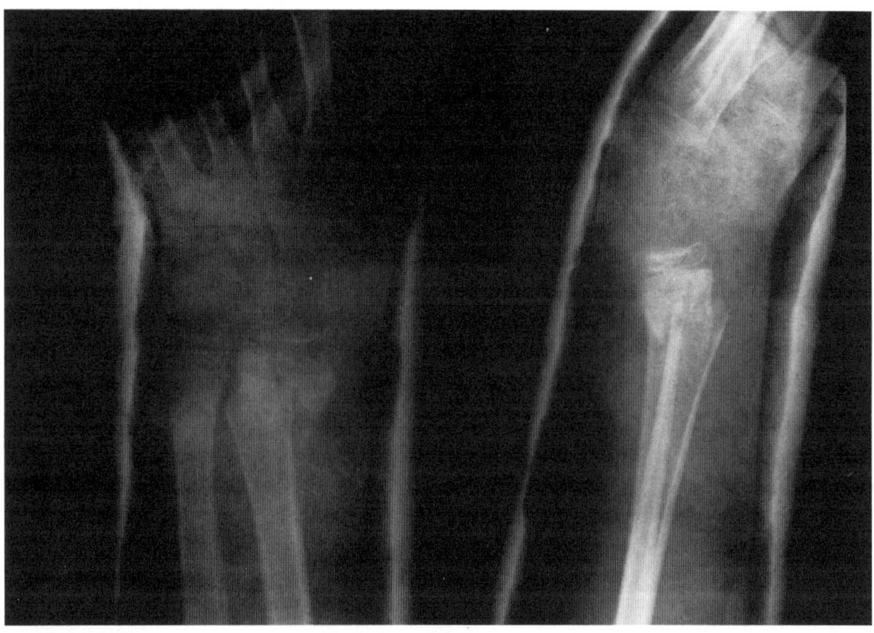

(a)

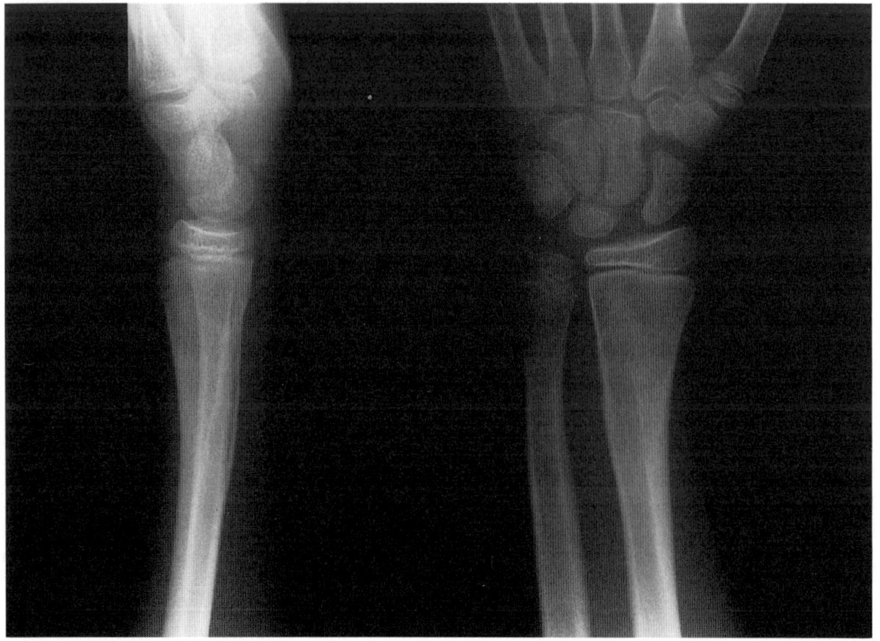

(b)

Fig. 10.11 Anteroposterior and lateral radiographs of a displaced fracture of the distal radius of a 5 year old: (a) 3 weeks after the fracture and (b) 1 year later showing remodelling.

tribute most to the overall length of bone; the proximal humerus, distal radius, distal femur and proximal tibia. The process may take up to 5 years and cannot therefore be relied upon to help those with less than 2 years of remaining growth. Remodelling will not help displaced intra-articular fractures, type IV epiphyseal injuries, malrotation and mid-shaft forearm fractures in those over 10 years if angulation is greater than 15° (Roberts 1986), varus or valgus angulation and those with gross shortening. Mid-shaft femoral fractures with less than 20° of coronal and 30° of sagittal angulation usually remodel to within 10% of the opposite side (Malkawi *et al.* 1986).

Overgrowth

The growth of long bone is influenced by the intrinsic tension within the growth plate and the periosteal sleeve. Disruption of the periosteal sleeve by a fracture and the subsequent increase in blood flow may play a part in the overgrowth that often accompanies fracture healing. Growth stimulation following a fracture is most active and consistent in 2- to 10-year-olds. It persists for 6 or more months after the fracture and the final difference in length is usually permanent. The amount of acceptable shortening during treatment in this age group is 1−2 cm. Over the age of 10 years the stronger muscles in the lower limb, particularly in the thigh, increase the risk of shortening if traction is inadequate or is discontinued too soon.

Progressive deformity

Damage to the growth plate, if complete, will result in growth arrest and progressive shortening (Fig. 10.10). If the growth plate is partially damaged, and this is more commonly the case, the result is progressive angular deformity. The outcome depends on the age of the child and whether it occurs in a one- or two-bone unit. Three types of partial growth arrest have been described (Bright 1984): type I peripheral (the most common), type II central and type III, a combined lesion which usually follows a type III or type IV growth plate injury. Before a plan of management can be made the diagnosis must be confirmed radiologically and the size of the bony bar determined. There should be no evidence of active infection and injured parts should have full-thickness skin cover. An estimation should be made of the eventual limb length discrepancy. As a rough guide, for the lower limbs, the distal femoral growth plate adds 9 mm per year and the proximal tibial growth plate 6 mm. The bony bar should be resected in type I and type II

lesions. In type III lesions, with less than 50% of the growth plate involved, the bar should be excised and the angular deformity (which may include an element of rotation) corrected by metaphyseal osteotomy or hemi-epiphyseal distraction. If more than 50% of the growth plate has been damaged the epiphysiodesis should be completed, angular deformity corrected and then a limb length equalization procedure performed.

Principles of management

Diagnosis

The history and examination should take place in calm surroundings and in an unhurried manner. It is important to ascertain whether the mechanism of the accident as described is consistent with the injury sustained. Older children can usually speak for themselves but it is essential that the history is also obtained from a responsible adult and non-accidental injury excluded. Displaced fractures are usually obvious. With undisplaced fractures the most reliable physical sign is local tenderness which indicates the region to be radiographed. At the initial consultation a general outline of the management of possible problems and complications should be discussed with the parents. Their first impressions are an important influence on how they view the way the injury is being treated and on their co-operation with follow-up.

Radiographs

The minimum that should be accepted is good quality anteroposterior and lateral radiographs of the affected bone including the joints above and below. If the clinical suspicion of a bony injury is not confirmed alternative views should be obtained. The radiolucent growth plate often causes problems so, if in doubt, radiographs of the opposite limb should also be obtained. Oblique views are particularly helpful in fully visualizing the nature of medial epicondyle and lateral condylar fractures of the distal humerus and also of fractures involving the ankle. Oblique views are also helpful with some diaphyseal fractures where the plane of displacement is 45° to that of the anteroposterior and lateral views. The opportunity to assess normal soft tissue shadows and haemarthroses should not be missed as the latter may be the only indication of an intra-articular fracture.

Principles of treatment

Undisplaced and minimally displaced fractures do not

require reduction. However, one must be careful of relying on remodelling to correct displaced fractures and it is wise to remember that 'what you get out of plaster depends on what you put into it'. The majority of undisplaced fractures can be treated successfully by closed reduction under general anaesthesia but regional anaesthesia has been shown to be an acceptable alternative for forearm fractures (Olney *et al.* 1988). As the periosteum is usually intact on the side to which the fracture has displaced this can be used to stabilize the fracture. Greenstick fractures, particularly in the diaphysis, may need to be completed in order to permit reduction. Traction is an alternative means of achieving reduction. Gallows traction is suitable for femoral shaft fractures and for infants under 2-years-old and Dunlop traction is suitable for supracondylar fractures of the humerus with considerable soft tissue swelling. Immobilization is generally obtained using a padded plaster cast with three-point moulding. Fractures of the clavicle need to be supported in a sling and those of the proximal humerus in a collar and cuff with use of gravity to assist reduction. Fractures of the shaft of the femur in children younger than 10-years-old are usually treated by skin traction. Alternatively, low velocity fractures may be managed after reduction in a one-and-a-half spica cast (Sugi & Cole 1987). Femoral shaft fractures in older children usually require skeletal traction.

The excellent primary management of a fracture may be ruined by poor follow-up. The parents should be given adequate instructions on how to detect complications such as increasing pain under the cast, swelling, coldness and discoloration distal to the cast. All displaced fractures should be radiographed at 1 week. Remanipulation of metaphyseal fractures 2-weeks-old or more is contraindicated because of the risk of damage to the growth plate. It is wise to review all epiphyseal fractures at 1 year.

Indications for open reduction

Because children's fractures can, in the majority of cases, be successfully treated by closed methods this does not mean that operative treatment is always contraindicated. Open reduction and internal fixation is indicated

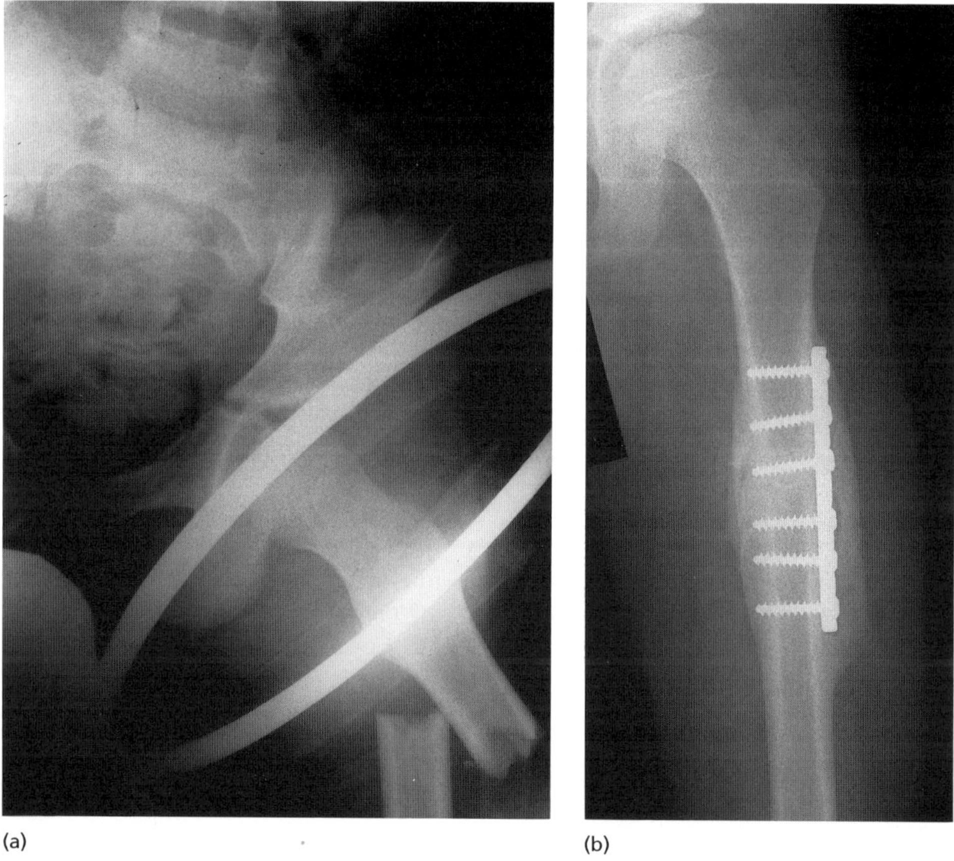

(a)(b)

Fig. 10.12 (a) Displaced fracture of the upper third of the femur in a 6-year-old; (b) 9 months later prior to removal of the 3.5 mm dynamic compression plate (DCP).

if conservative treatment cannot achieve acceptable results. This is often the case in children with multiple injuries or with head injury associated with spasticity. The more common indications are as follows:

1 Failed remanipulation of a forearm fracture in a child older than 10 years of age. Needless to say the remanipulation should be performed in an operating theatre so that surgery can proceed immediately. It is unacceptable practice to have to wake a child up and then reanaesthetize him or her on a separate occasion. In older children Monteggia fractures need open reduction.

2 Failed reduction or redisplacement of the proximal femoral shaft fracture with flexion, abduction and external rotation of the proximal fragment (Fig. 10.12). The likelihood of overgrowth following surgery is on balance less of a problem than malunion.

3 Open reduction of an avulsion of the anterior tibial spine is indicated if the fracture is not completely reduced by extending the knee.

4 Supracondylar fractures of the humerus associated with a vascular injury or swelling sufficient to prevent flexion of the elbow above 90°, and therefore maintenance of a closed reduction, can be stabilized either by closed reduction and parallel percutaneous Kirschner wire fixation from the lateral side or by open reduction using the posterior approach and crossed Kirschner wire fixation protecting the ulnar nerve.

5 Displaced type III epiphyseal fractures and all type IV (Fig. 10.9) epiphyseal fractures. In order to reduce the risk of avascular necrosis developing the soft tissue dissection should be kept to the minimum required to expose and reduce the fracture.

Following an open reduction and internal fixation the metalware should always be removed once solid fracture union has occurred.

Open fractures

The principles of management are the same as for open fractures in adults.

Acute complications

The most important immediate complications of children's fractures are vascular and nerve injury.

Vascular injury. A high index of suspicion is required to avoid the development of Volkmann's ischaemic contracture. The earliest symptom is severe unremitting pain made worse by passive stretching of the affected muscle groups. A vascular injury may either be a complication of the fracture itself, for example, an intimal tear in a kinked brachial artery associated with a supracondylar fracture of the humerus, or be due to a tight cast or Gallows traction strapping. The priority of management is either to reduce the fracture or release the extrinsic pressure by splitting the cast to the skin or releasing the traction binding. If the circulation fails to improve 'on the table' arteriography should be performed prior to vascular repair and open fasciotomy of all the fascial compartments in the limb.

Nerve injury. This is usually a traction lesion associated with an upper limb fracture. It is essential that the initial assessment of any fracture or dislocation includes an examination of peripheral nerves in the affected limb. The majority resolve spontaneously and only preventative measures to protect anaesthetic skin and the development of joint contractures are needed during the recovery phase.

Late complications

Overgrowth and progressive deformity following fracture have already been covered. The remaining significant late complication is that of malunion. This is usually the result of an overoptimistic expectation that remodelling will restore axial alignment in displaced diaphyseal fractures. This is commonly a problem in the forearm where the final restriction is twice the angular deformity.

References

Bright, R.W. Physeal injuries. In: Rockwood, C.A., Wilkins, K.E. & King, R.E. (eds) *Fractures in Children*. Lippincott: Philadelphia, 1984.

Bright, R.W., Burstein, A.H. & Elmore, S.M. Epiphyseal-plate cartilage. *J Bone Joint Surg* 1974; **56A**: 688–703.

Hensinger, R.N. *Standards in Pediatric Orthopedics: Tables, Charts and Graphs Illustrating Growth*. Raven Press: New York, 1986.

Malkawi, H., Shannak, A. & Hadi, S. Remodelling after femoral shaft fractures in children treated by the modified Blount method. *J Pediatr Orthop* 1986; **6**: 421–429.

Ogden, J.A. Injury to the growth mechanism. In: *Skeletal Injury in the Child*. Lea & Febiger: Philadelphia, 1982.

Olney, B.W., Lugg, P.C., Turner, P.L., Eyres, R.L. & Cole, W.G. Outpatient treatment of upper limb extremity injuries in childhood using intravenous regional anaesthesia. *J Pediatr Orthop* 1988; **8**: 576–579.

Peterson, C.A. & Peterson, H.A. Analysis of the incidence of injuries to the epiphyseal growth plate. *J Trauma* 1972; **12(4)**: 275–281.

Poland, J. Traumatic separation of the epiphysis in general. *Clin Orthop* 1965; **41**: 7–18.

Rang, M. Epiphyseal injuries. In: *Children's Fractures*. Lippincott: Philadelphia, 1983a.

Rang, M. Injuries of the perichondral ring. In: *Children's Fractures*. Lippincott: Philadelphia, 1983b.

Roberts, J.A. Angulation of radius in children's fractures. *J Bone Joint Surg* 1986; **68B**: 751−754.

Rogers, L.F. Radiology of epiphyseal injuries. *Radiology* 1970; **96**: 289−299.

Ryoppy, S. & Karaharju, E.O. Alteration of epiphyseal growth by an experimentally produced angular deformity. *Acta Orthop Scand* 1974; **45**: 490−498.

Salter, R.B. & Harris, W.R. Injuries involving the epiphyseal plate. *J Bone Joint Surg* 1963; **45A**: 587−622.

Sugi, M. & Cole, W.G. Early plaster treatment for fractures of the femoral shaft in childhood. *J Bone Joint Surg* 1987; **69B**: 743−745.

Weber, B.G. Fracture healing in the growing bone and in the mature skeleton. In: Weber, B.G., Brunner, Ch. & Freuler, F. (eds) *Treatment of Fractures in Children and Adolescents*. Springer-Verlag: New York, 1980.

11: Complications

Classification

P.J.GREGG

It cannot be stated too often that any patient present-ing with a fracture or dislocation must be examined as soon as possible for the presence of associated life-threatening injuries, and complications of the fracture or dislocation itself. In particular, immediate life-threatening complications, for example, shock, and limb-threatening complications, for example, associated vascular injury, must be looked for. All too frequently, even in the 1990s, the latter complication is missed or diagnosed late! It is convenient to classify complications into those which are *local* and those which are *general* (remote) and also according to whether they occur immediately, early or late.

Complications of fractures

Immediate complications

These include the following:
Local
  Skin (open fracture).
  Vascular.
  Neurological
    Nerve.
    Spinal cord and roots (see Chapter 18).
  Muscle.
  Viscera
    Abdominal.
    Thoracic.
General (remote)
  Multiple injuries.
  Haemorrhage; shock.
Skin damage (open fracture) is dealt with in Chapter 9; visceral injury is described in Chapter 7; and multiple injuries and shock are discussed in Chapters 7 and 6

respectively. Vascular injury and nerve injury are de-scribed in this chapter.

Early complications

Early complications of fractures are:
Local
  Sequelae of immediate complications
    Skin necrosis and gangrene.
    Compartment syndrome and Volkmann's
    ischaemia.
    Gas gangrene.
    Visceral complications.
  Venous thrombosis.
  Bone infection.
  Fracture blisters.
General (remote)
  Fat embolism.
  Pulmonary embolism.
  Pneumonia.
  Tetanus.
  Delirium tremens.
The more important of these are discussed in detail in this chapter.

Fracture blisters

Blistering of the skin is not unusual after fractures, especially in the region of the ankle, foot, lower leg and elbow. They appear during the first 24–48 hours after injury and result from traumatic oedema of the skin. They are particularly common after fracture of the os calcis (see Fig. 25.9). The blisters should be emptied by pricking with a sterile needle, then sprayed with an antibiotic spray and a non-stick dressing applied. Incisions through skin affected by fracture blisters are obviously best avoided if possible, but the author would not regard their presence as an absolute contraindication to surgery. The author has frequently carried out open reduction of fractures of the os calcis in the presence of fracture blisters without significant wound-healing problems.

Delirium tremens

Alcoholic patients not infrequently sustain injuries because of falls; they are then admitted to hospital where they find themselves suddenly separated from their regular supply of alcohol. It is not uncommon for them to suffer from delirium tremens and this should be considered as a possible cause of confusion and restlessness in these patients.

Late complications

In summary, these are:
Local
  Bone
    Malunion.
    Delayed and non-union.
    Growth disturbance.
    Chronic infection.
    Disuse osteoporosis.
    Refracture.
    Avascular necrosis.
  Joint
    Stiffness.
    Secondary osteoarthritis: avascular necrosis; intra-articular fracture.
  Nerve — tardy nerve palsy.
  Muscle and tendon
    Myositis ossificans.
    Late tendon rupture.
    Tendonitis.
  Reflex sympathetic dystrophy (Sudeck's atrophy, algodystrophy).
General (remote)
  Renal calculi.
  Accident neurosis.
Malunion, non-union, chronic infection of bone, avascular necrosis and reflex sympathetic dystrophy are described in this chapter. Where appropriate the remainder will be described in the chapters dealing with specific fractures.

Malunion

Strictly speaking, a fracture which unites with residual displacement is malunited. However, in clinical circumstances, the term malunion should be reserved for those fractures which have united with residual dis-

placement which produces a visible deformity and/or functional impairment. This complication of normal healing may result from imperfect reduction of the fracture or failure to stabilize a previously undisplaced or adequately reduced fracture. This complication will be considered further in relation to specific fractures.

Complications of dislocations

Complications of dislocations can be classified in a similar way:
Immediate local
  Skin (open dislocation).
  Vascular.
  Neurological.
  Ligamentous.
  Associated fracture.
Early local
  Joint infection.
Late local
  Joint stiffness.
  Joint instability.
  Recurrent dislocation.
  Secondary osteoarthritis.
  Reflex sympathetic dystrophy.
  Myositis ossificans.
  Avascular necrosis.
Ligamentous injury, joint instability and recurrent dislocation will be considered further in the chapters dealing with specific dislocations.

Vascular complications

S.D.PARVIN AND P.R.F.BELL

Major vascular injuries associated with orthopaedic trauma are rare and occur in approximately 0.1–0.6% of long bone fractures (Porter 1967, Connolly *et al.* 1971, Sher 1975). Individual experience gained in the management of such injuries is therefore limited. The majority occur as a result of road traffic accidents (Sher 1975) and may not be recognized initially. In a review of vascular injuries sustained during World War II, 68% of amputations performed on Americans were because of vascular damage; 40% of vascular injuries eventually came to amputation (DeBakey & Simeone 1946). By the time of the Korean war, urgent vascular reconstruction had become possible and the amputation rate was reduced to only 9% (Jahnke & Seeley 1953). The improvement in outcome is due to a number of factors including: earlier recognition of the injury, rapid vascular repair before fracture fixation and the increasing availability of appropriately trained vascular surgeons.

This chapter will place emphasis upon the early diagnosis of coexistent vascular injury, the avoidance of delay in restoration of the circulation, the common vascular injuries seen and upon techniques for their repair.

Arterial insufficiency

Fractures alone cause considerable blood loss, the extent of which may not be fully appreciated when there is a closed injury. Vascular injuries are usually more obvious when there is an open injury. Acute vascular insufficiency may be missed early on because the patient will be hypotensive with weak pulses and pale peripheries after the fracture. The majority of patients with combined orthopaedic and vascular trauma are young and every effort should be made to optimize the outcome by early recognition of the injury.

Local factors

The arteries most frequently involved in vascular trauma are those in close proximity to bone or those which are held in a semi-fixed position. The subclavian artery is at risk where it passes beneath the clavicle, against which it may be compressed by upward displacement of the first rib. The brachial artery adjacent to the humeral shaft is at risk from direct injury by fragments of bone. The supracondylar portion of the humerus may damage the brachial artery by stretching where it is relatively fixed by the collateral branches around the elbow joint. The common femoral and profunda femoris arteries may be damaged by fragments from a fractured neck of femur. Femoral shaft fractures may lead to stretching of the superficial femoral artery, particularly in the region of the adductor hiatus, or the artery may be damaged directly by bone fragments. The popliteal artery is particularly at risk where it is stretched across the popliteal fossa, being fixed by the collateral vessels around the knee.

The mixture of orthopaedic and vascular injuries may lead to damage to the collaterals in the region of the fracture. This shortens the time available to the vascular surgeon to complete the repair.

Outcome

The outcome of a vascular injury complicating a fracture or dislocation depends upon a number of factors:
1 Maintenance of blood supply.
2 Speed of operation.
3 Age.
4 Atherosclerosis.
5 Diabetes mellitus.

Maintenance of blood supply

In any vascular injury it is essential to re-establish the distal circulation as rapidly as possible. Sensory and motor nerve endings lose their conduction after about 30–60 minutes of ischaemia. Restoration of circulation within this period results in complete recovery. Ischaemia for longer than this may result in permanent nerve damage. Muscle, which has relatively high blood-flow requirements compared with nerves and bone, becomes oedematous after about 6 hours of ischaemia and this has been recommended as the longest time for which it can survive normally (Miller & Welch 1949). However, the time available depends upon the adequacy of the collateral circulation, the site of injury and associated destruction of surrounding tissue. Prolonged ischaemia increases the local swelling and may further limit an inadequate blood supply. Beyond 6 hours the muscles begin to undergo necrosis and subsequent recovery will be patchy and variable. If the ischaemia persists for 12–24 hours no tissues survive and gangrene develops.

Speed of operation

Provided that vascular reconstruction is performed rapidly there should be complete recovery. It is essential that this is done prior to fixation of the fracture. If grafting is indicated, the length of graft required must be estimated. Subsequent manipulation of the fracture is not normally a problem because artery and vein grafts are flexible and allow considerable stretching without disruption.

Age

The age of the patient is important because arteries become less resilient and more atheromatous with increasing age. The collateral circulation is not as good and patients are less able to cope with major vessel obstruction.

Atherosclerosis and diabetes mellitus

Diabetes mellitus leads to premature atheroma and peripheral vascular disease. The rigid calcified blood vessels are more at risk than the more supple vessels of younger patients. Whilst the collateral circulation may be better in diabetics, repair of the major vessels is more difficult.

Types of injury

Vascular injuries are of two types, where either the vessel has been breached (open) or where it remains in continuity (closed). Open injuries are:
1 Division.
2 False aneurysm.
3 Arteriovenous fistula.
Closed injuries are:
1 Compression.
2 Intimal tear.
3 Thrombosis.

Division

These vascular injuries are caused by vascular penetration by bone spicules. Recognition of the injury is easy when the fracture is open but may be missed when the fracture is closed. Retraction and spontaneous limitation of bleeding often fails because of the ragged or incomplete nature of the tear in the vessel. Venous injury is as common as arterial injury and it is as important to repair the veins as it is to repair the arteries (Figs 11.1 & 11.2).

False aneurysm

Occasionally, bleeding from partially divided vessels is contained by the surrounding tissues. When this occurs a pulsatile false aneurysm results (Fallon & Thomford 1970, Dolibois & Matrka 1975, Ebong 1978). This may

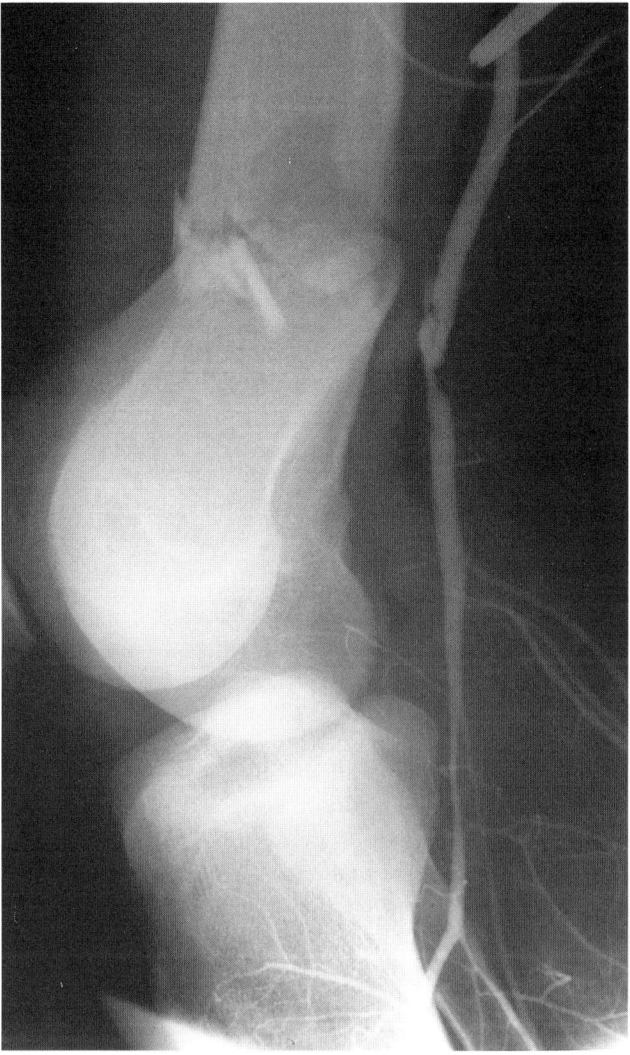

Fig. 11.1 There is disruption of the popliteal artery above the knee and compression of it behind the joint.

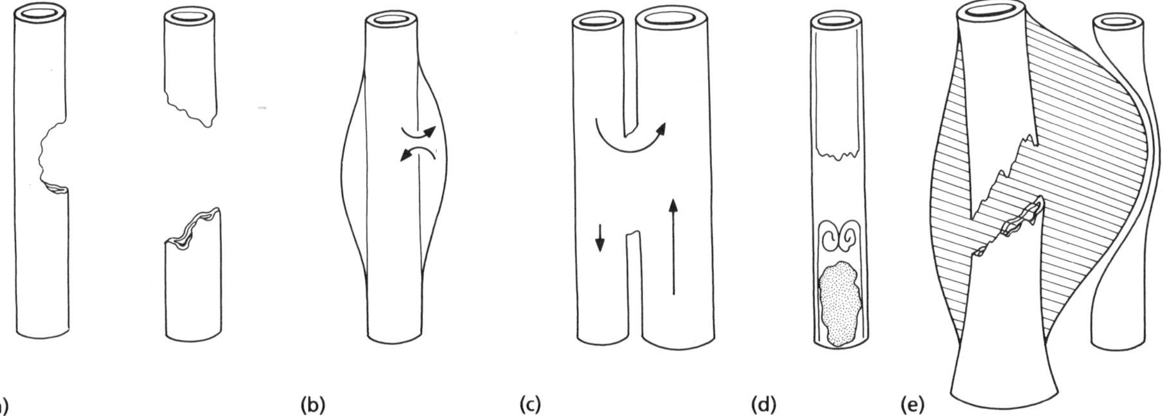

Fig. 11.2 Types of vascular injury. (a) Lacerated and divided arteries. (b) False aneurysm. (c) Arteriovenous fistula. (d) Intimal fracture with thrombosis. (c) Vascular compression by fracture haematoma.

rapidly expand, leading to true rupture, or it may be contained, leading to a stable aneurysm. Diagnosis is often not made until well after the injury and can be recognized by hearing a bruit over the site of the aneurysm (Fig. 11.2), or feeling a pulsatile mass.

Arteriovenous fistula

This occurs when there is damage to adjacent arteries and veins. It may pass unrecognized at the time of original injury, only to present some time later. The feeding artery enlarges and there is dilatation of the draining veins. Heart failure may ensue, particularly in the elderly patient. When recognized at the initial presentation it should be repaired (Fig. 11.2).

Compression

The haematoma resulting from the fracture itself, from the bony spicules or from pressure within closed compartments may result in vascular compression. Early reduction of the fracture with evacuation of the haematoma coupled with fasciotomy is required to prevent the development of ischaemic contracture (Figs 11.1 & 11.2).

Intimal tears

In these injuries the artery looks normal but the intima within is fractured and leads to thrombosis. Inspection of the outside of the vessel often reveals bruising of the adventitia. Intimal tears may be confused with spasm, but if there is any doubt the artery should be explored. Spasm, which was a popular concept in the past, should never be accepted without arteriography with papaverine, a vasodilator, to demonstrate the patency of the vessel (Fig. 11.2).

Thrombosis

Thrombosis may occur at the site of injury when there may be an intimal tear, or distal to the injury as a result of stasis. It is particularly important to recognize distal thrombosis because it is often impossible to clear with a balloon catheter. The best method of avoiding this complication is to restore the circulation as rapidly as possible, and to fill the distal circulation with heparinized saline while the repair is being performed (Fig. 11.2).

Diagnosis

The early recognition of a vascular injury complicating a fracture is of paramount importance because of the risk of limb loss due to gangrene in unsuspected cases.

Symptoms and signs

Symptoms of vascular injury include:
1 Pain.
2 Paraesthesiae.
3 Anaesthesia.
The signs are:
1 Pallor.
2 Paralysis.
3 Pulselessness.

An acutely ischaemic limb is painful but the pain is often difficult to differentiate from the pain of the fracture itself. Paraesthesiae and anaesthesia ensue rapidly if the circulation is not re-established, and indicate the need for rapid exploration and repair. Examination reveals a pale pulseless limb. Absence of pulses alone is of limited value as a sign because, in elderly patients, they may not have been present prior to the injury, and in all patients the peripheral vasoconstriction, which accompanies the blood loss secondary to the fracture, often makes pulses difficult to feel. Pallor is an unreliable sign alone because the patient may be hypotensive and anaemic as a result of bleeding around the fracture itself. Paralysis is a serious development which requires rapid re-establishment of the circulation if the limb is to be saved.

Non-invasive investigations

Simple serial observations of the limb with recording of pulses is the easiest way of assessing the distal circulation. Measurement of ankle or radial pressure with a Doppler probe will confirm the adequacy of the circulation when it is difficult to palpate distal pulses. This is not possible when the fracture involves the calf or forearm; invasive investigation is then required.

Arteriography

Where there is doubt about the diagnosis, and in order to define the anatomical level of the lesion, arteriography is indicated but it should not be allowed to delay surgery. When this is likely to occur, intraoperative arteriography, after exposure of the vessel proximal to the injury or after simple arterial puncture, is usually satisfactory. Intraoperative films have some advantages.

The contrast can be injected with inflow occlusion which provides better pictures than when a bolus injection is made into a more proximal vessel with continuing flow. Arteriography is particularly useful in the presence of a false aneurysm or arteriovenous fistula. Unsatisfactory results may occur when there is a lot of swelling around the fracture site (Grosz *et al.* 1973) with compression but no damage to the vessels. It should be stressed that speed is the most important requirement in the management of these patients, and that for the majority of cases intraoperative films are adequate.

Management

Emergency resuscitation

Haemostasis

Profuse haemorrhage from an open fracture site can be stopped by local pressure using a tourniquet above, or by application of clamps directly to, the bleeding vessel. Tourniquets lead to complete loss of circulation in the limb by compression of the collaterals as well as of the bleeding vessel. Subsequent removal of the tourniquet allows a bolus of ischaemic metabolites to return to the circulation. Tourniquets should therefore be reserved for severe uncontrollable haemorrhage and should be kept on for as short a time as possible. If there is difficulty in controlling bleeding, inflation of embolectomy catheters within the vessel, up or downstream from the injury, may help.

Ventilation and circulation

As in any patient requiring resuscitation attention must be paid to maintaining an adequate airway and to gaining rapid vascular access with a large-calibre cannula. Once stabilized, the patient with vascular trauma must be transferred for surgery as rapidly as possible. Rapid elevation of blood pressure may lead to recurrence of bleeding that has previously stopped as a result of hypotension and vessel retraction. Provided that the blood pressure is high enough to maintain renal perfusion, full replacement can wait until control of bleeding has been achieved in the operating theatre.

Antibiotics

An open fracture will almost certainly need treatment with broad-spectrum antibiotics to cover the perioperative period. In the absence of an open wound a patient with a complicating vascular injury also requires prophylactic broad-spectrum antibiotics, particularly if an artificial graft is to be used in its repair.

Surgery

The conservative management of potential vascular injuries associated with fractures is to be avoided because of the long-term consequences of failure to recognize a significant vascular injury. Surgery should be performed as soon as there is any suspicion of vascular insufficiency and, if appropriate, the fracture can be fixed at the same time. A combined vascular and orthopaedic surgical team is required so that immediate reduction of the fracture can be achieved to allow assessment of the vascular injury. The vascular surgeon should re-establish the circulation prior to fixation of the fracture. In the past the reverse has been recommended but the improvement in results that has occurred has been largely due to the expeditious return of circulation. It has been argued in the past that if the vascular injury is dealt with first it may be disrupted by subsequent manipulation of the fracture. However, Connolly (1971) has demonstrated that the disruptive resistance of a typical sound vascular repair is greater than 40 lb pull, indicating that primary vascular reconstruction is safe. Heparin-bonded shunts are available for bypassing a damaged arterial segment during fracture fixation if it is essential to do this first (Chitwood *et al.* 1981, Gainor & Metzler 1986).

Before inspecting the traumatized vessel it must be adequately exposed and local haemostasis must be secured. Silastic slings are passed around the vessel above the lesion and beyond it. If the injury is adjacent to a major division, as is the case in the popliteal artery below the knee, it may be necessary to expose and control each of the branches. This permits passage of an embolectomy catheter down each branch if required. Prior to clamping the vessel heparin should be given to prevent distal thrombosis. A dose of 5000 iu is sufficient and does not usually need to be reversed. If there is a lot of tissue trauma and bleeding, then systemic heparinization is best withheld. Distal thrombosis can then be avoided by local injection of heparinized saline (10 iu ml^{-1}).

The three main types of vascular injury are compression, laceration and intimal tear.

Compression

This may be due to pressure by a haematoma or displaced bone. Compression by a haematoma can be relieved by its evacuation with or without fasciotomy.

This permits an assessment of the cause of the haem-atoma and if there is a vascular injury, then it can be repaired. Relief of compression should result in a rapid recovery of the distal circulation if there is no significant vascular injury. If, however, the circulation does not improve, then an intimal fracture must be suspected. At this stage arteriography may be indicated to establish the site and extent of the damage. Alternatively, after heparinization of the patient, an arteriotomy may allow the passage of an embolectomy catheter to ensure distal patency.

Laceration

A lacerated artery must be exposed and isolated with silastic slings above and beyond the lesion. After hep-arinization, the extent of the damage is assessed and the ragged edges of lacerated arteries excised. The presence of forward and backbleeding is ascertained and, if absent, an embolectomy catheter is passed. Failure to achieve adequate backbleeding may mean that there is further damage distally or may be due to thrombosis secondary to stasis; an arteriogram is then indicated. If everything is satisfactory, the vessel is repaired (Fig. 11.3). There are three main methods of vascular repair:
1 *Suture.* Even if a short length of artery is removed it is often possible to suture the ends together. An obliquely cut vessel is easier to suture than one cut across at 90°, and interrupted sutures of fine Prolene (5/0 or 6/0) are used to join the ends.
2 *Vein patch.* If there is a longitudinal laceration in the vessel or if an arteriotomy has been performed to look for intimal damage, simple suture may result in stenosis and eventual thrombosis. In this situation a piece of vein is harvested, reversed, split longitudinally and

sewn in as a patch. The vein must either be taken from the contralateral limb or from the upper limb in the case of a leg injury to preserve the venous drainage of the injured limb (Fig. 11.4).
3 *Replacement.* Where damage is extensive, vascular replacement is indicated. Straight or bifurcated vein grafts can be used, either reversed or non-reversed after valve destruction. Bifurcated grafts are often indicated behind the knee after disruption of the popliteal trifur-cation, and sometimes in the antecubital fossa in brachial artery trauma (Fig. 11.5). When larger vessels have been damaged synthetic grafts such as Dacron or polytetrafluoroethylene may be required but these should be avoided, particularly in open wounds, be-cause of the risk of infection. They should also be avoided in young patients, in whom there may be a risk of occlusion in the long-term. If a short length of a larger artery is missing, then a piece of vein can be harvested, split longitudinally and sewn up end-to-end to create a vessel of large diameter (Fig. 11.6). Alternatively, several pieces of vein can be sewn together to provide a graft of large diameter. The vein graft is sewn in, end-to-end, using fine 6/0 or 7/0 Prolene sutures, depending upon the size of the artery.

Intimal tear

In this type of injury the vessel is mobilized with slings above and beyond the site of damage and a longitudinal arteriotomy is made through the contused part. The inside of the vessel is inspected for intimal fracture after the clot has been removed. Subsequent repair depends upon the severity of the injury. Repair may be by:
1 *Vein patch.* A local endarterectomy is performed and the distal flaps of intima are sewn down with fine 7/0

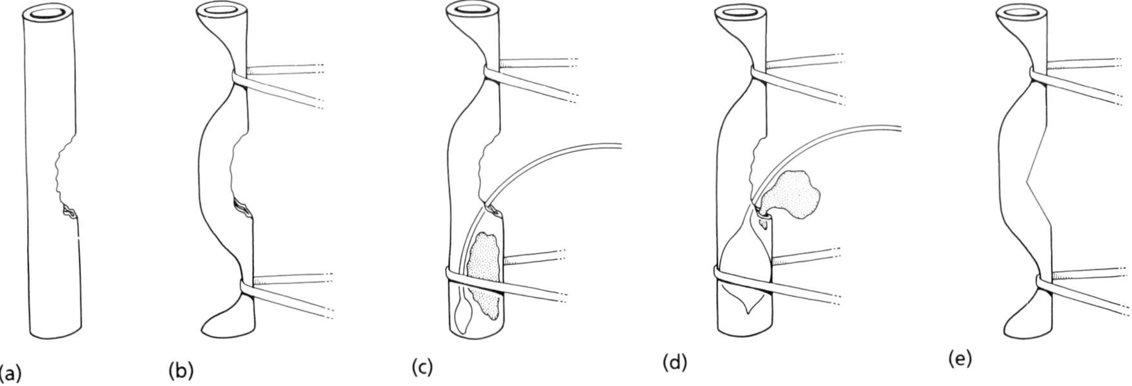

Fig. 11.3 Vascular injury; repair of laceration. (a) Arterial laceration. (b) Vessel isolated. (c) An embolectomy catheter is passed. (d) Clot is evacuated with return of backbleeding. (e) The edges are trimmed ready for repair.

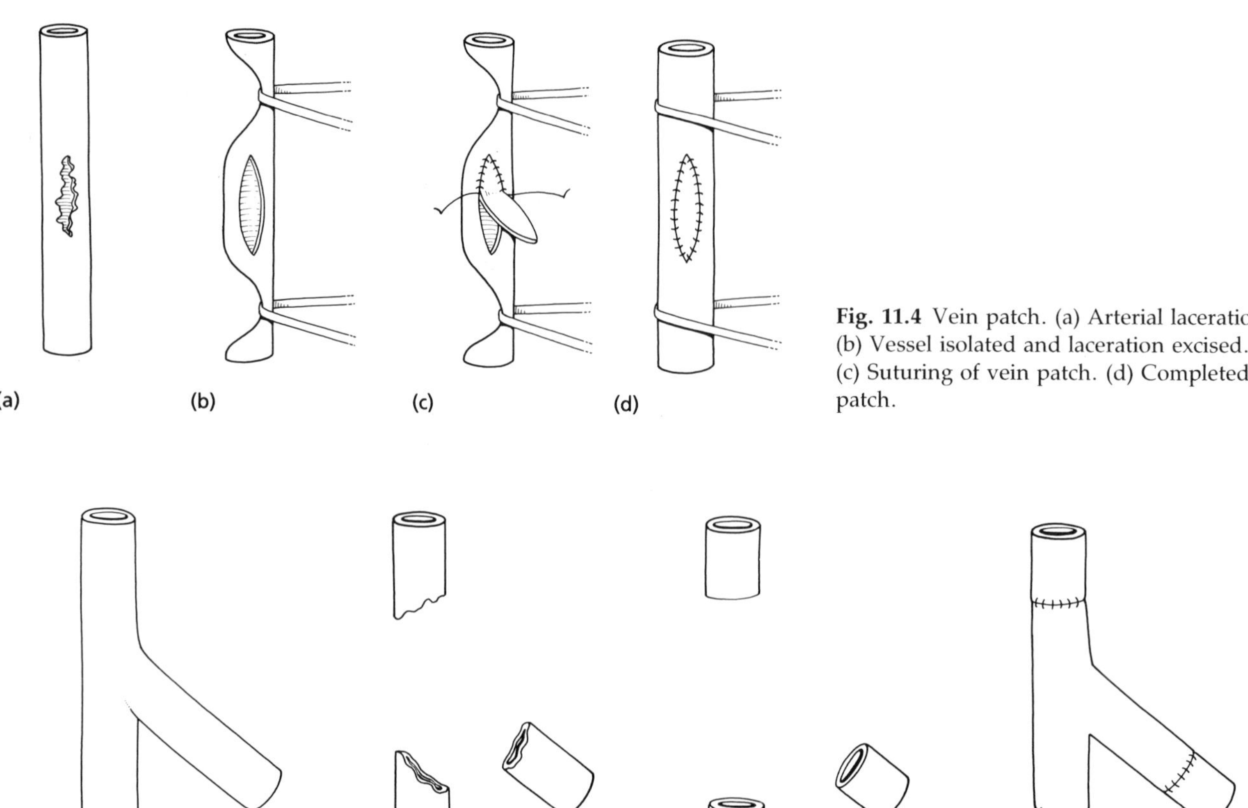

Fig. 11.4 Vein patch. (a) Arterial laceration. (b) Vessel isolated and laceration excised. (c) Suturing of vein patch. (d) Completed patch.

Fig. 11.5 Bifurcated graft. (a) Normal anatomy of bifurcation. (b) Damaged bifurcation. (c) Ragged edges excised. (d) Bifurcated vein graft sewn in after valve destruction.

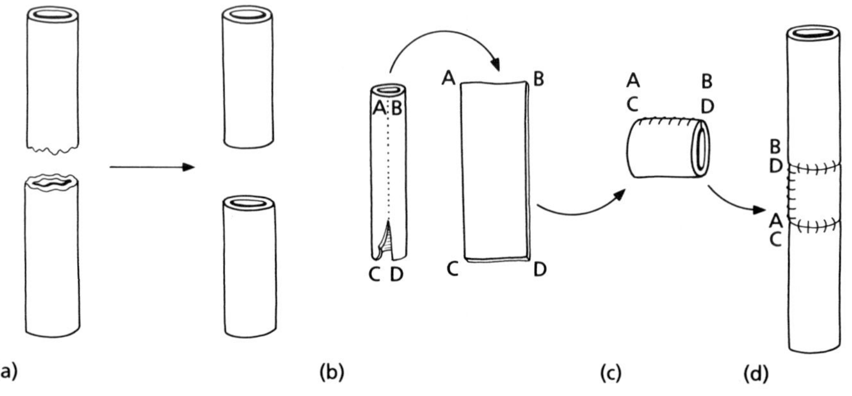

Fig. 11.6 Replacement. (a) Fractured vessel before and after debridement. (b) Vein for replacement is split longitudinally, and (c) sewn up transversely. (d) Completed vascular replacement.

Prolene sutures. The proximal flap is not important because the pressure of blood within the vessel will keep it pressed out against the outer layers of the vessel. The vessel is closed with the vein patch which is sewn in with Prolene sutures (Fig. 11.4).

2 *Replacement*. If the damage is extensive it is best to replace the vessel with a vein graft. This is sewn in end-to-end to the artery above and beyond the traumatized segment.

Arteriography

Once the vascular repair has been completed and the distal circulation has been restored it is essential to perform arteriography to ensure that there is adequate flow distally and that the anastomosis or vein patch has been performed adequately.

Fasciotomy

Fasciotomy is indicated either in the forearm or in the leg if there has been lengthy ischaemia of the muscles. It is much safer to perform a fasciotomy routinely than to leave it until the viability of the successfully revascularized limb is in doubt. Where available, compartment pressure monitoring may help in deciding which patients require it. There are five main compartments in the calf: anterior, peroneal, deep posterior, intermediate posterior and superficial posterior (Fig. 11.7). The easiest way to decompress all of them is to perform a middle-third fibulectomy. An alternative to this is two-thirds length medial and lateral incisions. The wounds should not be sutured but may be skin grafted at a later date.

Venous injury

Isolated arterial injury is unusual when associated with fractures. The veins running alongside the artery are comparatively fragile, are often damaged and may account for the majority of the bleeding. Ligation of all the veins in the area may lead to gross swelling of the limb postoperatively or in the long-term. Venous repair has been shown to be important in reducing limb oedema and in increasing the limb salvage rate (Alberty *et al.* 1981). It is therefore as important to repair the veins as it is to repair the arteries. Vascular clamps should be avoided as these cause intimal damage and increase the risk of subsequent venous thrombosis. If possible, the vein should be repaired with fine 7/o

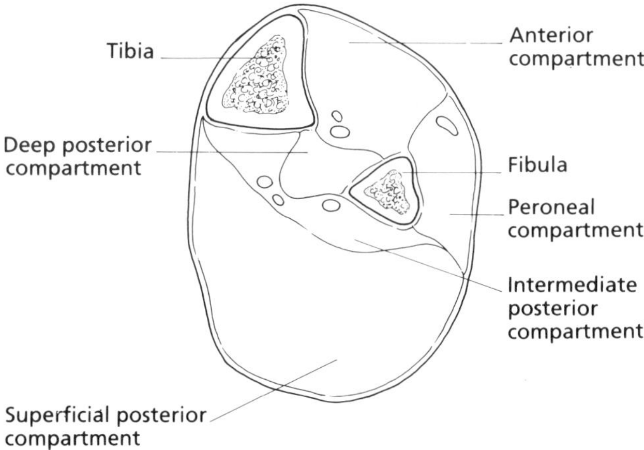

Fig. 11.7 Fasciotomy.

Prolene sutures after the bleeding has been stopped by simple pressure on the vein on either side of the laceration. Once the first stitch has been placed, tension on it often closes the hole and allows the rest of the suture line to be completed without the loss of much more blood. Where damage is severe ligation may be the only alternative available. Vein grafting or replacement in this situation often leads to thrombosis. Contralateral vein must always be used if replacement is required and it may be enlarged as in Fig. 11.6.

The bony injury

Internal fixation of the fracture is the treatment of choice for most fractures (Sher 1975). Some have recommended initial arterial repair with skeletal traction followed by internal fixation 1–2 weeks after the initial therapy (Rich *et al.* 1971). This approach is sensible when there is significant contamination of the wound. There is also evidence that the internal fixation achieved following or preceding vascular repair is often less than optimal because of the need to hurry and because of the risk of further tissue damage caused by mobilization of the bone ends (Connolly *et al.* 1971, Flint & Richardson 1983). Others have suggested rapid external fixation of the fracture followed by vascular repair (Holden 1979). Since the limb may be useless without adequate circulation the authors would recommend that arterial repair or bypass should *always* precede fracture immobilization, irrespective of how trivial the vascular injury may seem to be.

Postoperative care

Postoperative care of the vascular injury in an orthopaedic patient falls into two main areas:
1 Circulation
  (a) Distal pulses.
  (b) Swelling.
  (c) Anticoagulants.
  (d) Elevation.
2 Complications
  (a) Haemorrhage.
  (b) Thrombosis.
  (c) Contracture.
  (d) Infection.
  (e) Gangrene.
  (f) Claudication.

Circulation

General measures. It is essential to ensure the continued

adequacy of the circulation after vascular reconstruction. If the limb is covered in plaster of Paris then inspection holes should be left so that the pulses can be palpated distally and the colour of the extremity can be assessed. In most cases the distal part of the limb becomes hyperaemic and it is obvious that the circulation is adequate. Postoperative swelling is the rule after vascular reconstruction with or without orthopaedic injury, and can be limited to some extent by elevation.

Swelling. Swelling associated with diminishing pulses distally may indicate development of a compartment syndrome requiring fasciotomy.

Anticoagulants. Anticoagulants are not normally needed if adequate vascular reconstruction has been performed. If synthetic grafts have been used there is evidence that low dose aspirin ($175-300$ mg day^{-1}) may prolong graft patency by prevention of the accumulation of platelets on the surface of the graft.

Complications

Haemorrhage. This is a potential hazard after any vascular procedure and is avoided by meticulous attention to haemostasis prior to wound closure. It is helpful to close the wound over a suction drain to prevent accumulation of blood clot around the vascular repair. The presence of a drain may also give warning if sudden bleeding occurs after the patient has returned to the ward.

Thrombosis. Early thrombosis after vascular reconstruction usually indicates a technical error in the surgery. The patient should be returned to the operating theatre for re-exploration. Arteriography and further vascular reconstruction may be required.

Contracture. This occurs when there has been prolonged ischaemia in the muscles distal to the site of injury (Holden 1979). It should be avoidable if the vascular injury is repaired rapidly and a compartment syndrome is avoided by early fasciotomy. Delay of vascular reconstruction for any reason may lead to contracture, or even gangrene, if there is irreversible ischaemia of the muscles.

Infection. Infection is a particular hazard when employing synthetic grafts but any infected vascular anastomosis is liable to breakdown, leading to severe haemorrhage. Use of prophylactic antibiotics is indicated and these should be continued for several days after surgery until the wound is healing and the patient is no longer pyrexial.

Specific injuries

Subclavian artery

The subclavian artery is at risk after fracture of the first or second rib (Thomas *et al.* 1978), as are the brachiocephalic trunk, carotid, vertebral arteries and aorta (Livoni & Barcia 1982). Fractures of the lateral and posterior aspects of the first rib are more likely to be associated with vascular injury than are fractures of the anterior end. The likely mechanism of injury is from downward displacement of the posterior portion of the rib with upward displacement of the anterior portion, forcing the artery against the back of the clavicle.

Subclavian artery repair can be achieved by supra- or infraclavicular approaches. The artery can be replaced by Dacron or vein graft (Phillips *et al.* 1981) together with local resection of part of the first rib, if necessary. The association of vascular and severe brachial plexus injury has a poor prognosis but despite this, reconstruction should still be attempted.

Axillary artery

Axillary artery trauma may occur as a result of the fracture of the clavicle, posterior dislocation of the sternoclavicular joint or dislocation of the shoulder joint itself. In clavicular fractures the distal fragment is usually pulled downwards and forwards by the weight of the limb and the proximal fragment is pulled upwards and backwards into the belly of the trapezius so that compression of the underlying artery is avoided. When a vascular injury is present there is usually fracture of the first rib as well (Livoni & Barcia 1982).

Axillary artery trauma may complicate either a fracture of the surgical neck of the humerus or anterior dislocation of the shoulder joint (Theorides & de Keizer 1976, Hayes & Van Winkle 1983) (Fig. 11.8). At this level the cords of the brachial plexus surround the artery and are more often damaged than the artery itself. The vascular damage results either from direct injury by the bony spicule or from stretching of the artery during hyperabduction where it is relatively fixed by the anterior circumflex humeral artery. The collateral circulation around the shoulder joint is good but failure to recognize the injury or ligation of the axillary artery at this level may lead to an amputation rate as high as 40%.

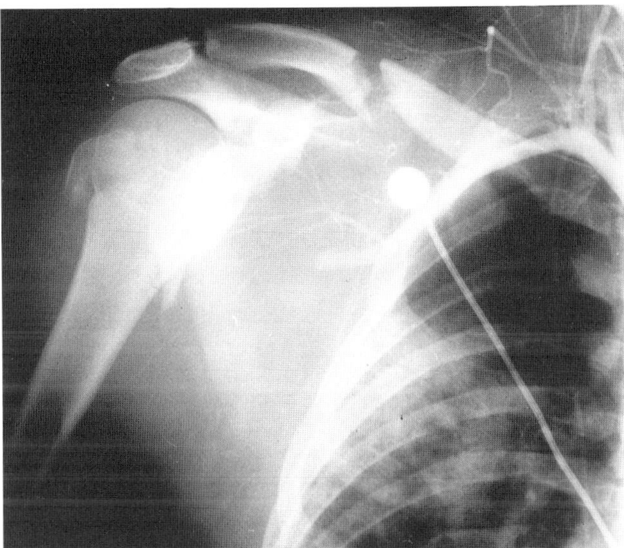

Fig. 11.8 The axillary artery is occluded, though apparently intact. A reversed saphenous vein graft was used to bypass the damaged segment.

Brachial artery

Fractures of the humeral shaft causing vascular injury are more common than those at the surgical neck (Fig. 11.9). Damage to the brachial artery above the origin of the profunda brachii artery is more important than beyond it because of the importance of this artery as a collateral. Most cases of brachial artery injury in this area involve the nerves as well; in one series less than 50% achieved normal limb function and there was an amputation rate of 30% (Gainor & Metzler 1986). Supracondylar fracture may lead to Volkmann's contracture if the vascular injury is missed. Early surgery is essential in this case and vascular spasm must be dismissed as a diagnosis when the distal pulses are absent.

Pelvic vessels

As many as 65% of patients who die as a result of pelvic fracture exsanguinate from related haemorrhage. Disruption of the iliac or femoral vessels is the major site of bleeding in 20% of these cases (Rothenberger *et al.* 1978b). The incidence of major vessel injuries secondary to pelvic fracture is approximately 1% (Rothenberger *et al.* 1978a). Patients are admitted in shock and require massive blood transfusion. Other intra-abdominal and urethral injuries are common. The majority of patients have multiple fractures affecting the pelvis. Venous injury is more common than arterial injury and bleeding is often equally severe. Early operation has been

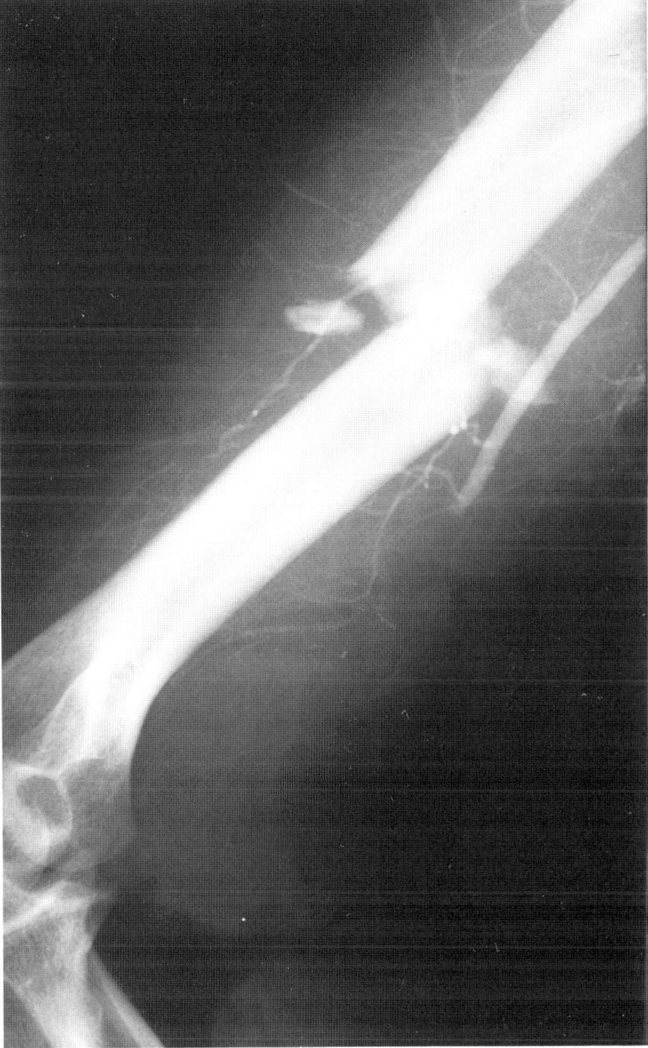

Fig. 11.9 There is an intimal fracture of the brachial artery. At exploration the vessel was apparently intact.

suggested in an attempt to reduce the mortality rate of 80% (Rothenberger *et al.* 1978a), but in the authors' experience release of the haematoma by laparotomy results in uncontrollable haemorrhage. Internal iliac artery ligation is recommended to control the bleeding but is not always effective. Conservative management permits tamponade of bleeding in closed injuries and is probably the best course. In open injuries uncontrolled haemorrhage is the main cause of death, and a combination of ligation of lacerated veins and repair of damaged arteries together with packing of the wound seems to hold out the best chance of success. Occasional injury to the femoral artery at the groin level may occur following operative fixation of an intertrochanteric fracture (Whitewell *et al.* 1978, Mauerhan *et al.* 1981).

Femoral vessels

Disruption of the femoral artery by the femoral shaft is usually associated with open fractures, but does occasionally occur with closed injuries (Isaacson *et al.* 1975). The mechanism of damage is thought to be either direct trauma by the bone ends or as a result of crushing of the vessel against the bone (Fig. 11.10). The commonest site of injury is at the level of the adductor hiatus. The diagnosis may be missed if there is a closed injury because up to 25% of patients have palpable distal pulses (Drapanas *et al.* 1970).

Popliteal artery

The popliteal artery and, in particular, the popliteal trifurcation is the most commonly injured vascular segment and still carries the highest morbidity (Fig. 11.11). There is often associated severe soft tissue trauma and this contributes to the poor outcome. Replacement of the popliteal trifurcation by a saphenous vein graft is the most commonly employed method of repair (Fig. 11.12). It has been suggested that at this level fasciotomy should be routine after vascular reconstruction (Dart & Braitman 1977).

Tibial vessels

The majority of fractures at this level are open and complex. Several factors are important in determining the outcome. Poor prognostic indicators include crushing injuries and segmental tibial fractures leading to

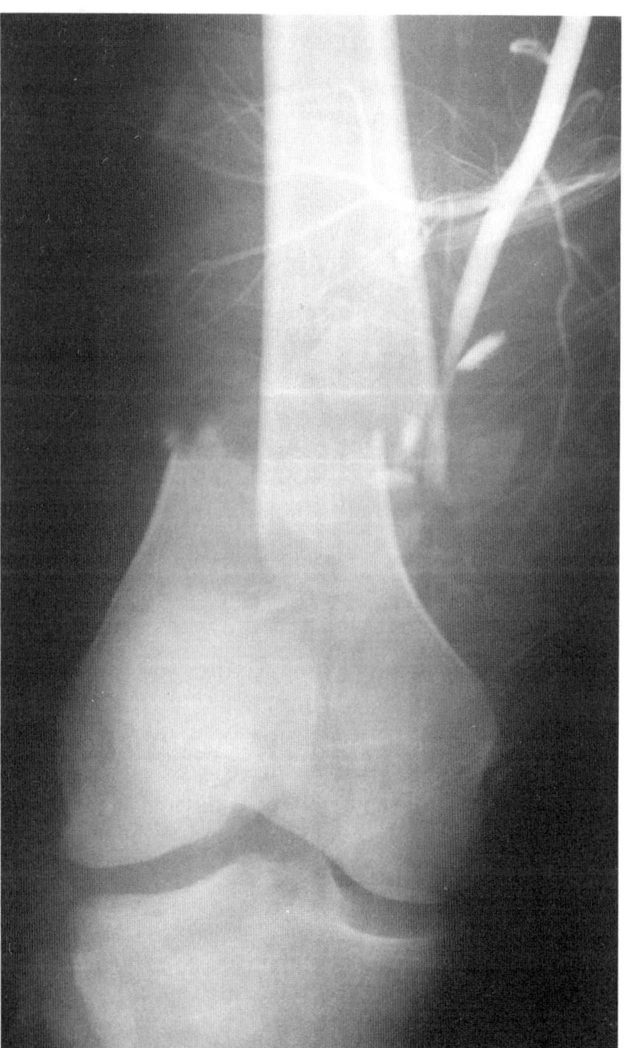

Fig. 11.10 The femoral artery was completely divided at the level of the adductor hiatus.

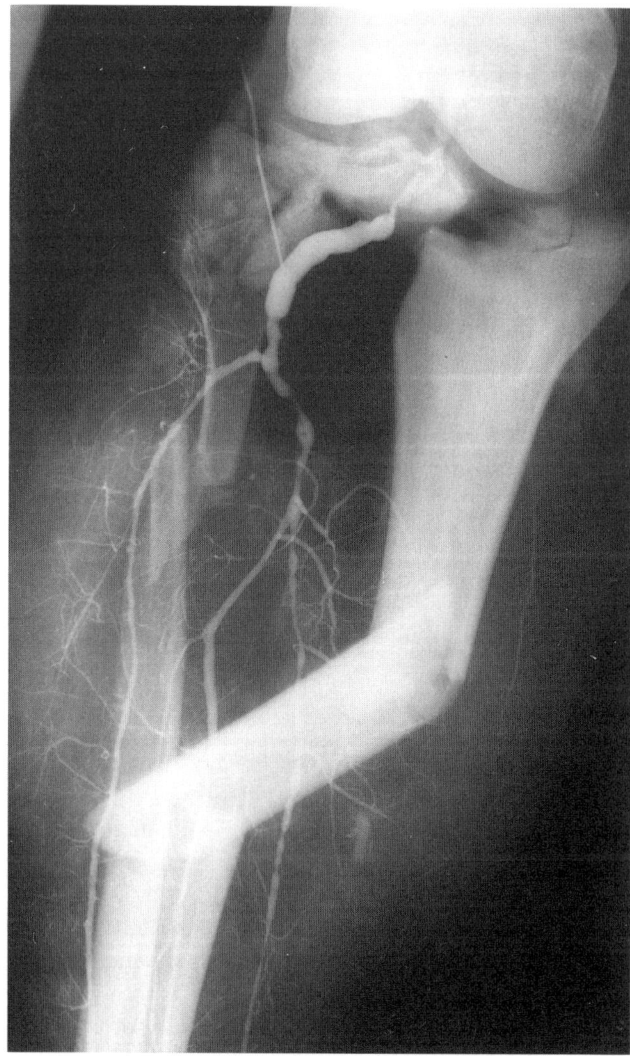

Fig. 11.11 There is severe damage to the popliteal trifurcation with thrombosis of the tibial and peroneal vessels in the calf.

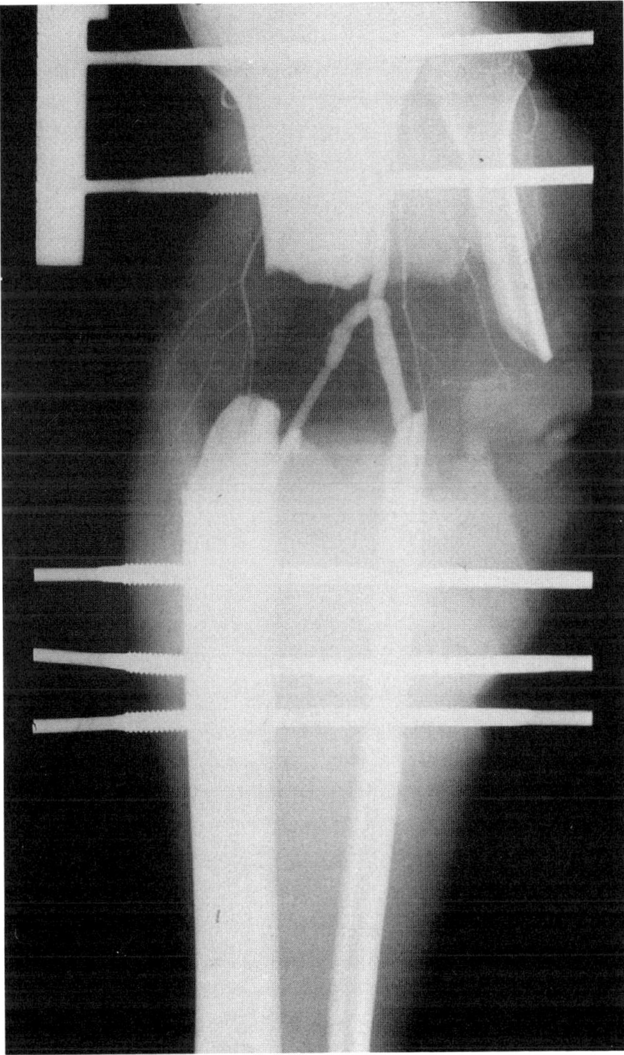

Fig. 11.12 The popliteal trifurcation has been replaced with an *in situ* branched saphenous graft from the contralateral limb.

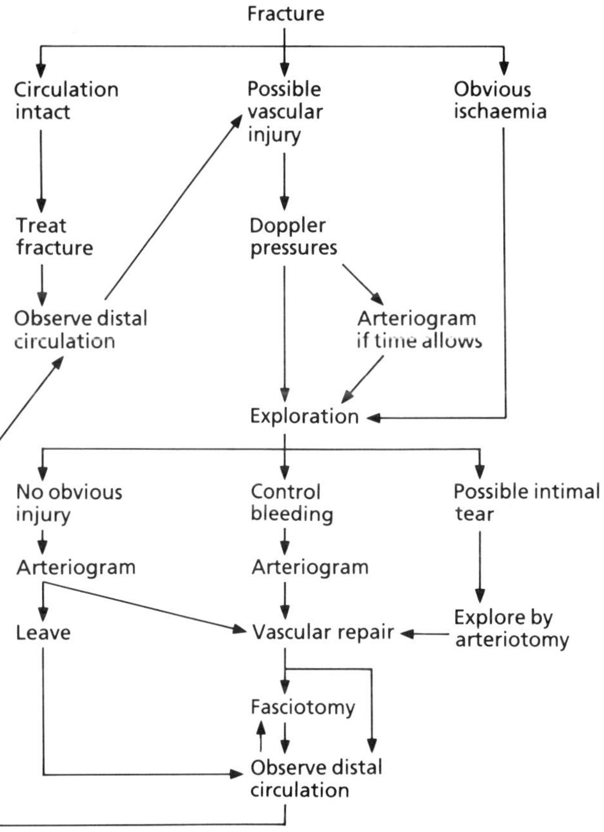

Fig. 11.13 Algorithm for the management of vascular injuries complicating orthopaedic trauma. Vascular repair precedes orthopaedic surgery.

massive soft tissue injury. Severe crushing leads to massive muscle necrosis. Favourable indicators include proximal tibial fractures and prompt revascularization (Rosental *et al.* 1975). Primary amputation is probably indicated when there has been complete disruption of

Table 11.1 Results of treatment of vascular injuries

Reference	Number	Amputation (%)	Useful (%)	Died	Site
Gainor & Metzler (1986)	10	3 (30)	7 (70)		Humeral shaft
Rothenberger *et al.* (1978a)	12			10	Pelvic vessels
Connolly *et al.* (1971)	7	1 (14)	6 (86)		Femoral artery
Flint & Richardson (1983)	14	0 (0)	14 (100)	0	Mid-femoral
Rosental *et al.* (1975)	21	4 (19)	7 (33)	1	Femoral shaft
Connolly *et al.* (1971)	6	3 (50)	2 (33)		Popliteal
Flint & Richardson (1983)	11	2 (18)	9 (82)		Popliteal
Flint & Richardson (1983)	16	12 (75)	4 (25)		Trifurcation
Alberty *et al.* (1981)	20	8 (40)			Trifurcation
Dart & Braitman (1977)	5	0 (0)	5 (100)		Trifurcation
Lange *et al.* (1985)	23	14 (61)	3 (13)		Tibial vessels

the posterior tibial nerve in adults and after severe crush injuries with a delay greater than 6 hours. In tibial injuries vascular replacement is almost always required, using vein graft from the other leg or from either arm. Fasciotomy should be carried out as a matter of course.

Results

Table 11.1 shows the results of treatment of vascular injuries; results vary with the site of the injury and the experience of the vascular surgeon. Improvements in outcome have usually been due to an earlier recognition of the injury coupled with a rapid and effective revascularization of the limb.

Figure 11.13 is an algorithm for the management of vascular injuries complicating orthopaedic trauma. When such an injury occurs the emphasis should be placed upon rapid assessment, combined care, arteriography in the event of doubt about the injury and, where required, restoration of the circulation as the first priority.

References

Alberty, R.E., Goodfried, G. & Boyden, A.M. Popliteal artery injury with fractural dislocation of the knee. *Am J Surg* 1981; **142**: 36–38.

Chitwood, W.R., Rankin, J.S., Bollinger, R.R. & Moylan, J.A. Brachial artery reconstruction using the heparin-bonded shunt. *Surgery* 1981; **89**: 355–358.

Connolly, J. Management of fractures associated with arterial injuries. *Am J Surg* 1971; **120**: 331.

Connolly, J.F., Whittaker, D. & Williams, E. Femoral and tibial fractures combined with injuries to the femoral or popliteal artery. *J Bone Joint Surg* 1971; **53A**: 56–68.

Dart, C.H. & Braitman, H.E. Popliteal artery injury following fracture or dislocation at the knee. *Arch Surg* 1977; **112**: 969–973.

DeBakey, M.E. & Simeone, F.A. Battle injuries of the arteries in World War II. *Ann Surg* 1946: **123**: 534.

Dolibois, J.M. & Matrka, P.J. False aneurysm of the brachial artery complicating closed fracture of the humerus. *Clin Orthop* 1975; **113**: 150–153.

Drapanas, T., Hewitt, R.L., Weichert, R.F. & Smith, A.D. Civilian vascular injuries: a critical appraisal of three decades of management. *Ann Surg* 1970; **172**: 351–360.

Ebong, W.W. False aneurysm of the profunda femoris artery following internal fixation of an intertrochanteric femoral fracture. *Injury* 1978; **9**: 249–251.

Fallon, G. & Thomford, N.R. False aneurysm of the superficial femoral artery associated with fracture of the femur. *Angiology* 1970; **21**: 120–123.

Flint, L.M. & Richardson, J.D. Arterial injuries with lower extremity fracture. *Surgery* 1983; **93**: 5–8.

Gainor, B.J. & Metzler, M. Humeral shaft fracture with brachial artery injury. *Clin Orthop* 1986; **204**: 154–161.

Grosz, C.R., Shaftan, G.W., Kottmeier, P.K. & Herbsman, H. Volkmann's contracture and femoral shaft fractures. *J Trauma* 1973; **13**: 129–131.

Hayes, J.M. & Van Winkle, G.N. Axillary artery injury with minimally displaced fracture of the neck of the humerus. *J Trauma* 1983; **23**: 431–433.

Holden, C.E.A. The pathology and prevention of Volkmann's ischaemic contracture. *J Bone Joint Surg* 1979; **61B**: 296–300.

Isaacson, J., Louis, D. & Costenbader, J.M. Arterial injury associated with closed femoral shaft fracture. *J Bone Joint Surg* 1975; **57A**: 1147–1150.

Jahnke, E.J. & Seeley, S.F. Acute vascular injuries in the Korean war: an analysis of 77 consecutive cases. *Ann Surg* 1953; **138**: 158–177.

Lange, R.H., Bach, A.W., Hansen, S.T. & Johansen, K.H. Open tibial fractures associated with vascular injuries: prognosis for limb salvage. *J Trauma* 1985; **25**: 203–208.

Livoni, J.P. & Barcia, T.C. Fractures of the first and second rib: incidence of vascular injury relative to type of fracture. *Radiology* 1982; **145**: 31–33.

Mauerhan, D.R., Maurer, R.C. & Effeney, D. Profunda femoris arterial laceration secondary to intertrochanteric hip fracture fragments. *Clin Orthop* 1981; **161**: 215–219.

Miller, H.H. & Welch, C.S. Quantitative studies on time factors in arterial injuries. *Ann Surg* 1949; **130**: 428.

Phillips, E.H., Rogers, W.F. & Gaspar, M.R. First rib fractures: incidence of vascular injury and indications for angiography. *Surgery* 1981; **89**: 42–47.

Porter, M.F. Arterial injuries in an accident unit. *Br J Surg* 1967; **54**: 100–105.

Rich, N.M., Matz, C.W., Hutton, J.E., Baugh, H. & Hughes, C.W. Internal versus external fixation of fractures with concomitant vascular injuries in Vietnam. *J Trauma* 1971; **11**: 463–473.

Rosental, J.J., Gaspar, M.R., Gjerdrum, T.C. & Newman, J. Vascular injuries associated with fractures of the femur. *Arch Surg* 1975; **110**: 494–497.

Rothenberger, D.A., Fischer, R.P. & Perry, J.F. Major vascular injuries secondary to pelvic fractures: an unsolved clinical problem. *Am J Surg* 1978a; **136**: 660–662.

Rothenberger, D.A., Fischer, R.P., Strate, R.G., Velasco, R. & Perry, J.F. The mortality associated with pelvic fractures. *Surgery* 1978b; **84**: 356–361.

Sher, M.H. Principles in the management of arterial injuries associated with fracture/dislocations. *Ann Surg* 1975; **182**: 630–634.

Theorides, T. & de Keizer, G. Injuries of the axillary artery caused by fractures of the neck of the humerus. *Injury* 1976; **8**: 120–123.

Thomas, A.N., Goodman, P.C. & Roon, A.J. Role of angiography in cervicothoracic trauma. *J Thorac Cardiovasc Surg* 1978; **76**: 633–638.

Whitewell, R., Wang, G.-J., Edwards, J.R. & Stamp, W.G. Late injuries to femoral vessels after fracture of the hip. *J Bone Joint Surg* 1978; **60A**: 541–542.

Nerve injuries

I.J.LESLIE

Nerve injuries may occur as a result of virtually any fracture or dislocation and, therefore, a neurological examination of the limb or trunk distal to the injury is mandatory in the initial assessment. Some injuries have a well-known association with nerve damage, e.g. a fracture of the shaft of the humerus producing a radial nerve palsy, or posterior dislocation of the hip producing a sciatic nerve palsy. However, some common fractures may just occasionally produce a neurological injury and a casual examination may miss the neurological deficit, e.g. a fractured clavicle producing a partial brachial plexus injury.

In the multiply injured, unconscious or uncooperative patient assessment may not be possible, but a high level of suspicion must be maintained until the deficit is positively excluded. Once a lesion is detected in the seriously injured patient it is still necessary to document the neurological abnormality even though it is essential to concentrate on the more serious problems (Fig. 11.14).

A nerve may be injured in one of the following ways:
1 Laceration.
2 Compression.
3 Stretching.
4 Ischaemia.
5 Radiation.
6 Heat or cold.
7 Chemicals.

In closed fractures or dislocations the nerve is commonly stretched or compressed, although ischaemic injuries can occur, such as in compartment syndromes. In open injuries the nerve may also be lacerated by sharp or even blunt instruments, e.g. a bullet wound.

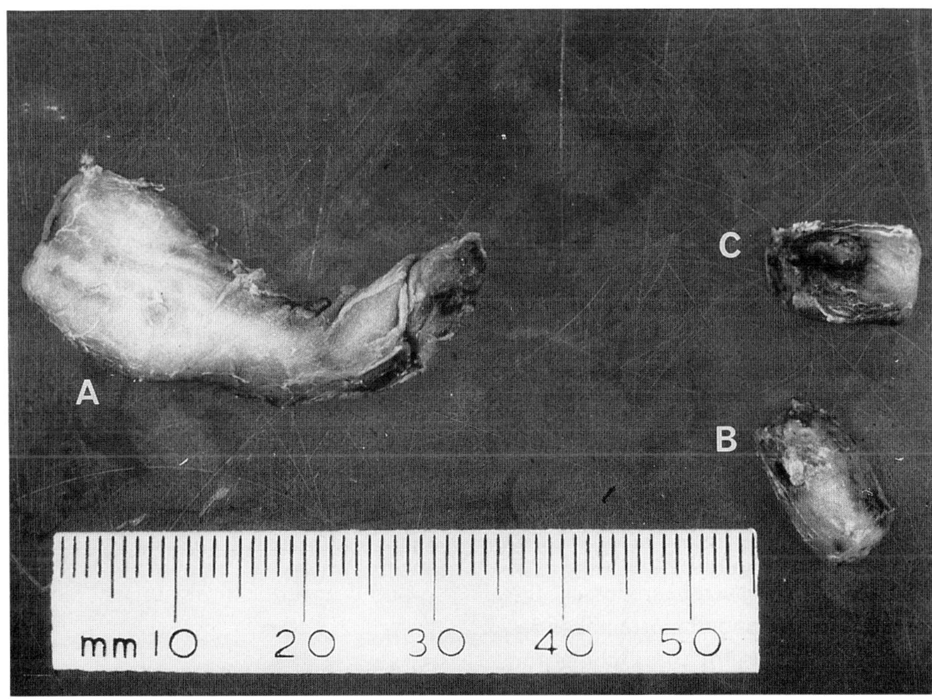

Fig. 11.14 A 12-year-old male suffered a severe head injury and a closed supracondylar fracture of the femur. Only when he regained consciousness, some 3 weeks later, was it possible to diagnose a sciatic nerve lesion. At 6 months, when no recovery had occurred, the nerve was explored. There had been a complete rupture of the nerve (neurotmesis/Sunderland 5th degree) with an 11 cm gap. The resected ends of the nerve are shown and the degree of damage is obvious. The nerve was repaired using a sural nerve graft.

When a nerve is crushed it remains in continuity; when stretched it may remain in continuity or may rupture completely. Therefore, in closed fractures it is still possible for the nerve ends to be completely separated following considerable stretching and eventual rupture.

Classification of nerve injuries

There are two major classifications in use. The most commonly used one is that of Seddon (1943) which divides the injury into three types.

1 *Neuropraxia*. This is the least serious injury and is a temporary local block of nerve conduction. It is associated with local demyelination of the nerve fibre. There is no loss of continuity of the axons, and the excitability of the nerve structures and the muscle tissue distal to the lesion is preserved. The conduction block persists until local myelin repair processes restore the local excitability of the nerve fibre and then conduction is restored over the damaged segment. Recovery takes place spontaneously over a period ranging from days to months. There is usually complete motor paralysis despite a lack of muscle wasting and the excitability of the muscle is preserved. There is often considerable sparing of the sensory and sympathetic functions. Resolution is usually complete with total restoration of motor and sensory function.

2 *Axonotmesis*. Axonal continuity is interrupted at the level of the lesion. The endoneural (Schwann) tubes remain intact; however, Wallerian degeneration takes place in the axons distal to the lesion. Electrical nerve conduction ceases and the excitability of the paralysed muscle is altered. There is total sensory and motor loss. Muscle wasting occurs and if the denervation is prolonged, then irreversible changes will take place in the muscle tissue. Regeneration of the axon takes place from the site of injury at a rate of approximately 1 mm day^{-1}. Since the endoneural tubes remain intact, the axons will generally regenerate down the original endoneural tube and are thus successful in reaching the correct sensory receptor or motor endplate. The time for functional recovery to occur depends on the distance between the site of injury and the distal end organ, and the final result will depend, to a large extent, on the permanent irreversible damage that has been done to these receptor organs during their time of inactivity.

3 *Neurotmesis*. This term is used where the entire nerve is completely severed and there is total loss of axonal continuity. However, the term can also be applied to lesions where there has been gross stretching and although the actual anatomical continuity of the nerve may be preserved, the scarring effectively blocks completely any axonal regeneration. The changes distal to the lesion are the same as those seen in axonotmesis and, therefore, in the early stages the two are indistinguishable. The distinction can only be made by operative inspection of the nerve or by waiting for recovery to occur in the axonotmesis. The endoneural tubes have now been completely disrupted and, therefore, when axonal regeneration does take place after surgical repair, then there will be considerable crossover resulting in the proximal axons reaching the incorrect distal end organ. Surgical repair is required in order to achieve any recovery and this creates a complex path for axonal growth, i.e. across the scar, suture gap or nerve graft.

Sunderland (1978) has proposed a more detailed classification which is based upon the pathological anatomy of the various tissue components of the nerve trunk (Fig. 11.15).

Type 1 — this corresponds to a neuropraxia.

Type 2 — this corresponds to axonotmesis.

Type 3 — there is loss of nerve conduction at the level of the injury and within the distal nerve segment. Axonal continuity is lost and the endoneural tube is destroyed but the perineurium remains intact. There is considerable scarring in the region of the injury and there is axonal misdirection when regeneration occurs. This lesion carries a poor prognosis and surgery may be required as the internal structures of the fascicles have been destroyed.

Type 4 — again, there is loss of axonal continuity as well as of the endoneural tubes and the perineurium. The epineurium remains intact. Once again there is axonal misdirection when regeneration occurs but on surgical inspection the nerve may still appear to have some degree of continuity.

Type 5 — there is transection or rupture of the entire nerve trunk. At operation the nerve ends will be completely separated and surgical coaptation is required in order to regain any recovery whatsoever.

Degeneration

Interruption of the continuity of the axon results in extensive changes throughout the nerve fibre. There is traumatic and retrograde degeneration, which occurs proximal to the site of injury, and Wallerian degeneration, which occurs distally.

Traumatic degeneration

This occurs in the region of the nerve just proximal to the injury. Here, the nerve fibre undergoes significant morphological and physiological changes which are

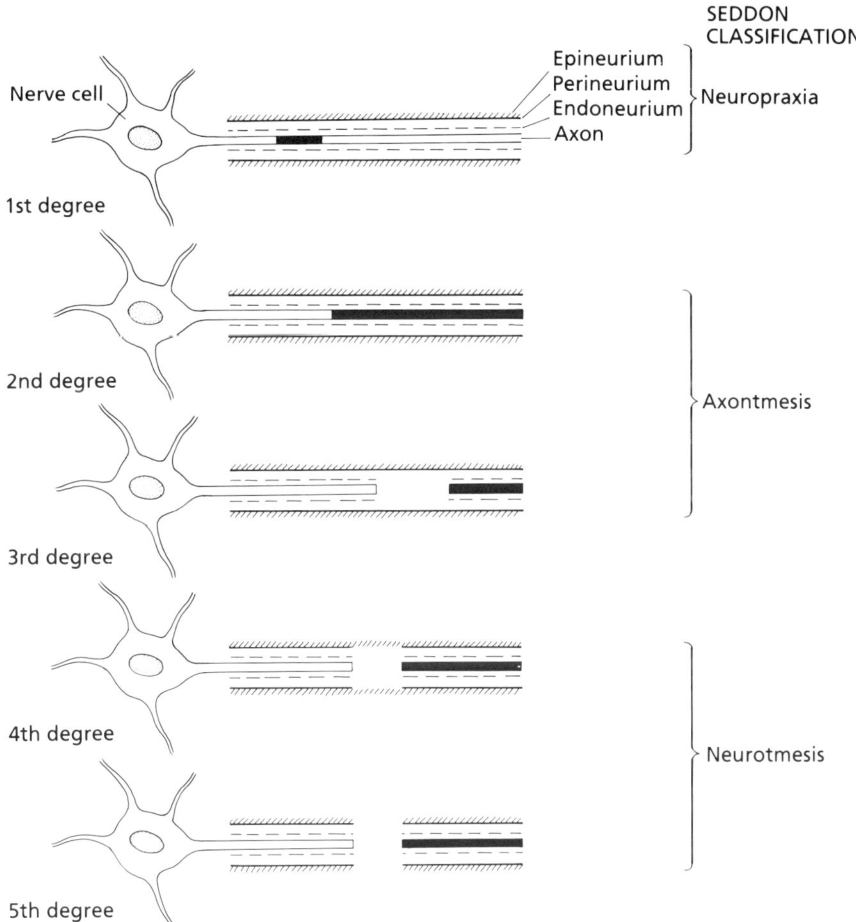

Fig. 11.15 Sunderland's classification of nerve injuries and their correspondence to Seddon's classification. (After Sunderland 1978.)

direct effects of the trauma. The severity depends on the cause of injury and it may affect either the first one or two internodal segments (1−2 mm) or, if the injury was severe, e.g. high-velocity bullet wound, then it may extend for 4 mm or more. The changes are similar to those seen in the distal segment but proximally they are reversible.

Retrograde degeneration

Retrograde degeneration refers to the changes seen in the cell body and the proximal axons after axonal continuity has been interrupted. This reaction, known as chromotolysis, is seen at a very early stage: the nucleus migrates to the periphery of the cell body and there is dispersal of the granules; it was first noted by Nissl towards the end of the last century. The number of cell bodies which are affected by this varies considerably. Some cell bodies remain unaffected while others undergo cell death. If regeneration is not possible, a large number of neurones degenerate. Even nerve cells which have a synapse with the injured nerve will show signs of degeneration and this is known as *transneuronal degeneration*.

Distal degeneration

Wallerian degeneration takes place in the axons distal to the injury. This degeneration advances progressively from the lesion towards the periphery. It seems that the integrity of a normal nerve is maintained by the stimulus of a neurotrophic factor which inhibits the lytic activities of the Schwann cell. This neurotrophic factor is synthesized within the nerve cell body and is carried along the axon by axoplasmic transport. After damage to a nerve, this flow is blocked at the site of injury, but distally this flow continues and there is progressive reduction in the concentration of this factor from proximal to distal. As the concentration falls below a critical level the Schwann cells are activated; they disrupt the axon and the myelin sheath. The myelin begins to fragment, starting from about the second day at the site of the lesion and spreads rapidly with the smallest fibres being affected first. This degeneration advances at the rate of about 250 mm day^{-1}. In the larger fibres it progresses at about 59 mm day^{-1}. Changes occur in the Schwann cells within 24 hours of injury and they start to multiply; mitotic activity is greatest when the Wallerian degeneration and the accumulation of debris are at their peak. The activity then drops off progressively and the Schwann cells tend to align longitudinally within the persisting basal laminae to form the 'bands of Büngner'; apparently these act as guidelines for the regenerating axons. The Schwann cell would appear to be able to digest axons and myelin debris and thus acts like a macrophage but it also tends to synthesize collagen fibrils that invade the scar.

The basal lamina, which covers the Schwann cell, forms a narrow tube along the whole fibre and runs from one cell to the next. This basal lamina together with the adjacent endoneural collagen fibrils is referred to as the Schwann tube or endoneural tube. During degeneration this basal lamina remains intact in the proximal and distal segments, forming the bands of Büngner which would appear to direct the regrowing axons.

Regeneration

A few days after the transection of the nerve, axons in the proximal stump produce a number of collateral and terminal sprouts which advance distally along the tube on the inside of the basal lamina. The time for these definite sprouts to appear is called the 'initial delay'. The mechanisms which trigger this phenomenon are unknown. The regenerating nerve trunk will organize itself into miniature compartments, each surrounded by new perineurium. This is seen in the first few months after transection, but is not seen a year later.

The process of regeneration may be divided into four stages:

1 Recovery of the nerve cell body from the retrograde effects of the injury.

2 Regeneration of the axons across the injured site and then along the bands of Büngner.

3 The reconnection of the appropriate axon to the correct end organ.

4 Maturation of the nerve fibres.

Recovery of the cell body

Protein synthesis commences in the neurone and this then allows the return of the axoplasmic transport system. The growth of the nerve fibres requires a continu-

ous supply of metabolites from the cell body and a diminution of this slows down the rate of growth. There is a time delay between the injury to the nerve and neuronal recovery. This is known as the latent period and it varies with the site and severity of the injury. An injury close to the cell body produces more severe retrograde damage and the cell body takes longer to recover; therefore axonal growth is delayed.

Regeneration of axons

Regeneration can be detected histologically in the proximal stump by the second day. During the first 2 weeks there is active axonal sprouting in the damaged zone with the axonal tip giving off one or more axonal outgrowths and collaterals arising at the level of the node of Ranvier. These act like pseudopodia: some retract and some progress.

When a nerve has been crushed, the basal lamina usually remains intact and the regenerating fibres cross the injury zone without much problem. However, in stretching injuries, the basal lamina may be completely disrupted and crossing of the damaged zone will be more difficult. If the nerve has been completely severed, then the gap becomes invaded by tissue of variable structure and density and the axons have significant difficulty in traversing this area. The density of axons completing their journey across the scar is often minimal, and is determined by the amount of scarring which is present, even after the nerve has been carefully sutured.

The rate of regeneration varies between 1 and 2.4 mm day^{-1} for sensory axons, and between 1.1 and 3.6 mm day^{-1} for motor axons (Sunderland 1978). The rate of regeneration depends on a number of factors: whether the basal lamina has been left intact or not, the distance between the injury and the cell body, the type and diameter of the fibre involved, and the age of the patient.

Maturation of the regenerated fibres

The axonal tip, which is advancing towards the receptor organ, is 'bare' and when it acquires a Schwann cell sheath, the axon becomes myelinated. The myelination process lags behind the axonal growth and seems to depend on the diameter of the axon. These and other complex changes are still in progress long after the neurone has established contact with its end organ, and therefore functional recovery occurs over a much longer period; even when sensation has been restored the maturation process continues. Functional recovery also depends on the density and pattern of innervation and on the arrest and reversal of the trophic changes in the end organ which resulted from the denervation.

Most nerve injuries associated with fractures are either due to crushing or stretching, or perhaps a combination of both. It is thus seen that where a nerve is crushed it has a better chance of recovery than where it is stretched; the worse prognosis is for nerves which have been completely severed.

Diagnosis

A diagnosis can only be made by being aware of the possibility of nerve injury following a fracture or dislocation. The history of the injury should be recorded in as much detail as possible; however, in many patients this will be difficult. It is important to realize that the patient may have had previous damage to the area and this should be taken into account.

Physical examination must include a careful assessment of the sensation proximal and distal to the injury. Fracture of the mid-shaft of the humerus may, of course, be associated with a traction injury of the brachial plexus. Some doctors assess sensory loss by asking the patient, 'Can you feel that?' as they brush the skin with their fingers. This is adequate if there is a negative response. However, if there is a positive response it still does not exclude neurological damage. The patient may still feel something but it could be grossly abnormal or, indeed, they may feel the finger moving their arm rather than the touch on the skin. If possible, it is important to compare the area with a known normal area. Differentiation between sharp and blunt is extremely helpful. However, the use of a hypodermic needle is incorrect because the tip is so sharp that it often penetrates the skin and causes bleeding before the sensation of pain is detected. A safety pin or, nowadays, a sterile disposable needle specifically designed for sensory testing should be used. Light touch sensation can be tested by using the tip of the examiner's finger or a piece of gauze or cotton wool. Vibration sensation can also easily be tested. The line of sensory loss should be mapped out on the patient and transferred to a drawing on the case-history sheet and/or a photograph taken.

Motor power is assessed and recorded using the Medical Research Council (MRC) muscle grading scale.

Grade 0 — paralysis.

Grade 1 — palpable contraction of muscle but no joint motion.

Grade 2 — muscle contraction producing active movement of the joint through its full passive range but with gravity eliminated.

Grade 3 — contraction of the muscle producing joint motion against gravity.

Grade 4 — contraction producing joint motion through its full passive range against gravity and moderate resistance.

Grade 5 — normal power.

It is also important to note the presence of sympathetic changes, e.g. absence of sweating, loss of papillary ridging and, in the case of brachial plexus injury, the presence of Horner's syndrome.

Patients may be able to perform trick movements, not, necessarily deliberately, and the examiner should be aware of these. A patient with a posterior interosseous nerve palsy will be able to dorsiflex the wrist but not the fingers or the thumb. The interphalangeal joint of the thumb may be extended by the use of intrinsic muscles in the absence of radial nerve function. Elbow flexion can occur against gravity by the use of the brachioradialis when the biceps and brachialis are paralysed. Abduction of the shoulder may be possible in some patients through the action of the rotator cuff in the presence of a deltoid paralysis.

The presence of a compartment syndrome should always be considered where there has been a crush injury, coma, unconsciousness resulting from drugs, or fractures. Nerve lesions may be due to the compartment syndrome and the diagnosis can be confirmed by intra-compartmental pressure measurement.

Electrophysiological studies may be helpful in differentiating neuropraxia from an axonotmesis or neurotmesis and may also be helpful in confirming a lack of neuronal recovery prior to late surgical exploration.

Treatment

Open injuries

Where there is evidence of neurological deficit associated with an open fracture or dislocation, it should be presumed that the nerve has been completely divided either by excessive stretching or by direct trauma. Operative exploration is therefore indicated. There may also be damage to the vascular structures.

The wound should be cleaned and debrided as necessary and then extended proximally and distally in the line of the neurovascular structures. The nerve may be easily identified and may be in continuity, in which case a note should be made of the structural damage using magnification. If it is not possible to find the nerve, then it has probably been transected or ruptured. It will then be necessary to identify the nerve in normal tissue away from the fracture site and to follow the nerve into the area. If the nerve has been cleanly transected, then a primary anastomosis is ideal. It will first be necessary to reduce the dislocation and stabilize it, if appropriate. In the presence of a fracture, there is little use in performing fine surgery, suturing the nerve and leaving the fracture mobile; therefore internal fixation is necessary prior to nerve anastomosis. In the fresh injury it is usually possible to approximate the nerve ends; however, in the humerus it is also possible to shorten that bone so that a nerve anastomosis can be made without undue tension. This, of course, will depend on the configuration of the fracture: it is easy to shorten a transverse fracture but much more difficult to do the same in a spiral fracture. Proceed with primary nerve repair only if local and general conditions are satisfactory.

Magnification should be used in the repair of a peripheral nerve and this can be in the form of loupes or an operating microscope. The nerve ends should be cleaned of blood clot and a small cuff of epineural fat resected at each end. The epineurium should be preserved. Fine suture material with a minimum size of 8/o is used for the epineural anastomosis having first orientated the fascicular bundles within the nerve ends. Where there is a definite pattern of fascicles, then orientation can be straight-forward. However, in oligofascicular patterns this may be extremely difficult and the orientation of blood vessels on the surface of the nerve will have to be used orientate, the ends. If two 8/o sutures will not hold the nerve ends approximated with the adjacent joint bent to a physiological position, then the tension is too great. A nerve graft will be necessary. However, conditions need to be ideal in order to perform nerve grafting and this is probably best left until the wound has completely healed and the viability of the surrounding tissue has been confirmed.

If the nerve ends cannot be approximated or if there has been a rupture with long segments of contused nerve at each end, then reconstruction should not be attempted at this stage, although the fracture should be internally fixed. It is important, however, to document, preferably with drawings, the extent of the nerve damage seen at operation. Some surgeons put a large suture through the end of the nerve for later identification; this should not be necessary as the nerve can usually be found by starting in normal tissue and working towards the injury. The soft tissues are allowed to heal and the patient should then be referred to a surgeon who is skilled in nerve grafting. With good internal fixation the joint can be mobilized early and the reconstruction can be undertaken when full mobility in the adjacent joint has been obtained.

Closed injuries

It is extremely important to document the neurological status of the limb prior to any attempt at reduction or relocation. The reduction of a dislocated joint may trap the nerve and lead to a subsequent loss of neurological function; this will obviously cause permanent damage if it remains undetected. Equally, the reduction of a

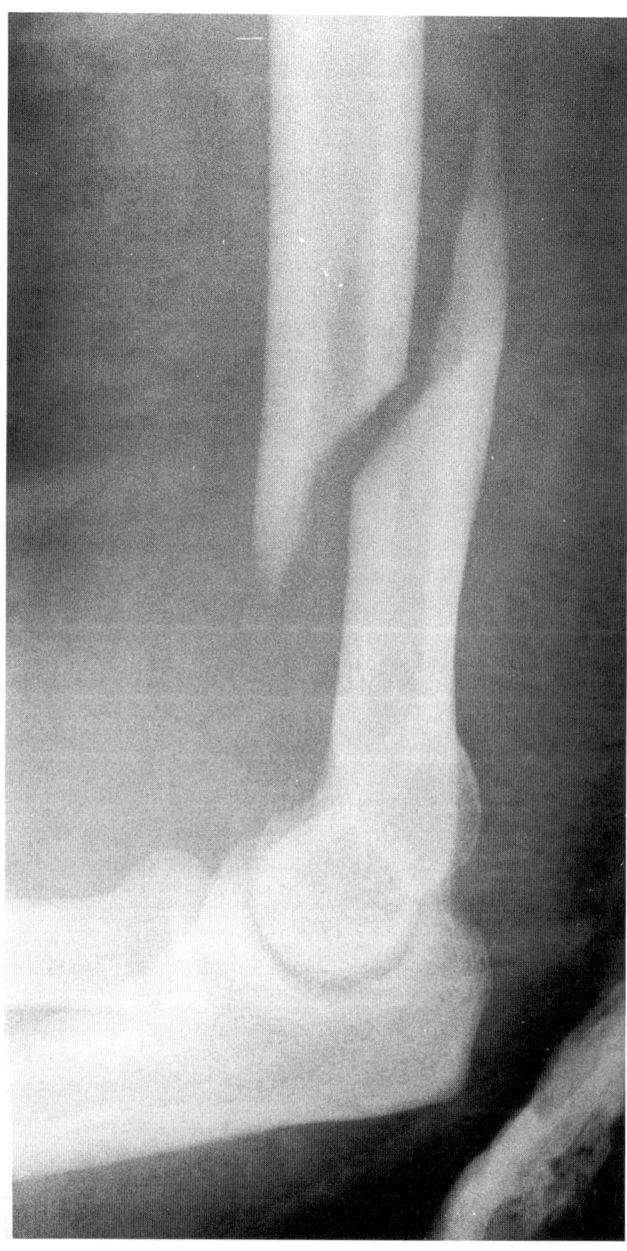

Fig. 11.16 An oblique fracture of the lower third of the humerus (a Holstein fracture). It is very liable to have the radial nerve within the fracture or even impaled on the sharp spike of the bone.

fracture may stretch the nerve over the end of the bone or, indeed, trap it within the fracture site and this is occasionally seen in an oblique fracture of the lower third of the humerus (Fig. 11.16). Any such deterioration in nerve function following reduction requires surgical exploration (Fig. 11.17).

The majority of nerve injuries associated with closed fractures are due to crushing and the prognosis is generally favourable. Recovery should be carefully monitored and a prediction made as to when the first sign of recovery should appear, e.g. with a fracture at the midshaft of the humerus the distance from that fracture to the proximal third of the brachioradialis can be measured, and if one estimates that the rate of nerve recovery is 1 mm day^{-1}, then, allowing for a latent phase, the brachioradialis muscle should be seen to commence some form of contraction at the appropriate stage. However, in dislocations and in some fractures there is a significant degree of traction and there may be nerve damage over a wide section so that recovery may not occur at all. It is not possible to predict this.

If recovery has not taken place according to the surgeon's estimation, then surgical exploration is indicated. Electrophysiological studies may be helpful to determine any subclinical neurological recovery which may assist in the decision, necessary at operation, to resect part of the nerve and put in a graft or to perform a neurolysis. If recovery is taking place, then further observation is necessary. If some recovery has occurred but then ceased, exploration and neurolysis may help.

Late exploration

An extensile exposure is required following the line of the peripheral nerve, which is first found in normal tissue proximal and distal to the area of injury, and careful dissection follows this nerve into the scarred region. Where there has been a total separation of the nerve ends, the nerve trunks usually head in different directions as they approach each other. The nerve stumps are resected until fascicles are seen bulging from the nerve. However, when there is a nerve lesion in continuity, it may be difficult to decide whether to perform a neurolysis or to resect the damaged segment. If there has been no clinical recovery whatsoever at 6 months and electrophysiological studies have confirmed these findings, then the nerve ends are resected back to the point when fascicles sprout from the transected end. Observation with magnification will reveal the amount of scar tissue present on a cross-sectional area of the nerve and it is important to resect the nerve until this scar tissue is at a minimum. Such resection usually precludes the ability to do a direct anastomosis. Nerve grafting is then required. If there has been a partial recovery but with failure to progress, then a neurolysis is performed using an operating microscope.

Nerve grafting

The graft is usually taken from the sural nerve in either or both legs. More recently strips of muscle, frozen then

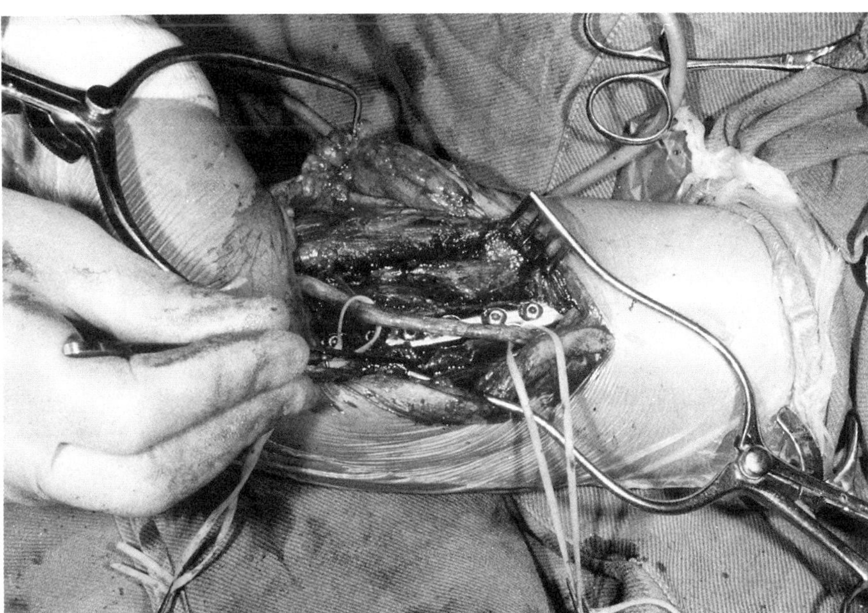

Fig. 11.17 A closed fracture of the shaft of the humerus was treated conservatively but during the first 48 hours a radial nerve palsy developed. At exploration that same day, the nerve was found trapped between the two fragments. An AO plate fixation was performed and the damaged nerve is seen lying free over the plate. The radial nerve made a complete recovery within 6 weeks.

thawed in water, have been used successfully to bridge nerve gaps. Whilst it would be ideal to accurately align fascicles and place one length of sural nerve between identical fascicles, this is not possible. The topographical pattern of a nerve changes very rapidly over short distances and after resection of a length of scarred nerve there will be no identifiable relationship between fascicles; therefore, all one can hope to do is to place the graft between the same portions of the nerve, i.e. the graft at the 3 o'clock position in the proximal end is attached to the distal end in the 9 o'clock position.

One end of the sural nerve is sutured, with one or two 10/0 nylon sutures, to the proximal end of the nerve trunk. The nerve graft is then placed between the two divided ends with the adjacent joints in full extension and the graft is transected at the appropriate length. One or two 10/0 sutures are used to position the nerve graft distally. During this time the remaining graft is kept in a moist swab. This process is repeated until the maximum number of cables have been fitted into the cross-sectional area of the nerve trunk. Following suture of all the cables the joint should be placed through its full range of motion so that no tension or displacement of the grafts is seen. Haemostasis must always be secured before closing the wound. Early mobilization can be commenced in view of the fact that no tension will be placed on the nerve graft.

Interfascicular nerve grafting has been shown to be quite successful and Millesi *et al.* (1976) have shown that even in radial nerve lesions 77% of patients can achieve very good functional results with either grade 4 or 5 muscle power.

Postreduction compression lesions

The importance of continued assessment of neurological function after reduction cannot be overemphasized. This is particularly true for the Colles' fracture in which the median nerve is often forgotten. An acute carpal tunnel syndrome can develop either as an immediate or as a late complication of a Colles' fracture. If it develops in the early phase, after reduction, then an urgent carpal tunnel decompression is required. These fractures usually occur in the elderly patient and if prolonged compression occurs in this age group the chances of complete recovery are minimal (Fig. 11.18).

Tendon reconstruction

Some nerve lesions produce a paralysis which can be corrected by tendon transfers which have a very good reputation. One example is the high radial nerve palsy which produces a wrist drop. The results of a flexor-to-extensor transfer in this group of patients are often successful and the surgeon may prefer to proceed straight to such a tendon transfer at 6 months rather than explore the nerve and wait for another 3–6 months for any signs of recovery. Even after nerve grafting a tendon transfer may be necessary to augment strength. Another example is the common peroneal nerve. After repair and/or grafting of this nerve the recovery is slow and unreliable. A tibialis posterior transfer through the interosseous membrane provides early dorsiflexion of the foot and quickly overcomes the annoying foot drop.

Early tendon transfer may be undertaken in these two

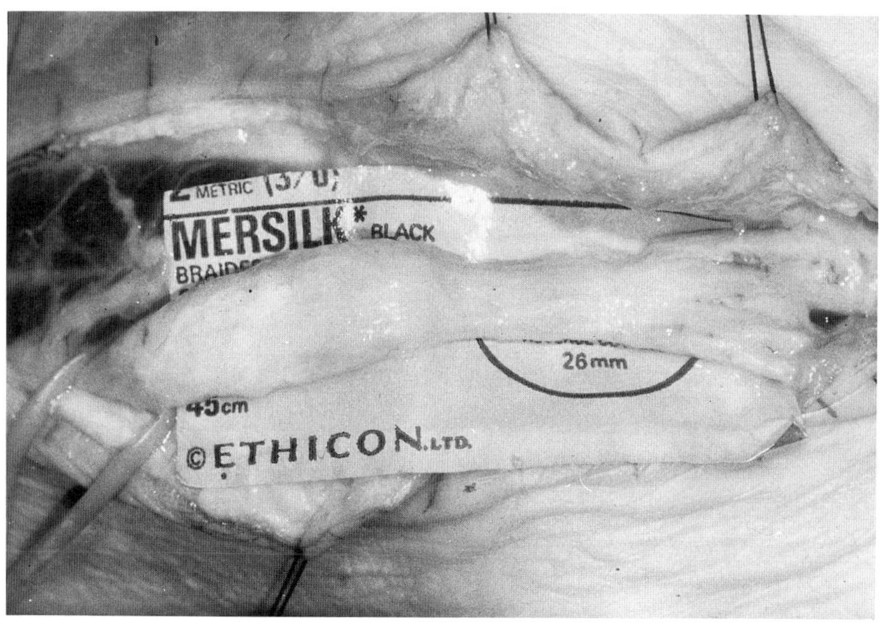

Fig. 11.18 A median nerve of the carpal tunnel has been severely compressed, secondary to a Colles' fracture some months previously. Recovery in this elderly patient did not occur. The narrowed segment indicates the area of compression.

situations when there has been a loss of neural tissue in an open fracture and neurotmesis associated with severe local tissue damage or infection.

Late tendon reconstruction is undertaken when there has been no recovery despite exploration, suture or grafting.

References

Millesi, H., Meissl, G. & Berger, A. Further experience with interfascicular grafting of the median, ulna and radial nerves. *J Bone Joint Surg* 1976; **58A**: 209–218.

Seddon, H.J. Three types of nerve injury. *Brain* 1943; **66**: 237–288.

Sunderland, S. *Nerve and Nerve Injury*. Churchill Livingstone: Edinburgh, 1978.

Compartment syndromes

M.J.ALLEN AND M.R.BARNES

Acute compartment syndromes following trauma are rare and, as a consequence, they continue to be misdiagnosed. Once the diagnosis has been made, urgent surgery is required to prevent significant limb morbidity. A greater awareness of such syndromes, repeated clinical assessment of the injured limb, the use of intra-compartmental pressure measurement and the appropriate prompt surgical intervention can prevent the development of serious sequelae.

Definition

A compartment may be defined as a closed space bounded by a relatively inelastic fascia and, on occasions, by bone. Within each compartment are to be found muscles, arteries, veins and nerves. Each compartment acts as a discrete pressure unit.

An acute compartment syndrome may be defined as a condition in which there is a build-up of pressure, within a closed osseofascial compartment, sufficient to reduce capillary blood perfusion below a level necessary for tissue viability (Mubarak & Hargens 1981). If this situation persists for several hours, irreversible muscle and nerve damage will result. At worst this may result in amputation or severe ischaemic contracture of the limb (Volkmann's) and at best it may result in minor contractures such as clawing of the toes. It should be noted that peripheral pulses will be present as the major blood supply to the limbs is uninterrupted, unless the compartment pressure exceeds the arterial pressure (a

rare occurrence). All the effects of raised compartment pressure take place at the capillary level.

Anatomical locations

Acute compartment syndromes can occur at a number of sites. The most common locations are in the lower leg (Seddon 1966, Matsen & Clawson 1975, Allen *et al.* 1985b), forearm (Seddon 1956, Eaton & Green 1975, Gelberman *et al.* 1981, Allen *et al.* 1985a, Shall *et al.* 1986) and thigh (Grosz *et al.* 1973, Allen *et al.* 1985b, Tarlow *et al.* 1986), although very rarely other sites such as the hand (Harris & Riordan 1954, Spinner *et al.* 1972, Salisbury *et al.* 1974, Halpern *et al.* 1979, Quigley *et al.* 1981), upper arm (Jenkins & Mintowt-Czyz 1986) or foot (Bonutti & Bell 1986) may be affected.

Lower limb

This comprises four compartments (Fig. 11.19) and is the most common site for acute compartment syndromes to occur. The deep posterior and anterior compartments are the ones most frequently at risk (Seddon 1966).

Forearm

Again, a common site for compartment syndromes. There are three compartments (Fig. 11.20): the superficial, and deep volar and the extensor. Further details of the anatomy of these compartments are discussed in relation to clinical signs later in the chapter.

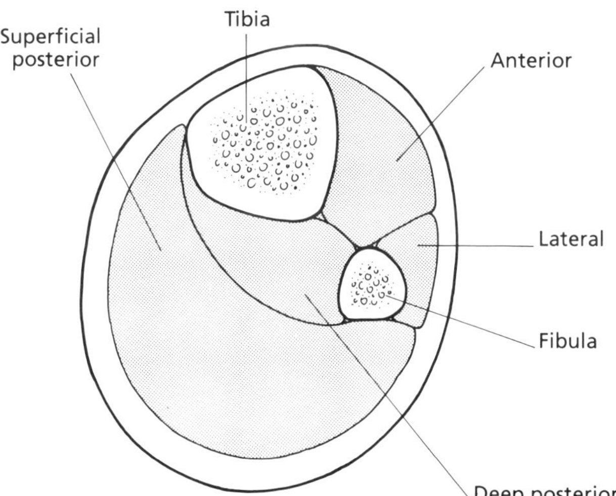

Fig. 11.19 Cross-section of the lower limb.

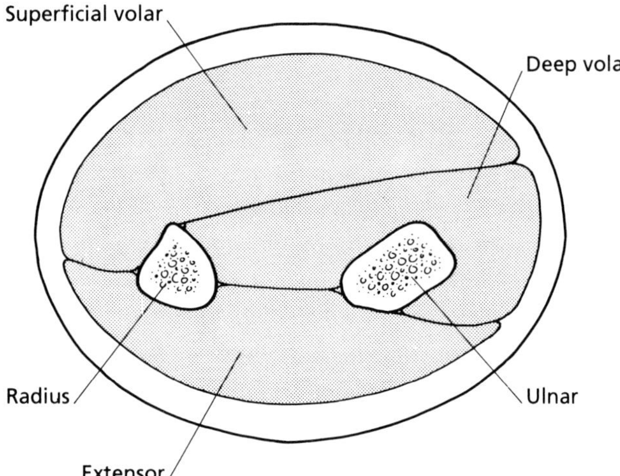

Fig. 11.20 Cross-section of the upper limb.

Aetiology

There are many and varied aetiological factors which may initiate or contribute to an acute compartment syndrome.

Soft tissue trauma

Severe soft tissue trauma, alone (Newmeyer & Kilgore 1976) or in combination with a fracture (Allen *et al.* 1985a), may be sufficient to precipitate the condition.

Fractures

Acute compartment syndromes occur most frequently following fractures with accompanying soft tissue damage (Rorabeck & MacNab 1976). Grossly comminuted and compound fractures are less likely to develop compartment syndromes as the limiting fascial envelopes are often disrupted, thereby decompressing the compartment (Blick *et al.* 1986).

Vascular trauma

Combined vascular and orthopaedic trauma carries a high risk of developing compartment syndromes following revascularization of the limb. This is especially so if the period of ischaemia of the limb prior to revascularization is long and there is an associated venous injury (Freedman & Knowles 1959, Gitlitz 1965, Husni 1967, Patman 1975, Allen *et al.* 1984).

Anticoagulant therapy

This will increase bleeding into a compartment after trauma, thus increasing the risk of developing a compartment syndrome (Neviaser *et al.* 1976). The author has seen at least three cases in which simple tears of the gastrocnemius muscle have been mistakenly diagnosed as deep vein thrombosis (DVT) and have been subsequently anticoagulated, resulting in the development of compartment syndromes (Hay *et al.* 1992).

Tight plaster casts and dressings

These can act either as a source of externally applied pressure (if overtight) or as an extra limiting envelope preventing the expansion of the compartment (Hardy 1979, Garfin *et al.* 1981, Brodell *et al.* 1986). Included in this category are air splints (Shakespeare *et al.* 1984, Werbel & Shybut 1986) and antishock trousers (Johnson 1981, Concannon 1982, Williams *et al.* 1982).

Prolonged limb compression

This is also called the 'Saturday night palsy'. Patients left lying with a limb trapped for many hours may develop a compartment syndrome when the trapped limb is released (Owen *et al.* 1979, Christensen & Klarke 1985). This situation is usually the result of alcohol or drug overdose (Barnes *et al.* 1992), but may also occur in conscious or unconscious patients who have been trapped for several hours (Mubarak & Owen 1975).

Traction

Traction will increase intracompartmental pressure (Shakespeare & Henderson 1982, Allen *et al.* 1985b) and in those patients at risk of developing a compartment syndrome careful observation is required if traction is used.

Burns

Circumferential burns associated with a traumatized limb may result in the development of a compartment syndrome. The resulting eschar reduces the normal elasticity of the skin and there may be an increase in free fluid.

Pathophysiology

Acute compartment syndromes usually occur fairly soon after injury but cases have been recorded of their occurring up to 72 hours after the initial insult (Allen *et al.* 1985a): the so-called lag period. A pressure of 50 mmHg in a compartment heralds the onset of such a syndrome (Fig. 11.21). The length of time for which the pressure remains above 50 mmHg will dictate whether or not the changes within the compartment are reversible. Experimental evidence shows that as the pressure within the compartment increases different components are affected. Muscle damage occurs at an early stage, as does damage to the nerves. Irreversible changes occur to both structures after 6–12 hours, depending on the pressure. Numerous hypotheses have been proposed to explain the pathophysiology of acute compartment syndromes and the exact answer to the problem is not yet known. There is no consensus as to what is a 'critical pressure level', above which permanent damage will be caused. Many authors (particularly in the United States) consider that any compartment exhibiting a pressure greater than 30 mmHg requires immediate surgical intervention. Others consider that the time factor is equally important — any rise above the 'normal' pressure will cause some damage eventually, as even a very small rise in pressure can reduce the capillary circulation.

In most cases the presence of oedema and/or blood within a space of restricted volume results in a rise in compartment pressure. Once the compartment pressure exceeds the pressure in the capillaries the microcirculation becomes compromised and results in inadequate capillary perfusion. A vicious circle is initiated as reduced capillary circulation causes further oedema of the muscle mass and extravasation of intracellular fluid into the extracellular space, which increases the compartment pressure even more.

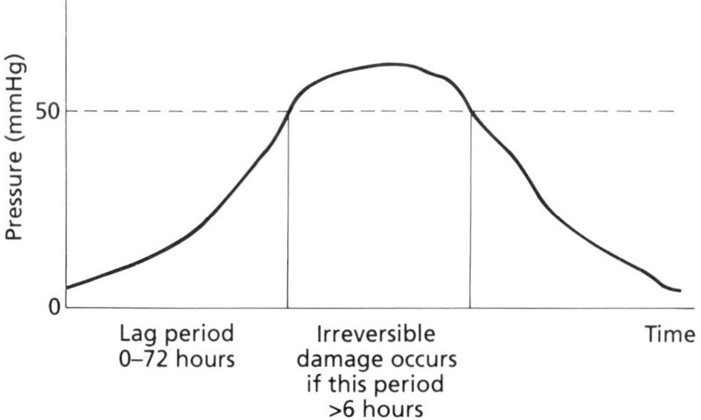

Fig. 11.21 Rise and fall in compartment pressure with time.

Clinical signs and symptoms

In all cases where a compartment syndrome exists the patient will be in considerable pain and the affected limb may be swollen. However, clinical signs and symptoms may be difficult or impossible to illicit in non-compliant or unconscious patients. The traditional clinical signs of a compartment syndrome have been based on the mnemonic of the '4 Ps' — Pain, Pallor, Paralysis and Pulselessness (Griffiths 1940, Mubarak & Hargens 1981). However, this concept is no longer valid. In particular it is important to note that the absence of pulses is indicative of arterial trauma and not a compartment syndrome. However, very occasionally compartment syndromes can cause the peripheral pulses to disappear if the compartment pressures are extremely high. Investigations of a pulseless limb should initially include an arteriogram, but if this is normal then a compartment syndrome should be considered as the cause.

On occasions it may be difficult to differentiate a compartment syndrome from other conditions such as vascular injury, neuropraxia, simple fracture or soft tissue injury. Repeated clinical evaluation of the limb should be made and if the clinical signs and symptoms are worsening then a compartment syndrome should be considered as very likely.

Pain

The most important indication of the possibility of a compartment syndrome is excessive pain or 'pain out of proportion to what is anticipated' (Matsen 1980). For example, the pain associated with a fracture should diminish following reduction and/or splintage. If the pain increases following the initial stabilization of the fracture, then a compartment syndrome should be considered as a possibility.

Swelling

The affected limb is swollen and the overlying skin appears tight and shiny. This may not be obvious through a plaster cast or dressing and, hence, can be easily missed. Swelling in the deep posterior compartment of the calf is impossible to detect as the compartment is deep to the gastrocnemius and soleus muscles. Similarly, swelling is not a feature of deep volar compartment syndromes of the forearm. If there is any doubt as to the possibility of such a syndrome being present, all dressings and plasters should be removed and the limb reassessed.

Pain on passive stretch

This is probably the best clinical sign of a compartment syndrome. Careful clinical examination will help to locate the compartment or compartments involved. This sign is often difficult to elicit in painful fractured limbs and is impossible to determine in unconscious patients.

Pain on passive stretch will not differentiate between a compartment syndrome and a vascular injury *per se*; other clinical signs, such as the presence or absence of peripheral pulses and the colour of the limb, have to be taken into account. If, however, the compartment pressure is above the arterial pressure, then the diagnosis will be difficult on clinical grounds.

Motor weakness

This may be indicative of a compartment syndrome but tends to be a rather late sign and should not be relied on for initial diagnosis. Weakness of the extensor hallucis longus would indicate the possibility of an anterior compartment syndrome (Fig. 11.22). Repeated clinical examination, carefully documenting muscle power (MRC grade 0–5), will enable suspected cases to be picked up early.

Sensory deficit

A sensory deficit in the distribution of the nerves passing through a compartment is a good indicator, assuming that there is no direct nerve damage. This sign can help to identify the compartments affected. For example, the deep branch of the peroneal nerve passes through the anterior compartment. If the pressure is raised there will be a sensory loss in the first web space and on the dorsum of the foot (Fig. 11.22). Repeated and careful neurological examination is required to pick up these changes.

Posture

The limb may take on a characteristic posture; this is especially true for the forearm (Fig. 11.23). The posture taken up allows for the maximum compartment volume to be achieved, thus minimizing the increase in pressure and allowing for maximum pain relief.

Clinical signs related to specific compartments

SENSORY CHANGES

Sensory changes will occur in relation to the specific nerves which pass through each of the compartments involved. Initially paraesthesia will be felt in relation to the sensory distribution of the nerve; this will be followed by complete anaesthesia (Table 11.2).

MUSCLE CHANGES

Pain with passive stretch of the muscles in the affected compartment can be elicited. There will also be pain associated with active movement of the muscles within the affected compartment (Table 11.3). Passive stretch pain is a far more reliable sign than weakness of active movement. Often changes may be subtle and a careful detailed examination is required.

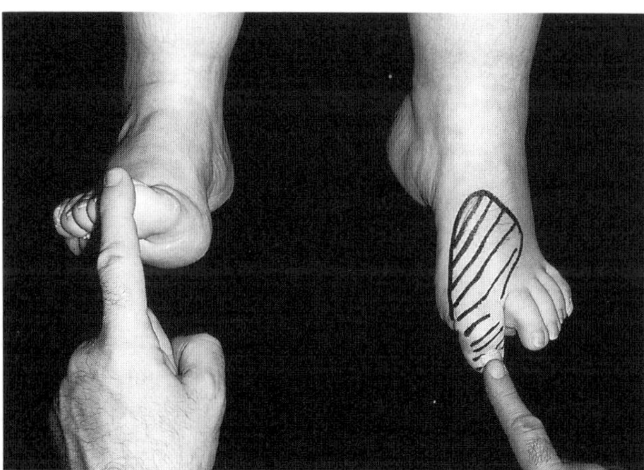

Fig. 11.22 Weakness of the extensor hallucis longus and area of sensory deficit in an anterior compartment syndrome.

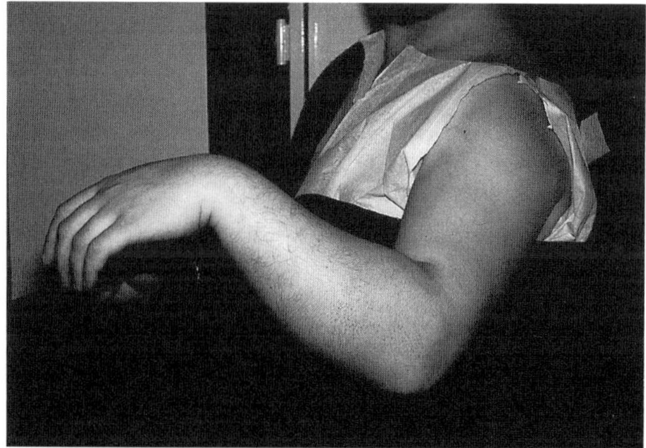

Fig. 11.23 Characteristic posture in volar compartment syndrome.

Table 11.2 Sensory changes in the lower limb

Compartment	Nerve	Sensory distribution
Anterior	Deep peroneal	1st web space
Deep posterior	Tibial	Plantar aspect of the foot
Superficial posterior	Sural	Lateral aspect of the ankle and foot
Lateral (peroneal)	Superficial peroneal	2nd and 3rd web spaces dorsum of the foot

Table 11.3 Muscle abnormalities in lower limb compartment syndromes

Compartment	Muscle group (nerve)	Movement causing passive stretch pain	Active movement reduced or lost
Anterior	Foot and toe dorsiflexors (Deep peroneal)	Plantarflexion of foot and toes	Foot and toe dorsiflexion
Deep posterior	Foot and toe plantarflexors Foot inversion	Dorsiflexion of foot and toes; foot eversion	Foot and toe plantarflexion; foot inversion
Superficial posterior	Foot plantarflexors	Foot and toe dorsiflexion	Plantarflexion
Lateral	Foot evertors	Foot inversion	Foot eversion

SWELLING

Tenseness and tenderness lateral to the tibial crest may be present in an anterior compartment syndrome. For the other compartments, particularly for the deep posterior compartment, swelling may not be as obvious.

Lower limb

The thigh is divided into two compartments (Table 11.4). The anterior compartment comprises the quadriceps and sartorius muscles which extend the knee; the major nerve of this compartment is the femoral. The posterior compartment comprises the hamstring muscle (knee flexors) supplied by the sciatic nerve and the adductor muscles supplied by the obturator nerve.

Table 11.4 Thigh compartments

Compartment	Muscles	Nerves
Anterior	Quadriceps Sartorius	Femoral
Posterior	Hamstrings Adductors	Sciatic Obturator

Anterior thigh compartment syndrome

The clinical signs of this syndrome are:
1 Pain on passive knee flexion.
2 Weakness of knee extension.
3 Sensory changes may be noted over the knee and medial aspect of the leg and foot, although the authors has never elicited this sign.
4 Tenseness over the anterior aspect of the thigh.
Compartment syndromes are far more common in the anterior than in the posterior thigh compartment and, indeed, the authors have never seen the latter.

Posterior thigh compartment syndrome

The clinical signs of this syndrome would include:
1 Pain on passive knee extension.
2 Weakness of knee flexion.
3 Neurological changes are thought to be rare due to the large size of the sciatic nerve. If the obturator nerve is involved, then sensory changes would occur on the medial aspect of the leg to the knee.

Forearm

This is composed of three compartments — superficial volar, deep volar and extensor.

Volar compartment syndrome

Clinically it is very difficult to differentiate between a superficial and a deep volar compartment syndrome. This is because the muscle groups of both compartments have a similar action and the two major nerves (ulnar and median) are situated along the fascial septa separating the two compartments and thus are not compartment-specific as in the lower limb. If a volar compartment syndrome is diagnosed it is mandatory that both compartments are surgically decompressed.

The clinical signs of a volar compartment syndrome are:

1 Pain on passive finger and wrist extension.
2 Pain on elbow extension.
3 Weakness of finger and wrist flexion.
4 Sensory loss over the palm and flexor aspects of the fingers and thumb.
5 Possible tenseness over the volar aspect of the forearm.
6 The fingers often assume a flexed posture, as does the elbow joint.
7 Paresis of the intrinsic muscles occur secondary to involvement of the median and ulnar nerves.

Extensor compartment syndrome

This is relatively rare. The major muscles in the extensor compartment are the wrist and finger extensors; the main nerve of the compartment is the posterior interosseous. The superficial radial nerve is located primarily in the volar compartment and thus, sensory changes are minimal.

The clinical signs of an extensor compartment syndrome are:

1 Pain on passive finger or wrist flexion.
2 Weakness of finger and wrist extension.
3 Tenseness over the compartment.

Pressure measurement

Intracompartmental pressure measurement is an important tool in the diagnosis of acute compartment syndromes as it offers certain important advantages over clinical assessment. A compartment syndrome will, by definition, always exhibit a raised pressure. Hence, pressure measurement makes diagnosis more certain. Pressure measurements can be carried out on unconscious or uncooperative patients in whom clinical signs may be difficult or impossible to assess. Each compartment can be individually measured and the exact location of the compartment or compartments involved can be established. This minimizes surgery since, before the advent of pressure measurements, all compartments were routinely decompressed.

Attempts have been made to measure compartment pressure since the end of the last century, but it was not until the advent of the needle technique of Whitesides *et al.* (1975) that a clinically useable method was implemented. The advantage of this method is that it uses widely available and cheap equipment, and it is still being utilized (Macey 1987). An even simpler technique is to use a central venous pressure (CVP) manometer (Brooker & Pezeshki 1979). However, both these techniques have two significant drawbacks: they do not provide a continuous permanent record of the pressure, and the accuracy of the technique is, to some extent, operator-dependent.

The introduction of the wick catheter (Mubarak *et al.* 1976), and later the slit catheter (Rorabeck *et al.* 1980), along with the infusion technique (Matsen *et al.* 1976) and the existence of reliable and rugged pressure transducers has enabled continuous accurate measurements to be made (Barnes *et al.* 1985); this is to be preferred to the above methods (Fig. 11.24). Both these catheters are designed to prevent the lumen from becoming blocked by tissue: the wick catheter does this by providing a fluid path to conduct the pressure from the tissues to the catheter; the slit catheter is designed to splay out at the end (Fig. 11.25) so that blockage cannot occur. Slit catheters are cheaper, simpler to make and easier to use, have a better frequency response and there is no wick to accidentally leave in the patient; hence, they are now the most widely used method of intracompartmental pressure measurement. In conjunction with a very slow (0.1 ml h^{-1}) infusion of heparinized saline patency is virtually guaranteed for up to 7 days.

Continuous pressure monitoring provides an objective assessment of the compartment pressures which can be easily read off the chart recorder. Both nurses

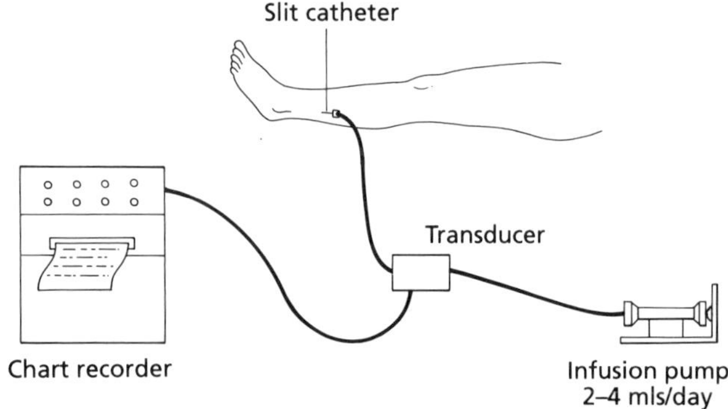

Fig. 11.24 Continuous pressure measurement technique.

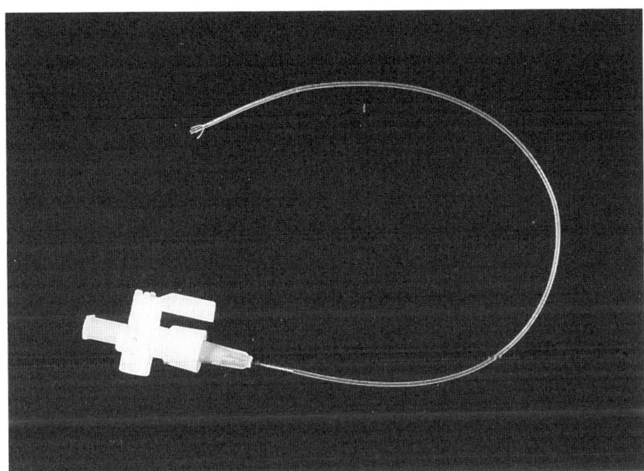

Fig. 11.25 Slit catheter.

and junior medical staff can be taught to interpret the recordings to provide an immediate assessment of the pressure. Trends can be readily identified. It is possible to see if the pressure is rising, falling or remaining stable and it is also possible to follow the rate at which these changes are occurring. These should always be taken in conjunction with the clinical findings. A rapidly increasing pressure in the region of 50 mmHg with worsening clinical signs (Table 11.5) would be an indication for immediate surgery. A pressure that had risen to 40 mmHg and then started to fall would be an indication to wait and see, providing the clinical signs mirrored the pressure trends. If the clinical signs do not fit with the pressure readings, then the measuring apparatus should be carefully checked (see 'Potential problems'). Pressure recordings also indicate the precise location of the compartment(s) involved, thus avoiding unnecessary surgery. However, it is strongly advised that if only some of the compartments of an affected limb are surgically decompressed, then those that have not undergone surgery should be monitored postoperatively.

Potential problems

1 Erroneously high pressures can occur if the catheter becomes blocked by a clot. Patency and correct location

of the catheter are best checked by squeezing the compartment. A squeeze will increase the pressure but upon release the pressure should fall immediately; if it does not a blocked catheter should be suspected (Fig. 11.26). A completely obstructed catheter may give a false high reading, particularly if an infusion is being utilized — the injection of fluid into a blocked catheter will cause the measured pressure to rise. This can only be identified by observing on a chart recorder the rate at which the pressure changes (Figs 11.27 & 11.28). A

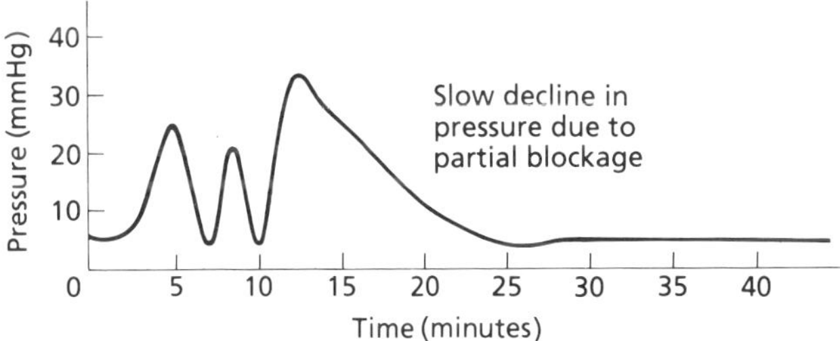

Fig. 11.26 Squeeze response with a blocked catheter.

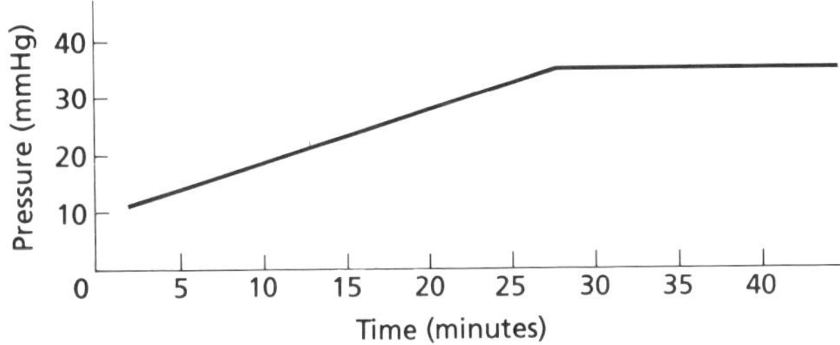

Fig. 11.27 Rise in pressure due to a blocked catheter and infusion.

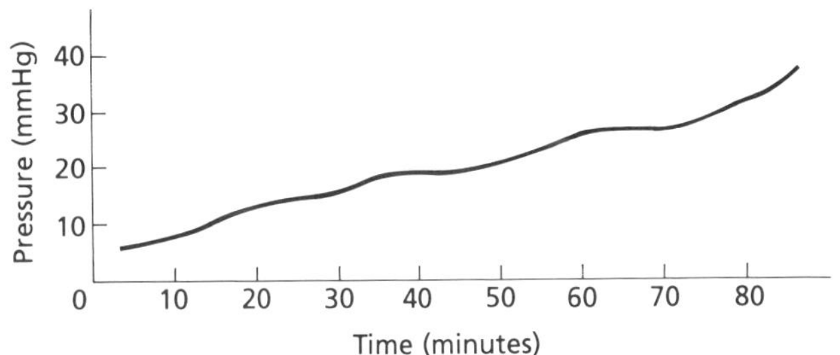

Fig. 11.28 Genuine rise in pressure.

Table 11.5 Worsening clinical signs

↑ Pain	↑ Analgesic requirements, inability to sleep
↑ Swelling	Limb becomes more tense
↑ Pain on passive stretch	Only a small amount of muscle stretch causes pain
↑ Motor weakness	MRC grade of muscle power begins to drop
↑ Sensory deficit	Initial partial sensory loss replaced by complete sensory loss
Classic posture	

completely blocked catheter will cause a much faster rise in pressure than a genuine physiological change.

2 Occasionally a catheter may become displaced owing to patient movement. If it falls out altogether then the pressure will return to zero, but if it is only slightly displaced, so that the end lies subcutaneously, then a false reading will occur.

3 One of the major problems that can occur is third-party interference with the measuring equipment. People are always tempted to 'twiddle' knobs; this can give rise to changes in sensitivity and scales, and therefore produce invalid recordings.

4 It is vital that the catheters are correctly located in the compartments. Placement in the deep posterior compartment in the calf and in the deep flexor in the forearm can be difficult.

Clinical problems in relation to pressure recording

Ideally, monitoring should be instituted as soon as possible following trauma as it has been shown (Allen *et al.* 1985b, Gibson *et al.* 1986) that the maximum pressures usually occur within the first few hours. Often, pressure monitoring is requested some time after injury and it is then impossible to tell whether the pressure is raised or whether it is on the rise or the fall of the curve (Fig. 11.21). In such cases account should always be taken of the clinical findings and the time at which the pressure is recorded after injury. If the pressure was recorded between 24 and 48 hours after injury and was found to be around 40 mmHg, then it is probable that the patient has had a compartment syndrome. Any surgical procedures done at this juncture would be too late and would not affect the eventual morbidity of the limb.

Great care has to be taken, however, if the patient is pyrexial and the limb warm; this indicates the possibility of necrotic infected muscle being present. Plain radiographs should be taken to look for gas in the soft tissue plains; large doses of intravenous antibiotics are commenced and immediate surgery should be undertaken in such cases. At surgery all dead muscle should be removed and a second examination should be made 24 hours later.

Technique

The basic technique is the same for all compartments. The slit catheter is inserted through an introducer into the compartment. The proximal end is attached, via three-way stopcocks and pressure tubing, to a pressure transducer; this entire system is filled with heparinized

saline to prevent blood clots from obstructing the catheter. For very long-term monitoring (greater than 24 hours) a slow infusion (0.1 ml h^{-1}) of saline (heparinized at 20 000 units l^{-1}) may also be used to ensure that the catheter remains patent.

The pressure transducer converts the pressure in the fluid-filled system into an electrical signal that can then be amplified, processed and displayed on a chart recorder so that trends can be easily identified. Monitoring can easily be carried out if the limb is to be put in plaster. The catheters are inserted and then simply threaded through the plaster cast as it is applied (Fig. 11.29). Once the danger period is over they can then be pulled out. Interpretation of the pressure recordings depends to some extent on the blood pressure. The figures given are for normotensive patients. If the patient is hypovolaemic then a compartment syndrome will occur at a lower pressure.

Lower leg

The anterior compartment is entered lateral to the tibial crest over the tibialis anterior muscle. The lateral compartment is approached from the lateral aspect of the leg, placing the cannula anterior to the fibula. The superficial posterior compartment is approached in the mid-line of the back of the calf, whereas the deep posterior compartment is entered on the posterior medial border of the tibia. Care has to be taken, when approaching this compartment, to avoid the long saphenous vein and the posterior tibial vessels (Fig. 11.30).

Forearm

To enter the superficial volar compartment the cannula

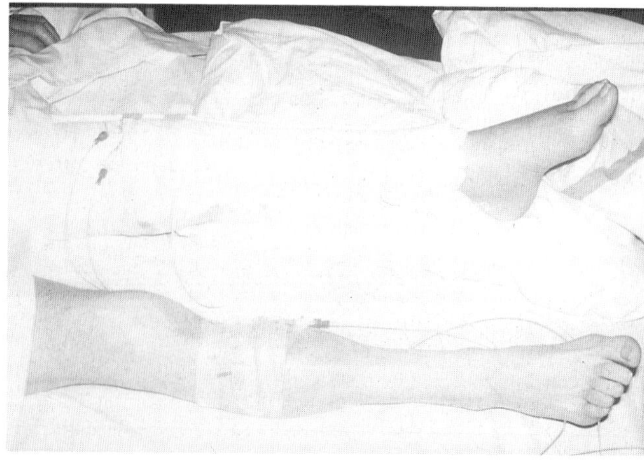

Fig. 11.29 Catheters threaded through a plaster cast.

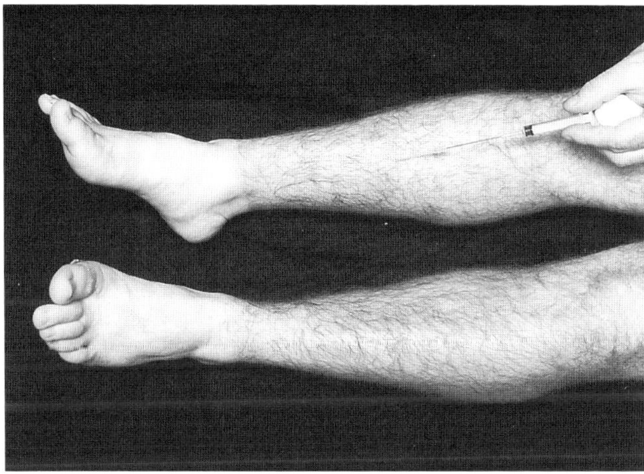

Fig. 11.30 Approach to the lower leg compartments.

is inserted in the mid-line of the flexor surface of the forearm at the junction of the proximal and distal two-thirds. For the deep volar compartment a cannula is inserted 1 cm volar to the subcutaneous border of the ulna, at the same level as for the superficial compartment. The extensor compartment is approached at the same level as the other two but from the extensor surface of the forearm (Fig. 11.31).

Interpretation of pressure measurements

The accepted value for capillary pressure is 30 mmHg, so any intracompartmental pressure above this value poses a threat to the capillary circulation. However, it has also been shown that there is no critical closing pressure for the capillaries and the process of reducing the blood supply to the tissues is a gradual one. As the compartment pressure increases above 30 mmHg

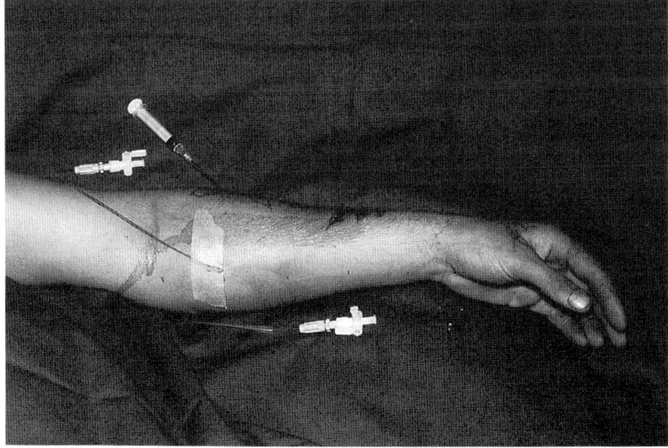

Fig. 11.31 Approach to the forearm compartments.

the blood supply is reduced; the higher the pressure, the greater the reduction. But time is also an important factor. Lower pressures for longer periods can be just as dangerous in causing permanent damage as can very high pressures for short periods.

A diagnosis of a compartment syndrome can be made on pressure readings alone in normotensive patients with an intracompartmental pressure of 50 mmHg (for a minimum time of 30 minutes to ensure that the reading is stable and accurate and not an artefact). If the pressure remains between 40 and 50 mmHg and is either stable or increasing, and remains at this level for more than 6 hours, then the patient is diagnosed as having a compartment syndrome. Patients with pressures between 30 and 40 mmHg are monitored carefully (particularly if the pressure is showing an upward trend) and a greater emphasis is placed upon clinical signs. Any pressure below 30 mmHg is considered to be normal and not indicative of a compartment syndrome.

Management

The diagnosis of a compartment syndrome is made after careful clinical examination and in conjunction with intracompartmental pressure monitoring if available. If pressures can be measured then the precise location of the affected compartments will be known. Once the diagnosis has been made urgent surgical decompression in the form of an open fasciotomy is required.

Surgery

Surgery should take the form of an open fasciotomy of the compartment or compartments involved (Sheridan & Matsen 1976). An open fasciotomy must be performed at all times to ensure that the skin does not act as a secondary envelope and restrict the expansion of the compartment.

Following surgery, closure of the wound should not be attempted, nor should tight dressings be applied as these can act as restricting envelopes and give rise to a secondary compartment syndrome. It is usual that the skin can be closed by delayed primary closure some 12–14 days after surgery. Rarely does the wound need skin grafting. An alternative technique is to apply serial steristrips daily to bring the wound edges together. If there is obvious muscle necrosis at the time of surgery, then adequate debridement is required and it is recommended that a further debridement is carried out some 24–48 hours later.

Technique

Lower limb fasciotomy

Before the advent of reliable pressure measuring techniques it was usual to decompress all four compartments. The safest and most reliable method is the double-incision fasciotomy described by Mubarak and Owen (1977) (Fig. 11.32). A longitudinal incision is made on both the medial and lateral aspects of the leg; this incision is extended proximally to just below the knee and distally to just above the ankle.

Anterolateral incision. Once the skin has been cut the fascia should be obvious. In the mid-part of the incision a small transverse incision is made in the fascia and the intermuscular septum between the anterior and lateral compartments is identified. A longitudinal incision is then made in the anterior compartment to decompress it. Associated haematomas are evacuated and bleeding vessels ligated.

In the posterior part of the incision the lateral compartment can likewise be decompressed. Care has to be taken not to damage the superficial peroneal nerve as it exits from the fascia at approximately the junction of the middle and lower thirds of the leg.

Posteromedial incision. This is similar to the above. The fascia is identified, as is the intermuscular septum. A longitudinal incision, placed anteriorly to the septum, will decompress the deep posterior compartment and an incision placed posteriorly will decompress the superficial posterior compartment.

An alternative technique that has been used is the 'fibulectomy-fasciotomy' where the fibula is removed and all four compartments are decompressed through a single incision (Ernst & Kaufer 1971). This is not recommended. With this technique adequate visualization of the muscles is not possible and proper debridement cannot be carried out.

With modern-day pressure measuring techniques it is possible to accurately locate the compartments involved and only fasciotomize those which show an increased pressure. If this is done, then the unoperated compartments must be measured after surgery.

Upper limb fasciotomy

The superficial volar compartment is approached via a longitudinal incision 2 cm to the ulnar side of the midline, extending from just below the elbow crease to the proximal wrist crease. The fascia is identified and decompressed.

The deep volar compartment is approached via the incision for the superficial compartment. The flexor carpi ulnaris is retracted medially and the superficial flexors are retracted laterally, giving access to the deep volar compartment fascia which may then be split. With this approach the ulnar nerve, which lies on the deep fascia, must be identified and retracted medially with the flexor carpi ulnaris (Fig. 11.33).

Missed compartment syndromes

An untreated acute compartment syndrome can lead to a variety of permanent problems, ranging from a minor neurological or muscular deficit, which the patient is hardly aware of (e.g. mild clawing of the toes), through the classical type of Volkmann's ischaemic contracture to gangrene which requires amputation. The outcome

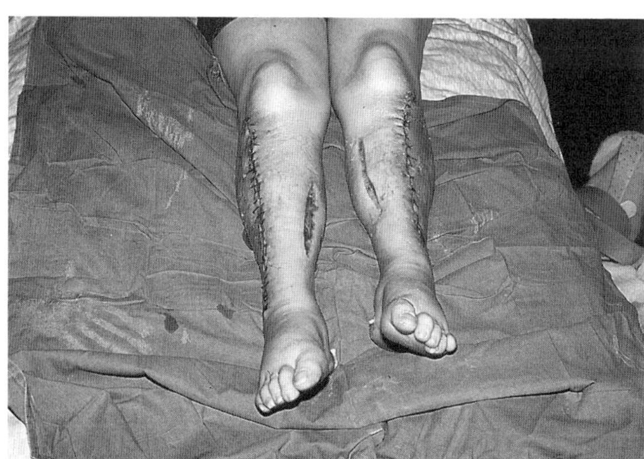

Fig. 11.32 Double-incision fasciotomy.

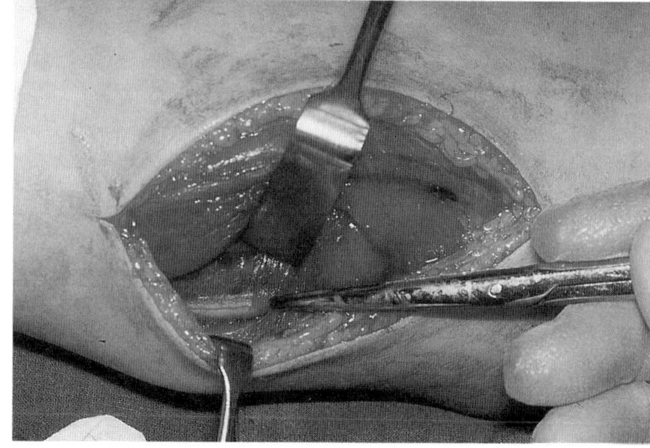

Fig. 11.33 Upper limb fasciotomy.

depends entirely on which compartments are affected and for how long. Once the diagnosis has been made urgent surgical decompression should be carried out.

Combined vascular and orthopaedic injuries

In those patients with combined injuries the potential for a compartment syndrome to develop, once revascularization has occurred, is great, especially if there has been a significant soft tissue injury, total venous interruption along with arterial occlusion and a delay in revascularizing the limb. Added to this, the further insult of orthopaedic surgery may cause additional soft tissue damage.

In order to minimize the delay it is recommended that a silastic shunt is introduced to restore arterial flow, following which the orthopaedic management can take place and then the operative arterial repair. The silastic shunt should be introduced into the proximal and distal ends of the artery and held in place with rubber clips. Once the orthopaedic and vascular surgery has taken place, then a prophylactic fasciotomy should be carried out; in the case of the lower leg all four compartments should be decompressed and in the case of the forearm all three compartments should be decompressed. An alternative would be to measure the compartment pressures following surgery for at least 48 hours.

Differential diagnosis

Numerous conditions may mimic a compartment syndrome (Table 11.6) and on occasions it may be difficult to differentiate between them on clinical grounds. The two conditions most likely to be confused with a compartment syndrome are arterial occlusion and neuropraxia. Measuring the compartment pressures will provide a reliable adjunct to the diagnosis.

Conclusions

Acute compartment syndromes are a relatively rare but important complication of orthopaedic injuries and if not recognized can lead to significant damage to a limb. There is no substitute for careful clinical examination and proper documentation of signs aided, if possible, by continuous intracompartmental pressure measurement. Once the diagnosis has been made prompt surgical decompression is required.

References

Allen, M.J., Nash, J.R., Ioannidies, T. & Bell, P.R.F. Major vascular injuries associated with orthopaedic injuries to the lower limb. *Ann R Coll Surg Engl* 1984; **66**: 101–104.

Allen, M.J., Steingold, R.F., Kotecha, M. & Barnes, M.R. The importance of the deep volar compartment in crush injuries of the forearm. *Injury* 1985a; **16**: 273–275.

Allen, M.J., Stirling, A.J., Crawshaw, C.V. & Barnes, M.R. Intracompartmental pressure monitoring of leg injuries. An aid to management. *J Bone Joint Surg* 1985b; **67B**: 53–57.

Barnes, M.R., Gibson, M.J., Scott, J., Bentley, S. & Allen, M.J. A technique for the long term measurement of intracompartmental pressure in the lower leg. *J Biomed Eng* 1985; **7**: 35–39.

Barnes, M.R., Harper, W.M., Tomson, C.R.V. & Williams, N.M.A. Gluteal compartment syndrome following drug overdose. *Injury* 1992; **23**: 274–275.

Blick, S.S., Brumback, R.J., Poka, A. *et al.* Compartment syndrome in open tibial fractures. *J Bone Joint Surg* 1986; **68A**: 1348–1353.

Bonutti, P.M. & Bell, G.R. Compartment syndrome of the foot. *J Bone Joint Surg* 1986; **68A**: 1449–1450.

Brodell, J.D., Axon, D.L. & McCollister Ewarts, C. The Robert Jones bandage. *J Bone Joint Surg* 1986; **68B**: 776–779.

Brooker, A.F. & Pezeshki, C. Tissue pressure to evaluate compartmental syndrome. *J Trauma* 1979; **19**: 689–691.

Christensen, K.S. & Klarke, M. Volkmann's ischaemic contracture due to limb compression in drug-induced coma. *Injury* 1985; **16**: 543–544.

Concannon, J.E. Antishock trousers. *J Fam Pract* 1982; **15**: 349–352.

Table 11.6 Differential diagnosis

Signs	Compartment syndrome	Arterial injury	Neuropraxia	Fracture and soft tissue	DVT
Increased pressure	+	−	−	−	−
Pain on passive stretch	+	+	−	±	±
Paresthesia	+	+	+	−	−
Paralysis	+	+	+	−	−
Pulses intact	+	−	+	+	+

+ Present; − absent.

Eaton, R.G. & Green, W.T. Volkmann's ischemia. A volar compartment syndrome of the forearm. *Clin Orthop* 1975; **113**: 58–64.

Ernst, C.B. & Kaufer, H. Fibulectomy-fasciotomy. An important adjunct in the management of lower extremity arterial trauma. *J Trauma* 1971; **11**: 365–380.

Freedman, B.J. & Knowles, C.H.R. Anterior tibial syndrome due to arterial embolism and thrombosis. Ischaemic necrosis of the anterior crural muscles. *Br Med J* 1959; **2**: 270–275.

Garfin, S.R., Mubarak, S.J., Evans, K.L., Hargens, A.R. & Akeson, W.H. Quantification of intracompartmental pressure and volume under plaster casts. *J Bone Joint Surg* 1981; **63A**: 449–453.

Gelberman, R.H., Garfin, S.R., Hergenroeder, P.T., Mubarak, S.J. & Menon, J. Compartment syndromes of the forearm: diagnosis and treatment. *Clin Orthop* 1981; **161**: 252–261.

Gibson, M.J., Barnes, M.R., Allen, M.J. & Chan, R.N.W. Weakness of foot dorsiflexion and changes in compartment pressures after tibial osteotomy. *J Bone Joint Surg* 1986; **68B**: 471–475.

Gitlitz, G.F. The anterior tibial compartment syndrome. A complication of a femoropopliteal bypass procedure. *Vasc Dis* 1965; **2**: 122–130.

Grosz, C.R., Shaftan, G.W., Kottmeier, P.K. & Herbsman, H. Volkmann's contracture and femoral shaft fractures. *J Trauma* 1973; **13**: 129–131.

Halpern, A.A., Greene, R., Nichols, T. & Burton, D.S. Compartment syndrome of the interosseous muscles; early recognition and treatment. *Clin Orthop* 1979; **140**: 23–25.

Hardy, A.E. Pressure recordings in patients with femoral fractures in cast-braces and suggestions for treatment. *J Bone Joint Surg* 1979; **61A**: 365–370.

Harris, C. & Riordan, D.C. Intrinsic contracture of the hand and its surgical treatment. *J Bone Joint Surg* 1954; **36A**: 10–19.

Hay, S.M., Allen, M.J. & Barnes, M.R. Acute compartment syndromes resulting from anticoagulant treatment. *Br Med J* 1992; **305**: 1474–1475.

Husni, E.A. The edema of arterial reconstruction. *Circulation* (suppl.) 1967; **33**: 169–173.

Jenkins, N.H. & Mintowt-Czyz, W.J. Compression of the biceps-brachialis compartment after trivial trauma. *J Bone Joint Surg* 1986; **68B**: 374.

Johnson, B.E. Anterior tibial compartment syndrome following use of MAST suit. *Ann Emer Med* 1981; **10**: 209–210.

Macey, A.C. Compartment syndromes in unconscious patients: a simple aid to diagnosis. *Br Med J* 1987; **294**: 1472–1473.

Matsen, F.A. *Compartmental Syndromes*. Grune & Stratton: New York, 1980.

Matsen, F.A. & Clawson, D.K. The deep posterior compartmental syndrome of the leg. *J Bone Joint Surg* 1975; **57A**: 34–39.

Matsen, F.A., Mayo, K.A., Sheridan, G.W. & Krugmire, R.B. Monitoring of intramuscular pressure. *Surgery* 1976; **79**: 702–709.

Mubarak, S.J. & Hargens, A.R. Compartment syndromes and Volkmann's contracture. W.B. Saunders: Philadelphia, 1981.

Mubarak, S.J. & Owen, C.A. Compartmental syndrome and its relation to the crush syndrome: a spectrum of disease. *Clin Orthop* 1975; **113**: 81–89.

Mubarak, S.J., Hargens, A.R., Owen, C.A., Garetto, L.P. & Akeson, W.H. The wick catheter technique for measurement of intramuscular pressure. A new research and clinical tool. *J Bone Joint Surg* 1976; **58A**: 1016–1020.

Neviaser, R.J., Adams, J.P. & May, G.I. Complications of arterial puncture in anticoagulated patients. *J Bone Joint Surg* 1976; **58A**: 218–221.

Newmeyer, W.L. & Kilgore, E.S. Volkmann's ischemic contracture due to soft tissue injury alone. *J Hand Surg* 1976; **1**: 221–227.

Owen, C.A., Mubarak, S.J., Hargens, A.R., Rutherford, L., Garetto, L.P. & Akeson, W.H. Intramuscular pressures with limb compression. *N Engl J Med* 1979; **300**: 1169–1172.

Patman, R.D. Compartmental syndromes in peripheral vascular surgery. *Clin Orthop* 1975; **113**: 103–110.

Quigley, J.T., Popich, G.A. & Lanz, U.B. Compartment syndrome of the forearm and hand: a case report. *Clin Orthop* 1981; **161**: 247–251.

Rorabeck, C.H. & MacNab, I. Anterior tibial-compartment syndrome complicating fractures of the shaft of the tibia. *J Bone Joint Surg* 1976; **58A**: 549–550.

Rorabeck, C.H., Castle, G.S.P. & Hardy, R. The slit catheter: a new device for measuring intracompartmental pressures. *Surg Forum Orthop Surg* 1980; **31**: 513–515.

Salisbury, R.E., McKeel, D.W. & Mason, A.D. Ischemic necrosis of the intrinsic muscles of the hand after thermal injuries. *J Bone Joint Surg* 1974; **56A**: 1701–1707.

Seddon, H.J. Volkmann's contracture: treatment by excision of the infarct. *J Bone Joint Surg* 1956; **38B**: 152–174.

Seddon, H.J. Volkmann's ischaemia in the lower limb. *J Bone Joint Surg* 1966; **48B**: 627–636.

Shakespeare, D.T. & Henderson, N.J. Compartmental pressure changes during calcaneal traction in tibial fractures. *J Bone Joint Surg* 1982; **64B**: 498–499.

Shakespeare, D.T., Henderson, N.J. & Sherman, K.P. Transmission of pressure into the human limb from pneumatic splints. *Injury* 1984; **16**: 38–40.

Shall, J., Cohn, B.T. & Froimson, A.I. Acute compartment syndrome of the forearm in association with fracture of the distal end of the radius. *J Bone Joint Surg* 1986; **68A**: 1451–1454.

Sheridan, G.W. & Matsen, F.A. Fasciotomy in the treatment of the acute compartment syndrome. *J Bone Joint Surg* 1976; **58A**: 112–115.

Spinner, M., Aiache, A., Silver, L. & Barsky, A.J. Impending ischemic contracture of the hand; early diagnosis and management. *Plast Reconstr Surg* 1972; **50**: 341–349.

Tarlow, S.D., Achterman, C.A., Hayhurst, J. & Ovadia, D.N. Acute compartment syndrome in the thigh complicating fracture of the femur. *J Bone Joint Surg* 1986; **68A**: 1439–1443.

Werbel, G.B. & Shybut, G.T. Acute compartment syndrome caused by a malfunctioning pneumatic-compression boot. *J Bone Joint Surg* 1986; **68A**: 1445–1446.

Whitesides, T.E., Haney, T.C., Harada, H., Holmes, H.E. & Morimoto K. A simple method for tissue pressure determination. *Arch Surg* 1975; **110**: 1311–1313.

Williams, Y.M., Knopp, R. & Ellyson, J.H. Compartment syndrome after anti-shock trouser application without lower extremity trauma. *J Trauma* 1982; **22**: 595–597.

Fat embolism and the fat embolism syndrome

J.C.STODDART

This condition shares many features with the adult respiratory distress syndrome (ARDS), but its onset is usually more easily recognized, its cause relatively well understood and its prognosis much better.

The distinction between fat embolism and the fat embolism syndrome should be recognized at the outset. Up to 90% of patients who have suffered major trauma, which includes bone injury, can be shown at autopsy to have fat droplet deposits in the lungs and elsewhere, without necessarily having shown any evidence of this phenomenon in life (Cole 1971, Editorial 1972). The fat embolism syndrome is much less common but it may present a threat to the patient's survival and always gives rise to identifiable symptoms (Niden & Aviado 1956, Gardner & Harrison 1957, Peltier 1969, 1984, Grosham *et al.* 1971, Editorial 1972).

Definition of the fat embolism syndrome

Fat embolism syndrome results from the liberation, transport and deposition of fat droplets, causing obstruction of small blood vessels in many organs and tissues. It is usually associated with major bone injuries; occasionally it may be identified after trivial bone injuries (Gurd 1971). The fat embolism syndrome has been described after trauma to adipose tissue, to the liver, the spleen and the pancreas, but in these instances it is probably more appropriate to group the cause in the ARDS category (Peltier 1969).

The distinction between fat embolism and the fat embolism syndrome is thought to be due to the total mass of fat which is released into the circulation from the traumatized tissues. It is believed that the fat droplets must exceed 8 μm in diameter before they can give rise to symptoms. The emboli are thought to block small arterioles and capillaries, after which they become coated with platelets and leukocytes. Plasma lipase converts the neutral fat to free fatty acids which damage the alveolar capillary cells and, together with lysed platelets, gives rise to the sequence of events described in Chapter 11 with the release of thromboxane, prostaglandin $F_{2\alpha}$, 5-hydroxytryptamine and histamine.

Alternative sources of fat emboli

Some investigators believe that the fat emboli do not always originate from bone marrow but may be formed by the coalescence of fat chylomicrons, normally present in plasma and less than 1 μm in diameter, through the increased secretion of corticosteroids and catecholamines which follows trauma (Peltier 1969). It is known that catecholamines can increase the level of circulating lipids, which are then converted to fatty acids. The fat embolism syndrome has been diagnosed following the use of high-dose corticosteroids (Gurd 1971, Mahley *et al.* 1972, Lessells 1981), but since these drugs are commonly given to patients who are suffering from acute cardiocirculatory failure due to trauma or sepsis, the relevance of these reports is questionable.

It is generally accepted that fat emboli contain mostly triglyceride fat, whereas coalesced chylomicrons or fat from adipose tissue contains cholesterol; this has only rarely been identified in embolic material. Occasionally, bone marrow cells and even spicules of bone have been identified in embolic material found in the lungs and elsewhere of patients who have died following injuries to the bony skeleton (Peltier 1984). Several attempts have been made to identify pathological quantities of fat and fat droplets in the plasma of patients suffering from the fat embolism syndrome, but these have not been generally successful (Grosham *et al.* 1971).

Whatever the origin of the fat may be, pathologists agree that if the patient survives for 7 days or more after the event, no fat emboli can be identified in the lungs or elsewhere, although stigmata of their recent presence may be found. These include small haemosiderin deposits surrounding cerebral arterioles and areas of microinfarction in the renal cortex. The respiratory evidence is usually obscured by the tissue reaction which is typical of ARDS.

Clinical features of the fat embolism syndrome

Classically these appear within 72 hours of the injury but they may not occur until after its surgical or manipulative treatment. The syndrome which occasionally follows the impaction of methylmethacrylate cement into the bone marrow may be identical. One of the most interesting aspects of the fat embolism syndrome is that it has never been known to develop twice in the same patient in spite of repeated orthopaedic manipulations of the original injury.

Presentation

Breathlessness, confusion, restlessness or coma are the most common presenting features, and grand mal seizures may occur. The patient usually has an irritating cough, with or without haemoptysis. Sudden cardio-vascular collapse during orthopaedic operations has been attributed to fat embolism. Occasionally it may present as failure to regain consciousness following orthopaedic manipulations performed under general anaesthesia. Focal neurological signs such as hemiplegia or paraplegia may appear but these are unusual and should cause the attendant to consider the possibility of more extensive intracranial damage. This should always be excluded before the treatment regimen described later is instituted, and a computerized axial tomography (CAT) scan may be necessary. The possibility of intra-cranial damage must always be considered if the patient has a history of transient loss of consciousness at the time of the injury or shortly afterwards. Although frank haematuria may be noted, this is unusual, but most patients with fat embolism syndrome have microscopic haematuria.

Pathophysiology of the fat embolism syndrome

One question which causes much debate is how fat droplets which are small enough to pass through the pulmonary capillaries can reach the left side of the heart and obstruct cerebral and renal vessels. Three possible explanations have been propounded. Of all patients who are submitted to autopsy examination 20% are found to have a potentially patent foramen ovale. It is suggested that widespread pulmonary fat emboli would cause pulmonary hypertension and a rise in the right ventricular and right atrial pressures. This could cause a right-to-left shunt, and allow emboli to reach the sys-temic circulation through the foramen ovale (Peltier 1969). Alternatively, it is proposed that there are pul-monary arteriovenous shunts which may be opened in the presence of raised pulmonary artery pressure (Peltier 1984). A third suggestion is that the fat chylomicrons coalesce in the pulmonary and systemic circulation in-dependently, due to hormonal influences, and no right-to-left shunt needs to be postulated.

Blood gas effects

A variable degree of hypoxia is always present, and some authorities have stated that the neurological effects of fat embolism are due to cerebral hypoxia. However, the level of oxygen desaturation is often not severe enough to explain the neurological symptoms. For ex-ample, a young patient with normal blood vessels does not become confused or comatose with a Pao_2 of 7.9 kPa or more. On the other hand, a patient who is very hypoxic may present with diffuse neurological symp-toms, of which confusion is the commonest, and which may improve when oxygen-enriched air is given. Cerebral fat embolism may cause confusion in the ab-sence of systemic hypoxia and vice versa. The early development of neurological signs is a feature which distinguishes fat embolism syndrome from ARDS.

The respiratory and neurological features of the syn-drome often appear concurrently but may be discrete. Dyspnoea, tachypnoea, bronchospasm and pulmonary oedema may occur separately or together. These symp-toms are often mistaken for bronchopneumonia, par-ticularly since the patient may also have an elevated temperature. At this stage, a chest radiograph shows the typical 'snowstorm' appearance but, later, the lung fields may be diffusely radiopaque.

Skin manifestations

A petechial rash is another feature of the syndrome, although this often appears without any systemic symptoms or signs. It is usually most noticeable on the chest wall, on the base of the neck and close to the inguinal ligaments, but it may become generalized and successive showers of petechiae may be recognized. The spots may also be noted in the lower conjunctival sac and, if the fundi are examined during the early phase, fat droplets are occasionally seen passing through the retinal vessels. The petechiae are 1−3 mm in diam-eter and are initially red but quickly turn brown. If a skin biopsy is taken fat droplets can be seen in the dermal capillaries. Fat droplets may occasionally be identified in sputum and in urine but these are not diagnostic features of the syndrome since both false positive and false negative findings are common.

Stress peptic ulcer

Patients with fat embolism syndrome are said to be at special risk of stress peptic ulceration. This has been attributed to mucosal infarction, but in the injured patient all the causes of stress ulceration are present.

Haematological features

Up to 50% of patients with fat embolism develop thrombocytopenia, and hypocalcaemia is also common (Peltier 1969, 1984). This latter finding is said to be due to the combination of calcium ions and the free fatty acids released as the emboli are hydrolysed. The hae-moglobin level may fall as much as 3 g dl^{-1} in 48 hours without obvious cause, although continued bleeding around closed fractures, into the gastrointestinal tract or into other occult sites is the more likely explanation. Usually, thrombocytopenia is an isolated finding but, occasionally, all the laboratory features of disseminated intravascular coagulation (DIC) are noted together with its clinical signs. At this stage the syndrome blends into DIC/ARDS with its additional problems.

The relationship between fat embolism and DIC is, at present, a matter for speculation since fat droplets *per se* do not activate the coagulation cascade. It is probable that the mechanisms which provoke fat embolism and DIC occur in parallel rather than being directly related, that is, they are separate manifestations of acute traumatic cardiocirculatory failure.

Clinical course of the fat embolism syndrome

The severity of the illness is largely related to the extent of the injuries and after very extensive fractures patients may succumb, within 24 hours of the incident, from diffuse embolic disease. However, trivial injuries may occasionally cause death from fat embolism. Some procedures have an ominous reputation; this is particularly the case with the open reduction and nailing of subcapital femoral neck fractures (Gossling & Pellegrini 1982, Peltier 1984).

Prognosis of fat embolism

The most challenging feature of the condition is its unpredictable nature, and the mortality rates quoted by different authorities range from 5 to 15% (Niden & Aviado 1956, Peltier 1984). A patient who presents with a florid rash, cyanosed, breathless and with a tachydysrhythmia may either improve steadily with only minimal treatment, or may progress inexorably downhill with a widening alveolar/asterial (Aa) gradient and die days later from intractable hypoxia, with evidence of multiple organ involvement.

The neurological effects of fat embolism have a good prognosis for functional recovery, provided that the patient's respiratory dysfunction is reversible. Patients who die in the acute phase of the disease are usually found to have many hundreds of petechial haemorrhages scattered throughout the cerebral white and grey matter and the basal nuclei. If the patient survives the immediate insult but dies days or weeks later, no gross areas of cerebral infarction are found. Patients who develop paraplegias or other focal signs have a less predictable prognosis.

Treatment of the fat embolism syndrome

Hypoxia is the most dangerous feature of this condition. As soon as the diagnosis is made the patient should be given 100% oxygen by facemask and the arterial oxygen tension should be monitored. The patient should preferably be admitted to the Intensive Therapy unit because rapid deterioration may occur and then controlled ventilation with added oxygen will be required. Baseline data should be obtained to identify the involvement of other organs, and a comprehensive neurological examination must be performed.

Pulmonary hypertension and pulmonary oedema

Pulmonary hypertension is an early manifestation of pulmonary fat embolism. This can be recognized clinically by auscultation when the second pulmonary sound is noted to be accentuated, or by means of a Swan Ganz catheter. Most patients have clinical and radiographic evidence of pulmonary oedema. Although this is usually due to the fat and its breakdown products, overenthusiastic intravenous fluid administration may also be involved. In either case, when the diagnosis is made, the patient should be given 20–40 mg frusemide intravenously and the arterial oxygen tension and Aa gradient should be measured after the subsequent diuresis. If these improve it may be advisable to give a second dose of frusemide. Every patient with the fat embolism syndrome should be maintained in perfect fluid balance until recovery has occurred.

Respiratory care

If oxygen by mask does not have the desired result, the patient should be sedated, intubated and ventilated. Intermittent positive pressure ventilation (IPPV) may be required for up to 10 days but, unless the patient develops a chest infection, tracheotomy should not be necessary since in many cases recovery is rapid and uncomplicated. However, if the Pao_2 continues to fall in spite of increasing the Pio_2 and adding positive end expiratory pressure, the prognosis is poor.

Other aids to treatment

The following list includes most of the agents which have been used to treat fat embolism.
1 Heparin — to speed lipolysis and reduce platelet adhesiveness (Ellis & Watson 1968).
2 Alcohol — to dissolve fat and act as a vasodilator (Gardner & Harrison 1957).

3 Aprotinin — to inhibit protein breakdown (Gurd 1970).

4 Corticosteroids — to reduce leukocyte aggregation, preserve lysosomal membranes and prevent the formation of vasodepressor kinins (Niden & Aviado 1956, Gardner & Harrison 1957).

5 Dextran 40 — to improve capillary flow (Editorial 1972).

6 Clofibrate — to reduce plasma lipids (Cole 1971).

Although few of the trials reported were well-controlled, none of these agents has been shown to produce any clearcut improvement and some may be positively harmful. Heparin may aggravate the syndrome by encouraging the breakdown of triglyceride fat to fatty acids, which provoke a more violent tissue response. Dextran 40 is contraindicated in the presence of renal impairment. Corticosteroids belong to the group of drugs whose actions consist almost entirely of side-effects; these include the encouragement of sepsis, pulmonary oedema and peptic ulceration. None of the published papers which attribute success to their use has demonstrated statistically significant improvement (Niden & Aviado 1956).

The prognosis for patients with fat embolism syndrome is very unpredictable. Treatment should be based upon fundamental principles which include maintenance of gas exchange, prevention or treatment of fluid overload and pulmonary oedema, and the avoidance of potentially harmful agents.

Prevention of fat embolism

With the present state of knowledge this desirable aim appears to be unattainable. Most orthopaedic surgeons believe that fracture manipulations should be applied as gently as possible and stabilization as early as possible, but there is still no substitute for careful monitoring and early resuscitation. Delayed recognition of fat embolism syndrome allows the complications of coma and infection to be added to what is still a dangerous condition.

References

Cole, W.G. Clofibrate and fat embolism: a double blind trial of the effects of clofibrate on sequelae to injury. *Br Med J* 1971; **2**: 148–149.

Editorial. Fat embolism. *Lancet* 1972; **i**: 672–673.

Ellis, H.A. & Watson, A.J. Studies on the genesis of traumatic fat embolism in man. *Am J Path* 1968; **53(2)**: 245–251.

Gardner, A.M.N. & Harrison, M H M. Report on the treatment of experimental fat embolism with heparin. *J Bone Joint Surg* 1957; **39B**: 538.

Gossling, H.R. & Pellegrini, V.D. Fat embolism syndrome. *Clin Orthop* 1982; **165**: 68–82.

Grosham, G.A., Kuczynski, A. & Rosborough, D. Fatal fat embolism following replacement arthoplasty for transcervical fractures of femur. *Br Med J* 1971; **1**: 617–619.

Gurd, A.R. Fat embolism: an aid to diagnosis. *J Bone Joint Surg.* 1970; **52B(4)**: 732–737.

Gurd, A.R. Pathogenesis and treatment of fat embolism. *J Bone Joint Surg* 1971; **53B(4)**: 756–757.

Lessells, A.M. Fatal fat embolism after minor trauma. *Br Med J* 1981; **282(1)**: 1586.

Mahley, R.W., Gray, M.E. & Lequire, V.S. Role of plasma lipoproteins in cortisone-induced fat embolism. *Am J Path* 1972; **66**: 43–47.

Niden, A.H. & Aviado, D.M. Effects of pulmonary embolism on the pulmonary circulation with special reference to arteriovenous shunts in the lung. *Circ Res* 1956; **4**: 67–79.

Peltier, L.F. Fat embolism: a current concept. *Clin Orthop* 1969; **66**: 241–242.

Peltier, L.F. Fat embolism. *Clin Orthop* 1984; **187**: 3–17.

Venous thromboembolism

P.D.TRIFFITT

Venous thrombosis has long been recognized as a clinical hazard. While often clinically 'silent', it is associated with one of the principal causes of death after injury: massive pulmonary embolism.

Pathogenesis

The classic triad of Virchow comprises vessel wall damage, circulatory statis, and increased coagulability of the blood. After trauma, statis appears to be more important than vessel wall injury (Sevitt 1974), while a hypercoagulable state associated with activation of Factor X and a fall in antithrombin III may be important (Lowe 1981). Both systemic and local leg vein fibrinolytic activity have been found to decrease after femoral fracture (Rawles *et al.* 1975). Thrombosis has been found in general to increase with age, obesity, level of oestrogen intake, pregnancy, malignancy, previous history of thromboembolism, varicose veins, immobility and various haematological disorders (Coon 1977, Janssen *et al.* 1987), but the roles of these various factors in thrombosis after trauma are not well defined. A factor of potential importance is a hypercoagulable state associated with activation of factor X and a fall in antithrombin III (Lowe 1981). Clinical studies are made difficult by the requirement to standardize fracture characteristics, making each subgroup small except in very large series (Hjelmstedt & Bergvall 1968).

Incidence

The incidence of deep venous thrombosis (DVT) after upper limb trauma appears to be very low, but it has been found to be high after various fractures of the lower limb. After fracture of the neck of the femur, Freeark *et al.* (1967) found a preoperative venographic incidence of 8% in the first 3 days rising to 15% thereafter up to the 12th day, frequently bilateral. Postoperative rates were between 24 and 38%, although the delay before repeat venography varied widely. Postoperative rates of 49% have been observed in the fractured limb by Hamilton *et al.* (1970), 57% by Borgström *et al.* (1965) and 40% by Culver *et al.* (1970). There was no significant difference between fractures treated by pinning or by hemiarthroplasty in the last study, and the common femoral vein was involved in 9% of cases. Powers *et al.* (1989) found a combined rate for both limbs of 46%. Fibrinogen uptake studies have given combined rates of 54% (Kakkar 1972) and 91% (Bergqvist *et al.* 1979).

Much less information is available on thrombosis after other lower limb fractures. After tibial fracture, Hjelmstedt and Bergvall (1968) found an overall venographic rate of 45%; many of these examinations being performed more than 2 months after the injury. These authors noted a significantly lower incidence of 12% in patients aged less than 25 years. After pelvic fractures, an incidence of 15% for thrombosis above the calf has been found with serial duplex-ultrasound screening (White *et al.* 1990), although most patients had more than one injury and had also received some form of prophylaxis.

After spinal trauma resulting in para- or tetraplegia, incidences of 72% and 100% have been found in small studies using the fibrinogen uptake method, the lower rate occurring in a group treated almost exclusively conservatively (Rossi *et al.* 1980, Myllynen *et al.* 1985, 1987). No thrombosis was detected in those immobilized without neurological injury, although a smallar proportion of these patients had been operated upon.

Clinical presentation

Deep venous thrombosis may present with local symptoms, by pulmonary embolism, or potentially by the development of postphlebitic syndrome. However, in the majority of cases thromboembolism is asymptomatic.

Locally, pain and local tenderness may develop, together with swelling and increased skin temperature. There may be a low-grade pyrexia. Passive dorsiflexion of the foot may increase pain in the presence of a calf thrombosis. The clinical presentation of pulmonary embolism covers a spectrum from virtually asymptomatic to sudden death. The classical clinical features are pleuritic chest pain with haemoptysis, pyrexia and a pleural friction rub. With pulmonary infarction there may be clinical and radiological pulmonary consolidation. The arterial oxygen tension is usually reduced and with more major embolism signs of right heart strain may appear on the electrocardiogram. Severe embolism is associated with hypotension and may result in circulatory arrest. Such an event has been reported to follow the preoperative exsanguination of a previously immobilized fractured limb (Pollard *et al.* 1983).

The postphlebitic syndrome is characterized by swelling and pain, which may be of a claudicant type, and venous ulceration. These features are the result of both chronic venous obstruction and the destruction of the venous valves in recanalized vessels, and may take several years fully to develop.

Diagnosis

Clinical diagnosis of DVT is notoriously unreliable (Negus *et al.* 1968, Kakkar *et al.* 1969, Culver *et al.* 1970, Hamilton *et al.* 1970). Contrast venography is generally regarded as the most accurate method, but its disadvantages have led to an extensive search for an alternative. In patients with trauma to the lower limb, difficulties for the various techniques available are posed by local treatment measures such as casts, traction apparatus and operative wounds.

Contrast venography

The veins of the lower limbs may be visualized by an injection of contrast medium into a vein on the dorsum of the foot, with or without the use of a tourniquet to assist the filling of the deep veins (Rabinov & Paulin 1972). By using a sufficient volume of medium the pelvic veins may be seen, or these vessels may be shown by femoral vein puncture (Lea Thomas 1972). Thrombi are diagnosed directly by the presence of filling defects within the vessel lumina, or indirectly by the absence of vessel filling, particularly if associated with an increased collateral circulation.

The soleal sinuses are difficult to image by this technique, and false positive results may arise from the emptying of such muscular veins into contrast-filled trunks, but the principal disadvantage of the method is its invasive nature, which precludes regular repetition. The use of non-ionic, low-osmolarity media has largely overcome the problem of the induction of thrombosis by the injection (Bettmann *et al.* 1987).

Fibrinogen uptake studies

Fibrinogen labelled with iodine-125 is injected intravenously and taken up by thrombi in the process of formation. The label remains *in situ* and may be detected by external scanning for up to 10 days (Atkins & Hawkins 1968, Negus *et al.* 1968, Kakkar *et al.* 1969, Browse 1972, Kakkar 1972). Diagnosis is based on a 15–20% increase in local isotope counts with respect to adjacent or contralateral areas; this increase persists for at least 24 hours. The method allows non-invasive monitoring of the venous system over a period of several days, but may give false negative results in the presence of an established thrombus. It is also unreliable in the locality of surgical wounds (Harris *et al.* 1976), and in the upper thigh the results may be subject to interference from circulating label in the major vessels. The positive predictive value of this method has been found to be poor in comparison with venography after proximal femoral fractures, and the negative predictive value is high only if the proximal results from the operated leg are excluded (Faunø *et al.* 1990). There is a potential risk of the transmission of infective agents from the fibrinogen pool.

Impedance plethysmography

This non-invasive technique is based on the changes in electrical resistance that occur with changes in blood volume in the calf. Increases in volume that occur with venous occlusion by a cuff around the thigh or with respiration are found to be reduced by prior occlusion by venous thrombi. This method is highly sensitive to the occlusion of proximal veins but much less so to that of distal veins, as this does not affect the main venous outflow from the limb (Harris *et al.* 1976). The results are also affected by both the distance between the electrodes and the presence of collaterals (Dmochowski *et al.* 1972, Wheeler *et al.* 1972).

Doppler ultrasonography

A beam of ultrasound is reflected from the blood cells. Stationary cells return a beam of the same frequency, while moving cells impart a shift which can be converted into an audible signal (Sigel *et al.* 1968, Strandness & Sumner 1972). As with plethysmography, the technique has a low sensitivity for calf vein thrombi and for non-occlusive proximal thrombi, and it is not possible to examine the pelvic veins (Sigel *et al.* 1972).

Real-time ultrasonography

Direct visualization of major veins using ultrasound may be used to assess their compressibility and therefore the presence of intraluminal clot. This method may be combined with Doppler analysis, a technique known as duplex scanning (Froehlich *et al.* 1989, White *et al.* 1990). On comparison with venography in symptomatic patients the sensitivity of these methods in the diagnosis of proximal thrombi has been reported to be 88–95%, with a specificity of 97–100% (O'Leary *et al.* 1988, Froehlich *et al.* 1989, Lensing *et al.* 1989, Monreal *et al.* 1989b, White *et al.* 1989), but its accuracy in the calf and in asymptomatic patients is low (Monreal *et al.* 1989b).

Plasma markers

The measurement of degradation products of factors involved in coagulation has been investigated for the diagnosis of venous thrombosis. In mixed populations of symptomatic in- and outpatients, the measurement of D-dimer, a breakdown product of crosslinked fibrin, has been found to have a sensitivity of 88–100% and a specificity of 47–68% when compared with venography (Heaton *et al.* 1987, Rowbotham *et al.* 1987, Chapman *et al.* 1990). This approach is more difficult in the trauma patient where coagulation is a normal part of the response to both the primary injury and to any subsequent operative intervention, and after elective orthopaedic surgical procedures such markers have not been found to discriminate accurtely those patients with DVT (Hoek *et al.* 1989, Jørgensen *et al.* 1990). Another potential drawback is that the method does not localize the thrombosis, although in general proximal thromboses have been found to generate significantly higher plasma levels of D-dimer (Rowbotham *et al.* 1987, Chapman *et al.* 1990). The importance of the location of the thrombosis with respect to subsequent embolism has yet to be confirmed in trauma patients and, in any event, distal thrombi diagnosed early may later propagate proximally (Kakkar 1972).

Treatment

The mainstay of treatment of thromboembolism is the use of anticoagulants in order to reduce the progression of the condition. Other techniques such as thrombectomy, fibrinolytic therapy and caval filters will not be discussed here, but anticoagulants merit further consideration in view of the question of the use of these agents in trauma patients in prophylaxis as well as in treatment.

Indications for anticoagulant therapy

The purposes of anticoagulant therapy are:
1 To reduce the incidence of significant pulmonary embolism.
2 To reduce the incidence of subsequent postphlebitic syndrome.

Despite the apparently high incidence of DVT after trauma to the lower limbs, the rate of *fatal* pulmonary embolism after modern fracture treatment of hip fractures, the only group extensively studied, is of the order of only 3% over the first 3–4 months (Sharnoff *et al.* 1976, Powers *et al.* 1989), and substantial studies are required to demonstrate any benefit of anticoagulants in this respect. Little is known about the incidence of postphlebitic syndrome, largely because it may take many years to develop (Aitken *et al.* 1987). Even the incidences of DVT after many types of injury are unknown. With this background it is impossible to give strict criteria for the use of anticoagulants. Patients treated with anticoagulants fall into three principal groups:
1 Those with a clinical DVT that is confirmed by another diagnostic technique.
2 Those that present with a pulmonary embolism without clinical evidence of DVT.
3 Those considered at high risk of developing DVT.

The first group essentially equates to the use of clinical examination as a screening procedure, while such subjective assessment is known to be very unreliable. Objective diagnostic methods should ideally be non-invasive if they are to be used as screening procedures, but the non-invasive methods available lack accuracy with regard to a distal thrombosis or the presence of a local surgical wound. While there is evidence that proximal thrombi give rise to the great majority of emboli (Moser & LeMoine 1981), this has yet to be confirmed in trauma patients, and distal thrombi may, in any event, be sufficient to give rise to the postphlebitic syndrome.

The second group represents those in whom a serious complication of thrombosis has already occurred, and in major cases resuscitation is at least difficult, if not of no avail. Thus, in the third group anticoagulants are given *before* thrombosis in an effort to avoid this problem, although this potentially entails the treatment of many patients who would not have developed thrombosis. While general factors such as age are found to be associated with an increased risk of thrombosis, patients with lower limb fractures may be considered, as a whole, to represent a high-risk group. The management of all such patients with prophylactic anticoagulants requires that such a measure is effective and safe. While various regimens have been found to reduce the incidence of DVT significantly, without an increase in other complications, thrombosis is not abolished, and such reductions are not equivalent to the demonstration of clinically significant reductions in the incidence of thrombotic sequelae. Such reductions have yet to be shown in trauma patients.

Anticoagulant prophylaxis

If it is decided that prophylaxis is warranted, the question arises as to the best method. At present, the evidence available from those studies using objective methods of diagnosis is limited to patients with fractures of the proximal femur.

Fractures of the proximal femur

In these patients, postoperative oral anticoagulation with phenindione has been found to reduce venographically proven DVT in previously ambulant patients who have been operated on within 48 hours of injury, but not in others (Hamilton *et al.* 1970); postoperative warfarin is similarly effective (Powers *et al.* 1989). Warfarin given from the day of admission in one study increased major haemorrhagic complications from 3% to 10% (Morris & Mitchell 1976). Aspirin commenced preoperatively reduces overall thrombosis rate (Snook *et al.* 1981) while postoperative aspirin reduces proximal thrombosis but not distal thrombosis (Powers *et al.* 1989). Prophylaxis from the time of admission with dextran or low doses of heparin ('minihep') reduces the overall rate of thrombosis as diagnosed by fibrinogen uptake (Bergqvist *et al.* 1979). The addition to dextran of dihydroergotamine, which causes venous constriction and may improve venous flow rate, does not appear to increase its efficacy (Fredin *et al.* 1985, Rørbæk-Madsen *et al.* 1988), while low molecular weight minihep has been found to be as effective (Pini *et al.* 1989) or less effective (Monreal *et al.* 1989a) than conventional minihep. Oral anticoagulation starting at the time of surgery with minihep cover for three days is less effective than continued heparin-dihydroergotamine prophylaxis (Schlag *et al.* 1986). Heparinoids have been found to be more effective than placebo (Agnelli *et al.* 1992) or dextran (Bergqivst *et al.* 1991). In general, these types of prophylaxis reduce the rate of thrombosis to approximately 25% and they have not been associated with significant haemorrhagic complications. Little is known about the occurrence of DVT after prophylaxis is discontinued and the patient discharged.

There is little evidence as to the effects of prophylaxis on *proven* pulmonary embolism. However, overall mortality in the first 4 months in one study was significantly reduced by phenindione, and the proportion of patients with major embolism at autopsy was similarly reduced (Sevitt & Gallagher 1959), although mortality was high in this early investigation. A reduction in embolism at autopsy has also been found with a controlled low-dose heparin regime (Sharnoff *et al.* 1976), although with the small numbers autopsied this effect did not reach statistical significance. Prospective ventilation–perfusion scanning has been undertaken by Monreal *et al.* (1989b), who found that conventional minihep abolished embolism, although a control group was not included.

A study documenting the rates of postoperative death over the first two months found that these did not differ between two groups treated with different prophylactic regimens, even though the rate of early venographic abnormality in one group was approximately one third of that found in the other (Bergqvist *et al.* 1991). This emphasizes the caution with which short-term studies of prophylaxis must be viewed.

Other methods of prophylaxis

Mechanical methods of prophylaxis include early mobilization, elevation of the lower limbs (Hartman *et al.* 1970) and use of various types of calf or foot compression device (Stranks *et al.* 1992), all of which are intended to increase the rate of venous return. After hip fracture there is evidence that delay before operative fixation, and therefore before mobilization, is associated with an increased risk of thrombosis (Hamilton *et al.* 1970).

A meta-analysis of anaesthesia for operative treatment of proximal femoral fractures has indicated that general anaesthesia is associated with a higher rate of DVT than regional anaesthesia, with an odds ratio of 4. However, the excess in overall postoperative mortality was marginal (Sorenson & Pace 1992).

References

Agnelli, G., Cosmi, B., Di Filippo, P., Ranucci, V., Veschi, F., Longetti, M., Renga, C., Barzi, F., Gianese, F., Lupattelli, L., Rinonapoli, E. & Nenci, G.G. A randomised, double-blind, placebo-controlled trial of dermatan sulphate for prevention of deep vein thrombosis in hip fracture. *Thromb Haemostas* 1992; **67**: 203–208.

Aitken, R.J., Mills, C. & Immelman, E.J. The postphlebitic syndrome following shaft fractures of the leg. A significant late complication. *J Bone Joint Surg* 1987; **69B**: 775–778.

Atkins, P. & Hawkins, L.A. The diagnosis of deep-vein thrombosis in the leg using ^{125}I-fibrinogen. *Br J Surg* 1968; **55**: 825–830.

Bergqvist, D., Efsing, H.O., Hallböök, T. & Hedlund, T. Thromboembolism after elective and post-traumatic hip surgery — a controlled prophylactic trial with dextran 70 and low-dose heparin. *Acta Chir Scand* 1979; **145**: 213–218.

Bergqvist, D., Kettunen, K., Fredin, H., Faunø, P., Suomalainen, O., Soimakallio, S., Karjalainen, P., Cederholm, C., Jensen, L.J., Justesen, T. & Stiekema, J.C.J. Thromboprophylaxis in patients with hip fractures: a prospective, randomized, comparative study between Org 10172 and dextran 70. *Surgery* 1991; **109**: 617–622.

Bettmann, M.A., Robbins, A., Braun, S.D., Wetzner, S., Dunnick, N.R. & Finkelstein, J. Contrast venography of the leg: diagnostic efficacy, tolerance, and complication rates with ionic and nonionic contrast media. *Radiology* 1987; **165**: 113–116.

Borgström, S., Greitz, T., van der Linden, W., Molin, J. & Rudics, I. Anticoagulant prophylaxis of venous thrombosis in patients with fractured neck of the femur. *Acta Chir Scand* 1965; **129**: 500–508.

Browse, N.L. The ^{125}I fibrinogen uptake test. *Arch Surg* 1972; **104**: 160–163.

Chapman, C.S., Akhtar, N., Campbell, S., Miles, K., O'Connor, J. & Mitchell, V.E. The use of D-Dimer assay by enzyme immunoassay and latex agglutination techniques in the diagnosis of deep vein thrombosis. *Clin Lab Haemat* 1990; **12**: 37–42.

Coon, W.W. Epidemiology of venous thromboembolism. *Ann Surg* 1977; **186**: 149–164.

Culver, D., Crawford, J.S., Gardiner, J.H. & Wiley, A.M. Venous thrombosis after fractures of the upper end of the femur. *J Bone Joint Surg* 1970; **52B**: 61–69.

Dmochowski, J.R., Adams, D.F. & Couch, N.P. Impedance measurement in the diagnosis of deep venous thrombosis. *Arch Surg* 1972; **104**: 170–173.

Faunø, P., Suomalainen, O., Bergqvist, D., Fredin, H., Kettunen, K., Soimakallio, S., Cederholm, C., Karjalainen, P., Vissinger, H. & Justesen, T. The use of fibrinogen uptake test in screening for deep vein thrombosis in patients with hip fracture. *Thromb Res* 1990; **60**: 185–190.

Fredin, H., Lindblad, B., Jaroszewski, H. & Bergqvist, D. Prevention of thrombosis after hip fracture surgery. *Acta Chir Scand* 1985; **151**: 681–684.

Freeark, R.J., Boswick, J. & Fardin, R. Posttraumatic venous thrombosis. *Arch Surg* 1967; **95**: 567–575.

Froehlich, J.A., Dorfman, G.S., Cronan, J.J., Urbanek, P.J., Herndon, J.H. & Aaron, R.K. Compression ultrasonography for the detection of deep venous thrombosis in patients who have a fracture of the hip. *J Bone Joint Surg* 1989; **71A**: 249–256.

Hamilton, H.W., Crawford, J.S., Gardiner, J.H. & Wiley, A.M. Venous thrombosis in patients with fracture of the upper end of the femur. *J Bone Joint Surg* 1970; **52B**: 268–289.

Harris, W.H., Athanasoulis, C., Waltman, A.C. & Salzman, E.W. Cuff-impedance phlebography and ^{125}I fibrinogen scanning versus roentgenographic phlebography for diagnosis of thrombophlebitis following hip surgery. *J Bone Joint Surg* 1976; **58A**: 939–944.

Hartman, J.T., Altner, P.C. & Freeark, R.J. The effect of limb elevation in preventing venous thrombosis. *J Bone Joint Surg* 1970; **52A**: 1618–1622.

Heaton, D.C., Billings, J.D. & Hickton, C.M. Assessment of D dimer assays for the diagnosis of deep vein thrombosis. *J Lab Clin Med* 1987; **110**: 588−591.

Hjelmstedt, Å. & Bergvall, U. Incidence of thrombosis in patients with tibial fractures. *Acta Chir Scand* 1968; **134**: 209−218.

Hoek, J.A., Nurmohamed, M.T., ten Cate, J.W., Büller, H.R., Knipscheer, H.C., Hamelynck, K.J., Marti, R.K. & Sturk, A. Thrombin-antithrombin III complexes in the prediction of deep vein thrombosis following total hip replacement. *Thromb Haemostas* 1989; **62**: 1050−1052.

Janssen, H.F., Schachner, J., Hubbard, J. & Hartman, J.T. The risk of deep venous thrombosis: a computerized epidemiologic approach. *Surgery* 1987; **101**: 205−212.

Jørgensen, L.N., Lind, B., Hauch, O., Leffers, A., Albrecht-Beste, E. & Konradsen, L.A.G. Thrombin-antithrombin III-complex and fibrin degradation products in plasma: surgery and postoperative deep venous thrombosis. *Thromb Res* 1990; **59**: 69−76.

Kakkar, V.V. The diagnosis of deep vein thrombosis using the ^{125}I fibrinogen test. *Arch Surg* 1972; **104**: 152−159.

Kakkar, V.V., Howe, C.T., Flanc, C. & Clarke, M.B. Natural history of postoperative deep-vein thrombosis. *Lancet* 1969; **ii**: 230−232.

Lea Thomas, M. Phlebography. *Arch Surg* 1972; **104**: 145−151.

Lensing, A.W.A., Prandoni, P., Brandjes, D., Huisman, P.M., Vigo, M., Tomasella, G., Krekt, J., ten Cate, J.W., Huisman, M.J. & Büller, H.R. Detection of deep-vein thrombosis by real-time B-mode ultrasonography. *N Engl J Med* 1989; **320**: 342−345.

Lowe, L.W. Venous thrombosis and embolism. *J Bone Joint Surg* 1981; **63B**: 155−167.

Monreal, M., Lafoz, E., Navarro, A., Granero, X., Caja, V., Caceres, E., Salvador, R. & Ruiz, J. A prospective double-blind trial of a low molecular weight heparin once daily compared with conventional low-dose heparin three times daily to prevent pulmonary embolism and venous thrombosis in patients with hip fracture. *J Trauma* 1989a; **29**: 873−875.

Monreal, M., Montserrat, E., Salvador, R., Bechini, J., Donoso, L., MaCallejas, J. & Foz, M. Real-time ultrasound for diagnosis of symptomatic venous thrombosis and for screening of patient at risk: correlation with ascending conventional venography. *Angiology* 1989b; **40**: 527−533.

Morris, G.K. & Mitchell, J.R.A. Warfarin sodium in prevention of deep venous thrombosis and pulmonary embolism in patients with fractured neck of femur. *Lancet* 1976; **2**: 869−872.

Moser, K.M. & LeMoine, J.R. Is embolic risk conditioned by location of deep venous thrombosis? *Ann Intern Med* 1981; **94**: 439−444.

Myllynen, P., Kammonen, M., Rokkanen, P., Böstman, O., Lalla, M. & Laasonen, E. Deep venous thrombosis and pulmonary embolism in patients with acute spinal cord injury: a comparison with nonparalyzed patients immobilized due to spinal fractures. *J Trauma* 1985; **25**: 541−543.

Myllynen, P., Kammonen, M., Rokkanen, P., Böstman, O., Lalla, M., Laasonen, E. & Vahtera, E. The blood F VIII : Ag/F VIII : C ratio as an early indicator of deep venous thrombosis during post-traumatic immobilization. *J Trauma* 1987; **27**: 287−290.

Negus, D., Pinto, D.J., Le Quesne, L.P., Brown, N. & Chapman, M. ^{125}I-labelled fibrinogen in the diagnosis of deep-vein thrombosis and its correlation with phlebography. *Br J Surg* 1968; **55**: 835−839.

O'Leary, D.H., Kane, R.A. & Chase, B.M. A prospective study of the efficacy of B-scan sonography in the detection of deep venous thrombosis in the lower extremities. *J Clin Ultrasound* 1988; **16**: 1−8.

Pini, M., Tagliaferri, A., Manotti, C., Lasagni, F., Rinaldi, E. & Dettori, A.G. Low molecular weight heparin (Alfa LMWH) compared with unfractionated heparin in prevention of deep-vain thrombosis after hip fractures. *Int Angiol* 1989; **8**: 134−139.

Pollard, B.J., Lovelock, H.A. & Jones, R.M. Fatal pulmonary embolism secondary to limb exsanguination. *Anesth* 1983; **58**: 373−374.

Powers, P.J., Gent, M., Jay, R.M., Julian, D.H., Turpie, A.G.G., Levine, M. & Hirsh, J. A randomized trial of less intense postoperative warfarin or aspirin therapy in the prevention of venous thromboembolism after surgery for fractured hip. *Arch Intern Med* 1989; **149**: 771−774.

Rabinov, K. & Paulin, S. Roentgen diagnosis of venous thrombosis in the leg. *Arch Surg* 1972; **104**: 134−144.

Rawles, J.M., Warlow, C. & Ogston, D. Fibrinolytic capacity of arm and leg veins after femoral shaft fracture and acute myocardial infarction. *Br Med J* 1975; **2**: 61−62.

Rørbæk-Madsen, M., Jakobsen, B.W., Pedersen, J. & Sørensen, B. Dihydroergotamine and the thromboprophylactic effect of dextran 70 in emergency hip surgery. *Br J Surg* 1988; **75**: 364−365.

Rowbotham, B.J., Carroll, P., Whitaker, A.N., Bunce, I.H., Cobcroft, R.G., Elms, M.J., Masci, P.P., Bundesen, P.G., Rylatt, D.B. & Webber, A.J. Measurement of crosslinked fibrin derivatives − use in the diagnosis of venous thrombosis. *Thromb Haemostas* 1987; **57**: 59−61.

Rossi, E.C., Green, D., Rosen, J.S., Spies, S.M. & Jao, J.S.T. Sequential changes in Factor VIII and platelets preceding deep vein thrombosis in patients with spinal cord injury. *Br J Haematol* 1980; **45**: 143−151.

Schlag, G., Gaudernak, T., Pelinka, H., Kuderna, H. & Welzel, D. Thromboembolic prophylaxis in hip fracture. *Acta Orthop Scand* 1986; **57**: 340−343.

Sevitt, S. The structure and growth of valve-pocket thrombi in femoral veins. *J Clin Pathol* 1974; **27**: 517−528.

Sevitt, S. & Gallagher, N.G. Prevention of venous thrombosis and pulmonary embolism in injured patients. *Lancet* 1959; **ii**: 981−989.

Sharnoff, J.G., Rosen, R.L., Sadler, A.H. & Ibarra-Isunza, G.C. Prevention of fatal pulmonary thromboembolism by heparin prophylaxis after surgery for hip fractures. *J Bone Joint Surg* 1976 **58A**: 913−918.

Sigel, B., Felix, R., Popky, G.L. & Ipsen, J. Diagnosis of lower limb venous thrombosis by Doppler ultrasound technique. *Arch Surg* 1972; **104**: 174−179.

Sigel, B., Popky, G.L., Wagner, D.K., Boland, J.P., Mapp, E.McD. & Feigl, P. A Doppler ultrasound method for diagnosing lower extremity venous disease. *Surg Gynecol Obstet* 1968; **127**: 339−350.

Snook, G.A., Chrisman, O.D. & Wilson, T.C. Thromboembolism after surgical treatment of hip fractures. *Clin Orthop* 1981; **155**: 21−24.

Sorenson, R.M. & Pace, N.L. Anesthetic techniques during surgical repair of femoral neck fractures. A meta-analysis.

Anesth 1992; **77**: 1095−1104.

Strandness, D.E. & Summer, D.S. Ultrasonic velocity detector in the diagnosis of thrombophlebitis. *Arch Surg* 1972; **104**: 180−183.

Stranks, G.J., MacKenzie, N.A., Grover, M.L. & Fail, T. The A-V Impulse System reduces deep-vein thrombosis and swelling after hemiarthroplasty for hip fracture. *J Bone Joint Surg* 1992; **74**B: 775−778.

Wheeler, H.B., Pearson, D., O'Connell, D. & Mullick, S.C. Impedance phlebography. *Arch Surg* 1972; **104**: 164−169.

White, R.H., Goulet, J.A., Bray, T.J., Daschbach, M.M., MacGahan, J.P. & Hartling, R.P. Deep-vein thrombosis after fracture of the pelvis: assessment with serial duplex-ultrasound screening. *J Bone Joint Surg* 1990; **72A**: 495−500.

White, R.H., McGahan, J.P., Daschbach, M.M. & Hartling, R.P. Diagnosis of deep-vein thrombosis using duplex ultrasound. *Ann Intern Med* 1989; **111**: 297−304.

Tetanus

J.C.STODDART

It is not known how many cases of tetanus occur in the world each year. World Health Organization (WHO) estimates range from 500 000 to 1 000 000 and the mortality rate is thought to be at least 60%. It is thus a major public health problem which, at the same time, should be preventable by immunization and attention to elementary details of hygiene.

In the United Kingdom there are fewer than 50 cases of tetanus per year and in the last year for which statistics are available only 18 cases were reported, of which 4 died. This is almost certainly not the total number of cases which occurred since, although tetanus is a notifiable disease, some cases are probably not reported and mild cases may not be recognized. However, since it is likely that, in the United Kingdom all of the deaths due to the disease were reported, the true mortality rate is probably less than 25%. With modern methods of treatment most of these deaths could be prevented. In the countries where tetanus is a common disease these methods cannot be provided but in the United Kingdom all cases of tetanus should be admitted to those few centres which have gained experience of the treatment of what is still a dangerous disease (Wainwright 1926, Adams *et al.* 1969).

Pathogenesis

Tetanus is caused by *Clostridium tetani*, a Gram-positive, anaerobic, spore-bearing organism which is found in soil and in the large intestine of many animals, often including man. The spores can live for many years in dust and are reactivated if they are inoculated into a suitable moist anaerobic environment. In favourable circumstances *C. tetani* produces two toxins: 'tetanolysin', which is unimportant, and 'tetanospasmin', which is responsible for the features of the disease. Tetanospasmin probably reaches the central nervous system from its site of inoculation by tracking in a retrograde fashion along motor, sensory and autonomic nerve trunks to the spinal cord and brain stem. It blocks inhibitory spinal reflexes, and by so doing causes hyperexcitability of motor nerves. If it reaches the hypothalamus it may interfere with control of the autonomic nervous system.

C. tetani grows best in wounds which are contaminated with road grit, soil or other foreign material and it is often found in mixed growth with anaerobic streptococci and other clostridia. Not infrequently, small gas pockets are found around the wound because of the coincidental presence of gas-producing bacteria.

Almost any type of injury can be followed by tetanus, although major injuries are usually treated and trivial injuries ignored. Table 11.7 shows the origin of the 21 cases of tetanus treated by the author in the last 16 years. Two patients who had undergone cholecystectomy at another hospital developed severe tetanus 18 and 20 days after the procedure (Lennard *et al.* 1984). The organism was not isolated from any of the instruments, dressings or suture material used during the operations, which were performed in widely separated operating rooms, and the origin is presumptive.

Other sites from which the disease commonly originates include the neonatal umbilicus, chronic middle ear disease, burns and retained products of conception.

Patients of any age may develop tetanus. Although prophylactic immunization has been practised for many years, patients who theoretically should have been immunized may be found either to have had an incomplete course of immunization or to have had none at all. Patients often have documentary evidence of complete primary immunization but have not had a booster injection within the recommended period of 7−10 years (Turner *et al.* 1958).

Clinical presentation

The symptoms and signs of tetanus are produced by spasm of voluntary muscles, which may be intermittent or may cause persistent painful muscle stiffness. Classically, the condition presents with trismus ('lock jaw') but other features may precede this sign. A 'sore throat', dysphagia or a sensation of choking are common; aching and stiffness of the facial, arm, leg or back muscles are also complained of. Non-specific symptoms are common; these include headache, sleeplessness, anxiety and restlessness which, in some cases, antedate the neuromuscular signs by up to 7 days. The first abnormal sign may be opisthotonus. (One of the patients treated by the author was in an orthopaedic ward after suffering a compound ankle fracture; the patient was seen to develop opisthotonus by a general practitioner who was a patient in the same ward. The ward staff dismissed the patient's symptoms as being a hysterical reaction to pain).

An opisthotonic spasm may be provoked by any external stimulus, which may be trivial (voice, other noises, movement of the bed, etc.), or it may be spontaneous. Typically, patients suddenly look terrified and may groan; they then take a deep breath and breathe out completely, moaning as they do so and, at the same time, arching the back acutely. Occasionally the extensor spasm is so acute that only patients' heels and the crown of the head touch the bed. In less severe cases it may be possible for the observer to pass a hand and arm between patients' backs and the mattress. On palpation the extensor muscles are found to be rigid. The spasm often lasts long enough for patients to become cyanosed and may recur at intervals from 5–15 minutes if untreated. The severity of spasms may be great enough to cause wedge fractures of vertebral bodies; rarely, one or both femoral necks may be fractured. Although patients usually have a rapid pulse rate, extreme bradycardia may occur during a spasm; between spasms the pulse rate and blood pressure are usually normal. Very occasionally, the spasms may affect flexor muscles predominantly (emprosthotonus) so that patients arch forward.

Diagnostic aids

There are no confirmatory tests of the disease and the diagnosis must be made on clinical grounds. Conditions which may be confused with tetanus include: poisoning with strychnine and organophosphorous insecticides; dystonic reaction to drugs, particularly phenothiazines (such as chlorpromazine and prochlorperazine) and metoclopramide (Maxolon, Primperan); and hysteria (Stoddart 1979b). The diagnosis of hysteria should only be made, if at all, after every possible cause has been eliminated.

Strychnine poisoning may be excluded by the history; if the patient survives its immediate effects, the signs of strychnine poisoning disappear within a few hours. Dystonic reactions to drugs may occasionally be very frightening and superficially may resemble tetanus, and this possibility must always be excluded. Such reactions usually occur only after several doses of the drug have been taken but, exceptionally, they may follow the first dose. Oculogyric crises and bizarre mouth and tongue movements, which are immediately abolished by the intravenous injection of benztropine (Artane), could make the diagnosis clear. Most patients who have dystonic reactions develop flexor rather than extensor spasms.

C. tetani is a non-pyogenic organism, and unless the patient has developed a chest infection or has cellulitis around the injury which caused the disease, high pyrexia is uncommon, although a moderate elevation of the body temperature (37.5–38°C) may be noted.

Patients with tetanus are almost always very frightened, particularly if they have experienced a major spasm. Those patients who are disinterested in their illness have probably not got the disease.

When the diagnosis is being considered the patient's immunization history must be obtained. It is most exceptional for a patient who has had a full course of immunization with a booster to develop the disease.

It has been reported that tetanus depresses the pseudocholinesterase level and that this can be used as a diagnostic test (Poratin *et al.* 1977), although this has not been the author's experience.

Classification of the disease

Tetanus is usually divided into three grades of severity:
1 Mild.
2 Moderate.
3 Severe.
Some clinicians add a fourth category which includes those patients who show signs of hypothalamic or dysautonomic involvement. This condition is described later.

The patient's prognosis and treatment regimen are initially based upon the grading of the disease. The two methods by which the severity of the infection is graded are based upon:
1 The interval which has elapsed between the injury and the first episode of muscle spasm (the incubation period).
2 The interval which has elapsed between the first symptom and the first spasm (the onset period).

The injury which caused the infection is found in only 60–70% of cases of tetanus and, in many of these, it is only discovered after the diagnosis has been made. Therefore, unless an obvious wound can be found and dated (for example, a penetrating wound of the foot made with a garden fork while manuring roses 5 days earlier), the incubation period is not very helpful. However, if such a history is obtainable and the incubation period is less than 7 days the disease will probably be very severe. If it is longer than this the severity may be expected to be less, but tetanus is a very unpredictable condition.

The onset period is more reliable as a predictor. If the interval between the first symptom and the first episode of spasm is less than 5 days, the illness will probably be very severe; if the interval is greater than this, it may be expected to be less severe. Patients who complain of painful muscle hypertonus or trismus without spasm and who have a relevant history which extends for 11–14 days will probably have only mild (though chronic) tetanus. Tetanus which is localized to one limb is well recognized; this tends to be mild but stiffness may persist for many weeks.

Cephalic tetanus has been described; it follows an infected wound in the distribution of one or more of the cranial nerves and is said to be particularly severe. The incubation period tends to be short (less than 5 days) and hypothalamic involvement is a prominent feature.

However mild or indeterminate the other signs may be, dysphagia must always be regarded seriously. A patient who has difficulty swallowing saliva, liquids or solids is at constant risk of aspiration asphyxia and usually requires a tracheostomy.

Investigations

The following investigations should be performed after admission to hospital and at appropriate intervals during treatment:
Full blood count.
Urea and electrolytes.
Plasma proteins.
Blood sugar.
Pseudocholinesterase.
Blood culture.
Urine and sputum culture.
Anaerobic cultures from suspected infection site(s).
Body weight before, during and after treatment.
Radiographs.
    Chest.
    Lumbar spine.
    Femoral neck.
    Soft tissue X-ray of the injury site (for gas and foreign
      material).

Treatment

The treatment regimen is determined by the severity classification, although tetanus is an unpredictable dis-

ease and both overestimates and underestimates of its severity and outcome are made. When the diagnosis is considered probable, the patient must be admitted to an Intensive Therapy unit for constant skilled observation. This may need to be maintained for several days before a definitive decision as to the presence or severity of the disease is made.

The treatment of grade 1 (minor) tetanus

Patients with grade 1 tetanus require:
Observation.
Sedation.
Bed rest.
Penicillin.
Wound debridement.
Active immunization.

Hyperacusis is a prominent feature of tetanus and patients should always be sedated and nursed in a quiet environment. The choice and dose of sedative drug depends upon its effects and, in particular, upon the patient's continued ability to protect the airway. In adults 10–15 mg diazepam emulsion is given intravenously 4- to 6-hourly. If patients are able to relax, remain awake and not be affected by the minimal noise and movement around them, then the dose is adequate. Overdosage must constantly be borne in mind. An intravenous infusion should be set up to guarantee access to the circulation in case of sudden deterioration, and to maintain fluid balance.

C. tetani is sensitive to penicillin and it is usual for patients with the infection to be given a 5- to 10-day course of this antibiotic. If they are allergic to penicillin, erythromycin should be given in its place. If the wound is also infected with pyogenic organisms it may be appropriate to give a broad-spectrum antibiotic.

The portal of entry is discovered in only 60–70% of cases and there is no evidence that those patients whose entry wound is excised have a shorter or less severe illness. However, if a typical wound is discovered it is sensible to explore and debride it and remove any foreign material. Wide excision is unnecessary, and it should never include disfiguring or amputative surgery, unless the area is grossly infected with pyogenic organisms or is necrotic.

Tetanus is not an immunizing disease: this is one of its more intriguing aspects. Two theories have been propounded as to why the infection does not confer immunity, while immunization is so effective. The first is that more of the toxin is required to produce immunity than to cause the disease; the second is that the toxin is bound to nerve tissue as soon as it is produced and does not activate the antibody-producing system (Turner *et al.* 1958, Stoddart 1979a). At present neither of these theories can be confirmed but every patient with tetanus must be actively immunized with three doses of tetanus toxoid.

The use of antisera

For many years the treatment of the established disease included the use of antitoxin (Vaishnava *et al.* 1966). Initially this was horse-based antiserum; more recently human antiserum has been made available. The complications of using horse antiserum are very common and include skin reactions, anaphylaxis and serum sickness. Human antiserum ('Humotet') is relatively free from side-effects but is expensive.

The author does not use any form of antiserum for patients with established tetanus since there is no recent evidence that such treatment modifies the duration or severity of the illness, and it may have untoward effects. Non-immune patients who are seen in the Casualty department with potentially contaminated wounds should be given 'Humotet' together with tetanus toxoid. Many experienced casualty officers rely upon the protective effect of penicillin and do not give passive immunization even in these circumstances.

The treatment of grade 2 (moderate) tetanus

This variety of the disease is most unpredictable and is often found to be much more severe than is first suggested by the history. The patient with grade 2 tetanus requires all of the treatment outlined in the previous section and, in addition, should have a tracheostomy with a cuffed tube inserted. The main distinction between these two grades of the disease is the presence of extensor (rarely, flexor) spasm, choking or intermittent dysphagia. The onset period (or incubation period) may also be shorter. Although the tracheostomy tube provides some protection against aspiration the patient may still become dangerously hypoxic during an opisthotonic spasm. If the patient's condition deteriorates further, a tracheostomy facilitates the application of controlled ventilation.

The treatment of grade 3 (severe) tetanus

The patient with untreated grade 3 tetanus is in danger of death from exhaustion, asphyxia and cardiocirculatory failure. The treatment includes all of the factors already mentioned together with continuous sedation, paralysis and IPPV. In some centres where these facilities are not available, grade 3 tetanus has to be treated by less effective methods which include continuous thiopentone or diazepam infusion. It is very difficult to maintain a safe level of sedation, the prevention of spasm and the avoidance of respiratory depression or asphyxia; this regimen should only be used if the sedation/paralysis regimen is unobtainable.

The natural history suggests that the duration of the disease is of the order of 3 weeks and any treatment programme should be based upon this estimate. On the other hand, the patient who survives this period should recover completely. Tetanus leaves no scars apart from those of its treatment and its complications.

Sedation and paralysis

For an adult patient the sedation/paralysis regimen which is used consists of:
Propofol — $10-20$ ml h^{-1} by infusion.
Morphine — $1-5$ mg h^{-1} by infusion.
Atracurium — $10-30$ mg h^{-1} by infusion.
Correspondingly smaller doses are used for children.

This combination has few cardiocirculatory side-effects, gives complete control of muscle spasm and appears to abolish the worst of the dysautonomic features of the illness. Access to the circulation for drugs and intravenous fluids is obtained via a subclavian venous catheter with its tip in the superior vena cava.

The course of treatment is continued for 20 days and then stopped. Recovery of consciousness may be delayed, but after a further 24 hours the patient is usually rousable and can breathe spontaneously. If episodic muscle spasms are still occurring, the regime is reapplied for a further 7 days and the patient then reassessed. One patient, out of the 21 reported, required a sedation/paralysis regime for 28 days before all spasms had subsided, although several have had generalized stiffness at the end of this period which occasionally persisted for several weeks.

Dysautonomic (hypothalamic) tetanus

This is the most feared complication of grade 3 tetanus. It is manifested by episodes of hyper- and hypotension, marked vasoconstriction and pilomotor erection, tachycardia, profuse sweating and variations in body temperature, usually occurring on the second and subsequent days after treatment has begun (Kerr *et al.* 1968). Not all patients with dysautonomic symptoms demonstrate all these features. Several deaths have been reported during episodes of this type, which are thought to be due to disturbed hypothalamic control of the autonomic nervous system. If signs of dysautonomia appear the patient should be given the maximal dose of a beta-adrenergic blocking agent such as propanolol or labetalol. These should be given for at least 7 days after the initial appearance of the symptoms or until all treatment has been suspended.

Most of the features of dysautonomia can be minimized by increasing the doses of the analgesic and sedative drugs. If a patient with tetanus develops a tachycardia or becomes hypertensive the dose of diazepam is increased and given more frequently. Only if this fails to control the cardiocirculatory disturbances is propanolol or labetalol given.

Nutritional problems

Tetanus is often described as a hypercatabolic disease. However, if patients with similar illnesses which cause prolonged paralysis, for example, paralytic polyneuritis, are compared, the weight loss is not disproportionate and can be explained largely on the basis of disuse muscle atrophy. If the patient with tetanus is not adequately sedated and paralysed and continues to have muscle spasms, or if a persistent pyrexia due to systemic infection develops, then an above-average amount of muscle will be lost.

As soon as the diagnosis has been made and treatment begun, an attempt must be made to maintain full nutrition. Frequently, the patient's gastric emptying is prolonged and usually bowel sounds are absent for the first 3−4 days; during this period the patient should be fed intravenously. A standard regimen, which provides 2000 calories and 120 g of protein, is given. Trace elements, vitamins and fat are included. When gastric emptying returns to normal, nasogastric feeds are poorly tolerated and the choice of feeding material is dictated by the patient's enteral tolerance. The nasogastric route is preferred to the parenteral route because it has fewer complications and also because it probably reduces the incidence of stress peptic ulceration. If delayed gastric emptying persists, the patient is given metoclopramide.

The blood sugar and plasma protein levels are monitored regularly so that the need for insulin and intravenous albumin supplements can be recognized. When the enteral route becomes available, insulin supplements are less frequently required. The commonest complication of enteral feeding is diarrhoea which can usually be controlled by changing the feeding material. However, constipation may also be a problem which should never be ignored, since it may lead to faecal impaction and, rarely, intestinal obstruction. Regular bowel evacuation must be maintained throughout the course of the illness.

The patient's fluid and electrolyte balance must be carefully controlled; the weighing bed facilitates the recognition of sudden changes in body weight, which are usually caused by increased insensible losses.

Miscellaneous problems

All patients in the Intensive Therapy unit are at risk of stress peptic ulceration and DVT, and they should routinely be given 5000 units of heparin bd subcutaneously and 50 mg ranitidine 8-hourly intravenously.

Long-term venous access for drug administration is often a problem and all intravenous lines must be inserted aseptically and given scrupulous care. The routine drugs are given continuously from syringe pumps and only exceptionally are drugs injected into the line. If other agents are required, the enteral route should be used whenever possible.

Apart from technical problems (including airway obstruction, ventilator disconnection, etc.), which should be avoidable, atelectasis, pneumonia and urinary tract infection are the greatest hazards of treatment because of the need for paralysis, tracheostomy, IPPV and catheterization. Septicaemia from intravascular lines and other invasive techniques is a potential problem which must be avoided. Sputum and urine must be taken for microbiological culture every second day, and chest radiographs should be taken when necessary. Antibiotics are not given prophylactically but if the patient shows clinical signs of infection a short course (5 days) of the appropriate antibiotic is given.

Patients who are paralysed for prolonged periods may develop muscle contractures and joint deformities, of which Achilles tendon shortening is the most obvious. These can be prevented by passive manipulation of all joints (including wrist and fingers) at least once every 4 hours.

Results

In this series (Table 11.7) 18 patients had grade 3 tetanus and three patients had grade 1 tetanus. Nineteen patients made a full recovery and had virtually no recollection of their stay in hospital, although two reported having vivid, but not frightening, dreams. Two patients died. One was a 77-year-old male with systemic lupus erythematosus who contracted tetanus from a skin abrasion. On admission to hospital he was in early chronic renal failure due to his underlying disease and after 2 weeks of treatment required haemodialysis. This was considered not to be in his best interests. The other was a 71-year-old male who had already had one myocardial infarction and who devel-

Table 11.7 Origin of tetanus

Origin	No. of cases
Trivial wounds	7
Extensive soft tissue injuries	4
Compound fractures	3
Clean surgical wounds	2
Varicose ulcer	1
Unknown	4

oped tetanus from an infected compound fracture. He had a second, fatal myocardial infarction 48 hours after admission to the Intensive Therapy unit.

Active immunization

The regimen of immunization which is given to all patients with tetanus is: an initial injection of 0.5 ml toxoid, followed 6 weeks and 6 months later by further 0.5 ml injections. Thereafter, boosters are required at 5- to 7-year intervals (Turner *et al.* 1958).

References

Adams, E.B., Laurence, D.R. & Smith, J.W.G. *Tetanus*. Blackwell Scientific Publications: Oxford, 1969.

Kerr, J.H., Corbett, J.L., Prys Roberts, C., Crampton-Smith, A. & Spalding, J.M.K. Involvement of the sympathetic nervous system in tetanus. *Lancet* 1968; **ii**: 236−241.

Lennard, T.W.J., Gunn, A., Sellers, J. & Stoddart, J.C. Tetanus after elective cholecystectomy and exploration of the common bile duct. *Lancet* 1984; **i**: 1466−1467.

Poratin, A., Acker, M. & Perel, A. Serum cholinesterase in tetanus. *Anaesthesia* 1977; **32**: 1009−1011.

Stoddart, J.C. The immunology of tetanus. *Anaesthesia* 1979a; **34**: 863−865.

Stoddart, J.C. Pseudotetanus. *Anaesthesia* 1979b; **34**: 877−881.

Turner, T.B., Velasco-Joven, E.A. & Prudovsky, S. Studies on the prophylaxis and treatment of tetanus. *Bull Johns Hopkins Hosp* 1958; **102**: 71−84.

Vaishnava, H., Goyal, R.Y., Neogy, C.N. & Mather, G.P. A controlled trial of antiserum in the treatment of tetanus. *Lancet* 1966; **ii**: 1371−1374.

Wainwright, J.M. Tetanus: its incidence and treatment. *Arch Surg* 1926; **12**: 1062−1063.

Gas gangrene

P.J.GREGG

The development of gas gangrene is one of the most serious complications of any open soft tissue injury. Although any wound may become infected with clos-tridial spores, which are widely distributed in the soil and environment, gas gangrene is, thankfully, uncommon following injuries resulting from civilian trauma. However, it must be remembered that cases still do occur, often following poor initial management of a wound or open fracture where basic principles have not been followed.

Wounds which are particularly at risk are those which have been heavily contaminated with soil from the outset and those where non-viable tissue remains after adequate exploration and debridement, and where non-viable tissue and foreign material remains after inadequate exploration and debridement! Under these circumstances the wound must never be closed primarily. Other wounds at risk are those around the hip and thigh, for example, after high thigh amputations, where spores of *Clostridium perfringens* may enter the wound from the patient's own faecal flora.

Most cases of gas gangrene result from *C. perfringens* (*welchii*) but *C. oedematiens*, *C. septicum* and, rarely, *C. histolyticum* may be implicated. These organisms are obligate anaerobes and cannot multiply in healthy tissues with high oxygen reduction potentials.

Presentation

The incubation period of clostridia is not long and symptoms and signs of the infection usually appear about 24 hours after surgery. The patient usually complains of pain and is also usually very unwell as a result of toxaemia caused by toxins secreted by the causative bacteria. The pulse rate is characteristically increased out of proportion to the rise in temperature. Shock, jaundice, severe haemolysis (resulting in haemoglobinaemia and haemoglobinuria) and acute renal failure may also develop. Local clinical signs which are suggestive of gas gangrene include oedema and a peculiar bronze discoloration of the overlying skin, which may also become mottled. A watery, foul-smelling exudate is also present. Gas formation in the tissues, which gives rise to palpable crepitus and is visible on radiographs, also develops. The presence of myositis and myonecrosis is confirmed at surgical exploration. The muscle is found to be oedematous, grey or dark red and ischaemic; contractility is absent and gas bubbles froth from the muscle fibres.

Diagnosis

Accurate diagnosis is essential to distinguish gas gangrene from more benign anaerobic cellulitis caused by coliform bacteria, anaerobic streptococci and anaerobic bacteroids. In anaerobic cellulitis the onset is more gradual: toxaemia is slight; gas formation is foul-smelling and abundant but there is no actual muscle invasion. Wound swabs, pus and blood cultures are obtained, before antibiotics are commenced, and these should be sent to the laboratory, without delay, in Stuart's transport medium. A Gram stain of pus will usually show non-motile Gram-positive bacilli which are thick and rectangular and without spores. *C. perfringens* is usually readily cultured using anaerobic techniques and also demonstrates a positive Nagler reaction. A zone of opacity is seen around each colony on a bacteriological plate containing lecithin; this zone is due to the release of triglycerides through the lecithinase activity of the alpha-toxin of the organism.

Management

The success of management depends on early diagnosis and prompt surgical treatment. Preoperative resuscitation may be required and should take the form of fluid, blood and electrolyte replacement. CVP monitoring and urinary output measurement may also be required. Surgery is absolutely essential in order to remove all infected and dead tissue. This surgery must be carried out immediately and involves the complete re-opening of the existing wound with a generous extension, as required, to give wide access to all gangrenous and infected muscles which must be excised. Care must be taken not to damage important neurovascular structures. The wound must be left open in its entirety and only very lightly packed. If massive gas gangrene is present, immediate amputation should be performed and the skin flaps left open. When the infection has been controlled, secondary suture is usually safe to perform 10 days later.

Antibiotics must also be given. Penicillin G is the antibiotic of choice and should be given in doses of 3 000 000 units 3-hourly intravenously. Gentamicin and flucloxacillin may also be given if there is superimposed Gram-negative and Gram-positive infection respectively. If the patient is allergic to penicillin, a cephalosporin or clindamycin should be used instead. Although some authorities also recommend administration of large doses of specific antitoxin, this practice, with its risk of anaphylaxis, has largely been abandoned.

Hyperbaric oxygen may be a useful adjunct for improving the general condition of the patient and for controlling the infection in extensive and difficult cases. The author has personal experience of the use of this form of treatment for patients treated in the compression chamber at the Royal Victoria Infirmary in Newcastle-upon-Tyne. The patient is placed in the compression chamber and breathes oxygen at 300 kPa absolute (200 kPa above ambient pressure) for 3–4 hours at a time; following this the patient undergoes a standard decompression. This procedure is repeated four times during the first 24 hours, twice in the second 24 hours and once in the third 24 hours. It must be remembered that there are potential complications associated with the use of this treatment. These include barotrauma, decompression sickness, convulsions, claustrophobia and oxygen toxicity. There are, however, several reports of the efficacy of hyperbaric oxygen treatment in gas gangrene (Roding *et al.* 1972, Holland *et al.* 1975, Tonjum *et al.* 1980, Welsh *et al.* 1980).

Conclusion

It goes without saying that prevention of gas gangrene must always be uppermost in the minds of surgeons treating patients who have sustained a wound which is at risk of this complication; for example, after farming accidents. Large doses of penicillin G should be given intravenously as soon as possible and, of course, should be followed by extensive and meticulous exploration and debridement of the wound, which must be left open.

References

Holland, J.A., Hill, G.B., Wolfe, W.G., Osterhout, S., Saltzman, H.A. & Brown, I.W. Experimental and clinical experience with hyperbaric oxygen in the treatment of clostridial myonecrosis. *Surgery* 1975; **77**: 75–85.

Roding, B., Groeneveld, P.H.A. & Boerema, I. Ten years of experience in the treatment of gas gangrene with hyperbaric oxygen. *Surg Gynecol Obstet* 1972; **134**: 579–585.

Tonjum, S., Digranes, A., Alho, A., Gjengsto, H. & Eidsvik, S. Hyperbaric oxygen treatment in gas-producing infections. *Acta Chir Scand* 1980; **146**: 235–241.

Welsh, F., Matos, L. & deTreville, R.T.P. Medical hyperbaric oxygen therapy. 22 cases. *Aviat Space Environ Med* 1980; **51**: 611–614.

Adult respiratory distress syndrome

J.C.STODDART

Respiratory failure is common, either as a presenting problem or as a complication of another serious illness or traumatic event. It is most often due to bronchopneumonia (including aspiration pneumonia), pulmonary oedema or direct pulmonary trauma. In this section a much less common condition will be described: namely, the adult respiratory distress syndrome (ARDS). Numerous synonyms have been used including shock lung, Da Nang wet lung, ventilator lung, interstitial pulmonary oedema, etc.

It has been known for many years that up to 30% of patients who die after extensive surgery and non-thoracic trauma do so from lung failure (Ashbaugh *et al.* 1967, Moore *et al.* 1969, Dowd & Jenkins 1972, Rinaldo & Rogers 1982). Although it had undoubtedly been described before this time, Ashbaugh *et al.* (1967) are usually credited with bringing ARDS to more general attention. Since that time it has been the subject of intense research and what follows is a brief summary of the present view.

ARDS occurs most commonly in patients with systemic sepsis who have undergone major surgery or suffered extensive physical injury, including burns (Rinaldo & Rogers 1982, Bernard & Brigham 1985). It may also complicate acute pancreatitis (Foulis *et al.* 1982) and pulmonary fat embolism (Dowd & Jenkins 1972), and a similar condition is occasionally recognized after cardiopulmonary bypass (Westaby 1987) or haemodialysis (Kaplow & Goffinet 1968, Arnaout *et al.* 1985, Knudsen *et al.* 1985).

Its clinical features include tachypnoea, hypoxia, reduced functional residual capacity and reduced compliance, with widespread pulmonary infiltrates on the chest radiograph.

Pathophysiology

The pulmonary lesion is initiated inside the alveolar capillaries (Jacob 1978, Rinaldo & Rogers 1982, Bernard & Brigham 1985). Tissue injury and endotoxins activate the complement cascade and combine to reduce pulmonary capillary blood flow. This permits the margination of polymorphonuclear leukocytes, which adhere to the capillary endothelium and release leukocyte membrane phospholipids and proteolytic enzymes (proteases) (Jacob 1978, Till *et al.* 1982, Tate & Repine 1983, Brigham & Meyrick 1984, Cohler *et al.* 1985, Solomkin *et al.* 1985). This process is associated with the appearance of oxygen free radicals (O_2^-, OH^-, peroxide) which are toxic to the endothelium (Sacks *et al.* 1978, Baldwin *et al.* 1986). Arachidonic acid is released; this is an intermediary in the formation of eicosanoids such as leukotrienes, which are permeability activators, and prostaglandins, which are vasoactive (Parratt & Sturgess 1977, Corrin 1980, Kadowtiz *et al.* 1981, Brigham 1985, Ball *et al.* 1986).

The results are transient pulmonary hypertension,

intravascular thrombosis and increased permeability of the pulmonary capillaries. This is followed by the accumulation of fluid in the pulmonary interstitium and alveoli.

The contribution of fibronectin (soluble and insoluble) to this series of events is uncertain (Saba *et al.* 1986). The coagulation cascade may also be activated, giving rise to disseminated intravascular coagulation (Hardaway 1973, Stoddart & Wardle 1974, Modig 1983).

Diagnostic features of the condition include the identification of protein and proteolytic enzymes in bronchial lavage fluid (Gorin *et al.* 1980, Arnaout *et al.* 1985, Bernard & Brigham 1985, Knudsen *et al.* 1985). The pulmonary artery wedge pressure is low. It was suggested that with pulmonary angiography, ARDS could be distinguished from other types of lung failure but this is not generally agreed upon (Greene *et al.* 1981).

The above description has emphasized the central place of the polymorphonuclear leukocyte. However, a similar condition may be seen in leukaemic patients and in others with extreme granulocytopenia; in this situation it is believed that other leukocytes may play a similar role (Braude *et al.* 1985, Laute *et al.* 1986, Ognibene *et al.* 1986). It is no longer believed that microaggregates from transfused blood play a significant part in the development of ARDS (Dorrington 1985).

It has been stated that there are 10 000—15 000 cases of ARDS in the United Kingdom each year with a mortality rate of 60—90% (Editorial 1986). This may be an overestimate, since the term is often used loosely and, by definition, ARDS does not occur in isolation; death is usually due to multiple organ failure rather than to hypoxia alone.

Treatment

The objectives of treatment are to achieve an acceptable (if not ideal) blood gas exchange with the smallest possible penalty. This usually involves controlled ventilation with oxygen-enriched air to maintain the arterial oxygen tension at, or above, 8.0 kPa (60 mmHg). Minimal positive end expiratory pressure (PEEP) is usually recommended (Suter *et al.* 1975, Gallagher *et al.* 1978). There is no evidence that the early application of intermittent positive pressure ventilation with PEEP delays or prevents the onset of ARDS (Pepe *et al.* 1984) and the disadvantages of PEEP are well known (Powers *et al.* 1973, Demling *et al.* 1975, Danek *et al.* 1980, Rounds & Brody 1984). Other methods of obtaining satisfactory gas exchange are being investigated; these include the use of reversed I:E (inspiratory:expiratory) ratios

(Cole *et al.* 1984) and high frequency ventilation (Wattwil *et al.* 1983, Berre *et al.* 1987). Although short-lived improvement in gas exchange has been reported, it has usually not been possible to apply such methods for the whole duration of the illness because of cardio-circulatory, or other, problems (Wattwil *et al.* 1983, Cole *et al.* 1984). Long-term extracorporeal membrane oxygenation (ECMO) has been tried and abandoned (Zapol & Snider 1980) but extracorporeal carbon dioxide removal and low frequency ventilation of the lungs with oxygen is still being assessed (Gattinoni *et al.* 1980).

Avoidance of fluid overload

Fluid overload must be avoided and dopamine and frusemide are given to cause a diuresis to help clear interstitial pulmonary oedema. Renal failure is common and haemodialysis and/or haemofiltration are then necessary. Haemofiltration may be useful in the early phase of the condition to correct an overload resulting from emergency resuscitation (Gotloib *et al.* 1984, Kaplan *et al.* 1984). These techniques are described elsewhere. In the established condition, central venous pressure or pulmonary wedge pressure monitoring may be unhelpful because these are affected by the application of controlled ventilation to poorly compliant lungs (Nadeau & Noble 1986).

Hypoalbuminaemia is common, from catabolism, starvation and redistribution (Deysine *et al.* 1973, Demling *et al.* 1979, Ellman 1984, Fleck *et al.* 1985). Patients are usually given 25–50 g albumin IV daily as plasma protein fraction; although much of this may exude into the pulmonary interstitium, a useful amount may remain in the circulating blood.

Antibiotics and other drugs

Patients are usually already receiving antibiotics but every effort should be made to avoid secondary bacterial infection. Evidence is accumulating that the incidence of secondary infection of the respiratory tract may be reduced by the prophylactic application of an antibiotic paste to the inside of the mouth, nasopharynx and stomach, combined with the simultaneous administration of an intravenous antibiotic (Stoutenbeek *et al.* 1984). Bacterial pneumonia is an important cause of morbidity and mortality in the Intensive Therapy unit and if this study is confirmed it will be a major contribution to care.

Experimentally, it has been demonstrated that some antibiotics in clinical use cause a disproportionate rise in plasma endotoxin (Shenep *et al.* 1985). The rate of rise was, in ascending order, from chloramphenicol through gentamicin to moxalactam. This work requires further clinical validation but its possible significance should be borne in mind, since endotoxin has been implicated as a causative factor of ARDS.

The results of a recent multicentre controlled trial have confirmed earlier work that corticosteroids are of no value and may be harmful (Sprung *et al.* 1984). Their use is no longer recommended in the manufacturer's data sheet. Because of the suspected involvement of complement and prostaglandins in the development of ARDS, prostaglandin inhibitors and non-steroidal anti-inflammatory drugs (NSAIDs) have been used both prophylactically and therapeutically but without long-term benefit (Brigham *et al.* 1980, Kerstein & Crivello 1980, Higgs & Flower 1981, Casey *et al.* 1982). A further problem derives from the fact that prostaglandin $F_{2\alpha}$ is released from renal arteriolar endothelium and may improve renal cortical blood flow in shock states; this effect is abolished by NSAIDs (Stiff & Clive 1983). At present, a multicentre trial of the use of prostaglandin E_1 (emprostonol) in ARDS is in progress, after its apparently successful use in some non-controlled trials (Richardson *et al.* 1984, Tokioka *et al.* 1985, Holcroft *et al.* 1986, Shoemaker & Appel 1986).

Treatment of the underlying cause

If the underlying cause of the condition is known it must be treated. It is particularly important to identify and treat intra-abdominal sepsis; repeated laparotomy or excisional surgery are often required. This should never be delayed because of the patient's physical status since, without effective treatment, a fatal outcome is inevitable.

References

Arnaout, M.A., Hakim, R.M., Todd, R.F., Dana, N. & Colten, H.R. Increased expression of an adhesion promoting surface glycoprotein in the granulocytopenia of hemodialysis. *N Engl J Med* 1985; **312**: 457–462.

Ashbaugh, D.G., Bigelow, D.B., Petty, T.L. & Levine, B.E. Acute respiratory distress in adults. *Lancet* 1967; **ii**: 319–321.

Baldwin, S.R., Simon, R.H., Grum, C.M., Ketai, L.H., Boxer, L.A. & Devall, J.J. Oxidant activity in expired breath of patients with adult respiratory distress syndrome. *Lancet* 1986; **1**: 11–14.

Ball, H.A., Cook, J.A., Wise, W.C. & Halushka, P.V. Role of thromboxane, prostaglandins and leukotrienes in endotoxic and septic shock. *Intensive Care Med* 1986; **12(3)**: 116–126.

Bernard, G. & Brigham, K. The adult respiratory distress syndrome. *Ann Rev Med* 1985; **36**: 195–205.

Berre, J., Ros, A.M., Vincent, P., Dufaye, J., Brimioulle, S. & Kahn, R.J. Technical and psychological complications of high frequency jet ventilation. *Intensive Care Med* 1987; **13**: 96–99.

Braude, S., Apperley, J., Krausz, T., Goldman, J.M. & Royston, D. Adult respiratory distress syndrome after allogenic bone marrow transplantation: evidence for a neutrophil independent mechanism. *Lancet* 1985; **1**: 1239–1242.

Brigham, K.L. Metabolites of arachidonic acid in experimental lung vascular injury. *Fed Proc* 1985; **44**: 43–45.

Brigham, K.L. & Meyrick, B. Interaction of granulocytes with the lungs. *Circ Res* 1984; **54**: 623–635.

Brigham, K.L., Padvoe, S.J., Bryant, D., McKeen, C.R. & Bowers, R.E. Diphenhydramine reduces endotoxic effects on lung permeability in sheep. *J Appl Physiol* 1980; **49(3)**: 515–520.

Casey, L.C., Fletcher, J.R., Zmidka, M. & Ramwell, P.W. Prevention of endotoxin induced pulmonary hypertension in primates by the use of a selective thromboxane synthetase inhibitor. *J Pharm Exp Therap* 1982; **222**: 441–446.

Cohler, L.F., Saba, T.M. & Lewis, E.P. Lung vascular injury with protease infusion. *Ann Surg* 1985; **202(2)**: 240–247.

Cole, A.G.H., Weller, S.F. & Sykes, M.K. Inverse ratio ventilation compared with PEEP in adult respiratory failure. *Intensive Care Med* 1984; **10(5)**: 227–232.

Corrin, B. Lung pathology in septic shock. *J Clin Path* 1980; **33**: 891–894.

Danek, S.J., Lynch, J.P., Weg, J.G. & Dantzker, D.R. The dependence of oxygen uptake on oxygen delivery in the adult respiratory distress syndrome. *Am Rev Resp Dis* 1980; **122**: 387–395.

Demling, R.H., Manohard, M., Will, J.A. & Belzar, F.O. The effect of plasma oncotic pressure on the pulmonary microcirculation after hemorrhagic shock. *Surgery* 1979; **86**: 323–328.

Demling, R.H., Staub, N.C. & Edmunds, L.U. Effect of end expiratory airway pressure on accumulation of extravascular lung water. *J Appl Physiol* 1975; **38**: 907–912.

Deysine, M., Lieblich, N. & Aufses, A.H. Albumin changes during clinical septic shock. *Surg Gynecol Obstet* 1973; **137(3)**: 475–478.

Dorrington, M.C. The present status of blood filtration. *Anaesthesia* 1985; **40**: 334–347.

Dowd, J. & Jenkins, L.C. The lung in shock — a review. *Can Anaesth Soc J* 1972; **19(3)**: 309–318.

Editorial. Adult respiratory distress syndrome. *Lancet* 1986; **i**: 301–303.

Ellman, H. Capillary permeability in septic patients. *Crit Care Med* 1984; **12**: 629–633.

Fleck, A., Raines, F., Hawker, F., Trotter, J., Wallace, P.I., Ledingham, I.McA. & Calman, K.C. Increased vascular permeability; a major cause of hypoalbuminaemia in disease and injury. *Lancet* 1985; **i**: 781–784.

Foulis, A.K., Murray, W.R., Galloway, D., McCartney, A.C., Lange, E., Veitch, J. & Whaley, K. Endotoxaemia and complement activation in acute pancreatitis in man. *Gut* 1982; **23**: 656–661.

Gallagher, T.J., Civetta, J.M. & Kirby, R.M. Terminological update: optimal PEEP. *Crit Care Med* 1978; **6**: 323–325.

Gattinoni, L., Agostini, A., Pesenti, A., Pelizzola, A., Ross, G.P., Langer, M. & Vesconi, S. Treatment of acute respiratory failure with low frequency positive pressure ventilation and extracorporeal removal of CO_2. *Lancet* 1980; **ii**: 292–294.

Gorin, A.B., Kohler, J. & De Nardo, G. Non invasive measurement of pulmonary transvascular flux in normal man. *J Clin Invest* 1980; **66**: 869–877.

Gotloib, L., Barzilay, E., Shustak, A. & Lev, A. Sequential hemofiltration in non-oliguric high capillary permeability pulmonary edema of severe sepsis: preliminary report. *Crit Care Med* 1984; **12**: 994–1000.

Greene, R., Zapol, W.M., Snider, M.T., Reid, L., Snow, R., O'Connell, R.S. & Novelline, R.A. Early bedside detection of pulmonary vascular occlusion during acute respiratory failure. *Am Rev Resp Dis* 1981; **124**: 593–601.

Hardaway, R.M. Disseminated intravascular coagulation as a possible cause of acute respiratory failure. *Surg Gynecol Obstet* 1973; **137**: 1–5.

Higgs, G.A. & Flower, R.J. Anti-inflammatory drugs and the inhibition of arachidonate lipoxygenase. In: Piper, P. (ed.) *Slow Release Substance of Anaphylaxis and Leukotrienes*. John Wiley & Sons: Bristol, 1981.

Holcroft, J.W., Vassar, M.J. & Weber, C.J. Prostaglandin E_1 and survival in patients with the adult respiratory distress syndrome. *Ann Surg* 1986; **203(4)**: 371–378.

Jacob, H.S. Granulocyte–complement interaction. *Arch Intern Med* 1978; **138**: 461–462.

Kadowtiz, P.J., Gruetter, C.A., Spannhaker, E.W. & Hyman, A.L. Pulmonary vascular response to prostaglandins. *Fed Proc* 1981; **40**: 1991–1996.

Kaplan, A.A., Longnecker, R.E. & Folkert, V.W. Continuous arteriovenous hemofiltration. *Ann Intern Med* 1984; **100**: 358–367.

Kaplow, L.S. & Goffinet, J.A. Profound neutropenia during the early phase of hemodialysis. *J Am Med Assoc* 1968; **205**: 1135–1137.

Kerstein, M.D. & Crivello, M. Reversal of histopathological pulmonary changes with indomethacin. *Surg Gynecol Obstet* 1980; **151**: 786–790.

Knudsen, F., Nielsen, A.H., Pedersen, J.O., Grimnet, N. & Jersild, C. Adult respiratory distress-like syndrome during hemodialysis: relationship between activation of complement, leukopenia and release of granulocyte elastase. *Int J Artif Organs* 1985; **8(4)**: 187–194.

Laute, M.D., Simon, R.H., Flint, A. & Keller, J.B. Adult respiratory distress in neutropenic patients. *Am J Med* 1986; **80**: 1022–1026.

Modig, J. The value of variables of disseminated intravascular coagulation in the diagnosis of adult respiratory distress syndrome. *Acta Anesth Scand* 1983; **27**: 369–373.

Moore, I.D., Lyons, J.H., Pierce, E.C., Morgan, A.P., Dunbar, P.A., MacArthur, J.H. & Dainman, G.J. (eds) *Post Traumatic Pulmonary Insufficiency*. WB Saunders: Philadelphia, 1969.

Nadeau, S. & Noble, W.H. Review: misinterpretation of pressure measurements from the pulmonary artery catheter. *Can Anaesth Assoc J* 1986; **33**: 352–363.

Ognibene, F.P., Martin, S.E., Parker, M.E., Schlesinger, T., Roach, P., Birch, C., Shelhamer, J.H. & Parrillo, J.E. Adult respiratory distress syndrome in patients with severe neutropenia. *N Engl J Med* 1986; **315**: 547–551.

Parratt, J.R. & Sturgess, R.M. The possible roles of histamine, 5-hydroxytryptamine and prostaglandin F_2 as mediators of the pulmonary effects of endotoxin. *Br J Pharm* 1977; **60**: 209–219.

Pepe, P.E., Hudson, L.D. & Carrico, C.J. Early application of positive end expiratory pressure in patients at risk for the adult respiratory distress syndrome. *N Engl J Med* 1984; **311**: 281–286.

Powers, S.R., Mannal, R., Neclerio, M., English, M., Marr, C., Leather, R., Ueda, H., Williams, G., Custead, W. & Dutton, R. Physiologic consequences of positive end expiratory pressure (PEEP) ventilation. *Ann Surg* 1973; **178(3)**: 265–272.

Richardson, A., Wells, F.C. & Branthwaite, M.K. Use of prostacyclin and ultrafiltration in adult respiratory distress syndrome. *Intensive Care Med* 1984; **10**: 107–109.

Rinaldo, J.E. & Rogers, R.M. Adult respiratory distress syndrome: changing concepts of lung injury and repair. *N Engl J Med* 1982; **306**: 900–909.

Rounds, S. & Brody, J.S. Putting PEEP in perspective. *N Engl J Med* 1984; **311**: 323–325.

Saba, T.M., Kilner, J.L. & Holam, J.M. Fibronectin and the critically ill patient: current status. *Intensive Care Med* 1986; **12**: 350–358.

Sacks, T., Moldow, C., Craddock, P.R., Bowers, T.K. & Jacob, H.S. Oxygen radicals mediate endothelial cell damage by complement-stimulated granulocytes. *J Clin Invest* 1978; **61**: 1161–1167.

Shenep, J.L., Barton, R.P. & Morgan, K.A. Role of antibiotic class in the rate of liberation of endotoxin during therapy for experimental gram negative bacterial sepsis. *J Infect Dis* 1985; **151(6)**: 1012–1018.

Shoemaker, W.C. & Appel, P.L. Effects of prostaglandin E$_1$ in adult respiratory distress syndrome. *Surgery* 1986; **99(3)**: 275–282.

Solomkin, J.S., Cotta, L.A. & Satoh, P.S. Complement activation and clearance in acute illness and injury; evidence for C$_5$ as a cell directed mediator of the adult respiratory distress syndrome in man. *Surgery* 1985; **97**: 668–678.

Sprung, C.L., Caralis, P.V., Marcial, E.H., Pierce, M., Gelbard, M.A., Long, W.H., Duncan, R.C., Tendler, M.D. & Karpf, M. The effect of high dose corticosteroids in patients with septic shock. *N Engl J Med* 1984; **311**: 1137–1143.

Stiff, J.S. & Clive, D.M. Role of prostaglandins and thromboxane in acute renal failure. In: Brenner, B.M. & Lazarus, M.G. (eds) *Acute Renal Failure*. WB Saunders: Philadelphia, 1983.

Stoddart, J.C. & Wardle, E.N. Post traumatic respiratory distress due to endotoxinaemia and intravascular coagulation. *Br J Anaesth* 1974; **46**: 892–896.

Stoutenbeek, C.P., Van Saene, H.K.F., Miranda, D.R. & Zandstra, D.F. The effect of selective decontamination of the digestive tract on colonization and infection rate in the multiple trauma patient. *Intensive Care Med* 1984; **10(4)**: 185–192.

Suter, P.M., Fairley, H.B. & Isenberg, M.I. Optimum end expiratory airway pressure in patients in acute pulmonary failure. *N Engl J Med* 1975; **292**: 284–289.

Tate, R.M. & Repine, J.E. Neutrophils and the adult respiratory distress syndrome. *Am Rev Resp Dis* 1983; **128**: 552–559.

Till, G.O., Johnson, K.S., Kunkel, R. & Ward, P.A. Intravascular activation of complement and acute lung injury. *J Clin Invest* 1982; **69**: 1126–1135.

Tokioka, H., Kobayashi, I., Ohta, Y., Wakabayashi, T. & Kosaka, F. The acute effects of prostaglandin E$_1$ on the pulmonary circulation and oxygen delivery in patients with the adult respiratory distress syndrome. *Intensive Care Med* 1985; **11**: 61–64.

Wattwil, L.M., Sjostrand, V.H. & Borg, U.R. Comparative studies of IPPV and HPPV with PEEP in critical care medicine. I. A clinical evaluation. *Crit Care Med* 1983; **11(1)**: 30–37.

Westaby, S. Organ dysfunction after cardiopulmonary bypass: a systemic inflammatory reaction initiated by the extracorporeal circuit. *Intensive Care Med* 1987; **13(2)**: 89–95.

Zapol, W.H. & Snider, M.T. Membrane lungs for acute respiratory failure: current status. *Am Rev Resp Dis* 1980; **121**: 907–909.

Delayed union, non-union and infected non-union

O.O.A.ONI, P.H.WORLOCK
AND P.J.GREGG

The process of fracture union cannot be precisely divided into stages. The point at which a fracture has achieved union is difficult to define precisely in practice. However, because the fractured bone is often strong enough for use before healing is complete, two clinical stages are recognized: namely, clinical union and consolidation.

A fracture is regarded as *clinically* united when there is no local tenderness on palpation nor pain on stressing. There is no detectable movement at the fracture site because of firm linkage of the fractured bone ends. However, these signs of clinical union may be present when a fracture is bridged by fibrocartilaginous tissue and not by bone. Therefore, only protected use of the injured limb may be allowed because of the possibility of angulation or refracture.

Clinical union precedes *radiological union* (defined as visible bridging callus and trabecular continuity) by several weeks (Watson-Jones & Coltart 1943). *Consolidation* or 'true repair' is deemed to have occurred when the radiographs show that the fracture has been bridged by well-formed bone and the fractured bone can be subjected to normal stresses. Weight-bearing is full, unprotected and pain-free following consolidation.

Although the point at which a particular fracture is regarded as united depends upon the observer, the average time a fracture is expected to take to unite, i.e. the healing time, has been defined (Perkins 1958, Brashear 1965). This healing time depends on factors such as age, type of bone and type of fracture (Table 11.8). In early childhood, callus is often visible radiologically within 2 weeks of injury and the fracture may be united by 6 weeks. By contrast, in adults a fractured long bone takes about 12 weeks on average to heal but often much longer. Fractures through cancellous bone unite more rapidly than fractures through the hard compact bone of the diaphysis.

Table 11.8 Approximate healing times (weeks) for fractures (From Perkins 1958)

	Spiral fractures, metaphyseal fractures	Transverse fractures, diaphyseal fractures
Upper limb		
Union	3	6
Consolidation	6	12
Lower limb		
Union	6	12
Consolidation	12	24

The healing times are halved in young children.

Delayed union and non-union

Delayed union

Delayed union occurs when it has taken longer than the expected time for a particular fracture to unite (Brashear 1965). However, the fracture may still show evidence that healing is progressing and that union could eventually occur without intervention.

Clinically, an ununited fracture produces pain of varying intensity when loaded, stressed or on palpation. There may be abnormal movement at the fracture site. There may be persistent oedema, tenderness and increased warmth in the soft tissues overlying the fracture. The fracture line is usually visible on plain radiographs, but there is no sclerosis or cavitation. Histologically, the fracture site is bridged by fibrous or fibrocartilaginous tissue (Sevitt 1981).

Non-union

In contrast to delayed union, true non-union is a specific pathological condition. The reparative processes have come to a halt and healing will not occur, regardless of how much time is allowed without intervention.

Clinically, non-union may present with little pain or warmth (as often observed in delayed union). There may be little movement at the fracture site, although progressive angulation can occur, particularly in weight-bearing bones. Radiologically, the fractured bone ends may be porotic or sclerotic and rounded with a well-defined fracture line (Fig. 11.34). The medullary cavity may be occluded by compact bone or there may be cavitation at the fracture cleft. There is a lack of progress towards union on serial radiographs, although a periosteal collar (Fig. 11.35) may be visible around the fracture fragments.

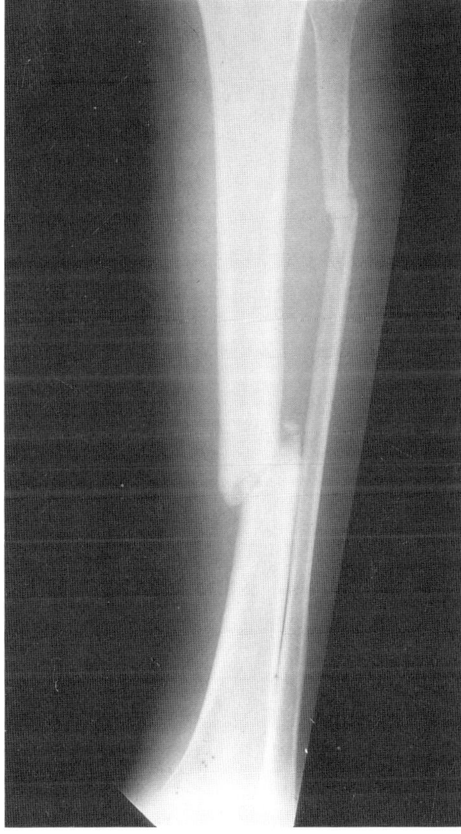

Fig. 11.34 Plain radiograph showing an atrophic non-union of the tibia.

Histologically, the fracture site is occupied by a variety of fibrous tissues in different stages of degeneration (Urist *et al.* 1954, Sevitt 1981) and some poorly formed osteoid may be observed in the midst of the fibrous tissues. The fractured bone ends appear avascular and may be covered by fibrocartilaginous tissues with the formation of a cyst in the fracture cleft: the so-called pseudoarthrosis (Fig. 11.36).

Other characteristics of non-union

Several workers have attempted to exploit bone scintigraphy as a prognostic indicator following fractures because radionuclide uptake may relate to new bone formation (Galasko 1975, 1984). However, the results have been conflicting. Some workers have classified fracture union into normal and delayed on the basis of a visual assessment of static scintigrams (Auchincloss & Watt 1982), but others have shown that all observed patterns of tracer uptake are represented in normal and slowly healing fractures (Gregg *et al.* 1983, 1984, Oni *et al.* 1989). Other investigators have demonstrated a

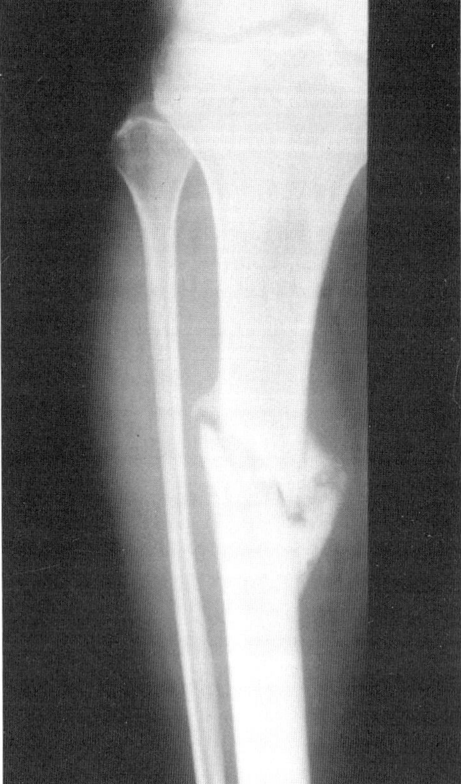

Fig. 11.35 Plain radiograph showing a hypertrophic non-union of the tibia.

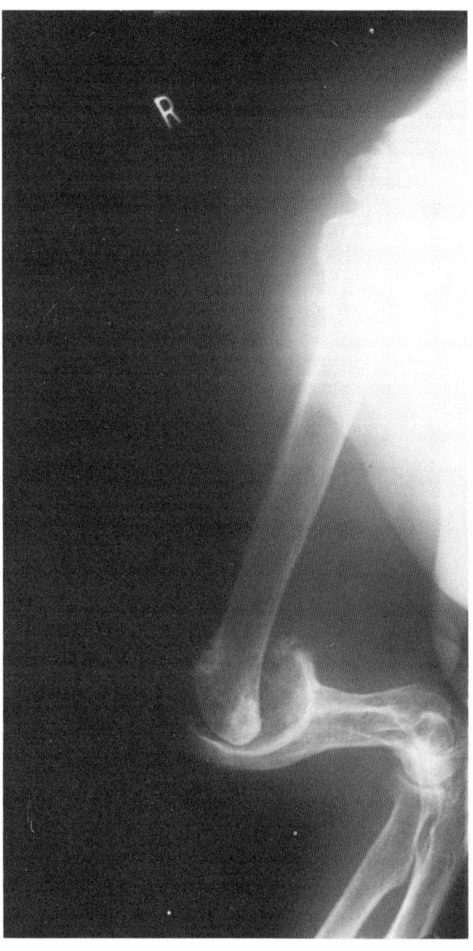

Fig. 11.36 Plain radiograph showing a pseudoarthrosis of the humerus.

close relationship between the rate of uptake at the fracture site relative to that at an adjacent control site (Jacobs *et al.* 1979) but the results have not been reproduced (Gregg *et al.* 1983, 1984). Similarly, while Illingworth and Schiess (1971) found no relationship between the speed of healing and uptake, Auchincloss and Watt (1982) did. Quantitative indices of radionuclide uptake (Smith *et al.* 1987) and of osteogenesis (Oni *et al.* 1989), which specifically identify slowly healing fractures, have recently been described. These new techniques require further evaluation before they can be recommended for widespread use.

Other workers have shown that, following intraosseous injection, a radiopaque dye does not cross the fracture line in non-union (Kaski 1971), whereas it does in normally healing fractures and in delayed union. The passage of dye from one fragment to the other apparently indicates that medullary continuity has been re-established; this does not occur in non-union. Gupta *et al.* (1980) described an additional feature in non-union, that is, pooling of dye at the injection site. However, recent work by Connolly *et al.* (1984) and by Oni *et al.* (1988) has cast some doubt on the reliability of this technique.

Osteophony, or the ability of bone to transmit sound, was offered as a possible diagnostic tool by Tillman as long ago as 1899. The ability of a bone to vibrate changes after fracture and during the healing process, and attempts have been made to use this to distinguish normal from slowly healing fractures. In the percussion–auscultation method, one end of the bone is struck and the sound is detected at the other end with a stethoscope (Misurya *et al.* 1987) or with a more sophisticated device (Sekiguchi & Hirayama 1979). Reliable diagnostic criteria have not yet been established. The impedance techniques utilize transducers to measure the frequencies of resonance produced in fractured bones (Campbell & Jurist 1971, Christensen *et al.* 1982). The results are inconsistent, partly because of damping by soft tissues and interstitial oedema. Finally, various centres have investigated the use of ultrasound (Floriani *et al.* 1967) in the diagnosis of slow healing of fractures, but the variability of the soft tissue interface decreases the accuracy of the method (Abendschein & Hyatt 1972).

The resistance of bone to stress, generally referred to as its stiffness, provides a mechanical measure of return to function after fracture (Frost 1964, Perren 1981). Changes in stiffness apparently reflect the gradual change in the nature of the fracture repair tissue with time (Lettin 1965). Hence, measurements of fracture stiffness have been used to assess fracture healing. Unfortunately, non-invasive methods, such as the radiological technique developed by Hammer *et al.* (1984), are inaccurate while the more reliable methods, such as the one proposed by Jernberger (1970), are unacceptably invasive.

Aetiology of non-union

The balance of evidence currently available suggests that local factors are more important in the causation of slow healing; only rarely have systemic factors been implicated. A number of factors related to the injury or treatment have been identified as contributing to slow healing and these have recently been reviewed by Oni (1987). The factors associated with injury include damage to the blood supply of the fracture fragments, high-energy injuries causing extensive soft tissue and periosteal damage, and open and multiple fractures. The factors associated with treatment include poor immobilization, distraction, open reduction and infection.

In spite of a voluminous literature, the aetiology of delayed and non-union remains unknown. The stimulus for bone formation in healing fractures is unknown but may be a chemical one (Trueta 1963, Urist 1965). Some workers, notably Hulth (1980, 1990), suggest a role for genetic mechanisms and others believe that feedback mechanisms, involving electrical (Yasuda 1954), nervous, endocrine (Koskinen 1967) and mechanical (Kenwright *et al.* 1987) factors, are important.

A fracture begins to heal as soon as the bone is broken (Tonna & Cronkite 1961). Within a week, new bone formation is histologically apparent even in fractures of adult diaphyseal bone (Fig. 11.37) and, as shown in Fig. 11.38, all the tissues of osseous origin, i.e. periosteum, marrow and cortex, are capable of contributing to the fracture callus. McKibbin (1978) proposed that two healing processes are involved (Fig. 11.39): a primary callus response mounted by the osseous tissues themselves, and a bridging callus response derived from the surrounding soft tissues. It is not known which of these healing processes are deranged in delayed and non-union.

Classification of non-union

Ununited fractures may be classified as:
1 Radiological
   (a) Hypertrophic.
   (b) Atrophic (hypotrophic).
2 Histological
   (a) Fibrous.
   (b) Cartilaginous.
   (c) Pseudoarthrosis.

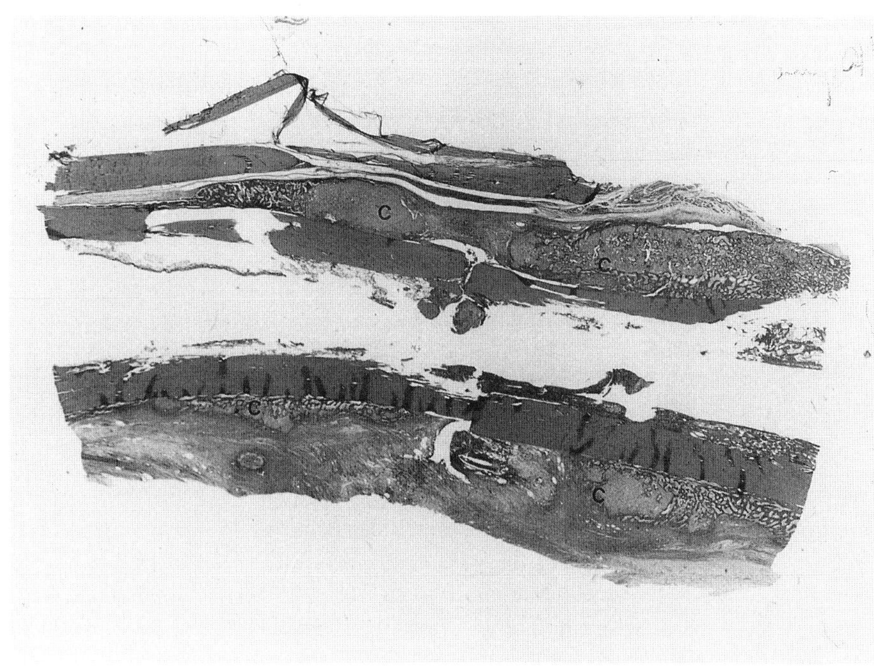

Fig. 11.37 Photomicrograph of a histological section of a healing osteotomy of the rabbit tibia 1 week after operation showing external callus formation.

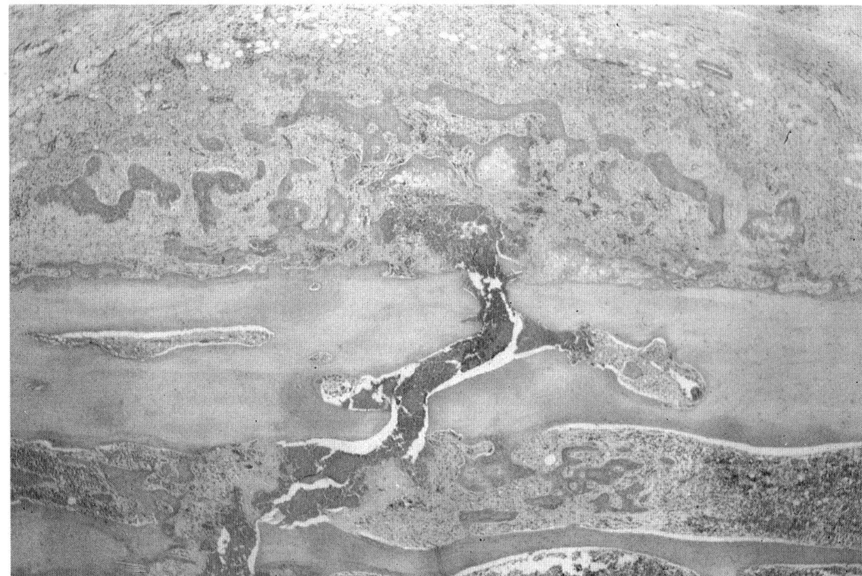

Fig. 11.38 Photomicrograph of a histological section of a healing human rib fracture showing callus surrounding the fractured bone ends.

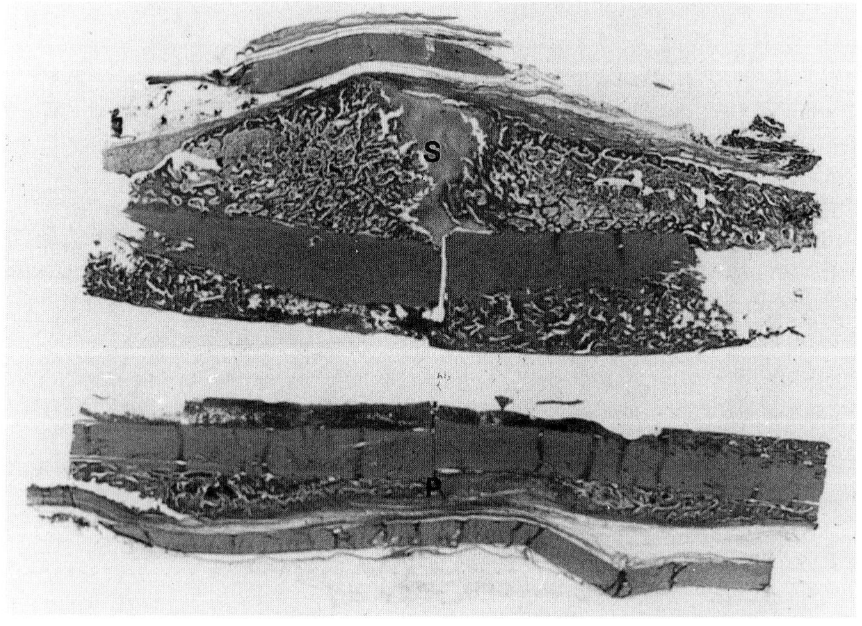

Fig. 11.39 Photomicrograph of a histological section of a healing osteotomy of the rabbit tibia showing McKibbin's primary (P) and secondary (S) callus responses.

3 Blood supply
  (a) Vascular.
  (b) Avascular.
4 Infection
  (a) Non-infected.
  (b) Previously infected.
  (c) Currently infected.

This classification is necessary for developing a rational treatment policy. The important factors in classification include the type of non-union, the vascularity, whether infection is present and whether there is an associated tissue defect or concurrent pathological change, such as malalignment, joint stiffness or osteoporosis.

Non-unions are often classified from their appearances on plain radiographs as hypertrophic or atrophic (hypotrophic).

In *hypertrophic non-union* (Fig. 11.40) a large amount of fracture callus is commonly observed, giving rise to the 'elephant foot' appearance. According to Charnley (1971), the function of the external callus is essentially a mechanical one. Consequently, the more movement there is at a fracture site, the more periosteal callus there will be formed as a result of the attempt to bridge the fracture gap as well as stabilize the fracture. The callus

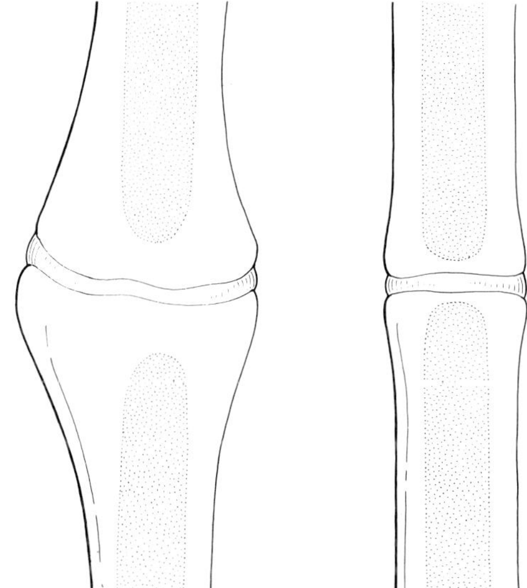

Fig. 11.40 Diagram showing different types of hypertrophic non-union.

is composed of bone, cartilage and fibrous tissue and the fracture will unite with minor adjustments to treatment (Frost 1989). On the other hand, a *hypertrophic* non-union may eventually progress to a *pseudoarthrosis* (Urist *et al.* 1954).

In the *atrophic* variety (Fig. 11.41) the bone ends are sclerotic, tapered and rounded-off and the medullary cavity is blocked (as it may also be in the hypertrophic variety). The affected bone itself is often porotic. There is very little periosteal new bone formation, possibly as the result of an inherent defect of bone repair. This type of non-union is considerably more resistant to treatment.

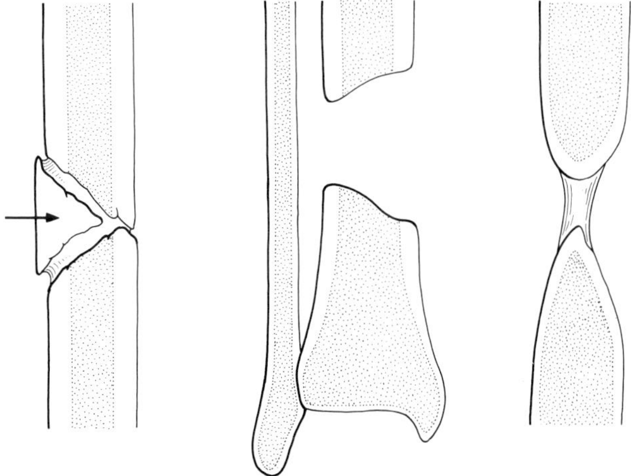

Fig. 11.41 Diagram showing different types of atrophic non-union.

HISTOLOGY

A non-union may be classified histologically as fibrous union, cartilaginous union or pseudoarthrosis.

In *fibrous union* the fracture site is bridged with scar tissue, which Sevitt (1981) believes can be converted to bone by applying a stimulus. In practice, some method of repetitive loading of the fracture is advocated (Sarmiento & Latta 1980). Others, notably Brighton *et al.* (1984), have used electrical stimulation.

A certain amount of cartilage is formed at the fracture site during normal healing (Ham & Cormack 1979) and this is normally converted to bone by a process of endochondral ossification. The cartilage may persist longer than usual in some fractures; the so-called *cartilaginous union*.

Inadequate immobilization could, in theory, cause shearing of the tissues at the fracture site. Some workers believe that this leads to inadequate vascularization at the fracture site with subsequent increased cartilage formation. Persistent motion then results in myxoid degeneration and liquefaction of the cartilage with the formation of a false joint or *pseudoarthrosis* (Sevitt 1981). However, the formation of a pseudoarthrosis may begin much earlier: Fig. 11.42 shows an experimental fracture of the adult rabbit tibia 2 weeks after operation where persistent motion at the fracture site has led to the formation of pseudosynovium; cartilage formation is not much in evidence. It is apparent from Fig. 11.39 that established pseudoarthrosis can be healed only after excision.

BLOOD SUPPLY

Although the results of different studies reveal adequate vascularization at sites of non-union (Ficat *et al.* 1984), some workers, notably Judet *et al.* (1958) and Weber and Cech (1976), have classified non-unions according to their probable vascularity as vascular or avascular.

The fractured bone ends are believed to be very well vascularized in the former and poorly vascularized in the latter. In the various texts adopting this classification, the term vascular non-union appears to be used interchangeably with hypertrophic non-union, and avascular non-union appears to be synonymous with atrophic non-union.

INFECTION

With regard to infection, non-unions may be classified as non-infected, previously infected or currently infected.

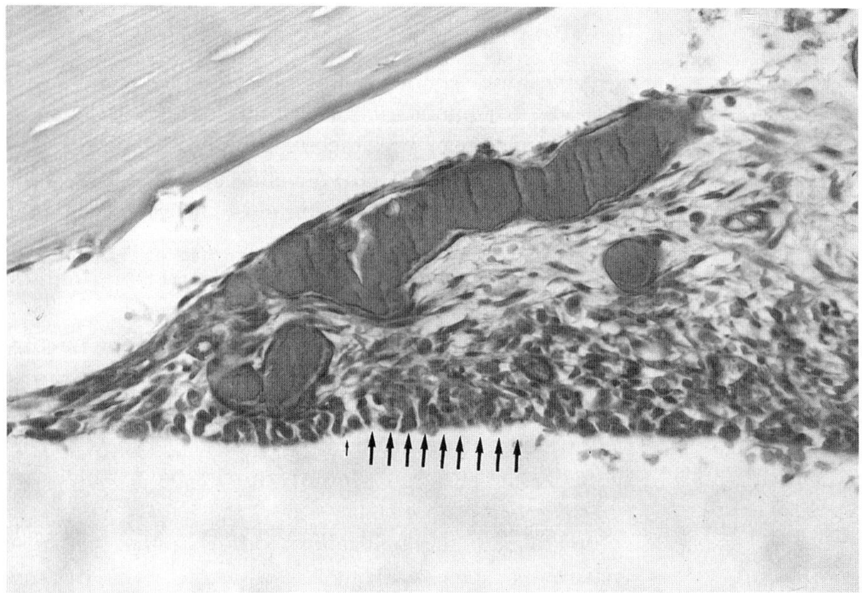

Fig. 11.42 Photomicrograph of a histological section of a healing osteotomy of the rabbit tibia showing pseudosynovium.

In the first variety the fracture site has never been infected. In the second variety the fracture site is free of infection at the time of treatment for non-union. The previous infection was probably responsible for the non-union and a large segment of each fragment may be relatively avascular. In addition, there may be a significant gap between the bone ends as a result of previous attempts to eradicate the infection. Hence, a *previously infected* non-union may be resistant to treatment even though the fracture is no longer infected.

In a *currently infected* ununited fracture there is evidence of continuing infection. Pus within the fracture cleft may impede the migration and differentiation of bone-forming cells and osteomyelitis may result in poor vascularization. Long segments of the fracture fragments may be affected and, therefore, an actively infected non-union poses formidable problems of management.

Associated pathological conditions

Slowly healing fractures are sometimes associated with other pathological conditions which may determine the prognosis or the method of treatment. Such pathological conditions include:
1 Tissue 'defects'
  (a) Bone.
  (b) Skin/soft tissues.
2 Malalignment
  (a) Angular.
  (b) Rotational.
  (c) Shortening.
3 Joint stiffness.
4 Sudek's syndrome — (reflex sympathetic osteodystrophy).

Tissue 'defects'

Ununited fractures are sometimes associated with gaps and defects within the tissues in their vicinity and this has been used for classification. The 'defect' may be in the bone or in the skin/soft tissues.

Bony defects result in significant fracture gaps which cannot be bridged by normal repair processes. Instead, the fracture site is invaded by fibrous scar tissue. These fractures require some form of bone grafting before they will heal.

Most of the repair tissue formed at the site of a fracture is derived from the osseous and extraosseous soft tissues; the hard tissue contributes only a small amount, if at all. Therefore, if a fracture site is denuded of soft tissue cover it is unable to unite. With regard to *skin* and *soft tissue defects*, split-thickness grafts will not survive on bare cortical bone. Therefore, granulation tissue covering may need to be encouraged by techniques such as decortication. Local, distant or free muscle or myocutaneous grafts may be required.

Malalignment

In addition to non-union, the fracture fragments may not be anatomically aligned in relation to each other. This may make internal fixation difficult or impossible. The malalignment may interfere with function after the fracture has eventually healed or may give rise to an objectionable appearance. Angular and rotational deformities may be readily corrected by operation but the restoration of length is often impossible without sophisticated manoeuvres.

Joint stiffness

Ununited fractures are frequently complicated by joint stiffness which manifests as a reduction in the range of joint motion. Joint stiffness may give rise to significant morbidity and disability even after the non-union has been successfully treated.

The causes of joint stiffness are many and include prolonged immobilization. Muscles, particularly after significant trauma, tolerate prolonged immobilization very badly. In addition, fractures are associated with soft tissue damage, local haemorrhage and interstitial oedema. With immobility, this fluid, which is normally removed by muscle activity, accumulates and encourages fibrin deposits within the soft tissues; these deposits are converted into fibrous tissue. This leads to fibrous adhesions between muscle and bone. Fibrosis within the joint capsule and muscles may make the eventual restoration of normal joint movement very difficult.

Haemarthrosis due to associated joint injury may result in fibrinoid deposits and adhesions within the joint and these will further restrict joint movement. Under these circumstances the nutrition of the articular cartilage by the synovial fluid is disturbed and this may lead to secondary osteoarthrosis.

Sudek's syndrome (reflex sympathetic osteodystrophy)

Slowly healing fractures are sometimes associated with an irritative lesion of the sympathetic nerves. The skin overlying the injured bone is atrophic and shiny and the adjoining joints are stiff. Plain radiographs show a characteristic patchy osteoporosis. The patient may complain of pain, particularly when the limb is touched or moved. Recovery from this condition is slow and may take several months.

Treatment

Much unproven dogma surrounds the treatment of ununited fractures; one extreme advocates rigid fixation and nothing else, while another favours prolonged immobilization with or without additional efforts to promote osteogenesis. Others, notably Boyd (1943) and Ilizarov (1984), believe that stable fixation, good apposition of fracture fragments and an environment which promotes osteogenesis are all necessary for success.

Principles

The goals of treatment are the achievement of union and the restoration of normal anatomy and function. Union may be achieved by removing the causes of the non-union, such as inadequate bone contact, distraction, bone defects, instability and/or inadequate local blood supply. Dead or infected bone and fibrocartilaginous union may need to be excised to allow contact between healthy bones. In many non-unions the fragments are displaced, angulated or overriding and these deformities may need to be corrected to achieve normal function. A non-union may have good, limited or poor osteogenic potential: in non-unions with limited potential, osteogenesis will need to be stimulated; in non-unions with poor osteogenic potential, petalling or shingling (Weber & Cech 1976) of the bone ends may be required. Joint stiffness may need to be treated by arthrolysis and osteoporosis by early mobilization. A good skin cover may need to be achieved before embarking on extensive bony procedures.

Methods

SURGICAL TREATMENT

To many surgeons delayed or non-union represents a failure of conservative treatment and, therefore, ununited fractures are frequently treated by surgical means.

Bone grafting

It has been known for over a century now that bone laid alongside an ununited fracture is able to stimulate its union. The graft provides a scaffold for 'creeping substitution' (Phemister 1947) by blood vessels and locally produced osteogenic cells. It also probably provides additional osteogenic cells and bone morphogenetic proteins (Urist 1965) which may induce the surrounding soft tissue (mesenchymal) cells to form bone.

In practice, bone grafts may be used to stimulate bony union, replace bony defects or aid the revascularization of avascular bone segments. The grafts may be obtained from cortical or cancellous bones. Massive cortical grafts were popularized by Campbell (1939) as onlay grafts and by Gill (1932) as sliding grafts (Fig. 11.43). Their main advantage is that they provide stability but they have poor osteogenic properties and are avascular. A further complication to watch out for is that fracture of the donor bed may occur; the tibia and the fibula are the most common sources.

Cancellous grafts implanted as corticocancellous strips around the ununited fracture (Fig. 11.44) are probably the most popular grafting technique used today. A cancellous graft is weak but cellular and, therefore, highly osteogenic. In addition, it is easily revascularized. The iliac crest and proximal tibia are the commonest sources. This method was initially popularized by Phemister (1914).

Osteosynthesis

In general, successful bone grafting requires good reduction, a sufficient amount of graft material and firm

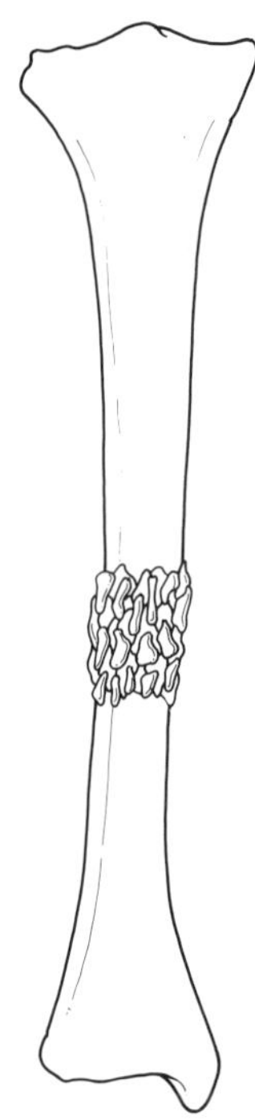

Fig. 11.44 Diagram showing cancellous bone grafts *in situ*.

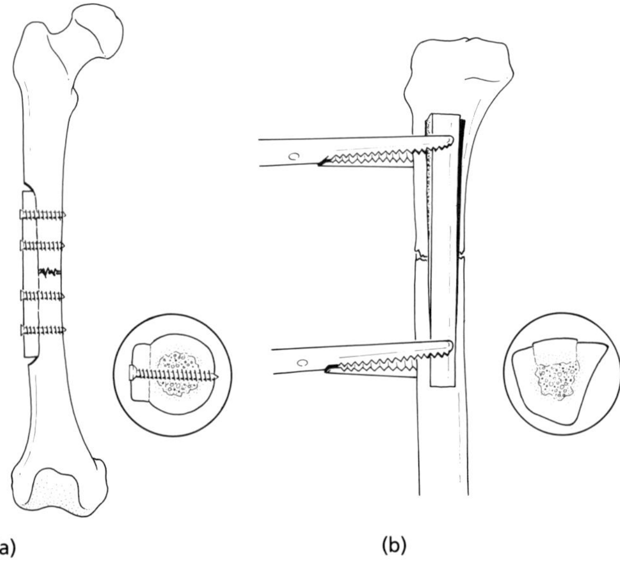

(a)　　　　　　　　　　　　　　(b)

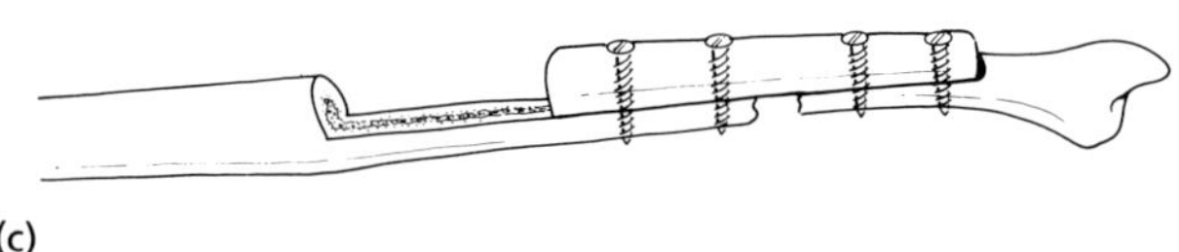

(c)

Fig. 11.43 Diagram showing (a) onlay, (b) inlay and (c) sliding grafts *in situ*.

stabilization, which is best achieved by conventional plating (Fig. 11.45) or intramedullary nailing (Fig. 11.46). Closed nailing has the advantage of not requiring a bone graft; the reamings from the marrow may provide a 'local internal' autogenous graft. Osteosynthesis has also been advocated to correct deformity and avoid further immobilization by plaster or other types of cast.

Other surgical methods

There are a number of miscellaneous procedures employed in the treatment of non-union at certain sites. Fibulectomy, with or without additional bone grafting, (DeLee *et al.* 1981) has been successfully employed in the treatment of non-union of the tibial shaft. The technique apparently improves stability at the fracture site.

NON-SURGICAL TREATMENT

Many modern writers appear to ignore the fact that ununited fractures can be, and commonly are, successfully treated by non-surgical means. The commonly used methods include casts and electrical stimulation (Patterson *et al.* 1980, Bassett *et al.* 1981, Brighton 1984, Connolly 1984).

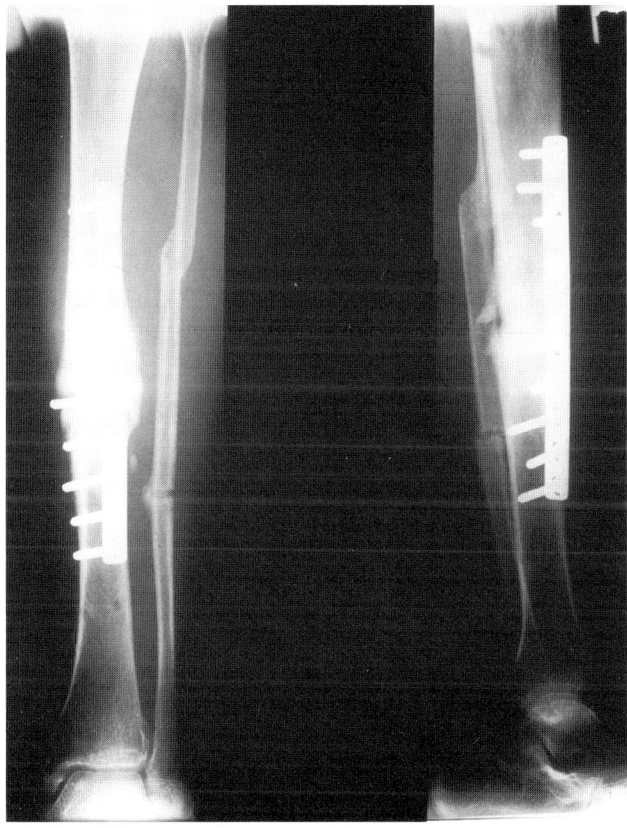

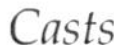

Fig. 11.45 Plain radiograph of a non-union of the tibia treated by plating.

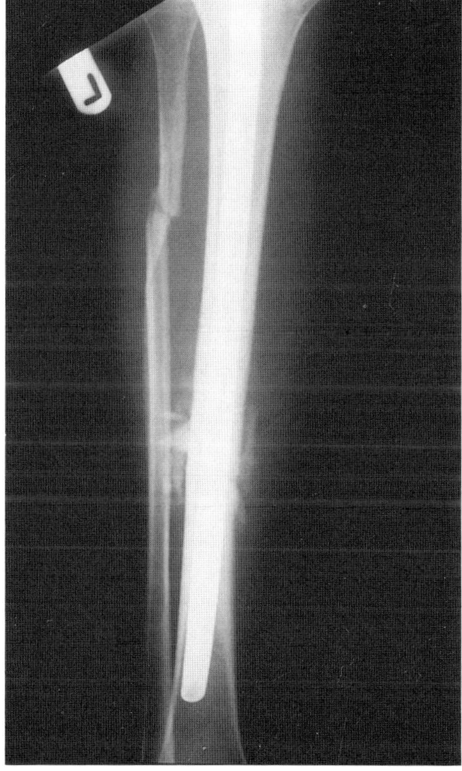

Fig. 11.46 Plain radiograph of a non-union treated by intramedullary nailing.

Casts

A patient who has invested some considerable time in conservative treatment may wish to continue with this if there was a possibility that the fracture will unite without surgical intervention. Recently, Oni *et al.* (1988) showed that most closed tibial shaft fractures which had not healed at the normal 20-week healing period did unite at 30 weeks after injury with continued cast treatment. However, prolonged immobilization may result in considerable morbidity; therefore, treatment by casts alone should be abandoned as soon as it becomes apparent that no further progress towards healing is occurring. At least, limited surgical intervention such as a fibulectomy to alter the mechanical environment or a bone graft alone (Reckling & Waters 1980) should be considered. The advantage of these methods is that they avoid the introduction of foreign material which may encourage infection.

Electrical stimulation

Where union is slow, in spite of adequate immobil-

ization, electrical stimulation may be considered. The hypertrophic non-union appears to be the most amenable.

The mechanism of action of electricity is uncertain but there are many hypotheses. Electricity is thought to stimulate osteogenesis by producing a change in the microenvironment at the fracture site in favour of calcification. Other workers have proposed that electricity realigns collagen molecules to make them attract calcium and phosphate ions. It has also been suggested that electricity activates the cyclic adenosine monophosphate (AMP) system.

Which form of electricity is the most efficient in stimulating or inducing osteogenesis is unclear. Success has been claimed for constant direct current, pulsing electromagnetic fields, slow pulsing asymmetrical direct current, alternating current and static fields (Connolly 1984). There are also differences in the techniques used to apply electrical stimulation. It is believed that invasive methods stimulate osteogenesis (Patterson *et al.* 1980) while non-invasive methods are inductive (Bassett *et al.* 1981). In invasive techniques (Fig. 11.47) electrodes, leads and power packs or a piece of Teflon electrect are

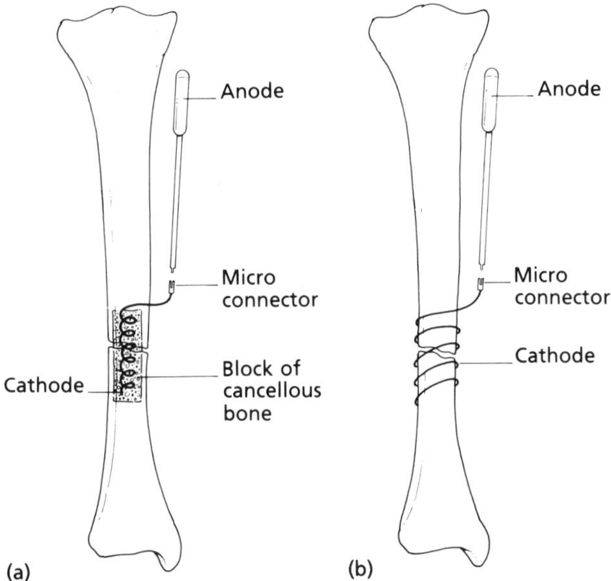

Fig. 11.47 (a) Diagram showing an implanted electrical stimulator of the invasive type.

implanted at the site of non-union. In the semi-invasive techniques (Fig. 11.48) only the cathode is inserted (Brighton 1984) and this can be done percutaneously. In the non-invasive inductive techniques (Fig. 11.49) the ununited fracture is left undisturbed and the currents are applied externally (Bassett *et al.* 1981). In spite of the voluminous literature on the subject, the true role of these expensive techniques in the management of non-union has not yet been established.

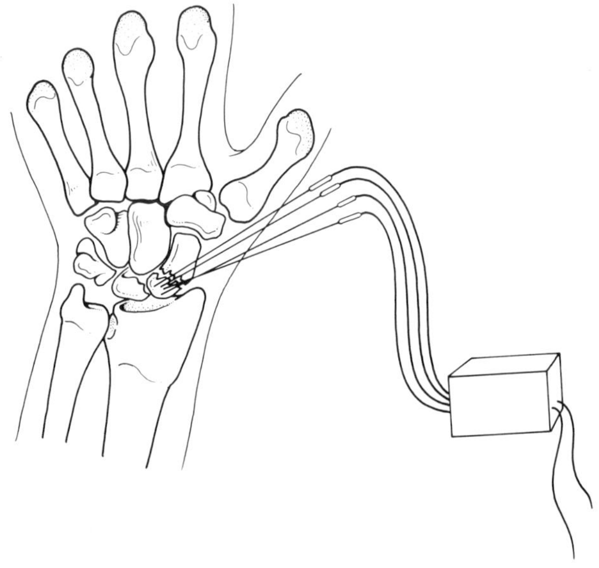

Fig. 11.48 Diagram showing an implanted electrical stimulator of the semi-invasive type.

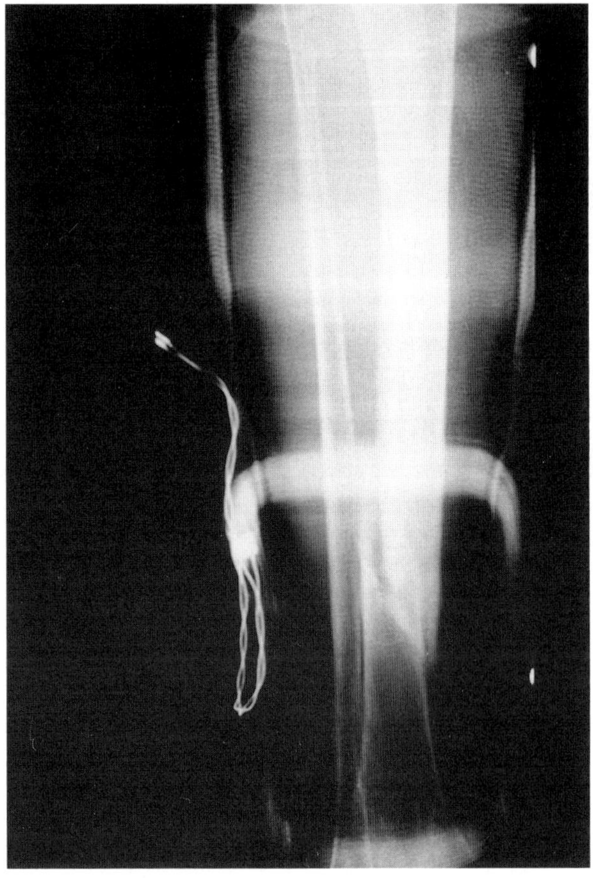

Fig. 11.49 Plain radiograph showing a non-invasive type of electrical stimulator.

Choice of treatment

Many factors need to be considered in the choice of treatment; these include:

1 *The patient* — what are the desired goals? Can the patient co-operate with the treatment regime? Are there other relevant disabilities?

2 *The limb* — what is the quality of the bone (and soft tissues)? Is there infection (or metal)? What is the state of the adjoining joints?

3 *The non-union* — what type is it? What is the osteogenic potential? What other associated lesions are there?

4 *The treatment* — what are the facilities available? What expertise is available?

The two most important investigations are plain radiographs, to determine the type of non-union and associated problems, and bone scintigraphy, to estimate the biological activity at the fracture site.

The decision to operate is relatively easy in cases of established non-union since no established non-union will unite without intervention. With atrophic non-union a bone graft is required but hypertrophic non-union may need only internal fixation. However, surgery for non-union is a major undertaking and certain considerations are essential before proceeding. First, since the procedure is likely to be extensive, it should not be undertaken lightly. Second, because the patient has probably been subjected to prolonged treatment and significant morbidity, it is advisable, where possible, to mobilize joints and re-educate muscles preoperatively. Third, 10% of patients with non-union will require two or more operations; therefore, it is most important that the surgeon determines preoperatively which biological mechanism should be stimulated. Finally, a 90% success rate is reported with bone grafting irrespective of whether or not fixation is used (Freeland & Mutz 1976, Reckling & Waters 1980). Therefore, the use of an implant is not essential unless it adds some positive factors to treatment.

The choice of treatment is more difficult in delayed union since the fracture is expected to unite eventually without surgical intervention. However, a number of factors should be taken into consideration before persevering with this line of treatment. First, the function of the affected limb may be so compromised that it may never be able to perform its normal functions properly again. Second, prolonged immobilization itself may increase morbidity by prolonging the recovery of function because of bone and muscle atrophy, joint stiffness and impaired local blood and lymphatic circulations. Third, there are financial and social costs associated with prolonged incapacity, particularly as most victims are young and are the 'breadwinners' of their families, and because the cost of prolonged treatment itself may be considerable.

Infected non-union

Despite many advances, the management of infected non-union (particularly of the tibia) presents a major challenge to any orthopaedic surgeon involved in post-trauma reconstruction. The objectives in management are to achieve:
1 Normal limb alignment and length.
2 Fracture healing.
3 Eradication of infection.
However, achieving such goals requires a logical multidisciplinary approach and, often, complex staged procedures are required. The five basic steps in the management of an infected non-union are:
1 Radically debride all infected/necrotic tissue.
2 Ensure effective antibiotic therapy.
3 Obtain stability of the fracture.
4 Obtain skin/soft tissue cover.
5 Obtain bone union.

Debridement

It is generally agreed that, in the management of an infected non-union, the first step is the removal of all infected or dead bone and soft tissue (Kelly 1984, Gustilo 1985, Cierny 1989b). All workers agree that debridement must be radical, but opinions differ as to the best method of ensuring that all dead tissue is resected. Kelly (1984) considers that visible bleeding is not a reliable sign and advocates the injection of a non-vital dye into the sinus track the day before operation. Tissue that remains stained is assumed to be non-viable and should be removed. Jenny *et al.* (1977) have described injecting a vital dye (Disulphine Blue) intravenously, which leaves dead tissue unstained.

Unfortunately, standard radiography, tomography and bone scanning are unreliable in distinguishing between living and dead bone (Wheat 1985). Both Cierny (1989a) and May *et al.* (1989) consider that tissue viability is best determined at operation by removing bone and soft tissue until active bleeding is seen. Cierny recommends resection of bone until there is uniform cortical and cancellous bleeding — the 'paprika sign' — while May *et al.* advocate the use of binocular loupe magnification.

Multiple cultures are taken during debridement surgery to allow adjustment of antibiotic regimes (see below). The wound is left open and further debridement performed 5–7 days later to ensure that all dead/infected tissue has been removed. Although time-consuming and tedious, meticulous and radical debridement remains the keystone of management (Kelly 1984).

Antibiotic therapy

Before debridement surgery an attempt should be made to determine the infecting organism. This may require a formal biopsy of the deeper part of the wound or fracture site. Once bacteria have been isolated, antibiotic sensitivities should be determined and treatment commenced with high-dose, appropriate antibiotics. Cierny (1989a) recommends that antibiotics are given for 5 days before the first debridement. Multiple cultures are taken at debridement surgery and antibiotics are adjusted as necessary on the basis of the organisms isolated and their sensitivities. Prolonged antibiotic therapy after debridement should be avoided if possible. Once the debrided wound is clean and biologically healthy, the rationale for systemic antibiotic therapy disappears.

Gentamicin — Polymethyl-methacrylate beads (Septopal) can be used to ensure high local levels of antibiotic in the debrided wound. Such beads have the added advantage of filling the resultant dead space (Cierny 1989b). Walenkamp *et al.* (1986) have demonstrated that *in vivo* the half-life of the gentamicin in the beads was between 5.7 and 10 days. Concentrations of gentamicin in the wound exudate were more than 300 times that of the serum concentration. It is usual to remove the beads 10—14 days after insertion, by which time 40—70% of the available gentamicin will have leached out of the beads. It is important to realize that very high local levels of gentamicin can only be achieved with the wound closed. Such a situation is often difficult to ensure in the initial management of an infected non-union. However, suitable techniques are available to achieve reliable skin and soft tissue cover at an early stage (see below).

Fracture stability

The importance of achieving and maintaining fracture stability, when managing an infected non-union, has been stressed by Burri (1975) in his extensive clinical review. The hypothesis that stability will favourably affect the outcome in established post-traumatic osteitis was studied experimentally by Rittmann and Perren (1974). They performed tibial osteotomies in sheep and fixed the osteotomies with plates of varying stiffness, giving three grades of stability. *Staphylococcus aureus*, in high concentrations, were injected into the wounds until infection ensued. Rittman and Perren concluded that rigid fixation of the osteotomy offered favourable conditions for bone healing and that the stabilizing effect of the implant outweighed the possible disadvantages of the foreign body effect.

Both Burri (1975) and Gustilo (1985) recommend the retention of an existing implant in an infected non-union if it is providing stability. If an implant is loose, then it should be removed. In such a situation, or where the infected non-union is unstable and has never undergone osteosynthesis, then some new means of stabilization must be found. The use of external fixation is widely favoured, particularly when the tibia is involved (Kelly 1984, Gustilo 1985, Jupiter *et al.* 1988). However, Gustilo (1985) recommends the use of plates as the first choice for stabilization of the femur, with intramedullary nails as the second choice.

When the external fixator is applied, the opportunity must be taken to correct the length and alignment of the bone. The use of an external fixator (or other implant) allows joint mobility to be regained and/or preserved.

The major problem of pin-track sepsis can be reduced by a careful insertion technique (Green 1983). Skin necrosis is prevented by adequate incisions for pin insertion and heat necrosis of bone is avoided by pre-drilling of the bone. Motion at the pin—skin interface can be reduced by the use of bulky, antiseptic-soaked dressings. Pins should be inserted, if possible, into subcutaneous areas of bone and the transfixation of muscle should be avoided.

It has been shown that the stability of the external fixator can be improved by increasing the number of pins, increasing the pin diameter, increasing the distance between pins and aligning the fixator as close to the bone as possible (Chao & Pope 1982). A unilateral external fixator is the easiest to apply and allows access to soft tissues. Such a frame can be modified to allow a small amount of axial movement, which seems important for fracture healing (Goodship & Kenwright 1985). However, in an infected non-union (particularly where there is a bone defect) movement at the fracture site should be avoided until infection has been eradicated. A more rigid frame is thus required initially and this can be achieved by using triangular or quadrilateral frames (Ackroyd 1989). Once the infection is under control, such frames can be progressively reduced in complexity and rigidity to encourage bone union.

Whatever method of skeletal stabilization is chosen, it will have to be maintained until radiological evidence of bone union, with resolution of infection, is seen.

Skin/soft tissue cover

There are four basic techniques for achieving skin and soft tissue cover of the debrided wound: secondary healing, local delayed closure, transposition flaps and free tissue transfer.

The use of secondary healing, when dealing with an infected non-union, is reserved for cases where an open cancellous bone graft is planned (the Papineau technique) to obtain bone union (see below). In all other cases, soft tissue reconstruction and closure should be performed when the debrided wound is clean. Cierny (1989b) recommends that soft tissue reconstruction should be performed 4—6 days after the final debridement.

Delayed primary closure may be performed when there is no skin loss. If there is a skin defect, the undermining of skin edges to achieve closure may result in compromising skin viability (Clifford 1989). Delayed closure is most likely to be useful on the humerus and femur, where a soft tissue envelope surrounds the bone completely.

Transposition flaps have been widely used to obtain skin cover and the last 30 years have seen major advances in flap design and management (Jackson 1976). The traditional tubed pedicle flap has now been superceded by newer techniques, as has the cross-leg flap. The cross-leg flap is, however, simple and may yet have a role in situations where there is no ready access to sophisticated plastic surgery techniques.

Modern transposition flaps are based on an understanding of the axial nature of skin blood flow and must be based on the deep fascia or supported by vascularized muscle (Clifford 1989). In the tibia, for instance, the proximal third can be covered by a gastrocnemius muscle flap, the middle third by a soleus muscle flap and the distal third by a fasciocutaneous flap (as initially described by Ponten in 1981).

Free flaps, based on a microsurgical vascular anastasmosis, are indicated at any site where the conditions of adjacent tissues prevents the use of a transposition flap. The two commonly used skin flaps are the groin flap, based on the superficial epigastric artery (MacGregor & Jackson 1972), and the delto-pectoral flap, based on the perforating branches of the internal mammary artery (Bakamjian 1965).

Soft tissue defects which expose large bone defects or areas of devascularized bone are best covered by a free muscle flap. The latissimus dorsi flap, based on the thoraco-dorsal artery, is widely used (Bailey & Godfrey 1982). This flap may be raised with overlying skin, as a free myocutaneous flap, or as a free muscle flap to be covered with a split-skin graft.

Large soft tissue defects with bone loss can be reconstructed in a simple procedure by transfer of a free composite flap consisting of skin, muscle and bone. The iliac osteocutaneous flap, based on the deep circumflex iliac artery (Taylor *et al.* 1979), provides a segment of straight iliac crest, 6—8 cm long, and overlying skin. Bone defects which are longer than 8 cm require a vascularized fibular graft. The osteoseptocutaneous fibular flap (Wei *et al.* 1986) provides a vascularized fibula and area of overlying lateral skin.

Bone healing

The technique used to obtain bone union depends to a large extent on the size of the defect to be bridged. Defects of less than 6 cm can often be bridged by cancellous bone grafts (Green & Dlabal 1983). For defects over 6 cm other techniques are preferred because of the delay in remodelling and formation of cortical bone.

There are essentially four techniques available to obtain bone union.

1 *Open cancellous bone grafting*. This is also known as the Papineau technique (1973). After debridement, the wound dressings are changed daily until healthy granulation tissue covers the defect. Cancellous bone graft is then harvested and packed into the defect, up to the level of the skin. Lortat-Jacob (1989) recommends avoiding the creation of an extensive, superficial defect at initial debridement as this makes it difficult to retain the bone graft in position. As soon as there is a layer of granulation tissue covering the bone graft, split-skin grafting is performed.

The technique requires that the wound is clean and sufficiently vascularized in order to support adequate granulation tissue. It is a time-consuming procedure and it may be months before the bone graft incorporates and remodels sufficiently to permit weight-bearing. The skin cover is also less durable. Nevertheless, it is a safe and simple technique for patients in whom a flap is unsuitable.

2 *Cancellous bone grafting under a flap*. The use of a transposition or free flap to cover a skin/soft tissue defect provides a vascular environment, suitable for cancellous bone grafting. The flap should have healed before bone grafting, which should be delayed for 3—4 weeks after flap construction (May *et al.* 1989). Care must be taken to avoid damage to the vascular pedicle of the flap when it is raised for insertion of the bone graft. The cancellous bone graft packed under such a vascularized flap generally revascularizes and incorporates quickly. Nevertheless, protected weight-bearing must be maintained until graft remodelling has occured.

3 *Distraction histogenesis*. This is also known as the Ilizarov technique and has been used in the Soviet Union since the 1950s (Paley 1988). The technique involves cutting through the cortex (corticotomy) of the bone, at a site distant from the defect, and slowly transporting this segment (along with the overlying soft tissue envelope) towards the bone defect, using a modified external fixator. This technique obviates the need for additional bone graft or flap cover.

The technique only requires a single reconstructive procedure after debridement. The length and alignment of the bone are controlled by the external fixator while distraction proceeds. Theoretically, a bone defect of any length can be closed by this technique. Nevertheless, the whole procedure is time-consuming and protected weight-bearing is necessary until the corticotomy-woven bone remodels and the defect unites. Further procedures may be necessary to encourage union at the defect site, even when the gap is closed.

4 *Free vascular bone grafts*. As described above, bone defects of less than 6—8 cm can be bridged by an iliac osteocutaneous flap. However, Salibian *et al.* (1987) have reported problems with the shape and strength of free iliac bone grafts and with the positioning of the graft and overlying skin in the defect.

For bone defects longer than 6–8 cm, a vascularized fibular graft is recommended (May *et al.* 1989). In an infected non-union of the tibia, if the ipsilateral fibula is intact, then this fibula can be raised on its peroneal vascular pedicle and transferred as a 'fibula–protibia' operation (Chacha *et al.* 1981). The fibula responds well to progressive weight-bearing and hypertrophies within 12–16 weeks from transfer (Sowa & Weiland 1987). Such a procedure is contraindicated when the peroneal artery is the only blood supply to the foot.

In other situations, a fibular osteoseptocutaneous flap is used, as described above. The shape, size and length of the fibula allows bridging of most defects. The overall success rate is high (Wood & Cooney 1984) and bone union can usually be expected within 3–5 months. However, the technique requires access to centres with microvascular expertise. The operative procedure is lengthy and there are significant risks when it is performed in a situation where only one major artery is intact in the limb.

Conclusion

Management of infected non-union remains a difficult and time-consuming problem for the orthopaedic surgeon. Both patient and surgeon must understand the implications of 'travelling the road' to reconstruction, if triumphs of technique over reason are to be avoided. Once a reconstruction programme has begun, a logical and analytical approach to all facets of the problem must be followed, based on the principles of eradicating infection, obtaining soft tissue cover and bridging the bone defect, as has been described.

References

Abendschein, W.F. & Hyatt, G.W. Ultrasonics and physical properties of healing bone. *J Trauma* 1972; **12**: 297.

Ackroyd, C.E. External fixation. In: Coombs, R.H. & Fitzgerald, R.H. (eds) *Infection in the Orthopaedic Patient*. Butterworth: London, 1989.

Auchincloss, J.M. & Watt, I. Scintigraphy in the evaluation of potential fracture healing: a clinical study of tibial fractures. *Br J Radiol* 1982; **55**: 707.

Bailey, B.N. & Godfrey, A.M. Latissimus dorsi muscle free flaps. *Br J Plast Surg* 1982; **35**: 47–52.

Bakamjian, V.Y. A two-staged method for pharynoesophageal reconstruction with a primary pectoral skin flap. *Plast Reconstr Surg* 1965; **36**: 173–184.

Bassett, C.A.L., Mitchell, S.N. & Gaston, S.R. Treatment of ununited tibial diaphyseal fractures with pulsing electromagnetic fields. *J Bone Joint Surg* 1981; **63A**: 511.

Boyd, H.B. The treatment of difficult and unusual non-unions: with special reference to bridging of defects. *J Bone Joint Surg* 1943; **25**: 535.

Brashear, H.R. Diagnosis and prevention of non union. *J Bone Joint Surg* 1965; **47A**: 174.

Brighton, C.T. The semi-invasive method of treating nonunion with direct current. *Orthop Clin North Am* 1984; **15**: 33.

Burri, C. *Post-Traumatic Osteomyelitis*. Hans Huber: Berne, 1975.

Campbell, J.N. & Jurist, J.M. Mechanical impedance of the femur: a preliminary report. *J Biomech* 1971; **4**: 319.

Campbell, W.C. Onlay bone graft for ununited fractures. *Arch Surg* 1939; **38**: 313.

Chacha, P.B., Ahmed, M. & Daruwalla, J.S. Vascular pedicle graft of the ipsilateral fibula for non-union of the tibia with a large defect. *J Bone Joint Surg* 1981; **63B**: 244–253.

Chao, E.Y.S. & Pope, M.H. The mechanical basis of external fixation. In: Seligson, D. & Pope, M.H. (eds) *Concepts in External Fixation*. Grune & Stratton: New York, 1982.

Charnley, J. *The Closed Treatment of Common Fractures*. Churchill Livingstone: Edinburgh, 1971.

Christensen, A.B., Tougaard, L., Dyrbye, C. & Vibe-Hansen, H. Resonance of the human tibia. Method, reproducibility and effect of transection. *Acta Orthop Scand* 1982; **53**: 867.

Cierny, G. The staging of adult osteomyelitis. In: Coombs, R.H. & Fitzgerald, R.H. (eds) *Infection in the Orthopaedic Patient*. Butterworth: London, 1989a.

Cierny, G. Managing the debridement defect. In: Coombs, R.H. & Fitzgerald, R.H. (eds) *Infection in the Orthopaedic Patient*. Butterworth: London, 1989b.

Clifford, R.P. Skin cover in open tibial fractures. In: Bunker, T.D., Colton, C.L. & Webb, J.K. (eds) *Frontiers in Fracture Surgery*. Martin Dunitz: London, 1989.

Connolly, J.F. Electrical treatment of non-union. Its use and abuse in 100 consecutive fractures. *Orthop Clin North Am* 1984; **15**: 89.

Connolly, J.F., Chakkalakal, D. & Kelbel, M. Clinical and experimental use of intraosseous venography to assess fracture union. In: Arlet, J., Ficat, R.P. & Hungerford, D.S. (eds) *Bone Circulation*. Williams & Wilkins: Baltimore, 1984.

Danis, R. *Theorie et pratique de l'osteosynthese*. Masson: Paris, 1949.

DeLee, J.C., Heckman, J.D. & Lewis, A.G. Partial fibulectomy for ununited fractures of the tibia. *J Bone Joint Surg* 1981; **63A**: 1390.

Ficat, P., Horvath, E., Durroux, R., Boussaton, M. & Senve, J.N. Bone circulation in fractures and pseudarthroses. In: Arlet, J., Ficat, R.P. & Hungerford, D.S. (eds) *Bone Circulation*. Williams & Wilkins: Baltimore, 1984.

Floriani, L.P., Debevoise, N.T. & Hyatt, G.W. Mechanical properties of healing bone by the use of ultrasound. *Surg Forum* 1967; **18**: 468.

Freeland, A.E. & Mutz, S.B. Posterior bone grafting for infected ununited fracture of the tibia. *J Bone Joint Surg* 1976; **58A**: 653.

Frost, H.M. *Mathematical Elements of Lamellar Bone Remodelling*. CCT, Springfield, 1964.

Frost, H.M. The biology of fracture healing. Part II. An overview for clinicians. *Clin Orthop* 1989; **248**: 294.

Galasko, C.S.B. The pathological basis for skeletal scintigraphy.

J Bone Joint Surg 1975; **57B**: 353.

Galasko, C.S.B. In: Galasko, C.S.B. & Weber, D.A. (eds) *Radio-nuclide Scintigraphy in Orthopaedics*. Churchill Livingstone: Edinburgh, 1984.

Gill, A.B. Treatment of ununited fracture of the bones of the forearm. *Surg Clin North Am* 1932; **12**: 1535.

Goodship, A. & Kenwright, J. The influence of induced micromovement upon the healing of experimental tibial fractures. *J Bone Joint Surg* 1985; **67B**: 650−655.

Green, S.A. Complications of external skeletal fixation. *Clin Orthop* 1983; **180**: 109−116.

Green, S.A. & Dlabal, T.A. The open bone graft for septic non-union. *Clin Orthop* 1983; **180**: 117−124.

Gregg, P.J., Barsoum, M.K. & Clayton, C.B. Scintigraphic appearance of the tibia in the early stages following fracture. *Clin Orthop* 1983; **175**: 139.

Gregg, P.J., Clayton, C.B., Fenwick, J.D., Ions, G.K., Miller, S.W.M. & Smith, S.R. Static and sequential dynamic scintigraphy of the tibia following fracture. *Injury* 1984, **17**: 95.

Gupta, R.C., Kumar, S. & Gupta, K.K. A clinical evaluation of osteomedullography in diaphyseal fractures. *J Trauma* 1980; **20**: 507.

Gustilo, R.B. Current concepts in the management of infected fractures. In: Uhthoff, H.K. (ed.) *Current Concepts of Infections in Orthopaedic Surgery*. Springer−Verlag: Berlin, 1985.

Ham, A.W. & Cormack, D.H. *The Histophysiology of Cartilage, Bone and Joints*. Lippincott: Philadelphia, 1979.

Hammer, R., Edholm, P. & Lindholm, B. Stability of union after tibial shaft fracture. *J Bone Joint Surg* 1984; **66B**: 529.

Hulth, A. Fracture healing: a concept of competing factors. *Acta Orthop Scand* 1980; **51**: 5.

Hulth, A. Current concepts of fracture healing. *Clin Orthop* 1990; **249**: 265.

Ilizarov, G.A. Treatment of pseudoarthroses and defects of the long tubular bones using distraction stress and compression stress with author's apparatus for transosseous osteosynthesis. *Sci Publ Kniiekot Inst* (Kurgan, USSR) 1984; **9**: 48.

Illingworth, G.I. & Schiess, F.A. Strontium 87m in the prognosis of fractures of the tibia. *Proc R Soc Med* 1971; **64**: 633.

Jackson, I.T. Flaps: design and management. In: Calman, J. (ed.) *Recent Advances in Plastic Surgery I*. Churchill Livingstone: Edinburgh, 1976.

Jacobs, R.R., Jackson, R.P., Preston, D.F., Williamson, J.A. & Gallagher, J. Dynamic bone scanning in fractures. *Injury* 1979; **12**: 455.

Jenny, G., Kempf, I., Jaegar, J.H. *et al*. Coloration vitale au bleu de disulphine dans la cure chirurgicale de l'infection osseuse. *Rev Chir Orthop* 1977; **63**: 531−636.

Jernberger, A. Measurement of stability of tibial fractures. A mechanical method. *Acta Orthop Scand Suppl* 1970; **135**: 1−88.

Judet, R., Judet, J. & Roy-Camille, . La vascularisation des pseudarthroses des os long. *Rev Chir Orthop* 1958; **44**: 381.

Jupiter, J.B., First, K., Gallico, G.G. *et al*. The role of external fixation in the treatment of post-traumatic osteomyelitis. *J Orthop Trauma* 1988; **2**: 79−93.

Kaski, P. Osteomedullography of the tibia. Intraosseous phlebography with compression of the soft tissue veins. *Acta Radiol Suppl* 1971; **312**.

Kelly, P.J. Infected non-union of the femur and tibia. *Orthop Clin North Am* 1984; **15**: 481−490.

Kenwright, J., Richardson, J.P., Goodship, A.E., Evans, M.,

Kelly, D.J., Spriggins, A.J., Newman, J.H., Burroughs, J.J., Harris, J.D. & Rowley, D.I. Effect of controlled axial micromovement on healing of tibial fractures. *Lancet* 1976; **iii**: 1185.

Koskinen, E.V.S. Effect of endocrine factors on callus development in experimental fractures. *Symp Biol Hung* 1967; **7**: 315.

Lettin, A.W.F. The effects of axial compression on the healing of experimental fractures of the rabbit tibia. *Proc Roy Soc Med* 1965; **58**: 882.

Lortat-Jacob, A. The Papineau technique. In: Coombs, R.H. & Fitzgerald, R.H. (eds) *Infection in the Orthopaedic Patient*. Butterworth: London, 1989.

May, J.W., Jupiter, J.B., Weiland, A.J. *et al*. Clinical classification of post-traumatic tibial osteomyelitis. *J Bone Joint Surg* 1989; **71A**: 1422−1428.

MacGregor, I.A. & Jackson, I.T. The groin flap. *Br J Plast Surg* 1972; **22**: 3−16.

McKibbin, B. The biology of fracture healing of long bones. *J Bone Joint Surg* 1978; **60B**: 150.

Misurya, R.K., Khare, A., Mallick, A., Sural, A. & Vishwakarma, G.K. Use of tuning fork in diagnostic auscultation of fractures. *Injury* 1987; **18**: 63.

Oni, O.O.A. *Delayed Union of Fractures of the Shaft of the Adult Tibia: A Clinical and Experimental Study*. MD thesis: University of Leicester, 1987.

Oni, O.O.A., Pearse, M., Graebbe, A. & Gregg, P.J. Prediction of the healing potential of closed adult tibial shaft fractures by bone scintigraphy. *Clin Orthop* 1989; **245**: 239.

Oni, O.O.A., Stafford, H. & Gregg, P.J. An investigation of the routes of venous drainage from the bone marrow of the human tibial diaphysis. *Clin Orthop* 1988; **230**: 237.

Paley, D. Current techniques of limb lengthening. *J Pediatr Orthop* 1988; **8**: 73−92.

Papineau, L.J. L'excision — greffe avec fermeture retardee de liberee dans l'osteomyelite chronique. *Nouve Presse Med* 1973; **2**: 2753−2755.

Patterson, D.C., Lewis, G.N. & Cass, C.A. Treatment of delayed union and non-union with an implanted direct current stimulator. *Clin Orthop* 1980; **148**: 117.

Perkins, G. *Fractures and Dislocations*. Athlone Press: London, 1958.

Perren, S.M. Physical and biological aspects of fracture healing with special reference to internal fixation. *Clin Orthop* 1979; **138**: 175.

Phemister, D.B. The fate of transplanted bone and regenerative power of its various constituents. *Surg Gynecol Obstet* 1914; **19**: 303.

Phemister, D.B. Treatment of ununited fractures by onlay bone grafts without screw or tie fixation and without breaking down the fibrous union. *J Bone Joint Surg* 1947; **29**: 946.

Ponten, B. The fasciocutaneous flap: its use in soft tissue defects of the lower leg. *Br J Plast Surg* 1981; **34**: 215−220.

Reckling, F.W. & Waters, C.H. Treatment of non-union of fractures of the tibial diaphysis by posterolateral cortical cancellous bone grafting. *J Bone Joint Surg* 1980; **62A**: 936.

Rittmann, W.W. & Perren, S.M. *Cortical Bone Healing After Internal Fixation and Infection*. Springer-Verlag: Berlin, 1974.

Salibian, A.H., Anzel, S.H. & Salyer, W.A. Transfer of vascularised grafts of iliac bone to the extremities. *J Bone Joint Surg* 1987; **69A**: 1319−1327.

Sarmiento, A., Latta, L.L. *Closed Functional Treatment of Fractures*. Springer-Verlag: Berlin, 1981.

Sekiguchi, T. & Hirayama, T. Assessment of fracture healing by vibration. *Acta Orthop Scand* 1979; **50**: 391.

Sevitt, S. *Bone Repair and Fracture Healing in Man*. Churchill Livingstone: Edinburgh, 1981.

Smith, M.A., Jones, E.A., Strachan, R.K., Nicoll, J.J., Best, J.J.K., Tothill, P. & Hughes, S.P.F. Prediction of fracture healing in the tibia by quantitative radionuclide imaging. *J Bone Joint Surg* 1987; **68B**: 441.

Sowa, D.T. & Weiland, A.J. Clinical applications of vascularised bone autografts. *Orthop Clin North Am* 1987; **18**: 257–273.

Taylor, G.I., Townsend, P. & Corlett, R. Superiority of the deep circumflex iliac vessels as the supply for free groin flaps. *Plast Reconstr Surg* 1979; **64(6)**: 745–759.

Tillman, H. *Textbook of Surgery*, Vol I. Appleton: New York, 1899.

Tonna, E.A. & Cronkite, E.P. Cellular response to fracture; studies with tritiated thymidine. *J Bone Joint Surg* 1961; **43A**: 352.

Trueta, J. The role of vessels in osteogenesis. *J Bone Joint Surg* 1963; **45B**: 402.

Urist, M.R. Bone formation by autoinduction. *Science* 1965; **150**: 893.

Urist, M.R., Marzet, R. Jr. & McLean, F.C. The pathogenesis and treatment of delayed union and non-union. A survey of eighty-five ununited fractures of the shaft of the tibia and one hundred control cases with similar injuries. *J Bone Joint Surg* 1954; **34A**: 931.

Walenkamp, G.H.I.M., Vree, T.B. & Van Rens, T.J.G. Gentamicin — PMMA beads. Pharmacokinetic and nephrotoxicological study. *Clin Orthop* 1986; **205**: 171–183.

Watson-Jones, R. & Coltart, W.D. Slow union of fractures with a study of 804 fractures of the shafts of the tibia and femur. *Br J Surg* 1943; **30**: 260.

Weber, B.G. & Cech, O. *Pseudarthrosis*. Hans Huber: Berne, 1976.

Wei, F.C., Chen, H.C., Chuang, C.C. *et al*. Fibula osteoseptocutaneous flap: anatomic study and clinical applications. *Plast Reconstr Surg* 1986; **78(2)**: 191–199.

Wheat, J. Diagnostic strategies in osteomyelitis. *Am J Med* 1985; **78**: 218–224.

Wood, M.B. & Cooney, W.P. Vascularised bone segment transfers for management of chronic osteomyelitis. *Orthop Clin North Am* 1984; **15**: 461–472.

Yasuda, L. On the piezoelectric activity of bone. *J Jap Orthop Surg Soc* 1954; **28**: 267.

Post-traumatic reflex sympathetic dystrophy

D.P.CONLAN

The term 'reflex sympathetic dystrophy' encompasses several clinical syndromes that are characterized by burning pain, hyperaesthesiae, oedema, hyperhydrosis and trophic changes of skin, muscle and bone (Bonica 1979). The synonym 'algoneurodystrophy' (Greek, algos = pain) was introduced by French rheumatologists in the nineteenth century. The alternative terms 'post-traumatic dystrophy' and 'algodystrophy' have been generated by those authorities who question the involvement of the sympathetic nervous system.

Historical perspective

In 1864 Mitchell, as a result of his experience in the American Civil War, coined the term 'causalgia' (Greek, kausis = heat; algos = pain) for the pain syndrome associated with injuries of major mixed nerves (Mitchell *et al*. 1864). In 1940 Homans acknowledged that, in some cases, there was no gross evidence of nerve injury and applied the term 'minor causalgia' to patients in whom there was thought to be covert damage to a sensory nerve.

Although Volkmann was the first to recognize post-traumatic rarefaction of bone, it was Sudeck (1900) who described the full clinical and radiological features of 'post-traumatic acute atrophy of bone'. The term 'Sudeck's atrophy' should therefore be reserved for those cases in which characteristic bone demineralization is evident.

The shoulder–hand syndrome was first described by Steinbrocker (1947) and most commonly occurs in older patients after myocardial infarction, cerebrovascular accident or with cervical radiculopathy. Such patients suffer from a typical 'frozen shoulder' in addition to reflex sympathetic dystrophy of the upper limb.

Classification

Thus, several clinical syndromes have been given different designations by virtue of the predominant clinical features or precipitating factor. In order to rationalize the situation, Lankford suggested classification of reflex sympathetic dystrophy into the causalgias (due to direct nerve trauma) and the post-traumatic dystrophies (Lankford & Thompson 1977) (Table 11.9). It is implicit in this system that the terms 'major' and 'minor' reflect

Table 11.9 Lankford's classification of reflex sympathetic dystrophy

	Type of injury
Causalgias	
Major	Mixed nerve
Minor	Sensory nerve
Traumatic dystrophies	
Major	Major skeletal injury, e.g. a fracture
Minor	Soft tissue injury, e.g. a sprain

the extent of the precipitating tissue damage and not the severity of the symptoms.

Pathogenesis

Three conditions are thought to be required for reflex sympathetic dystrophy to develop. These are:
1 A precipitating event.
2 A diathesis or predisposition.
3 An abnormal sympathetic response.

Precipitating causes

Causalgia is most commonly precipitated by a high-velocity injury, resulting in incomplete division of a peripheral nerve. The overall prevalence of causalgia has been estimated at between 3 and 5% of such injuries and is more commonly seen following trauma in the proximal part of the limb; damage to the sciatic nerve accounts for 40% and damage to the median nerve accounts for a further 35% of cases. In more than two-thirds of patients who subsequently develop causalgia, characteristic symptoms appear within the first week of the injury; late onset, a month or more after the injury, occurs in only 5%. It is claimed that early debridement and vascular repair reduces the risk of subsequently developing causalgia.

Of the other reflex sympathetic dystrophies, although a specific precipitant cannot be found in up to 35% of cases, accidental trauma is the most commonly identified cause and accounts for a further 30%.

Fractures of the wrist and hand most frequently trigger the condition and, indeed, features consistent with reflex sympathetic dystrophy have been reported in up to 37% of patients 2 months after a Colles' fracture (Atkins *et al.* 1990). Other important antecedent events include hand and foot surgery, cerebral or spinal cord injury, vertebral crush fractures and surgical laminectomy. Reflex sympathetic dystrophy of the knee has also recently been recognized as an uncommon, but refractory, complication of knee injuries. It may also explain some cases of unaccountable postoperative pain following total knee replacement and other surgical procedures on the knee (Katz *et al.* 1986, Katz & Hungerford 1987).

There is, however, no correlation between the severity of the precipitating event and the incidence of post-traumatic dystrophy, severity of symptoms and subsequent prognosis. Even relatively minor trauma such as cuts, sprains and even venepuncture can precipitate this condition.

Predisposing factors

The prevalence of reflex sympathetic dystrophy is greater amongst patients who have a history of ischaemic heart disease, hypertension, cerebrovascular and peripheral vascular disease. A positive association with cigarette smoking and type IV hyperlipidaemia has been reported.

There is also a widely held belief that psychological factors, particularly depression, hysteria and hypochondriasis, may be a significant cause of pain dysfunction. However, it remains to be established whether such findings are inherent traits or are secondary to the pain syndrome.

Sympathetic dysfunction

Leriche (1916) was the first authority to implicate the sympathetic nervous system in the disease process. Since then a number of autonomic theories have been advocated. In 1943 Livingston proposed that dystrophic pain was due to chronic stimulation of a peripheral nerve, giving rise to a hyperexcitable state of the internuncial neuronal pool. Subsequently, Doupe *et al.* (1944) suggested that the condition was due to the generation of abnormal synapses or 'ephapses' between afferent pain fibres and the sympathetic outflow. In the 'gate control theory of pain' Melzack and Wall (1965) proposed that the transmission of pain impulses in the small 'C' fibres are modulated in the spinal cord by other afferent impulses and descending control. Despite continued debate over the details this theory helps to explain the variable relationship between injury and clinical response and has, therefore, gained widespread acceptance.

The involvement of the sympathetic nervous system in this condition is by no means universally accepted (Tahmoush *et al.* 1983). Goris *et al.* (1987) implicated toxic oxygen radicals in the pathogenesis and it has also been suggested that microthrombosis in the affected extremity may be the underlying cause (Ecker 1985).

General clinical features

In the severe intractable case three phases are recognizable, although in mild cases the condition may resolve before stage II or III is reached.

Stage I — the acute (vasodilatation) phase

The patient complains of burning or non-specific aching pain, which is felt superficially in the periphery of the extremity. It is generally more intense in the fingertips and the hollow of the palm, or in the toes and sole of the foot. The skin is oedematous, often with accelerated nail and hair growth. There is evidence of vasomotor instability with increased blood flow and a rise in skin temperature, typically of 2–6°C.

Stage II — the dystrophic (vasoconstriction) phase

Typically, the pain and skin sensitivity becomes more intense, but remains localized distally. Dysaesthesiae are now characteristic, environmental temperature changes may either aggrevate or relieve the pain and somatosensory and emotional stimuli frequently exacerbate the condition. Oedematous tissues become indurated, the nails become cracked and brittle, and hair loss occurs. The skin often appears cyanotic and is cool and hyperhydrotic. Movements are markedly limited and painful and muscular atrophy ensues. Radiographs at this stage show characteristic demineralization.

Stage III — the atrophic phase

Whilst the pain spreads proximally and may involve the contralateral limb, skin hypersensitivity typically decreases. The skin is thin and shiny, but blood flow and skin temperature return to normal. Movements remain limited and joints become refractory to mobilization due to advanced muscle wasting, fascial thickening and pericapsular fibrosis.

Clinical features in children

Prior to 1978 less than 10 cases of reflex sympathetic dystrophy had been reported in children. The prevalence of the condition in children and adolescents is now thought to be more common than was previously recognized (Silber & Majd 1988).

Symptoms are often milder than in adults and trophic skin changes are rare. Radiographs are frequently normal, even in the established case, and bone scintigraphy may be normal or, in contrast to adults, shows decreased uptake in the affected extremity. Because of the insidious and atypical presentation the condition may not be considered in children and a diagnosis of psychiatric disturbance or malingering may be made. When recognized, the response to analgesics and physiotherapy and the long-term prognosis is much better than in adults.

Diagnosis

Patients with reflex sympathetic dystrophy thus exhibit a spectrum of clinical manifestations depending on the severity and stage of the condition. Kozin *et al.* (1981) therefore suggested four clinical diagnostic categories:

1 Definite reflex sympathetic dystrophy
  (a) Pain and tenderness in an extremity.
  (b) Signs or symptoms of vasomotor instability.
  (c) Swelling (usually associated with dystrophic skin changes).
2 Probable reflex sympathetic dystrophy — pain and tenderness in an extremity and *either* signs and symptoms of vasomotor instability *or* swelling (often with dystrophic skin changes.
3 Possible reflex sympathetic dystrophy — signs or symptoms of vasomotor instability *and/or* swelling (no pain, but often tenderness).
4 Doubtful reflex sympathetic dystrophy
  (a) Unexplained pain in an extremity.
  (b) No vasomotor instability or swelling.
  (c) Often no tenderness present.
As the clinical picture may well be ill defined, further investigation in support of the diagnosis is often of value.

Radiography

The most obvious radiological finding is diffuse osteoporosis of cancellous bone, but this is not present in all cases and is seen with simple disuse atrophy of bone.

High resolution, fine detail radiography is a useful research technique and has demonstrated more specific features. In addition to generalized demineralization and periarticular soft tissue swelling, there is periarticular and juxta-articular accentuation of bone loss and cortical bone resorption occurs in the subperiosteal, endosteal and intracortical zones. There may also be juxta-articular and subchondral erosive changes.

Bone scintigraphy

As an aid to diagnosis three-phase static and dynamic ^{99m}-technetium scintigraphy has a reported sensitivity and specificity of up to 97% (Mackinnon & Holder 1984). Typically positive static scintigrams demonstrate increased periarticular activity involving multiple joints in the affected extremity. Dynamic studies are considered positive when there is asymmetrical blood flow in the limb.

Thermography

Electronic infrared thermography is a valuable aid in the diagnosis of reflex sympathetic dystrophy, but is not widely available. Liquid crystal contact thermography has also been used to assess skin temperature and is a useful screening test. It is generally accepted that an increase or decrease of 0.6°C between the two extremities constitutes an abnormal thermographic pattern.

Other diagnostic procedures

There are no characteristic biochemical changes associated with reflex sympathetic dystrophy. Synovial histology is non-specific. Synovial oedema, hyperplasia and fibrosis are accompanied by capillary proliferation and perivascular inflammatory changes in the established case.

Treatment

Whilst it is generally accepted that physiotherapy has an important role to play in the management of patients with reflex sympathetic dystrophy, to date there have not been any controlled clinical studies to confirm or refute this teaching. Forced passive movements and extreme temperatures should be avoided, but the judicious use of active movement regimens, wax therapy, splinting and occupational therapy is thought to be helpful.

For patients refractory to physiotherapy, transcutaneous electrical nerve stimulation may be beneficial. It is believed to act by enhancement of large fibre activity; this stimulates the substantia gelatinosa of the spinal cord which is inhibitory to the transmission of afferent pain impulses.

Regional sympathetic blockade using local anaesthetics is commonly used as a diagnostic test and therapeutically in cases refractory to more conservative measures. In 1974 Hannington-Kiff described intravenous sympathetic blockade using the false neurotransmitter guanethidine sulphate. Following the insertion of an intravenous cannula, the affected limb is exsanguinated and a tourniquet is then inflated to 100 mmHg above systolic blood pressure. A solution containing 15 mg of guanethidine, 100 mg lignocaine, 500 units of heparin and normal saline to a total volume of 20 ml is injected and the cuff is kept inflated for 15 minutes. This technique has the advantage of producing complete sympathetic blockade for up to 4 days and long-term palliation can be achieved in 60–80% of cases by one or more blocks administered at weekly intervals.

The current indication for surgical sympathectomy is for a patient with established reflex sympathetic dystrophy who has responded to treatment by regional sympathetic blockade but who has not achieved lasting benefit following four blocks. Paravertebral sympathetic ganglionectomy used in these circumstances can give complete relief in 60–90% of cases; failure is associated with incomplete denervation and long-standing disease. Chemical sympathectomy with 6% aqueous phenol produces sympathetic interruption for several weeks and is a useful alternative in high risk cases.

The use of steroids, beta blockade and calcitonin therapy have been advocated by some authorities, but the results are less predictable and unfavourable side-effects more common.

Prognosis

Reflex sympathetic dystrophy may follow a benign course, remain virtually subclinical and resolve spontaneously. Conversely, it can become chronic, severely incapacitating and refractory to treatment. Following early diagnosis and treatment the outlook is significantly improved.

References

Atkins, R.M., Duckworth, T. & Kanis, J.A. Features of algodystrophy after Colles' fracture. *J Bone Joint Surg* 1990; **72B**: 105–110.

Bonica, J.J., Liebeskind, J.C. & Albe-Fessard, D.G. Causalgia and other reflex sympathetic dystrophies. In: Bonica, J. *et al.* (eds) *Advances in Pain Research and Therapy*, Vol. 3. Raven Press: New York, 1979.

Doupe, J., Cullen, C.H. & Chance, G.O. Post-traumatic pain and the causalgic syndrome. *J Neurol Neurosurg Psych* 1944; 7: 33–48.

Ecker, A. Contact thermography in diagnosis of reflex sympathetic dystrophy: a new look at pathogenesis. *Thermology* 1985; 1: 106–109.

Goris, R.J., Dongen, L.M. & Winters, H.A. Are toxic oxygen radicals involved in the pathogenesis of reflex sympathetic dystrophy? *Free Rad Res Commun* 1987; 3: 13–18.

Hannington-Kiff, J.G. Intravenous regional sympathetic block with guanethidine. *Lancet* 1974; i: 1019–1020.

Homans, J. Minor causalgia: a hyperesthetic neurovascular syndrome. *N Engl J Med* 1940; **222**: 870–874.

Katz, M.M. & Hungerford, D.S. Reflex sympathetic dystrophy affecting the knee. *J Bone Joint Surg* 1987; **69B**: 797–803.

Katz, M.M., Hungerford, D.S., Krackow, K.A. & Lennox, D.W. Reflex sympathetic dystrophy as a cause of poor results after total knee arthroplasty. *J Arthro* 1986; 1: 117–124.

Kozin, F., Soin, J.S., Ryan, L.W., Carrera, G.F. & Wortmann, R.L. Bone scintigraphy in the reflex sympathetic dystrophy syndrome. *Radiology* 1981; **138**: 437−443.

Lankford, L.L. & Thompson, J.E. Reflex sympathetic dystrophy, upper and lower extremity: diagnosis and management. *American Academy of Orthopaedic Surgeons Instructional Course Lecture* 1977; **26**: 163−178.

Leriche, R. De la causalgie envisagée comme une névrite du sympathique et de son traitment par la dénudation et l'excision des plexus nerveux périartériels. *Presse Méd* 1916; **24**: 178−180.

Livingston, W.K. *Pain Mechanisms*. Macmillan: New York, 1943.

Mackinnon, S.E. & Holder, L.E. The use of three-phase radionuclide bone scanning in the diagnosis of reflex sympathetic dystrophy. *J Hand Surg* 1984; **9A**: 556−563.

Melzack, R. & Wall, P.D. Pain mechanisms: a new theory. *Science* 1965; **150**: 971−979.

Mitchell, S.W., Morehouse, G.R. & Keen, W.W. *Gunshot Wounds and Other Injuries of Nerves*. Lippincott: Philadelphia, 1864.

Silber, T.J. & Majd, M. Reflex sympathetic dystrophy syndrome in children and adolescents. Report of 18 cases and review of the literature. *Am J Dis Child* 1988; **142**: 1325−1330.

Steinbrocker, O. The shoulder hand syndrome. Associated painful homolateral disability of the shoulder and hand with swelling and atrophy of the hand. *Am J Med* 1947; **3**: 402−407.

Sudeck, P. Uber die akute entzundliche Knockenatrophie. *Arch F Klin Chir* 1900; **62**: 147−156.

Tahmoush, A.J., Malley, J. & Jennings, J.R. Skin conductance, temperature and blood flow in causalgia. *Neurology* 1983; **33**: 1483−1486.

Avascular necrosis

P.J.GREGG

Avascular necrosis of bone is a well-recognized complication of fractures at certain sites. The fractures which are most commonly associated with the development of this complication are intracapsular fractures of the proximal femur, fractures of the waist of the scaphoid and neck of the talus and four-part fractures of the proximal humerus. Avascular necrosis of the head of the femur and lunate may also occur after dislocation of the hip and lunate respectively. The management of this complication at specific sites will be dealt with later in the book (see Chapters 12, 16, 20 & 25) and only general comments will be made in this section.

Use of the term avascular necrosis is appropriate in these situations because the necrosis of bone almost certainly results from interruption of the blood supply to one or other of the fracture fragments at the time of the fracture. The term avascular necrosis is often used inappropriately in the author's opinion for non-traumatic cases of bone necrosis where it is far from proven that the cause is, in fact, due to an interruption of the blood supply of the bone. The reason that avascular necrosis develops after certain fractures is due to the particular relationship between the blood supply to one of the fracture fragments and the site of the fracture; this is probably best exemplified by an intracapsular fracture of the proximal femur. Most of the blood supply to the femoral head passes in vessels which are intimately related to the cortex of the intracapsular portion of the femoral neck (retinacular vessels) and within the medullary cavity of the femoral neck (metaphyseal vessels); these vessels are therefore at risk of damage when the neck of the femur is fractured.

It is necessary to review briefly the pathology of avascular necrosis of bone for a proper understanding of the indications and limitations of the available imaging techniques which are currently available for the diagnosis of this condition. The primary event in avascular necrosis of bone is the death of cells within the affected bone and marrow. These cells include the osteocytes and haematopoietic and fat cells of the marrow. Death of these cells occurs shortly ($<$ 24 hours) after the occurrence of the fracture which interrupts the blood supply. Following death, the cells undergo lysis which results in the loss of nuclear staining of the affected cells when histological sections of affected bone are viewed down a microscope. It should be noted that loss of osteocyte nuclear staining, resulting in empty lacunae, may not be complete until 4−6 weeks after fracture. In the early stages following the development of avascular necrosis, no change in density and no other abnormality will be observed on plain radiographs because the total mineral content of the bone remains unchanged, unless the patient is immobilized for a period of time (for example, on traction after sustaining an injury of the hip). In the latter situation the rest of the skeleton will undergo disuse osteoporosis but the necrotic area of bone will not be affected because of the absence of a blood supply. This results in a relative increase in density of the affected bone.

Following the primary event of cellular death, there may be a series of secondary events which constitute a repair phase. Cells in the surrounding normal bone may proliferate and, along with blood vessels, may invade the necrotic area. Some of the cells differentiate into osteoblasts which lay down seams of new bone on the surface of pre-existing dead trabeculae: so-called 'creeping apposition'. This process results in an absolute increase in the amount of mineral present within the affected area and, if sufficiently great, may lead to the characteristic absolute increase in density which may be observed on a standard radiograph (Fig. 11.50). In other parts, cells differentiate into osteoclasts which resorb pre-existing dead trabeculae prior to the laying

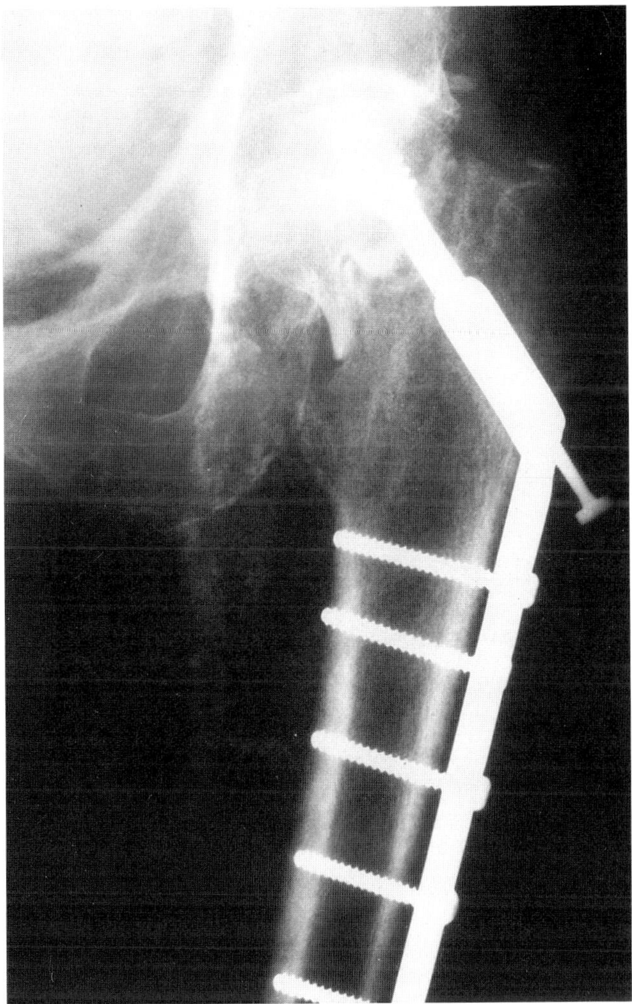

Fig. 11.50 Anteroposterior radiograph of the left hip of a patient who had sustained an intracapsular fracture of the proximal femur and was treated with a sliding hip screw system. Note the absolute increase in density of the femoral head and the presence of a non-union.

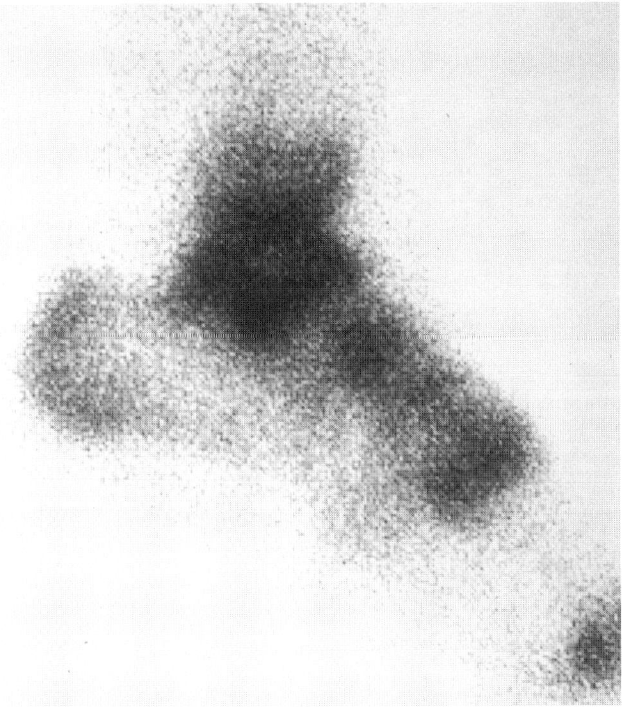

Fig. 11.51 Lateral scintigram of the ankle of a patient who had previously sustained a fracture of the neck of the talus. Note the generalized increased uptake of ^{99m}Tc-methylene diphosphonate (normal response to fracture) and a possible 'cold spot' in the centre of the body of the talus (arrow). (Reproduced with permission from Galasko, C.S.B. & Isherwood, I. (eds) *Imaging Techniques in Orthopaedics.* (Springer-Verlag: Berlin, 1989.)

down of new bone: so-called 'creeping substitution'. This process may lead to areas of decreased density which may be observed on a plain radiograph.

At some stage during the repair process a fracture may occur within the affected bone. This fracture may be situated in the subchondral region or may be deeper within the affected bone (Fig. 11.51); in the latter case there is usually an extension into the subchondral region. It is important to mention at this stage that it is the development of this fracture which leads to the onset of symptoms (usually pain), the development of joint surface irregularity and the progression to secondary degenerative osteoarthritis. In the early stages of avascular necrosis the condition is entirely asymptomatic.

It must be remembered that plain radiographs cannot distinguish normal living bone from dead bone before any repair process has begun, unless the affected part is immobilized; nor can they distinguish normal living bone from revascularized dead bone before new bone formation has taken place. Therefore, dense does not always equal dead!

Standard radiography

Plain radiography is still the standard method for confirming the diagnosis of avascular necrosis of bone which causes symptoms and for the detection of symptomless areas of avascular necrosis. The latter is particularly important in order to give both the patient and, if relevant, the patient's solicitor an accurate prognosis as soon as possible after injury in those instances where the development of avascular necrosis is a real possibility; for example, after a traumatic dislocation of the hip in a young active individual. The basic radiographic abnormality is one of altered density but, less often, it may be a decrease. The radiographic changes which can be seen as a result of avascular necrosis are basically the same regardless of which bone is affected; these changes were well described as long ago as 1930 by Phemister.

In some cases, particularly in patients who have avascular necrosis of bone and are asymptomatic because fracture of the necrotic bone had not occurred, the plain radiographs may be entirely normal. It is well recognized that there is often a long delay between the causative fracture and the appearance of an abnormality which can be seen on a radiograph. In the case of the femoral head this delay may be as long as 3–4 years or more. The reason for this delay is probably that a considerable alteration in bone mineral content, particularly in cancellous bone, must develop before a radiographic charge may be detected (Borak 1942, Bachman & Sproul 1955, Edelstyn *et al.* 1967).

If revascularization occurs it may not be associated with any new bone formation, or the new bone formation may be insufficient to increase the local mineral content to an extent that it can be recognized as an abnormality on the radiograph. It is well known, for example, that even after an area of avascular necrosis has been 'repaired' fully, including extensive new bone formation, no abnormality may be detected on the radiograph (McCallum & Walder 1966). For these reasons additional investigations are required in the presence of a normal initial plain radiograph.

Skeletal scintigraphy

It has been shown that, in an experimental animal model, it is possible to detect areas of bone and marrow necrosis by skeletal scintigraphy using ^{99m}Tc-labelled phosphate compounds and a gamma camera. It was also found that abnormalities could be detected on a scintigram at a much earlier stage than was possible using standard radiographs (Gregg 1977, Gregg & Walder 1980). The abnormality observed on a scintigram was an area of increased uptake of the radioactive tracer producing a 'hot spot'. The pathological basis for this 'hot spot' was probably the new bone formation associated with the repair of some of these lesions (Gregg 1977). It is therefore of value to obtain a skeletal scintigram of patients suspected of having avascular necrosis of bone when plain radiographs are found to be normal (Fig. 11.52). However, it should be emphasized that the abnormal scintigram is probably also dependent on the establishment of a repair process in the nature of revascularization and subsequent new bone formation, and that if this does not occur then the scintigram will also be normal. Thus, a normal scintigram does not rule out the possibility of the presence of avascular necrosis.

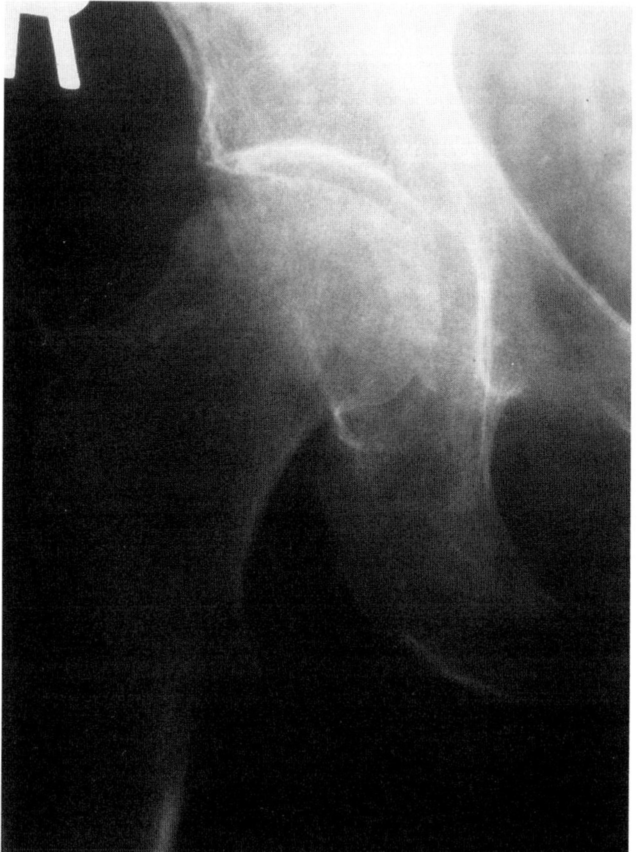

(a)

(b)

Fig. 11.52 (a) Normal radiograph of the hip of a patient with osteonecrosis of the femoral head. (b) Scintigram of both hips. Note the increased uptake of ^{99m}Tc-labelled methylene diphosphonate in the right femoral head. (Reproduced with permission from Galasko, C.S.B. & Isherwood, I. (eds) *Imaging Techniques in Orthopaedics*. Springer-Verlag: Berlin, 1989.)

Because the uptake of radioactive tracer in bone probably only occurs in the presence of an adequate blood supply (Hughes 1980), it is possible that, in the presence of avascular necrosis where revascularization has not occurred, a 'cold spot' may be detected on the scintigram due to the lack of tracer uptake. It may be useful, therefore, to obtain a scintigram in the early stages following fracture or dislocation to investigate this possibility. However, in the author's experience, these 'cold spots' are often ill defined when compared with the more obvious 'hot spots' associated with an area of repairing avascular necrosis of bone (Fig. 11.53) and false positive

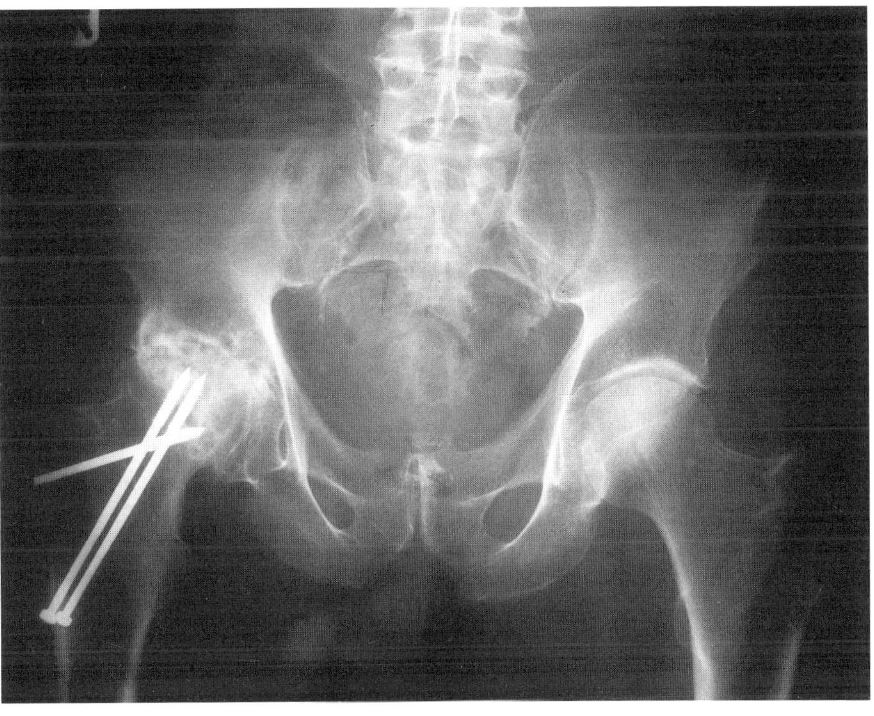

(a)

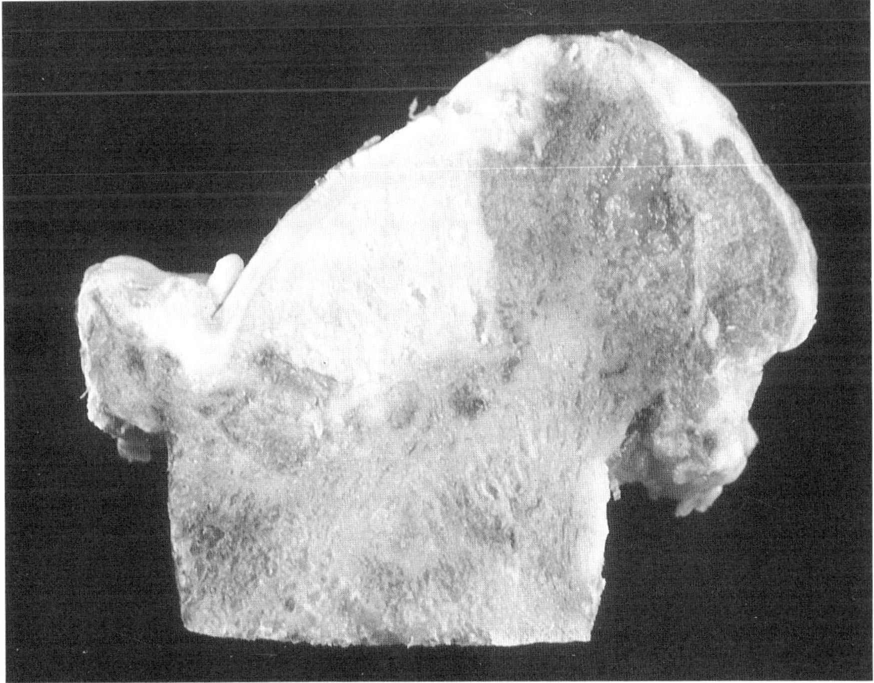

(b)

Fig. 11.53 (a) Anteroposterior radiograph of the pelvis of a patient who had sustained an intracapsular fracture of the proximal femur some years previously. This had been treated by multiple pin fixation. Note the increased radiological density of the femoral head and the collapse and irregularity of the articular surface. (b) Section of the femoral head showing the macroscopic appearance of avascular segment (wedge-shaped light area) which has collapsed into the rest of the femoral head following fracture of subchondral bone.

and false negative scintigrams are, therefore, not uncommon. Some workers have devised methods of measuring the amount of tracer uptake in the abnormal site and comparing this with the contralateral normal side by defining uptake ratios and, in this way, they claim to be able to detect avascular necrosis of bone. This method has been applied mostly to avascular necrosis of the femoral head after an intracapsular fracture of the proximal femur (Stromqvist *et al.* 1987).

Patients with avascular necrosis of bone are not usually symptomatic unless a fracture has occurred through the necrotic bone and results in collapse and/or irregularity of the articular surface overlying the affected bone. The subchondral fracture and resulting articular surface irregularity are not always well defined on standard radiographs. In these circumstances high quality tomograms and, on occasions, arthrograms will usually reveal the subchondral fracture. In the author's experience computerized axial tomography scanning rarely produces additional useful information in the diagnosis of avascular necrosis of bone.

Magnetic resonance imaging (MRI) is probably the most sensitive technique for the detection of bone ischaemia of the femoral head for those who have access to this technique (Mitchell *et al.* 1986, Markisz *et al.* 1987). A chronological pattern of segmental MRI signal features may allow the staging of bone ischaemia (Mitchell *et al.* 1987). Early bone ischaemia is associated with retention of the normal fat signals throughout the affected area, except for a low signal rim; in advanced disease there is a low signal throughout the necrotic area. This late effect is probably due to the replacement of fatty marrow by fibrous tissue. More work and experience with MRI in the early diagnosis of avascular necrosis of bone after trauma is still required before its precise role can be clearly established. The author has, however, found it a useful pointer to the presence of avascular necrosis of the femoral head in the early stages after trauma when other imaging techniques have been negative (Fig. 11.54).

Management

Patients who have sustained fractures or dislocations, known to be associated with the development of avascular necrosis of bone, should be investigated along the lines outlined previously as soon after injury as possible in order to detect the presence of this complication. This is particularly important at sites where the presence of avascular necrosis has potentially serious clinical consequences, for example, the femoral head. This will allow an accurate prognosis to be given to the patient

and also, where applicable, to the patient's solicitor who may be preparing a case for compensation. At this early stage plain radiographs will usually be normal and, although bone scintigraphy may suggest the presence of a 'cold spot', in the author's experience this is difficult to detect with certainty. Therefore, the author's preference, particularly in the case of the femoral head, is to obtain an MRI as soon as possible. This does not present a problem in the case of a traumatic dislocation of the hip, but in the case of the intracapsular fracture of the proximal femur it will usually not be possible to obtain this until the metalware used for internal fixation has been removed. In any event, patients at risk of developing avascular necrosis as a late complication should be reviewed annually by clinical examination and standard radiography.

The presence of avascular necrosis may also be associated with non-union of the fracture and, in this situation, treatment is directed at obtaining union of the fracture. For non-union and avascular necrosis following fractures of the scaphoid and neck of the talus, this will usually involve simple autogenous bone grafting and some form of internal fixation. For non-union of intracapsular fractures of the proximal femur in association with avascular necrosis of the femoral head, some form of replacement arthroplasty, either hemi or total, will usually be required. For younger patients some consideration may have to be given to further internal fixation of the fracture and to supplementing this with simple autogenous bone grafting or a muscle—pedicle bone graft (see Chapter 20).

For those patients whose fractures have united but show evidence, from the use of imaging techniques, that avascular necrosis of bone is present, management depends on whether or not the patient has symptoms. In the absence of symptoms there is no place for further intervention. Not all patients with avascular necrosis of, for example, the femoral head, go on to experience significant symptoms and there is, therefore, no place for imposing on them treatment modalities for which there is no evidence that they affect the natural history of the process. In the author's opinion there is no place for restricting such patients to no or partial weight-bearing for prolonged periods of time, and there is no place for performing vascularized grafts or drilling procedures on a prophylactic basis. Those patients who experience symptoms, most usually pain, do so because of the development of a fracture in the necrotic sub-chondral bone; this leads to collapse and irregularity of the articular surface of the affected half of the joint. For practical purposes, these patients are suffering from secondary degenerative osteoarthritis and treatment is

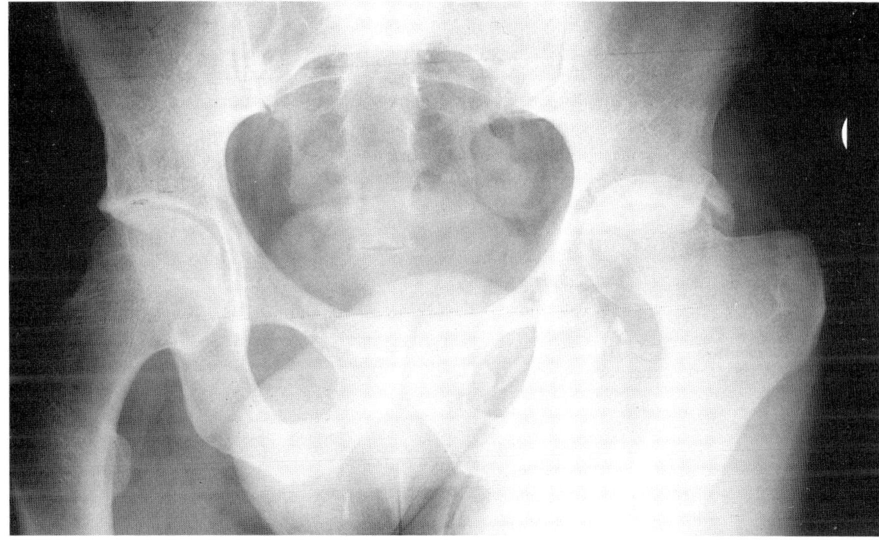

(a)

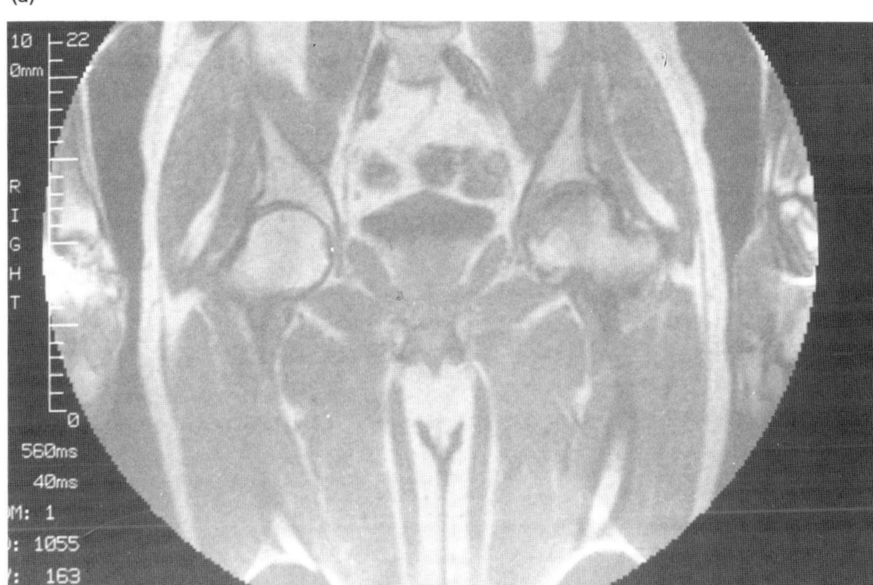

(b)

Fig. 11.54 (a) Anteroposterior radiograph of the pelvis showing a posterior dislocation of the left hip. (b) MRI scan of both hips performed 12 weeks after injury at a time when plain radiographs were normal. Note the reduced signal in the superior half of the left femoral head, producing an obvious dark area (arrow).

the same as that which is available for osteoarthritis of that particular joint, taking into account the age of the affected patient.

References

Bachman, Al. & Sproul, E.E. Correlation of radiographic and autopsy findings in suspected metastases in the spine. *Bull NY Acad Med* 1955; **31**: 146−148.

Borak, J. Relationship between clinical and roentgenological findings in bone metastases. *Surg Gynecol Obstet* 1942; **75**: 599−604.

Edelstyn, G.A., Gillespie, P.J. & Grebbell, F.S. The radiological demonstration of osseous metastases: experimental observations. *Clin Radiol* 1967; **18**: 158−162.

Gregg, P.J. *Caisson Disease of Bone. Studies Relating to the Aetiology, Early Diagnosis and Natural History of Caisson Disease of Bone.* MD thesis: University of Newcastle-upon-Tyne, 1977.

Gregg, P.J. & Walder, D.N. Scintigraphy versus radiography in the early diagnosis of experimental bone necrosis; with special reference to caisson disease of bone. *J Bone Joint Surg* 1980; **62B**: 214−221.

Hughes, S.P.F. Radionuclides in orthopaedic surgery. *J Bone Joint Surg* 1980; **62B**: 141−150.

Markisz, J.A., Knowles, R.J.R., Altchek, D.W., Shneider, R., Whalen, J.P. & Cahill, P.T. Segmental patterns of avascular necrosis of the femoral heads: early detection with MR imaging. *Radiology* 1987; **162**: 717−720.

McCallum, R.I. & Walder, D.N. Bone lesions in compressed air workers. *J Bone Joint Surg* 1966; **48B**: 207−235.

Mitchell, D.G., Rao, V.M., Dalinka, M.K., Spritzer, C.E., Alavi, A., Steinberg, M.E., Fallon, M. & Kressel, H.Y. Femoral head avascular necrosis: correlation of MR imaging, radiographic staging, radionuclide imaging, and clinical findings.

Radiology 1987; **162**: 709–715.

Mitchell, M.D., Kundel, H.L., Steinberg, M.E., Kressel, H.Y., Alavi, A. & Axel, L. Avascular necrosis of the hip: comparison of MR, CT and scintigraphy. *Am J Roentgenol* 1986; **147**: 67–71.

Phemister, D.B. Repair of bone in the presence of aseptic necrosis resulting from fractures, transplantations and vascular obstruction. *J Bone Joint Surg* 1930; **12**: 769–787.

Stromqvist, Hansson, L.I., Nilsson, L.T. & Thorngren, KG. Prognostic precision in post-operative ^{99m}Tc-MDP scintimetry after femoral neck fracture. *Acta Orth Scand* 1987; **58**: 494–498.

PART 2
SPECIFIC INJURIES
BY REGION

12: The Shoulder

Introduction

P.G.STABLEFORTH

Injuries of the shoulder region can cause permanent disability from disturbance of the comfort, mobility, strength and stability needed for effective hand positioning and function. Patients with multiple injuries and those with pre-existing lower limb disorders may have additional problems if pain, weakness or instability hamper transfer or crutch-walking mobility.

Patterns of injury

Most closed injuries follow low-violence falls on the level, and occur in isolation. Although transient nerve damage is not uncommon, most usually after gleno-humeral dislocation, damage to other adjacent structures is rare. Local soft tissue damage with contusion and swelling may, however, be followed by organization of periarticular exudate and often leads to shoulder stiffness.

An important, but smaller, group of injuries follow the more major violence of traffic accidents or falls from a height; these may occur with other complex multiple injuries that need priority treatment. Locally, there may be brachial plexus injury (with acromio-clavicular disruption) or intrathoracic visceral or chest wall damage (in association with scapula fractures) and damage to the articular surfaces may lead to permanent disability.

Age distribution

Children and adolescents usually sustain clavicle or proximal humeral fractures from side falls onto the shoulder. These injuries are also seen in late adolescent or early adult life, but subcoracoid dislocation from a sports injury and posterior dislocation from seizures are quite common, and both low- and high-violence acromio-clavicular disruptions, the latter with brachial plexus injury, are seen most frequently in this age group.

Supraspinatus tendon injury usually occurs in young adult males, while biceps tendon rupture, usually a marker of rotator cuff degeneration, affects older males.

The benign undisplaced, or little displaced, proximal humeral fracture usually follows a fall onto the shoulder by an elderly osteoporotic female patient, but a similar fall of a middle-aged, male or older female may cause one of the most complex and severe proximal humeral injuries and lead to life-long pain, stiffness and functional disability.

Signs and symptoms of shoulder injury

Injuries of the clavicle or acromio-clavicular joint cause severe local pain and swelling; the shoulder is often more comfortable if the elbow of the injured side is cradled in the other hand.

Proximal humeral fractures cause rapid swelling of the shoulder region, but bruising may be delayed and appear in the mid or lower arm; shoulder movement is inhibited by pain and the arm is more comfortable when supported.

Whilst subcoracoid dislocation is usually obvious from the 'squaring' of the shoulder contours and acromial prominence, deformity is rarely a feature of posterior dislocation, though pain on movement and an inability to rotate the forearm off the chest are usually evident.

If after injury there is marked shoulder swelling, severe pain and total inhibition of movement, but good quality biplanar radiographs show no bone or joint damage, supraspinatus tendon rupture should be suspected; the diagnosis is almost certain if the patient cannot maintain 80° flexion at the shoulder after joint aspiration and the instillation of 10–15 ml of 1% bupivacaine.

Scapular fractures cause deep, upper thoracic pain and tenderness. Blade fracture alone produces a swelling that outlines the scapular shape; those fractures that involve the glenoid produce subdeltoid swelling and pain with inhibition of shoulder joint movement.

Radiographic investigation

Good quality radiographs of the shoulder region are essential if injuries, particularly dislocations, are not to be missed. An anteroposterior radiograph of the gleno-humeral joint (a frontal view with the beam laterally angled 35° to the frontal plane) and an axial view of the scapula (at 90° to this) are the essential minimum, and can be taken with the patient sitting and the arm resting in a sling. The transaxillary view of the 70° abducted arm is also very useful.

Clavicle

H.K.KALYAN AND W.A.WALLACE

Introduction

Fractures of the clavicle have been thought to unite uneventfully and predictably. Yet an understanding of the need for bone-to-bone contact and a knowledge of the unique mechanics of fractures of the distal third of the clavicle, associated with rupture of the coracocla-vicular ligaments, will enable the doctor to identify cases where non-union and potential malunion may occur. It is widely believed, and correctly so, that conservative treatment is the cornerstone of treatment of fractures of the clavicle. However, it is important to emphasize that certain definite indications for operative management do exist. It is important for the modern orthopaedist to regard fractures of the clavicle with the same careful consideration given to fractures of other long bones such as the tibia.

Surgical anatomy

The clavicle is an almost horizontally placed strut that articulates at its inner end with the sternum and at its outer end with the acromion, thereby connecting the chest to the upper extremity. It maintains the width of the shoulders by holding the shoulder upwards, back-wards and outwards during rest and motion, and adds to the stability of the shoulder by acting as a strut or something to push against (Post 1989). It augments the strength of the arm-trunk mechanism, especially when the arm is at or above the horizontal position, which is clinically borne out by the fact that excision of the whole or a major part of the clavicle causes medial displacement of the shoulder, with a resultant weaken-ing and instability.

It derives its name from the Latin word clavis (key) (Dameron & Rockwood 1984), whose diminutive, cla-vicula, refers to a musical symbol of a similar shape. It has two curves when seen from above, being convex anteriorly in its medial one-third and convex posteriorly in its lateral two-thirds, with the weakest point being at the transition of the two curves. This is the most common location of fracture. The double curve affects the cross-sectional anatomy of the clavicle, the inner one-third being prism-shaped and the outer two-thirds being flattened. As the shoulder is abducted, the distance between the acromion and the sternoclavicular joint decreases; this shortening is permitted by the curved shape of the clavicle and the rotation of the bone during elevation.

It lies subcutaneously throughout its length, which predisposes it to direct injury. The clavicle lies in close proximity to major neurovascular structures. Lying behind and below are the great vessels passing to the upper limb from the thoracic outlet and the anterior roots of the brachial plexus. The medial and lateral cords of the brachial plexus lie directly below the middle third of the clavicle, and are separated from the bone by the thin subclavius muscle and clavipectoral fascia. The subclavius muscle protects the neurovascular bundle from injury in fractures of the mid-portion of the clavicle which are not grossly displaced. However, the proximity of the first rib results in a narrow space for these important neurovascular structures and compromise of the costoclavicular interval can easily result in neuro-vascular damage, as is discussed later in this chapter.

The clavicle also serves as a bony framework for the attachment of major muscles, including the sternoclei-domastoid and the anterior portion of the trapezius from above and the clavicular origin of the pectoralis major and anterior portion of the deltoid muscles below. The clavicle is certainly not a surplus part of the skel-eton, as has been suggested by some authors in the past.

Classification

Allman (1967) classified fractures of the clavicle into three groups.
Group I — includes fractures of the middle one-third, where the clavicle is unsupported by ligaments. This group constitutes the most frequent site of injury and is said to account for 80% of all clavicular fractures

(Neer & Rockwood 1984). The area of greatest frequency of fracture is just medial to the coracoclavicular ligament.

Group II — includes fractures of the distal clavicle lateral to the coracoclavicular ligament. The clavicle fractures less frequently in this portion as it is well supported by ligaments, the outer fragment being fixed to the acromion, and the inner fragment to the coracoid process by the coracoclavicular ligament. These distal or interligamentous fractures account for 15% of clavicular fractures (Neer & Rockwood 1984). *Neer* (1963) has further classified distal clavicular (group II) fractures into two types (Fig. 12.1), depending on the status of the ligaments:

Type 1 fractures are those in which the coracoclavicular ligament remains intact, with little tendency for displacement. It occurs most frequently (75% of group II fractures) and has a good prognosis.

Type 2 fractures are those in which the coracoclavicular ligament is ruptured and detached from the medial fragment which, in turn, has a marked tendency to displace upwards (Fig. 12.2). The type 2 fracture of Neer has specific features and problems in management and is considered in detail later in this chapter. Subsequently, Neer (Neer & Rockwood 1984) expanded his classification to include:

Type 3 fractures which are those which involve the articular surface. They are of significance because they may be easily overlooked, and may be a cause of disabling post-traumatic arthritis.

Group III — involves the medial end of the clavicle and is the least common. If the supporting costoclavicular ligament remains intact there is little or no resultant displacement. This group comprises the remaining 5% of clavicular fractures.

Thompson (1989) of Baltimore developed a classification system in 1985, which was publicized at the 4th International Conference on Surgery of the Shoulder in New York in 1989. This comprehensive classification is illustrated in Fig. 12.3 and is designed to predict problem adult clavicular fractures and develop a treatment option that would prevent non-union. The classification system recognizes five locations on the clavicle and subclassifies each of these into three categories, known as modifiers A, B and C:

Location 1 is the acromio-clavicular joint.

Location 2 is the lateral one-third of the clavicle.

Location 3 is the middle one-third.

Location 4 is the medial one-third.

Location 5 is the sternoclavicular joint.

'A' indicates <100% displacement.

'B' indicates >100% displacement.

'C' indicates neurovascular compression.

In his own study, Thompson recognized that type 3B fractures, although accounting for only 3% of all clavicular fractures, account for about 90% of non-unions. He carried out an exhaustive review of the English-language literature and found that of the 111 non-unions from 11 research papers that he could classify according to this model, 84% were type 3B, which closely matched his own findings. This led him to recommend primary open reduction and internal fixation (ORIF) for this fracture, if it could not be converted to a type 3A.

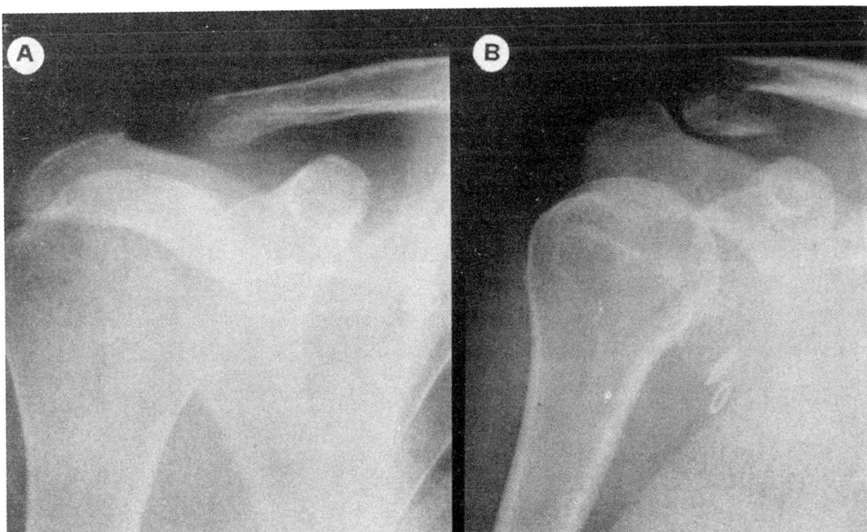

Fig. 12.1 Radiographs depicting Neer's classification of fractures of the distal portion of the clavicle: types 1 (A) and 2 (B).

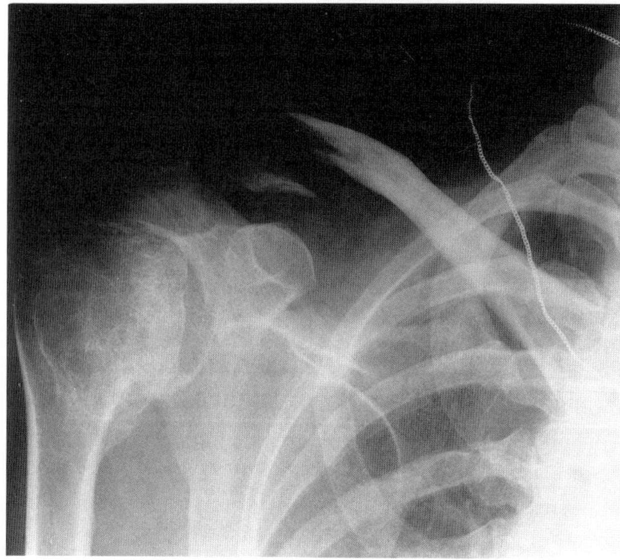

Fig. 12.2 Neer type 2 fracture showing upward displacement of the medial fragment and detachment of the ligaments.

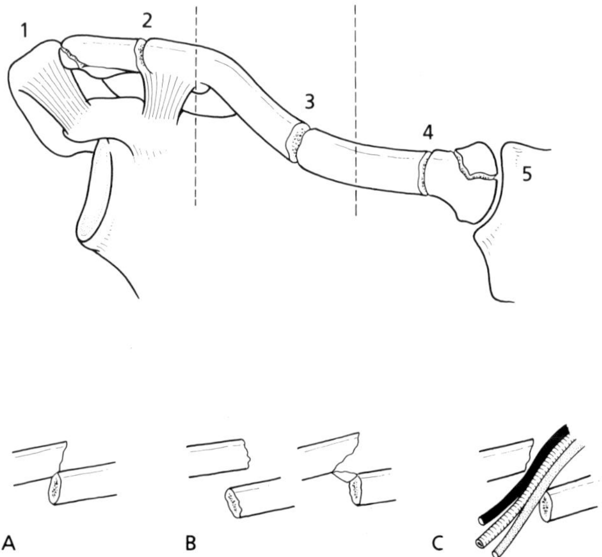

Fig. 12.3 Thompson's classification of clavicular fractures. Types 1–5 with displacements A–C.

Mechanism of injury and biomechanics

The most common mechanism of clavicular fracture has been assumed for a long time to be due to a fall on the outstretched hand (Fig. 12.4a) (Sharrard 1979, Kessel 1982, Apley & Solomon 1982). However, other authors (Fowler 1962, Sankarankutty & Turner 1975) have linked clavicular fractures with direct trauma to the shoulder (Fig. 12.4b).

Stanley *et al.* (1988) studied the history of injury in 150 consecutive patients with clavicular fractures and analysed the mechanics of injury, both clinically and biomechanically. They found that 94% of patients sustained their fractures as a result of a direct injury to the shoulder region, with 10% having tell-tale skin grazing over the point of the shoulder to substantiate their findings, whereas only 6% stated that they had fallen on to the outstretched hand.

To substantiate their clinical findings, they carried out a biomechanical analysis of clavicular impact loading and found that, apart from uniaxial tension, three basic mechanisms can raise the local stress levels in slender bones sufficiently to initiate crack propagation and subsequent fracture. These are bending, torsion and compressive buckling with resultant bowing. The freedom of motion afforded to the clavicle by the sternoclavicular joint makes pure bending an unlikely mechanism of fracture during clavicular impact loading. Similarly, the available rotation about the long axis of the clavicle (about 50°) virtually eliminates torsion as a mechanism. This leaves the most likely mechanism for clavicular fractures as compressive loading by a force transmitted along its long axis following the abutment of the acromion with the ground or another solid object. Elastic buckling of the clavicle was seen to occur when the compressive force is approximately equal to body weight. The typical curvature and geometrical changes along the axial length of the clavicle are likely to reduce the critical buckling load. Further, the critical force required to produce a fracture will depend upon the speed at which the body makes contact with the surface, the time taken for the collision, the direction of the applied force and the weight of the person.

If forces coming into play when falling on the outstretched arm are analysed (Fig. 12.4a), it is found that the impact force vector F is directed along the humerus. If this force is resolved into its three mutually perpendicular components (Fx, Fy and Fz) along and perpendicular to the axis of the clavicle, then it becomes apparent that Fx, which is the compressive force along the long axis of the clavicle, is only likely to be of sufficient magnitude to produce a fracture in cases where the outstretched arm is in the coronal plane relative to the body. When the force is applied along the axis of the arm, however, the forces are such that dislocation of the shoulder is the more likely outcome.

In contrast, if there is a direct blow to the shoulder, it is possible for the entire impact force to be transmitted along the clavicular axis, via the acromion process, so that components Fy and Fz are zero. In this case, critical

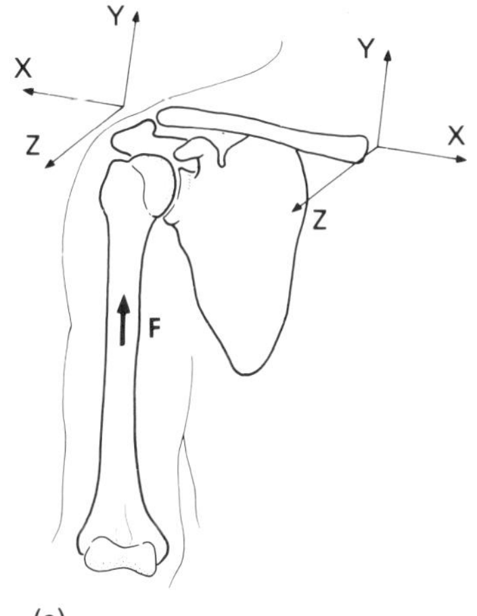

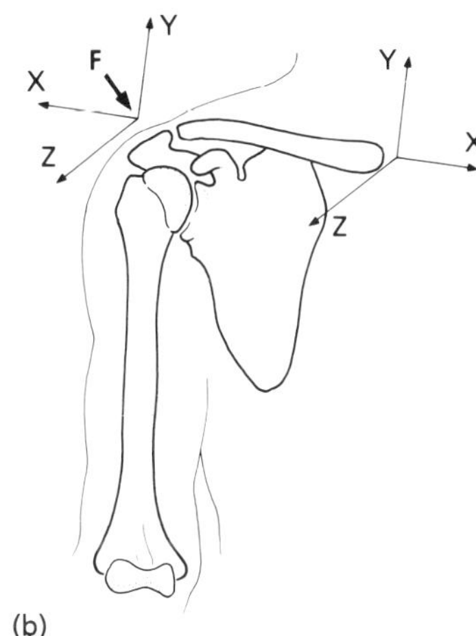

Fig. 12.4 (a) and (b) Mechanism of injury. The bold arrow (F) shows the direction of the force producing the injury.

buckling is reached at values close to the body weight and fracture results (Fig. 12.4b).

The authors further suggest that even in the 6% of patients who describe a fall onto the outstretched hand, the patient's body weight and falling velocity are such that movement is not arrested at this point, but the fall continues with the shoulder becoming the upper limb's next contact point with the ground. A biomechanical analysis of the forces involved has indicated that with a direct injury, the critical buckling load will be exceeded at a compressive force equivalent to the body weight and this results in a clavicular fracture.

Clinical features

The signs of fracture of the clavicle in adults are similar to those of any fracture in general. The patient usually holds the arm against the chest, and the shoulder appears to be slumped downward and inward. The area over the fracture site is swollen and tender. Overlying bruising may result from tearing of the underlying soft tissues and is a useful guide to the severity of displacement.

It is mandatory in all cases of a suspected fracture of the clavicle to look for and document the presence or absence of the distal pulses and peripheral nerve function on the affected side.

Radiology

In all cases of a suspected fracture of the clavicle, a routine anteroposterior view and 45° oblique view with the tube directed from below cephalad (Neer & Rockwood 1984) are recommended. If the diagnosis of fracture is in doubt, an additional radiograph may be required 7–10 days after the injury (Post 1989).

Rarely, tomograms or computerized tomography (CT) scans are necessary for an accurate diagnosis of fractures involving the articular surfaces of the acromio-clavicular or sternoclavicular joints, or to distinguish fractures of the medial end of the clavicle from sternoclavicular joint dislocations (Neer & Rockwood 1984, Post 1989).

Specific radiography for fractures of the distal end of the clavicle is discussed separately.

Treatment of the acute fracture

Conservative treatment

There is no doubt that the majority of clavicular fractures can be successfully treated closed. However, for a bone that is known to heal predictably, it seems surprising that more than 200 methods of treatment for fractures of the clavicle have been described (Zenni *et al.* 1981, Neer & Rockwood 1984). In 1954, Nicoll stated that 'the fractured clavicle cannot really be immobilized except perhaps by a shoulder spica incorporating the head' which emphasizes the point that displaced fractures of the clavicle cannot be reduced and maintained in a perfect position by closed methods. However, malunion of the clavicle rarely results in unacceptable cosmesis and uniformly excellent functional results can be anticipated in the majority of patients. It is important to avoid the temptation to treat a fracture of the clavicle by open reduction merely because a patient objects to a bony prominence at the fracture site. Surgery should be reserved for carefully selected indications which are discussed in the next section.

Virtually all methods of conservative treatment described so far fall into two major groups (Neer & Rockwood 1984): *those that merely support the shoulder* (e.g. sling, sling and swathe or Velpeau bandage) and *those that attempt to maintain a reduction achieved by closed means* (e.g. figure-of-eight bandages, Billington yoke (basically a plaster of paris figure-of-eight), adhesive dressing of Sayre and various types of modified shoulder spicas). Materials also vary and include plaster of paris, plastic, leather, muslin and metal.

The two most common methods of conservative treatment will be discussed here: namely, the broad arm sling and the figure-of-eight bandage. The authors personally prefer to use the method most widely practised in Britain, that is, the simple broad arm sling, and use the following regimen.

The sling is used under the clothes for comfort for 2 weeks and then outside the clothes for a further 2 weeks (Fig. 12.5), with a return to normal everyday activities as soon as possible thereafter and a return to contact sports at 12 weeks. As far as children under 16 years of age are concerned, it is the authors' practice to halve the above treatment times for those under 16 with category A fractures, but to make it slightly longer for displaced fractures. Using this treatment regime, non-union and other complications are uncommon, but patients are usually quite uncomfortable during the first 3 weeks of treatment when they have difficulty sleeping at night because of pain. Many patients prefer to sleep upright in an armchair for the first 3 or 4 nights and strong analgesia is recommended. Fracture clinic attendances are usually only required at the beginning of treatment and 3 weeks later, and further attendance is necessary only in the event of a problem or ongoing discomfort.

The figure-of-eight bandage, or a modification of it (Fig. 12.6), has been a more widely used method of conservative treatment in Europe and North America, and has been advocated in the hope that it would reduce and maintain the position of the displaced fracture. There is doubt about its efficacy for reducing malunion but it is generally felt to be more comfortable. However, the figure-of-eight bandage does have certain specific disadvantages. It must be tightened regularly (every 1 or 2 days), and Nicoll (1954), who used a sling for his own patients, which gave consistently good functional results, remarked that 'The usual compromise is that the patient attends daily to have his splint, strapping or bandage adjusted, thereby maintaining a reasonable degree of reduction for about a couple of hours a day (Sundays excepted)' — an eloquent criticism of other methods. Mullick (1967) showed, by the use of serial radiography, that these bandages do not in actual

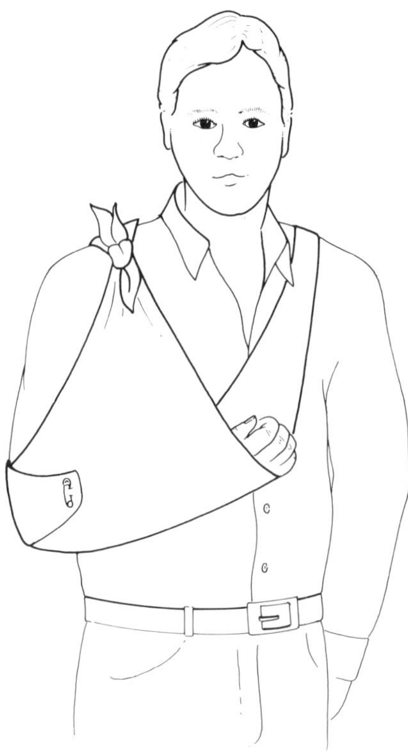

Fig. 12.5 Broad arm sling worn over the clothes for 2–4 weeks after clavicular fracture.

fact maintain the position of a displaced fracture and, in some cases, the displacement may be made worse (Sankarankutty & Turner 1975). Stanley and Norris (1988) carried out a study of 140 consecutive patients with fractures of the clavicle reviewed 3–12 months after injury. They found no statistical difference in the time taken to achieve full recovery in two groups of patients matched for age and sex and treated with either a figure-of-eight bandage or a broad arm sling. Fowler (1962) pointed out that chafing and pressure from the figure-of-eight bandage may cause more discomfort than the fracture, and Piterman (1982) described the development of an axillary pressure sore in a patient whose figure-of-eight bandage had been applied too tightly. Post (1989) has pointed out that a patient who complains of swelling or tingling in the hands should be instructed to (i) hold the hands on the hips with the arms abducted from the body, or (ii) to lie back with the arms outward towards the overhead position, or (iii) to hold the hands clasped on top of the head. This minimizes the compression of the arterial circulation against the hard edge of the splint in the axilla, helps retraction and maintains the proper length of the bone. The senior author of this section has had one patient suffer an

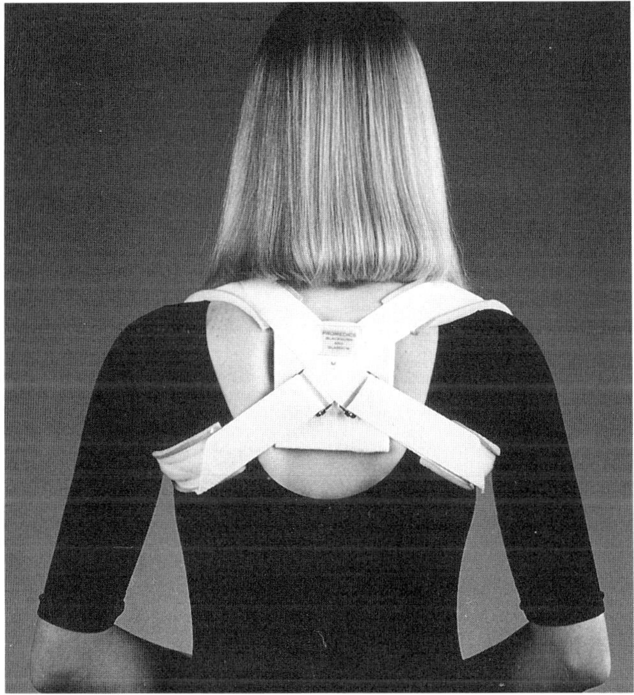

Fig. 12.6 Specially designed brace on the figure-of-eight principle.

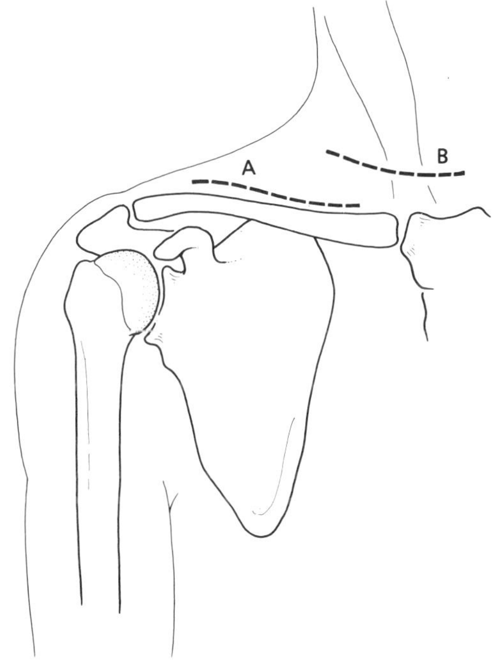

Fig. 12.7 Incisions, (A) and (B), for fixation of clavicular fractures. The low 'thyroid' incision (B) results gives a cosmetically acceptable scar.

extensive brachial vein thrombosis following the use of a figure-of-eight bandage.

Non-union is also seen more frequently when this method of treatment is used (Stanley & Norris 1988).

Surgical treatment

Several techniques of osteosynthesis of the clavicle have been employed, including intramedullary fixation using threaded or smooth pins or wires, cerclage wiring, plate and screw fixation and external fixation.

ORIF

Open reduction of acute clavicular fractures should be carried out with the utmost discretion, as it has often been the cause of ugly keloid scars and, indeed, has been incriminated as the most common cause of clavicular non-union (Neer 1960, Rowe 1968). The different skin incisions used for ORIF are shown in Fig. 12.7. However, ORIF does have a place in the treatment of acute clavicular fractures in the following specific situations:

1 *Severe angulation or comminution of a fracture in the middle third of the clavicle* causing compromise of the integrity of the skin overlying the fracture site. This is the commonest indication in the authors' experience.

Although Thompson (1989) recommended immediate ORIF for all type 3B fractures, it is clear that a number unite without surgery. The authors consider cautiously use of ORIF for these fractures, and only if the patient is over 16 years of age. Severe pain, not relieved by simple conservative treatment, is a relatively strong indication.

2 *Neurovascular compromise*, which is not resolved by closed reduction of the fracture, is an indication for immediate open reduction and the fracture should be anatomically reduced and internally stabilized. Vascular exploration and repair is carried out prior to fixation only if there is no radial pulse after manual reduction.

3 *Neer type 2 fractures of the distal clavicle* (considered later) present a strong case for open reduction.

4 *Multiple injuries*. ORIF of the clavicle is justified in the presence of a flail shoulder girdle with scapular fractures, to stabilize the skeleton rigidly and allow easier nursing and management.

5 *Inability of a patient to tolerate prolonged immobilization, or for relief of pain.* Such situations may arise because of Parkinson's disease, a seizure disorder or neuromuscular disease. It may also be indicated in drug addicts to avoid resumption of narcotics for pain.

INTRAMEDULLARY FIXATION

Technique

The surgical technique is quite simple and the essential steps are as follows. The fracture site is exposed by making a transverse incision centred around the fracture, and an intramedullary implant is passed in a retrograde fashion out through the medullary canal of the lateral fragment to emerge posteriorly near the conoid tubercle of the clavicle. It is then delivered through a small stab incision. The fracture is reduced and the pin, which must be threaded and should preferably have a head (i.e. a Knowles pin), is now passed anterograde and drilled across the fracture into the medial fragment. If a threaded implant is used, the threaded part must not be left across the fracture lest it cause distraction, and with subsequent movement it will be more likely to break. A check radiograph is taken to verify the position of the pin and fragments, and the redundant part of the pin is cut off beneath the skin.

Results

Neviaser *et al.* (1975) reported excellent results with no complications in 11 cases, including seven fresh fractures and four non-unions, treated using a small Knowles pin. They highlighted that all patients, followed for a minimum of 1 year and a maximum 20 years after injury, had no operative or postoperative complications, regained a range of movement equal to the normal side and returned to their previous occupational and recreational activities with no difficulty.

They reported that the design of the Knowles pin permits a compressive force to be applied to the fracture site instead of the distracting force that results from use of completely threaded pins, medial migration is prevented by the hub of the Knowles pin, and the time of external postoperative immobilization is 6 weeks and could even be shortened in view of the secure fixation. They had never found the need to remove the implant subsequently.

Paffen and Jansen (1978) reported 73 fractures treated by open reduction and intramedullary Kirschner (K)-wire fixation, with or without supplemental cerclage wires, in their review of 1400 clavicular fractures and had found a non-union rate of only 3%. Zenni *et al.* (1981) reported 25 cases treated by open reduction and intramedullary fixation in a series of 800 clavicular fractures and found excellent results in terms of healing and function without there being undue risk of non-union or postoperative infection.

Complications

The known complications following intramedullary fixation of clavicular fractures include distraction of the fracture site by fully threaded implants owing to the curvature of the bone and the narrow medullary canal, pin-track infection, pin breakage, non-union and pin migration.

Although pin migration is relatively rare, the disastrous consequences when it does occur make it necessary to formulate guidelines for their use. Lyons and Rockwood (1990) reviewed 37 reports from the literature regarding migration of pins used in operations around the shoulder girdle, and published some spectacular and alarming results. Pins migrated from the site of insertion around the shoulder girdle to an extraordinary variety of locations including major vascular structures, the heart itself, the lung and mediastinum, the cervicodorsal junction of the spine, where the tips traversed the intervertebral foramen to enter the spinal canal, the trachea, breast, proximal part of the arm, abdomen and spleen. Perhaps the most dramatic migration of all was the passage of a pin that had been used to fix a fracture of the shaft of the left clavicle, which travelled through the pharyngeal tissue into the right orbit and resulted in an acute, painful exophthalmos. The authors made several recommendations on the basis of their review:

1 Pins must be used with the utmost caution, if at all, in the shoulder girdle.

2 The ends of the pins must be bent or have restraining devices, such as the nut of the Hagie pin or the hub of the Knowles pin, to prevent or delay migration.

3 Radiographs should be obtained intraoperatively, or immediately postoperatively, to document the placement of the pins and follow-up radiographs must be obtained every 4 weeks until all pins have been removed. If they show any migration they should be removed at once, regardless of symptoms.

4 The patient must be carefully instructed about returning for follow-up evaluation and for later removal of the pins, and must be followed clinically and by serial radiographs until the completion of treatment, when all pins should be removed.

PLATE AND SCREW FIXATION

In appropriate cases the Association for Osteosynthesis (AO) group (Müller *et al.* 1979) recommends ORIF with either the six-hole semi-tubular plate or the small (3.5 mm) dynamic compression plate (DCP). More recently the 'pelvic reconstruction plate' has become popular for clavicle fractures.

Certain points need to be emphasized with regard to surgical technique. The AO group (Müller *et al.* 1979) recommended the supraclavicular incision for a surgical approach because it is more aesthetic, with the curved infraclavicular incision to be used only if it is unavoidable. The senior author of this section now regularly uses a low thyroidectomy type incision with much improved cosmetic results. Because of the contours of the clavicle, bending and contouring of the plate is normally necessary. The periosteum must be stripped sparingly at the fracture site but the plate can be applied extraperiosteally, away from the fracture. The plate should be applied to the superior surface of the clavicle, taking great care in drilling and placing the screws to avoid injury to the subclavian vein and underlying thoracic contents. Closed suction drainage for 24 hours is mandatory to avoid the possibility of a large haematoma close to the airway. Ali Khan and Lucas (1978) have emphasized the need to meticulously close the soft tissues in layers, especially the platysma, to achieve a painless, linear scar. They recommended mobilization at 2 weeks post-operatively. Correctly executed, rigid plating can give good fixation and overcome the drawbacks of other procedures.

Major complications include infection, non-union and a painful keloid scar. It is common for the plated area to become tender after union of the fracture and plate removal is often required after 9 to 12 months because of this discomfort.

External fixation

Advantages over ORIF

Schuind *et al.* (1988) reported that, in cases where operative fixation of fractures of the clavicle was indicated, external fixation offers considerable advantages, which include the following:

1 For open fractures and septic non-unions there is an increased risk of deep infection if internal fixation is used. External fixation allows easy access to soft tissues and the care of other injuries is facilitated.

2 Because of a reduction of periosteal stripping in the operative procedure, devascularization of the bone is slight.

3 Because of the cortical structure of the clavicle the anchorage of the external fixator pins is excellent, allowing good stabilization of the fracture and rapid healing of the bone, while early active mobilization of the shoulder and upper limb is permitted.

4 The dangers of intramedullary fixation are avoided. Transarticular implantation of an intramedullary device

is not used, so there is no risk of secondary osteoarthritis of the acromio-clavicular joint.

5 Removal does not require a second operation.

Technique

The patient, under general anaesthesia, is placed supine on the operating table with a sandbag placed under the cervico-thoracic region and the head turned towards the opposite side. The fracture site is exposed through a short linear transverse incision. The periosteum is not stripped; any soft tissue interposition is removed taking extreme care to avoid damage to the neurovascular bundle and pleural dome, and then the fracture site is reduced. Pre-drilling is carried out and two threaded pins are inserted into each fragment. In the medial fragment pins are placed in an ascending anteroposterior or almost horizontal direction to avoid the pleural dome, and in the lateral fragment they are placed in a superoinferior and anterior or almost vertical direction. The pins are then fixed using a simple rod and clamps in a half-frame configuration (Fig. 12.8). Postoperatively, mobilization can be started within 24–48 hours.

Results

Schuind *et al.* (1988) used the Hoffmann external fixator as a technique of osteosynthesis for the clavicle in 20 patients with acute injuries and non-union in adults, and reported no neurovascular or pleural complications. Two patients had superficial infection of the skin around

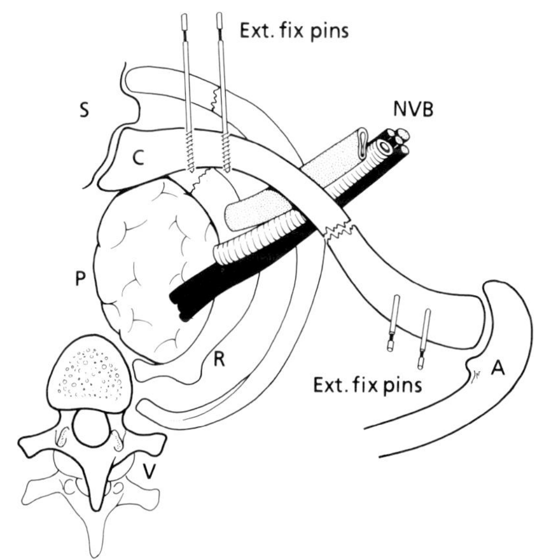

Fig. 12.8 Surgical technique for implantation of the external fixator pins.

the pins, but in all patients the fracture united satis-factorily with restoration of normal clavicular length and configuration and they regained normal shoulder motion. Scars were satisfactory in 19 out of 20 patients, only one required plastic surgery. On average, the external fixator was removed after 51 days.

Fractures of the distal clavicle with displacement

Historically, the clavicle has been thought to be invincible and fractures of the collarbone have been expected to unite with or without treatment, with even gross deformity being compatible with normal function and comfort. Although Smith (1847) recognized the problems of this injury more than 100 years ago, it was Neer who, in 1960, emphasized the fracture of the distal clavicle as one with a high propensity for non-union and prolonged disability. He identified the incriminating lesion as a fracture lateral to the coracoid tubercle and associated with a detachment of the coracoclavicular ligaments from the medial fragment. Depending upon the integrity of these ligaments, he identified two types of distal clavicular fractures, and later added a third type, as described earlier.

Incidence

Distal clavicular fractures comprise 10% of all clavicular fractures (Neer 1963, Heppenstall 1975, Edwards, Kavanagh & Flannery 1992). Type 1 injuries occur more frequently, in the ratio 3:1 (Neer 1963, Heppenstall 1975).

Pathological anatomy

The conoid and trapezoid parts of the coracoclavicular ligament attach along the entire length of the flat part of the clavicle, from the conoid tubercle medially to the capsule of the acromio-clavicular joint laterally. They allow rotary motion of the clavicle in its long axis and this is associated with scapular rotation. Tilting of the acromio-clavicular joint occurs during these movements. Disruption of these ligaments is the anatomical reason for the displacement of these fractures (Fig. 12.9).

In type 2 fractures there are four displacing factors acting in unison to retard union (Neer 1963), namely:
1 *The trapezius muscle*: the clavicular head of the trapezius attaches to the entire outer third of the bone and draws the large medial fragment upwards and backwards within the substance, often resulting in muscle interposition. Further, the outer end of the medial frag-

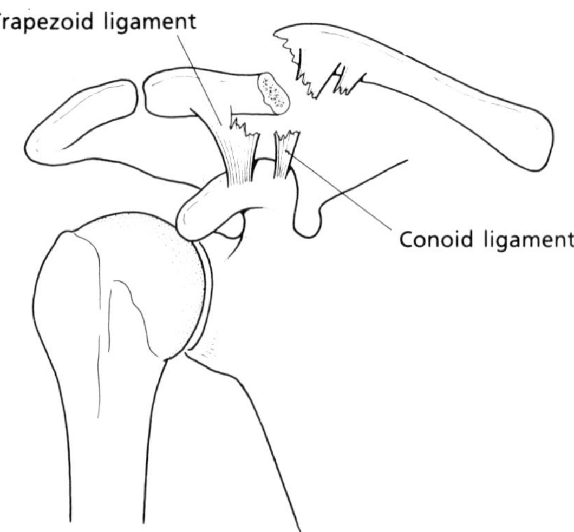

Fig. 12.9 Pathological anatomy of Neer type 2 fractures. Disruption of the coracoclavicular ligaments results in displacement of the fracture site.

ment often causes tenting of the overlying skin.
2 *The weight of the arm*: as the scapula and the arm descend, the outer fragment, which remains attached to the lateral portion of the trapezoid ligament and the acromion, is displaced downward and forward.
3 *Trunk muscles attaching to the humerus and scapula*: these displace the outer fragment medially toward the apex of the thorax.
4 *Rotatory displacement*: the intact attachment of the scapular ligaments to the outer fragment may cause its rotation by as much as 40° with movement of the arm.

Mechanism of injury

Type 1 fractures usually result from a relatively mild lateral impacting force which displaces the outer fragment slightly cephalad.

Type 2 fractures are caused by a violent force applied to the point of the shoulder (Neer 1963, Stanley & Norris 1988) or by a fall from a height (Heppenstall 1975); the humerus and scapula are driven downwards. The displacement of the humerus and scapula against the chest wall may cause multiple fractures of the ipsilateral upper ribs (Neer 1963) (Fig. 12.10). Other associated injuries include avulsion of the coracoid process and head and neck injuries (Neer & Rockwood 1984).

Radiograph evaluation

Routine posteroanterior views and the 45° cephalad oblique view, taken with the patient supine, do not always demonstrate the problem. Neer (1963) described

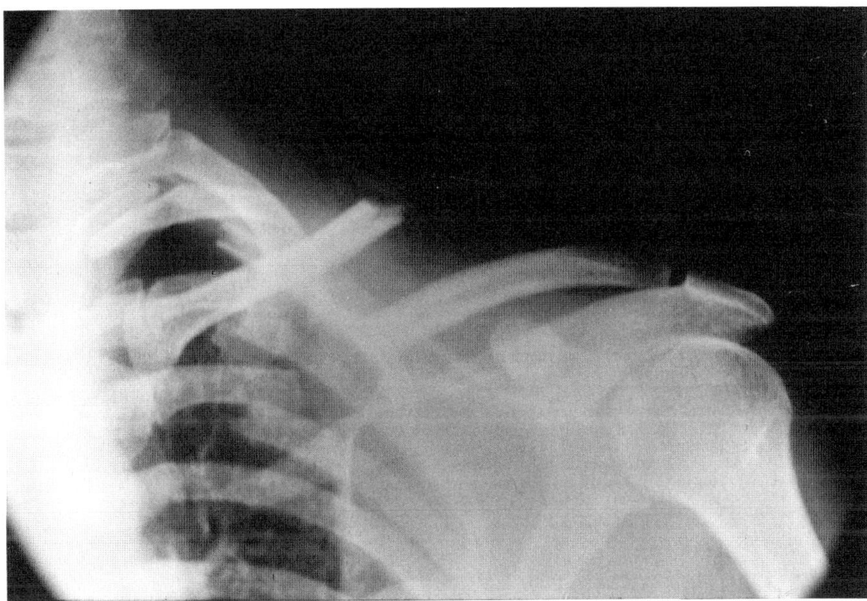

Fig. 12.10 Fractures of the ribs associated with a clavicular shaft fracture. This is a severe injury.

the following radiographic studies to determine the integrity of the coracoclavicular ligaments and study the fracture displacement:

1 Posteroanterior view to include both shoulders on a single large film with the patient erect and holding a 4.5 kg (10 lb) weight in each hand. Widening of the distance between the proximal fragment and the coracoid on the injured side is evidence of ligamentous detachment (Fig. 12.11).

2 Anterior 45° oblique view, with the patient erect and the injured shoulder against the plate, and with the tube directed from below cephalad, gives a lateral view of the scapula and clearly demonstrates the posterior displacement of the medial fragment and shows the gap (Fig. 12.12).

3 Posterior 45° oblique view, with the patient erect and the injured shoulder against the plate, also reveals this information (Fig. 12.13).

It is important to note that in usual shoulder radiographs the distal clavicle cannot be clearly evaluated since it appears too dark from overexposure. Proper exposure for the distal clavicle and acromio-clavicular joint is half that for the shoulder joint and small fragments can only be noted on good quality radiographs.

Treatment

Closed reduction and external support

Type 1 fractures usually heal uneventfully with conservative treatment, which should be in the form of a simple sling.

Several authors have reported the high incidence of delayed union, non-union and prolonged disability in Neer type 2 fractures treated conservatively. Neer (1963) noted that although these lesions are uncommon, they accounted for one-half of a series of ununited clavicles following closed treatment. He carried out a long-term follow-up of 23 patients with type 2 fractures and considered union to be delayed when there was no radiological evidence of bony bridging 3 months after injury, and non-union to be characterized by a lack of bony bridging 12 months after the injury with eburnation of the fracture surface. Based on these criteria he reported eight delayed unions and four non-unions in 12 conservatively treated patients compared with none in the seven patients treated by internal fixation. Heppenstall (1975) also abandoned this method of treatment after finding a high incidence of non-union and recommended ORIF as the preferred method. Kavanagh *et al.* (1985) studied 30 Neer type 2 fractures which were followed up for an average of 2 years: half were treated non-operatively and half by ORIF. They reported 40% non-unions and 40% delayed non-unions in the non-operative group compared with 100% healing by bone in the operated group; this led them to conclude that ORIF was the treatment of choice for these fractures. Edwards *et al.* (1992) further expanded on this series and reported 30% of patients with non-union and 45% with delayed union in the conservatively managed group of 23 patients compared with a 100% union rate in the same number of patients 6–10 weeks post-surgery.

Conservative treatment for type 2 fractures carries

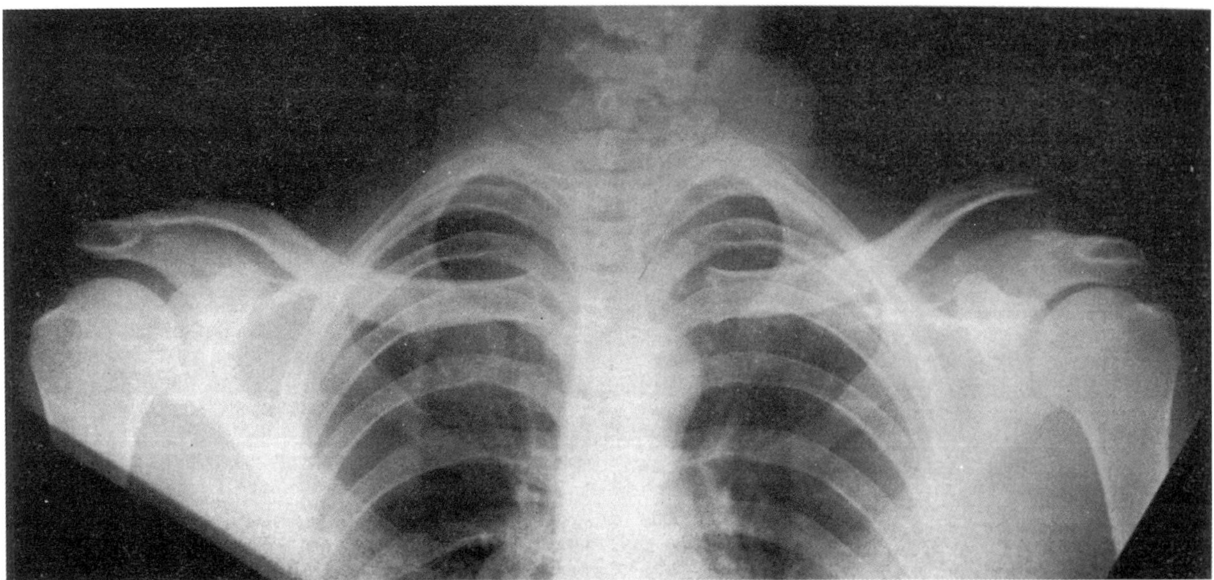

Fig. 12.11 Stress radiographs (patient erect and holding weights).

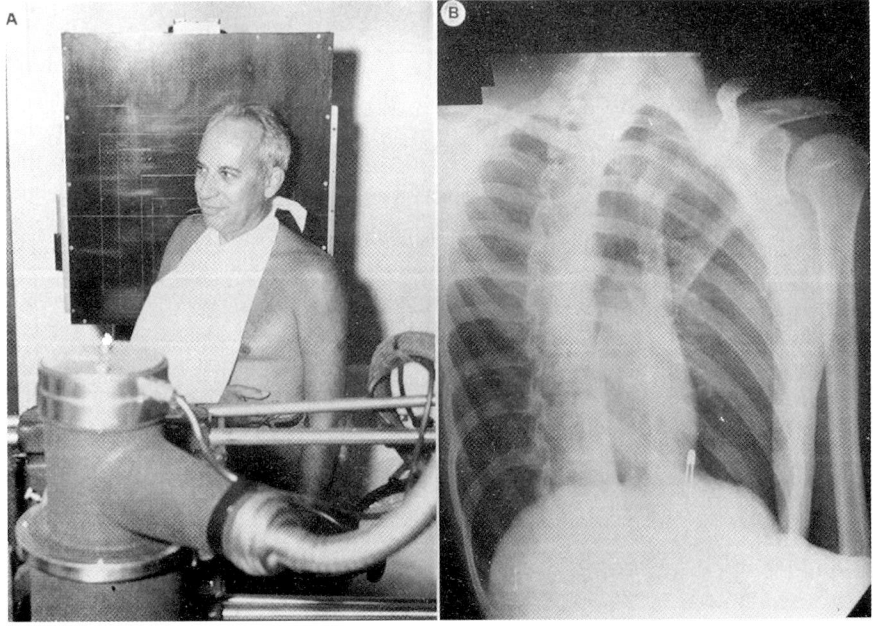

Fig. 12.12 Anterior 45° oblique view of the right shoulder with the patient erect.

such a high failure rate that the authors no longer recommend it.

Neer found that, in a group receiving closed treatment, the period of disability for those engaged in heavy work was from 7 months to 1 year. Shoulder discomfort, difficulty in sleeping on the affected side and shoulder stiffness presented persistent problems. Patients with non-union of the fracture experienced local weakness and fatigued easily. Kavanagh *et al.* (1985) reported that pain at the outer end of the clavicle required surgery to stabilize the bone in one patient while four others complained of an aching pain on lifting. Edwards *et al.* (1992) reported severe pain, painful limitation of abduction due to impingement and shoulder stiffness in the patients with delayed union, two of whom had to be dealt with surgically at a later date.

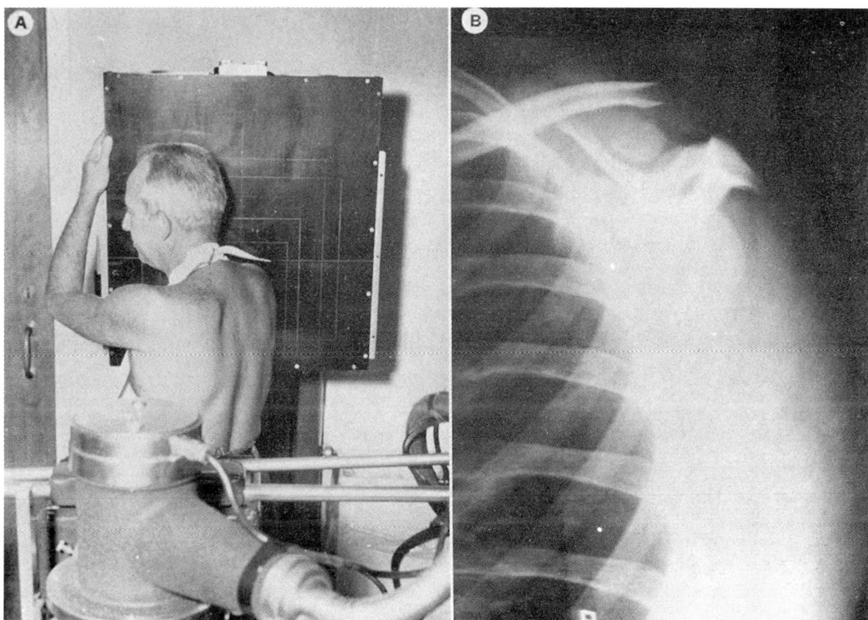

Fig. 12.13 Posterior 45° oblique view of the right shoulder with the patient erect.

Excision of the outer end of the clavicle

Simple excision of the outer end of the clavicle produces more problems than it solves (Heppenstall 1975). The outer fragment retains a valuable ligamentous attachment to the coracoid, and if excision is carried out without reconstruction of the coracoclavicular ligaments the clavicular shaft becomes even more unstable, displaces upwards and may become symptomatic by impinging on the scapula and soft tissues, perhaps requiring additional re-resection later.

Occasionally, a Weaver–Dunn procedure may be performed (Post 1989) to control the high-riding medial fragment from a chronically displaced clavicle. If this is not possible, a transfer of the coracoid to the lateral end of the clavicle with its active short head of biceps and coracobrachialis may be performed as a salvage procedure (Post 1989).

Neer (1963) performed excision with reconstruction of the ligament using a silk suture in one case and temporary stabilization of the shaft by transacromial medullary wires in three cases, but reported only one satisfactory late result. The preservation of the outer fragment offers the obvious advantage of the opportunity for bone-to-bone repair and is the vastly preferred option.

The only real place for excision of the outer end of the clavicle is in the type 3 fracture of Neer (Neer & Rockwood 1984), which has led to symptomatic arthritis. Here again it is vital to leave the coracoclavicular ligament intact. Interestingly, osteolysis of the lateral end of the clavicle, commonly seen in weight-lifters, is thought to be due to repeated microtrauma which can produce small fractures of this type.

ORIF

ORIF is the treatment of choice of Neer type 2 fractures (Fig. 12.14a) and is best undertaken within 48 hours of fracture. The best form of fixation is, as yet, unresolved and methods used have included coracoclavicular screws (Edwards *et al.*, personal communication) and transacromial K-wire fixation (Neer 1963, Neviaser *et al.* 1975, Edwards *et al.* 1992). Neer and others (Neer 1963, Allman 1967, Heppenstall 1975) have recommended the retrograde passage of two wires outward from the fracture site and through the distal fragment and acromion to protrude from the skin; following this the fracture is reduced and held as the wires are inserted back into the medial fragment. The wires are then bent over with pliers and are cut off beneath the skin to minimize the risk of migration. Reconstruction of the ligaments is not considered necessary in recent fractures (Neer 1963). The patient's hospital stay does not usually exceed 2–3 days and the patient can be discharged with a sling. Light use of the arm within the sling is permitted, but excessive shoulder motion must be prevented, since scapular motion will cause rotation and tilting at the fracture site, increasing the chance of a pin complication (Heppenstall 1975). The wires are kept in position for 6–8 weeks and then they are removed.

The authors' preferred method is by peroperative

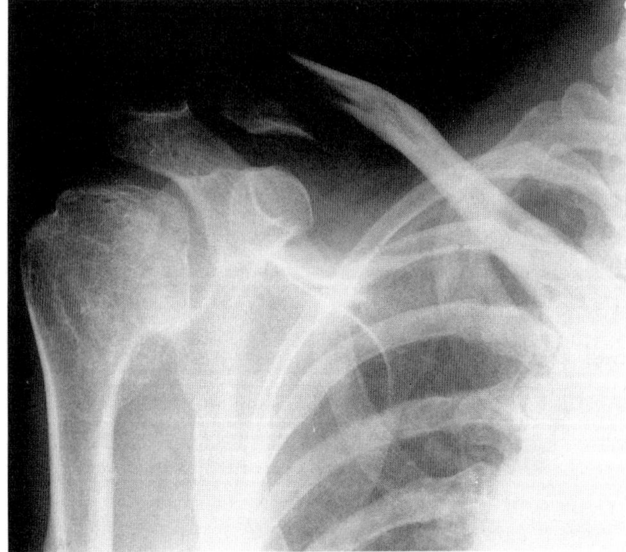

(a)

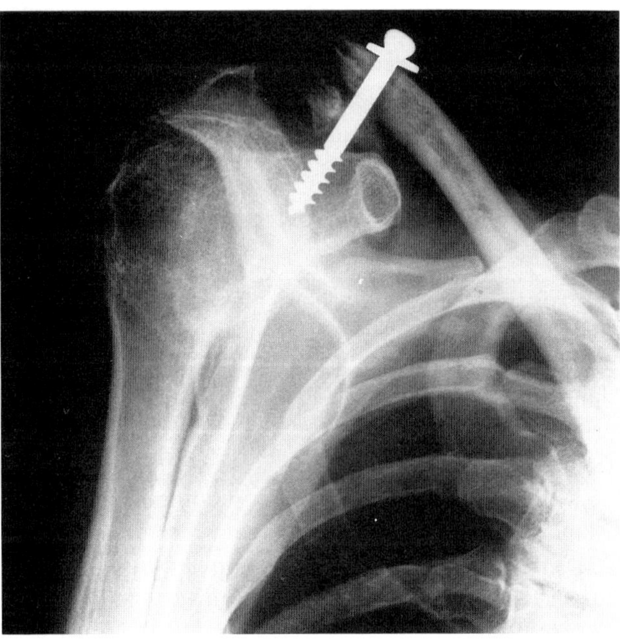

(b)

Fig. 12.14 (a) Preoperative radiograph (Neer type 2).
(b) Postoperative radiograph showing fixation with a
coracoclavicular screw.

stabilization of the reduced fracture with one stout
K-wire while a coracoclavicular (4.5 mm or 6.5 mm) AO
cancellous screw with a washer is inserted and checked
with radiography on the table; the K-wire is then
removed before the wound is closed. Accurate placement of the coracoclavicular screw is difficult but, if
placed properly as shown in Fig. 12.14b, this provides
excellent stabilization of the fracture. Radiological

union, applying Neers criteria (Neer 1963), usually
occurs in 6 to 10 weeks (Kavanagh *et al.* 1985, Edwards
et al. 1992).

The AO group (Müller *et al.* 1979) recommends that
transverse fractures of the distal clavicle just medial to
the acromio-clavicular joint, with or without joint involvement, are best fixed by a combination of a tension-
band wire and a malleolar screw, which is inserted
across the acromio-clavicular joint in a lateral to medial
direction. They recommend that the coracoclavicular
ligaments should be either repaired or replaced. If they
are sutured, one must suture the conoid ligament with
the arm in maximum abduction and the trapezoid ligament with the arm in maximum adduction, to take the
slack off the ligaments as they are being sutured. The
authors do *not* support this method, which causes excessive damage to the acromio-clavicular joint.

Complications of ORIF include superficial pin-track
infection, pin migration and breakage. Operation scars
commonly develop keloid and these may need corrective
plastic surgery later.

However, the predictable union, shortened disability
time and good anatomical and functional results make
this the best treatment for Neer type 2 fractures at the
present time.

Fractures of the medial end of the clavicle

This is the least common location for fractures of the
clavicle. Articular surface involvement may be undetected at the time of original injury and may be a cause
of subsequent post-traumatic arthritis.

Treatment

In acute cases, a supportive sling is all that is needed. If
secondary post-traumatic arthritis of the sternoclavicular joint develops, excision of the inner end of the
clavicle may be carried out (Neer & Rockwood 1984). In
doing so, it is important to leave most of the costoclavicular ligament intact and to transfer the head of the
sternocleidomastoid into the dead space in order to
reduce the risk of haematoma formation and the tendency of the stump to ride upwards.

Complications

Neurovascular complications

Neurovascular complications, although uncommon, are
potentially dangerous and can occur when any injury or
deformity causes an encroachment of the space between

the clavicle and the first rib. Mechanical compression or angulation of the subclavian vessels, brachial plexus or carotid artery are the common mechanisms responsible for neurovascular involvement associated with clavicular injuries.

Pathogenesis (Howard & Shafer 1965)

At the time of the fracture the pressure of displaced bone fragments may lead to neurovascular compression. On the other hand, stretching of the brachial plexus at the time of injury may cause a neuropraxia or axonotmesis. Therefore, it is important to enquire into the mechanism of injury.

Massive callus formation about a hypertrophic union or pseudoarthrosis at a non-union site may cause local pressure to the nerves and vessels.

Symptoms

These are classified into two general groups (Howard & Shafer 1965): (i) obstruction of the carotid artery at the medial end of the clavicle causing symptoms of syncope and (ii) compression of the subclavian vessels and/or brachial plexus between the clavicle and first rib causing neurological or vascular symptoms in the arm or hand. It is believed that the presence of an anomalous cervical rib predisposes the patient to this problem.

Diagnosis

Every case of a fracture of the clavicle must be examined carefully for distal neurovascular compromise in the ipsilateral limb. Early reduction and adequate immobilization may often solve the problem.

If the brachial plexus is injured, it may be the result of compression or stretching. Evaluation must be guided by history, physical findings, electromyograms and nerve conduction studies.

If vascular compromise is present because of a thoracic outlet syndrome, Adson's test, the costoclavicular manoeuvre, the attention test, downward traction on the upper extremity and the hyperabduction test must be carried out in an attempt to determine the site of compression.

Treatment

Initially, an attempt should be made to reduce the fracture by the closed method and to immobilize it adequately using a simple figure-of-eight splint. If there is no relief of neurovascular compression by closed reduction, prompt elevation of the depressed fragment must be carried out using ORIF and, at the same time, stabilizing the fracture. Posterior dislocation of the medial end of the clavicle can cause pressure on the common carotid artery and is an indication for immediate open reduction. If large vessels are torn in the subclavian region, immediate surgical exploration and vascular repair is warranted, but the subclavian vein is very thin walled and the company of a vascular surgeon at the time of operation can be very reassuring! This is followed by ORIF of the clavicular fracture site.

In long-standing cases of compression due to exuberant callus on the non-union mass, resection of the callus may be carried out along with brachial plexus exploration and neurolysis. If resection of the clavicle does not restore the radial pulse, the subclavian artery should be explored to eliminate local compression by scar tissue or the presence of an intimal tear. If the clavicle has a satisfactory appearance and is stable, enlargement of the costoclavicular space and neurovascular decompression can be accomplished by resection of the first rib and partial resection of the scalenus anterior muscle.

Non-union

Incidence

Although the clavicle is the most frequently fractured bone, comprising 5–10% of all fractures, non-union of the clavicle is rare, the reported incidence being 0.1–1.9% (Manske & Szabo 1985).

Diagnosis

SYMPTOMS

Not all non-unions of the clavicle are symptomatic. Symptomatic patients may complain of moderate to severe pain and/or grating from motion at the fracture site with the use of the ipsilateral shoulder. More commonly, the patient complains of impaired function or weakness of the shoulder which is severe enough to affect work or sporting activities. The deformity may cause pressure on the neurovascular structures in the costoclavicular space, leading to paraesthesia in the distal part of the extremity. Others may be bothered by the cosmetic appearance of the affected shoulder (Fig. 12.15). Surgical treatment should be reserved only for symptomatic cases, with the rare exception being made for the treatment of a painless cosmetic deformity in young females.

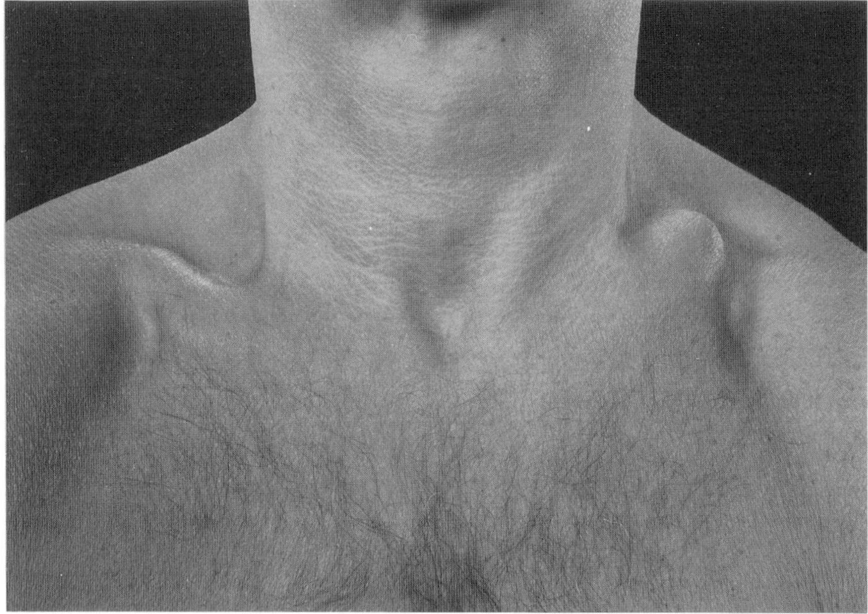

(a)

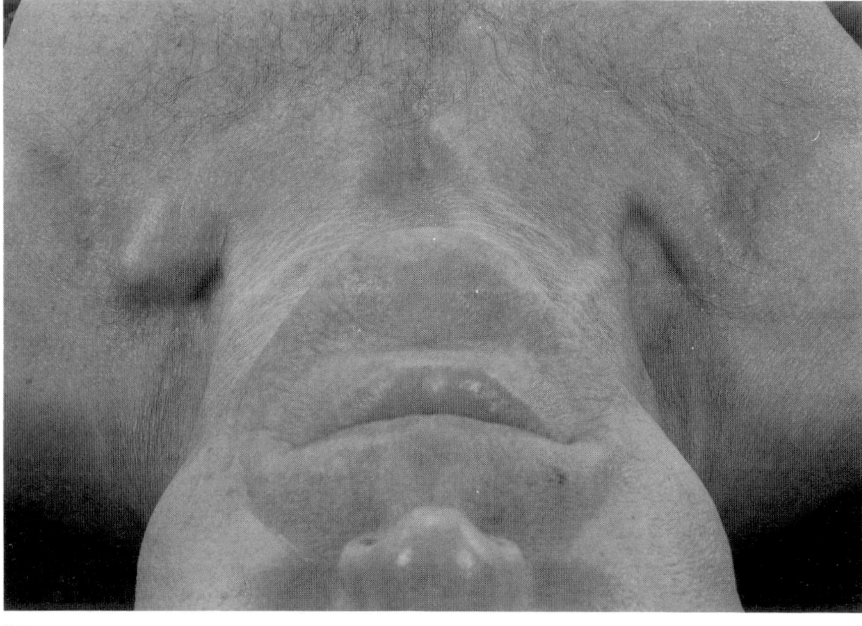

(b)

Fig. 12.15 Clinical appearance of clavicular non-union (left clavicle).

SIGNS

Most clavicular non-unions are *easily* diagnosed clinically by eliciting pain on stressing the fracture, local tenderness at the fracture site and abnormal mobility.

RADIOLOGICAL APPEARANCE

The time at which a clavicular fracture can be declared a non-union has not been clearly defined. Many authors have stated that an ununited clavicular fracture is one that has no demonstrable healing at 16 weeks (Manske & Szabo 1985).

The routine posteroanterior and 45° anterior oblique views are carried out to establish the type of non-union (Fig. 12.16). The radiological types of non-union are similar to those seen in any long bone and include atrophic non-union, with little or no evident callus, and hypertrophic non-union, in which callus production is excessive. Sometimes a true pseudoarthrosis may exist,

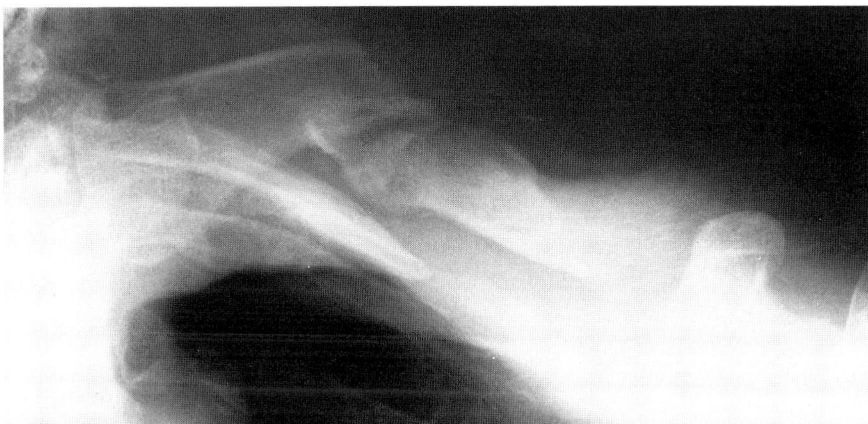

Fig. 12.16 Radiological appearance of clavicular non-union.

with a smooth rounding of the fracture ends, or there may be a gap non-union, because of the resorption of bone adjacent to the fracture, with obliteration of the medullary canal and with an intervening gap sometimes up to 3 cm in size (Neer 1960).

Factors predisposing to non-union

Primary ORIF

ORIF has, over the years, acquired a bad reputation because it is reported to be a cause of non-union. Neer (1960), in a review of 2235 patients with mid-shaft clavicular fractures, found a 0.1% incidence of non-union in those treated non-operatively and a 4.6% incidence following operative treatment, thereby indicating that primary operative treatment of clavicular fractures was a strong risk factor for non-union. Rowe (1968) analysed a series of 690 fractures and reported a non-union rate, following closed treatment, of 0.8%, whereas the rate following open reduction was 3.7%. However, it is important to put these results in their correct perspective. Zenni *et al.* (1981) pointed out that Neer's and Rowe's series included fractures in children, who normally have an infinitesimal incidence of non-union. More importantly, most of the techniques that had been used to fix clavicular fractures required extensive soft tissue stripping and, in the past, many were complicated by infection. Indeed, Rowe (1968) stated that since the adoption of intramedullary fixation, which causes significantly less surgical trauma, he had encountered no postoperative non-union. Further, Manske and Szabo (1985) pointed out that the fractures which were treated surgically were often the more difficult fractures. Non-rigid fixation without supplemental bone grafting and inadequate immobilization may have certainly led to non-union in the past. The message here is

to exercise prudence in the selection of cases for ORIF, to carry out the operation with the utmost respect for the soft tissues and to aim to achieve rigid fixation in these patients. For atrophic non-unions, autogenous bone grafting is recommended but in the authors' experience this is not necessary for hypertrophic non-unions.

Severity of trauma and degree of displacement

Severe trauma results in cases with gross comminution and/or displacement of the fracture site, with or without associated multiple injuries. Jupiter and Leffert (1987) considered the amount of displacement in the middle third of the clavicle in particular. They suggested that there was more instability of the fragment because of the more extensive damage to the soft tissue which, in turn, increased the risk of non-union. Thompson (1989) identified his type 3B fractures (see p. 333), accounting for 90% of non-unions, and made a case for primary ORIF of these fractures.

Soft tissue interposition

This is a major contributing factor in fractures that proceed to non-union. One of the fragments is often found impaled in the trapezius muscle and this is usually confirmed surgically (Manske & Szabo 1985).

Refracture

Wilkins and Johnston (1983) found that patients who sustained a refracture in the area of a previously united fracture had a predilection to non-union. They suggest that healing of a refracture may be compromised by the ability of the already altered microvascular anatomical pattern to respond to the re-injury.

Other factors, which are common predisposing factors to non-union of other bones, include: *insufficient length or stability of immobilization*, and *open fractures*; these often lead to non-union complicated by infection.

Treatment

Not all non-unions require surgery. Surgical treatment is only indicated if it is significantly symptomatic. The surgical options are:

1 *Plate and screw fixation.* Several authors have reported that rigid compression fixation with a plate and screws and autogenous iliac bone graft for the treatment of non-union have resulted in excellent functional results with a high rate of radiological union (Pyper 1978, Wilkins & Johnston 1983, Manske & Szabo 1985, Jupiter & Leffert 1987). It has been recommended that the iliac bone graft be placed posteriorly away from the neuro-vascular bundles and subcutaneous surfaces (Neer & Rockwood 1984). Manske and Szabo (1985) reported that 10 patients treated by this method had clinically united by 10 weeks after surgery with no operative or postoperative complications and had a full, painless range of motion of the ipsilateral shoulder with an acceptable cosmetic result. Jupiter and Leffert (1987) pointed out that the apex of the deformity in most patients with non-union of the middle third of the clavicle is directed superiorly. Therefore, when the plate is placed superiorly on the bone, it functions as a tension-band and would theoretically be effective since it is sufficiently rigid to withstand both the bending and torsional forces at the middle third of the clavicle. They reported that the high success with plate fixation in this and other series supports these theoretical advantages. Pyper (1978), in a small series of three patients, reported a successful outcome by AO compression plating without the need for supplemental bone graft in two of the patients. Further advantages of this method are the lack of need for additional external immobiliz-ation and a shortened rehabilitation time. Clearly, this is the most proven preferred method of treatment for clavicular non-unions at the present time.

2 *Intramedullary fixation.* Although frequently recom-mended in the past (Watson-Jones 1955, Taylor 1969, Marsh & Hazarian 1970), the outcome following intra-medullary fixation techniques is not uniformly suc-cessful (Wilkins & Johnston 1983). Also, it has the disadvantages of requiring a period of prolonged sup-plemental immobilization and consequent increased morbidity postoperatively, in addition to its other dis-advantages. Neviaser *et al.* (1975), however, reported that the method of intramedullary fixation using a Knowles pin provided a secure compression fixation and allowed union without complications in all cases.

3 *External fixation.* Schuind *et al.* (1988) used external fixation in five patients with delayed union or symp-tomatic non-union and reported that all patients united without secondary refracture or complications.

4 *Partial resection of the clavicle or resection of the non-union site.* This method has a very limited place in the management of clavicular non-union, except perhaps to relieve neurovascular compression at the thoracic outlet.

Malunion

Some degree of malunion, resulting from routine con-servative treatment of the fractured clavicle, is common-place and is usually compatible with acceptable cosmesis and good function. However, sometimes an exaggerated cosmetic bump on the dropped shoulder, from shorten-ing and angular deformity at the fracture site, may be a worrying unsightly abnormality, especially for young females. In these cases, either a simple 'bumpectomy' can be performed or more complex osteotomy and re-alignment with lengthening of the clavicle can be per-formed using internal fixation with a plate and the addition of iliac bone graft around the raw bone site (Post 1989). However, it is important to involve the patient closely in the decision to operate, and the wise surgeon will only operate if pushed to do so by the patient and after appropriate advice about potential scars and complications has been given. If a long oblique osteotomy is used, then lengthening of the clavicle is usually fairly straightforward (Fig. 12.17), but it is the proximity of the brachial plexus and major vessels which is the main concern and these should, of course, be carefully protected during surgery.

Post-traumatic arthritis

This is most commonly seen following type 3 fractures of the distal clavicle (Neer & Rockwood 1984) which involve the acromio-clavicular joint. Arthritis of the sternoclavicular joint is much less common. An articular surface injury is difficult to demonstrate using routine radiographs and is often overlooked at the time of injury. The patient usually presents with ongoing pain many months or years after the injury as a typical case of acromio-clavicular joint arthritis. Radiographic studies should include a radiograph of the opposite side for comparison and a CT scan can be beneficial. If an injection of 1% lignocaine into the acromio-clavicular joint gives a satisfactory relief of pain, it is an indication that excision of the joint will be beneficial. Excision of

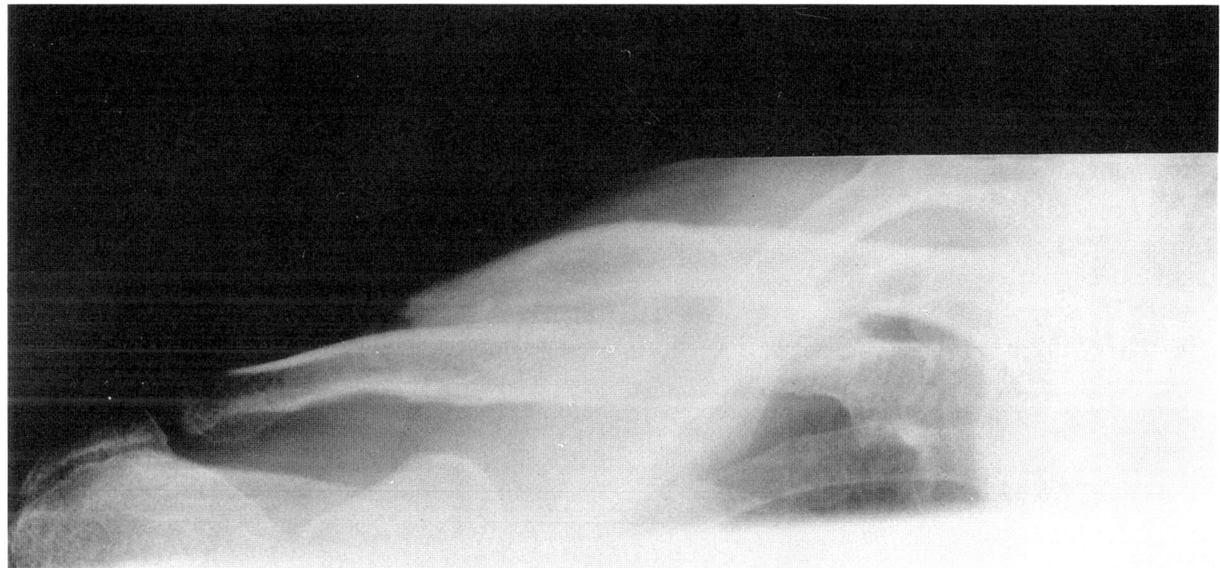

(a)

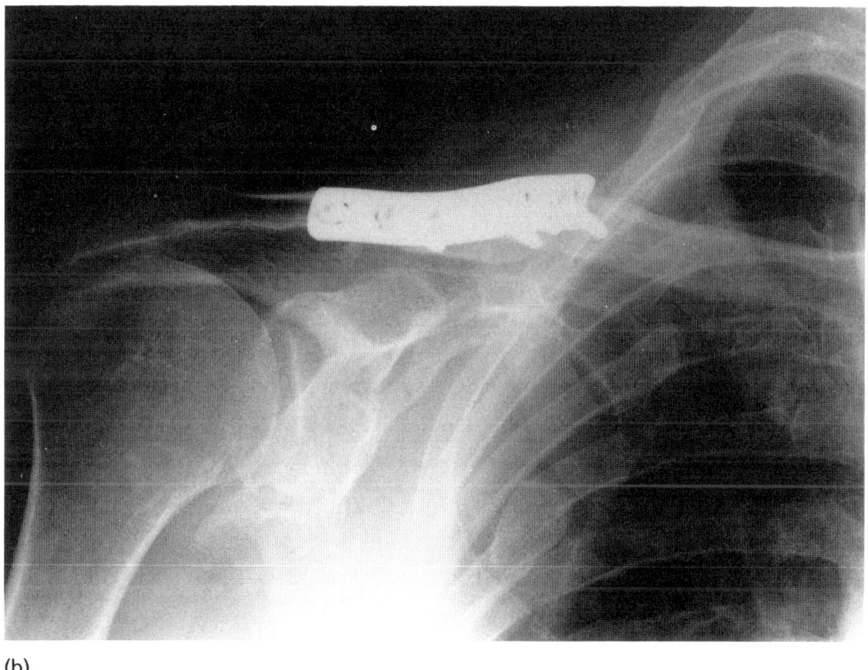

(b)

Fig. 12.17 Treatment of a malunion (a) with oblique osteotomy, lengthening and the application of a 3.5 mm AO plate and bone graft (b).

the lateral 1 cm of clavicle should be carried out, keeping the coracoclavicular ligaments intact for best results.

Fractures of the clavicle in children and neonates

The clavicle is the most frequently fractured bone in children and more than 80% of these fractures occur in the shaft. The frequency of the fracture in children, and the special features that it exhibits prior to skeletal maturity, makes it imperative to include a special section on childhood clavicular fractures.

Growth and development (Dameron & Rockwood 1984)

Most authors classify the central portion of the clavicle

as membranous bone. Cartilaginous growth plate areas develop at the medial and distal ends of the shaft, with the plate at the sternal end dominating the longitudinal growth of the clavicle.

The clavicle is unique as it is the first bone in the embryo to ossify. Ossification begins in two different areas which fuse into one mass on, or about, the 45th day or when the crown–rump measurement is 19 mm. This ossification centre contributes to growth up to 5 years of age. A secondary ossification centre appears routinely on radiographs at the sternal end of the clavicle, but only rarely does the secondary ossification centre at the acromial end become apparent on radiographs.

Ogden *et al.* (1979) have reported that the sternal epiphysis contributes to 80% of the growth in length of the clavicle. This epiphysis begins to ossify at 12–19 years and fuses with the clavicle at 22–25 years. The sternal epiphysis is not usually seen on plain radiographs and can barely be noted on tomograms. The late fusion of the medial clavicular epiphysis is important since many so-called dislocations of the sternoclavicular joint, even in adults up to 25 years of age, may, in reality, be unrecognized physeal injuries.

Clavicle fractures in the newborn

The clavicle is the most frequent fractured bone during parturition (Oppenheim *et al.* 1990) and the incidence has been reported as between 2 and 7 fractures per 1000 live births. Oppenheim *et al.* (1990) carried out a retrospective review of 21 623 live births over a 5-year period and found the overall incidence of clavicular fractures to be 2.7 per 1000 live births. Based on their extensive studies, they came up with some interesting conclusions with regard to the risk factors for fractures of the clavicle in the newborn.

Risk factors

The vertex of the fetus is simply too large to negotiate the maternal pelvis easily and, consequently, excessive pressure is placed on the shoulder by the symphysis pubis (Fig. 12.18). Since the left occipito-anterior position is the most common presentation, a majority of the burden falls on the right shoulder, explaining why the right clavicle is more likely to be fractured than the left; this is supported statistically. Also, an association was found between fractures of the clavicle, heavy neonates and shoulder dystocia. A heavy neonate is more likely to experience shoulder dystocia and consequent birth injury. Further, shoulder dystocia makes the use of

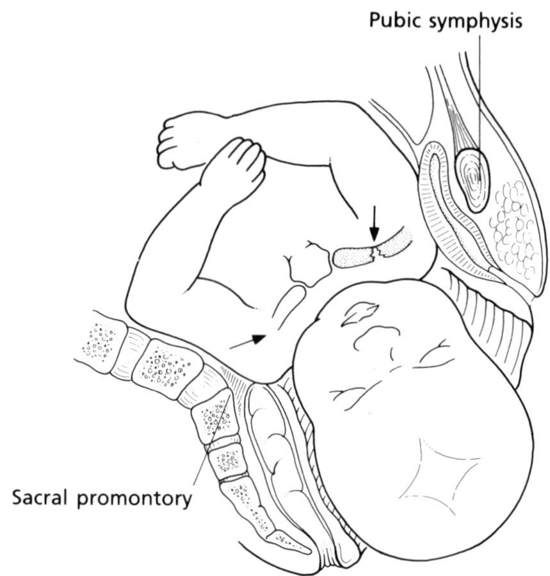

Fig. 12.18 Mechanism of clavicular fracture in a vertex delivery complicated by clavicular fracture.

forceps more likely, which, in turn, increases the incidence of birth trauma. These findings led the authors to suggest that the incidence of clavicular fractures in the newborn may be decreased by identifying the large fetus and minimizing shoulder dystocia. This depends on good prenatal care. Dameron and Rockwood (1984) reported an incidence of 160 fractures of the clavicle per 1000 breech deliveries and linked the high incidence to the difficulty experienced by the obstetrician in delivering the extended arms and shoulders.

Diagnosis

Typically, a neonate with a fracture of the clavicle presents with a pseudoparalysis (Dameron & Rockwood 1984) or reluctance to actively move the affected extremity. It must be clearly differentiated from brachial plexus injuries, traumatic separation of the proximal humeral epiphysis, humeral shaft fractures, dislocation of the shoulder (Kessel 1982) and acute osteomyelitis around the shoulder, especially in the proximal humerus. Fractures of the clavicle are almost always of the greenstick variety and may sometimes only become apparent 2–3 weeks later by the presence of a palpable mass of exuberant callus around the fracture site. The diagnosis, once suspected, is confirmed radiographically by a plain posteroanterior chest radiograph.

Complications

Brachial plexus injuries have similar risk factors to

fractures of the clavicle and have been shown to be associated with larger neonates, shoulder dystocia, the use of forceps and abnormal presentations (Kessel 1982). They are caused by excessive tension on the brachial plexus, owing to wide separation of the head and shoulder, and throw a particular strain on the C5 and C6 nerve roots. Oppenheim *et al.* (1990) found that one in 19 clavicular fractures was associated with a brachial plexus injury. Hence, it is of vital importance to carry out a thorough neurological examination in all newborn cases with fracture of the clavicle. The prognosis for nerve recovery, however, is good and uneventful recovery is the rule.

Treatment

Treatment for the fracture is gentle handling and rest, with careful turning and lifting to avoid pain. Healing easily occurs by 1–2 weeks without any additional treatment.

Clavicle fractures in children

Clinical features

Clavicular fractures in children between 2–12 years is usually of the greenstick variety and may be undiagnosed until visible or palpable callus appears. If, however, the fracture is displaced, the clinical signs are more obvious, with the shoulder drooping downwards, forwards and inwards and with the affected arm held under the elbow with the opposite hand.

Torticollis is often an accompanying feature with the chin turned towards the uninjured side and the head tilted towards the injured side, ostensibly in an attempt to relax the pull of the sternocleidomastoid. Goddard *et al.* (1990) presented five cases of children with atlanto-axial rotatory fixation (AARF) or subluxation and with an associated fracture of the clavicle. They postulated that the rotatory fixation was a direct result of the trauma which produced the fracture. It is important to recognize this association and to pay particular attention to torticollis in children with clavicular fractures. The doctor must be absolutely satisfied that the radiographs are indeed normal and must not assume that the torticollis is due to protective sternocleidomastoid spasm related to the clavicular fracture. The diagnosis of concomitant AARF must be established early, by fluoroscopy, spot films or, if there is any lingering doubt, by a CT scan. The incidence of these cases is undoubtedly low but prompt diagnosis is necessary since treatment instituted early can lead to a permanent resolution of the deformity without surgical intervention.

Radiographic features

In a suspected clavicular fracture in a child, radiographic investigations should include routine posteroanterior and 45° anterior oblique views to determine the presence of a fracture and the degree of displacement, if any. Fractures of the medial end are easily missed because they are often incomplete and may be obscured by the second rib. It is important to differentiate traumatic fractures (Dameron & Rockwood 1984) from:

1 Ossification centres in the epiphyses on the sternal and acromial ends of the clavicle.

2 Congenital pseudoarthroses. This condition is usually differentiated from a traumatic fracture by the absence of a history of trauma, by a lack of early callus formation and by its predominance in the distal portion of the central one-third of the bone. The pseudoarthrosis typically has smooth hypertrophic bone ends, and usually only the right clavicle is affected.

3 Cleidocranial dysostoses. The clavicle is the most frequently involved bone. Usually the distal portion, but less commonly the entire clavicle, and very uncommonly the sternal segment, is absent. Central clavicular deficiency is characteristic in that the ends of the bone adjacent to the defect are attenuated and taper gradually and progressively towards the defect. Again, there is no history of trauma and no callus formation is seen.

Complications

Neurovascular. Although childhood fractures heal with abundant callus, it rarely encroaches upon the costo-clavicular space sufficient to cause neurovascular compression. Usually, the thickened periosternum protects against vascular lesions from bony fragments in children. If injuries to the subclavian artery or vein do occur, appropriate vascular surgery must be instituted promptly.

Malunion. Although malunion, with resultant foreshortening from healing in a bayonet position, occurs frequently, it presents no problem, nor does angular deformity because the remodelling potential of the clavicle in children is incredible.

Non-union. Non-union in children is extremely rare. When it occurs it is most likely to be due to a missed congenital pseudoarthrosis.

Refracture. This is usually the result of a second episode of trauma. Unlike in the adult, its occurrence does not delay satisfactory healing.

Treatment

Despite the many methods of treatment described, fractures of the clavicle in children heal quickly with an excellent prognosis for normal function and with few, if any, complications.

The younger the child, the shorter is the period of immobilization required. For children under 2 years, clinical union usually occurs in less than 2 weeks; in the 2–12 year age group it occurs in 2–3 weeks; and from 12 years to maturity 3–4 weeks of immobilization may be needed. The tendency for complete fracture and displacement also increases with age, since in younger children the thick periosteal cover and more flexible associated structures protect the bone from complete breakage.

Whenever possible, ambulatory treatment in a figure-of-eight splint is preferred. For younger children this can be fashioned from three to four layers of roller sheet wadding pulled into a piece of 5 cm cotton tubular stockinet. For older children and teenagers a commercially available figure-of-eight harness may be used. The figure-of-eight harness may not immobilize the fracture very effectively, but its main purpose is to remind the patient to hold the shoulder up and back. If the patient allows the shoulder to slump forwards, the support cuts into the anterior axillae and acts as a memory aid! It should therefore be tightened after 2–3 days and again 1 week after the injury.

Sometimes, other forms of conservative treatment may be effectively employed. For example, a sling may be substituted for a figure-of-eight splint in older co-operative children with incomplete fractures; this has the advantage of greater comfort. On the other hand, in active or uncooperative teenagers, a shoulder spica may be used as a safer method of immobilization.

Surgery is rarely, if ever, required for childhood fractures of the clavicle. Open fractures and neurovascular injuries present a case for operative treatment (Dameron & Rockwood 1984). Post (1989) reported a case where open reduction was used in a case of bilateral severely displaced Allman group I fractures, in which the right medial clavicle pierced the platysma and trapezius while the whole delto-trapezius aponeurosis was avulsed from the clavicle. However, he used only a single suture to hold the reduction, repaired the aponeurosis and did not find the need to internally fix the fracture.

References

Ali Khan, M.A. & Lucas, K.J. Plating of fractures of the middle third of the clavicle. *Injury* 1978; **9**: 263–267.

Allman, F.L. Jr. Fractures and ligamentous injuries of the clavicle and its articulation. *J Bone Joint Surg* 1967; **49A**: 774–784.

Apley, A.G. & Solomon, L. *Apley's System of Orthopaedics and Fractures* 6th edn. Butterworth: London, 1982.

Dameron, T.B. Jr. & Rockwood, C.A. Jr. Fracture of the shaft of the clavicle. In: Rockwood, C.A. Jr., Wilkins, K.E. & King, R.E. (eds) *Fractures in Children*. Lippincott: Philadelphia, 1984.

Fowler, A.W. Fracture of the clavicle. *J Bone Joint Surg* 1962; **44B**: 440.

Edwards, D.J., Kavanagh, T.G. & Flannery, M.C. Fracture of the distal clavicle: a case for fixation. *Injury* 1992; **23**: 44–46.

Goddard, N.J., Stabler, J. & Albert, J.S. Atlanto-axial rotatory fixation and fracture of the clavicle: an association and a classification. *J Bone Joint Surg* 1990; **72B**: 72–75.

Heppenstall, R.B. Fractures and dislocations of the distal clavicle. *Orthop Clin North Am* 1975; **6(2)**: 477–479.

Howard, F.M. & Shafer, S.J. Injuries to the clavicle with neurovascular complications. *J Bone Joint Surg* 1965; **47A**: 1335–1346.

Jupiter, J.B. & Leffert, R.D. Non-union of the clavicle: associated complications and surgical management. *J Bone Joint Surg* 1987; **69A**: 753–760.

Kavanagh, T.G., Sankar, S.D. & Phillips, H. Complications of displaced fractures (type II Neer) of the outer end of the clavicle. *J Bone Joint Surg* 1985; **67B**: 492–493.

Kessel, L. *Clinical Disorders of the Shoulder*. Churchill Livingstone: Edinburgh, 1982.

Lyons, F.A. & Rockwood, C.A. Current concepts review: migration of pins used in operations on the shoulder. *J Bone Joint Surg* 1990; **72A**: 1262–1267.

Manske, D.J. & Szabo, R.M. The operative treatment of midshaft clavicular non-unions. *J Bone Joint Surg* 1985; **67A**: 1367–1371.

Marsh, H.O. & Hazarian, E. Pseudarthrosis of the clavicle. *J Bone Joint Surg* 1970; **52B**: 793.

Müller, M.E., Allgöwer, M., Schneider, R. & Willenegger, H. (eds) Fractures of the clavicle. In: *Manual of Internal Fixation: Techniques Recommended by the AO Group* 2nd edn. Springer-Verlag: New York, 1979.

Mullick, S. Treatment of midclavicular fractures. *Lancet* 1967; **i**: 499.

Neer, C.S.II Non union of the clavicle. *J Am Med Assoc* 1960; **172(10)**: 1006–1011.

Neer, C.S.II Fractures of the distal clavicle with detachment of the coracoclavicular ligaments in adults. *J Trauma* 1963; **3**: 99–110.

Neer, C.S.II & Rockwood, C.A. Jr. Fractures and dislocations of the shoulder. In: Rockwood, C.A. Jr. & Green, D.P. (eds) *Fractures in Adults* 2nd edn. Lippincott: Philadelphia, 1984.

Neviaser, R.J., Neviaser, J.S., Neviaser, T.J. & Neviaser, J.S. A simple technique for internal fixation of the clavicle. *Clin Orthop* 1975; **109**: 103–107.

Nicoll, E.A. Annotation: miners & mannequins. *J Bone Joint Surg* 1954; **36B(2)**: 171–172.

Ogden, J.A., Conologue, G.J. & Bronson, M.L. Radiology of postnatal skeletal development. III. The clavicle. *Skel. Radiol* 1979; **4**: 196−203.

Oppenheim, W.L., Davis, A., Grasdon, W.A., Dorey, F.J. & Davlin, L.B. Clavicle fractures in the newborn. *Clin Orthop* 1990; **250**: 176−180.

Paffen, P.J. & Jansen, E.W.L. Surgical treatment of clavicular fractures with K-wires: a comparative study. *Arch Clin Neder* 1978; **30**: 43−53.

Piterman, L. The fractured clavicle. *Aust Fam Physician* 1982; **11**: 614.

Post, M. Current concepts in the treatment of fractures of the clavicle. *Clin Orthop* 1989; **245**: 89−101.

Pyper, J.B. Non-union of fracture of the clavicle. *Injury* 1978; **9**: 268−270.

Rowe, C.R. An atlas of anatomy and treatment of mid-clavicular fractures. *Clin Orthop* 1968; **58**: 29−42.

Sankarankutty, M. & Turner, B.W. Fractures of the clavicle. *Injury* 1975; **7**: 101−106.

Schuind, F., Pay-Pay, E., Adrianne, Y., DonkerWelcke, M., Rasquin, C. & Burny, F. External fixation of the clavicle for fracture or non-union in adults. *J Bone Joint Surg* 1988; **70A**: 692−695.

Sharrard, W.J.W. *Paediatric Orthopaedics and Fractures* 2nd edn. Blackwell Scientific Publications: Oxford, 1979.

Smith, R.W. *A Treatise on Fractures in the Vicinity of Joints.* Hodges & Smith: Dublin, 1847.

Stanley, D. & Norris, S.H. Recovery following fractures of the clavicle treated conservatively. *Injury* 1988; **19**: 162−164.

Stanley, D., Trowbridge, E.A. & Norris, S.H. The mechanism of clavicular fracture: a clinical and biomechanical analysis. *J Bone Joint Surg* 1988; **70B**: 461−464.

Taylor, A.R. Non-union of fractures of the clavicle: a review of thirty-one cases. *J Bone Joint Surg* 1969; **51B**: 568.

Thompson, J.S. ORIF uniquely suited to displaced midthird clavicle fractures. *Orthopaedics Today* 1989; **14**: 1.

Watson-Jones, R. *Fractures and Joint Injuries*, Vol. 2. Churchill Livingstone: Edinburgh, 1955.

Wilkins, R.M. & Johnston, R.M. Ununited fractures of the clavicle. *J Bone Joint Surg* 1983; **65A**: 773−778.

Zenni, E.J., Kreig, J.K. & Rosen, M.J. Open reduction and internal fixation of clavicular fractures. *J Bone Joint Surg* 1981; **63A**: 149−151.

Acromio-clavicular joint

J.J.DIAS AND P.J.GREGG

Introduction

The management of the dislocated acromio-clavicular joint remains controversial and the role of surgical reconstruction of this joint has not yet been clearly defined. The exact incidence of injury to the acromio-clavicular joint is not known. Three-quarters of the patients in most studies sustained their injury during contact sport or during a road traffic accident (Allman 1967, Scott & Orr 1973) and most of the patients were male; there was a male:female ratio of 4:1. Most patients were in their early thirties (Nevaiser 1968, Deerhake & Olix 1975).

Anatomy

The acromio-clavicular joint is a planar joint. Its joint capsule is reinforced by superior and inferior acromio-clavicular ligaments, of which the former is the stronger structure. It contains an intra-articular cartilaginous disc that starts degenerating by the third decade (Fig. 12.19). Urist (1946) documented that the joint surface was obliquely disposed in 49% of normal radiographs whilst it was vertical in 36%. It has been suggested that the obliquity of the joint surface may predispose to traumatic disruption.

The acromio-clavicular joint is stabilized by the coracoclavicular ligaments (Fig. 12.19) which prevent medial displacement of the scapula. The trapezoid component restricts backward rotation whilst the conoid restricts forward rotation of the scapula. The main movement taking place at the joint is rotation in the long axis of the clavicle (Copeland & Kessel 1979).

Pathology

The mechanism of injury is assumed to be forcible depression of the acromion due to a fall onto the point

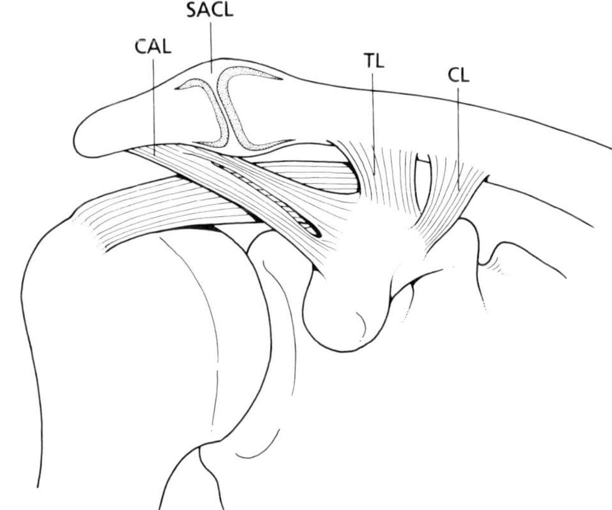

Fig. 12.19 The acromio-clavicular joint showing the intraarticular disc and reinforced by superior (SACL) and inferior acromio-clavicular ligaments. The trapezoid (TL) and conoid (CL) components of the coracoclavicular ligament are demonstrated as is the coracoacromial ligament (CAL).

of the shoulder. However, in most studies on this injury, the patients have been unable to state exactly how the injury was sustained.

The pathology in acute dislocation of this joint is well documented (Horn 1954). The following structures give way in sequence: (i) the superior attachment of the intra-articular disc and the superior acromio-clavicular ligament from its distal attachment, (ii) the lateral end of the clavicle is shelled out of the inferior periosteum, (iii) the coracoclavicular ligaments and the clavipectoral fascia are torn and, in very severe cases, (iv) the entire clavicular attachment of the deltoid is stripped off with an associated longitudinal tear in the trapezius between the clavicular and acromial attachments.

Symptoms and signs

Following an injury to the shoulder (usually during contact sport such as rugby or football) the patient presents with pain and swelling in the region of the shoulder. Acute tenderness can be elicited over the acromio-clavicular joint. If no step can be palpated over the superior aspect of the acromio-clavicular joint then the patient has probably merely sprained this joint. A slight step would suggest a subluxation, although a radiographic assessment would be necessary to establish the severity of the injury. An obvious step suggests a joint dislocation (Fig. 12.20). The lateral end of the clavicle is prominent. Resisted flexion of the elbow with the arm by the side of the patient contracts the deltoid muscle. This can affect the dislocation in one of three ways: (i) the joint may reduce if the clavicular attachment of the deltoid is intact, (ii) there may be no change in the dislocated position or (iii) the lateral end of the clavicle may become more prominent, suggesting an associated tear of the clavicular attachment of the deltoid. This test (Bannister 1983) helps to determine the severity of the dislocation.

Radiographic diagnosis and classification

This injury is best appreciated on a standard postero-anterior radiographic view with a 15° cephalad tilt (Zanca 1971). Suspending 4.5 kg (10 lb) weights from the wrists and repeating this radiographic view may reveal an occult dislocation.

The classification of this injury (Fig. 12.21) into three grades — a sprain, a subluxation and a dislocation — proposed by Tossy *et al.* (1963) on weight-bearing radiographs, and later re-emphasized by Allman (1967), reflects the pathology of this injury. Patients presenting with localized tenderness over the acromio-clavicular

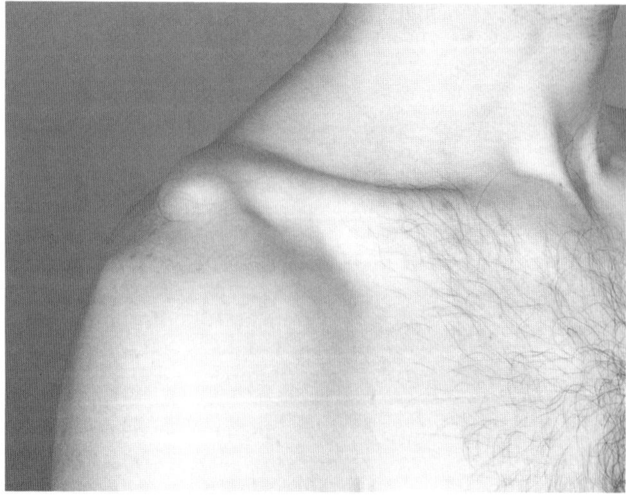

Fig. 12.20 Clinical appearance of a dislocated acromio-clavicular joint.

joint and in whom the orientation of the lateral end of the clavicle to the acromion is similar to the contralateral side, are considered to have sprained this joint. Those presenting with a slight deformity and in whom radiographs reveal a subluxation of the joint in comparison to the other side, are considered to have sustained a subluxation. Those in whom the lateral end of the clavicle no longer articulates with the acromion have dislocated this joint. The classification mentioned earlier does not define the severity of dislocation.

It is possible (Bannister 1983) to distinguish three patterns of acromio-clavicular dislocation on a special weight-lifting radiographic view designed to contract the anterior deltoid (a 3.6 kg (8 lb) weight held with the elbow flexed and the arm next to the body). This view establishes whether: (a) the joint reduces from its dislocated position, indicating that the deltoid attachment to the clavicle is essentially intact; or (b) the joint remains in its dislocated position; or (c) the degree of dislocation increases, indicating that the clavicular attachment of the deltoid is stripped off (Fig. 12.21).

Early management

There is no controversy regarding the early management of a sprained (type I) or subluxed (type II) acromio-clavicular joint. The injured upper limb is supported in a broad arm sling for the initial 2–3 weeks and this is followed by gentle mobilization of the shoulder, within the limits of pain. Full functional recovery is usual.

The treatment of acute dislocation (type III) remains controversial. In 1946, Urist reviewed 101 previous

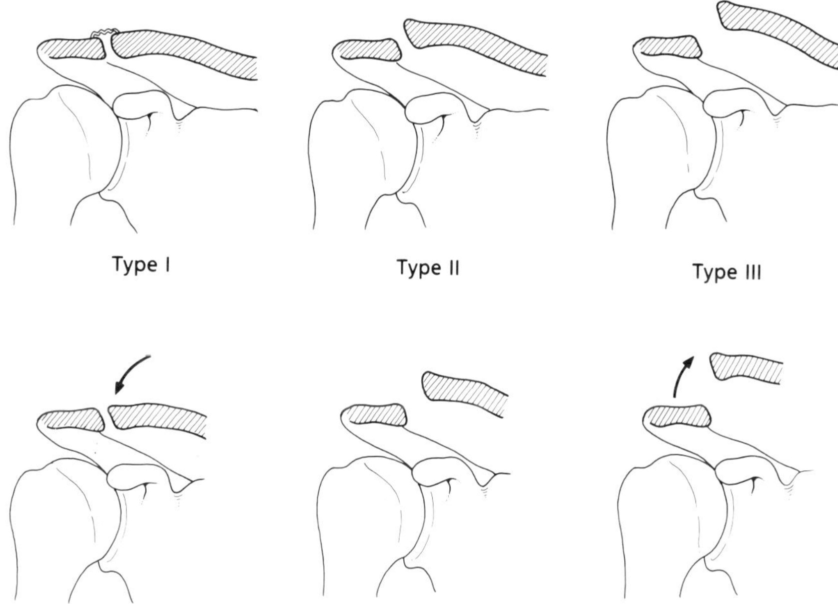

Fig. 12.21 The classification of acromio-clavicular joint injuries: type I, a sprain; type II, a subluxation; and type III, a dislocation. (After Tossy *et al.* 1963, Allman 1967.) The dislocations can be subdivided on a special 'weight-lifting view' into those in which (IIIa) the joint reduces from its dislocated position, or (IIIb) the joint remains in its dislocated position, or (IIIc) the degree of dislocation increases, indicating that the clavicular attachment of the deltoid is stripped off.

papers and reported between 10 and 20% unsatisfactory results following conservative management. It was generally assumed that an untreated dislocation results in serious functional disability and a variety of surgical procedures to stabilize the joint have been described. These procedures may involve acromio-clavicular transfixation (Phemister 1942, Bargren & Erlangers 1970), rigid coracoclavicular fixation (Bosworth 1941) or reconstruction of the coracoclavicular ligaments using the coracoacromial ligament, conjoint tendon or Dacron tape (Vargas 1942, Nevaiser 1968, Deerhake & Olix 1975).

However, none of the surgical methods have been consistently shown to improve on the outcome following conservative management. One-third of acromio-clavicular transfixations and about 16% of coracoclavicular fixations using a screw or a loop were reported as unsatisfactory (Bannister 1983). In addition, surgery itself may extend the associated muscular lesion and in one-third of cases the reduction achieved surgically was subsequently lost.

The few prospective studies comparing conservative and surgical management have been unable to demonstrate that early surgical intervention led to improved results. Imatani *et al.* (1975) compared 12 conservatively treated patients with 11 patients who had either acromio-clavicular transfixation or a coracoclavicular screw. They used an exacting scoring system to assess the results and were unable to establish any significant differences between the two groups. Bannister (1983) reported on 58 cases of acromio-clavicular dislocation,

28 of which had been treated with coracoclavicular screw fixation. The results were satisfactory in 90% of the conservatively treated cases and in 82% of the operated patients. In addition, patients treated conservatively returned to work and sport quicker than those treated surgically. Therefore, most acromio clavicular dislocations can be treated conservatively in a broad arm sling for the initial painful period, followed by shoulder mobilization.

Is there a place for surgical reconstruction?

It is possible that in severe dislocation surgical stabilization may be indicated. Such a dislocation may be one in which (i) the distance between the upper border of the acromion and the upper border of the clavicle was greater than 20 mm and/or (ii) the acromio-clavicular distance increased on weight-lifting (type IIIc), indicating disruption of the clavicular attachment of the deltoid.

Bannister (1983) found that in 13 patients with severe dislocation, the only difference in those treated surgically ($n = 7$) to those treated conservatively ($n = 5$) was that four of the latter group had mild pain in the region of the acromio-clavicular joint in contrast to two patients in the operated group. In the authors' own study (Dias & Gregg 1987, Dias *et al.* 1987) four patients were identified who satisfied the first criterion (the second was not assessed). None of these patients had significant discomfort or functional disability at about 5 years following injury. The role of surgical reconstruction remains debatable and the decision to operate is an individual one for the surgeon. It is the authors' opinion, however, that perhaps the only indication for acute reconstruction is when the lateral end of the clavicle is so displaced that it tents the skin and may compromise skin viability.

Surgical technique

The patient is placed supine on the operating table with the head supported on a ring and turned away from the injured side. A small sandbag is placed medial to the scapula in order to stabilize it. The operating table is then tilted head-up to approximately 30° and the hips and knees are flexed as appropriate. The arm is draped free as for other procedures on the shoulder.

This region of the shoulder can be adequately exposed through an incision centred over the acromio-clavicular joint and directed towards the coracoid process. It extends from 2 cm above the acromio-clavicular joint to approximately 1 cm below the coracoid process. Incision of the deep fascia immediately reveals the lesion. At this stage, care must be taken to avoid extending the damage to the soft tissues, in particular the deltoid attachment to the clavicle. Exploration of the lesion usually reveals that the intra-articular disc is attached to the acromion. This disc may be degenerate but, if possible, should be retained. Having carefully determined the extent of the lesion the reconstruction must be planned. This involves three steps: repair of the coracoclavicular ligaments, repair of the acromio-clavicular joint, and a method of retaining the reduction (Fig. 12.22).

1 Repair of the coracoclavicular ligament is usually difficult because the ligament is often torn in its substance and the ends are shredded. If possible, the ligament should be repaired by direct suture, which may need to be passed through drill holes in the clavicle and coracoid. This repair may need to be reinforced using a synthetic material such as Dacron tape, which may be looped under the coracoid and through a drill hole in the clavicle. Roper and Levack (1982) reported on 15 dislocations that were treated early in this manner. Synthetic material such as Dacron tape often leads to erosion of both the clavicle and the coracoid process, around which it is looped (Takagishi *et al.* 1990).

2 Repair of the acromio-clavicular joint with interrupted box sutures, using strong absorbable sutures, should then be done. This repair may need to be reinforced by either (i) transferring the acromial attachment of the coracoacromial ligament to the distal end of the clavicle and fixing it with a small screw and washer (Fig. 12.22)

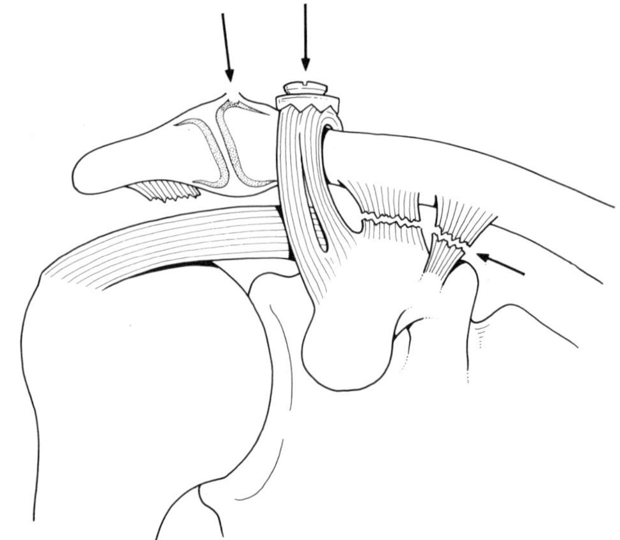

Fig. 12.22 The three arrows identify the superior rupture of the capsule of the acromio-clavicular joint, the usual mid-substance tear of the coracoclavicular ligaments and the transfer of the coracoacromial ligament (fixed with a small screw and washer). The capsule can be sutured with box sutures and reinforced by transferring the coracoacromial ligament. The coracoclavicular ligaments may be repaired with sutures which may need to be passed through drill holes in the clavicle and coracoid. This repair may need to be reinforced with a prosthetic (Dacron) tape passed under the coracoid and through drill holes in the clavicle.

or fixing it through drill holes in the lateral end of the clavicle, or (ii) securing the lateral end of the clavicle to an intact coracoacromial ligament through three sets of drill holes placed approximately 1 cm apart in the lateral part of the clavicle. The latter technique has the advantage of holding the clavicle forward (Vukov 1990).

3 If, at this stage, the joint is still unstable one might decide to reinforce the fixation by temporary internal fixation using (i) a transacromial wire or screw, (ii) a coracoclavicular screw or (iii) a tension-band wire. If a wire is used the outer end must be bent in order to avoid migration. These methods of internal splintage need to be removed at about 6 weeks, before mobilizing the shoulder in order to allow movement of the acromio-clavicular joint.

Postoperative management

The arm is nursed in a broad arm sling to support the weight of the upper limb. Passive movement (abduction to 90° and external rotation to 30°) is initiated at 2 weeks if no internal fixation has been used. Assisted mobilization, progressing to resistive exercises, is started at 4 weeks. The patient usually regains a full arc of shoulder movement. If internal fixation has been used, early mobilization is restricted to external rotation exercises. At around 6 weeks the internal fixation is surgically removed and formal exercises are started.

Late management

In some patients it has been suggested that the injured acromio-clavicular joint may be a source of considerable pain and crepitus, although limitation of shoulder joint movement is uncommon. Pain in the region of the joint, which worsens on continued abduction, suggests the diagnosis. Ballottment may be demonstrated in the sagittal and transverse planes.

If the symptoms can be relieved by local injection of lignocaine, the patient could be offered surgical excision of the lateral 1 cm of the clavicle. While this is a satisfactory procedure in most instances, the results can occasionally be disappointing and Gillespie (1964) reported unsatisfactory results in 14 out of 30 patients. In the authors' experience this procedure has not yet been required.

Surgical technique

The position of the patient and the incision are similar to that described earlier. An incision is made at the lateral end of the clavicle, in line with the acromio-clavicular joint, and is extended for 1 cm in line with the trapezius muscle proximally and for a similar distance into the deltoid muscle distally. The scar tissue and the periosteum of the lateral end of the clavicle are reflected medially in a single layer by sharp dissection and the use of the periosteal elevator. The lateral end of the clavicle (1–1.5 cm) is then excised using an oscillating saw. The rough edges are smoothed down and the capsule is sutured over a vacuum drain. The conjoint tendon, with or without the coracoid tip, may be transferred to the clavicle to prevent elevation of the lateral end (Weaver & Dunn 1972).

The need for late surgical reconstruction of the acromio-clavicular joint is rare and the problems encountered during surgery have been well described. Copeland and Kessel (1979) stressed the need to divide the clavicular attachment of the trapezius muscle in order to allow the reduction of the clavicle. The method of late reconstruction may involve: (i) transfer of the coracoacromial ligament, (ii) transfer of the tip of the coracoid process with its attached muscles to the clavicle, or (iii) the use of synthetic materials, e.g. Dacron

tape. Rigid coracoclavicular fixation, as recommended by Bosworth (1941), should perhaps be avoided.

Late results

Reports on the long-term results following conservative or surgical management of this injury are scarce and are summarized in Table 12.1. These studies demonstrate that results following conservative treatment are comparable to, if not better than, those following surgery. The authors' own study (Dias *et al.* 1987) on the long-term results of acromio-clavicular injuries also suggests that significant disability is uncommon following conservative management in a broad arm sling, followed by shoulder mobilization. The only patient with functional disability which led to a change of occupation had a painful subluxation. The rest of the patients with subluxations ($n = 8$) and all those with initial dislocation ($n = 44$) did not have any significant impairment of function. However, many (24 out of 44) had slight discomfort and 10 patients expressed some difficulty in carrying a heavy load (a packed suitcase).

Table 12.1 Review of literature on long-term results

Reference	Patients (n)	Mean follow-up* (years)	Poor results†
Conservative treatment			
Scott & Orr (1973)	50	10 (?)	2‡
Rosenhorn & Pedersen (1974)	13	7 (2–10)	1
Glick *et al.* (1977)	35	3 (1–10)	1‡
Bjerneld *et al.* (1983)	33	6 (2–?)	2
Dias *et al.* (1987)	53	5.3 (4.5–6.9)	1
Total	184		7
Surgical treatment			
Ejeskar (1974)§	54	9.6 (6–12)	4
Smith & Stewart (1979)‖	86	4.4 (1–16)	9
Vandekerckhove *et al.* (1985)§	41	5.7 (1.7–12.2)	3
Total	181		16

* Values in ( ) indicate the range of years over which there was follow-up.
† Poor result: pain or limitation of movement leading to a change in occupation or ‡ needing further surgery.
§ Coracoclavicular wiring.
‖ Resection of the clavicle and K-wire transfixation.

Radiographic outcome

In the authors' review a radiographic assessment of the dislocated acromio-clavicular joint suggested that the joint usually became stable spontaneously. This was reflected by the following observations:

1 The position of the joint improved in 48% of patients with dislocation. Of the 44 initial dislocations, 23 were still considered to be dislocated at review, 20 were subluxed and one was normal. Such improvement following conservative management has also been reported by others.

2 The coracoclavicular distance did not increase significantly on weight-bearing radiographs (Table 12.2).

3 In this study, 59% of the patients had ossification in the region of the coracoclavicular ligaments. This was minor, spurs from the coracoid or clavicle and small discrete ossicles in the region of the ligaments (Fig. 12.23), in 16 patients and major, complete or almost complete bridging between the coracoid process and the clavicle (Fig. 12.24), in 10.

4 Finally, the contour of the lateral end of the clavicle had changed in all but four patients. In 30 it had expanded (Fig. 12.25), probably reflecting new bone formation within the stripped inferior periosteum. In 10 it had undergone atrophy (Fig. 12.26), appearing tapered when compared with that of the opposite side (Dias *et al.* (1987).

Conclusion

The prolific literature on the treatment of this injury suggests that comparable results are obtained regardless of the method of management. Surgery is not only unable to improve the results of conservative management but also exposes the patients to possible complications. Ejeskar (1974) reported an 18% complication rate following coracoclavicular loop fixation in 54 patients. On the other hand, one can confidently expect a satisfactory outcome following conservative management of acromio-clavicular joint injuries with spon-

Table 12.2 Radiographic assessment of acromio-clavicular joint dislocations at a mean of 5.6 years after injury

	Normal* (*n* = 1)	Subluxed* (*n* = 20)	Dislocated* (*n* = 23)	Total
Coracoclavicular distance (mm)†				
At rest	1.75	6.10	6.10	
Loaded	2.25	7.84	7.20	
Increase	0.50	1.74	1.10	
Change in the lateral end of the clavicle				
None	1	2	1	4
Expanded	0	16	14	30
Atrophied	0	2	8	10
Ossification in the coracoclavicular ligament				
None	1	8	9	18
Minor	0	6	10	16
Major	0	6	4	10

* Normal, subluxed and dislocated refer to the position of the involved joint at the time of review.
† Mean distance from the unaffected side.

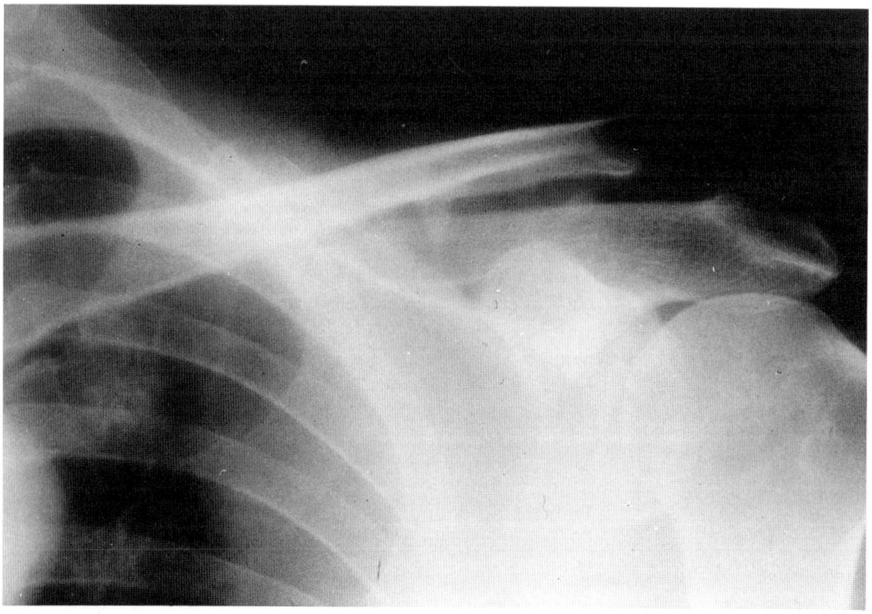

Fig. 12.23 Minor ossification in the coracoclavicular ligament. A small spur is seen arising from the inferior aspect of the clavicle, while a discrete ossicle is visible in the trapezoid ligament.

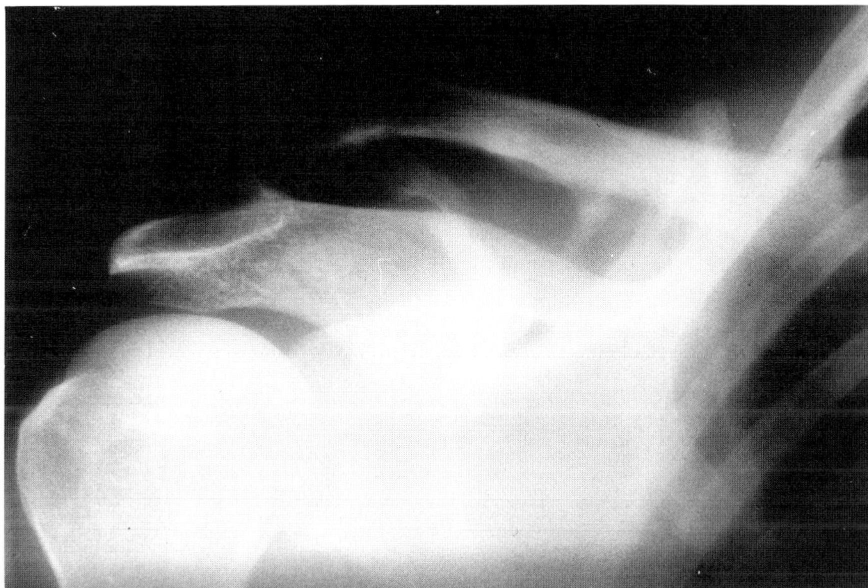

Fig. 12.24 Major ossification in the coracoclavicular ligament. There is complete bridging in line with the trapezoid ligament, while there is almost complete bridging of the coracoid process and the clavicle in line with the conoid ligament.

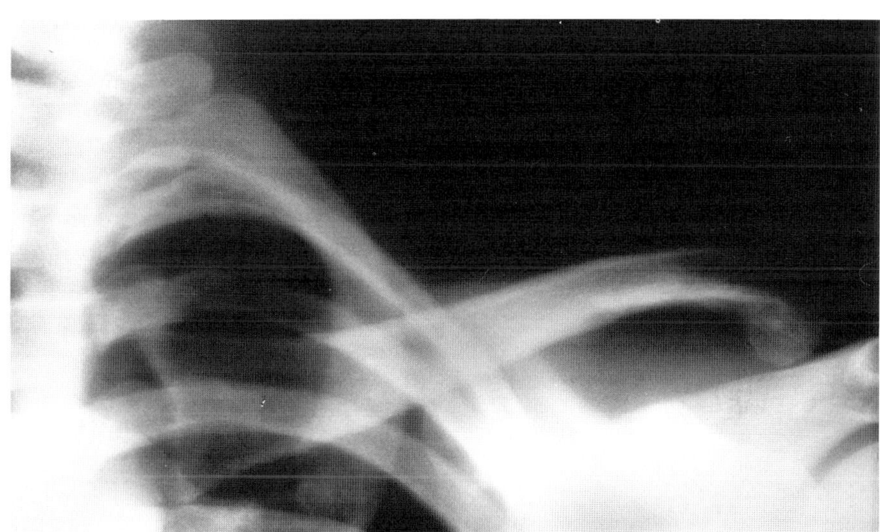

Fig. 12.25 There is expansion of the lateral end of the clavicle with new bone formation on the inferior aspect.

taneous improvement in the position of the joint in about half the patients.

Until a specific surgical procedure is shown to consistently produce better results in a clearly defined type of dislocation, conservative management must remain the treatment of choice for most acromio-clavicular joint injuries.

References

Allman, F.L. Fractures and ligamentous injuries of the clavicle and its articulation. *J Bone Joint Surg* 1967; **49A**: 774–784.

Bannister, G. *The Management of Complete Acromio-clavicular Dislocation. A Randomised Prospective Controlled Trial Comparing Early Movement with Coraco-clavicular Screw Fixation.* Mch, Orth. thesis: University of Liverpool, 1983.

Bargren, J.H. & Erlangers, D. Biomechanics and comparison of two operative methods of treatment of complete acromio-clavicular dislocation. *Clin Orthop* 1970; **130**: 267–272.

Bjerneld, H., Hovelius, L. & Thorling, J. Acromioclavicular separations treated conservatively: a five year follow-up study. *Acta Orthop Scand* 1983; **54**: 743–745.

Bosworth, B.M. Acromioclavicular separation. A new method of repair. *Surg Gynecol Obstet* 1941; **73**: 866–871.

Copeland, S. & Kessel, L. Disruption of the acromio-clavicular joint: surgical anatomy and biological reconstruction. *Injury* 1979; **11**: 208–214.

Deerhake, R.H. & Olix, M.L. Stabilisation in acromio-clavicular disruption. *J Sports Med* 1975; **3**: 218–227.

Dias, J.J. & Gregg, P.J. Management of acromio-clavicular joint

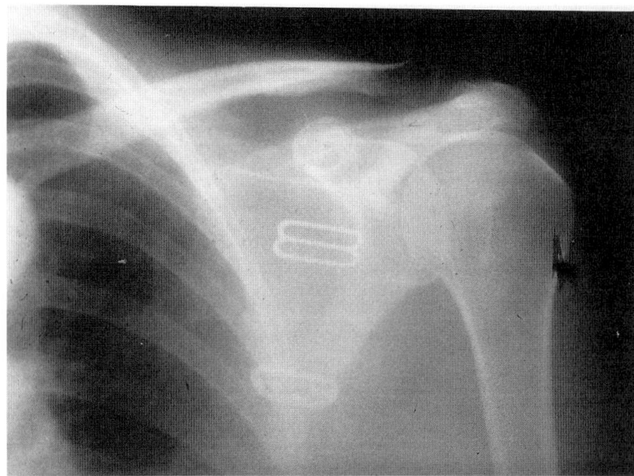

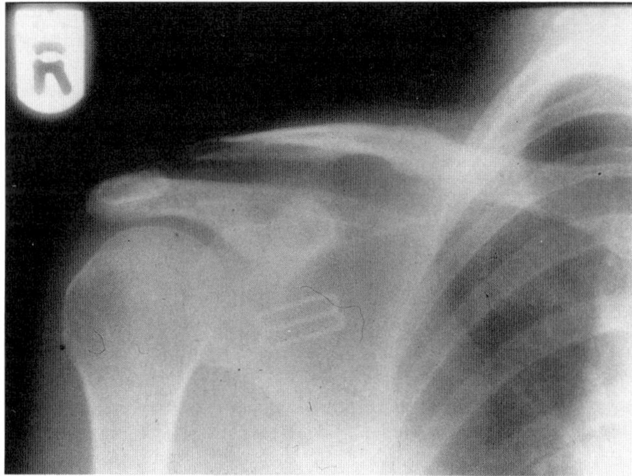

Fig. 12.26 Atrophy of the lateral end of the right clavicle.
On the involved side the lateral end appears tapered when
compared with that of the contralateral normal side.

injury. *Semin Orthop* 1987; **2(4)**: 239–245.

Dias, J.J., Steingold, R.F., Richardson, R.A., Tesfayohannes, B.
& Gregg, P.J. Five year review of conservatively treated
acromio-clavicular joint injuries. *J Bone Joint Surg* 1987; **69B**:
719–722.

Ejeskar, A. Coracoclavicular wiring for acromio-clavicular joint
dislocation: a ten year follow-up study. *Acta Orthop Scand*
1974; **45**: 652–661.

Gillespie, H.S. Excision of the outer end of the clavicle for
dislocation of the acromio-clavicular joint. *Can J Surg* 1964;
7: 18–20.

Glick, J.M., Milburn, L.J., Haggerty, J.F. & Nishimoto, D.
Dislocated acromio-clavicular joint. Follow-up study of
thirty-five unreduced acromio-clavicular dislocations. *Am J
Sports Med* 1977; **5**: 264–270.

Horn, J.S. The traumatic anatomy and treatment of the acute
acromio-clavicular dislocations. *J Bone Joint Surg* 1954; **36**:
194–201.

Imatani, R.J., Hanlow, J.J. & Cady, G.W. Acute complete

acromio-clavicular separation. *J Bone Joint Surg* 1975; **57A**:
328–331.

Nevaiser, J.S. Acromioclavicular dislocation treated by transference of coracoacromial ligament. *Clin Orthop* 1968; **58**:
57–68.

Phemister, D.B. The treatment of dislocation of the acromio-
clavicular joint by open reduction and threaded wire fixation. *J Bone Joint Surg* 1942; **24**: 166–168.

Roper, B.A. & Levack, B. The surgical treatment of acromio-
clavicular dislocations. *J Bone Joint Surg* 1982; **64A**: 597–599.

Rosenhorn, M. & Pedersen, E.B. A comparison between conservative and operative treatment of acute acromio-clavicular
dislocation. *Acta Orthop Scand* 1974; **45**: 50–59.

Scott, J.C. & Orr, M.M. Injuries to the acromio-clavicular joint.
Injury 1973; **5**: 13–18.

Smith, M.J. & Stewart, M.J. Acute acromio-clavicular separations: a 20 year study. *Am J Sports Med* 1979; **7**: 62–71.

Takagishi, K., Yonemota, K., Tsukamoto, Y. & Yamamoto, M.
Treatment of complete acromioclavicular dislocation using
synthetic materials. In: Post, M., Morrey, B.F. & Hawkins,
R.J. (eds) *Surgery of the Shoulder*. CV Mosby: St Louis, 1990.

Tossy, J.D., Mead, N.C. & Sigmoid, H.M. Acromioclavicular
separations: useful and practical classification for treatment.
Clin Orthop 1963; **28**: 111–119.

Urist, M.R. Complete dislocations of the acromio-clavicular
joint. *J Bone Joint Surg* 1946; **28**: 813–837.

Vandekerckhove, B., Van Meirhaeghe, J., Van Steenkiste, M.,
De Groote, W., Verbeke, R. & Vertongen, P. Surgical treatment of acromio-clavicular dislocations: long-term follow-
up study. *Acta Orthop Belg* 1985; **51**: 66–79.

Vargas, L. Repair of complete acromioclavicular dislocation,
utilizing the short-head of the biceps. *J Bone Joint Surg* 1942;
24: 772.

Vukov, V. Clinical experience with a new way of clavicle
fixation in acromioclavicular injuries. In: Post, M., Morrey,
B.F. & Hawkins, R.J. (eds) *Surgery of the Shoulder*. CV Mosby:
St Louis, 1990.

Weaver, J.K. & Dunn, H.K. Treatment of acromioclavicular
injuries, especially complete acromioclavicular separation.
J Bone Joint Surg 1972; **54A**: 1187–1194.

Zanca, P. Shoulder pain: involvement of acromio-clavicular
joint: analysis of 1000 cases. *Am J Roentgenol* 1971; **112**:
493–506.

Sternoclavicular joint

W.A.WALLACE

Introduction

Acute dislocations of the sternoclavicular joint occur as
a result of either direct or indirect trauma to the shoulder
girdle. There is an additional group of patients, however, who develop anterior subluxation or partial dislocation of the sternoclavicular joint with minimal
trauma and these will also be discussed. Dislocation of
the sternoclavicular joint is rare. In a series of 1603
injuries about the shoulder girdle, reviewed by Rowe

and Marble in 1958, they noted that dislocation of the gleno-humeral joint had occurred in 85% of cases, acromio-clavicular dislocation in 12% and sternoclavicular dislocation in only 3%. This was later confirmed by Rockwood (1975) who identified these injuries as forming only 2.5% of all dislocations in the region of the shoulder.

Surgical anatomy

The sternoclavicular joint (Fig. 12.27) is the only true articulation between the upper extremity and the bony skeleton. The area of the articular surface on the medial end of the clavicle is considerably larger than that on the sternum. Both surfaces are covered by fibrocartilage and are separated by an intra-articular disc which is partly responsible for stabilizing the joint. The shape of the two joint surfaces differ, with the medial end of the clavicle having a concave anteroposterior surface and a convex superoinferior contour while the sternum has only a slightly concavity. This results in a saddle type of joint with little inherent stability. The stabilizing ligaments for the sternoclavicular joint are the anterior and posterior sternoclavicular ligaments, the superior interclavicular ligament and the costoclavicular ligament, lying some distance lateral to the joint but conferring considerable stability to it. It seems that the weaker anterior part of the joint capsule is more easily injured than the posterior part, and this explains why anterior dislocation is much more common than posterior dislocation (Rockwood & Green 1975, Post 1978). The clavicle ossifies early in fetal development but the secondary centre at the sternal end does not appear before the 18th year and may not unite until the 25th year. Therefore, when a patient under the age of 25 years sustains an acute injury to the sternoclavicular joint, it is very likely that the injury is *not* a true dislocation but, more probably, a Salter–Harris type 1 epiphyseal injury (Post 1978).

Mechanisms of injury and biomechanics

The sternoclavicular joint functions like a ball-and-socket joint in that the joint moves in all planes, including rotation (Inman *et al.* 1944). During normal motion of the shoulder the sternoclavicular joint moves through 30–35° of elevation, 35° of flexion and extension and 45–50° of rotation around its long axis (Rockwood & Odor 1989) as shown in Fig. 12.28.

In 1961, Cave stated that the costoclavicular ligaments stabilized the clavicle by resisting the upward pull of the clavicular head of the sternomastoid and the lateral

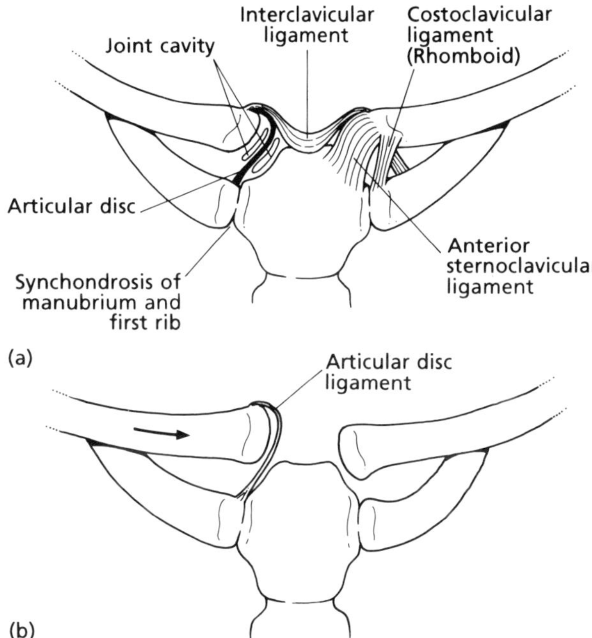

Fig. 12.27 Anatomy of the sternoclavicular joint.

pull of the clavicular portion of the pectoralis major muscle. Even after division of the capsule, the anterior and posterior sternoclavicular ligaments and the intra-articular disc, the joint remained stable until the costoclavicular ligament itself was divided. Bearn, in 1967, in an elegant series of post-mortem biomechanical experiments showed that the capsule and its reinforcing ligaments were the chief factors in preventing upward displacement of the medial end of the clavicle when stress was applied to the outer end of the clavicle. Upward displacement of the clavicle is not, however, the normal direction of displacement which occurs when this joint dislocates.

The most frequent cause of injury is a relatively minor abduction and hyperextension injury to the arm in a patient with generalized joint laxity. The patient often reports that the sternoclavicular joint is felt to 'pop' and suddenly the clavicle becomes prominent anteriorly at its medial end. An acute anterior dislocation produced by severe trauma occurs only rarely and is usually sustained in a road traffic accident when the whole shoulder girdle is levered backwards across the upper chest, forcing the clavicle anteriorly out of the joint. This is associated with severe pain, extensive soft tissue damage and obvious excessive mobility of the medial end of the clavicle. The more common cause of an acute injury occurs with a heavy fall onto the shoulder that causes the shoulder to be compressed and rolled forward. The resultant force on the medial end of

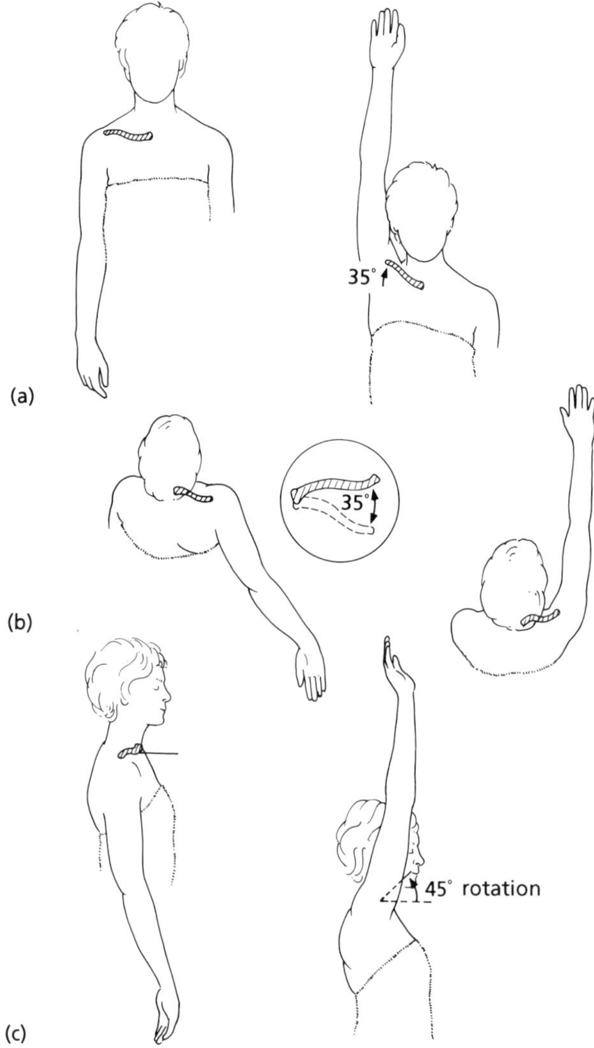

Fig. 12.28 The normal range of movement of the sternoclavicular joint. (Redrawn from Rockwood and Odor 1989). (a) Vertical, (b) horizontal angulation.

the clavicle, pushing it backwards, causes a posterior displacement of the clavicle at the sternoclavicular joint. A few cases have been reported of direct trauma to the medial end of the clavicle causing a posterior dislocation.

Classification and clinical features

Three types of dislocation of the sternoclavicular joint are recognized and are described in the order of their perceived frequency: spontaneous anterior subluxation (with minimal trauma), acute traumatic posterior dislocation and acute traumatic anterior dislocation.

Spontaneous anterior subluxation with minimal trauma

This injury is relatively common and the author has experience of over 30 cases. It usually occurs in teenagers or young adults. The medial end of the clavicle is noted to become prominent after a simple overhead action with the arm, such as occurs in playing tennis or taking part in gymnastics, swimming or other sports. A number of patients cannot recall any injury and did not feel any discomfort when the swelling appeared, while others can recall a distinct episode of injury and a sudden onset of pain. The anterior subluxation only occurs when the shoulder is elevated and pushed into external rotation or extension. The joint is then noted to bulge anteriorly and usually a click is heard. Approximately 30% of these cases are bilateral and over 80% of those affected have evidence of generalized joint laxity (Rockwood & Odor 1989). The resulting chronic instability is an inconvenience for some patients while for others, such as those with strong sporting interests or with a career in the armed forces, the instability is reported to be significantly disabling.

Acute traumatic posterior dislocation (Fig. 12.29)

This uncommon but important injury has been dealt with on only three occasions by the author. It occurs either from a heavy fall at rugby or American football or as the result of a road traffic accident. The medial end of the clavicle becomes displaced posteriorly behind the sternum and locks in this position. Because of the local pressure of the displaced clavicle on the underlying trachea, these patients may develop airway obstruction and require urgent or emergency treatment to avoid this. The clinical signs are usually obvious if sought. The doctor simply palpates the clavicle from its lateral to its medial end. In the early stages a depression is seen and felt just lateral to the sternoclavicular joint. Later, after soft tissue swelling has occurred, palpation of the clavicle close to the sternum results in a palpable boggy swelling which results from the intact, but taut, clavicular head of the pectoralis major muscle with an underlying haematoma. The patient is usually in severe pain, and is aware of some pressure on the throat.

Acute traumatic anterior dislocation

This injury is also rare (the author has treated only one case) and usually occurs from severe trauma, such as a fall from a tree or a horse, or from a road traffic accident. There is usually an obvious swelling with a bony de-

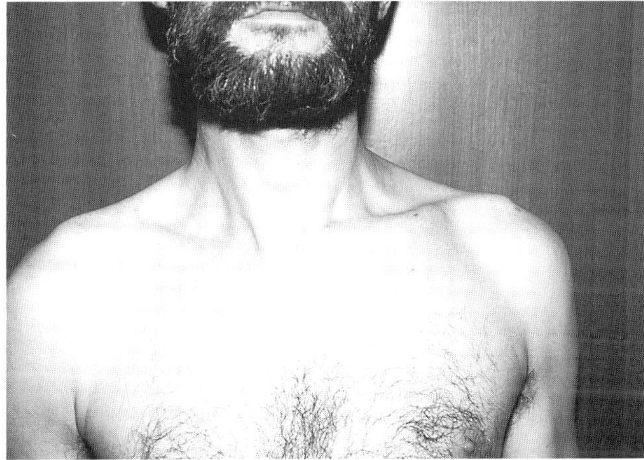

(a)

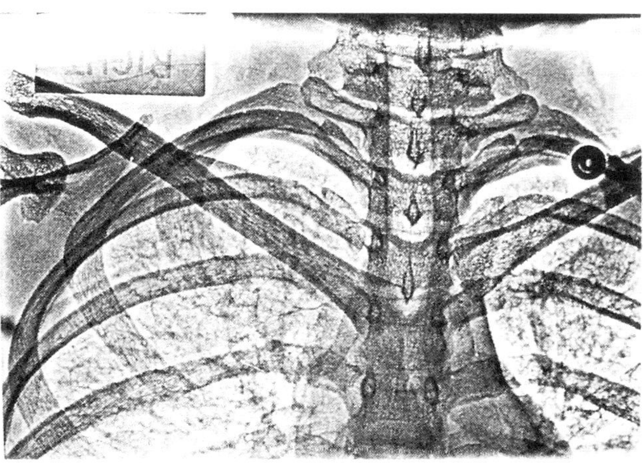

(b)

Fig. 12.29 (a and b) Acute traumatic posterior dislocation.

formity on the front of the upper chest and the medial end of the clavicle is dramatically mobile on palpation (Fig. 12.30). In this situation, because the clavicle has come forward, there is less likely to be respiratory obstruction.

Radiology

The diagnosis of a sternoclavicular dislocation is essentially a clinical diagnosis. This is fortunate because until the 1980s imaging of the sternoclavicular joint was difficult. Good quality anteroposterior radiographs will show the vertical relationship of the joint but, as this is usually not disturbed when a dislocation or subluxation occurs, anteroposterior radiographs are of little help. A technique has been described by Rockwood and Green (1975) in which the X-ray beam is directed upward at 40° from the vertical, with the patient lying flat and the X-ray tube focused on the manubrium. If this view is

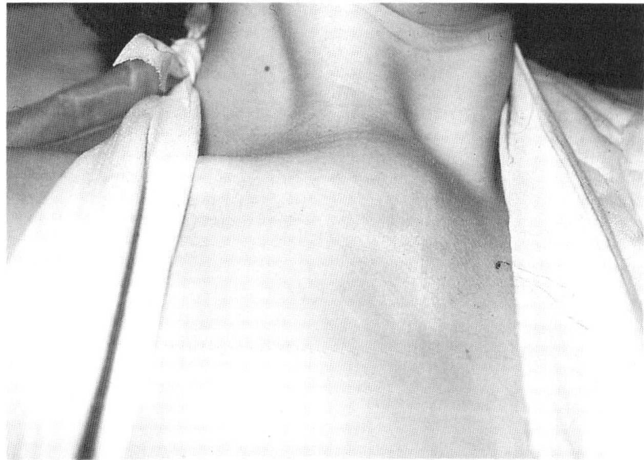

Fig. 12.30 Anterior clavicle dramatically mobile on palpation.

taken exactly as described, any anterior dislocation will be identified by the medial end of the clavicle appearing above the interclavicular line, and a posterior dislocation will be shown if the medial end of the clavicle is found to lie below the interclavicular line (Fig. 12.31). Although, in theory, CT scans should be the answer, they are also difficult to interpret in this clinical situation and undoubtedly the most effective investigation is a CT scan with three-dimensional reconstruction, if this is available. The majority of acute injuries will, in the author's view, continue to be diagnosed and managed on the basis of a careful clinical examination, and not on radiology.

Treatment of acute traumatic injuries

Although these acute injuries are much rarer than the spontaneous subluxation cases, they require careful evaluation and treatment.

Acute traumatic posterior dislocation

This injury should be considered an orthopaedic emergency. The patient should be kept comfortable, if possible sitting up at an angle of 30° with a backrest. High concentrations of oxygen should be given using a face-mask. It is unwise to give strong opiate analgesia for fear of causing respiratory depression. The patient should be reassured and the surgeon should immediately call for anaesthetic assistance and, if possible, for the help of a cardio-thoracic surgeon. The routine ABC (Airway Breathing Circulation) trauma evaluation should be carried out to ensure that all other life-threatening injuries are recorded and, where appropriate, treated. The patient should then be taken to the operating theatre as an emergency case, anaesthetized

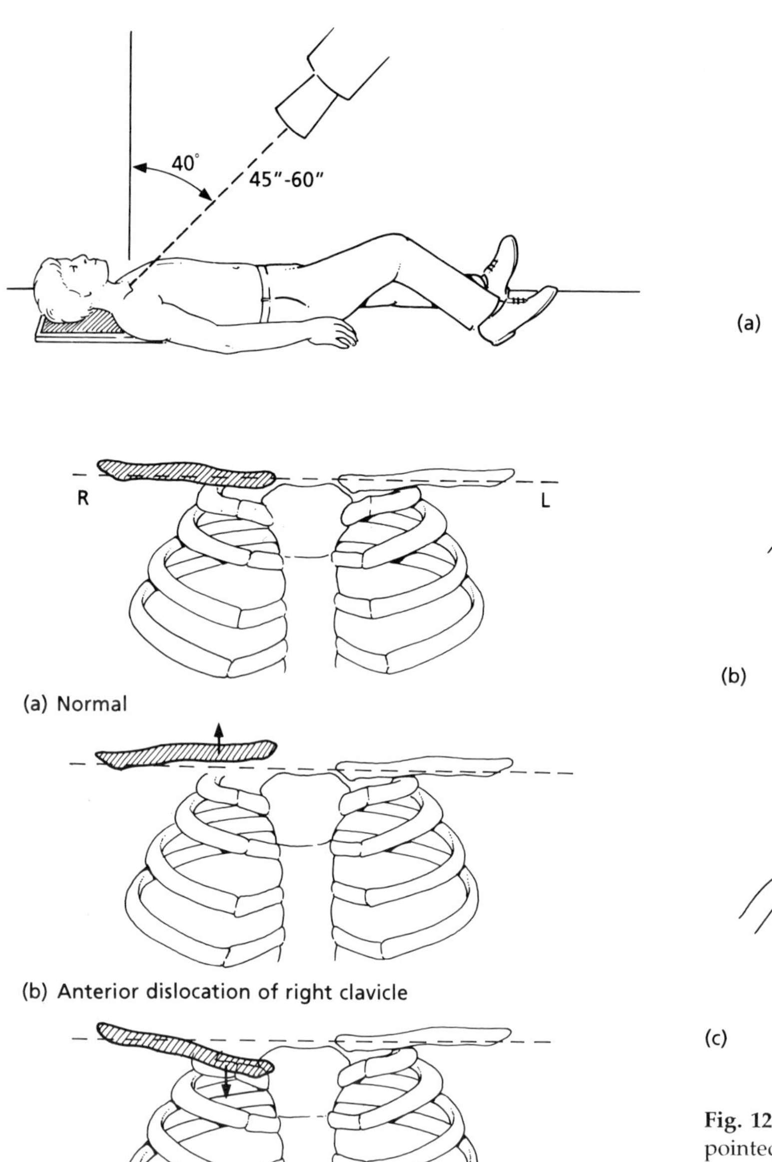

Fig. 12.31 (a and b) Rockwood and Green 40° upward tilt view showing displacement in relation to the inter-clavicular line.

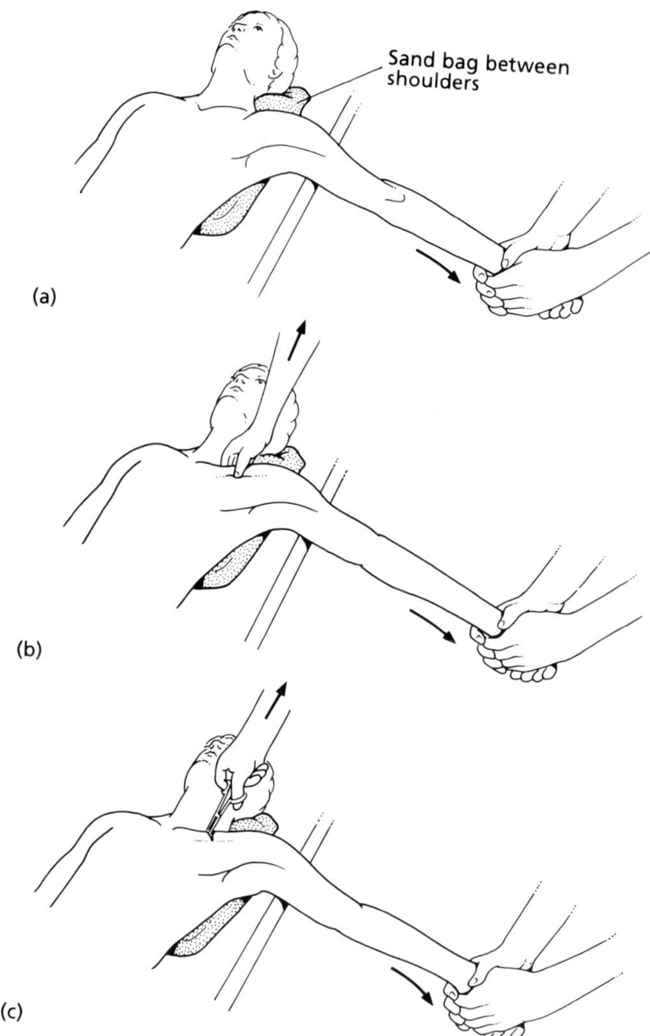

Fig. 12.32 Medial end of the clavicle grasped with a sharp pointed towel clip.

using a general anaesthetic with endotracheal intubation, and laid supine on the operating table with a sandbag under the upper thoracic spine. The front of the upper chest should now be prepared for surgery with a full sterile preparation and draping, leaving exposed the whole of the sternum and the whole length of both clavicles. The palpable part of the medial end of the clavicle should be grasped firmly, through the skin, with a towel clip (Fig. 12.32) and the clavicle manipulated laterally, upwards and forwards. If closed reduction is

successful, an obvious clunk will be heard and, in the author's experience, this is usually quite stable. In cases treated with delayed surgery, closed reduction is less easy or impossible (Selesnick *et al.* 1984). Open reduction is then indicated. Although it should be kept in mind that if the patient is under 25 years the injury might be an epiphyseal injury, rather than a dislocation, this is only of academic importance because the operative steps are similar, irrespective of the exact nature of the injury. The author's preference is for a low transverse (thyroidectomy type) neck incision which is associated with a cosmetically more acceptable scar. The surgical approach is described in the clavicle section of this chapter. Usually the medial end of the clavicle has buttonholed through the periosteum at the back of the clavicle and all that is necessary is to enlarge the tear in the periosteum, reduce the medial end of the clavicle and repair the torn soft tissues. *If excessive bleeding occurs, the surgeon should immediately open the chest with a mid-line sternotomy in order to control bleeding* — hence the presence of a cardio-thoracic surgeon in the operating theatre is a wise precaution. Deaths have occurred on the operating table from this injury *and* from its surgical treatment. There is no place for the use of metal implants for stabilizing the repair of the dislocated joint as these commonly cause complications (Rockwood & Odor 1989). If it is difficult to maintain a reduction, an artificial ligament (i.e. the Leeds Keio ligament) has been found by the author to be a valuable aid to effecting a stabilization. Before closing, two vacuum drainage tubes should be inserted to ensure that there will be no postoperative respiratory obstruction from a haematoma. These should be kept in place for at least 48 hours. Postoperatively, the shoulder should be splinted with a figure-of-eight bandage and the arm supported in a broad arm sling for 4 weeks. Re-injury to the shoulder should be avoided for at least 12 weeks.

Acute traumatic anterior dislocation

This injury is not an emergency as acute respiratory obstruction does not occur in this situation. The author has experience of only one case and surgical treatment was indicated because of severe pain, gross instability and, as a consequence, great difficulty in using the affected arm. Again, the injury may reflect an epiphyseal injury rather than a true dislocation, but the management is the same for both. The operation can be carried out on a routine trauma operating list. The surgical management is similar to that for acute posterior dislocation (but less dangerous) and, again, the surgeon will find the medial end of the clavicle has buttonholed out of its surrounding periosteal sheath. The tear in the soft tissues should be enlarged and the clavicle reduced, with reduction being easily maintained by repairing the rent in the soft tissues with absorbable sutures (Fig. 12.33). Postoperatively, a broad arm sling is used for comfort for 3 weeks and the arm can then be mobilized by the patient, with no physiotherapy required. Conservative treatment may have a place in treatment in the elderly, when a figure-of-eight bandage should be considered, mainly for comfort only.

Treatment of chronic anterior subluxation

The subject of surgical treatment for recurrent anterior subluxation of the sternoclavicular joint has stimulated heated controversy in orthopaedic circles. Surgical treat-

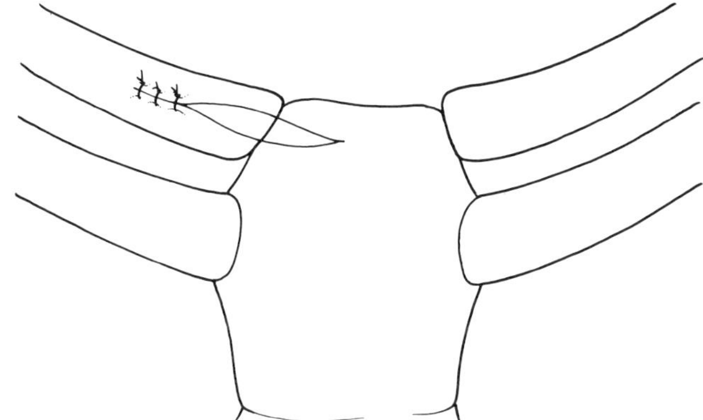

Fig. 12.33 Repair of an acute traumatic anterior sternoclavicular dislocation.

ment carries well-recognized risks with a number of deaths reported to be associated with attempts to stabilize the joint (Selesnick *et al.* 1984). Rockwood and Odor (1989) have reported on the outcome of 37 patients followed up for an average of 8 years. They found that 29 patients, treated conservatively, tended to become asymptomatic with time, while the eight patients who had been treated operatively all continued to have symptoms and a scar; the worst outcome occurred in the three patients who had had a resection of the inner end of the clavicle.

Other surgeons have a different experience. Eskola *et al.* (1989) from Finland studied 12 patients who had had disabling symptoms from chronic (anterior) sternoclavicular dislocations which were treated surgically. It would appear that the majority of these patients had the same recurrent anterior subluxation problems as Rockwood's series had included. Eskola reported good results in four out of eight patients treated with fascial loops around the first rib and the clavicle, with and without tendon grafts. The other four patients, who were treated by surgical excision of the medial end of the clavicle, all did badly and had given up their manual jobs at the time of review. This poor result from excision of the medial end of the clavicle accords with the author's experience of two patients who have never returned to work after medial clavicular excision, and it is the author's view that resection of the medial end of the clavicle should no longer be carried out. Booth and Roper (1979) have reported a series of five athletic females, aged 15–20 years, with chronic anterior subluxation who were stabilized with a dynamic repair using a strip of sternal periosteum attached to the sternomastoid muscle proximally. This strip was looped around the first rib, passed through a hole in the clavicle and sutured back to its parent muscle as shown in Fig. 12.34. Good results were obtained in four of the five cases.

In the author's view there remains a small but definite group of younger patients with chronic recurrent anterior subluxation of the sternoclavicular joint who cannot play sport or are unable to carry out normal manual work. This represents only about 20% of those with chronic anterior subluxation. The author has used his own operation to stabilize the medial end of the clavicle, but not all the patients are improved and, to date, there is only a 3-year follow-up on eight cases. The operation is carried out as follows. Under general anaesthesia, with the patient supine on the operating table, a sandbag is placed under the upper thoracic spine. The upper half of the chest and the neck are exposed. A low thyroidectomy incision (Fig. 12.35) is carried through skin and platysma down to the sternomastoid muscle. The sternal head of the sternomastoid is divided just above the manubrium and reflected superiorly. Using careful blunt dissection, the retrosternal soft tissues are eased off the back of the sternoclavicular joint and the manubrium. A 3-cm broad copper retractor is passed into the retrosternal space to protect the major vessels and the trachea. Using a 5-mm-diameter drill, one hole is drilled through the manubrium and one through the medial clavicle (Fig. 12.36). A length of fascia lata strip is passed through the sternoclavicular joint and then through the holes in the manner shown in Fig. 12.37. The ligament

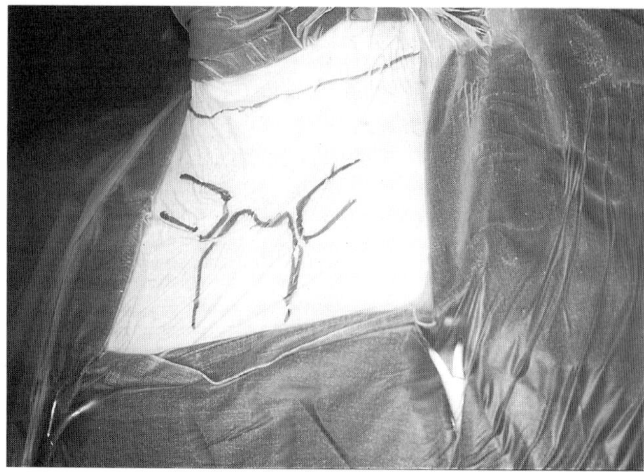

Fig. 12.35 A low thyroidectomy incision for exposure of the sternoclavicular joints.

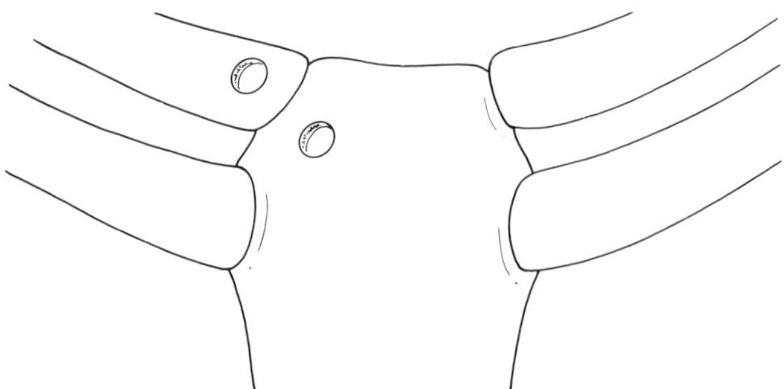

Fig. 12.36 Holes drilled through the clavicle and manubrium.

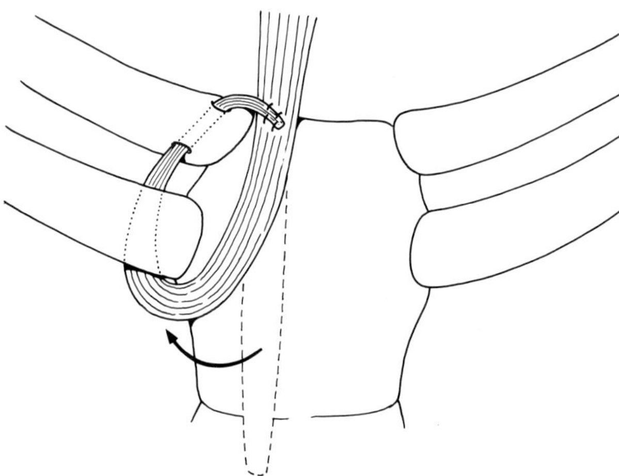

Fig. 12.34 Stabilization of the sternoclavicular joint with sternal periosteum and sternomastoid muscle. (Redrawn from Booth & Roper 1979.)

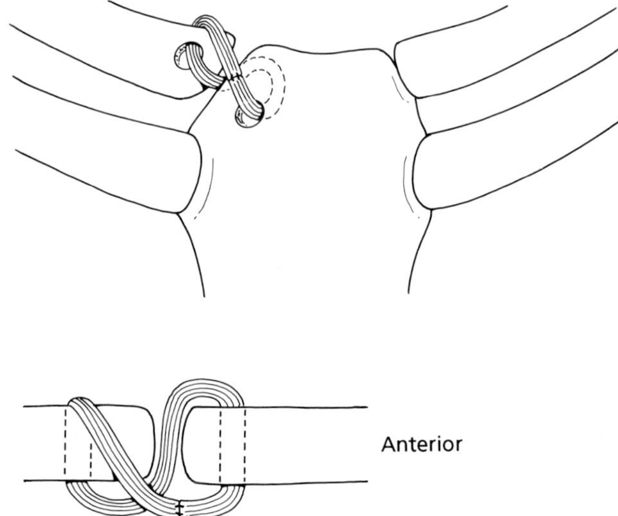

Fig. 12.37 Fascia lata graft passed through pre-drilled holes.

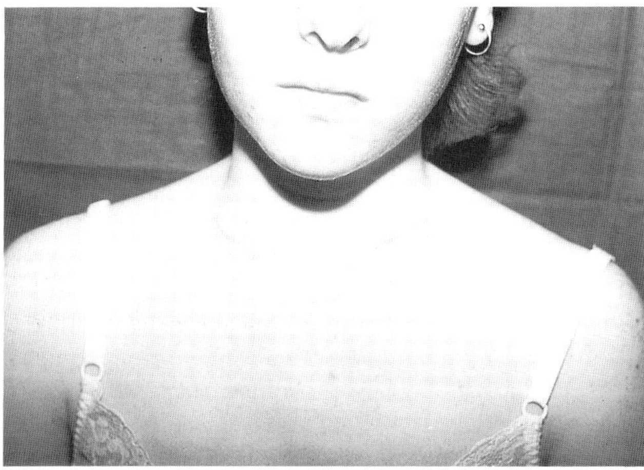

Fig. 12.38 The post-operative scar after sternoclavicular stabilization.

is pulled taught and anchored with non-absorbable suture material. After inserting two suction drains into the retrosternal space, the sternomastoid is repaired, the platysma is closed and suture clips are used to close the skin wound. The final cosmetic outcome is satisfactory with an almost invisible scar (Fig. 12.38), but there is usually a residual lump at the site of the sternoclavicular joint and there can be a loss of up to 40° of elevation of the arm. It is therefore important to offer this form of surgery to only those who are significantly disabled. Of the eight patients treated in this way six are sufficiently improved to be satisfied with their surgical treatment. This remains an operation which should be reserved for the orthopaedic surgeon with a special interest in the shoulder.

References

Bearn, J.G. Direct observations on the function of the capsule of the sternoclavicular joint in clavicular support. *J Anat* 1967; **101**: 159–170.

Booth, C.M. & Roper, M.A. Chronic dislocation of the sternoclavicular joint: an operative repair. *Clin Orthop* 1979; **140**: 17–20.

Cave, A.J.E. The nature and morphology of the costoclavicular ligament. *J Anat* 1961; **95**: 170–179.

Eskola, A., Vainionpaa, S., Vastamaki, M., Slatis, P. & Rokkanen, P. Operation for old sternoclavicular dislocation: results in 12 cases. *J Bone Joint Surg* 1989; **71B**: 63–65.

Inman, V.T., Saunders, J.B.deC. & Abbott, L.C. Observations on the shoulder joint. *J Bone Joint Surg* 1944; **26**: 1–30.

Post, M. In: *The Shoulder: Surgical and Nonsurgical Management*. Lea & Febiger: Philadelphia, 1978.

Rockwood, C.A. Dislocations of the sternoclavicular joint. In: *Instructional Course Lectures*, The American Academy of Orthopaedic Surgeons, Vol. 24, CV Mosby: St Louis, 1975.

Rockwood, C.A. & Green, D.P. In: *Fractures*, Vol. 1. Lippincott: Philadelphia, 1975.

Rockwood, C.A. & Odor, J.M. Spontaneous atraumatic anterior subluxation of the sternoclavicular joint. *J Bone Joint Surg* 1989; **71A**: 1280–1288.

Rowe, C.R. & Marble, H.C. Sternoclavicular dislocations. In: Cave, E.F. (ed.) *Fractures and Other Injuries*. Year Book Medical: Chicago, 1958.

Selesnick, F.H., Jablon, M., Frank, C. & Post, M. Retrosternal dislocation of the clavicle. *J Bone Joint Surg* 1984; **66A**: 287–291.

Gleno-humeral joint

W.A.WALLACE AND G.H.EL-SOBHI

Introduction

The gleno-humeral joint is the site of more dislocations than any other. This is partly because of its structure and shape but also because the upper limb is frequently stressed into abnormal positions at work, during sporting activities and at the time of accidents. *Shoulder dislocation* occurs when the ball of the humeral head displaces away from the cartilage of the glenoid and usually locks in that displaced position for a period of time. The condition of *shoulder subluxation* is a less severe form of dislocation where the humeral head only partially displaces from its socket, does not lose contact with the articular surface of the glenoid and the head does not 'lock' in the displaced position. In patients under 40 years who develop shoulder pain on movement — felt as pain in the region of the belly of the deltoid muscle — the first diagnosis which should spring to the mind of the examining doctor is 'Is this shoulder unstable and is the pain a symptom of subluxation or dislocation?'.

Surgical anatomy

In order to provide as large a range of movement as possible, the gleno-humeral joint has minimal bony mechanical constraints. The joint is formed by a ball, the humeral head, sitting on a flat saucer, the glenoid, which is deepened by the glenoid labrum attached around the margins of the glenoid rim (Fig. 12.39). The capsule of the joint is strengthened by three areas of thickening on its anterior surface: these are the gleno-humeral ligaments which are also attached to the glenoid labrum. Figure 12.40 demonstrates these gleno-humeral ligaments and highlights how they help to stabilize the humeral head within the shoulder joint. The normal shoulder has a glenoid which lies almost perpendicular

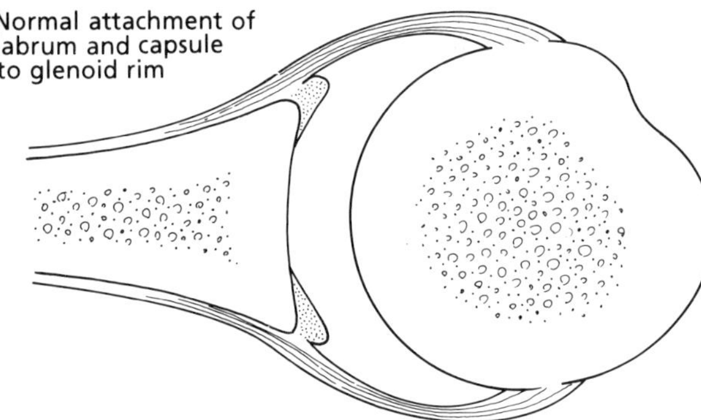

Fig. 12.39 The gleno-humeral joint. The joint is formed by a ball, the humeral head, sitting on a flat saucer, the glenoid, which is deepened by the glenoid labrum.

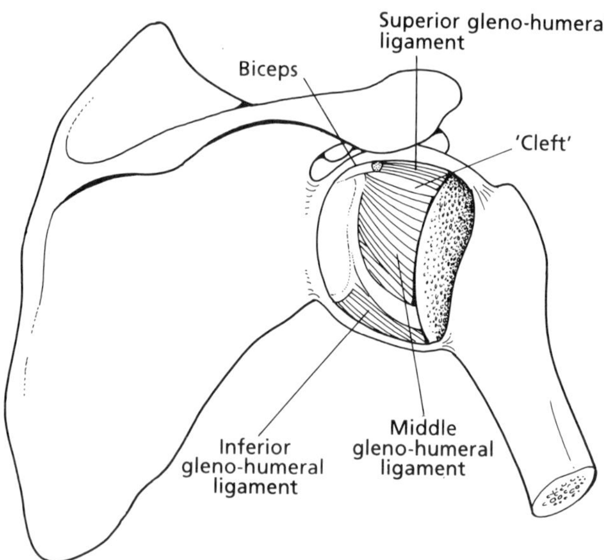

Fig. 12.40 The gleno-humeral ligaments as seen from posteriorly.

to the blade of the scapula. The flat blade of the scapula is angled at about 35° forwards from the coronal plane and the humeral head is normally retroverted about 30° to match this scapular position. There is some evidence that a reduction in the humeral retroversion angle (below about 30°) is associated with an increased risk of anterior dislocation (Pieper 1987).

Mechanisms of injury and biomechanics in acute dislocations

The most common cause of an *anterior shoulder dislocation* is trauma to the outstretched arm, with the arm in a position of abduction and external rotation. This is the most vulnerable position of the shoulder and results in an indirect traction injury to the inferior gleno-humeral ligament complex. The effect is either to stretch the inferior gleno-humeral ligament alone (resulting in capsular laxity) or to both stretch the inferior gleno-humeral ligament and avulse the anterior inferior glenoid labrum from its attachment to the anterior glenoid rim (producing the typical Bankart lesion) as shown in Fig. 12.41. In either situation, the result is damage to the soft tissue sling which normally holds the humeral head in joint, thus resulting in a potential for instability in the future. It is important to recognize this mechanism as also being the cause of the condition loosely described as a 'sprained shoulder' where the patient often complains that the shoulder was injured during sport — it was painful and felt stiff immediately afterwards and required physiotherapy to loosen it up. Many of these patients go on to develop typical instability symptoms long-term. Less than 5% of anterior dislocations are related to epileptic fits.

Posterior dislocation of the shoulder is much less common than anterior dislocation in a ratio of 1 : 40 (Matsen *et al.* 1990). In acute cases the shoulder is injured when the arm is pushed backwards while the shoulder is in the flexed position, but it is uncommon for the patient to be able to describe the mechanism accurately. Up to 40% of posterior dislocations, however, occur secondary to a fit — either an epileptic seizure or an electric shock. In a number of cases of posterior dislocation due to epileptic fits the patient gives no previous history of a fit because the shoulder dislocation is the first presentation of the condition — either occurring with the first fit or revealing the occurrence of previously unrecognized nocturnal fits.

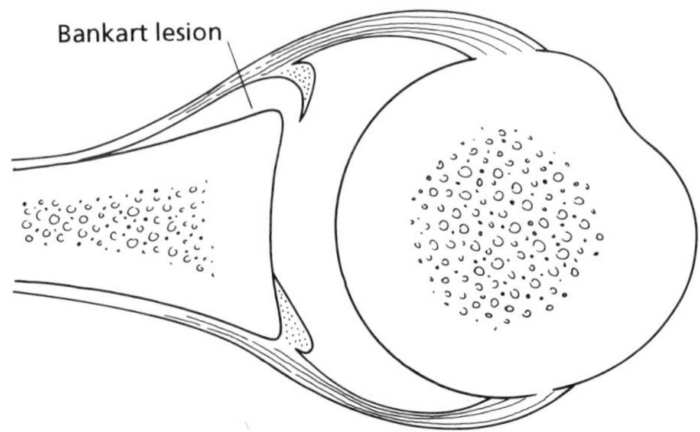

Fig. 12.41 The typical Bankart lesion.

Diagnosis of acute shoulder dislocation

Anterior shoulder dislocation is usually easy to diagnose because the symptoms of severe pain in the shoulder, and the signs of marked deformity in the shoulder region with flattening of the deltoid and an 'epaulette' appearance of the shoulder (rather like the appearance of Joan Collins' shoulder pads) are typical (Fig. 12.42). The patient is often confused about the direction of the dislocation because although the shoulder is dislocated anteriorly, the displaced humeral head tends to push the scapula outwards unnaturally at the back: hence the frequent statement by the patient that the shoulder dislocated backwards when the radiograph showed an anterior dislocation. While the shoulder is dislocated the arm is useless and the patient often reports that the arm has 'gone dead'. Often pins and needles are felt in the hand or the hand feels numb. It is important at this stage to check the neurovascular status of the arm, particularly the axillary and radial nerves, and, in addition, the radial pulse as these are the most commonly damaged structures that may complicate this injury. The brachial plexus may also sustain a traction injury. Although these nerve injuries in themselves do not preclude a closed reduction of the dislocation, the wise surgeon will avoid litigation by meticulously recording any nerve deficit before attempting a reduction of the joint. The typical radiographic appearance of an anterior dislocation of the shoulder is shown in Fig. 12.43.

Acute inferior dislocation is rare. The mechanism is similar to an acute anterior dislocation but the humeral head drops inferiorly and locks in that position. The patient is then stuck with the arm up in the air (luxatio erecta) and is unable to move or to reduce it. Such a patient is seen in Fig. 12.44 together with the corresponding radiograph (Fig. 12.45). A general anaesthetic is recommended to facilitate the reduction of this dislocation.

Unfortunately, *acute posterior shoulder dislocations* are much less obvious and a large number (as many as 50%) are missed at the first presentation. Again, there is shoulder pain and loss of function but the appearance of the shoulder is fairly normal with no 'epaulette' sign. The two clinical signs which establish the diagnosis are:

1 Loss of all external rotation of the arm (often with over 30° of fixed internal rotation).

2 A fullness and palpable 'lump' felt posterior to the shoulder — just below the spine of the scapula (Fig. 12.46).

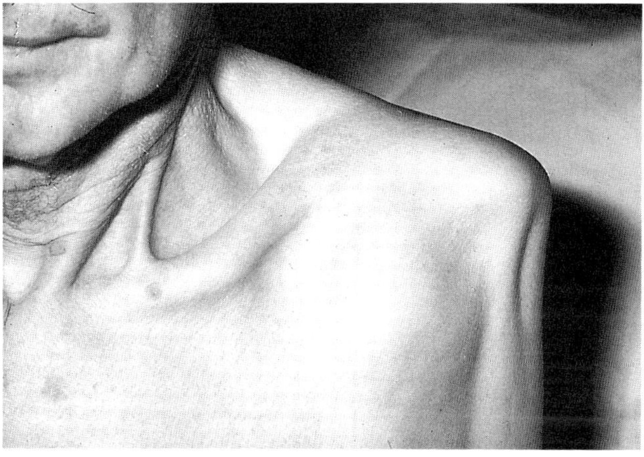

Fig. 12.42 The clinical appearance of an acute anterior dislocation of the gleno-humeral joint.

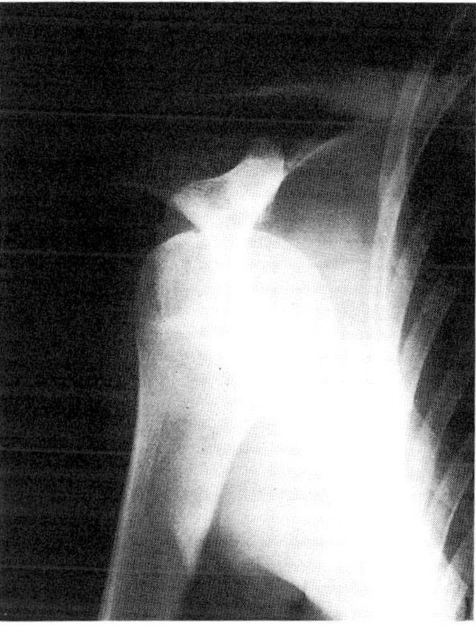

Fig. 12.43 The typical radiological appearance of an acute anterior dislocation of the shoulder.

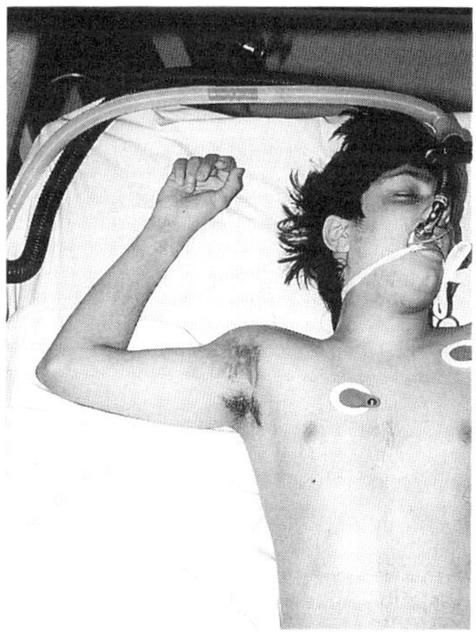

Fig. 12.44 The clinical appearance of luxatio erecta.

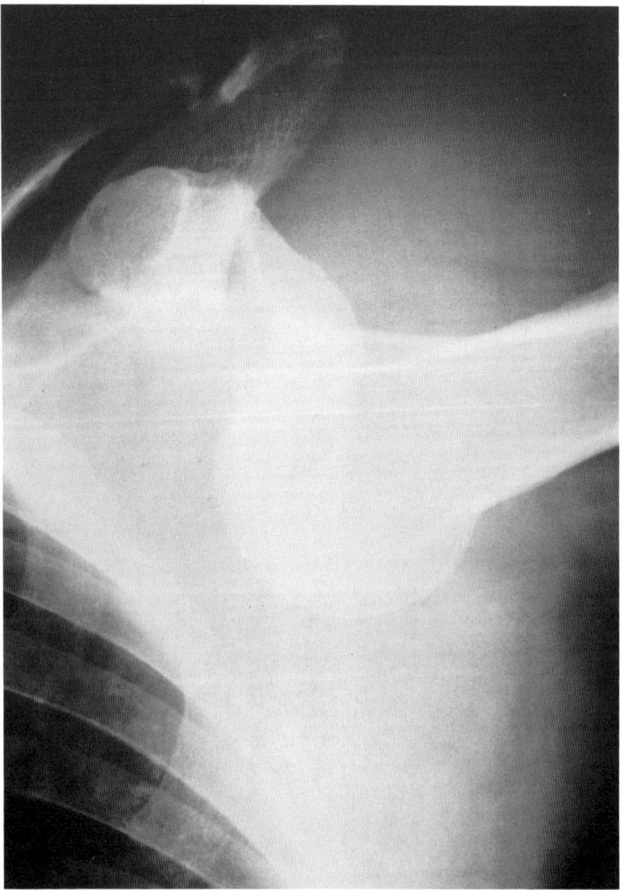

Fig. 12.45 Radiograph of luxatio erecta.

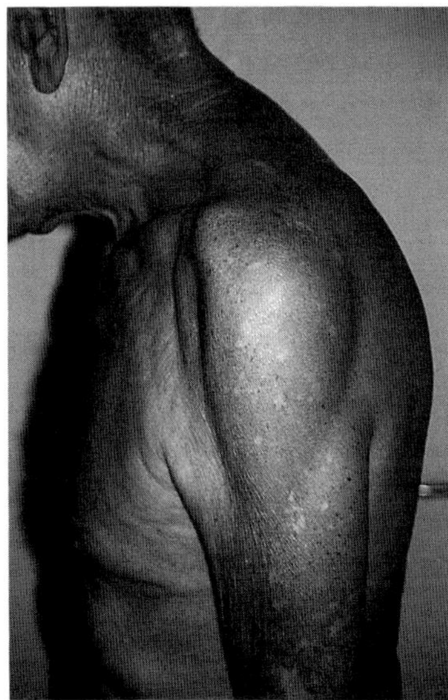

Fig. 12.46 The clinical appearance after posterior shoulder dislocation — a 'lump' under the pine of the scapula.

Radiography of the suspected shoulder dislocation

Although an anterior dislocation of the shoulder should be diagnosed clinically, it should also be confirmed radiologically. The reasons for this are: (i) some surgeons do not always believe another doctor's assessment; (ii) future management depends on an accurate knowledge of whether the head dislocated anteriorly or posteriorly; and (iii) rarely, patients may dislocate in different directions on separate occasions — first posteriorly and later anteriorly. All patients with suspected dislocation of the shoulder should be radiographed in two planes. The anteroposterior view is easy and often clearly demonstrates that the shoulder is out of joint because of the loss of congruity of the joint surfaces (see Fig. 12.43). It is possible, however, to miss a posterior shoulder dislocation on the anteroposterior view and a second view, the modified axial view (Wallace & Hellier 1983), is obtained by the technique demonstrated in Fig. 12.47; this will provide a radiograph which is easily interpreted by the junior doctor. Figure 12.48 shows a typical radiograph from a modified axial view of an anterior dislocation.

Management of an acute anterior dislocation

Anterior dislocations should be reduced as quickly as possible because they are very painful. Two methods of reduction are recommended: the 'hanging arm' method and the Hippocratic method. The gentlest method of reducing the dislocation is by the 'hanging arm' method described by Stimson in 1912. The patient lies prone on an examination couch or a trolley and a weight (2−3 kg) is hung from the wrist. As the arm hangs, the muscles relax and eventually, after 15−20 minutes, the shoulder clicks back into joint. This method is successful in about 30% of acute cases. If it fails, the patient should be sedated with 10−20 mg of Diazepam and the Hippocratic method shown in Fig. 12.49 should be used. A description of this method follows.

> The surgeon places his unshod foot in the patient's axilla, the patient's arm is then pulled downwards with the surgeon's foot producing countertraction in the axilla. A firm pull is then applied to the arm for up to 5 to 10 minutes during which the muscles in the region of the shoulder slowly relax. The humeral head will eventually suddenly slip back into joint.

The traditional Kocher's manoeuvre was first introduced when no anaesthetics were available and is a forceable rotational reduction. It is dangerous as it can convert a

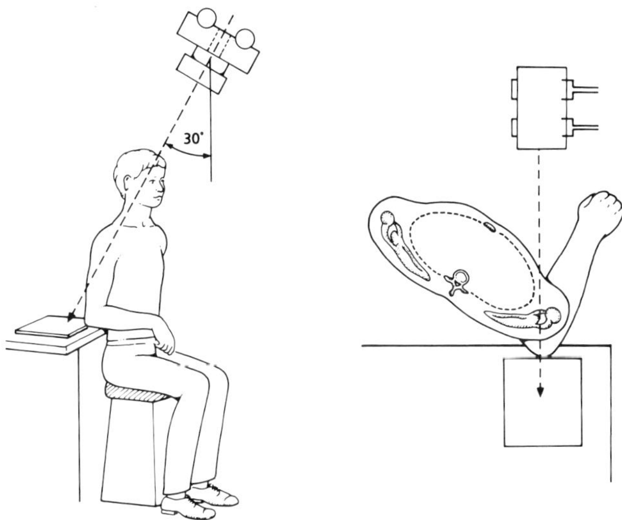

Fig. 12.47 The Wallace—Hellier modified axial view is taken using this technique.

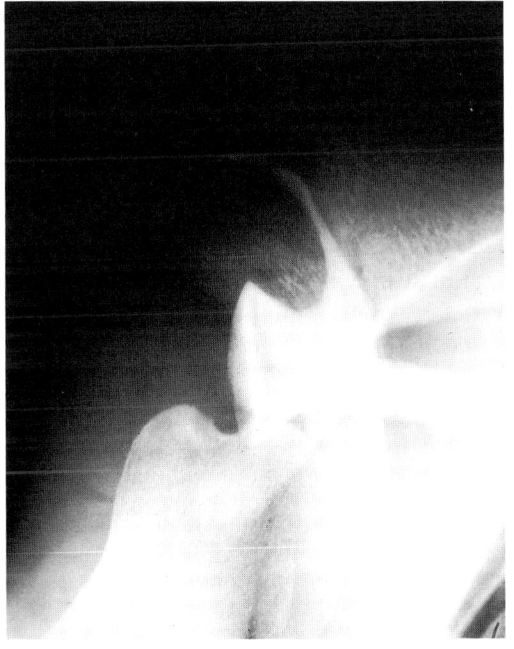

Fig. 12.48 A typical radiograph of a modified axial view in a patient with an anterior dislocation.

simple dislocation into a complex fracture—dislocation leading to permanent long-term disability — a complication seen by the senior author on three occasions. For this reason the Kocher manoeuvre should now be abandoned for the safer technique first described by Hippocrates in the fourth century BC.

Three common problems may trap the unwary. First, a very muscular patient who sustains a dislocation may

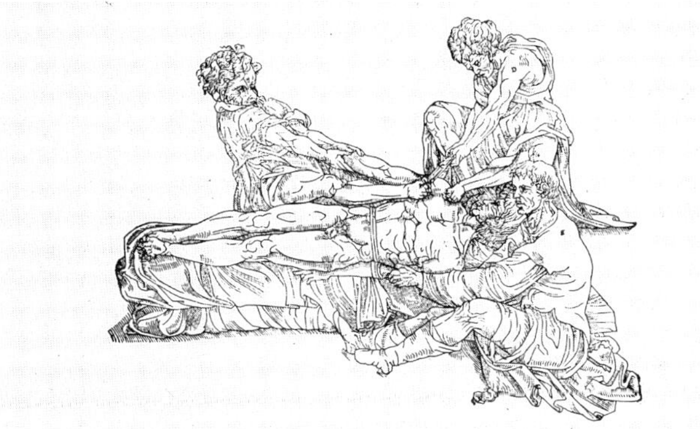

Fig. 12.49 The Hippocratic method of reduction of anterior shoulder dislocation.

have so much muscle spasm that a reduction under sedation is not possible. Secondly, if the dislocation is associated with a fracture *or* if the dislocation has been out for longer than 1 hour a reduction under a full general anaesthetic is strongly recommended. Finally, before reducing an elderly female's dislocated shoulder, double check with relatives that the dislocation is indeed an acute one. It is very embarrassing to struggle unsuccessfully in an attempt to reduce such a dislocation only to be told later by a friend or relative 'Oh, Mrs Smith's shoulder hasn't been right for five years you know, she injured it then in a fall.'

Aftercare following an acute anterior dislocation

After reduction of the shoulder a second radiograph, to confirm the reduction, is essential. Although clinically it may not be essential, medico-legally it is. The arm should then be treated with either a broad arm sling and a body bandage (Fig. 12.50) or a Gilchrist-type sling (Gilchrist 1967) as shown in Fig. 12.51. The period of immobilization depends on the age of the patient. Patients over 40 years only require 1 week's immobilization and they should then be mobilized very actively with outpatient physiotherapy supervision. For patients under 40 years there is considerable argument about the duration of immobilization: some authorities recommended only 3 weeks, others recommend 4 weeks, while some published evidence supports a period of 5—6 weeks for the top-class athlete (Yoneda *et al.* 1982). In sportsmen and women the senior author uses strict immobilization for 4 weeks (Wallace 1990). For recurrent dislocations, the damage has already been done to the shoulder and will not be improved by prolonged immobilization and a maximum of 1 week in a sling is all that is required.

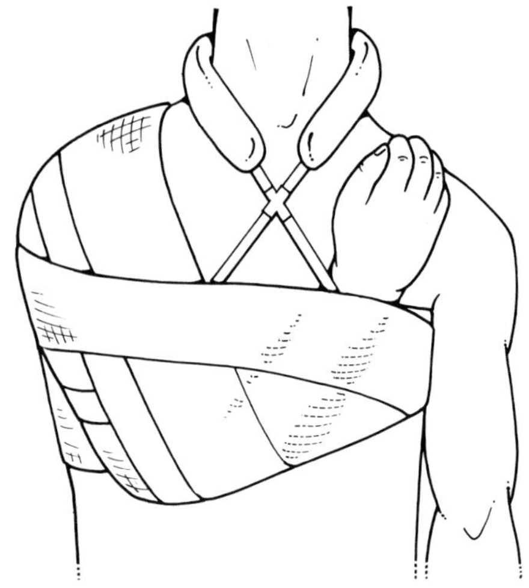

Fig. 12.50 Treatment of a shoulder after reduction in a broad arm sling and body bandage.

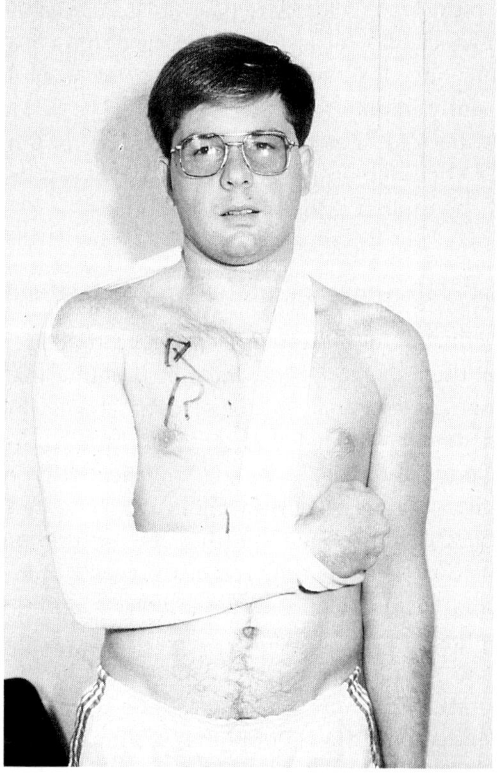

Fig. 12.51 Treatment of a shoulder after reduction in a Gilchrist-type sling.

Management of an acute posterior dislocation

Before the surgeon considers reducing a posterior dislocation of the humeral head, a careful assessment of the radiographs is required. In these injuries there is usually significant damage to the anterior part of the articular surface of the humeral head. If the damage is only a small dent then a manipulative reduction is indicated. If there is loss of up to one-third of the humeral head, transfer of the subscapularis tendon into the head defect, as described by McLaughlin (1963), is indicated, and if there is loss of 30–50% of the humeral head then a hemiarthroplasty of the shoulder is recommended (Hawkins *et al.* 1987).

The average orthopaedic surgeon deals with this injury only occasionally and caution is required when carrying out any manipulation for fear of fracturing the humeral neck and causing further disability. Because this injury is frequently missed it is essential to identify from the history when the dislocation first occurred. If the dislocation is less than 6 weeks old then a careful manipulative reduction is the best management. If the injury is more than 6 weeks old then probably an open reduction should be carried out. These patients should be managed by manipulation under general anaesthesia only. The patient is placed in the lateral position on the operating table and the manipulation should be carried out as follows.

> With the elbow bent to 90°, the arm is internally rotated to 'unlock' the humeral head which is trapped behind the glenoid. The surgeon's other hand is then used to apply direct pressure to the back of the humeral head while the shoulder is being distracted in 45° to 90° of abduction. The arm is now gently externally rotated and rocked to ease the damaged humeral head over the posterior lip of the glenoid. Once the arm can be passively externally rotated to 30° the dislocation is probably reduced but this would also occur if the surgeon was unlucky enough to have fractured the humeral neck — a well recognized complication of this manipulation. A check X-ray on the operating table is therefore mandatory.

Aftercare following an acute posterior dislocation

In patients who have minimal damage to the humeral head and where closed reduction is possible, the shoulder must be held reduced in the postoperative period in a spica for 6 weeks. Such a spica is shown in Fig. 12.52 with the elbow held in 90° flexion and the shoulder in 40–60° of external rotation.

In patients treated with the McLaughlin operation or a hemiarthroplasty, a standard broad arm sling is all that is required after operation.

Recurrent instability of the shoulder

Recurrent instability can present in two forms: either as recurrent *dislocation* episodes (requiring manipulative reduction of the shoulder by either a doctor or the patient), or recurrent *subluxation* episodes where the humeral head partially dislocates on the glenoid but does not come out of joint completely and the humeral head does not lock in the displaced position. A subluxation does not therefore require a manipulation to reduce the displacement. Recurrent subluxation produces symptoms of momentary episodes of pain in the shoulder and arm and a resulting disability. Shoulder subluxation occurs more commonly in patients with joint laxity and it is therefore necessary to clarify what is meant by laxity and instability.

Laxity and instability

Different people have different degrees of suppleness of their joints. In children it is common to have very

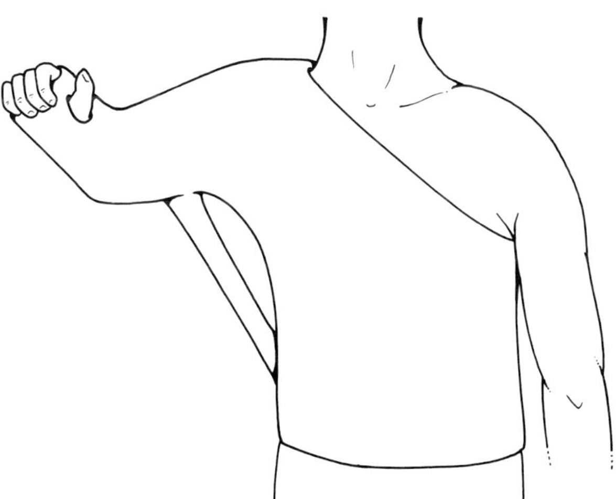

Fig. 12.52 A typical spica used for immobilization after a posterior dislocation has been reduced.

mobile joints while those in middle age tend to have stiffer, less mobile joints. For every patient with shoulder symptoms it is important to check the inherent joint laxity. The best system in current use to identify 'generalized joint laxity' is the assessment described by Beighton *et al.* (1973) where the following signs are sought:

1 Hypermobility of the thumb — thumb can touch forearm (1 point/side).
2 Hyperextension of the fifth metacarpophalangeal joint — bends back to 90° (1 point/side).
3 Hyperextension of the elbow — greater than 10° hyperextension (1 point/side).
4 Hyperextension of the knee — greater than 10° hyperextension (1 point/side).
5 Bend down with knees straight and place palms of hand on floor (1 point).

If the assessment identifies 4 points or more in an adult and 6 points or more in an adolescent or child, then that individual is considered to have generalized joint laxity and this is likely to affect the shoulders as well as the other joints.

If a shoulder is *lax* it may be possible to push the shoulder out of joint painlessly but the joint does not dislocate during normal use. This is a relatively common finding which is quite different from a shoulder being *unstable*, when the shoulder tends to come out of joint during normal use and is *painful*.

Shoulder instability can only occur in three directions: anteriorly, posteriorly or, more rarely, inferiorly. If the shoulder is unstable in only one direction this is called unidirectional instability, while instability in more than one direction is considered to be a multidirectional instability. The shoulder cannot normally be unstable superiorly because of the constraints of the coraco-acromial ligament and the acromion. However, this does not mean that the humeral head does not 'try' to displace upwards, thus abutting against the coraco-acromial ligament in some shoulder instabilities. Such a situation is common and gives rise to 'the painful arc syndrome of shoulder instability' (Fig. 12.53). Any patient under 40 years of age with a painful arc between 70 and 120° of elevation should be considered as possibly having an unstable gleno-humeral joint.

Expected outcome from surgery for shoulder instability in the 1990s

Surgical treatment of recurrent anterior dislocation of the shoulder became popular in the 1940s, although it had been described, using cauterization, as far back as the times of Hippocrates in the fourth century BC. The

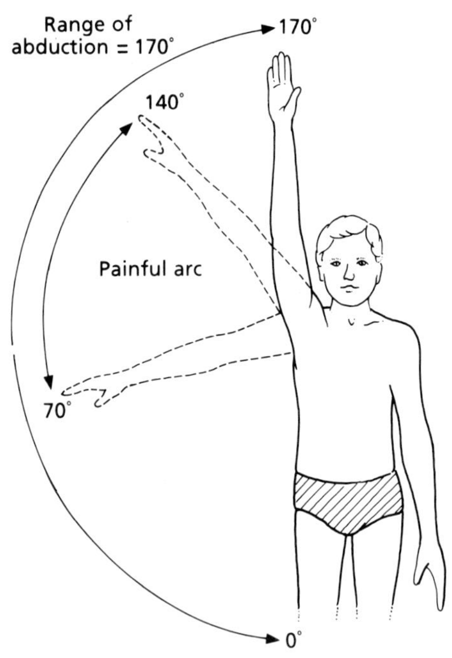

Fig. 12.53 The painful arc syndrome of shoulder instability.

main purpose of the operation was simply to keep the shoulder in joint and prevent the shoulder from recurrently dislocating. A successful result from surgery was considered to have been obtained if the shoulder did not dislocate again after surgery, although some shoulders were obviously still painful, intermittently subluxing and not quite right. Bankart reported his results from the Bankart operation used for recurrent anterior dislocation in 1939. In the 1970s attitudes towards the expected outcome from surgery were changed significantly when Rowe (Rowe *et al.* 1978), from Boston published the results from 145 patients treated with the Bankart operation. He emphasized the need to consider the outcome of shoulder stabilization surgery, not only in terms of stopping recurrent dislocation but also with regard to returning the shoulder to complete stability without any subluxation symptoms and with a near normal range of movement. The goal-posts have therefore now been moved, in that a 'good' result in the past may have been recorded for a patient transformed from a dislocating shoulder to a subluxing shoulder but that is no longer the case. As a consequence, the reports of the outcomes from stabilization operations before 1978 must be judged with considerable reservation.

The results from shoulder stabilization operations should now be graded in scientific reports as:
Recurrent dislocation > recurrent subluxation —

improved (previously good).
Recurrent dislocation > no instability* — cured (previously excellent).
Recurrent subluxation > more stable — improved.
Recurrent subluxation > no instability* — cured.

The other factor which must be taken into account is the changing expectations of patients with regard to the outcome of surgery. In the past, the patient was happy if the shoulder simply stopped dislocating after a shoulder stabilization operation. This is no longer the case; today, most patients expect a fully mobile pain-free shoulder which will allow them to return to their previous sports of swimming, rugby, karate, rock-climbing or even javelin throwing (Wallace 1990). The surgeon who decides to operate on these patients must use operations and techniques which will permit the patient to return to such activities, *or* must tell the patient very clearly before surgery about the limitations of any planned shoulder stabilization operation according to the surgeon's own past experience of the outcome from patients who have been operated on.

Pathogenesis of recurrent anterior dislocation of the shoulder

There are two main types of unstable shoulder (Matsen *et al.* 1990): TUBS is a *t*raumatic, *u*nilateral dislocation which usually has a *B*ankart lesion and is best treated with *s*urgery; AMBRI is a dislocation which is *a*traumatic, often *m*ultidirectional, usually *b*ilateral and which should be treated with *r*ehabilitation exercises and only if conservative measures fail should surgery be considered with an *i*nferior capsular shift operation described by Neer and Foster (1980). Unidirectional recurrent anterior dislocation of the shoulder usually follows a traumatic injury — either an acute anterior dislocation or a momentary anterior subluxation. Beware the shoulder 'sprain' which occurs either at rugby or at soccer; this is usually the consequence of a momentary subluxation or dislocation. The effect of an acute anterior dislocation in the younger patient (<40 years) is firstly to stretch the anterior capsular structures (in particular the inferior gleno-humeral ligament — IGHL) and then, usually, to cause a Bankart lesion — the stripping of the anterior inferior glenoid labrum from the front of the glenoid rim and the capsule and periosteum from the front of the neck of the scapula (Fig. 12.54). The

---

* A trace of apprehension in elevation and external rotation is permitted. Excellent or good gradings are as defined by Rowe *et al.* 1978.

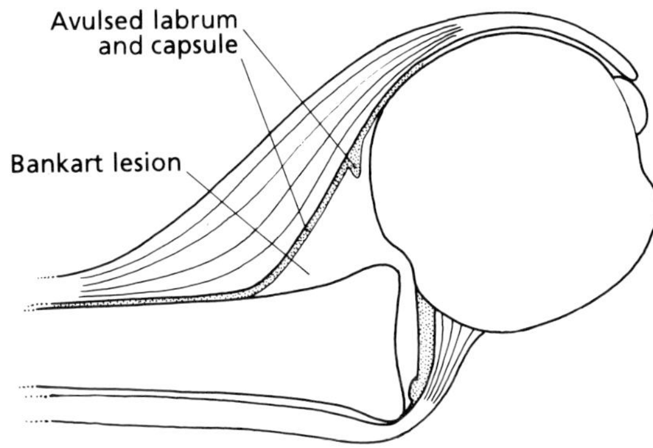

Fig. 12.54 The pathology associated with an acute anterior dislocation.

effect of dislocation in the older patient (>40 years) is different; usually, at this age, the anterior capsule of the shoulder is torn (Reeves, 1966). The damage to the shoulder in those over 40 years of age usually heals and recurrence of the dislocation is rare, while in those under 40 the stretched IGHL tends to remain slightly lax and the Bankart lesion does not usually heal spontaneously; therefore recurrence is common. The most helpful study of the development of recurrent dislocation and subluxation after one acute dislocation is that by Simonet and Cofield (1984). Their findings are summarized in Tables 12.3–12.5.

These findings are important in influencing both the initial management of the dislocation and the decision to carry out further treatment. As a general rule, the patient with recurrent anterior dislocation must earn his or her stabilization operation and surgical stabilization should usually only be offered if: (i) the patient has sustained at least three dislocation episodes, or (ii) the patient has chronic instability symptoms which last more than 12 months and restrict the patient's

Table 12.3 Age-related outcome from one acute anterior dislocation of the shoulder (From Simonet & Cofield 1984)

Outcome	<20 years	20–40 years	>40 years
Normal (no recurrence of subluxation or dislocation)	5/32 (16%)	22/43 (51%)	37/41 (90%)
Symptomatic instability (without recurrence)	6/32 (19%)	4/43 (9%)	4/41 (10%)
Recurrence of dislocation	21/32 (65%)	17/43 (40%)	0/41 (0%)

Table 12.4 Effect of sport on outcome from one acute anterior dislocation of the shoulder <30 years only (From Simonet & Cofield 1984)

Outcome	Sports injury	Non-sports injury
Recurrence of dislocation	27/33 (82%)	8/27 (30%)

Table 12.5 Effect of restriction of normal activities (including sport) on outcome from an acute anterior dislocation of the shoulder <30 years only (From Simonet & Cofield 1984)

Outcome	Restriction <6 weeks	Restriction >6 weeks
Stable shoulder without surgery	5/33 (15%)	15/27 (56%)

ability to carry out normal activities, including sport. Although it is commonplace for orthopaedic surgeons in the United Kingdom to advise a restriction of sporting activity after shoulder stabilization operations, it is the senior author's view that it is the surgeon's responsibility to return the patient's shoulder to its pre-injury state and allow sport to be carried out thereafter. This will mean considerable attention to detail at surgery if the operation is to be successful. Experience in both North America and Scandinavia has confirmed that such aims are quite realistic.

Chronic instability symptoms

What complaints does a patient with recurrent subluxation of the shoulder have? If the shoulder is unstable the patient will sometimes clearly say 'I feel the shoulder jump out of joint' or 'In some positions my shoulder seems to catch'. The patient is usually right and if there is no clear cut history of an earlier dislocation, then it is important to explore the past history carefully for an earlier episode of possible acute traumatic subluxation. A useful question to ask the patient about these episodes of shoulder discomfort is 'Does your hand ever feel funny or develop pins and needles at the same time?' If so, it is likely that the problem is indeed a recurrent shoulder subluxation. Some patients with recurrent instability report a temporary paralysis or loss of power of the whole arm while throwing, the dead arm syndrome, and this is, again, a valuable feature to be sought in the history. Apprehension, perceived by the patient as pain, is a valuable symptom. The patient will report 'In some positions of my arm during sport, my shoulder suddenly becomes painful or catches.' In recurrent dislocation of the shoulder the direction of the dislocation is usually obvious clinically, from the history or from radiographs taken at the time of the dislocation episodes. Not so for recurrent subluxation. There are few pointers from the history to guide the surgeon to the direction in which the subluxation might be occurring. It is therefore important for the surgeon to examine the chronically unstable shoulder very carefully to establish clinically the direction in which instability is most likely to be taking place.

Shoulder assessment for instability: anterior, posterior and multidirectional

It should be assumed that all patients with shoulder pain or a sensation of instability might have an unstable shoulder, and the following tests for laxity and instability should be carried out.

The anterior and posterior drawer tests for shoulder laxity (Fig. 12.55)

These tests are based on a similar principle to the drawer tests for the assessment of the cruciate ligaments in the knee and have been well described by Gerber and Ganz (1984). The humeral head is grasped by the examiner in one hand and the other hand is used to locate the tip of the coracoid anteriorly and the spine of the scapula posteriorly. The humeral head is then pushed either forwards or backwards while axial loading is applied (i.e. pushing the head in the direction of the glenoid). At the same time, the scapula is stabilized

while the patient is encouraged to relax. The amount of movement has been graded (Fig. 12.56) by Hawkins and Saddemi (1990) as:

Grade 1 — translation of the humeral head across the glenoid to the glenoid rim.

Grade 2 — translation of the humeral head over the rim, but spontaneous reduction upon release of the applied stress.

To these can be added:

Grade 3 — translation of the humeral head over the rim of the glenoid with the head remaining dislocated even when the applied stress is removed.

There does appear to be a relationship between joint laxity, as assessed by this method, and recurrent instability symptoms, but it must again be emphasized that not all lax joints are unstable.

The apprehension test for anterior instability (Fig. 12.57)

The patient is best examined sitting and facing a large mirror. The problem shoulder is passively abducted to

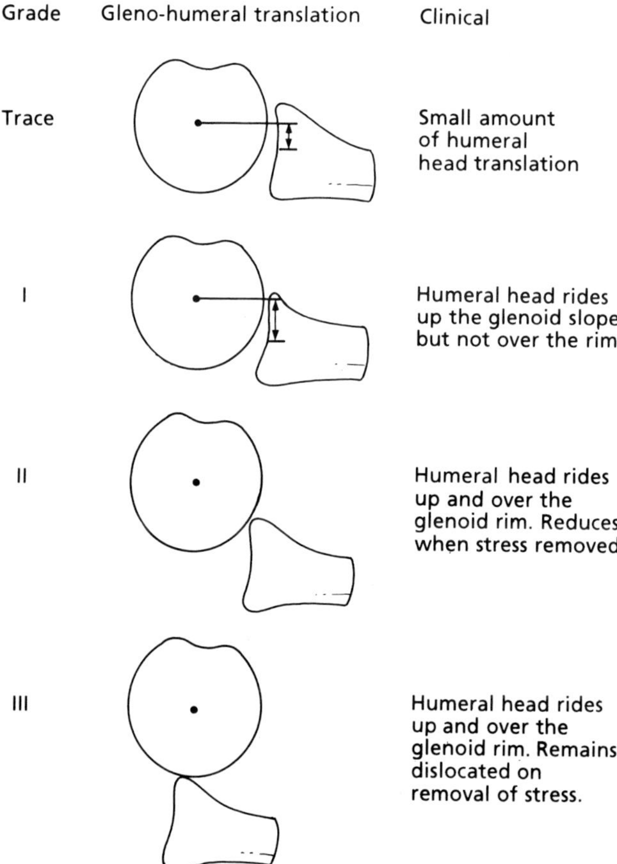

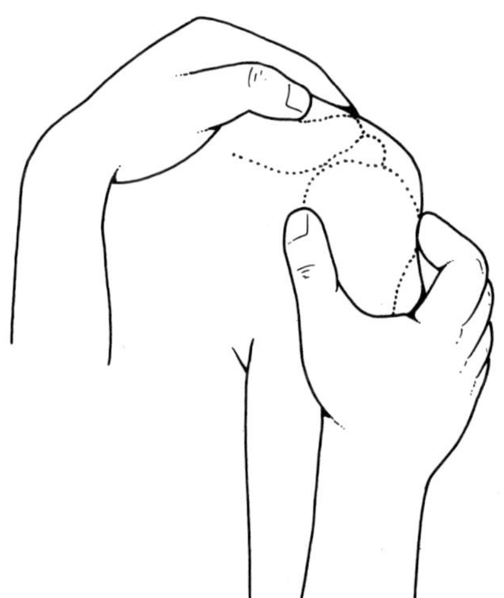

Fig. 12.55 The anterior and posterior drawer tests for shoulder laxity.

Fig. 12.56 Grading of the anterior and posterior drawer test. (Redrawn from Hawkins and Saddemi 1990.)

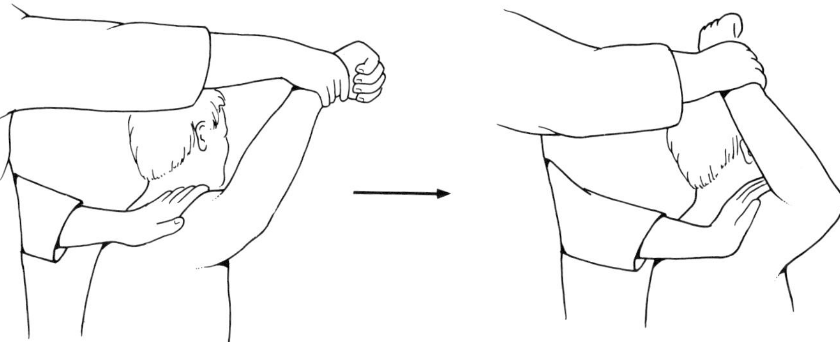

Fig. 12.57 The apprehension test for anterior instability.

90° with the elbow flexed at 90° and is then passively externally rotated by the examiner into full external rotation with one hand controlling the patient's wrist while the other hand stabilizes the shoulder girdle. The patient's arm is then pushed into the fully stressed position with firm forward pressure applied to the back of the humeral head by the examiner's other hand, while the patient's face is studied for apprehension and the anterior shoulder muscles are examined to observe any muscle spasm. The arm is then lifted higher under stressed external rotation and then lowered, putting the externally rotated shoulder through a range of 60–140° of abduction in order to identify any part of the abduction arc which might produce additional apprehension. During this test there is a risk of provoking an anterior dislocation if the shoulder is grossly unstable, and if this is suspected it is probably wise not to stress the shoulder too much! The normal shoulder should now be examined and stressed in the same way and then the two sides compared to see if, on the problem side, there is a loss of the passive range of external rotation — an important sign of mild apprehension.

The sulcus sign for inferior laxity of the shoulder (Fig. 12.58)

This has been described by Neer and Foster (1980). The patient is seated, with arms hanging downwards on either side of the chair, and is asked to relax. The examiner applies a downward traction on the arm by holding the wrist and distracting the arm downwards, firmly but not roughly. If the shoulder is inferiorly unstable a sulcus will appear under the acromion — between the acromion and the humeral head which will be both visible and palpable (Fig. 12.58). It is important to note that this test only identifies laxity of the shoulder; it does not identify subluxation and there are many patients with laxity, according to the sulcus sign, who are free of symptoms and do not have an unstable

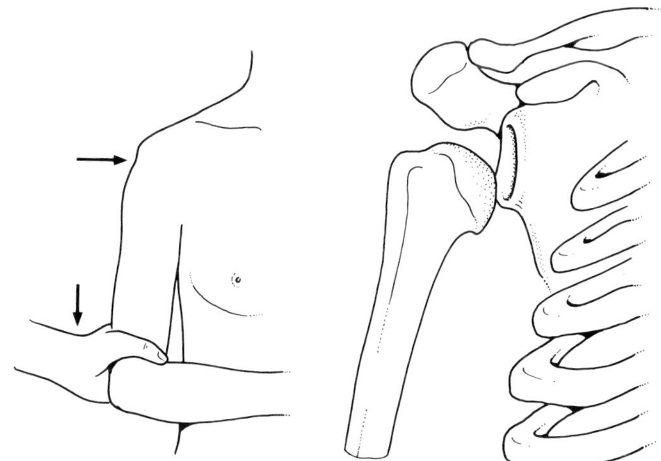

Fig. 12.58 The sulcus sign of inferior laxity of the shoulder.

shoulder. The presence of the sulcus sign does, however, alert the examiner to the fact that there is a joint laxity problem and that the shoulder may require a different management policy. Inferior shoulder joint laxity is usually a bilateral clinical finding, the symptomatic side being slightly more lax than the asymptomatic side.

The posterior stress test for posterior instability (Fig. 12.59)

The patient is examined lying supine on an examination couch. The arm is brought passively into 90° elevation in flexion. For examination of a right shoulder, the examiner's left hand is placed behind the gleno-humeral joint, i.e. under the shoulder blade. The humeral head is then pushed posteriorly by holding the elbow with the examiner's right hand and applying an axial loading to the humerus with the elbow at a right angle, i.e. by pushing along the arm from the elbow, trying to push the humeral head backwards out of joint. If the joint is

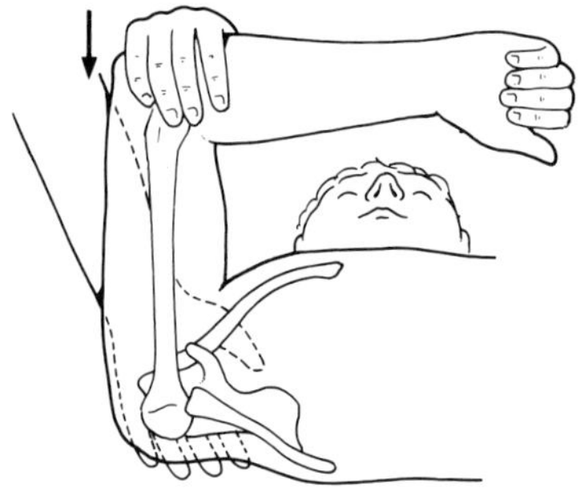
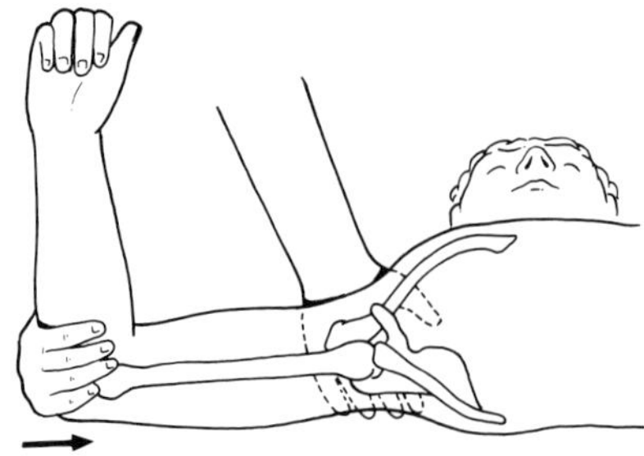

Fig. 12.59 The posterior stress test for posterior instability.

posteriorly unstable it will sublux posteriorly at this stage and the examiner's left hand may feel this happening. However, it may not be picked up at this stage. The shoulder is now extended from its 90° flexed position with the shoulder axially loaded by the examiners right hand, i.e. the examiner continues to push hard along the length of the humerus while extending the shoulder to a position of 90° of abduction. If the shoulder was posteriorly subluxed initially, as it is extended it will jump back into joint and a clunk will be both felt and heard. Again, in the grossly unstable shoulder, there is a definite risk of producing a complete posterior dislocation using this stress test.

These four tests are very valuable in the assessment of the problem shoulder. If the patient is unstable in one direction (either anteriorly or posteriorly) then the patient has a unidirectional instability, but if the patient is unstable anteriorly and posteriorly then the instability is multidirectional and, in general, the condition is more difficult to treat. If a positive sulcus sign is present the shoulder is more likely to have a multidirectional instability.

Further investigations for instability

All patients should have good quality radiographs: one anteroposterior view in external rotation and one axial view. In addition, two special views, an anteroposterior view in 60° of internal rotation (Adams 1948) and a Stryker view, are valuable in picking up the Hill–Sachs (Hill & Sachs 1940) or Broca (Broca & Hartman 1890) lesion which is a bony defect or dent in the humeral head. The other lesion typically found in 85% of anterior dislocation patients is the Bankart lesion — an avulsion of the capsule and glenoid labrum from the anterior inferior portion of the glenoid rim (Rowe *et al.* 1978). Usually this can be picked up only on an arthrogram (preferably a double-contrast CT arthrogram), a magnetic resonance imaging (MRI) scan or by arthroscopy.

There is only an indication for these more specialized investigations when the diagnosis of instability is not definite, or when there have been recurrent episodes of trouble with the shoulder and it has not been possible either to make a diagnosis or to be sure in which direction the shoulder is subluxing. Finally, if the diagnosis is still in doubt it may be necessary to perform an examination under anaesthetic (EUA); this should be carried out by an orthopaedic surgeon with experience of shoulder instability.

EUA

The EUA is an important part of the assessment of a patient with instability, but the principles of the examination are poorly understood. In order for a dislocation of the shoulder to occur, the patient must not only have displaced the humeral head, but also the muscles around the shoulder must lock it there by secondary muscle spasm. During anaesthesia it is usual for the muscles to be relaxed by the anaesthetic and, therefore, the humeral head will not lock in its displaced position. The examiner must, during the examination, re-create the forces of normal muscle contraction around the shoulder by providing an axial loading along the humerus (similar to that produced during the posterior stress test). The examination should start with the arm placed in 120° of abduction in the coronal plane. The arm is then hyperextended, externally rotated and axially loaded; this will dislocate or sublux the shoulder if it is anteriorly unstable. The arm is then brought anteriorly into the saggital plane, while still being axially loaded. If the shoulder is dislocated it will suddenly reduce with a loud clunk and a visible jerk. If the shoulder is only subluxed, the examiner will feel and may hear a click as the head of the humerus rides over the anterior glenoid rim. To check for posterior instability, the reverse manoeuvre is carried out starting with the arm in 90° of abduction, but in the saggital plane.

Classification of shoulder instabilities

The classification of chronic instability of the shoulder reported here is that used by the senior author, although it is recognized that there are many others. Firstly, the direction of instability is identified: anterior, posterior or multidirectional. Next, the degree of instability is ascertained: is the joint subluxing or intermittently dislocating, or even locked in the dislocated position? Then the association with trauma is clarified. This is most relevant for the first episode of instability of the shoulder. Was there a definite *and significant* injury that first brought on the symptoms? If the answer is yes then the instability is 'traumatic'. If there was only a minor injury, such as throwing a ball or reaching up to a shelf, then the instability is 'atraumatic'. Finally, is the instability voluntary (i.e. actively produced by the patient) or involuntary (i.e. the subluxation or dislocation episodes occur without the patient actively producing them)?

By using this classification the main groups of patients with instability can be identified as:

1 Traumatic involuntary anterior instability.
2 Atraumatic involuntary anterior instability.
3 Traumatic involuntary posterior instability.
4 Atraumatic involuntary posterior instability.
5 Multidirectional instability.
6 Voluntary (or habitual) instability.

Treatment of shoulder instabilities

Treatment of traumatic involuntary anterior instability

If the shoulder is subluxing and not frankly dislocating a course of *rotator cuff strengthening exercises* should be tried first. The supraspinatus muscle will be built up with isometric and isokinetic abduction exercises, the infraspinatus with external rotation exercises with the elbow flexed to 90° and the arm by the side, and the subscapularis similarly but with internal rotation exercises. In general, exercises should be restricted to below shoulder level as subluxation is usually precipitated by elevation of the arm above shoulder level and there is usually no problem with the range of movement of the shoulder in these patients. The patient should be warned that some multigym activities (i.e. 'Pec Deck' exercises) do stress the shoulder and provoke, rather than help, anterior instability; patients should be given physiotherapy or medical guidance about which exercises are most appropriate for their instability.

If subluxation or dislocation episodes continue to recur, despite conscientious non-operative treatment

for more than 9 months, *and* the instability is unidirectional, then surgical stabilization of the shoulder should be considered. What is the best operation? The results from 12 different operations have been reviewed (Wallace 1993), and for the sporting person with anterior instability the best have been identified as the Bankart operation, with a 94–97% success rate (Rowe *et al.* 1978, El-Sobhi 1991), and the Bristow operation, with between 71 and 94% success depending on the surgeon (Hovelius 1984, Gazielly *et al.* 1987). There is currently great enthusiasm for carrying out arthroscopic shoulder stabilization; however, in the majority of series at present the success rate of arthroscopic operations is significantly less than for the standard open operation.

The shoulder stabilization operation most often carried out in Britain has been the Putti-Platt operation described by Osmond-Clarke (1948), but not only is its published success rate only around the 70% level, but those surgeons with a special interest in shoulder surgery seem to see many more failures from this one procedure than from any other, as shown in Table 12.6. It is relevant to note that Hovelius (1979) abandoned the Putti-Platt operation because of the poor results he identified when reviewing patients 2 years after surgery.

At present, the Bankart operation, as described by Rowe *et al.* (1978), is the gold standard for shoulder stabilization surgery and remains the operation of choice. It is, however, a technically difficult operation and if, at operation, the anterior glenoid rim should fracture major technical difficulties can occur. The Bankart operation can now be carried out much more easily with the use of suture anchors such as the Mitek anchor (Wallace 1990). The operation is carried out in the 'deckchair' position with a sandbag under the

Table 12.6 Recurrence of dislocation after shoulder stabilization surgery (From Hawkins & Hawkins 1985, McAuliffe *et al.* 1988)

	Number of recurrences	
Previous operation	Hawkins & Hawkins (1985)	McAuliffe *et al.* (1988)
Putti-Platt	42	38
Magnuson-Stack	13	–
Bristow	7	–
Staple capsulorrhaphy	5	–
Bankart	–	5
Capsular shift	–	1
Posterior repair	1	1
Moseley	1	–
Gallie	1	–

scapula on the operation side (Fig. 12.60). The surgical approach is either through an 8-cm anterior vertical skin incision or, in the female, through a bra-strap incision (Fig. 12.61). The approach is through an anterior delto-pectoral approach with pre-drilling of the coracoid before it is osteotomized (Fig. 12.62). The subscapularis is tagged medially with two stay sutures and divided 3 cm from its lateral insertion, avoiding damage to the underlying capsule (Fig. 12.63). The arm is fully externally rotated and the capsule is divided at the level of the glenoid labrum (Fig. 12.64). Inspection of the anterior glenoid rim will usually identify a Bankart lesion (in 85% of cases) and, if present, the soft tissues on the front of the glenoid rim are mobilized (Fig. 12.65). Three Mitek anchor holes are drilled into the anterior rim of the glenoid and three No. 2 Mitek anchors with No. 2 Ethibond sutures attached are inserted (Fig. 12.66). These sutures are then used to reattach the anterior capsule to the anterior glenoid rim in a mattress configuration with minimal shortening of the capsule (Fig. 12.67) and are reinforced anteriorly by 'double breasting' the medial flap of labrum and periosteum (Fig. 12.68). If no Bankart lesion is found, the glenoid labrum should be left intact and the anterior capsule (including the IGHL) should be sutured with a modest plication incorporating an inferior capsular shift (Neer & Foster, 1980). Upon completion of the capsular repair at least 40° of external rotation should be possible on the operating table. Closure involves an end-to-end repair of the subscapularis with a No. 1 absorbable suture and reattachment of the coracoid with an AO small cancellous screw (35 × 4.0 mm). The delto-pectoral interval is closed with two loose absorbable sutures and skin closure is carried out in two layers with a subcuticular 2/0 Prolene suture for skin.

This operation is particularly appropriate for athletes

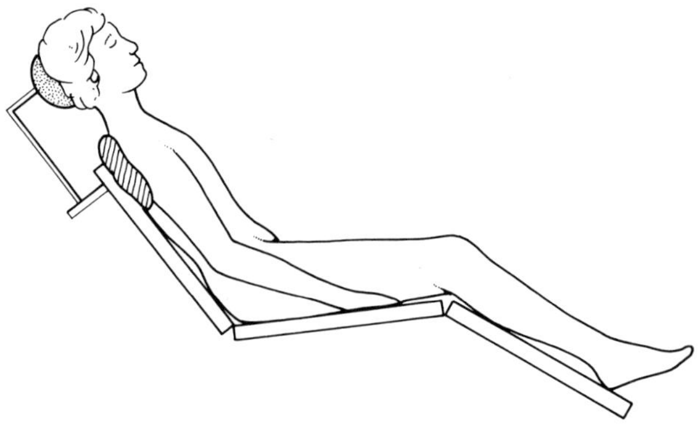

Fig. 12.60 The 'deck chair' position for anterior shoulder surgery.

who need a near full range of external rotation in abduction as the operation provides this regularly within the first year of surgery. El-Sobhi (1991) has demonstrated just how successful this operation is in returning athletes to their chosen sports. However, for some sports, such as javelin throwing, karate, canoeing, pitching in baseball and bowling in cricket, full external rotation of the shoulder may be essential. Even with the Bankart operation up to 20° of external rotation may be lost, and such competitive athletes should be warned that there is a small risk that surgery may end their sporting career in these particular sports.

The next most satisfactory operation is the Bristow procedure which, again, has produced excellent results in sportsmen and women in experienced hands (Gazielly *et al.* 1987). However, the surgeon must ensure that the coracoid transfer is made flush with the face of the glenoid and attached to the inferior third of the glenoid, as highlighted by Hovelius (1984), for the best results. Arthroscopic Bankart-type repairs have become the

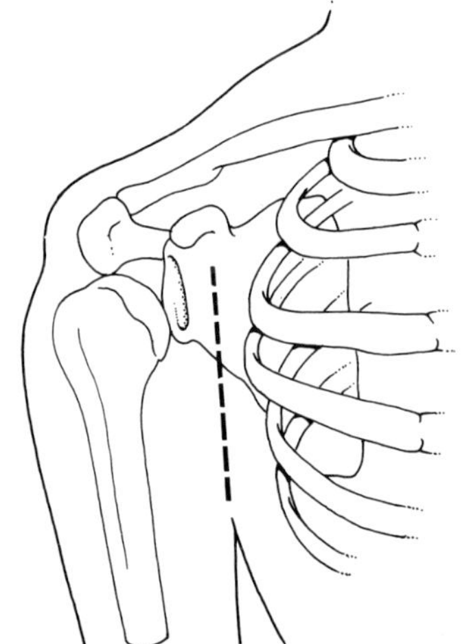

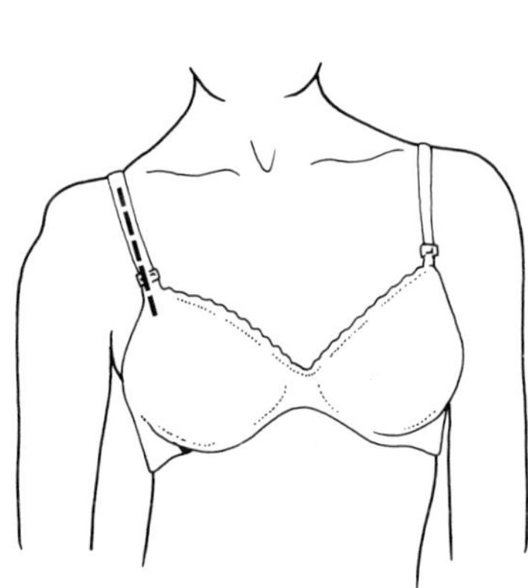

Fig. 12.61 The skin incision — vertical or bra-strap.

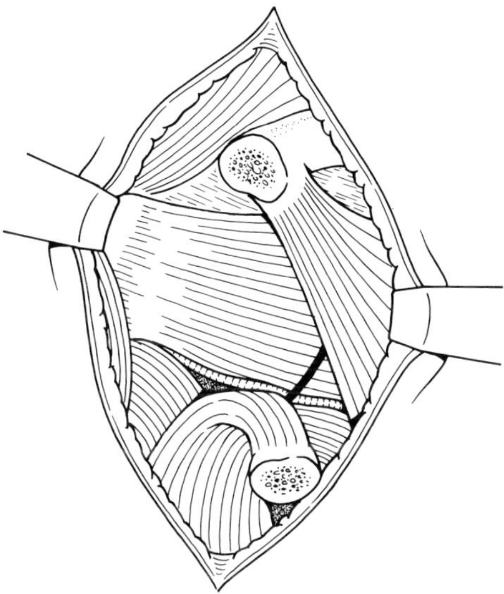

Fig. 12.62 Coracoid osteotomy.

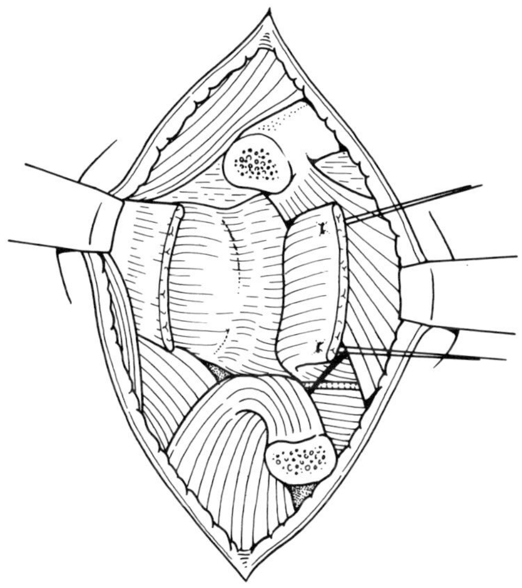

Fig. 12.63 Division of subscapularis and application of stay sutures.

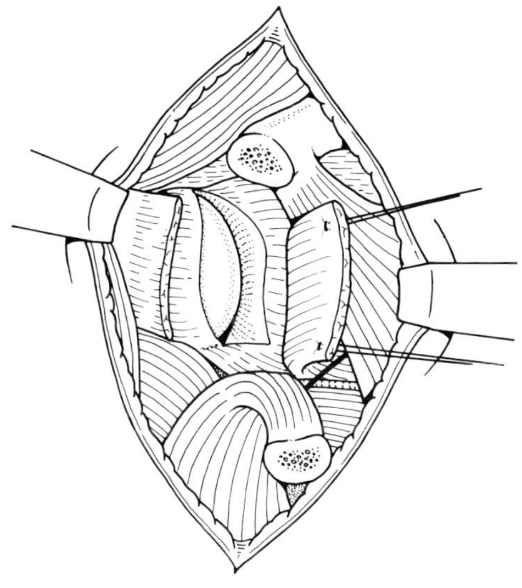

Fig. 12.64 Anterior capsule divided at the level of the glenoid labrum.

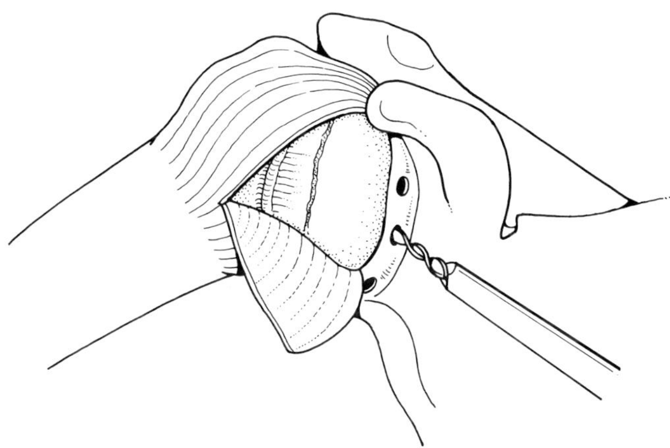

Fig. 12.65 The medial soft tissues are elevated.

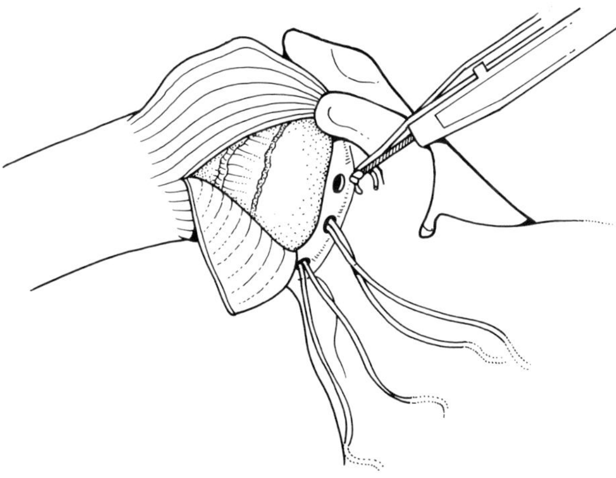

Fig. 12.66 Three Mitek anchors holes are drilled and three × No. 2 Ethibond sutures are inserted with anchors.

vogue in the United States and are becoming increasingly popular in Europe. They have the advantage of a minimal scar but depend, to a much greater extent, on the expertise of the surgeon and they require sophisticated equipment. The early, reported success rates of around 80% (with instability assessed) are slightly poorer than the open procedures discussed above and have been shown to deteriorate with time. They *do not* allow an earlier return to sport and, if early return to sport is the most important factor, then a standard

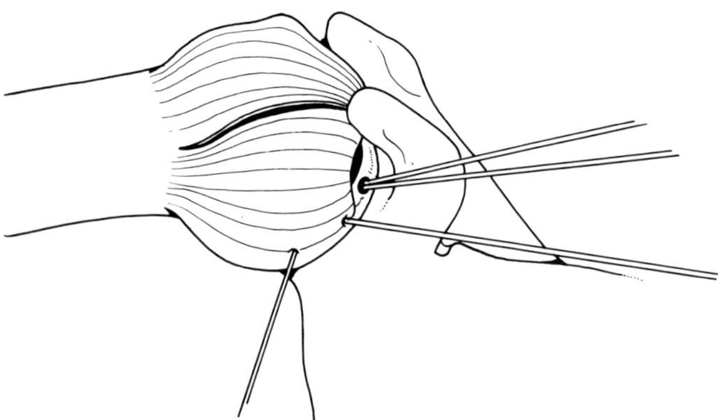

Fig. 12.67 Re-attachment of the capsule with an Ethibond mattress suture arrangement.

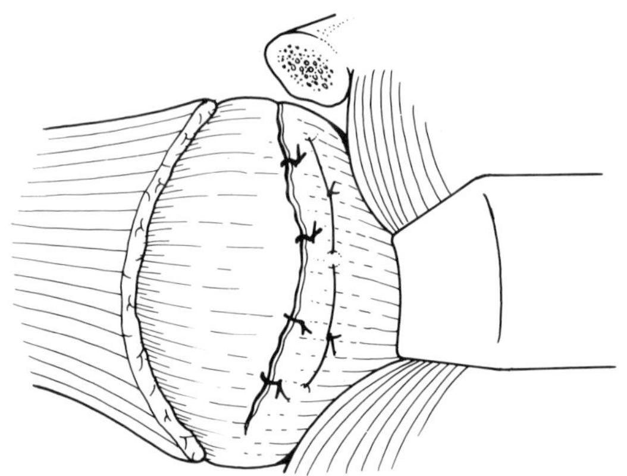

Fig. 12.68 The medial flap can be double breasted over the front of the repair.

Bankart operation, which allows a return to full contact sport at 4 months, remains the operation of choice.

Treatment of atraumatic involuntary anterior instability

Patients with atraumatic instability give *no significant* history of trauma and usually report a gradual onset of symptoms. The authors are seeing an increasing number of young athletes with this problem and it is now recognized that in addition to joint laxity being a recognized predisposing factor, so also is a repeated stretching injury (or microtrauma) to the shoulder as occurs in swimming (Kennedy *et al.* 1978, Richardson *et al.* 1980), racquet sports, gymnastics and throwing sports. These patients do not usually develop a true Bankart lesion but they do stretch the anterior capsule of the shoulder and, in particular, the IGHL. For minor degrees of instability, avoidance of the activity causing the instability is recommended together with rotator cuff strengthening exercises, but for established instability an anterior capsular operation, through the same approach as for a Bankart operation, is required. In general, an anterior cruciate-type capsulorrhaphy, as described on p. 384, is indicated, addressing the laxity and sometimes in conjunction with an inferior capsular shift. Unfortunately, the surgical results are less satisfactory in this group, dropping, in the senior author's hands, to around 75% cure rate.

Treatment of traumatic involuntary posterior instability

Frank posterior dislocation is uncommon and accounts for only 2–3% of all acute dislocations. The most common presentation is a locked posterior dislocation, which is often missed. There have been a number of series which have reported such injuries (Hawkins *et al.* 1987, Meadows & Wallace 1987).

Recurrent traumatic posterior subluxation is much more common (Norwood & Terry 1984). The patient often complains of pain and instability with the arm in forward flexion, adduction and internal rotation and, although trauma appears to be the predisposing factor in this group, most patients have a significant element of joint laxity in the opposite shoulder and in their other joints generally. Management of this group focuses on non-operative treatment with strengthening exercises, particularly to the infraspinatus muscle, and rehabilitation for at least 9 months. In people under 16 years, surgery should never be considered — physiotherapy is the management of choice. About one-third of adult patients do not respond to this regime, and for them a posterior surgical procedure is indicated.

Recommended operations for posterior shoulder instability

Before surgery it is important to establish two points:
1 Is the problem a pure posterior instability only?
2 Is the glenoid retroversion excessive? (Normal retroversion = 7°.)
If the diagnosis is pure posterior instability and glenoid retroversion is excessive, the senior author uses a posterior glenoid osteotomy as described by Kretzler and Scott (1982), with a posterior capsular plication. If not, a posterior soft tissue procedure is used: either a capsular and muscle plication or a posterior inferior capsular shift with muscle plication.

The operative steps are as follows. The patient is positioned on the unaffected side in the lateral position. A vertical skin incision, crossing the spine of the scapula

(Fig. 12.69), gives the best cosmetic result. The posterior third of the deltoid is detached from the spine of the scapula and elevated, protecting the axillary nerve (Fig. 12.70). The infraspinatus muscle is divided, and elevated with stay sutures just medial to the glenoid, leaving the posterior capsule intact (Fig. 12.71). Too much retraction will damage the nerve to the infraspinatus and should be avoided. The capsular layer is then opened and the posterior neck of the glenoid exposed. If a glenoid osteotomy is chosen, the scapular neck is divided with an oscillating saw 5–10 mm medial to the glenoid face and parallel with it. The glenoid is then tilted through an angle of 20–30° and an iliac crest triangular bone block is inserted to maintain the anterior tilt (Fig. 12.72). The arm is held in full external rotation while a posterior capsular repair and a 'double breasting' of the infraspinatus is carried out with absorbable sutures. In the authors' experience it is impossible to repair these posterior structures too tightly and a plaster spica should be used postoperatively for 4 weeks to protect the repair. Although Kretzler and Scott (1982) have reported a success rate of 93% for posterior glenoid osteotomies, the authors' success rate, despite a careful selection of patients, is only around 70%.

Treatment of atraumatic involuntary posterior instability

Alarm bells should ring when a patient presents with no history of trauma and with a shoulder which is posteriorly subluxing or dislocating. This is the most common presenting feature of a patient with voluntary

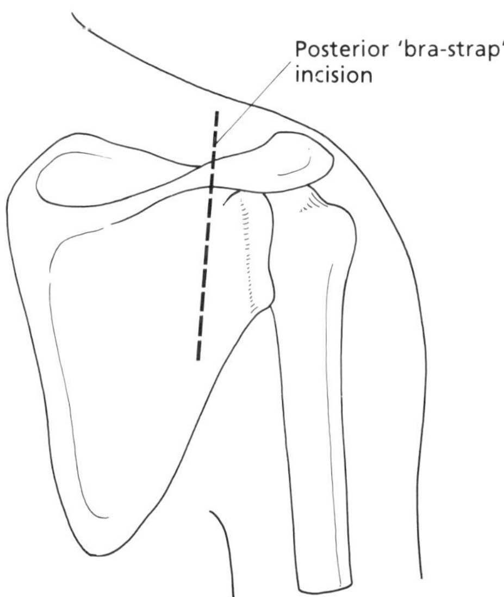

Fig. 12.69 Vertical skin incision for the posterior approach to the shoulder.

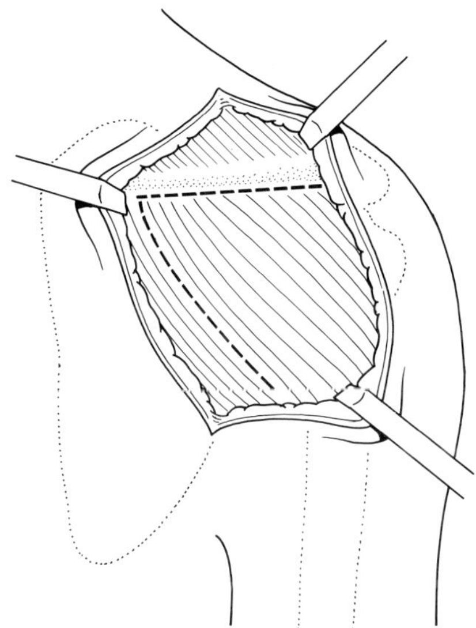

Fig. 12.70 The posterior third of the deltoid is elevated.

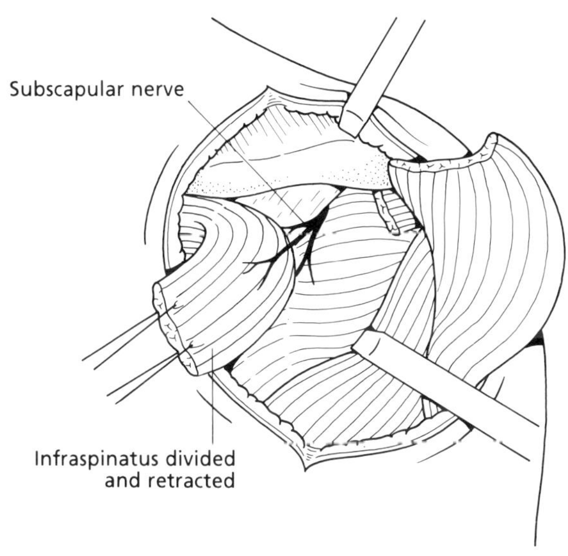

Fig. 12.71 The infraspinatus muscle is divided and elevated leaving the posterior capsule intact.

instability, and this diagnosis must be excluded before further management of the patient is undertaken. Having excluded voluntary instability (although this may not be easy to do), the first line of treatment is conservative with a retraining programme, supervised by an experienced physiotherapist, combined with rotator cuff strengthening exercises. Again, patients under 16 years should not be offered surgery. Approximately 30% of adult patients fail to respond to this regime. For those with a significant ongoing disability, the senior author advises surgery using a posterior capsular plication, as described above, with or without an inferior

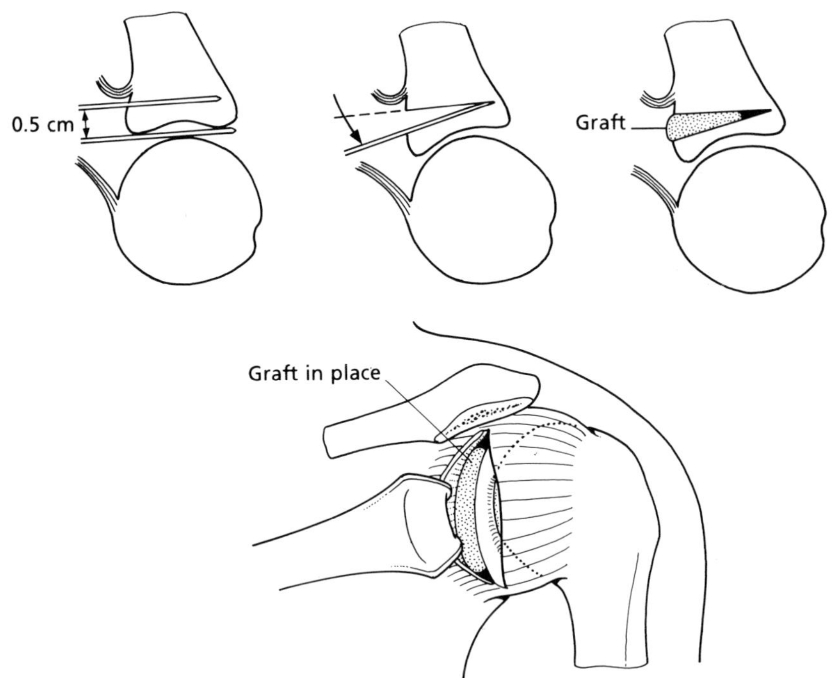

Fig. 12.72 Glenoid osteotomy with anterior tilt and insertion of iliac crest bone graft.

capsular shift. The success rate of such surgery in the senior author's hands is between 60 and 70%.

Treatment of multidirectional instability

Patients who have instability in more than one direction provide a major treatment challenge. Athletes, particularly swimmers and gymnasts, if they develop this problem often have to retire early from their sporting careers. Generalized joint laxity is frequently a predisposing factor, so that examination of the wrists, thumbs, elbows and knees should automatically be carried out to detect hyperextensibility. The first line of treatment is a conservative regime of strengthening of the rotator cuff muscles with up to 1 year of physiotherapy and avoidance of activities which provoke the subluxation episodes. Sport may have to be discontinued during the treatment period. It has been the experience of some shoulder surgeons that certain multigym exercises (particularly those which stretch the anterior shoulder capsule, as occurs with movements with the arms elevated to 90° while the arms are pushed backwards into full extension and external rotation) have been responsible for producing this kind of instability; it is also more common in butterfly swimmers (Richardson *et al.* 1980).

If multidirectional instability continues for more than 12 months and causes a significant ongoing disability, then surgery can be considered. Neer, in New York, has devised an 'inferior capsular shift' operation for multidirectional instability (Neer & Foster 1980). Recurrence of instability is not uncommon after this procedure — up to 30% in the senior author's experience. It is essential that the patient is warned about this before surgery. Again, this operation should be resisted in patients under 16 years.

Recommended operations for multidirectional shoulder instability

The surgical approach is similar to that for the Bankart operation. After dividing the subscapularis the surgeon must decide whether to mobilize the shoulder capsule from the lateral (humeral) side or from the medial (glenoid) side. The authors favour a medial mobilization only if the glenoid labrum requires surgical attention, and this is probably best decided by a previous arthroscopy. If there is no labral detachment then a lateral mobilization is preferred as this will allow a much tighter capsular repair. Having exposed the whole of the anterior shoulder capsule, any defect in the rotator interval — the interval between the supraspinatus and the subscapularis — is repaired.

A T-shaped incision is made in the capsule (Fig. 12.73) to create two flaps: a small superior flap and a large inferior flap (Fig. 12.74). The inferior flap is mobilized all round the inferior part of the humeral neck and this is made easier by extreme external rotation of the arm. It is possible to divide the capsule posteriorly halfway up the back of the humeral neck. It is important that this is done under vision and that the surgeon has a

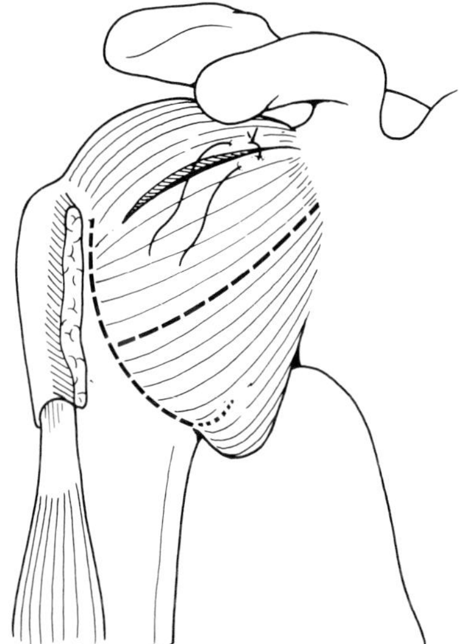

Fig. 12.73 The 'T' incision in the capsule for an inferior capsular shift.

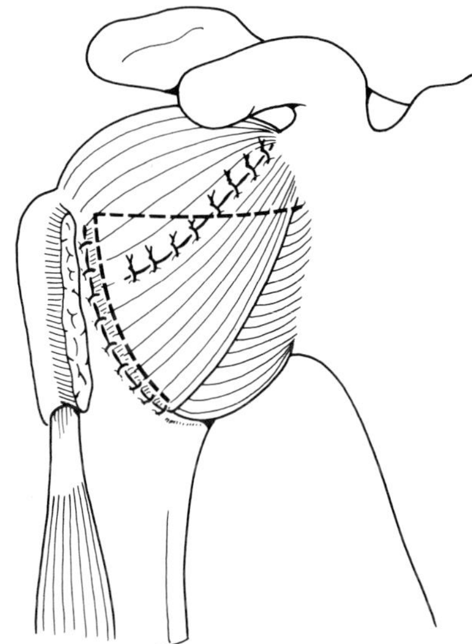

Fig. 12.75 The inferior capsular flap is sutured to the under surface of the subscapularis.

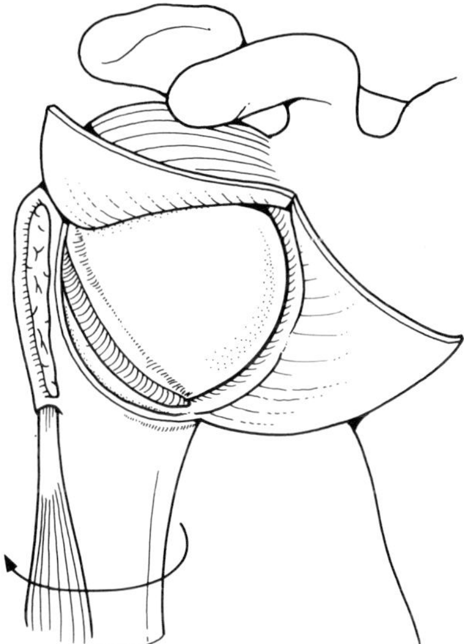

Fig. 12.74 The small superior and large inferior capsular flaps.

good knowledge of anatomy. During this operation the axillary nerve may be only 5 mm away from the surgeon's knife! After full mobilization, the arm is brought into flexion and the inferior flap is pulled as high up on the humeral neck as possible, and sutured to the local soft tissues (Fig. 12.75). The superior flap is then pulled down inferiorly, crossing the superior flap in a cruciate manner, and is sutured over the top. The result is that the posterior capsule is pulled anteriorly and tightened and the redundant inferior recess is ablated. After routine closure, the patient is immobilized in a broad arm sling and body bandage for up to 4 weeks. Mobilization is then carried out only slowly, concentrating on strengthening exercises. A return to sport is prohibited for 9 months. If there is a Bankart lesion present at surgery, a similar procedure is carried out but on the medial side, with a combination of a Bankart operation and an inferior capsular shift procedure, completed again in a cruciate manner.

Treatment of voluntary (habitual) instability

This condition should not be treated surgically. Patients should be encouraged to understand that the disability is, in part, due to their own tendency to put the shoulder joint out of position. It should then be managed with an intensive rehabilitation programme. If this fails, patients should be referred to a surgeon with a special interest in this condition.

Conclusions

Shoulder instability is becoming an increasingly important problem in young people because of a greater exposure to sports and trauma and because of an increasing expectation by patients that their upper limbs should be good enough for them to participate in all forms of sport. The success rates for treatment are very high for traumatic anterior instability but fall off significantly for other instabilities. They are so poor for voluntary instability that surgery should no longer be undertaken for such patients, except by specialist shoulder surgeons who have an in-depth understanding of all the problems associated with this group of patients.

References

Adams, J.C. Recurrent dislocation of the shoulder. *J Bone Joint Surg* 1948; **30B**: 26–38.

Bankart, A.S.B. The pathology and treatment of recurrent dislocation of the shoulder joint. *Br J Surg* 1939; **26**: 23–29.

Beighton, P., Solomon, L. & Soskolne, C.L. Articular mobility in an African population. *Ann. Rheum Dis* 1973; **32**: 413–418.

Broca, A. & Hartman, H. Contribution a l'étude des luxations de l'epaule. *Bull Soc Anat Paris*, 5me serie 1890; **4**: 312.

El-Sobhi, G.H. *Surgical Stabilisation of Anterior Instability of the Shoulder — Evaluation and the Medium Term Results of the Boytchev and Bankart Operations for Traumatic Instability, and the Bone Block Operation Specifically for Patients with Epilepsy.* MD thesis: University of Al-Azhar, 1991.

Gazielly, D.F., Godeneche, J.L. & Welsh, R.P. Shoulder stabilisation in athletes by coracoid process transfer. In: Takagishi, N. (ed.) *The Shoulder*. Professional Postgraduate Services: Japan, 1987.

Gerber, C. & Ganz, R. Clinical assessment of instability of the shoulder — with special reference to anterior and posterior drawer tests. *J Bone Joint Surg* 1984; **66B**: 551–556.

Gilchrist, D.K. A stockinette-Velpeau for immobilisation of the shoulder girdle. *J Bone Joint Surg* 1967; **49A**: 750–751.

Hawkins, R.H. & Hawkins, R.J. Failed anterior reconstruction for shoulder instability. *J Bone Joint Surg* 1985; **67B**: 709–714.

Hawkins, R.J. & Saddemi, S.R. Mini-symposium: the shoulder. (iv) Shoulder instability. *Curr Orthop* 1990; **4**: 242–252.

Hawkins, R.J., Neer, C.S., Pianta, R.M. & Mendoza, F.X. Locked posterior dislocation of the shoulder. *J Bone Joint Surg* 1987; **69A**: 9–18.

Hill, H.A. & Sachs, M.D. The grooved defect of the humeral head. A frequently unrecognized complication of dislocation of the shoulder joint. *Radiology* 1940; **35**: 690–700.

Hovelius, L. Operative treatment of recurrent anterior shoulder dislocation with the Bristow–Laterjet procedure. In: Bateman, J.E. & Welsh, R.P. (eds) *Surgery of the shoulder*. CV Mosby: Toronto, 1984.

Hovelius, L., Thorling, J. & Fredin, H. Recurrent anterior dislocation of the shoulder. Results after the Bankart and Putti-Platt operations. *J Bone Joint Surg* 1979; **61A**: 566–569.

Kennedy, J.C., Hawkins, R. & Krissof, W.B. Orthopaedic manifestations of swimming. *Am J Sports Med* 1978; **6**: 309–322.

Kretzler, H. & Scott, D.J. Posterior glenoid osteotomy for posterior dislocation of the shoulder. In: Bayley, I. & Kessel, K. (eds) *Shoulder Surgery*. Springer-Verlag: Berlin, 1982.

Matsen, F.A., Thomas, S.C. & Rockwood, C.A. Anterior glenohumeral instability. In: Rockwood, C.A. & Matsen, F.A. *The Shoulder*. WB Saunders: Philadelphia, 1990.

McAuliffe, T.B., Pangayatselvan, T. & Bayley, I. Failed surgery for recurrent anterior dislocation of the shoulder. *J Bone Joint Surg* 1988; **70B**: 798–801.

McLaughlin, H.L. Locked posterior subluxation of the shoulder — diagnosis and treatment. *Surg Clin North Am* 1963; **43**: 1621.

Meadows, T. & Wallace, W.A. Missed posterior dislocation of the shoulder. In: Takagishi, N. (ed.) *The Shoulder*. Professional Postgraduate Services; Japan, 1987.

Neer, C.S. & Foster, C.R. Inferior capsular shift for involuntary inferior and multi-directional instability of the shoulder. *J Bone Joint Surg* 1980; **62A**: 897–908.

Norwood, L.A. & Terry, G.C. Shoulder posterior subluxation. *Am J Sports Med* 1984; **12**: 25–30.

Osmond-Clarke, H. Habitual dislocation of the shoulder. The Putti-Platt operation. *J Bone Joint Surg* 1948; **30B**: 19–25.

Pieper, H.G. Correction of pathological amount of humeral retrotorsion in operative treatment of recurrent shoulder dislocation. In: Takagishi, N. (ed.) *The Shoulder*. Professional Postgraduate Services: Japan, 1987.

Reeves, B. Arthrography in acute dislocation of the shoulder. *J Bone Joint Surg* 1966; **48B**: 182.

Richardson, A.B., Jobe, F.W. & Collins, H.R. The shoulder in competitive swimming. *Am J Sports Med* 1980; **8**: 159–163.

Rowe, C.R., Patel, D. & Southmayd, W.W. The Bankart procedure — a long-term end result study. *J Bone Joint Surg* 1978; **60A**: 1–16.

Simonet, W.T. & Cofield, R.H. Prognosis in anterior shoulder dislocation. *Am J Sports Med* 1984; **12**: 19–24.

Stimson, L.A. *A Practical Treatise on Fractures and Dislocations* 7th edn. Lea & Febiger: Philadelphia, 1912.

Wallace, W.A. Sporting injuries of the shoulder. *J R Coll Surg Edinb* 1990; **35** (Suppl.): S21–S26.

Wallace, W.A. Recurrent anterior dislocation of the shoulder. In: Bentley, G. (ed.) *Rob & Smith's Operative Surgery — Orthopaedics* 4th edn. Butterworth: London, 1991a.

Wallace, W.A. The shoulder. In: Colton, C.L. & Hall, A.J. (eds) *Atlas of Orthopaedic Surgical Approaches*. Butterworth: London 1991b.

Wallace, W.A. Recurrent instability of the shoulder and its management. In: Kelly, I.G. (ed.) *The Practice of Shoulder Surgery*. Butterworth Heinemann: Oxford 1993.

Wallace, W.A. & Bunker, T.D. Management of proximal humeral fractures. In: Bunker, T.D., Colton, C.L. & Webb, J.K. (eds) *Frontiers in Fracture Management*. Martin Dunitz: London, 1989.

Wallace, W.A. & Hellier, M. Improving radiographs of the injured shoulder. *Radiography* 1983; **49**: 229–233.

Yoneda, B., Welsh, P. & Macintosh, D.L. Conservative treatment of shoulder dislocation in young males. In: Bayley, I. & Kessel, L. (eds) *Shoulder Surgery*. Springer-Verlag: Berlin, 1982.

Proximal humerus

P.G.STABLEFORTH AND W.A.WALLACE

Fractures and fracture–dislocations of the proximal humerus form some 5% of all bone and joint injuries. There are two peaks of fracture incidence: the first is in late adolescent or young adult life when young males sustain displaced extracapsular fractures from falls at speed or from a height; the second, which is much larger, occurs in the sixth and seventh decades when there is a preponderance of undisplaced fractures in females following simple falls on the level (Fig. 12.76).

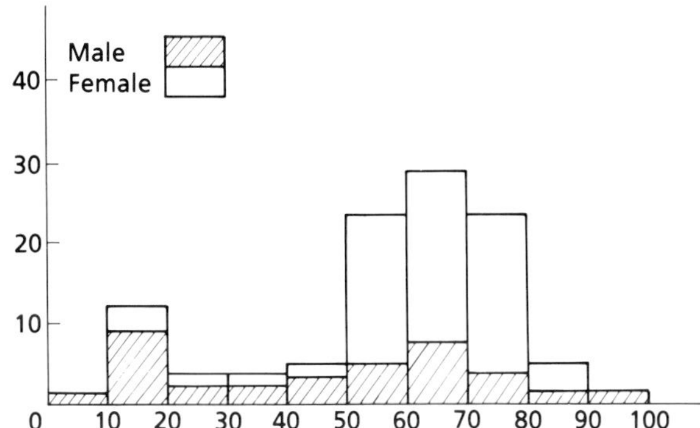

Fig. 12.76 Incidence of proximal humeral fracture by age and sex.

The most complex fractures, the displaced three- and four-segment injuries, are, however, usually seen in males aged 40–60 years and in females between 50 and 70 years old.

Fracture classification

Management of proximal humeral fractures is simplified by the use of the four-segment classification (Codman 1934, Neer 1970, 1975) which takes account of the soft tissue attachments of the major bone segments (Fig. 12.77). With this system fracture displacements and the viability of the articular segment can be predicted with some confidence (Fig. 12.78).

Radiographic examination

Good quality biplanar radiographs are essential for the correct diagnosis of fracture type and displacement (Neer 1970). A true anteroposterior radiograph of the shoulder joint (a frontal view with the beam angled 35° to the frontal plane) and an axial view of the scapula (with the beam at 90° to the anteroposterior view) are the essential minimum and can be taken with the arm resting in a broad arm sling (Fig. 12.79); the transaxillary lateral view of the 70° abducted arm is also very useful but may be impossible to obtain in the conscious recently injured patient. For more complex or old injuries CT scanning techniques can be of great help in surgical planning.

Complications and associated injuries

Most proximal humeral injuries are isolated injuries. Shoulder pain, swelling and muscle spasm are immediate and severe; subsequent organization of the fracture haematoma with adhesions and capsular contracture is

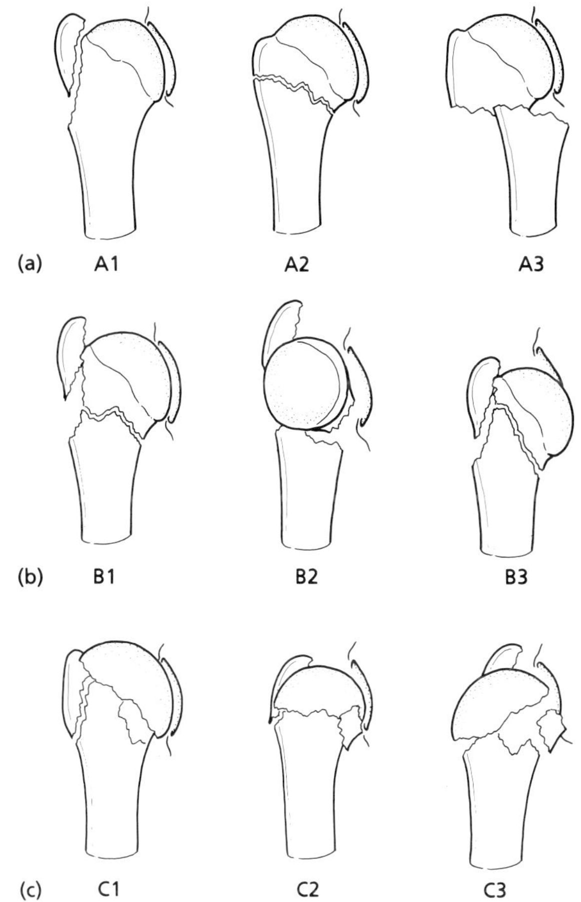

Fig. 12.77 AO modification of the four-segment classification. (a) Two-segment, (b) three-segment and (c) four-segment extra-articular fractures.

a common cause of shoulder stiffness. Bruising may be delayed and may be more obvious around the elbow.

Local neurovascular complications are uncommon. Damage to an atherosclerotic circumflex or axillary vessel may occasionally occur with a displaced two-segment fracture. Infraclavicular brachial plexus injury sometimes, and rib cage and intrathoracic injury rarely, complicate displaced three- or four-segment fractures (Table 12.7). Compromise of the blood supply of the articular segment is a common complication of four-segment fractures.

Principles of management

Some 85% of proximal humeral fractures are not significantly displaced, are stable and do not require surgical treatment (Neer 1970, Jacob et al. 1984). In the remaining 15%, one or more of the major segments is displaced and the soft tissues are disrupted; for these injuries

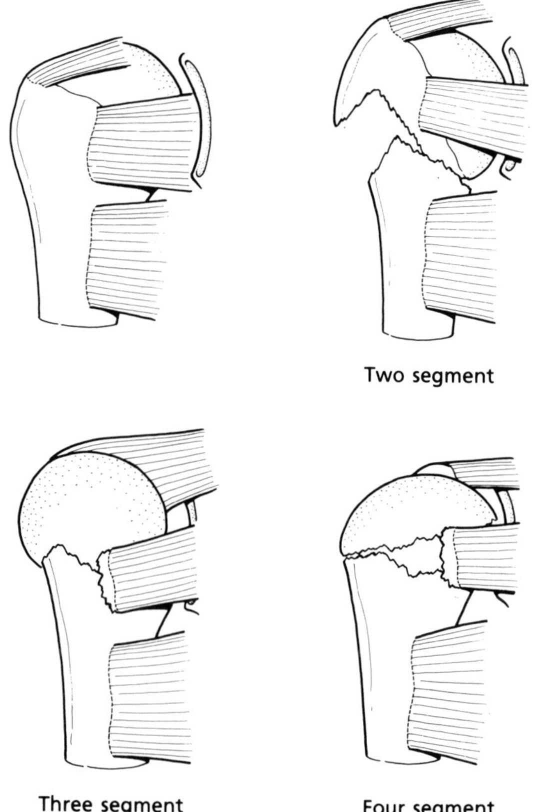

Fig. 12.78 The four-segment classification. Diagram to show the direction of pull of the three groups of muscles, bicipital groove group, subscapularis and supraspinatus, in the different fractures.

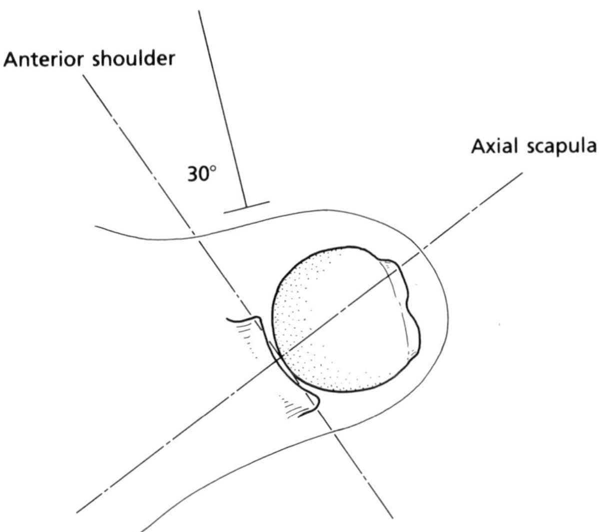

Fig. 12.79 Neer's 'trauma series' views of the proximal humerus. The patient can sit with the arm supported in a sling.

Table 12.7 Incidence of injuries found with proximal humeral fractures

Associated injuries	Incidence (%)
Brachial plexus injury	8
Axillary vessel damage	5
Pneumothorax	2
Colles' fracture	5
Lower limb fracture	5

fracture manipulation or surgical reconstruction may be needed to correct malalignments and restore articular congruence, to prevent bony impingements and to allow early movement after fracture stabilization.

Whilst management will depend principally on the fracture type and displacement, consideration must also be given to the patient's age and general health and to the presence of intercurrent disease (Table 12.8). Many elderly patients, who are otherwise fit and previously independent, are entirely suitable candidates for surgical reconstruction whilst some who were socially dependent or uncooperative are not.

The results of surgical reconstruction are not uniformly good, and a fairly satisfactory outcome may follow non-operative management, so that surgery should only be undertaken if the necessary surgical skills are available and a vigorous postoperative regimen can be followed by patient and therapist (Kraulis & Hunter 1976, Sturznegger *et al.* 1982, Paavolainen *et al.* 1983, DesMarchais & Morais 1984, Hagg & Lundberg 1984, Stableforth 1984, Willems & Lim 1985). A suggested surgical plan is set out in Table 12.9.

Although a dislocated humeral head needs reduction, the dislocation does not, by and large, otherwise affect the principles of management of associated fractures.

Standard AO techniques are used for screw or plate fixations, but these are less popular in the 1990s.

Bone defects created by fracture reduction should always be packed with cancellous bone taken from a discarded humeral head or from the usual donor sites. Neither K-wires nor cortical screws hold well in osteoporotic bone; in patients over 65 years old, an intramedullary locked nail or two Rush pins and tension bands (Robinson & Christie 1993) may give more predictable fixation.

If K-wires are used for fracture fixation, their free ends must always be bent to prevent medial migration.

Wire tension-bands are difficult to control and a strong non-absorbable suture (e.g. No. 5 Ethibond) is easier to use; these sutures can conveniently be threaded through a large-bore needle and passed though a pre-drilled

Table 12.8 Intercurrent disorders found with proximal humeral fractures

Intercurrent disorders	Incidence (%)
Dementia	15
Cardiac ischaemia	10
Intercurrent infection	5
Terminal illness	3

Table 12.9 Suggested surgical plan for displaced proximal humeral fractures

Two-segment extra-articular fractures
Closed reduction and percutaneous K-wire or external skeletal fixation or
open reduction and T-plate fixation

Greater tuberosity or anatomical neck fractures
Open reduction and screw fixation

Three-segment fractures
Open reduction, K-wires, bone graft and tension-band fixation

Four-segment intracapsular fractures
Open reduction, bone graft and T-plate fixation (younger patients)
Neer reconstruction with humeral head prosthesis (older patients)

track. Tension-band sutures are, whenever possible, passed through bone and not through cuff tendons; they should secure tuberosity to shaft as well as tuberosity to tuberosity.

Surgical approaches

For open surgery on proximal humeral fractures the anterior delto-pectoral approach (Wallace 1991) is the most generally useful and appropriate. A superior approach under the anterior acromion (Neer 1972, Gschwend 1984) has some advantages for the experienced surgeon when dealing with complex three- or four-segment injuries, isolated greater tuberosity fractures or posterior fracture-dislocations. This is particularly appropriate for open reduction and internal fixation when the surgeon wishes to carry out the minimum of dissection, thus preserving the blood supply to the proximal humerus (minimal fixation).

Access to the front and to the top of the proximal humerus is improved if the patient is 'chaired', so as to sit up some 50–70° on the operating table, and a sandbag is placed behind the medial edge of the scapula to tilt the patient and stabilize the shoulder joint. The upper limb is draped free and the patient positioned so that the arm can be brought into extension over the edge of the table.

Anterior delto-pectoral approach

The skin incision runs from the acromio-clavicular joint down over the coracoid to the lower border of the pectoralis major muscle. The cephalic vein is identified and reflected laterally and the delto-pectoral interval developed. The long head of the biceps is followed proximally to lead to the tuberosities and the cuff interval. Access is improved by partial distal detachment of the deltoid tendon, division of the proximal 1 cm of the pectoralis major tendon and arm flexion at the shoulder. Exposure of the top of the humerus is much improved if the upper surface of the lateral end of the clavicle is cleared and if its anterior quarter and deltoid attachment are osteotomized and reflected laterally. At the end of the operation the bone fragment is secured by strong sutures passed around or through drill holes in the shaft of the clavicle (Fig. 12.80).

Superior approach

In this modified approach a skin crease incision extends from 3 cm below the clavicle up over the acromio-clavicular joint to end 2–3 cm below the scapular spine; the skin flaps are reflected to expose the upper deltoid fibres, the outer end of the clavicle, the supraclavicular fossa and the trapezius (Fig. 12.81). The deeper incision now bisects the angle between the trapezius and clav-

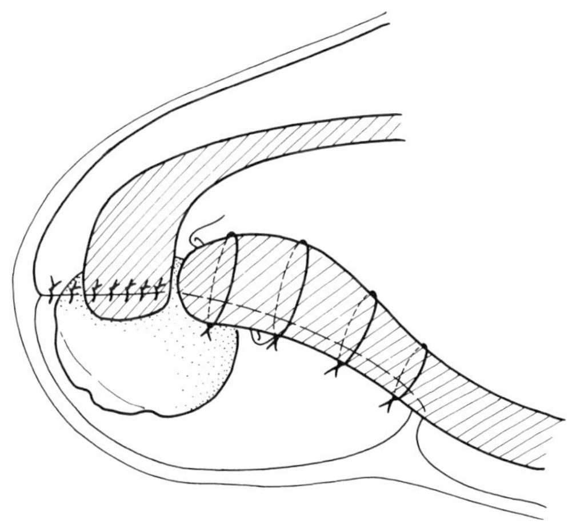

Fig. 12.80 With the extended anterior approach a strong repair, without compromise of the deltoid, is possible if strong non-absorbable sutures are placed round the clavicle to secure the anterior fragment.

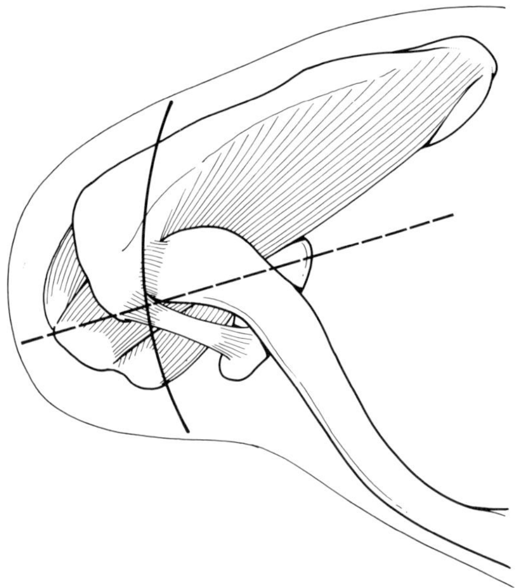

Fig. 12.81 The superior approach. A skin crease incision gives the best scar; the deeper incision bisects the angle between the clavicle and anterior border of the trapezius.

icle, passes over the front of the acromio-clavicular joint and upper acromion and splits the upper two fingers' breadth of the deltoid along the line of its fibres. The periosteum of the acromion is 'petalled' and reflected forwards with the deltoid as a thick flap to expose the upper aspect of the shoulder and subacromial bursa; the anterior quarter of the acromion can be undercut and removed to improve the exposure. At the end of

the procedure the anterior and posterior flaps of periosteum and muscle are secured together with strong nonabsorbable sutures.

With either the anterior or superior approach the coracoacromial ligament is divided for access if there is a greater tuberosity fracture.

Undisplaced fractures

Fractures in which no segment of the complex is more than 1 cm (one-third of a shaft diameter) displaced, or more than 45° rotated, do not require manipulation. It must be remembered, however, that some fractures are unstable, and that secondary displacement can occur up to 10 days after injury. Delayed retraction of the greater tuberosity fracture with subcoracoid dislocation is well recognized but delayed displacement of three- and four-segment fractures may also occur (Fig. 12.82).

It is wise to repeat the radiographs 7–10 days after injury.

Displaced two-segment fractures

The humerus is shortened and the shaft displaced anteromedially.

In an ambulant patient the weight of the hanging arm, with the wrist supported in a collar-and-cuff sling, may allow an adequate, if incomplete, fracture reduction to occur over 5–7 days. If the patient is bedfast or if reduction does not occur, it can often be achieved by manipulation under anaesthesia, though interposed

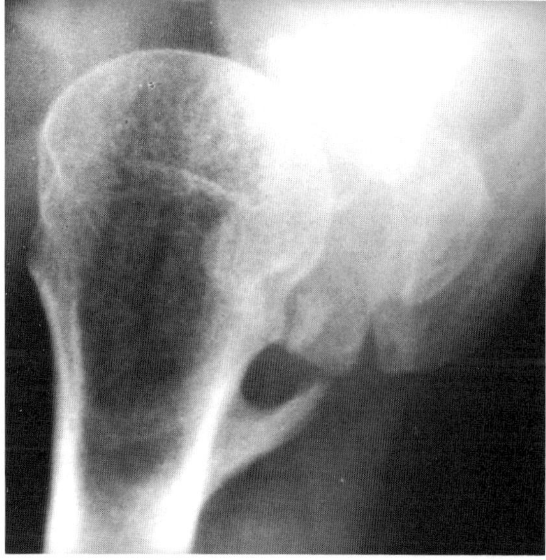

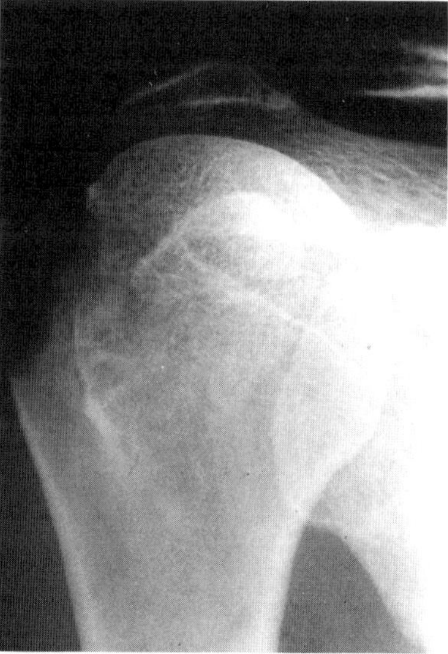

Fig. 12.82 The greater tuberosity avulsion was not seen in the postreduction films of this subcoracoid dislocation. Functional recovery was poor. Radiographic examination at 1 year shows the displacement of the supraspinatus origin.

soft tissue may sometimes prevent reduction. However, 35–40% of these fractures will redisplace if they are not fixed surgically. An 'irreducible' fracture can sometimes be aligned following percutaneous K-wire or Ex-fix pin 'capture' and manipulation; otherwise, it may need open reduction.

Unstable reduced fracture segments can be controlled by percutaneous K-wires or by external or internal fixation.

Percutaneous K-wire fixation

A power drill is used to pass two or three long 3-mm-diameter K-wires, under radiographic control, obliquely across the fracture from below upwards and backwards to pierce the cortex behind the humeral head or, less safely, drilled from the edge of the greater tuberosity downwards and forwards to emerge at the anteromedial aspect of the humeral shaft. Good image intensification is necessary if this method is used. The protruding ends of the wires are bent over to prevent medial migration. Only very gentle shoulder mobilization is possible until the wires have been removed after 3–4 weeks. In patients over 65 years old the wires often loosen and migrate in the osteoporotic bone with loss of fracture reduction. Some surgeons do not permit mobilization of the shoulder for the first three weeks to reduce the risk of pin loosening.

External skeletal fixation

This technique is of particular value in a patient who is bedfast or has sustained multiple injuries. Displaced fracture segments are 'captured' with fixation pins which are then used for fracture manipulation (Kristiansen & Kofoed 1987, Kristiansen 1989). Schanz pins are the most secure, but stout K-wires or small threaded pins can be used. A single axis or biplane fixation frame is applied and secured (Fig. 12.83).

Open reduction and T-plate fixation

The delto-pectoral approach is used. The long head of the biceps is identified and followed to the intertuberous groove; the bone ends are cleared and the fracture is reduced with the biceps tendon used as the guide to rotation. K-wires are used to provide temporary fracture control. A T-plate is applied to the anterolateral surface of the upper humerus and is secured proximally by two fully threaded screws inserted across the humeral head, and distally by screws gripping at least six cortices of the upper shaft. Proximal fixation is much more secure if a further cortical screw can be passed into the calcar humerale just below the humeral head (Fig. 12.84). Range-of-movement exercises are started at once.

Rush pin and tension band fixation

Either the delto-pectoral or superior approach is used. The fracture is reduced. Short splits, one anterior and one posterior, are made in the lateral part of the supra-spinatus tendon. Through these the edge of the articular surface at its junction with the greater tuberosity is exposed. Rush pins are then passed through broach

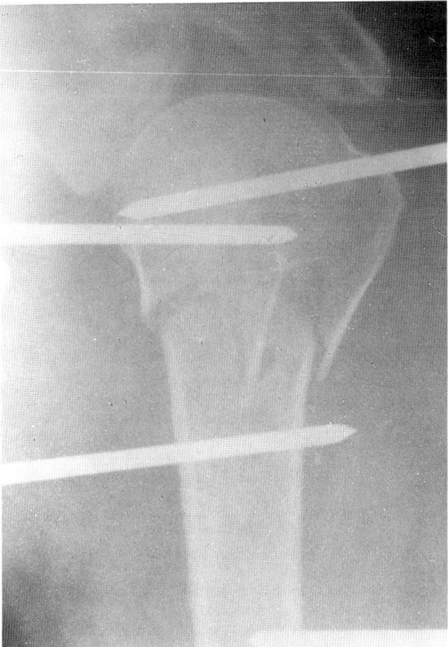
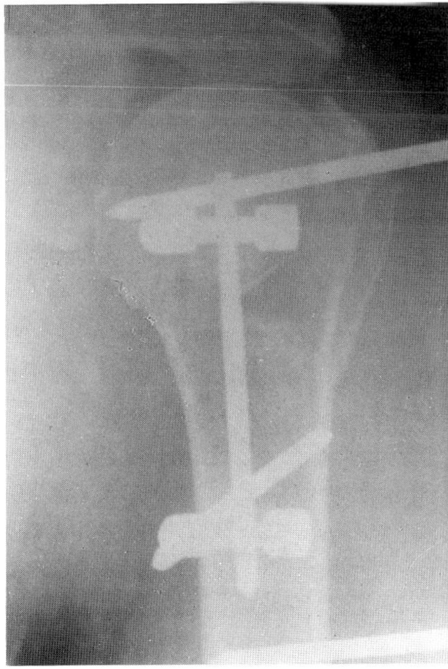

Fig. 12.83 A four-segment fracture has been reduced and stabilized with guide wires and a rectangular frame.

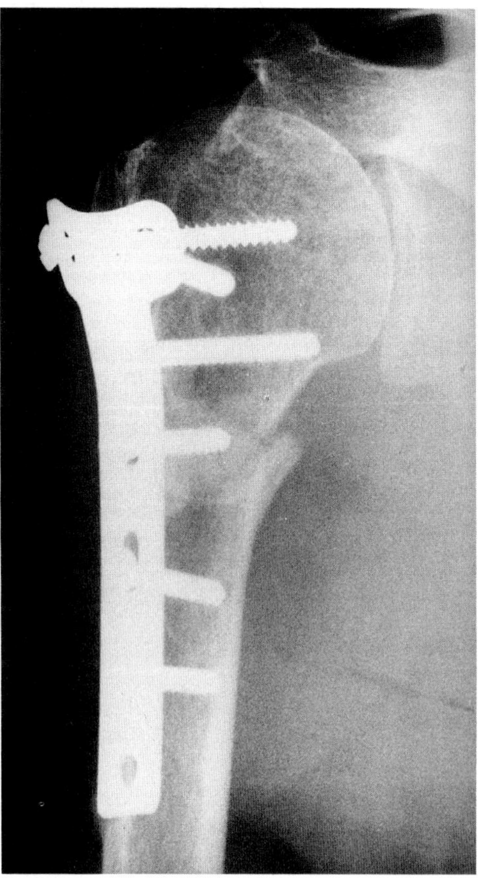

Fig. 12.84 A cortical screw holds the calcar humerale and provides much more secure fixation of the proximal fragment.

holes and across the fracture site into the distal medullary canal. A figure-of-8 tension suture is passed under the cuff tendon and the Rush pin hooks, then over the lateral side of the fracture and through a hole drilled in the lateral cortex of the distal fragment. The fracture is impacted and the suture tensioned with the arm in some abduction. A range of movement exercises is started at once.

Displaced three-segment fractures

Malrotation of the articular segment occurs as a consequence of the pull of whichever cuff muscle remains attached through its tuberosity segment. If, as is more usual, the greater tuberosity is separated from the head, the unopposed subscapularis will pull on the lesser tuberosity and rotate the articular segment so that its cancellous surface looks forwards. With the less common lesser tuberosity detachment the supraspinatus will rotate the head so that its cancellous surface looks backwards.

Open reduction; bone graft; K-wire and tension-band fixation

Through an anterior or superior approach the coracoacromial ligament is divided, and the long biceps tendon is followed to the tuberosities and cuff interval. The detached tuberosity is drawn aside and the articular segment gently rotated into the correct orientation, positioned so that its medial edge rests correctly on the calcar. It is stabilized by two K-wires drilled from the tuberosity−head junction down to the medial cortex below the fracture line. The detached tuberosity is temporarily aligned and a radiograph taken to confirm the reduction and orientation. Any defects are then packed with cancellous bone before the tuberosity is finally reduced and secured by figure-of-eight tension-band sutures, which are inserted to pass between the tuberosities and to the shaft below the fracture (Fig. 12.85). Active-assisted and passive flexion exercises are started at once, but rotation is delayed for 7−10 days.

Displaced four-segment intracapsular fractures

The articular segment has no muscle attachments, may be totally free of soft tissue attachments and may lie in almost any orientation; it may be in the axilla or subcoracoid, but even if not dislocated it rarely faces the glenoid (Fig. 12.86). The lesser tuberosity is pulled medially to lie at the front of the glenoid margin, and the greater tuberosity is pulled upwards and backwards to lie behind the shoulder joint with its cancellous surface facing forwards.

If the articular segment is undamaged and potentially viable, then fracture reconstruction, bone grafting and

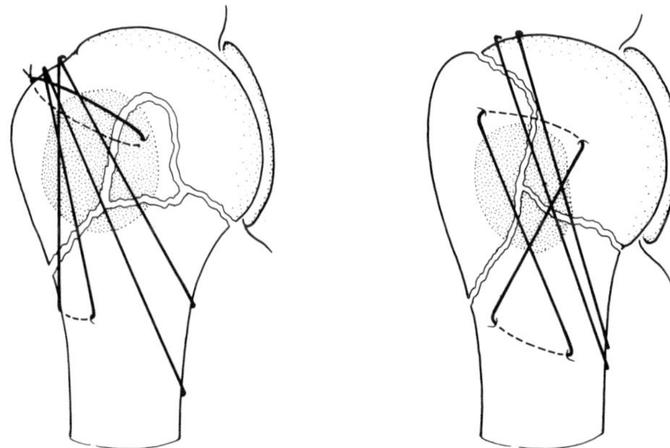

Fig. 12.85 Diagram to show the fixation of a three-segment fracture by bone graft, K-wire and figure-of-eight tension-band fixation.

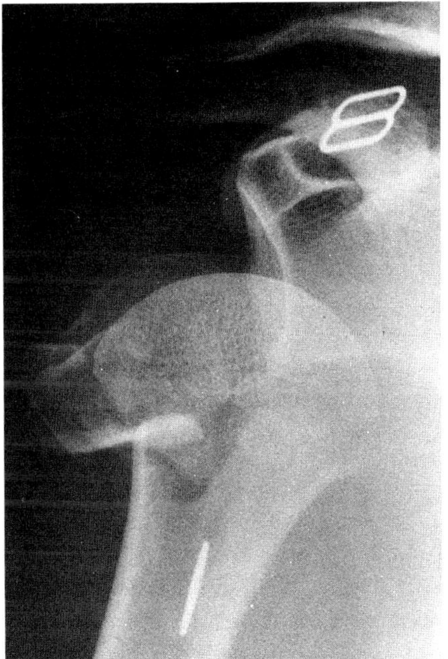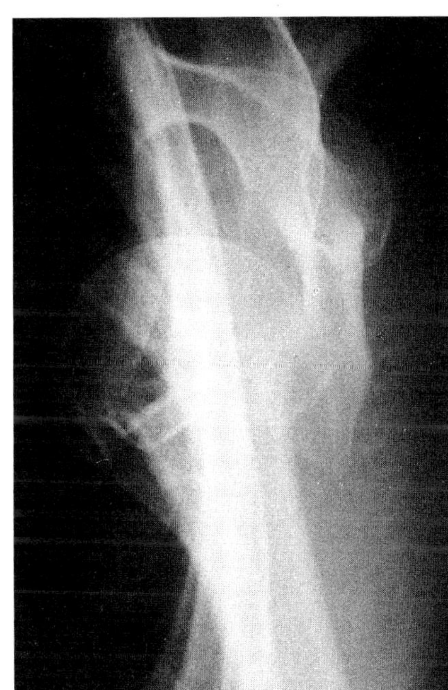

Fig. 12.86 A displaced four-segment fracture–dislocation in a 45-year-old female. The articular segment is undamaged.

stabilization should be considered, particularly in younger patients. A humeral head with articular cartilage damage or a comminuted fracture, or totally devoid of soft tissue attachments, is probably best removed and replaced by a humeral head prosthesis; proximal reconstruction with humeral head replacement is the easiest and quickest option in older patients (Neer 1963, 1970, Tanner & Cofield 1983, Stableforth 1984).

Neer reconstruction of the proximal humerus

The delto-pectoral approach is used with the long head of the biceps as the guide to the anatomy. If radiographic examination shows the articular segment to be sub-coracoid or axillary it is usually lying amongst the axillary vessels and branches of the brachial plexus; its removal needs care and if it should seem particularly inaccesible it can perhaps be left, as neurological recovery is not dependent on its removal. The arm is gently extended to expose, and allow clearance of, the open end of the humeral shaft. A prosthesis of the same thickness as the discarded humeral head, and with the largest stem that will pass down the medullary cavity, is tapped gently into the humeral shaft in 35–40° retroversion (the lateral fin then usually aligns with the bicipital groove).

Humeral length must be restored and the prosthesis should be inserted so that its upper surface lies 4–5 mm proud of the greater tuberosity; it should not be hammered down to rest on the calcar (Fig. 12.87). The two

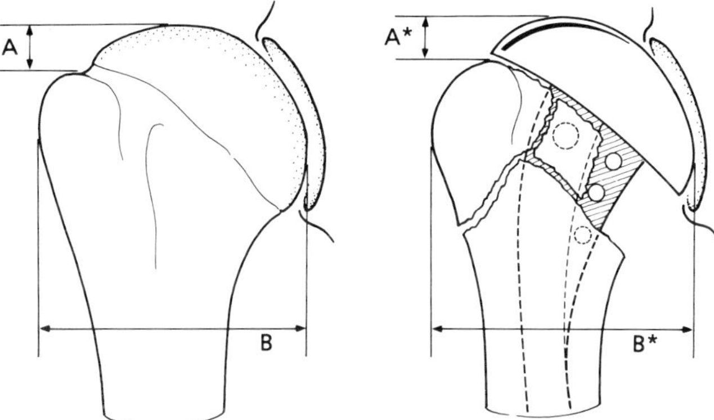

Fig. 12.87 Proximal humeral reconstruction using a Neer prosthesis. The distance from the tuberosity to the top of the prosthesis (A/A*), and from the tuberosity to the medial edge of the prosthesis (B/B*) should be the same on sound and injured sides.

tuberosities are drawn across the lateral side of the prosthesis and if the 'fit' seems satisfactory they are released and the grip of the prosthesis in the shaft is checked; an unstable implant can be cemented in position or impacted in the medullary cavity with cancellous bone taken from the discarded humeral head.

The glenoid is inspected and irrigated, and the cuff tendons are finally secured in correct tension by sutures passed through the tuberosity fragments and through drill holes in the upper humeral shaft. Alignment and stability are checked and the wound is closed with firm deltoid reattachment. The arm is supported in a broad sling.

Range-of-movement pendulum and active-assisted flexion exercises are started at once and rotation is started after 5–7 days.

Open reduction and internal fixation of four-segment fractures

If the articular segment has retained soft tissue attachments and can be reduced, proximal humeral reconstruction should be considered.

The extended delto-pectoral or the superior approaches give good access. Fracture capture and reduction is as described for the three-segment injury, but great care must be taken to avoid dissection or disturbance of the calcar humerale at the inferior angle of the articular segment.

A stable reconstruction is needed to allow early mobilization and to protect the blood supply of the articular segment. A T-plate gives good but bulky fixation. In the 1990s there has been a swing towards anatomical fixation, with the packing of any voids with cancellous bone, which then allows stable 'minimal' fixation with screws or with 3 mm-diameter K-wires and tension band sutures (Jacob *et al.* 1991, Stableforth 1994) (Fig. 12.88).

Complications of surgery

Shoulder stiffness

Stable internal fixation with grafting of bone defects and secure deltoid reattachment are vital as stiffness from the organization of periarticular exudate leads to subdeltoid fibrosis and obliteration of the normal axillary capsular recess. This can only be avoided by early range-of-movement exercises. Severe stiffness may follow postoperative soft tissue calcification, though this uncommon complication is usually only seen in patients whose fractures are explored more than a week after injury.

Fracture malunion or non-union

These complications may result from poor surgical technique, and attention to detail is important. Although fracture stabilization may be difficult, most malunions arise from incomplete fracture reduction or from failure to graft bone defects.

Intraoperative radiographs are a useful check on surgical progress (Fig. 12.89).

Late reconstruction of malunions is difficult and time-consuming. In some patients malposition may lead to subacromial impingement, and coracoacromioplasty

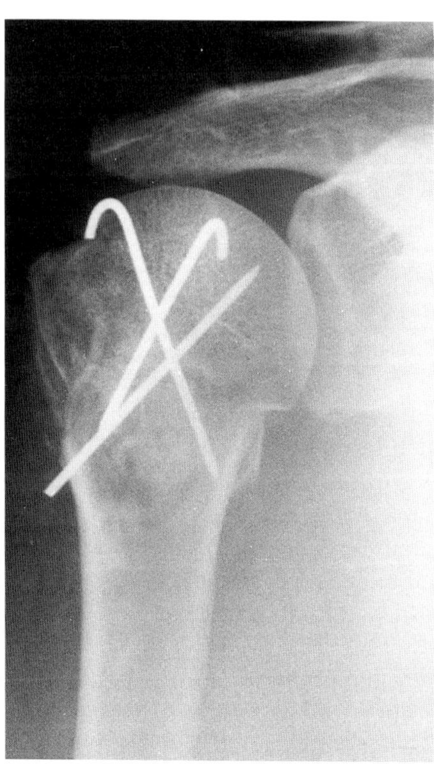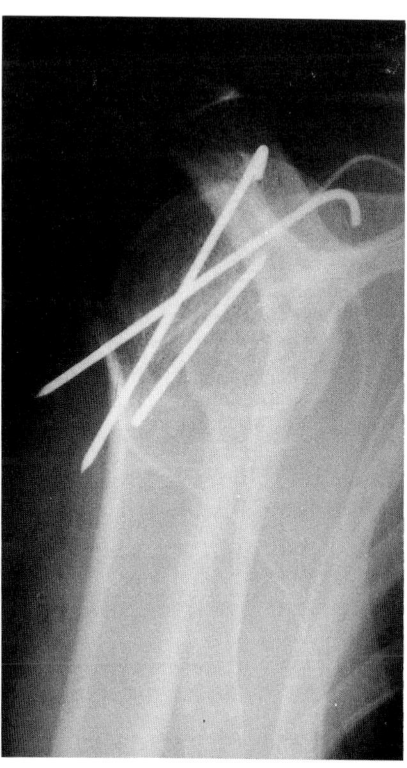

Fig. 12.88 Same patient as in Fig. 12.85. The proximal humerus has been reconstructed and stabilized with bone graft, K-wires and strong tension sutures (radiolucent). The blood supply to the articular segment was preserved.

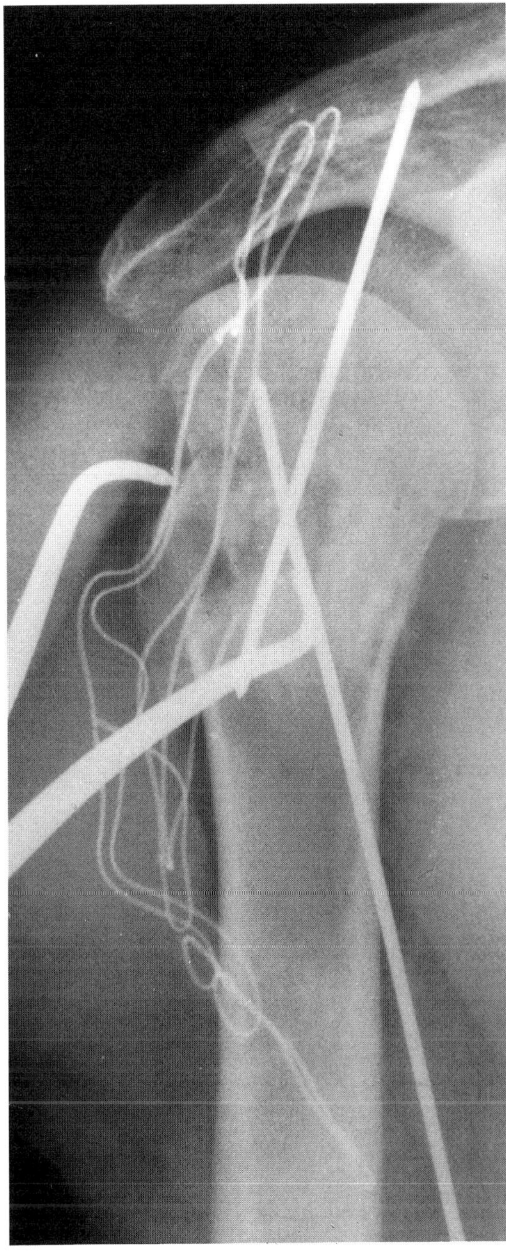

Fig. 12.89 Intraoperative radiograph showing good alignment of the articular defect; note the use of K-wires for temporary fracture control, and the large defect that needs bone grafting for fracture stability.

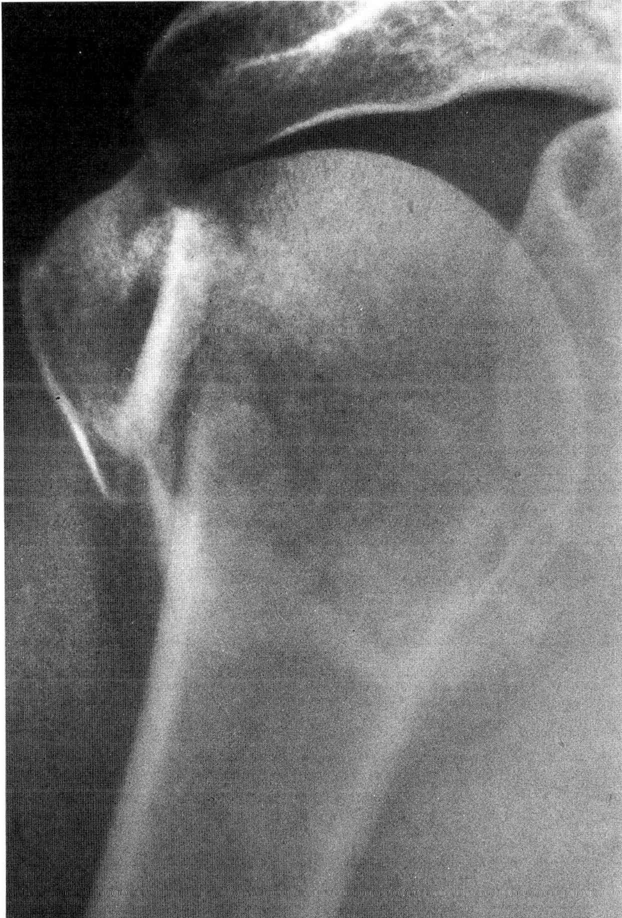

Fig. 12.90 The greater tuberosity in this three-segment fracture has rotated on its soft tissue hinge and impacted against the acromion.

gives satisfactory pain relief and increased mobility; however in other patients it may be necessary to explore the fracture and separate the segments with an osteotome before realignment and stabilization can be effected. In these cases the blood supply of the articular segment may be jeopardized and a prosthetic replacement may be necessary.

Careful preoperative investigation of segment displacements, possibly by CT scanning techniques, can be invaluable in surgical planning.

Avascular necrosis

Necrosis of the articular segment may follow soft tissue stripping at injury or surgical damage to the branches of the circumflex humeral vessels as they enter the humeral head. Prosthetic replacement of the humeral head may be needed.

Greater tuberosity fractures

The greater tuberosity may be pulled away from its bed particularly with subcoracoid dislocation. It may be the only displaced segment in a multisegment fracture, or may be displaced with other segments in a more complex proximal humeral injury.

Displacement may occur initially or may be delayed for up to 10 days after injury, and may range from a rotation of the bony supraspinatus insertion on an intact posterior soft tissue hinge to a total and widely displaced avulsion of the greater tuberosity, which is then retracted to lie above and behind the shoulder joint. A displaced tuberosity may cause subacromial impingement with painful restriction of movement (Fig. 12.90), whilst total avulsion of the supraspinatus from its humeral attachment causes a loss of external rotation and elevation at the shoulder.

Most avulsed tuberosity fragments with subcoracoid dislocation will realign with reduction of the dislocation. Tuberosities that remain rotated or displaced after injury can sometimes be reduced by elevation of the arm into external rotation and abduction under anaesthesia, and then transfixed with a 3-mm-diameter K-wire passed percutaneously under radiographic control.

An irreducible or unstable greater tuberosity should be exposed through the superior approach, anatomically reduced and fixed with one or two cancellous screws with washers or with a tension band wire or suture. The arm should be rested in a sling, and a range-of-movement exercises can be started at once if the proximal humerus is otherwise stable.

References

Codman, E.A. *The Shoulder, Rupture of the Supraspinatus Tendon and Other Lesions in or about the Subacromial Bursa.* T. Todd: Boston, 1934.

DesMarchais, J.E. & Morais, G. Treatment of complex fractures of the proximal humerus by Neer arthroplasty. In: Bateman, J.E. & Welsh, R.P. (eds) *Surgery of the Shoulder.* CV Mosby: St Louis, 1984.

Gschwend, N. A surgical approach to rotator cuff tears. In: Bateman, J.E. & Welsh, J.E. (eds) *Surgery of the Shoulder.* CV Mosby: St Louis, 1984.

Hagg, O. & Lundberg, B. Aspects of prognostic factors in comminuted and dislocated proximal humeral fractures. In: Bateman, J.E. & Welsh, R.P. (eds) *Surgery of the Shoulder.* CV Mosby: St Louis, 1984.

Jacob, R.P., Kristiansen, B., Mayo, K., Ganz, R. & Müller, M.E. Classification and aspects of treatment of fractures of the proximal humerus. In: Bateman, J.E. & Welsh, R.P. (eds) *Surgery of the Shoulder.* CV Mosby: St Louis, 1984.

Jacob, R.P., Miniachi, A., Anson, P.S., Jaberg, H., Osterwalder, A. & Ganz, R. Four part valgus impacted fractures of the proximal humerus. *J Bone Joint Surg* 1991; **73B**: 295−298.

Kraulis, K. & Hunter, G. The results of prosthetic replacement in fractures of the upper end of the humerus. *Injury* 1976; **8**: 129.

Kristiansen, B. External fixation of displaced proximal humeral fractures. *Injury* 1989; **20**: 196−199.

Kristiansen, B. & Kofoed, H. External fixation of displaced fractures of the proximal humerus. Technique and preliminary results. *J Bone Joint Surg* 1987; **69B**: 643−647.

Neer, C.S. Prosthetic replacement of the humeral head. Indications and operative technique. *Surg Clin North Am* 1963; **43**: 1581−1597.

Neer, C.S. Displaced proximal humeral fractures. Part 1. Classification and evaluation. *J Bone Joint Surg* 1970; **52A**: 1077−1089.

Neer, C.S. Anterior acromioplasty for the chronic impingement syndrome. *J Bone Joint Surg* 1972; **54A**: 41−50.

Neer, C.S. In: Rockwood, C.A. & Green, D.P. (eds) *Fractures and Dislocations.* Lippincott: Philadelphia, 1975.

Paavolainen, P., Bjorkenheim, J.M. & Slatis, P. Operative treatment of severe proximal humeral fractures. *Acta Orthop Scand* 1983; **54**: 374.

Robinson, C.M. & Christie, J. The two part proximal humeral fracture. A review of operative treatment using two techniques. *Injury* 1993; **24**: 123−125.

Stableforth, P.G. Four part fractures of the proximal humerus. *J Bone Joint Surg* 1984; **66B**: 104−109.

Stableforth, P.G. Open reduction and internal fixation of displaced four segment fractures of the proximal humerus. *Operat Tech Orth* 1994; **4**: 26−30.

Sturznegger, M., Fornaro, E. & Jacob, R.P. Results of surgical treatment of multifragmented fractures of the humeral head. *Acta Orthop Trauma Surg* 1982; **100**: 249−259.

Tanner, M.W. & Cofield, R.H. Prosthetic arthroplasty for fractures and fracture dislocations of the proximal humerus. *Clin Orthop* 1983; **179**: 116.

Wallace, W.A. In: Colton, C.L. & Hall, A.H. (eds) *Atlas of Orthopaedic Surgical Approaches.* Butterworth-Heinemann: Oxford, 1991.

Willems, W.J. & Lim, T.E.A. Conservative treatment of fracture dislocations of the upper end of the humerus. *J Bone Joint Surg* 1985; **67B**: 373.

Rotator cuff

P.G.STABLEFORTH

Injuries may affect any part of the cuff, but supraspinatus lesions are the most common, the most persistent and the most disabling (Kessel & Watson 1977). Thinning and degeneration of the cuff becomes more common with advancing age, and whilst an injury in the fit young adult is usually a strain lesion of healthy tissues, that in an older patient is more often quite an extensive tear of a thinned and degenerate cuff.

Strain lesions in younger patients are most commonly partial and surface tears; a few fibres near the tendinous insertion are 'teased' apart after a single sudden overload or after a series of smaller repetitive stresses at work or sport. There may be immediate intense pain or, later, aching discomfort with use; 'release pain' — sharp pain that is experienced as a sudden movement is completed — is a common complaint. Most of these lesions heal if shoulder activity is reduced and local physical treatment, and a short course of non-steroidal anti-inflammatories, is prescribed. Subacromial injection of steroid and local anaesthetic should be delayed for 6–8 weeks for fear of tendon rupture, but may finally relieve symptoms and allow a return to full activity.

In a few patients stress or impingement symptoms continue and if release pain or a painful arc syndrome is only briefly eased by subdeltoid local anaesthetic, then injection, decompression by coracoacromial ligament division or undercutting anterior acromionectomy should be considered.

Complete rupture of a normal cuff is uncommon and usually follows a fall in which the arm is wrenched as the patient tries to grasp an overhead support. Tears of an asymptomatic but thinned cuff in a 30- to 40-year-old, or a degenerate cuff in an older male, may follow an unguarded strain or a simple fall on the level. The shoulder is swollen and all movements are totally and painfully inhibited. Biplanar radiographs are normal. The shoulder should be aspirated and 10–15 ml of local anaesthetic injected; if the patient is then pain-free but cannot maintain the 80° flexed arm, cuff rupture is probable (Brown 1949). This can be confirmed, if necessary, by shoulder arthrography, an MRI scan or, in experienced hands, by arthroscopy.

For younger patients with a healthy cuff early exploration and cuff repair will usually result in a comfortable and robust shoulder. In older patients, and particularly in those whose radiographs show calcification or another cuff abnormality, the surgical result is less certain (Wolfgang 1974). Although delay allows muscle atrophy with tendon retraction and fibrosis, initial treatment by analgesics, protected use and graded exercises is usually the better option. If shoulder pain or weakness persists, surgical exploration and cuff-plasty should be considered.

Exploration and acute cuff repair

The superior approach or the Neer anterior acromioplasty (Neer 1972) is used. Reflection of the anterior deltoid exposes the outer wall of the subdeltoid bursa (not the cuff, with which it is sometimes confused!), which is divided to reveal the tear. The anterior acromion, with its attached coracoacromial ligament, is divided by an oblique osteotomy that runs 45° backwards and downwards, and is removed to decompress the tendons. As the arm is rotated and abducted, a longitudinal or L-shaped tear is usually seen just behind the biceps tendon; the torn edge is freshened and repaired with fine non-absorbable sutures, or is reattached to the cleared inner edge of the greater tuberosity by sutures, passed through drill holes, to emerge laterally. The wound is closed with drainage. The arm is supported in a broad arm sling on a flexion wedge and active-assisted exercises are started cautiously.

Biceps tendon rupture

This is usually seen in middle-aged male manual workers and, occasionally, in young athletes after injury, perhaps after a fall onto a braced arm or after an unguarded arm strain at work or sport. It may also follow lesser repetitive strains (O'Donoghue 1970).

There may be localized shoulder pain with arm use or a complaint of arm weakness, and examination shows tenderness over the bicipital groove or a lump in the lower arm; resisted elbow flexion with forearm supination produces stress or release pain. Pain often eases in a few weeks, with or without treatment, but acute onset or continuing symptoms in a younger patient may warrant surgical exploration of the upper arm and suture of the long head of the biceps to the coracoid (early) or tenodesis in the bicipital groove (delayed) to restore arm comfort, strength and appearance (O'Donoghue 1970, Mariani et al. 1988).

References

Brown, J.T. Early assessment of supraspinatus tears; procaine infiltration as a guide to treatment. *J Bone Joint Surg* 1949; **31B**: 423–425.

Kessel, L. & Watson, M. The refractory painful arc syndrome. *J Bone Joint Surg* 1977; **59B**: 166–172.

Mariani, E.M., Cofield, R.H., Askew, L.J., Li, G. & Chao, E.Y.S. Rupture of the tendon of the long head of biceps brachii. *Clin Orthop* 1988; **228**: 223–239.

Neer, C.S. Anterior acromioplasty for the chronic impingement syndrome. *J Bone Joint Surg* 1972; **54A**: 41–50.

O'Donoghue, D.H. *Treatment of Injuries to Athletes*. WB Saunders: Philadelphia, 1970.

Wolfgang, G.L. Surgical repair of tears of the rotator cuff of the shoulder. *J Bone Joint Surg* 1974; **56A**: 14–26.

Scapula

P.G.STABLEFORTH

Scapular fractures may follow falls onto the shoulder, often with shoulder dislocation, or may be caused by high-violence injuries of the upper thorax or shoulder region. They are much more common in males, with a peak incidence in the fourth and fifth decades (Rowe 1963, Aston & Gregory 1973, Wilber & Evans 1977). Low-violence injuries may split the glenoid vertically and lead to continuing gleno-humeral instability. The fractures that follow long falls or major traffic accidents may result in severe shoulder stiffness from local soft tissue damage or major glenoid fracture; there may be associated rib fractures and intrathoracic or brachial plexus damage. The outcome of the scapular injury is more related to gleno-humeral instability or incongruity and to soft tissue injury than to the extent or complexity of the scapular fracture (Fig. 12.91).

Major scapular fractures

These fractures usually follow high-speed injury. As-sociated multiple fractures and life-threatening ab-dominal or chest injuries are common and take priority in treatment (Armstrong & Van der Spuy 1984). Scapular blade fracture alone is common, but in some 15% of cases the glenoid is split transversely and in a further 10% of cases there is a fracture of the scapular blade and neck.

A scapular blade fracture causes severe pain and a haematoma which outlines the blade. If the scapular neck is fractured the glenoid and proximal humerus may drop inferiorly and flatten the shoulder contour. A transverse fracture of the blade, neck and glenoid will produce marked swelling with total painful inhibition of shoulder movement.

Identification of these fractures may be delayed by concern about life-threatening injury and many do not

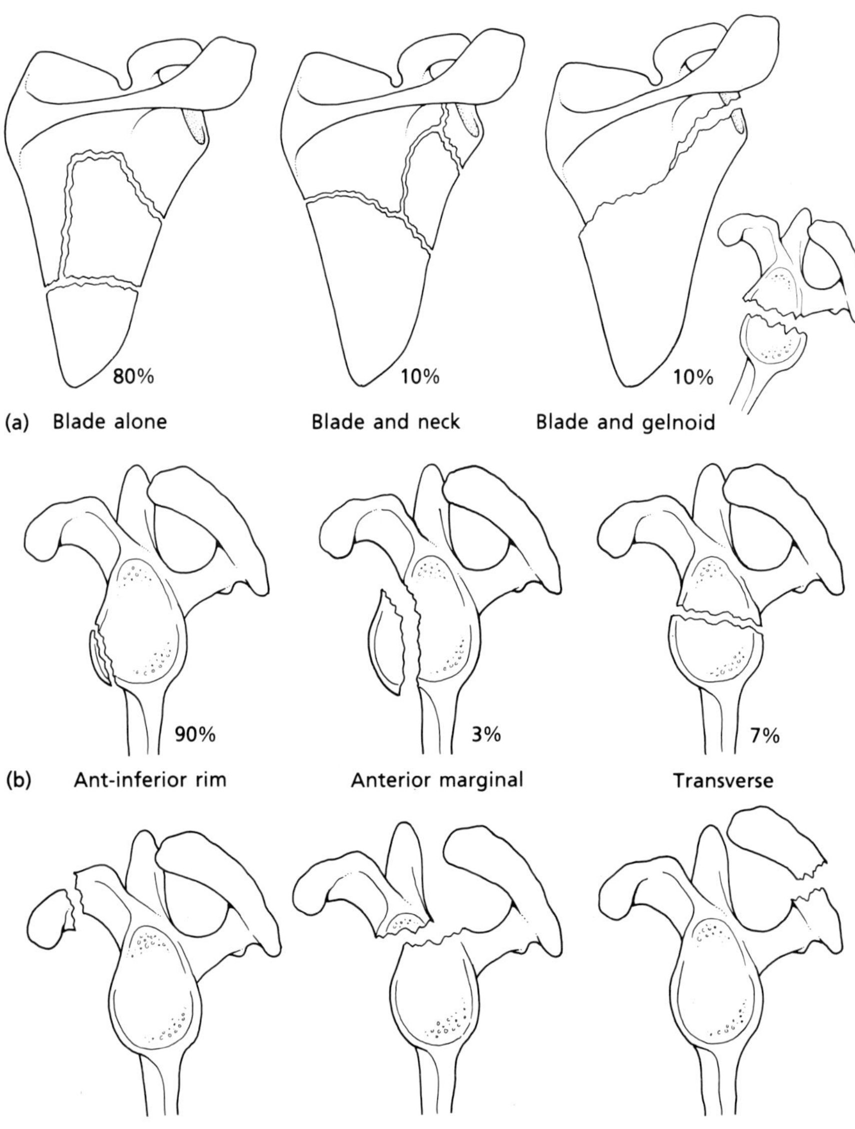

Fig. 12.91 (a) Scapular blade fractures. (b) Glenoid fractures. (c) Scapular process fractures (rare).

require intervention. A scapular neck fracture with gross malrotation, or a glenoid fracture causing a widely split or stepped articular surface, may need open reduction and internal fixation (Rowe 1963, Ideberg 1984). Surgical access is usually best through the posterior approach. The patient lies on the uninjured side and the arm is draped free. The transverse skin incision overlies the lateral half of the scapular spine; the deltoid muscle is detached from the spine of the scapula and posterior acromion to reveal the infraspinatus. The suprascapular nerve, deep to the infraspinatus, and the axillary nerve, passing from below the infraspinatus to the deltoid, should not be disturbed. The infraspinatus tendon is divided vertically and the muscle reflected upwards and medially to reveal the back of the scapular neck. The capsule is incised to allow inspection of the joint, the fracture is reduced to restore a smooth articular surface and is then fixed with plate or screws.

Vertical glenoid fractures

Of glenoid fractures 75−80% are anteroinferior marginal shear fractures, usually with a labral avulsion or tear following acute traumatic subcoracoid dislocation. A marginal fragment may become trapped and will then need removal or reattachment to allow congruous and stable reduction. A larger anterior marginal fracture may be caused by a fall onto the point of the shoulder and may need reattachment to prevent recurrent instability.

Acromial fractures

These rare injuries follow a hard fall onto the point of the shoulder; there may be a brachial plexus injury. An ugly step may require reduction and temporary K-wire transfixion, or a painful non-union may sometimes need excision.

Coracoid fractures

A transverse upper blade fracture may occasionally run from the suprascapular notch to the glenoid and detach the coracoid. Coracoid avulsion may occur in high-grade athletes; whilst it is usually ignored, coracoid reattachment will restore muscle power.

References

Armstrong, C.P. & Van der Spuy, J. The fractured scapula; importance and management based on a series of 62 patients. *Injury* 1984; **15**: 324−329.

Aston, J.W. & Gregory, C.F. Dislocation of the shoulder with significant fracture of the glenoid. *J Bone Joint Surg* 1973; **55A**: 1531−1533.

Ideberg, R. Fractures of the scapula involving the glenoid fossa. In: Bateman, J.E. & Welsh, R.P. (eds) *Surgery of the Shoulder*. CV Mosby: St Louis, 1984.

Rowe, C.R. Fractures of the scapula. *Surg Clin North Am* 1963; **43**: 1565−1571.

Wilber, M.C. & Evans, E.B. Fractures of the scapula. *J Bone Joint Surg* 1977; **59A**: 358−362.

13: The Arm

I.H.THOMAS

Introduction

Fractures of the shaft of the humerus are uncommon. In a 5-year period (1984–1989) 252 cases, representing approximately 1% of all the fractures seen in the fracture clinic, were treated at the Leicester Royal Infirmary. The humerus is subjected to a variety of forces in occupational, sport and road traffic accidents which result in a diverse range of fracture patterns. As a general rule fractures of the humerus heal readily and minor degrees of malunion (angular, rotational and shortening) which could not be accepted in other long bones do not cause loss of function or cosmetic deformity. Furthermore, stiffness in the shoulder or elbow is an infrequent long-term complication.

Anatomical aspects

Knowledge of the anatomy of the arm is necessary in order to be able to understand the response of the humerus to injury and to treat these fractures properly.

The shaft of the humerus extends from just above the insertion of the pectoralis major to the supracondylar ridges just proximal to the olecranon fossa. The upper half of the shaft is circular in cross-section and flattens out distally, rotating slightly so that the lateral epicondyle lies posterior to the medial epicondyle (30° to the coronal plane). The humerus has three borders and three surfaces.

The anterior border extends from the greater tuberosity to the coronoid fossa below, the lateral border extends from the back of the greater tuberosity to the lateral supracondylar ridge and the medial border extends from the lesser tuberosity to the medial supracondylar ridge. The anterolateral surface lies lateral to the insertion of the pectoralis major and includes the insertion of deltoid, the distal third of the musculospiral groove and the origin of brachioradialis. The anteromedial surface covers proximally the insertions of the

latissimus dorsi, teres major and coracobrachialis and the area occupied by the medial part of the origin of brachioradialis and the medial head of the triceps. The posterior surface includes the musculospiral groove and the medial and lateral heads of the triceps. Contrary to popular belief, the radial nerve, profunda artery and its branches do not lie in the musculospiral groove but are separated from bone by a layer of muscle at least 1 cm thick. In the upper part of the groove lies the medial head of the triceps and lower down lies the lateral part of the origin of brachialis.

Medial and lateral intermuscular septa divide the arm into anterior and posterior compartments. The anterior (flexor) compartment contains the coracobrachialis, biceps brachii and brachialis. The brachial artery, the vein, median and ulnar nerves all lie medial to the biceps. The musculocutaneous nerve lies between the two fused heads of the coracobrachialis. The posterior (extensor) compartment contains the three heads of the triceps, the radial nerve and its associated vessels. The distal third of the radial nerve pierces the lateral intermuscular septum, comes to lie in contact with the humerus and, at this point, is relatively fixed (Holstein & Lewis 1963). In a small proportion of individuals a medial supratrochlear spur of variable size is present and from this a fibrous band arises to be inserted into the medial epicondyle (Struthers 1854). This band lies anterior to the medial intermuscular septum, and the brachial artery and/or the median nerve pass anteriorly beneath the band. They are vulnerable to injury when fractures occur at this level in the same way as the femoral artery is at risk in the adductor hiatus.

As in fractures of the shaft of the femur an understanding of the attachments of muscles, which may, by unopposed contraction, displace a fracture, is essential (Fig. 13.1). The proximal fragment of fractures above the insertion of pectoralis major may rotate into abduction and internal rotation due to action of the rotator cuff. Below the insertion of pectoralis major and above the

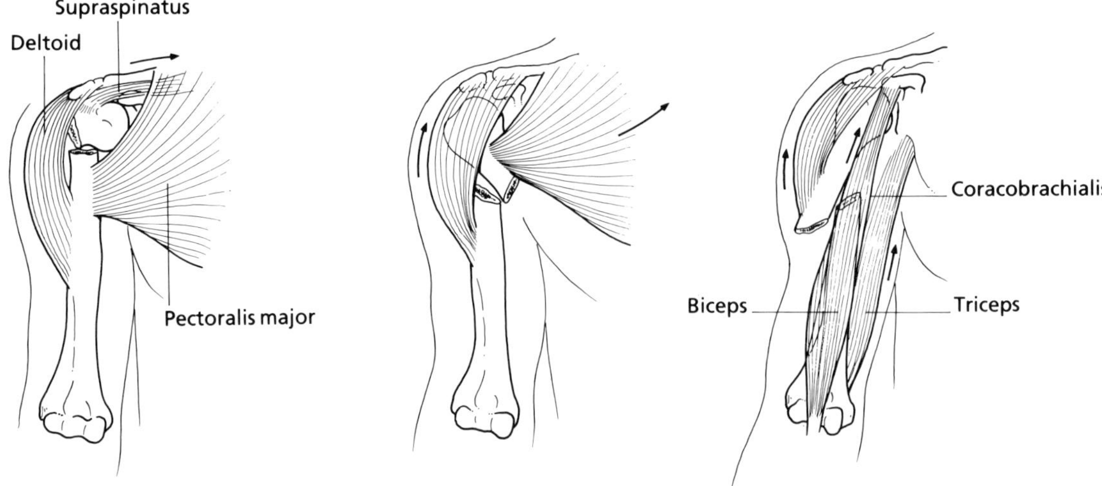

Fig. 13.1 Fracture displacement with respect to site: the effect of unopposed muscle action.

insertion of deltoid the proximal fragment is adducted by the pectoralis, latissimus dorsi and teres major. The deltoid displaces the distal fragment laterally. Fractures distal to the insertion of deltoid may be displaced by contraction of the deltoid (abduction of the proximal fragment), biceps and coracobrachialis (shortening). Fractures sited further down the shaft may be displaced by gravity or by the position in which the elbow or forearm is held. For example, overenthusiastic support of the upper limb in a broad arm sling may result in flexion, adduction and shortening of the fracture.

Diagnosis

This is made by obtaining the relevant details of the mechanism of the injury and by careful examination of the entire upper limb including the shoulder girdle. Attention must be paid to the neurological and vascular status of the limb. In high energy injuries vascular complications are usually obvious but nerve damage, including damage to the brachial plexus, may be missed, particularly if the patient has a significant head injury. A general examination of the patient should be performed and all the positive and negative clinical findings recorded. The radiographic examination must include, in addition to anteroposterior and lateral views of the whole bone, views of the shoulder and elbow.

With respect to the classification of humeral shaft fractures, Müller *et al.* (1990) stated 'a classification is useful only if it considers the severity of the bone lesion and serves as a basis for treatment and for the evaluation of the results'. The AO classification achieves this aim but for practical purposes the author has found the descriptive classification shown in Table 13.1 to be useful.

Table 13.1 Classification of fractures of the shaft of the humerus

Open/closed	
Site	Proximal to pectoralis major insertion
	Distal to pectoralis major insertion
	Distal to deltoid insertion
Complete/incomplete	
Configuration	Transverse
	Oblique
	Spiral
	Longitudinal
	Comminuted
	Segmental
Pathological	Congenital
	Acquired:
	Tumour (benign/malignant)
	Infection
	Atrophy
	Metabolic
Complications	Vascular
	Nerve
	Soft tissue loss
Other injuries	Regional:
	Shoulder
	Elbow
	Forearm
	Wrist and hand
	General

Management

Factors which influence the prognosis of humeral shaft fractures, and hence determine how an individual fracture should be treated, include the site, type, degree of displacement, whether the fracture is open or closed, the presence or absence of complications (local and general), age and likely compliance with the given method of treatment. Charnley (1950) considered that these fractures are perhaps the easiest of all major long bone fractures to treat by conservative methods and it is now generally accepted that the majority of closed humeral shaft fractures should be treated by closed methods (Ruedi *et al.* 1974, Sarmiento *et al.* 1977). Several different cast techniques have been used with considerable success over the last 50 years and these offer a range of options for any individual case.

Closed methods

It is rarely necessary to reduce a fracture of the humeral shaft formally by manipulation. Treatment by closed methods does, however, require close supervision of the fracture. In particular, weekly radiographs should be taken for the first 3–4 weeks or more frequently as indicated. A very common finding is the development of varus and anterior angulation. Fortunately accurate alignment is not essential for a satisfactory result (Klenerman 1966, Hunter 1982). It has been shown that not only will the musculature of the arm hide anterior angulation of 20–30° of varus and 2–3 cm of shortening but also, once the fracture has healed, function will not be significantly compromised.

The hanging cast

During the first half of this century fractures of the humeral shaft were associated with the highest rates of non-union for any long bone fracture. Following Caldwell's introduction of the hanging cast technique in 1933 the non-union rate had dropped to less than 2% by 1940 (Caldwell 1940). The method was not as widely used in the United Kingdom largely because of the influence of Charnley who considered that the mechanical principles of the method were open to serious criticism. Apart from the risk of distraction, longitudinal alignment using gravity is only effective when the patient is erect (Fig. 13.2). The cast is suspended from the wrist and the way this is done will determine what happens at the fracture. It will be flexed if the suspension is shortened and extended if the suspension is lengthened. If the forearm is internally rotated the fracture will fall into valgus and into varus if externally rotated. Moving the suspension point closer to the elbow will reduce the weight of traction and all these manoevres can be used to correct angular and longitudinal displacement. The shoulder should be mobilized within the first week, or as soon as the initial pain and discomfort has eased, by pendulum exercises.

'Sugar-tong' cast or U-slab

Charnley's main criticism of the hanging cast was that it readily produced overdistraction of the fracture. This is reduced by using a 'sugar-tong' cast which consists of a slab of plaster applied, over adequate layers of padding, from the axilla, distally to the elbow and laterally up

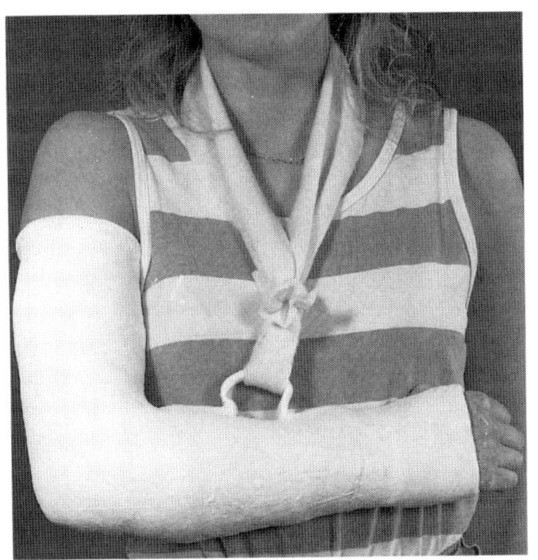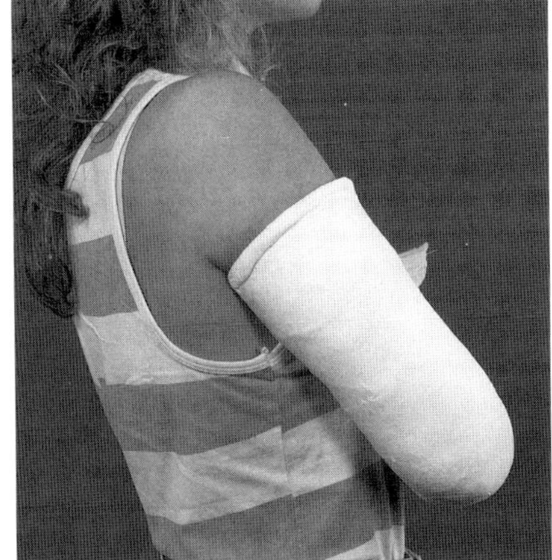

Fig. 13.2 The hanging cast. (a) Front view. (b) Side view.

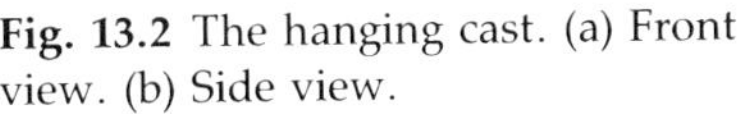
(a)   (b)

over the arm to cover the deltoid, and moulded whilst drying (Fig. 13.3). The wrist is suspended with the elbow at or slightly above 90° of flexion and the whole arm is immobilized in a Velpeau bandage or is simply protected inside clothing. Should the reduction be lost once swelling in the arm has subsided it is a simple matter to reapply the cast with moulding. At 2–3 weeks pendulum exercises of the shoulder and elbow extension and flexion exercises (within the limits of the cast) should be started.

Functional humeral brace

The concept of functional bracing, developed for fractures of the tibia, has been successfully used for treating fractures of the humerus (Sarmiento *et al*. 1977). The technique works on the principle that a sleeve firmly applied to the arm compresses the soft tissues around the humerus and, hence, maintains the reduction of the fracture. The brace is cut using templates from sheets of Orthoplast or polypropylene. To avoid the necessity of regular early adjustments it is advised that the fracture is initially treated in a 'sugar-tong' cast until the swelling and oedema has settled. On about day 10–14 the functional brace may be fitted. This should extend from the acromion and axilla proximally to the epicondyles distally and is shaped around the elbow to allow the joint to move through its full range. At first a non-removable brace is applied and the arm rested in a sling with the elbow in 90° of flexion. Active assisted movement of the shoulder and elbow should be started as soon as comfort allows. On about the fifth week the brace may be converted to a removable one until union has taken place. Good results have also been reported with use from the outset of an adjustable prefabricated brace (Zagorski *et al*. 1988).

Thoraco-brachial spica cast

This has been used in the initial management of comminuted fractures and later changed, once union is noted radiographically to be proceeding satisfactorily, to one of the simpler methods already described. The method has obvious disadvantages in that the cast is difficult to apply well and places significant limitations on the patient. A fracture requiring this method could nowadays be stabilized by an external fixator.

Skeletal traction

Skeletal traction is indicated in the rare circumstance where the patient has to be nursed supine, as in the case of an associated spinal injury, and where there is a contraindication to operative fixation, for example the presence of an extensive wound, soft tissue loss and if, for technical reasons, it is not possible to apply an external fixator. Traction is applied through either a tensioned Kirschner wire or a Steinman pin placed transversely through the olecranon or distal humerus (transcondylar). The traction should be set up in an

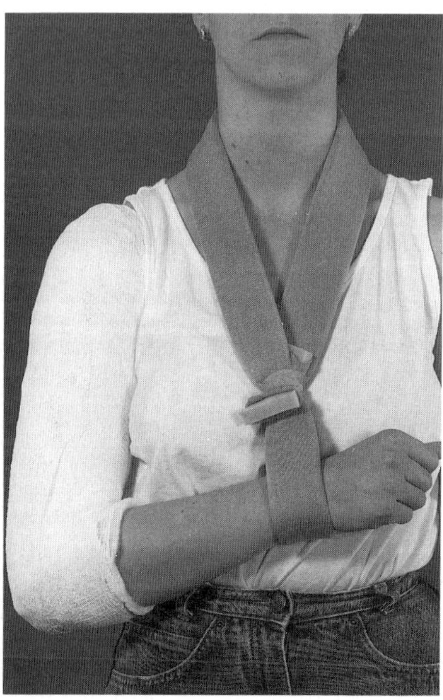
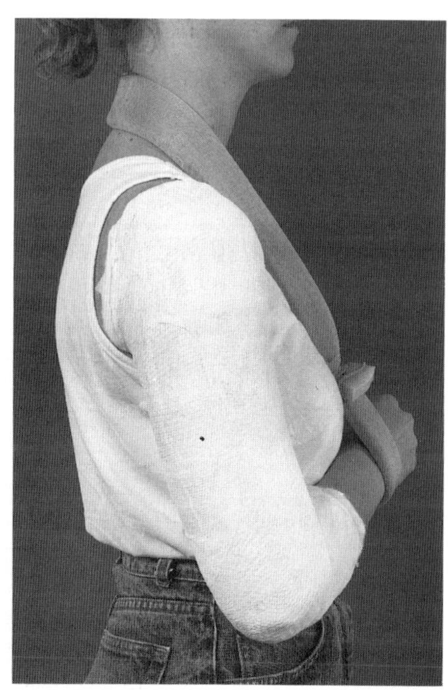

(a)   (b)

Fig. 13.3 'Sugar-tong' cast or U-slab. (a) Front view. (b) Side view.

operating theatre and if the olecranon site is used the wire or pin should be inserted from the medial side at the point where the olecranon joins the ulna. The insertion wound should be large enough to ensure that the ulnar nerve is not injured. A screw may be inserted into the olecranon instead but this is not as mechanically sound as a wire or pin. The elbow is then flexed to 90°, the forearm suspended by light traction and lateral traction applied through the olecranon. Alternatively, the traction may be applied overhead with the shoulder flexed to 90° and the forearm supported horizontally in a sling. In the absence of a neurological complication of the fracture the hand and wrist should be actively mobilized from the outset. If a peripheral nerve lesion is present the wrist and hand should be treated with appropriate splintage and passive movements.

Operative methods

Although the majority of humeral shaft fractures can be successfully treated by closed methods there are circumstances in which operative stabilization of a fracture is necessary (Table 13.2). Bilateral fractures are very disabling if treated by closed methods and fixation of at least the dominant arm improves the patient's ability to look after him- or herself. Sometimes stabilizing a humeral shaft fracture makes it easier to manage a patient with a severe chest injury or multiple injuries. It is often the case that these circumstances lead to a less-than-optimal result for the humeral shaft fracture treated by closed methods. A satisfactory reduction may not be achieved in long spiral fractures because these are often associated with soft tissue interposition, commonly of either of the two heads of biceps or brachialis. If the position is accepted delayed union is inevitable and

Table 13.2 Indications for open reduction and internal fixation

---

Bilateral humeral shaft fractures

Fracture of humerus associated with multiple injuries or severe chest wall injury

Vascular injury

Radial nerve injury

Failure to obtain and maintain a satisfactory reduction
   Soft tissue interposition
   Distracted transverse fracture
   Distal periarticular fracture

Fracture associated with separate fracture of (i) elbow or shoulder or (ii) extending into a joint

Pathological fracture

---

this not infrequently proceeds to atrophic non-union. Similarly, overdistracted transverse fractures which are not reduced by decreasing the weight of the cast should be considered for surgery. Distal periarticular fractures, particularly a short oblique fracture just proximal to the olecranon fossa, can be difficult to reduce and maintain by closed treatment. Open fractures should be managed by thorough debridement and delayed wound closure. Once the decision has been made to treat a given fracture by operative means the most appropriate method must be selected.

Plate osteosynthesis

AO techniques (Müller *et al.* 1991) have now been universally adopted. It is, however, important to bear certain points in mind when using AO methodology on the humerus. Interfragment screw fixation should always be protected from bending, shear and torque

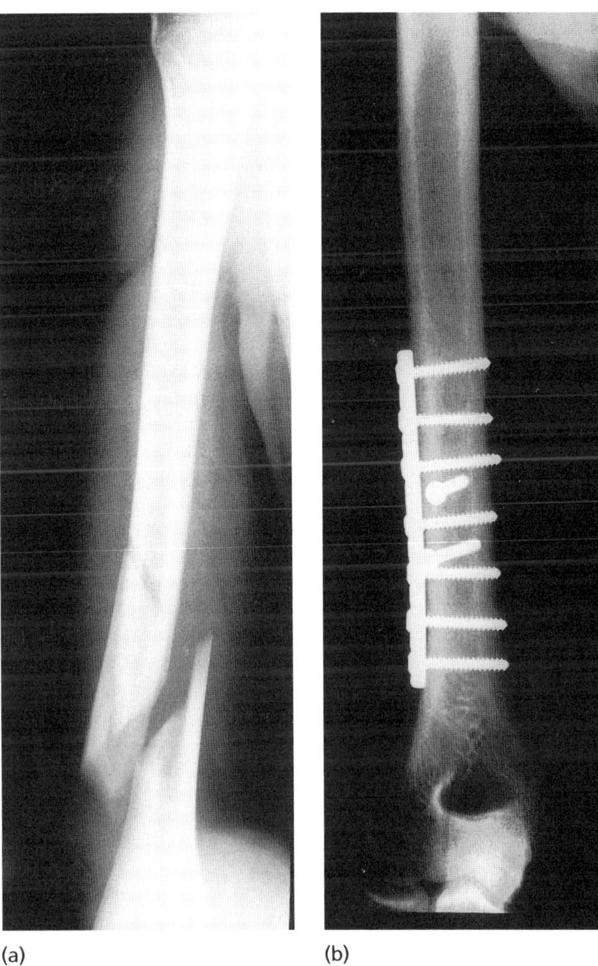

(a)   (b)

Fig. 13.4 Interfragmentary screw and plate fixation of humeral shaft fracture. (a) Preoperative radiograph. (b) Postoperative radiograph.

forces by a neutralization plate (Fig. 13.4). Another reason for doing this is the risk of producing longitudinal fissure fractures. Short oblique and transverse fractures should be treated by axial compression. Although from a mechanical point of view the plate should be placed posteriorly in patients with a mobile elbow, there are practical reasons for not doing so in the upper two-thirds. The bone can be easily exposed by Henry's anterolateral approach and this avoids the medial neurovascular bundle and the radial nerve posteriorly (Henry 1973). The plate can be applied to the anterolateral surface and the biomechanical rule 'bent' because the humerus is not a weight-bearing bone. In the distal third a posterior triceps splitting approach is advised because the posterior surface of the humerus is flat, the neurovascular bundle, which is moving anteriorly into the antecubital fossa, is avoided and the plate can be placed more distally without compromising elbow movement. The position of the radial nerve in the middle and distal thirds should always be considered when making this approach. There are also occasions with distal shaft fractures when medial and lateral plates, one-third semi-tubular, 3.5 mm dynamic compression plate (DCP) or reconstruction plates, are required and these can be applied through the posterior approach. If when plating a humeral shaft fracture there is any doubt about the blood supply to any of the fragments it is sensible to place a cancellous bone graft around the fracture site. This is particularly so in the case of high energy injury with periosteal stripping or if this is done while mobilizing and reducing the fracture.

Intramedullary fixation

Although open reduction and plate fixation is the most common form of stabilization by operation, humeral shaft fractures may be stabilized by intramedullary devices. The issues are whether multiple, flexible rods should be used or the device inserted by the anterograde or retrograde method and whether a rigid nail should be locked with screws. There is good evidence that anterograde insertion of Rush rods and Küntscher nails is associated with a high complication rate in the shoulder, mainly of subacromial impingement and interference with the rotator cuff (Foster *et al.* 1985, Brumback *et al.* 1986). Hackethal 'stacked nailing' has been popular in mainland Europe for many years. The multiple flexible rods are introduced retrogradely and tight stacking ensures stability at the fracture site (Durbin *et al.* 1983). This method is suitable for fractures in the middle third of the humerus and although the rods fan out into the humeral head the more proximal

the fracture the less secure the fixation. Humeral Ender's nails have also been successfully used (Fig. 13.5) (Hall & Pankovich 1987). The advent of locking humeral nails has provided an alternative to plate synthesis or external fixation for the management of severely comminuted shaft fractures (Seidel 1989). Proximally inserted locking nails, in addition to resulting in protrusion above the femoral head producing subacromial impingement, damage to the humeral circumflex arteries during insertion of the locking screws, weakness of the shoulder abduction and forward flexion, can be complicated by difficulties in obtaining satisfactory perioperative radiology resulting in the iatrogenic fracture (Habernek & Orthner 1991, Robinson *et al.* 1992). Retrograde insertion has to some extent reduced these complications (Ingman & Walters 1994). It cannot be stated too often

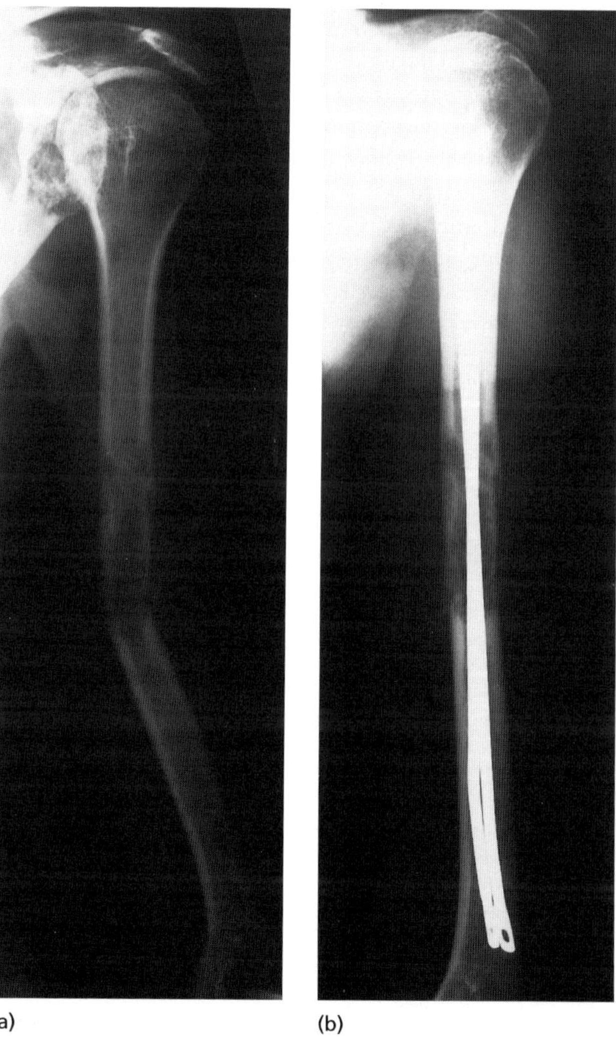

(a)   (b)

Fig. 13.5 Ender's nailing of pathological fracture of humeral shaft. (a) Preoperative radiograph. (b) Postoperative radiograph.

that all methods of operative treatment of humeral fractures are technically demanding and careful attention to detail is essential in order to avoid error. The principal indications for the use of intramedullary fixation are (1) an impending or pathological fracture, (2) a severely comminuted shaft fracture and (3) as part of the management of a multiply injured patient.

External fixation

The specific indications for applying an external fixator include severely comminuted fractures, fractures associated with bone loss, open fractures with large wounds or skin and soft tissue loss and fractures associated with a burn or vascular injury. Although there are significant advantages in using such a device in these circumstances, particularly relating to the access to skin and wounds, the complications specific to the method should be borne in mind. Whilst inserting the screws, nerves or blood vessels may be damaged, muscles and tendons impaled and screw track infections may occur. The benefits are that the devices are easily adjusted and can be used to suspend a limb. Because of anatomical constraints the sites available for inserting the screws are limited and may be divided into three zones (Green 1981). Half pins (screws engaging both cortices) can only be used in the upper and middle thirds. In the distal third transcondylar pins can be used only if the ulnar nerve is identified and protected.

UPPER THIRD

The important structures to be considered are the brachial artery and median and ulnar nerves which lie medial to the shaft. In the upper part, just distal to the surgical neck, the radial nerve also lies medially and then separates from the main vascular bundle passing to the posterior aspect and separated from the bone by the medial head of triceps. The musculocutaneous nerve and cephalic vein lie anteriorly. Half pins should be placed in the lateral aspect of the humerus, which lies in the sagittal plane when the humerus is internally rotated and the forearm lies across the abdomen.

MIDDLE THIRD

The radial nerve winds round the posterior surface and anterolateral border of the shaft. The brachial artery and nerves remain on the medial side but the ulnar nerve begins to separate from the main neurovascular bundle. The musculocutaneous nerve becomes the lateral cutaneous nerve of the forearm and remains anteriorly

placed. Half pins should be inserted through the lateral aspect but only with direct observation of the radial nerve. If this is ignored there is a substantial risk of winding the nerve round the pins as they are inserted.

DISTAL THIRD

The radial nerve lies on the anterolateral border of the junction of the middle and distal thirds and comes to lie anteriorly just proximal to the condylar expansion. The median nerve and brachial artery lie anterior and medial to the shaft and are separated from it by the brachialis. The ulnar nerve passes posteriorly past the medial border of the humerus to lie posteromedially and medially above the elbow joint. Half pins may be placed from the lateral to medial epicondyle or posteriorly in the mid-line. Full pins may, if necessary, be inserted in the transcondylar plane. In general, stability can be achieved with half pins and a monolateral frame or bar. Aseptic technique and good pin track care substantially reduce problems associated with pin track infection. The shoulder and elbow should be mobilized as soon as the condition of the skin and soft tissues permit.

Complications

Vascular injury

This is one of the true orthopaedic emergencies and delay in treatment, if it does not result in loss of the arm, may significantly compromise wrist and hand function in the long term. The average orthopaedic surgeon will encounter very few of these injuries in a working lifetime and so expert vascular surgical assistance is essential. Angiography is not always necessary because in the majority of cases the arterial injury is in close proximity to the fracture. However, this may not be the case if there is an element of distraction in the mechanism of the injury. Spasm of the brachial artery for practical purposes does not occur and all these injuries should be explored. It is, almost without exception, stated in the general texts that the fracture must be stabilized first. It is in fact much more important, and particularly so in the arm, to restore the circulation if there is likely to be any delay in stabilizing the fracture. An adequate arterial repair should stand up to the gentle manipulations required to reduce the fracture under direct vision. Stabilization of the fracture can then take place at a comfortable pace.

Radial nerve injury

Fractures of the shaft of the humerus are more commonly associated with a peripheral nerve injury than are any other fractures. Of neuropathies resulting from fractures 60% occur to the radial nerve and approximately 10–15% of all humeral fractures are complicated by an immediate radial nerve paralysis (Kettlekamp & Alexander 1967, Pollock *et al.* 1981, Omer 1982). Although this complication is usually made obvious by the presence of a wrist drop, it is easy to miss in a patient with life-threatening multiple injuries. It is essential that these patients are reassessed within the first 24–48 hours. Secondary nerve paralysis may occur after over-energetic attempts to reduce the fracture, by trapping the nerve between the fractured bone ends during closed reduction, during the excision of an open fracture, during open reduction or during the insertion of screws for external fixation.

The nerve is vulnerable in a middle third fracture although it is separated from the bone by the long and medial heads of triceps and the lateral origin of brachialis. In the distal third, as the nerve pierces the lateral intermuscular septum, it is in contact with the bone and is relatively fixed (Whitson 1954). At this point the nerve may be injured and trapped between the ends of a short oblique or spiral fracture. It is often stated that the nerve is more prone to damage at these two sites than with fractures elsewhere but there is no evidence to support this (Whitson 1954, Garcia & Maeck 1960, Packer *et al.* 1972, Shah & Bhatti 1983). There is no clear consensus regarding the role of early exploration of the nerve. The only clear indication for this at presentation is when nerve injury accompanies an open fracture.

The prognosis of the lesion depends on the type and age of the patient (Seddon 1947). In the majority of cases the injury is due to stretching or to contusion which results in an axonotmesis or in a neuropraxia. This is invariably the case in secondary paralysis. Sensory sparing may be regarded as evidence against division of the nerve (neurotmesis). However, neurotmesis and axonotmesis are clinically indistinguishable initially because distal degeneration of the axons occurs in both cases. Division of the nerve has been reported in between 5 and 20% of cases. Fortunately, the surgeon can expect spontaneous recovery in about 85% of primary lesions and in all secondary injuries. There is usually evidence of recovery of the neuropraxia by the time the fracture has healed. Regeneration of an axonotmesis and neurotmesis takes place at the rate of 1 mm per day. Since it is reasonable to assume that the site of the nerve injury more or less corresponds to the fracture site and because the motor branch to brachioradialis enters the muscle 2 cm above the lateral condyle it is possible to calculate the interval before recovery may be expected to be detectable. The advantage of pursuing an expectant policy of management is that unnecessary surgery is avoided. There is no convincing evidence that early exploration confers any benefit over observation (Brown 1970, Packer *et al.* 1972, Pollock *et al.* 1981, Bostman *et al.* 1986).

Suggested management plan

Immediate measures should be taken to prevent secondary joint contractures developing in the hand and wrist. Passive stretching is supplemented with static extension splinting of the wrist and dynamic extension splinting of the fingers and thumb (Fig. 13.6). If at 6 weeks there is no clinical evidence of recovery electromyographic (EMG) examination of brachioradialis should be performed. If this indicates recovery the lesion is most probably neuropraxia. However, if there is evidence of denervation a further examination is required 6 weeks later. At that stage there should be indication of recovery in an axonotmesis. If there is no EMG evidence of recovery at 6 months the nerve should be explored. The results of secondary suture at this stage are as satisfactory as those of primary suture.

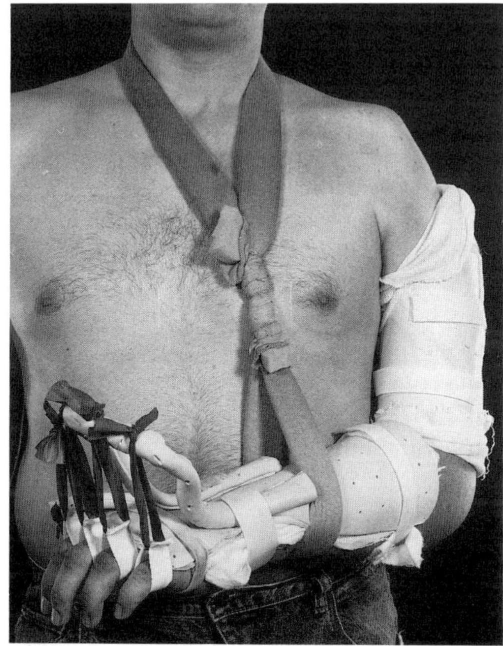

Fig. 13.6 Static extension splintage of the wrist and dynamic extension splintage of the fingers and thumb for radial nerve injury.

If the decision to operate is delayed until 1 year after the injury the risk of failure increases because of permanent degeneration of the motor endplates which occurs at about 18 months. Secondary reconstruction by tendon transfers is indicated if there is no functional recovery 1 year after injury or 6 months after nerve repair.

TENDON TRANSFERS TO RESTORE WRIST, THUMB AND FINGER EXTENSION

The principles governing tendon transfer have been well described and are summarized as follows (Lamb 1981):

1 No muscle under the power of four on the Medical Research Council (MRC) scale should be transferred since one grade is usually lost following transfer.

2 The amplitude of the transferred musculotendinous unit should be capable of the function required. No motor unit should be transplanted into two tendons of different amplitude of excursion.

3 The blood and nerve supply to the transposed unit must not be compromised.

4 The line of pull between the origin of the transferred unit and its new insertion should be as straight as possible.

5 The joints must be normally supple.

In a radial nerve palsy above the elbow joint extension of the wrist, thumb and fingers is lost along with abduction of the thumb. The muscles available to restore lost function are pronator teres and the wrist flexors. The classical Jones transfer (Lamb 1981) consists of detaching pronator teres from its insertion into the radius and reattaching it to the tendons of extensor carpi radialis longus and brevis. Flexor carpi ulnaris is transferred around the ulnar border of the forearm into the extensor compartment and is inserted in an oblique fashion moving distally from ulnar to radial aspects through buttonholes in the finger extensor tendons and finally into extensor pollicis longus. The final part of the Jones transfer involves the transposition of palmaris longus into the long thumb abductor. A variant of this is to transfer palmaris longus into /extensor pollicis longus which thus acts as both extensor and abductor (Riordan 1974). These methods have the advantage of preserving a wrist flexor (flexor carpi radialis). However, palmaris longus is absent in approximately 10% of individuals and in these cases flexor carpi radialis should be used. Since flexor carpi ulnaris has an important role in normal hand and wrist function an alternative to its sacrifice is to transfer flexor digitorum superficialis to the middle and ring fingers through the intraosseous membrane

proximal to pronator quadratus to power the paralysed finger and thumb extensors (Boyes 1960).

Postoperatively the wrist and hand should be immobilized in a cast for 4 weeks with the wrist extended, the thumb extended and abducted and the metacarpophalangeal joints flexed to 40°. At the end of week 4 the cast is changed to dynamic splintage for a further 2 weeks and then intensive physiotherapy is started to re-educate the transferred motor units. As a general rule the functional results of tendon transfer for radial nerve palsy are amongst the most rewarding of all tendon transfers.

Non-union

Radiological union of humeral shaft fractures usually occurs within 12 weeks of injury. It is generally accepted that a state of delayed union is present if there is no clinical evidence of union at 8 weeks; however, adequate closed methods of treatment should be continued for at least 16 weeks. It is prudent to wait until 6 months have passed before declaring that a fracture will never unite (Rosen 1990). Non-unions are probably caused by interference with the blood supply at the time of fracture or subsequently during treatment. They may occur if there is uncontrolled movement at the fracture site, if fragments are separated either by overdistraction or soft tissue interposition and in segmental fractures. Infection is an uncommon cause of non-union and is associated with open fractures or following operative treatment.

The method of closed treatment used does not appear to have much bearing on the risk of non-union (Table 13.3) but the site of fracture may do. The non-union rate has been reported to be highest in proximal third fractures and lowest in distal third fractures (Table 13.4). Intramedullary nailing, either open or closed, is more likely to result in a non-union than is stabilization by a plate (Table 13.5). If a decision is made to treat a fracture primarily by operation it is essential that the fracture is properly reduced and that the stabilization is rigid. Distraction is more likely to occur in intramedullary fixation, particularly if the closed method is used.

Once a state of non-union has been accepted the decision must be made as to whether or not to treat it and by what method. An aggressive surgical approach is required but it must be realized that pain-free non-unions do not automatically require surgery. The factors to be taken into consideration include the age and general state of health of the patient. Osteoporosis is a significant problem in the elderly and in those on steroids or on haemodialysis. These patients tend to heal slowly, the donor sites for autogenous bone grafts do

Table 13.3 Incidence of non-union following different methods of closed treatment

Method	Incidence (%)	Reference
Hanging cast	1.9	Thompson *et al.* (1965)
	6.5	Mann and Neal (1965)
U-slab	0	Klenerman (1966)
	5	Mast *et al.* (1975)
Functional	1	Zagorski *et al.* (1988)

Table 13.4 Effect of fracture site on incidence of non-union following closed treatment

Site	Klenerman (1966)	Mann and Neal (1965)
Proximal third	11.0%	17.2%
Middle third	11.3%	7.7%
Distal third	5.9%	5.8%

Table 13.5 Incidence of non-union following surgical treatment

Method	Incidence (%)	Reference
Intramedullary nailing		
Rush pins and Küntscher nail	11	Fenyo (1971)
Rush pins	8.3	Stern *et al.* (1984)
Hackethal stacked rods	8	Durbin *et al.* (1983)
Ender's nails	1	Hall and Pankovich (1987)
Plate osteosynthesis	2.9	Bell *et al.* (1985)
	2.9	Griend *et al.* (1986)
	0	Foster *et al.* (1985)

not yield good quality bone and, if used, allograft resorption may compromise the result. Surgical treatment will require considerable co-operation from the patient and is contraindicated in dementia, poorly controlled psychosis and alcoholism. In these circumstances, even if function is compromised, it is safer in the long term to splint the arm with a lightweight removable brace.

The objectives of treatment are to correct the deformity if present, but complete restoration of the axis of the humerus is not essential, to secure union and to restore movement of the shoulder and elbow. Pre-existing infection should be treated by a combination of aggressive debridement, irrigation and dependent drainage. Local antibiotic therapy (with the appropriate antibiotics after identification of the organism(s) present) should be applied in the form of impregnated beads and systemic antibiotics should also be given. A fibrous non-union does not always have to be taken down but pseudarthroses should be excised. Once the local environment has been controlled rigid internal fixation is required and autogenous cancellous graft should be applied. Rigid fixation obviates the necessity of external splintage and allows early mobilization once the operative wound has healed.

Pathological fracture

Metastatic deposits not infrequently result in pathological fractures of the humeral shaft. Localized pain often precedes the fracture, which is usually simple and undisplaced (Parish & Murray 1970). The treatment of these fractures must be approached on an individual basis depending on the extent of bone destruction, regional osteoporosis, location of the fracture, general condition of the patient and overall prognosis. The only absolute contraindication to treatment is impending death. It is well-established that surgical stabilization is the most effective method of relieving pain, easing nursing care and maximizing the patient's ability to look after himself or herself (Sim & Pritchard 1982, Flemming & Beals 1986).

The arguments for and against plating versus intramedullary fixation are clearer in pathological fractures. In these circumstances retrograde closed nailing is a less traumatic procedure than open plating, the risk of radial nerve injury is reduced and stabilization is often more satisfactory. The distal humerus is approached posteriorly through a triceps splitting incision. An oval slot is cut through the posterior cortex at a position 1 cm proximal to the olecranon fossa and, under image intensification control, the distal shaft is reamed by hand to 10 mm. Then two to three prebent 3.5 mm Ender's nails are inserted and directed so that the tips diverge into the humeral head. The elbow is splinted at 90° for 10 days, during which time the shoulder may be mobilized, and then active mobilization of both joints is started.

References

Bell, M.J., Beauchamp, C.G., Kellam, J.K. & McMurty, R.Y. The results of plating humeral shaft fractures in patients with multiple injuries. *J Bone Joint Surg* 1985; **67B**: 293–296.

Bostman, O., Bakalim, G., Vainionpaa, S., Wilppula, E., Patiala, H. & Rokkaner, P. Radial palsy in shaft fractures of the humerus. *Acta Orthop Scand* 1986; **57**: 316–319.

Boyes, J.H. Tendon transfers for radial palsy. *Bull Hosp J Dis* 1960; **21**: 97–105.

Brown, P.W. The time factor in surgery of upper-extremity peripheral nerve injury. *Clin Orthop* 1970; **68**: 14−21.

Brumback, R.J., Bosse, M.J., Poka, A. & Burgess A.R. Intramedullary stabilization of humeral shaft fractures. *J Bone Joint Surg* 1986; **68A**: 960−970.

Caldwell, J.A. Treatment of fractures of the humerus by hanging cast. *Surg Gynecol Obstet* 1940; **70**: 421−425.

Charnley, J. Fractures of the shaft of the humerus. In: *The Closed Treatment of Common Fractures* 3rd edn. Churchill Livingstone: Edinburgh, 1950.

Durbin, R.A., Gottesman, J.J. & Saunders, K.C. Hackethal stacked nailing of humeral shaft fractures. *Clin Orthop* 1983; **179**: 168 174.

Fenyo, G. On fractures of the shaft of the humerus. *Acta Chir Scand* 1971; **137**: 221−228.

Flemming, J.E. & Beals, R.K. Pathological fracture of the humerus. *Clin Orthop* 1986; **203**: 258−260.

Foster, R.J., Dixon, G.L., Bach, A.W., Appleyard, R.W. & Green, T.M. Internal fixation of fractures and non-unions of the humeral shaft. *J Bone Joint Surg* 1985; **67A**: 857−864.

Garcia, A. & Maeck, B.H. Radial nerve injuries in fractures of the shaft of the humerus. *Am J Surg* 1960; **99**: 625−627.

Green, S.A. *Complications of External Fixation: Causes, Prevention and Treatment*. Charles C. Thomas: Springfield, 1981.

Griend, R.V., Tomasin, J. & Ward, E.F. Open reduction and internal fixation of humeral shaft fractures. *J Bone Joint Surg* 1986; **68A**: 430−433.

Habernek, H. & Orthner, E. A locking nail for fractures of the humerus. *J Bone Joint Surg* 1991; **69A**: 558−567.

Hall, R.F. & Pankovich, A.M. Ender nailing of acute fractures of the humerus. *J Bone Joint Surg* 1987; **69A**: 558−567.

Henry, A.H. Exposures in the upper limb. In: *Extensive Exposure* 2nd edn. Churchill Livingstone: Edinburgh, 1973.

Holstein, A. & Lewis, G.B. Fractures of the humerus with radial nerve paralysis. *J Bone Joint Surg* 1963; **45A**: 1381−1388.

Hunter, S.G. The closed treatment of fractures of the humeral shaft. *Clin Orthop* 1982; **164**: 192−198.

Ingman, A.M. & Waters, D.A. Locked intramedullary nailing of humeral shaft fractures. *J Bone Joint Surg* 1994; **76B**: 23−29.

Kettlekamp, D.B. & Alexander, H. Clinical review of radial nerve injury. *J Trauma* 1967; **7(3)**: 424−432.

Klenerman, L. Fractures of the shaft of the humerus. *J Bone Joint Surg* 1966; **48B**: 105−111.

Lamb, D.W. Reconstructive procedures in the disabled hand. In: Lamb, D.W. & Kuczynski, K. (eds) *The Practice of Hand Surgery*. Blackwell Scientific Publications: Oxford, 1981.

Mann, R.J. & Neal, E.G. Fractures of the shaft of the humerus in adults. *South Med J* 1965; **58**: 264−268.

Mast, J.W., Spiegel, P.J., Harvey, J.P. & Hamson, C. Fractures of the humeral shaft: a retrospective study of 240 adult fractures. *Clin Orthop* 1975; **112**: 254−262.

Müller, M.E., Allgower, M., Schneider, R. & Willenegger, H. Fractures of the humerus. In: *Manual of Internal Fixation, Techniques Recommended by the AO−ASIF Group* 3rd edn. Springer-Verlag: Berlin, 1991.

Müller, M.E., Nazarian, S., Koch, P. & Schatzker, J. *The AO Classification of Fractures*. Springer-Verlag: Berlin, 1990.

Omer, G.E. Results of untreated peripheral nerve injuries. *Clin Orthop* 1982; **163**: 15−19.

Packer, J.W., Foster, R.R., Garcia, A. & Grantham, S.A. The humeral fracture with radial nerve palsy: is exploration warranted? *Clin Orthop* 1972; **88**: 34−38.

Parish, F.F. & Murray, J.A. Surgical treatment of secondary neoplastic fractures: a retrospective study of 96 patients. *J Bone Joint Surg* 1970; **52A**: 665−686.

Pollock, F.H., Drake, D., Bovill, E.G., Day, L. & Trafton, P.J. Treatment of radial neuropathy associated with fractures of the humerus. *J Bone Joint Surg* 1981; **63A**: 239−243.

Riordan, D.C. Radial nerve paralysis. *Orthop Clin North Am* 1974; **2**: 283−287.

Robinson, C.M., Bell, K.M., Court-Brown, C.M. & McQueen, M.M. Locked nailing of humeral shaft fractures. *J Bone Joint Surg* 1992; **74B**: 558−562.

Rosen, H. The treatment of non-union and pseudoarthrosis of the humeral shaft. *Orthop Clin North Am* 1990; **21(4)**: 725−742.

Ruedi, T., Moshfegh, A., Pfeiffer, K.M. & Allgower, M. Fresh fractures of the shaft of the humerus: conservative or operative treatment? *Reconstr Surg Traumatol* 1974; **14**: 65−74.

Sarmiento, A., Kinman, P.B., Galvin, E.G., Schnitt, R.H. & Phillips, J.G. Functional bracing of fractures of the shaft of the humerus. *J Bone Joint Surg* 1977; **594**: 596−601.

Seddon, H.J. Nerve lesions complicating certain closed bone injuries. *J Am Med Assoc* 1947; **135(11)**: 691−694.

Seidel, H. Humeral locking nail: a preliminary report. *Orthopaedics* 1989; **12**: 219−226.

Shah, J.J. & Bhatti, N.A. Radial nerve paralysis associated with fractures of the humerus. A review of 62 cases. *Clin Orthop* 1983; **172**: 171−176.

Sim, F.H. & Pritchard, D.J. Metastatic disease in the upper extremity. *Clin Orthop* 1982; **169**: 83 94.

Stern, J., Mattingly, D.A., Pomeroy, D.L., Zenni, E.J. & Kreig, J.K. Intramedullary fixation of humeral shaft fractures. *J Bone Joint Surg* 1984; **60A**: 639−646.

Struthers, J. On the supra-condyloid process. In: *Anatomical and Physiological Observations*. Sutherland & Knox: Edinburgh, 1854.

Thompson, R.G., Compere, E.L., Schnute, W.J., Compere, C.L., Kernaham, W.T. & Keagy, R.D. The treatment of humeral shaft fractures by the hanging cast method. *J International Coll Surg* 1965; **43**: 52−60.

Whitson, R.O. Relation of the radial nerve to the shaft of the humerus. *J Bone Joint Surg* 1954; **36A**: 85−88.

Zagorski, J.B., Latta, L.L., Zych, G.A. & Finnieston, A.R. Diaphyseal fractures of the humerus: treatment with prefabricated braces. *J Bone Joint Surg* 1988; **70A**: 607−610.

14: The Elbow

R.HORNBY

Introduction

The elbow joint normally has a wide range of motion and tolerates injury and immobilization badly. Thus, in most injuries in this region, the surgical aim must be to achieve early return of function. Fortunately, with the majority of injuries, which are relatively minor, this can be obtained by non-operative methods. There is, however, a minority of unstable fractures which have a poor outcome despite satisfactory reduction, if the reduction has to be maintained at the expense of prolonged immobilization. Successful stable internal fixation, on the other hand, allows early movement and spectacularly good results. Hidden within this group is a subset of highly comminuted fractures which defy the skill of the most accomplished fracture technician, whose best efforts may do no more than produce an improved overall appearance in the fracture assembly, but lack the pain-relieving rigidity which is essential for satisfactory rehabilitation, and thus result in a final outcome which is worse than if no operation had been attempted. Experience in recognizing which fractures are operable and which are not can seldom be gained quickly because of the relative infrequency of these injuries. Comminuted, intercondylar fractures are possibly the most tantalizing in this regard.

Myositis ossificans is peculiarly troublesome in relation to fractures and dislocations of the elbow and there appears to be some relationship between its onset and delayed surgical intervention. Injudicious operation after a week or so of conservative treatment may be jeopardized by this soft tissue complication and premature physiotherapy for stiff elbows, after simple dislocation, may also be complicated by myositis. For obvious reasons, controlled trials have not been possible and the separate elements of passive motion, secondary trauma and the degree of primary muscle and bone damage contributing to this fortunately rare problem have not yet been quantified.

Anatomy

The elbow joint (Fig. 14.1) is adapted to provide pronation and supination and a wide range of flexion and extension. Loss of pronation can partly be compensated by shoulder abduction, but a range from $30°$ to $130°$ approximately is required for feeding and toilet activity. The radius and ulna glide round the fixed axis which lies at the centre of the circular capitellum and trochlea. These articulations are set anterior to the line of the humeral shaft, thus allowing room for the elbow flexors at the limit of full flexion. When the elbow is in full extension the axis of the elbow joint is tilted away laterally from the line of the humeral shaft by about $6°$, i.e. approximately half the carrying angle. This geometry brings the forearm back into line with the humerus as the elbow is flexed. From an engineering point of view, the elbow behaves as a third-class lever in flexion, with the applied force acting between the fulcrum and the load. In extension, the triceps acts as a first-class lever, but has a similarly low mechanical advantage because of the short lever arm. In fact, the majority of joint forces at the elbow are due to muscle actions rather than to the externally applied load, because the muscles pass so close to the joints and work at such a mechanical disadvantage that they normally function under high tension.

The concentric axes of the trochlea and capitellum can readily be discerned on a lateral radiograph of the elbow. Any distortion of these surfaces such as, for example, in the upward displacement of the capitellum, inevitably restricts the range of movement available by acting, in this case, as a flexion block. The need for perfect reduction of joint surface anatomy after displaced fractures is thus evident, as also is the disappointing loss of motion seen after relatively minor displacements which may persist with conservative treatment. In normal subjects the elbow can experience forces of several times the body weight. Analysis of extension

413

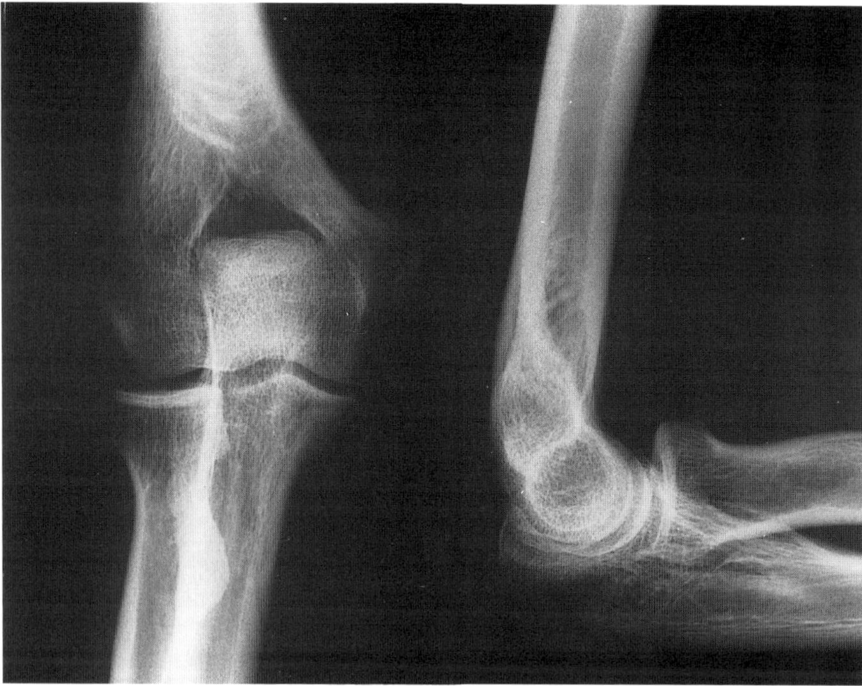

Fig. 14.1 Radiograph of a normal elbow.

forces demonstrate that the triceps can exert 2 kN which acts on the olecranon. Repair of olecranon fractures must be able to withstand this high load if displacement is not to occur (Amis 1990, Basmajian 1978).

Three types of injury loading may occur when a person falls on an outstretched hand. These mechanisms may occur in combination or in isolation. The most commonly encountered mechanism is abduction combined with hyperextension loading. A fall on the outstretched hand generates an axial force and a bending moment resisted by the elbow structures, and results in a force couple of medial soft tissue tension and lateral joint surface compression. The result may be a posterolateral dislocation or subluxation of the elbow, a tear of the medial ligament or a compression fracture of the capitellum or radial head. Less commonly the whole lateral condyle is sheared off by the lateral compression and the medial ligament and radial head remain unscathed.

A fall on to the point of the flexed elbow produces a high load between the crest of the articular surface of the olecranon and the trochlea of the humerus. Depending upon the relative bone quality this may result in a fracture of the olecranon (the usual pattern) or the olecranon itself may withstand the injury and act as a wedge which is driven into the distal humerus producing a T or Y fracture pattern and separating the medial and lateral joint masses. In the case of the olecranon fracture, simultaneous contraction of the triceps muscle may produce wide separation.

When the elbow is forcibly hyperextended, the proximal end of the ulna is forced into the olecranon fossa where it acts as a fulcrum to produce a supracondylar fracture through the weakest part of the humerus. This pattern of fracture is seen most commonly in children, where the capsular and ligamentous structures are relatively stronger than the distal humeral bone, but it is uncommon in adults who are more likely to sustain a dislocation. In fact, pure hyperextension is rare and is usually combined with axial compression forces. Scrutiny of the radiographs of adult dislocations, however, usually demonstrate some medial or lateral displacement implying transverse as well as axial loading. The pattern of injury where the elbow is dislocated posterolaterally and the medial epicondyle is displaced, sometimes into the joint, is, however, rarely encountered in adults. When a patient has sustained an elbow injury the probable mechanism of injury is more often discernible from the radiographs than from the history. Before beginning treatment, the surgeon should consider how the fracture, or dislocation, pattern was probably generated. This intellectual exercise, apart from making fracture surgery more interesting, may suggest an obvious mechanism of reduction and/or stability and may provoke the surgeon to re-examine the patient and/or the radiographs to seek evidence of occult injury which was not evident at the first encounter.

Fractures of the lower end of the humerus

Epicondylar fractures

Although fracture of the medial epicondyle (Fig. 14.2) is occasionally encountered in the adult, the injury is much less common than in children. A displaced fracture may occur in association with posterolateral elbow dislocation and, as in children, the fragment may occasionally be caught in the joint. A direct blow to the medial side of the elbow may result not only in a fracture of the medial epicondyle but also in a coincidental injury to the ulnar nerve. Avulsion fractures are more likely to be displaced, whereas direct-blow fractures are more often comminuted.

Patients usually present with a painful swollen elbow and an appropriate history of injury. Ulnar nerve signs may be elicited, but symptoms are less commonly volunteered. Minimally displaced fractures may be treated by a brief period of rest followed by mobilization. Even when displaced, provided the fragment is not in the elbow joint, early motion may give satisfactory results, even if fibrous union occurs. Ulnar nerve symptoms usually regress spontaneously. Even when the fragment is caught in the elbow, surgery may even be avoided by using galvanic stimulation of the flexor muscles to withdraw the offending fragment! Thus, surgical treatment which gives an equally good result cannot be said to be strictly necessary. If surgery is undertaken, however, it should be carried out after a careful preoperative evaluation of the ulnar nerve function, and the ulnar nerve should be identified and carefully protected. Nothing less than anatomical reduction and rigid internal fixation with a lag screw is acceptable.

Fracture of the lateral epicondyle of the humerus is nearly always part of a dislocation of the elbow in the adult. Most often there is no more than the thin flake of bone avulsed from the cortex of the humerus and symptomatic treatment is all that is necessary.

Fractures of the capitellum

Fracture of the capitellum (Fig. 14.3) most often occurs as a result of a fall on the outstretched arm. In some instances no clear radiographic evidence may be discernible at the time of injury, but there may be local tenderness which is subsequently followed by radiographic evidence of impaction of bone and/or avascular change in the subchondral bone surface of the capitellum. Such cases are, however, extremely rare. Somewhat less uncommon is the vertical, shearing fracture, in a coronal plane, associated with varying amounts of

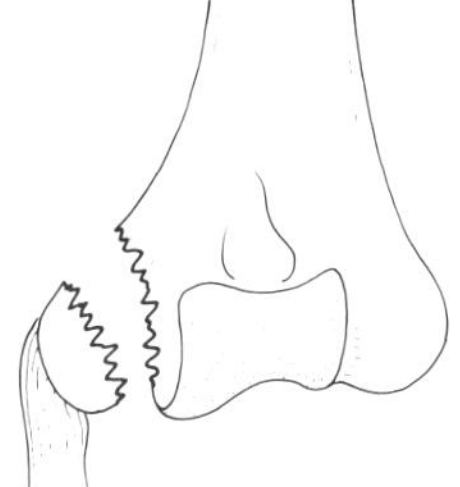

Fig. 14.2 Fracture of the medial epicondyle of the humerus.

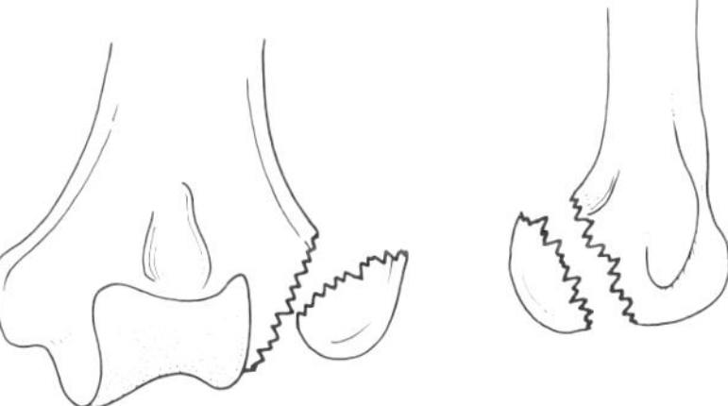

Fig. 14.3 Fracture of the capitellum.

underlying subchondral bone. Most often, the fracture line is a clearly discernible vertical, flat cleavage-plane through the anterior third of the capitellum with a few millimetres of subchondral bone underlying the articular fragment (Hahn 1853, Wilson 1933). When displaced, these fractures can be readily treated by open reduction using a posterolateral approach, securing the fragment with a small lag screw directed from back to front. Rotational stability may be obtained by the addition of a Kirschner (K) wire or a second screw but care must be taken not to produce fragmentation of the capitellum. Occasionally the articular cartilage shears off in a circumferential manner from the anterior aspect of the capitellum, taking with it only a thin sliver of subchondral bone. These fractures are difficult to recognize even on good quality radiographs and late diagnosis is therefore not uncommon. In this instance, excision of the fragments is usually appropriate and, indeed, internal fixation, even in the cases recognized early, may not be feasible. Minimally displaced capitellar fractures can be treated entirely conservatively provided that the surgeon is confident that there is no block to elbow motion. A useful approach is to aspirate the haemarthrosis and instil local anaesthetic into the elbow joint. If, after a suitable delay whilst the anaesthetic takes its effect, full range of motion can be obtained, then the patient should be encouraged to continue active movement in the elbow and should be provided with analgesics. The use of a sling is best avoided. If there is evidence of a mechanical block, however, open reduction and internal fixation is the best policy (Fig. 14.4). It should be stressed that displacement in a capitellar fracture almost always occurs superiorly. The fracture fragment may be completely detached within the joint but more often it has a slender synovial connection at its superior margin. The fragment is inherently unstable and closed treated of displaced fractures is futile (Keon-Cohen 1966, Alvarez *et al.* 1975).

Fractures of the medial and lateral condyles

Isolated fracture of the lateral condyle (Fig. 14.5) in the adult is analogous to the fracture of the lateral mass seen more commonly in children. Although the fracture may extend in part into the trochlea, the sulcus is usually left intact and elbow stability is not seriously threatened.

Fracture of the medial condyle (Fig. 14.6) extending to the depths of the trochlear sulcus destabilizes the elbow. Where the ulna is widely displaced medially or laterally, along with the trochlear fragment, collateral ligament injury occurs on the contralateral side: strictly speaking such injuries are fracture-dislocations (Patrick 1956). Associated ulnar nerve lesions may occur at the time of injury, or may arise in tardy form after malunion of displaced lateral condylar injuries.

In practice, isolated condylar fractures of the humerus are uncommon in adults and open reduction often reveals unsuspected hairline cracks in the adjacent condyle or supracondylar zone. From a practical point of view they are best considered along with T-Y inter-condylar injuries and supracondylar fractures, with which they show common mechanisms of injury and problems of surgical management.

Except for undisplaced fractures, isolated condylar separation is best managed by early open reduction with rigid internal fixation and a prompt mobilization programme. The presence of an intact supracondylar element to which the free fragment may be anchored makes the task much simpler than in more complex injuries where the lower end of the humerus is entirely separate from the shaft. Two simple lag screws, inserted from the appropriate side, are usually sufficient to provide rigid fixation which allows the patient to move the elbow, unencumbered by splintage, within 48 hours of injury. Near-normal function can be expected in most cases.

Supracondylar and transcondylar fractures

The condyles of the humerus are suspended from the shaft by a transverse plate of dense bone which is very thin anteroposteriorly and which may even be fenestrated. Fractures which separate the shaft from the condyles are generally described as supracondylar fractures and because of the tortuous line of capsular attachment are partly intra- but mainly extracapsular. A much rarer variety, which is slightly more distal and entirely within the capsule, has been described as transcondylar (Bryan 1981). Apart from being even more difficult to manipulate than the commoner type, perhaps because

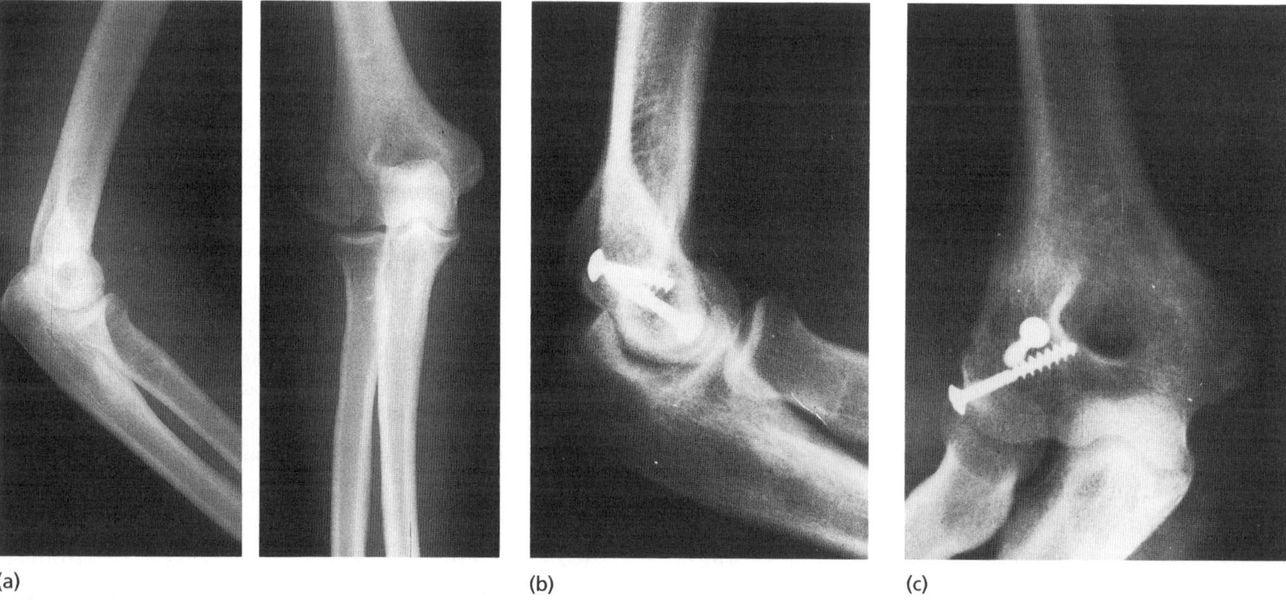

(a)   (b)   (c)

Fig. 14.4 (a), (b) and (c) Radiographs of a displaced fracture of the capitellum treated by open reduction and fixation with two lag screws.

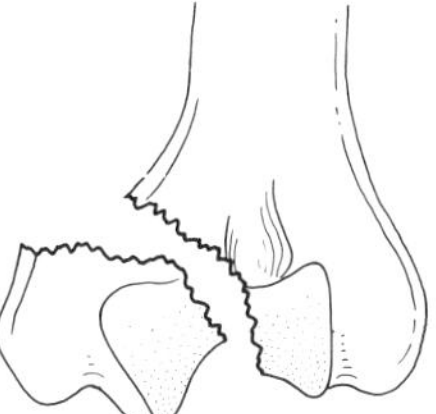

Fig. 14.5 Fracture of the medial condyle of the humerus.

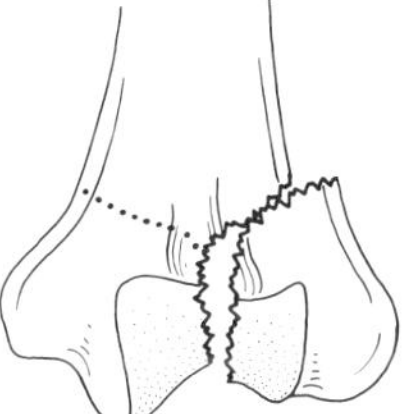

Fig. 14.6 Fracture of the lateral condyle of the humerus. The dotted line shows a commonly associated fracture.

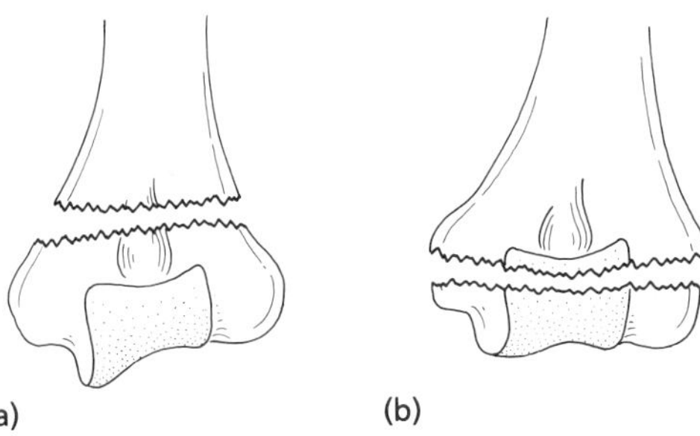

(a)   (b)

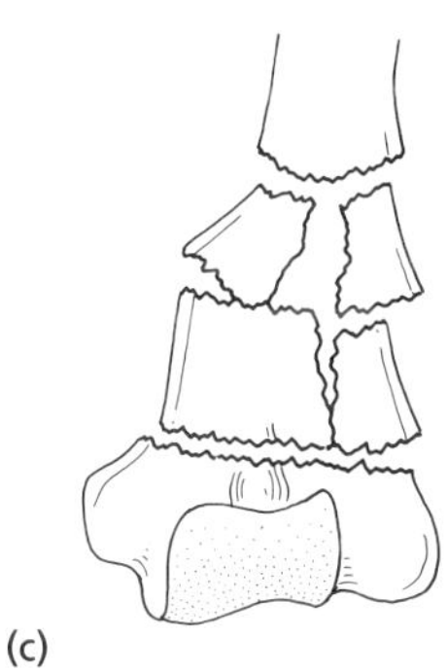

(c)

Fig. 14.7 Supracondylar fractures. (a) Common type of simple supracondylar fracture (extra-articular). (b) Rare, distal type of 'transcondylar' fracture (intra-articular). (c) Comminuted (complex) supracondylar fracture.

of the smaller fragment size, they have no other particular distinguishing features and their separate identity appears to serve little purpose. These injuries will therefore be considered under the heading of supracondylar fractures.

Supracondylar injuries (Fig. 14.7) are usually classified according to the believed mechanism of injury, i.e. flexion or extension, and by the associated extent of comminution.

Extension type

As in the case of comparable injuries seen in children, the history is usually one of a fall on the outstretched hand. Simple hyperextension of the elbow on a fixed humerus or forearm may produce the same result and both mechanisms may be associated with 'in-out' penetration of skin by the bone ends. When the fracture occurs as a result of direct trauma to the elbow, open injury is even more common. The anterior periosteal hinge is ruptured along with a variable amount of soft tissue involving capsule, periosteum and brachialis muscle. The sharp anterior edge of the proximal humeral fragment places the median nerve and brachial artery at risk and the radial nerve may even be trapped on the lateral side. The posterior soft tissue hinge usually remains intact and the distal fragment is displaced proximally by the action of triceps and the proximal fragment is brought into a flexion attitude by combined action of the forearm muscles. The resulting deformity is therefore very similar to that observed with a posterior

dislocation of the elbow, from which it may be distinguished clinically by persistence of the normal relationships between the olecranon and the epicondyles, if the examiner is able to palpate the elbow before the onset of swelling. Soft tissue injury in these cases is often severe (Fig. 14.8) and even if the brachial artery escapes direct trauma, Volkmann's ischaemic contracture is a recognized risk.

Flexion type

A direct blow on the posterior aspect of the flexed elbow is the usual mechanism of injury in this much less common variety of supracondylar fracture. The fracture is almost always displaced and perforation of dorsal skin and underlying triceps is not uncommon. In both types of supracondylar fracture internal fixation of the fracture is usually the method of choice.

After a closed reduction under image intensifier control, pins are passed percutaneously through medial and lateral condyles into the humeral shaft. This method usually provides sufficient stability to allow early movement. Undisplaced extension-type injuries may be managed conservatively by a short period of splintage in a lateral slab for 10 days with a subsequent vigorous

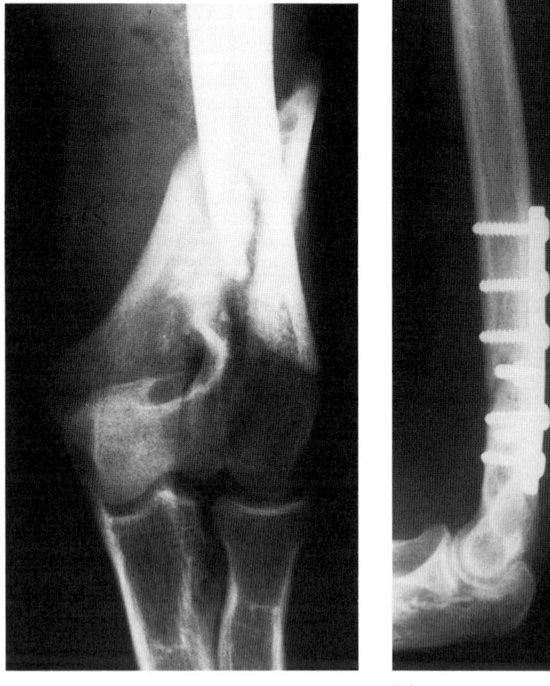

(a)   (b)

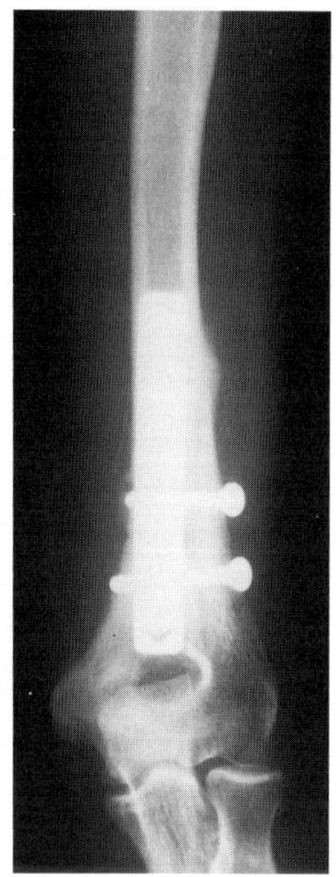

Fig. 14.8 (a) and (b) Radiograph of 'high' supracondylar fracture, 'extension' type, with vertical distal split, managed by lag screws and posterior plate.

physiotherapy programme. If, for some reason, a surgical approach to displaced fractures is not feasible, extension injuries may be treated by closed manipulation using the method described for the same injury in children. Similar precautions for adequacy of circulation and careful monitoring must be followed. The use of radiolucent plaster-substitute gives more useful radiographic information than traditional plaster-of-Paris splintage. Conservative methods are associated with a high incidence of late displacement and joint stiffness. In elderly patients, where pinning might otherwise have been considered, it is often best to compromise and reduce the fracture by a combination of traction and manipulation and to immobilize the elbow afterwards in some degree of flexion, ignoring the X-ray appearance and encouraging active motion.

Comminuted supracondylar injuries reflect an increased level of violence and carry a greater risk. Although the general principles, as outlined above for simple fracture patterns, may be applicable, all too often the surgeon is faced with a choice between treating the elbow as a 'bag of bones', ignoring the X-ray appearance and encouraging early mobilization, or, on the other hand, attempting a daunting open reduction in an attempt to achieve stability and thus facilitate pain-free movement at an earlier stage. A compromise solution which may be applicable in young patients is to use traction via an olecranon screw or pin to maintain humeral alignment at the same time as encouraging

elbow movement. Careful attention should be paid to varus and valgus tilt of the articular fragment (Dunlop 1939, Smith 1972).

Technical details of internal fixation of comminuted supracondylar fractures are considered in the following section on intercondylar injuries.

Intercondylar fractures

The humeral condyles may be separated by the wedge-like action of the olecranon crest when a direct blow is applied to the flexed elbow — the Y pattern. Alternatively, the humeral condyles may be wrenched off the shaft by hyperextension and then be split apart by the articular crest adjacent to the olecranon process which is jammed into the olecranon fossa — the T pattern (Fig. 14.9). Associated comminution is a feature of more violent injuries. As in the 'side-swipe' fracture, which is incurred when the elbow, protruding through the open window of a motor vehicle, strikes a hard object at speed, soft tissue injury may be extensive, but primary nerve injury, paradoxically, is rare in closed injuries.

Undisplaced fractures

Undisplaced intercondylar and supracondylar fractures are seen most often in elderly patients and may be treated by application of a lateral splint for 10 days followed by a mobilization programme. Soft tissue

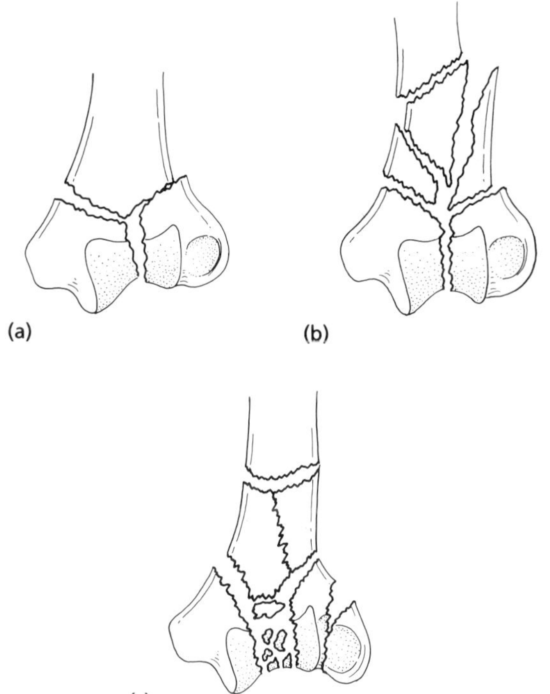

Fig. 14.9 Intercondylar fractures. (a) Simple intercondylar T fracture. (b) Simple intercondylar T fracture with supracondylar comminution. (c) Complex supracondylar T fracture with comminution of articular surface — usually most obvious in the trochlea.

damage is minimal and a good outcome is usual, apart from loss of extremes of flexion and extension.

Simple displaced fractures

Adequate radiographs are essential to the primary management of intercondylar injuries (Fig. 14.10). Unfortunately, films obtained in hospital Accident and Emergency departments often fail to clarify the precise extent and nature of the fracture pattern. In fact, it may not be until further views are obtained under anaesthesia, when traction can be applied to the arm, that a clear understanding of the degree of comminution can be obtained. The young adult with good bone texture and only two large articular fragments constitutes the ideal patient for operative treatment. Ideally, such intervention should be carried out as early as possible. The aim of operation is to restore the integrity of the condylar elements and joint surface and then to secure the reconstructed joint fragment to the humeral shaft with a compression lag screw to fix medial and lateral condyles and either narrow compression plates or two oblique lag screws to secure the medial and lateral supracondylar

pillars. With modern implants postoperative pain is rapidly abolished and early restoration of motion is the norm. Anatomical reduction of these displaced fractures cannot usually be obtained or maintained by non-operative means. Prolonged immobilization of a displaced fracture leads inevitably to pain and stiffness (Bickel & Perry 1963, Brown & Morgan 1971).

Complex displaced fractures

Comminution of intercondylar T-Y fractures increases the difficulty of their surgical management (Fig. 14.11): comminution in the region of the trochlea is more troublesome than in the supracondylar zone. Provided that the articular fragments are neither too small nor too numerous, accurate reconstruction of the joint surface may yet be feasible by the use of AO techniques. Usually trochlear comminution is the core problem. Interfragmentary compression along the axes of the condyles is only practicable if there is no gap in the joint surface and if the medial and lateral end-fragments are large enough to accept screw heads and/or threads. Free bone grafts, fashioned to match the articular gap, may be required to maintain requisite spacing of the capitellum and trochlear anatomy.

In general, bone texture deteriorates with age. Extreme osteoporosis may therefore preclude any thoughts of operative treatment in elderly patients in whom the fracture may have to be managed as a 'bag of bones' with active motion being encouraged as soon as pain allows. In Robert Jones' (1921) original description, the elbow was splinted in maximum tolerable flexion after a token attempt at manipulative 'improvement' of the fracture. Active extension of the elbow was then encouraged as the acute effects of injury settled down. In the writer's experience a more useful functional range of movement is likely to be obtained if the elbow is held at a right angle in the first instance, with progressive lengthening of a collar-and-cuff sling as the patient attempts active flexion and extension. This method avoids too much loss of reach and an active range between 60° and 90° is commonly obtained. The results are particularly gratifying in elderly patients. In younger patients to whom surgery is not appropriate the arm may be suspended in overhead traction via an olecranon screw. The screw is inserted into the posterior aspect of the ulna at the level of the coronoid. The patient is encouraged to mobilize the elbow and once the fracture begins to show signs of clinical union and cannot be readily displaced, traction may be discontinued and the patient fitted with a hinged brace (Desault 1811, Eastwood 1937).

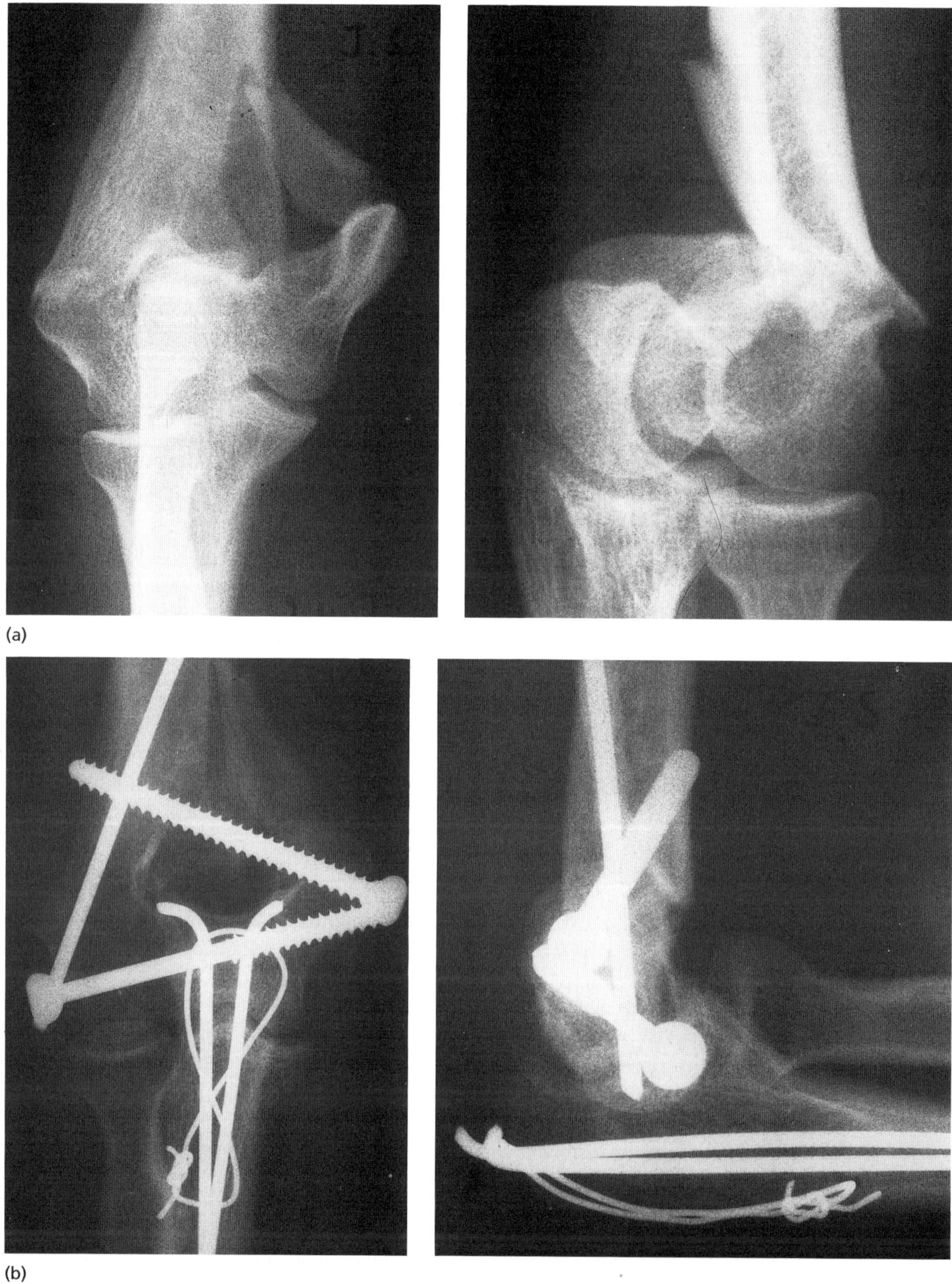

Fig. 14.10 (*Above* and *opposite*.) (a) Radiographs of a closed intercondylar fracture: two main articular fragments plus supracondylar comminution. (b) After open reduction and internal fixation, via olecranon.

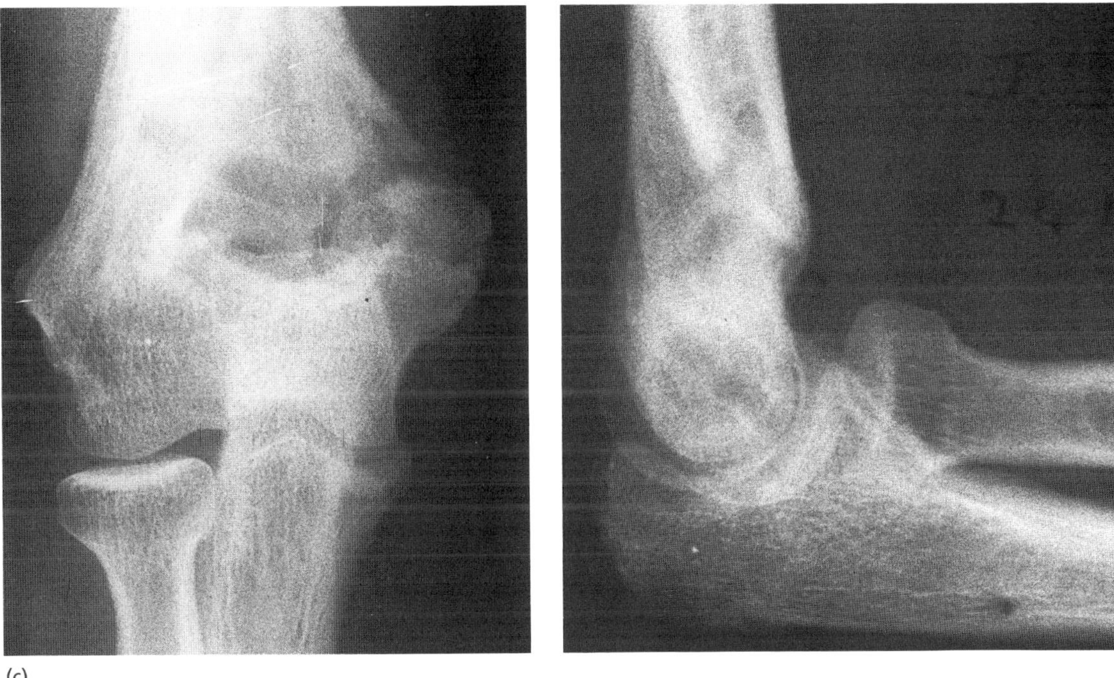

Fig. 14.10 (*Continued.*) (c) After removal of implants — full elbow movement.

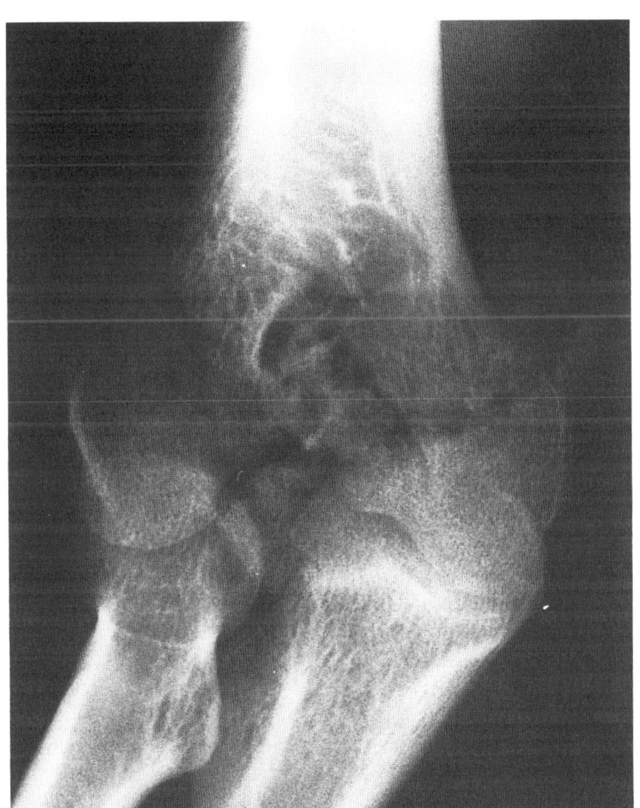

Fig. 14.11 Radiograph of complex intercondylar fracture — note the comminution of the central part of the articular surface.

Unless operation is otherwise contraindicated or deemed futile on account of osteoporosis and/or excessive comminution, early surgical treatment is recommended. Recognition of potentially operable fractures and their separation from the hopelessly complex is, at best, an inexact art which can only be learned from experience. This is best obtained by theoretical and practical instruction in the principles of fracture surgery and by assisting surgeons who have extensive personal knowledge of the full range of modern fixation techniques in this context. Time spent in preoperative rehearsal of all steps of the procedure and in the thoughtful assessment of the radiographs is strongly encouraged. If the films do not allow tracing of all fracture lines they are probably not of sufficient quality to allow the surgeon to decide whether operation is feasible! Computerized tomography (CT) scanning may clarify difficult cases where fracture overlap is present. In general, once a decision has been made to operate, further delay is unwise.

Interventions delayed for more than 1 week are prone to myositis ossificans. Open fractures require urgent management (Fig. 14.12): they may be treated according to identical principles as for closed injuries, provided that adequate soft tissue cover is obtainable after wound treatment. In such cases, early stabilization of the fractures gives better results than attempts at delayed reduction some days after debridement.

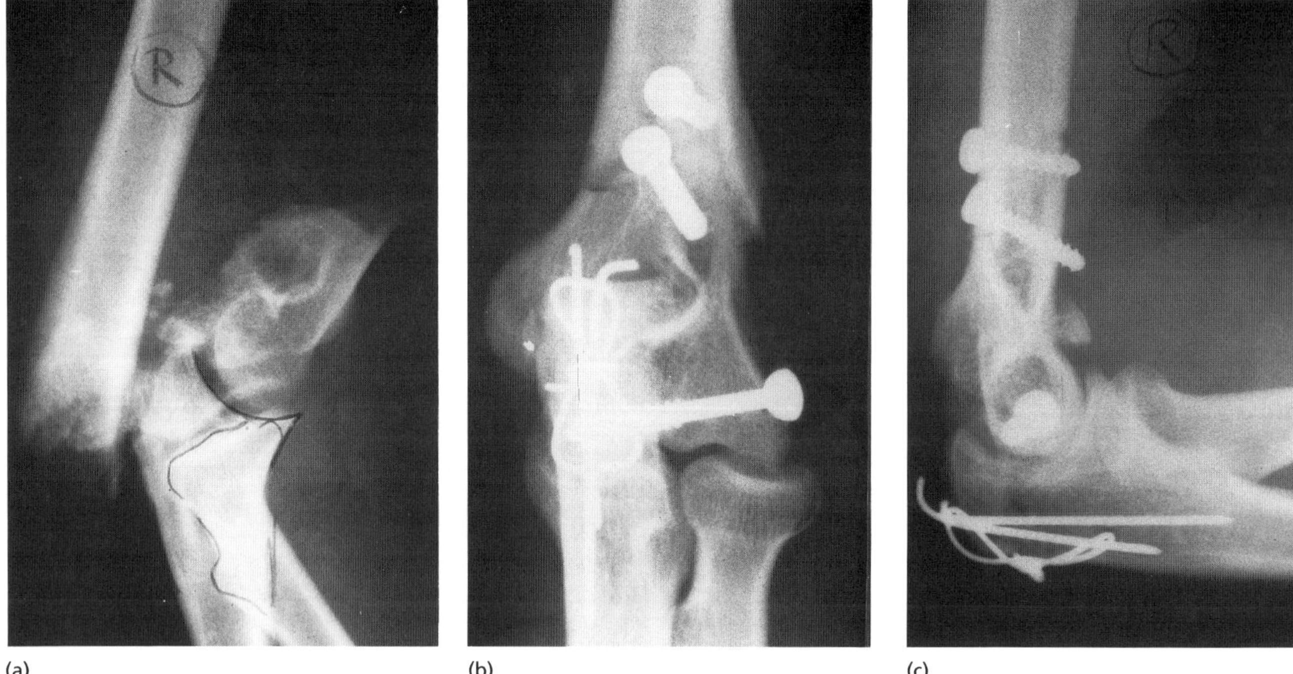

(a)   (b)   (c)

Fig. 14.12 (a) Radiograph of an open, contaminated T fracture with extensive soft tissue injury and skin loss. Note avulsion of the tip of the olecranon and absence of part of the lateral condyle. (b) After minimal internal fixation to restore joint surface. (c) The reduction was protected by a period of traction.

PRACTICAL ASPECTS

The distal humerus is approached through a posterior incision, slightly to the medial side of the mid-line. The patient is best placed either in the lateral position with the elbow flexed over a folded towel and the forearm hanging down, or prone with the shoulder abducted and the upper arm supported on a thin board which must not be pushed too far laterally to prevent full elbow flexion. The presence of associated injuries in the same limb may influence the particular choice of positioning.

Supracondylar fractures may be adequately exposed by a posterior approach in which the triceps is turned down on a distally based triangular flap with muscle-splitting of the deeper layer. With the elbow fully flexed this gives reasonable access to the distal end of the humeral condyles, but for complex fractures involving the articular surface the writer prefers the transolecranon approach. Although this prolongs the operation somewhat and has the theoretical risk of additional distortion in the olecranon, the improved access more than justifies the increased complexity. In either approach, identification and protection of the ulnar nerve is a necessary preliminary to dissection (Van Gorder 1940, Cassebaum 1952). The olecranon is divided transversely at the level

of the joint with an oscillating saw which stops short of the articular surface. The osteotomy is then completed with an osteotome which is used as a lever. The aim is to sever the olecranon without loss of articular surface. Prior axial drilling of the olecranon to accept a cancellous screw facilitates the later repair. The first step is to reconstruct the articular surfaces of the medial and lateral humeral condyles. These are usually held with preliminary K-wire fixation and are then transfixed with a compression lag screw. The next step is to secure the articular elements to the shaft either by small compression plates with screws on the medial and lateral pillars or by axial intramedullary screws. It is particularly important to avoid blocking the olecranon fossa with metalware or bone fragments which limit extension. Medial/lateral 'axial' screw fixation requires somewhat less extensive dissection than plates. When the supracondylar fracture is comminuted, however, plating is clearly more appropriate. Modern reconstruction plates which can be bent in all planes have considerably increased the scope of this type of internal fixation. Schatzker and Tile (1987) have elaborated on technical aspects of this fracture and the logical approach to choosing appropriate treatment.

Increasing familiarity breeds a healthy respect for these fractures and experience will quickly lead the surgeon to recognize limitations in employing the theory. Occasionally, despite the best efforts, an apparently successful internal fixation will not withstand the early mobilization programme for which it was designed. In such sad cases, stability should be augmented by a cast-brace or by traction and the primary aim of early active movement continued (Södergård 1992).

Dislocation of the elbow

Dislocation of the elbow is seen less often in adults than in children. This is usually presumed to be a result of the deepening of the semi-lunar notch of the ulna with maturity. Dislocations of the elbow are usually classified according to the resulting disposition of the combined radius and ulna in relation to the distal humerus. In the great majority (80–90%) the forearm elements are displaced posteriorly on the humerus, with varying degrees of medial or lateral shift. Apparently pure medial or lateral dislocations are occasionally seen but the anterior type is extremely rare. Even rarer are dislocations in which the proximal ends of the ulna and radius are spread apart with disruption of the superior radial ulnar joint and dislocation of the elbow joint. Dislocation of the superior radio-humeral joint (Monteggia injury) and isolated ulnar dislocation are usually associated with forearm fractures and are outside the scope of this chapter (Stimson 1980).

Posterior dislocation

In most cases the elbow is dislocated by hyperextension of the elbow, often in association with axial compression — a fall on the outstretched hand (O'Driscoll 1992). The distal humerus is levered out of the semi-lunar notch and tears off the anterior joint capsule, adjacent periosteum and the overlying brachialis muscle origin. Clinically, the dislocation may be obvious if the injury is fresh, when the posterior shift of the olecranon leaves a hollow at the back of the elbow and the anterior shift of the humeral condyles creates a bulge anteriorly. The distorted relationships of these bony points may be readily recognized in the slightly flexed joint. When anterior soft tissue damage is severe and/or if soft tissue swelling has intervened, palpation from these classical diagnostic features may be less rewarding.

Radiographs of dislocated elbows, even when taken in planes at right angles, often produce oblique views because the limb is held in an unusual position and the radiographer is unable to get any accurate bearing. Two such views are a minimum (Fig. 14.13) and further

projections may be necessary if associated fractures are not to be missed. Such injuries, particularly of the medial epicondyle, are not infrequent and the surgeon should make a conscious effort to look for these so as to minimize the risk of error.

Reduction of posterior dislocation of the elbow

Before reduction is attempted the state of circulation in the limb and the function of the three major nerve trunks should be observed and recorded. Neurovascular injuries are usually mild and are best managed by prompt gentle reduction. Spasm in the muscles around the elbow develops rapidly after posterior dislocation and in muscular individuals is a hindrance to reduction without anaesthesia. The beguilingly simple reductions achieved on the sports-field are usually accomplished before this troublesome spasm has become established; pristine humeral condyles can be guided safely back into position without excessive force. In cases seen more than 1 hour after injury, analgesia is a humane, and anaesthesia a sensible, context to a closed gentle reduction attempt which is almost always successful. Numerous descriptions of reduction techniques are found in the orthopaedic literature, with several suggestions available to assist the single-handed operator without benefit of anaesthetic help. They may be regarded as first-aid manoeuvres for extreme circumstances rather than optimal advice (Parvin 1957, Meyn & Quigley 1974).

Complete muscular relaxation, obtained under regional or general anaesthesia, facilitates reduction. Grasping the forearm in one hand, the surgeon holds the supracondylar humeral region in the other and applies traction to the flexed elbow to disengage the distal humerus from the coronoid. Medial/lateral shift is next corrected before final reduction is attempted. Maintaining the traction on the joint, the thumb of the proximally placed hand is pressed over the displaced olecranon tip which is then pushed anteriorly at the same time as the fingers are pressing the distal humerus in the opposite direction. Depending on the relative size of the patient's elbow and the surgeon's hands, the above technique may need to be modified by engaging an assistant to apply forearm traction while the surgeon uses both hands to apply the force couple to the displaced bony elements. Reduction can usually be felt as it occurs.

The joint should then be moved through as full a range as possible and the stability of reduction assessed. When fracture fragments are displaced into the joint (most often the medial epicondyle), they may cause a

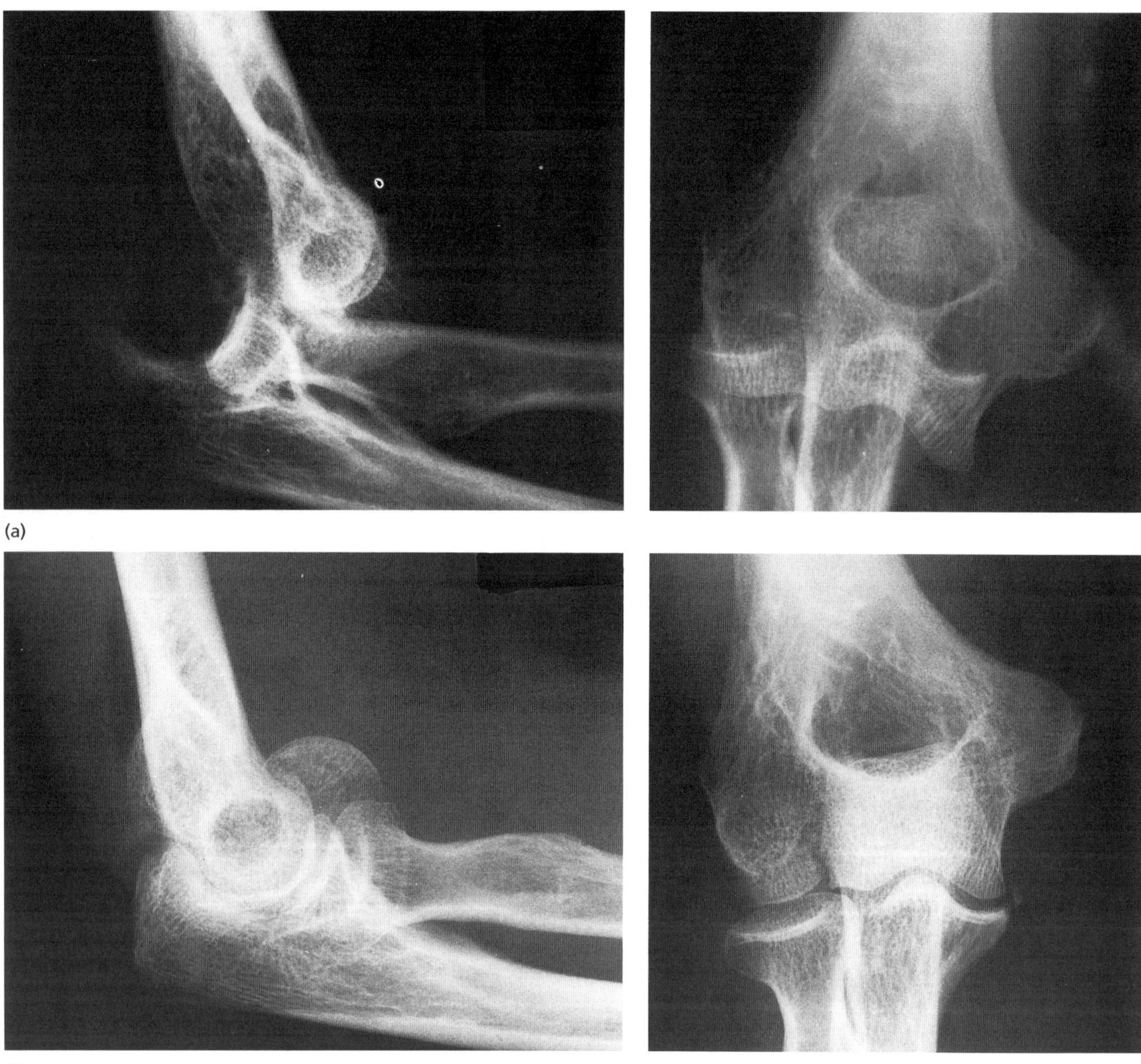

(a)

(b)

Fig. 14.13 (a) Radiographs showing posterior dislocation of the elbow. (b) 'Postreduction' views reveal a displaced fracture of the capitellum.

mechanical obstruction to movement, but this is not a reliable sign and good quality radiographs in antero-posterior and lateral projections are necessary before a satisfactory reduction can be confirmed. On reversal of anaesthesia, the neurovascular examination should be repeated.

Unless the elbow is unstable, active mobilization should begin as soon as pain and swelling allow. A sling provides comfort and warns others that the limb is injured, but prolonged use is harmful. Simple dis-location of the elbow is not, in fact, as benign as had

formerly been believed. In one series of adult dis-locations 60% of patients reported symptoms, one-third of patients reported pain and 15% were limited by more than 30° of flexion contracture. The longer the period of immobilization the greater the flexion contracture and the more severe the residual pain. Early active mobiliz-ation is essential for good outcome (Mehlhoff *et al.* 1988).

In the first few days after reduction a careful check must be kept on the circulatory and neurological state of the limb, and admission to hospital with high elevation of the arm is advisable in cases where severe swelling occurs. Active movement is the essence of aftercare for elbow injuries and is best supervised in a Physiotherapy department.

The difficult problem of late reduction has been reviewed by Mahaisavariya (1993).

Unusual forms of elbow dislocation

Lateral dislocation (Fig. 14.14) is usually associated with a greater degree of soft tissue injury and with greater displacement than medial dislocation. Some degree of contact often remains. The displacement can usually be reduced by longitudinal traction plus medial → lateral pressure on the proximal forearm as appropriate.

Anterior dislocation and 'divergent' elbow dislocation are both extreme rarities. Anterior dislocation is caused by a blow on the back of the flexed elbow driving the olecranon forwards to the humeral condyles. Reduction is said to be simple — by pushing the ulna in the reverse path. The triceps may be completely torn and vascular injury is not infrequent (Oury *et al.* 1972).

'*Divergent*' dislocation is a description applied to two very unusual injuries. In the first type the proximal ends of the radius and ulna are split apart with rupture of the soft tissue between them and then they come to lie on the medial and lateral sides of the distal humerus. Reduction is achieved by axial traction and medial/lateral compression of the separated elements. A second, less uncommon, variant is described in which posterior dislocation of the ulna occurs but, apparently as a result of overpronation, the radial head is displaced anteriorly in relation to the humeral condyles. The effect is that, on the lateral radiograph, the proximal ends of the radius and ulna lie on opposite sides of the humerus (Stimson 1890). Stabilization, if necessary, by operative repair of soft tissue damage would appear to be a sensible step prior to early mobilization.

The trapped medial epicondyle

The possibility that the medial epicondyle has been fractured and caught within the elbow joint should be considered as a possibility, at least, in every elbow dislocation, especially in children. The presence of a mechanical block preventing smooth motion after reduction should alert the surgeon to this possibility. Even when movement is apparently normal, careful inspection of good quality anteroposterior and lateral post-reduction radiographs should always involve a conscious identification of the medial epicondyle. If it is not in its normal location, where is it? In the joint? Although trapped medial epicondylar fragments have been extracted from the elbow by electrical stimulation of the elbow flexors, a direct surgical reduction with some form of internal fixation is more widely practised. Even this may not be necessary, however, if the elbow is stable (Purser 1954).

Recurrent dislocation of the elbow

This condition, comparable to recurrent dislocation of the shoulder, is fortunately less common. In some instances the explanation may be found in a failure to recognize residual subluxation, failure to recognize non-union of a fractured coronoid process or underestimation of anterior soft tissue damage. In other cases no obvious cause may be found. Osborne and Cotterill (1966) have drawn attention to a posterolateral defect in the elbow capsule and ligaments in recurrent dislocation

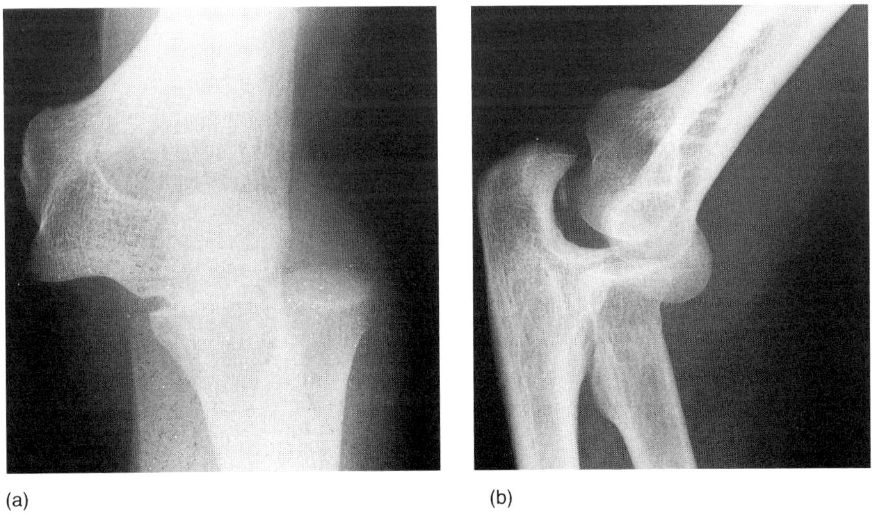

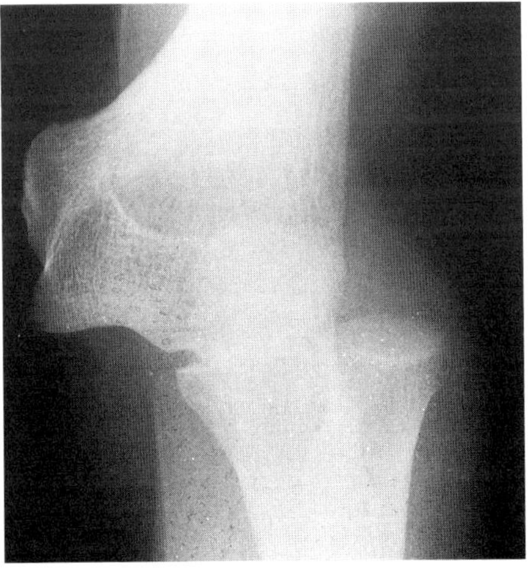

Fig. 14.14 (a) and (b) Radiographs showing lateral dislocation of the elbow.

(a)　　　　(b)

and have suggested that repair of this defect is a critical element in surgical treatment. Others have stressed the importance of medial collateral ligament tension (Osborne & Cotterill 1966, Edmonson 1987, Schwab *et al.* 1980).

Neurovascular injury after dislocation of the elbow

Approximately one in 25 elbow dislocations shows some degree of associated vascular injury (Linscheid & Wheeler 1965). The brachial artery is usually damaged at joint-level. In most cases circulatory deficits improve once reduction has been obtained and direct pressure on the artery removed. In other cases, however, the vessel may have been torn or have suffered damage in the tunica intima and ischaemia may only become obvious with the passage of time. The possibility of Volkmann's ischaemia should always be borne in mind when treating elbow injuries and adequacy of circulation should be given first priority. Expert radiological and vascular surgical help should be sought whenever ischaemia is suspected. The diagnosis, assessment and management of Volkmann's ischaemia is discussed in Chapter 8.

For the most part, nerve injuries which complicate dislocation of the elbow involve the median or ulnar nerves. These lesions are generally detectable at the time of dislocation and may be managed conservatively with careful clinical and electrophysiological monitoring. If spontaneous recovery does not occur at the predicted time, exploration may be indicated. Earlier exploration of nerves may be appropriate, however, in particular circumstances: (i) if a neurological deficit begins, or gets worse after reduction; or (ii) there is painful, 'rubbery' block to movement suggesting nerve entrapment within the joint. If the nerve is found to be compressed within the joint, prompt relocation may be helpful; if the nerve has been excessively stretched, however, less dramatic benefit is likely (Hallet 1981).

Heterotopic calcification

Minor degrees of post-traumatic calcification in and around the elbow joint are not uncommon, being seen in medial and lateral ligaments and in the anterior capsule. A more serious and fortunately now less common problem is myositis ossificans arising within the injured brachialis muscle. Formerly it was seen after injudicious late operation on the elbow, following delayed and unusually difficult closed reductions and in societies where passive motion was used in a misguided attempt to accelerate recovery of function. Nowadays,

the incidence of this complication is very low, but no comparable improvement has been seen with regard to effective treatment.

Possibly the best that the surgeon can do is to recognize that the complication is occurring and limit movement of the joint until the ossification mass is mature. This means, in effect, splinting the elbow in about 45° of flexion until the local pain, heat and tenderness have subsided and the initially amorphous mass in the anterior soft tissues shows mature trabeculation and a smooth surface on lateral radiographs. The writer has seen little or no convincing evidence that any form of treatment improves the ultimate outcome. Even extensive resection of the mature bone mass, several months after injury, seldom results in much functional improvement.

It is likely that most present-day examples are manifestations of severe damage to the soft tissues and periosteum in the area immediately deep to the brachialis muscle and, therefore, they are more often associated with fracture-dislocation than with pure dislocation.

The surgeon's suspicions will be alerted by the paradoxical increase in signs of local pain, heat, redness and swelling several days after elbow injury, when a diminution would normally be expected. Calcification is usually detectable as a 'cloud' on the anterior soft tissues in a lateral radiograph obtained within 3 weeks of injury in most instances (Thompson & Garcia 1967, Mohan 1972).

Fractures of the head and neck of the radius

In contrast to similar injuries in children, adult fractures of the radial head occur more often than fractures of the radial neck. The peak incidence is around 30 years of age and is predominant in females. Usually a history of a fall on to the outstretched hand, with or without valgus strain, is obtained. The presence of medial collateral ligament injury suggests, in some cases at least, that the mechanism of injury probably involved lateral subluxation of the elbow.

Fractures of the radial head

Minor fractures of the radial head may be clinically silent and may pass unnoticed. Comminuted injuries with associated haemarthrosis and painful muscle spasm are easily recognized. Fractures with minimal displacement may be difficult to recognize on X-ray if the radiographic projection misses the plane of the fracture cleft. However, a positive 'fat-pad sign' is usually in evidence.

Radial head fractures (Fig. 14.15) comprise three groups: (1) undisplaced vertical split fractures; (2) displaced vertical split fractures; and (3) comminuted head fractures (Mason 1954, Murphy & Siegel 1977, Smith & Lee 1978).

All group 1 and most group 2 fractures may be managed conservatively. Relief of pain by aspiration of the haemathrosis and instillation of local anaesthetic into the elbow joint is a simple and effective way of identifying the minority of displaced fractures where operative treatment may be required. If, when pain has been eliminated, there is found to be a mechanical block to rotation, the offending group 2 fragment should be excised or, if it is big enough to accept screws, anatomically reduced and held by lag technique (Fig. 14.15). Small AO screws or the neat double-threaded screw designed by Herbert for scaphoid fractures may be countersunk to leave a smooth contour to the radial head.

If no block is present, early active exercises are begun forthwith and even after operation they should be commenced within 48 hours of surgery. Prolonged splintage leading to capsular adhesions is to be deprecated. In the case of comminuted group 3 fractures, the writer's preference is for early aspiration of the joint and insertion of a long-acting anaesthetic which usually allows early mobilization. The fact that the radial head fragments are moving within the confines of the annular ligament probably explains the relatively congruous 'reduction' obtained by this method and the functional range of forearm rotation which is usually obtained. In some instances, however, fragments may be widely spread within the joint and must be excised. If radiographs demonstrate such large fragments, which are clearly destined to obstruct elbow motion, prompt excision is indicated. Thereafter, early mobilization as described above should be encouraged. In heavy manual workers, primary excision of the radial head in the case of comminuted fractures may lead to proximal migration of the radius, with secondary pain arising from the distal radial ulnar joint as well as from elbow problems.

Where coincident medial collateral ligament rupture has occurred, early excision of the radial head may produce disastrous elbow instability. In such cases every effort should be made to preserve the length of the radius until such times as the medial structures have healed. If osteoarthritis occurs as a late consequence of damage to the radial head, the choice of treatment lies between excision of the head and replacement arthroplasty using a metal or silastic prosthesis (Knight 1993).

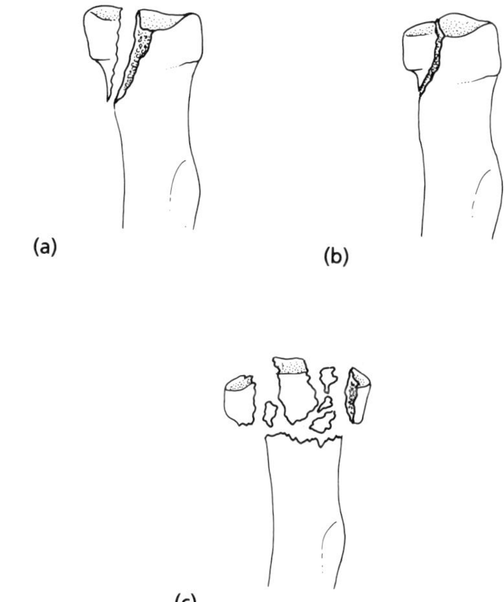

Fig. 14.15 Radial head fractures. (a) 'Split' or 'wedge' fractures: here shown slightly displaced — part of the head is intact. (b) Impacted fracture, often slightly comminuted — part of the head is intact. (c) Comminuted fracture — no part of the head is intact.

Radial head excision may give excellent pain relief and improve motion; when carried out as a late procedure, distal radio-ulnar joint symptoms are less troublesome. The use of radial head prostheses as a primary treatment after excision is not yet fully established, but secondary use of the silastic prosthesis to treat symptoms of proximal radial migration seems to be a logical salvage operation (Taylor & O'Connor 1964, Swanson *et al.* 1981).

When primary excision of the radial head has to be performed for mechanical obstruction, it is important that the excision should be complete. Partial excision gives poor results and a perioperative X-ray to confirm adequacy of clearance is a wise precaution.

Fractures of the radial neck

Undisplaced fractures or fractures tilted 20° or less may be managed by non-operative means. The painful haematoma is aspirated and replaced with local anaesthetic, and active movement begun. A sling may be a comfort in the first 48 hours, but should be discarded as quickly as possible in order to maximize joint range.

Displacement greater than 20°, especially associated with transverse shift of the fragment, may be associated with some limitation of elbow movement and require more active intervention. Occasionally, the degree of angulation may be reduced by manual pressure over the radial head as the anaesthetized forearm is rotated. Anatomical repositioning is unlikely to be obtained by this method, but an acceptably small tilt may be achieved. Severely displaced radial neck fractures, particularly if associated with dislocation of the elbow, require open surgical treatment. Although not inevitable, avascular necrosis is a frequent complication of attempts to reduce and hold displaced radial neck fractures. This has led some surgeons to a policy of surgical excision of the head. Although it is known that the operation should be carried out within 48 hours of injury, that completeness of excision must be confirmed on perioperative X-rays, and that operations carried out after this golden period have a prohibitive risk of myositis ossificans, no properly controlled studies are available to help make the choice between open reduction and primary excision, and between excision and prosthetic replacement.

Complaint of wrist pain after radial head and neck fractures is not uncommon. Although in most cases this is believed to be a referred phenomenon related to dual innervation of the superior and inferior joints, in some, where the radius has been shortened, there is clear evidence of proximal migration of the radius and thus implicit subluxation of the distal joint as described above. There is, however, a small group of patients in whom the distal radio-ulnar joint is injured at the same time as the radial head fracture occurs. Routine examination of the wrist in patients with elbow injuries will lead the surgeon to try and preserve the length of the radius in these rare cases and to consider prosthetic replacement more strongly in those fractures where the radial head has to be excised (Curr & Coe 1946, Essex-Lopresti 1951).

Fracture of the coronoid process of the ulna

The importance of this injury is the need to recognize that it exists and that it may be a cause of instability after elbow dislocation. In most cases, minor avulsions by anterior capsular traction heal spontaneously. In situations where large fragments are pulled off, screw fixation allows earlier mobilization (Fig. 14.16).

Fractures of the olecranon

The olecranon is the point of application of the triceps extensor mechanism and fractures at this site have several features in common with those of the extensor mechanism of the knee, in which the patella is fractured. Whereas some fractures are sustained as a result of

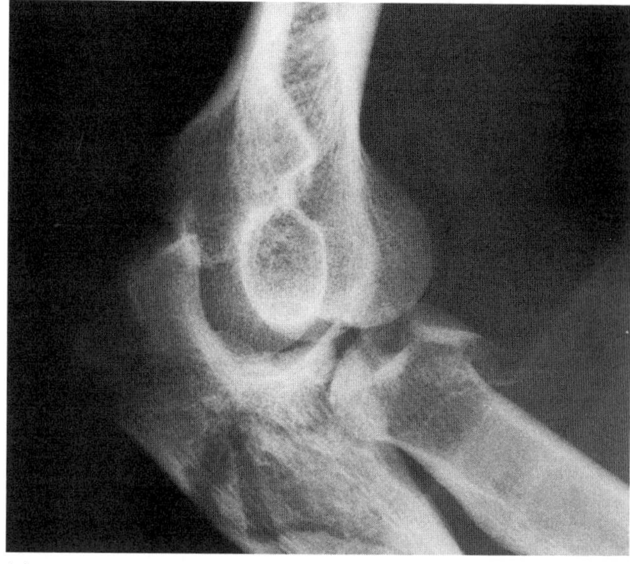

(a)

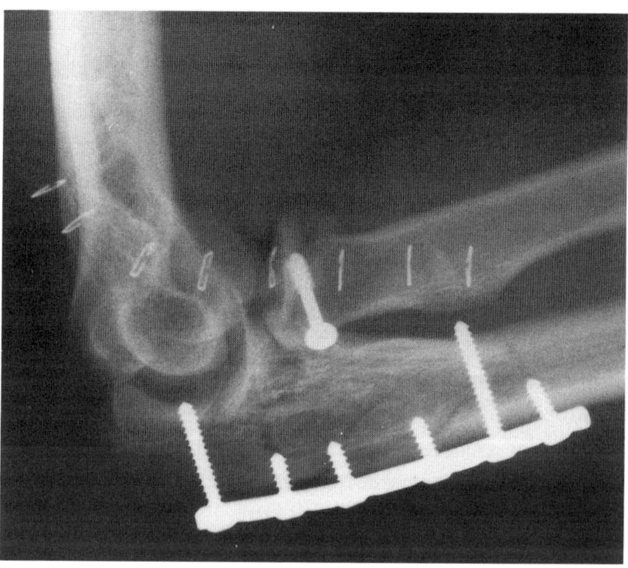

(b)

Fig. 14.16 (a) Radiograph of complex fracture of the olecranon and 'wedge' fracture of the radial head. (b) Postoperative film: the proximal olecranon screw has been placed obliquely and does not penetrate the joint!

direct violence, often with resulting comminution, others appear to represent pure tensile failure and are simple transverse fractures which readily lend themselves to anatomical reduction. Fracture of the olecranon does not necessary imply loss of active extensor power, provided that superficial and/or collateral fibres of the triceps tendon remain intact. Such undisplaced fractures may be treated by early active motion once it has been demonstrated that the patient has active extension against gravity. Most olecranon fractures, however, are displaced and the triceps mechanism is rendered temporarily ineffective. The skin and soft tissue coverage of the olecranon is thin and open fractures are therefore common. The literature on olecranon fractures is replete with 'new' methods of treatment and expressions of dissatisfaction with previous experience. Non-operative management has included attempts at reduction by extension splintage, which is followed by the inevitable loss of ultimate flexion, and the opposite policy of active mobilization of the elbow with no attention being paid to reduction. A compromise approach in which the elbow is rested in a splint or sling in 45° of flexion for 10 days, followed by active motion in the 0—90° range for 4 weeks is one which the writer still prefers in the case of elderly osteoporotic patients in whom operative treatment is inappropriate. The central criticism of non-operative treatment, however, is that prolonged splintage devoted to maintaining reduction leads to elbow stiffness and that long fibrous union, which develops after mobilization, does not provide strong enough elbow power for a manual worker.

The olecranon was the first structure to which open reduction and internal fixation of a fracture was applied, when Joseph Lister used a forerunner of the currently popular tension-band wire loop technique in 1884 (Keon-Cohen 1966), and, as for the patella, the extensive literature is disproportionate to its small size.

Ideally, operative treatment for a displaced fracture would maintain anatomical reduction of the articular surface and would be strong enough to allow early active motion of the elbow without fear of redisplacement. As yet, there is no single method which satisfies these criteria and which can be applied to all types of olecranon fractures and an eclectic approach, matching technique to fracture type is necessary.

Classification

Fractures of the olecranon (Fig. 14.17) can be classified as:

1 Transverse.
2 Oblique.
3 Comminuted with/without coronoid process and radial head fractures.

For best results operative treatment should be carried out within 48 hours of injury. At that stage, haematoma is not yet organized and the fracture surfaces may be cleared to allow hairline quality of reduction. Access is obtained through a vertical, posterior incision, placed slightly to the medial side of the ulnar crest allowing good access to the fracture area and identification and protection of the ulnar nerve. If the patient is positioned

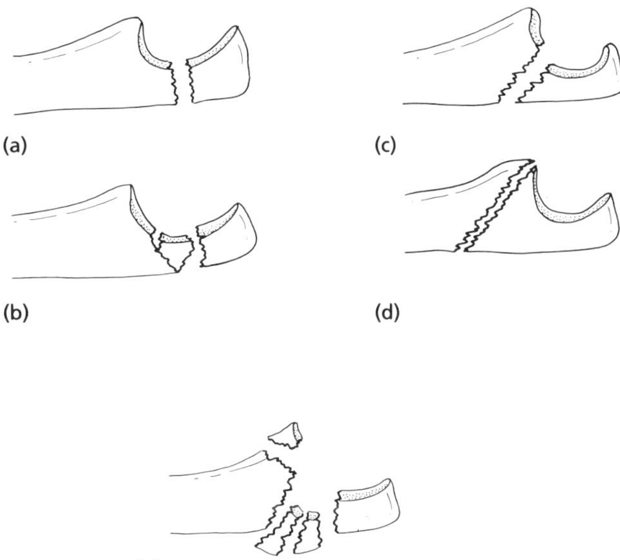

Fig. 14.17 Classification of olecranon fractures. (a) Transverse fracture. (b) Transverse fracture with depressed articular fragment. (c) Oblique 'proximal' fracture. (d) 'Distal' type of oblique fracture — unsuitable for tension-band fixation. (e) Comminuted olecranon fractures may extend into the coronoid process and proximal shaft of the ulna.

on the contralateral side, gravity will assist the surgeon in extending the fracture and thus producing a reduction. When the elbow is flexed, the fracture opens to allow inspection of the articular surface and evacuation of the clot.

Transverse fractures

These fractures cross the articular surface at the deepest point of the trochlear notch. An unusual variant is the almost entirely extra-articular variety in which the tip of the olecranon is avulsed.

The use of long intramedullary screws has now given way to tension-band wiring in most centres. If screws are to be employed, they must be long enough and have a sufficiently wide thread to engage the inner surface of the cortex of the ulnar shaft and they should be reinforced at the fracture site, to withstand fatigue failure from cyclical bending stresses. It should be remembered, however, that screw fixation achieves maximum tightness at the moment of insertion and, thereafter, any change will be in the direction of loosening. In contrast, tension-band methods result in increased axial compression of the fracture during elbow flexion, which further improves the stability of the reduction and fixation. When the tension-band method is used, however, the wires must be strong and stout and the bone texture of the ulna must be strong enough to withstand the high tensile forces. The two parallel K-wires are driven through the reduced fracture into the ulnar shaft for 3–4 cm. Strong flexible wire, at least 1.3 mm in diameter, is passed deep to the triceps and proximal to the K-wires and is then passed superficially over the ulna in a figure-of-eight manner and back through a drill hole in the strong bone of the ulnar crest distal to the fracture. When the wire is tightened a traction-absorbing element is formed on the superficial aspect of the olecranon. The proximal ends of the K-wires are then cut short and bent back on themselves to form a complete 'U' shape which can be impacted through small vertical slits in the triceps tendon and then embedded in the proximal fragment (Fig. 14.18). If this step is omitted there is a definite risk of their being systematically pulled proximally by the triceps tendon each time the elbow is extended.

It is important to recognize the presence of depressed joint fragments in these injuries. Where possible, such fragments should be elevated to restore a smooth joint surface, otherwise the bone loss should be made up with grafts so as not to reduce the volume of the trochlear notch during compression manoeuvres. When minimal joint surface has been lost a gap may be simply left, provided that overall contour is preserved by anatomical reduction of overlying cortical elements.

Fractures which extend into the coronoid process are likely to be associated with anterior dislocation of the ulna. Such distally placed fractures are not always controllable by tension-bands and are more safely managed by the use of screws and plates.

Oblique fractures

These injuries lend themselves ideally to bicortical screw fixation; one or more screws is placed approximately at right angles to the fracture to engage the opposite cortex. A clearance hole should be drilled in the proximal fragment and screw thread-lengths should be such that threads do not cross the fracture line. If only one screw can be inserted it is wise to protect the fixation with a figure-of-eight tension-band loop in order to absorb tensile stress and allow safe early active movement.

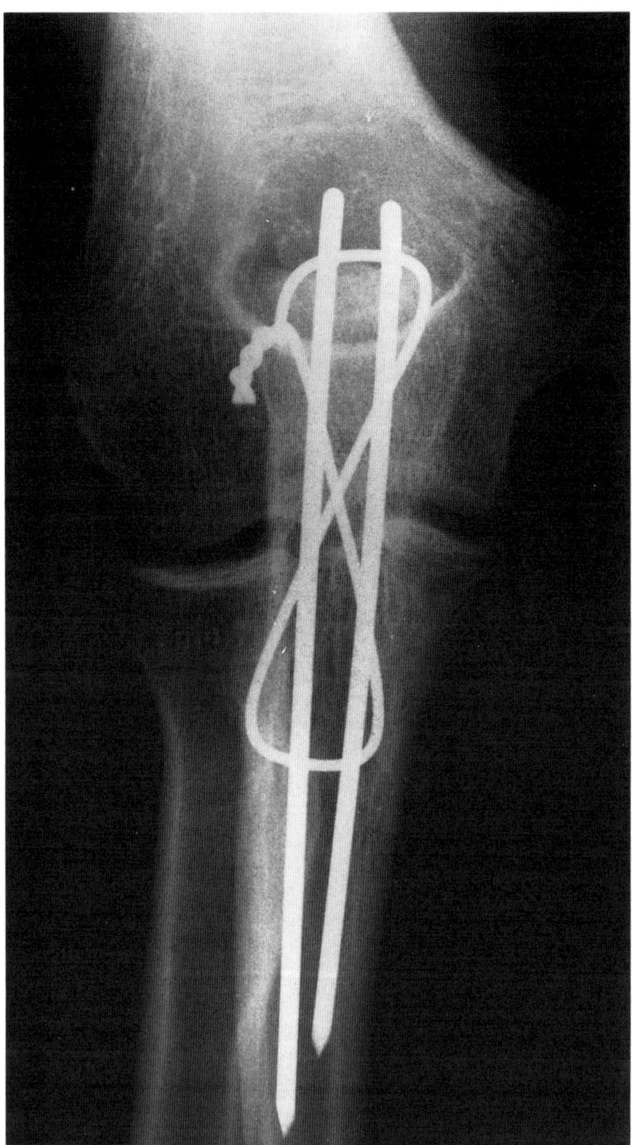

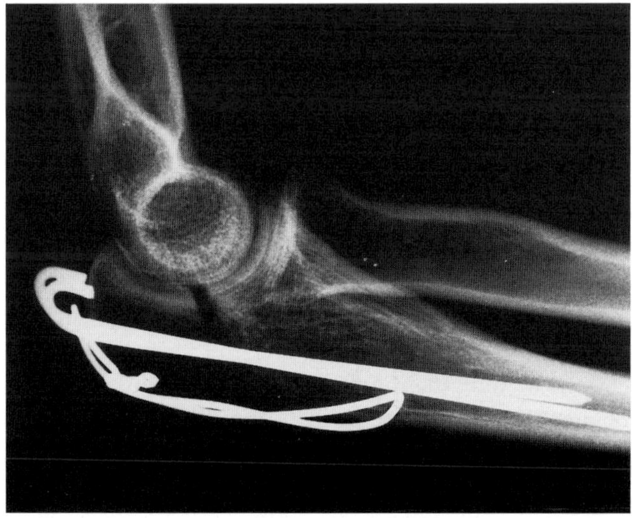

Fig. 14.18 (*Right.*) Postoperative radiographs of transverse fracture of the olecranon treated by tension-band method: tightening of the flexible wire has temporarily opened the articular surface which comes under intermittent compression as the elbow is actively flexed — compatible with excellent outcome.

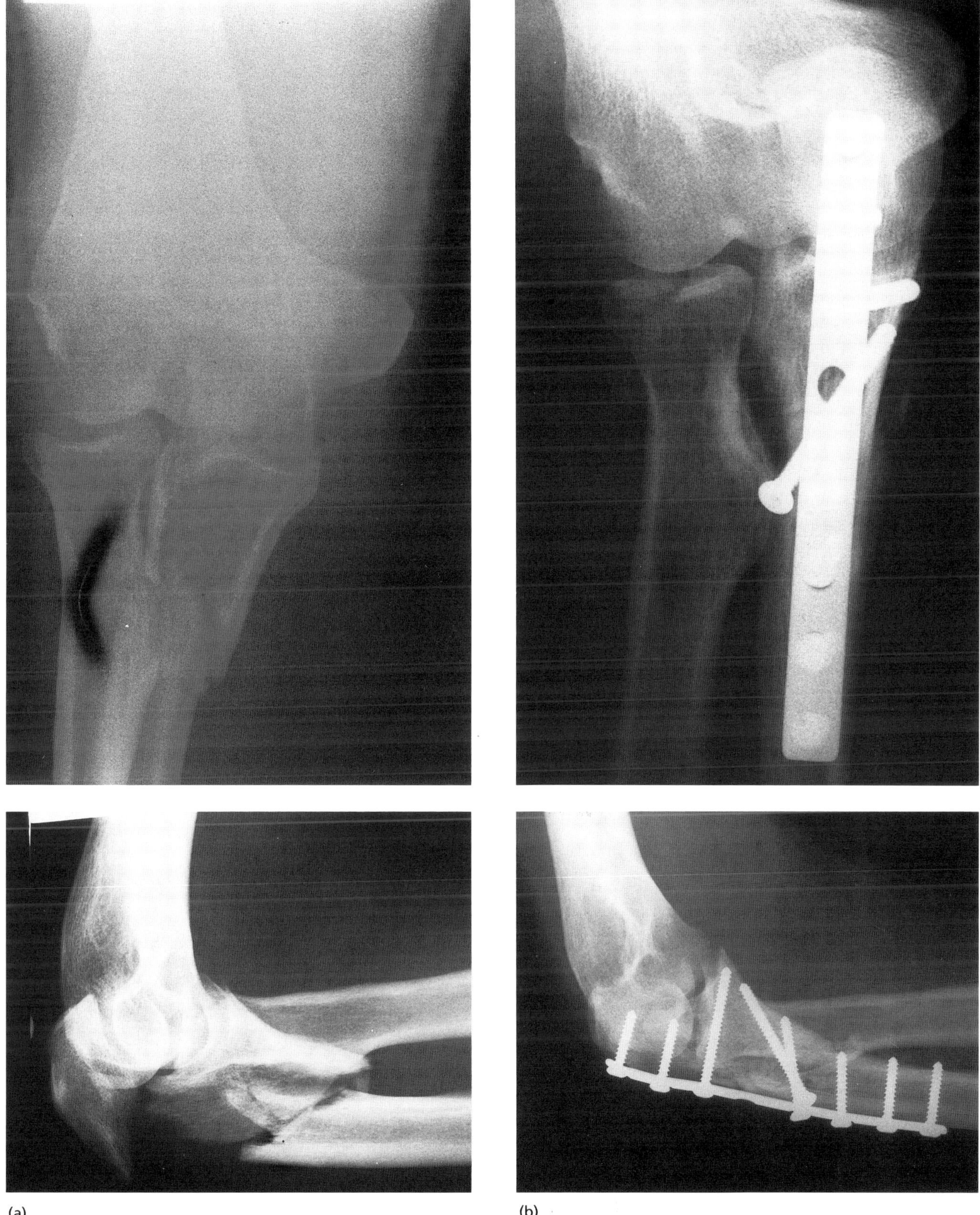

(a)

(b)

Fig. 14.19 (a) Radiographs showing complex fracture of the olecranon. (b) Postoperative films demonstrate use of interfragmentary compression and neutralization plate — plus an impacted fracture of the radial head.

Comminuted fractures

These injuries represent a higher level of fracture violence and the degree of comminution may be extreme. Internal fixation of these injuries requires a delicate technique if accurate reduction is to be obtained and soft tissue attachments to the small fragments preserved. The delegation of such operations to relatively inexperienced surgeons, who traditionally may have found these subcutaneous injuries to be an attractive challenge, is to be deprecated, as follow-up studies have shown (Helm *et al.* 1987).

In highly comminuted injuries involving the proximal half of the olecranon, and if elbow stability is not in question, the fragments may be excised and the triceps sutured directly to the ulna via drill holes in the distal fragment (Fig. 14.19).

If the comminution is capable of undergoing anatomical reduction, fractures at, or proximal to, the deepest part of the trochlear notch may be managed by tension-band and K-wire fixation after careful preliminary assembly of the smaller elements. The use of a neutralization plate to protect such tenuous fixation is often a useful addition however. When the fracture involves the coronoid process, simple tension-band principles cannot be applied and a strong plate to resist bending and twisting moments is mandatory. Reduction and fixation of the coronoid elements is the first step in these difficult operations and it may be necessary to use multiple fine K-wires to maintain temporary stability of the many small fragments until the whole assembly can be stabilized by compression. When the cortical shell cannot be restored, compression with tension-band and axial wires is clearly not appropriate and a dorsal buttress plate is therefore preferable.

Postoperatively, the elbow is held at 90° flexion in a padded splint with the arm elevated. Most fractures can then be managed by active exercises. Extremely comminuted fractures and those which extend into the proximal ulnar shaft should be treated with care and it is wise to protect such patients, with a cast-brace, from the risk of secondary displacement (Müller *et al.* 1965, Schatzker & Tile 1987).

Pseudarthrosis

The incidence of non-union after operative treatment is low and requires treatment only if the patient has relevant complaints. Non-union after conservative treatment is the expected outcome, but is rarely painful. When symptoms demand, the application of a cancellous bone graft and a buttress plate is usually effective (Rowe 1965).

References

Alvarez, E., Patel, M.R., Nimberg, G. & Pearlman, H.S. Fractures of the capitellum humeri. *J Bone Joint Surg* 1975; **57A**: 1093–1096.

Amis, A.A. Biomechanics: upper limb. Part I. *Curr Orthop* 1990; **4**: 21–26.

Basmajian, J.V. *Muscles Alive* 4th edn. Williams & Wilkins: Baltimore, 1978.

Bickel, W.E. & Perry, R.E. Comminuted fractures of the distal humerus. *J Am Med Assoc* 1963; **184**: 553–557.

Brown, R.F. & Morgan, R.G. Intercondylar T-shaped fractures of the humerus. *J Bone Joint Surg* 1971; **53B**: 425–428.

Bryan, R.S. Fractures about the elbow in adults. American Academy of Orthopaedic Surgeons. *Instructional Course Lectures* **30**: 200–223. CV Mosby: St Louis, 1981.

Cassebaum, W.H. Operative treatment of T & Y fractures of the lower end of the humerus. *Am J Surg* 1952; **83**: 265–270.

Curr, J.F. & Coe, W.A. Dislocation of the inferior radio-lucent joint. *Br J Surg* 1946; **34**: 74–77.

Desault, P.J. *A Treatise on Fractures, Luxation and Other Affections of the Bones* 2nd edn. Kumber & Conrad: Philadelphia, 1811.

Dunlop, J. Transcondylar fractures of the humerus in childhood. *J Bone Joint Surg* 1939; **21**: 59–73.

Eastwood, W.J. The T-shaped fracture of the lower end of the humerus. *J Bone Joint Surg* 1937; **19**: 364–369.

Edmonson, A.S. In: Crenshaw, A.H. (ed.) *Campbell's Operative Orthopaedics* 7th edn. CV Mosby: St Louis, 1987.

Essex-Lopresti, P. Fractures of the radial head with distal radioulnar dislocation. Report of two cases. *J Bone Joint Surg* 1951; **33B**: 244–247.

Hahn, N.F. Fall von ein besonderes Varietat der Frakturen des Ellenbogens. *Z Wundarzt Geburtshelfe* 1853; **6**: 185–189.

Hallet, J. Entrapment of the median nerve after dislocation of the elbow. A case report. *J Bone Joint Surg* 1981; **63B**: 408–412.

Helm, R., Hornby, R. & Miller, S. The complications of surgical treatment of displaced fractures of the olecranon. *Injury* 1987; **18**: 48–50.

Jones, R. Sir (ed.) *Orthopaedic Surgery of Injuries.* Oxford Medical Publications, Oxford 1921.

Keon-Cohen, B.T. Fractures of the elbow. *J Bone Joint Surg* 1966; **48A**: 1623–1639.

Knight, D.J., Rymaszewski, L.A., Amis, A.A. & Miller, J.H. Primary replacement of the fractured radial head with a metal prosthesis. *J Bone Joint Surg* 1993; **75B**: 572–576.

Linscheid, R.L. & Wheeler, D.K. Elbow dislocations. *J Am Med Assoc* 1965; **194**: 1171–1176.

Mahaisavariya, B., Laupattarakasem, W., Supachutikul, A., Taeseri, H. & Sujaritbudhungkoon, S. Late reduction of dislocated elbow. *J Bone Joint Surg* 1993; **75B**: 426–428.

Mason, M.L. Some observations on fractures of the head of the radius with a review of one hundred cases. *Br J Surg* 1954; **42**: 123–132.

Mehlhoff, T.L., Noble, P.C., Bennett, J.B. & Tullos, M.D. Simple dislocation of the elbow in the adult. *J Bone Joint Surg* 1988; **70A**: 244–249.

Meyn, M.A. & Quigley, T.B. Reduction of posterior dislocation of the elbow by traction on the dangling arm. *Clin Orthop* 1974; **103**: 106–108.

Mohan, K. Myositis ossificans traumatica of the elbow. *Int Surg* 1972; **57**: 475–578.

Müller, M.E., Allgower, M. & Willenegger, H. *Technique of Internal Fixation of Fractures*. Springer-Verlag: Berlin, 1965.

Murphy, W.A. & Siegel, M.J. Elbow fat pads with new signs and extended differential diagnosis. *Radiology* 1977; **124**: 659–665.

O'Driscoll, S.W., Morrey, B.F., Korinek, S. & An, K.-N. Elbow subluxation and dislocation: A spectrum of instability. *Clin Orthop* 1992; **280**: 186–198.

Osborne, G. & Cotterill, P. Recurrent dislocation of the elbow. *J Bone Joint Surg* 1966; **48B**: 340–346.

Oury, J.H., Roe, R.D. & Laning, R.C. A case of bilateral anterior dislocations of the elbow. *J Trauma* 1972; **12**: 170–173.

Parvin, R.W. Closed reduction of common shoulder and elbow dislocations without anaesthesia. *Arch Surg* 1957; **75**: 972–975.

Patrick, J. Fracture of the medial epicondyle with displacement into the elbow joint. *J Bone Joint Surg* 1956; **28**: 143–147.

Purser, D.W. Dislocation of the elbow and inclusion of the medial epicondyle in the adult. *J Bone Joint Surg* 1954; **36B**: 247–249.

Rowe, C.R. Management of fractures in elderly patients. *J Bone Joint Surg* 1965; **47A**: 1043–1059.

Schatzker, J. & Tile, M. *The Rationale of Operative Fracture Care*. Springer-Verlag: Berlin, 1987.

Schwab, G.H., Bennett, J.B., Woods, G.W. & Tullos, H.S. Biomechanics of elbow instability. The role of the medial collateral ligament. *Clin Orthop* 1980; **146**: 42–52.

Smith, D.N. & Lee, J.R. The radiological diagnosis of post-traumatic effusion of the elbow joint and its clinical significance: 'The displaced fat pad sign'. *Injury* 1978; **10**: 115–119.

Smith, F.M. *Surgery of the Elbow* 2nd edn. WB Saunders: Philadelphia, 1972.

Södergård, J., Sandelin, J. & Bostman, O. Mechanical failures of internal fixation in T and Y fractures of the distal humerus. *J Trauma* 1992; **33**: 687–690.

Stimson, L.A. *A Treatise on Fractures*. Henry C. Lea & Son: Philadelphia, 1890.

Swanson, A.B., Jaeger, S.H. & Rochelle, D.L. Comminuted fractures of the radial head. The rôle of silicone implant replacement arthroplasty. *J Bone Joint Surg* 1981; **63A**: 1039–1049.

Taylor, T.K.F. & O'Connor, B.T. The effect upon the inferior radio-ulnar joint of excision of the head of the radius in adults. *J Bone Joint Surg* 1964; **46B**: 83–88.

Thompson, H.C. III & Garcia, A. Myositis ossificans (aftermath of elbow injuries). *Clin Orthop* 1967; **50**: 129–134.

Van Gorder, G.W. Surgical approach in supracondylar 'T' fractures of the humerus requiring open reduction. *J Bone Joint Surg* 1940; **22**: 278–292.

Wilson, P.D. Fractures and dislocations in the region of the elbow. *Surg Gynecol Obstet* 1933; **56**: 335–359.

15: The Forearm

A.J.CARR AND P.H.WORLOCK

Introduction

This chapter deals with fractures of the shafts of the radius and ulna, of either both bones or one bone. Shaft fractures of the forearm bones require special attention. It is essential to maintain the complex interdependent rotational movements of the radius and ulna if full forearm movement is to be retained. Even slight malunion may result in loss of function.

The radius and ulna are in contact only at their ends and lie approximately parallel in the forearm. Proximally they are held together by the capsule of the elbow joint and the annular ligament. Distally they are joined by the capsule of the wrist joint, the anterior and posterior radioulnar ligaments and the triangular ligament of the ulna. The ulna is a relatively straight bone but the shape of the radius is much more complex. Sage (1959) described the anatomy of these bones and emphasized the importance of maintaining their shape in fracture treatment. The fibres of the interosseous ligament run obliquely between the radius and ulna. The strength of this ligament and the oblique arrangement of its fibres are essential to the dynamic relationship of the two bones.

The radius and ulna are subject to muscle forces which create deforming forces when the bones are fractured. They are joined by the supinator, pronator teres and pronator quadratus muscles. The forearm muscles that have their origin on the volar side of the ulna and insert on the radial side of the wrist or hand exert a pronating force. The abductor pollicis longus and brevis and the extensor pollicis longus muscles have their origin on the ulna and insert on the radial side of the dorsum of the wrist and tend to exert a supinating force.

In fractures of the radius distal to the insertion of supinator and proximal to the insertion of pronator teres, the two fragments of the radius are pulled in opposite directions by the opposing forces of these two muscles. In fractures of the radius distal to pronator teres, the force of supinator and biceps is somewhat neutralized by the pronator teres and the proximal fragment lies in less external rotation (Fig. 15.1). These complex forces make closed treatment very difficult.

Management

Closed methods of treatment

The need for early accurate reduction of fractures of the radius and ulna has long been understood. Charnley (1961) described the basic principles underlying the maintenance of the reduced fracture position. This requires an understanding of the rotational forces involved in forearm movement, particularly pronation and supination. Hughston (1957), Anderson *et al.* (1975) and Dodge and Cady (1976) all report poor results from the closed treatment of these fractures. Some reports of early functional bracing have suggested that this method may have some advantages over other methods of closed treatment (Sarmiento *et al.* 1975). Closed methods are acceptable in the skeletally immature, where there remains sufficient potential for bone remodelling to occur. However, in the majority of children from the age of 11 or 12 years open methods should be considered for displaced fractures (Voto *et al.* 1990) (Fig. 15.2).

Open methods of treatment

Early attempts at some form of internal fixation began with the use of Kirschner wires (Böhler 1936), but still required prolonged periods of plaster immobilization. Even with the advent of plate fixation the materials and techniques used did not provide for a sound and stable anatomical reduction. Patients needed long periods in plaster and the outcome was often less than perfect. Knight and Purvis (1949) reported high rates of non-union and forearm stiffness. In addition to plate fixation,

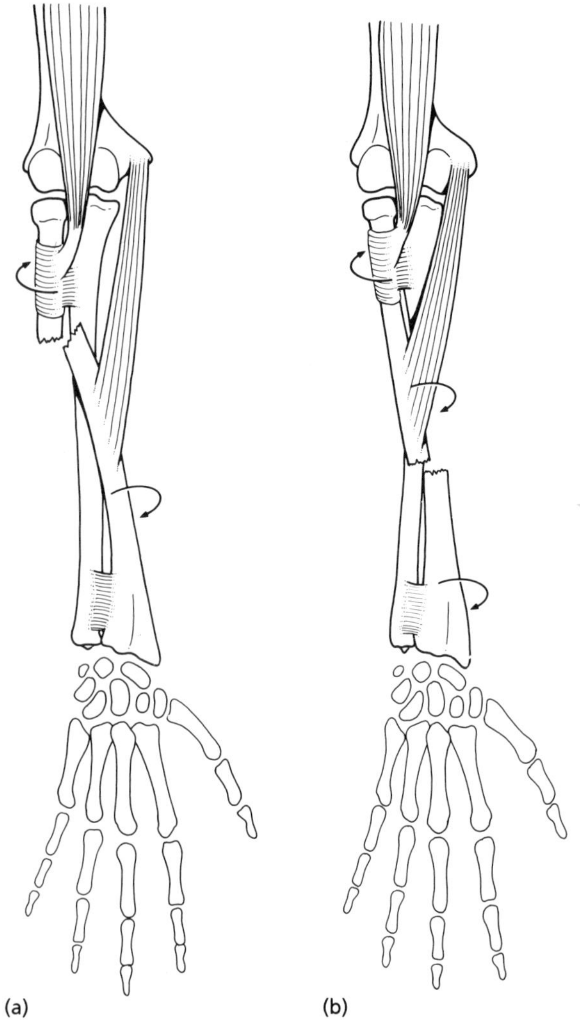

(a)   (b)

Fig. 15.1 (a) Fracture of the upper shaft of the radius between the insertion of the supinator and pronator teres muscles. The proximal fragment is supinated and the distal fragment pronated. (b) Fracture of the middle or lower part of the radius between the insertions of the pronator teres and the pronator quadratus. The proximal fragment is supinated, but to a lesser extent than in fractures above the insertion of the pronator teres.

intramedullary devices were also employed (Smith & Sage 1957) (Fig. 15.3). Unfortunately, these systems may fail to restore the axial alignment of the forearm bone and tend to overstraighten the radius. Such factors inevitably produce a reduced range of forearm movement. Murray *et al.* (1964) described the use of non-slotted dual plates. Comparison of the use of dual plates and single compression plates showed less infection and radio-ulnar synostosis occurred with the single plates (Teipner & Mast 1980). In 1981, Rosacker and Kopta reported 54 patients treated with various devices

for fractures of both bones of the forearm. They used either conventional plates, compression plates or intramedullary rods, and found that the best results were obtained for fractures that were accurately reduced. The compression plate was found to provide anatomical reduction in the highest proportion of cases (Fig. 15.4).

The Association for Osteosynthesis/Association for the Study of Problems of Internal Fixation (AO/ASIF) group have long recommended accurate anatomical reduction of the fracture with a plate, used either with static axial compression (for transverse fractures) or in a neutralization mode after primary interfragmentary compression with a lag screw (for oblique or spiral fractures) (Fig. 15.5). Malunion rates of less than 5% have been reported (Petrie & Tile 1974, Anderson *et al.* 1975). This compares well with a non-union rate of 20% expected with closed methods of treatment.

Classification

A classification of fractures is useful only if it considers the severity of the bony problem and also serves as a basis for the treatment and evaluation of results. The AO classification (Fig. 15.6) divides all long-bone segment fractures into three types and then into three groups and three subgroups. This arrangement is in ascending order of severity according to the morphological complexity of the fracture.

The underlying principle of treatment is to restore function. The anatomical alignment of the bones must be returned to normal. Restoration of length will prevent subluxation or dislocation of the proximal or distal radio-ulnar joints. Restoration of rotational alignment is necessary for normal pronation and supination of the forearm.

Indications for surgery

Fractures of both bones

The case for non-operative treatment is weak and open reduction is recommended. Plate fixation is the preferred method of fixation. External fixation is rarely indicated. This is technically demanding, particularly for the radius, and should be avoided. Certain open comminuted fractures of the ulna are suitable for treatment with a small external fixator.

Single bone fractures

The non-operative treatment of displaced single bone fractures gives poor results. Unless the fracture

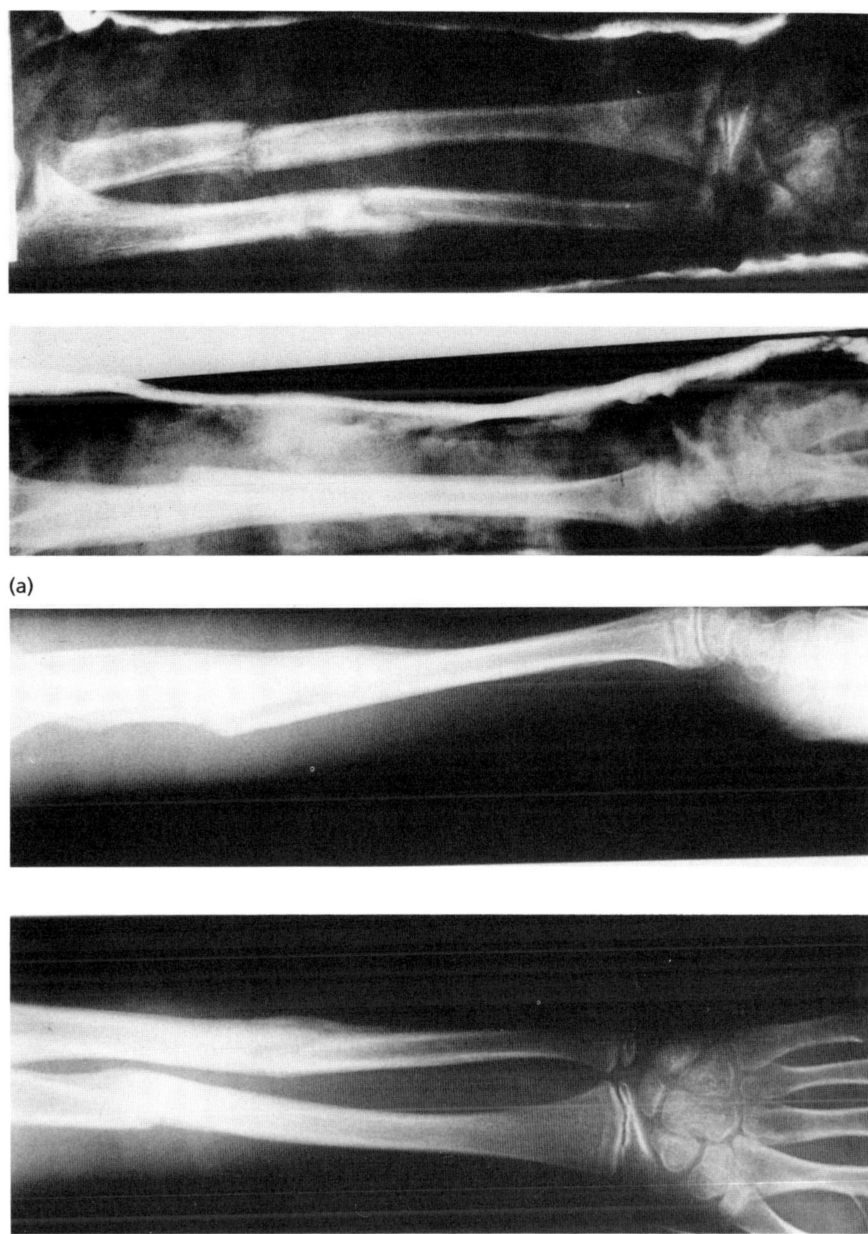

Fig. 15.2 Radiographs of (a) mid-shaft fractures of the radius and ulna, and (b) malunion of mid-shaft fractures following conservative treatment.

(a)

(b)

reduction is perfect there may be permanent subluxation of the proximal or distal radio-ulnar joint and this will result in significant limitation of movement.

Galeazzi fracture

This is a fracture of the radius with distal radio-ulnar subluxation (Fig. 15.7). Internal fixation of the radius restores the radial length, which allows accurate reduction of the distal radio-ulnar joint. No further specific treatment is required for the dislocation in the majority of cases. If the distal ulna or styloid process has been fractured, then open reduction and screw fixation is sometimes necessary. Wound closure is usually possible for closed fractures. Mobilization can be started after 48 hours unless the distal radio-ulnar joint remains unstable, in which case cast immobilization in forearm supination is required for 6 weeks.

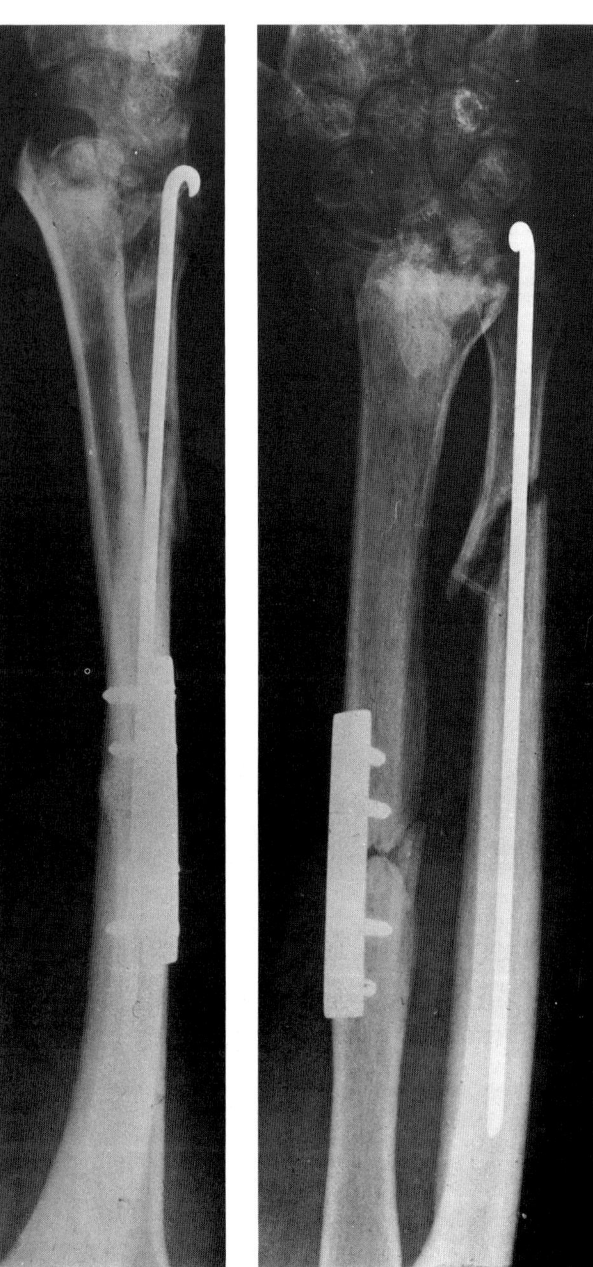

Fig. 15.3 Radiograph demonstrating intramedullary fixation of forearm fractures.

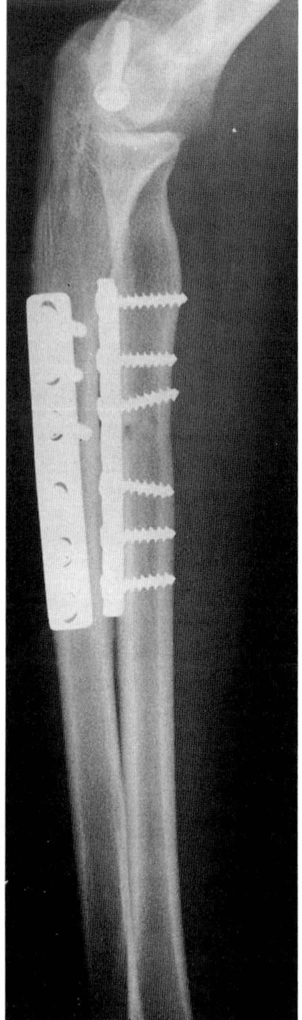
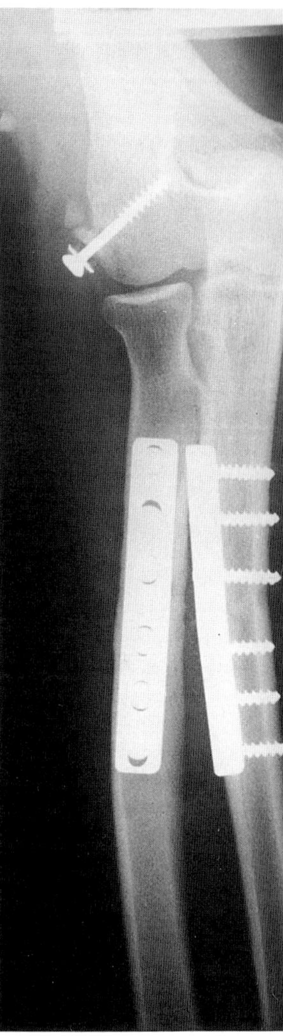

Fig. 15.4 Radiograph of a fractured radius and ulna to demonstrate internal fixation with dynamic compression plates.

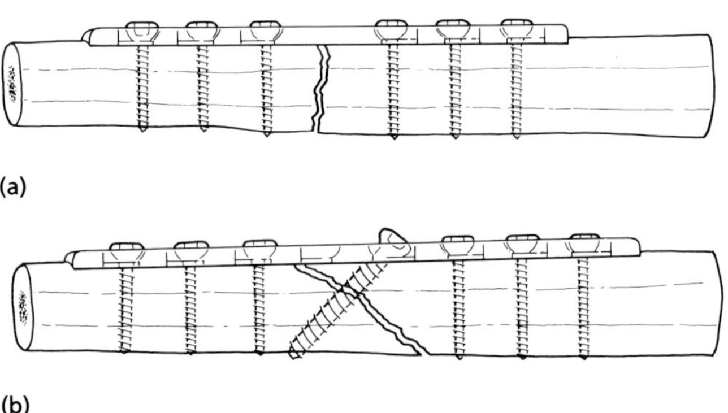

(a)

(b)

Fig. 15.5 (a) Fixation of a transverse fracture with a dynamic compression plate. (b) Fixation of an oblique fracture with an interfragmentary lag screw and a neutralization plate.

Monteggia fracture

This is a fracture of the ulna with associated proximal radio-ulnar dissociation (Fig. 15.8). Open and accurate anatomical reduction is essential. In the majority of cases reduction and fixation of the ulnar fracture results in stable reduction of the radial head. If the radial head is stable, then mobilization can begin after 48 hours. If the radial head is unstable in extension and reduction

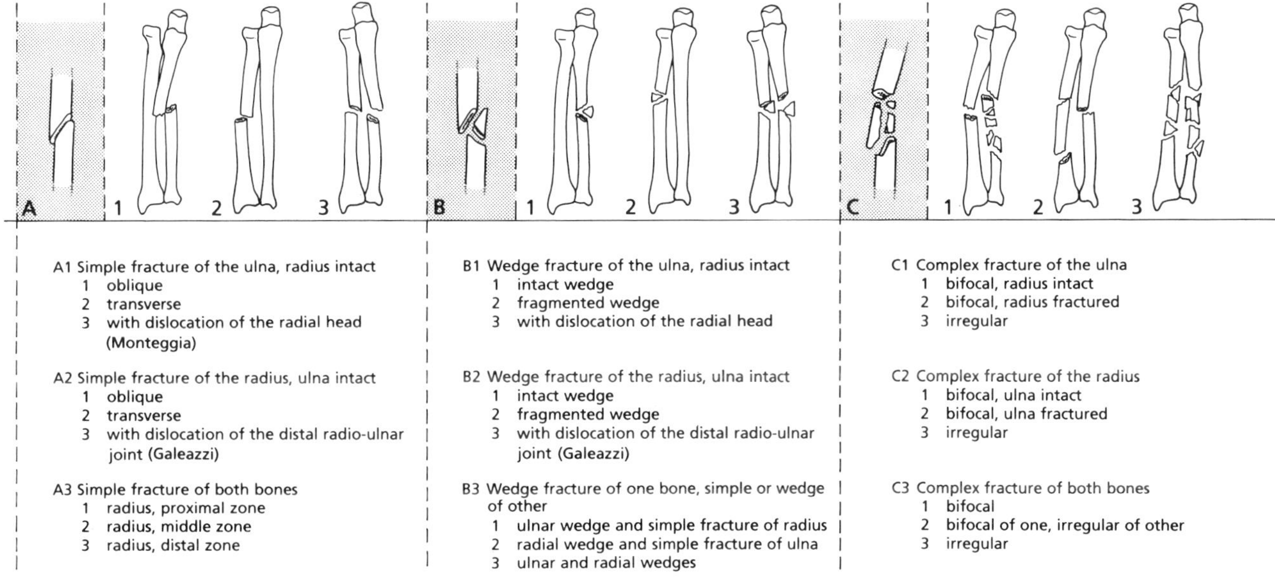

A1 Simple fracture of the ulna, radius intact
1 oblique
2 transverse
3 with dislocation of the radial head (Monteggia)

A2 Simple fracture of the radius, ulna intact
1 oblique
2 transverse
3 with dislocation of the distal radio-ulnar joint (Galeazzi)

A3 Simple fracture of both bones
1 radius, proximal zone
2 radius, middle zone
3 radius, distal zone

B1 Wedge fracture of the ulna, radius intact
1 intact wedge
2 fragmented wedge
3 with dislocation of the radial head

B2 Wedge fracture of the radius, ulna intact
1 intact wedge
2 fragmented wedge
3 with dislocation of the distal radio-ulnar joint (Galeazzi)

B3 Wedge fracture of one bone, simple or wedge of other
1 ulnar wedge and simple fracture of radius
2 radial wedge and simple fracture of ulna
3 ulnar and radial wedges

C1 Complex fracture of the ulna
1 bifocal, radius intact
2 bifocal, radius fractured
3 irregular

C2 Complex fracture of the radius
1 bifocal, ulna intact
2 bifocal, ulna fractured
3 irregular

C3 Complex fracture of both bones
1 bifocal
2 bifocal of one, irregular of other
3 irregular

Fig. 15.6 The classification employed by the AO group.

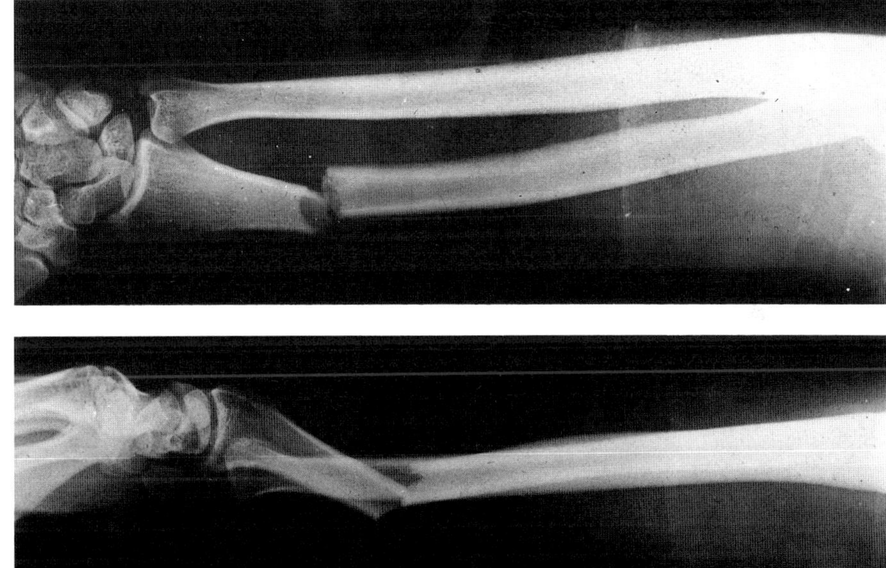

Fig. 15.7 Radiograph of a Galeazzi fracture.

of the ulnar fracture cannot be improved, then a cast-brace limiting extension may be required postoperatively. In less than 10% of cases the radial head cannot be reduced after fixation of the ulnar fracture. The proximal radius should then be exposed by extending the ulnar incision proximally. Usually, this failure of reduction is caused by soft tissue interposition, most commonly a torn section of the annular ligament. Rarely, the supinator muscle and radial nerve are also trapped. This fracture is notorious for producing late elbow stiffness, and early mobilization, possibly with continuous passive motion, is important to reduce stiffness.

Isolated fracture of the ulna shaft

These fractures are usually caused by a direct blow ('nightstick fracture') and management has been the subject of controversy. Fracture union can be expected when conservative methods are used, and Sarmiento *et al.* (1975) report good results using below-elbow

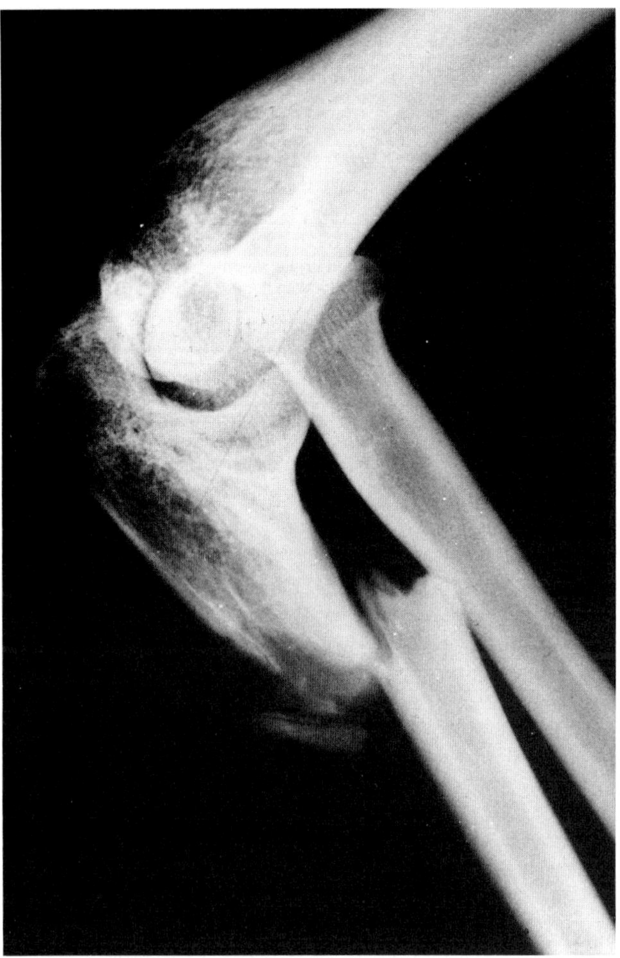

Fig. 15.8 Radiograph of a Monteggia fracture.

casts. Union can be delayed, particularly with proximal fractures where the deforming forces are greater. Operative treatment has the advantage of preventing the need for prolonged splintage, but has the disadvantage of the potential introduction of sepsis, the production of a stress riser and the possible need for a second operation to remove the plate.

Open fractures

Open fractures require open reduction and stable internal fixation, for the same reasons as do closed fractures. Moed *et al.* (1986) report low rates of sepsis for open fractures treated with early wound debridement and internal fixation. For heavily contaminated wounds with severe fracture comminution, external fixation may be the only method of providing stable reduction of the fracture. Accurate reduction is more difficult to achieve with external fixation than with internal fixation (Fig. 15.9).

Timing of surgery

In forearm fractures open reduction is the treatment of choice and early surgery is preferable. Early surgery is technically easier with respect to both the surgical approach and the ease of fracture reduction. Smith and Sage (1957) reported that delayed surgery improved the rate of primary bone union. This finding is disputed (Schatzker & Tile 1987) and we advocate early reduction and fixation. Rarely, delay may be necessary in patients with significant soft tissue contamination.

Surgical technique

The patient should be positioned supine on the operating table with the arm resting on an arm board and the shoulder in 90° of abduction. A lateral or prone position can be used for the arm on the arm board. The authors use a tourniquet for closed fractures, but for open fractures prefer not to use a tourniquet unless bleeding prevents adequate identification of the tissues.

Surgical approaches

The ulna

The standard approach to the ulna is subcutaneously (Fig. 15.10). Using this route the whole length of the bone can be exposed. It is preferable to avoid a skin incision directly over the subcutaneous crest of the ulna.

The radius

Anterior approach (of Henry)

The authors prefer this anterior approach to the radius for surgery to the proximal and distal thirds. The approach can be extended proximally or distally and permits exposure of the whole length of the radius if necessary. If the proximal third of the radius is approached, then the radial nerve is well protected within the supinator muscle. This is a particularly important consideration during subsequent surgery for plate removal. The flat anterior surface of the radius in its lower third allows easy application of a plate. The anterior surface of the upper and middle thirds is compressive rather than tensile. However, application of plates on this surface does not appear to compromise the end result. Useful landmarks are the biceps tendon and the styloid process of the radius. The fascia is incised between the brachioradialis and flexor carpi radialis muscles. The antebrachii lateralis nerve lies

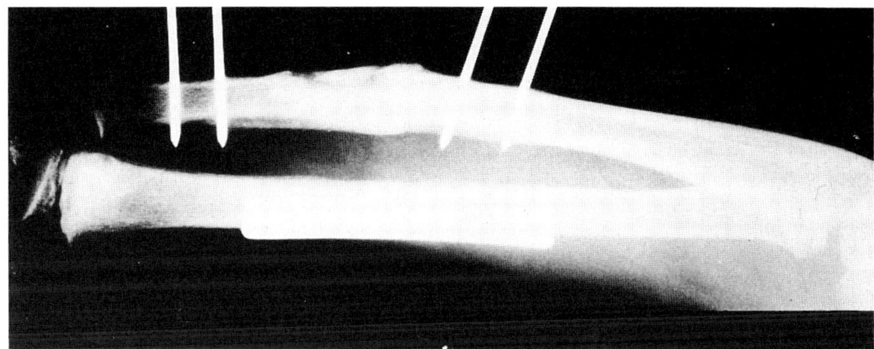

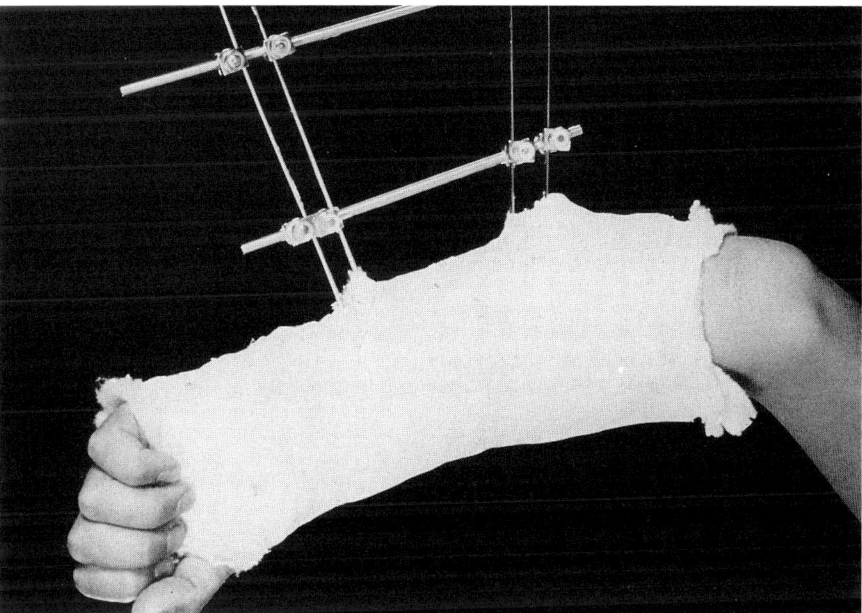

Fig. 15.9 Illustration of the use of an external fixator.

subcutaneously and the superficial branch of the radial nerve lies along the brachioradialis muscle. Several branches of the radial artery pass laterally and these must be ligated. The radial artery and veins are retracted medially. The insertion of the pronator teres muscle should be preserved if possible. Proximally, the supinator muscle is incised at its insertion and retracted laterally with the deep branch of the radial nerve within it (Fig. 15.11).

Posterior approach

For middle-third fractures the approach of Thompson (1918) can be used; it is not suitable for distal-third fractures where the plate may interfere with extensor tendons, particularly to the thumb. Useful landmarks are the lateral epicondyle of the humerus and Lister's tubercle. The fascia between the extensor carpi radialis brevis and the extensor digitorum communis is incised to expose the radius. In the distal part of the incision abductor pollicis longus and extensor pollicis brevis emerge obliquely and plates can be inserted beneath them. Proximally, the radial nerve should be identified entering and leaving the supinator. A posterior approach to the upper third of the radius was described by Boyd in 1940. The major problem with this approach is the proximity of the radial nerve, which can easily be damaged at the point where it leaves the supinator muscle. Useful landmarks are the lateral epicondyle of the humerus and the styloid process of the ulna. The anconeus muscle should be detached along with the extensor carpi ulnaris and the supinator from their insertions into the ulna until the radius is exposed (Fig. 15.12).

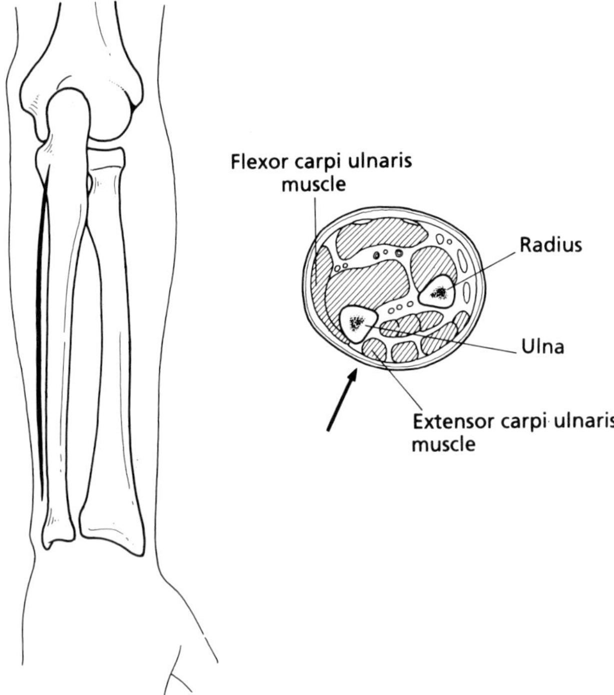

Fig. 15.10 The skin incision for a fracture of the ulna. The cross-section demonstrates the surgical approach between the flexor and extensor carpi ulnaris muscles.

Lateral approach

The radius can be approached laterally in its middle and distal thirds. The approach is between the extensor digitorum communis and the extensor carpi radialis brevis muscles.

Techniques of plate application

Care must be taken to prevent stripping of the soft tissue attachments and blood supply to the periosteum. Compression of the fracture provides the most fixation, either with plates under static compression or with interfragmentary screws supplemented by a neutral-ization plate. Transverse or short oblique fractures are best managed with dynamic compression plates (DCP). If the fracture is sufficiently oblique, as may be the case with spiral or comminuted fractures, then interfrag-mentary screw fixation should be used. During plate fixation it is important that the soft tissues around the fracture are protected as much as possible and that the blood supply to the fracture fragments is maintained.

Choice of implant

The 3.5-mm DCP is recommended for use in adults. Six cortices of fixation should be obtained on both sides of the fracture (see Fig. 15.4). The length of the plate used will depend on the type and degree of comminution of the fracture. In children, a 2.7-mm DCP can be employed. If an external fixator is to be used then a unilateral frame is usually sufficient. Two or three pins are required on each side of the fracture. The authors do not recommend external fixation of the radius.

Site of plate application

The ulnar plate should be applied on the medial border (Fig. 15.13). If the anterior approach is used for fractures of the radius the plate should be placed on the anterior surface for upper- and lower-third fractures. For middle-third fractures the plate may be applied to the anterior or lateral surfaces. If a posterior approach is used then the plate is applied to the posterolateral or lateral surfaces.

Bone grafting

Iliac crest bone grafts should be used when there has been significant bone loss or when anatomical reduction is impossible owing to comminution or where the stability of the fixation is in doubt. Problems may arise if bone graft is placed next to breaches in the inter-osseous membrane because cross-union may occur between the radius and ulna. If bone loss has been extensive, then plate fixation may be inappropriate and stabilization with an external fixator employed. The breach in cortical bone length may then be filled with corticocancellous bone graft from the iliac crest or with a vascularized bone graft from the fibula. Bone grafting can be undertaken as soon as soft tissue healing permits. This approach should be used as a salvage procedure when plate fixation is impossible.

Wound closure

Wounds should be closed over a suction drain. When two incisions have been made closure of one wound may be difficult because of swelling of the forearm muscles and soft tissues. The deep fascia should not be closed and the authors recommend extending the fascial incision proximally and distally to prevent the develop-ment of compartment syndrome. If the wound cannot be closed without undue tension then it should be left open. Secondary closure is usually possible after 5 or 7

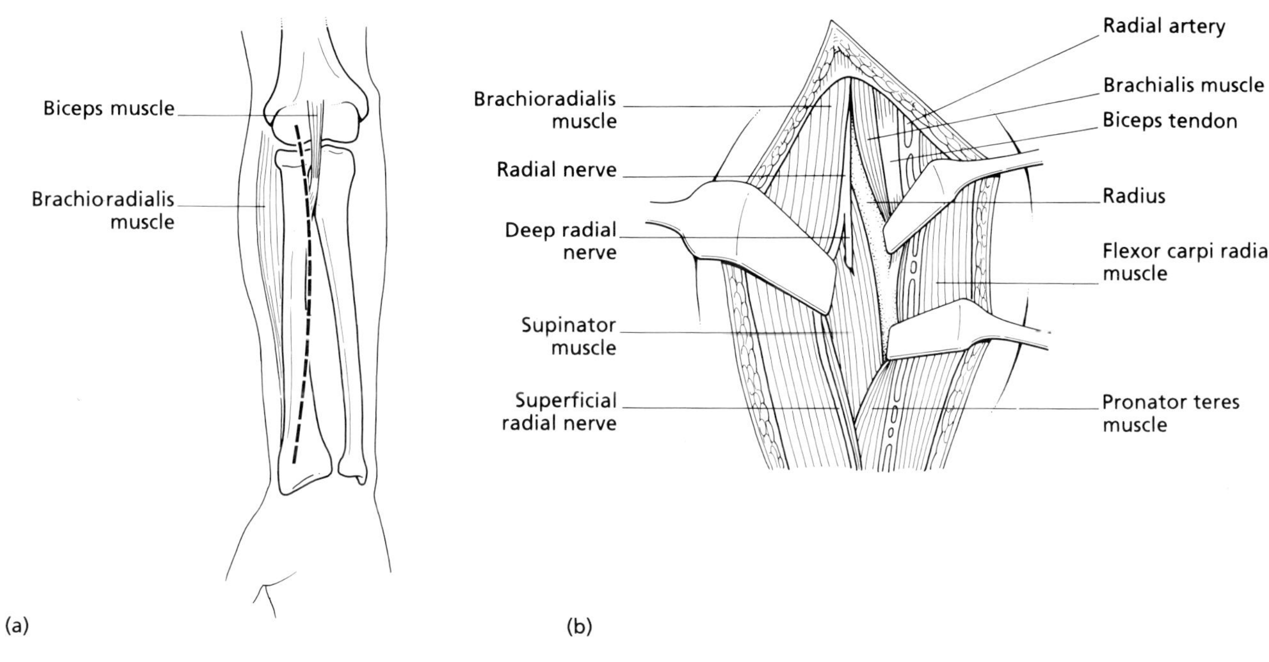

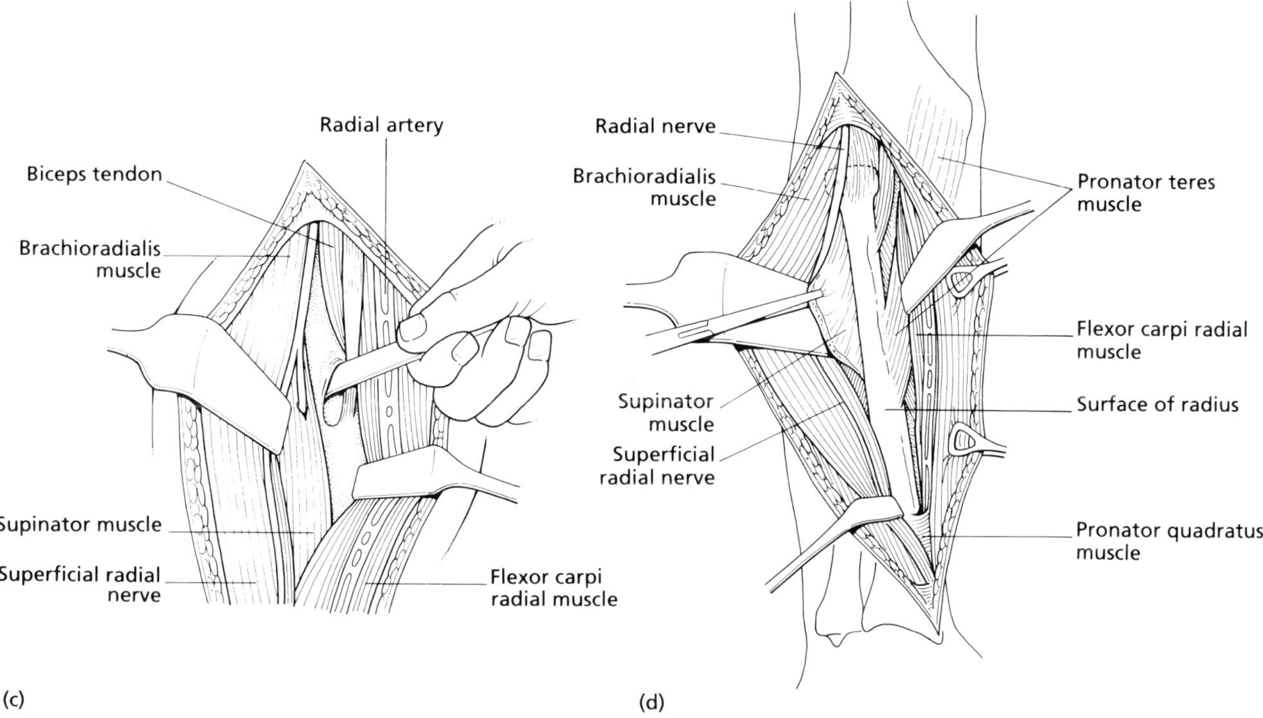

Fig. 15.11 Anterior approach to the radius. (a) Skin incision. (b) Position of the radial nerve entering the supinator muscle. (c) The radial nerve is protected during dissection of the supinator from the upper third of the radius. (d) Extensile exposure; the entire shaft of the radius can be exposed.

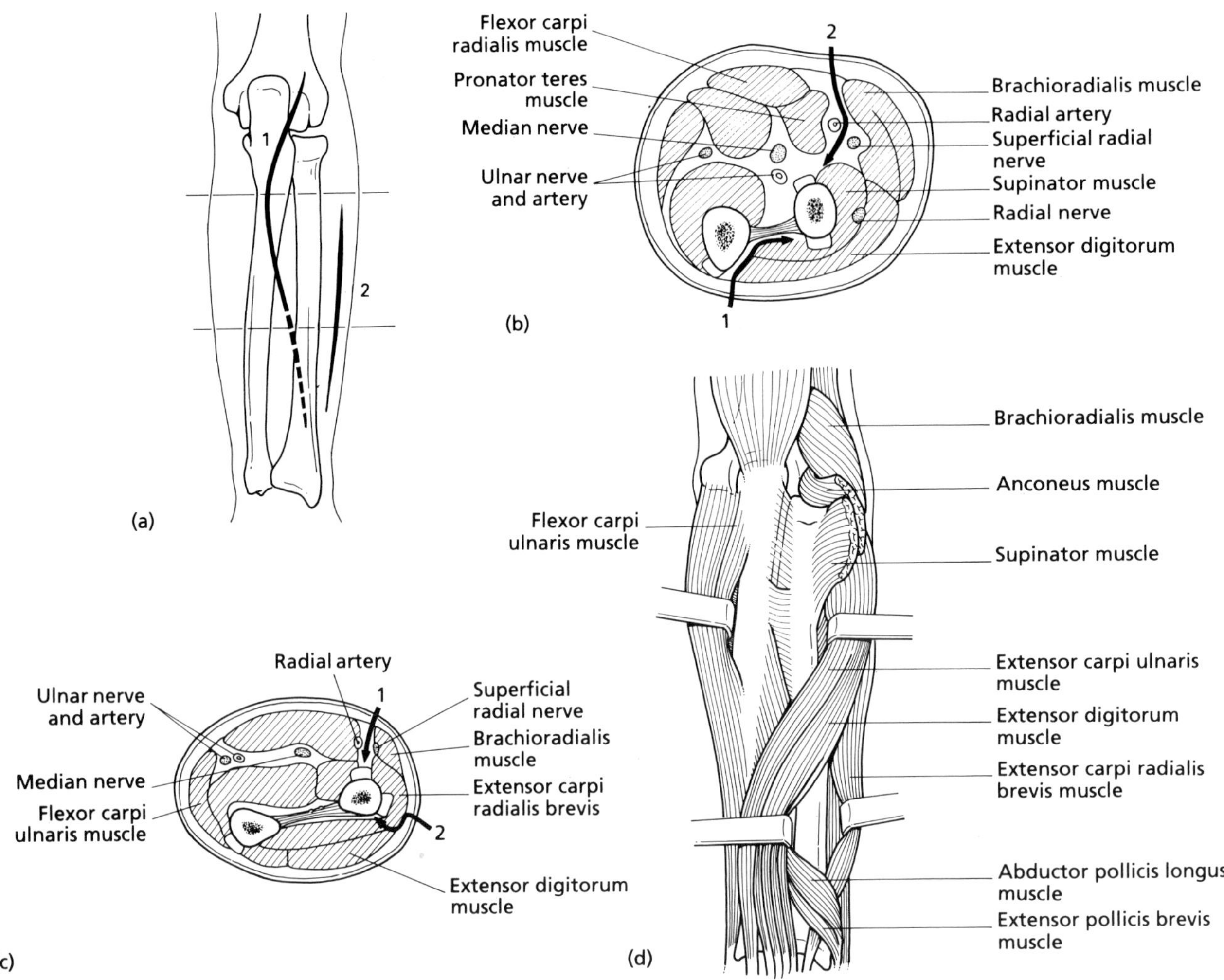

Fig. 15.12 Posterior and lateral approaches to the forearm. (a) (1) Extensile exposure method of Boyd and Thompson; (2), approach to the middle and distal third of the radius between extensor digitorum communis and extensor carpi radialis brevis. (b) Cross-section through the proximal third of the forearm to illustrate the proximal dorsal approach to the radius (1). The anterior approach of Henry is also shown (2). (c) Cross-section through the middle third of the forearm to illustrate the anterior (1) and lateral (2) approaches to the radius. (d) The extensile posterior approach to the radius of Boyd and Thompson. The supinator muscle has been partly detached and reflected with the posterior interosseous nerve.

days. If one wound is to be left open, this should be the radial wound which has more soft tissue underlying the skin. There are few cosmetic problems associated with delayed primary closure. Many more problems arise from closing wounds under too much tension. Tissue necrosis is then common and may result in infection of the implant and delayed or non-union.

Postoperative care

If a stable fixation has been achieved then the arm is wrapped in a wool and crepe dressing with a plaster back slab. This can be reduced after 48 hours of elevation.

Movements may then begin under supervision. The patient should be instructed to use the arm for light work but to avoid any heavy lifting. Follow-up should be at monthly intervals. The average time for union is between 8 and 12 weeks. Delays may arise if there has been comminution at the fracture site. If the fracture fixation is not completely stable then a removable above-elbow cast should be applied. The assessment of healing is based on the absence of pain at the fracture site and on the absence of any radiological signs of loosening: irritation callus, bone resorption at the fracture site or screw loosening.

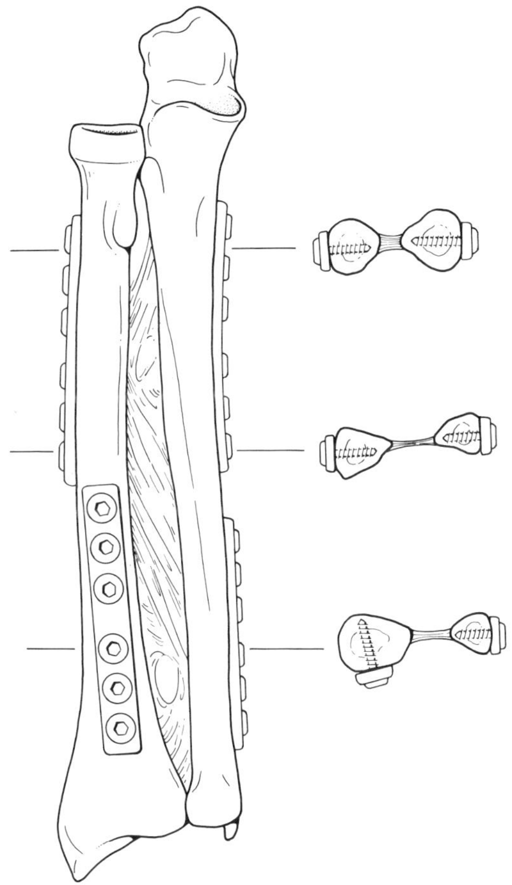

Fig. 15.13 The sites of plate application on the radius and ulna.

Complications

Radio-ulnar synostosis

Radio-ulnar synostosis occurs in between 1 and 8% of fractures (Botting 1970). Tile and Petrie (1969) reported an incidence of 3.3%, Anderson *et al.* (1975) 1.2%, and Teipner and Mast (1980) 4.8%. It is a more common complication of open or severely comminuted fractures, and is also more common with open than closed methods of treatment (Fig. 15.14). Schatzker and Tile (1987) believe that delayed open reduction further increases the risks of this complication, and immediate primary surgery is recommended. Bone grafting close to a ruptured interosseous membrane may also increase the risk of synostosis occurring.

Infection

Infection is an uncommon complication of internal fixation of forearm fractures with plates. It is more common with contaminated open fractures. The authors believe that early fixation involving peroperative antibiotic prophylaxis and meticulous operative technique gives the best chance of avoiding this complication.

Neurovascular

Neurovascular complications are more likely to occur following plate fixation of the radius. The posterior interosseous nerve is vulnerable in approaches to the proximal third of the radius and an anterior approach minimizes the risk of damage to the nerve. The anterior interosseous branch of the median nerve may also be damaged by fracture-reducing forceps.

Plate removal

Plates should not be removed routinely. Complication rates as high as 40% have been described following plate removal (Langkamer & Ackroyd 1990). Problems have arisen with refracturing. Neurological damage is more common after removal of radial plates than ulnar plates. However, plates may need to be removed if there is pain, particularly owing to irritation of the tissues by a subcutaneous ulnar plate or the lower screws of a radial plate. If plates are to be removed then this

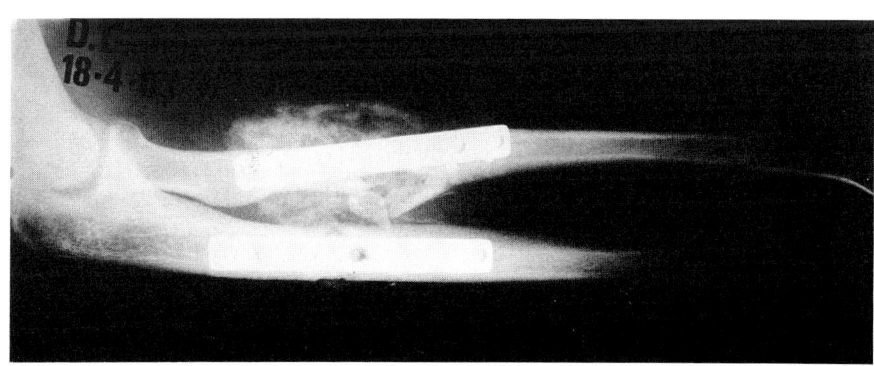

Fig. 15.14 Radiograph to demonstrate radio-ulnar synostosis following plate fixation of fractures of the radius and ulna.

should occur after at least 24 months. Perren (1988) has described early temporary osteoporosis around plate implants. Other authors have described a significant rate of refracture when plates are removed too early (Hidaka & Gustillo 1984).

References

Anderson, L.D., Sish, T.D., Tooms, R.E. & Park, W.I. Compression plate fixation in acute diaphyseal fractures of the radius and ulna. *J Bone Joint Surg* 1975; **57A**: 287–297.

Botting, T.D. Post-traumatic radio-ulnar cross-union. *J Trauma* 1970; **10**: 16–24.

Böhler, J. *Treatment of Fractures*. Wright: Bristol, 1936.

Boyd, H.B. Surgical exposure of the ulna and proximal third of the radius through one incision. *Surg Gynecol Obstet* 1940; **71**: 86.

Charnley, J. *Closed Treatment of Common Fractures*, 3rd edn. Churchill Livingstone: Edinburgh, 1961.

Dodge, H.S. & Cady, G.W. Treatment of fractures of the radius and ulna with compression plates. *J Bone Joint Surg* 1976; **54A**: 1167–1176.

Hidaka, S. & Gustillo, R.B. Refracture of bones of the forearm after plate removal. *J Bone Joint Surg* 1984; **66A**: 1241–1243.

Hughston, J.D. Fractures of the distal radial shaft, mistakes in management. *J Bone Joint Surg* 1957; **39A**: 249–264.

Knight, R.A. & Purvis, G.D. Fractures of both bones of the forearm in adults. *J Bone Joint Surg* 1949; **31A**: 755–764.

Langkamer, V.G. & Ackroyd, C.E. Removal of forearm plates. A review of the complications. *J Bone Joint Surg* 1990; **72B**: 601–604.

Moed, B.R., Kellam, J.F., Foster, R.J., Tile, M. & Hansen, S.T. Jr. Immediate internal fixation of open fractures of the forearm. *J Bone Joint Surg* 1986; **68A**: 1008–1017.

Murray, W.R., Lucas, D.B. & Inman, V.T. Treatment of non-union of fractures of the long bones by two plate method. *J Bone Joint Surg* 1964; **46A**: 1027–1048.

Perren, S.M. Early temporary porosis of bone induced by internal fixation implants. *Clin Orth* 1988; **232**: 139–151.

Petrie, D. & Tile, M. Fractures of radius and ulna — an end result study following the use of compression plates. *J Bone Joint Surg* 1974; **54B**: 762.

Rosacker, J.A. & Kopta, J.A. Both bone fractures of the forearm: a review of surgical variables associated with union. *Orthopaedics* 1981; **4**: 1353–1356.

Sage, F.P. Medullary fixation of fractures of the forearm. *J Bone Joint Surg* 1959; **41A**: 1489–1516.

Sarmiento, A., Cooper, J.S. & Sinclair, W.F. Forearm fractures. *J Bone Joint Surg* 1975; **57A**: 297–304.

Schatzker, J. & Tile, M. *The Rationale of Operative Fracture Care*. Springer: Berlin, 1987.

Smith, H. & Sage, F.P. Medullary fixation of forearm fractures. *J Bone Joint Surg* 1957; **39A**: 91–98.

Teipner, W.A. & Mast, J.W. Internal fixation of forearm diaphyseal fractures: double plating versus single compression (tension-band) plating — a comparative study. *Orthop Clin North Am* 1980; **3**: 381–391.

Thompson, J.E. Anatomical methods of approach in operations on the long bones of the extremities. *Ann Surg* 1918; **68**: 309.

Voto, S.J., Weiner, D.S. & Leighley, R.N. Redisplacement after closed reduction of forearm fractures in children. *J Pediatr Orthop* 1990; **10**: 79–84.

16: The Wrist

G.HOOPER, J.J. DIAS AND P.J. GREGG

Introduction

The word 'wrist' is thought to derive from an old Teutonic word meaning to twist or bend. The structure of the wrist allows the hand to be moved freely and then stabilized on the forearm in its various functional positions.

The wrist consists of a number of joints that work together as a functional unit. These include the radiocarpal joint, the ulnocarpal structures and the intercarpal articulations; functionally, the distal radioulnar articulation could be regarded as part of the forearm complex rather than as part of the wrist but as it is so frequently involved in wrist injuries it will be included in this chapter. Distally, the wrist ends at the carpometacarpal joints but its proximal extent is not clearly defined and extra-articular injuries of the distal radius are usually regarded as wrist injuries.

A knowledge of the anatomy of the various components of the wrist is necessary for an understanding of wrist injuries and the important features are noted below.

Distal radioulnar joint

The head of the ulna articulates with the ulnar notch of the radius and the proximal cartilaginous surface of the triangular fibrocartilage. The synovial membrane of the joint extends proximally as a pouch and the fibrous capsule is reinforced by weak anterior and posterior ligaments. The triangular fibrocartilage is attached at its base to the ulnar notch and at its apex to the styloid process of the ulna. It is thin in the centre and is often perforated, particularly in later life (Palmer & Werner 1981).

Radiocarpal joint

The proximal convex surface of the carpus articulates with the concave surface of the radius and the triangular cartilage. When the wrist is in the neutral position only the scaphoid bone and part of the lunate are in contact with the radius, the rest of the lunate being in contact with the triangular cartilage and the triquetrum with the joint capsule. In ulnar deviation the triquetrum comes to lie opposite the triangular cartilage.

The articular surface of the radius shows differently orientated and shaped articular facets for the scaphoid and lunate, since these carpal bones have different arcs of rotation and, moreover, do not move as a solid block but displace relative to each other during wrist movements.

The capsule of the radiocarpal joint is thick on the volar aspect and much thinner dorsally where, however, it is reinforced by the fibrous tissue of the extensor tendon compartments. Ligaments strengthen the capsule, the main ones being:
1 The radial collateral ligament.
2 The ulnocarpal complex (see below).
3 The dorsal radiocarpal ligament.
4 The volar radiocarpal ligaments, consisting of superficial fibres and three important deeper ligaments (radioscaphocapitate, radiolunate and radioscapholunate).

Ulnocarpal complex

This consists of the triangular cartilage, the ulnocarpal meniscus, the ulnar collateral and ulnolunate ligaments and the palmar wall of the sheath of the extensor carpi ulnaris tendon (Palmer & Werner 1981). The apex of the triangular cartilage is attached to the styloid process of the ulna and blends with the ulnocarpal meniscus which, together with the ulnar collateral ligament arising from the styloid process, inserts into the triquetrum, hamate and base of the metacarpal bone of the little finger. On the palmar surface of the wrist the complex is firmly attached to the triquetrum but dorsally its attachments are weak, except where it blends with the sheath of the extensor carpi ulnaris tendon. The complex stabil-izes the head of the ulna and acts as a cushion between the head and the carpus.

The ligaments of the wrist are summarized in Table 16.1 and the most important ligaments are illustrated in Figs 16.1 & 16.2. Ligaments may be classed as *extrinsic*, between the radius or ulna and the carpus, or between the carpus and the metacarpals, or *intrinsic*, between the carpal bones themselves. It should be noted that the lunate has a number of strong volar ligamentous attach-ments, but the lunocapitate articulation is not supported by strong ligaments (Mayfield *et al.* 1976, Taleisnik 1976).

The carpus

It is no longer adequate to think of the carpus as two transverse rows of bones, bridged by the scaphoid bone and held together with short interosseous ligaments to form a solid block moving as a whole. A series of subtle intercarpal displacements occur in normal wrist move-ments, to allow the maximal range of movements with stable positioning of the hand on the forearm. These movements are dictated by the contour of the intercarpal articular surfaces and the ligamentous attachments to the bones.

Taleisnick (1976) has developed the concept of the

Table 16.1 The ligaments of the wrist

> *Intrinsic*
> Short
>   Volar
>   Dorsal
>   Interosseous
> Intermediate
>   Lunotriquetral
>   Scapholunate
>   Scaphotrapezial
> Long
>   Volar intercarpal ('V')
>   Dorsal intercarpal
>
> *Extrinsic*
> Distal
>   Carpometacarpal.
> Proximal
>   Radiocarpal
>   Radial collateral
>   Dorsal radiocarpal
>   Volar radiocarpal: Radioscaphocapite
>   Radiolunate
>   Radioscapholunate
>   Ulnocarpal
>   Ulnocarpal complex

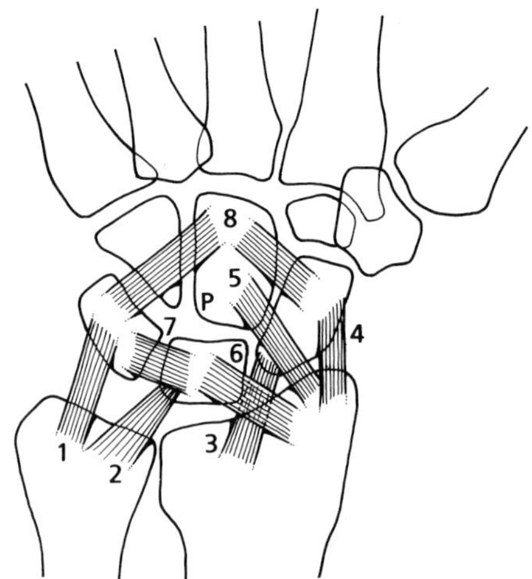

Fig. 16.1 The major volar ligaments of the wrist. Extrinsic ligaments: (1) ulnocarpal meniscus, (2) ulnolunate, (3) radioscapholunate, (4) radial collateral, (5) radioscaphocapite, (6) radiolunate. Intrinsic ligaments: (7) lunotriquetral, (8) volar intercarpal (V or deltoid). P is the space of Poirier.

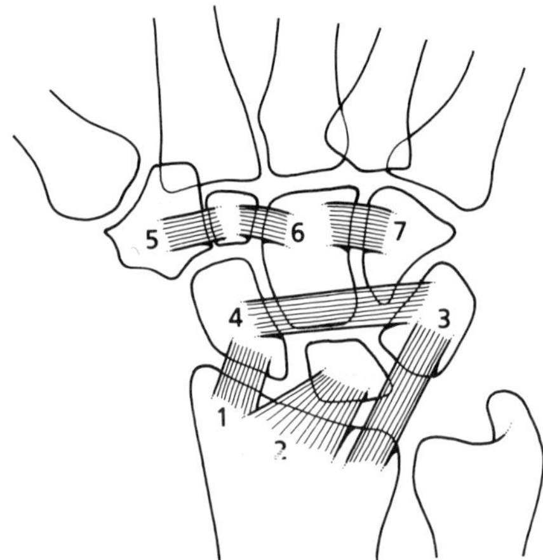

Fig. 16.2 The major dorsal ligaments of the wrist. Extrinsic ligaments: (1) radioscaphoid, (2) radiolunate, (3) radiotriquetral (these are fascicles of the dorsal radiocarpal ligament). Intrinsic ligaments: (4) dorsal intercarpal, (5) trapeziotrapezoid, (6) trapeziocapitate, (7) capitohamate.

carpus as a group of three longitudinal columnar struc-tures, each subserving a particular carpal function (Fig. 16.3); there is a central column for flexion and extension and two lateral columns to allow rotational movements of the mobile radial and ulnar components of the hand. He sees the distal carpal row (hamate, capitate, trapezoid and trapezium, which are firmly bound to each other and to the metacarpal bases by ligaments) and the lunate as forming the central column. During flexion and extension of the wrist the capitate moves within

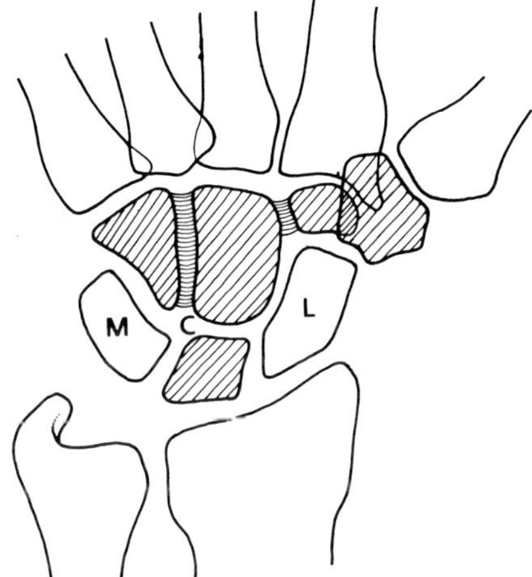

Fig. 16.3 The columnar concept of the carpus. L is the lateral column, C the central column and M the medial column.

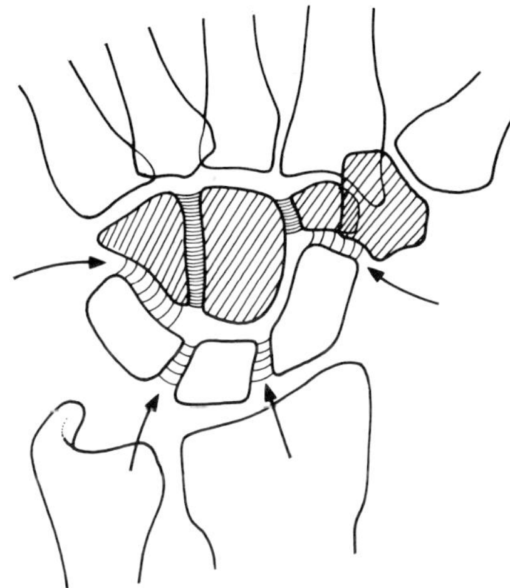

Fig. 16.4 The ring concept of the carpus. The hatched bones form the relatively rigid distal half of the ring. Arrows indicate potential sites of disruption of the ring.

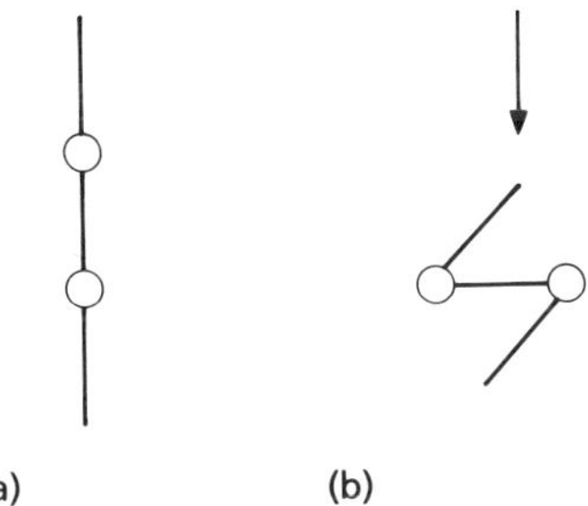

Fig. 16.5 (a) A longitudinal link system will collapse in (b) a Z-shape when stress is applied.

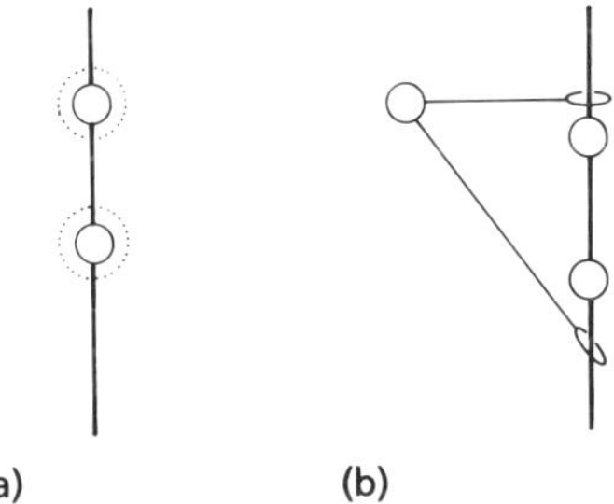

Fig. 16.6 The tendency to Z-collapse is resisted by (a) carpal ligaments (dotted lines) and (b) the scaphoid with its attached ligaments acting as a 'slider-crank' mechanism.

the cup of the lunate and compressive forces are transmitted along the central column in gripping actions of the hand. The scaphoid bone and the scaphoid–trapezium–trapezoid (STT) articulation form the lateral (radial) column which is involved in prehension and precision grip between the index finger and the thumb. The medial (ulnar) column is formed by the triquetrum and the triquetro-hamate articulation and extends the rotation of the forearm into the carpus. This concept of the carpal arrangement is particularly helpful in classifying the various types of carpal instability (see p. 465).

An alternative to the columnar concept has been proposed by Lichtman *et al.* (1981) who described the carpal bones as forming a ring (Fig. 16.4). The distal half of the ring formed by the hamate, capitate, trapezium and trapezoid is fixed to the metacarpal bones while the proximal half (scaphoid, lunate and triquetrum) is mobile. This ring concept accords well with the distribution of the intrinsic ligaments of the carpus and can also be used for classification of the various carpal injuries and instabilities. Distortion or disruption of the mobile proximal part of the ring causes the displacements of its components, relative to the distal half, that are seen in such injuries.

It is the soft tissue attachments to bones that give stability to the wrist, not the shapes of the bones themselves. The central column acts as a mobile longitudinal link mechanism between the distal radius and the metacarpal bones, into which the long extensors and flexors of the wrist are inserted. Such a system is potentially unstable to longitudinal stresses and, unless balanced by static or dynamic forces, will tend to collapse in a Z-shaped deformity with flexion or extension of the intercalated segment (the lunate) (Fig. 16.5). In the normal

wrist the scaphoid acts as a slider-crank between the links (Fig. 16.6) to prevent this (Linscheid *et al.* 1972) and damage to the scaphoid or its ligamentous attachments is a common cause of carpal instability and collapse (Fisk 1970).

Wrist movements

The axis of all wrist movements is located in the neck of

the capitate (Youm & Flatt 1979). All movements are associated with intercarpal displacements that are dicated by the shape of the carpal bones and their ligamentous attachments.

Palmarflexion occurs mainly at the mid-carpal level (Sarrafian *et al.* 1977). Dorsiflexion is also initiated at this level but, as the radioscaphocapitate ligament tightens, it causes the scaphoid to dorsiflex along with the attached lunate. The capitate and lunate therefore remain coaxial in dorsiflexion.

Ulnar deviation occurs at the radiocarpal level but radial deviation occurs at the mid-carpal level. During ulnar deviation the proximal carpal bones and the scaphoid dorsiflex; in radial deviation they palmarflex and the scaphoid bone appears foreshortened on radiographs (Fig. 16.7). The radioscaphocapitate ligament acts as a sling around which the scaphoid rotates during ulnar and radial deviation of the wrist. When there is disruption of the ligamentous attachments between the scaphoid and lunate ('scapholunate dissociation') the scaphoid can move independently of other carpal bones and tends to assume a palmarflexed position (see p. 466).

Classification of wrist injuries

Wrist injuries are classified by their anatomical site: the distal radius, the radiocarpal joint, the distal radioulnar joint and the carpus. More than one of these may be involved in severe injuries.

The injuries considered in this chapter are:

1 Fractures of the distal end of the radius
  (a) with dorsal displacement (Colles' fracture).
  (b) With volar displacement (Smith fracture).
2 Radiocarpal injuries
  (a) Dorsal fracture−subluxations.
  (b) Volar fracture−subluxations.
  (c) Fractures of the radial styloid.
3 Injuries of the distal radioulnar joint
  (a) Fractures involving the joint.
  (b) Fractures of the styloid process of the ulna.
  (c) Dislocation of the head of the ulna.
4 Carpal injuries
  (a) Ligamentous injuries and carpal instability.
  (b) Isolated fractures of carpal bones.
  (c) Carpal dislocations and fracture−dislocations.
5 Wrist injuries in childhood.

Diagnosis of wrist injuries

History

The history will indicate the force involved and possibly the position of the wrist at the moment of injury. Most wrist injuries are caused by forced dorsiflexion, resulting in compression of the dorsal structures and distraction of volar components. Frequently there is an element of rotation as well, either of the hand on the forearm or of the forearm on the fixed hand. Flexion injuries are less common. Rarely, the wrist may be crushed in the

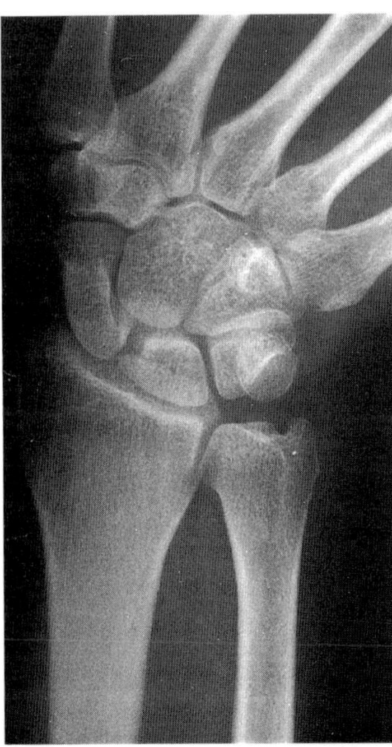
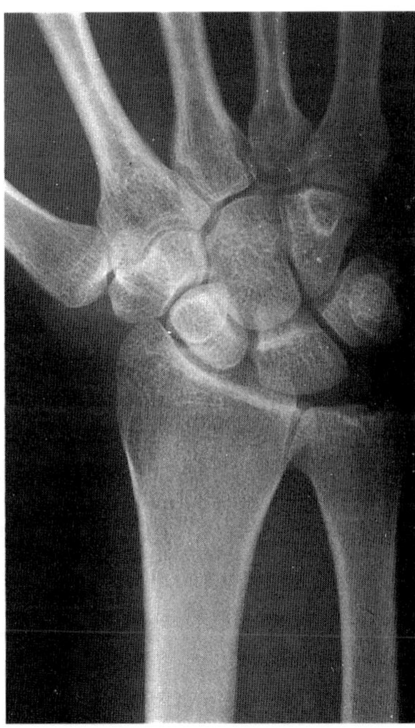

Fig. 16.7 When the wrist is radially deviated the scaphoid bone becomes palmarflexed within the carpus.

anteroposterior plane by direct forces that tend to flatten the arch of the carpus (Garcia-Elias *et al.* 1985).

Specific enquiry should be made about previous wrist injuries, hand dominance, occupation and leisure pursuits.

Physical examination

Swelling, bruising and deformity may be obvious on inspection. Characteristic gross deformities, such as a 'dinner fork' appearance, demand immediate radiological assessment without further examination, other than a rapid check of peripheral vascular and neurological function. However, many wrist injuries have less obvious signs, with perhaps only slight local swelling and tenderness.

In the non-swollen wrist many structures are palpable and even visible, allowing fairly precise definition of the anatomical location of any tenderness. The bony points that can be examined easily include the radial and ulnar styloid processes, Lister's tubercle, the tuberosities of the scaphoid and trapezoid bones at the base of the thenar eminence, the scaphoid bone in the floor of the anatomical snuff-box, the pisiform bone, the hook of the hamate, the head of the ulna and the distal radioulnar joint.

Active movements should be checked first. Dorsiflexion and palmar flexion can be compared in the two wrists by asking the patient to place the two hands together in the 'prayer' position and then abduct the arms. The backs of the hands are placed together to check palmar flexion. These are not true active movements, since the uninjured hand pushes against the injured one, but the patient can voluntarily limit any painful movement. Radial and ulnar deviation are compared in the two hands in the neutral position with respect to flexion−extension. Pronation and supination are tested with the elbows held against the trunk.

With some carpal subluxations particular movements may cause a painful snap in the wrist which the patient should be asked to demonstrate, if possible.

Wrist laxity should be assessed in suspected ligamentous injuries, provided that the examination can be carried out without causing severe pain. The normal wrist should be examined first as many people have quite marked wrist laxity. The forearm is stabilized by holding it just proximal to the wrist and the examiner moves the carpus in the dorso-volar and radioulnar planes. Clicking, snapping or palpable (and sometimes visible) subluxations may be identified in certain positions of the wrist. Any pain experienced with particular movements is noted.

Radiological examination

This is mandatory in suspected wrist injuries but the interpretation of radiographs calls for a great deal of experience. A surgeon familiar with the assessment of wrist injuries is inclined to forget that to junior medical staff in accident and emergency units the wrist radiograph may present a difficult challenge, particularly if the films are not of good quality. Subtle radiological changes are often overlooked and it is not unusual for gross injuries that are obvious to the experienced eye to be missed as well. In assessing wrist problems, as with so many other injuries, the doctor who first sees the patient must have a high index of suspicion and the willingness to seek further advice if the best treatment is to be given at an early stage.

Radiographs must be of high quality. The primary requirements are for anteroposterior and lateral views with the wrist in neutral flexion−extension. If a scaphoid fracture is suspected, then pronation-oblique and supination-oblique views should be added.

The history and physical findings will dictate whether more specialized views are needed. These include the carpal tunnel view (Hart & Gaynor 1941), the carpal bridge view to show abnormalities on the dorsum of the wrist (Lentino *et al.* 1957), views of the hook of the hamate (Polivy *et al.* 1985) and views of the tuberosity of the trapezium (Palmer 1981). If instability is suspected it is useful to take films with the fist clenched to provide a dynamic load. Static collapse patterns may be obvious on standard films but additional views in radial and ulnar deviation will demonstrate alteration in the normal intercarpal movements. Dynamic displacements of intercarpal joints may be seen on films taken when the wrist is placed in the appropriate position, but are better assessed by video-radiographs of a series of standard wrist movements and of movements that produce symptoms in the wrist.

Because of superimposition of the carpal bones it may be difficult to identify fractures in complex fracture−dislocations of the carpus. In this situation it is often useful to take views of the carpus with traction applied at the time of reduction, as these will often demonstrate small fragments that would otherwise be overlooked.

Wrist arthrography (Palmer *et al.* 1983) will show any abnormal flow of contrast between compartments, indicating ligamentous tears, and is best combined with video-radiography. Other special techniques that can be helpful in certain circumstances include tomography and computerized axial tomography (CAT) scanning. Isotope bone scanning will demonstrate lesions, such as occult fractures, bone cysts, early degenerative changes and Kienböck disease, that may not be visible on plain films. The role of magnetic resonance imaging (MRI) in wrist injuries is currently being evaluated; it seems to be especially helpful in demonstrating soft tissue changes and the vascularity of bone (Imaeda *et al.* 1992).

Fractures of the distal end of the radius

Fractures with dorsal displacement (Colles' fracture)

A Colles' fracture is a fracture of the distal radius within 3.75 cm of the distal articular surface of the radius with dorsal displacement of the distal fragment. Colles described this fracture, its management and outcome in detail in 1814 (Colles 1814). It is the commonest wrist fracture in adults, especially in the elderly, and leads to huge demands on outpatient clinic and physiotherapy services.

Nature of injury

The fracture usually occurs as the result of a fall onto the outstretched hand. The radiographic appearance of the fracture suggests that the volar surface of the radius fails in tension. The fracture line is clean without any comminution and the periosteum is torn on the volar surface. The dorsal surface of the radius fails in compression and shear and the fracture line is often comminuted. Impaction of the cancellous bone may occur. A varying extent of the dorsal periosteum remains intact, depending on the severity of the injury. It has been demonstrated that the less the dorsiflexion of the wrist at the moment of impact, the smaller is the force required to fracture the distal radius, and the greater is the chance of an intra-articular fracture. A greater force is required to fracture normal bone than that required to fracture osteoporotic bone.

Damage to the adjacent soft tissues also occurs, depending on the magnitude and direction of the forces of impact. Tearing of the volar periosteum has already been mentioned. The articular cartilage of the wrist joint sustains a crushing injury, the ligaments of the wrist may be stretched or torn and traumatic synovitis may occur within tendon sheaths. In addition, the median and, less commonly, the ulnar and radial nerves may be injured at the moment of impact. Apart from the nerve lesions, it is difficult to assess the degree of soft tissue injury following a Colles' fracture. Associated soft tissue injury is an important factor in relation to continuing symptoms after the fracture has healed. This, however, is not commonly appreciated by those treating this very common fracture.

While a Colles' fracture can occur in any age group (before skeletal maturity a similar injury results in a distal greenstick fracture of the diaphysis or metaphysis, or a Salter–Harris type II injury of the distal epiphysis of the radius), it is most common in the sixth decade and occurs predominantly in females. It has been demonstrated that 75% of elderly (>55 years of age) patients with this fracture have osteoporosis (Dias *et al.* 1987b). It is also known that these patients are at greater risk of sustaining a femoral neck fracture (Gay 1974). Osteoporosis not only predisposes to a fracture after minimal trauma but also increases the amount of collapse at the fracture, owing to the crushing of cancellous bone at the time of injury. In addition, probably by reducing the ability to resist deforming forces in the healing phase, osteoporosis facilitates the progression of the bony deformity.

Classification

Numerous classifications of this injury have been proposed; the most common are that of Gartland and Werley (1953) and the more cumbersome Frykman (1967) classification, which is based on the presence or absence of an intra-articular extension and an ulnar styloid fracture. Both these features rarely influence management. The authors, therefore, prefer to consider this fracture as being either undisplaced or displaced, depending on whether a reduction was needed.

UNDISPLACED FRACTURES

Patients without a clinical deformity are considered to have an undisplaced fracture. In some of these patients, especially those who are plump, minimal bony deformity may be present on radiographs (Fig. 16.8). Any undisplaced intra-articular extension can be disregarded.

DISPLACED FRACTURES

Patients with a clinical deformity are considered to have a displaced fracture requiring reduction (Fig. 16.9). Displaced fractures can be further divided into three types as follows:

1 The displacement is only at the metaphyseal fracture line; any intra-articular extension is essentially undisplaced.

2 The displacement has occurred at both the metaphyseal region and in the intra-articular fracture (arbitrarily taken as a >2 mm gap or step at the fracture site).

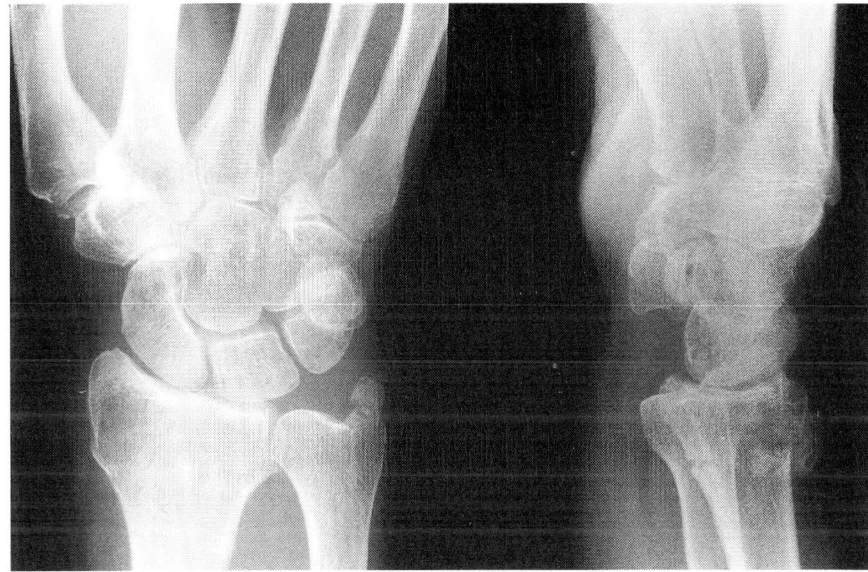

Fig. 16.8 A minimally displaced Colles' fracture. On the posteroanterior radiograph a transverse fracture of the distal radius is seen. There is no obvious radial tilt or shortening, nor is there any radial shift. The fracture does not enter either the radiocarpal joint or the distal radioulnar joint. There is a fracture of the body of the ulnar styloid with very slight displacement. On the lateral projection the distal radius fragment has tilted back with a loss of the normal 11° forward tilt. There is some comminution of the dorsal cortex. Note how the lunate is already facing dorsally.

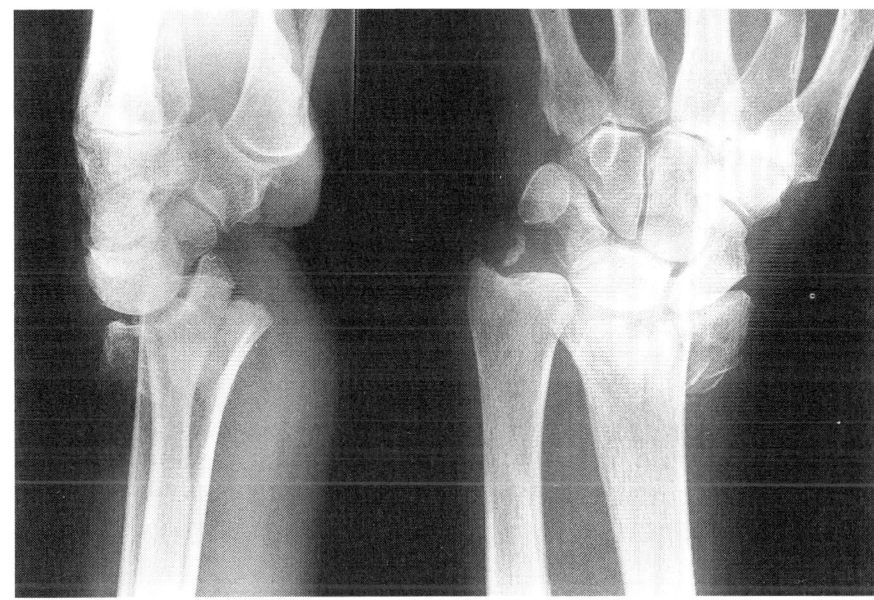

Fig. 16.9 A displaced Colles' fracture. On the posteroanterior radiograph a transverse fracture of the distal radius is seen. There is obvious radial tilt and shortening with the radial styloid now lying proximal to the distal articular surface of the ulna. There is a marked radial shift. It is difficult to establish whether the fracture line extends into either the radiocarpal joint or the distal radioulnar joint. There is a fracture of the tip of the ulnar styloid with very considerable displacement. On the lateral projection the distal radius fragment has tilted back. The gap between the scaphoid and lunate appears normal.

The integrity of the scapholunate ligament must be established.

3 There is gross comminution of the metaphyseal region involving a large area of the dorsum only, or also involving some of the volar cortex, and resulting in an unstable fracture.

For patients with a displaced fracture one further factor must be taken into account in planning the management and that is the quality of bone. Osteoporosis would preclude most attempts at internal fixation.

Signs and symptoms

The patient, usually a female in her sixties, presents with a painful and swollen wrist following a fall onto an outstretched hand. Local tenderness over the distal radius can be elicited. The deformity, which is not always present, is as described by Colles in 1814.

The posterior surface of the limb presents a considerable deformity; for a depression is seen in the forearm, about an inch and a half above the end of this bone, while considerable swelling occupies the wrist and the metacarpus. Indeed, the carpus and the base of the metacarpus appear to be thrown backward so much, as on first view to excite a suspicion that the carpus has been dislocated forward (dinner fork deformity).

...The extremity of the ulna is seen projecting towards the palm and the inner edge of the limb...If the surgeon proceeds to investigate the nature of this injury he will find the end of the ulna admits of being readily moved backwards and forwards.

In addition, specific examination should be carried out to determine injury to the soft tissues, especially the median and ulnar nerves. Clinical examination must also include the elbow, shoulder and neck, as any or all of these regions may be injured by the fall (e.g. fracture of the neck of the humerus).

Radiographic evaluation

A posteroanterior and a lateral view usually provides enough information regarding the site of the fracture, the extent of comminution and the presence of any intra-articular fracture. In addition, a fracture of the ulnar styloid (33% of patients) or the head of the ulna can also be demonstrated.

The displacement of the distal fragment can be measured on the posteroanterior and lateral views (Fig. 16.10). The distal fragment can displace as follows: dorsal angulation, dorsal shift, radial angulation, radial shift, impaction or shortening and supination.

In the normal wrist the distal articular surface of the radius is angled so that it faces palmarwards (volar tilt) by a mean of 11° (range 0–20°). Any change in this forward inclination can be seen and measured on the lateral radiograph. The lateral view establishes that the distal fragment has tilted dorsally (as opposed to the volar tilt in a Smith fracture or the volar shift of an intra-articular Barton fracture).

In a normal wrist the distal end of the radius is angled towards the ulna by 26° (range 18–35°). The radial length (the difference between the levels of the distal articular surface of the ulna and the tip of the radial styloid) is usually 11 mm (range 7–14 mm). The displacement of the distal fragment is represented on a posteroanterior radiograph as a change in angulation and radial length. In addition, any lateral translation (radial shift) of the distal fragment can be noted.

These radiographs should also be carefully reviewed to exclude any carpal injury, in particular scapholunate ligament disruption with an increase in the gap between the scaphoid and lunate.

Treatment

The classic method of treatment is closed reduction of the fracture and immobilization in a plaster of Paris below-elbow cast, with the wrist in slight palmar flexion and ulnar deviation until the fracture has healed.

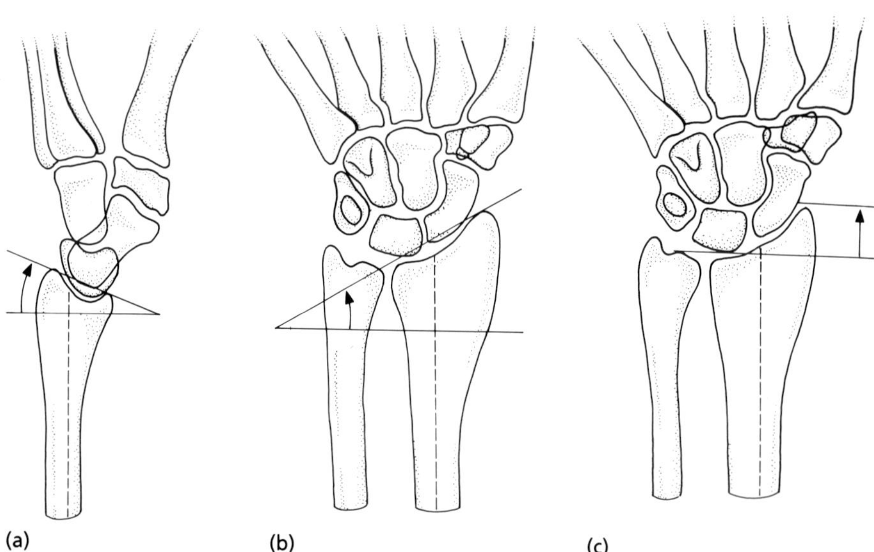

(a)   (b)   (c)

Fig. 16.10 The normal orientation of the distal articular surface of the radius. (a) On the lateral projection the distal articular surface is tilted volarwards by a mean of 11°. (b) On the posteroanterior projection the distal articular surface of the radius is tilted by a mean of 26° towards the ulna. (c) The tip of the radial styloid lies on average 11 mm distal to the distal articular surface of the ulna.

UNDISPLACED FRACTURES

In undisplaced fractures, the authors believe that the only reason for immobilization is to ease the discomfort. Such a fracture, regardless of any intra-articular extension, is essentially stable and is unlikely to displace significantly (Fig. 16.11). It has been demonstrated that 'undisplaced' fractures can safely be treated without immobilization (Dias *et al.* 1987c). This leads to a rapid resolution of swelling and recovery of function (Fig. 16.12).

The authors' present policy is to provide patients with a removable wrist splint and encourage them to remove the splint and use the hand, within the limits of comfort, from the very outset. Patients are reassured regarding the stability of the fracture and are warned that the discomfort could last for the initial 2 weeks. They are also told that the hand might feel weaker than normal. In particular, they are told to be careful with hot cups of tea etc. where they might put themselves or others at risk of scalding.

Patients are reviewed at around 3 weeks after injury, at which stage a careful assessment of wrist movement and strength is made. The clinical deformity is noted and, if repeat radiographs demonstrate marked deterioration of the position of the fracture, a manipulation under anaesthesia may be needed. However, the authors have not yet had to manipulate an undisplaced fracture treated in this manner.

These patients usually recover 75% of their wrist movement within 5 weeks (Fig. 16.12). If they were treated in a conventional plaster cast for 5 weeks they would require at least 3 months to regain a similar range of wrist movement and strength (Dias *et al.* 1987c).

Displaced fractures in poor quality bone

In these patients a clinical deformity exists which requires correction. The fracture needs to be reduced under a local, regional or general anaesthetic. It is important to ensure that the patient does not experience any unneccessary pain during reduction as this will make the reduction more difficult and might result in accepting a less than optimal position. A regional intravenous anaesthetic or a general anaesthetic is advisable.

The patient lies supine with the arm abducted to 90° and the elbow flexed to 90° so that the forearm lies parallel to the patient's body. Axial traction is applied by grasping the thumb and radial two fingers. Counter-traction is provided by an assistant pulling on the arm just above the elbow. This results in disimpaction of the fracture and correction of the radial deviation and radial

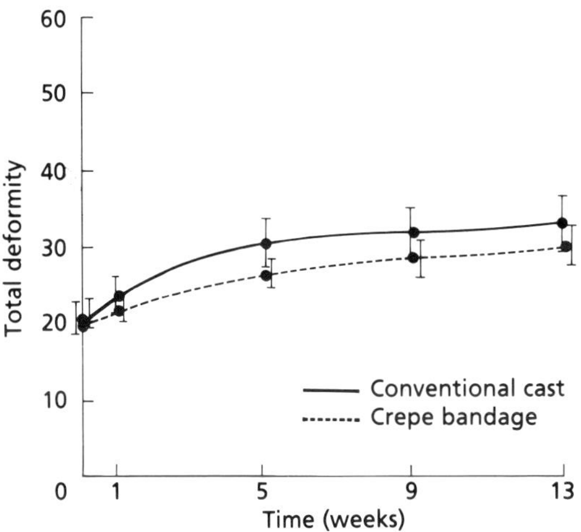

Fig. **16.11** The graph demonstrates the progression of the bony deformity in the healing phase in 47 patients with minimally displaced fractures treated conventionally and in 50 patients with similar fractures treated in a crepe bandage. The tilt of the distal fragment of the radius worsened by a mean of 5°. There was no significant difference between the two groups. (After Dias *et al.* 1987c.)

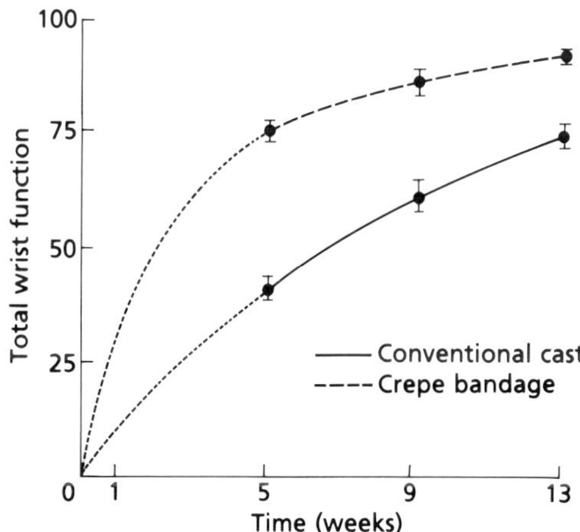

Fig. **16.12** The graph demonstrates the recovery of wrist movement in a group of 97 patients (47 treated conventionally and 50 treated in a crepe bandage). (After Dias *et al.* 1987c.)

shift of the distal fragment.

The dorsal tilt is then reduced by initially increasing the dorsiflexion of the distal fragment, in order to align the dorsal cortical surfaces, following which the distal fragment is flexed, thereby correcting the dorsal tilt and dorsal shift. Finally, the wrist is moulded by placing the flat of one hand under the volar surface proximal to the fracture while the other hand, over the dorso-radial aspect of the distal fragment, pushes it into flexion and ulnar deviation. The whole manoeuvre must be gentle so as not to extend the soft tissue component of the injury. Special care must be taken if the skin is fragile to avoid superficial avulsion of the skin. For a superlative and detailed description of the principles and method of reduction of the Colles' fracture the reader is referred to Charnley's account of the closed manipulation of fractures (Charnley 1974).

Adequacy of reduction, in the absence of marked swelling, may be assessed by the clinical appearance of the hand: absence of radial deviation of the wrist, absence of the prominent ulnar styloid and absence of the dinner fork deformity. Careful palpation may reveal the absence of the dorsal step between the proximal and distal fragments. The radial styloid, which is usually 1 cm distal to the ulnar styloid, provides information regarding correction of the radial length of the distal fragment. Posteroanterior and lateral radiographs are usually obtained to confirm the adequacy of the reduction.

Once the fracture has been reduced, the forearm is put into a below-elbow cast with moulding as described. The wrist is usually in neutral or in slight palmar flexion and ulnar deviation. The plaster cast is retained for 5–6 weeks. At 3 weeks the patient is reviewed and radiographs are obtained to determine whether significant re-displacement has occurred.

During the healing period the three main concerns are: (i) to promote resolution of any swelling, (ii) to promote functional recovery, and (iii) to prevent deformity of the wrist.

RESOLUTION OF SWELLING

Following adequate initial treatment the injured arm is placed in a broad arm sling for the first few days, and the patient is cautioned against leaving the hand in a dependent position. The patient has to be informed to return immediately if pain or swelling fails to subside after even a short period (around 1 hour) of high elevation, as the plaster may require splitting. If the injury was severe and marked swelling is anticipated, the patient may need admission and overhead elevation of the affected limb under close monitoring. The need for this, however, is uncommon. A carefully applied plaster cast should avoid any local constriction caused by injudicious finger pressure. In any event, if the injury was severe, the plaster should be split along the dorso-ulnar region and any underlying padding must also be cut to expose underlying skin. The plaster must be split along its entire length to avoid a proximal constriction. Subsequently, this cast may be reinforced or replaced after the resolution of swelling.

RECOVERY OF FUNCTION

The second concern is to regain function as quickly as possible. The patient is advised to use the hand, within the limits of comfort, from the very outset. When the cast has been removed, active exercises are demonstrated and the patient is encouraged to use the hand as normally as possible. At this stage reassurance needs to be given that (i) the stiffness of the wrist, (ii) the weakness of the hand and (iii) the ulnar styloid discomfort, especially on forearm rotation, is not uncommon and usually gets better with time. The patient should be followed-up in 2–4 weeks, depending on the stiffness of the wrist, in order to determine whether supervised physiotherapy is needed. If there is persistent significant swelling of the wrist and fingers or if non-compliance is anticipated, the patient should be referred for supervised physiotherapy immediately. Active shoulder movements should also be encouraged to prevent stiffness.

THE DEFORMITY

The third concern is to prevent deformity. Colles, in 1814, pointed out that the deformity could recur even in a splint if it were loose. It has been shown that a plaster cast, regardless of its extent or the position of the forearm in it, does not prevent the tendency of the deformity to recur. This recurrence is very gradual and the deformity, as seen on radiographs obtained at 2 weeks, may be such that it is considered to be acceptable. The progression of deformity, however, continues long after the plaster cast has been removed (Fig. 16.13). Osteoporotic bone, especially, results in a greater recurrence of the deformity and probably reflects the impaired ability of the healing osteoporotic bone to withstand axial loading (Dias *et al.* 1987c).

The radial deviation and the radial shift recur completely. A dorsal tilt of less than 20° may also recur completely. However, a dorsal tilt of the distal radius of greater than 20° usually heals in a better position after reduction. It would therefore appear that in elderly patients, with an initial deformity of less than 20° of dorsal tilt, reduction does not achieve any significant improvement (Dias *et al.* 1987c). These patients are usually left with a hand which is slightly radially deviated and in which the ulnar styloid is prominent.

Displaced fractures in good quality bone

In the young patient with a displaced fracture the injury is usually more severe and one can expect greater swell-

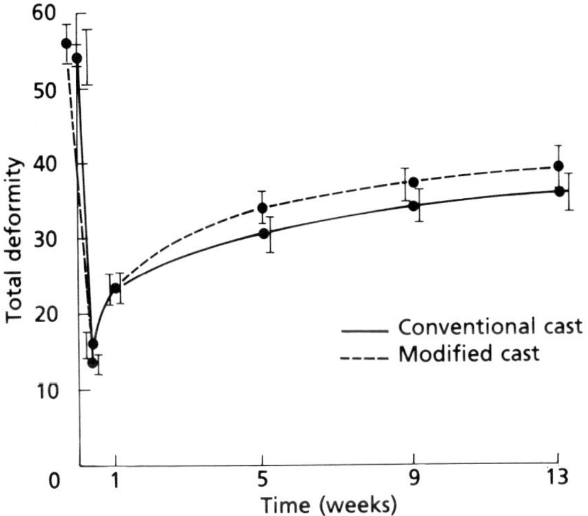

Fig. 16.13 The graph demonstrates the progression of the bony deformity in the healing phase in 47 patients with displaced fractures treated conventionally and in 43 patients with similar fractures treated in a modified cast which allowed early wrist movement. The deformity in both groups of patients tended to recur, not only while the wrist was in a plaster cast but even after plaster immobilization had ceased. (After Dias *et al.* 1987c.)

ing. The injured limb must, therefore, be closely monitored and every effort (high elevation and use of an incomplete plaster cast) must be made to prevent the complications of swelling. Also, the good bone quality means that any reduction achieved is likely to be maintained in the healing phase. The displaced Colles' fracture in the young patient, therefore, merits greater

effort in achieving an accurate reduction.

In a young patient with a displaced and unstable Colles' fracture, and in whom the comminution is either extensive or involves the volar surface too, external fixation may be considered in order to regain the length and hold the wrist during the healing phase. If there is an intra-articular fracture into the radiocarpal joint, with either opening of the fracture line or depression of one or more articular fragments, the possibility of scapholunate ligament injury must also be considered.

If possible, the distal pins should be introduced into the metaphysis in order to leave the wrist joint free to mobilize. This, however, is rarely possible and the distal pins may need to be introduced into the second or third metacarpal bones, thereby immobilizing the wrist during the healing phase of 6–8 weeks.

SURGICAL TECHNIQUE

The fracture is reduced by axial distraction using Chinese finger traps (Fig. 16.14). Once the position, as seen on the image intensifier, is considered to be acceptable two proximal and two distal pins are introduced. The distal pins are introduced into the proximal ends of the index and middle metacarpals. The index metacarpal pin is introduced into its dorso-radial surface while the middle metacarpal pin is introduced perpendicular to the plane of the hand. The proximal pins are introduced into the shaft of the radius, as close to the fracture line as possible. One pin is introduced in the plane of the index metacarpal pin and another is introduced in the

Fig. 16.14 The deformity is corrected by distraction using finger traps. The corrected position is maintained by a four-bar, four-pin external fixator. In the diagram each distal pin is shown in a separate metacarpal but both may be placed in the index metacarpal, provided that a 90° separation is maintained. Although the apparatus can be assembled and tightened with distraction, it is usually preferable to translocate the distal fragment palmarwards and release the distraction immediately before tightening the external fixator. (After Cooney *et al.* 1979.)

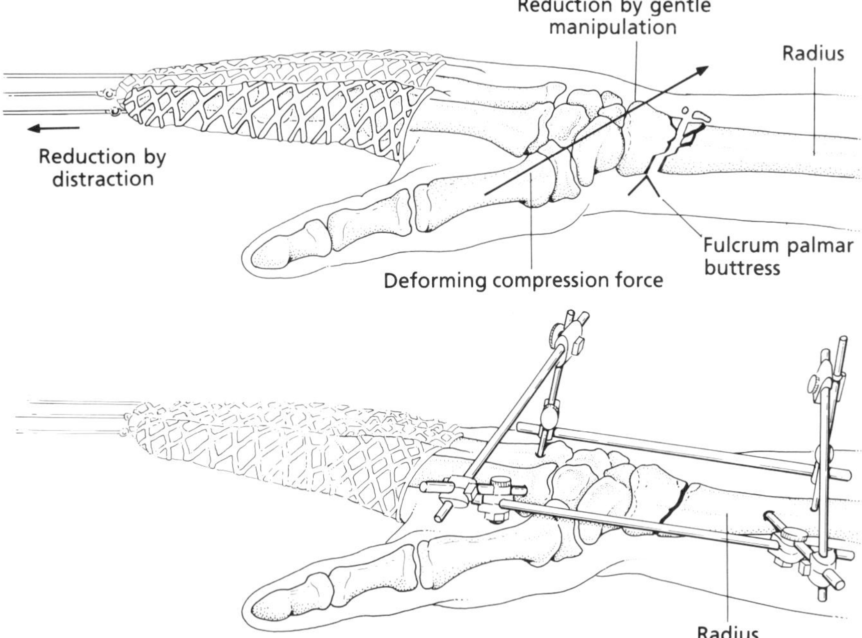

plane of the middle metacarpal pin. Care must be exercised in order to avoid damage to the superficial division of the radial nerve during introduction of the pins into the radius. A four-bar frame is then constructed using the mini Hoffman or a similar fixator. Before the bars are locked into position, the axial distraction is decreased to allow bone apposition in an optimal position, as determined on an image intensifier. The postoperative treatment is similar to that for conservatively managed Colles' fractures (Cooney *et al.* 1979).

A unilateral frame may also be constructed using two parallel pins inserted into the proximal index metacarpal and two pins inserted in the distal radius proximal to the fracture. All pins should lie in the same plane.

Some fixators are now available which allow some movement at the wrist during the healing phase. The value of such fixators is uncertain.

When there is a considerable loss of cancellous bone volume because of compaction the need for cancellous bone graft must be considered. If required, this is best introduced through a short longitudinal dorsal incision between the extensor pollicis longus and the extensor digitorum.

Complications

The most common complications of a Colles' fracture are malunion and wrist stiffness (Cooney *et al.* 1980a).

Malunion

As a Colles' fracture is most frequently seen in postmenopausal osteoporotic females, it is difficult to prevent malunion by any form of external splintage. In addition, the poor bone quality and degree of comminution often precludes most methods of internal or external fixation. Most patients with displaced fractures will be left with radially deviated hands with a prominent ulnar styloid. A persistent dinner fork deformity is uncommon. If the pain in the distal radioulnar joint, on forearm rotation, is particularly bothersome one might need to excise the ulnar head, as described by Darrach (1927).

Stiffness

Stiffness of the wrist results from bony deformity and periarticular adhesions secondary to the soft tissue component of the injury. Careful splintage and elevation, to promote the resolution of swelling, together with early mobilization of the wrist and hand, within the limits of comfort, promotes a rapid recovery of function. In displaced fractures the stiffness might persist for a long time and may take more than a year to resolve.

Some patients develop reflex sympathetic dystrophy following a Colles' fracture. This leads to progressive stiffness of the wrist and fingers and to other well-recognized symptoms and signs (see Chapter 11).

Carpal tunnel syndrome

Approximately one in seven patients with a Colles' fracture will have some clinical evidence of compression of the median nerve at the wrist. This is probably due to an injury to the median nerve at the time of impact or is secondary to the oedema within the carpal tunnel. These patients are usually older (in their mid-sixties). In most instances the symptoms resolve within 6 months. If no improvement occurs, or if the symptoms persist beyond 6 months, nerve conduction studies should be carried out to confirm the diagnosis and a formal decompression of the carpal tunnel must be considered (Stewart *et al.* 1985).

The ulnar nerve at the wrist and the superficial division of the radial nerve may develop signs of irritation. These usually improve spontaneously.

Rupture of the extensor pollicis longus tendon

A rupture of the extensor pollicis longus tendon usually occurs between 5 and 12 weeks after injury. The tendon ruptures over the dorsum of the distal radius, where it turns around the Lister's tubercle. It is probably caused by compromised vascularity of the tendon at this site and/or attrition of the tendon, over a bony spur, following the fracture. The displacement of the fracture is usually minimal and this would favour a vascular etiology. The patient presents with a sudden inability to extend the interphalangeal joint of the thumb. The treatment, if the patient regards the inability to extend the interphalangeal joint of the thumb as disabling, consists of transferring the extensor indicis proprius tendon (divided at the level of the neck of the index metacarpal) to the distal stump of the extensor pollicis longus tendon at the level of the middle of the thumb metacarpal.

Shoulder stiffness

This is not an uncommon complication of Colles' fracture and is probably caused by injury to the shoulder at the time of the fall. All patients with this fracture are encouraged to put their shoulders through a full range of movement from the outset in order to prevent any stiffness. Very occasionally, refractory stiffness may occur as a component of reflex sympathetic dystrophy: the shoulder—hand syndrome (Frykman 1967).

Intercarpal collapse

It has been suggested that a change in the orientation of the distal articular surface of the radius results in a dorsal intercalated segment carpal instability (DISI). Indeed, Taleisnik and Watson (1984) reported corrective osteotomies of the distal radius in 13 patients with this complication with a resolution of symptoms. It has been demonstrated that the magnitude of any change in the radiolunocapitate angle is directly proportional to the change in the volar angulation of the distal radius after such a fracture. The scapholunate angle is similarly dependent on the radial angulation of the distal radius (Dias & McMohan 1988). Whether these changes are, to some extent, responsible for the functional disability following Colles' fractures and whether it represents true ligamentous instability is unknown.

Other complications

Trigger finger, DeQuervain's stenosing tenovaginitis and Dupuytrens disease have all been documented following Colles' fracture (Stewart *et al.* 1985). Depending on the magnitude of articular surface disorganization and of cartilage injury, the patient may develop secondary degenerative wrist arthritis.

The long-term disability after Colles' fractures in the elderly

There is very little information in the literature regarding the long-term disability after Colles' fractures in the elderly. Smaill (1965) reviewed 41 out of 97 patients with such fractures over 5 years after injury and demonstrated that although over half had a cosmetic deformity, most patients had very good wrist movement and were satisfied. In a recent (personal series) 6-year review of elderly patients with Colles' fractures who had been studied prospectively, 19.1% of the patients had moderate or severe pain and 17.2% had wrist stiffness, although only 10.6% said they were bothered by the pain and only 2.4% were bothered by the stiffness. The appearance of the hand concerned 4.7%, although 23.4% had moderate radial deviation of the hand. The range of movement in all cases was better than 75% of that of the opposite side with a mean of 96.2%. The deformity did not correlate with the range of movement.

The disability, however, was considerable; 32.9% had difficulty opening jars and 24.7% could not wring a cloth as a consequence of the wrist fracture. They also had difficulty lifting a full kettle (15.9%) or a full saucepan (20.2%).

It would appear, therefore, that although patients with a Colles' fracture recover their range of wrist and forearm movement almost completely, one in four patients with a Colles' fracture will have persisting disability which would interfere with their ability to perform daily tasks.

Conclusion

Colles' fracture is one of the most common fractures, especially in the elderly osteoporotic female. Malunion is common, but providing adequate emphasis is given to functional recovery, the outcome need not be as poor as it has been in the past. Undisplaced fractures do not require immobilization; this results in rapid recovery of function without the complications of a plaster cast.

Fractures with volar displacement (Smith fracture)

This type of fracture is said to result from a fall on the back of the hand with the wrist flexed, but can also be caused by a direct blow on the dorsum of the hand with the wrist flexed; the frequency of this injury in motorcyclists would tend to indicate that the latter mechanism is quite common.

Classification

There is some confusion about the nomenclature and classification of fractures of the distal end of the radius with volar displacement. Thomas (1957) described three types of Smith fracture:

Type 1 — an extra-articular fracture occurring mainly in older females; this is the classic 'reversed Colles' fracture' (Fig. 16.15).

Type 2 — an anterior marginal fracture of the distal articular surface of the radius with volar and proximal displacement of the entire carpus (Fig. 16.16).

Type 3 — the same type of fracture as type 1 but occurring in younger people and believed to be caused by a blow on the knuckles as occurs in motorcycle accidents. Since the mechanism of injury may be difficult to ascertain, there is probably little significance in distinguishing between type 1 and type 3 fractures.

In considering this group of injuries a clear distinction should be made between extra-articular fractures and

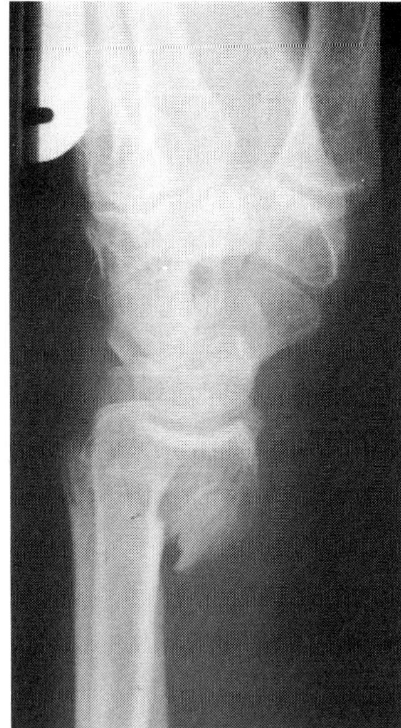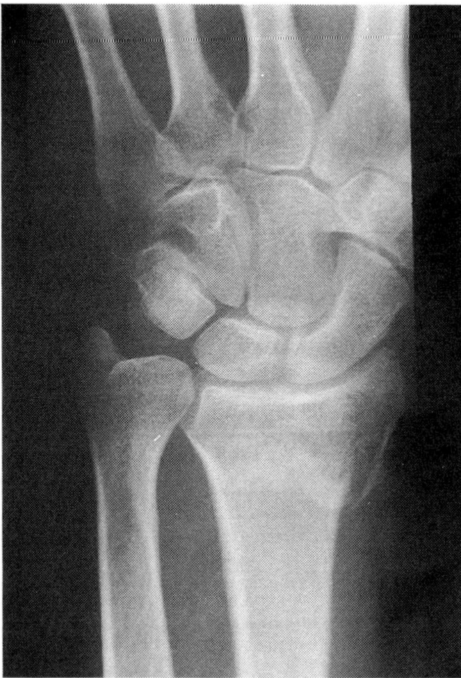

Fig. 16.15 A type 1 Smith fracture.

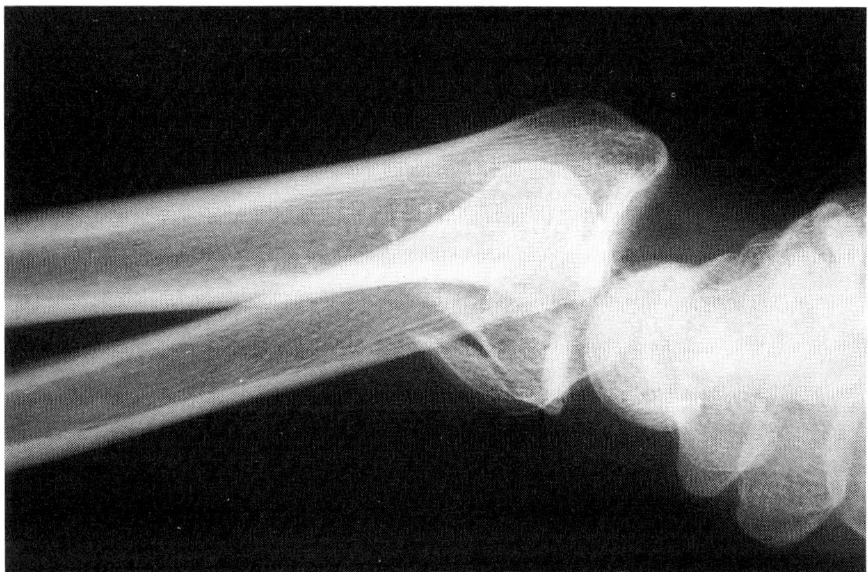

Fig. 16.16 A type 2 Smith fracture.

intra-articular fractures with subluxation of the carpus. A dorsal lip fracture of the distal end of the radius, with or without dorsal shift of the carpus, is known as the Barton fracture. Barton's name is also associated with the opposite, less common, injury (i.e. a Thomas type 2 Smith fracture, 'reverse Barton fracture') (Ellis 1965, De Oliveira 1973). These fracture—subluxations will be discussed separately in the subsequent section and only the extra-articular fracture of the distal end of the radius

with volar displacement (Thomas type 1 and type 3) will be considered here.

Clinical and radiological features

As with any wrist injury there is pain, tenderness and swelling. The hand is displaced in a palmar direction but this may not be very apparent if there is much swelling.

Radiographs confirm the volar shift of the distal articular surface of the radius (Fig. 16.15).

Treatment

Under appropriate anaesthesia the fragments are first disimpacted by longitudinal traction. Then, while gripping the patient's forearm with one hand, the surgeon uses the thenar eminence of the other hand to reduce the fracture by pressing over the volar surface of the distal end of the radius and supinating the patient's hand. There is no need to bring the wrist into dorsiflexion.

Stable fractures can be held in a moulded forearm cast but there is a tendency for displacement to occur as swelling goes down and it is preferable to apply an above-elbow cast with the forearm held in supination for the first 2–3 weeks. Protection in a cast for 6 weeks is usually sufficient.

Most of these fractures can be treated conservatively but if it proves difficult to maintain reduction the fracture may be stabilized using a buttress plate (Fig. 16.17) (Ellis 1965, Fuller 1973) (see p. 463).

Complications

These are the same as those encountered in fractures of the distal end of the radius with dorsal displacement.

Radiocarpal injuries

Fracture–subluxations

These may be in a dorsal or volar direction, depending on the direction of force and the configuration of the fracture. Fractures of the radial and ulnar styloid processes are frequently associated.

Dorsal

The dorsal rim fracture with dorsal subluxation (Barton fracture) (Fig. 16.18) is caused by forced pronation of the forearm on the fixed dorsiflexed wrist. Typically, the injury occurs in a young person involved in a high-energy accident such as a fall from a height. The dorsal displacement is obvious clinically and confirmed by radiographic examination. Reduction is straightforward but may be unstable, particularly if the wrist is held palmarflexed (Taleisnik 1985) (Fig. 16.19), and it may be necessary to hold the carpus on the radius with percutaneous Kirschner (K) wires or external fixation.

Volar

Dislocation in a volar direction is usually associated with a fracture of the distal end of the radius that may involve the volar lip (reverse Barton fracture) (Fig. 16.20)

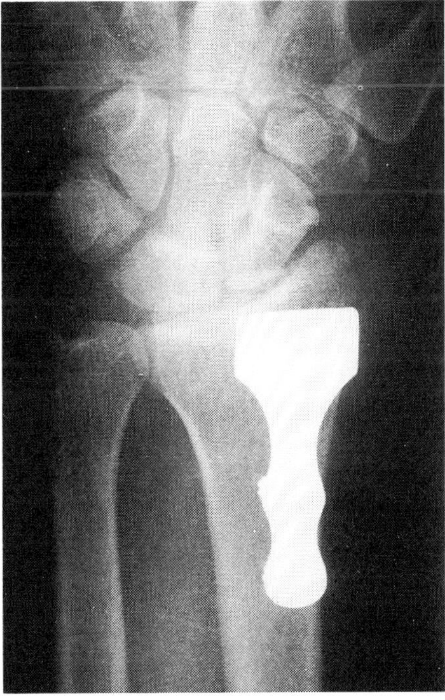
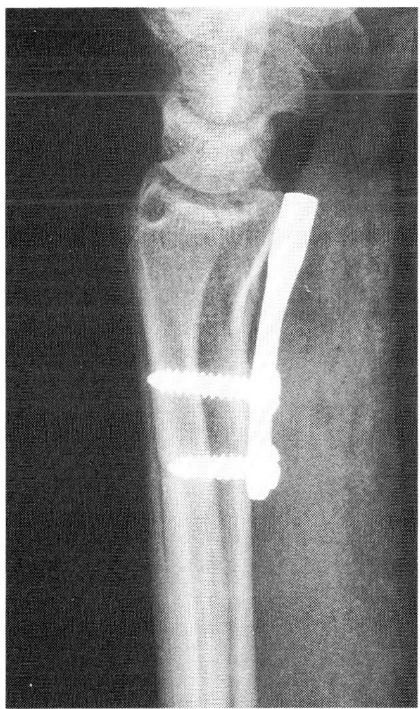

Fig. 16.17 A buttress plate applied to a type 2 Smith fracture.

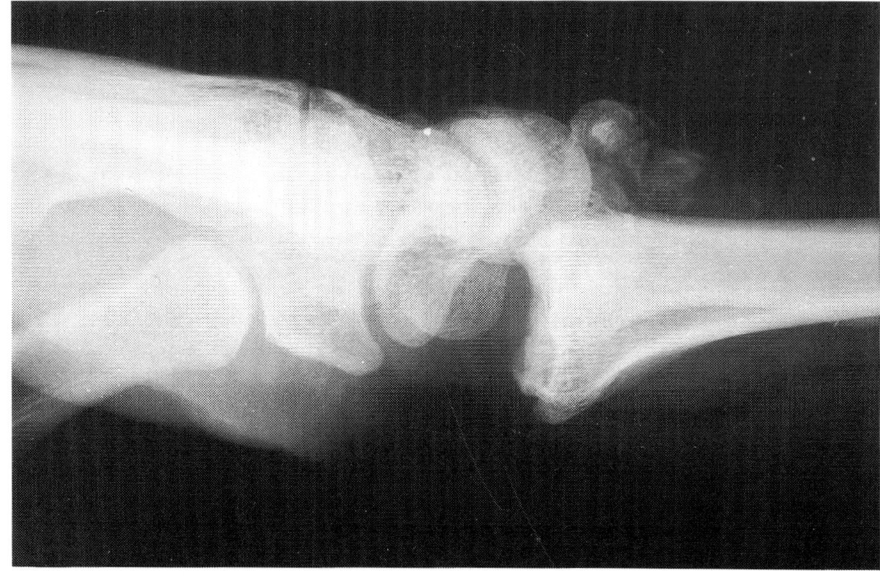

Fig. 16.18 Dorsal radiocarpal dislocation with lip fracture.

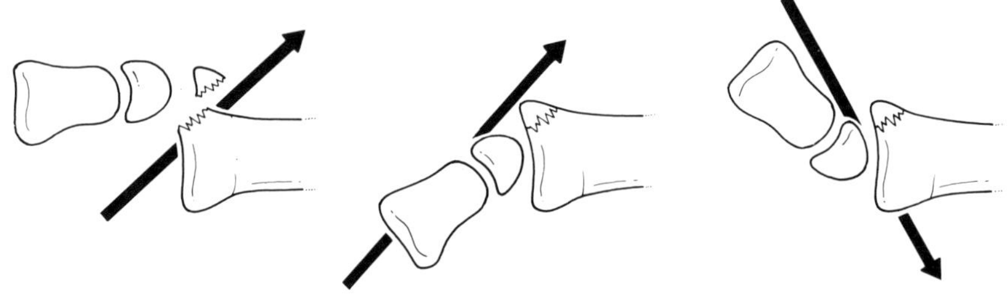

Fig. 16.19 Reduction of the dorsal radiocarpal dislocation is unstable when the wrist is flexed. The wrist must be dorsiflexed. The reverse holds true for palmar carpal dislocations.

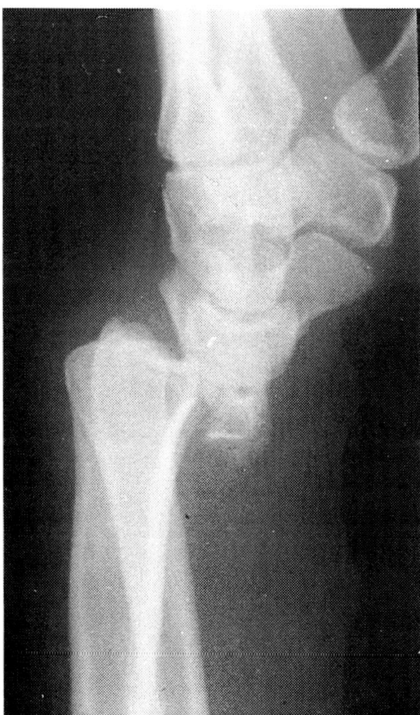
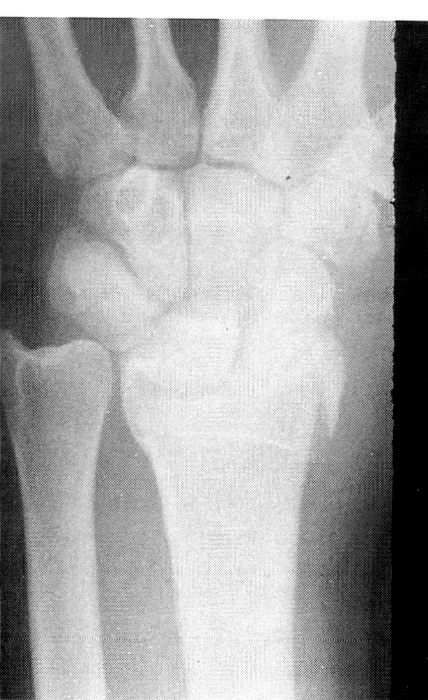

Fig. 16.20 Volar radiocarpal dislocation with lip fracture.

or, more commonly, most of the articular surface (Thomas type 2 variety of Smith fracture) (Fig. 16.16).

Like the dorsal fracture−subluxation these are high-energy injuries occurring in young people, probably caused by forced supination of the forearm on the fixed dorsiflexed wrist. The physical and radiographic features are diagnostic. Reduction is straightforward but these are unstable injuries. If there is a volar lip fracture the radiocarpal joint should be stabilized with K-wires after reduction. The sheared volar surface of the distal end of the radius should be stabilized with a buttress plate, such as the Ellis plate (Ellis 1965, Fuller 1973). The fracture is exposed through a longitudinal incision radial to the tendon of the flexor carpi radialis, and part of the pronator quadratus muscle is detached, if necessary. The plate is contoured to the curve of the distal radius and fixed with screws proximally, the broad distal part of the plate holding the fracture reduced. A protective forearm cast is worn for 4−6 weeks.

Fractures of the radial styloid process

This fracture (Fig. 16.21) is now most commonly the result of a fall on the outstretched hand, the mechanism probably being direct impact of the scaphoid on the articular surface of the radius. Formerly, the injury was often the result of a backfire causing a starting crank-handle to jerk backwards suddenly (Edwards 1926).

Tenderness and swelling are noted over the radial styloid process. The diagnosis is confirmed by radiographic examination, although the fracture may not be seen clearly on lateral films. The carpus should be scrutinized carefully for evidence of ligamentous disruption, which is sometimes associated with this injury.

Reduction is rarely necessary. The wrist is protected in a forearm cast for 5−6 weeks. There may be some stiffness and discomfort in the wrist for a while after this injury, probably as a result of associated ligamentous damage.

Stabilization with K-wires may be advisable if there is a large displaced fragment.

Injuries of the distal radioulnar joint

Fractures and ligamentous injuries of the distal radioulnar joint usually occur in association with fractures of the distal radius, and the joint is less commonly injured in isolation (Vesely 1967). Often, such injuries will also involve the ulnocarpal complex which, as mentioned in the anatomical introduction to this chapter, is part of the radiocarpal joint.

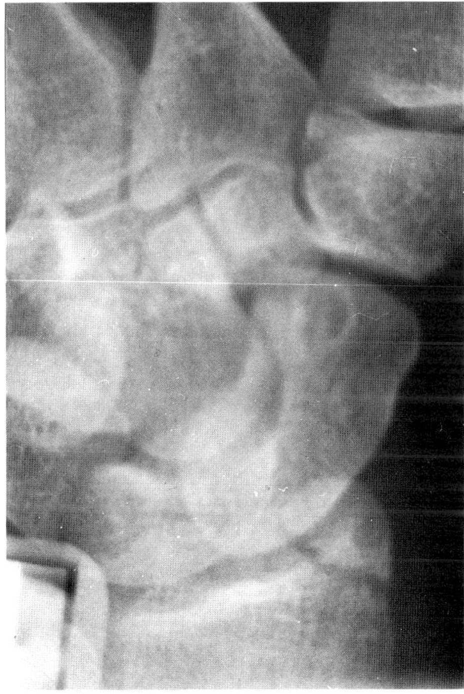

Fig. 16.21 Fracture of the radial styloid.

Fractures involving the distal radioulnar joint

Fractures of the distal end of the radius often have an intra-articular component involving the radioulnar joint. When this occurs in a Colles', Smith or Barton fracture it is important to ensure that the distal radio-ulnar joint is congruent after reduction but beyond that there is no specific treatment required.

Isolated fractures of the head or neck of the ulna, involving the articular surface of the radioulnar joint, are uncommon. Open reduction and internal fixation to restore the articular contour should be considered. This is not always feasible if there are a number of small fragments and the alternative is to excise the head of the ulna. As always, this must be done with care to avoid the complication of instability of the distal end of the ulna.

Fractures of the styloid process of the ulna

Again, these are frequent associations of fractures of the distal end of the radius and do not call for specific treatment in addition to that of the main fracture. Nevertheless, the presence of a fracture of the styloid process is indicative of significant additional ligamentous damage. The triangular fibrocartilage is attached near the base of the styloid process, so a fracture near the base usually means that there has been loss of this support between the radius and ulna. Fortunately, the fibro-cartilage usually heals while the fracture of the distal end of the radius is supported in a cast.

A fracture of the styloid process, occurring as an isolated injury, should be treated by supporting the wrist in supination until the fragment unites. Fractures through the distal half of the styloid process are not usually associated with major ligamentous disruption and should be treated symptomatically.

An ununited fracture is not in itself a cause of persistent wrist symptoms and should not be treated simply by excision of the fragment. A careful assessment of the patient's symptoms should be made and this may involve wrist arthrography and CAT scanning. It is most likely that symptoms arise from ligamentous damage that may necessitate reconstruction, especially if the head of the ulna is unstable. The ulnar head should only be removed if there is demonstrable articular damage that is believed to be responsible for the patient's symptoms. It is important not to excise the triangular fibro-cartilage simply because a leak of dye has been demonstrated through its central part, as this may be a normal finding in the older person (Menon *et al.* 1984). Radical removal of the fibrocartilage without stabilizing the head of the ulna will cause symptomatic instability of the radioulnar joint.

Dislocation of the head of the ulna

In association with other injuries

Acute dislocations can occur in association with fractures of the shaft of the radius (Galeazzi fracture) (Fig. 16.22) or of the head of the radius (Essex-Lopresti fracture) (Essex-Lopresti 1951). These are examples of fractures in which it is vital to have X-ray views of both ends of the bones if errors in management are to be avoided.

The distal radioulnar joint is usually reduced satisfactorily when the Galeazzi fracture is reduced and internally fixed, and it is only necessary to protect the joint for a few weeks to ensure satisfactory ligamentous healing. Excision of a badly shattered radial head is likely to cause further displacement of the radioulnar joint in the Essex-Lopresti fracture and it is probably advisable to stabilize the head of the ulna in its correct relationship to the radius with K-wires if the radial head must be removed.

There is sometimes slight subluxation of the radio-ulnar joint with fractures of the shaft of the ulna. This is seldom a problem, but significant displacement would be an indication for restoration of the normal anatomy of the ulna by internal fixation.

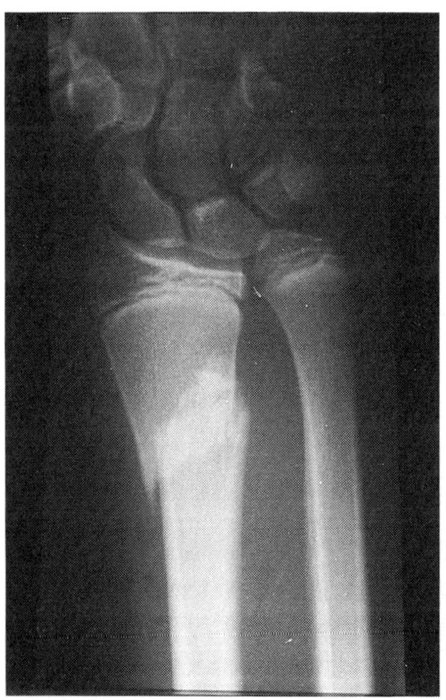
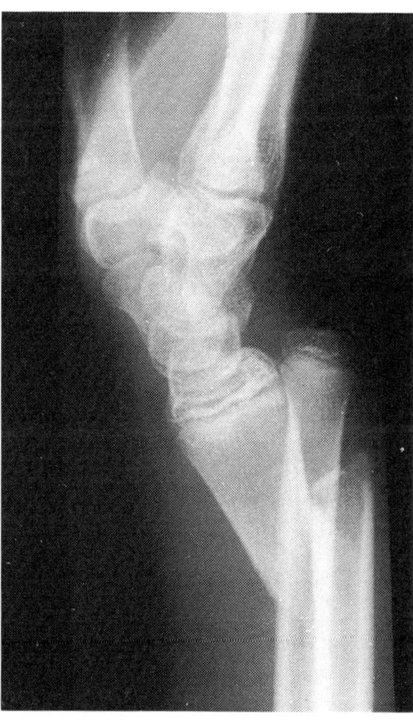

Fig. 16.22 Dislocation of the head of the ulna in a Galeazzi-type fracture–dislocation. Internal fixation of the fracture of the radius and open reduction of the head of the ulna is usually necessary.

Isolated injuries

Acute isolated traumatic dislocations of the distal radio-ulnar joint are quite uncommon. They are usually caused by falls or twisting injuries, such as may occur during sporting activities. The dislocation of the head of the ulna may be in a palmar (Fig. 16.23) or dorsal direction (Dameron 1972) although, since the radius rotates about the fixed ulna, one should really speak of dislocation of the radius on the ulna.

These injuries are sometimes overlooked, despite the clinical presentation, because of a failure to interpret the radiographs correctly. The appearance may be dismissed as the result of an unusual projection of the wrist on the film.

On examination the wrist is painful and deformed. Dorsal dislocation or subluxation results in dorsal prominence of the distal end of the ulna. The presentation is usually more dramatic when the head of the ulna is dislocated palmarwards because the wrist may be locked in the supinated position.

Acute dorsal subluxation is treated by reduction of the head of the ulna, holding it in position in an above-elbow cast, which is applied with the forearm in supination and moulded over the wrist. The cast should be retained for 6 weeks. Late injuries may need ligamentous reconstruction or even removal of the head of the ulna and ligamentous stabilization.

Acute palmar dislocation may be reduced by increasing the supination of the wrist (Rose-Innes 1960). Reduction is usually stable but should be held in an above-elbow cast with the forearm in pronation for 2–3 weeks; thereafter a forearm cast should be worn for another 3 weeks. Late injuries are less commonly seen, in contrast to dorsal subluxations. Open reduction is usually necessary.

Carpal injuries

Carpal instability

The arrangement of the carpus and its stabilizing ligaments has been discussed earlier in the chapter. It will be recalled that stability in the carpus and the direction of intercarpal movements depend largely on the ligaments attached to the bones. Disruption of these ligaments, by injury or disease, may cause profound alterations in the mechanics of the wrist.

Ligamentous injuries are frequently the result of falls on the outstretched hand since, in this position, the important volar radiocarpal ligaments are put on the stretch. Many such injuries are simple sprains that will settle with symptomatic treatment, but when ligaments are significantly stretched or disrupted the carpus may become unstable and the individual bone malaligned.

Classification

There are two primary types of instability:
1 *Static:* The carpus assumes an abnormal alignment

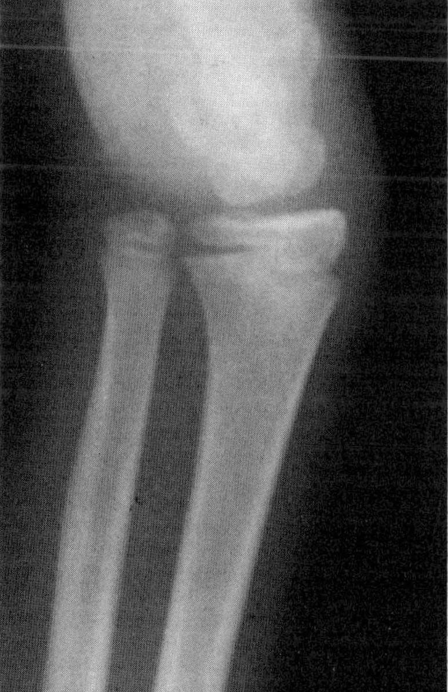
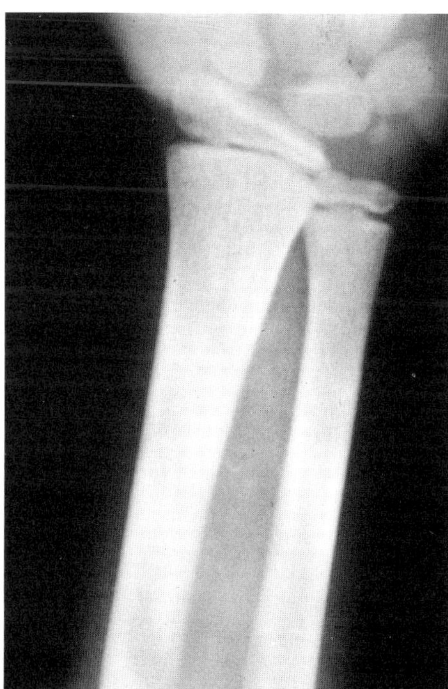

Fig. 16.23 Acute volar dislocation of the head of the ulna.

that cannot be actively altered by the patient. Paradoxically, although termed an instability, this alignment is a stable position assumed by the carpal bones after removal of the controlling influence of the ligaments.

2 *Dynamic*. The alignment of the carpus suddenly alters from normal to abnormal on a certain movement of the wrist, which is often associated with an audible, palpable and painful snap.

The various patterns of instability may be considered in terms of the three-column concept of the carpus (p. 464). It will be recalled that the arrangement of the carpus can be considered as a central column, consisting of the lunate and distal row of carpal bones, and lateral and medial columns consisting of the scaphoid and triquetrum respectively (Fig. 16.1).

In many forms of instability the link mechanism of the central column collapses in a Z-deformity (Fig. 16.3). The lunate may assume either a dorsiflexed or palmarflexed position. Because the lunate is the 'intercalated segment' of the central column the two types of collapse have been termed dorsal intercalated segment instability (DISI) (Fig. 16.24) and volar intercalated segment instability (VISI) (Fig. 16.25) respectively. In about 75% of cases a DISI collapse pattern is seen (Linscheid *et al.* 1972).

A Z-collapse is often associated with loss of the sliding-link control of the scaphoid on the central column because of damage to the ligaments connecting the lateral and central columns, or the presence of an unstable scaphoid fracture or nonunion. A scapholunate diastasis may be manifest radiologically as an abnormal gap between the scaphoid and lunate on an anteroposterior view of the wrist (the 'Terry-Thomas' sign) (Fig. 16.26) (Frankel 1977). Normally, this gap should not be greater than 2 mm or not wider than any other intercarpal space. In the static form of scapholunate dissociation the scaphoid assumes a flexed position in the carpus and does not extend when the wrist is ulnar deviated. In the dynamic form the scaphoid suddenly displaces into a flexed position when the wrist is loaded (e.g. by gripping) and assumes a normal position when the wrist is relaxed.

Scaphocapitate diastasis and STT instability have been described but these other forms of lateral column instability are very rare (Taleisnik 1985).

A central Z-collapse may also follow disruption of the ligaments connecting the medial and central columns, without scapholunate dissociation. When there is triquetro-lunate dissociation (most commonly a result of rheumatoid arthritis of the wrist, rather than trauma) a static VISI deformity follows because the lunate is then solely under the control of the scaphoid, which tends to assume a palmarflexed position. A rupture of the ulnar limb of the palmar intercarpal ('V') ligament (Fig. 16.5) causes triquetro-hamate dissociation, which results in a dynamic mid-carpal instability of either the DISI or VISI form; typically, the distal row of the carpus shifts dorsally or palmarwards as the wrist is ulnar or

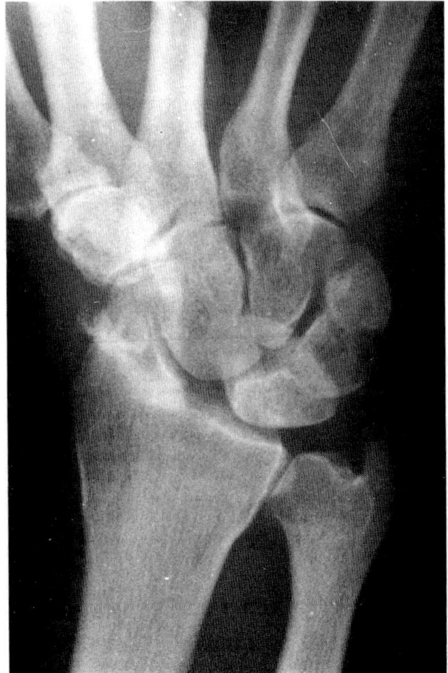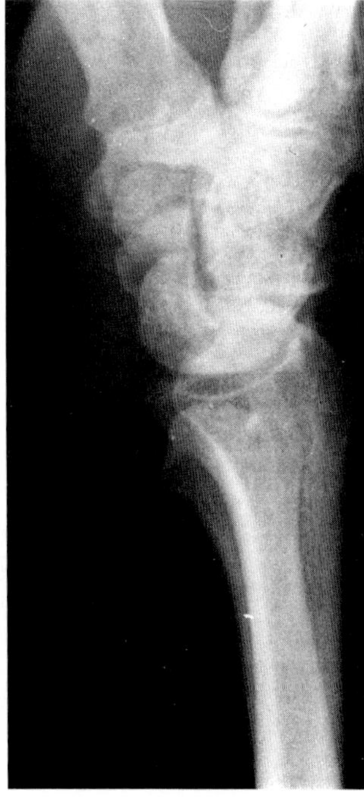

Fig. 16.24 DISI following an old scaphoid fracture. Note the widening of the scapholunate gap.

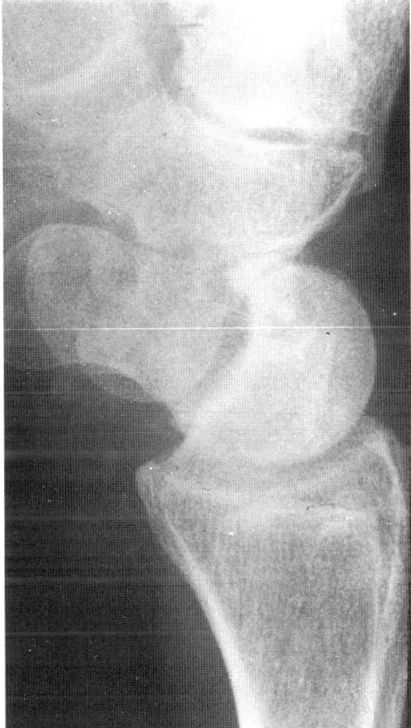
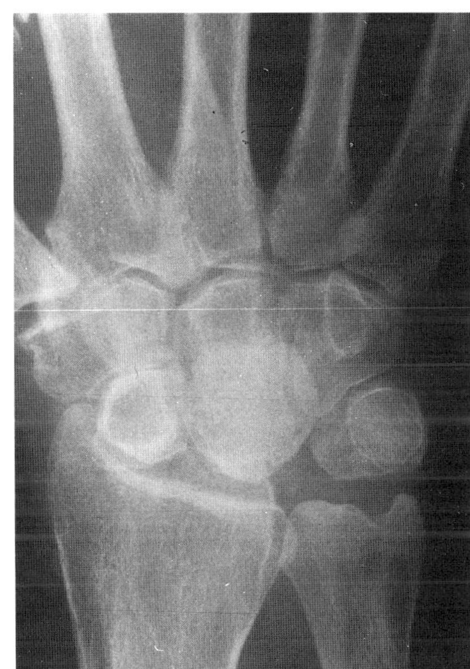

Fig. 16.25 An extreme example of VISI.

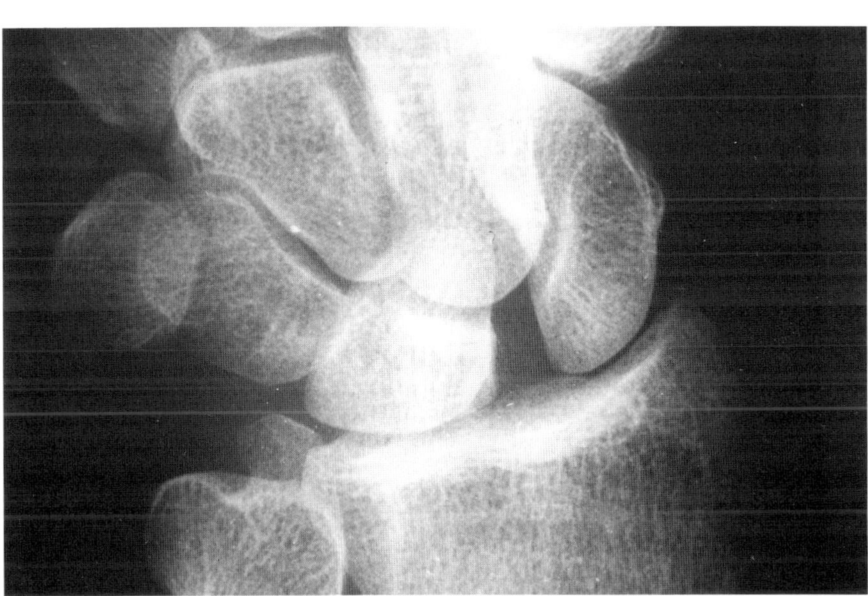

Fig. 16.26 Scapholunate dissociation (the 'Terry-Thomas' sign).

radially deviated, often with the characteristic painful snap of a dynamic instability (Figs 16.27 & 16.28) (Lichtman *et al.* 1981).

Finally, there is a group of proximal instabilities in which there is no primary intracarpal pathology. They are caused by disruption of the radiocarpal ligaments (again, frequently due to rheumatoid arthritis), or by malunion of fractures of the distal end of the radius, resulting in reversal of the usual palmar orientation of the articular surface.

The carpus is 'slung' from the distal end of the radius by the volar ligaments and, when these are disrupted, the carpus as a whole tends to migrate in an ulnar direction and comes to articulate with the head of the ulnar and the triangular fibrocartilage (Rayhack *et al.* 1987). Rarely, ligamentous laxity can result in volar or dorsal subluxation but these are more often caused by fractures and fracture–dislocations of the radiocarpal joint.

When a malunion of the distal end of the radius

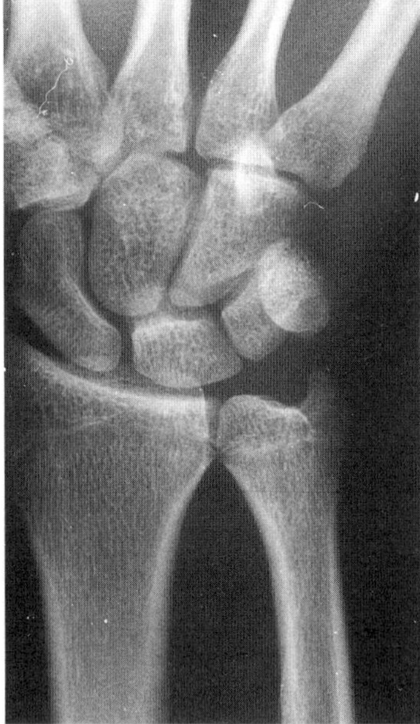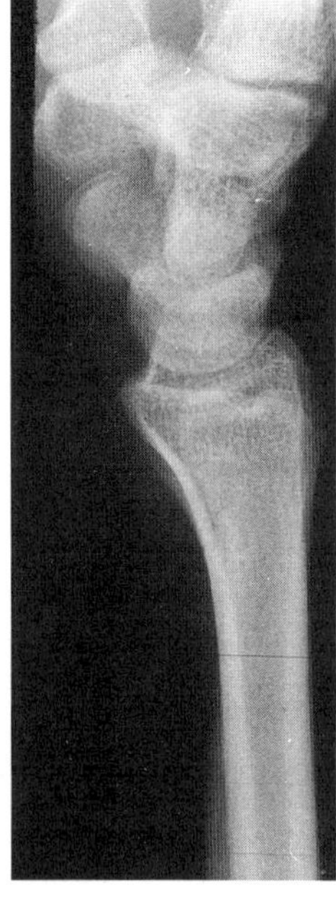

Fig. 16.27 This patient complained of a painful snap from the wrist. Anteroposterior and lateral films with the wrist in the neutral position show no significant abnormality.

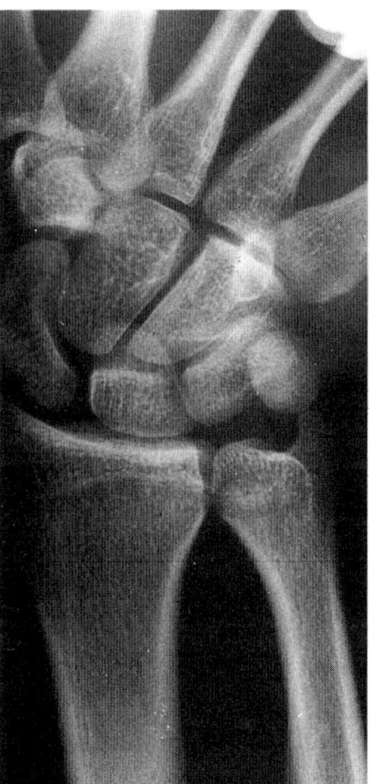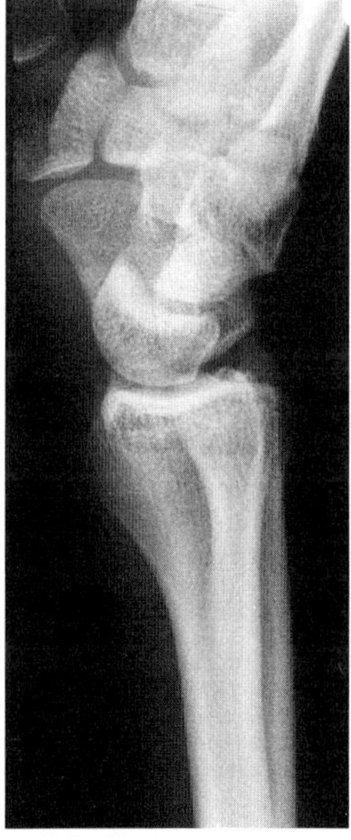

Fig. 16.28 The snap occurred when the wrist was ulnar deviated with the fist clenched. Films now show overlap of the hamate on the triquetrum and a typical DISI collapse pattern. This is an example of a dynamic medial (triquetro-hamate) instability.

causes the articular surface to be directed dorsally there may be a DISI pattern of alignment between the proximal and distal rows of the carpus. This probably represents a compensatory realignment rather than true instability (Linscheid *et al.* 1972), although a dynamic DISI pattern is sometimes produced on ulnar deviation of the wrist (Taleisnik & Watson 1984). It should be stressed that scapholunate dissociation is the most common reason for instability after a fracture of the distal end of the radius, with or without malunion.

In summary, the various forms of carpal instability are:

Lateral
  Scapholunate.
  Scaphotrapezial.
  Scaphocapitate.
Medial
  Triquetro-hamate.
  Triquetro-lunate.
Proximal
  Radiocarpal.
  Mid-carpal.

Diagnosis

Although acute, dynamic forms of instability are usually symptomatic, causing sudden painful snapping in the wrist, many patients with chronic, static types of instability have no complaints, or only a vague sense of weakness, especially on gripping. Later, there may be pain in the wrist because of the onset of secondary osteoarthritic changes.

On clinical examination there may be an obvious malalignment of the wrist, but this is uncommon. The scaphoid may be palpable in an abnormally flexed position and, in static deformities, will remain flexed when the wrist is ulnar deviated. In dynamic forms of instability the painful snap may be visible and palpable. Many patients demonstrate laxity in the other, uninjured wrist.

Adequate radiographic examination is essential for the assessment of wrist instability. Dynamic instabilities can be identified if films are taken when the wrist is in the position of instability. Films should be taken with the fist clenched to load the wrist. Video-radiography is extremely useful in displaying abnormal intercarpal translations. Acute tears of the carpal ligaments are often demonstrable by arthrography. Static deformities are usually readily seen on plain films. On the lateral view the axes of the capitate, lunate and radius should be co linear and the scaphoid axis should be some 30–60° flexed to this line; alterations in these axes can usually be identified quite easily. Features such as a scaphoid non-union, malunion of the distal end of the radius and secondary osteoarthritic changes will be obvious. Sometimes, there may be a fairly rapid appearance of radioscaphoid osteoarthritis after scapholunate dissociation, while the radiolunate articulation is unaffected. This characteristic appearance, which has been termed the scapho lunate advanced collapse (SLAC) wrist, is believed to be due to the fact that the radiolunate joint remains congruent, since the articular surface of the lunate is part of a sphere, whereas the displaced scaphoid is not congruent within the elliptical scaphoid fossa on the radius (Watson & Ballet 1984).

Treatment

Very careful assessment of the patient's problem is required before treatment is recommended. The site of the instability must be clearly identified. The form of treatment is dependent upon whether the instability is acute or chronic, static or dynamic and associated with other problems such as non-union of the scaphoid or secondary arthritic changes in the wrist.

SCAPHOLUNATE INSTABILITY

It may be possible to reduce an acute scapholunate dissociation and maintain reduction in a padded cast with appropriate moulding, but open reduction is more reliable. A dorsal exposure is used, torn ligaments repaired and the scaphoid restored to its normal alignment by inserting K-wires through it and into the lunate and capitate (Green & O'Brien 1978).

Many methods of stabilizing chronic scapholunate instability by ligamentous reconstruction have been described but, like ligamentous reconstructions elsewhere, there is a tendency for the deformity to recur. For this reason a limited intercarpal arthrodesis is now more favoured. It might seem logical to fuse the scapholunate joint but satisfactory fusion is difficult to achieve. STT arthrodesis is technically easier and will produce the same effect of stabilizing the lateral column on the central column (Watson & Hempton 1980, Goldner 1982, Kleinman et al. 1982, Eckenrode et al. 1986, Watson et al. 1986). The disadvantage is that the range of movement of the wrist is decreased, and there is a theoretical risk of increased wear on the radioscaphoid articulation.

TRIQUETRO-LUNATE AND MID-CARPAL INSTABILITY

Acute triquetro-lunate sprains are treated by resting the wrist in a cast. Ligamentous reconstruction or intercarpal fusion may be indicated for chronic injuries (Reagan et al. 1984).

Ulnar mid-carpal instability, caused by a tear of the ulnar limb of the 'V' ligament, is seldom identified after an acute injury. The patient usually presents later with a snapping wrist. Symptoms can often be controlled by a simple splint that prevents ulnar deviation. If this is not successful then triquetro-hamate arthrodesis should be considered (Lichtman et al. 1981). Like other intercarpal arthrodeses, this has the disadvantage of some loss of movement of the wrist.

INSTABILITIES ASSOCIATED WITH SCAPHOID NON-UNION OR OSTEOARTHRITIC CHANGES

Static central column collapse due to scaphoid non-union is corrected at the time of grafting the scaphoid by ensuring that the length of the scaphoid is restored.

Procedures to correct carpal instability are not indicated when there are degenerative changes within the carpus or affecting the radiocarpal joint. Treatment is aimed towards relieving the patient of any symptoms caused by the osteoarthritic process. If arthrodesis is necessary it may be possible to limit it to the intercarpal or radiocarpal joints (Watson et al. 1981), but extensive changes will necessitate complete wrist fusion.

Isolated fractures of the carpal bones

Most fractures of carpal bones are associated with some degree of ligamentous damage that may be more important than the fracture itself. Some carpal fractures occur as part of complex fracture—dislocations of the wrist and these will be considered later. In this section only isolated injuries will be discussed but any apparently isolated fracture should be assessed with the possibility in mind that it represents a greater injury to the carpus: perhaps a fracture—dislocation that has reduced spontaneously before radiographic examination.

Scaphoid

ACUTE FRACTURES

Scaphoid fractures (Fig. 16.29) are common, accounting for approximately 1% of fractures seen in Accident departments. They usually occur in young, active males in the course of occupational or sporting activities. The injury is most often the result of a fall on the outstretched hand with the wrist dorsiflexed and supinated. In this position the proximal pole is stabilized against the

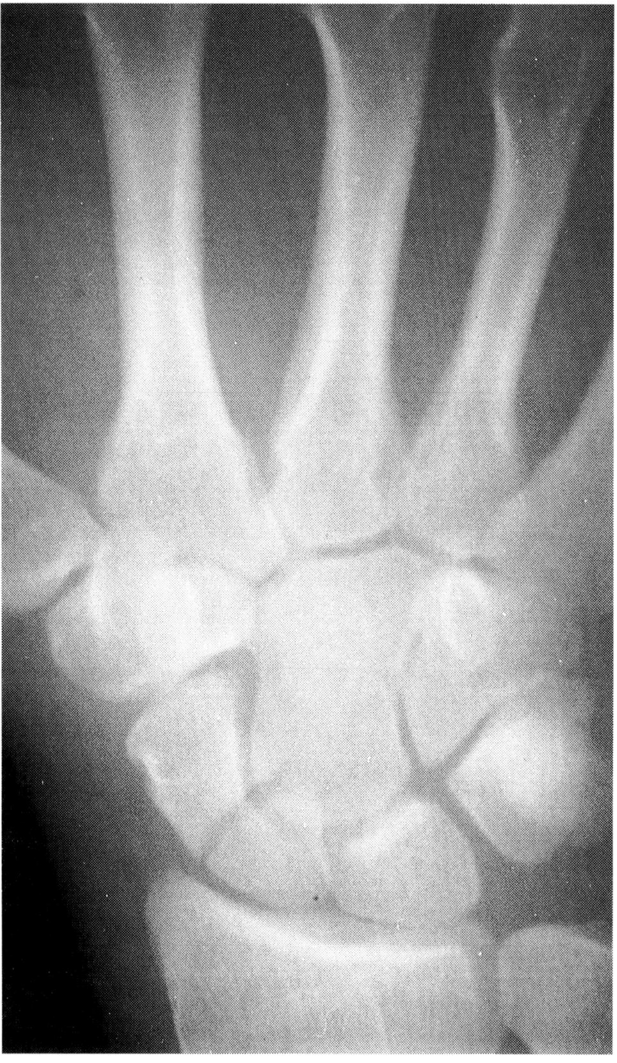

Fig. 16.29 A transverse, undisplaced fracture of the waist of the scaphoid bone.

radius and force is applied to the distal pole, the dorsal lip of the radius acting as an anvil against the dorsal aspect of the scaphoid (Weber & Chao 1978, Mayfield 1980). The more ulnar deviated the wrist at the moment of injury, the more proximal the fracture. In about 15% of patients the injury is result of a direct force in the first web, for example, by a starting handle kick-back or a blow from a motorcycle handlebar or steering wheel; this causes a vertical, shearing type of fracture that is slower to unite than transverse fractures (Leslie & Dickson 1981). Fractures of the scaphoid tuberosity (Fig. 16.30) represent avulsions of the bony attachment of the transverse carpal ligament (Prosser *et al.* 1988).

The clinical signs of a scaphoid fracture are discomfort and, sometimes, swelling in the anatomical snuff-box. Radiographic examination is mandatory in a patient with the relevant history and these clinical signs.

There are four standard radiographic views in the 'scaphoid series': posteroanterior, lateral and two oblique views taken in 45° pronation and 45° supination. The study by Leslie and Dickson (1981) showed that 95% of fresh fractures were identified on these films alone by relatively inexperienced doctors working in an accident and emergency department. This excellent rate was increased to 98% when the films were subsequently scrutinized by an experienced radiologist. The fractures that were *not* well seen on initial films were incomplete infractions that have an excellent prognosis for healing, even without treatment. Thus, it is unlikely that a scaphoid fracture will be missed in the accident and emergency department *provided that radiographs are taken and scrutinized*; if a fracture is not seen it is probably one with a good prognosis. The spectre of the fracture that is not seen on radiographs in the accident and emergency department and which progresses to inevitable non-union because of the lack of treatment, has been overemphasized: most patients who present with established non-union either did not seek treatment at the time of the initial injury or did not have a radiographic examination (Warren-Smith & Barton 1988).

The standard teaching is that patients with 'suspected' scaphoid fractures should be treated with a forearm cast for 10 days and then have a further radiographic examination, the assumption being that the fracture will have become more visible. It is perfectly reasonable to treat a patient in this way for symptomatic relief of pain, although a supportive bandage is probably just as effective and less inconvenient (Sjølin & Andersen 1988).

About a third of scaphoid fractures do become more visible in the first 2–3 weeks after injury, because of bone absorption. It may also be that some fractures that were not well seen on initial films show up better on subsequent films because these were taken with the wrist in slightly different positions. The radiological visibility of a scaphoid fracture depends on the angle of the fracture relative to the incident angle of the X-ray beam. The fracture will be well seen when the beam is parallel to it, but is less visible if it lies at an angle to the beam (Fig. 16.31). For example, as the long axis of the scaphoid lies in some 45° flexion to the axis of the arm, it is necessary to take a film with the wrist dorsiflexed and in ulnar deviation in order to show a fracture that is transverse to the axis of the scaphoid. Such considerations are probably not important in the diagnosis of a fresh fracture of the scaphoid, which is nearly always visible on the original scaphoid series of films, but they

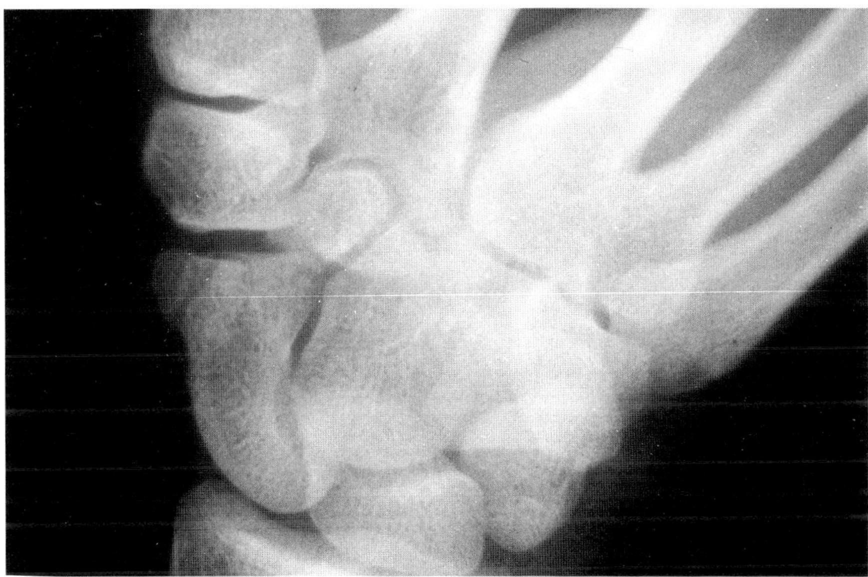

Fig. 16.30 A fracture of the tuberosity of the scaphoid.

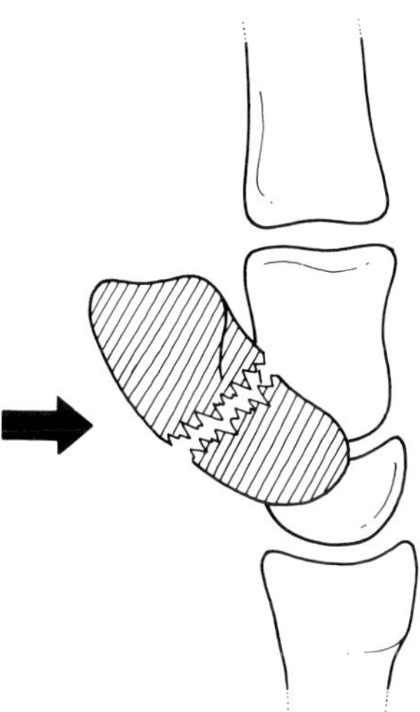

Fig. 16.31 The visibility of a fracture line in the scaphoid bone depends upon the inclination of the X-ray beam to the fracture. In this example the fracture would be more clearly seen on a film taken with the wrist dorsiflexed.

become more important when attempting to assess radiological union.

The scaphoid fat pad lies between the radial collateral ligament and the tendons of the abductor pollicis longus and extensor pollicis brevis. It shows as a radiolucent stripe on plain posteroanterior films of the wrist. Oedema or haematoma causes radial displacement or distortion of the stripe and this may be an indication of an occult scaphoid fracture (Cetti & Christensen 1982).

Classification

Most classifications of scaphoid fractures are based on the site and direction of the fracture line (Fig. 16.32). Both these factors have some bearing on the prognosis for union but this also depends on other factors, such as instability and displacement of the fracture and local soft tissue damage.

Dickson (1988) analysed 1105 fresh fractures from six large series and reported the frequency of the site of fracture to be: tuberosity, 10%; distal third, 11%; waist, 72%; and proximal pole, 6%. Russe (1960) reported the direction of the common waist fractures to be: horizontal oblique, 35%; transverse, 60%; and vertical oblique, 5%. In general, healing will be slower and less certain the more proximal the fracture and the more vertical the fracture line (Leslie & Dickson 1981).

The role of the scaphoid blood supply in healing is unclear. In common with other short bones, the scaphoid is supplied by a number of vessels (Gelberman & Menon 1980). These enter the scaphoid via ligamentous attachments around the tuberosity and along the dorsal ridge between articular surfaces. In about one-third of scaphoid bones there are no vascular foramina in the proximal half, which must derive its blood supply via intramedullary vessels from the distal half (Obletz & Halbstein 1938). Thus, one-third of fractures through the waist and proximal pole of the scaphoid will result in avascularity of the proximal fragment. Since many fractures are stable the blood supply is probably rapidly re-established, but it is apparent that avascular changes

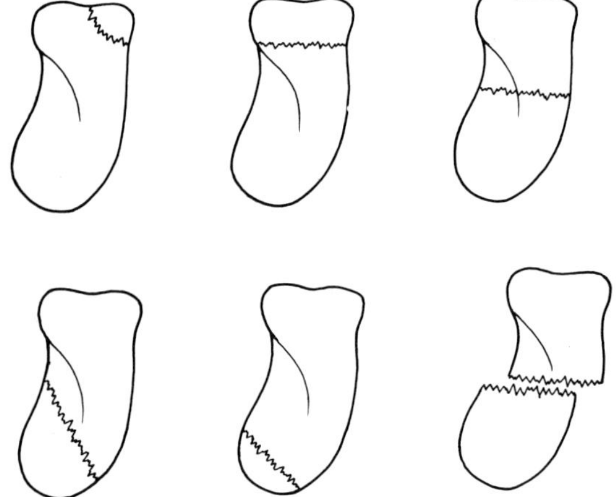

Fig. 16.32 Patterns of acute scaphoid fractures. Those on the bottom row have a higher incidence of delayed and non-union than those on the top row.

may follow in some unstable fractures or if non-union occurs.

Treatment

Conservative treatment is by cast immobilization of the wrist. A large number of different regimes have been described, the variables being the position of the wrist, the use of short or long arm casts, whether the thumb is incorporated in the cast or left free and time of immobilization. Of all these variables it is the last, time of immobilization, that is the most important.

London (1961) noted that eight different positions of the wrist had been recommended by various authorities, indicating that the position of the wrist was of no great significance. There is no evidence that extending the cast above the elbow confers any advantage in terms of healing time or rate of non-union and the same can be said for incorporating the thumb in the cast.

The average time to radiographic union in conservatively treated fractures is about 9 weeks (Leslie & Dickson 1981). Fractures of the tuberosity and distal pole take less time to unite, but vertical oblique fractures of the waist and fractures of the proximal pole take up to 3 weeks longer. Fractures in teenagers take less time to unite than fractures in young adults. Taking these factors into account, it is possible to predict the likely time to union of any given fracture and the required period of time in a cast. There is no reason to treat a fresh scaphoid fracture for any longer than 12 weeks in a cast; if there is a radiologically obvious gap at the fracture site at that time it should be regarded as a non-union and treated as such. Most scaphoid fractures will have

healed within 8–12 weeks of injury and it is premature to internally fix fractures that have not healed by 6 weeks, as is sometimes recommended.

It is difficult to decide when an acute scaphoid fracture has united. The most reliable radiographic sign of union is the presence of trabeculae crossing the fracture line, but mention has been made of the difficulty in obtaining radiographs that show the fracture line without overlap of the scaphoid fragments, and such films are necessary if trabeculae crossing the fracture line are to be seen clearly. Another sign of union in an acute fracture has been described by Russe (1960) who noted that bands of increased density in the bone at the site of the fracture were an indication of union, rather than of delayed union. (In an old fracture these bands are *not* indicative of union.)

Dias *et al.* (1988) found that there was considerable disagreement between experienced clinicians who were asked to assess radiographs taken 12 weeks after injury for signs of scaphoid union. When each observer was asked to look at the same films 2 months later there was poor agreement between the first and second opinions. These findings should be borne in mind when considering published statistics for scaphoid union. It is reasonable to take the decision to discontinue immobilization after 8–12 weeks if there is no tenderness in the scaphoid region and if there is no clear radiographic gap at the fracture line, but a final opinion about healing should be based on radiographs taken at least 3 months later.

The non-union rate in most large published series of conservatively treated fractures is around 5% (Dickson 1988). A significant factor in the occurrence of non-union is displacement of the fracture. Obvious displacement on initial films (Fig. 16.33) may be an indication of a more extensive carpal injury associated with ligamentous disruption or other carpal fractures, and in this situation operative fixation of the scaphoid fracture may be needed as primary treatment (see p. 474). Increasing displacement of the fracture during conservative treatment is also an indication for operative treatment.

There is a tendency towards early operative treatment of all scaphoid fractures by internal fixation to spare young, working males from a prolonged period of treatment in plaster, which carries at least a 5% chance of non-union. This is a reasonable policy, but results of this form of treatment in a large series of patients have not yet been published, so there is no evidence that early surgery is superior to conservative methods in terms of union rate or freedom from complications.

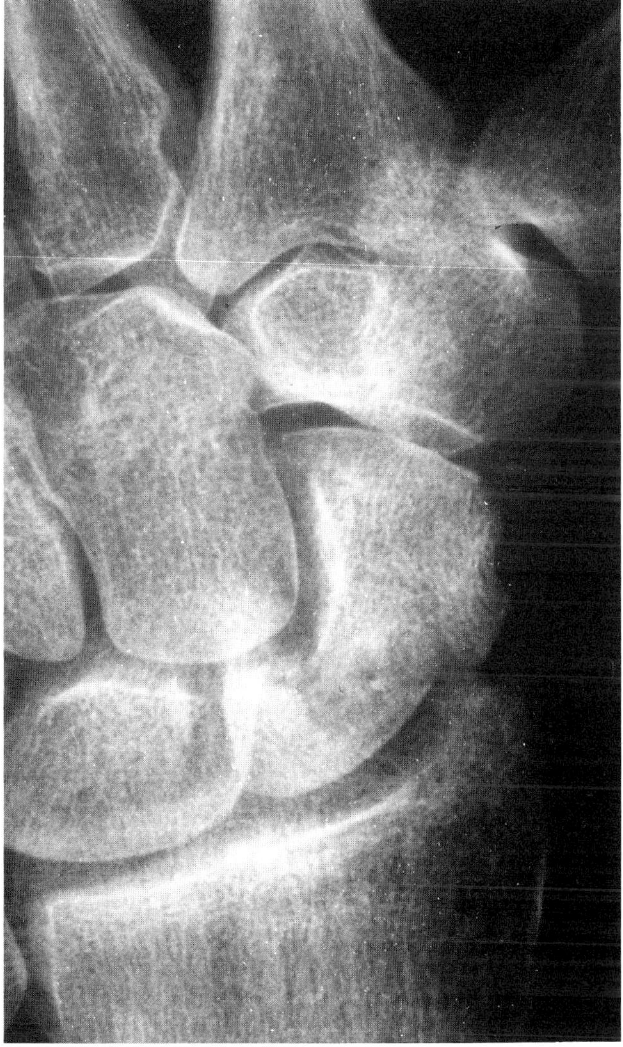

Fig. 16.33 A displaced scaphoid fracture.

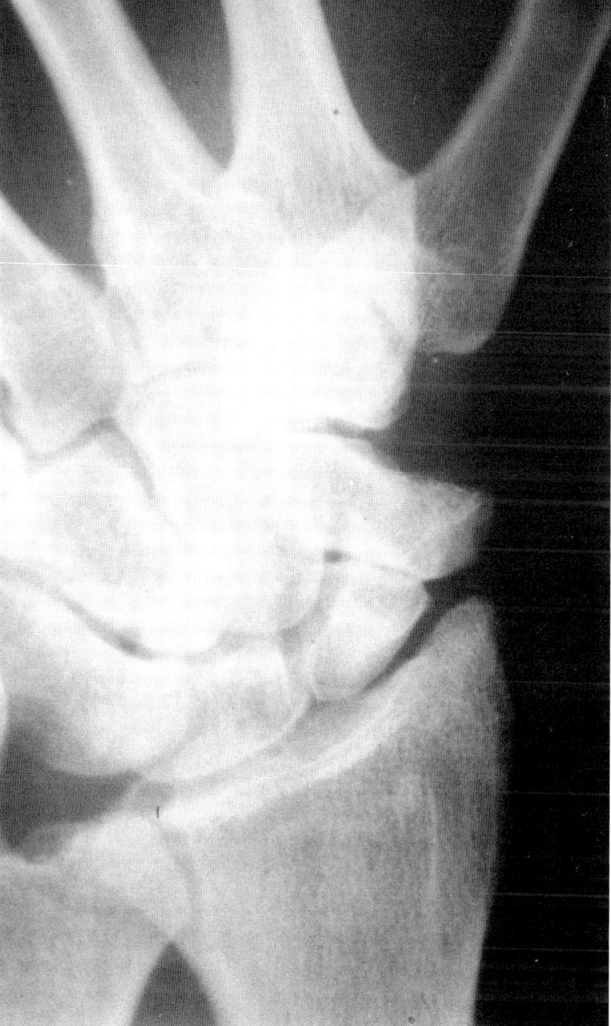

Fig. 16.34 An established scaphoid non-union. There is beaking of the radial styloid process, indicating early degenerative change.

SCAPHOID NON-UNION

The natural history of scaphoid non-union (Fig. 16.34) is largely unknown. At least 5% of adequately treated fresh fractures will fail to unite but few patients who are seen with non-unions will have received adequate treatment at the time of injury (Warren-Smith & Barton 1988). It is not uncommon to hear that the injury was dismissed as a sprain by the patient or a medical advisor and that radiographic examination was omitted or, if the fracture was recognized, the patient failed to comply with treatment. Patients with scaphoid non-unions are often unaware of any problem in the wrist until it is brought to light by a further injury or a radiographic examination for some other purpose. Frequently, the

possibility of a previous injury is denied, even though the radiographic changes are clearly of long standing. This suggests that there must be many people with scaphoid non-unions who never come to medical attention and presumably have no significant symptoms. Not every non-union goes on to cause carpal instability and degenerative changes, although studies of patients with *symptomatic* non-unions indicate that degenerative changes tend to increase with time and are correlated with the severity of symptoms (Mack *et al.* 1984, Ruby *et al.* 1985, Düppe *et al.* 1994). However, it is not unusual to encounter a patient with marked degenerative changes and no complaints (Fig. 16.35). It is therefore wise to treat the patient and not the non-union.

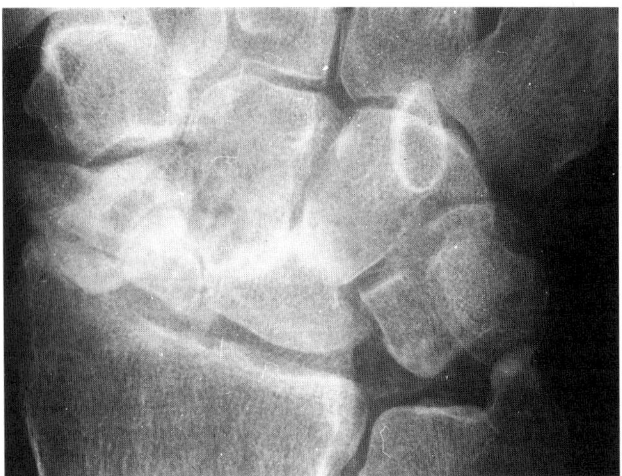

Fig. 16.35 A scaphoid non-union of long standing, with marked degenerative changes within the carpus. The patient did not recall any previous injury and denied any discomfort.

Patients with scaphoid non-unions tend to fall into one of four groups:

1 Patients with acute fractures that fail to unite within the expected time should be treated surgically by internal fixation and bone grafting, rather than waiting to see if symptoms develop. It is wise to allow the patient to mobilize the wrist out of a cast for about 3 weeks before surgery.

2 People with asymptomatic non-unions which are identified by chance do not require treatment but follow-up should be offered.

3 It is not uncommon for someone with an old non-union to sustain a further wrist injury, usually a sprain but sometimes of more significance, which draws attention to the scaphoid injury. The recent injury should be treated on its merits and most wrists will become asymptomatic again. The relationship of residual symptoms, if any, to the non-union should be carefully considered before recommending any active treatment.

4 Patients with established scaphoid non-union and who develop symptoms require treatment but the type of treatment depends on the severity of symptoms in relation to the patient's everyday activities and the radiological changes in the wrist.

Treatment

The usual symptoms caused by scaphoid non-union are aching, pain, weakness and restriction of movement. There is no procedure that will restore lost movement, but the other symptoms can be helped by surgical treatment.

In the absence of significant arthritic changes, the standard treatment of a non-union is by bone grafting, usually supplemented by some form of internal fixation. Internal fixation alone is not adequate for non-union, although it has been used for delayed union (Leyshon *et al.* 1984). A cancellous bone graft inserted through an anterior approach has been popular, but this does not correct the 'humpbacked' deformity that often occurs when there is an element of carpal instability and there is resorption of the anterior margins of the fracture. In this situation it is better to insert a corticocancellous graft that will restore the scaphoid to its former length and stabilize the carpus (Fig. 16.36). Fisk (1982) recommends using the styloid process, which he removes through a snuff-box exposure and inserts anterolaterally into the scaphoid. A popular alternative is a wedge graft from the iliac crest inserted through an anterior exposure (Russe 1960, Mulder 1968). Before inserting a graft it is most important to freshen the bone ends and this gives an opportunity to assess the vascularity of the fragments; the white, non-bleeding surface of an avascular proximal pole is obvious and is associated with a poorer prognosis for union (Green 1985).

Additional stabilization by internal fixation is wise. K-wires are not ideal as they do not provide stability by compression. Lag screws are suitable but the threaded part of the screw may be too long and strut the fragments apart, especially if the proximal fragment is small. The Herbert screw system (Herbert & Fisher 1984) overcomes this problem by having short threads of different pitches at either end of the screw so that it will grip into small fragments and also produce compression across the graft when tightened (Fig. 16.37). The scaphoid is exposed through an anterior approach and a jig is placed around it to ensure accurate drilling and placement of the screw after the graft has been inserted. It is necessary to open the scaphotrapezial joint to put on the jig and this is a cause for concern as it may predispose to later degenerative changes, although these have not been a problem so far. When the proximal fragment is very small, the screw can be inserted freehand via a dorsal exposure.

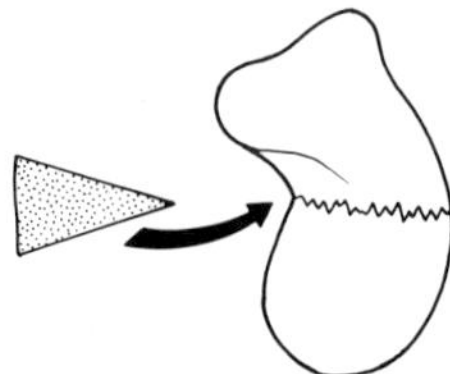
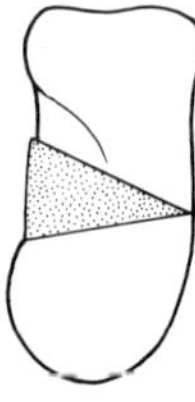

Fig. 16.36 It is necessary to insert an anterior wedge graft to lengthen the scaphoid in order to overcome carpal collapse.

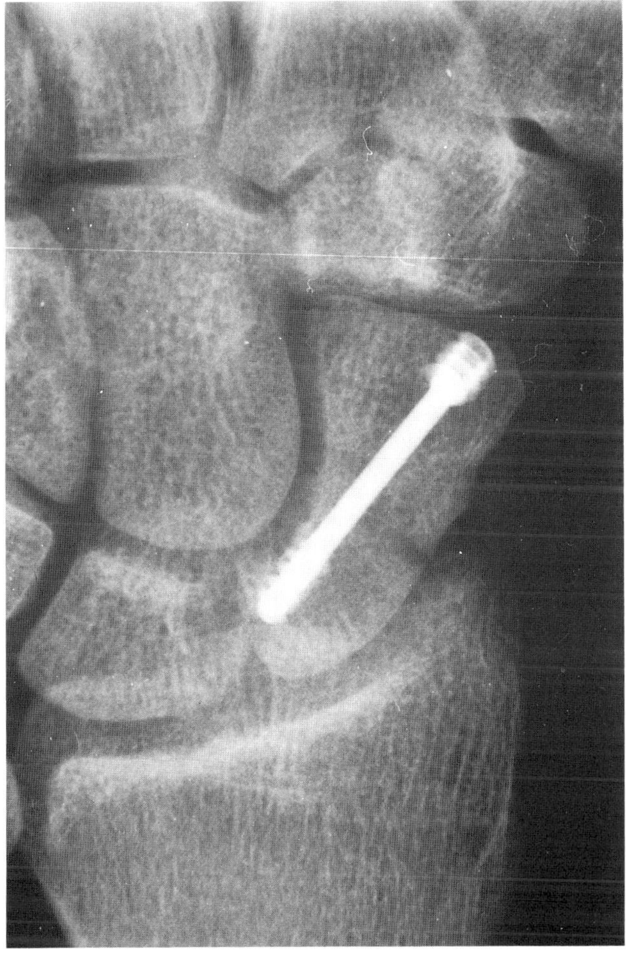

Fig. 16.37 The Herbert screw used to stabilize a grafted scaphoid non-union.

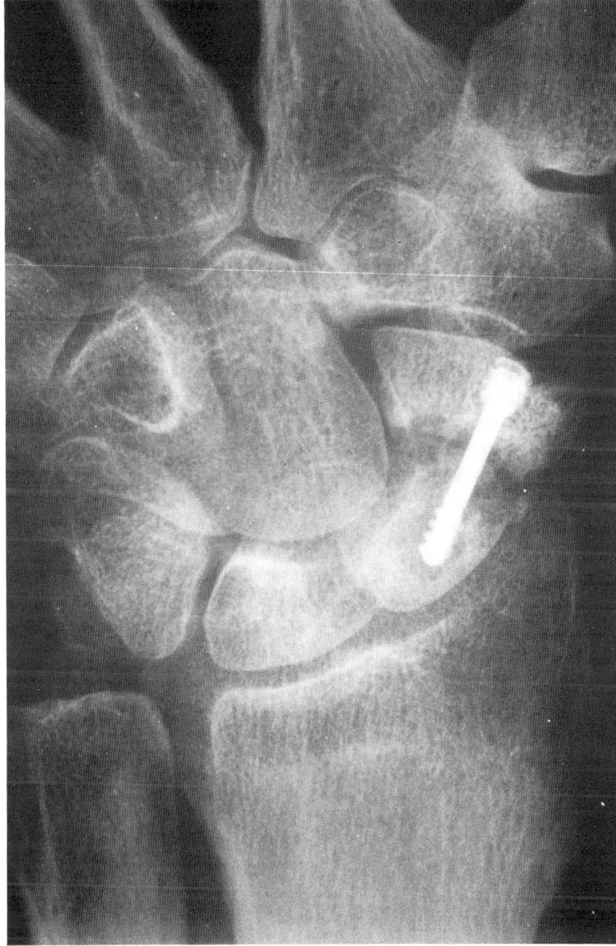

Fig. 16.38 A failed Herbert screw procedure. Note the lucent zone around the proximal end of the screw. The patient had no complaints.

After grafting alone, a cast must be worn for 12—16 weeks but if internal fixation is used this is not necessary and the cast may be discarded when the immediate postoperative discomfort has eased.

Operations to obtain union are not always successful; the overall rate of union is 70—80% (Cooney *et al.* 1980). These figures must be regarded as approximate since it is very difficult to follow-up young males, many of whom are notoriously non-compliant with treatment. The same comments about assessing radiological union of fresh fractures also apply to the assessment of non-unions that have been grafted and it may well be that the reported rates of union are something of an overestimate.

Most surgeons who use additional internal fixation have noted that patients frequently claim that the wrist is symptom-free even when the bone has failed to unite and the fixation is clearly loose (Fig. 16.38). It remains to

be seen what the natural history of these wrists will be.

Operations designed to achieve union by grafting are not adequate when there are degenerative changes in the wrist, as the pain will not be relieved. Radial styloidectomy (Mazet & Hohl 1960) is sometimes helpful if arthritic changes are limited to the articulation between the scaphoid and the radial styloid process, and particularly if the patient has impingement pain on radial deviation. The ununited scaphoid should be grafted and stabilized to prevent the distal scaphoid fragment displacing over the cut surface of the radius.

Simple excision of the ununited proximal pole, especially if it is avascular and fragmented, has been recommended for non-union but is probably not advisable if there are arthritic changes. Proximal row carpectomy (Nevaiser 1983) has its advocates when there are marked arthritic changes but is not widely favoured as it tends to produce weakness in the wrist. A more certain solution is arthrodesis, either partial or complete, depending on the extent of the arthritis. Most patients with a non-union and arthritic changes will need a fusion extending from the radius to the bases of the index and long metacarpal bones. The ulnar side of the carpus, the distal radioulnar joint and the joints at the base of the thumb are excluded from the fusion.

In the Bentzon procedure a flap of soft tissue is placed between the scaphoid fragments, the object being to obtain a pain-free pseudoarthrosis. This can be combined with excision of the radial styloid process. Clearly, this procedure will not prevent the carpal collapse that is so often a long-term consequence of scaphoid non-union but, despite this, the results appear to be very satisfactory many years later (Boeckstyns *et al.* 1985).

It is possible to replace the whole of the bone by an acrylic or silicone rubber prosthesis, but such a prosthesis can act only as a spacer and as there are no ligamentous attachments the normal complex intercarpal movements will not be regained. There may be a place for partial replacement of the scaphoid with a silicone implant when the proximal pole is avascular (Zemel *et al.* 1984, Jones 1985).

It is not known why some scaphoid non-unions are associated with avascular necrosis of the proximal pole (Fig. 16.39) while others are not, although it is generally thought that the anatomical arrangement of the blood supply is a major factor. Very rarely, the scaphoid undergoes total avascular necrosis and collapse (Bray & McCarroll 1984). This condition, Preiser disease (Fig. 16.40), is analogous to Kienböck disease of the lunate (see p. 477); like Kienböck disease the cause is unknown, although trauma is thought to be a significant factor. Treatment is symptomatic and arthrodesis of the wrist may prove necessary.

Dorsal chip fractures

The dorsal chip fracture (Fig. 16.41) is the carpal injury that is next in frequency to fracture of the scaphoid. It is often difficult to be sure from which bone the fragment has derived because it can seldom be identified on the anteroposterior view and is seen only as a displaced chip on the lateral view. Most are probably from the triquetrum but such chips can be detached from the dorsum of the radius and most of the carpal bones. Dorsal triquetral fractures are often said to be the result of ligamentous avulsions caused by falls with the wrist in flexion. However, they may also result from a chisel action of the ulnar styloid process on the dorsum of the triquetrum when the wrist is dorsiflexed (Levy *et al.* 1979, Garcia-Elias 1987).

Treatment is by simple support of the wrist in a cast until symptoms settle. The fracture may fail to unite but this does not give rise to long-term problems (Bartone & Grieco 1956).

Lunate

Acute fractures of the lunate are seldom identified and their true incidence is uncertain. Most fractures are not well seen on standard films and tomography is necessary if such an injury is suspected. If a fracture is identified it should be treated by application of a scaphoid-type cast

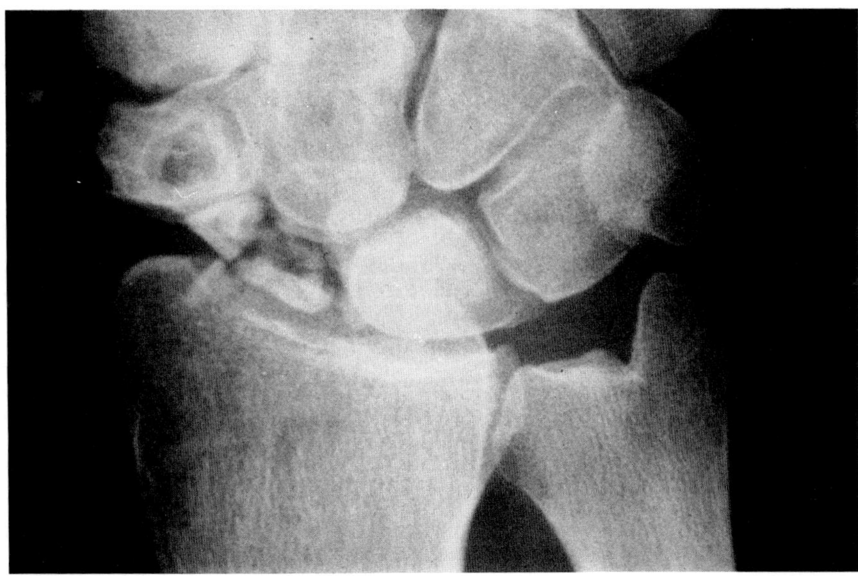

Fig. 16.39 Scaphoid non-union with avascular collapse of the proximal pole.

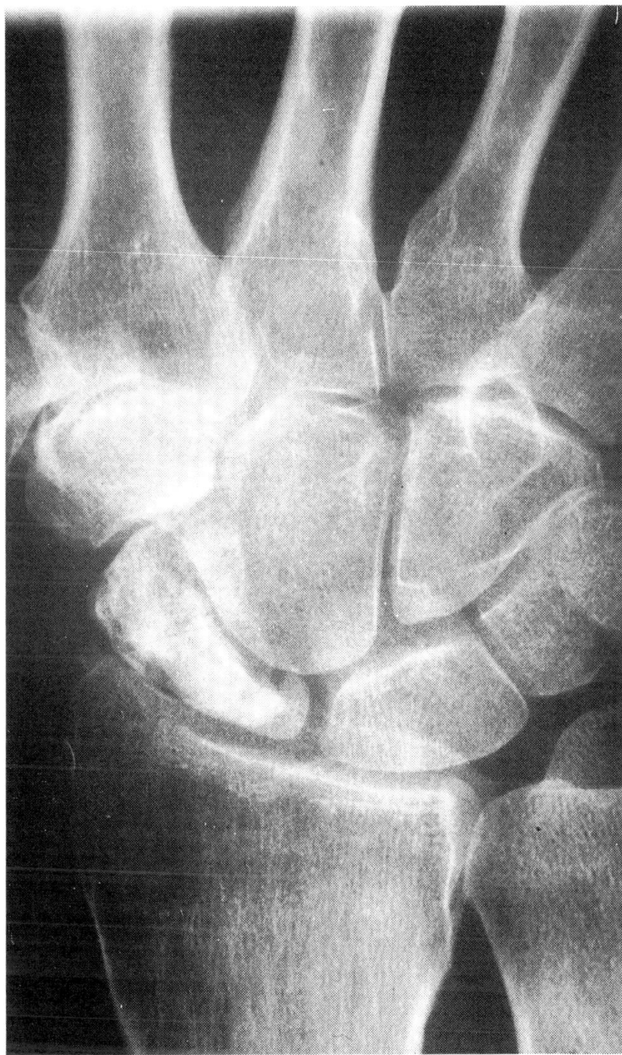

Fig. 16.40 Total avascularity of the scaphoid bone — Preiser disease.

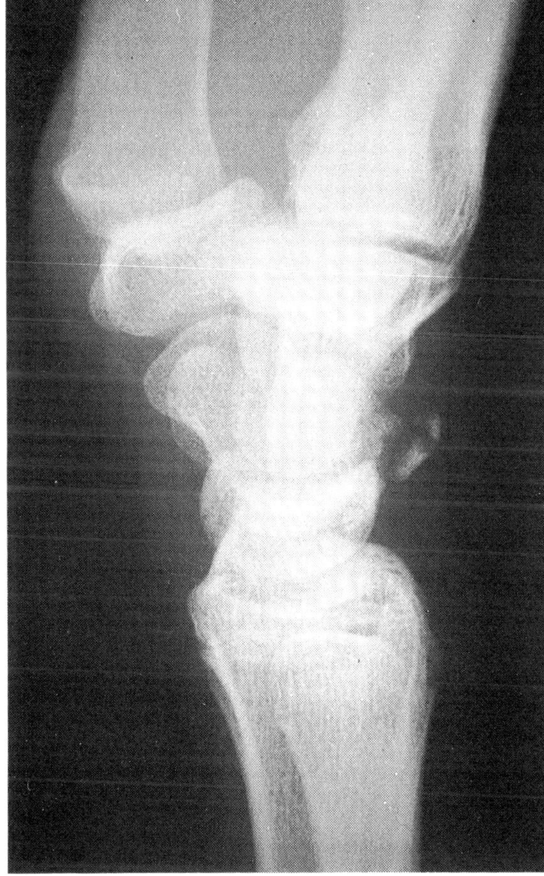

Fig. 16.41 Dorsal chip fracture from the carpus.

for at least 8 weeks. The prognosis is good in adolescents but avascular necrosis is a not uncommon complication in older people.

It is possible that unrecognized microfractures precipitate avascular necrosis of the lunate (Kienböck disease, lunatomalacia) (Fig. 16.42) in many cases (Beckenbaugh *et al.* 1980), but other factors are also important. There must be some alteration in the blood supply of the lunate (Gelberman *et al.* 1980). Nutrient vessels usually enter the bone from both dorsal and volar aspects. The arrangement of vessels within the bone is variable (Lee 1963) and it is possible that osteochondral fractures of the proximal pole can cause devascularization of part of the bone. It is interesting that avascular necrosis is seldom a complication of lunate dislocations (White & Omer 1984).

Many people with Kienböck disease have a relative shortening of the ulna with respect to the radius (ulnaminus variant), and this is postulated as a cause of increased stress on the lunate in repeated loading of the wrist. It is important that films taken to demonstrate the relative lengths of the radius and ulna are taken in a standard way (Palmer *et al.* 1982).

Avascular necrosis may be discovered by chance on radiographs taken for another reason, but in some people it is symptomatic, causing aching pain and weakness of the wrist. The radiographic changes may be staged:

I — minimal or absent changes on radiographs, but increased uptake on bone scan.

II — increased density with minimal collapse.

III — avascular changes with lunate collapse and changes in carpal alignment.

IV — as above with perilunate osteoarthritis.

Many people with Kienböck disease have little trouble in the long term (Kristensen *et al.* 1986) so the type of treatment depends on the severity of symptoms and the

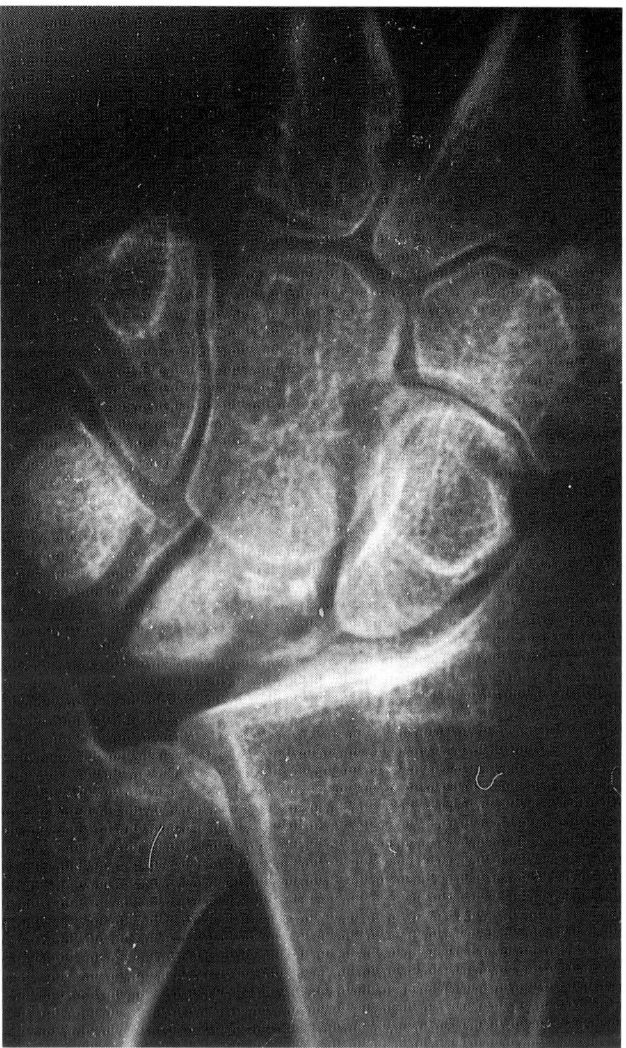

Fig. 16.42 Kienböck disease (grade III).

stage of the disease. Ulnar lengthening (Armistead *et al.* 1982) or radial shortening (Almquist & Burns 1982) is recommended in stage I and II disease if symptoms fail to respond to a period of rest in a cast. In stage III disease the lunate may be simply excised (Kawai *et al.* 1988) or excised and replaced with either an 'anchovy' of rolled-up tendon or a silicone rubber implant (Lichtman *et al.* 1982). Recent reports of 'silicone synovitis' have caused some surgeons to restrict the use of silicone implants in younger patients with heavy demands on their wrists (Alexander *et al.* 1990). Painful stage IV disease is usually treated by wrist arthrodesis but excision and replacement may be an alternative if arthritic changes are not too marked and the patient is not engaged in heavy manual work.

In addition to the above, some surgeons would also carry out a STT fusion (Watson *et al.* 1985), either to unload the lunate in stage II disease or stabilize the carpus in stage III.

Triquetrum

Two main types of injury occur. The dorsal chip fracture has been described above. The body of the triquetrum may be fractured by compression or impingement of the hamate on the dorsum of the bone when the wrist is dorsiflexed and ulnar deviated (Bryan & Dobyns 1980). This is an uncommon injury. Views of the wrist in several planes may be needed to identify the fracture, which is usually undisplaced. It is treated by supporting the wrist in a cast for 4–6 weeks. In contrast to the dorsal chip fracture, most fractures of the body of the triquetrum unite satisfactorily (Bartone & Grieco 1956).

Pisiform

The pisiform is rarely fractured. The mechanism of injury is a heavy fall directly on the bone. When an uninjured wrist is palmarflexed the pisiform can be gripped on either side and moved freely; acute discomfort with this manoeuvre should lead the examiner to suspect an injury of the pisiform. It may be difficult to see the fracture on radiographs and repeated views in different planes may be necessary.

Recent fractures are treated by a simple protective splint or cast. Symptoms usually settle rapidly. The later onset of degenerative changes in the pisotriquetral joint can give discomfort on strong gripping and if this is a problem the pisiform should be excised subperiosteally (Helal 1978).

Trapezium

Fractures of the trapezium fall into two main groups: fracture of the body of the trapezium, usually involving the trapeziometacarpal joint (Cordrey & Ferrer-Torells 1960, Jones & Ghorbal 1985); and fracture of the volar ridge of the trapezium, to which is attached the transverse carpal ligament (Palmer 1981). As with any carpal fracture, there may be associated carpal ligament injuries.

The body of the trapezium is usually broken by a longitudinal force transmitted through the adducted thumb, causing a longitudinal split in the bone with comminution (Fig. 16.43). On physical examination there is pain and swelling in the anatomical snuff-box, with discomfort on moving the thumb. Closed reduction can be achieved by longitudinal traction on the thumb but open reduction may be needed if the articular fragment remains malaligned. The metacarpal and tra-

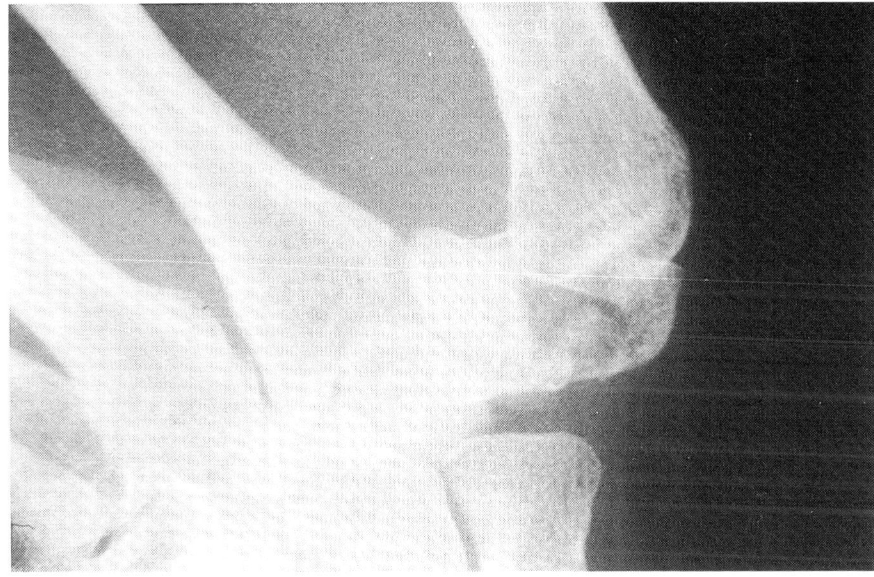

Fig. 16.43 Fracture of the trapezium.

pezium can be retained in the reduced position by K-wires driven through the thumb metacarpal into an adjacent bone, as for the Bennett fracture (Fig. 16.44). Stabilization of the trapezium by wires (Cordrey & Ferrer-Torrells 1960) or screws (Freeland & Finley 1984) is only feasible if the fragments are large. The wires are retained for 3–4 weeks and then active mobilization is started.

A fracture of the palmar trapezoidal ridge or tuberosity is usually the result of a fall on to the base of the thenar eminence causing direct trauma to the bone or avulsion of the transverse palmar ligament. The injury is easily missed unless there is a high index of suspicion and adequate films, including a good carpal tunnel view, are available. Palmar (1981) described two types of fracture:

Type 1 — a fracture through the base of the process which, being through cancellous bone, usually heals with rest in a thumb cast.

Type 2 — a fracture at the tip of the process which often goes on to non-union and may require excision.

Long-term tenderness at the base of the thenar eminence is common after trapezial ridge fractures and is probably due to concomitant soft tissue injury.

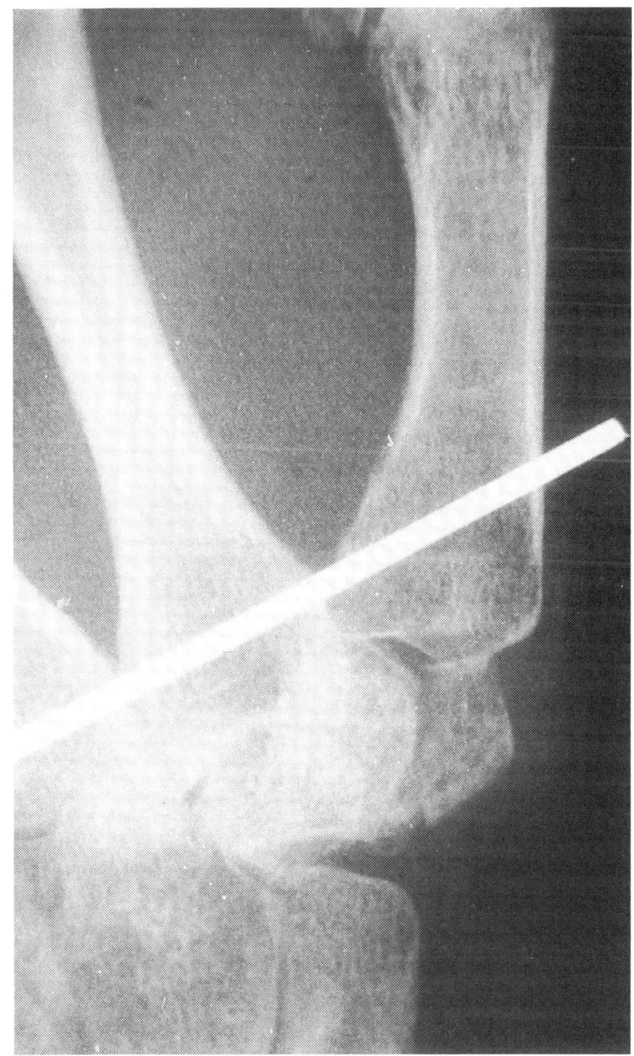

Fig. 16.44 (*Right.*) Stabilization after reduction of this trapezium fracture was attained by driving a K-wire between the thumb and index metacarpal bones.

Trapezoid

Isolated fractures of the trapezoid are extremely rare. Almost invariably, a fracture of this bone is part of a more extensive injury, most commonly a fracture—dislocation involving the index finger metacarpal. These injuries are discussed on p. 486.

Hamate

There are two main types of hamate fracture (Bowen 1973): fractures of the body, which includes those involving the proximal pole and the distal articular surface; the latter may be associated with subluxation of the metacarpal base. The second group is fracture of the hook of the hamate.

Fractures through the body may be caused by forces transmitted along the little finger metacarpal (Fig. 16.45). The hook is broken by a direct fall on the base of the hypothenar eminence or a direct blow from the butt or grip of a sports implement, such as a golf club or tennis racquet (Stark *et al*. 1977).

A fracture of the hamate should be suspected if there is an appropriate history and local discomfort on the ulnar border of the wrist, with or without swelling. Careful radiographic examination, repeated if necessary, is required to show either type of fracture: oblique films or tomograms may be needed to show fractures of the body; the hook of the hamate is visualized by carpal tunnel views (Hart & Gaynor 1941) and an oblique projection with the hand in 45° supination and the wrist radially deviated and dorsiflexed. Tomograms or a CT scan (Egawa & Asai 1983, Polivy *et al*. 1985) may be needed if the fracture is strongly suspected but not seen on standard radiographs.

Fractures of the body of the hamate usually heal uneventfully with protection for 4—6 weeks. Acute fractures of the hook of the hamate may heal with similar treatment, but are most often not identified until some weeks to months after the injury, when symptomatic non-union is present (Carter *et al*. 1977). Excision of the ununited hook is then recommended (Stark *et al*. 1977) and gives good results.

The ulnar nerve is closely related to the hook of the hamate in the Guyon canal and delayed palsy of the deep branch of the ulnar nerve has been reported after hamate fractures (Baird & Freidenberg 1968), particularly those involving the hook. Treatment is by decompression of the nerve and excision of the fragment. Attritional rupture of the flexor tendons to the ring and little fingers has also been described (Crosby & Linscheid 1974).

Capitate

The capitate may be fractured alone or in combination with other injuries; the latter type of fracture is considered on p. 485.

The mechanism of injury in isolated fractures is uncertain but may involve a direct blow to the wrist. This is an uncommon fracture, usually through the waist of the bone (Fig. 16.46), and it may not be seen on initial films. Further films should be taken a week or so later if the injury is suspected and, sometimes, traction views are helpful. Patients sometimes present with established non-union of the capitate.

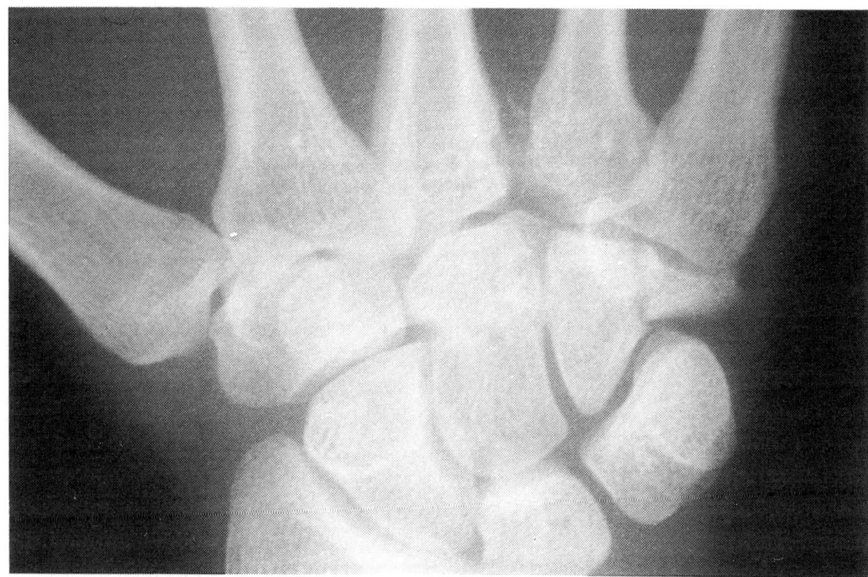

Fig. 16.45 A fracture of the body of the hamate.

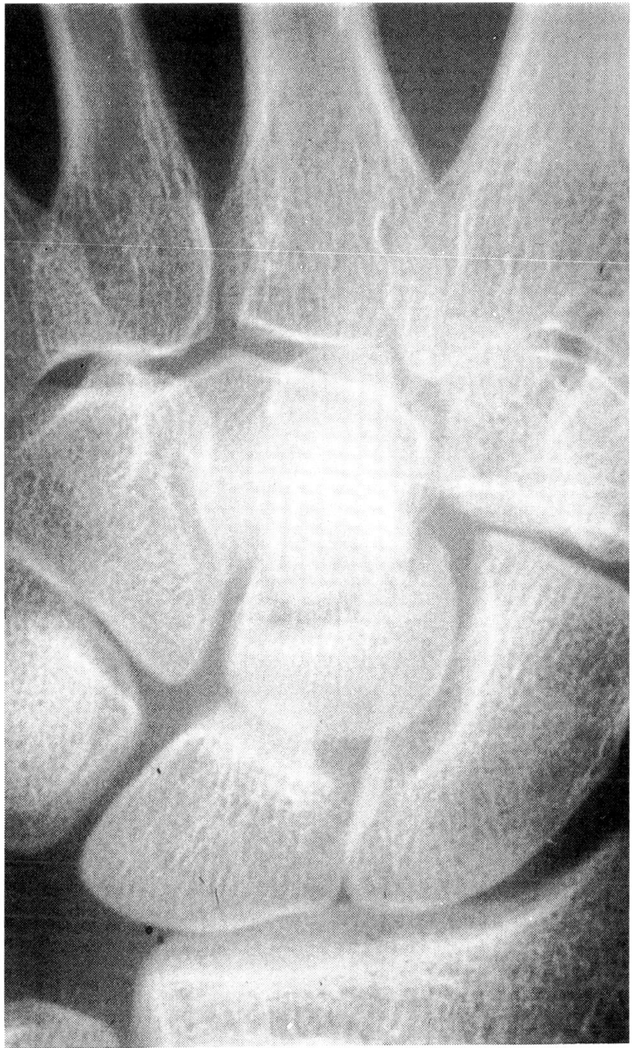

Fig. 16.46 A fracture of the waist of the capitate.

The blood supply of the capitate enters through the waist of the bone and avascular necrosis of the proximal pole after injury has been described (Vander Grend *et al.* 1984), although the condition is more commonly idiopathic and not associated with a fracture (Bolton-Maggs *et al.* 1984).

Acute fractures, if recognized, should be treated with 4–6 weeks rest in a forearm cast (Adler & Shaftan 1962). Established non-union is treated by bone grafting, taking care to restore the length of the carpus with an intercalary block of bone (Rand *et al.* 1982).

Intercarpal osteoarthritis is not uncommon in the long term after capitate fractures and is treated by appropriate intercarpal arthrodesis. Excision of the proximal pole has been recommended for established avascular necrosis with collapse (Kimmel & O'Brien 1982). The resulting space is filled with an 'anchovy' of rolled-up tendon, and an intercarpal fusion to prevent late carpal collapse should be considered.

Carpal dislocations and fracture–dislocations

These are uncommon injuries (Russell 1949). Most carpal fractures and dislocations affect the 'vulnerable zone' which lies between a 'lesser arc' around the lunate and a 'greater arc' crossing the scaphoid, capitate, hamate and triquetrum (Johnson 1980) (Fig. 16.47). The variety of injuries that may occur and their apparent complexity seems bewildering at first, but one can classify almost all carpal dislocations and fracture–dislocations within one of the following groups:

1 Lesser arc injuries — perilunate and lunate dislocations.

2 Greater arc injuries — perilunate fracture–dislocations with fractures through one or more of the bones adjacent to the lunate. The most common variety is the trans-scaphoid perilunate fracture–dislocation with dorsal displacement of the carpus.

3 Variants of injuries within the 'vulnerable zone' — these include fracture–dislocations associated with fractures of the radial styloid process, the 'scapho-capitate syndrome' and dislocation of the scaphoid with or without other bones.

4 Dislocations of other individual carpal bones.

5 Other intercarpal dislocations and fracture–dislocations — these are injuries outside the 'vulnerable zone' and would include such rarities as STT dislocation and crush injuries of the wrist that cause longitudinal disruption of the carpus.

The lunate is the key to the classification of carpal dislocations and fracture–dislocations. It is centrally

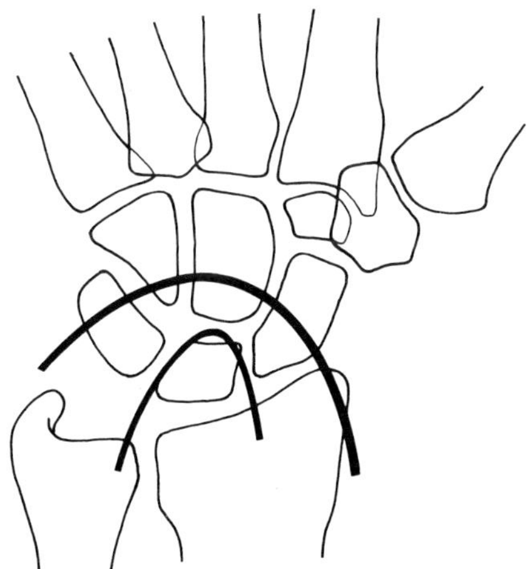

Fig. 16.47 The greater and lesser arcs of the carpus. Most injuries affect the region between the two.

placed and well anchored by ligaments, particularly by volar attachments to the radius (Figs 16.5 & 16.6). Strong forces that dorsiflex and radially deviate the wrist may tear the ligaments that attach the lunate to surrounding carpal bones without damaging the radiolunate ligaments. Because of the direction of the forces involved, pure carpal dislocations, without fracture, are usually perilunate and dorsal. Sometimes, the carpus rebounds into its normal position and pushes the lunate into the carpal tunnel (Mayfield *et al.* 1980); this apparent dislocation of the lunate from the carpus is the end-stage of a perilunate dislocation. These pure lunate and perilunate dislocations account for virtually all lesser arc injuries. Injuries along the greater arc are perilunate dislocations that are associated with fractures of bones adjacent to the lunate.

DIAGNOSIS

The clinical presentation of most dislocations and fracture–dislocations is similar, with pain, swelling and limited wrist movements after injury. Depending on the displacement and the swelling there may or may not be a visible and palpable deformity. Symptoms of acute median nerve compression are not uncommon (Stewart & Cross 1968). Such signs should draw immediate attention to the wrist and indicate the need for radiographic assessment, yet it is not uncommon for these injuries to be overlooked. There are two main reasons for this: firstly, patients may have other, life-threatening injuries that overshadow the wrist problem or make it impossible for them to call attention to it; and secondly, radiographs may be taken but are misinterpreted as showing no injury.

Lesser arc injuries — lunate and perilunate dislocations

Mayfield *et al.* (1980) studied the onset of perilunar instability in cadaver wrists by applying increasing loads with the wrist in dorsiflexion, ulnar deviation and supination. They identified four stages of increasing instability:

1 Scapholunate dissociation caused by tearing of the scapholunate and radioscaphoid ligaments.

2 Dorsal perilunate dislocation.

3 Dorsal perilunate dislocation with triquetro-lunate disruption.

4 Volar dislocation of the lunate with return of the carpus to its normal position relative to the radius.

Fresh dorsal perilunar dislocations and volar dislocations of the lunate (Fig. 16.48a & b) are treated by closed manipulative reduction and stabilization of the

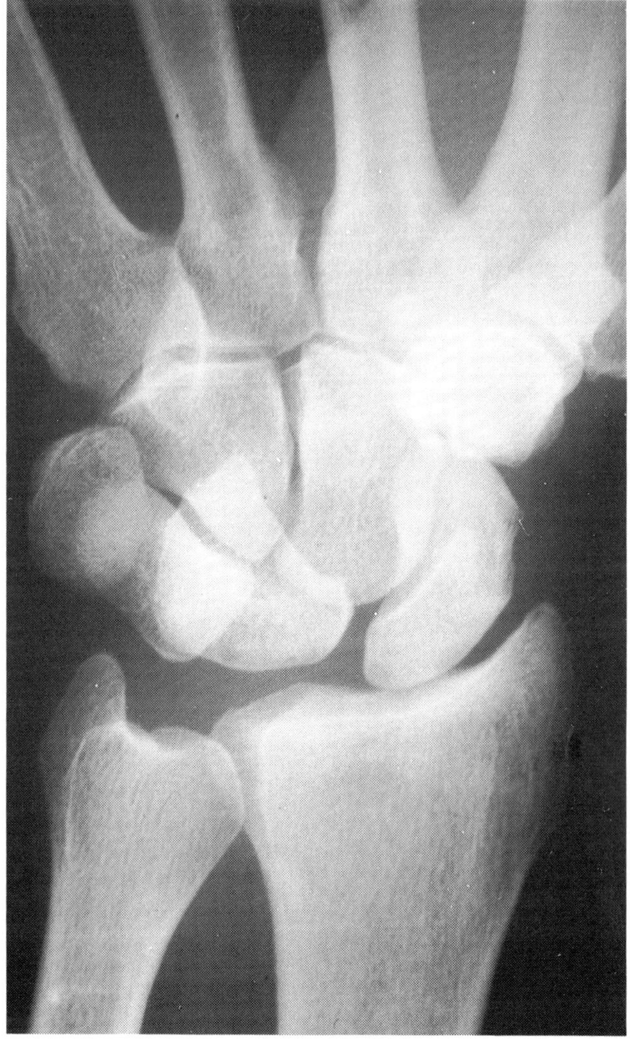

(a)

Fig. 16.48 (*Above* and *opposite*.) Anterior dislocation of the lunate. (a) The characteristic wedge shape of the lunate on the anteroposterior view.

carpus with 1.1-mm-diameter K-wires. The dorsal perilunate dislocation can usually be reduced by traction on the hand, followed by dorsiflexion and then gradual palmar flexion and pronation to bring the capitate into the cup of the lunate, the lunate being stabilized by the surgeon's thumb to prevent displacement. A similar sequence of manoeuvres is used to reduce a volar dislocation of the lunate, which is thumbed back into position as the wrist is dorsiflexed. At this point the carpus may displace dorsally off the radius into the position of perilunate dislocation.

One should not rely on a cast alone to maintain reduction as the ligamentous disruption makes the carpus very unstable. Supplementary stabilization of the carpus with K-wires is necessary. These can be

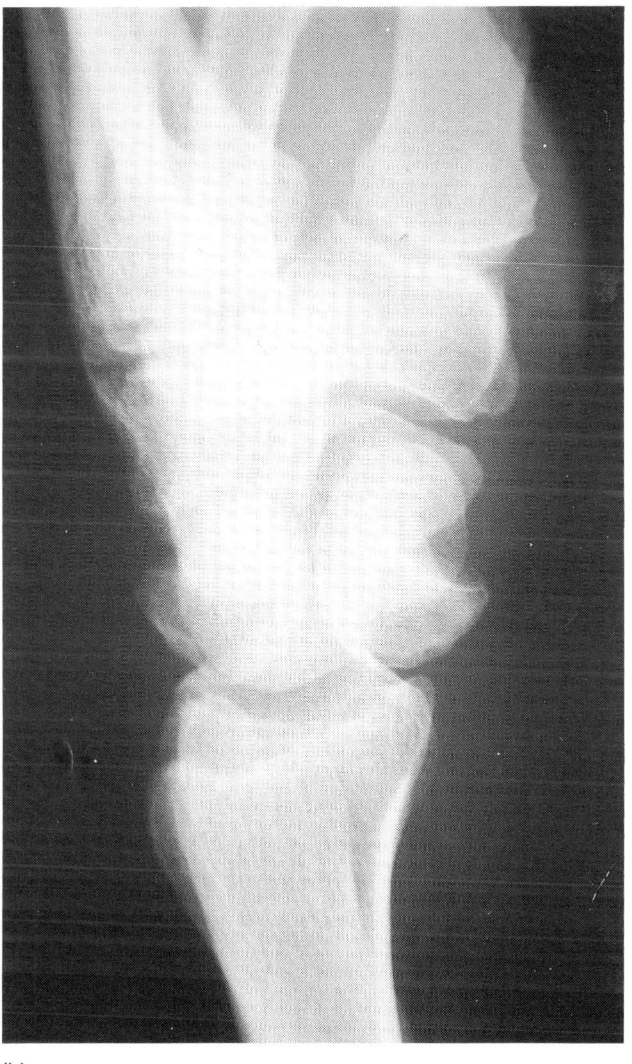

(b)

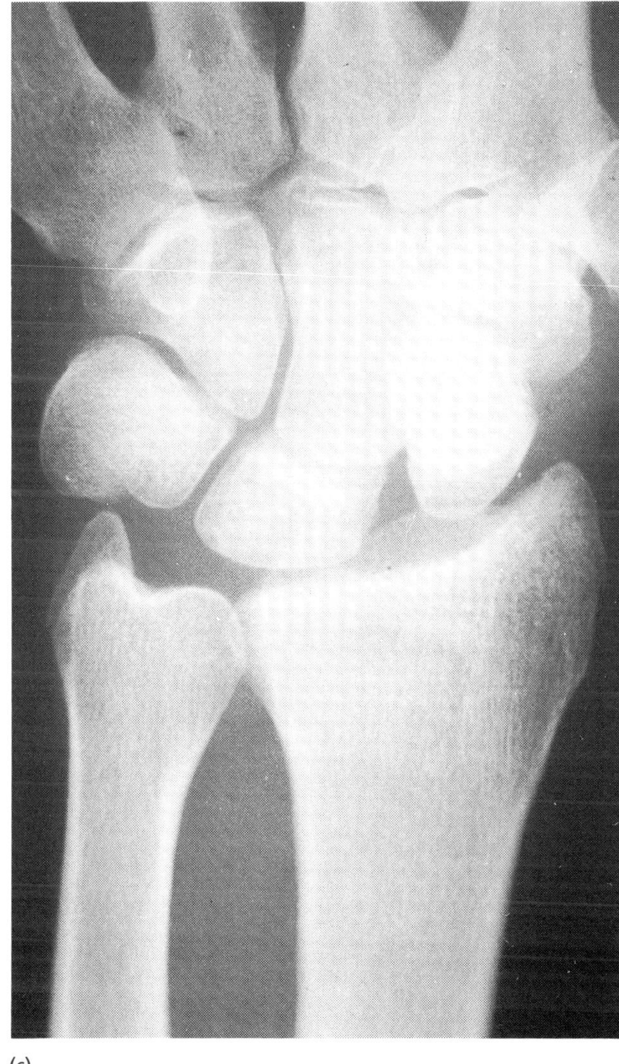

(c)

Fig. 16.48 (*Continued.*) (b) The lateral view. (c) After closed reduction — note scapholunate dissociation, indicating the need for ligamentous repair.

inserted percutaneously, but marked carpal dissociation after reduction is an indication for open reduction and stabilization (Green & O'Brien 1978, Adkinson & Chapman 1982). In fact, postreduction films almost invariably show scapholunate dissociation (Fig. 16.48c) which should be reduced under direct vision through a dorsal exposure and held with K-wires which are retained for 6–8 weeks. A forearm cast is worn for 12 weeks.

Acute carpal tunnel syndrome may necessitate decompression. A longer exposure than usual is made and this gives an opportunity to repair the rent in the volar capsule that is found when the lunate displaces anteriorly.

Open reduction is necessary if the dislocation is ir-

reducible, and open reduction using both volar and dorsal incisions may be needed if reduction has been delayed for any reason.

Avascular necrosis of the lunate is uncommon after dislocations that have been reduced soon after injury. The blood supply of the lunate is derived, in part, from vessels that enter it via the volar radiolunate ligament, which remains intact even when the lunate is displaced.

Volar perilunate dislocations (Fig. 16.49) (Saunier & Chamay 1981) and dorsal lunate dislocations (Bilos & Hui 1981) are exceptionally rare and are probably the result of hyperflexion injuries. Their treatment follows the lines described above, the main consideration being the restoration of normal intercarpal relationships.

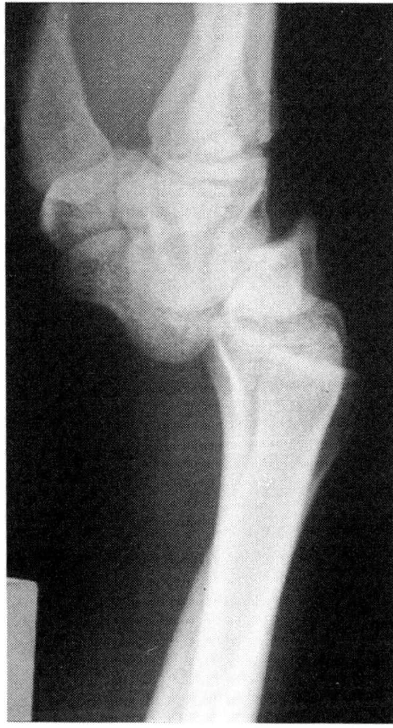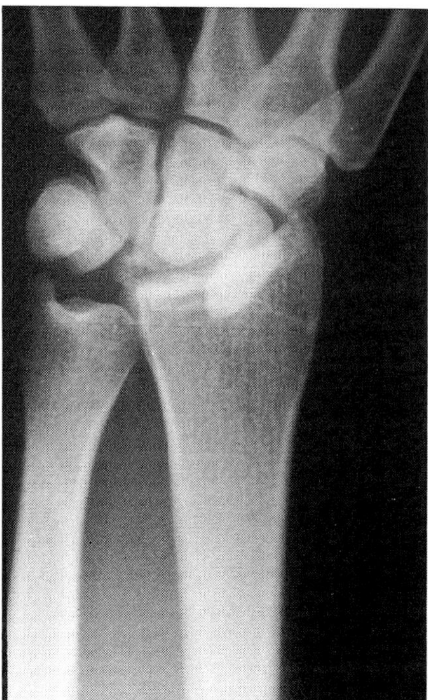

Fig. 16.49 Volar perilunate dislocation.

Greater arc injuries — Trans-scaphoid perilunate fracture–dislocation

In the most common type of greater arc injury, a dorsal perilunate dislocation is accompanied by a fracture through the waist of the scaphoid, the proximal part of the scaphoid remaining attached to the lunate (Fig. 16.50).

Reduction of the dislocation is usually straightforward but the scaphoid fracture is invariably displaced or will become so, so internal fixation is necessary. This can be done via a volar approach through the sheath of the flexor carpi radialis tendon. The Herbert screw can be used for fixation (Viegas *et al.* 1987) but the technique is more difficult than for a simple scaphoid fracture or non-union (Herbert & Fisher 1984). An alternative is to insert the screw freehand through a dorsal exposure of the scaphoid and this should be done if the proximal fragment is small. Instead of the Herbert screw, the broken scaphoid can be stabilized by parallel K-wires driven percutaneously across the fracture site under direct vision; either a dorsal or volar exposure can be used. Good impaction of the fracture is seldom achieved and this may be a contributory factor to non-union and avascular necrosis of the proximal pole of the scaphoid, which frequently follow this injury. A further option is to use a lag screw for internal fixation. This is best inserted through a snuff-box exposure but this does not allow good visualization of the mid-carpal dislocation;

also, the proximal pole of the scaphoid is sometimes too small to be gripped by the screw threads without strutting the fracture surfaces apart.

Acute carpal tunnel syndrome is not uncommon after this injury and may need urgent decompression. This may dictate the surgical exposure of the scaphoid.

Whatever form of scaphoid fixation is chosen, it is usually necessary to maintain the correct carpal relationships after reduction by additional percutaneous K-wires (Fig. 16.51). The wires are removed after about 8 weeks but a forearm thumb spica cast must be worn for a few weeks longer. Secondary fixation and grafting of the scaphoid should be considered if it fails to unite but, not uncommonly, the wrist is surprisingly asymptomatic even when there is obvious non-union with collapse of the scaphoid.

The other forms of greater arc injury are rare. They are dealt with in a similar manner to a dorsal trans-scaphoid perilunate fracture–dislocation but the other fractures may need additional fixation with K-wires or, in the case of small osteochondral fractures, they can be excised.

Variants of injuries within the 'vulnerable zone'

The most common types are perilunate dislocations or fracture–dislocations which are associated with a fracture of the radial styloid process. The dislocation is usually trans-styloid (Fig. 16.52). Treatment follows the

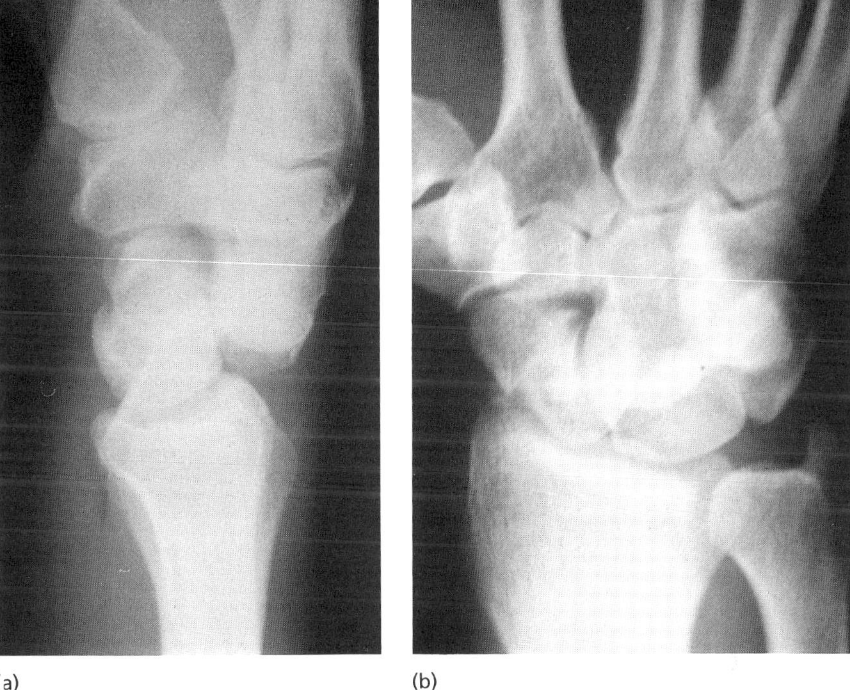

Fig. 16.50 Trans-scaphoid perilunate
dislocation. (a) Lateral view.
(b) Anterior view.

(a)

(b)

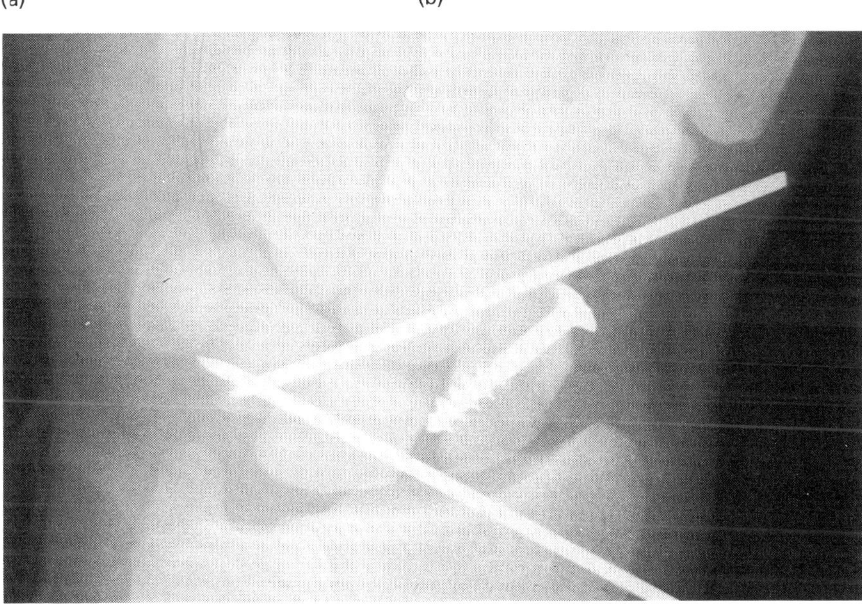

Fig. 16.51 A trans-scaphoid perilunate
dislocation after reduction, internal
fixation of the scaphoid with a lag
screw and stabilization of the carpus
with K-wires.

general lines given above, with open reduction of the
dislocation and internal fixation of fractures.

The 'scaphocapitate syndrome' is a fracture of the
waist of the scaphoid occurring together with a fracture
through the capitate, the proximal fragment of which is
rotated 180°. This injury can occur as part of a perilunate
fracture–dislocation. The fracture of the capitate is
easily overlooked and a traction view, after reduction of
the dislocation, is helpful in identifying it. Both scaphoid and capitate fractures should be fixed after reduction, using K-wires or small screws (Meyers *et al.*

1971). Alternatively, the displaced fragment of the
capitate can be excised (Fenton 1956), and this should
be done as a primary procedure if there has been a
delay in recognizing the capitate fracture.

Dislocation of the scaphoid, with or without dislocation of the lunate, is rare (Brown & Muddu 1981,
Maki *et al.* 1982, Kupfer 1986). The direction of dislocation is volar or radial. Closed reduction has been
successful in most reported cases, but additional stabilization by K-wires is sensible.

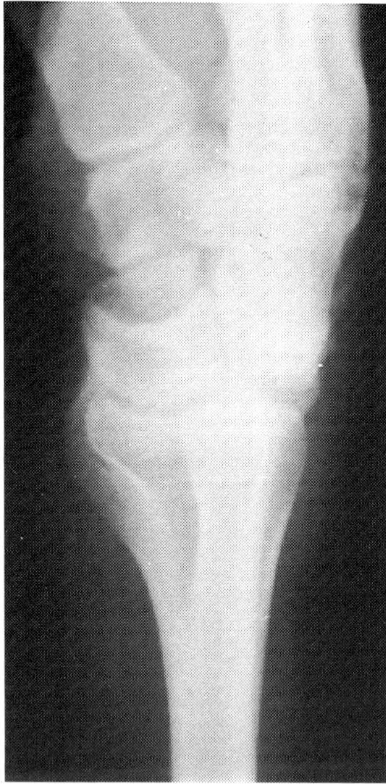 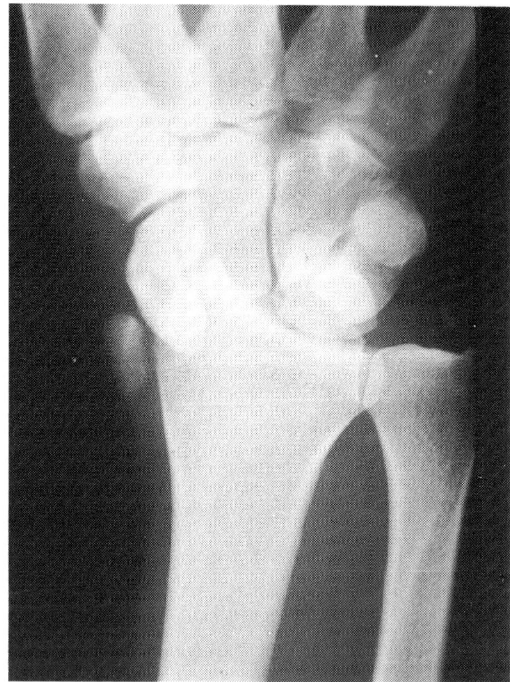

Fig. 16.52 A trans-styloid perilunate dislocation.

Dislocation of other individual carpal bones

These are all rare injuries, mostly described in case reports and reviews of preceding literature.

TRAPEZIUM

Volar dislocations are more common than dorsal dislocations and the injury is often open (Siegel & Hertzberg 1969, Boe 1979). Excision has been recommended if the bone is devoid of soft tissue attachments. If possible, however, it should be reduced by open or closed means, as appropriate, and stabilized by wires. Complications include avascular necrosis and stiffness of the trapezio-metacarpal joint.

TRAPEZOID

True dislocation is rare. The direction of dislocation is usually dorsal (Stein 1971) and closed reduction may be successful. Volar dislocations (Goodman & Shankman 1984, Kopp 1985) require open reduction, which may be achieved through a dorsal exposure in recent injuries.

It is more common to find that a large fragment of the trapezoid has dislocated dorsally with the index metacarpal bone. Reduction is unstable and supplementary K-wire fixation is necessary.

OTHER BONES

Isolated dislocations of the pisiform (Immerman 1948), hamate (Duke 1963, Gunn 1985), triquetrum (Bieber & Weiland 1984) and capitate (Lowrey *et al.* 1984) are very rare. Open reduction and K-wire stabilization is needed for most of these injuries, although the pisiform may be excised (Helal 1978).

Other intercarpal dislocations

STT

This joint is very rarely dislocated, although subluxations may occur (Gibson 1983, Kuur & Boe 1986). Treatment is by open reduction and temporary K-wire stabilization or, in late cases, by arthrodesis. Chronic instability of this joint may be a forerunner of osteoarthritic changes.

CARPAL ARCH INJURIES

A severe crush injury, for example, from a power press, can flatten the transverse carpal arch. Typically, the line of disruption passes through the capitohamate and pisotriquetral articulations, causing malrotation of the ulnar two digits (Fig. 16.53) (Primiano & Reet 1974).

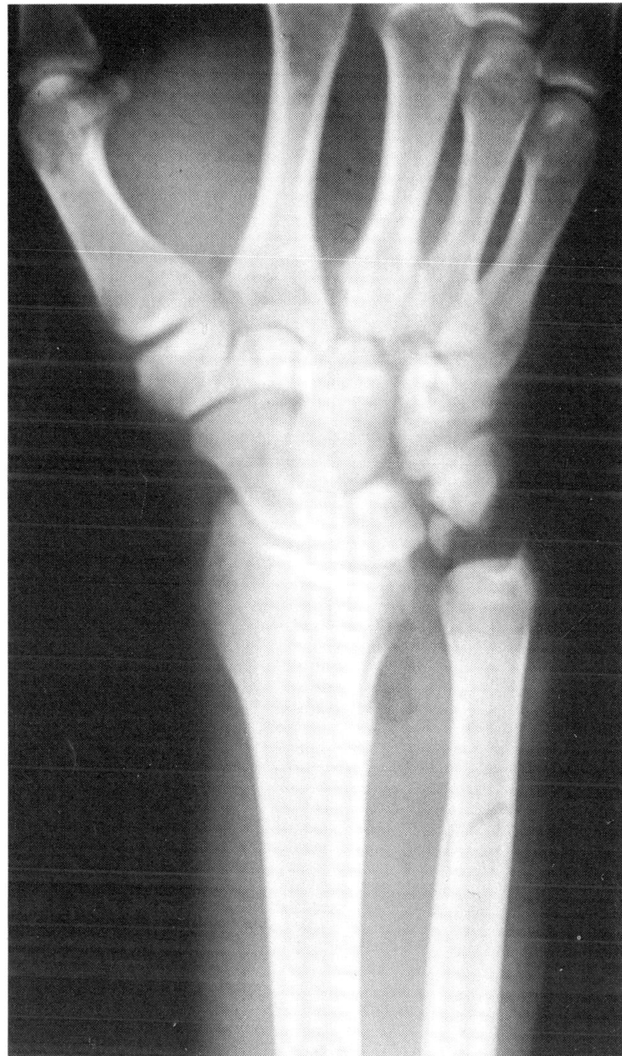

Fig. 16.53 Longitudinal disruption of the carpus caused by a crushing injury.

There is often a bursting laceration of the thenar eminence. Closed reduction may be successful in early cases (Garcia-Elias *et al.* 1985) but it may be necessary to stabilize the carpus with K-wires.

The wrist injury is part of a major crush of the hand and it may be associated with acute compression of the median or ulnar nerves, or compartmental syndrome of the intrinsic muscles. These complications demand urgent treatment by decompression. In addition, the hand should be elevated and splinted in the correct position of immobilization.

Wrist injuries in childhood

Fractures of the distal radius and ulna are common in childhood but carpal fractures and dislocations are quite rare. The usual explanation for this is that the carpal bones in childhood are still largely cartilaginous and resilient, so that the bones of the distal part of the forearm tend to fail before the carpus.

Fractures of the distal radius and ulna

The common types are:
1 Fractures involving the epiphyses.
2 Compression (torus) fractures.
3 Greenstick fractures.
4 Complete fractures.
Fractures may involve one or both bones. If both bones are involved the fractures are frequently not the same type.

MECHANISM

Almost all the common wrist injuries are caused by a fall on the outstretched hand with the wrist extended. There may be an additional element of pronation or supination.

DIAGNOSIS

The child is in pain and unwilling to move the limb. Gentle palpation will localize the pain at the site of injury. If deformity is present it is almost always of the 'dinner fork' type and palpation will not be necessary to make the diagnosis.

Neurovascular problems are rare but should be excluded. Nerve injuries are usually a result of neuropraxia of the median or ulnar nerves but, rarely, a nerve may be trapped between the bone ends (Prosser & Hooper 1986).

Radiographic examination will demonstrate the bony injury, but will not indicate the degree of displacement (which may have been considerable) at the moment of injury.

Fractures involving the epiphysis

These occur most commonly between the ages of 6 and 12 years. Most are Salter−Harris type II injuries of the distal radial epiphysis. The displacement is almost invariably dorsal or dorsolateral (Fig. 16.54).

Closed reduction under appropriate anaesthesia is straightforward, although unnecessary in injuries with minimal displacement. A split above-elbow cast is applied after reduction and the position is held by gentle moulding of the cast, rather than by putting the wrist in flexion. The cast is completed about 5 days after

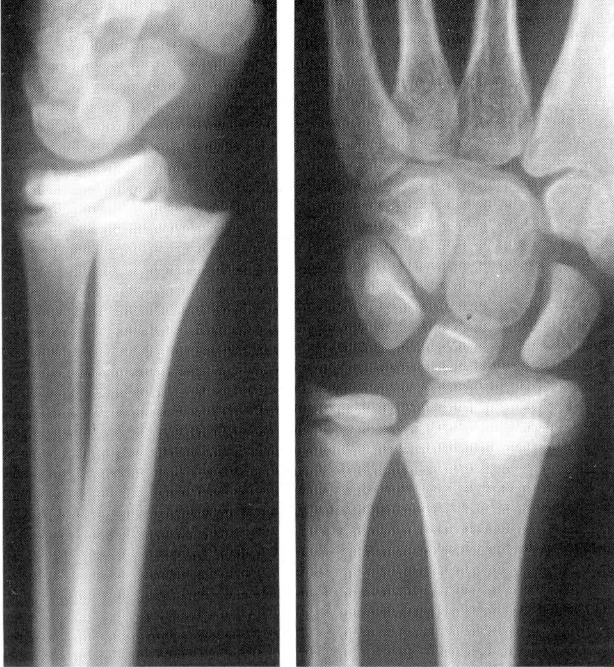

Fig. 16.54 Displacement of the distal radial epiphysis.

injury, when any swelling has settled, and is retained for 5 weeks. A check radiographic film is taken 1 week after reduction, but re-displacement of a properly reduced radial epiphysis is uncommon. Remanipulation is seldom required and should be avoided more than 1 week after injury for fear of damage to the growth plate. Remodelling of a displaced epiphysis is usually rapid, even near the age when growth plate closure is imminent.

Open reduction is needed in rare cases when the epiphysis cannot be reduced. It is usually found that a flap of periosteum has become interposed between the bone ends and must be extracted. The reduced epiphysis is stabilized with an oblique K-wire.

Growth disturbances are uncommon after epiphyseal injuries of the distal radius (Aitken 1935). Radial lengthening is usually feasible if premature fusion has occurred.

Compression fractures

In these common injuries the bone buckles as a result of axial loading (Fig. 16.55). Usually the buckling is most obvious dorsally. These are sometimes called torus fractures because of the fancied resemblance to the raised band around an architectural column.

The only treatment required is simple protection in a forearm splint for a couple of weeks.

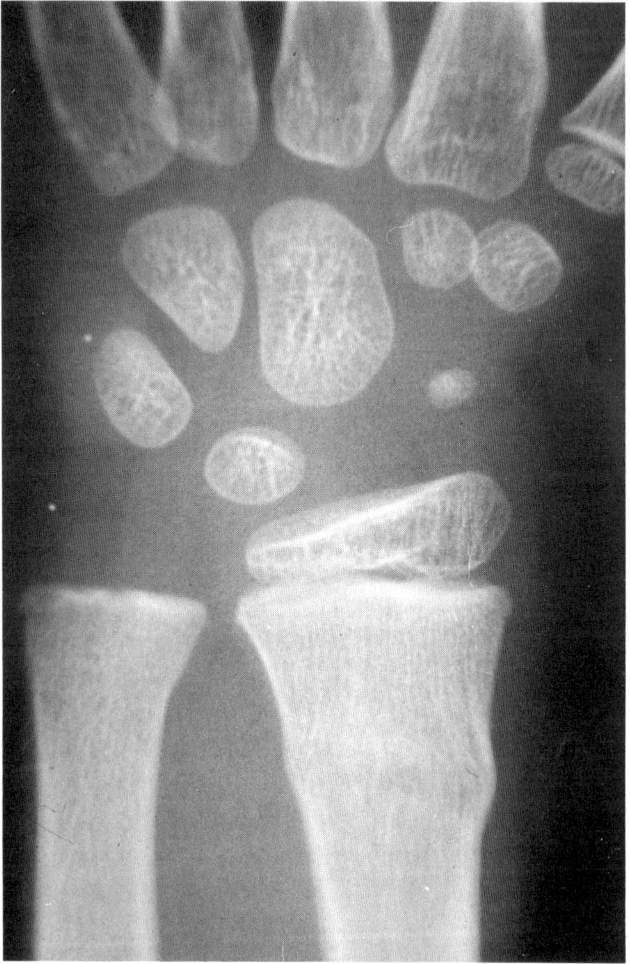

Fig. 16.55 Buckle fracture of the distal radius.

Greenstick fractures

As with any greenstick fracture, there is disruption of the periosteum and bone on the tension (convex) surface of the fracture, but this does not extend to the compression (concave) side. The distal fragment is dorsally angulated in the majority of cases.

The angulation associated with greenstick fractures is very likely to increase in the cast, even after satisfactory reduction (Fig. 16.56). This is due to several factors: the soft tissue on the intact side acts as a tension-band; gravity may cause sagging at the fracture site, depending on the position of the forearm in the cast; and the action of the brachioradialis muscle may increase dorsal angulation if the forearm is pronated.

There is some controversy about the amount of angulation that is acceptable in the distal forearm, as well as the best method of preventing an increase in deformity. Since it is generally accepted that the radiological deformity may be no reflection of the angulation at the

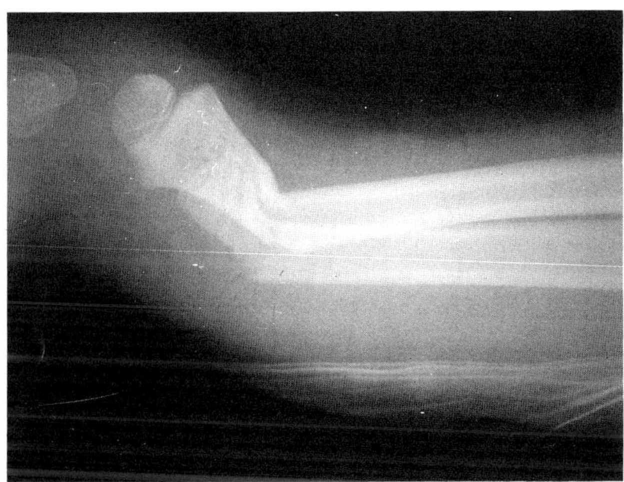

Fig. 16.56 Greenstick fracture of the distal radius. This displacement may recur even after satisfactory reduction.

moment of injury, and also that there is a tendency for deformity to increase during cast immobilization, it is best to err on the side of overtreatment and reduce all fractures with an angulation greater than 15°. Since recurrent deformity is less likely after a complete fracture, many authorities recommend completing the fracture at the time of reduction. The disadvantage of doing this is that the fragments may become displaced and more difficult to hold reduced, although this is probably not such a serious concern as it would be with a fracture of the mid-shaft of the radius or ulna. In practice, it is not usually necessary to complete a distal radial fracture. Most fractures can be held reduced by applying three-point moulding (Fig. 16.57) to an above-elbow cast with the forearm in either pronation or supination, depending on the angulation: if the distal fragment is angulated dorsally the forearm should be pronated, but if the fragment is angulated volarwards the forearm should be supinated (Evans 1951).

Reduction is carried out under general anaesthetic. The cast is split immediately after application and completed when any swelling has gone down. It is changed at 2 weeks and it is usually possible to correct any recurrent angulation up to this time, if need be. A cast is retained for 6 weeks but it may be changed to a forearm type at 4 weeks, in most cases.

Complete fractures

Treatment follows the principles outlined for greenstick fractures. The main problem with this type of injury is difficulty in reduction, usually because of the soft tissue hinge on one side of the fracture (Fig. 16.58), but some-

times because of soft tissue interposition.

Reduction of a displaced fracture can only be achieved by increasing the deformity to overcome the action of the soft tissue hinge (Fig. 16.58). Thereafter, the arm is placed in an above-elbow split cast with appropriate moulding, as for a greenstick fracture.

If reduction cannot be obtained and the bone ends remain out of contact, it usually indicates that soft tissue is interposed between the bone ends and open reduction is then required. The fracture is held reduced by a K-wire driven from the radial styloid process.

COMPLICATIONS

Complications of distal radial fractures in children are rare but include compartment syndrome, growth arrest (after epiphyseal injuries), infection (after open injuries), malunion and refracture (Davis & Green 1976).

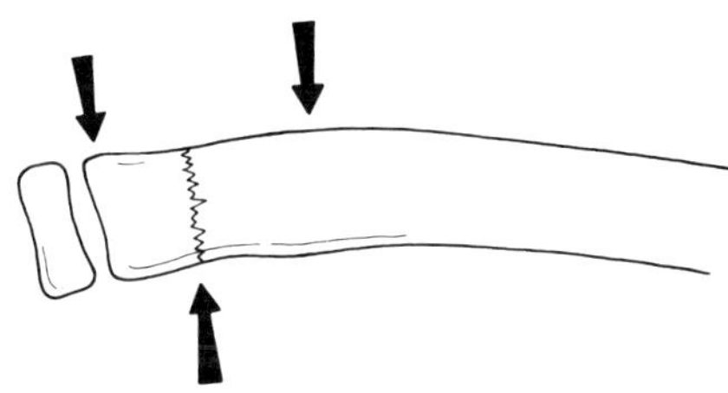

Fig. 16.57 It is necessary to apply three-point moulding to maintain reduction of distal forearm fractures.

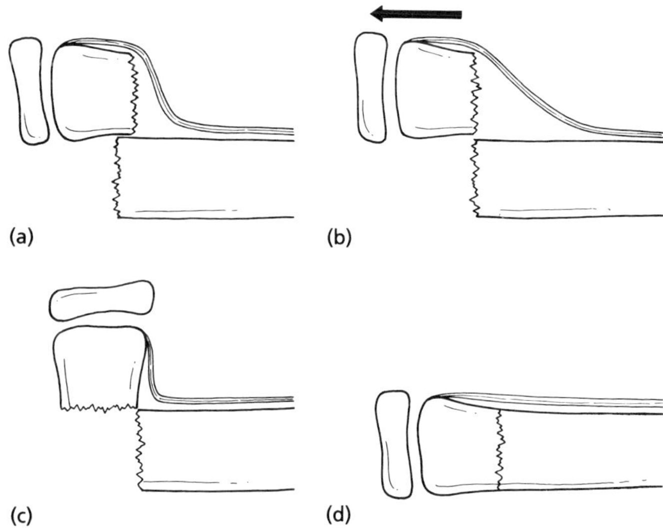

(a)

(b)

(c)

(d)

Fig. 16.58 (a) There is always a dorsal soft tissue hinge when a complete radial fracture is displaced dorsally. (b) Longitudinal traction will tighten the soft tissue hinge and reduction will be impossible. (c) The deformity must first be *increased* to slacken the hinge, (d) allowing the distal fragment to be reduced.

Dislocations of the distal radioulnar joint

These injuries can occur in childhood. The diagnosis and management does not differ from that described for injuries in adults.

Carpal injuries

Fractures

Fracture of the scaphoid is rare before the age of 10 years but, thereafter, is not too uncommon (Vahvanen & Westerlund 1980, Greene *et al*. 1984). The distal part of the bone is most often broken and displacement is uncommon. Treatment follows the general lines described for adults. Delayed union can occur, particularly if there is any delay in diagnosis and treatment, but union will usually take place if immobilization is continued for a long period. Non-union is very rare but bone grafting is usually successful (Southcott & Rosman 1977).

Fractures of the capitate also occur and a non-union, necessitating a bone graft, has been reported in a 13-year-old (Minami *et al*. 1987).

Dislocations and fracture–dislocations

These are extreme rarities. A trans-scaphoid perilunate fracture–dislocation has been described in a 10-year-old (Peiro *et al*. 1981).

Carpal instability

A 7-year-old child with chronic scapholunate dissociation has been reported (Gerard 1980). Ligamentous reconstruction was carried out.

References

Adkinson, J.W. & Chapman, M.W. Treatment of acute lunate and perilunate dislocations. *Clin Orthop* 1982; **164**: 199–207.

Adler, J.B. & Shaftan, G.W. Fractures of the capitate. *J Bone Joint Surg* 1962; **44A**: 1537–1547.

Aitken, A.P. The end result of the fractured distal radial epiphysis. *J Bone Joint Surg* 1935; **17**: 302–308.

Alexander, A.H., Turner, M.A., Alexander, C.E. & Lichtman, D.M. Lunate silicone replacement arthroplasty in Kienböck's disease: a long-term follow-up. *J Hand Surg* 1990; **15A**: 401–407.

Almquist, E.E. & Burns, J.F. Radial shortening for the treatment of Kienböck's disease — a 5- to 10-year follow-up. *J Hand Surg* 1982; **7**: 348–357.

Armistead, R.B., Linscheid, R.L., Dobyns, J.H. & Beckenbaugh, R.D. Ulnar lengthening in the treatment of Kienböck's disease. *J Bone Joint Surg* 1982; **64A**: 170–178.

Baird, D.B., Freidenberg, Z.B. Delayed ulnar nerve palsy following a fracture of the hamate. *J Bone Joint Surg* 1968; **50A**: 570–572.

Bartone, N.F. & Grieco, R.V. Fractures of the triquetrum. *J Bone Joint Surg* 1956; **38A**: 353–356.

Beckenbaugh, R.D., Shives, T.C., Dobyns, J.H. & Linscheid, R.L. Kienböck's disease: the natural history of Kienböck's disease and consideration of lunate fractures. *Clin Orthop* 1980; **149**: 98–106.

Bieber, E.J. & Weiland, A.J. Traumatic dorsal dislocation of the triquetrum: a case report. *J Hand Surg* 1984; **9A**: 840–842.

Bilos, J. & Hui, P.W. Dorsal dislocation of the lunate with carpal collapse. *J Bone Joint Surg* 1981; **63A**: 1484–1486.

Boe, S. Dislocation of the trapezium (multangulum majus). *Acta Orthop Scand* 1979; **50**: 85–86.

Boeckstyns, M.E.H., Kjaer, L., Busch, P. & Holst-Neilsen, F. Soft tissue interposition arthroplasty for scaphoid nonunion. *J Hand Surg* 1985; **10A**: 109–114.

Bolton-Maggs, B.G., Held, B.H. & Ravell, P.A. Bilateral avascular necrosis of the capitate: a case report and review of the literature. *J Bone Joint Surg* 1984; **66B**: 557–559.

Bowen, T.L. Injuries of the hamate bone. *Hand* 1973; **5**: 235–238.

Bray, T. & McCarroll, H. Preiser's disease: a case report. *J Hand Surg* 1984; **9A**: 730–732.

Brown, R.H.L. & Muddu, B.N. Scaphoid and lunate dislocation: a report on a case. *Hand* 1981; **3**: 303–307.

Bryan, R. & Dobyns, J.H. Fractures of the carpal bones other than the lunate and navicular. *Clin Orthop* 1980; **149**: 107–111.

Carter, P.R., Eaton, R.G. & Littler, J.W. Ununited fracture of the hook of the hamate. *J Bone Joint Surg* 1977; **59A**: 583–588.

Cetti, R. & Chirstensen, S.E. The diagnostic value of displacement of the fat stripe in fracture of the scaphoid bone. *Hand* 1982; **14**: 75–79.

Charnley, J. *The Closed Treatment of Common Fractures*. Churchill Livingstone: Edinburgh, 1974.

Colles, A. *Edinb Med J* 1814; **10**: 182–186.

Cooney, W.P., Dobyns, J.H. & Linscheid, R.L. Complications of Colles' fractures. *J Bone Joint Surg* 1980a; **62A**: 613–619.

Cooney, W.P., Dobyns, J.H. & Linscheid, R.L. Nonunion of the scaphoid: analysis of the results from bone grafting. *J Hand Surg* 1980b; **5**: 343–354.

Cooney, W.P., Linscheid, R.L. & Dobyns, J.H. External pin fixation for unstable Colles' fractures. *J Bone Joint Surg* 1979; **61A**: 840–845.

Cordrey, L.J. & Ferrer-Torrells, M. Management of fractures of the greater multangular. *J Bone Joint Surg* 1960; **42A**: 1111–1118.

Crosby, E.B. & Linscheid, R.L. Rupture of the flexor profundus tendon of the ring finger secondary to ancient fracture of the hook of the hamate. Review of the literature and report of two cases. *J Bone Joint Surg* 1974; **56A**: 1076–1078.

Dameron, T.B. Traumatic dislocation of the distal radioulnar joint. *Clin Orthop* 1972; **83**: 55–63.

Darrach, W. Fractures of the lower extremity of the radius: diagnosis and treatment. *J Am Med Assoc* 1927; **89**: 1683–1685.

Davis, D.R. & Green, D.P. Forearm fractures in children. Pitfalls and complications. *Clin Orthop* 1976; **120**: 172–184.

De Oliveira, J.C. Barton's fractures. *J Bone Joint Surg* 1973; **55A**: 586–594.

Dias, J.J. & McMohan, A. Effect of Colles' fracture malunion on carpal alignment. *J R Coll Surg Edinb* 1988; 234–236.

Dias, J.J., Taylor, M., Thompson, J., Brenkel, I.J. & Gregg, P.J. Radiographic signs of union of scaphoid fractures. *J Bone Joint Surg* 1988; **70B**: 299–301.

Dias, J.J., Wray, C.C. & Jones, J.M. The radiological deformity of Colles' fractures. *Injury* 1987a; **18**: 304–308.

Dias, J.J., Wray, C.C. & Jones, J.M. Osteoporosis and Colles' fractures in the elderly. *J Hand Surg* 1987b; **12B**: 57–59.

Dias, J.J., Wray, C.C., Jones, J.M. & Gregg, P.J. The value of early mobilisation in the treatment of Colles' fractures. *J Bone Joint Surg* 1987c; **69B**: 463–467.

Dickson, R.A. Scaphoid fractures: conservative management. In: Barton, N.J. (ed.) *Fractures of the Hand and Wrist*. Churchill Livingstone: Edinburgh, 1988.

Duke, R. Fractures of the hamate bone. *J Bone Joint Surg* 1963; **45B**: 744.

Düppe, H., Johnell, O., Lundborg, G., Karlsson, M. & Redlund-Johnell, L. Long-term results of fracture of the scaphoid. *J Bone Joint Surg* 1994; **76A**: 249–252.

Eckenrode, J.F., Louis, D.F. & Green, T.L. Scapho-trapezio-trapezoid fusion in the treatment of chronic scapholunate instability. *J Hand Surg* 1986; **11A**: 497–502.

Edwards, H.C. Mechanism and treatment of backfire fracture. *J Bone Joint Surg* 1926; **8**: 701–717.

Egawa, M. & Asai, R. Fracture of the hook of the hamate: report of six cases and the suitability of computerized tomography. *J Hand Surg* 1983; **8**: 393–398.

Ellis, J. Smith's and Barton's fractures. A method of treatment. *J Bone Joint Surg* 1965; **47B**: 724–727.

Essex-Lopresti, B. Fractures of the head of the radius with distal radioulnar dislocation. *J Bone Joint Surg* 1951; **33B**: 244–247.

Evans, E.M. Fractures of the radius and ulna. *J Bone Joint Surg* 1951; **33B**: 548–561.

Fenton, R.L. The naviculo-capitate fracture syndrome. *J Bone Joint Surg* 1956; **38A**: 681–684.

Fisk, G.R. Carpal instability and the fractured scaphoid. *Ann R Coll Surg Engl* 1970; **46**: 63–76.

Fisk, G.R. Injuries of the wrist. In: Wilson, J.N. (ed.) *Watson-Jones Fractures and Joint Injuries* 6th edn. Churchill Livingstone: Edinburgh, 1982.

Frankel, V.H. The Terry-Thomas sign. *Clin Orthop* 1977; **129**: 321–322.

Freeland, A.E. & Finley, J.S. Displaced vertical fractures of the trapezium treated with a small cancellous lag screw. *J Hand Surg* 1984; **9A**: 843–845.

Frykman, G. Fractures of the distal radius including sequelae — shoulder–hand–finger syndrome. Disturbance in the distal radio-ulnar joint and impairment of nerve function. A clinical and experimental study. *Acta Orthop Scand Suppl* 1967; **108**.

Fuller, D.J. The Ellis plate operation for Smith's fracture. *J Bone Joint Surg* 1973; **55B**: 173–178.

Garcia-Elias, M. Dorsal fractures of the triquetrum — avulsion or compression fractures? *J Hand Surg* 1987; **12A**: 266–268.

Garcia-Elias, M., Abanco, J., Salvador, E. & Sanchez, R. Crush injury of the carpus. *J Bone Joint Surg* 1985; **67B**: 286–289.

Gartland, J.J. Jr. & Werley, C.W. Evaluation of healed Colles' fractures. *J Bone Joint Surg* 1953; **33A**: 895–907.

Gay, J.D.L. Radial fracture as an indicator of osteoporosis: a 10-year follow-up study. *Can Med Assoc J* 1974; **111**: 156–157.

Gelberman, R.H. & Menon, J. The vascularity of the scaphoid bone. *J Hand Surg* 1980; **5**: 508–513.

Gelberman, R.H., Bauman, T.D., Menon, J. & Akeson, W.H. The vascularity of the lunate bone and Kienböck's disease. *J Hand Surg* 1980; **5**: 272–278.

Gerard, F.M. Post traumatic carpal instability in a young child. *J Bone Joint Surg* 1980; **62A**: 131–133.

Gibson, P.H. Scaphoid-trapezium-trapezoid dislocation. *Hand* 1983; **15**: 267–269.

Goldner, J.L. Treatment of carpal instability without joint fusion — current assessment. *J Hand Surg* 1982; **7**: 325–326.

Goodman, M.L. & Shankman, G.B. Update: palmar dislocation of the trapezoid — a case report. *J Hand Surg* 1984; **9A**: 127–131.

Green, D.P. The effect of avascular necrosis on Russe bone grafting for scaphoid nonunion. *J Hand Surg* 1985; **10A**: 597–605.

Green, D.P. & O'Brien, E.T. Open reduction of carpal dislocations: indications and operative techniques. *J Hand Surg* 1978; **3**: 250–265.

Greene, M.H., Hadied, A.M. & LaMont, R.L. Scaphoid fractures in children. *J Hand Surg* 1984; **9A**: 536–541.

Gunn, R.S. Dislocations of the hamate bone. *J Hand Surg* 1985; **10B**: 107–108.

Hart, V.L. & Gaynor, V. Roentgenographic study of the carpal canal. *J Bone Joint Surg* 1941; **23**: 382–383.

Helal, B. Racquet player's pisiform. *Hand* 1978; **10**: 87–90.

Herbert, T.J. & Fisher, W.E. Management of the fractured scaphoid using a new bone screw. *J Bone Joint Surg* 1984; **66B**: 114–123.

Imaeda, T., Nakamura, R., Miura, T. & Makino, N. Magnetic resonance imaging in scaphoid fractures. *J Hand Surg* 1992; **17B**: 20–27.

Immerman, E.W. Dislocation of the pisiform. *J Bone Joint Surg* 1948; **30A**: 489–492.

Johnson, R.P. The acutely injured wrist and its residuals. *Clin Orthop* 1980; **149**: 33–44.

Jones, K.G. Replacement of the proximal portion of the scaphoid with spherical implant for post-traumatic carporadial arthritis. *J Hand Surg* 1985; **10B**: 217–226.

Jones, W.A. & Ghorbal, M.S. Fractures of the trapezium. *J Hand Surg* 1985; **10B**: 227–230.

Kawai, H., Yamamoto, K., Yamamoto, T., Tada, K. & Kaga, K. Excision of the lunate in Kienböck's disease. *J Bone Joint Surg* 1988; **70B**: 287–292.

Kimmel, R.B. & O'Brien, E.T. Surgical treatment of avascular necrosis of the proximal pole of capitate: a case report. *J Hand Surg* 1982; **7**: 284–286.

Kleinman, W.B., Steichen, J.B. & Strickland, J.W. Management of chronic rotary subluxation of the scaphoid by scaphotrapezio-trapezoid arthrodesis. *J Hand Surg* 1982; **7**: 125–136.

Kopp, J.R. Isolated palmar dislocation of the trapezoid. *J Hand Surg* 1985; **10A**: 91–93.

Kristensen, S.S., Thomassen, E. & Christensen, F. Kienböck's disease — late results by non-surgical treatment. *J Hand Surg* 1986; **11B**: 422–425.

Kupfer, K. Palmar dislocation of the scaphoid and lunate as a unit: case report with special reference to carpal instability and treatment. *J Hand Surg* 1986; **11A**: 130–134.

Kuur, E. & Boe, A.M. Scaphoid-trapezium-trapezoid subluxation. *J Hand Surg* 1986; **11B**: 434–435.

Lee, M. The intraosseous arterial pattern of the carpal lunate bone and its relation to avascular necrosis. *Acta Orthop Scand* 1963; **33**: 43–55.

Lentino, W., Lubetsky, H.W., Jacobson, H.G. & Poppel, M.H. The carpal-bridge view: a position for the roentgenographic diagnosis of abnormalities in the dorsum of the wrist. *J Bone Joint Surg* 1957; **39A**: 88–90.

Leslie, I.J. & Dickson, R.A. The fractured carpal scaphoid: natural history and factors influencing outcome. *J Bone Joint Surg* 1981; **63B**: 225–230.

Levy, M., Fischel, R.E., Stern, G.M. & Goldberg, I. Chip fractures of the os triquetrum. The mechanism of injury. *J Bone Joint Surg* 1979; **61B**: 355–357.

Leyshon, A., Ireland, J. & Trickey, E.L. The treatment of delayed union and non-union of the carpal scaphoid by screw fixation. *J Bone Joint Surg* 1984; **66B**: 124–127.

Lichtman, D.M., Alexander, A.H., Mack, G.R. & Gunther, S.F. Kienböck's disease — update on silicone replacement arthroplasty. *J Hand Surg* 1982; **7**: 343–347.

Lichtman, D.M., Schneider, J.R., Swafford, A.R. & Mack, G.R. Ulnar midcarpal instability — clinical and laboratory analysis. *J Hand Surg* 1981; **6**: 515–523.

Lidstrom, A. Fractures of the distal end of the radius. A clinical and statistical study of end results. *Acta Orthop Scand Suppl* 1959; **41**.

Linscheid, R.L., Dobyns, J.H., Beabout, J.W. & Bryan, R.S. Traumatic instability of the wrist. *J Bone Joint Surg* 1972; **54**: 1612–1632.

London, P.S. The broken scaphoid bone: the case against pessimism. *J Bone Joint Surg* 1961; **43B**: 237–244.

Lowrey, D.G., Moss, S.H. & Wolff, T.W. Volar dislocation of the capitate. *J Bone Joint Surg* 1984; **66A**: 611–613.

Mack, G.R., Bosse, M.J., Gelberman, R.H. *et al*. The natural history of scaphoid non-union. *J Bone Joint Surg* 1984; **66A**: 504–509.

Maki, N.J., Chuinard, R.G. & D'Ambrosia, R. Isolated complete radial dislocation of the scaphoid. A case report and review of the literature. *J Bone Joint Surg* 1982; **64A**: 615–616.

Mayfield, J.K. Mechanism of carpal injuries. *Clin Orthop* 1980; **149**: 45–54.

Mayfield, J.K., Johnson, R.P. & Kilcoyne, R.F. The ligaments of the wrist and their functional significance. *Anat Rec* 1976; **186**: 417–428.

Mayfield, J.K., Johnson, R.P. & Kilcoyne, R.F. Carpal dislocations: pathomechanics and progressive perilunar instability. *J Hand Surg* 1980; **5**: 226–241.

Mazet, R. & Hohl, M. Radial styloidectomy and styloidectomy plus bone graft in the treatment of old ununited scaphoid fractures. *Ann Surg* 1960; **152**: 296–302.

Menon, J., Wood, V.E., Schoene, H.R., Frykman, G.K., Hohl, J.C. & Bestard, E.A. Isolated tears of triangular fibrocartilage of wrist: results of partial excision. *J Hand Surg* 1984; **9A**: 527–530.

Meyers, M.H., Wells, R. & Harvey, J.P. Naviculocapitate fracture syndrome: review of the literature and a case report. *J Bone Joint Surg* 1971; **53A**: 1383–1386.

Minami, M., Yamazaki, J., Chisaka, N., Kato, S., Ogino, T. & Minami, A. Nonunion of the capitate. *J Hand Surg* 1987; **12A**: 1089–1091.

Mulder, J.D. The results of 100 cases of pseudarthrosis in the scaphoid bone treated by the Matti-Russe operation. *J Bone Joint Surg* 1968; **50B**: 110–115.

Nevaiser, R.J. Proximal row carpectomy for post-traumatic disorders of the carpus. *J Hand Surg* 1983; **8**: 301–305.

Obletz, B.E. & Halbstein, B.M. Non-union of fractures of the carpal navicular. *J Bone Joint Surg* 1938; **20**: 424–428.

Owen, R.A., Melton, L.J., Ilstrup, D.M., Johnson, K.A. & Riggs, B.L. Colles' fracture and subsequent hip fracture risk. *Clin Orthop* 1982; **171**: 37–43.

Palmer, A.K. Trapezial ridge fractures. *J Hand Surg* 1981; **6**: 561–564.

Palmer, A.K. & Werner, F.W. The triangular fibrocartilage complex of the wrist — anatomy and function. *J Hand Surg* 1981; **6**: 153–162.

Palmer, A.K., Glisson, R.R. & Werner, F.W. Ulnar variance determination. *J Hand Surg* 1982; **7**: 376–379.

Palmer, A.K., Levinsohn, E.M. & Kuzma, G.R. Arthrography of the wrist. *J Hand Surg* 1983; **8**: 15–23.

Peiro, A., Martos, F., Mut, T. & Aracil, J. Trans-scaphoid perilunate dislocation in a child. *Acta Orthop Scand* 1981; **52**: 31–34.

Polivy, K.D., Millender, L.H., Newberg, A. & Phillips, C.A. Fracture of the hook of the hamate: a failure of clinical diagnosis. *J Hand Surg* 1985; **10A**: 101–104.

Primiano, G.A. & Reet, T.C. Disruption of the proximal carpal arch of the hand. *J Bone Joint Surg* 1974; **56A**: 328–332.

Prosser, A.J. & Hooper, G. Entrapment of the ulnar nerve in a greenstick fracture of the ulna. *J Hand Surg* 1986; **11B**: 211–212.

Prosser, A.J., Brenkel, I.J. & Irvine, G.B. Articular fractures of the distal scaphoid. *J Hand Surg* 1988; **13B**: 87–91.

Rand, J., Linscheid, R.L. & Dobyns, J.H. Capitate fractures. A long term follow-up. *Clin Orthop* 1982; **165**: 209–216.

Rayhack, J.M., Linscheid, R.L. & Dobyns, J.H. Post traumatic ulnar translocation of the carpus. *J Hand Surg* 1987; **12A**: 180.

Reagan, D.S., Linscheid, R.L. & Dobyns, J.H. Lunotriquetral sprains. *J Hand Surg* 1984; **9A**: 502–514.

Rose-Innes, A.P. Anterior dislocation of the ulna at the inferior radio-ulna joint. *J Bone Joint Surg* 1960; **42B**: 515–521.

Ruby, L.K., Stinson, J. & Belsky, M.R. The natural history of non-union of the scaphoid. A review of fifty-five cases. *J Bone Joint Surg* 1985; **67A**: 428–432.

Russe, O. Fracture of the carpal navicular: diagnosis, non-operative treatment and operative treatment. *J Bone Joint Surg* 1960; **42A**: 759–768.

Russell, T.B. Intercarpal dislocations and fracture–dislocations: a review of fifty-nine cases. *J Bone Joint Surg* 1949; **31B**: 524–531.

Sarrafian, S.K., Melamed, J.L. & Goshgarian, G.M. Study of wrist motion in flexion and extension. *Clin Orthop* 1977; **126**: 153–159.

Saunier, J. & Chamay, A. Volar perilunar dislocation of the wrist. *Clin Orthop* 1981; **157**: 139–142.

Siegel, M.W. & Hertzberg, H. Complete dislocation of the greater multangular (trapezium): a case report. *J Bone Joint Surg* 1969; **51A**: 769–772.

Sjølin, S.J. & Andersen, J.C. Clinical fracture of the carpal scaphoid — supportive bandage or plaster cast immobilization? *J Hand Surg* 1988; **13B**: 75–76.

Smaill, G.B. Long-term follow-up of Colles' fracture. *J Bone Joint Surg* 1965; **47B**: 80–85.

Southcott, R. & Rosman, M.A. Non union of carpal scaphoid fractures in children. *J Bone Joint Surg* 1977; **58B**: 20−23.

Stark, H.H., Jobe, F.W., Boyes, J.H. & Ashworth, C.R. Fracture of the hook of the hamate in athletes. *J Bone Joint Surg* 1977; **59A**: 575−582.

Stein, A.H. Dorsal dislocation of the lesser multangular. *J Bone Joint Surg* 1971; **53A**: 377−379.

Stewart, H.D., Innes, A.R. & Burke, F.D. The hand complications of Colles' fractures. *J Hand Surg* 1985; **10B**: 103−106.

Stewart, M.J. & Cross, H. The management of injuries of the carpal lunate with a review of sixty cases. *J Bone Joint Surg* 1968; **50A**: 1489.

Taleisnik, J. The ligaments of the wrist. *J Hand Surg* 1976; **1**: 110−118.

Taleisnik, J. *The Wrist*. Churchill Livingstone: New York, 1985.

Taleisnik, J. & Watson, H.K. Midcarpal instabilities caused by malunited fractures of the distal radius. *J Hand Surg* 1984; **9A**: 350−357.

Thomas, F.B. Reduction of Smith's fracture. *J Bone Joint Surg* 1957; **39B**: 463−470.

Vahvanen, V. & Westerlund, M. Fractures of the carpal scaphoid in children. *Acta Orthop Scand* 1980; **51**: 909−913.

Vander Grend, R., Dell, P.C., Glowczewskie, F., Leslie, B. & Ruby, L.K. Intraosseous blood supply of the capitate and its correlation with aseptic necrosis. *J Hand Surg* 1984; **9A**: 677−680.

Van der Linden, W. & Ericson, R. Colles' fracture. How should its displacement be measured and how should it be immobilized? *J Bone Joint Surg* 1981; **63A**: 1285−1288.

Vesely, D.G. The distal radio-ulnar joint. *Clin Orthop* 1967; **51**: 75−91.

Viegas, S.F., Bean, J.W. & Schram, R.A. Transscaphoid fracture/ dislocations treated with open reduction and Herbert screw internal fixation. *J Hand Surg* 1987; **12A**: 992−999.

Warren-Smith, C.D. & Barton, N.J. Non-union of the scaphoid: Russe graft vs Herbert screw. *J Hand Surg* 1988; **13B**: 83−86.

Watson, H.K. & Ballet, F.L. The SLAC wrist: scapholunate advanced collapse pattern of degenerative arthritis. *J Hand Surg* 1984; **9A**: 358−365.

Watson, H.K. & Hempton, R.F. Limited wrist arthrodesis. Part I: the triscaphoid joint. *J Hand Surg* 1980; **5**: 321−327.

Watson, H.K., Goodman, M.L. & Johnson, T.R. Limited wrist arthrodesis. Part II: intercarpal and radiocarpal combination. *J Hand Surg* 1981; **6**: 223−233.

Watson, H.K., Ryu, J. & DiBella, A. An approach to Kienböck's disease: triscaphe arthrodesis. *J Hand Surg* 1985; **10A**: 179−187.

Watson, H.K., Ryu, J. & Akelman, E. Limited triscaphoid intercarpal arthrodesis for rotatory subluxation of the scaphoid. *J Bone Joint Surg* 1986; **68A**: 345−349.

Weber, E.R. & Chao, E.Y. An experimental approach to the mechanism of scaphoid waist fractures. *J Hand Surg* 1978; **3**: 142−148.

White, R.E. & Omer, G.E. Transient vascular compromise of the lunate after fracture−dislocation or dislocation of the carpus. *J Hand Surg* 1984; **9A**: 181−184.

Youm, Y. & Flatt, A.E. Kinematics of the wrist. *Clin Orthop* 1979; **149**: 21−32.

Zemel, N.P., Stark, H.H., Ashworth, C.R., Rickard, T.A. & Anderson, D.R. Treatment of selected patients with an un-united fracture of the proximal part of the scaphoid by excision of the fragment and insertion of a carved silicone-rubber spacer. *J Bone Joint Surg* 1984; **66A**: 510−517.

17: The Hand

P.D.BURGE

Introduction

Injuries to the hand cause substantial morbidity and time loss from work. Between one-fifth and one-quarter of patients presenting at Accident departments have injuries to the hand (Clark *et al.* 1985). Data from many countries indicate that approximately 30% of work-related injuries affect the hand (Blair & McCormick 1985). Tubiana (1985) found that, in France, hand injuries accounted for one-quarter of all days lost from work and for one-third of permanent partial disabilities.

The aim of management of a hand injury is the restoration of movement, strength and dexterity. In the hand, perhaps more than in other parts of the musculo-skeletal system, the quality of the primary treatment determines whether the maximal potential for recovery will be achieved. If opportunities are missed on the day of injury, or inappropriate treatment is given, the chance of restoring hand function may be lost. Hand injuries are common; potentially serious lesions may present as apparently trivial lacerations or soft tissue injuries, to trap the inexperienced or the unwary. The aphorism 'there is no such thing as a minor hand injury' should not be forgotten.

Assessment

The first responsibility of the doctor treating hand injury is to ensure that no life-threatening injury is present. Injury to the hand seldom represents immediate danger to the patient, but more serious injuries must be excluded. The injured motorcyclist may have a ruptured spleen as well as a Bennett's fracture.

Although the dramatic appearance of the injured hand invites immediate examination, the surgeon must resist this temptation. The history may uncover vital information which cannot be obtained by other means, especially with regard to the mechanism of injury. Was the hand cut or crushed? If injured in machinery, what type of machine and how? Has it passed between rollers and, if so, were they hot? What gap is normally present between the rollers? For how long was the hand trapped? What cut the hand? Was the blade sharp or blunt? What type of saw? Were the fingers flexed or extended at the moment of injury? Has an avulsion injury occurred? Has material been injected into the finger with high pressure? The replies given to these questions may prompt others, with the aim of identifying the extent and nature of tissue damage and contamination.

The patient's occupation, general health and social circumstances may influence the management and response to treatment. Close co-operation with post-operative care is essential for some methods of treatment in the hand. Simpler methods must be chosen in those who cannot or will not co-operate.

Examination

Physical examination

Wounds and displaced fractures are usually obvious. As in other parts of the skeleton, damage to the soft tissues is at least as important as damage to bone, but is easy to overlook. The critical step in diagnosis is to *consider the possibility* of nerve injury, for example. It is then a straightforward matter to exclude it by systematic examination. The only safe rule is to assume that all the structures in the vicinity of a wound have been injured, until proved otherwise either by adequate examination or by surgical exploration. In most instances, simple clinical tests will provide a provisional diagnosis. In intoxicated, unconscious or very young patients, surgical exploration will be necessary. Exploration should take place under sterile conditions in an operating theatre: probing the wound in the Accident department seldom provides useful information and may introduce infection.

Bruising or swelling may indicate an underlying fracture or joint injury. Careful palpation around an injured joint should be accompanied by a mental picture of the underlying bones, ligament attachments and tendon insertions, and a search for localized tenderness by gentle palpation with a blunt object such as a pen-top.

Prompt correction of deformity is desirable to restore circulation and remove pressure on the skin, but no manipulation should be carried out until the state of the nerves and circulation has been determined and recorded. If X-ray facilities are available without delay, a radiograph should be taken before reduction, for it may provide valuable evidence of injury to articular surfaces, ligament attachments and tendon insertions.

Joint laxity may be demonstrated by appropriate stress examinations and documented with a stress radiograph. Laxity may be masked by muscle spasm due to pain and it may be necessary to give a local anaesthetic before a proper examination is possible. However, the state of the nerves and the vessels should be determined and recorded before the anaesthetic is administered.

The excellent discussion of examination of the hand by Lister (1993) is strongly recommended to all those who treat the injured hand.

Radiographic examination

The two essential steps in radiographic examination are to obtain the appropriate films and to inspect them thoroughly. Because of superimposition of the metacarpals on the lateral projection, the standard X-ray of the hand in many hospitals comprises anteroposterior and oblique views. However, a lateral view is necessary for accurate assessment of angulation of metacarpal fractures. These may be supplemented by further oblique views if necessary. Injuries in the finger, especially fractures around joints, are not shown adequately on the standard anteroposterior and oblique films; a *true lateral* view of the finger must be obtained and supplemented by oblique views if necessary (Fig. 17.1).

The importance of examining the entire radiograph cannot be overemphasized. Once a fracture is seen, the radiograph should be scrutinized for other injuries. Common associated injuries should be remembered; for example, carpometacarpal (CMC) dislocation may accompany fractures of the metacarpal shaft (Fig. 17.2).

Anaesthesia

Most procedures in the adult hand can be performed under some form of local anaesthesia (Ramamurthy & Hickey, 1993). Digital and metacarpal block are appropriate for many procedures in the fingers and thumb. Local anaesthetic may be injected into the web, but infiltration into the finger more distally should be

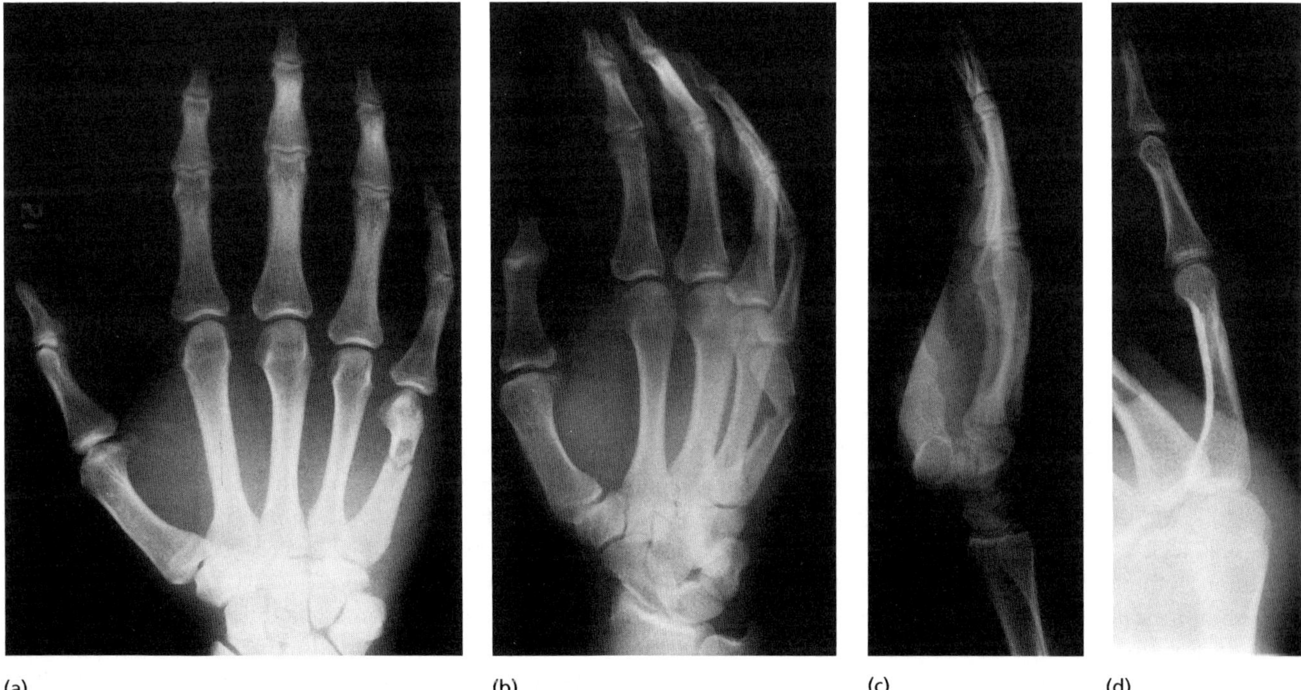

(a)   (b)   (c)   (d)

Fig. 17.1 Standard radiographs of the hand. (a) Anteroposterior. (b) Oblique. (c) Lateral. There is superimposition of the metacarpals but angulation of the metacarpal fracture is best assessed on this view. (d) True lateral radiograph of a finger.

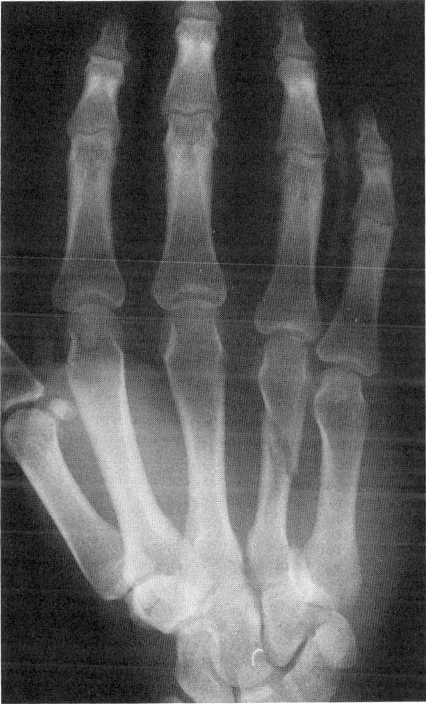 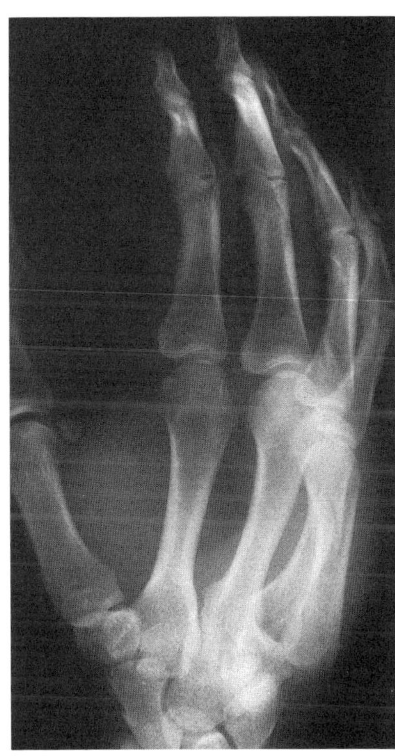

Fig. 17.2 (a) The fracture of the ring metacarpal is obvious; the dislocation of the little finger CMC joint may be missed unless the entire radiograph is scrutinized and other views obtained (b).

(a)

(b)

avoided as it may compromise the circulation in this relatively unyielding area.

Ulnar nerve block at the wrist is an excellent method of anaesthesia for manipulations in the little finger. Local anaesthetic is infiltrated beneath the tendon of flexor carpi ulnaris, having first aspirated to ensure that the needle is not within the ulnar artery. The subcutaneous tissues are infiltrated from this point around the ulnar border of the wrist to block the dorsal branch of the ulnar nerve. Anaesthesia on the radial side of the hand can be provided by blocking the median and radial nerves just proximal to the wrist (Fig. 17.3).

Persistent parasthesiae, which occur rarely after local anaesthetic blocks, probably result from fascicular damage by the needle or from intraneural injection of local anaesthetic. For this reason, a short-bevel needle should be used for blocks of large nerves. If parasthesiae occur when the needle is introduced, it should be repositioned before injection.

Intravenous regional block (Bier's block) is a convenient, easily administered and reliable technique but it carries the ever-present risk of fatal toxic reactions due to unexpected tourniquet deflation and release of anaesthetic into the systemic circulation. It requires immediate access to resuscitation facilities, access to the systemic circulation via a cannula in an uninjured limb and a responsible assistant whose sole task is to super-

vise the tourniquet. Prilocaine is a suitable local anaesthetic agent. Bupivacaine should not be used because of its tendency to bind to myocardial cells.

Brachial plexus block by the axillary route is the ideal form of anaesthetic for most procedures on the hand and forearm. It gives good analgesia and provides postoperative paresis, avoiding the risk of disruption of nerve and tendon repairs which can occur if the patient struggles during recovery from general anaesthesia. Brachial plexus block is technically demanding and an experienced operator is required if a significant failure rate is to be avoided. The supraclavicular technique of brachial plexus block carries a risk of pneumothorax and should not be used for day-case surgery.

Management of open hand injuries

The management of open fractures of the hand follows the principles applied to open fractures elsewhere in the body, but its practice is somewhat different because of the special functional significance of many of the structures in the hand.

The aim in treatment of an open fracture is the creation of an environment which will favour rapid wound healing without infection and allow the earliest return of function. Every effort should be made to obtain primary wound healing and avoid the formation of

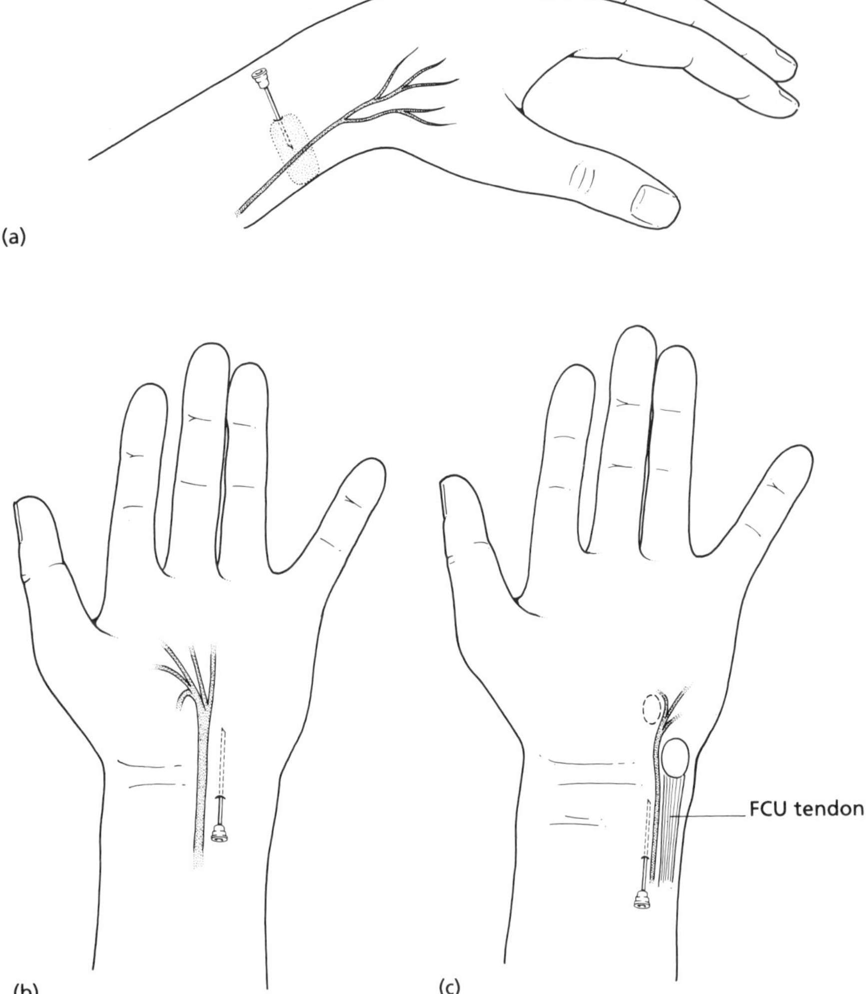

Fig. 17.3 Wrist block anaesthesia.
(a) Radial. (b) Median; the short-bevel
needle is introduced through the volar
forearm fascia just ulnar to the
palmaris longus tendon. (c) Ulnar.

granulation tissue, which is always accompanied by fibrosis.

The order of priorities in management of open fractures is wound excision and irrigation, stabilization of the skeleton, vascular repair, repair of other structures and skin closure. If possible, the first three of these should be completed within 8 hours of injury, before contamination has progressed to bacterial proliferation.

The mainstay of wound cleansing is thorough irrigation, using a gentle jet of saline to explore the crevices of the wound and flush out foreign material. Strong pulsatile irrigation may propel such material further into the wound and should be avoided. Hydrogen peroxide has a vigorous action which may damage the delicate tissues in the hand; the author prefers to use saline. Serious open injuries require several litres of irrigation, which may be conveniently provided from an intravenous fluid bag and suitable tubing.

Thorough wound excision as practised in the thigh or forearm is not possible in the hand. Apart from some fat and muscle, the tissues are essential for function. Skin excision is not necessary unless the edges are badly damaged or clearly non-viable. Viability is best judged by capillary refill and by bleeding from the cut edge. There is no spare skin on the hand; if the survival of an area of skin is uncertain, the options are to excise it and resurface the area or to leave it and reinspect 2–3 days later. If excision does not compromise the plan for wound closure (direct or by means of a flap), smaller areas of dubious skin should be removed. If the viability of a large area is in doubt, it may be left in place and inspected 3–4 days later, when its condition will be apparent. However, this approach carries a greater risk of infection; it must be weighed against the risk of excising valuable skin which might otherwise survive.

Badly crushed and contaminated nerves and tendons

should be cleaned as much as possible, but often a compromise must be made because these structures cannot be sacrificed without unacceptable loss of function. Suprising recovery is sometimes exhibited by nerves which appeared badly damaged.

Skeletal stability is a prerequisite for proper management of the soft tissue injury. In fact, the worse the injury, the more pressing is the need for a stable skeleton. Reduction and stabilization of fractures realigns the neurovascular structures and restores length, thereby reducing dead space available for collection of haematoma. It improves venous and lymphatic return, stabilizes the soft tissue planes to allow capillary proliferation with revascularization of injured tissues and allows gentle early restoration of motion. Stability must be provided at the earliest opportunity. On the day of injury, fractures can usually be reduced easily. After a few days, oedema and contraction of the soft tissue make reduction much more difficult.

Kirschner (K) wire fixation generally provides adequate stability and has the definite advantage that it requires a minimum of additional dissection. The main disadvantage of K-wiring is the relative insecurity of fixation, but it is usually sufficient to allow some early mobilization. The fixation can be enhanced by interosseous wiring or by external fixation, using K-wires and methylmethacrylate cement or a purpose-built external fixator. External splintage alone provides insufficient stability for most open fractures in the hand. On occasion, the rigid fixation offered by screws and plates has definite advantages, but the risk of additional dissection must be considered. In a study of 140 open fractures, Duncan *et al.* (1993) found, as expected, a strong correlation between the severity of soft-tissue injury and the final range of motion. Grade I, II and IIIa fractures which required additional incision and dissection for application of internal fixation, fared less well than comparable injuries in which no such dissection was needed.

Vascular insufficiency is often a consequence of severe fracture displacement and can be corrected by reduction. If ischaemia persists, the injured vessels should be repaired. Vein grafts are often necessary to bridge the defect created by excision of damaged vessel ends.

Nerves and tendons which have been divided cleanly may be repaired primarily provided that wound healing without infection can be expected. In contaminated but otherwise simple injuries, repair of these structures is best undertaken as a secondary procedure, when the risk of infection has passed. In more complex injuries, however, meticulous wound debridement and primary or delayed primary repair of all injured structures is frequently the best approach (Fig. 17.4). Secondary surgery in these hands is often difficult and may be hazardous. In addition, secondary repair of one structure may interfere with the rehabilitation of others.

Primary wound closure is appropriate if the wound is clean with healthy margins, or if it can be made so by excision and irrigation, and if it is less than 8–10 hours old. If necessary, flap coverage can be provided, but the surgeon must be quite certain that the excision is adequate and that the risk of infection is minimal. Many wounds which need flap cover are neither clean nor tidy and it is safer to apply a flap after 2–3 days delay, when it is clear that the wound margins are viable and beginning to heal without infection, lest a valuable flap be lost because of infection. When there is any doubt about the ability of the wound to heal without infection, it should be left open and closure performed 2–3 days later. Tendon and nerve repair can be performed at this stage if necessary, together with skin cover by means of local or distant flaps.

Every effort must be made to achieve skin cover within 3–5 days, otherwise exposed tendons and bone dry out and die, granulation tissue with its bacterial flora develops and fibrosis begins at the wound margins. If the condition of the wound is unsuitable for flap cover at 2–3 days, tendon and bone should be covered with vascularized soft tissues, if possible, and split skin graft applied to the remainder. Definitive skin cover by means of a flap can then be applied when the danger of infection has passed. Godina (1986) showed that the infection rate for free flaps applied within 72 hours for grade 3 open limb injuries was 1.5% of 134 flaps, whereas after 72 hours the infection rate rose to 17.5% of 167 cases. It is, therefore, desirable that the surgeon who will be providing skin cover is consulted on the day of injury. Cogent arguments in favour of early free flap cover of major hand defects are presented in a discussion by Lister (1993), to which the reader is referred.

The concept of primary repair of all injured structures has been analysed and refined by Büchler and Hastings (1993), who point out that a combination of injuries to several structural systems does not behave as the sum of its components. They define *isolated* injuries as those involving a single structural system at one level (e.g. extensor tendon laceration, closed fracture); in this context a simple skin laceration is disregarded. A *combined* injury involves two or more systems (e.g. open fracture with extensor tendon injury, division of flexor tendon, digital nerve and digital artery). The concept of primary repair is well established and generally appropriate for isolated injuries. In combined injuries, however, the

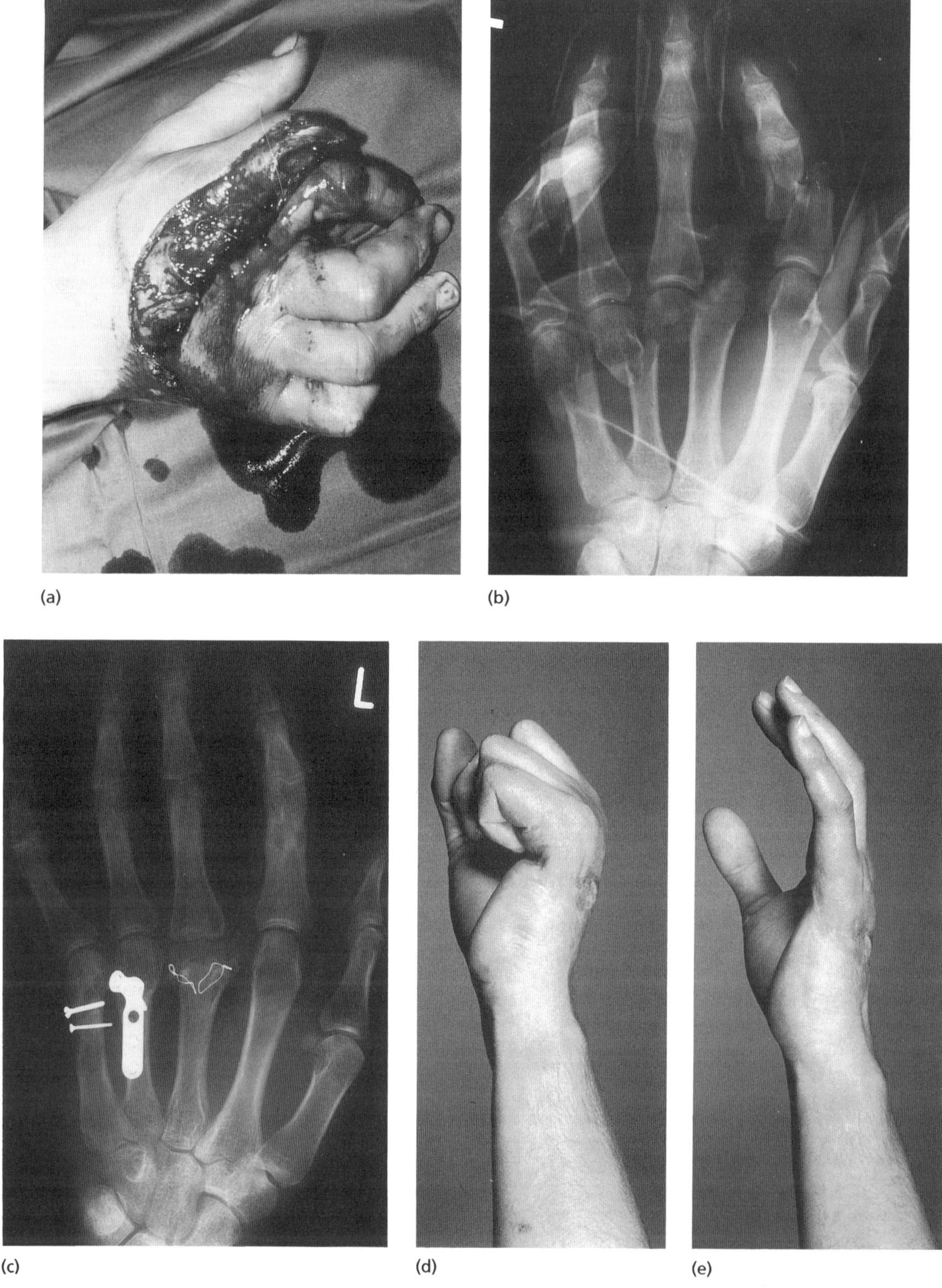

Fig. 17.4 (a)−(c) Cut−crush injury requiring skeletal stabilization prior to revascularization of middle, ring and little fingers with skin-graft cover of the dorsum of the hand. Thorough wound excision and primary repair of all injured structures is preferable for this type of injury. Silicone implant arthroplasty was necessary in the middle MP joint. (d)−(e) Movement at 2 years after injury.

surgeon must consider how interactions between the involved structures may affect their function and recognize that these effects may extend to involve uninjured systems in the hand, especially if the function of gliding structures is not maintained by early motion.

So far as the skeletal elements (bone, muscle, tendon, joint) are concerned, therefore, the primary treatment should allow immediate mobilization of the digit and this requirement takes precedence over the desire to repair all injured structures primarily. If it is not possible to achieve a flexor tendon repair secure enough for immediate motion, for example, secondary tendon reconstruction is preferable. Stable skeletal fixation is clearly an essential foundation in the management of combined injuries. The reader is referred to the excellent discussion by Büchler and Hastings (1993).

Principles of fracture management in the hand

Fractures of the bones of the hand heal rapidly; non-union is rare. It is perhaps surprising that these injuries are so often followed by loss of function and it is instructive to consider why this is so. Leaving aside the problems which follow nerve and tendon injury, almost all residual disability after hand fractures is due either to *loss of motion* or to *malunion*.

Swelling and stiffness of the hand are inter-related. Swelling increases the resistance of the tissues to movement; immobility encourages the formation of oedema because lymphatic drainage is inhibited. Persistent swelling is associated with fibrous adhesions between the numerous tissue planes which glide upon one another as the fingers move. Swelling is such an important factor in production of stiffness that it is essential to understand its formation and how its effects may be minimized.

Swelling is an increase in the interstitial fluid volume (IFV) of the hand. The control of IFV is mediated by local factors, activated by changes in transmural vascular pressure or by changes in interstitial pressure and composition (Aukland & Nicolaysen 1981). The chief factors which influence IFV are the capillary pressure, the surface area of the capillary bed, the colloid osmotic pressure (due to interstitial fluid protein) and the rate of lymph flow.

Under normal circumstances, the transcapillary hydrostatic pressure exceeds slightly the colloid osmotic pressure of plasma protein, so that water is filtered though the capillary wall into the interstitium and is subsequently returned to the circulation through the lymphatics.

The normal hand is relatively resistant to oedema in the dependent position. Large variations in IFV which might otherwise occur as a result of the rise in venous pressure are counteracted by local feedback mechanisms which provide an 'oedema safety factor' of about 15 mmHg. The safety factor represents the capacity of the tissue to buffer increases in capillary filtration forces and prevent oedema; it is due in part to increased lymphatic flow, in part to local vascular responses which limit the rise in capillary pressure and in part to changes in osmotic pressure as a consequence of increased capillary filtration.

The acute inflammatory response to injury is accompanied by increased capillary permeability to protein, which passes into the interstitial fluid and, by its osmotic effect, draws water into the interstitial space. This phenomenon is an inevitable consequence of injury but may be modified considerably by other factors, of which the most important is capillary pressure. Once inflammatory oedema has begun, the safety factor is lost and the hand is quite sensitive to changes in capillary pressure. Holding the injured hand in the dependent position can increase swelling dramatically.

Protein and water are cleared from the interstitial space by the lymphatic system. Filling of lymphatics and transport along them is a passive process that depends largely on local pressure differences generated by movement of the tissues. Movement serves not only to clear oedema fluid from the interstitial space but also maintains the relative motion of the gliding tissue planes and prevents their adhesion.

Elevation and active movement are, therefore, essential components of the management of the injured hand and must not be prevented unless absolutely necessary. If the hand must be immobilized, the joints should be placed in the position which is least likely to result in permanent loss of motion. The position of safe splintage is wrist extension, metacarpophalangeal (MP) joint flexion and interphalangeal (IP) joint extension (James 1970).

Swelling tightens the dorsal skin and pulls the MP joints into extension. The wrist and IP joints tend to flex, producing the characteristic posture of the untreated swollen hand (Fig. 17.5). These positions quickly become fixed. The tendency for the MP joints to become fixed in extension is a consequence of their anatomy. In the sagittal plane the metacarpal head is cam-shaped (Fig. 17.6). The collateral ligaments are slack in extension and allow radial and ulnar deviation, a fact which can be demonstrated in the reader's hand. In flexion, the ligaments are taut and provide stability during grip.

If the MP joints of the swollen hand are immobilized

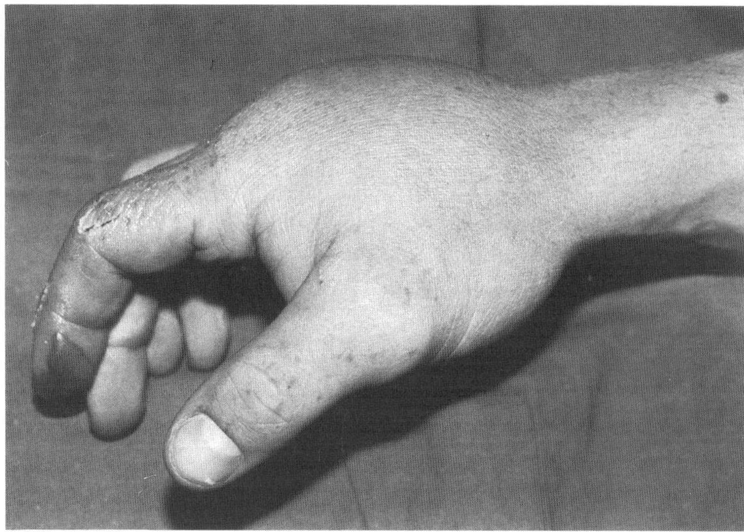

Fig. 17.5 Gross swelling owing to multiple metacarpal shaft fractures.

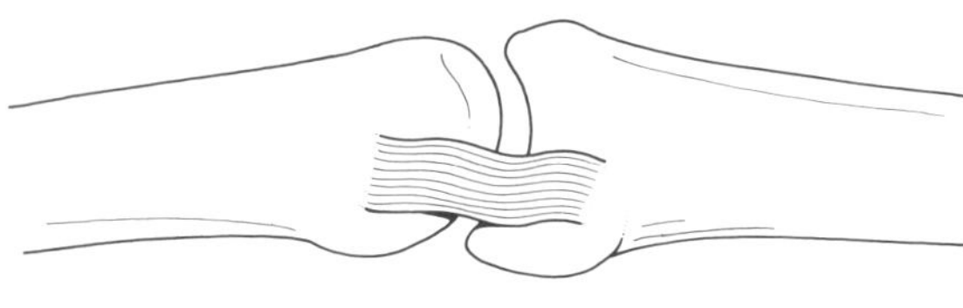

(a)

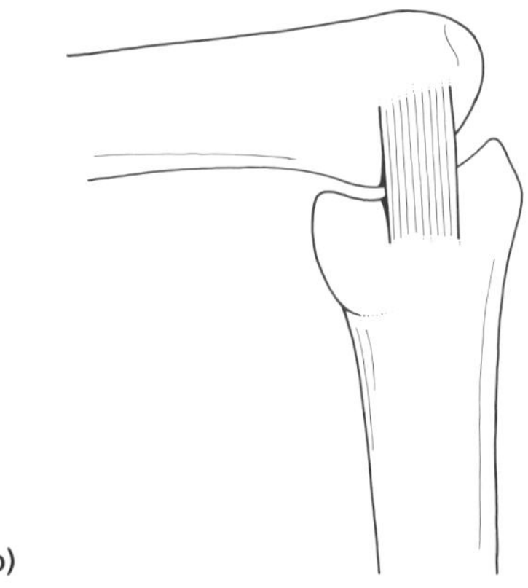

(b)

Fig. 17.6 The collateral ligaments of the MP joint are (a) slack in extension and (b) taut in flexion, owing to the cam shape of the metacarpal head in the sagittal plane.

in extension, the slack collateral ligaments become swollen and shorten. When the hand is subsequently mobilized, the shortened ligaments will prevent flexion over the cam of the metacarpal head. Permanent loss of MP joint flexion may follow only 2 weeks of immobilization of a swollen hand in extension. The MP joints should be immobilized in flexion to maintain the length of the collateral ligaments. This is the *position of safe splintage* (Fig. 17.7).

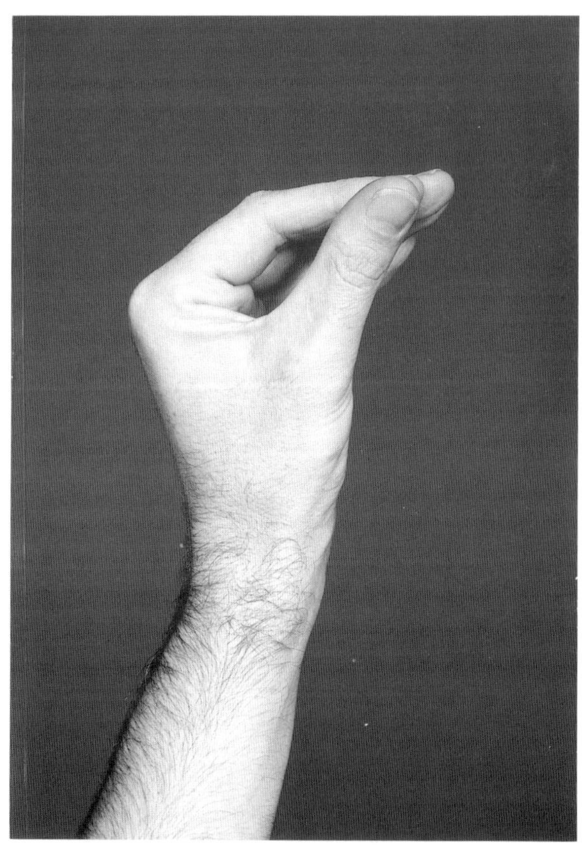

Fig. 17.7 The position of safe splintage.

The position of safe splintage of the IP joints is near to full extension. Contracture of the palmar plate or accessory collateral ligaments may occur if the proximal interphalangeal (PIP) joint is immobilized in flexion. Such contracture is difficult to treat, partly because active extension forces at the IP joints are relatively weak. If these joints are immobilized in extension, dorsal capsular adhesions may form but can usually be overcome by the strong flexors during the mobilization period.

The wrist should be positioned in moderate extension to facilitate flexion of the MP joints. If the wrist is at neutral or in flexion, the MP joints tend to drift into extension.

Various methods of splintage may be employed to maintain the position of safe splintage. Dorsal and palmar slabs offer the best control of joint position. A single palmar slab usually fails because it slips distally, extending the MP joints and allowing the IP joints to flex. The 'boxing glove' bandage, applied as recommended by James (1970), is an effective alternative.

Whichever method is chosen, it is essential to make a conscious effort to hold the MP joints well flexed and the wrist extended. Circular bandaging alone is insufficient; several lengths of bandage should pass from the radial and ulnar borders of the hand and wrist over the dorsum of the phalanges to maintain MP joint flexion. If an attempt is made to exaggerate the position of safe splintage as the plaster sets, the correct posture will usually be obtained.

If extreme difficulty in maintaining a safe position by external splintage is anticipated (e.g. severe burns), K-wires may be passed across the flexed MP joints (Fig. 17.8), or alternatively across both IP joints.

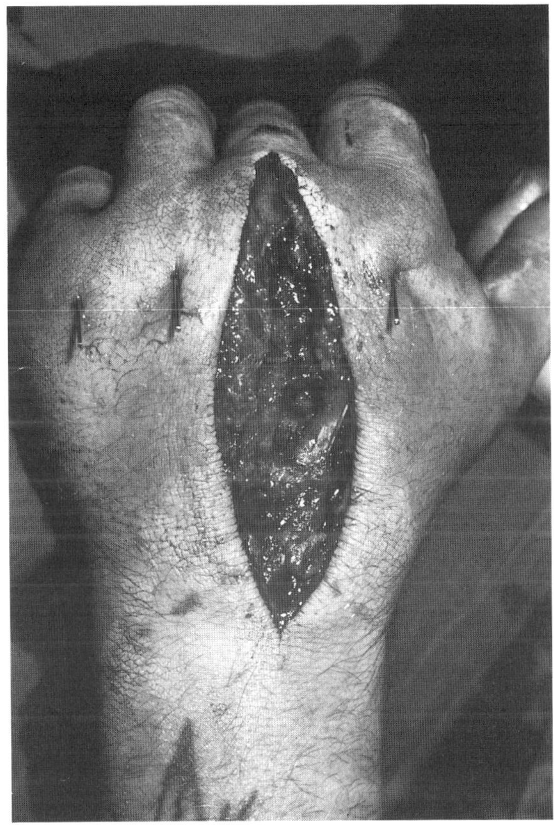

Fig. 17.8 Severe swelling was expected after this high-pressure grease injection injury from the palm into the dorsum of the hand. The position of safe splintage is maintained by K-wires passed across the flexed MP joints.

Fractures of the distal phalanx

Fractures of the distal phalanx make up about half of all fractures of the hand, no doubt because of the exposed position of the fingertips.

Most injuries of the tuft and shaft of the distal phalanx are the result of crushing: open fractures, injury to the nail-bed and soft tissue damage are frequent. Although the fracture may be comminuted, significant displacement or angulation are unusual because of the support provided by the soft tissues. The fascial bands, which separate the distal pulp into fibrofatty compartments, attach to the spade-like tuft of the distal phalanx and stabilize the bone fragments from the palmar aspect, while the nail-bed supports the bone dorsally. However, injury to soft tissues and swelling within the fibrofatty compartments contribute to the severe pain which crush injuries may cause.

Treatment of the soft tissue injury dominates the management of crush fractures of the distal phalanx (Fig. 17.9). Open fractures must receive proper wound care and irrigation. Prophylactic antibiotic treatment may reduce the risk of infection (Sloan *et al*. 1987). Reduction of the fracture is seldom possible or necessary. A padded protective splint provides pain relief, but it should accommodate swelling and must not compress the soft tissues. Motion of the PIP joint should not be restricted. Movement of the distal interphalangeal (DIP) joint may begin as soon as discomfort will allow, usually within 3 weeks. Occasionally there is sufficient damage to the support structures to permit angulation or displacement of a transverse fracture of the shaft of the distal phalanx (Fig. 17.10). These injuries require debridement of the soft tissues and may need K-wire fixation of the fracture.

Fractures of the distal phalanx are frequently accompanied by injury of the nail-bed, which is contiguous with the dorsal periosteum (Zook *et al*. 1980). Dramatic relief of pain usually follows drainage of a subungual haematoma, most easily accomplished with a red-hot paper-clip. Injuries of the nail-bed are often underestimated and their treatment neglected (Fig. 17.11). Crush injuries may cause ragged lacerations of

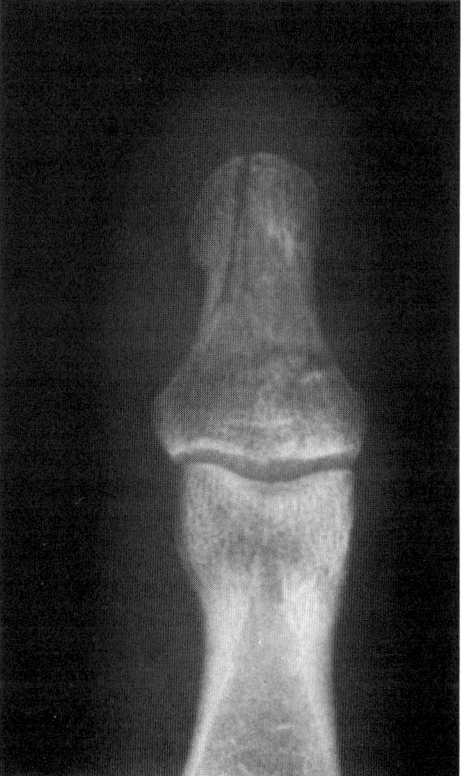

Fig. 17.9 Crush fracture of the distal phalanx.

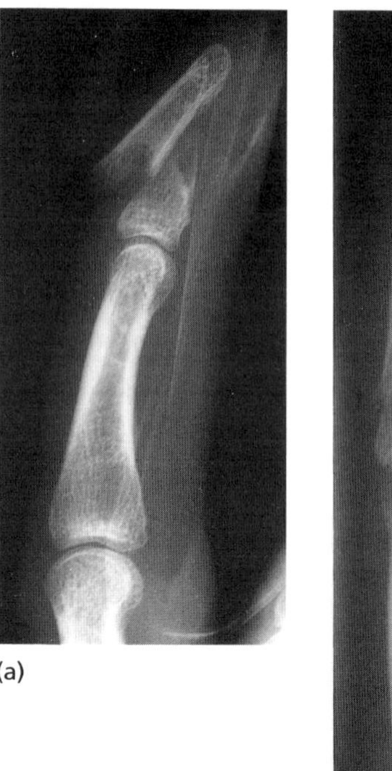

(a)

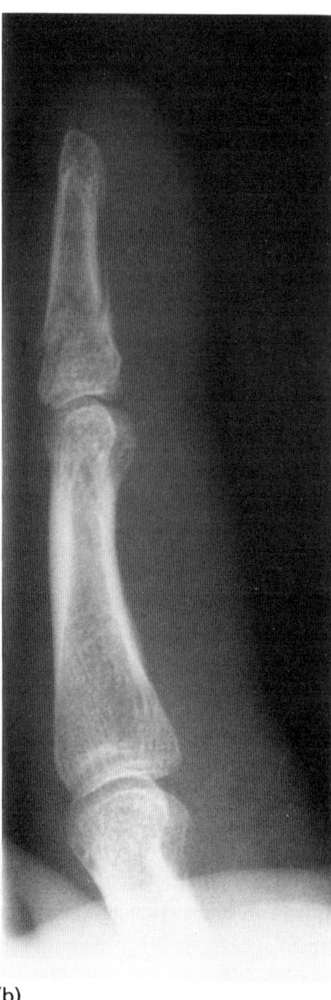

(b)

Fig. 17.10 (a) Transverse fracture of the distal phalanx; (b) the reduction is held by splintage in this case, but K-wire fixation may be necessary.

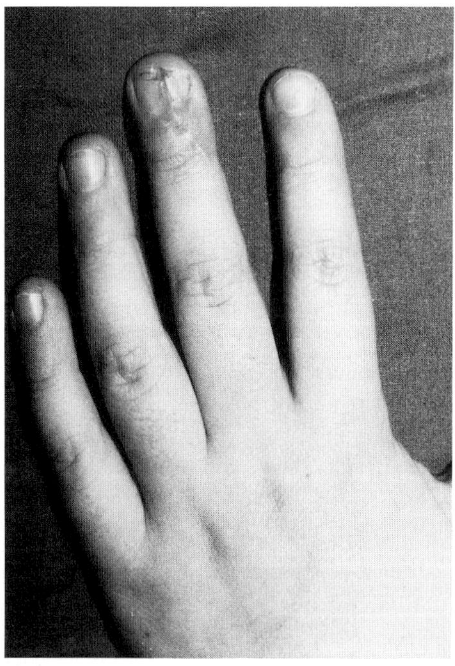

Fig. 17.11 Late result of unrepaired nail-bed laceration.

the nail-bed and although some late deformity of the nail is inevitable, it can be reduced substantially by a careful repair of the nail-bed with fine (6/o or 7/o) sutures under loupe magnification (Zook *et al.* 1984). Injury to the eponychial fold may cause adhesion between its surfaces, leading to a longitudinal split in the nail. If the nail is uninjured, it may be cleaned and replaced to maintain the eponychial fold and mould the healing nail-bed, securing it with a suture through the tip of the finger. Alternatively, a piece of non-adherent gauze or silicone sheet may be used.

Fractures of the base of the distal phalanx

Fractures of the base of the distal phalanx may be divided into three groups: (i) tendon avulsions; (ii) fracture−dislocations; and (iii) epiphyseal separations.

Tendon avulsion fractures

These most often affect the dorsal lip of the distal phalanx. Forcible flexion of the extended finger results in avulsion of a flake of bone at the insertion of the terminal tendon of the dorsal aponeurosis (Fig. 17.12). The fragment is usually small, but it may form up to 30% of the articular surface. Loss of active extension results in the deformity known as *mallet finger*.

The treatment of closed mallet finger injuries should be approached with several facts in mind (Stark *et al*. 1962). The results of treatment by splintage are not uniformly good, but a residual extension lag causes very little functional impairment in most patients. Splintage of the PIP joint in flexion, while theoretically desirable in order to slacken the lateral bands, may cause permanent flexion contracture of the proximal joint, especially in older patients. Secure repair of a ruptured tendon or fixation of a small bone fragment is difficult to achieve. Operative repair often results in loss of distal joint flexion and may be complicated by poor skin healing, especially if the dorsal skin is subjected to pressure from a splint. Lastly, pain and tenderness of the dorsal skin are the rule but, in patients treated by splintage, these symptoms almost invariably resolve after 6–9 months.

Although some authors have recommended operative management the difficulties outlined above have led the majority of surgeons to treat mallet finger by splintage of the distal joint in extension for 6–10 weeks. Various types of splint are available; the Stack splint (Stack 1969) is convenient, but padded metal and other splints can be used provided that the DIP joint is held in extension (Fig. 17.13).

Successful use of the Stack splint demands attention to the details of fitting and instruction of the patient. The DIP joint must be held in a slight hyperextension but not enough to cause blanching of the dorsal skin, which occurs at approximately 50% of the total range of hyperextension (Rayan & Mullins 1987). The splint must not apply excessive force to the fragile dorsal skin. It may be necessary to pad the palmar surface of the splint to hold the DIP joint in the correct position. Skin maceration can be controlled by daily cleaning and powdering of the skin. The patient may safely remove the splint for this purpose, provided that the distal joint is held extended.

Crawford (1984) analysed the results of treatment of 166 mallet fingers with the Stack splint for 8 weeks. Eighty-five percent of patients with tendon injury and 82% with avulsion fractures had a residual extension lag of 10° or less. Good results were achieved most often when splintage began within 10 days, but splintage was still worthwhile up to 2 months after injury. There was no loss of flexion. Many of the poor results occurred in non-compliant patients.

Imbalance of the extension forces in the digit may produce swan-neck deformity in those patients with late mallet finger who also have hyperextension of the PIP joint. If the deformity causes disability, the extension forces may be rebalanced by tenotomy of the central slip, originally described by Fowler. In 20 patients,

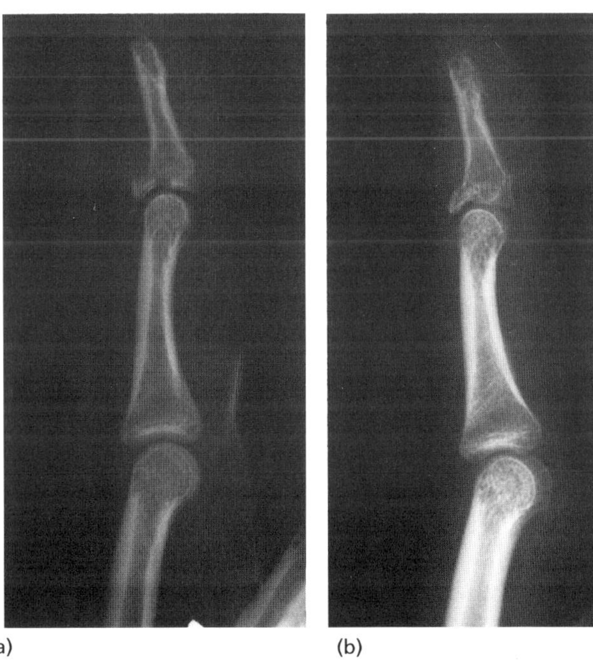

(a)　　　　(b)

Fig. 17.12 (a) Extensor tendon avulsion fracture of the distal phalanx. (b) After 6 weeks splintage.

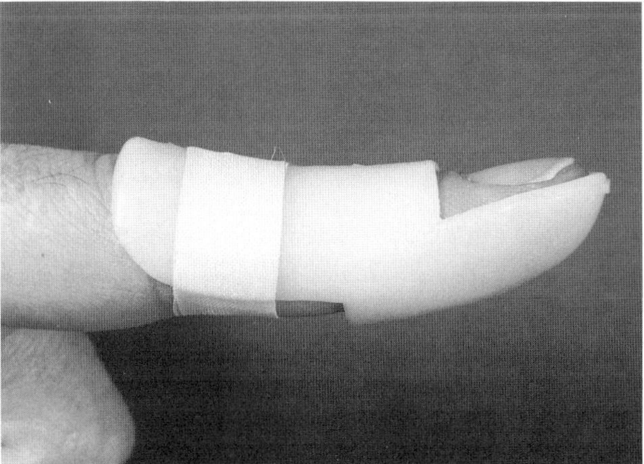

Fig. 17.13 Stack mallet finger splint.

Grundberg and Reagan (1987) improved the DIP joint lag from 37° to 9° and PIP joint hyperextension from 10° to an average 2° PIP joint extension lag by central slip tenotomy. The procedure appears to carry minimal morbidity and does not seem to produce a boutonnière deformity.

Avulsion of the insertion of the profundus tendon is less common than mallet finger, but more often misdiagnosed (Fig. 17.14). It occurs when the strongly flexed finger is forcibly extended, typically when the patient attempts to grasp the jersey of an opponent at rugby. In three-quarters of cases the ring finger is affected.

The injury is often dismissed as a sprained finger and the patient may not present until he notices loss of active DIP joint flexion, some days or weeks later. In the early stages, there is pain and tenderness on the palmar aspect of the DIP joint. There may be fullness of the flexor sheath in the finger or the palm. Unlike mallet finger, there is no characteristic deformity and the diagnosis will be missed unless the examiner tests specifically for active flexion of the distal joint.

Profundus tendon avulsion has been classified by Leddy and Packer (1977):

Type I — retraction to the palm. The long and short vincula are torn.

Type II — retraction to the level of the PIP joint. The long vinculum is intact. There may be a small bone flake visible on a true lateral radiograph of the finger.

Type III — avulsion of a large bone fragment. The A4 pulley prevents retraction proximal to the neck of the middle phalanx.

Untreated, profundus avulsion results in a 'superficialis finger', with normal motion at the MP and PIP joints but loss of active flexion of the distal joint. There is slight weakness of grip but the disability is modest unless the patient (e.g. a violinist) has some specific requirement for distal joint flexion.

Reattachment of the tendon offers restoration of active motion of the distal joint and adds flexion power to the digit. However, there is a definite risk of tendon adhesion and loss of PIP joint motion which must be considered carefully and explained to the patient preoperatively. In some instances, and especially in older patients, it is safer to leave the finger alone and perform an arthrodesis later if instability of the distal joint is troublesome.

When the tendon has retracted to the palm (type I) it rapidly becomes fixed and contracted. Loss of blood supply of the profundus tendon, damage to the vincular system at the PIP joint and the manipulation necessary to rethread the tendon though the digital sheath increase the risk of adhesion in this type. Reattachment to the distal phalanx is usually possible within 7 days of injury, but after that the difficulty and risk of PIP joint stiffness increase.

If the tendon has been held up at the level of the PIP joint (type II), it is often possible to reattach it, even after a delay of 2–3 months. The tendon, with or without a small bone fragment, may be reattached to the base of the distal phalanx with a suture or wire tied over a button on the dorsum of the finger. It may be necessary to trim the swollen tendon stump before it will pass

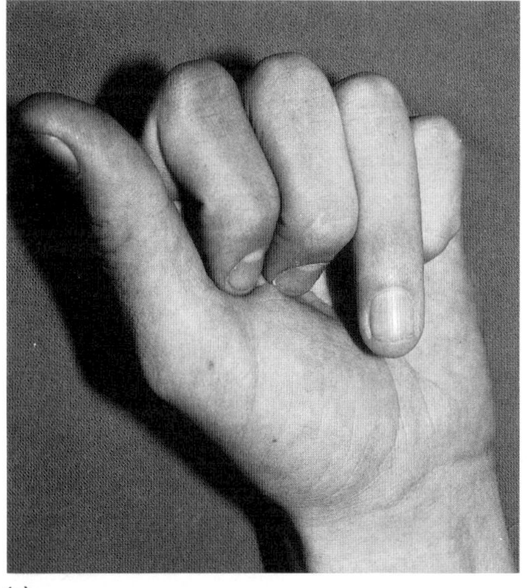

(a)

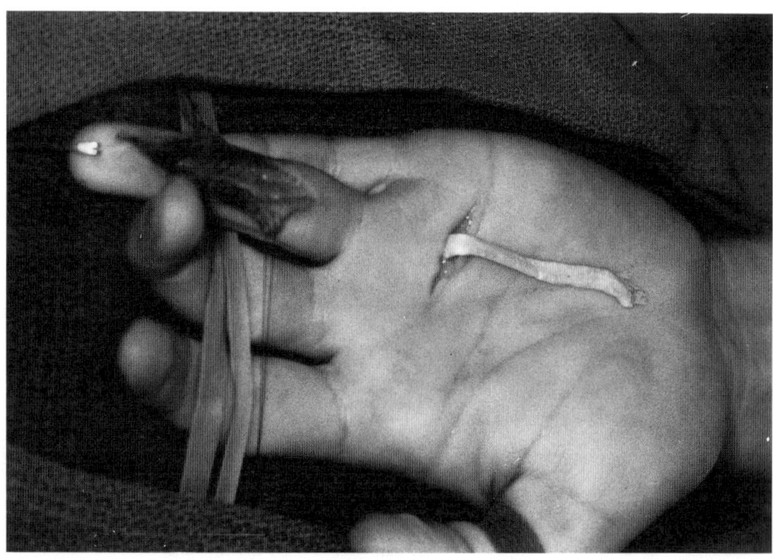

(b)

Fig. 17.14 (a) Loss of active DIP joint flexion due to avulsion of the profundus tendon insertion. (b) The tendon retrieved from its retracted position in the palm.

under the A4 pulley. It is, of course, essential to preserve at least part of this pulley.

Type III injuries (Fig. 17.15) are treated by reattachment of the large bone fragment to the distal phalanx with a K-wire or interosseous wire, depending on the configuration of the fracture.

Fracture–dislocations of the DIP joint

Fractures involving more than 40% of the articular surface of the distal phalanx are often associated with subluxation or dislocation of the DIP joint. The injury is usually the result of a blow to the end of the finger, from a cricket ball, for example. Dorsal fracture with palmar dislocation is more common than the reverse. The subluxation is maintained by the unopposed action of the profundus tendon.

A number of authors (Stark 1970, Hamas *et al.* 1978) have recommended operative reduction and internal fixation of the fracture wherever possible, on the grounds that precise reduction is necessary to avoid pain, loss of motion and late degenerative arthritis.

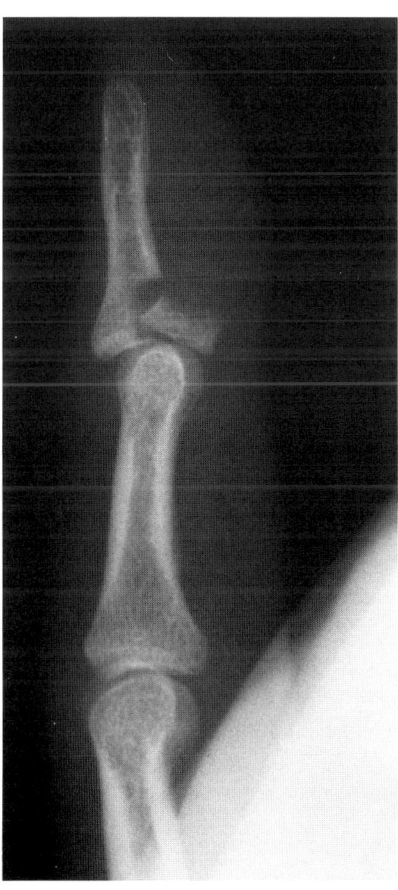

Fig. 17.15 Type III profundus avulsion fracture. The size of the fragment prevents retraction through the pulley system.

However, operative techniques are difficult, unreliable and prone to the complications of poor skin healing, splitting of small bone fragments and difficulties of exposure which may require section and repair of the ulnar collateral ligament.

Other authors (Wehbe & Schneider 1984, Steel 1988) have found surprisingly good results after non-operative management. Their studies indicate that fracture–dislocation is much less disabling at the DIP joint than it is at the PIP joint. The articular surfaces may exhibit considerable remodelling (see Fig. 17.12). Pain and late degenerative change were rare. Although a dorsal lump and some loss of motion were often present, they were consistent with excellent function.

The author prefers to treat patients with mild to moderate subluxation with the mallet finger type of splintage for 4 weeks, followed by mobilization. Care is taken to avoid excessive hyperextension which can increase the subluxation. The patients are warned about a lump on the dorsum of the finger and told that discomfort and stiffness will improve gradually over 6 months. DIP joint fusion is reserved for those very few cases in which persistent pain interferes with function.

If there is gross subluxation or dislocation which cannot be improved by splintage, the joint is reduced and transfixed with a K-wire for 3–4 weeks.

When the injury presents 2 weeks or more after injury, there is little prospect of improving the position by splintage. These patients are managed by gentle active motion, protecting the digit in a splint between exercise sessions. Open reduction and internal fixation is reserved for the rare case of a young patient with a single large bone fragment and is only undertaken when the surgeon is confident of achieving stable fixation (Fig. 17.16).

Epiphyseal separations

Epiphyseal separations of the distal phalanx occur in two age groups (Weiland *et al.* 1988). In the preadolescent child there is a type I or type II separation which is usually an open injury resulting from hyperflexion of the fingertip. The extensor tendon remains attached to the epiphysis and holds it extended. The profundus tendon flexes the distal fragment (Fig. 17.17).

The nail and nail-bed retain their attachment to the metaphysis and may be torn from the proximal nail-fold, coming to lie superficial to the nail-fold skin (Fig. 17.18). The injury is more serious than it might seem; the tendon attachments perpetuate the deformity and may cause malunion. Barton (1979) found residual mallet deformity in three out of four cases. Infection is liable to

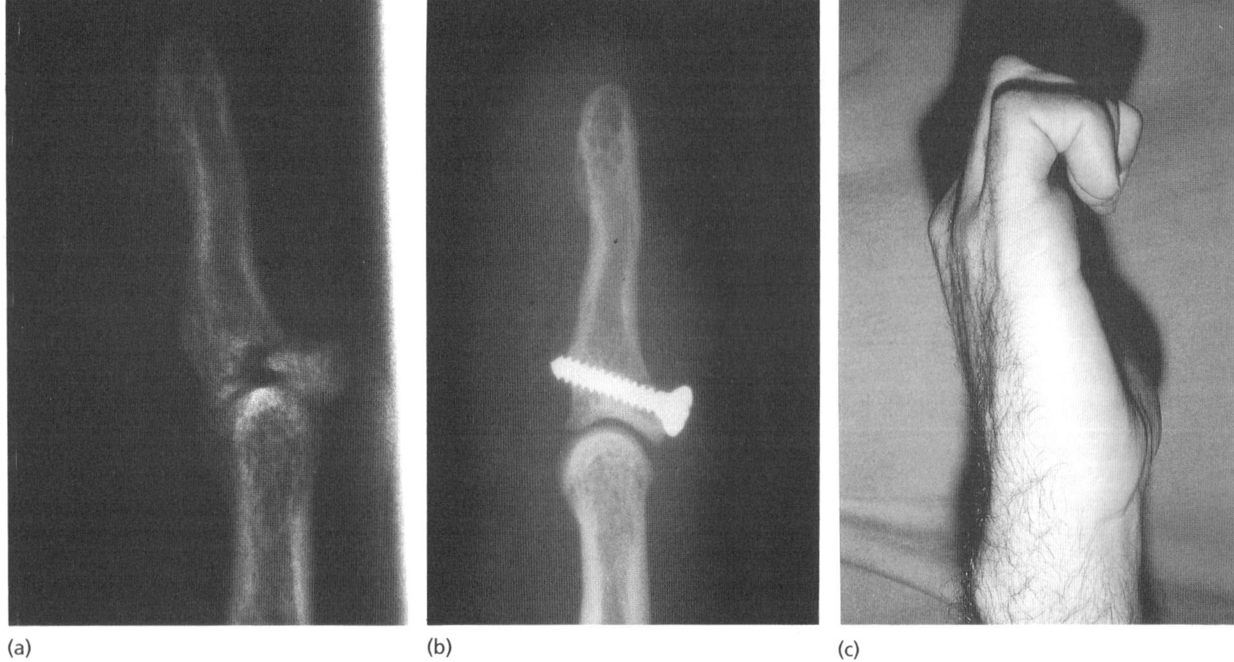

Fig. 17.16 (a) Extensor tendon avulsion fracture with a large single fragment. (b) Successful lag screw fixation can provide excellent function and restoration of the joint surface if the fragment is large enough. (c) Movement on the 12th postoperative day.

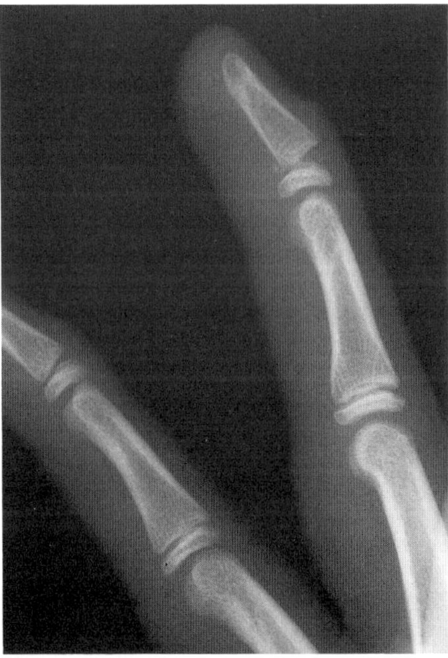

Fig. 17.17 Fracture separation of the distal phalangeal physis. The deformity is maintained by the extensor tendon attachment to the epiphysis and the flexor attachment to the metaphysis.

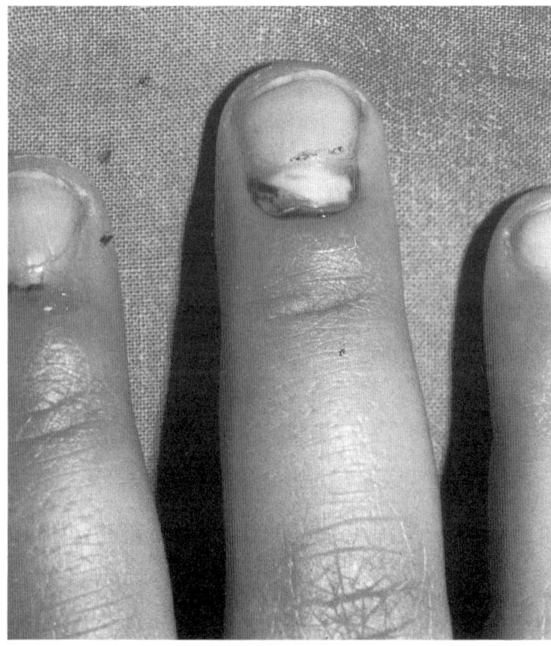

Fig. 17.18 Proximal part of the nail avulsed from the nail-fold and lying on the eponychial skin.

occur, with the potential for further damage to the epiphysis and the nail-bed.

Seymour (1966) indicated the importance of the nail in stability of the injury after reduction. There was difficulty in controlling the position in six patients in whom the proximal portion of the nail was removed and infection occurred in three. Infection also occurred in three out of five patients treated by K-wire fixation.

The nail-plate should therefore be preserved. After thorough irrigation and minimal debridement, the nail-plate should be replaced in the nail-fold and stabilized with a suture at each corner. This manoeuvre usually results in adequate reduction and stability of the fracture. The finger is supported with a splint and the position checked by X-ray, which should be repeated at 1 and 2 weeks. If the injury is unstable, a single fine K-wire can be placed across the centre of the epiphysis.

In the adolescent, hyperflexion produces a type III epiphyseal separation which is an avulsion injury similar to the bony type of mallet finger which occurs in adults. It should receive the same treatment.

Fractures of the middle and proximal phalanges

Displaced phalangeal fractures are a frequent cause of disability in the hand. James (1962) found that stiffness of the IP joints was common and that flexion contractures of the PIP joints were present in almost all of 58 cases of unstable phalangeal fracture. Strickland *et al.* (1982) confirmed that return of total active movement (TAM — normal 260°) correlated with displacement of non-articular phalangeal fractures without tendon injury (undisplaced 88%, minimally displaced 80%, markedly displaced 74% of normal TAM). TAM was 79% overall for fractures without tendon injury but only 49% for those with complete extensor tendon division.

The phalanges are enveloped by complex flexor and extensor tendon systems, from which they are separated by a thin layer of periosteum. There is no muscle padding and only a thin layer of fat beneath the skin. Relatively minor changes in length or alignment of the skeleton may upset the mechanics of the tendon systems. Adhesion between bone and tendon prevents gliding and limits active motion of the IP joints. The palmar surface of the phalanges is the floor of the flexor sheath; residual displacement of the fracture may restrict the excursion of the tendons. Passive motion may be restricted in the early stages by swelling of the finger and later by adhesion or contracture of the collateral ligaments and palmar plates. For these reasons, the fingers are rather intolerant of injury and easily stiffen. For the

same reasons, they are intolerant of operative assault, a fact which underlies the dilemmas often encountered in treating phalangeal fractures.

The outcome of treatment of phalangeal fractures is influenced by the type of patient, the nature of the fracture and method of management (Strickland *et al.* 1982). The surgeon can only control the last of these, but must give consideration to the others because features of the patient and the fracture may indicate the most appropriate treatment, provide a prognosis and warn of pitfalls in management. Features of the patient which affect the outcome include age, patient understanding and motivation, associated diseases and socioeconomic factors. Displacement, stability, joint involvement and associated soft tissue injury are features of the fracture which strongly influence the final result. Aspects of management include prompt recognition of the injury with proper care of the soft tissues, maintenance of a stable reduction, mobilization as early as possible and prompt treatment of complications. Stiffness is much more likely if the fracture is immobilized for more than 3 weeks (Wright 1968, Strickland *et al.* 1982). It should be noted that stability and absence of local tenderness are the most useful signs of fracture healing; radiographic evidence of union lags several weeks behind the clinical signs (Fig. 17.19).

Phalangeal fractures exhibit characteristic deformities which depend upon the type of force which produced the fracture and on the pull of muscles and tendons which insert into the bones. The relative importance of these factors has been debated in the literature and probably varies from one fracture to another. The typical deformity of a fracture of the shaft of the proximal phalanx is angulation with its apex toward the palmar surface of the bone (Fig. 17.20). The proximal fragment is flexed by the attachment of the interosseous muscles. Loss of stability of the proximal phalanx allows the finger to collapse in 'Z' fashion under the influence of the flexor and extensor insertions on the middle phalanx.

In passing we should note that the terminology of angular deformity in the plane of finger flexion is confused. Angulation of a fracture of the shaft of the proximal phalanx with its apex on the palmar surface of the bone is termed palmar angulation by some authors (Green & Rowland 1981) and dorsal angulation by others. In this chapter, the convention will be followed of placing the proximal fragment in the anatomical position and then describing the direction of angulation of the distal fragment relative to the proximal one. The typical proximal phalanx fracture described above therefore has *dorsal* angulation of the distal fragment with respect to the proximal.

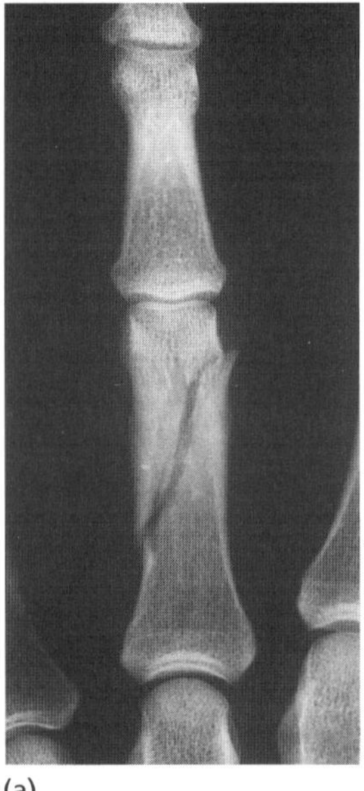

(a)

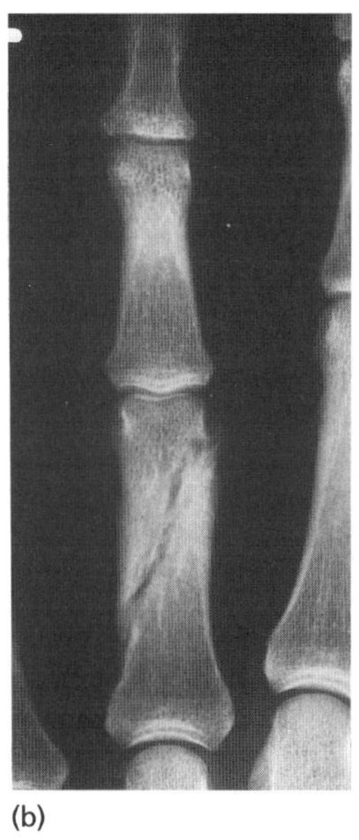

(b)

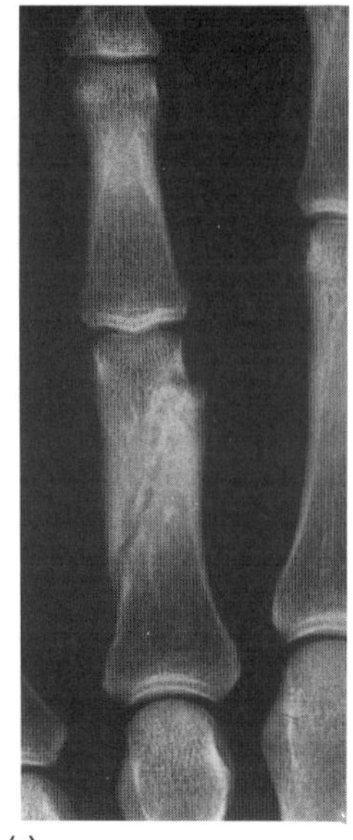

(c)

Fig. 17.19 Radiographic evidence of union of phalangeal shaft fractures appears later than the clinical signs: (a) day 1; (b) 7 weeks; (c) 16 weeks. The fracture was stable and non-tender at 3 weeks.

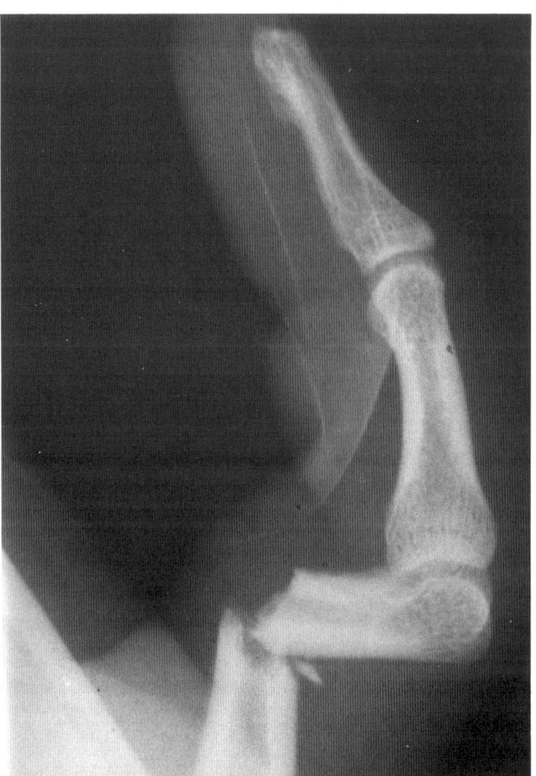

Fig. 17.20 Angulation with the apex towards the palmar surface is termed *dorsal* angulation.

Angulation of fractures of the middle phalanx is influenced by the action of the central slip at the base and by the long insertion of the superficialis tendon which extends over the proximal three-quarters of the bone. Fractures at the base of the middle phalanx tend toward palmar angulation while those at the neck angulate dorsally.

Rotational displacement is a subtle but important consequence of spiral and some oblique fractures. A high index of suspicion must be maintained when the mechanism of injury or the configuration of the fracture suggest a rotational injury has occurred. Rotational deformity is obvious when the fingers are able to flex, producing overlap of the fingers (Fig. 17.21). The flexed fingers do not, as is sometimes stated, all point to the tubercle of the scaphoid. It is usually the ring finger which points directly to the tubercle; the other digits lie parallel to the ring finger. When pain and swelling prevent flexion, one must rely on examining the plane of the fingernail of the injured finger in comparison to the adjacent digits and those of the other hand.

Classification

It is helpful to classify phalangeal fractures into articular and extra-articular fractures. Displaced articular fractures usually demand open reduction and internal fixation. The numerous methods of management which have been recommended for extra-articular phalangeal fractures attest to the fact that no single method has proved suitable for all fractures. A frequent conflict arises between the need to maintain reduction of an unstable fracture and the requirement for early active motion. No one method can resolve this conflict for every fracture. The surgeon must select the most appropriate method for a particular fracture in a particular patient, remembering to consider the soft tissues as well as the bone. The goal in treatment of hand fractures

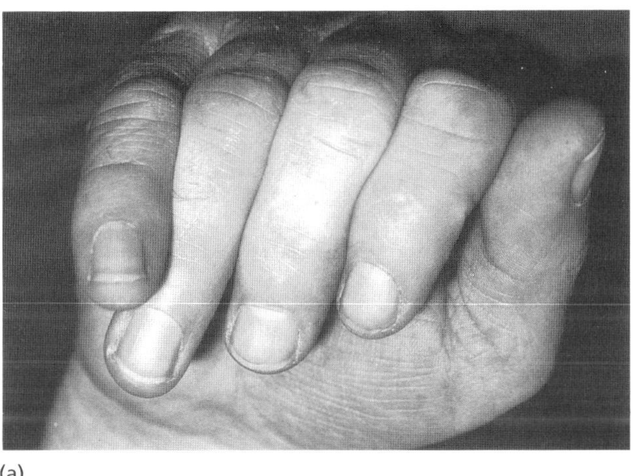

(a)

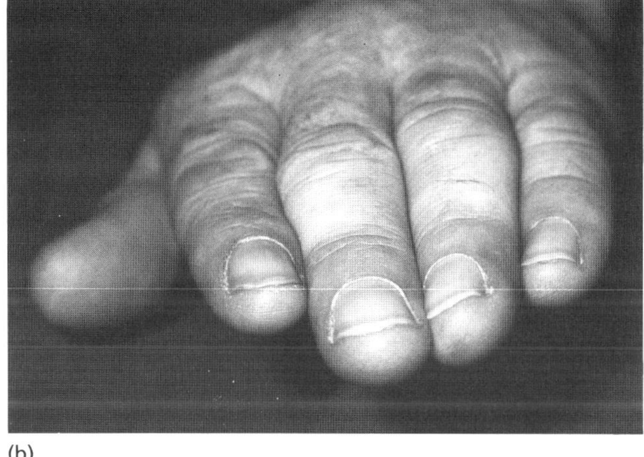

(b)

Fig. 17.21 (a) Rotational malalignment due to spiral proximal phalangeal fracture is obvious when the fingers are flexed. (b) Rotation may be assessed by comparing the plane of the fingernail with other digits; in this case, the ring finger is pronated.

is not just a healed fracture but a supple, mobile, sensitive and stable digit that performs well and adds to hand function' (Büchler & Fischer 1987).

The main treatment methods available are: protected active motion, closed reduction and splintage, traction, closed reduction and percutaneous pinning, external fixation and open reduction with internal fixation.

PROTECTED ACTIVE MOTION

Fractures which are undisplaced or in a stable position consistent with normal function can be managed simply and safely by protected active motion. Barton (1984) states that about 75% of phalangeal fractures can be treated in this way. Protection is provided by taping the injured finger to an adjacent digit and unresisted active motion is begun immediately, within limits imposed by pain (Fig. 17.22). The patient is given instructions about exercise and cautioned about movement against resistance. Review at 5–7 days will detect further displacement before healing of the fracture makes intervention difficult. A clear relationship between the duration of immobilization and the final range of motion was demonstrated by Wright (1968). In a series of 529 patients, full function was regained by 81% of stable fractures treated by immediate mobilization but by only 50% of stable fractures immobilized for 3 weeks.

CLOSED REDUCTION AND EXTERNAL SPLINTAGE

Displaced phalangeal fractures need to be reduced. Even a modest degree of displacement, which in the metacarpals may be consistent with normal function, is likely in the phalanx to alter the mechanical balance in

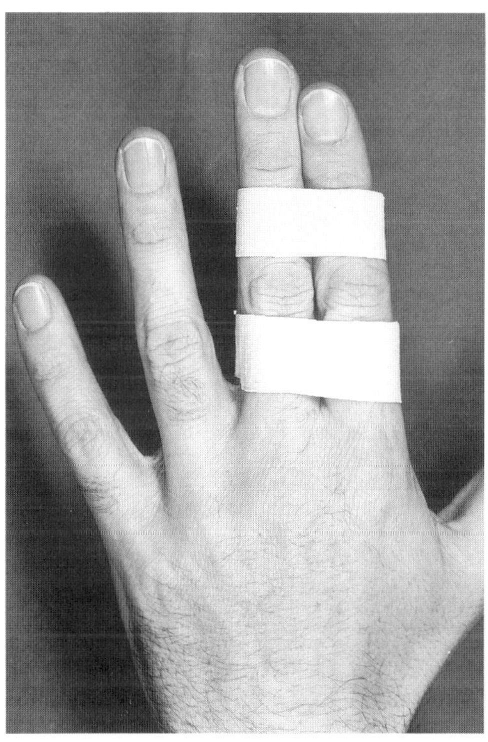

Fig. 17.22 'Buddy' taping for early protected movement.

the dorsal aponeurosis and may restrict the excursion of the flexor tendons, whose sheath is contiguous with the phalangeal periosteum. Most displaced phalangeal fractures can be reduced to a stable position by manipulation if it is performed with 12 hours of injury. After that time, swelling makes reduction more difficult. The intact periosteal hinge can be used to control the reduction and prevent overcorrection. After reduction, these fractures are generally not stable enough for immediate motion and require some type of external splintage until fracture healing has produced some stability, usually at about 3 weeks.

Early authors recommended immobilization of the finger in flexion, a position in which the fracture is usually most stable. However, this advantage is definitely outweighed by the risk of PIP joint flexion contracture which may result if the joint is immobilized in more than 20° flexion. James (1962) defined the *position of immobilization* of the hand, sometimes called the position of safe splintage. The MP joints are flexed at least 70° to hold the collateral ligaments out at their full length and prevent the shortening which may cause permanent loss of flexion if the joints are immobilized in extension for as little as 2 weeks. The PIP joints tend to become stiff in flexion, probably because of fibrosis of the palmar plate and contracture of the accessory collateral ligaments and they should therefore be immobilized in full extension. Adhesion of the dorsal aponeurosis to the fracture may cause stiffness of the PIP joint in extension, but it can usually be overcome by the strong finger flexors, whereas the relatively weak extensor mechanism has great difficulty in correcting a flexion deformity.

Fractures of the middle phalanx can often be controlled by splintage of the DIP and PIP joints, leaving the MP joint free, using a short length of padded aluminium splint taped to the palmar surface of the finger (Fig. 17.23a). It is both unnecessary and dangerous to bend the splint over the finger tip and tape it to both surfaces of the finger, as is sometimes illustrated, because of the risk of soft tissue compression and skin necrosis.

For fractures of the proximal phalanx, the MP joint must be immobilized and most authors agree that the wrist should also be splinted. Wrist motion alters the tension in the flexor and extensor tendons and may transmit deforming forces to the fracture. The splint must be bent at the level of the distal palmar crease in order to flex the MP joint and if the wrist is left free, a very short length of splint remains for secure fixation to the palm. The wrist is immobilized in moderate extension to slacken the finger extensors and facilitate flexion of the MP joints. A plaster cast is the most practical method of immobilization for the wrist and it may be extended as a palmar slab to support the fingers. The slab is liable to break unless it is strengthened by a longitudinal ridge of plaster. Alternatively, the finger may be taped to a length of padded aluminium splint incorporated in the cast. The strength of the splint is increased considerably by bending the edges upwards to form a U-shape (Fig. 17.23b). Control of the fracture is improved if an adjacent digit is included; this can often be achieved conveniently for fractures of the ring and little fingers by an ulnar gutter splint, leaving the other digits free (Fig. 17.24).

TRACTION

Various methods of traction via skin, pulp, nail and bone have been devised for phalangeal fractures but none has become popular. Sliding or elastic traction is difficult to apply and maintain and associated complications include skin necrosis, tethering of the dorsal aponeurosis and joint stiffness. However, Fitzgerald and Khan (1984) described a method of fixed traction

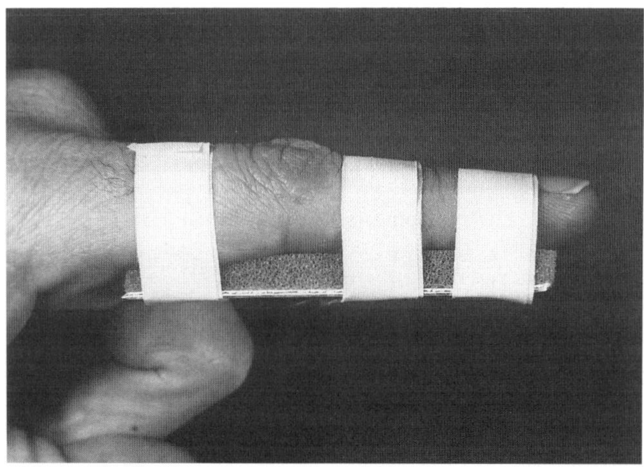

(a)

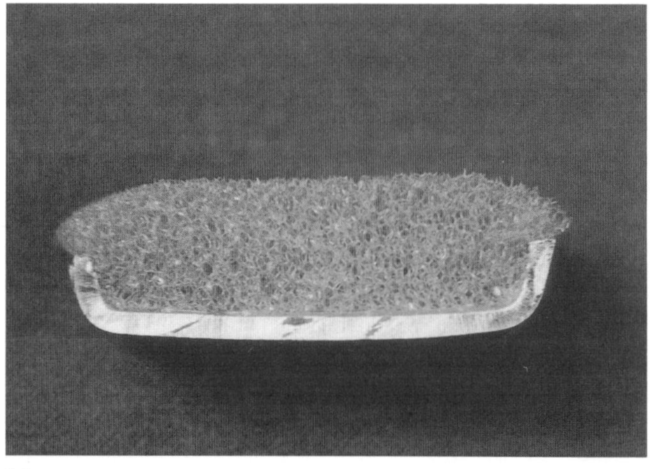

(b)

Fig. 17.23 (a) A padded aluminium splint is useful for splintage of the phalanges and IP joints. (b) Its rigidity is increased by bending the edges into a shallow U-shape.

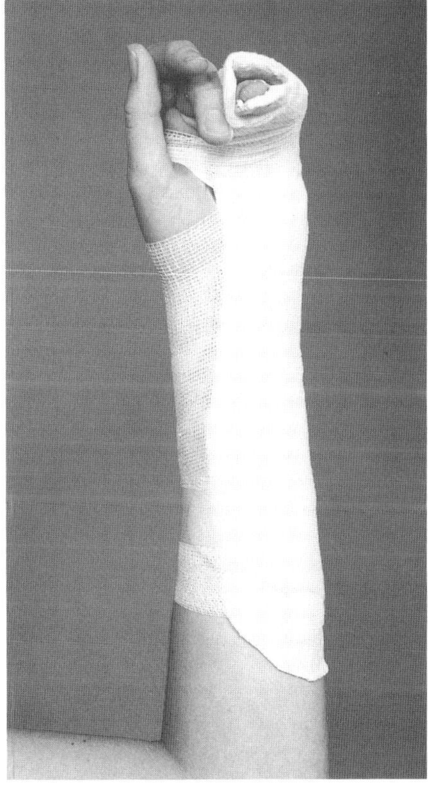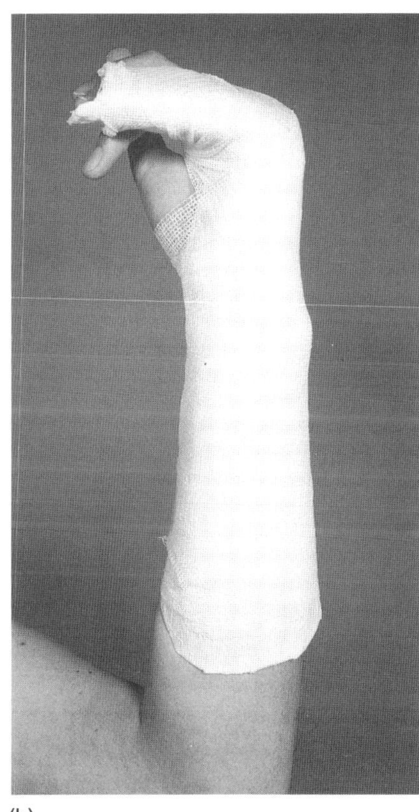

(a) (b)

Fig. 17.24 (a) and (b) Ulnar gutter splint for fractures of the ring and little fingers, allowing function of the other digits.

over a padded aluminium splint for phalangeal shaft fractures and reported restoration of full movement in 16 out of 18patients with no complications. After skin traction was applied to the finger and fastened to the end of the splint in extension, the finger was flexed. advocates of traction emphasize that it is used not to reduce the fracture but simply to maintain the position after reduction.

EXTERNAL FIXATION

Where a comminuted fracture, or one with bone loss, must be held out to length, external fixation provides a safer and more practical alternative, as well as allowing movement of adjacent joints (Ashmead *et al.* 1992). It has been used when K-wire fixation is inadequate or when internal fixation is inappropriate because of comminution, though it has found wider application for metacarpal than for phalangeal fractures. Purpose-built external fixators are available commercially, or fixation can be custom-made from K-wires and methylmethacrylate cement (Scott & Mulligan 1980, Riggs & Cooney 1983). The strength of the fixation increases with the number of pins and their diameter (Stuchin & Kummer 1984). It is difficult to place pins in the

phalanges without tethering the dorsal aponeurosis, but in the severe injuries for which external fixation is indicated, this disadvantage is outweighed by the stability which is achieved. The spring-tensioned external fixation device devised by Fahmy and Harvey (1992) is a useful addition to the armarmentarium.

CLOSED REDUCTION AND PERCUTANEOUS PIN FIXATION

This is a safe and versatile technique which is frequently the next choice of management when a fracture cannot be controlled by splintage. The pins can be placed with the minimum of additional trauma and the complications of open reduction are avoided. If satisfactory reduction cannot be achieved by closed manipulation, open reduction will be required; however, the greater risks of open reduction dictate that closed reduction and pin fixation should be employed whenever possible.

The technique of pin fixation depends on the configuration of the fracture. Transverse and short oblique fractures require a wire passing longitudinally. Joshi (1976) introduced a K-wire through the base of the proximal phalanx, just distal to the articular surface, and reported satisfactory results in 55 out of 61 patients.

Passage of the wire through the flexed PIP joint has been described but seems undesirable because of the risk of flexion deformity.

Belsky *et al.* (1984) reported good results in 90 out of 100 displaced proximal phalanx fractures treated by percutaneous pin fixation. For transverse and short oblique fractures of the neck, shaft and base, the fracture is reduced by traction and flexion of the MP and PIP joints. A K-wire mounted in a T-handle chuck is passed to one side of the extensor tendon, into the metacarpal head and across the flexed MP joint into the medullary canal of the proximal phalanx, up to the subchondral bone of the condyles (Fig. 17.25). An essential part of the technique is immobilization of the fractured digit and an adjacent finger using a snugly fitting cast extending from the forearm to the DIP joints, otherwise motion of the MP joint may cause irritation or even breakage of the wire. This is an excellent technique which can be performed under wrist block anaesthesia without the need for power instruments.

Spiral and long oblique fractures may be stabilized by transverse fine K-wires inserted along the mid-axial line (Fig. 17.26). Green and Anderson (1973) found 18 out of 21 patients recovered full movement when treated in this fashion for 3 weeks, followed by 3 weeks buddy taping.

The main disadvantage of percutaneous pin fixation is the difficulty of obtaining a good reduction and accurate pin placement. The technique is awkward without an experienced assistant because two hands are required to hold the reduction and a third hand is needed to pass the wires. A power drill is essential, preferably fitted with a chuck which can be released with one hand. Cannulated reduction forceps (Fig. 17.27) are helpful in holding the reduction of spiral and oblique fractures while the wire is inserted (Blalock *et al.* 1975, Glasgow & Lloyd 1981). If such a clamp is not available, the surgeon may be able to maintain the reduction and at the same time hold the point of a suitably sized intravenous needle against the surface of the bone. The needle acts as a drill guide, prevents slipping of the wire on the cortex, and allows a less-experienced assistant to pass the wire while the surgeon controls its direction. Percutaneous fixation is usually strong enough to permit early protected movement with taping to an adjacent finger. However, it is frequently impossible to achieve satisfactory motion until the pins are removed because of tethering of the dorsal aponeurosis and skin. The pins may be cut off beneath the skin, in which case local anaesthesia is necessary for their removal. Alternatively, the ends may be left protruding though the skin. Mild drainage from the pin sites is not uncommon but usually responds to immobilization and antibiotics or, if necessary, to removal of the pin. Persistent infection after removal of a pin is rare.

OPEN REDUCTION AND INTERNAL FIXATION

This is necessary when satisfactory position and stability cannot be achieved by closed methods. The most

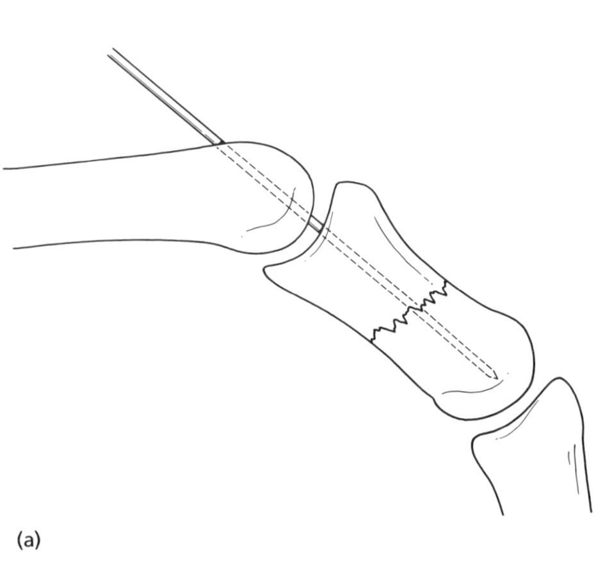

(a)

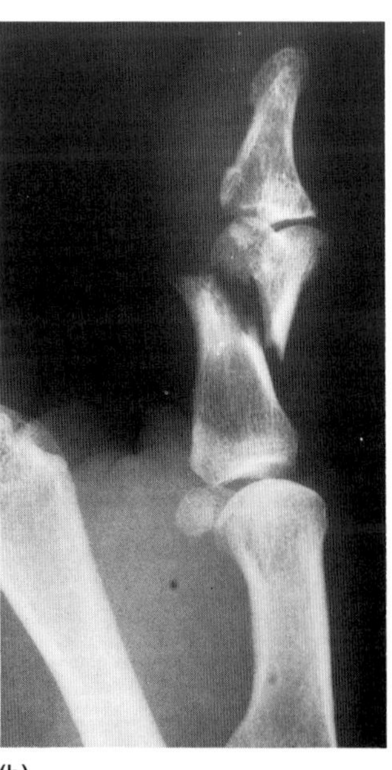

(b)

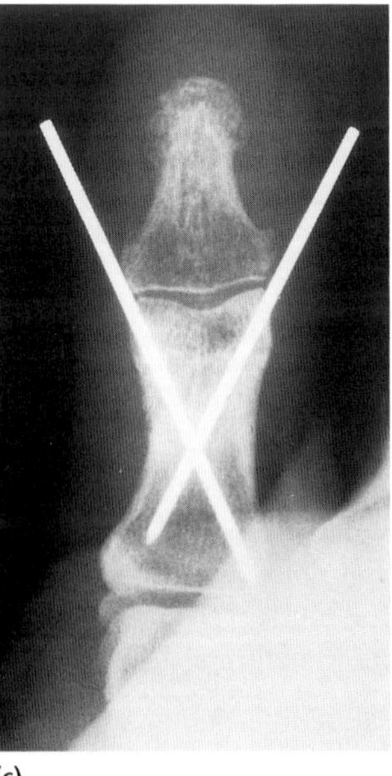

(c)

Fig. 17.25 Percutaneous pin fixation. (a) Transverse fracture of the proximal phalanx fixed by longitudinal K-wire passed across the flexed MP joint. (b) Crossed pin fixation of thumb proximal phalanx fracture.

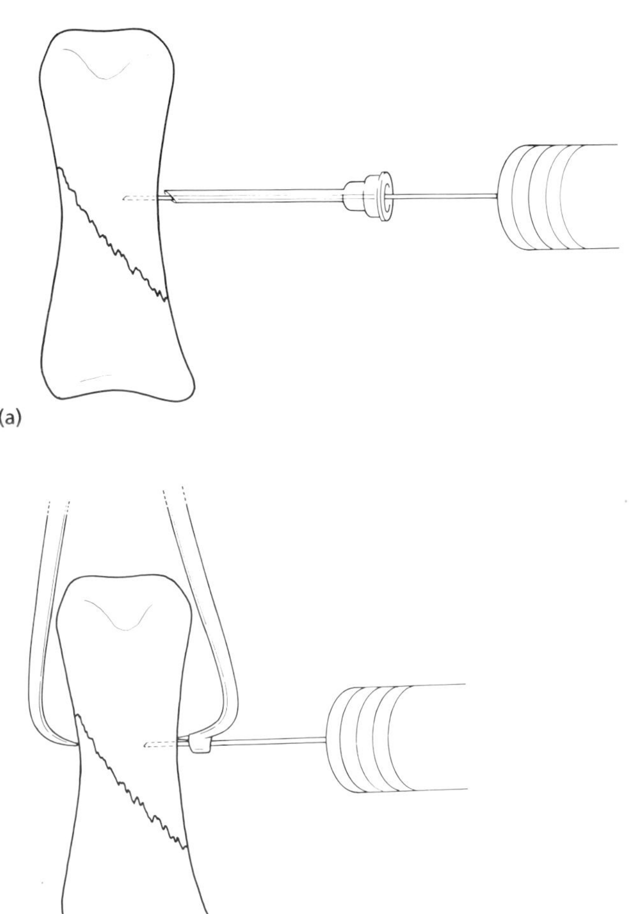

(a)

(b)

Fig. 17.26 Percutaneous pin fixation of oblique phalangeal fracture. (a) Reduction and 14 gauge needle held by the surgeon while the assistant passes the wire. The reduction can only be checked *after* pin insertion. (b) Use of cannulated reduction forceps allows confirmation of reduction *before* the pins are inserted.

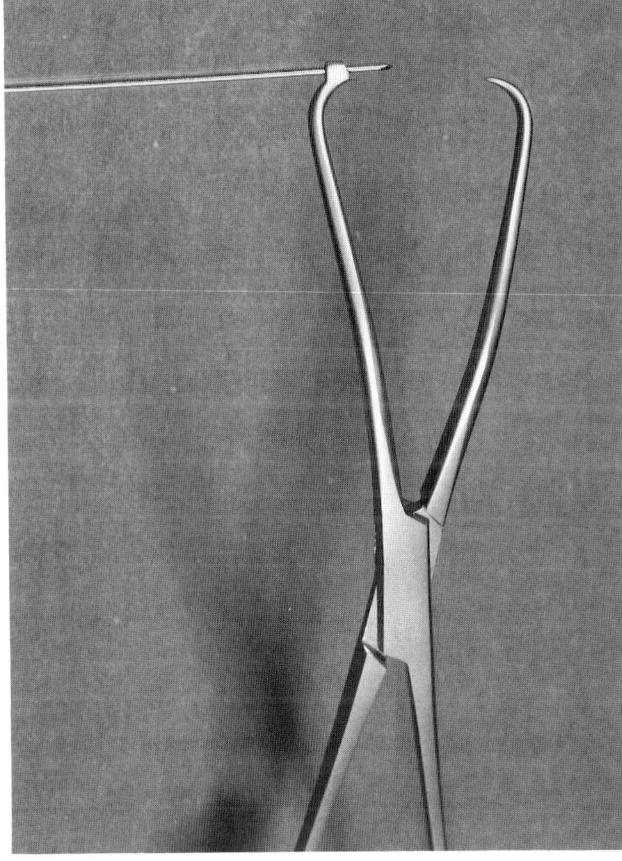

Fig. 17.27 Cannulated reduction forceps which are helpful for percutaneous pin fixation.

frequent indication is a displaced articular fracture, where precise reduction and early motion offer the best chance of recovery of joint function (Steel 1978). Open reduction may also be required for unstable extra-articular fractures when reduction is prevented by soft tissue interposition or by delay in treatment, or when satisfactory internal fixation cannot be achieved by closed methods. Other indications are fractures with associated nerve or tendon injury, most open fractures and digits requiring revascularization.

The potential benefits of accurate reduction and stable fixation must be balanced against the risks of additional injury to the soft tissues which inevitably accompanies open reduction and internal fixation. The delicate soft tissues must be handled carefully with minimal strip-

ping of periosteum, protection of neurovascular structures and gentle manipulation of fracture fragments. The use of magnifying loupes is strongly recommended. The extra soft tissue injury inflicted by surgery is justified only if its effects can be overcome by immediate active motion, otherwise disabling loss of digital motion may occur. Adhesion between extensor mechanism and bone is particularly liable to occur over the proximal phalanx, where a large surface of bone is enveloped by the dorsal aponeurosis.

The factors which need to be considered when selecting a method of internal fixation include:
1 Fracture configuration.
2 Nature of the soft tissue injury.
3 Relative strength of fixation technique.
4 Transfixion/tethering of mobile soft tissues.
5 Extent of dissection required for insertion.
6 Need for another operation to remove metal.
7 Effect of the fixation technique on fracture healing.
The best technique is the simplest one which provides adequate stability for early active motion.

K-wire fixation

This is a popular and versatile technique for internal fixation and can be applied to almost any fracture configuration. It provides stability rather than rigid fixation and immediate mobilization is frequently impeded by the need for protective splintage as well as by tethering of the soft tissues. K-wires may be passed longitudinally or obliquely for transverse fractures and transversely for oblique fractures. Crossed oblique K-wires may, however, hold apart the surfaces of transverse fractures unless the fragments are firmly impacted while the wires are driven across the fracture.

Interosseous wiring

Interosseous wiring (Lister 1978) is an excellent technique for fixation of transverse phalangeal fractures which is stronger than crossed K-wires and gives better compression at the fracture site (Massengill *et al.*

1982). A 26 gauge wire loop is passed through drill holes 5 mm either side of the fracture; the holes are made with a fine K-wire and should be placed just dorsal to the mid-axis of the phalanx so that the wire acts as a tension-band. The K-wire is drilled obliquely across one fragment, the fracture reduced and the wire loop tightened. The K-wire is then driven into the second fragment to provide additional control of rotation and angulation (Fig. 17.28a). The fixation is strong enough to allow immediate unresisted active motion. Lister (1978) reported recovery of 80% of normal joint motion in 44 phalangeal fractures. Intraosseous wiring may also be employed for fixation of small articular or juxta-articular fragments, passing the wire loop through the fragment and adjacent bone (Fig. 17.28b). Alternatively, the wire can be passed around the attached ligament or tendon if the fragment is small or comminuted. Tension-band wiring of phalangeal fractures has also proved to be a reliable technique capable of supporting early active motion (Greene *et al.* 1987).

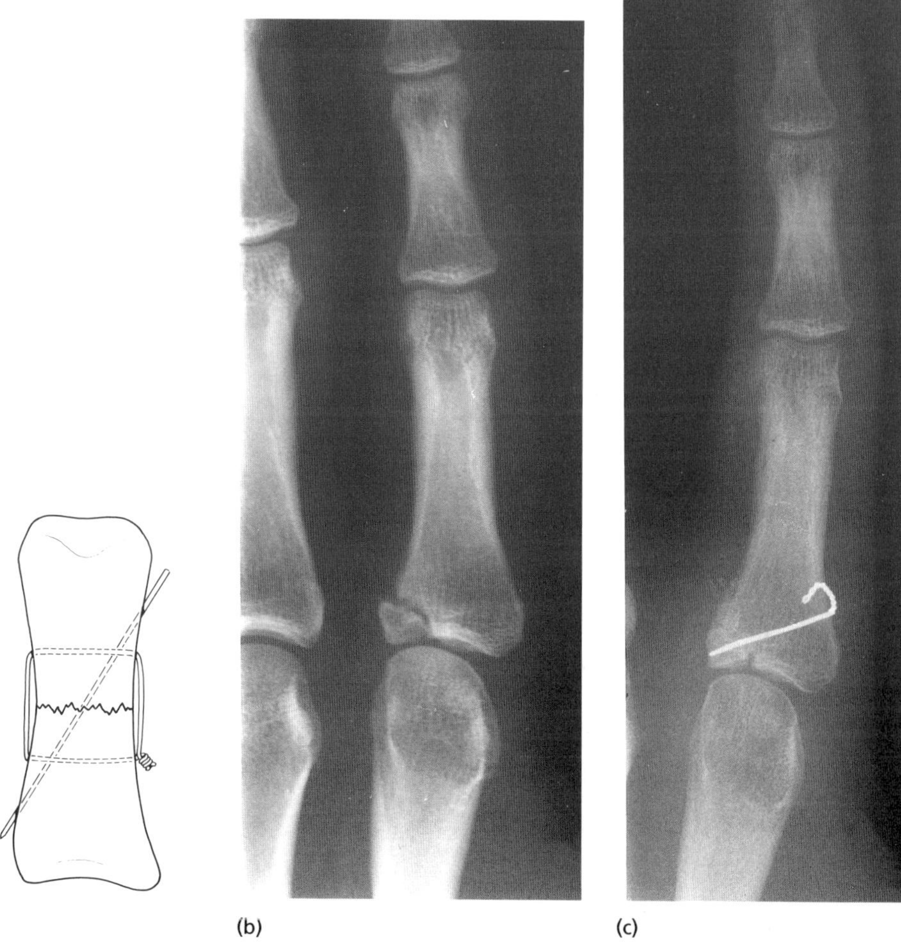

(a)   (b)   (c)

Fig. 17.28 Interosseous wire fixation technique. (a) Shaft fractures. (b) and (c) Ligament avulsion fractures.

Plate and screws

The principles advocated by the AO group for large bone fractures, namely anatomical reduction, rigid fixation and early motion, have been extended to the hand by the development of a small plate and screws (Segmuller 1977, Büchler & Fischer 1987, Heim & Pfeiffer 1987). Increasing experience has led many authors to emphasize the limited indications and potential complications of these techniques, especially with respect to phalangeal fractures (Steel 1978, Dabezies & Schutte 1986, Diwaker & Stothard 1986, Jabalay & Freeland 1986, Ford *et al.* 1987, Hastings 1987). However, for a few difficult fractures, e.g. condylar fractures of the proximal phalanx, interfragmentary screw fixation does offer the best chance of restoring finger function (Fig. 17.29).

The small bone size, delicate soft tissue envelope and absence of muscle padding of the fingers do not constitute a good environment for plates and most authors advise against their use in the phalanges. Stern *et al.* (1987) recorded complications in six out of nine of phalangeal fractures treated by plating. The main indications for screw fixation are articular fractures (Fig. 17.30) and oblique fractures where the length of the fracture is greater than twice the diameter of the shaft (Fig. 17.31). Small bone fragments should be at least three times larger than the thread diameter of the screw.

The operative technique is demanding and the margin for error very narrow; there is usually only one opportunity to drill, tap and insert a screw correctly. If the hole is misplaced or the thread damaged, there is seldom room to drill another and the entire fixation may be compromised. If the fixation is insecure, the final result is almost invariably worse than if a simpler treatment had been adopted initially.

The results of screw fixation depend on precise, gentle operative technique and meticulous aftercare. Excellent results can be obtained in ideal circumstances, but there is greater risk of complications than with simpler methods. Flexion contracture of the PIP joint, adhesion of the dorsal aponeurosis to the fracture and loss of flexion are the main complications (Ford *et al.* 1987). Particular care should be taken to prevent PIP joint contracture by active and passive exercise, supplemented by splintage in extension during sleep. Adherence of the dorsal aponeurosis is a particular problem after internal fixation of the proximal phalanx. It is characterized by an extension lag at the PIP joint, often without fixed contracture. The results of tenolysis are poor, probably because of the large area of bone covered by aponeurosis at this level and the relative weakness of the extensors compared with the flexors (Green 1986). The earlier active movement is commenced, the better the ultimate range of motion is likely to be; active

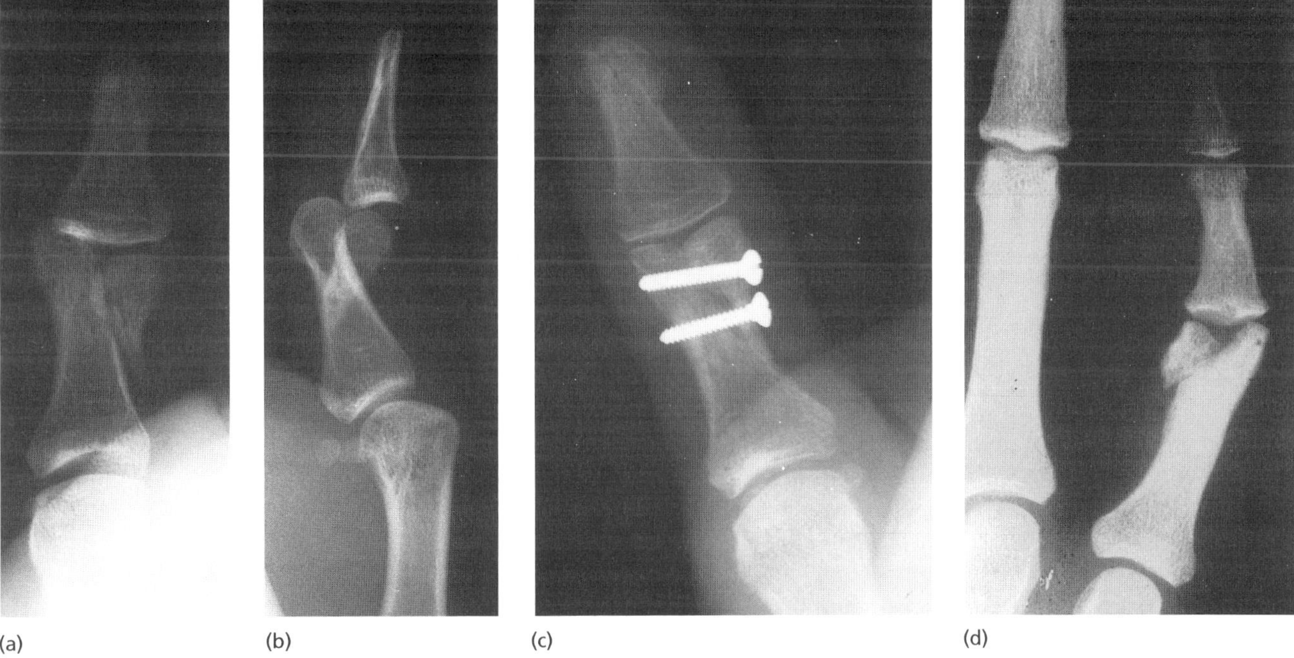

(a) (b) (c) (d)

Fig. 17.29 (a) and (b) Condylar fracture of thumb proximal phalanx with rotation of the condylar fragment and some articular surface comminution. (c) Open reduction and internal fixation with two interfragmentary screws. (d) Untreated condylar fracture 15 months after injury.

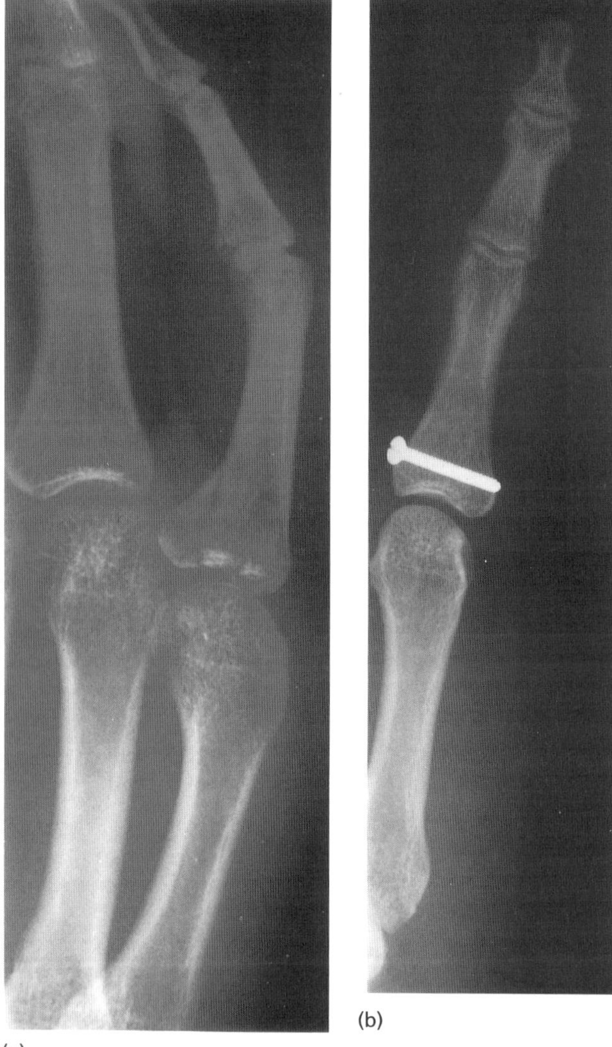

(a)

(b)

Fig. 17.30 (a) Displaced articular fracture at the base of the proximal phalanx. (b) Open reduction and interfragmentary screw fixation.

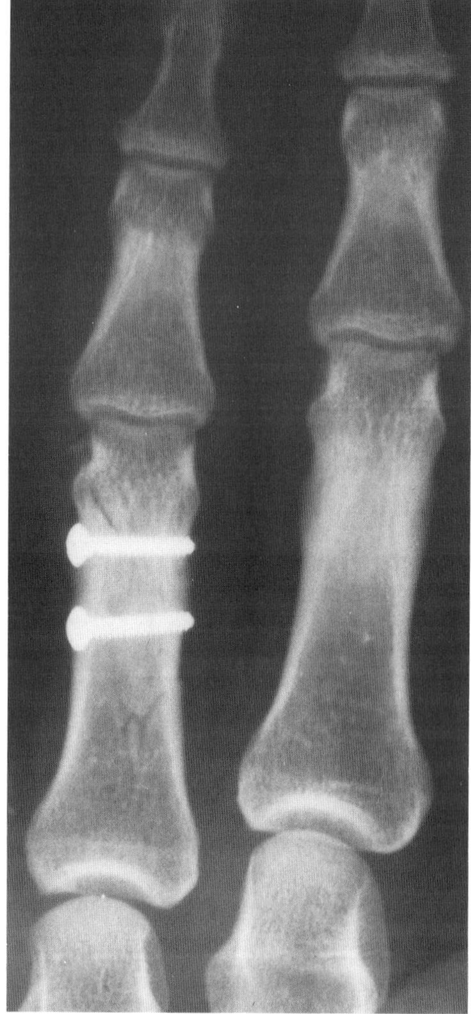

Fig. 17.31 Open reduction and screw fixation of an oblique proximal phalanx fracture with rotatory displacement.

movement should be started as soon as possible and certainly within 48 hours. The author's experience with continuous passive motion, applied in the recovery room and continued for 24–48 hours, suggests that it minimizes swelling, maintains passive joint motion and makes resumption of active motion easier than after 48 hours immobilization. However, conclusive data on the use of continuous passive motion is not currently available.

Plate fixation of phalanges is probably only indicated in rare cases when there is severe comminution or bone loss adjacent to a joint. The minicondylar plate designed by Büchler and Fischer (1987) provides stable fixation of the articular fragments and fixes them to the shaft by means of a plate along the lateral side of the phalanx.

Screw and plate fixation is considerably more difficult in the hand than in larger bones and the potential for complications is greater. The author believes that these techniques should be used only by surgeons who are experienced in hand surgery, who are familiar with the techniques of internal fixation of large bones and who have received specific instruction from an experienced colleague or at a 'hands-on' course on small bone fixation.

Intramedullary fixation

This type of fixation using a Steinmann pin was described by Grundberg (1981), who devised a method of insertion which avoids damage to adjacent joints. The size of the medullary canal is determined with a Steinmann pin and a pin one size larger is used to ream the proximal and distal fragments, starting with the sharp end and finishing with the blunt end to avoid penetration of the subchondral bone. The blunt end is then introduced into the proximal fragment and the end cut off so that 1 cm protrudes in a phalanx and 1.5 cm in a metarcarpal. The fracture is distracted and the distal fragment manipulated over the end of the pin, which may need to be shortened to allow reduction. The fracture is then impacted to lock the fragments and prevent rotation. Union occurred in 17 out of 18 phalangeal fractures with no infections, even though 14 fractures were open with a high proportion of crushing injuries.

The stability provided by various internal fixation methods has been analysed for fractures of the metacarpals and the proximal phalanges (Massengill *et al.* 1982, Black *et al.* 1985). Data from these studies allow the fixation techniques to be ranked in order of increasing strength for *transverse fractures* as follows:
Crossed K-wires.
Intraosseous wire plus K-wire.
Tension-band wiring plus K-wire.
Plate applied to tension surface.
Plate applied to tension surface plus lag screw.
For *oblique fractures* the order of increasing strength is:
Multiple K-wires.
Two lag screws.
Two lag screws plus neutralization plate.

Plates applied to the compression surface of the bone without interfragmentary screws offer only the strength of the plate itself. Plates applied to the dorsal surface of the metacarpals provide strength against flexion forces which is almost equal to that of the intact bone.

Extra-articular fractures of the phalanges

Extra-articular fractures which are undisplaced are best treated with immediate protected mobilization with taping to an adjacent digit. Further displacement is unlikely provided that vigorous activity is avoided, but the patient must be instructed about exercises and should be examined at the end of the first week to check that displacement has not occurred.

Transverse fractures of the shaft of the proximal phalanx angulate dorsally owing to flexion of the proximal fragment by the interossei. Since the periosteum forms the dorsal surface of the flexor tendon sheath, malunion may restrict the excursion of the flexor tendon as well as interfere with the dorsal aponeurosis. Reduction to within 1–2 mm can usually be achieved by manipulation under metacarpal block. The fracture is stable if the PIP joint is flexed, but immobilization in excessive flexion may lead to flexion contracture of the

PIP joint. If the reduction appears stable with the PIP joint at 30° flexion, the fracture may be immobilized in this position by taping the finger to a length of padded metal splint incorporated in a short-arm cast. Internal fixation is preferable if the fracture is unstable or if excessive flexion is required to maintain reduction. Passage of a longitudinal K-wire across the flexed MP joint and along the medullary canal of the proximal phalanx (see Fig. 17.30) is simpler and safer than open reduction with internal fixation and the results are at least as good (Belsky *et al.* 1984).

Spiral fractures of the phalangeal shaft are the result of rotational injury. Shortening of the fracture is accompanied by rotation which may be quite difficult to detect initially but later produces troublesome overlap of digits (Fig. 17.32). It is extremely difficult to maintain correct rotational alignment by external splintage; time may be wasted by repeated attempts at non-operative treatment, leaving the surgeon with a difficult decision between taking down a partially healed fracture or correcting malalignment by subsequent osteotomy. The author believes that rotational displacement is an indication for internal fixation, which can usually be achieved with percutaneous transverse K-wires provided that the fracture is no more than 5 days old. Open reduction and lag screw fixation may be required after this time. Spiral fractures without malrotation should be watched closely; rotation is seen best during finger flexion, but if flexion is prevented by pain one must rely on comparing the plane of the fingernail with that of its neighbours (Fig. 17.21).

Rotational malunion of the proximal phalanx may be corrected by osteotomy, which can be made at the site of the fracture or in the metacarpal (Fig. 17.33). Malunion with lateral angulation as well as rotation can only be corrected at the fracture but there is a greater risk of stiffness in the PIP joint than if osteotomy is performed in the metacarpal (Fig. 17.34). For pure rotational deformity up to 25°, it is safer to make the osteotomy through cancellous bone at the base of the metacarpal (Weckesser 1965). It may be fixed with K-wires or with a small T-plate.

Fracture of the neck of the proximal phalanx occurs in young children and usually results from a crushing injury. The condyles rotate dorsally but the deformity is masked by swelling; the degree of displacement may be underestimated unless a true lateral radiograph is taken. Inadequate reduction results in a block to flexion by the proximal fragment (Fig. 17.35). There is no physis at the distal end of the phalanx and remodelling of these injuries is slow and incomplete. Accurate reduction and K-wire fixation is required. Dixon and Moon (1972)

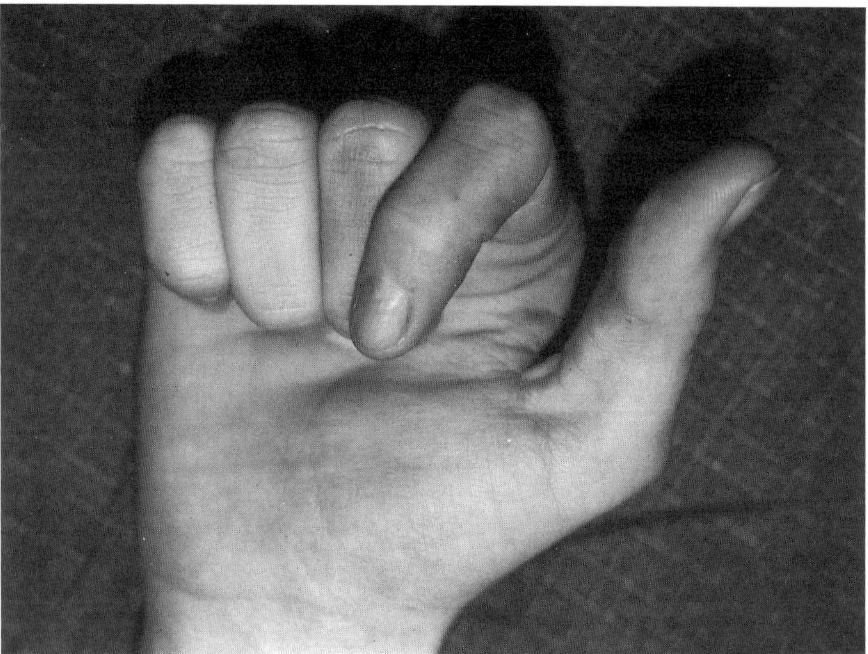

Fig. 17.32 Cross-over deformity due to rotatory malunion of the proximal phalanx.

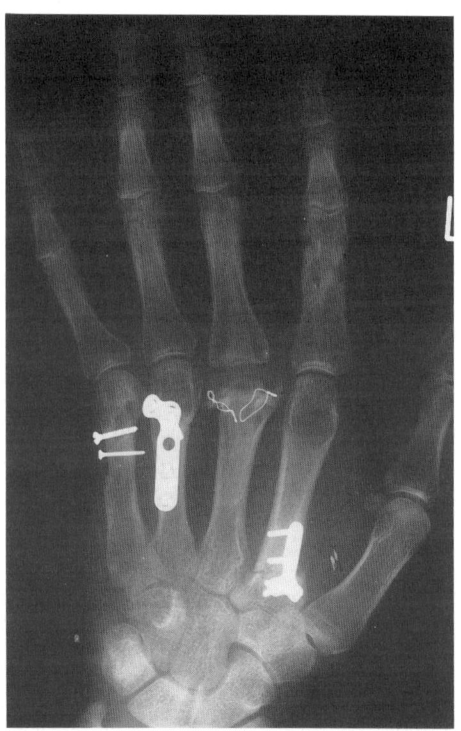

Fig. 17.33 Correction of rotatory malunion of the proximal phalanx by osteotomy at the base of the metacarpal. Use of a plate allows early motion and safeguards the alignment.

recommend that a needle inserted percutaneously may be used to manipulate the distal fragment. Inability to reduce the fracture is one of the few indications for open reduction in the child's hand, for unless the deformity is corrected full IP joint flexion is unlikely. Correction of malunion by osteotomy carries a risk of stiffness; it is safer to remove the offending bone from the palmar aspect of the neck of the proximal phalanx, recreating the subcondylar fossa (Simmons & Peters 1987).

A similar block to flexion may follow a long oblique fracture of the proximal phalanx, which may unite with shortening so that a palmar spike of bone on the proximal fragment impinges on the middle phalanx and blocks flexion of the PIP joint. Removal of the spike will usually restore adequate flexion.

Fractures of the base of the proximal phalanx often exhibit marked dorsal angulation which is underestimated by oblique radiographs and is difficult to see on lateral films because of overlap of other digits (Fig. 17.36). It occurs most often in the little finger, where a claw posture results with secondary flexion contracture of the PIP joint. Deformity can be prevented by prompt recognition and treatment. Severe angulatory malunion may be corrected by opening or closing wedge osteotomy through the fracture (Froimson 1981).

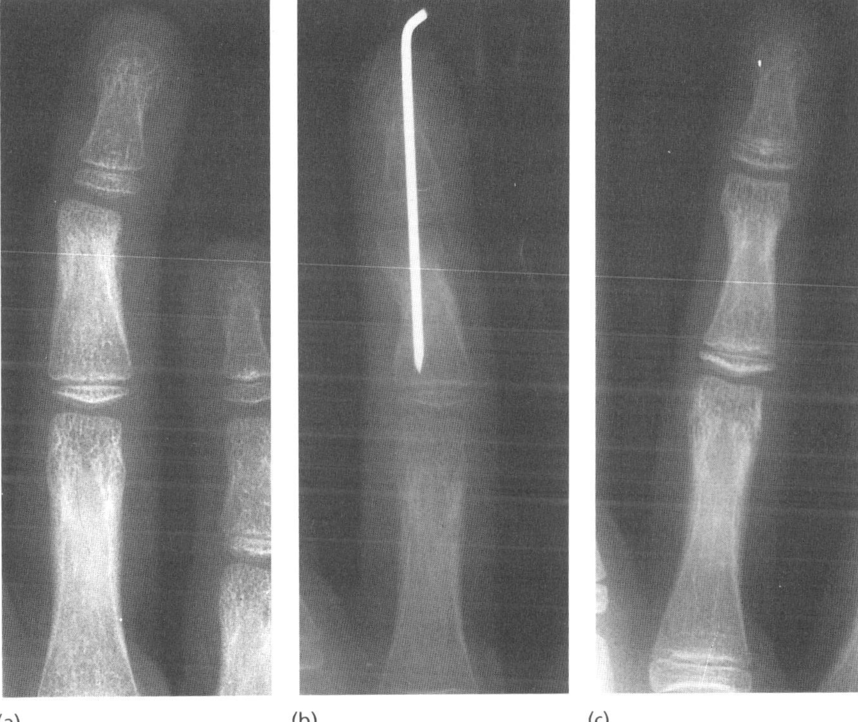

Fig. 17.34 Correction of angular malunion of the middle phalanx (a) by closing wedge osteotomy and (b) K-wire fixation. (c) After 18 months.

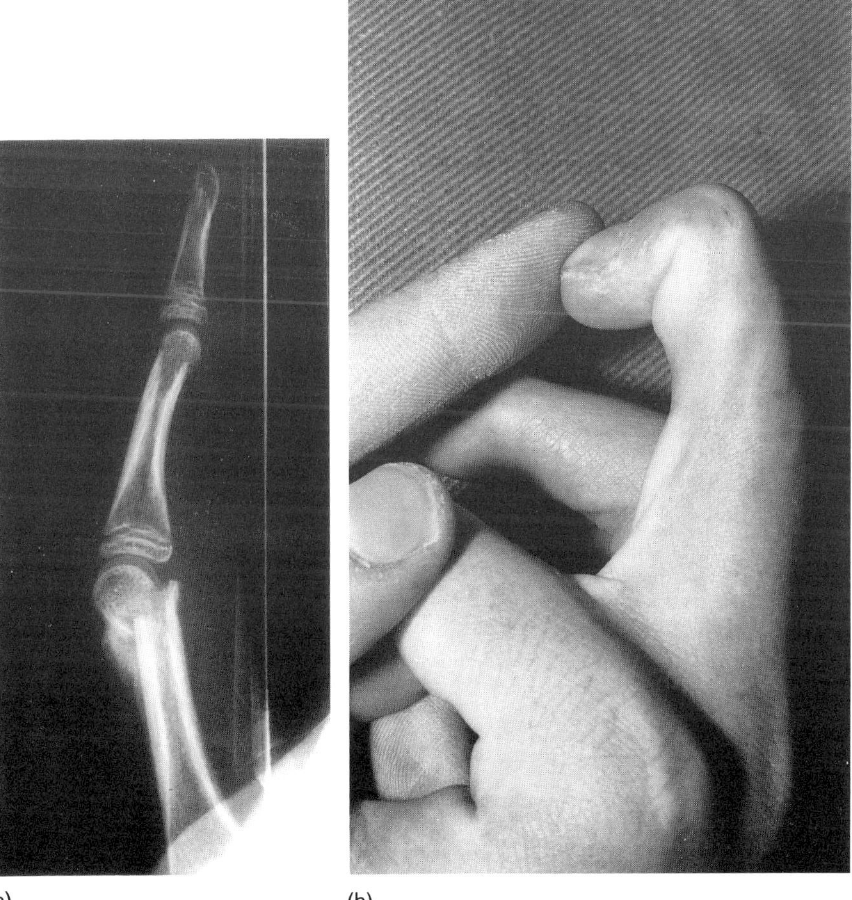

Fig. 17.35 (a) Palmar bone block to PIP joint flexion resulting from malunion of a fracture of the neck of the proximal phalanx. (b) Long-standing bone block to PIP joint flexion with compensatory excessive DIP joint flexion.

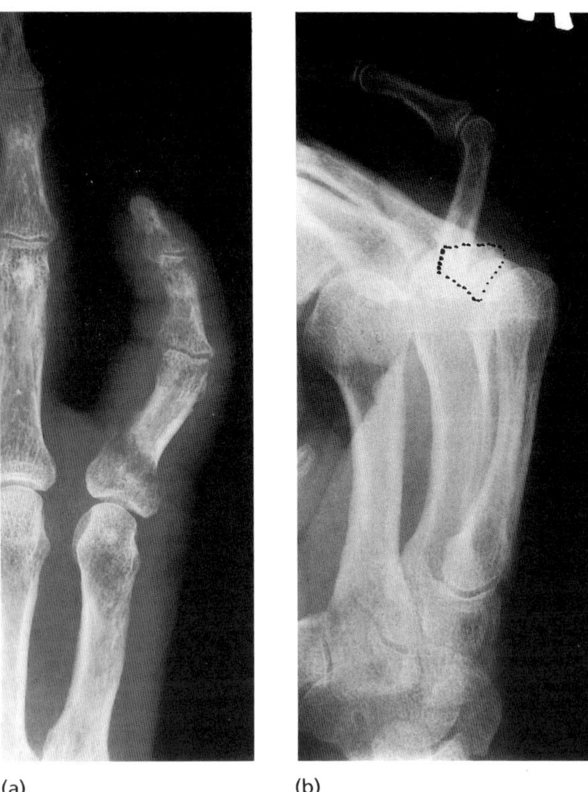

Fig. 17.36 (a) Dorsal angulation of a fracture of the base of the proximal phalanx. Oblique radiographs underestimate the deformity; (b) a true lateral view is required.

Articular fractures

The aim in treatment of articular fractures is restoration of stability, articular congruity and motion. In theory, open reduction with stable internal fixation and early movement are the best means of achieving these aims, but technical considerations limit their use to fragments which are large enough for secure fixation, i.e. at least three times the core diameter of the screw. Open reduction and insecure fixation is worse than non-operative treatment, since the penalties of operative treatment are incurred without the benefits.

Where comminution precludes open reduction and internal fixation, the options include acceptance of the position and early protected motion, traction, external fixation, reduction and transarticular pin fixation, and limited open reduction/internal fixation supported by external fixation. Barton (1989) has emphasized that articular fractures are tolerated better at the DIP and MP joints than at the PIP joint. Stiffness at the distal joint has a small effect on overall hand function; fractures of the base of the distal phalanx often show remarkable remodelling of the joint surface. Fractures of the base of the proximal phalanx also behave relatively well.

If alignment is satisfactory, if the patient can demonstrate perhaps 30° of active motion, and if the configuration of the fracture precludes internal fixation, early protected motion often provides a better result than might be expected, at least so far as the DIP and MP joints are concerned. O'Rourke *et al.* (1989) showed that only four out of 54 patients had significant pain at an average of 11 years after intra-articular fractures of the phalanges. However, the long term results of these injuries are unknown.

Undisplaced articular fractures are best treated by immediate protected mobilization, but must be supervised to detect displacement during the first 2 weeks. Displaced articular fractures usually produce deformity and permanent loss of motion unless the surfaces are restored anatomically by open reduction and internal fixation. At the PIP joint, some loss of motion is common however the injury is treated, but perfect reduction, stable fixation and early motion offers the best chance of good joint function.

Condylar fractures may involve one or both sides of the head of the middle and proximal phalanges. It may be possible to obtain precise reduction and fixation by percutaneous pinning, but this is frequently very difficult; imperfect reduction should not be accepted because it seldom results in good joint function (Fig. 17.29d). Unicondylar fractures may be exposed via a dorsal approach, opening the interval between the central slip and the lateral band. It is essential to obtain a good view of the joint surface and the lateral aspect of the neck of the phalanx. Injury to the central slip must be avoided. The fracture is reduced and provisional fixation obtained with a bone clamp or fine K-wire. One or two interfragmentary screws (1.5 or 2.0 mm) provide the most secure fixation (Fig. 17.29) and avoid the tethering of the transverse retinacular ligament and lateral band which tends to occur with K-wires and which may prevent immediate active movement. It may be necessary to release a portion of the origin of the collateral ligament to make room for the screw head. Active movement must begin as soon as the soft tissues are stable, preferably within 24 hours. An extension splint worn at night for 3–4 weeks helps to prevent flexion contracture of the PIP joint. Bicondylar fractures are difficult to treat. If displacement is minimal, a short period of immobilization followed by protected motion is the safest management. The condylar plate designed by Büchler and Fischer (1987) may be used for internal fixation of displaced bicondylar fractures (Fig. 17.37), but the potential risks of plating phalangeal fractures should be kept in mind.

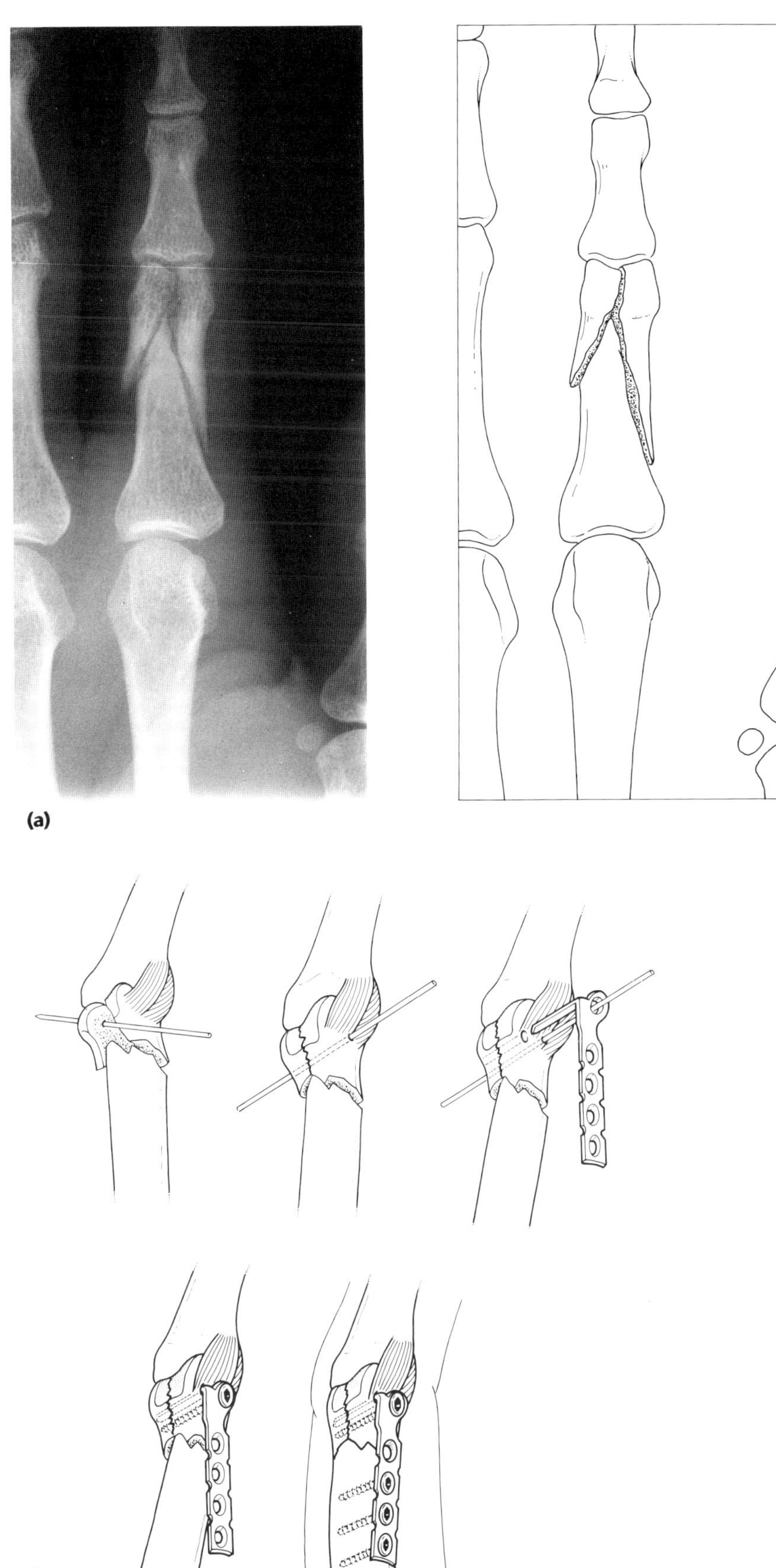

Fig. 17.37 (a) Bicondylar fracture of the proximal phalanx. (b) Condylar blade-plate designed by Büchler and Fischer. (Redrawn with permission from SYNTHES AG, Switzerland.)

Epiphyseal injuries of the phalanges

Epiphyses are located at the proximal but not the distal ends of the phalanges. The patterns of injury can often be predicted from the insertion of tendons and ligaments about the epiphysis (O'Brien 1991). For example, the collateral ligaments of the MP joint insert into the epiphysis at the base of the proximal phalanx, probably accounting for the occurrence of Salter–Harris type III injuries at this site. At the base of the middle phalanx, the PIP joint collateral ligament has fibres which attach to the metaphysis as well as to the epiphysis; type III injuries are rare. The central slip and terminal tendon of the dorsal aponeurosis are attached to the epiphyses of the respective phalanges, where type III injuries are commonly seen. However, type III injuries seldom occur on the flexor surface because the corresponding flexor tendons are attached to the metaphyses.

Type II injuries occur as a result of hyperextension or abduction stress. The little finger, thumb and ring finger are the digits most often involved. In the little finger, the injury is due to abduction force and there may be marked ulnar deviation (Fig. 17.38), almost justifying the description 'extra-octave' fracture (Rang 1974). Ulnar nerve block at the wrist provides excellent anaesthesia for manipulation of this injury and is well-tolerated by most older children. Manipulation is impossible in the extended position because the collateral ligaments of the MP joint are slack. However, if the MP joint is flexed, the collateral ligaments tighten and stabilize the proximal fragment for manipulation. Alternatively, a pencil may be placed in the web and used as a fulcrum around which the base of the proximal phalanx may be levered. The reduction is stable and simply requires immobilization in an ulnar gutter splint for 2 weeks, followed by protected mobilization with buddy taping.

Displaced type III and IV epiphyseal injuries justify open reduction and fixation because of the articular surface irregularity which is usually present.

PIP joint

The PIP joint is a hinge joint. The convex bicondylar head of the proximal phalanx articulates with the base of the middle phalanx, which has matching biconcave surfaces separated by a vertical median ridge.

The head of the proximal phalanx lies in a three-sided box comprising the collateral and accessory collateral ligaments on each side and the volar plate beneath (Eaton 1971). The cord portion of the collateral ligament arises from a depression just dorsal to the mid-axial line of the head of the proximal phalanx and inserts into the

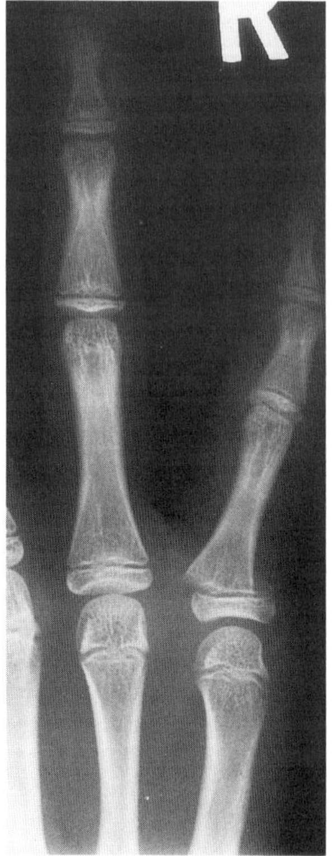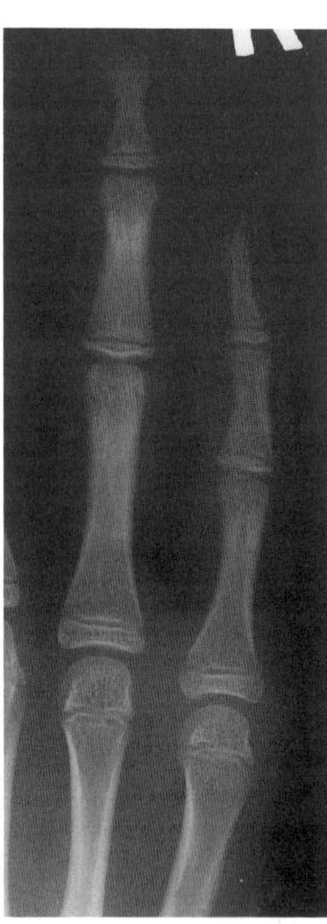

(a)   (b)

Fig. 17.38 (a) Abduction ('extra-octave') fracture of the little finger proximal phalanx. (b) After reduction.

volar lateral tubercle at the base of the middle phalanx. The accessory collateral ligament runs obliquely from the head of the proximal phalanx into the volar plate. The volar plate is a tough fibrocartilaginous structure which acts as a static restraint to hyperextension (Bowers *et al.* 1980). It has strong attachments to the volar corners of the middle phalanx, where fragments of bone may be avulsed. The central portion of the volar plate has a rather tenuous attachment to the periosteum of the base of the middle phalanx (Fig. 17.39). The central portion becomes thinner proximally, but at each side the volar plate has a long fibrous attachment to the proximal phalanx at the distal margin of the A2 pulley. These 'check-rein ligaments' prevent hyperextension of the PIP joint. Displacement of the PIP joint cannot occur unless the box-like ligaments are disrupted in at least two planes (Eaton 1971).

Ligament injuries to the PIP joint may be dorsal, lateral, palmar or combined. In each case, there is a spectrum of severity from the simple PIP joint sprains common in athletes to dislocation. The physical examination should locate points of tenderness accurately, using palpation with a fine blunt object, and assess the

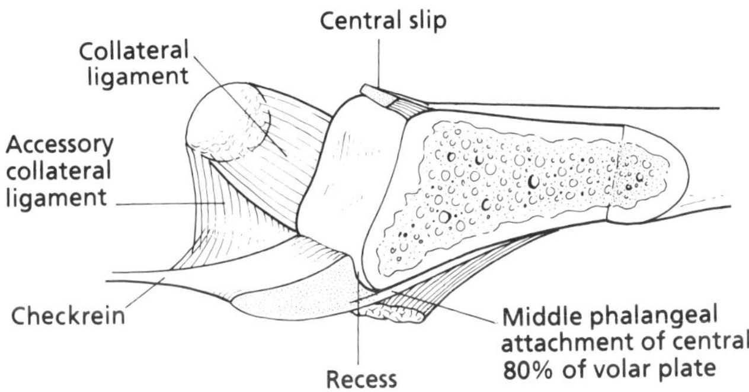

Fig. 17.39 Anatomy of the PIP joint volar plate. (After Bowers *et al*. 1980.)

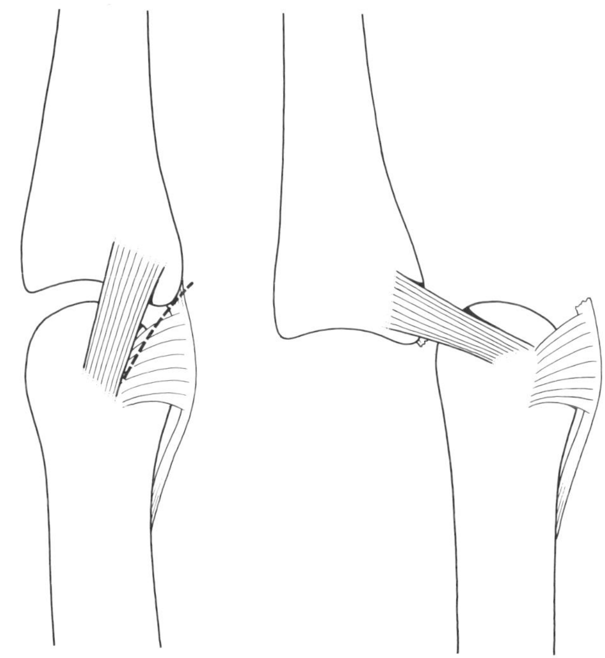

Fig. 17.40 Dorsal dislocation of the PIP joint. The volar plate is torn distally and the tear extends proximally along the fibres of the collateral ligament.

integrity of the extensor mechanism, collateral ligaments and volar plate. Finally, the joint should be observed for instability or deviation during active motion, under digital nerve block if necessary (Eaton 1971).

Dorsal dislocation

Dorsal dislocation of the PIP joint is the result of hyperextension stress which produces a distal tear of the volar plate or avulsion of a small bone fragment from the base of the middle phalanx (Bowers *et al*. 1980). The tear extends longitudinally within the collateral ligament, allowing the base of the middle phalanx to dislocate dorsally, but the collateral ligaments are seldom ruptured and the joint is stable to lateral stress after reduction (Fig. 17.40).

Most dorsal dislocations achieve satisfactory movement and stability with minimal treatment after reduction. Splintage in 10° flexion for 7–10 days provides comfort but the aim of treatment is early restoration of movement. The patient should be warned that swelling, discomfort and stiffness may persist for several months. The presence of a small volar lip avulsion fracture at the base of the middle phalanx does not jeopardize stability of this injury or affect its management.

Chronic laxity of the volar plate is a rare sequel to hyperextension injury. Bowers (1981) suggests that it may develop when multiple hyperextension injuries occur or where the acute lesion is ignored or splinted in extension. The finger adopts a 'swan-neck' posture with hyperextension at the PIP joint and flexion at the DIP joint, but mechanical difficulty initiating PIP joint flexion is usually the reason for consultation. As the finger is flexed, the PIP joint 'hangs up' in hyperextension, snapping down into flexion as the voluntary effort is increased (Fig. 17.41). Repair of the attenuated volar plate, if possible, or construction of a new static restraint to hyperextension is required. Tenodesis using one slip of the superficialis tendon is a simple and reliable technique (Curtis 1982). One slip is divided proximally, leaving its insertion intact, passed obliquely across the palmar aspect of the PIP joint and sutured into a drill-hole in the mid-axial line of the proximal phalanx.

Open dislocation of the PIP joint is usually associated with a transverse wound at the level of the PIP joint (Vicar 1988). The substantial risk of infection and stiffness may be underestimated, especially if it is not appreciated that the wound communicates with the joint and the tendon sheath. Stern and Lee (1985) found that the best results followed thorough debridement in the operating theatre, antibiotic treatment and temporary K-wire fixation. Patients managed in the emergency room by closed reduction and suture had a high incidence of infection and stiffness.

Palmar dislocation

This type of dislocation of the PIP joint is much less common than dorsal dislocation, but may be irreducible or unstable (Fig. 17.42). Failure to recognize and treat this injury is usually followed by a severe flexion contracture or boutonnière deformity. A rotary force ruptures one collateral ligament and the volar plate, allowing the head of the proximal phalanx to buttonhole through

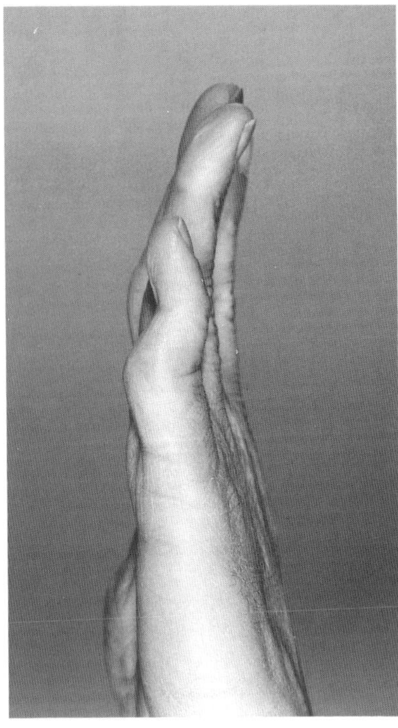

(a)

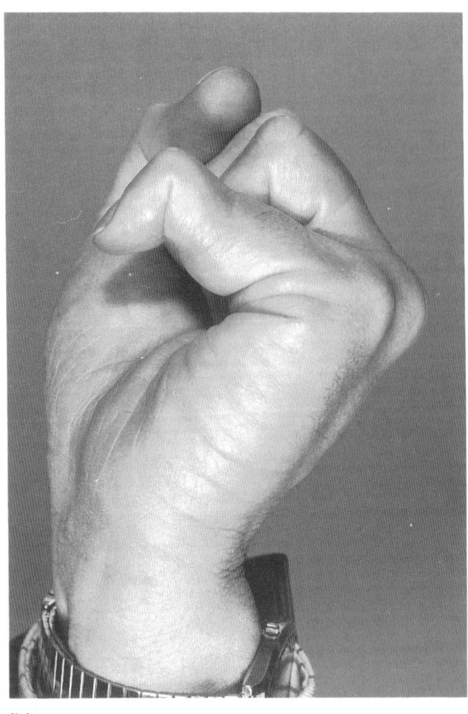

(b)

Fig. 17.41 (a) and (b) Swan-neck deformity resulting from chronic volar plate laxity.

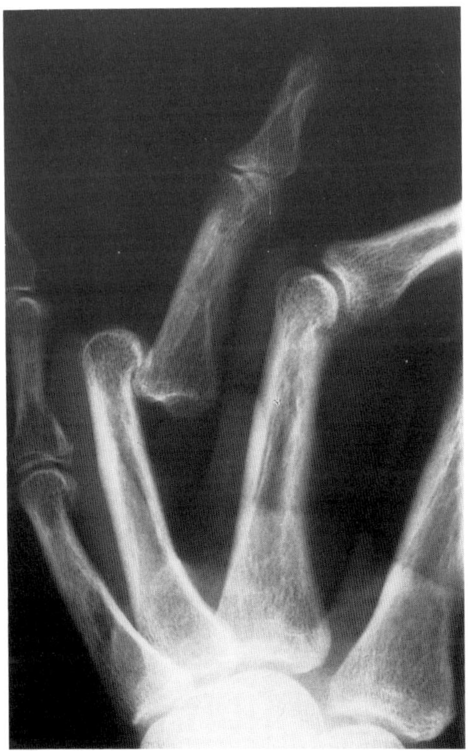

Fig. 17.42 Palmar dislocation of the PIP joint.

the dorsal aponeurosis, usually between the central slip and the lateral band (Spinner & Choi 1970). These structures may prevent reduction, or the central slip may be ruptured (Peimer *et al.* 1984).

Flexion of the MP joint will slacken the lateral band and may permit reduction if it cannot be achieved in the extended position. After reduction, the presence of active PIP joint extension will indicate whether the central slip is intact, in which case immobilization in extension for 2 weeks is appropriate, followed by active flexion with dynamic and/or static splintage to prevent development of a flexion contracture. The combination of central slip, volar plate and collateral ligament rupture permits rotation around the intact collateral ligament with palmar subluxation of the middle phalanx. Peimer *et al.* (1984) recommend open reduction and repair of these structures when displaced intra-articular fractures, irreducibility or fixed contracture are present. Otherwise, percutaneous pin fixation in extension will allow healing of the central slip.

Boutonnière deformity

This deformity is a consequence of injury of the dorsal aponeurosis at the level of the PIP joint. Extension of the IP joints depends upon the co-ordinated and balanced action of the central slip and the lateral bands which extend the PIP and DIP joints respectively. The relative length of these structures ensures that full extension of the PIP and DIP joints is achieved simultaneously; lengthening of the central slip, either by closed rupture or avulsion of its bony insertion, together with palmar migration of the lateral bands, results in boutonnière deformity with flexion of the PIP joint and hyperextension of the distal joint (Fig. 17.43). Closed injury of the PIP joint may disrupt the central slip and tear the triangular ligament, which normally holds the two lateral bands in the correct relationship over the PIP joint. The injury presents with a painful, swollen PIP joint but usually without the typical deformity, which only becomes apparent over the next few days. The diagnosis is made from the presence of local tenderness at the central slip insertion and the inability to extend

the PIP joint actively. Lack of active extension may, however, be due merely to pain and digital nerve block may be required to allow adequate examination. If the PIP joint cannot be held extended, then the central slip has been torn *and* palmar migration of the lateral bands has occurred. However, if the lateral bands remain in the normal position, they can maintain full extension of both IP joints despite rupture of the central slip. Therefore, the proximal phalanx should be stabilized by the examiner and the PIP joint flexed to 40°; if it can be extended actively from this position, the central slip is intact (Elson 1986, Riordan 1988). The radiograph may show a fragment of bone avulsed from the central slip insertion (Fig. 17.44).

The boutonnière deformity develops as the lateral

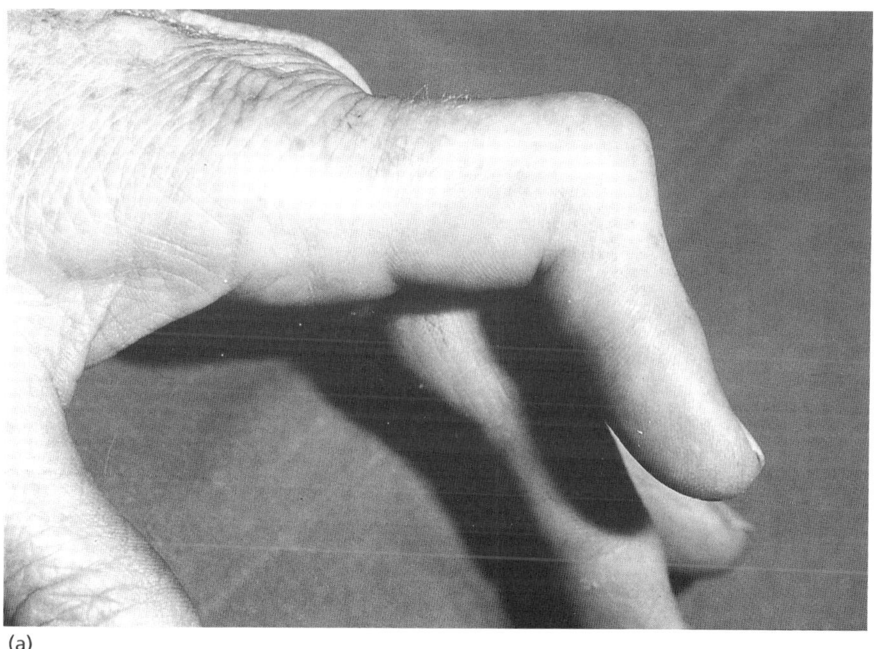

(a)

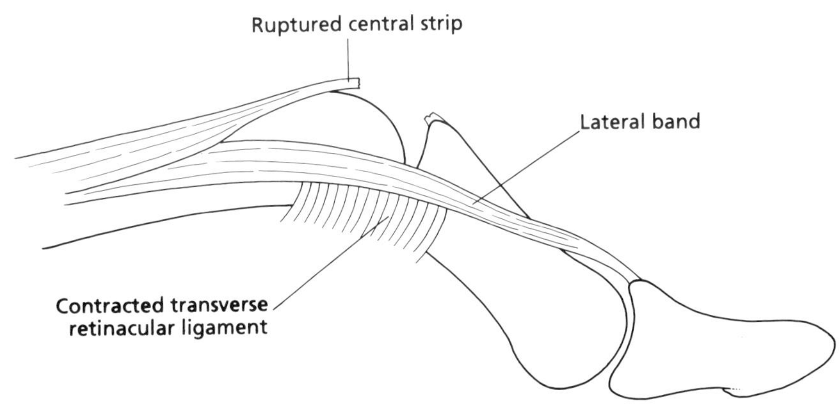

(b)

Fig. 17.43 (a) Boutonnière deformity. (b) Central slip rupture with palmar migration of the lateral bands and contracture of the transverse retinacular ligaments.

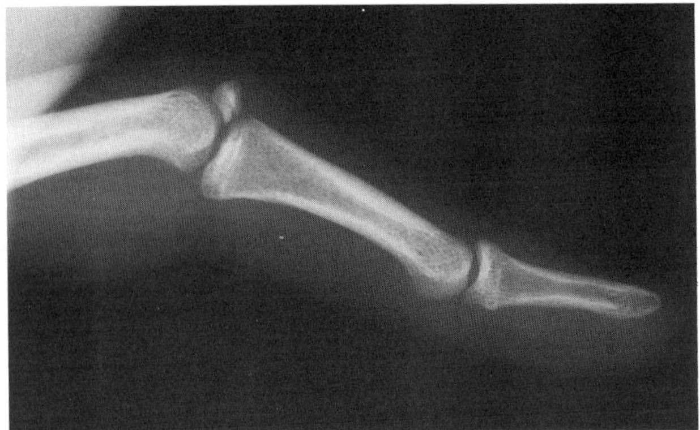

Fig. 17.44 Avulsion fracture of the central slip insertion.

bands slip over the sides of the PIP joint, where they may act as flexors, and their palmar subluxation is fixed by contracture of the transverse retinacular ligaments. The entire extension force of the dorsal aponeurosis is transferred to the distal joint, resulting in hyperextension which later becomes fixed owing to contracture of the oblique retinacular ligaments.

Treatment of boutonnière injuries is difficult and patients should be warned that full digital movement may not be regained. The essence of treatment is to hold the PIP joint in full extension, to allow the central slip to heal at the correct length and to prevent palmar migration of the lateral bands (Souter 1967). In the case of acute closed ruptures, this position can be maintained by external splintage; active flexion of the distal joint is encouraged in order to draw the extensor mechanism distally and maintain mobility of the lateral bands. It is quite difficult to splint a swollen PIP joint in extension and yet allow distal joint motion; frequent supervision and adjustment of the splint is necessary. Small central slip avulsion fractures may be treated in the same manner, but large fragments should be reattached operatively.

Unfortunately, many boutonnière injuries present late with fixed contracture. Dynamic splintage or serial static splintage is required to correct the PIP joint flexion deformity and active flexion exercises of the distal joint are performed to overcome the loss of passive flexion. Early diagnosis and prompt treatment of this injury is most desirable.

Lateral dislocations

Such dislocations involve rupture of one collateral ligament and the volar plate. After reduction, early protected motion is appropriate provided that the joint surfaces are congruous on X-ray and lateral deviation does not occur during flexion and extension. If instability with deviation occurs during movement, the collateral ligament should probably be repaired. Incongruity after reduction is likely to be due to soft tissue entrapment within the joint and this requires operative release and repair (Eaton 1971).

Lateral strains

Lateral strains of the PIP joint are frequent in athletes. Protected active movement with buddy taping for 2–3 weeks is sufficient treatment. The collateral ligament is the primary restraint to lateral angulation stress at the PIP joint. Partial or complete disruption of the collateral ligaments results from adduction or abduction stress. Pain, swelling and stiffness often persist for several months but late instability is rare. Most authors recommend that these injuries are treated non-operatively. Kiefhaber *et al.* (1986) showed that the collateral ligament fails at the proximal end with rupture of the palmar and, subsequently, the dorsal fibres, followed by separation between the collateral and accessory collateral ligaments and finally by rupture of the volar plate. More than 20° angulation on lateral stress was associated with complete rupture, but some joints with less than 20° opening also had complete tears. No studies are available to indicate whether conservative or operative treatment is superior.

Dorsal fracture–dislocation

A dorsal fracture–dislocation of the PIP joint is the result of hyperextension combined with axial compression (Fig. 17.45). When the fracture involves more than 40% of the base of the middle phalanx, the joint is unstable because of loss of a portion of the articular surface and because the fragments carry the insertion of the collateral ligament (Lubahn 1988).

Dorsal fracture–dislocation is a deceptive injury, presenting with a joint which is swollen but not obvi-

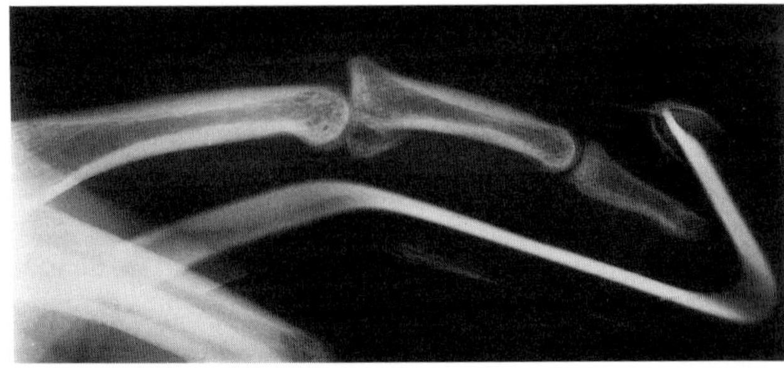

Fig. 17.45 Dorsal fracture–dislocation of the PIP joint.

ously displaced, and the diagnosis may be missed on an oblique radiograph — a true lateral view is essential. It is a serious injury and a complete range of movement is seldom regained. The aim of treatment is to maintain congruous reduction of the joint; it is the relationship of the proximal phalanx to the intact dorsal fragment which is important, not the position of the volar fragments.

If the reduction is stable in flexion, the technique of extension block splintage can be employed (McElfresh *et al*. 1972). Attention to detail is essential for successful use of this method. A dorsal padded aluminium splint is incorporated into a forearm cast and the splint is bent to block extension at the position of least flexion which is compatible with a congruent reduction, usually about 50°. Active flexion is encouraged. The proximal phalanx must be held against the splint with tape, otherwise the patient may flex the MP joint and allow the PIP joint to extend (Fig. 17.46). The splint may be protected against accidental bending by a stout length of tape fixed between its tip and the anterior surface of the cast. Each week the block can be decreased by 10—15°, provided

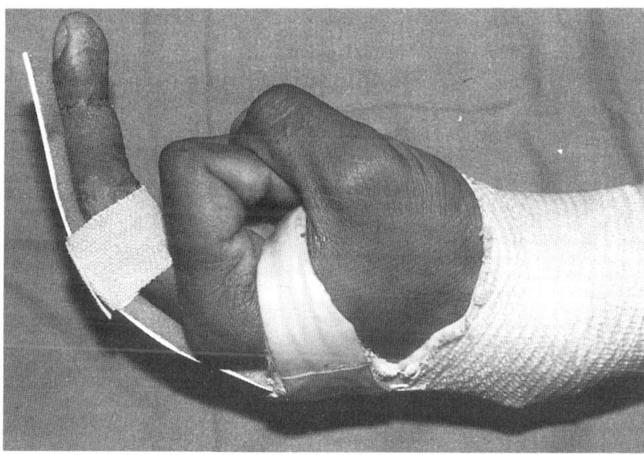

(a)

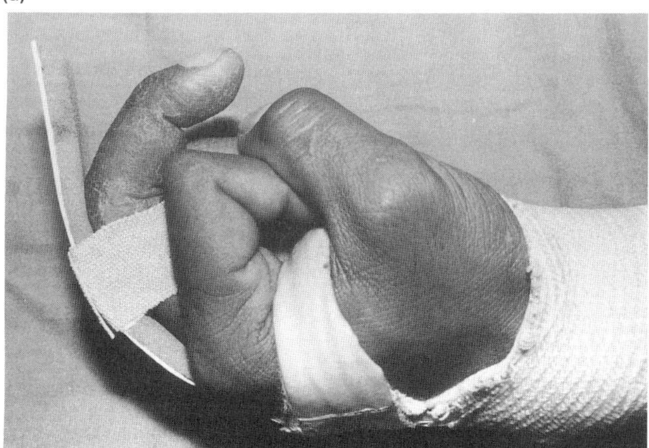

(b)

Fig. 17.46 (a) and (b) Extension-block splintage.

that congruity is maintained on the lateral radiograph. The splint may be discarded after 4—6 weeks and replaced by buddy taping for another 2—3 weeks.

Open reduction is needed if a congruent reduction cannot be obtained in flexion, which is usually the case when the fragment comprises more than 40% of the articular surface. In theory, precise reduction and fixation of the palmar fragments would restore stability and congruity, but the small size of the fragments makes this difficult in practice. If one or two large fragments are present, open reduction and internal fixation can be achieved through a palmar or dorsal approach.

In the presence of comminution, the options include attempted open reduction and internal fixation, traction, transarticular pin fixation and external fixation (Fahmy 1992). Stern *et al*. (1987) reported 20 cases of comminuted fracture of the base of the middle phalanx. Fractures treated by splintage became stiff. In no case managed by traction or by open reduction was articular congruity restored or full motion regained. External fixation devices which incorporate a dorsal translation force and which allow early movement may offer some advantages in these difficult injuries (Hastings & Carroll 1988).

An alternative technique for restoring the damaged volar articular surface is volar plate arthroplasty (Eaton & Malerich 1980). The bone fragments are excised and the volar plate is advanced into a transverse groove created in the defect in the base of the middle phalanx (Fig. 17.47). A wire or synthetic monofilament suture is passed through drill holes in the middle phalanx and tied over a button on the dorsum of the finger. Release of the collateral ligaments is usually necessary in late cases. After immobilization for 2 weeks with a transarticular K-wire, the joint is mobilized in an extension-block splint for a further 2 weeks. If a flexion contracture is present at 5 weeks, dynamic splintage should be applied, because otherwise a permanent contracture may result (Dray & Eaton 1988).

MP joints of the fingers

The MP joints are protected from injury by the strong collateral ligaments and by support from adjacent digits. The volar plate has firm attachments to the proximal phalanx but is thin and weak proximally, lacking the fibrous 'check—reins' of its counterpart at the PIP joint. The collateral and accessory collateral ligaments insert into the edges of the volar plate and form a 'ligament box' similar to the PIP joint. The lateral edges of the volar plate are continuous with the deep transverse metacarpal ligament which links the joint to adjacent

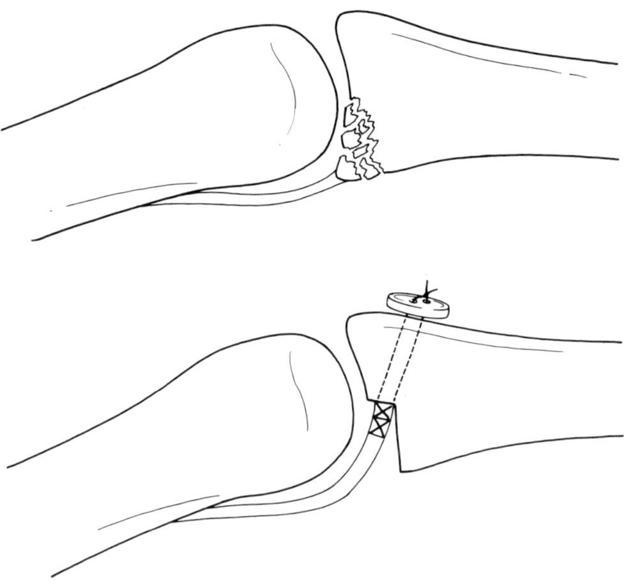

Fig. 17.47 Volar plate arthroplasty. Bone fragments are excised and the free edge of the volar plate is advanced into a transverse groove in the base of the proximal phalanx.

rays. The primary stabilizing structures are the collateral ligaments. The volar plate resists hyperextension and only contributes to lateral stability when it is taut in the extended position (Minami *et al.* 1985).

Dorsal dislocation of the MP joint is uncommon (though it is the most common finger dislocation in children). The index finger is the digit most often affected, followed by the little finger. The middle and ring fingers are protected by adjacent digits and are only dislocated if the border digit is also injured (Hall *et al.* 1985). The mechanism of injury is forced hyperextension, tearing the thin proximal attachment of the volar plate. The collateral ligaments are not usually disrupted.

Simple dislocation

A simple dislocation of the MP joint is characterized by marked hyperextension (60–80°), the base of the proximal phalanx lying with its articular surface in contact with the dorsum of the metacarpal head. The torn volar plate is draped over the head of the metacarpal but does not block reduction. Inappropriate manipulation, especially longitudinal traction, may flip the volar plate onto the dorsum of the metacarpal head and convert the injury into a complex dislocation (McLaughlin 1965). The dislocation should be reduced with the wrist flexed, to slacken the flexor tendons, and accomplished by direct pressure over the dorsum of the base of the

proximal phalanx in a distal and palmar direction, pushing it back over the metacarpal head.

Complex dislocation

This occurs in the MP joint when the volar plate becomes interposed between the base of the proximal phalanx and the metacarpal head. It is characterized by modest (20–40°) hyperextension with slight flexion of the IP joints (Fig. 17.48). The metacarpal head is prominent in the palm, where it may blanch the palmar skin, and the skin distal to this is puckered by palmar fascial fibres attached to the base of the proximal phalanx. On the dorsum, a hollow is palpable just proximal to the base of the phalanx. There may be an osteochondral fracture of the metacarpal head (Becton *et al.* 1975).

The primary block to reduction of a complex dislocation is the volar plate, attached distally to the base of the proximal phalanx and lying dorsal to the metacarpal head (McLaughlin 1965, Green & Terry 1973). One attempt at closed manipulation is justified, but open reduction is usually required.

Farabeuf (1876) described open reduction through a dorsal approach. Many surgeons adopted a palmar approach after the classic paper by Kaplan (1957), who described a case in which dorsal release of the volar plate failed and a palmar approach was necessary to release the metacarpal head which was trapped by the palmar aponeurosis. In cadaver studies, Kaplan found that the metacarpal head passed between the superficial transverse ligament of the palmar aponeurosis and the natatory ligament running transversely, and between the flexor tendons and the lumbrical muscle running longitudinally. Whilst the palmar approach gives direct access to these structures, it may be questioned how often they prevent reduction after release of the volar plate, which is undoubtably the chief culprit (McLaughlin 1965). Release of the volar plate may be difficult through a palmar approach because it is relatively inaccessible, lying on the dorsum of the metacarpal head. Furthermore, the digital nerves are easily injured where they are pressed tightly against the skin by the metacarpal head.

A dorsal approach to complex MP joint dislocation is simpler, quicker and avoids the risk of digital nerve injury. Becton *et al.* (1975) reported reduction in 13 cases by longitudinal incision of the volar plate through a dorsal approach. In three cases reduction had been attempted unsuccessfully though a palmar approach and in two of these a digital nerve had been injured. The extensor tendon is split in the mid-line, exposing the base of the proximal phalanx and entering the cavity

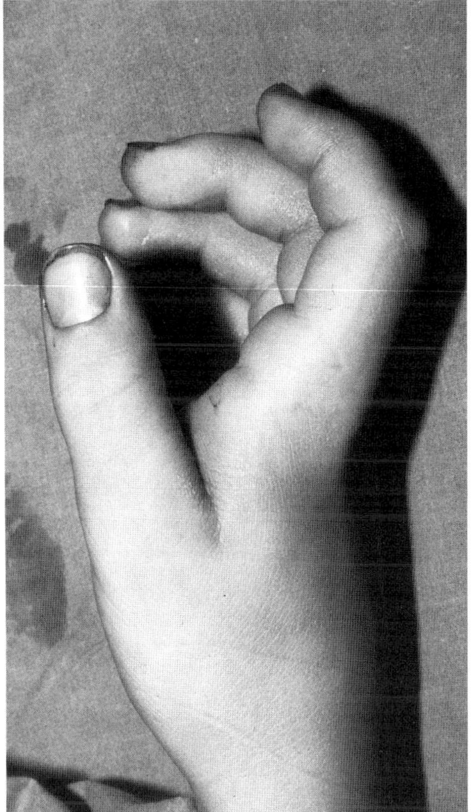
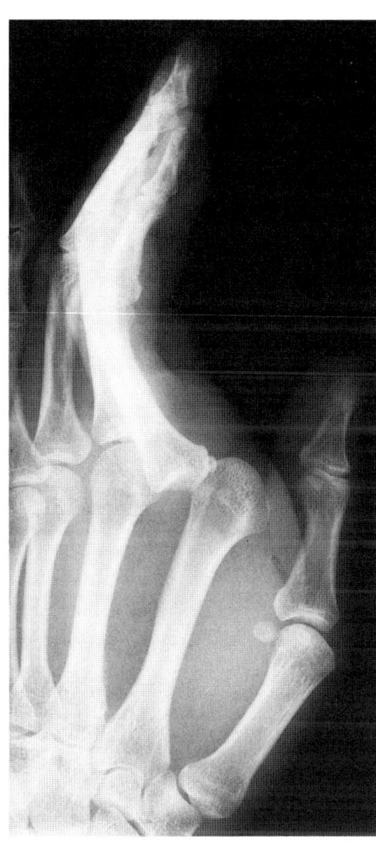

Fig. 17.48 Complex dorsal dislocation of the MP joint. (a) Hyperextension of the MP joint. (b) Lateral radiograph.   (a)   (b)

previously occupied by the metacarpal head. The volar plate forms the floor of this cavity, where its fibrocartilaginous surface may be mistaken for the metacarpal head which lies immediately anterior to it. A longitudinal incision in the volar plate allows the two halves to slip back over the head of the metacarpal. A further advantage of the dorsal approach is that osteochondral fractures (seven out of 13 in Becton's series) may be identified and dealt with. In the event that reduction cannot be obtained through the dorsal approach, an additional palmar incision may be made, but this has not so far been necessary in the author's experience.

The MP joint is stable after reduction. Immobilization is unnecessary and may be harmful, since McLaughlin (1965) found that return of MP joint movement was inversely proportional to the duration of immobilization. Redislocation or late instability do not seem to occur in the fingers, though injury to the volar plate of the thumb MP joint may lead to hyperextension and swan-neck deformity.

Complex volar dislocation

Such a dislocation of the MP joint is rare and usually requires open reduction because of entrapment of the volar plate or dorsal capsule (Moneim 1983, Khuri & Fay 1986).

Locking

Locking of the MP joint may be acute, chronic or intermittent. It is characterized by a history of forced active flexion, e.g. gripping a rope, and by a 20−40° flexion deformity which cannot be corrected passively. Full active flexion is preserved (Feldon & Belsky 1987). In patients over the age of 50, the usual cause is an osteophyte on one side of the volar aspect of the metacarpal head (Fig. 17.49) which catches the volar plate or accessory collateral ligament (Goodfellow & Weaver 1961). Oblique views may be required to demonstrate the osteophyte. In younger patients, the collateral ligament may be trapped over a bony prominence on the side of the metacarpal head. Less common causes of locking include loose bodies, malunited articular fractures and

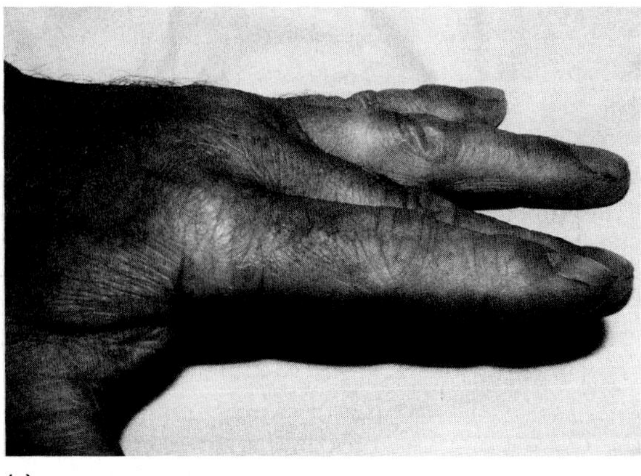

(a)

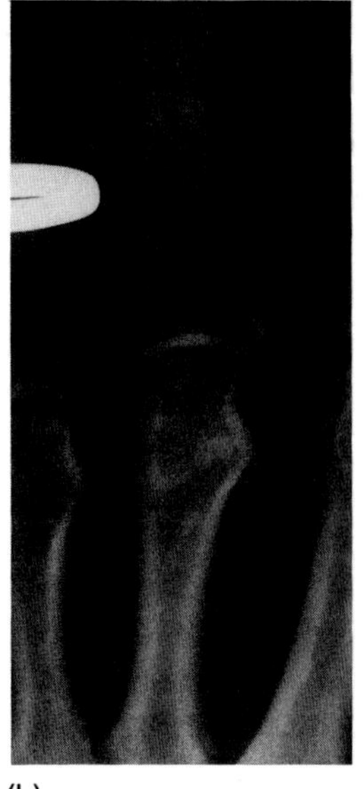

(b)

Fig. 17.49 (a) Locking of the middle finger MP joint. (b) An osteophyte on the metacarpal head is the most usual cause.

entrapment of an interosseous tendon on an exostosis (Rankin & Uwagie-Ero 1986). The definitive treatment is exploration of the joint and removal of the cause of excision of an osteophyte or release of the accessory collateral ligament. Closed reduction may be achieved by manipulation (Guly & Azam 1982) or by distension of the joint under local anaesthetic to force the ligaments and capsule away from the metacarpal head, a manoeuvre attributed to Millender (see Feldon & Belsky 1987). Forceful manipulation may cause damage to the joint and should be avoided.

Fractures of the metacarpals

Fractures of the metacarpal head

These are uncommon. McElfresh and Dobyns (1983) reviewed 103 intra-articular metacarpal head fractures and classified them according to the configuration of the fracture. The second metacarpal was affected more often than the others, probably because of its border position and rigid basal joint. Epiphyseal injuries (four cases) were Salter−Harris type III with little displacement and were all in patients over the age of 11 years. All four healed without complication after splintage. Collateral ligament avulsion fractures occurred in 17 patients. These fractures may not be demonstrated on the standard radiographs, but can be seen on the Brewerton view in which the MP joints are flexed to 65°, the dorsum of the fingers placed flat on the X-ray plate and the beam angled at 15° from the ulnar side of the hand (Lane 1977). Most collateral ligament fractures are not

displaced sufficiently to cause instability of the joint and do not merit internal fixation. However, if the fragment is markedly displaced or involves a substantial portion of the articular surface, it should be reduced and fixed with a K-wire or small lag screw. Osteochondral fractures (eight cases) may be associated with dorsal dislocation of the MP joint (Becton *et al.* 1975) or be caused by a tooth during a clenched fist injury. Small displaced fragments should be removed.

Oblique fractures in the sagittal plane (22 cases) resulted in loss of MP joint motion if the fracture healed with displacement. The oblique fracture line allows the distal fragment, which carries most of the articular surface, to slide proximally, leaving an intra-articular spike of proximal fragment protruding. Rotational deformity may occur (Fig. 17.50). These fractures should be reduced and stabilized with K-wires or small lag screws. Transverse fractures distal to the collateral ligament insertion (Fig. 17.51) developed avascular necrosis of the metacarpal head in three out of four cases and led to pain and loss of motion.

The most frequent type of injury was the comminuted fracture (28 cases), generally caused by crushing and associated with other fractures in the hand. McElfresh and Dobyns (1983) recommend internal fixation for fractures when the fragments are large, displaced and few in number, but stress that the procedure is difficult and seldom achieves normal movement. Immobilization for 2−3 weeks followed by protected movement was advised for comminuted fractures with minimal displacement and also for injuries at the other extreme, where the degree of comminution precluded internal

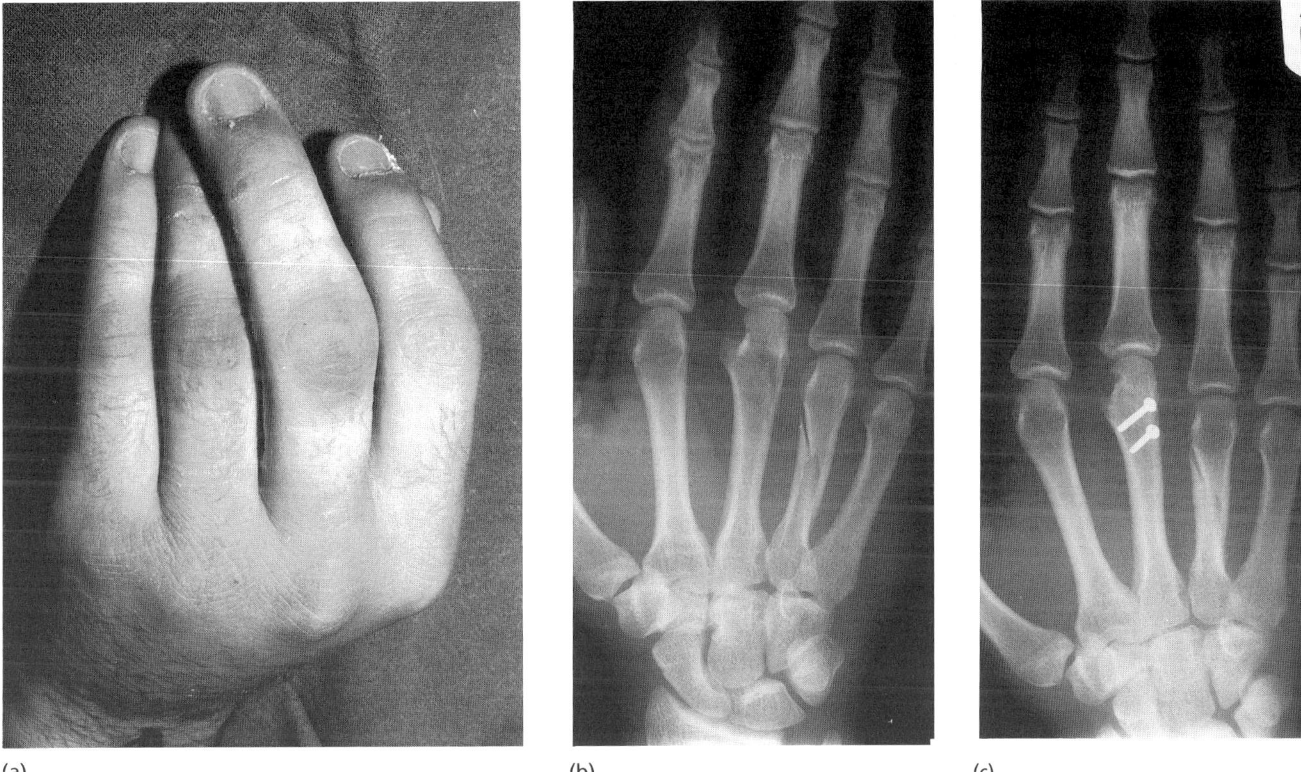

(a)   (b)   (c)

Fig. 17.50 (a) and (b) Oblique fracture of the metacarpal head with rotational displacement of the middle finger; there was no rotation of the ring metacarpal fracture. (c) Correct rotation was restored by open reduction and lag screw fixation; satisfactory MP joint motion resulted despite comminution of a portion of the metacarpal head.

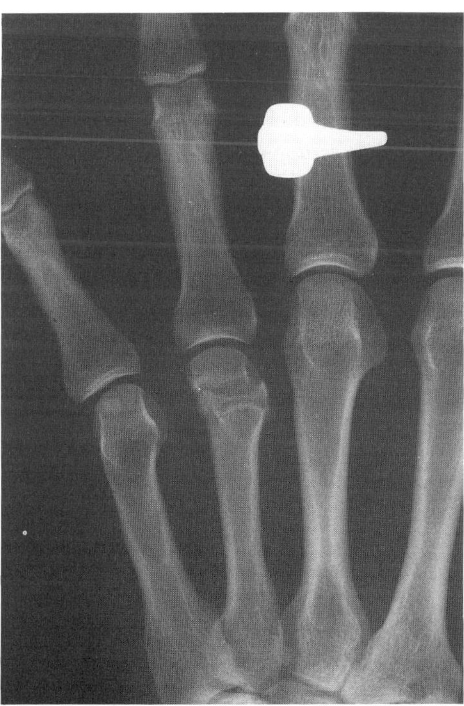

Fig. 17.51 Healing transverse fracture of the metacarpal head.

fixation. If there is loss of bone substance with destruction of both surfaces of the MP joint, primary silastic arthroplasty will usually provide better function than arthrodesis, with perhaps 20–50° movement, depending upon damage to the soft tissues (see Fig. 17.4). However, the long-term outlook for these implants is unknown; arthrodesis or excision arthroplasty may eventually be necessary.

Fractures of the metacarpal neck

Fractures of the metacarpal neck are the most common hand fractures and are usually the result of a direct blow to the knuckle. There is angulation with the apex dorsally, where it forms a prominence, and flattening of the knuckle which is most noticeable with the fingers flexed. The fractures are most frequent in the ring and little fingers (Fig. 17.52), where residual angulation is, in many cases, compatible with normal function because of the mobility of the CMC joints of these digits. However, the CMC joints of the index and middle fingers allow no such movement. Angulation greater than 15° may cause uncomfortable protrusion of the metacarpal head in the palm and should be corrected.

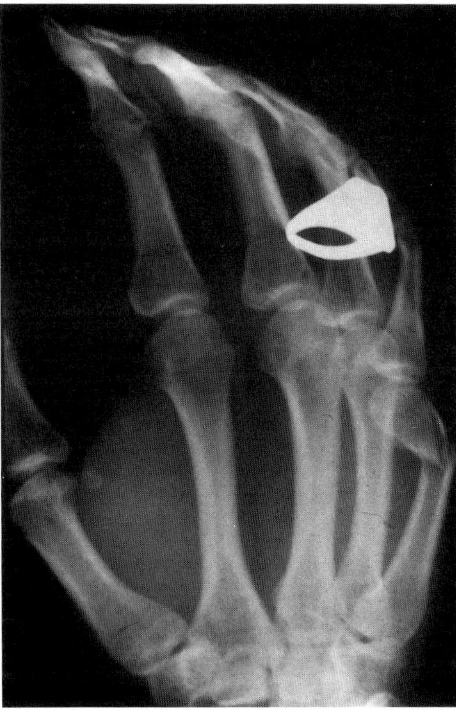

Fig. 17.52 Boxer's fracture of the little metacarpal neck.

The amount of angulation of the ring and little metacarpals which can be accepted without loss of function has been the subject of much discussion in the literature. Many authors adopt the conservative approach supported by the data of Hunter and Cowan (1970), who did not attempt reduction unless the angulation was over 40° and who were prepared to accept angulation up to 70° if reduction was not easily obtained. The results were uniformly satisfactory and the patients resumed work, many as firemen and policemen, within 4 weeks. Barton (1984) treats these injuries with a crepe bandage and without reduction unless the angulation is greater than 50°. However, Green and Rowland (1991) recommend intervention if the angulation exceeds 15°.

The wide range of angles accepted in the literature may be partly explained by different methods of measurement of the neck/shaft angle of the metacarpal. Lowdon (1986) has emphasized that, because of the metacarpal arch, the lateral profile of the little metacarpal is best seen on an oblique (pronated lateral) radiograph. The average neck/shaft angle of intact little metacarpals was 26°. When angulation at the fracture was expressed as an increase over the normal angle, rather than as the total neck/shaft angle, Lowdon (1986) found an average angulation of 16.8° and only four fractures with angulation greater than 30° in a series of 74 patients.

The author's management of metacarpal neck fractures

in the little finger is influenced by the angulation on the pronated lateral radiograph, the degree of pain, the presence of rotational deformity (which is rare) and an assessment of the patient's compliance (Hall 1987). The indications for reduction and fixation are extreme angulation, complete separation of the head from the shaft, a displaced articular component of the fracture and rotational displacement. Apart from these rare indications, the position is accepted and the initial treatment simply directed at relief of pain with an ulnar gutter splint or buddy taping. The nature of the injury is explained to the patient, who is told that function of the hand will be normal but there may be a minor alteration in the appearance of the ulnar side of the hand. If a splint has been used, it is removed after 7–10 days and active movement encouraged.

Reduction can be achieved, if necessary, by flexing the MP and PIP joints to 90° and applying pressure directed dorsally over the base of the middle phalanx. However, this position should *never* be used to maintain the reduction because of the risk of PIP joint flexion contracture and skin necrosis over the dorsum of the joint. A plaster splint applied with the IP joints extended and the MP joints flexed can be moulded with gentle pressure over the metacarpal shaft dorsally and beneath the metacarpal head (Green & Rowland 1991), but in the author's experience it is seldom possible to maintain a good reduction in this way because of the limited purchase on the distal fragment and the inherent instability of the fracture resulting from comminution of the volar cortex. The few fractures of the little metacarpal which require reduction are unstable and require internal fixation. Percutaneous K-wires may be placed obliquely, longitudinally or transversely. Transverse wires may be used to impale the injured metacarpal to its neighbour proximal and distal to the fracture (Lamb *et al.* 1973), or the ends of the wires may be left long and bonded together with a longitudinal wire and bone cement (Dickson 1975).

Fractures of the index and middle metacarpal necks with angulation less than 15° should be immobilized with a palmar splint to relieve pain, and the position checked by radiographs within the first week, since these fractures heal rapidly and correction of malalignment soon becomes difficult. If the angulation is greater than 15°, closed reduction and percutaneous fixation is indicated.

Fractures of the shaft of the metacarpals

Fractures of the shaft of the metacarpals may be transverse, oblique, comminuted, multiple or associated with bone loss. The three main problems in management are shortening, angulation and rotational deformity. In most closed fractures, shortening is resisted by the deep transverse metacarpal and interosseous ligaments. Loss of up to 5 mm length is compatible with normal function. The support is greater for the middle and ring fingers than for the border digits or thumb, where functionally significant shortening occurs more easily (Fig. 17.53).

The management of undisplaced fractures of the metacarpal shafts is directed simply at protection and relief of pain, using buddy taping or splintage as necessary and allowing active movement to begin as soon as possible. A close watch should be kept for rotatory malalignment which can occur despite apparently good radiographic alignment. Provided that the fracture is protected against further displacement, the only significant complication is loss of motion which is nearly always due to inappropriate or excessive immobilization.

Transverse fractures of the metacarpal shaft are usually the result of a direct blow. The pull of the interosseous muscles, which pass anterior to the fracture, produces angulation with the apex towards the dorsum (Fig. 17.54). Angulation greater than 10° of the index or middle

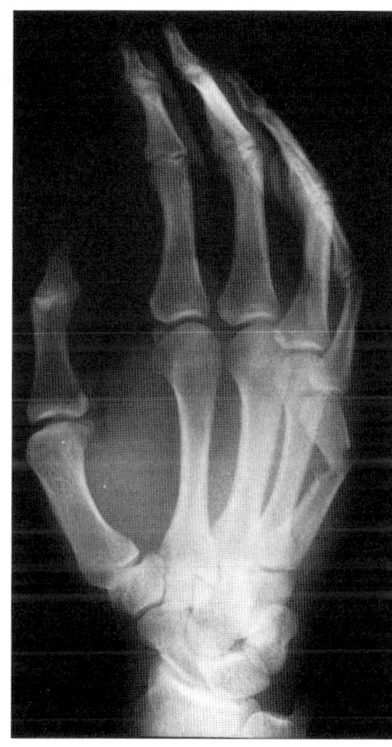

Fig. 17.54 Palmar angulation of transverse metacarpal fracture.

metacarpals may cause prominence of the metacarpal head in the palm and should be corrected. The functional consequences of angulation are much less in the ring and little fingers, which have mobile CMC joints. Up to 30° angulation of the ring and little metacarpals is compatible with good function but the dorsal prominence is unsightly and many patients dislike it. In the author's opinion, angulation which will lead to an obvious deformity is an indication for reduction.

Closed reduction of transverse fractures is usually straightforward. The use of dorsal and palmar splints to provide three-point fixation may suffice but it is difficult to control angulation by external splintage in the swollen hand and percutaneous pin fixation is more reliable.

Percutaneous pins may be inserted transversely, obliquely or longitudinally. Transverse pins, one or two distally and one proximally, may be used to impale the fractured metacarpal to its intact neighbour (Lamb *et al.* 1973). The proximal pin may be omitted in the index and middle metacarpals because the rigid CMC joint stabilizes the proximal fragment. Although the pins pass through the interosseous muscles, in practice this does not restrict mobilization and long-term problems with the interossei do not seem to occur. In the case of multiple metacarpal fractures, extra stability may be provided by bonding the protruding ends of the wires together with a longitudinal K-wire and bone cement (Dickson 1975). Transverse pinning will control rotation as well as angulation and shortening.

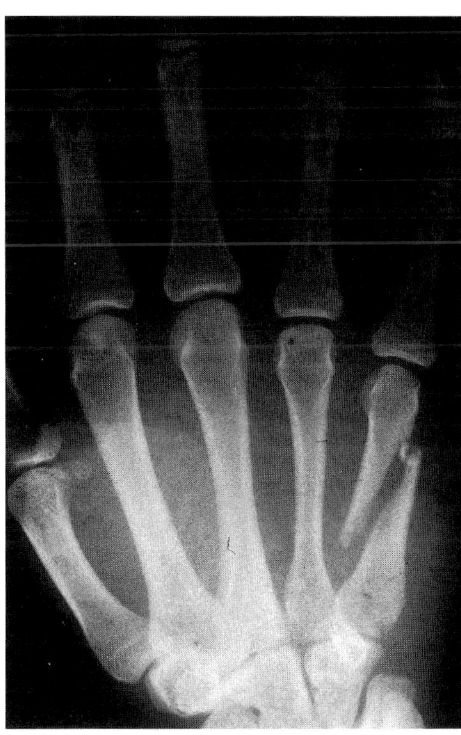

Fig. 17.53 Oblique fracture of the little metacarpal; lack of soft tissue support on the ulnar side may allow functionally significant shortening.

Longitudinal pins may be inserted through the head of the metacarpal and, with the wrist flexed, passed out through the skin at the wrist until the end of the wire is buried within the head of the metacarpal (Green & Rowland 1991). It is necessary to immobilize the wrist to prevent skin irritation by the pins. This technique does not control rotation and therefore external splintage should be added if there is any question of rotational instability.

Oblique fractures are usually caused by rotatory forces transmitted through the finger, which acts as a lever. These fractures are liable to shortening, which is frequently associated with rotational displacement; significant angulation is unusual. Malrotation of 5° may cause 1.5 cm of finger overlap during flexion. Open reduction is frequently necessary to achieve accurate alignment. K-wires may be used for fixation, but once the fracture is open there is very little additional risk in applying rigid internal fixation, which ensures an anatomical reduction and permits immediate active movement without the soft tissue tethering which usually occurs with pins.

Multiple metacarpal shaft fractures present a substantial risk of malunion and permanent loss of finger motion (Fig. 17.55). These injuries are often the result of crushing or other violent trauma. The possibility of associated CMC joint injury should always be considered in patients with multiple metacarpal fractures and the appropriate lateral and oblique radiographs should be obtained. Extensive injury to the soft tissues and loss of support from adjacent metacarpals leads to gross displacement which, in the presence of severe swelling, is difficult to control with either external splintage or pinning. Skeletal stability is essential so that soft tissue healing is facilitated and active movement can begin as soon as possible to prevent adhesion between the gliding surfaces within the hand.

Several studies have confirmed that open reduction and fixation by the AO technique is safe and reliable for multiple metacarpal fractures (Fig. 17.56), provided that the principles and recommended technique (see below) are followed closely (Segmuller 1977, Hastings 1987). However, external fixation may be preferred in severely contaminated wounds. It may be used in combination with other methods of fixation such as K-wires or interfragmentary screws, or employed for temporary stabilization until the condition of the wound allows definitive internal fixation (Freeland 1987).

Comminuted fractures may be managed non-operatively if there are multiple fragments with little displacement. Moderate comminution does not preclude

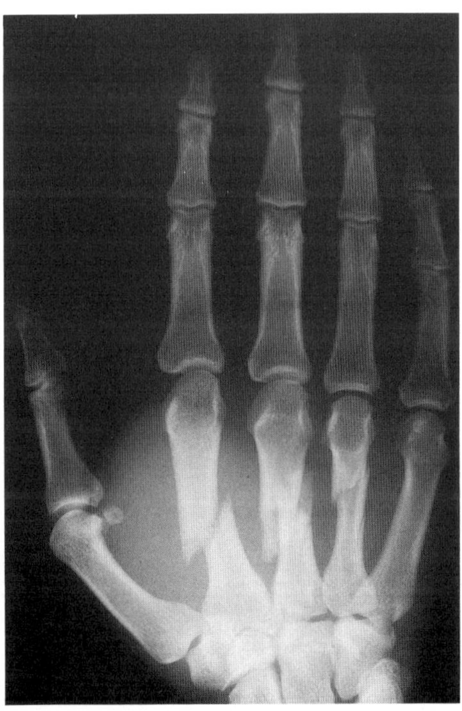

Fig. 17.55 Multiple metacarpal shaft fractures.

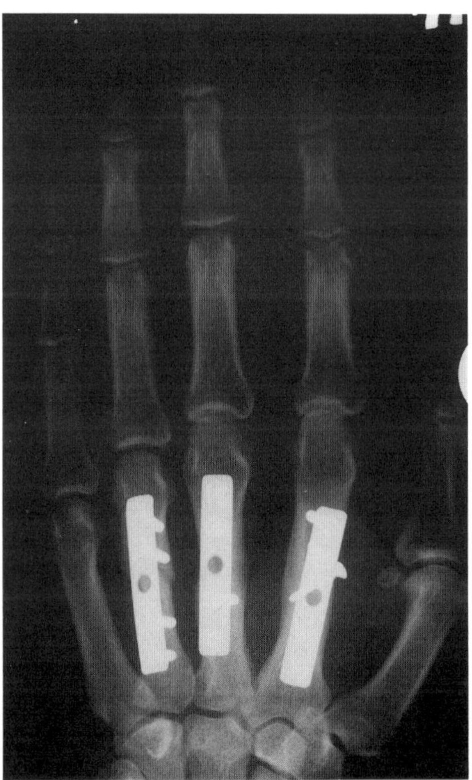

Fig. 17.56 Open reduction and internal fixation with AO plates and screws.

plate fixation, with grafting of any bone defects, but extensive comminution is best managed by transmetacarpal pin fixation to maintain length. Open fractures with bone loss require operative stabilization to allow adequate treatment of the soft tissues. Skeletal length can be maintained by 'spacer' wires bent from a length of K-wire (Fig. 17.57) until the tissues are ready for bone grafting.

Open reduction and internal fixation of metacarpal shaft fractures

Accurate closed reduction and percutaneous pin fixation is an excellent method of treatment for the majority of metacarpal shaft fractures because it interferes very little with the soft tissues and the risk of complications is small (Green & Rowland 1991). If open reduction is required a variety of fixation techniques are available, including oblique K-wires, intramedullary Steinmann pins (Grundberg 1981), tension-band wiring (Greene *et al*. 1987), and fixation with screws and plates (Segmuller 1977).

The use of plates and screws in the metacarpals is less hazardous than in the phalanges because the soft tissue envelope is thicker and because the extensor mechanism is simpler and less prone to adhesion. The particular advantage of plate fixation is anatomical reduction with fixation which is stable enough to allow immediate unresisted active motion (Freeland *et al*. 1986). The biomechanical studies of Black *et al*. (1985) indicate that fixation of a transverse metacarpal shaft fracture with a dorsal quarter-tubular plate and 2.7 mm screws is four

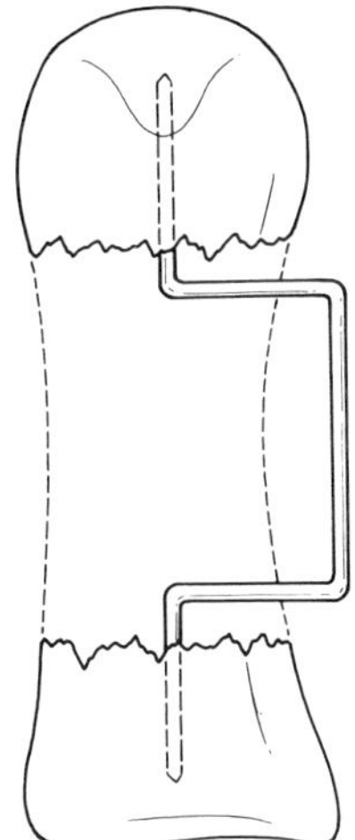

Fig. 17.57 Use of a temporary 'spacer' wire to maintain length in cases of bone loss.

to six times stronger than wire fixation and approaches the rigidity and strength of the intact bone.

Primary internal fixation is appropriate for most severe open hand injuries because it provides a stable foundation for repair and healing of skin, vessels, nerves and tendons. It can be applied to grade I and grade II open fractures provided that wound care is meticulous with excision of all contaminated and non-viable tissue. It is also the best form of fixation for complete or incomplete amputations, where revascularization is dependent on a stable skeleton (Fig. 17.4). In grade III open injuries with severe contamination, internal fixation may be delayed to avoid additional dissection and risk of infection; external fixation or K-wires are used for temporary stabilization (Freeland 1987). When there is a risk of adhesion of partially injured but functionally competent tendons or joints, stable internal fixation will allow early active movement.

Ford *et al*. (1987) recorded uniformly satisfactory results after plate and screw fixation in 22 patients with multiple or unstable metacarpal fractures. Movement was commenced within 7 days. In six patients, the final TAM was less than 220°, but in these cases there was associated tendon or joint injury. There were no infections or non-unions. Dabezies and Schutte (1986) obtained an average of 252° TAM in 27 cases of metacarpal shaft fracture in which motion was begun within 24 hours of operation. All fractures healed without infection or loss of position.

Indications for open reduction and internal fixation of metacarpal shaft fractures include:
1 Multiple metacarpal fractures.
2 Fractures with associated soft tissue injuries requiring a stable skeleton for healing and rehabilitation.
3 Segmental fractures and those with bone loss.
4 Isolated displaced transverse fractures when closed reduction cannot be achieved.
5 Oblique fractures with rotational malalignment.

The isolated displaced metacarpal shaft fracture is a relative indication for open reduction and internal fixation. Simpler methods such as percutaneous pin fixation should be employed if adequate closed reduction can be obtained. Screw or plate fixation is the most appropriate method for the displaced oblique fracture with rotational malalignment when accurate closed reduction is impossible.

Problems with screw and plate fixation are usually due to incorrect patient selection or faulty operative technique. Interfragmentary screws will not provide sufficient stability of spiral or oblique fractures unless the fracture is long enough to accommodate at least two screws. Otherwise, a neutralization plate should be added. Small bone fragments will splinter unless the fragment is at least three times the thread diameter of the screw. Plates applied to the dorsal surface of the metacarpals function as tension-band devices so long as there is stable apposition of the palmar cortices. If the palmar cortices are not in contact, the plate will be subject to bending stress rather than tensile stress, and there will be the risk of implant failure and non-union. A stronger plate must be used in this situation and the bone defect should be grafted.

Correct rotational alignment is especially difficult to achieve in multiple comminuted metacarpal fractures; intact digits are not available for comparison and the correct rotation is not apparent from the reduction. When flexed, the fingers should lie parallel, with the ring finger pointing to the scaphoid tubercle.

CMC joint injury

Dislocation of the CMC joints of the fingers may involve one or more joints, with or without fracture of the articular surfaces or fracture of adjacent metacarpal bones. The displacement is usually dorsal and the little finger ray is the one injured most frequently, though numerous types of multiple dislocation have been reported (Kleinman & Grantham 1978, Resnick *et al*. 1985, Berg & Murphy 1986, Rawles 1988).

The CMC joints of the index and middle rays allow virtually no movement owing to their interlocking articular surfaces and strong ligaments. The base of the ring metacarpal articulates with the radial facet of the hamate and has 10–15° flexion/extension. The little CMC joint allows 15–20° flexion as well as some rotation, allowing the palm to be cupped and aiding opposition of the thumb to the little finger. The deep branch of the ulnar nerve runs close to the palmar aspect of the ring and little CMC joints, where it may suffer injury or operative damage (Peterson & Sacks 1986).

Single CMC joint dislocations may result from blows to the hand or from falls, causing flexion and axial loading of the metacarpal. The little ray is most often involved. Disruption of several joints, especially the strong index and middle joints, requires high-energy trauma such as crush or road-accident injury. These patients frequently have multiple injuries. The severity of injury produces gross swelling which masks the deformity.

CMC joint dislocations are easily overlooked (Henderson & Arafa 1987). Factors which contribute to this include obliteration of deformity by swelling, inadequate radiographs or their incorrect interpretation and the presence of multiple injuries. It cannot be overemphasized that severe swelling of the wrist after a violent injury almost always conceals a serious CMC or carpal injury. The minimum radiographic examination comprises anteroposterior, true lateral and oblique views in 30° pronation and supination from the lateral position. Further oblique views and tomograms may be necessary (Fig. 17.58). A pitfall is the frequent combination of a displaced metacarpal fracture with CMC joint dislocation in an adjacent ray; the fracture catches the eye and the dislocation is missed (see Fig. 17.2).

Undisplaced articular fractures of the CMC joints may be treated satisfactorily with external splintage alone. Fracture–subluxation of the little finger CMC joint is a relatively frequent injury which is sometimes called 'reverse Bennett's fracture' because of its similarity to fracture–subluxation of the thumb CMC joint (Fig. 17.59). The fracture line runs obliquely across the metacarpal base, leaving the radial fragment attached to the base of the ring metacarpal and hamate by the strong intermetacarpal ligaments and allowing the remainder of the metacarpal to displace in an ulnar and dorsal direction. The sloping surface of the hamate, the obliquity of the fracture line and the pull of the extensor carpi ulnaris tendon all contribute towards redisplacement after reduction (Bora & Didizian 1974). Closed reduction can usually be achieved without difficulty using a combination of traction and direct pressure but external splintage alone is insufficient and percutaneous pin fixation is required. The aim is restoration of the relationship between the metacarpal shaft and the hamate; slight displacement of the intra-articular fracture may be accepted. The indications for open reduction are failed closed reduction, due to gross swelling, soft tissue interposition or late presentation, and open injuries.

Although Petrie and Lamb (1974) found symptoms in only one patient out of 23 with untreated little finger CMC joint fracture–subluxation after an average of 4.5 years, other authors believe that persistent subluxation leads to pain and weakness of grip in a proportion of patients. Partial resection of the metacarpal base to prevent impingement has been reported to relieve pain and improve grip, whilst preserving some CMC joint motion (Black *et al*. 1987). However, arthrodesis would appear to be more predictable and some useful movement of the little ray remains because of residual motion at the triquetro-hamate joint (Clendenin & Smith 1984)

Multiple CMC joint dislocations are difficult to hold in the reduced position by external splintage because of the swelling which usually occurs. Percutaneous pin fixation may be possible but it can be difficult to achieve in the presence of swelling and may be blocked by

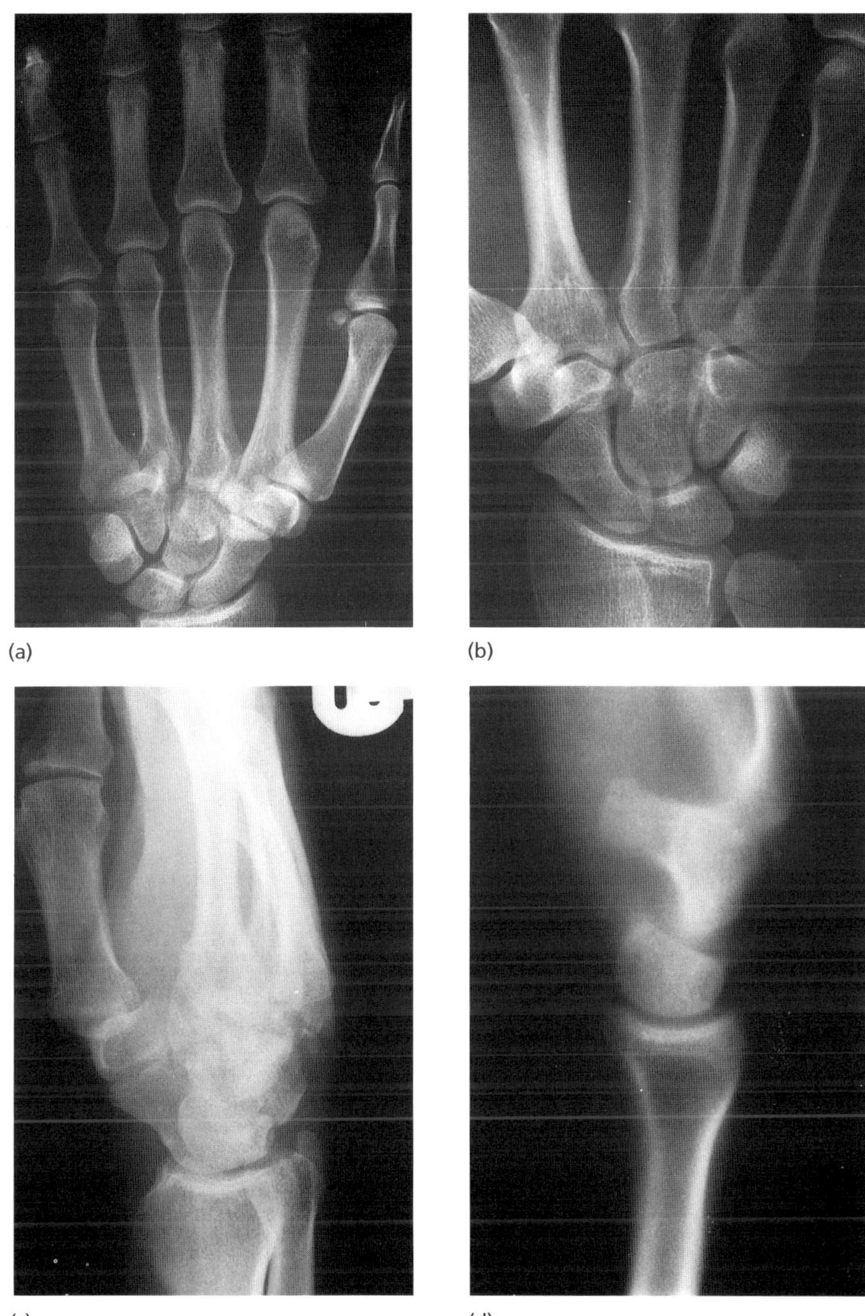

Fig. 17.58 (a) Anteroposterior view of ring and little CMC fracture—dislocation. There is loss of congruity, compared to (b) a normal radiograph. (c) Pronated lateral view. (d) Lateral tomography.

interposition of soft tissues such as the extensor carpi radialis brevis tendon (Ho *et al*. 1987). Multiple pins are required and they tend to interfere with movement of the extensor tendons if the ends are left long. The potential for stiffness of the fingers in these severe injuries demands mobilization as soon as possible. Open reduction with fixation by buried K-wires, together with screw fixation of associated metacarpal fractures and large intra-articular fragments, permits

early movement and also ensures an accurate reduction (Rawles 1988).

Injuries of the thumb

Fractures of the thumb metacarpal

Fractures of the thumb metacarpal are commonly the result of direct blows or axial compression force. Most

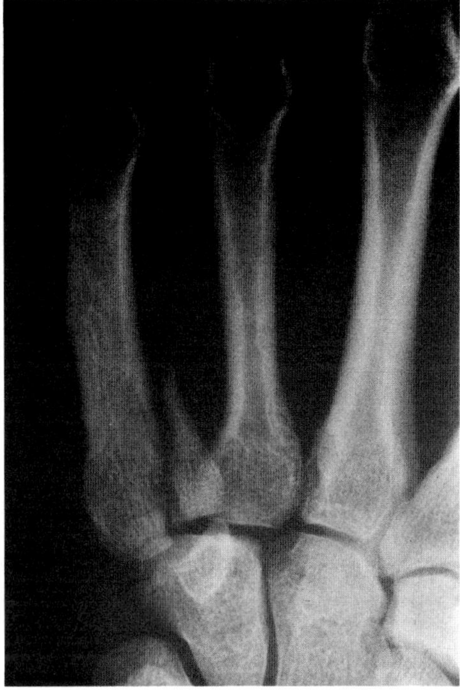

Fig. 17.59 Oblique articular fracture of the base of the little metacarpal — 'reverse Bennett's fracture'.

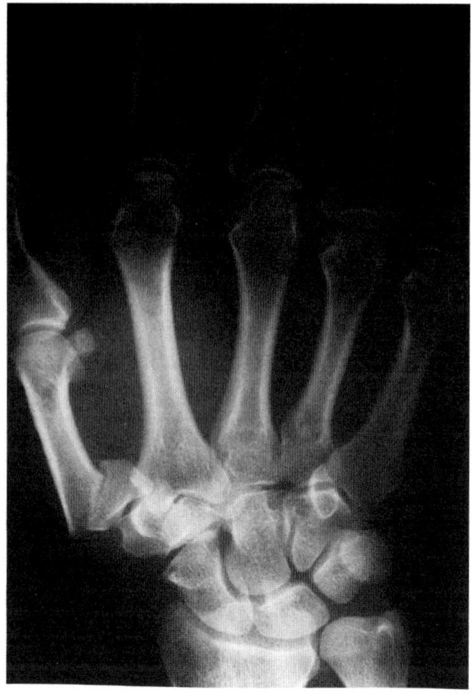

Fig. 17.60 Oblique extra-articular fracture of the thumb metacarpal.

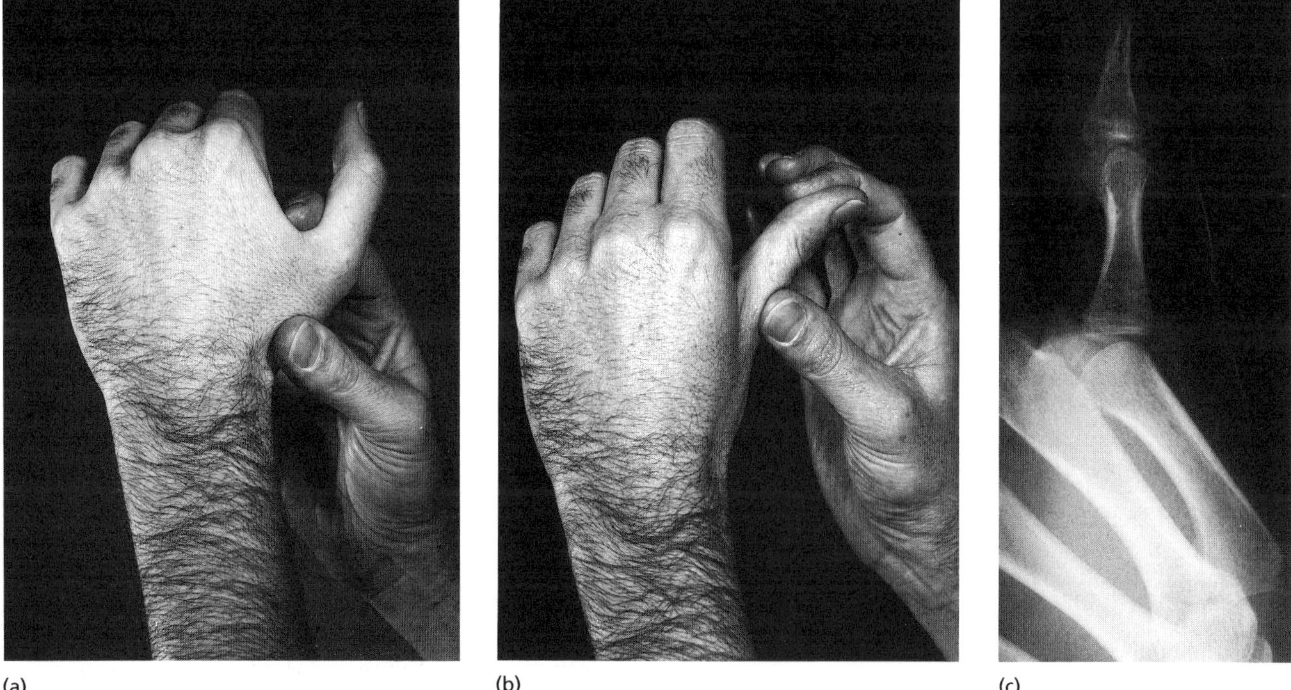

(a) (b) (c)

Fig. 17.61 Position for reduction of fractures at the base of the thumb. (a) Correct — the CMC joint is extended and abducted, the MP joint is slightly flexed. (b) and (c) Incorrect — the CMC joint is adducted and the MP joint is hyperextended.

fractures occur at the base of the metacarpal. Extra-articular fractures may be transverse or oblique (Fig. 17.60). The distal fragment angulates into flexion and adduction, occasionally leading to dynamic collapse of the thumb with hyperextension at the MP joint and weak pinch. Good reduction can almost always be achieved by manipulation. However, residual angulation of 30° is consistent with excellent function because of compensatory motion at the CMC joint. Immobilization for 3–4 weeks in a thumb spica cast is sufficient. During application of the cast, a conscious effort must be made to provide extension at the fracture and not at the MP joint, otherwise flexion occurs at the fracture and the deformity is accentuated (Fig. 17.61). Percutaneous pin fixation may be used if external splintage fails to hold the reduction.

Intra-articular fractures are of two types: Bennett's fracture–dislocation, and comminuted intra-articular fractures.

Bennett's fracture

The saddle-shaped surfaces of the trapeziometacarpal joint permit multiaxial movement. Cooney *et al*. (1981) found an average of 53° flexion/extension, 42° abduction/adduction and 17° axial rotation. Stability of the joint depends mainly on the stout palmar ligament which passes between the anterior lip of the metacarpal base and the trapezium. Bennett (1886) described a fracture–dislocation in which the fracture passed obliquely across the articular surface, leaving an articular fragment attached to the palmar ligament and allowing the remainder of the metacarpal base to dislocate laterally and proximally (Fig. 17.62).The displacement is perpetuated by the pull of the abductor pollicis longus tendon and the intrinsic muscles.

Standard X-rays of the hand may not show the injury adequately. The Robert view (forearm fully pronated, shoulder internally rotated and thumb abducted) will provide a true anteroposterior view of the CMC joint (Robert 1936).

There is disagreement in the literature concerning the consequences of residual articular irregularity after Bennett's fracture. Very few patients present for treatment of osteoarthritis of the CMC joint after Bennett's fracture. Cannon *et al*. (1986) reviewed the literature on treatment of thumb CMC joint osteoarthritis and found that only seven out of 456 cases were known to be associated with Bennett's fracture.

Gedda (1954) observed a correlation between residual displacement and disability in a study of 60 patients with closed treatment after a mean follow-up of 7.5

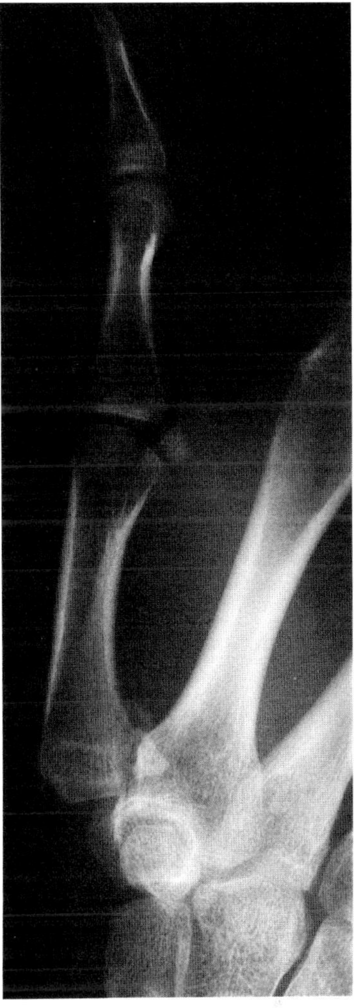

Fig. 17.62 Bennett's fracture–dislocation.

years. In 29 patients treated by open reduction and internal fixation, there was less pain and fewer degenerative changes were present in the radiographs, but the length of follow-up of this group was shorter. However, Griffiths (1964) found only one patient with symptoms and four with osteoarthritis in a series of 38 patients after an average follow-up of 6.8 years. Cannon *et al*. (1986) conducted a detailed review of 25 patients 5–16 years after Bennett's fracture. Although 21 patients had lost motion at the CMC joint, only two had significant symptoms. Salgeback *et al*. (1971) showed that mild residual deformity was frequent and apparently well tolerated. However, after follow-up averaging 26 years in 17 patients treated conservatively, Livesley (1990) found consistent loss of movement and strength, though only seven patients reported symptoms. Degenerative arthritis was present in 16 patients. It is fair to conclude, therefore, that an incongruent reduction leads to stiffness, weakness and radiographic signs of osteoarthritis, even though few patients seem to complain of these problems later on.

Many methods of treatment have been recommended for Bennett's fracture. Closed reduction of the subluxation is usually achieved without difficulty by longitudinal traction, extension and pressure over the base of the metacarpal. It is, however, quite difficult to maintain the reduction by external splintage. The injury is inherently unstable, the pull of the long abductor causes redisplacement and the effect of a moulded cast is soon lost as the swelling diminishes. Excessive pressure over the base of the metacarpal may damage the skin (Fig. 17.63). A common error is extension of the thumb at the MP joint rather than at the CMC joint, causing adduction and subluxation of the metacarpal (Fig. 17.61).

In the author's opinion, Bennett's fracture cannot be controlled reliably by external splintage and, therefore, percutaneous pin fixation should be the first line of management. The reduction is obtained as described above and a K-wire is passed across the base of the metacarpal into the trapezium (Wagner 1950). Alternatively, the wire may be passed from the thumb to the index metacarpal or placed just proximal to the base of metacarpal and into the carpus to act as a buttress against subluxation. The position of the fracture is then checked by X-ray. What constitutes an adequate reduction depends on the age of the patient, the size of the fragment and the surgeon's view of the consequences of residual articular irregularity (see above). If the position is judged to be inadequate and there is a single large fragment, the fracture may be exposed through a curved radio-volar incision and anatomical reduction obtained (Gedda & Moberg 1953, Heim & Pfeiffer 1987). The fracture may be fixed with K-wires, an interfragmentary screw or an interosseous wire. In the case of small or multiple fragments, open reduction is unlikely to improve on the results of percutaneous pin fixation.

Rolando (1910) described a comminuted fracture in which the metacarpal base is separated into two fragments, a large dorsal fragment and a volar fragment of the type found in Bennett's fracture (Fig. 17.64). There is no uniformly satisfactory method of treating comminuted fractures of the base of the thumb metacarpal. The

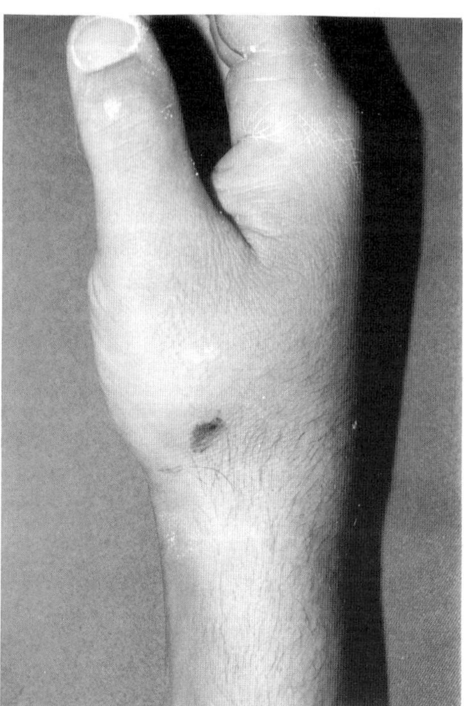

Fig. 17.63 Skin necrosis resulting from excessive pressure from a cast applied for Bennett's fracture.

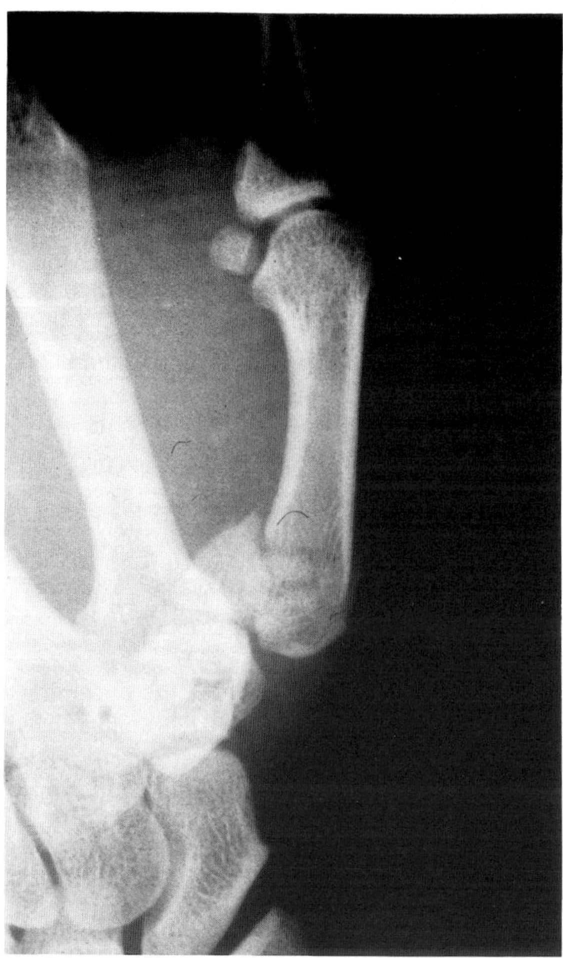

Fig. 17.64 Comminuted fracture of the base of the thumb metacarpal.

configuration described by Rolando is amenable to open reduction and internal fixation, but in most instances the fracture is more comminuted and internal fixation is precluded by the small size of the fragments or by extensive comminution. Percutaneous pin fixation seldom provides sufficient stability for early motion and considerable joint stiffness may result. Spangberg and Thoren (1963) employed the principle of ligament-otaxis by skeletal traction via a K-wire placed obliquely across the metacarpal to correct the varus angulation and shortening. The wire is passed at an angle 45° to the shaft, emerging through the thumb web, and traction is applied by an elastic band attached to an outrigger incorporated in a cast (Fig. 17.65). The proximal end of the wire is bent to an acute angle and engages the cortex of the metacarpal. Plaster is omitted from the web and early movement is allowed. Radiographs are taken at intervals during the first 14 days and adjustments of the force and direction of traction are made as necessary (Breen *et al.* 1988). If traction fails to provide reasonable alignment of the articular surface, it may be better to accept some shortening and angulation and allow active movement as soon as possible (Green & Rowland 1991). Büchler *et al.* (1991) performed open reduction, internal fixation, bone grafting of metaphyseal defects and neutralization by a quadrilateral external fixation frame placed between thumb and index metacarpals. Nine out of 10 patients achieved a good result.

Dislocation of the thumb CMC joint

Dislocation without fracture (Fig. 17.66) is less frequent than Bennett's fracture. It results from longitudinal force along the metacarpal shaft with the CMC joint flexed. The volar ligament is ruptured and there is potential for late subluxation or instability, leading to degenerative change (Eaton & Littler 1973). Reduction is usually straightforward, but it is essential to ensure that a congruous reduction is maintained during the healing period. If there is any doubt about the stability of the reduction or if radiographs demonstrate incongruity, the joint should be transfixed with one or two K-wires. Watt and Hooper (1987) reviewed 12 patients, in seven of whom a stable reduction was obtained on the day of injury and held in a cast. All seven had stable pain-free joints after an average of 3 years, but five patients who presented late (after 3–21 days) had pain and in four the joint was unstable.

Instability of the CMC joint may be demonstrated by an anteroposterior stress radiograph with the radial surfaces of the thumbs pressed together (Eaton & Littler

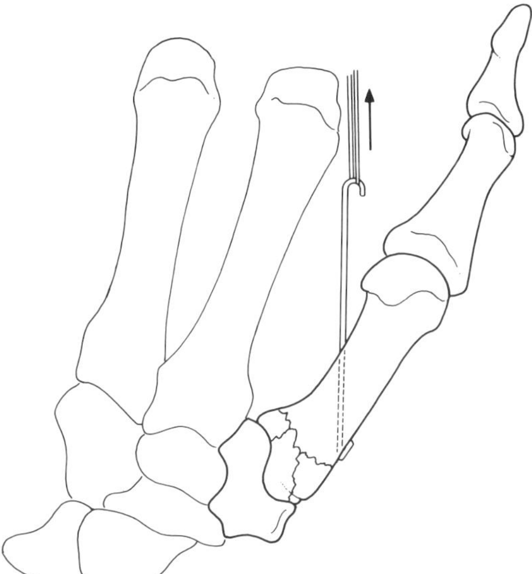

Fig. 17.65 Skeletal traction for comminuted fractures of the thumb metacarpal base.

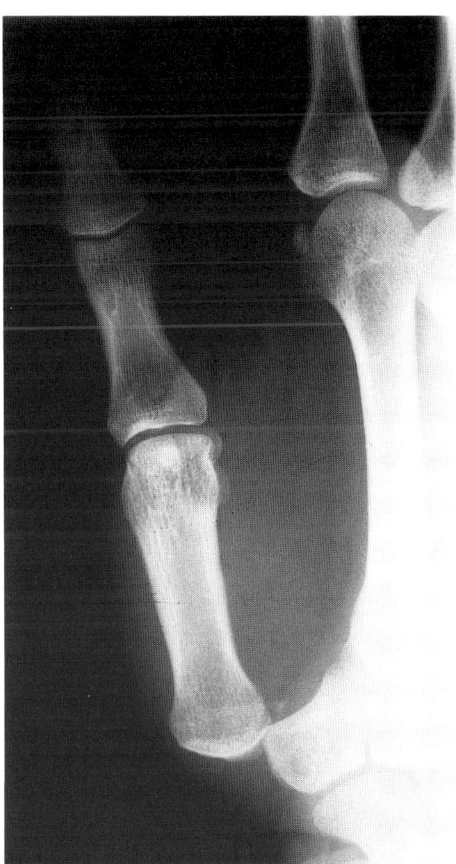

Fig. 17.66 Dislocation of the thumb CMC joint.

1973). The treatment of painful instability or subluxation depends on the state of the articular surfaces. Ligament reconstruction using a strip of the flexor carpi radialis tendon is appropriate if there is no degenerative change (Eaton & Littler 1973). Eaton *et al.* (1984) reported consistent pain relief and stability at an average of 7 years after ligament reconstruction, though most of these patients had idiopathic rather than post-traumatic instability. Arthrodesis is necessary if painful instability is accompanied by degenerative change (Eaton & Littler 1969).

Injuries of the thumb MP joint

The primary stabilizers of the MP joint of the thumb are the collateral ligaments and volar plate; additional dynamic stability is provided by the adductor pollicis via its insertion into the base of the proximal phalanx. The adductor also sends fibres into the ulnar side of the dorsal aponeurosis, forming the adductor aponeurosis which lies directly over the ulnar collateral ligament. The range of motion available at the MP joint varies from one individual to another. Coonrad and Goldner (1968) recorded an average of 75° flexion, 20° hyperextension and 10° abduction/adduction in a series of 1000 normal thumbs.

Rupture of the ulnar collateral ligament

This is caused by forced abduction stress, with or without hyperextension. The extent of the injury varies from a strain of the ligament without loss of stability to disruption of the collateral ligament, palmar plate and dorsal capsule. Common causes of this injury are motorcycle accidents, falls onto the outstretched thumb and skiing accidents. A stable ulnar collateral ligament is necessary to resist the forces generated during pinch against the index finger. Laxity of the ligament is associated with a weak painful pinch and predisposes to degenerative arthritis of the MP joint.

Tears of the ulnar collateral ligament may be partial or complete. Both types present with pain and swelling of the MP joint with tenderness maximal on the ulnar side of the joint. Complete tears of the ulnar collateral ligament heal poorly and most authors agree that operative repair is required. Stener (1962) recognized that the ligament, which is usually torn from its insertion on the proximal phalanx, frequently slips around the proximal free edge of the adductor aponeurosis as the aponeurosis slides distally at the moment of injury. The aponeurosis is interposed between the torn end of the ligament and its site of attachment to the proximal phalanx, pre-

venting healing (Fig. 17.67). This lesion was present in 25 out of 39 cases explored by Stener (1962); a similar ratio has been found by others.

The integrity of the ligament can be determined by applying radial deviation stress and comparing the range of abduction with the opposite side (Fig. 17.68). It is often necessary to relieve pain and spasm by regional block or local infiltration of the ligament before an adequate examination is possible. A clear increase in laxity *compared to the opposite side* is good evidence of rupture of the ulnar collateral ligament and operative repair is indicated. However, the amount of laxity which indicates a complete tear is uncertain. Smith (1977)

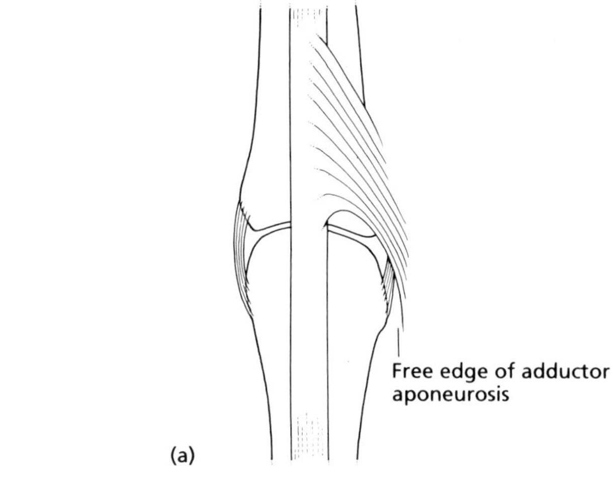

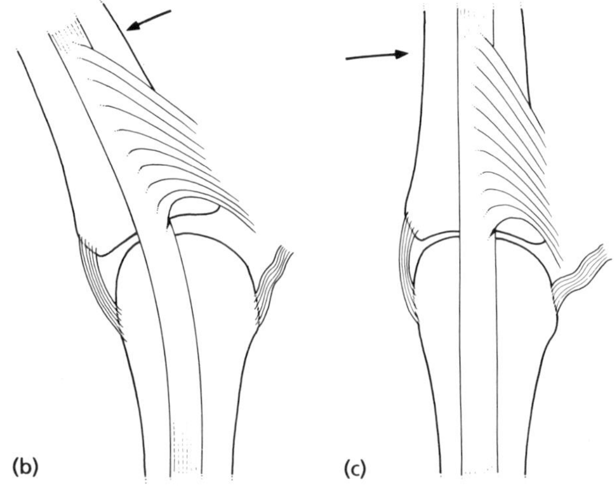

Fig. 17.67 Stener lesion of the thumb MP joint. (a) The ulnar collateral ligament lies deep to the adductor aponeurosis. (b) The aponeurosis slides distally at the moment of injury, allowing the distal torn end of the ligament to flip over the free edge of the aponeurosis and become trapped superficial to it (c).

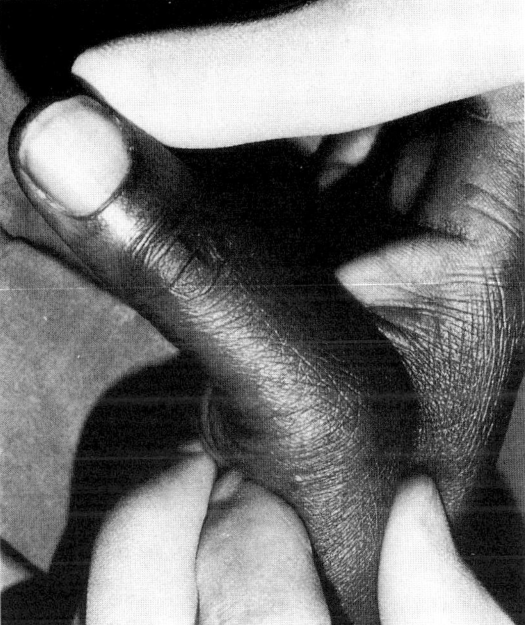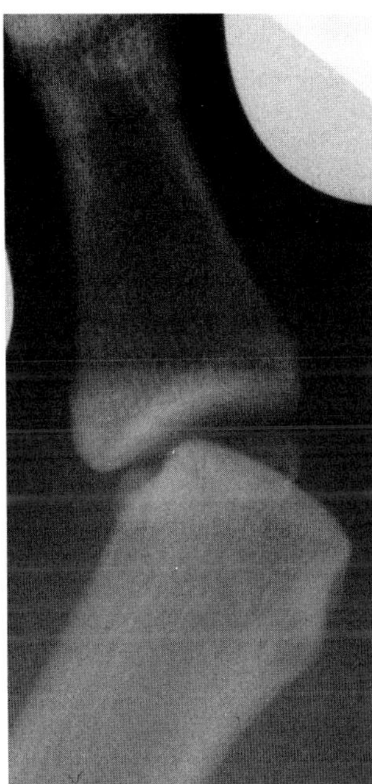

Fig. 17.68 (a) and (b) Stress examination of the thumb MP joint.

quotes 45°; Bowers and Hurst (1977) suggest 10° more than the uninjured side. Palmer and Louis (1978) prefer to test the joint in flexion, having found in cadaver studies that an intact palmar plate prevented excessive opening in extension. Louis *et al.* (1986) found a Stener lesion at the time of operation in 20% of cases during the period when testing was performed in extension, but when the decision to operate was based on testing in flexion, the incidence of Stener lesions rose to 70%. However, care must be taken to avoid rotation when stress testing is performed in flexion.

Repair of the ulnar collateral ligament is performed through a slightly curved dorso-ulnar incision centred on the MP joint. A branch of the superficial radial nerve often crosses the incision and should be avoided. If a Stener lesion is present, the distal end of the collateral ligament is usually found to be turned back upon itself, immediately beneath the subcutaneous fat. The free proximal edge of the adductor aponeurosis is identified and the aponeurosis incised longitudinally. The edges may be marked with stay sutures. Beneath the aponeurosis lies the ulnar aspect of the MP joint. The ulnar collateral ligament is identified and its margins cleared of haematoma and fibrin. The ligament is usually torn at its distal insertion, which is on the palmo-ulnar corner of the base of the proximal phalanx. This area is exposed and the bone surface roughened. The ligament may be repaired by suture to the adjacent periosteum and soft tissues; frequently, however, this material is of poor quality and it is necessary to pass the suture into bone.

A weaving suture of 3/0 or 4/0 synthetic monofilament suture is placed in the ligament stump and the ends passed through oblique drill-holes in the base of the proximal phalanx to exit on its radial surface, where the suture is tied over a button. If monofilament suture is employed, it can be removed after 4 weeks simply by cutting one end flush with the skin and pulling on the other end; a pull-out suture is unnecessary. The author prefers to protect the repair with an oblique transarticular K-wire because it is otherwise impossible to splint the thumb in abduction without undue stress on the repair. The volar plate and dorsal capsule may be repaired with fine non-absorbable sutures and the adductor aponeurosis is also repaired. A forearm cast extending to the tip of the thumb is applied.

The wire is removed after 4 weeks and the thumb protected for another 4 weeks by a thermoplastic splint which is removed for exercises. Strong pinch should be avoided for at least 8 weeks. Moderate loss of MP joint motion is frequent but not disabling: in this joint, stability is more important than movement.

The treatment of late instability of the thumb MP joint is controversial. After 2 weeks, the chance of direct ligament repair lessens as the ligament shortens and it is difficult to obtain a secure repair. Smith (1977) recommended reconstruction of the ligament with a strip of palmaris longus tendon for injuries more than 3 weeks old, provided that the joint surfaces are normal; the tendon graft is passed through drill holes in the bone on each side of the joint. Neviaser *et al.* (1971)

provided dynamic stability by distal advancement of the tendon of adductor pollicis; this procedure is probably best reserved for support of a static ligament reconstruction. In the presence of degenerative arthritis, arthrodesis is an excellent procedure which provides stable pain-free pinch. Very little disability results from loss of MP joint movement provided that there is good motion at the basal joint.

Tears of the radial collateral ligament

These account for about a quarter of MP joint collateral ligament injuries (Camp *et al.* 1980). There is no counterpart of the Stener lesion on the radial side of the joint and the ligament may tear at either end. Pinch is normal but there is swelling, pain with motion and tenderness of the prominent radial aspect of the metacarpal head. Pain occurs when pressure is placed on the radial side of the thumb, particularly when pushing against a surface with the hand flat. Excessive ulnar deviation occurs on adduction stress. Camp *et al.* (1980) treated eight patients with repair of the radial collateral ligament, advancement of the abductor pollicis brevis into the proximal phalanx and repair of the abductor aponeurosis, and observed good results in each case.

Avulsion fractures of the base of the proximal phalanx

In the thumb these represent injury to the insertions of the respective collateral ligaments. Provided that displacement of the fragment does not occur, healing with satisfactory stability will take place (Fig. 17.69). Fractures with displacement of 2 mm or less may be splinted in a cast extending to the tip of the thumb for 3 weeks, followed by protection in a removable splint for a further 3 weeks. If there is more than 2 mm displacement, the fragment should be reduced operatively and fixed with a K-wire, interosseous wire (Lister 1978) or small lag screw, depending on its size.

Dislocation

Hyperextension injury of the thumb MP joint may cause strain or rupture of the palmar plate as well as dorsal dislocation. Dislocation of the thumb MP joint is similar in many respects to dislocation of the index and little finger MP joints. It results from forcible hyperextension and may be simple or complex, the latter resulting from interposition of the palmar plate, and the management is the same as in the index finger, including a dorsal approach for release of the trapped palmar plate. After reduction the stability of the collateral liga-

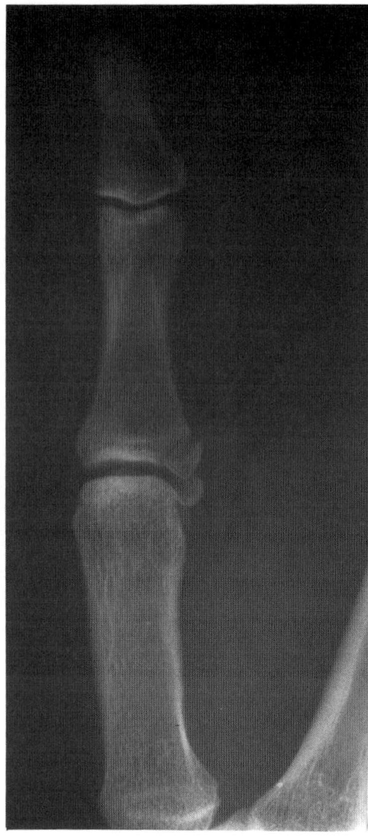

Fig. 17.69 Avulsion of the insertion of the ulnar collateral ligament of the thumb MP joint.

ments should be checked; complete rupture is dealt with as described above.

Strains of the palmar plate may be distinguished from ruptures by comparing the range of hyperextension with the opposite thumb (Stener 1963), using a local anaesthetic block if necessary. Strains require only symptomatic treatment. Complete ruptures should be immobilized with the MP joint in 15–20° flexion for 3–4 weeks to encourage healing of the palmar plate at its correct length. Hyperextension injuries occasionally lead to hyperextension laxity and dynamic collapse of the thumb skeleton with hyperextension of the MP joint and flexion at the IP and CMC joints (Fig. 17.70). Capsulodesis or tenodesis of the MP joint will prevent hyperextension and correct the deformity. Arthrodesis should be employed if the articular surfaces are degenerate.

Condylar fractures of the thumb metacarpal and proximal phalanx should be treated in the same manner as the corresponding similar injuries in the fingers, using open reduction and internal fixation for displaced fractures.

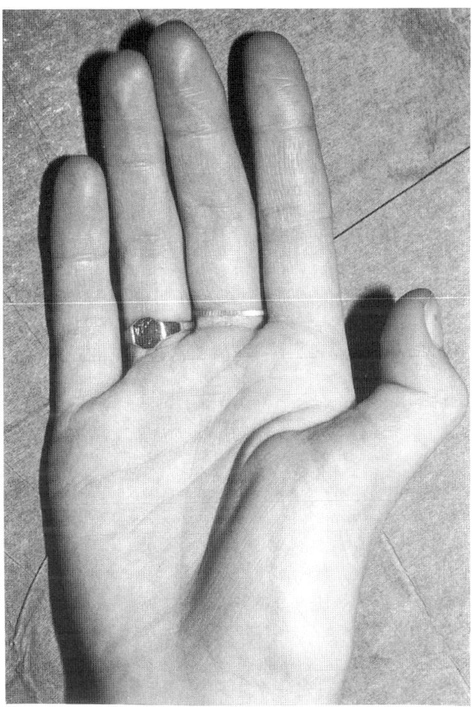

Fig. 17.70 Dynamic instability of the thumb resulting from chronic volar plate laxity. The deformity was corrected by palmar capsulodesis of the MP joint.

References

Ashmead, D., Rothkopf, D.M., Walton, R.L. & Jupiter, J.B. Treatment of hand injuries by external fixation. *J Hand Surg* 1992; **17A**: 956–964.

Aukland, K. & Nicolaysen, G. Interstitial fluid volumes; local regulatory mechanisms. *Physiol Rev* 1981; **61**: 566–643.

Barton, N. Conservative treatment of articular fractures in the hand. *J Hand Surg* 1989; **14A**: 183–193.

Barton, N.J. Fractures of the hand in children. *Hand* 1979; **11**: 134–143.

Barton, N.J. Fractures of the hand. *J Bone Joint Surg* 1984; **66B**: 159–167.

Becton, J.L., Christian, J.D., Goodwin, H.N. & Jackson, J.G. A simplified technique for treating complex dislocation of the index metacarpophalangeal joint. *J Bone Joint Surg* 1975; **57A**: 698–700.

Belsky, M.R., Eaton, R.G. & Lane, L.B. Closed reduction and internal fixation of proximal phalanx fractures. *J Hand Surg* 1984; **9A**: 725–729.

Bennett, E.H. On fracture of the metacarpal bone of the thumb. *Br Med J* 1886; **11**: 12–13.

Berg, E.E. & Murphy, D.F. Ulnopalmar dislocation of the fifth carpometacarpal joint — Successful closed reduction: review of the literature and anatomic re-evaluation. *J Hand Surg* 1986; **11A**: 521–525.

Black, D.M., Mann, R.J., Constine, R. & Daniels, A.U. Comparison of internal fixation techniques in metacarpal fractures. *J Hand Surg* 1985; **10A**: 466–472.

Black, D.M., Watson, H.K. & Vender, M.I. Arthroplasty of the ulnar carpometacarpal joints. *J Hand Surg* 1987; **12A**: 1071–1074.

Blair, S.J. & McCormick, E. Prevention of trauma; cooperation toward a better working environment. *J Hand Surg* 1985; **10A**: 953–958.

Blalock, H.S., Pearce, H.L., Kleinert, H. & Kutz, J. An instrument designed to help reduce and percutaneously pin fractured phalanges. *J Bone Joint Surg* 1975; **57A**: 792–794.

Bora, F.W. & Didizian, N.H. The treatment of injuries to the carpometacarpal joint of the little finger. *J Bone Joint Surg* 1974; **56A**: 1459–1463.

Bowers, W.H. The proximal interphalangeal joint volar plate. II. A clinical study of hyperextension injury. *J Hand Surg* 1981; **6**: 77–81.

Bowers, W.H. & Hurst, L.C. Gamekeeper's thumb. Evaluation by arthrography and stress roentgenography. *J Bone Joint Surg* 1977; **59A**: 519–524.

Bowers, W.H., Wolf, J.W. Jr., Nehil, J.L. & Bittinger, S. The proximal interphalangeal joint volar plate. I. An anatomical and biomechanical study. *J Hand Surg* 1980; **5**: 79–88.

Breen, T.F., Gelberman, R.H. & Jupiter, J.B. Intra-articular fractures of the basilar joint of the thumb. *Hand Clin* 1988; **4**: 491–501.

Büchler, U. & Fischer, T. Use of a minicondylar plate for metacarpal and phalangeal periarticular injuries. *Clin Orthop* 1987; **214**: 53–58.

Büchler, U. & Hastings, H. Combined injuries. In: Green, D.P. (ed.) *Operative Hand Surgery*. Churchill Livingstone: New York, 1993.

Büchler, U., McCollam, S.M. & Oppikofer, C. Comminuted fractures of the basilar joint of the thumb: combined treatment by external fixation, limited internal fixation, and bone grafting. *J Hand Surg* 1991; **16A**: 556–560.

Camp, R.A., Weatherwax, R.J. & Miller, E.B. Chronic post-traumatic radial instability of the thumb metacarpophalangeal joint. *J Hand Surg* 1980; **5**: 221–225.

Cannon, S.R., Dowd, G.S., Williams, D.H. & Scott, J.M. A long-term study following Bennett's fracture. *J Hand Surg* 1986; **11B**: 426–431.

Clark, D.P., Scott, R.N. & Anderson, I.W.R. Hand problems in an Accident and Emergency Department. *J Hand Surg* 1985; **10B**: 297–299.

Clendenin, M.B. & Smith, R.J. Fifth metacarpal/hamate arthrodesis for post-traumatic osteoarthritis. *J Hand Surg* 1984; **9A**: 374–378.

Cooney, W.P., Lucca, M.J., Chao, E.Y. & Linscheid, R.L. The kinesiology of the thumb trapeziometacarpal joint. *J Bone Joint Surg* 1981; **63A**: 1371–1381.

Coonrad, R.N. & Goldner, J.L. A study of the pathological findings and treatment in soft tissue injury of the thumb metacarpophalangeal joint. *J Bone Joint Surg* 1968; **50A**: 439–451.

Crawford, G.P. The moulded polyethylene splint for mallet finger deformities. *J Hand Surg* 1984; **9A**: 231–237.

Curtis, R.M. Injuries to joints. In: Flynn, J.E. (ed.) *Hand Surgery* 3rd edn. Williams & Wilkins: Baltimore, 1982.

Dabezies, E.J. & Schutte, J.P. Fixation of metacarpal and phalangeal fractures with miniature plates and screws. *J Hand Surg* 1986; **11A**: 283–288.

Dickson, R.A. Rigid fixation of unstable metacarpal fractures using transverse K wires bonded with acrylic resin. *Hand* 1975; **7**: 284–286.

Diwaker, H.N. & Stothard, J. The role of internal fixation in closed fractures of the proximal phalanges and metacarpals in adults. *J Hand Surg* 1986; **11B**: 103–108.

Dixon, G.L. & Moon, N.F. Rotational supracondylar fractures of the proximal phalanx in children. *Clin Orthop* 1972; **83**: 151–156.

Dray, G.J. & Eaton, R.G. Dislocations and ligament injuries in the digits. In: Green, D.P. (ed.) *Operative Hand Surgery.* Churchill Livingstone: New York, 1993.

Duncan, R.W., Freeland, A.E., Jabalay, M.E. & Meydrech, E.F. Open hand fractures: an analysis of the recovery of active motion and of complications. *J Hand Surg* 1993; **18A**: 387–394.

Eaton, R.G. *Joint Injuries of the Hand.* Charles C. Thomas: Springfield, 1971.

Eaton, R.G. & Littler, J.W. A study of the basal joint of the thumb. Treatment of its disabilities by fusion. *J Bone Joint Surg* 1969; **51A**: 661–688.

Eaton, R.G. & Littler, J.W. Ligamentous reconstruction for the painful thumb carpometacarpal joint. *J Bone Joint Surg* 1973; **55A**: 1655–1666.

Eaton, R.G. & Malerich, M.M. Volar plate arthroplasty for the proximal interphalangeal joint: a ten-year review. *J Hand Surg* 1980; **5**: 260–268.

Eaton, R.G., Lane, L.B., Littler, J.W. & Keyser, J.J. Ligament reconstruction for the painful thumb carpometacarpal joint: a long-term assessment. *J Hand Surg* 1984; **9A**: 692–699.

Elson, R.A. Rupture of the extensor hood of the finger: a test for early diagnosis. *J Bone Joint Surg* 1986; **68B**: 229–231.

Fahmy, N.R.M. & Harvey, R.A. The S-Quattro in the management of fractures of the hand. *J Hand Surg* 1992; **17B**: 321–331.

Farabeuf, L.H.F. De la luxation du pouce en arrière. *Bull Soc Chirurgie* 1876; **11**: 21–62.

Feldon, P. & Belsky, M.R. Degenerative diseases of the metacarpophalangeal joints. *Hand Clin* 1987; **3**: 429–445.

Fitzgerald, J.A. & Khan, M.A. The conservative management of fractures of the shafts of the phalanges of the fingers by combined traction-splintage. *J Hand Surg* 1984; **9B**: 303–306.

Ford, D.J., El-Hadidi, S., Lunn, P.G. & Burke, F.D. Fractures of the phalanges: results of internal fixation using 1.5 mm, and 2.0 mm AO screws. *J Hand Surg* 1987; **12B**: 28–33.

Freeland, A.E. External fixation for skeletal stabilisation of severe open fractures of the hand. *Clin Orthop* 1987; **214**: 93–100.

Freeland, A.E., Jabalay, M.E. & Hughes, J.L. *Stable Internal Fixation of the Hand and Wrist.* Springer-Verlag: New York, 1986.

Froimson, A.L. Osteotomy for digital deformity. *J Hand Surg* 1981; **6**: 585–589.

Gedda, K.O. Studies on Bennett's fracture: anatomy, roentgenology and therapy. *Acta Chir Scand Suppl* 1954; **193**: 1–114.

Gedda, K.O. & Moberg, E. Open reduction and osteosynthesis of the so-called Bennett's fracture in the carpometacarpal joint of the thumb. *Acta Orthop Scand* 1953; **22**: 249–257.

Glasgow, M. & Lloyd, G.J. The use of modified AO reduction forceps in percutaneous fracture fixation. *Hand* 1981; **13**: 214–216.

Godina, M. Early microsurgical reconstruction of complex trauma of the extremities. *Plast Reconstr Surg* 1986; **78**: 293–294.

Goodfellow, J.W. & Weaver, J.P.A. Locking of the metacarpophalangeal joints. *J Bone Joint Surg* 1961; **43B**: 772–777.

Green, D.P. Complications of phalangeal and metacarpal fractures. *Hand Clin* 1986; **2**: 307–328.

Green, D.P. & Anderson, J.R. Closed reduction and percutaneous pin fixation of fractured phalanges. *J Bone Joint Surg* 1973; **55A**: 1651–1653.

Green, D.P. & Rowland, S.A. Fractures and dislocations in the hand. In: Rockwood, C.A., Green, D.P. & Bucholz, R.W. (eds) *Fractures in Adults* 3rd edn. Lippincott: Philadelphia, 1991.

Green, D.P. & Terry, G.C. Complex dislocation of the metacarpophalangeal joint. *J Bone Joint Surg* 1973; **55A**: 1480–1486.

Greene, T.L., Noellert, R.C. & Belsole, R.J. Treatment of unstable metacarpal and phalangeal fractures with tension band wiring techniques. *Clin Orthop* 1987; **214**: 78–84.

Griffiths, J.C. Fracture of the first metacarpal bone. *J Bone Joint Surg* 1964; **46B**: 712–719.

Grundberg, A.B. Intramedullary fixation for fractures of the hand. *J Hand Surg* 1981; **6**: 568–573.

Grundberg, A.B. & Reagan, D.S. Central slip tenotomy for chronic mallet finger deformity. *J Hand Surg* 1987; **12A**: 545–547.

Guly, H.R. & Azam, M.A. Locked finger treated by manipulation. *J Bone Joint Surg* 1982; **64B**: 73–75.

Hall, R.F. Jr. Treatment of metacarpal and phalangeal fractures in noncompliant patients. *Clin Orthop* 1987; **214**: 31–36.

Hall, R.F. Jr., Gleason, T.F. & Kasa, R.F. Simultaneous closed dislocations of the metacarpophalangeal joints of the index, long, and ring fingers: a case report. *J Hand Surg* 1985; **10A**: 81–85.

Hamas, R.S., Horrell, E.D. & Pierret, G.P. Treatment of mallet finger due to intra-articular fracture of the distal phalanx. *J Hand Surg* 1978; **3**: 361–363.

Hastings, H. II. Unstable metacarpal and phalangeal fractures — treatment with screws and plates. *Clin Orthop* 1987; **214**: 37–52.

Hastings, H. & Carroll, C. Treatment of closed articular fractures of the metacarpophalangeal and proximal interphalangeal joints. *Hand Clin* 1988; **4**: 503–527.

Heim, U. & Pfeiffer, K.M. *Internal Fixation of Small Fractures* 3rd edn. Springer-Verlag: New York, 1987.

Henderson, J.J. & Arafa, M.A. Carpometacarpal dislocation. An easily missed diagnosis. *J Bone Joint Surg* 1987; **69**: 212–214.

Ho, P.K., Choban, S.J., Eshman, S.J. & Dupuy, T.E. Complex dorsal dislocation of the second carpometacarpal joint. *J Hand Surg* 1987; **12A**: 1074–1076.

Hunter, J.M. & Cowan, N.J. Fifth metacarpal fractures in a compensation clinic population. *J Bone Joint Surg* 1970; **52A**: 1159–1165.

Jabalay, M.E. & Freeland, A.E. Rigid internal fixation in the hand: 104 cases. *Plast Reconstr Surg* 1986; **77**: 288–298.

James, J.I.P. Fractures of the proximal and middle phalanges of the fingers. *Acta Orthop Scand* 1962; **32**: 401–412.

James, J.I.P. The assessment and management of the injured hand. *Hand* 1970; **2**: 97–105.

Joshi, B.B. Percutaneous internal fixation of fractures of the proximal phalanges. *Hand* 1976; **8**: 86–92.

Kaplan, E.B. Dorsal dislocation of the metacarpophalangeal joint of the index finger. *J Bone Joint Surg* 1957; **39A**:

1081–1086.

Khuri, S.M. & Fay, J. Complete volar metacarpophalangeal joint dislocation of a finger. *J Trauma* 1986; **26**: 1058–1060.

Kiefhaber, T.R., Stern, P.J. & Grood, E.S. Lateral stability of the proximal interphalangeal joint. *J Hand Surg* 1986; **11A**: 661–669.

Kleinman, W. & Grantham, S.A. Multiple volar carpometacarpal joint dislocation of the medial four carpometacarpal joints in a child and review of the literature. *J Hand Surg* 1978; **3**: 337–382.

Lamb, D.W., Abernathy, P.A. & Raine, P.A.M. Unstable fractures of the metacarpals: a new method of treatment by transverse wire fixation to intact metacarpals. *Hand* 1973; **5**: 43–48.

Lane, C.S. Detecting occult fractures of the metacarpal head: the Brewerton view. *J Hand Surg* 1977; **2**: 131–133.

Leddy, P.J. & Packer, J.W. Avulsion of the profundus insertion in athletes. *J Hand Surg* 1977; **2**: 66–69.

Lister, G. Intraosseous wiring of the digital skeleton. *J Hand Surg* 1978; **3**: 427–435.

Lister, G. *The Hand: Diagnosis and Indications* 3rd edn. Churchill Livingstone: Edinburgh, 1993.

Lister, G. Free and composite skin flaps. In: Green, D.P. (ed.) *Operative Hand Surgery*. Churchill Livingstone: New York, 1993.

Livesley, P.J. The conservative management of Bennett's fracture-dislocation: a 26 year follow-up. *J Hand Surg* 1990; **15B**: 291–294.

Louis, D.S., Huebner, J.J. Jr. & Hankin, F.M. Rupture and displacement of the ulnar collateral ligament of the metacarpophalangeal joint of the thumb. Preoperative diagnosis. *J Bone Joint Surg* 1986; **68**: 1320–1326.

Lowdon, I.M. Fractures of the metacarpal neck of the little finger. *Injury* 1986; **17**: 189–192.

Lubahn, J.D. Dorsal fracture dislocations of the proximal interphalangeal joint. *Hand Clin* 1988; **4**: 15–24.

Massengill, J.B., Alexander, H., Langrana, N. & Mylod, A. A phalangeal fracture model — quantitative analysis of rigidity and failure. *J Hand Surg* 1982; **7**: 264–270.

McElfresh, E.C. & Dobyns, J.H. Intra-articular metacarpal head fractures. *J Hand Surg* 1983; **8**: 383–393.

McElfresh, E.C., Dobyns, J.H. & O'Brien, E.T. Management of fracture dislocation of the proximal interphalangeal joints by extension block splinting. *J Bone Joint Surg* 1972; **54A**: 1705–1711.

McLaughlin, H.L. Complex 'locked' dislocation of the metacarpophalangeal joint. *J Trauma* 1965; **5**: 683–688.

Minami, A., An, K.N., Cooney, W.P., Linscheid, R.L. & Chao, E.Y. Ligament stability of the metacarpophalangeal joint: a biomechanical study. *J Hand Surg* 1985; **10A**: 255–260.

Moneim, M.S. Volar dislocation of the metacarpophalangeal joint. Pathologic anatomy and report of two cases. *Clin Orthop* 1983; **176**: 186–189.

Neviaser, R.J., Wilson, J.N. & Lievano, A. Rupture of the ulnar collateral ligament of the thumb (gamekeeper's thumb). Correction by dynamic repair. *J Bone Joint Surg* 1971; **53A**: 1357–1364.

O'Brien, E.T. Fractures of the hand and wrist region. In: Rockwood, C.A., Wilkins, K.E. & King, R.E. (eds) *Fractures in Children*. Lippincott: Philadelphia, 1991.

O'Rourke, S.K., Gaur, S. & Barton, N.J. Long-term outcome of articular fractures of the phalanges: an eleven year follow-up. *J Hand Surg* 1989; **14B**: 183–193.

Palmer, A.K. & Louis, D.S. Assessing ulnar instability of the metacarpophalangeal joint of the thumb. *J Hand Surg* 1978; **3**: 542–546.

Peimer, C.A., Sullivan, D.J. & Wild, D.R. Palmar dislocation of the proximal interphalangeal joint. *J Hand Surg* 1984; **9A**: 39–48.

Peterson, P. & Sacks, S. Fracture-dislocation of the base of the fifth metacarpal associated with injury to the deep motor branch of the ulnar nerve: a case report. *J Hand Surg* 1986; **11A**: 525–527.

Petrie, P.W.R. & Lamb, D.W. Fracture-subluxation of the base of the fifth metacarpal. *Hand* 1974; **6**: 82–86.

Ramamurthy, S. & Hickey, R. Anaesthesia. In: Green, D.P. (ed.) *Operative Hand Surgery*. Churchill Livingstone: New York, 1993.

Rang, M.C. *Children's Fractures* 2nd edn. Lippincott: Philadelphia, 1974.

Rankin, E.A. & Uwagie-Ero, S. Locking of the metacarpophalangeal joint. *J Hand Surg* 1986; **11A**: 868–871.

Rawles, J.G. Dislocations and fracture-dislocations of the carpometacarpal joints of the fingers. *Hand Clin* 1988; **4**: 103–112.

Rayan, G.M. & Mullins, P.T. Skin necrosis complicating mallet finger splinting and vascularity of the distal interphalangeal overlying skin. *J Hand Surg* 1987; **12A**: 548–552.

Resnick, S.M., Greene, T.L. & Roeser, W. Simultaneous dislocation of the five carpometacarpal joints. *Clin Orthop* 1985; **192**: 210–214.

Riggs, S.A. & Cooney, W.P. External fixation of complex hand and wrist fractures. *J Trauma* 1983; **23**: 332–336.

Riordan, D.C. Tendon trauma and reconstruction. In: Dobyns, J.H., Chase, R.A. & Amadio, P.C. (eds) *1988 Year Book of Hand Surgery*. Year Book Medical Publishers: Chicago, 1988.

Robert, P. La radiographie de la articulation trapeziometacarplen et les arthroses de cette jointre. *Bull Mem Soc Radiol Med France* 1936; **24**: 687–690.

Rolando, S. Fracture de la base du premier metacarpien: et principalement sur une variété non encore decrite. *Presse Med* 1910; **33**: 303–304.

Salgeback, S., Eiken, O., Carstam, N. & Ohlsson, N. A study of Bennett's fracture with special reference to fixation by percutaneous pinning. *Scand J Plast Reconstr Surg* 1971; **5**: 142–148.

Scott, M.M. & Mulligan, P.J. Stabilizing severe phalangeal fractures. *Hand* 1980; **12**: 44–50.

Segmuller, G. *Surgical Stabilisation of the Skeleton of the Hand*. Williams & Wilkins: Baltimore, 1977.

Seymour, N. Juxta-epiphyseal fractures of the terminal phalanx of the finger. *J Bone Joint Surg* 1966; **48B**: 347–349.

Simmons, B.P. & Peters, T.T. Subcondylar fossa reconstruction for malunion of fractures of the proximal phalanx in children. *J Hand Surg* 1987; **12A**: 1079–1082.

Sloan, J.P., Dove, A.F., Maheson, M., Cope, A.N. & Welsh, K.R. Antibiotics in open fractures of the distal phalanx? *J Hand Surg* 1987; **12B**: 123–124.

Smith, R.J. Post-traumatic instability of the metacarpophalangeal joint of the thumb. *J Bone Joint Surg* 1977; **59A**: 14–21.

Souter, W.A. The boutonnière deformity. A review of 101 patients with division of the central slip of the extensor expansion of the fingers. *J Bone Joint Surg* 1967; **49B**: 710–721.

Spangberg, O. & Thoren, L. Bennett's fracture: a method of

treatment with oblique traction. *J Bone Joint Surg* 1963; **45B**: 732–736.

Spinner, M. & Choi, B.Y. Anterior dislocation of the proximal interphalangeal joint. *J Bone Joint Surg* 1970; **52A**: 1329–1336.

Stack, H.G. Mallet finger. *Hand* 1969; **1**: 83–89.

Stark, H.H. Troublesome fractures and dislocations of the hand. In: *American Academy of Orthopaedic Surgeons Instructional Course Lecture*, Vol. 19. CV Mosby: St Louis, 1970.

Stark, H.H., Boyes, J.H. & Wilson, J.N. Mallet finger. *J Bone Joint Surg* 1962; **44A**: 1061–1068.

Steel, W.M. The AO small fragment set in hand fractures. *Hand* 1978; **10**: 246–253.

Steel, W.M. Articular fractures. In: Barton, N.J. (ed.) *Fractures of the Hand and Wrist*. Churchill Livingstone: Edinburgh, 1988.

Stener, B. Displacement of the ruptured ulnar collateral ligament of the metacarpophalangeal joint of the thumb. A clinical and anatomical study. *J Bone Joint Surg* 1962; **44B**: 869–879.

Stener, B. Hyperextension injuries to the metacarpophalangeal joint of the thumb. *Acta Chir Scand* 1963; **125**: 275–293.

Stern, P.J. & Lee, A.F. Open dorsal dislocations of the proximal interphalangeal joint. *J Hand Surg* 1985; **10A**: 364–370.

Stern, P.J., Roman, R.J., Kiefhaber, T.R. & McDonough, J.J. Pilon fractures of the proximal interphalangeal joint, *J Hand Surg* 1991; **16A**: 844–850.

Stern, P.J., Wieser, M.J. & Reilly, D.G. Complications of plate fixation in the hand skeleton. *Clin Orthop* 1987; **214**: 59–65.

Strickland, J.W., Steichen, J.B., Kleinman, W.B., Hastings, H. &

Flynn, N. Phalangeal fractures. Factors influencing digital performance. *Orthop Rev* 1982; **11**: 39–50.

Stuchin, S.A. & Kummer, F.J. Stiffness of small-bone external fixation methods: an experimental study. *J Hand Surg* 1984; **9A**: 718–724.

Tubiana, R. Incidence and cost of injuries to the hand. In: Tubiana, R. (ed.) *The Hand*. WB Saunders: Philadelphia, 1985.

Vicar, A.J. Proximal interphalangeal joint dislocations without fractures. *Hand Clin* 1988; **4**: 5–13.

Watt, I. & Hooper, G. Dislocation of the trapezio-metacarpal joint. *J Hand Surg* 1987; **12B**: 242–245.

Wagner, C.J. Method of treatment of Bennett's fracture dislocation. *Am J Surg* 1950; **80**: 230–321.

Weckesser, E.C. Rotational osteotomy of the metacarpal for overlapping fingers. *J Bone Joint Surg* 1965; **47A**: 751–756.

Wehbe, M.A. & Schneider, L.H. Mallet fractures. *J Bone Joint Surg* 1984; **66A**: 658–669.

Weiland, A.J., White, G.M. & Moore, J.R. Epiphyseal fractures. In: Barton, N.J. (ed.) *Fractures of the Hand and Wrist*. Churchill Livingstone: Edinburgh, 1988.

Wright, T.A. Early mobilisation of fractures of the metacarpals and phalanges. *Can J Surg* 1968; **11**: 491–498.

Zook, E.G., Guy, R.J. & Russell, R.C. A study of nail bed injuries. Causes, treatment and prognosis. *J Hand Surg* 1984; **9A**: 247–252.

Zook, E.G., Van Beek, A.L. & Russell, R.C. Anatomy and physiology of the perionychium: a review of the literature and anatomical study. *J Hand Surg* 1980; **5**: 528–536.

18: The Spine

Cervical spine

T.McSWEENEY

In this section the more common injuries of the neck are considered with the aim of providing an overall view of their medical and surgical management. The seriousness of these injuries varies from a 'sprain' to a fracture–dislocation and the resulting disability depends largely on the extent of the bony and ligamentous damage but, more significantly, on the severity of any neurological impairment. Great forces are required to produce neurological impairment in a normal cervical spine despite the almost horizontal disposition of the facet joints, so that only a small number of injuries are complicated by damage to the spinal cord or nerve roots. While the greatest damage occurs at the time of injury, the potential for increasing the neurological deficit by faulty management or injudicious surgery must be recognized. Because of the obvious implications greater emphasis will be placed on the treatment of those injuries with neurological signs but similar principles apply to the uncomplicated spinal injury.

Mechanism of injury

The anatomical arrangement of the cervical spine allows for a great range of mobility and this is especially noticeable in children and in slender-necked individuals. Most injuries result from indirect violence transmitted through the head in relation to the relatively fixed cervico-thoracic junction. Alternatively, forces applied to the trunk may cause excessive neck movement which is sufficient, in either case, to transgress the normal range. Commonly, the injury results from a combination of simultaneously acting forces in which one vector predominates. These external forces are modified by factors including the position of the neck at the time of injury, the varying strength of the bones and ligaments at different ages and whether the protective muscles are 'on guard' in anticipation of injury. Pure deforming forces include rotation, compression, shear, flexion (ante flexion, lateral flexion), and hyperextension (deflexion, retroflexion). The term 'extension' is used in the conventional sense as meaning the opposite of flexion. This may be confusing as the term is also applied to distraction forces which imply an increase in length; in this context it is the opposite of compression.

Direct injuries are less common and are caused by heavy blows on the neck resulting in fractures of the posterior arch. Missile injuries are included in this group.

Classification

Various classifications have been proposed, notably those of Roaf (1960), Whitley and Forsyth (1960), Selecki and Williams (1970) and Denis (1983). Radiological terminology is often at variance with experimental and clinical concepts and initial radiographs may fail to reveal serious ligamentous injuries unless special studies are made. White and Panjabi (1978) suggest that 'families' of injuries may result from similar or identical forces. The mechanism of injury can usually be deduced from the history and circumstances of the accident, the clinical findings (location of bruise marks, facial injuries, scalp wounds) and a careful study of the radiographs. This is an important mental exercise and should obviate failure in diagnosis.

Most of the injuries will fall into four main groups:
1 Flexion, including lateral flexion and flexion–rotation injuries.
2 Hyperextension, and extension–rotation injuries.
3 Compression or axial loading fractures.
4 A miscellaneous group including distraction injuries and those where the mechanism of injury is not readily apparent.

It is vital to distinguish between injuries in which the

predominant force is one of flexion and hyperextension injuries. If an extension injury is mistaken for a flexion injury and the neck is immobilized in hyperextension, this will increase the deformity and may hazard the spinal cord. Similar remarks apply to certain distraction injuries in the upper cervical spine where excessive traction will lead to the patient being 'hanged by mistake'.

In cadaveric experiments, Roaf (1960) was unable to produce a rupture of 'normal' spinal ligaments by hyperextension or hyperflexion. When a rotational or a shearing force was employed, ligamentous rupture and dislocations were readily produced. Selecki & Williams (1970) were critical of the (mainly) two-segment spinal unit used in Roaf's experiments, preferring to use the entire intact cervical spine. They stressed the importance of compression forces while agreeing that other components of the injury can often be demonstrated. It is generally agreed that cadaveric experiment can be misleading, and that radiographs show the resting position rather than the dynamics of the original displacement.

Stability

A fundamental consideration in the treatment of these injuries is an early decision on the stability of the cervical spine. Despite an immense amount of experimental work and clinical experience, there remains much confusion about this concept. In general terms, a stable fracture is one without ligamentous disruption. For example, the minor wedge fracture of a vertebral body following flexion−compression forces is a stable injury because the posterior ligaments are intact. In contrast, severe bursting injuries of the vertebral bodies, resulting from axial loading, may be unstable initially, although the ligamentous structures may be intact.

The term 'unstable' should be regarded as a relative one and is more properly applied to the acute stage of injury rather than as an indicator of ultimate stability. In the immediate post-injury phase, the spine is stable if the segments will not displace or angulate under physiological loads including active muscle contraction and normal nursing routines. Some would not agree with this, contending that it is prudent to regard all cervical injuries as potentially unstable until some weeks have elapsed from the time of injury. The spine can be regarded as stable at a later stage if there is no progressive deformity in the upright position and if there is no increasing neurological impairment. Others would regard all spinal injuries with immediate neurological impairment as unstable. It is difficult to reconcile this

with the central cord syndrome following extension injuries in spondylotic spines, or with injuries in congenital fusion of vertebral bodies where the spine often remains stable. In discussing the results of conservative treatment, Cheshire (1969) defined stability as 'the absence of movement between any pair of vertebrae, with or without pain or other clinical manifestations, when lateral X-rays of the cervical spine are taken in flexion and extension at the conclusion of treatment'. The study is interesting in a general context. There were 257 cases available for analysis; eliminating those patients in whom there was no possibility of late instability and those in whom early surgery was performed (only 12 cases), there remained 160 conservatively treated cases. In all the main groups, except one, the late instability rate was between 4.8 and 7.2%. The exception was in a group of 19 patients who had sustained anterior subluxations (flexion−rotation injuries). Four of these patients showed late instability: an incidence of 21%.

Nicoll (1949) offered a classification of dorso-lumbar fractures which distinguished stable from unstable injuries . This was later modified by Holdsworth (1963) to include the cervical spine and to introduce the concept of the 'posterior ligamentous complex'. This complex included the interspinous and supraspinous ligaments, the ligamenta flava and the capsules of the facet joints. The term is particularly applicable to the mid and lower cervical spine. Here the ligaments are weaker and the small posterior facet joints are almost horizontal, as distinct from the stronger ligaments and the vertically disposed articular processes of the thoraco-lumbar spine. Holdsworth believed that damage to this ligamentous complex was largely responsible for instability. It has been shown, however, that surgical division of the posterior ligamentous complex does not cause immediate instability, unless there is accompanying damage to the posterior longitudinal ligament or to the posterior annulus (disc).

In clinical practice, the author has assumed that damage to the posterior complex alone (a rare injury) may account for minor subluxations of the facet joints, many of which are stable initially, but that the commoner injury includes damage to the posterior longitudinal ligament or posterior annulus, or both, thus rendering the spine unstable. With this reservation the author believes that the notion is useful and pragmatically valid.

More recently, Denis (1983) formulated a classification of thoraco-lumbar injuries based on a description of a three-column spine. This important study addresses the spinal, as well as the neurological, injury and it goes a long way to identify the complex biomechanical problems. In the three-column theory, the anterior column is formed by the anterior longitudinal ligament, the anterior part of the vertebral body and the anterior annulus. The posterior column includes Holdsworth's posterior ligamentous complex as well as the bony posterior arch. The all-important middle column is formed by the posterior wall of the vertebral body, the posterior annulus and the posterior longitudinal ligament. The anterior column is compressed and the posterior column is distracted during flexion. The opposite happens in hyperextension (deflexion) when the posterior column is compressed and there is simultaneous distraction of the anterior column. In compression injuries the middle column remains intact and, acting as a hinge, allows the deforming force to bear on the anterior column and produce a wedge-shaped appearance of the vertebral body on lateral radiographs. The posterior height of the vertebral body is maintained. In contrast, bursting fractures result from failure of both anterior and posterior columns under axial loading. There is deformity and loss of depth of the vertebral body including its posterior wall, often with retropulsion and splaying of the posterior arch. In fracture−dislocations there is failure of all three columns under compression, rotation or shear. It will be appreciated that while the three-column concept is more pertinent to the thoracolumbar region, it forms a helpful basis when deciding on the stability of cervical injuries.

A number of biomechanical studies on cadaveric spines were conducted by White *et al.* (1975), in which it was found that under 'normal' conditions only very little movement was permitted between adjacent vertebrae. The angular movement between the vertebrae was 11° or less and the horizontal translation never exceeded 3 mm. Measurements exceeding these figures provide useful guidelines to instability. However, it should be noted that these measurements are only useful when there is obvious ligament damage and they do not apply to children or to patients with advanced spondylotic changes.

Bony injuries tend to stabilize with time and almost always heal by bone. In contrast, ligamentous injuries, where rotation plays a major role, heal badly, if at all, so that late pain and deformity are not uncommon.

When considering the stability of the spinal column, many have reflected on the parallel problem of instability of the spinal cord. Baker (1989) points out that deterioration in the injured spinal cord is almost certainly multifactorial and that under-oxygenation is a crucial element. He has shown that in the early post-injury stages the vertical position ('sitting up') may lead to hypotension and increasing neurological impairment.

Baker is also concerned about the safety of some of the measures used to secure stability, postulating that untimely intervention may lead to autoregulatory failure and diminished cord perfusion. Presumably the injured spinal cord is more vulnerable to diminished oxygen supply than the intact cord.

Pathology of spinal cord and nerve root injury

The neuropathology of the damaged spinal cord varies with the magnitude of the injuring force and the time of survival. Knowledge of the sequential events of the early post-injury phase is largely based on animal experiments which involve measurable compressive forces rather than the part torsional, part compressive damage associated with the clinical injury. The historical background to the subject has been reviewed by Dohrmann (1972).

In the model developed by Allen (1911) graduated weights were dropped through a hollow calibrated tube onto the spinal cord of laminectomized cats. The apparatus has been modified over the years; both the histological examination and the biochemical analysis have been greatly improved. There is general agreement that in experimental injuries the changes begin in the central grey matter with rupture of capillaries and diapedesis of red cells. The venules distend and areas of haemorrhage and ischaemia lead to infarction of the grey matter. The area of central haemorrhagic necrosis appears to be self perpetuating for a time and, in the more serious injuries, it may spread rostrally and caudally over many segments (Fig. 18.1). The changes soon extend into the more central white fibres with chromatolysis, oedema and vacuolation. A localized tissue anoxia (Kelly *et al.* 1970) and various toxic substances have been identified (Ducker *et al.* 1971, Osterholm & Matthews 1972). Pringle (1992) believes that on clinical grounds there would seem to be little doubt that the injured cord is vulnerable to hypotension and possibly hypoxia for many weeks following injury.

The immediate post-traumatic phase is followed by resorption and organization so that the damaged areas are replaced by a gliocollagenous scar. The injured long tracts show ascending and descending changes similar to the Wallerian degeneration of peripheral nerves, but occurring at a much slower rate. Hydromyelia and cyst formation may appear at a distance from the major injury (Fig. 18.2). In incomplete lesions many fibres escape and the glial scarring is more localized.

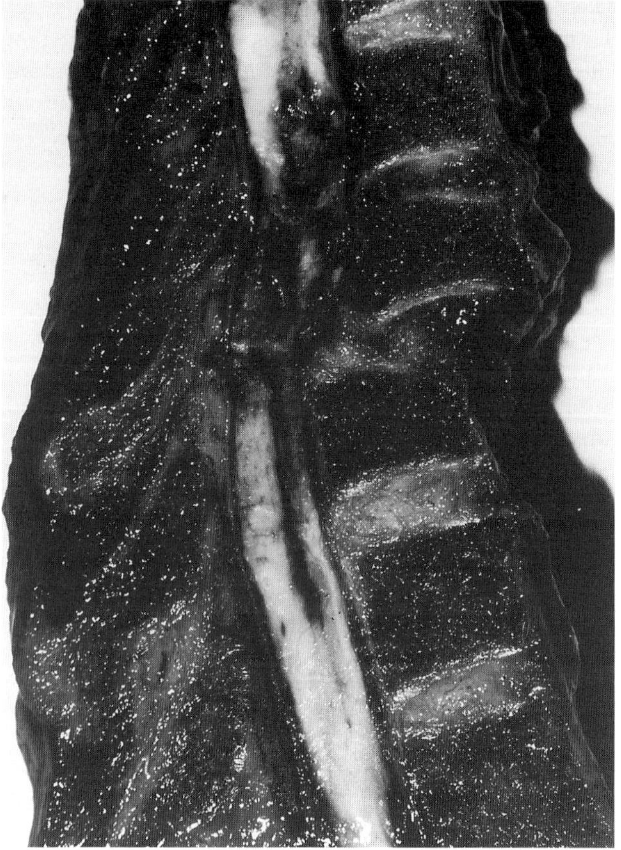

Fig. 18.1 Fracture–dislocation of the mid-cervical region showing the local damage and longitudinal extent of the injury.

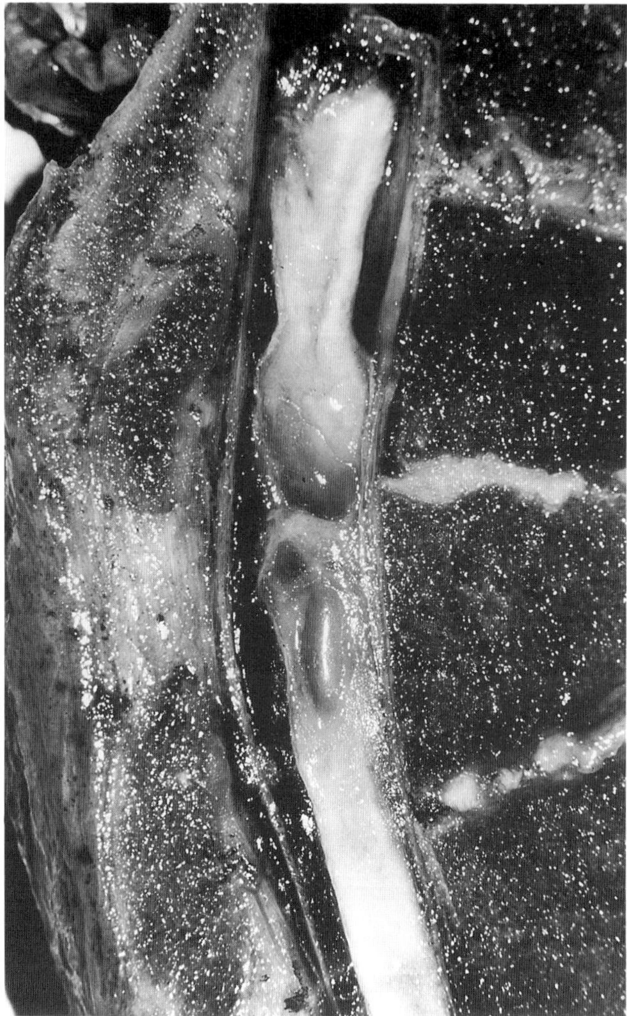

Fig. 18.2 Cyst formation and gliosis 15 years after incomplete cord lesion.

Effects of neurological injury

The results of the spinal injury, which are reflected in the paralysis of voluntary muscles and sensory impairment, require no detailed description. The effects on the autonomic nervous system, however, are less well understood. These include alterations in vasomotor and respiratory control and the emergence of unusual reflex patterns (Frankel *et al.* 1975) as well as the phenomenon of autonomic hyper-reflexia (Head & Riddoch 1917, Guttmann & Whitteridge 1947). There is disturbance of endocrine function and of bone metabolism. The loss of calcium and hydroxyproline leads to osteoporosis and a negative calcium balance. The loss is greatest during the first 6 months and exceeds that in patients confined to bed for other reasons. Heterotopic ossification may be related to autonomic dysfunction. Body temperature regulation is disturbed and this is an important consideration in varying climatic conditions. The effects are greatest in the cervical region and less marked below the mid-thoracic level where the autonomic outflow is reduced. There is an immediate loss of sphincter control in most serious cord injuries; the outcome for bowel and bladder function depends on the completeness, or otherwise, of the lesion, and on the skill in the total management of the patient.

Incomplete lesions may be classified into five main subgroups, recognizing that diagnosis is often difficult in the early days after injury, and that the classification does not offer an absolute prognostic index.

1 *Subtotal syndrome.* There is partial preservation of motor and sensory function below the level of injury. Rapid improvement during the first week implies a normal, or near normal, return of function. A similar, but transient, syndrome has been described by Torg *et al.* (1986) and by Ladd and Scranton (1986). The sensory effects include tingling, burning pain and impaired sensation with a varying degree of muscle weakness. The tempo of recovery is more rapid than in the usual subtotal syndrome, and recovery commences within 10–15 minutes. Pain in the neck is unusual; the 32 patients described by Torg and colleagues (1986) were mainly, but not exclusively, American football players. The author has encountered a number of similar cases in rugby players, trampoline accidents and in horse-riding injuries; four of these patients had congenital fusions of the cervical vertebrae. The hallmark of the syndrome is a statistically significant spinal stenosis. The syndrome has been attributed to neuropraxia of the spinal cord, produced by pressure or direct impact with transient abolition of axonal function. In this potentially dangerous situation it seems reasonable to preclude the individual from participation in contact sports. The advice is not always taken.

2 *Anterior cord syndrome.* This is associated with varying degrees of muscle paralysis with loss of pain and temperature appreciation. Posterior column function is generally not affected so that deep pressure sensation, and the sense of joint position and vibration are spared. The syndrome is attributed to compression or destruction of the anterior part of the cord. A similar picture accompanies thrombosis of the anterior spinal artery. The prognosis is bleak.

3 *Posterior cord syndrome.* This rare syndrome may follow every type of spinal injury but, classically, it occurs in hyperextension injuries with fractures of the posterior elements and in stab wounds (Lipschitz & Block 1962). There is no loss of muscle power or of thermal discrimination. Deep pain, proprioception and vibration are impaired. The prognosis is good but the patient is left with some degree of ataxia.

4 *Brown–Séquard syndrome.* This follows disproportionate damage to the cord as occurs in lateral flexion injuries, fractures of the lateral masses and open wounds (Lipschitz & Block 1962, Lipschitz 1976). The greater motor loss, the impaired sense of joint position and the loss of two-point discrimination are on the side of the injury. There is loss of pain and temperature appreciation on the opposite side of the body with minimal motor loss below the level of injury.

5 *Central cord syndrome.* This is the commonest of the incomplete syndromes and while it is usually associated with hyperextension injuries in older patients, it may occur in any type of spinal injury. There is a flaccid paralysis of the hands and a spastic paresis of the lower limbs in typical cases.

Injury to nerves

Any associated nerve injury assumes a much greater significance in the cervical region than elsewhere in the spinal column, and particularly so when the cord lesion is irrecoverable. Early reduction may considerably reduce the final neurological deficit, as has been shown by Braakman and Vinken (1967, 1968), and this equates with the author's experience. Primary brachial plexus injuries and root avulsions may follow severe lateral flexion injuries and imply a poor prognosis.

Comment

This cursory account does not necessarily explain the effects of the clinical injury where stretching and tearing of white fibres is a primary feature of severe torsional forces. Nevertheless, there is ample evidence to suggest that the major damage is central and, in effect, is similar to the central cord syndrome of cervical trauma. Raynor and Koplik (1985) have suggested that the recognized syndromes are not due to different mechanisms but represent a progression in the magnitude of the applied force with increasing severity of injury. Thus, gradations may be seen between the central cord syndrome, followed by the anterior cord syndrome and various incomplete lesions, culminating, in more severe cases, with the complete motor and sensory paralysis of physiological transection. It must be appreciated that incomplete cord lesions can be expected to make some neurological recovery, and that the paralysis following foraminal root compression, while aided by prompt reduction, tends to lessen in many cases.

Psychological effects

The long-term consequence of a serious spinal cord injury is a study in its own right and will be briefly considered in the section on rehabilitation. Even with lesser injuries there is often a prolonged period of anxiety and surgeons are only too familiar with the disability following many so-called whiplash injuries. Immediately after a serious cord injury there is usually a state of mental shock in which the patient does not seem to comprehend the gravity of the situation. This gives way to a gradual recognition which varies with age, intelligence and pre-accident personality. At this stage, the surgeon should discuss the implications and proposed procedures truthfully and sympathetically with the patient in the light of a clinical assessment. At the same time, the patient's relatives should be fully informed. To do this effectively requires experience, empathy and a little imagination, as well as an extension of understanding well beyond the framework of other traumatic conditions.

Clinical features

Injuries to the neck vary in severity and, to some extent, the incidence is governed by environmental factors, notably the increase in traffic accidents and recreational activities. As with all victims of trauma, the history and circumstances of the accident should alert the examiner to the likely patterns of injury. Pain and stiffness in the neck, swelling and loss of contour, spasm of the neck muscles producing an unusual posture, or a complaint of electric shock-like sensations in the limbs should arouse suspicion. In the unconscious patient the respiratory pattern, failure to produce a reflex withdrawal on painful stimuli, areflexia and flaccidity may provide useful clues. In practice, that overused phrase 'a high index of suspicion' has a special emphasis here.

A new dimension is added when the injury is accompanied by neurological impairment and the account which follows is mainly concerned with these injuries. The paralysis is usually instantaneous, some become paralysed in transit and, in a minority, the paralysis may be of gradual onset despite impeccable treatment. The latter form a thought-provoking subgroup, often with medico-legal implications.

Assessment and early management

The initial assessment of the injured patient has been discussed in Chapters 5 and 6, and in this section some repetition is unavoidable. Respiratory function is often so precarious in severe neck injuries that any additional embarrassment may be fatal. In ideal circumstances all the seriously injured should be examined by a doctor experienced in trauma care so that priorities are established. These include maintenance of the airway, arrest of haemorrhage with circulatory support and evaluation of associated injuries. These latter are uncommon in recreational accidents but cervical injuries are often missed in the multiply injured victim of road traffic and industrial accidents.

Respiratory aspects

Clinical experience and experimental studies (Kelly *et al.* 1970, Ducker *et al.* 1971) suggest that oxygenation is a vital factor in the survival of damaged neurological tissue and, conversely, that ischaemia and hypoxia are contributory causes in the failure of neurological recov-

ery. For this reason the author stresses that immediate attention should be paid to the airway and adequate oxygenation provided by a facemask. Has the patient vomited? Are fractures of the mandible or facial skeleton causing obstruction?

The presence of diaphragmatic breathing can be visually confirmed from the end of the bed by the relative immobility of the chest wall, the flaring of the lower ribs and the passive movements of the abdomen. Extreme anxiety associated with distended neck veins, absent breath sounds and tracheal deviation suggest a tension pneumothorax. This requires immediate relief by the insertion a large-bore needle into the second or third intercostal space in the mid-clavicular line. Palpation may reveal surgical emphysema or the paradoxical movement of a flail segment. Radiographs should help to confirm the nature of other intrathoracic lesions and the need for chest tube drainage or more extensive surgery.

Spirometric readings are repeated at frequent intervals (Fig. 18.3); a tidal volume of less than 800 ml is a cause for concern. Blood gas analysis is seldom an urgent requirement in uncomplicated cases, but when there are multiple injuries it is imperative to obtain a baseline assessment. A Pao_2 of less than 70 mmHg or a $Paco_2$ above 45 mmHg indicates the need for endotracheal intubation and ventilatory support. Nasopharyngeal and bronchial suction should be performed with caution as there is a danger of cardiac arrest or severe bradycardia. Prophylactic atropine is advised before these manoeuvres are carried out.

Respiratory care

Injuries in the upper cervical cord may be accompanied by temporary impairment in diaphragmatic function. Such injuries are often neurologically incomplete so that a short period of intermittent positive pressure ventilation (IPPV) is followed by spontaneous respiration.

With advances in cardiopulmonary resuscitation and the increased competence of ambulance crews, more patients now survive high cord lesions. Extensive damage above the C4 level leads to permanent ventilatory impairment and the need for some form of life-long respiratory support. The management of these tragic cases is beyond the scope of this chapter; the pioneering work of Glenn *et al.* (1980) and Glenn and Phelps (1985) should be consulted. The medical and philosophical problems have been described in papers from the Mersey Regional Spinal Injury Centre (Gardner *et al.* 1985, 1986).

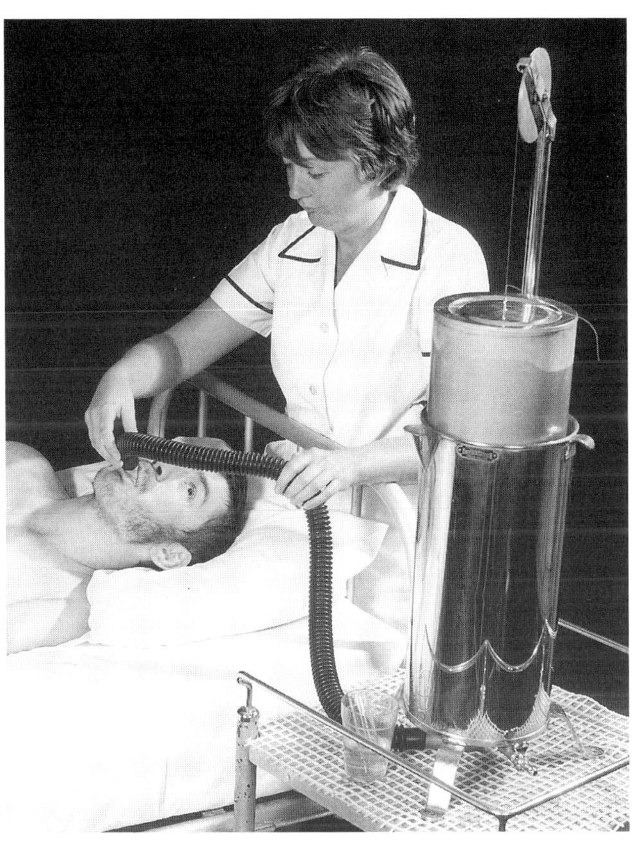

Fig. 18.3 Spirometric readings are a useful guide to respiratory function.

In the more usual cases the impairment in respiration is greatest in mid-cervical injuries and lessens at successively lower levels. Chest therapy should commence on admission and should be supervised by an experienced therapist. The patient is instructed and assisted in performing deep inspirations aided by percussion, manual vibration and gentle slapping of the chest (Fig. 18.4). The lower costal margin is manually stabilized by the physiotherapist and the patient is instructed to cough 'on command' while the chest is compressed (Fig. 18.5). Round-the-clock supervision is imperative and chest therapy sessions should follow each change of posture. All ward staff and relatives must be instructed in these procedures. Humidification is an aid in preventing respiratory complications and antibiotic therapy is advised in high-risk patients only. Endotracheal intubation will usually tide the patient over the early critical period. A preliminary lateral radiograph of the neck is recommended and the situation should be discussed with the anaesthetist.

Tracheotomy is seldom indicated, and then only for severe accompanying chest or head injuries. It is probably less dangerous than long continued endotracheal intubation, but both procedures carry special risks including that of tracheal stenosis.

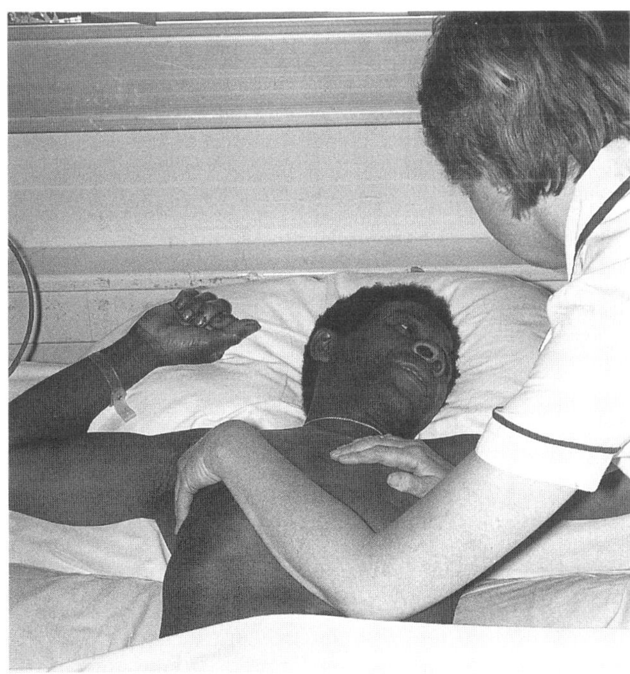

(a)

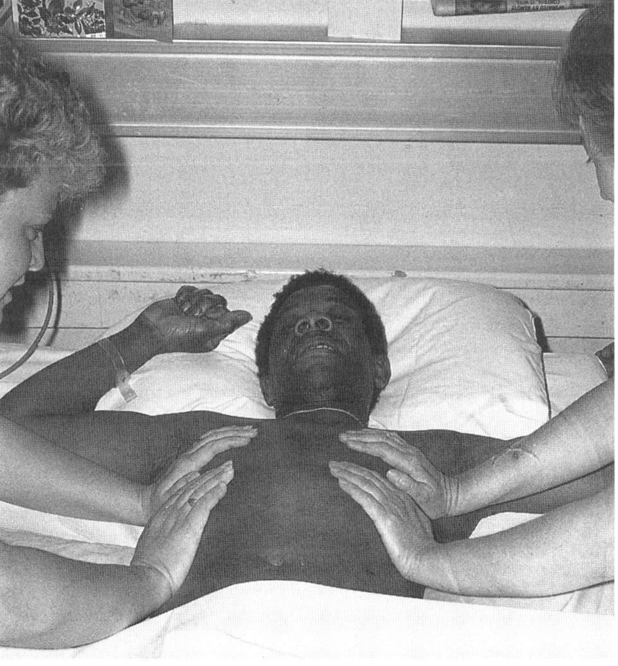

(b)

Fig. 18.4 (a) Round-the-clock chest therapy helps to obviate the need for tracheotomy in most patients. (b) Gentle percussion of the chest wall.

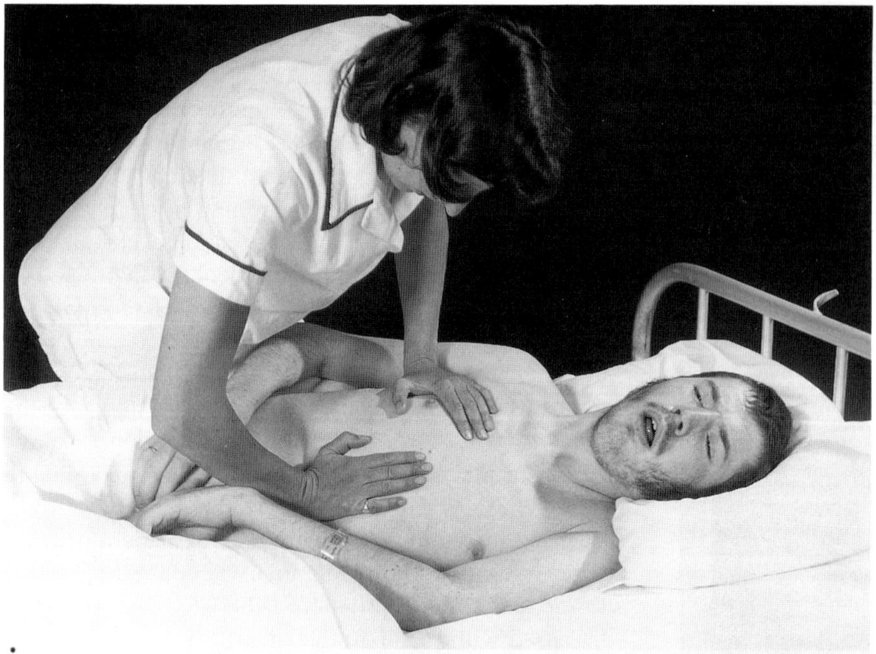

Fig. 18.5 The chest wall is stabilized while the patient coughs on command.

Circulatory support

In most serious injuries, blood loss and shock are synonymous. 'Shock' may be present without significant blood loss in patients with cord impairment. This is especially true of cervical injuries where a state of 'spinal shock', characterized by a slow pulse and a falling systolic pressure, may confuse the unwary. The hypotension follows on the sudden temporary failure of sympathetic control and the loss of the vasoconstrictor effect on the vascular bed. Vagal preponderance reduces the heart rate, adding to the circulatory impairment. Dopamine and other vasopressive drugs are of doubtful value and many of these patients are overtransfused. When the patient has suffered severe additional injuries the fall in blood pressure is often extreme. A clinical assessment of the amount of blood loss is made and an appropriate transfusion is arranged. Frequent auscultation of the lungs is necessary as large volumes of fluid may precipitate pulmonary oedema.

Care of the skin and joints

Various mechanical turning beds, notably the Egerton—Stoke Mandeville and the Keene Roto-rest bed, are now in common use. They should not be regarded as a substitute for good nursing care. In default of a mechanical bed, the patient is nursed on a foam mattress, at least 15 cm in depth, which rests on a firm base. The patient is turned at 2-hourly intervals using a log-rolling technique while the neck is carefully controlled. Pillows are placed under and between the legs to prevent pressure sores and foot pillows guard against equinus deformity. The upper limbs are supported on pillows while the patient is in the supine position. The arms are abducted to 45° with the elbows extended. The arms are alternatively held suspended in a roller towel when the patient lies in the lateral position. Daily washing of the skin is essential and areas of redness or abrasions are noted. Synthetic fabrics should be avoided as they lead to excessive moisture and maceration of the skin. Natural sheepskin may be used with confidence.

These remarks may appear prosaic and of greater concern to the nursing staff, but the team approach is of the utmost importance and the overlap of duties between nurses, physiotherapist and occupational therapist cannot be overemphasized. While each has his or her special responsibility there is no place for rigid demarcation in the treatment of these patients.

All paralysed joints are put through a full range of movement following each turn or at 2-hourly intervals during the early weeks. Pericapsulitis of the shoulders is a real threat in older patients and is often helped by local hydrocortisone injections. The unopposed action of the biceps quickly leads to incorrigible contracture of the elbows unless the arms are kept in extension. The hands often develop a curious oedema which may not readily respond to elevation or other measures. Even pressure is applied using a modified 'boxing glove' bandage (Fig. 18.6). The finger joints are put through a

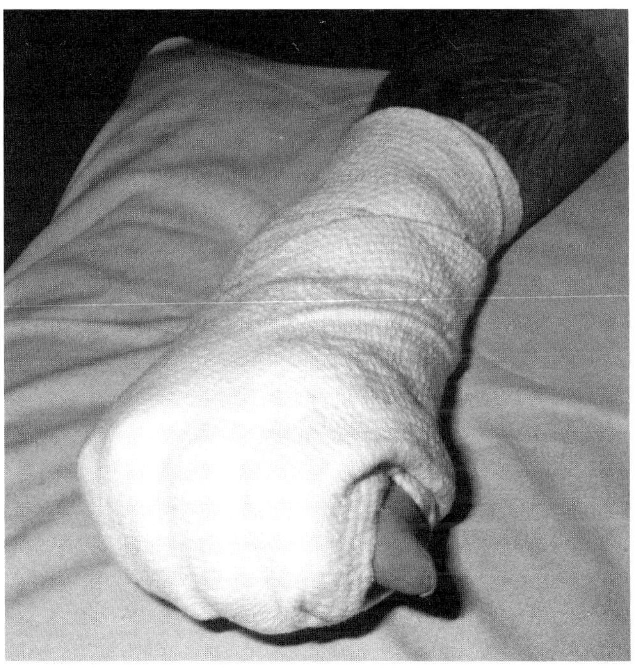

(a)

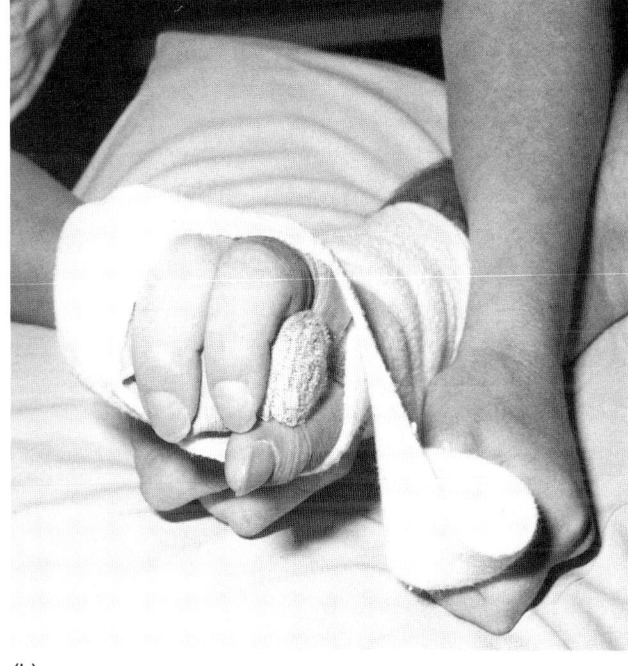

(b)

Fig. 18.6 (a) 'Boxing glove' bandage and elevation of the arm to lessen oedema. (b) Change and reapply at intervals to prevent sores.

full range of movement and the impairment in sensation requires that the bandages are frequently removed. The wrists are maintained in dorsiflexion by the intermittent use of light cock up splints. Some weeks later the hands are bandaged over a cotton wool pad with the metacarpophalangeal joints flexed almost to 90° and the interphalangeal joints to between 10° and 30°. This will encourage a useful tenodesis effect. At this stage mechanical hand-exercise machines are useful (Fig. 18.7).

Early urological care

Retention with overflow will follow most spinal injuries unless the bladder is drained. As a rule, there is no urgency to pass a catheter during the first 24 hours; at this time there is relative suppression of renal function and the bladder is toneless. Exceptions must be made (i) when an injury to the urinary tract is suspected, (ii) if the patient has taken a large amount of fluid immediately before the accident, and (iii) when a large transfusion is necessary because of associated injuries.

In most instances and when the fluid intake is controlled, a regimen of 8-hourly intermittent catheterization is advised. This is performed with a full aseptic ritual, using a non-touch technique and a disposable catheter (Fig. 18.8). The initial catheterization should be performed by one of the medical staff.

When a large transfusion in anticipated (as in (iii) above) it is wise to use an indwelling balloon catheter for monitoring purposes and to adopt the intermittent regimen as soon as possible. Eight-hourly catheterization is appropriate for a daily fluid intake of 1500 ml. As the fluid intake is increased, a less rigid regimen is appropriate. When an indwelling catheter is required, the fluid intake is increased to 3 l, the urine is acidified and antibiotic therapy is advised.

In young women, a modified suprapubic catheterization is now often favoured until reflex micturition is established.

The prognosis and quality of life largely depend on a well-regulated follow-up. Parsons (1992) in describing contemporary management of the neuropathic bladder reflects on the improved survival of these patients and the rarity of renal complications.

Associated injuries

Dislocations are promptly reduced and long bone fractures are realigned and immobilized on pillows or on well-padded splints. Definitive surgery may be undertaken later, usually by internal fixation. Computerized tomography (CT) is essential in the unconscious patient and when an intracranial injury is suspected. Abdominal injuries present a difficult diagnostic problem.

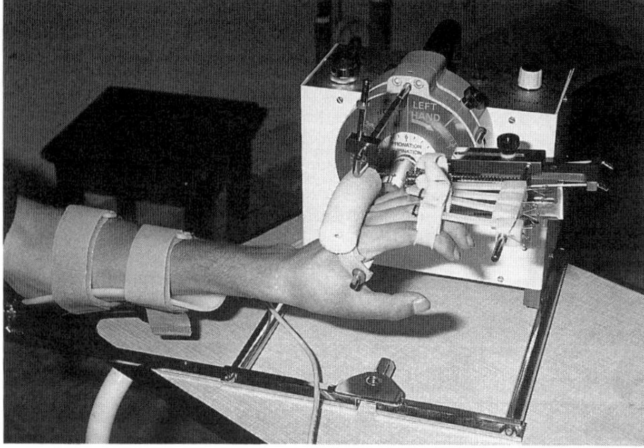

Fig. 18.7 Mechanical aid for finger movements at a later stage.

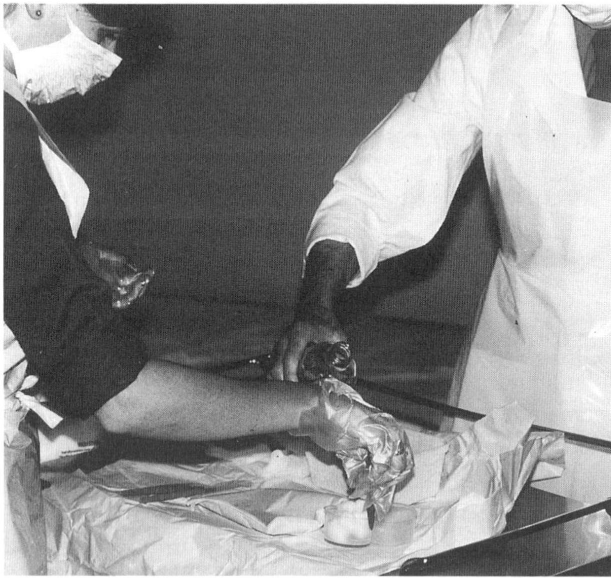

Fig. 18.8 Aseptic technique for catheterization.

Nausea, vomiting, excessive facial sweating and shoulder-tip pain should arouse suspicion. Abdominal guarding is not a feature. Peritoneal lavage is helpful in establishing the diagnosis. Bowel sounds may be present for many hours after injury but some degree of ileus is inevitable and is often most marked 48 hours later. Food should not be given and oral fluids are withheld or restricted. A nasogastric tube should be passed. Intestinal bleeding and acute gastric ulcers complicate a minority of cases; cimetidine or similar H_2 antagonists are useful.

Pharmacology

In the immediate post-injury phase there is a loss of electrical activity, membrane dysfunction and leakage across the blood/spinal cord barrier.

As the axoplasm fragments, secondary processes, including ischaemia and lowering oxygen tension, supervene. Many agents, including naloxone, nimo-dipine and thyrotropin-releasing hormones, have been investigated in the hope of interrupting, or otherwise modifying, this sequence of events. Foremost among these are the glucocorticoids which, in animal experiments, have been shown to limit the oedema and histological changes in the contused spinal cord.

By analogy with the reported beneficial effect of steroids in cerebral oedema, methylprednisolone has been advocated in the acute phase of spinal cord injury. Early experience was disappointing, but it now appears that the conventional dosage was too small, and in the author's cases the risks of sepsis and haematemesis appeared unacceptably high, particularly in the older age group (central cord syndrome).

A multicentre, double-blind randomized clinical trial was undertaken by an American study group (Bracken *et al.* 1985). No significant difference in neurological recovery was observed at 1 year, using 1 g bolus doses of methylprednisolone followed by 1 g daily for 10 days. Meanwhile, further experimental evidence suggested that the dose of methylprednisolone was too low. In a second trial (Bracken *et al.* 1990) methylprednisolone was given to 162 patients in an initial bolus of 30 mg per kilogram of body weight followed by infusion at 5.4 mg kg^{-1} h^{-1} for 23 hours. Patients who started treatment within 8 hours of injury showed a significant improvement in motor function, sensation to pin prick and touch at 6 months. In a second group naloxone was given to 154 patients as a bolus of 5.4 mg kg^{-1} followed by a 23-hour maintenance dose of 4.0 mg kg^{-1} h^{-1}. No significant improvement was noted over 171 patients who received a placebo.

It was concluded that, in patients with an acute spinal cord injury treatment with methylprednisolone in the dose used in the study improves neurological recovery when the medication is given in the first 8 hours. While the results of this trial are encouraging, further clinical experience is awaited with interest.

A further impetus to pharmacological research is supported by a pilot study on the clinical use of mono-sialotetrahexosyl-ganglioside (GM-1) undertaken at the Shock Trauma Centre of the Maryland Institute of Emergency Medical Services in Baltimore (Geisler *et al.* 1991). The study comprised 34 patients, of whom 16 were included in the GM-1 group and 18 in a placebo group. All patients were treated in accordance with the protocol in use at the Shock Trauma Centre, which included prompt surgical decompression of neural elements if closed spinal realignment failed to relieve the compression.

The GM-1-treated group improved more than the placebo-treated group, but the study sample was not large enough to permit a simultaneous analysis of the timing of intervention, the level of severity of injury, management-related variables or other categories of patients.

The authors report a greater than expected neurological recovery at 1 year, and suggest further studies to confirm the clinical benefit and safety of GM-1.

Other aspects

Assessment, resuscitation and diagnosis are a continuous process in which the anxiety of the patient and relatives should not be forgotten. The Accident department is not normally the setting for protracted explanations, but the surgeon should not shirk responsibilities; the projected treatment and its aims should be outlined. In the more serious cases (complete lesions) it is as well to remember that the prognosis remains in doubt for many weeks and that improvement is likely in incomplete lesions. Truthfulness based on experience is essential in answering leading questions. These are seldom posed by the patient but, understandably, the relatives may enquire and are entitled to a sympathetic and more candid account. Relatives will appreciate that a fuller explanation will follow provided that the initial discussion is factual and honest.

Neurological examination

The initial neurological assessment should be performed in a quiet area. It should be done in an unhurried and systematic manner and should be carefully documented. A prepared proforma is useful. The conscious patient may be all too aware of the extent of the paralysis, but difficulties arise when the patient is intoxicated or has suffered a head injury.

The history from the patient or witnesses may indicate the mechanism of injury and establish whether the onset of the paralysis was immediate or delayed. In general terms, paralysis of gradual onset has a better prognosis. At this stage, joint movement rather than the action of individual muscles is tested, with allowance being made for inhibition due to pain or apprehension.

The relative dryness of the skin, localized sweating, nasal congestion and conjunctival redness are usual features at this stage. There is often a zone of hyperpathia at the junctional area or the patient may complain of painful sensations in the territory of a single nerve root. This is helpful in defining the sensory level. Each sensory modality, including light touch, pin prick, vibration and joint position sense, is noted. Particular attention is necessary in testing for sensory preservation over the sacral area and in the perineum. To this end, the patient may be gently rolled onto the side while an assistant controls the neck. Sacral sparing is a hopeful sign and suggests an incomplete lesion. Two important cutaneous reflexes are now tested. The bulbocavernosus reflex (S2/S4) is elicited by squeezing the glans penis or compressing the clitoris, while noting the contraction (or otherwise) of the bulbocavernosus muscle and anal sphincter. The anal skin reflex (anal wink) is evoked when the skin around the anus is stimulated with a pin. Both reflexes are in abeyance following serious cord injuries and, with other signs, are manifestations of 'spinal shock'. This phenomenon, implying the transient suppression of nervous function below the level of transection, was described by Hall (1841). There is considerable controversey about this subject (Guttmann 1976) but it is generally agreed that in complete transverse lesions these cord-mediated reflexes reappear within 24−48 hours. At the same time the unpredictable nature of neurological recovery or deterioration after spinal cord injury should be noted. Temporary or permanent ascent of the paralysis, dramatic recovery within days or weeks of an apparently complete lesion and a modest improvement in neurological states over some years are relatively familiar phenomena.

The favourable prognosis in incomplete cord lesions has already been mentioned. Neurological deterioration may occur because of redisplacement of the vertebral column or manifest compression by displaced disc or bone. Surgical intervention is often indicated, having excluded other causes of deterioration.

If there is no evidence of sensory sparing or return of voluntary muscle power below the level of spinal cord injury and when an anal skin reflex is present or a positive bulbocavernosus reflex can be elicited, then the cord lesion is complete. Not all clinicians would accept this statement in its dogmatic form, but in the author's experience, patients judged to have sustained a complete lesion by these criteria do not make a useful functional recovery below the level of cord injury.

The neurological examination is repeated at frequent intervals without tiring the patient and it is wise to request independent findings from an experienced colleague. Many experienced observers would agree that the ultimate functional recovery is more accurately reflected by the degree and extent of the neurological impairment shortly after the injury than by the type of bony injury or displacement. Equally so, if the cord lesion is incomplete from the outset, then the prognosis is much better.

Certain key muscles offer a useful guide. The response of deltoid and biceps (C5); wrist extensors (C6); triceps, pronators and flexor carpi radialis (C7); finger flexors (C8); and intrinsic muscles of the hand (T1) should be noted. Joint movement is less well defined in the lower limbs where individual muscles are innervated from more than one spinal segment. Familiarity with the contour of the dermatomes is important when investigating the sensory disturbance. The extent of the C4 dermatome and the fact that it becomes continuous with T2/T3, over the front of the chest, and with T3/T4, over the scapular area, should not be overlooked. Reference to a pictorial atlas is an advantage and the recently revised *Aids to the Examination of the Peripheral Nervous System* (Guarantors of *Brain* 1986) is especially informative. It is a sad reflection that some of these serious injuries may not be recognized on the first examination (Ravichandran & Silver 1982); this carries the risk of increasing the neurological deficit, quite apart from the medico-legal implications. Prejudgement because of intoxication, the presence of intracranial or associated injuries, minimal or misinterpreted neurological signs and failure to insist on appropriate radiographs are the common causes of misdiagnosis. Another unpardonable error in the initial examination is to attribute an inappropriate muscle response on command, or an unfamiliar pattern of sensory loss, to hysteria or another imaginary cause.

Prevention of deep vein thrombosis

Pulmonary embolism is a major risk in the early weeks after a serious spinal injury. Anticoagulant therapy should be maintained for 10–12 weeks; passive movement of the limbs, use of full length antithrombotic stockings and the avoidance of constipation are important measures.

Radiology

The surgeon should be present during the preliminary radiological examination in the Accident department and should be available for consultation with the radiologist when more detailed investigations are required. A lateral radiograph of the cervical spine is the first essential and in the unconscious patient this is combined with a radiograph of the skull when a CT scan is anticipated. Only high-quality pictures are acceptable

and these must include the cervico-cranial and the cervico-thoracic areas. Magnetic resonance imaging (MRI) has presented a remarkable advance in diagnosis especially in patients presenting neurological features or equivocal radiographic findings.

Effacement of the normal lordosis (with due allowance for age) is suspicious (Fig. 18.9), as is interruption of the harmonious outline of the bony canal. Unusual angulation of a vertebral body demands further radiological investigation. Transoral views will display the atlanto-axial area. The superimposed shoulder shadows may obscure the lower cervical vertebrae; this can be overcome by downward traction on the arms (Fig. 18.10).

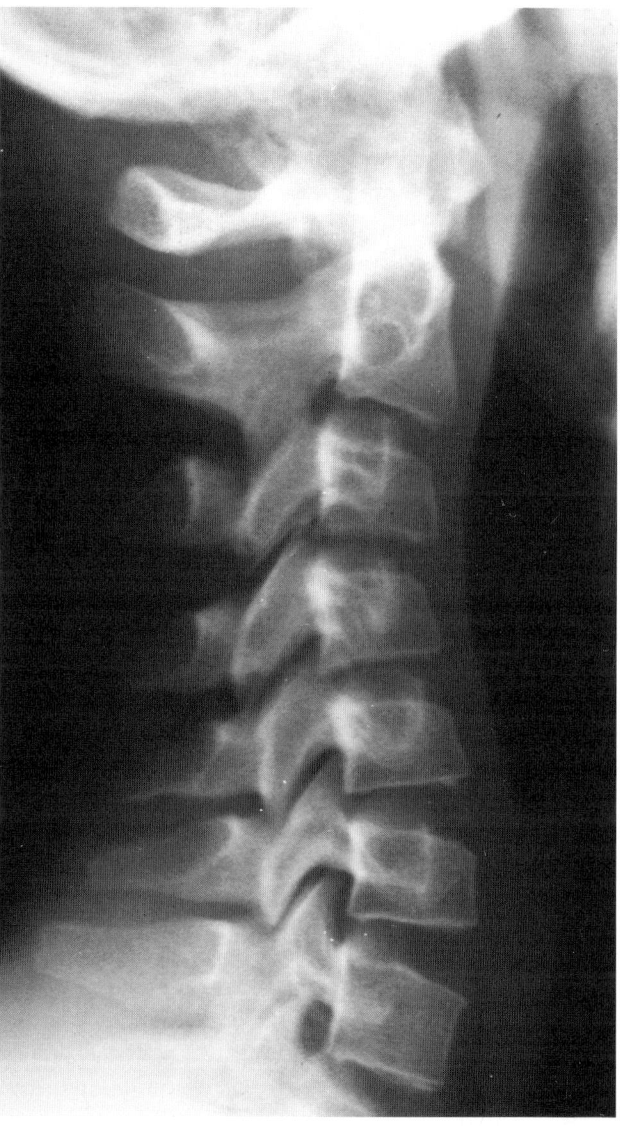

Fig. 18.9 Loss of the harmonious outline of the bony canal should arouse suspicion. This patient has sustained a severe whiplash injury.

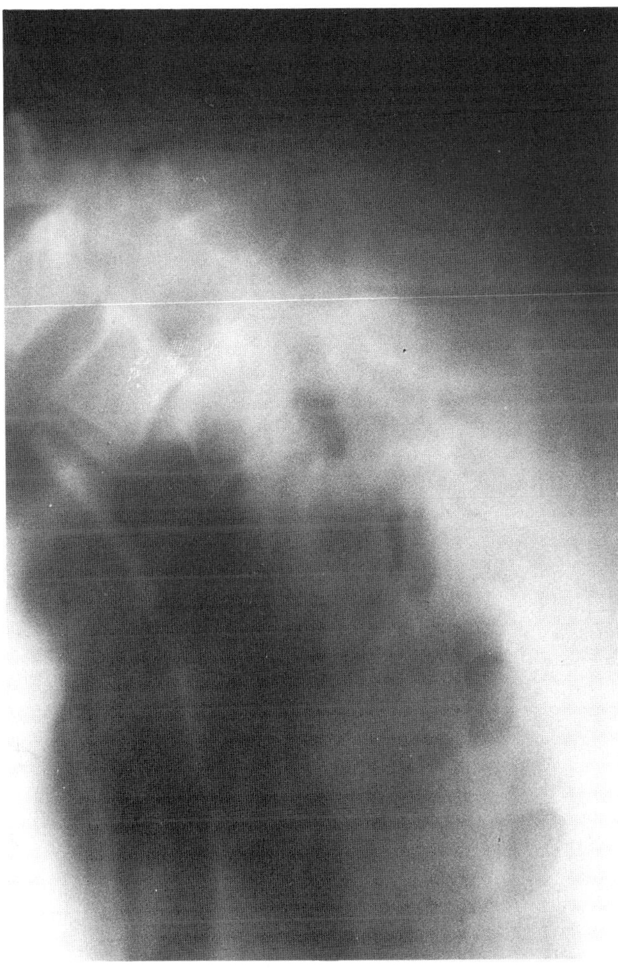

Fig. 18.10 Pain and muscle spasm cause elevation of the shoulder girdles. Sustained downward traction on the arms helps to overcome this and will help to display the cervico-thoracic junction.

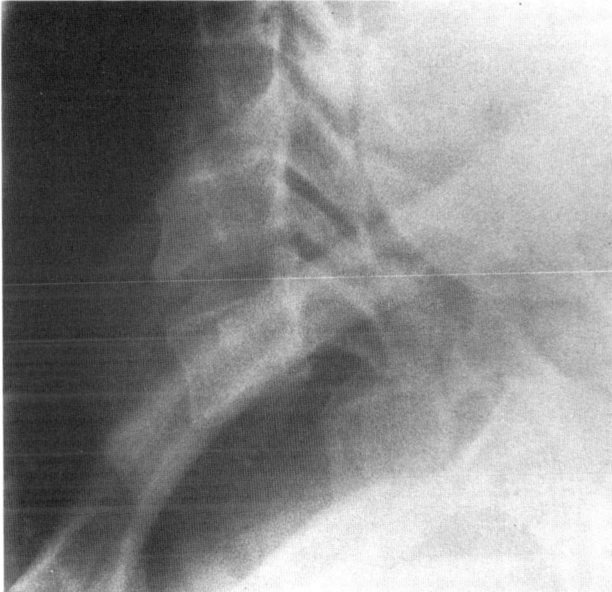

Fig. 18.11 Abduction elevation of the arm is useful in displaying this injury, which is frequently overlooked.

The swimmer's view (Scher & Vambeck 1977) is an additional help (Fig. 18.11). Fractures of the odontoid and dislocations of C7 on T1 are frequently missed when these simple precautions are neglected.

Severe ligamentous injuries may occur without overt bony damage and luxations may spontaneously reduce during transit. A large pre-vertebral shadow (the haematoma) may be the only indication as to the severity of the injury (Fig. 18.12). Penning (1980) measured the normal pre-vertebral soft tissue width from C1 to C7. He estimated the upper limits of 'normal' (in millimetres) as C1 (10), C2 (5), C3 (7), C4 (7), C5 (6) and C7 (20). No correction was made for radiological magnification of about 1.3. Weir (1975) concluded that a pre-vertebral soft tissue shadow of over 5 mm at C3 provided indirect evidence of injury. Undue widening of the interspace between the spinous processes (Fig. 18.13)

suggests damage to the posterior ligamentous complex (Webb *et al.* 1976).

The anteroposterior radiographs are examined for deviation of a spinous process and for widening of the interspinous distance. Tilting of an articular process or compression fractures of the facet joints are often accompanied by a scoliotic angulation. Fractures of the laminae may be observed.

The hypermobility of the cervical spine in children is confusing (Cattell & Filtzer 1965) but a short period of recumbency followed by dynamic views will usually clarify the position. Step formation and hypermobility at the C2/3 level has been mistaken for subluxation (Fig. 18.14). The child may present after an injury when muscle spasm may compound the problem. Traction in recumbency for a few days is advised with a careful radiological follow-up. True subluxation does occur, usually in older children, as evidenced by a large pre-vertebral shadow and later calcification or ossification in the interspinous ligament between C2 and C3 (Fig. 18.15).

Congenital anomalies, including variants of the Klippel–Feil syndrome, absence of the odontoid and developmental atlanto-axial instability, may present for the first time after an injury (Fig. 18.16). Acute neurological impairment of variable progression may follow comparatively trivial injuries in such cases.

The supine oblique views described by McCall *et al.* (1973) will display deformation of the intervertebral

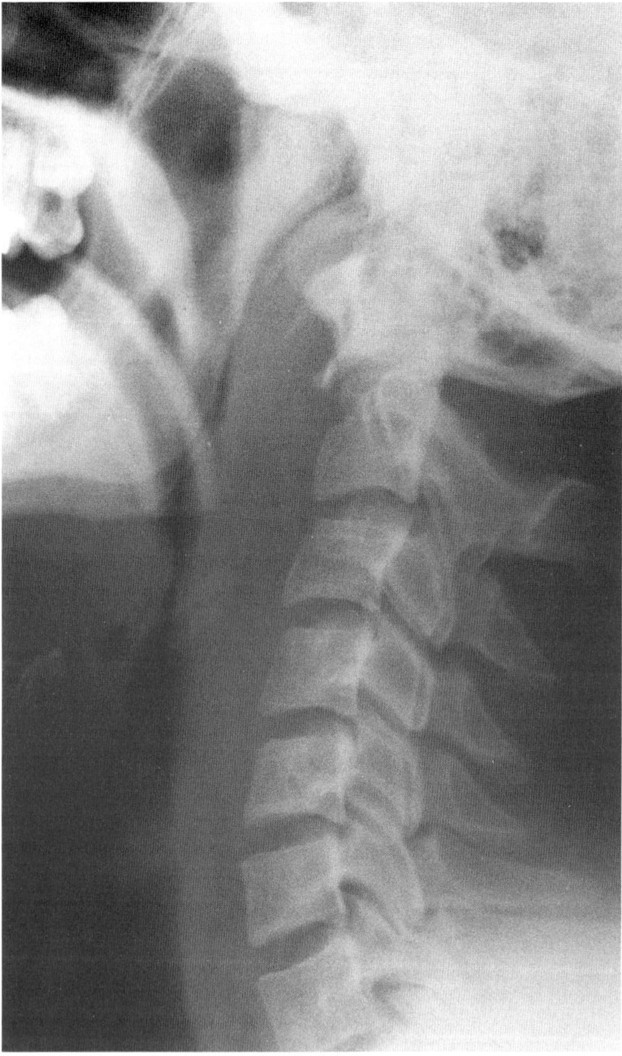

Fig. 18.12 A large pre-vertebral haematoma requires further investigation (note the fracture of the odontoid process).

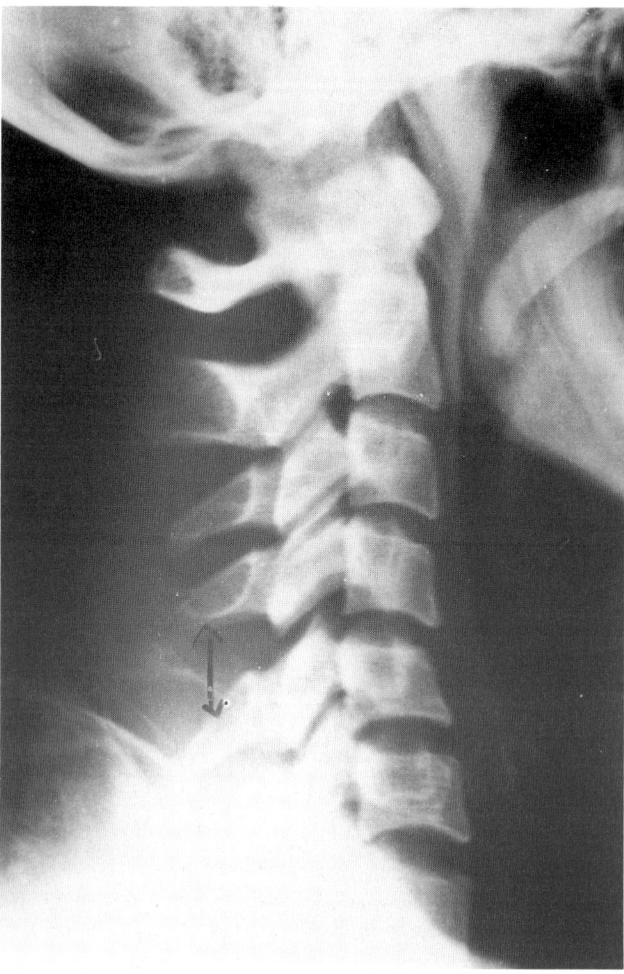

Fig. 18.13 Widening of the interspinous space suggests the probability of a ligamentous injury.

foramina and are useful in lateralizing luxations of the facet joints (Fig. 18.17). They have the merit that the patient's neck need not be moved during the procedure.

The basic radiographs will display most of the common injuries of the cervical spine and these should be carefully reviewed before imaging techniques are arranged. A CT scan is especially helpful in demonstrating the bony posterior arch and the size and shape of the spinal canal (Fig. 18.18). In 'burst' fractures, retropulsion and encroachment of bony fragments are readily depicted. The indication for contrast enhancement (metrizamide) CT in the acute phase of injury remains controversial, but it should be considered when the findings of conventional radiography are not in keeping with the patient's clinical signs.

MRI is the best method of identifying soft tissue damage following spinal column injury. Herniated disc material and bony fragments can be accurately located, but the most significant advance offered by the technique is that the nature and degree of damage to the spinal cord can be assessed.

Clinical features and treatment of the vertebral column injury

The foregoing account has emphasized the neurological aspects of spinal trauma, but it should be remembered that most of these injuries are unassociated with a neural deficit. The aim in both circumstances is to ensure a stable column by the simplest method, avoiding neurological mishaps or late deformity. There are differences of opinion on how this should be achieved. Interpretation of the findings requires close communication

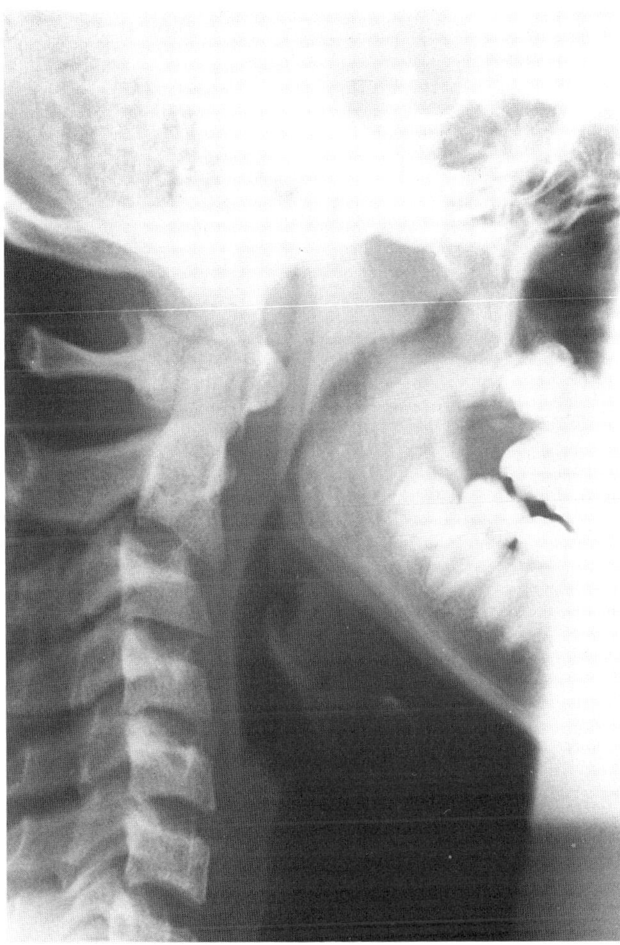

Fig. 18.14 Hypermobility of C2 on C3 in a 10-year-old male patient. Symptoms resolved in 24 hours when further radiographs showed a normal appearance.

between the radiologist and the surgeon. Irreversible damage to the cord can usually be recognized. In contrast, the correlation between potential sources of cord compression and the presenting neurological signs must be made with caution.

The less severe injuries, including sprains and so-called whiplash injuries, are not considered in detail here. They form a large part of orthopaedic practice, often with medico-legal overtones. They require appropriate sedation, immobilization in a collar and early physiotherapy directed towards strengthening the neck muscles. A factual explanation predicated on a careful analysis of the clinical features and the radiographs is essential.

In more severe injuries, the conservative school would argue that natural stability will be achieved in a reasonable time following realignment of most injuries involving bone. The time factor and late pain are important

considerations and for these reasons many surgeons advocate early fusion where the ultimate stability is in doubt. The decision is easier in predominantly ligamentous injuries where the consensus favours early localized fusion; similar remarks apply to late instability.

Much of the controversy centres round the treatment of those injuries associated with neurological impairment and the notion of what constitutes a complete neurological lesion. Alan Hardy, with a vast experience of these injuries, has often posed the question 'How complete is complete?' Many authorities believe that it is impossible to know with certainty the extent of the cord damage in the first 48 hours or the real significance of intraspinal bony fragments or extruded disc material and advise early decompression. The author has found this approach to be disappointing in a limited personal experience and has not been convinced that the marginal improvement in neurological gains following 'decompressions' in other series are rightly attributable to the intervention. Most experienced surgeons will recall anecdotal cases where decompression has been followed by a remarkable recovery but the author knows of no large series which unequivocally supports the more aggressive approach. Paradoxically, late decompression has given satisfactory results in selected cases. The more widespread and critical analysis of MRI findings may help to identify the indications for surgical intervention (Silberstein *et al.* 1992). Accepting that in most cases the greatest damage to the spinal cord occurs at the moment of injury, then the need for exploration would be clarified were it possible to estimate the *degree* of cord compression (by disc or bony fragment) and its effect on the neurological outcome.

Immediate measures

Sprains, whiplash injuries, minor compression fractures and hyperextension injuries in older patients presenting with a central cord syndrome may be treated by immobilization of the neck in an inflatable collar or similar device. Isolated fractures of spinous or transverse processes may be treated in the same way, provided that other associated cervical injuries are excluded.

In almost all other injuries, skull traction should be applied (Fig. 18.19). Dislocations, fracture—dislocations and distortions of a vertebral body require prompt reduction or realignment.

Various types of skull calipers are available (Fig. 18.20). The characteristics and limitations of the individual instruments have been described by Minns and Sutton (1985). Crutchfield calipers (Crutchfield 1954, 1966) are useful as temporary measures and where later

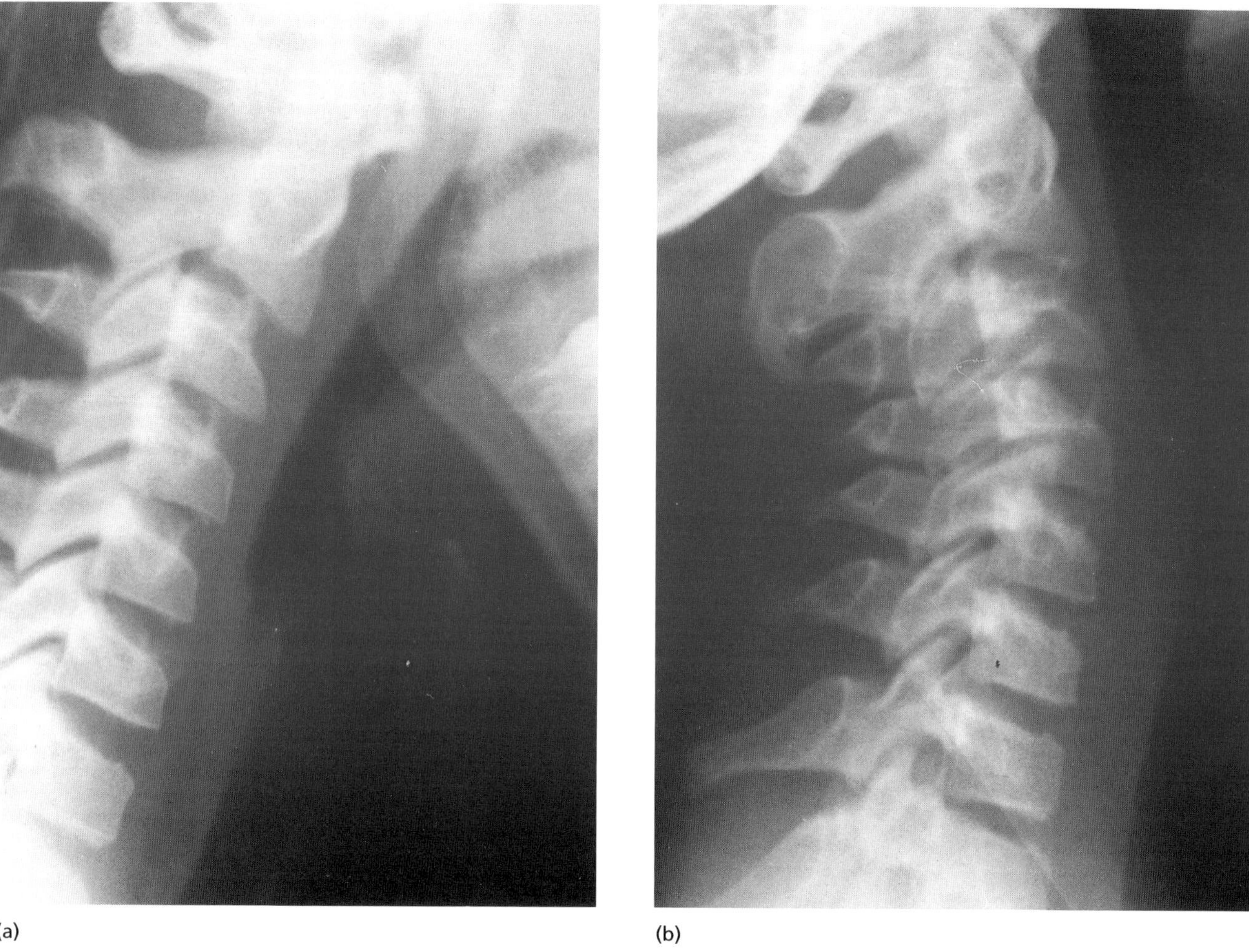

Fig. 18.15 (a) A more severe injury. Discomfort and restriction of movement persisted for many weeks. (b) Radiographs at 3 months showed ossification in the interspinous ligament.

application of a halo is anticipated. The Cone type of caliper (Cone & Turner 1937) is favoured by many; the author's personal preference is for the Gardner–Wells spring-loaded instrument (Gardner 1973). Immediate application of a halo is favoured by some surgeons in selected cases. The author prefers to use skull calipers until investigations are complete and a definitive decision can be made (Fig. 18.21).

Individual injuries

There are good reasons for separately discussing injuries of the upper cervical spine (above C3) from those of the mid and lower cervical regions (McSweeney 1992). Some of the injuries above C3 are immediately fatal. Many escape neural damage but if this occurs, there is no set pattern of neurological impairment. Often, a bizarre and widespread paralysis is quickly reversed and cranial

nerve palsies may confuse the picture (Grundy *et al.* 1984). In the absence of a neurological deficit, occipital or postauricular pain may be incorrectly attributed to the head injury. The injuring force is commonly applied directly through the base of the skull to the C1–C2 complex. Apart from acute atlanto-axial dislocations and displaced fractures near the waist of the dens, many of these will heal spontaneously, given efficient immobilization.

Atlanto-occipital dislocation

The real incidence of this injury is unknown, largely because rigor mortis obscures the instability between the head and neck at autopsy. Bucholz and Burkhead (1979) described the *post mortem* findings in nine cases and discussed the mechanism of injury. There are reported cases of 22 survivors (Ramsay *et al.* 1986), at

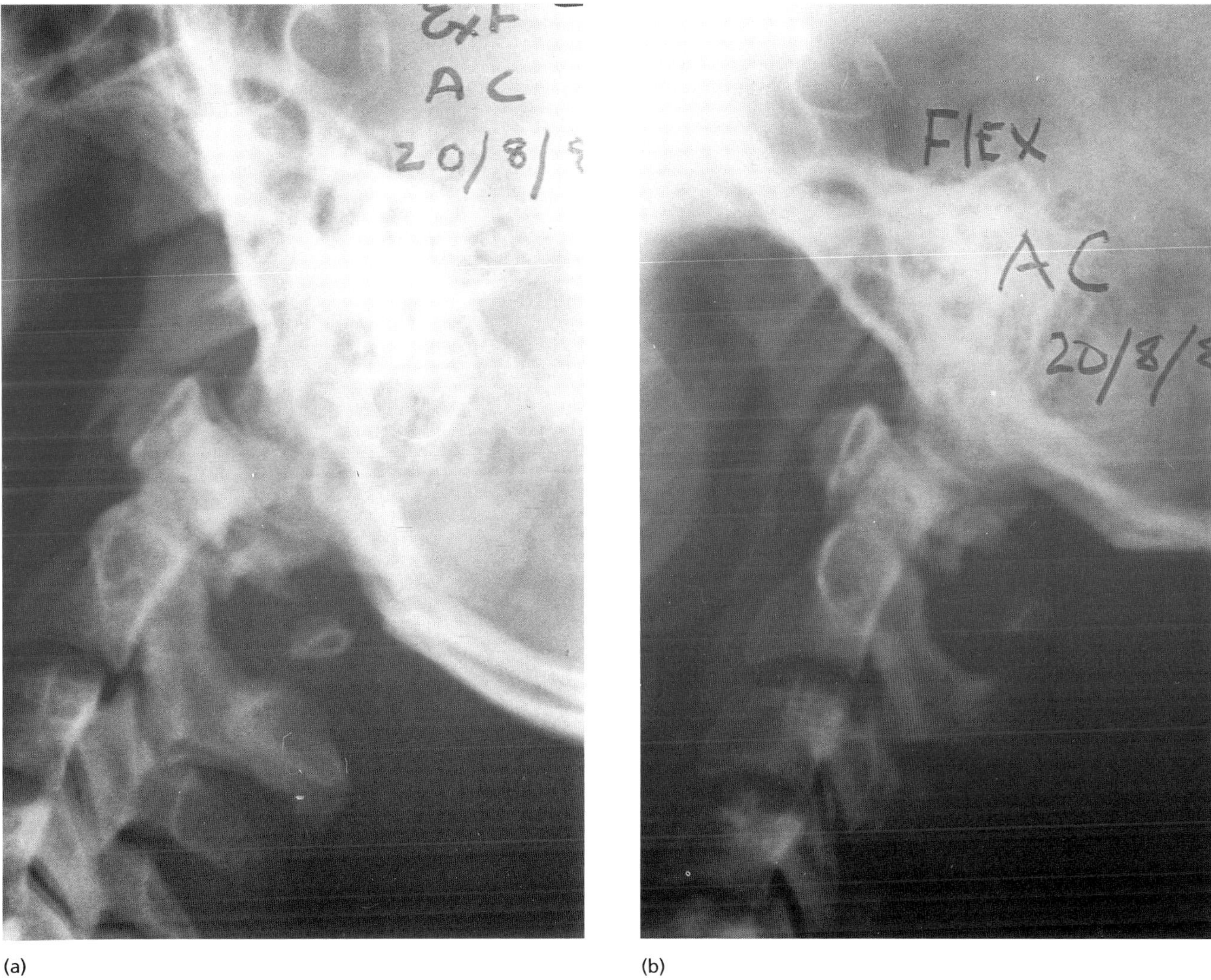

(a)

(b)

Fig. 18.16 (a) Congenital aplasia of the atlas. There was one episode of transient paresis following a fall from a horse. The admission radiograph shows posterior displacement of the skull. (b) Flexion of the head under sedation resulted in early neurological recovery. The injury was observed over an uneventful 3-year period. Fusion was not advised despite a minor degree of posterior instability.

least three of whom had no localizing neurological signs at the initial examination. Other cases have presented with respiratory impairment, bradycardia and a spastic tetraparesis resembling the cruciate paralysis described by Bell (1976). A large retropharyngeal haematoma and the distraction produced by skull traction should arouse suspicion (Fig. 18.22). Following a period of light skull traction and general supportive measures, a posterior occipito-cervical fusion is the treatment of choice. In some cases, reduction under general anaesthesia has been achieved within a few days of injury.

Unilateral dislocation may occur in association with injuries of the C1–C2 complex, and occipito-cervical fusion has been satisfactory (Fig. 18.23). Most of the survivors have made a satisfactory recovery.

Fractures of the atlas

Isolated fractures of the posterior arch are caused by hyperextension and axial loading. Confusion may arise with congenital anomalies (Fig. 18.24). The fracture is usually bilateral and occurs near the grooves for the vertebral vessels; the great occipital nerve may be injured. A pre-vertebral haematoma is not a feature. Immobilization in a collar for 8 weeks is normally sufficient to secure healing.

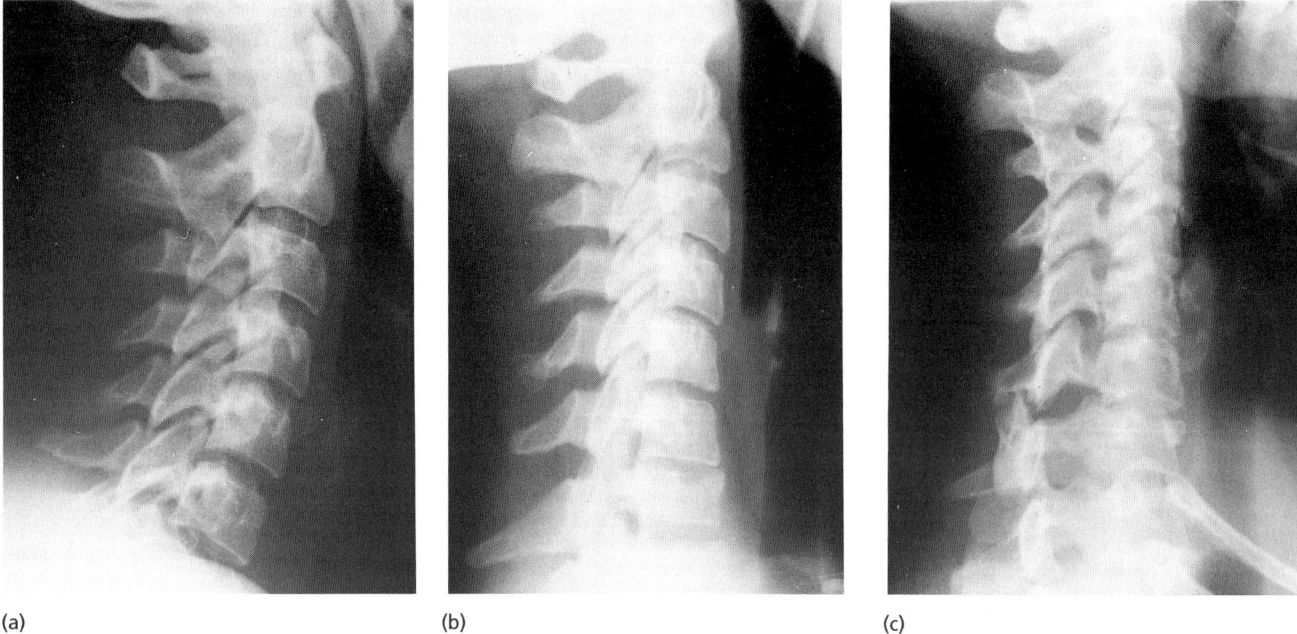

(a)   (b)   (c)

Fig. 18.17 (a) Radiograph inadequate, displays spine to C6. (b) Anterior marginal fracture of C7. (c) Supine oblique views show distortion of the intervertebral foramen and subluxation of the facet joints.

Many of these 'isolated' fractures are associated with more serious injuries in the cervical spine, especially with odontoid fractures and fractures at a lower level. This is an important consideration in the management of the associated injury. For example, a displaced fracture near the waist of the odontoid process may require posterior atlanto-axial fixation. It would be unwise to attempt this until any accompanying arch fracture has been soundly united (Fig. 18.25). Bursting fractures of the atlantal ring vary in severity and, since the fragments are displaced centrifugally, damage to the spinal cord or to the vertebral vessels is uncommon. Jefferson, whose name is rightly associated with these injuries, described four cases and reviewed the literature in 1920. In subsequent papers he described the treatment and the historical background (Jefferson 1940, 1960).

The ring may fracture at two, three or four points and fractures of the lateral masses may occur, depending on the severity of the axial force. Anteroposterior transoral views show splaying of the lateral masses and offer a convenient method of determining the total lateral displacement at the atlanto-axial joints (Fig. 18.26). Combined displacement of over 5 mm suggests disruption of the transverse ligament. The degree of severity may be further assessed by the extent of local bruising in the suboccipital region, the size of the pre-vertebral shadow, two-plane tomography and MRI.

Skull traction for 2 weeks, followed by immobilization in a collar, is usually sufficient for minimally displaced fractures. Frequent radiographic monitoring is recommended. More severely displaced fractures require skull traction in recumbency for a minimum of 8 weeks; the weights should be sufficient to prevent recurring displacement. Absolute reduction is seldom achieved. A halo-jacket is then applied and worn for 4–6 weeks. At this stage, dynamic radiographs are required to determine the stability of the atlanto-axial joint. Most of these injuries are stable at the end of this period, presumably because the alar ligaments are intact and a firm fibrosis surrounds the atlanto-axial joints. An associated fracture of the odontoid will complicate the picture.

Rupture of the transverse ligament

The normal joint space between the dens and the posterior aspect of the anterior atlantal arch does not exceed 3 mm in adults, and displacement of over 5 mm is generally accepted as pathological (Fig. 18.27). Primary rupture of the transverse ligament may follow a heavy blow to the back of the head and is believed to be commoner in older people. Watson-Jones (1955) pointed out that when there is an associated fracture of the dens there is less danger of cord compression. The ligament may rupture at its mid-point or be avulsed with a small flake of bone from the lateral mass on either side.

The presenting features include bruising of the scalp

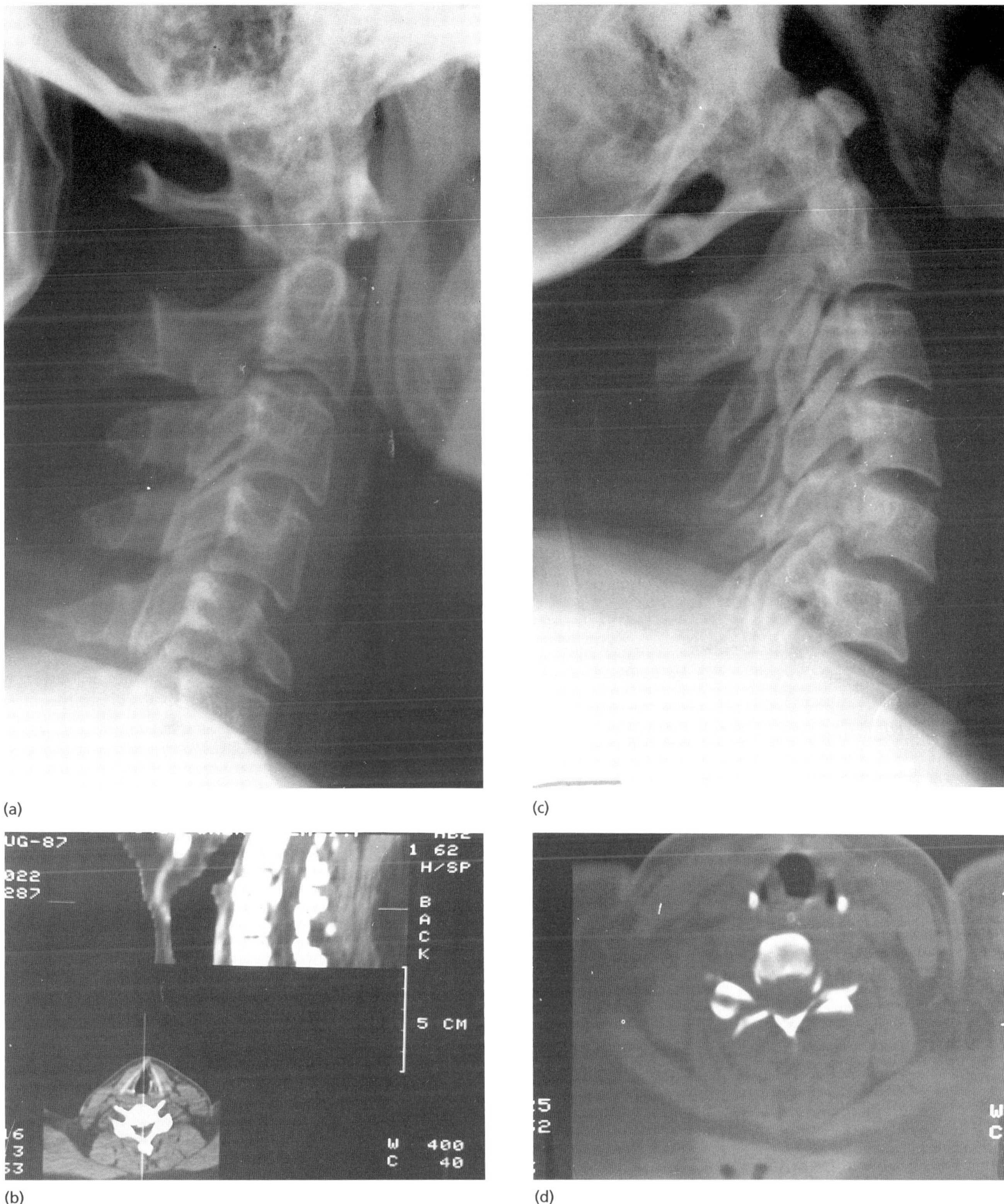

(a)

(b)

(c)

(d)

Fig. 18.18 (a) 'Tear drop' fracture of C5 with retropulsion. (b) A CT scan reconstruction shows stenosis resulting from displaced fragments. (c) Unilateral facet dislocation of C5/6. (d) A CT scan reveals a fracture of the laminae and dislocation of the right facet joint.

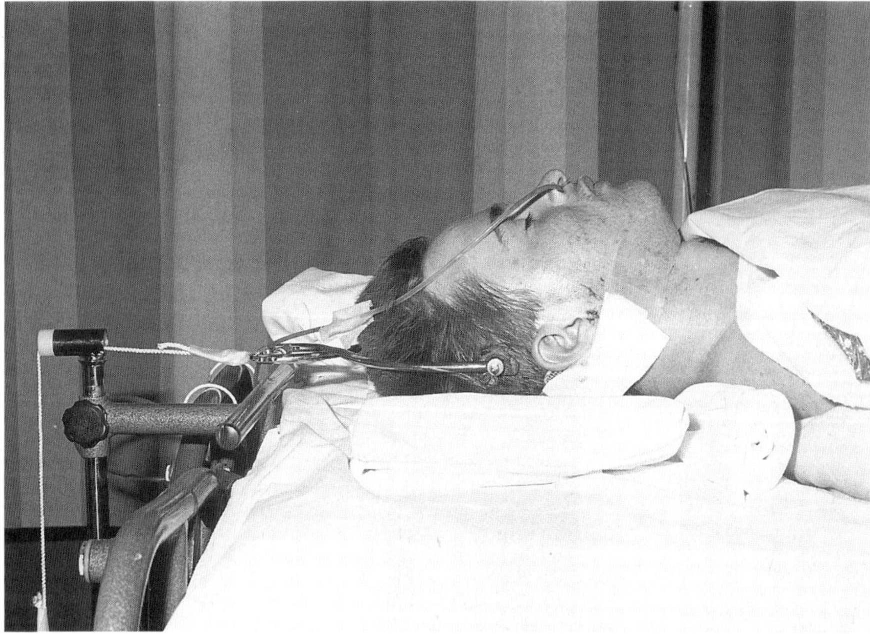

Fig. 18.19 Skull traction. The head end of the bed is then elevated.

over the occipital region, pain in the upper part of the neck and immobility due to extreme local muscle spasm. The neurological picture is variable and often quickly improves when the neck is extended with reduction of the subluxation.

Radiography can be misleading. The standard lateral radiograph is made with the head slightly flexed because of the overhang of the occiput. This position will normally demonstrate the displacement, whereas the injury may be missed if the patient is lying with the head and neck extended. In such cases suspicion is aroused by the presence of a bony flake near the lateral mass or by an otherwise unexplained enlargement of the pre-vertebral shadow. CT scanning in the plane of the atlas is especially helpful and avoids the danger of overflexing the neck.

Atlanto-axial stabilization is obligatory. The dislocation is reduced on skull traction which is kept in position throughout the operative procedure. The wires encircling the atlantal arch should pull the atlas backwards (overcorrection is impossible provided that the odontoid is intact) and should be firmly secured around the spinous process of the axis. Cancellous bone strips are safer than the conventional bone block in such cases and radiographs should be available during the operation (see p. 568 and p. 588). A halo-vest is used post-operatively and stability is confirmed by dynamic views before dispensing with the orthosis.

Fractures of the odontoid process

The clinical features may be unremarkable and confined to pain over the occiput and in the upper part of the neck. There may be no neurological signs, but these may develop after a few hours. Other patients may present with a widespread motor pareses and sensory impairment. These features are often influenced by the position of the head as noted many years ago by Elliot and Sachs (1912). There is often a delay in diagnosis because of unconsciousness, intoxication or associated injuries. Earlier reports (Osgood & Lund 1928) suggest a high mortality and frequent failure of bony union.

Bony union of the dens, like fractures of the femoral neck, depends on the site of the fracture, the degree of displacement and its timely reduction. The vascularity of the normal bone is ensured by a well-developed arterial arcade (Schiff & Parke 1973) but this is compromised following injury, and particularly so when the supporting ligaments are damaged.

Anderson and d'Alonzo (1974) classified these injuries according to their anatomical level. Type I is a small avulsion fracture at the tip of the dens. It is an uncommon and normally benign injury which requires support in a collar until healing is secured. Type II injuries occur at the base of the dens or between the base and the waist of the bone. Failure of union leading to atlanto-axial instability is common (Figs 18.28 & 18.29). Type III

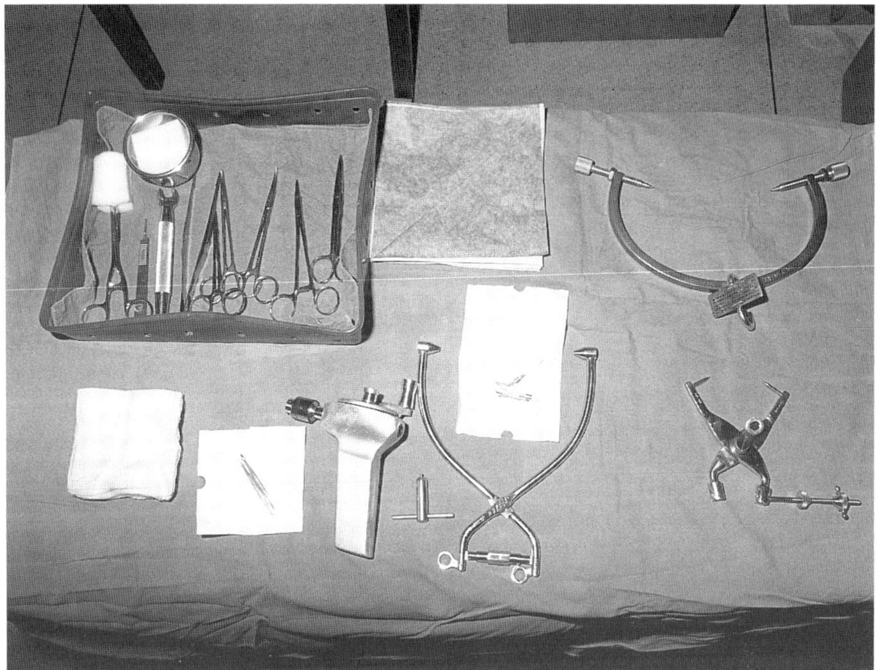

Fig. 18.20 (a) Calipers in common use: Cone, Crutchfield and Gardner–Wells. (b) The use of all calipers requires careful supervision and familiarity!

(a)

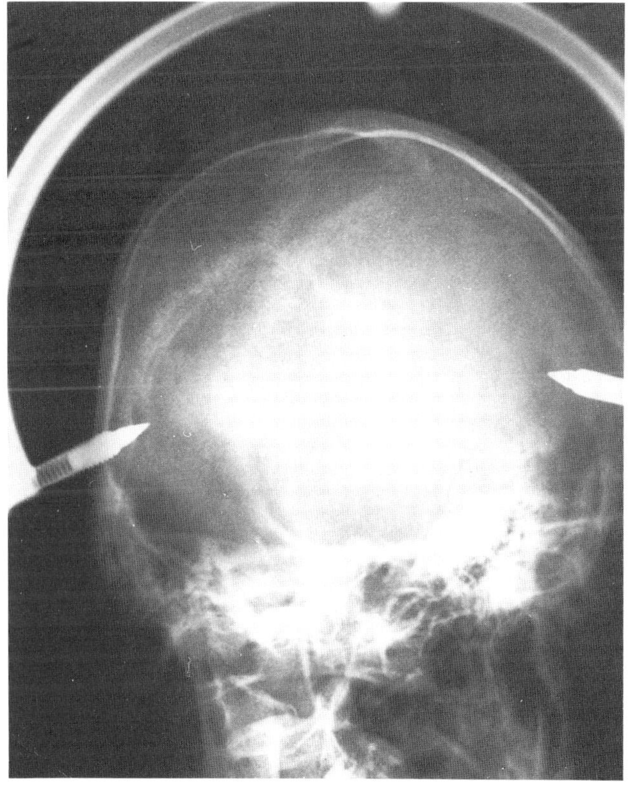

(b)

fractures involve the cancellous bone of the axis; non-union is uncommon except in severely displaced injuries. Skull calipers are applied as an initial measure, thus allowing for a full clinical and radiological assessment on which subsequent treatment is based. Type II fractures and displaced type III fractures are immobilized in a halo-vest 7–10 days later. A more satisfactory reduction may then be achieved by horizontal adjustment of the halo. Undisplaced type III injuries may be managed in a collar after the initial period of recumbency, but frequent radiographic control is essential.

Flexion–extension radiographs are made after 4 months. A firm fibrous union may be acceptable in older patients. In the younger age group, failure of trabeculation across the fracture line or the demonstration of C1/2 instability is an indication for posterior atlanto-axial fusion. Some surgeons advocate an earlier fusion for displaced type II fractures. Anterior stabilization procedures and screw fixation have been described. They are more liable to lead to neurological complications and, in the author's opinion, carry a substantial morbidity (Fig. 18.30). Lateral atlanto-axial fusion using bilateral transarticular screws (du Toit 1976) may have a special place when there are associated anomalies, as in the absence of the posterior arch. A review of the contemporary management of these injuries was undertaken by the Cervical Spine Research Society and reported by Clark and White (1985).

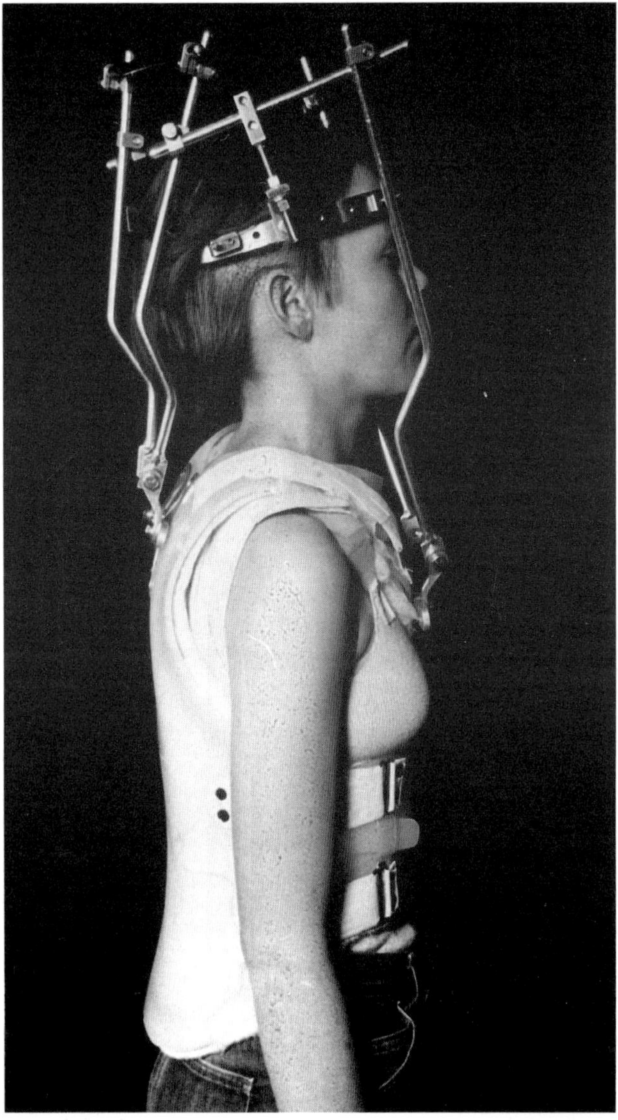

Fig. 18.21 Application of a halo-vest is preferably deferred for a few days until all appropriate investigations are complete.

Children

Fractures in young children occur at the synchondrosis between the odontoid process and the body of the axis below the superior articular facets. They comprise the largest number of cervical fractures up to the age of 7 years and in traffic accidents are often accompanied by acute atlanto-axial subluxation. The fracture unites readily when properly immobilized. A Minerva cast or halo-jacket is worn for 12 weeks and remodelling occurs even in incompletely reduced fractures (Blockey & Purser 1956). Acute atlanto-axial subluxations are

reduced by extension over a pillow. In exceptional cases, maintenance of the reduced position is extremely difficult so that internal fixation is advised (Fig. 18.31).

Atlanto-axial rotatory injuries

The primary function of the atlanto-axial joint is to permit free rotation of the head. Security largely depends on muscle tone and the strength of the surrounding ligaments. Two varieties of displacement may occur, varying in severity from the mild rotatory deformity seen in childhood to the dangerous fixed deformity described by Fielding and Hawkins (1977). The common childhood deformity may follow a trivial injury and is sometimes associated with upper respiratory tract infections (Watson-Jones 1932). Diagnosis is suggested by tilting of the head to one side with rotation to the opposite side ('cock robin' appearance). Spontaneous recovery with or without gentle intermittent halter traction is the rule. The early diagnosis of rotatory fixation in children has been discussed by Johnson and Fergusson (1986).

An unexpected glancing blow to the head may damage the atlanto-axial ligaments which fail to heal unless appropriately immobilized (Fig. 18.32). In adults the untreated deformity gradually becomes fixed so that the patient cannot correct the tilt of the head to the neutral position. As the pain and spasm increase, the asymmetry between the odontoid and the lateral masses of the atlas may not be seen in transoral radiographs. For this reason, some patients have been unjustly labelled as hysterical.

Cineradiography demonstrates that both bones move as a unit and CT scanning will usually confirm the diagnosis. Manipulation is dangerous, and for these rare injuries a period of skull traction, which may help to correct some of the deformity, is advised. This is followed by posterior atlanto-axial fusion.

Traumatic spondylolisthesis of the axis

The fracture passes through the neural arch (pedicles) of the axis and is commonly bilateral so that anterior displacement of the axis on the third cervical vertebra may or may not occur (Fig. 18.33). There is an interesting historical background to this injury (Schneider *et al.* 1965) and its association with judicial hanging. Wood-Jones (1913) reviewed the subject from a study of two groups of specimens in the Hunterian Museum. He concluded that a subaural knot usually resulted in fractures at the base of the skull. In contrast, a submental knot produced bilateral arch fractures — the 'ideal

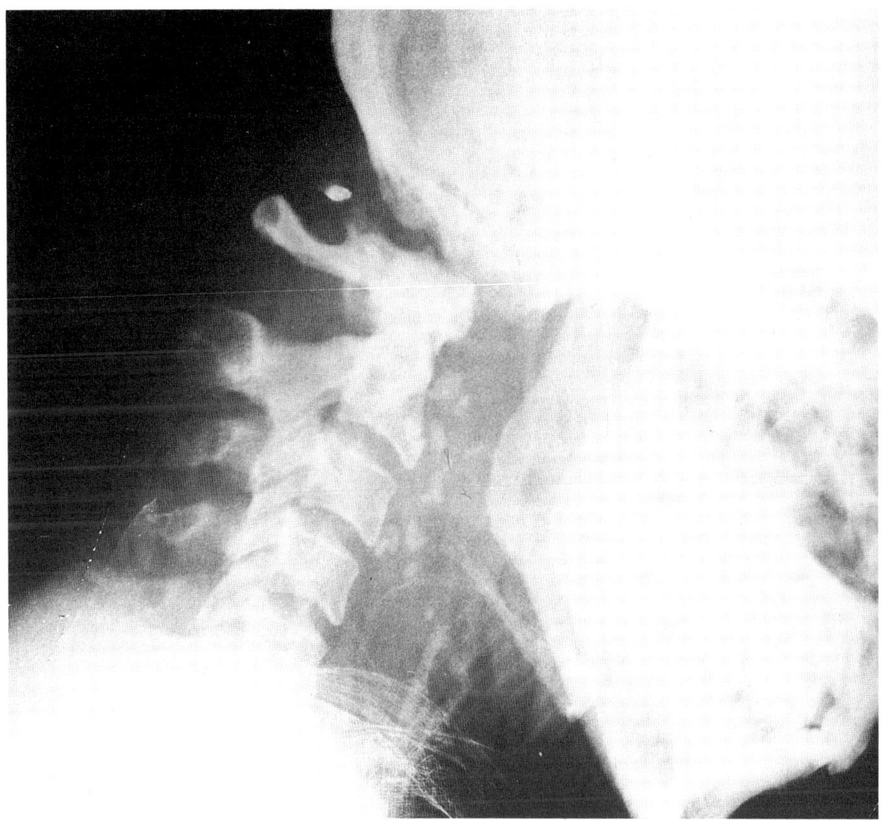

Fig. 18.22 Atlanto-occipital dislocation is usually accompanied by a severe head injury but is not necessarily fatal.

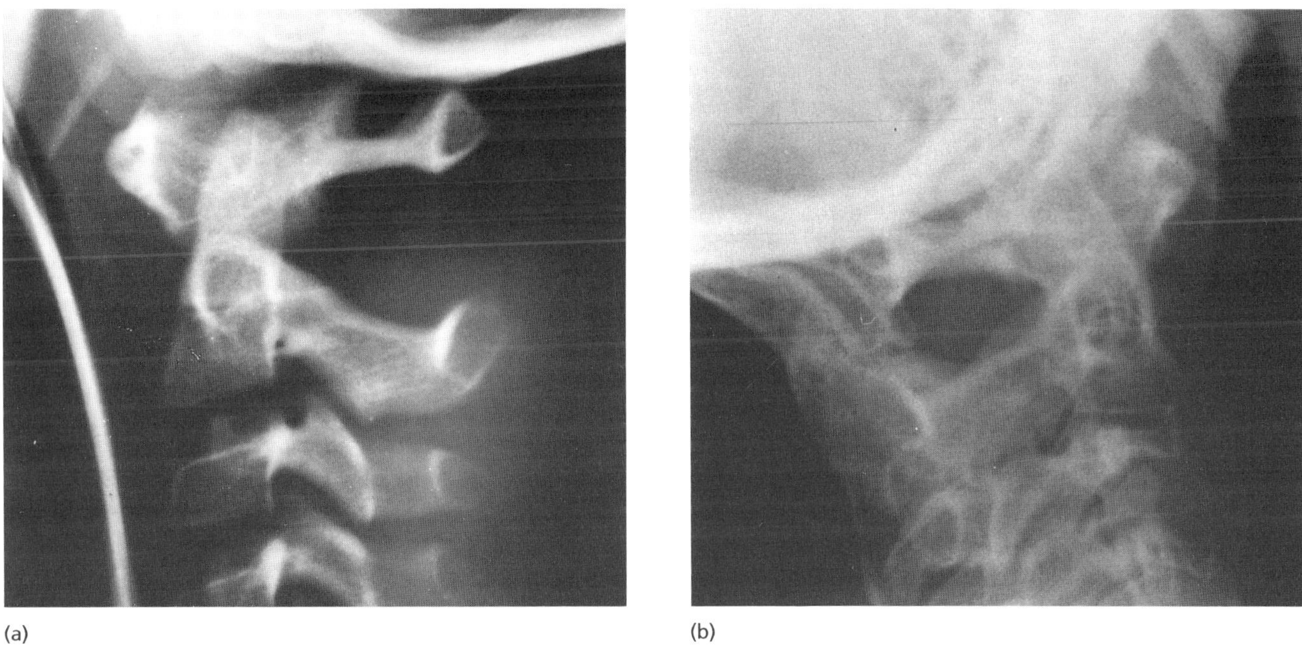

(a)　　　　(b)

Fig. 18.23 (a) Unilateral atlanto-occipital dislocation with presumed rupture of the transverse ligament. (b) Gradual improvement in the neurological picture (including cranial nerve palsies) following skull traction and occipito-cervical fusion.

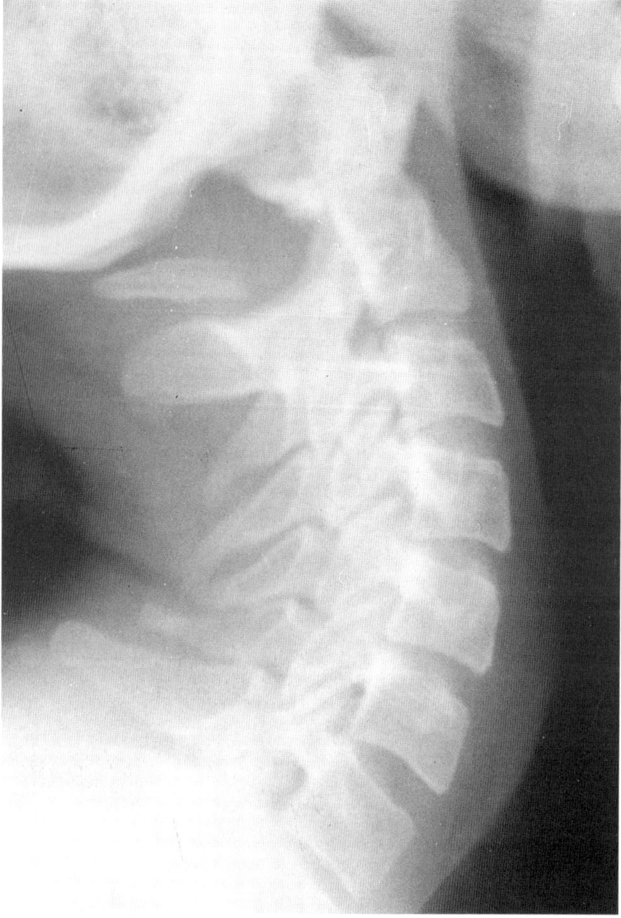

Fig. 18.24 A deficient posterior arch; not a fracture.

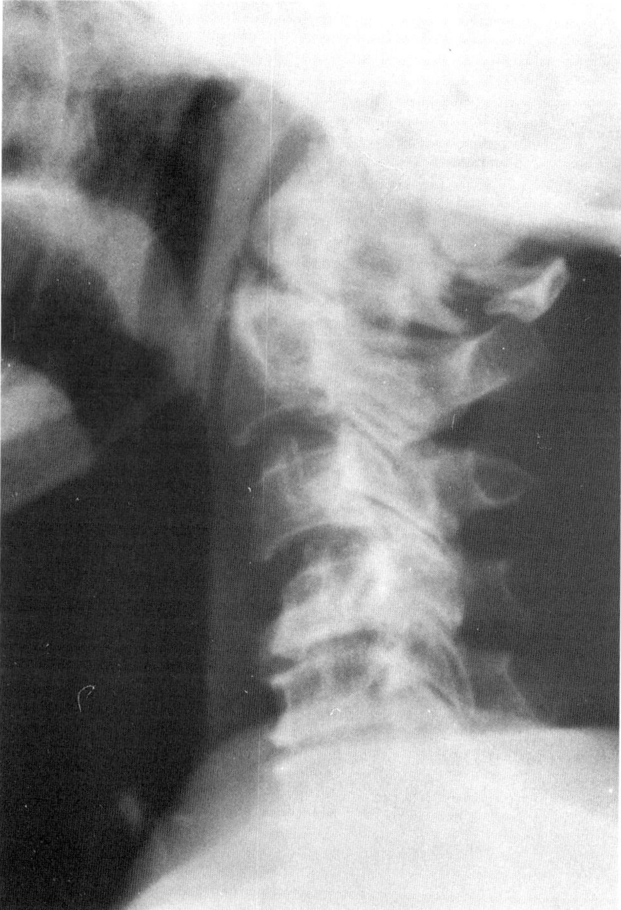

Fig. 18.25 Type II fracture of the odontoid and fracture of the posterior arch. Surgery should be delayed until the arch fracture has united.

lesion'. Thus, the eponym 'hangman's fracture' has come to be associated with this injury.

The true hangman's fracture is caused by hyperextension and distraction, whereas the modern counterpart follows on severe axial loading and extension. Most of these injuries result from traffic accidents in which the victim strikes the face or forehead against the interior of the car. Any neurological features may be transient but in some cases permanent neurological impairment occurs.

The standard lateral radiograph will display this fracture, which should be suspected in all serious facial injuries. Minimally displaced fractures may be safely treated in a collar. The position of more severely displaced fractures can usually be improved by light skull traction (not exceeding 2 kg) followed by fixation in a halo-jacket. Union is usually complete at 12 weeks. Late instability is uncommon, and when it occurs the poss-

ibility of subluxation of the posterior facet joints should be considered. This would require posterior fusion from C1 to C3. Some authors favour an anterior fusion (DeLorme 1967, Cornish 1968).

Pseudosubluxation in children

Clinical hypermobility of the cervical spine in children is well recognized. Bailey (1952) reported on the frequent appearance of forward displacement of C2 on C3 on the radiographs of normal children when the neck is flexed. This gives rise to the suspicion of subluxation. Cattell and Filtzer (1965) reported similar findings from the Children's Hospital in Baltimore. Diagnostic difficulties arise when there is a history of injury. Rapid remission of symptoms following rest and token immobilization of the neck usually clarifies the diagnosis. However, true subluxation may occur as evidenced by an enlarged

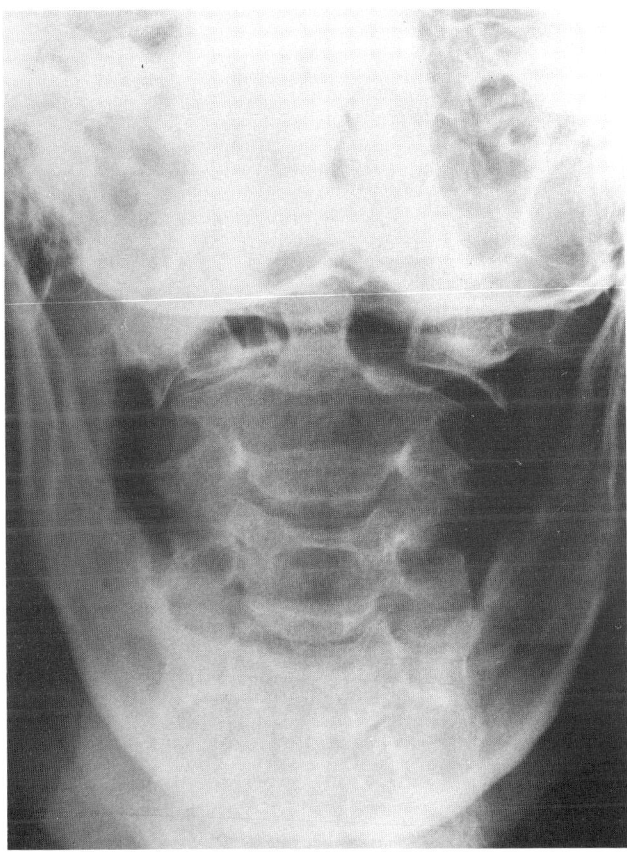

Fig. 18.26 Jefferson fracture.

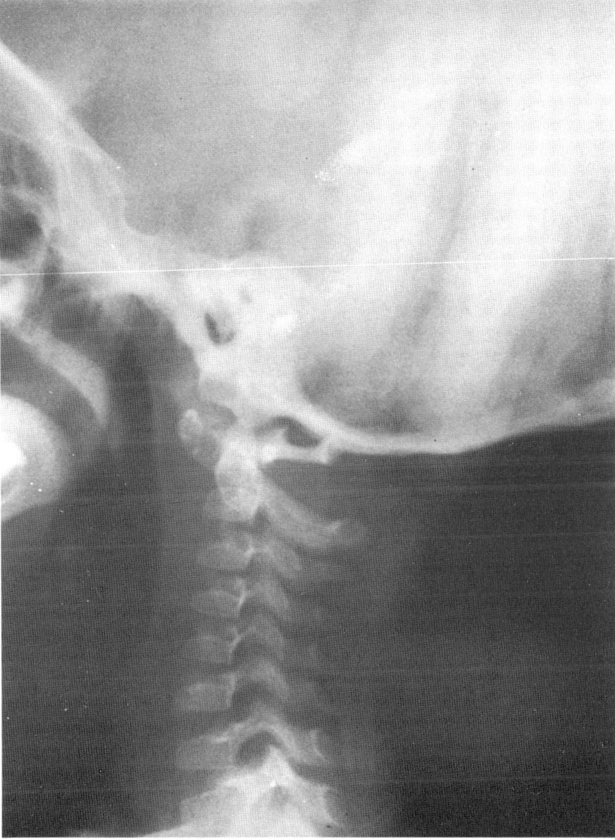

Fig. 18.27 Rupture of the transverse ligament in a child. This was easily reduced but remained unstable, and required atlanto-axial fusion 2 years later.

pre-vertebral shadow shortly after injury with continuing pain and spasm. Late calcification in the interspinous ligament is the hallmark of more severe injuries. Rarely, persistent pain dictates the need for localized posterior fusion (Fig. 18.34).

Injury to the anomalous cervical spine

There are a number of developmental abnormalities of varying biomechanical and pathological significance in the cervical spine (Fig. 18.35). Most of these malformations occur in the upper part and are often associated with minor anomalies at a lower level. The importance of recognizing these anomalies is that relatively trivial injuries may be followed by neurological impairment. Included in this group are absence and hypoplasia of the odontoid (Giannestras *et al.* 1964), atlanto-axial instability in Down's syndrome (Burke *et al.* 1985), and variations of the Klippel–Feil syndrome (Hensinger *et al.* 1974). Apart from these suboccipital abnormalities there are a number of occipital dysplasias which cause

instability at the cranio-cervical junction. The clinical aspects and diagnosis of these conditions have been reviewed by Spillane (1957) and Wadia (1967). Many of the anomalies are symptomless but some develop progressive, often asymmetrical, neurological manifestations. In others, injury plays a major role in the onset of pyramidal tract signs. Transitory weakness of the lower limbs, clumsiness of the hands and disassociated sensory loss on sudden flexion of the neck have long been recognized in association with these anomalies. Atlanto-axial instability frequently accompanies these abnormalities and is a major factor in the development of the neurological features.

Atlanto-axial instability

It will be perceived that atlanto-axial instability may follow a number of congenital and acquired conditions, and that injury plays a major part in the development of symptoms (Fig. 18.36). When anterior atlanto-axial subluxation is regarded as the main deformity, it can be

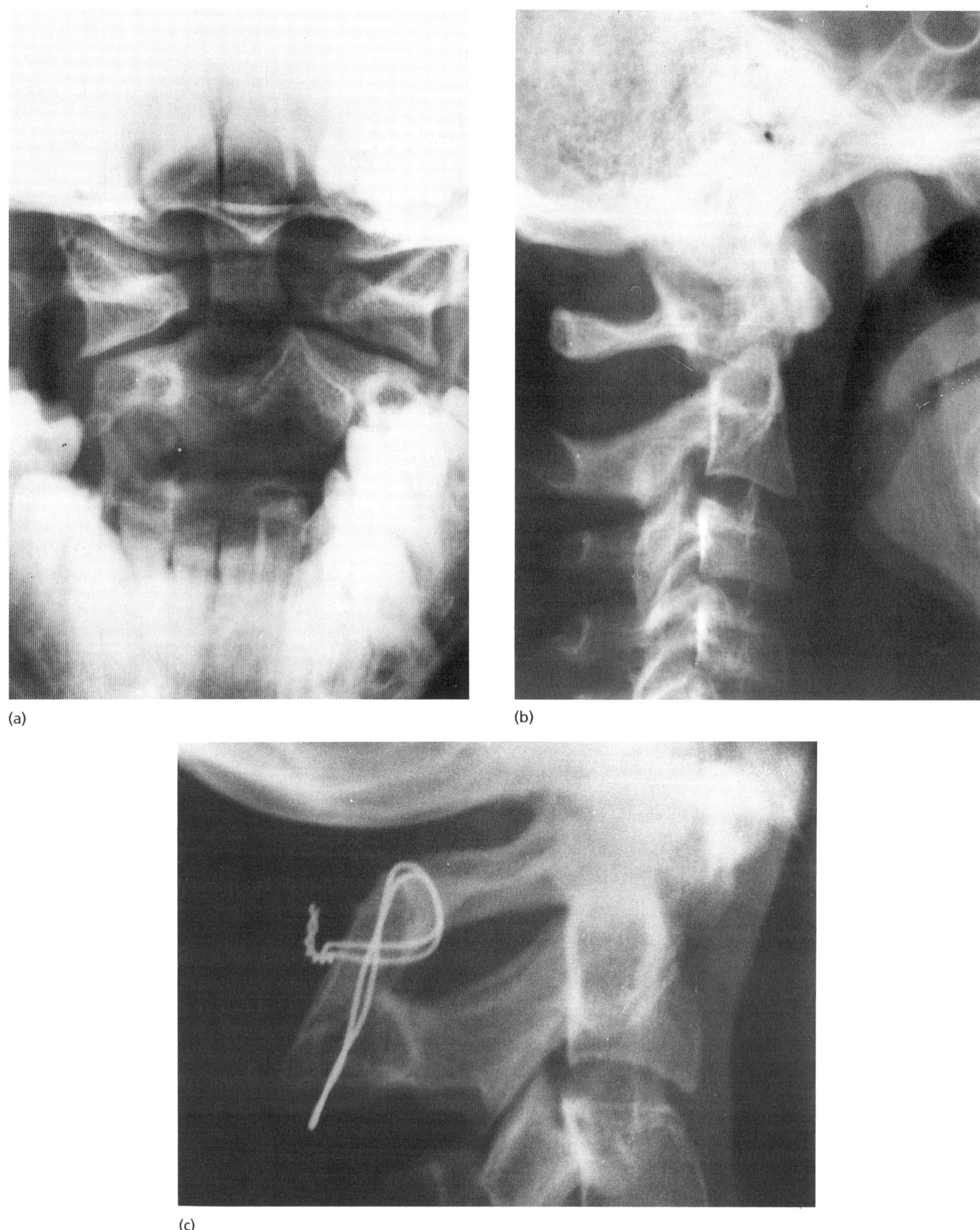

Fig. 18.28 (a) Type II fracture of the odontoid. (b) Ununited at 10 weeks. (c) Atlanto-axial fusion.

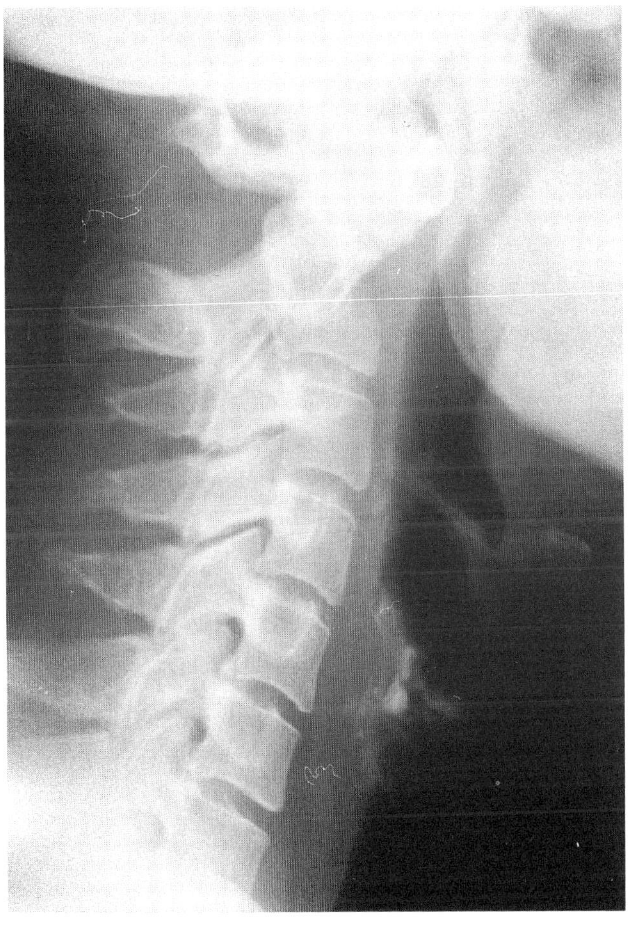
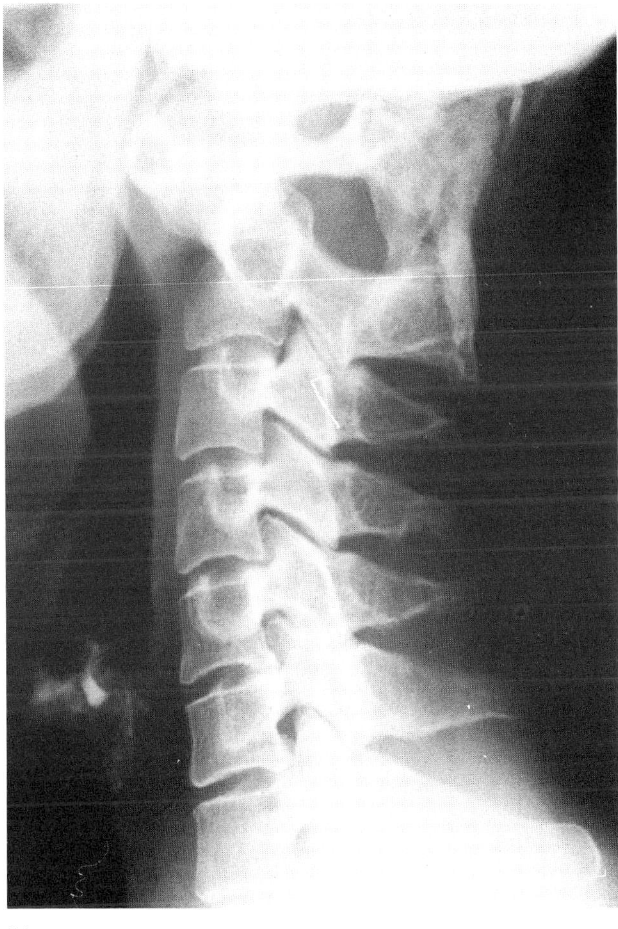

(a)   (b)

Fig. 18.29 (a) Old ununited fracture of the odontoid with anterior instability. This case was referred because of increasing neurological signs. (b) Occipito-cervical fusion with improvement in the neurological deficit.

appreciated that increasing ligamentous laxity will permit lateral, rotatory and posterior luxations. At a later stage, destruction of the articular facets will lead to vertical migration of the dens — a common finding in severe rheumatoid arthritis. Not all cases progress in this manner and many remain symptomless.

The potential dangers have been recognized for many years. Hutchinson (1868) described a patient who had sustained a fracture of the odontoid process and noted the gradual onset of paralysis. Elliot and Sachs (1912), Khan and Yglesias (1935) and Bachs *et al.* (1955) reported on the delayed myelopathy associated with this condition. More recent reports amply confirm the risk of neurological deterioration.

The decision to fuse the upper cervical spine in these situations is an extremely difficult one. It should be based on a full clinical assessment, on a careful study of the radiographs and on the natural history of the disease process or injury. Unfortunately, our knowledge of the natural history of many of the associated conditions, notably in the mucopolysaccharide disorders, is far from complete. For example, major surgery in variants of the Morquio–Brailsford syndrome (Melzak 1969, Beighton & Craig 1973, Stevens *et al.* 1991) and in the Klippel–Feil disorder should be approached with extreme caution. In contrast, the decision is straightforward in an otherwise healthy individual when progressive myelopathy or an acute neurological emergency follows on an ununited fracture of the dens with instability. In many instances a conservative approach with limitation of athletic activities is justified. This should be remembered in the management of Down's syndrome and selected rheumatoid patients (Jeffreys 1980, Burke *et al.* 1985). The absolute indication for stabilization is significant neurological deterioration in an otherwise healthy patient. Prophylactic surgery should be considered in the light of the inherent risks, the available technical facilities and the experience of the

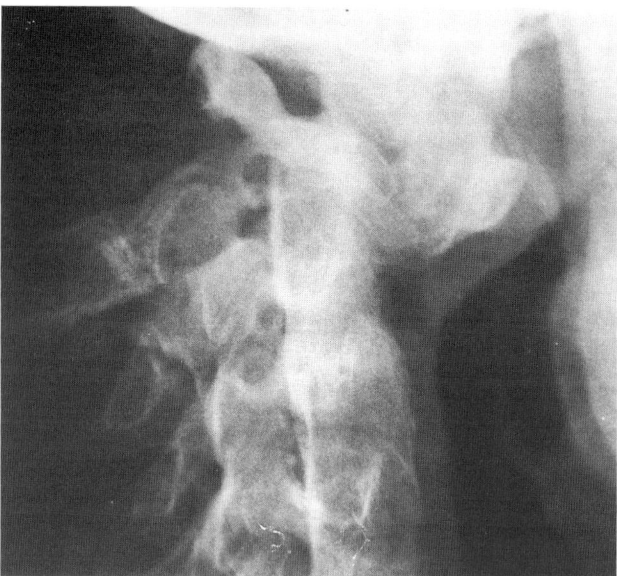

Fig. 18.30 Attempted anterior fusion (bone graft) for a fracture of the odontoid. This was immobilized in a soft collar but there was subsequent malunion. Surprisingly, there was no neurological impairment despite gross deformity.

operator. The author favours posterior fusion for manifest instability, after discussing the lack of a reasonable alternative with the patient and relatives.

Various methods of atlanto-axial fusion by a posterior approach have been described, conspicuously those of Mixter and Osgood (1910), Gallie (1939) and McGraw and Rusch (1973). In contemporary techniques a 20 gauge wire looped on itself, or a strong nylon ribbon (McSweeney 1980), is passed deep to the posterior arch of the atlas and drawn backwards. The wire secures a corticocancellous bone graft to the prepared surface of the axis and atlantal arch. In certain circumstances cancellous bone slivers are more acceptable. It is essential to 'reduce' the subluxation preoperatively and to maintain the reduced position by skull traction (or halo-jacket fixation) during the operation.

Intraoperative radiography is indispensible; the reduction may be altered during transportation or during induction of anaesthesia. The procedure is not applicable in hypoplasia or absence of the posterior arch, or in seriously displaced irreducible subluxations. It should be employed with circumspection in posterior subluxations where occipito-cervical fusion may be more appropriate. There is no absolute rule for deciding how much displacement can be safely tolerated; Howard Steel's 'rule of thirds' is helpful. He defined the area of the vertebral canal at this level into one-third odontoid, one-third cord and one-third 'space'. This latter represents a safety zone (Steel 1968) in which displacement may occur without cord impingement, and it is ap-

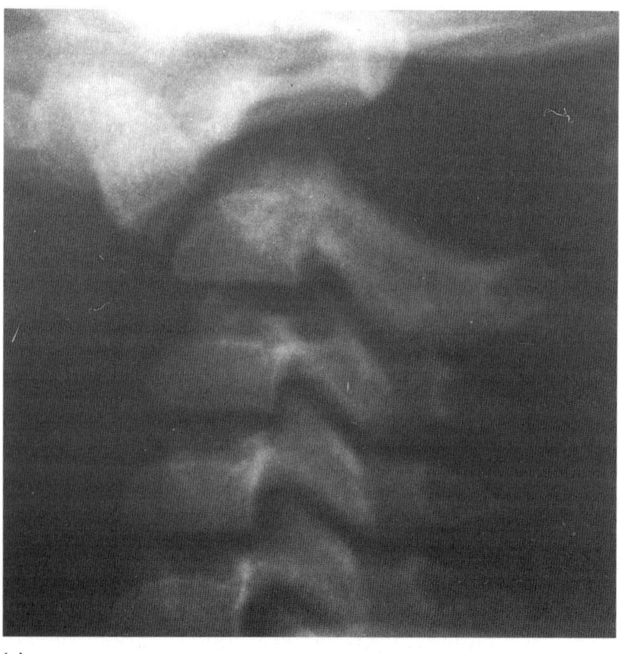

(a)

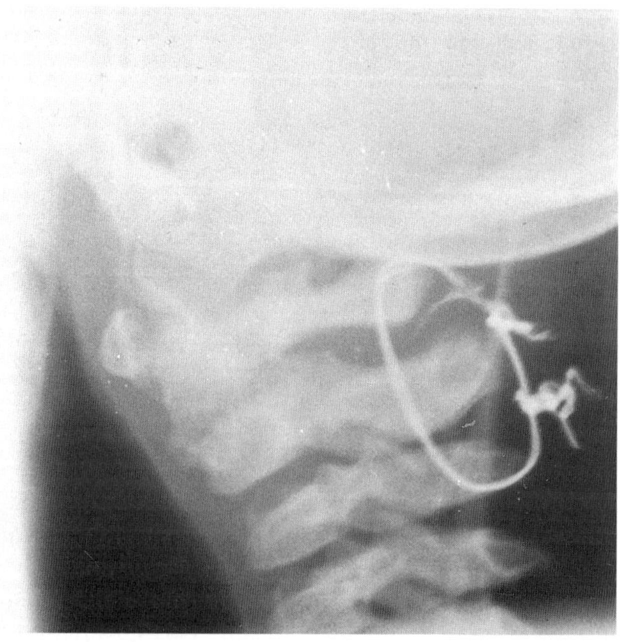

(b)

Fig. 18.31 (a) Atlanto-axial dislocation in a child. Nursing and immobilization were extremely difficult. (b) Atlanto-axial fixation was ultimately followed by bony union.

proximately equivalent to the transverse diameter of the adult odontoid (about 1 cm). The postoperative management is important. A cervico-thoracic brace or extended Philadelphia collar is generally favoured and is satisfactory, provided that the fixation is technically secure. Because of the limitations of many neck orthoses (Johnson *et al*. 1981) the author prefers to employ a halo-vest postoperatively for 3−4 months.

Occipito-cervical fusion

This useful procedure has been criticized because it limits rotation of the head to a greater extent than does atlanto-axial fusion. The author is not convinced that the additional restriction of movement is a critical functional handicap. The operation is indicated for instability when the arch of the atlas is deficient, where bone has been removed for neurological procedures, for irreducible posterior displacements and when a satisfactory preoperative reduction cannot be secured. The author used the plaster bed method of immobilization for many years (McSweeney 1978), following the operative technique described by Newman and Sweetnam (1969). The method was found to be eminently satisfactory but the author now favours the earlier mobility afforded by a halo-jacket.

Ransford *et al*. (1986) describe a method of posterior rigid internal fixation for the myelopathy associated with anterior pathology in the atlanto-axial region. In

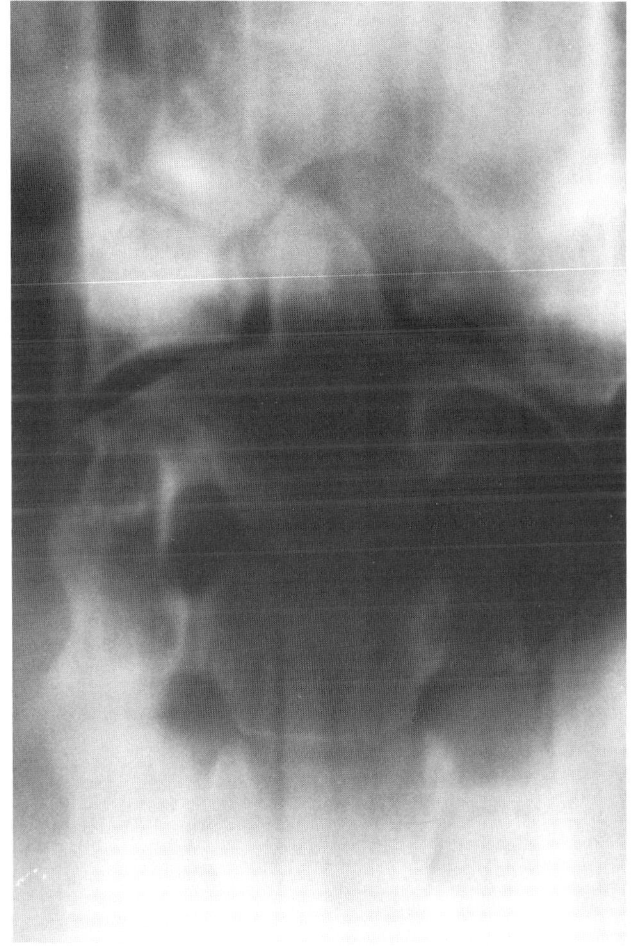

(a)

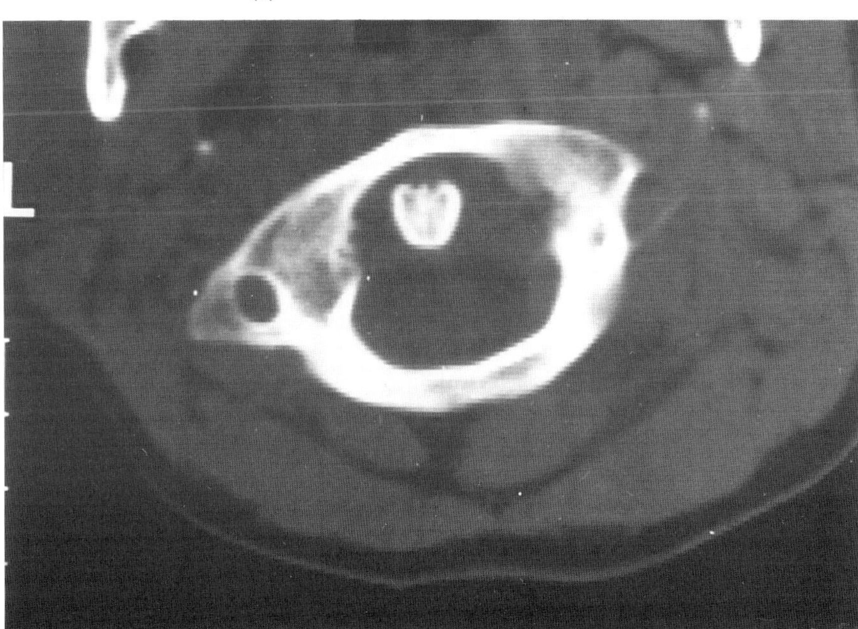

(b)

Fig. 18.32 (a) Rotatory subluxation following a glancing blow to the head. (b) Confirmed by a CT scan. Complete reduction followed a period of skull traction. (Courtesy of R.G. Pringle.)

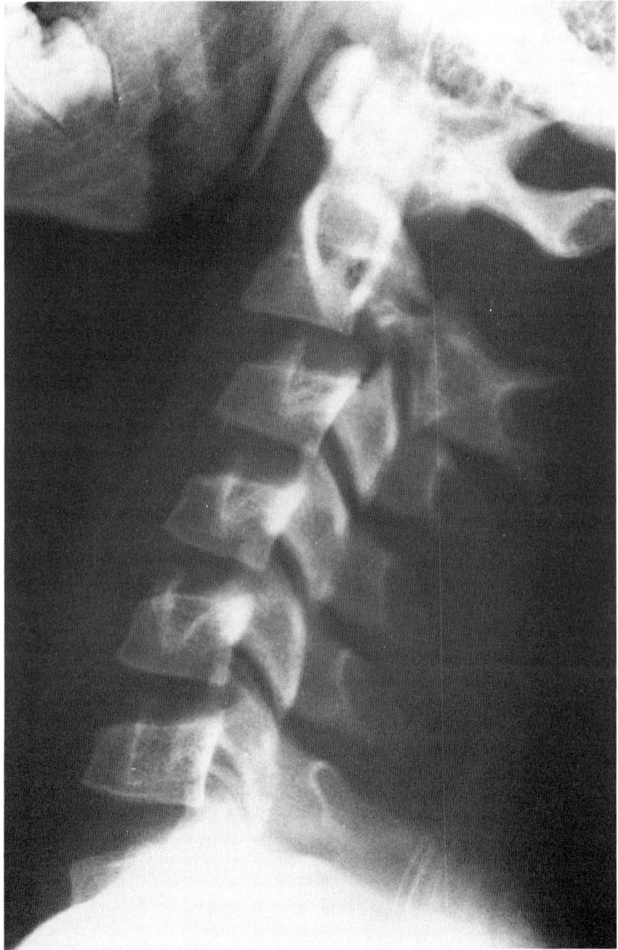

Fig. 18.33 Fracture through the neural arch of the axis. Most of these fractures unite spontaneously.

these difficult cases the authors recommend transoral decompression with excision of the odontoid, immediately followed by placement of a conforming Wisconsin (or Luque) rod wired to the occiput and upper cervical spine. Cancellous grafts are then applied to the decorticated bone.

Other approaches to the upper cervical spine

Only in exceptional circumstances is anterior surgery advised for post-traumatic disorders of the upper cervical spine. The reader is referred to the important descriptions by Fang and Ong (1962), Bonney and Williams (1985) and Crockard (1988). Anterolateral approaches have been described by Whitesides and Kelly (1966) and by Andrade and MacNab (1969). It must be said that these approaches are hazardous and are not advised for the occasional operator. Acrylic cement is not normally recommended for post-traumatic conditions where bony fusion is the ultimate aim.

Injuries of the mid and lower cervical spine

Most of these injuries are caused by indirect violence transmitted through the head or trunk (see p. 551) and any accompanying neurological impairment usually follows a well-recognized pattern. It is convenient to have a working classification and to appreciate that while there are many exceptions, there is a correlation between the neural deficit and the type of vertebral injury. The following classification is suggested:

1 Flexion–rotation injuries (facet luxations and dislocations).
2 Hyperextension (retroflexion, deflexion) injuries.
3 Compression (axial loading) injuries.
4 A miscellaneous group (gunshot, stab, ankylosing spondylitis and other pathological fractures; iatrogenic).

The first few hours after injury are crucial. The importance of adequate oxygenation and immobilization of the neck have been mentioned. Radiographs may show dislocations and disruption of the vertebral bodies which must be promptly realigned. Skull callipers are applied, the patient is reassured and appropriate sedation is arranged. The exceptions are the hyperextension injury of older patients presenting with a central cord syndrome, minor compression injuries of the vertebral bodies and isolated fractures of the transverse or spinous processes which may be safely treated in a supporting collar.

In the account which follows an eclectic approach is advocated; procedures applicable to a patient who has escaped neurological injury may not be appropriate for another patient who has been rendered tetraplegic but who has a similar radiographic injury.

Flexion–rotation injuries

Bilateral facet dislocation

This injury is commonly associated with severe cord damage and often leads to complete and irrecoverable tetraplegia. Despite serious encroachment on the diameter of the spinal canal some patients escape neural damage, presumably because of a capacious canal or because of the decompressing effect of an associated laminar fracture. The posterior ligamentous complex, the intervertebral disc and the posterior longitudinal ligament are disrupted. The anterior longitudinal ligament is stripped off the vertebral bodies and may be torn. A lateral radiograph will show more than half

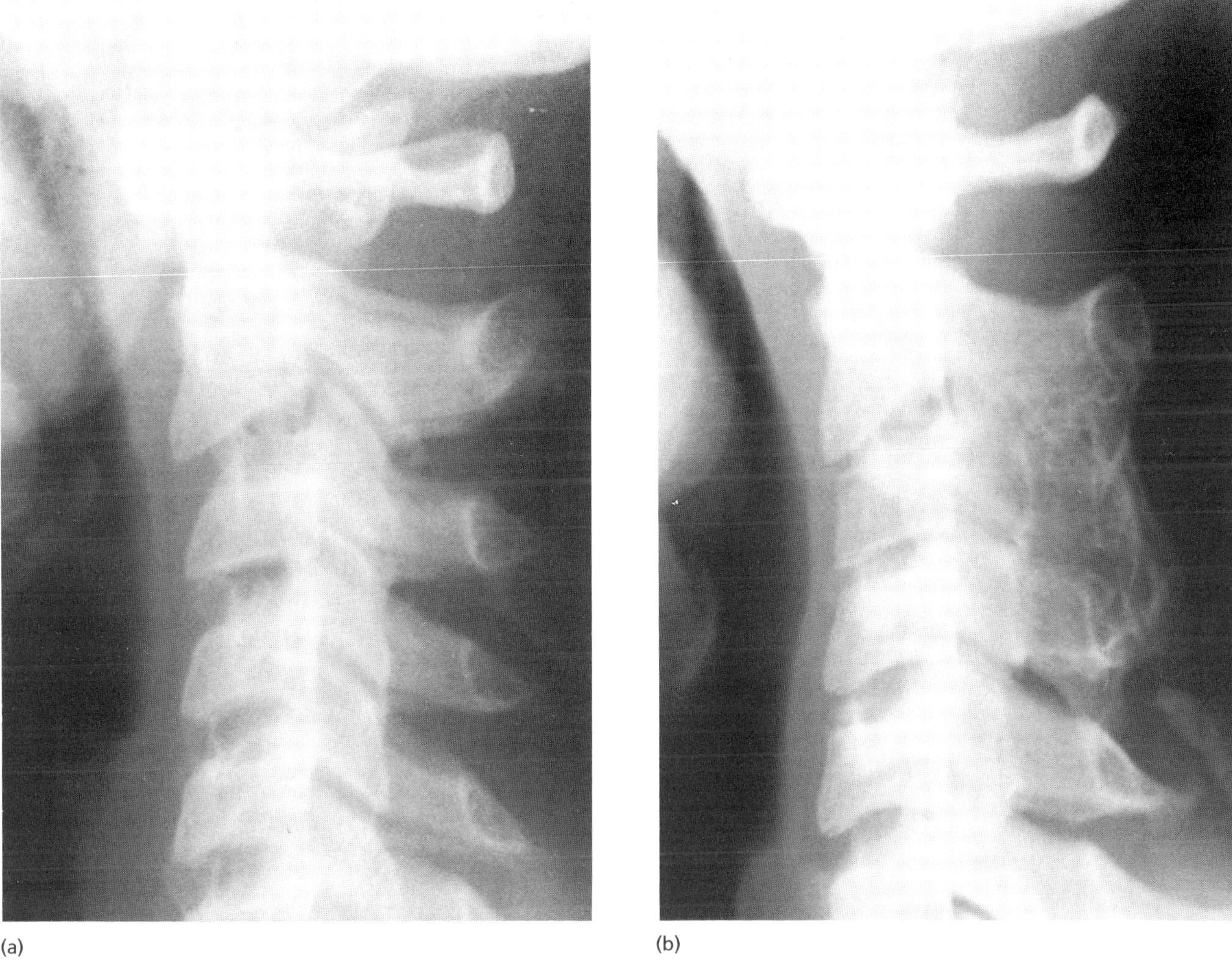

(a)

(b)

Fig. 18.34 (a) Subluxation of C2 on C3 with persistent pain, uncomfortable clicking and restricted movement. (b) Posterior fusion relieved the symptoms.

the anteroposterior vertebral body depth displaced forwards (Beatson 1963). The role of the intervertebral disc in flexion–rotation injuries has given rise to considerable controversy. Disc derangements in association with spinal injuries have been noted and reviewed (Bohlman 1979), but the relevance in the individual patient is often far from precise. Much depends on the time from injury, the degree of disc extrusion and the diameter of the spinal canal.

Any difficulty in reducing the dislocation or an increase in the neurological deficit should alert the surgeon to the possibility of a significant disc prolapse (Eismont *et al*. 1991). Similar remarks apply to unilateral facet dislocations and to subluxations.

In such circumstances MRI or CT is required (Robertson & Ryan 1992). A large fragment judged to have the potential to cause cord compression requires prompt removal through an anterior approach. If alignment has not already been secured, then open reduction and posterior fusion is indicated.

The results of anterior decompression have been encouraging, but not uniformly satisfactory, which is understandable in the light of the multifactorial nature of neurological deterioration. Closed reduction is usually achieved by graduated skull traction or by repositioning under general anaesthesia and a muscle relaxant. Open reduction may be necessary in dislocations below C6 and when there is a time lapse.

Reduction by graduated skull traction is generally advised. Traction is commenced in the line of the deformity so that the neck is brought into increasing flexion. The weights are gradually increased from 4.5 kg (10 lb) to a maximum of 23 kg, depending on the appearance as shown on serial lateral radiographs. The

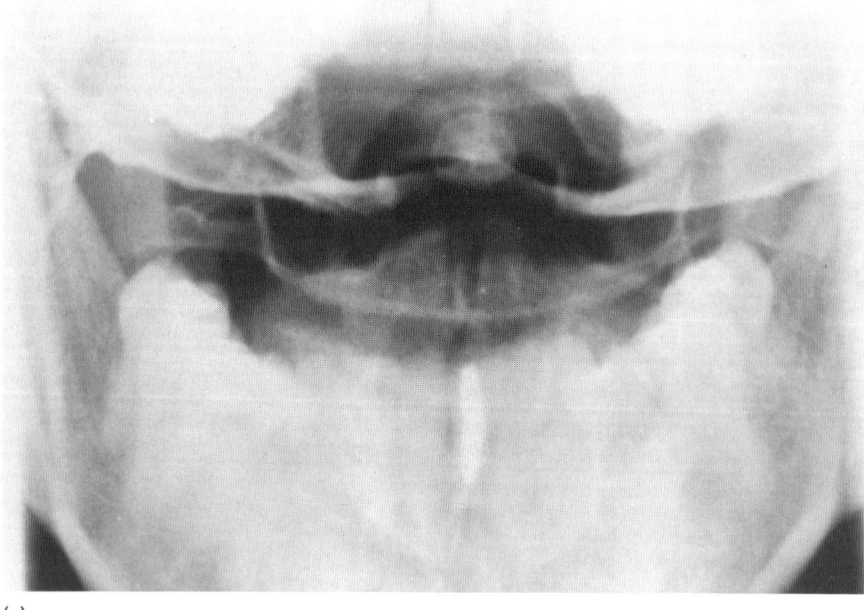

(a)

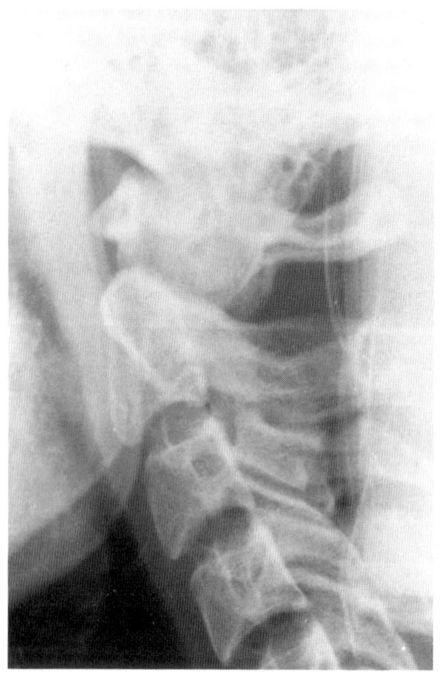

(b)

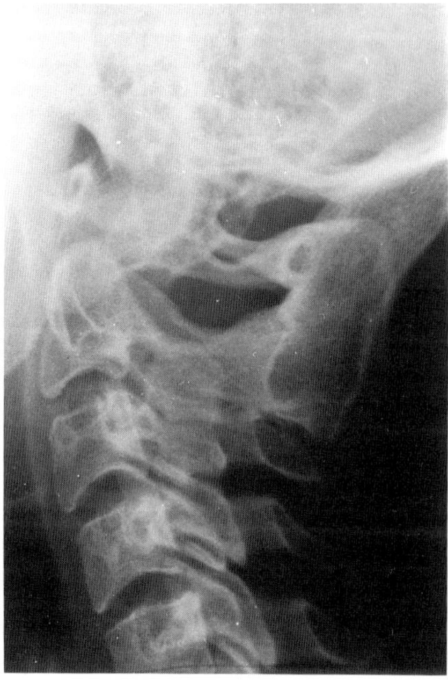

(c)

Fig. 18.35 (a) Os odontoideum.
(b) Increasing tetraparesis following
a trampoline injury. (c) Occipito-
cervical fusion was followed by
complete recovery.

head end of the bed is raised. As the facets commence to distract, the supported neck is brought into a greater degree of flexion. When adequate distraction has been achieved and confirmed by lateral radiographs, the neck is allowed to extend over a small pillow. This should not be permitted until the facets are 'overperched', that is, until the leading edges are just separated and in line. Once reduction has been achieved, the weights are reduced to 2–3 kg and the degree of extension is checked radiologically.

The aim is to secure reduction in under 3 hours, during which time the patient is observed for any neurological deterioration and is instructed to report any unusual symptoms. While the patient is comfortable and the radiographic appearances confirm progressive distraction, it is reasonable to extend the period up to 8 hours.

Some surgeons, including the author, favour manipulation as the first choice, and when graduated traction is not successful within a reasonable time. The method

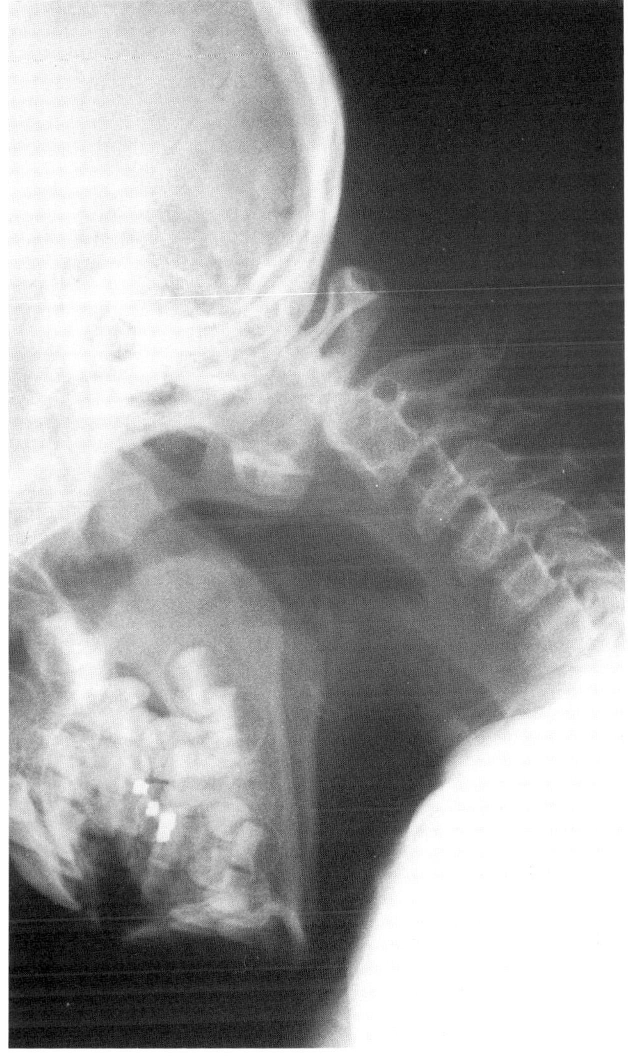

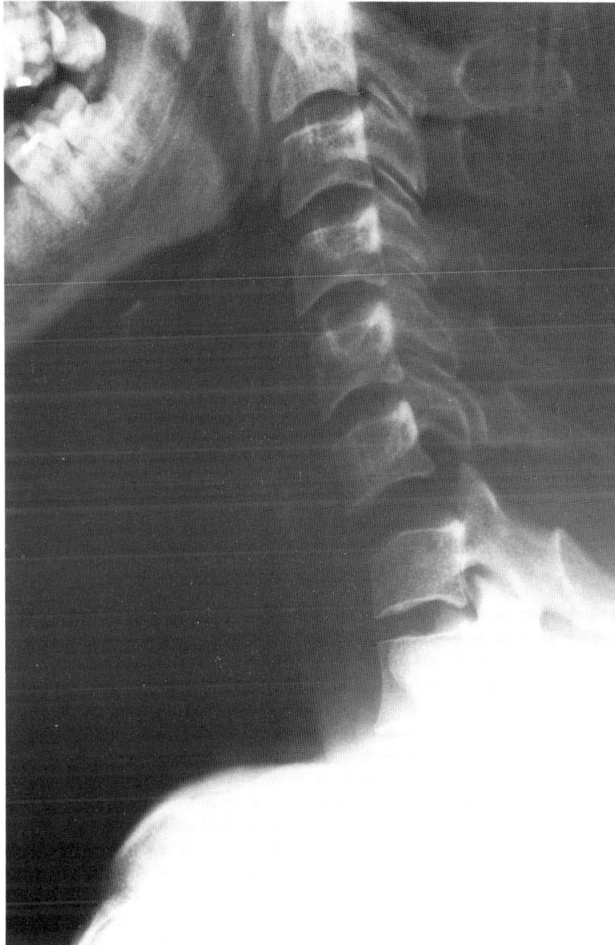

Fig. 18.37 Bilateral dislocation on skull traction. Facets are tip-to-tip so that deflexion (extension) may commence.

Fig. 18.36 Atlanto-axial instability in Down's syndrome. The child has been under supervision for 5 years without any evidence of neurological deficit.

has remained popular in Europe since the time of Malgaigne but is decidedly unpopular in North America, despite the important descriptions of Walton (1893) and Taylor (1924). The technique has gradually improved with better radiographic control and Evans (1961) emphasized the value of good muscular relaxation. Attention to detail is important. The recommended procedure requires full muscular relaxation and, to this end, endotracheal anaesthesia, without extending the neck, is combined with a muscle relaxant. An absolute rapport between the anaesthetist and the surgeon is essential so that traction is commenced when full muscular relaxation has been secured. Serial radiographs or image intensification is required. Traction is commenced in the line of deformity or in the neutral

position and the neck is gradually flexed. In some instances it may be necessary to rotate and laterally flex the neck before unlocking is achieved. Gentleness is the essence of these manoeuvres and, in this context, 'reposition' would be more descriptive than the inelegant term 'manipulation' with its implied use of force (McSweeney 1975). As soon as the facets are tip-to-tip, and therefore unlocked, the neck is allowed to extend and token traction is maintained (Fig. 18.37). The method is ideal for reducing dislocations from C3 to C6 and, when successful, has the merit of speedily relieving pressure on the spinal cord. It is not recommended when there is another major injury in the cervical spine, in patients seen a week after injury and in elderly patients. It is unlikely to succeed in injuries below C6.

Dislocations at the cervico-thoracic junction are uncommon and often missed (Evans 1983). The cord injury is usually complete. When the dislocation is not associated with fractures at the C7-T1 level, and a complete lesion is present for 24 hours, Evans suggests that no attempt should be made to reduce the dislocation. If the cord lesion is incomplete, reduction should only be undertaken by an experienced surgeon.

Failure to reduce the dislocation by closed methods should logically lead to open reduction by the posterior approach. Many surgeons would proceed to open reduction as an immediate measure, emphasizing that the procedure is safer under direct vision, and that a fusion can be performed at the same time. More than half of these injuries will heal by spontaneous anterior fusion between the vertebral bodies. When there is an accompanying spinal cord injury it is the author's policy to maintain light skull traction for 6–8 weeks after reduction, by which time callus formation over the front of the adjacent vertebral bodies may be seen. This is a reassuring sign. Flexion–extension radiographs are made at 3 months and, unless there is evidence of instability, immobilization is continued in a well-fitting collar for a further 3 months. This regimen applies in particular to patients who have sustained a cord injury. Some will improve following reduction but, unfortunately, others will remain almost completely paralysed. In the author's view the period of enforced recumbency allows for a better readjustment to the neurological damage and encourages earlier urological and bowel training.

If there are no neurological signs, a good case can be made for early posterior fusion in bilateral dislocations, while recognizing that many will stabilize in the fullness of time. Early fusion has many advocates and it would be difficult to discredit this approach when economic factors are considered. When an open reduction has been performed it must always be accompanied by bony fusion. Anterior fusion is not attractive in such cases; it creates another area of potential instability, unless the bone block remains absolutely secure in the postoperative period.

Unilateral facet dislocation

This injury results from flexion–rotation forces which tear the facet joint capsule on the dislocated side as well as the interspinous ligament. This is a stable injury which may be associated with nerve root pressure. The patient may present some days after injury with neck stiffness and pain in the upper limb. More often than not, reduction by closed methods is singularly difficult and should not be attempted if 3–4 weeks have elapsed. If nerve root impingement is not a feature, then the injury may be left to stabilize.

Confusion arises with more severe injuries which appear radiographically to be very similar. Some of these may have originated as a bilateral facet dislocation which has 'spontaneously' reduced in transit. Others are associated with damage to the intervertebral disc and posterior longitudinal ligament. In both cases, neurological impairment is the rule; there may be a complete cord lesion but, more commonly, there is an asymmetrical compression leading to a Brown–Sequard syndrome. Reduction is easy, but redislocation (even on traction) is common, indicating that this is an unstable injury. As a general rule, these injuries require early posterior fusion.

Radiological differentiation between stable and unstable facet dislocations is not easy, but the injury should be regarded as unstable in patients with signs of cord impairment. It has been found that the 45° supine oblique views (McCall *et al.* 1973) display the line of the facet joints and the outlines of the intervertebral foramina to the cervico-thoracic junction. In this projection, lateralization is straightforward and there is no need to rotate the patient's neck. The anteroposterior view will show deviation of the spinous process corresponding to the side of the dislocation. In a true lateral projection, less than half of the anteroposterior depth of the vertebral body is displaced forward.

Anterior subluxations

Stringa (1964), Cheshire (1969) and Evans (1976) reported on a group of injuries, the unstable nature of which is easily overlooked (Fig. 18.38). The greater part of the articular surfaces of the facet joints are in contact and appear normal on extension radiographs. The pathological anatomy is similar to that in dislocation but the damage to the posterior ligamentous complex is less severe (Fig. 18.39). Increasing deformity may occur following an injury or, more commonly, the patient becomes aware of a forward angulation of the neck (Fig. 18.40). Spasm of the neck muscles causes increasing discomfort. Progressive neurological impairment has been reported. These anterior subluxations have been described as 'hidden flexion injuries' (Webb *et al.* 1976) and an attempt has been made to delineate the group in which early fusion is required. Four localizing features were recognized; (i) loss of the normal cervical lordosis due to muscle spasm, (ii) widening of the interspinous space, (iii) partial overriding of the facet joints, and (iv) a minor compression fracture of the vertebral body. This fracture may only present as a small protuberance at, or near, the upper and anterior aspect of the vertebral body at the level of injury, or in the body below.

Posterior fusion is advised and this usually involves

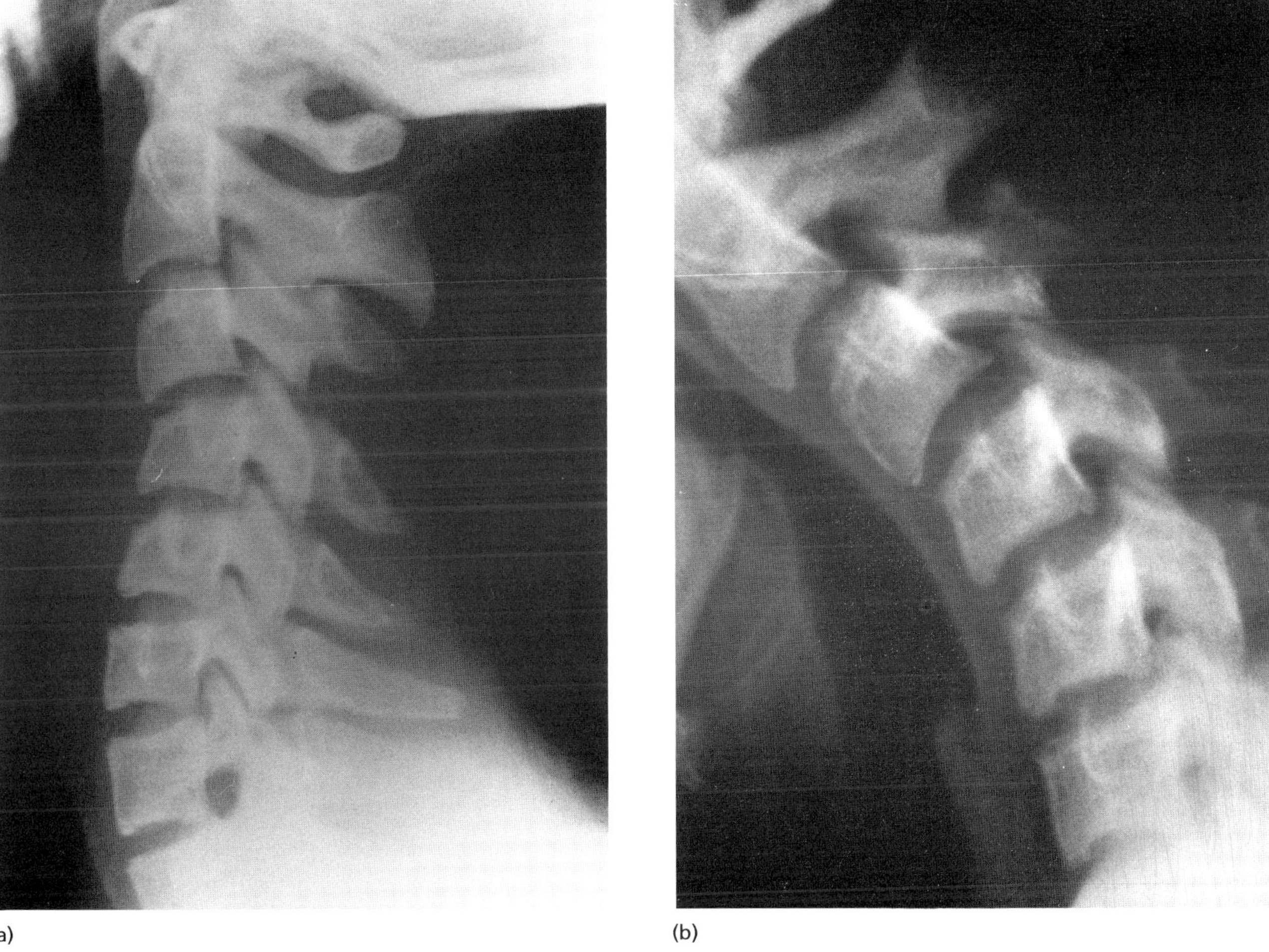

(a)   (b)

Fig. 18.38 (a) The Radiograph was considered to be normal despite widening of the C3/4 interspace. (b) Progressive deformity occurred within 2 months.

one segment. It is important to establish that the ligaments of adjacent segments are intact and to extend the fusion accordingly.

Hyperextension injuries

The pattern of hyperextension injuries varies with the magnitude of the injuring force and with the flexibility of the spine. Thus, in older patients, a comparatively trivial fall may be associated with a profound but slowly recovering paralysis. A bony injury may not be immediately apparent on conventional radiographs, but more careful examination often shows avulsion fractures at the anterior margins of the vertebral bodies or, more significantly, anterior widening of an intervertebral disc space. At the other extreme, a younger patient may sustain bilateral fractures of the articular processes with

forward displacement of the vertebral body and irrecoverable tetraplegia (Fig. 18.41). The hyperextension injury of older patients is associated with degenerative changes (spondylosis) in the cervical spine. Because of the presumed absence of an overt bony injury, it was customary to refer to these cases as 'tetraplegia without bony injury'. While it is now known that some bony or ligamentous injury is almost invariably present, the severity varies from a rupture of the anterior longitudinal ligament to a transverse tear of an intervertebral disc with fractures of the posterior elements. Following Thorburn's description (Thorburn 1887) there has been much experimental work and speculation as to the genesis of the cord injury. The reader is referred to the interesting work of Taylor and Blackwood (1948) and Burke (1971), as well as to the more recent accounts by Merriam *et al.* (1986) and McMillan and Silver (1987).

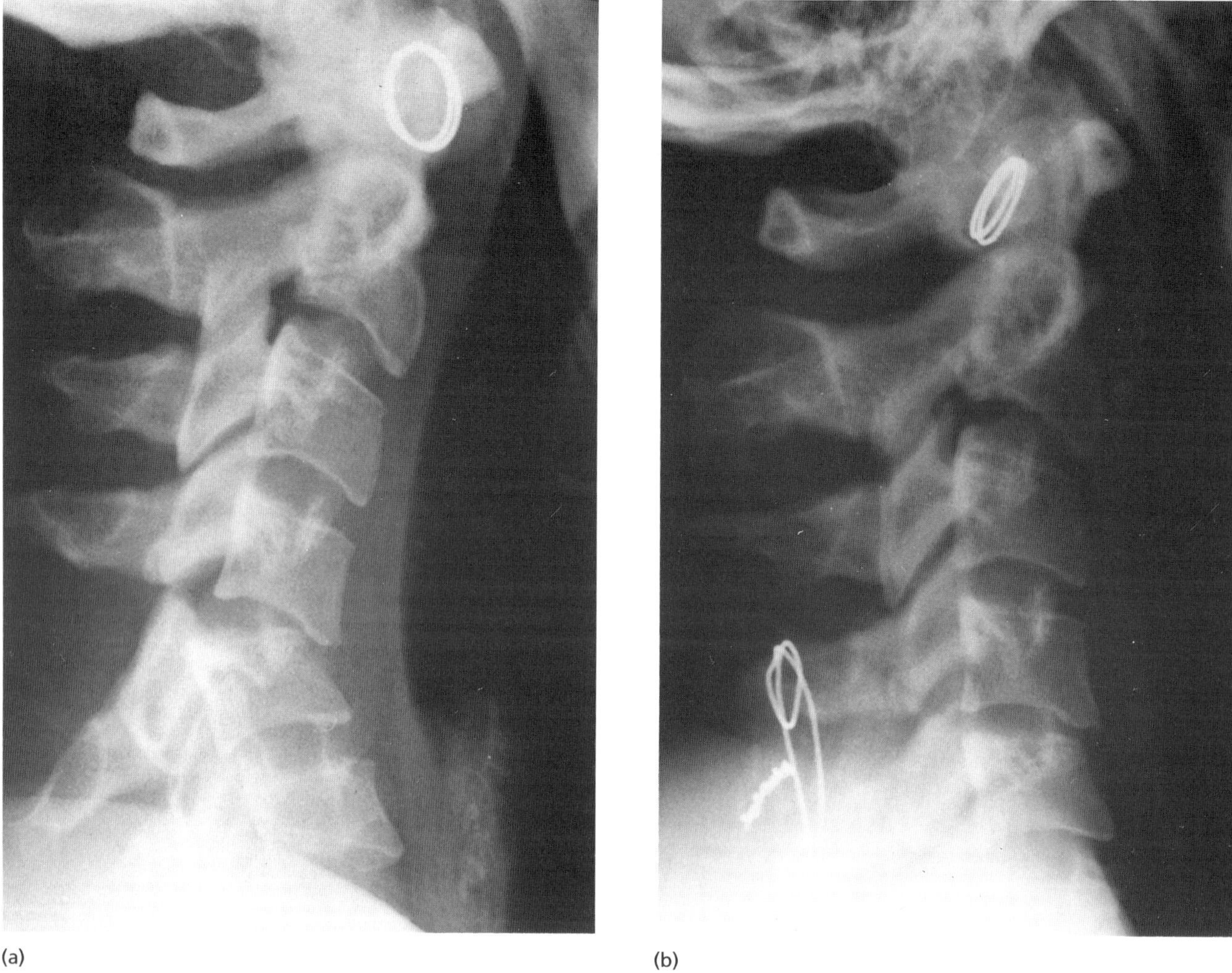

Fig. 18.39 (a) The patient sustained an anterior subluxation of C4 on C5. This was easily reduced but subluxation recurred while on traction. (b) Posterior fusion.

The stereotype syndrome in older patients is well recognized and follows damage to the soft, highly vascular central area of the spinal cord. Experimental work has shown that this area is most vulnerable to injury (Ducker *et al*. 1971) and that the damage is not necessarily irreversible. The transverse and longitudinal extent of the damage is reflected in the clinical picture, which ranges over a number of incomplete syndromes (see p. 554).

In a representative case there is impairment in lower limb sensation and voluntary muscle control with a profound paresis of the upper limbs, notably affecting the small muscles of the hands. This latter aspect is usually attributed to anterior horn cell damage. Hyperpathia, with a prolonged after-reaction, is a distressing feature in the early weeks. This excessive sensory response is often most marked over the shoulders and in the hands. The painful inhibition of movement leads to severe shoulder joint stiffness, resembling a pericapsulitis, and may contribute to the oedema and stiffness of the hands. Sphincter disturbance is present during the early weeks but tends to lessen. Recovery commences in the lower limbs and the majority of these patients are able to walk within a few weeks. Impaired proprioception may lead to an unsteady gait and to reliance on visual appreciation. Weakness in the upper limbs may persist for many months so that the arms hang limply by the sides. The prehensile function of the hands often remains seriously impaired and while the musculature slowly improves, this is offset by stiffness the contractures of the finger joints. Every effort should be made to mobilize these unfortunate patients once the lower limb weakness commences to improve. A collar is advised for comfort and to guard against exten-

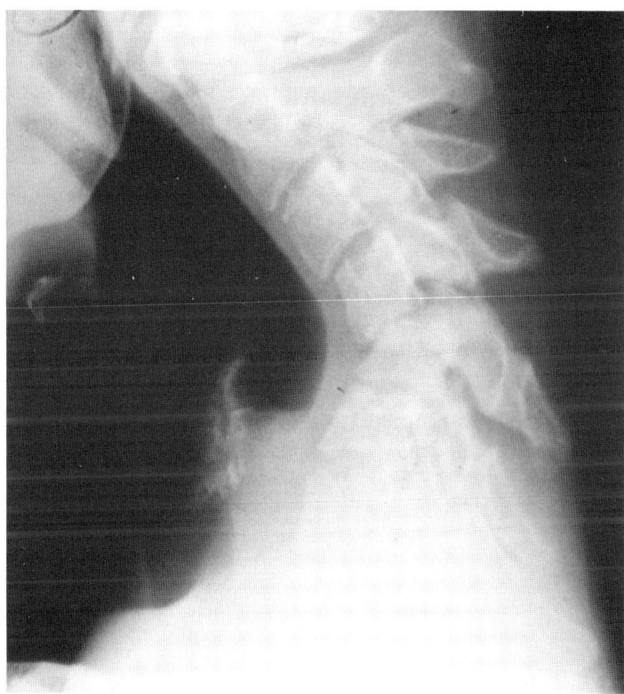

Fig. 18.40 Severe deformity following an unrecognized anterior subluxation. Progressive neurological signs only partially lessened following posterior fusion. Moderate lower limb spasticity did not improve.

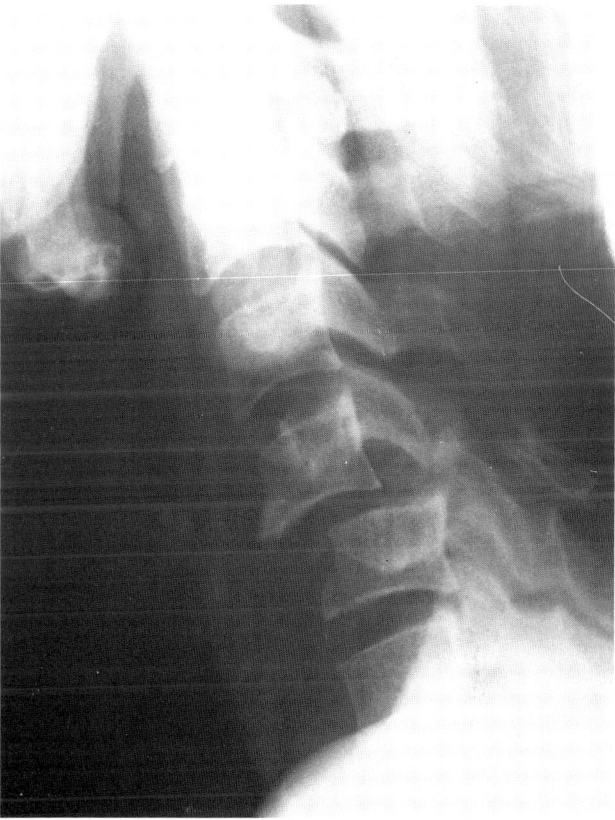

Fig. 18.41 Hyperextension injury of C5 on C6. Note the fracture near the base of the spinous process, with fracture of the facets.

sion of the neck. Almost all these injuries quickly stabilize but radiographic monitoring is important. Surgical fusion is seldom required, and then only for manifest instability.

In contrast, the severe hyperextension injury of younger patients is often accompanied by a complete cord lesion. Road traffic accidents and gymnastic injuries, associated with severe facial wounds, account for the majority of cases. Gross swellings of the neck and difficulty in swallowing are usual features (Fig. 18.42). The radiographs in a typical case will show forward displacement of the vertebral body and fractures of the facets or pedicles, often with a fracture near the base (rather than the tip) of the spinous process. The mechanism of this injury has been described by Whitley and Forsyth (1960) and by Forsyth (1964). As the head and neck are forcibly hyperextended, the posterior elements are so crowded together as to fracture the facets or laminae and these, acting as a fulcrum, cause rupture of the anterior longitudinal ligament. As the force continues, the head moves through an arc travelling backwards and downwards. With further continuation of the force the head will finally be travelling with a forward momentum. As the anterior ligament ruptures, the continuing force displaces the vertebral body for-

wards, so that it finally comes to rest in an anteriorly displaced position. The forwardly displaced body may be mistaken for a flexion injury. This led Burke (1971) to describe the appearance as a hyperextension 'masquerading' as a flexion injury (Fig. 18.43). Posterior displacement of a vertebral body is a rare, and almost invariably fatal; the injury is sometimes associated with fractures of the hyoid bone.

All grades of severity may be encountered in hyperextension injuries and their unstable nature may not be realized unless the clinical features are correlated with the radiographic findings. The neck must not be allowed to extend and the alignment of even severely displaced injuries is improved by skull traction in the neutral or slightly flexed position. Bony union is normally achieved in 6–8 weeks, during which time the patient should remain recumbent. In the author's experience a halo-vest arrangement is unsatisfactory. Failure to reduce the forward displacement rarely requires open reduction through an anterior approach combined with posterior fusion.

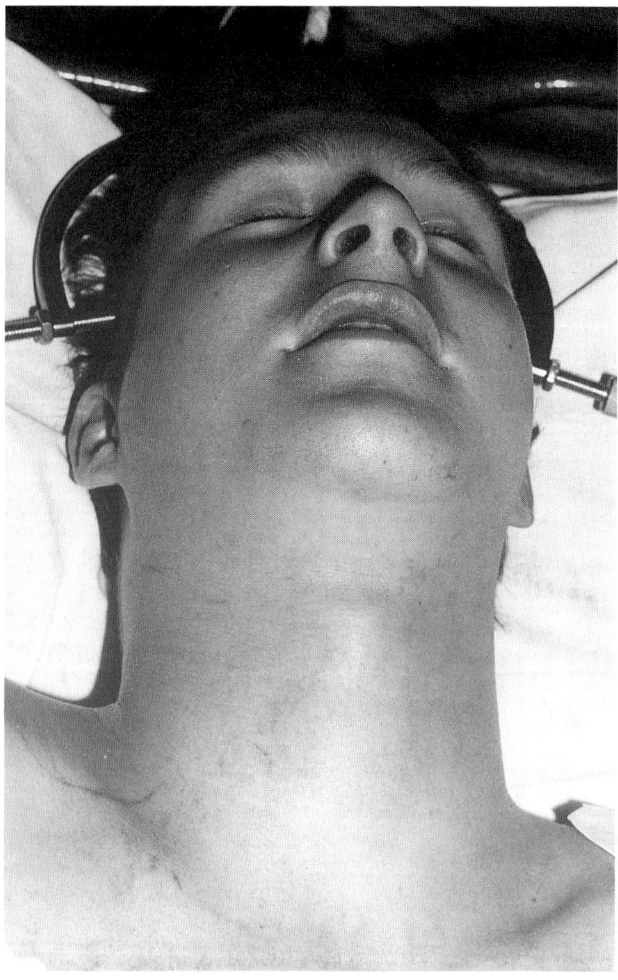

Fig. 18.42 Gross swelling of the neck is common in hyperextension injuries.

It will be appreciated that similar hyperextension injuries may occur in the Klippel–Feil syndrome, in ankylosing spondylitis and in congenital fusion of vertebral bodies. Hairline crack fractures in these conditions are easily 'missed' in the initial radiographs, often with disastrous results. These injuries behave like long bone fractures with the same potential for angulation and displacement unless efficiently immobilized (Fig. 18.44).

Axial loading injuries

These injuries are often combined with a flexion force, so that a diversity of fracture patterns may be encountered. Minor wedge-shaped compression of a vertebral body is characteristic of less severe injuries. Apart from discomfort and stiffness in the neck there may be no physical signs. The posterior ligaments are intact and the fracture is a stable one, merely requiring immobilization in a collar until the symptoms disappear. In more severe accidents (diving into shallow water, traffic accidents) the wedging is greater, the anterior inferior part of the vertebral body is 'pinched off' and the posterior part is driven backwards towards the spinal canal (Fig. 18.45). These notorious injuries are often associated with a complete cord lesion and have been aptly described as 'teardrop' fractures. Pure axial loading causes a bursting or exploding fracture of the vertebral body. Many authorities consider these as stable injuries because the posterior ligamentous complex is presumed to be intact. In the author's experience most of these injuries are unstable, and unless adequately immobilized they quickly deform into a severe kyphotic angulation.

These severe injuries ('teardrop' and bursting fractures) should be nursed initially on skull traction. The alignment is usually improved but there is seldom a corresponding change in the neurological picture. Bony union can be anticipated in most of these cases. When the neurological deficit is incomplete the author prefers to maintain skull traction in the knowledge that many incomplete lesions will continue to improve. When the expected recovery plateau has been reached, there is sometimes a place for anterior decompression guided by the MRI and CT studies. Bohlman (1980) has shown the benefit of such procedures.

A more controversial situation arises when the neurological lesion appears to be complete from the outset and shows no improvement. This is often so in teardrop and severe axial loading fractures. Early surgical intervention, designed specifically for the individual patient and based on evidence of external compression of the dura, has been recommended. It is difficult to avoid advocating a personal philosophy but the author's limited experience of anterior decompression has been uniformly discouraging. Other surgeons take a more hopeful view and advocate anterior decompression in those cases where there is evidence of cord impairment. They argue that incomplete lesions will show a greater degree of improvement, and that it is impossible to know with certainty the extent of the cord damage within the first 48 hours in lesions presumed to be complete. In the latter case, patients have little to lose by exploration, other than the operative risks which are not inconsiderable (Osti *et al.* 1989).

There is an inherent difficulty in assessing the effectiveness of any form of treatment in cord injury. Has improvement resulted because of the intervention, or in accord with the natural history of the particular lesion? Hard statistical evidence in such diverse lesions is most

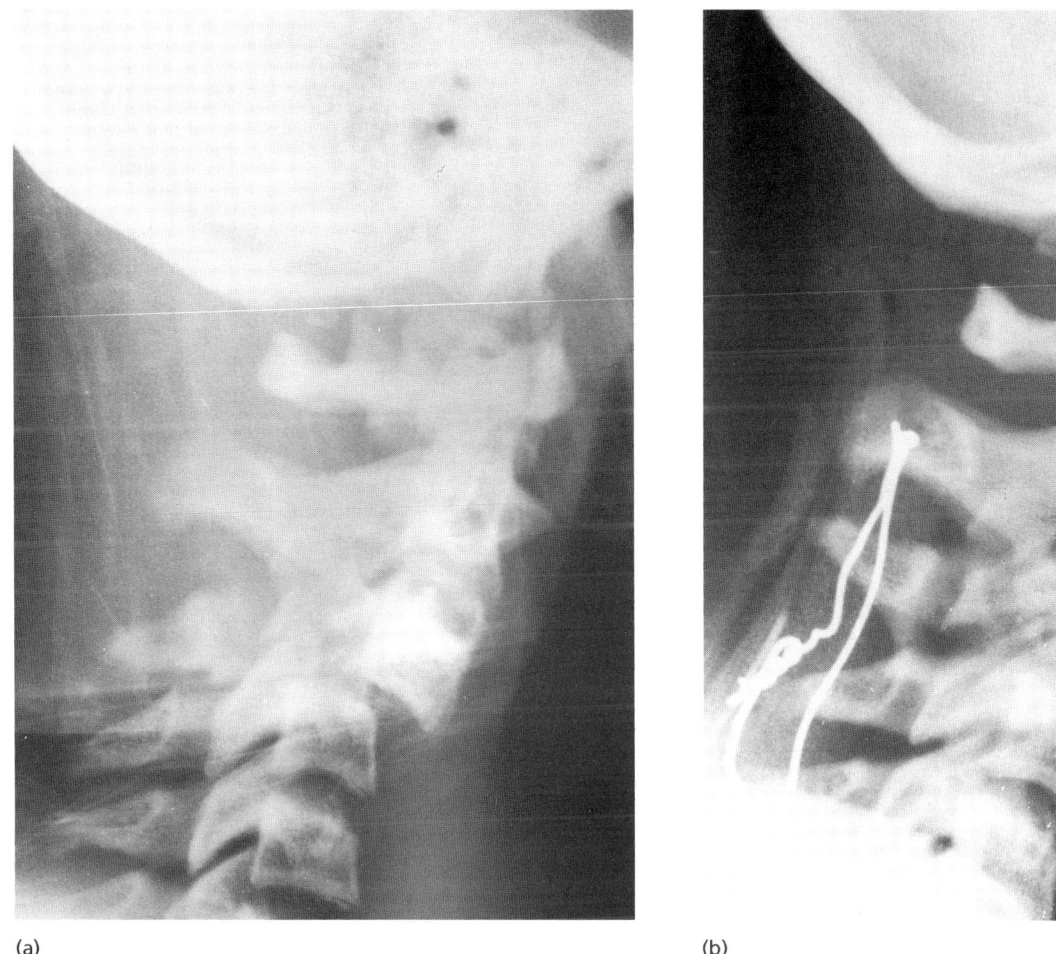

(a)   (b)

Fig. 18.43 (a) Hyperextension fracture–dislocation of C3 on C4 following a trampoline injury; complete tetraplegia occurred. (b) Fusion following reduction; there was no neurological improvement.

elusive. The case for decompression in the acute phase of injury has been forcefully described by Schneider (1951), Pierce (1969), Norrel (1971), Ransohoff (1977) and others. It is hoped that a carefully executed one-stage anterior decompression with simultaneous stabilization will prove more satisfactory than conservative measures. A convincing series is awaited.

Comment on operative procedures

It is not proposed to describe in detail the operations used to stabilize the mid and lower cervical regions. Accounts are available in the standard textbooks of operative surgery and the various methods have been reviewed by Jeffreys (1980). Only an outline is mentioned here. Skull (preferably) or halo traction is in place and intraoperative radiography is advised to define the level of injury (Fig. 18.46). Posterior fusion is

probably the most popular method. A mid-line incision is carried down to the appropriate spinous processes, releasing the muscles by sharp dissection, and following the sinuous course of the median raphe. A fishtail osteotome is used to sweep the muscles to the lateral aspect of the facet joints. In dislocations the obstructing tip(s) of the facet joints may require removal with a rongeur. An angled power drill is used to produce a hole in the thickest part of the spinous process for passage of a 20–22 braided steel wire. One end of the wire is passed through the interspinous space and looped under the lower spinous process. It is then tightened with a wire twister. There is little advantage in wiring grafts onto the laminae, as was the custom. A power drill carrying a large burr is used to decorticate the laminae and spinous processes; this is augmented by use of a fine nibbling forceps. Thin slivers of iliac cortico-cancellous grafts are placed over the prepared

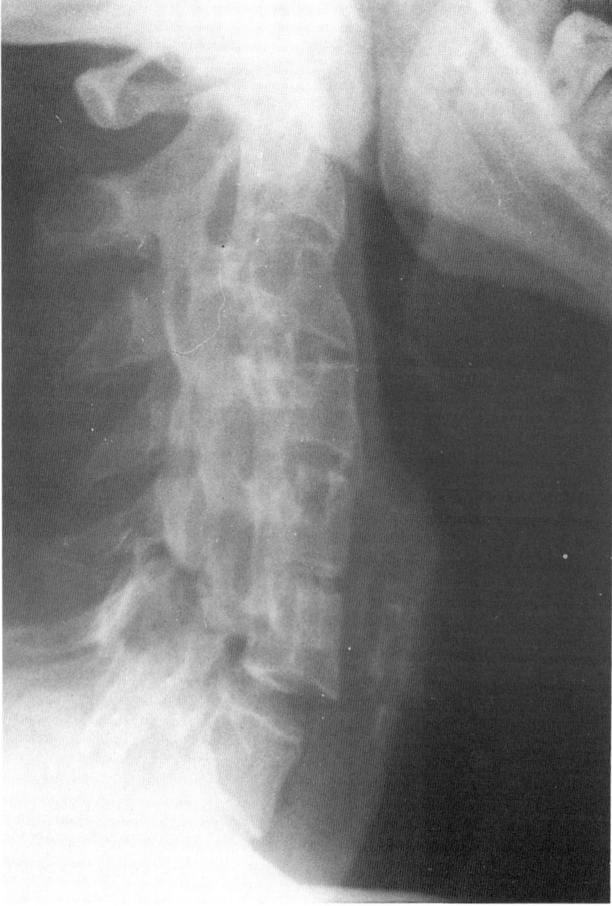

Fig. 18.44 Fracture in ankylosing spondylitis: a 'long bone' fracture.

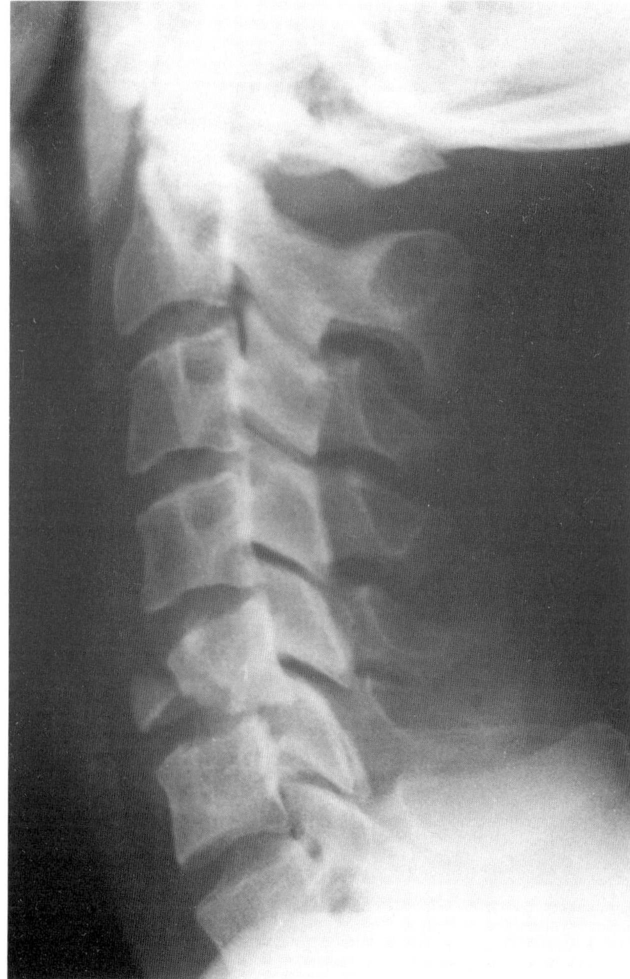

Fig. 18.45 Teardrop fracture of C5; complete neurological lesion.

area. Dove has modified the Luque principle of segmental wiring for the internal fixation of many spinal disorders including difficult fractures and dislocation of the cervical spine (Fig. 18.47).

Anterior fusion and decompression is performed through a transverse incision on the right side of the anterolateral aspect of the neck 5 cm above the clavicle. The mid-cervical fascia is incised along the anterior border of the sternomastoid muscle, which is then retracted laterally with the carotid sheath. The interval between the carotid artery and the oesophagus is developed by blunt (finger and gauze) dissection down to the pre-vertebral fascia. The longus colli muscles are identified and the longitudinal ligament is exposed and incised, keeping strictly to the mid-line. The author's practice is to incise the annulus and, having removed the greater part of the disc with curettes and pituitary

forceps, to excavate a space which will accept a horse-shoe-shaped bone graft. This is taken from the iliac crest and is 8 mm in height, 16 mm wide and 15 mm deep; it should be slightly larger than the bed. Head traction is applied as the graft is countersunk and then released (McSweeney 1978).

Rigid internal fixation of the posterior elements has the attraction of minimal postoperative immobilization. Various techniques have been described, notably those of Camille (1976), Murphy and Southwick (1983) and Magerl (1983). The author finds it difficult to accept that these have a distinct advantage in the average traumatic case. In general, metallic fixation should not be used in anterior procedures because of the risk of oesophageal erosion, and methylmethacrylate, sometimes recommended for posterior fusion, fails to bond permanently and has a high risk of infection.

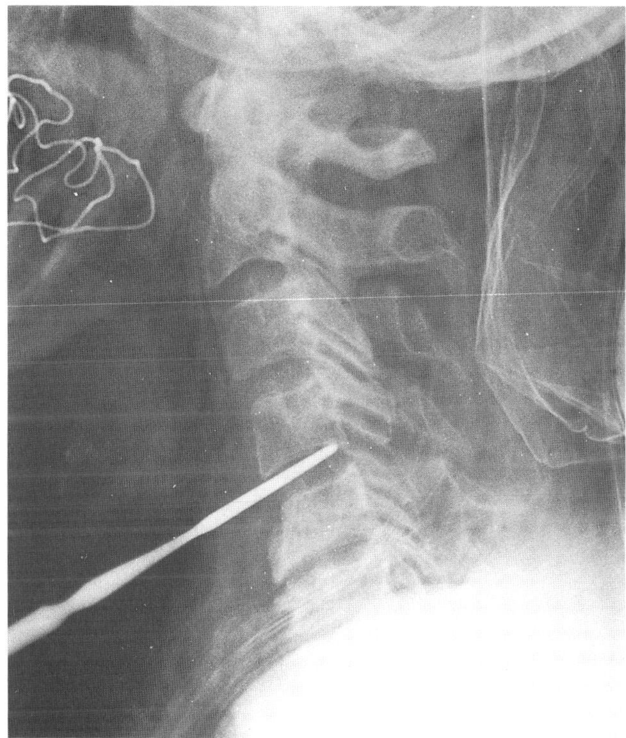

Fig. 18.46 Intraoperative radiography defines the level of injury.

Miscellaneous group

Mention has been made of some of these injuries and of the fact that fused vertebrae of ankylosing conditions or congenital fusions behave like fractures of long bones. Ankylosing spondylitis presents a special problem because of the accompanying respiratory embarrassment, and the tendency to develop pressure sores. Skull calipers are applied and overdistraction is avoided. The patient is nursed in the semi-sitting position and the neck is immobilized in a degree of flexion consistent with the pre-existing deformity. There is a great danger in attempting to improve the posture by extending the neck. Most of these injuries will unite within a few weeks but frequent radiographic monitoring is advised. An occasional patient develops a pseudoarthrosis, and if callus formation is delayed or is otherwise unusual, there should be little delay in advising a posterior fusion. Neurological deterioration is uncommon when the fracture can be immobilized in a good position. A rapid worsening in the paralysis should suggest an epidural haemorrhage. MRI is invaluable in this situation, which calls for decompression by laminectomy followed by posterior fusion.

Stab wounds do not affect stability and seldom demand exploration. Massive broad-spectrum antibiotic therapy and tetanus prophylaxis are required. Similar measures apply to most civilian gunshot wounds. Wounding by high-velocity bullets and war wounds, which are almost always contaminated, require debridement and exploration. Persistent and intractable pain is a common sequence to many of these injuries, irrespective of the neurological lesion.

Severe damage to the spinal cord may occur in young children without there being any evidence of bony injury. The paralysis is permanent and a severe scoliosis is almost inevitable. The author has observed a number of the children over a period of 15–20 years; late radiographs show no evidence of a bony injury. In other cases a bony injury may occur remote from the level of paralysis. A vascular cause is usually postulated but a severe 'stretch' injury of the cord, following the changes in the relative length of the spinal canal and spinal cord, is an alternative explanation. This can occur in extreme ventroflexion of the entire axial skeleton (Breig 1960) and may have been the explanation in one of the cases observed by the author (McSweeney 1979).

Despite the intimate anatomical relationship, injury to the vertebral artery in fracture–dislocation of the neck has only rarely been described (Louw *et al.* 1990). Realignment, rather than direct arterial surgery, would appear to be the treatment of choice. Transient neurological symptoms have been described but the potential for more serious neurological impairment or a fatal outcome must be recognized (Louw *et al.* 1990). Simulated paraplegia, usually of short duration, is an occasional problem in Spinal Injury units. A unit with 50 beds may expect to see at least one case each year. Watson (1982) reported seven cases among 2000 admissions over a 30-year period but in the author's experience the incidence is higher. In contrast, simulated tetraplegia is extremely rare; the author can recall only two cases, both of whom slowly improved, making a full recovery with regard to the motor paralysis.

There are inherent dangers in making the diagnosis of a factitious paralysis following a spinal injury, however trivial. The diagnosis should be reserved until all organic causes have been excluded and the response to treatment is known. Among the inconsistencies are preservation of sphincter function, unless the condition enters a chronic phase. When the disorder does not respond to a forceful, yet sympathetic, explanation a prolonged period of inpatient rehabilitation, as described by Delargy *et al.* (1986) may be successful. This often serves as a 'face saver' and offers the patient a 'cure' which would otherwise be difficult to explain.

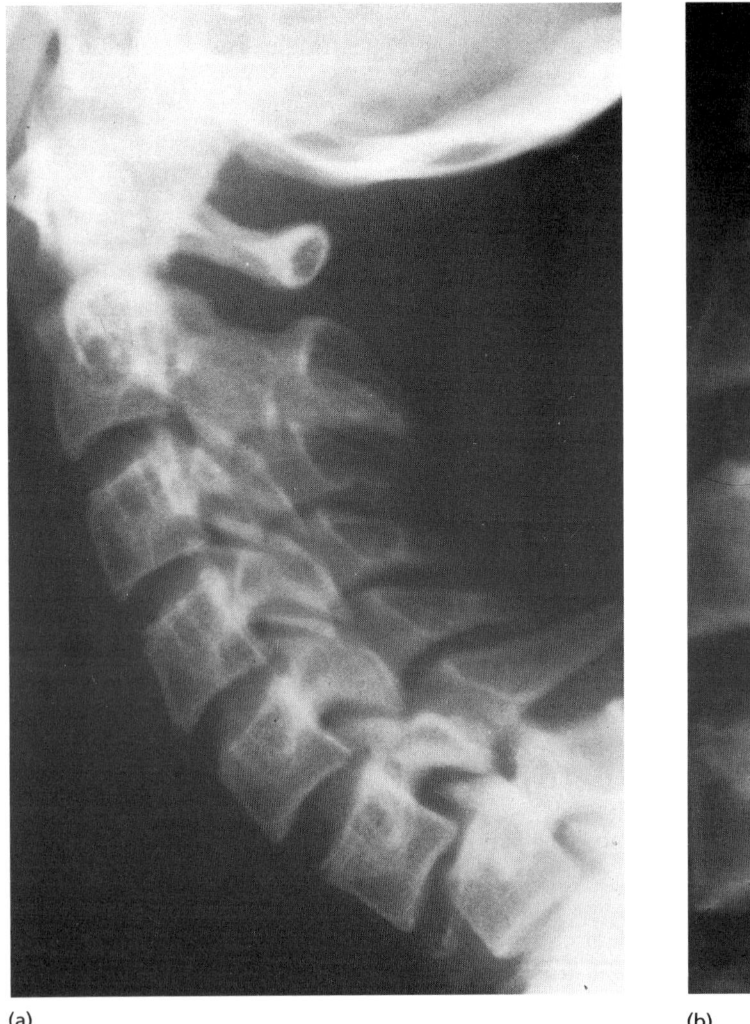
(a)

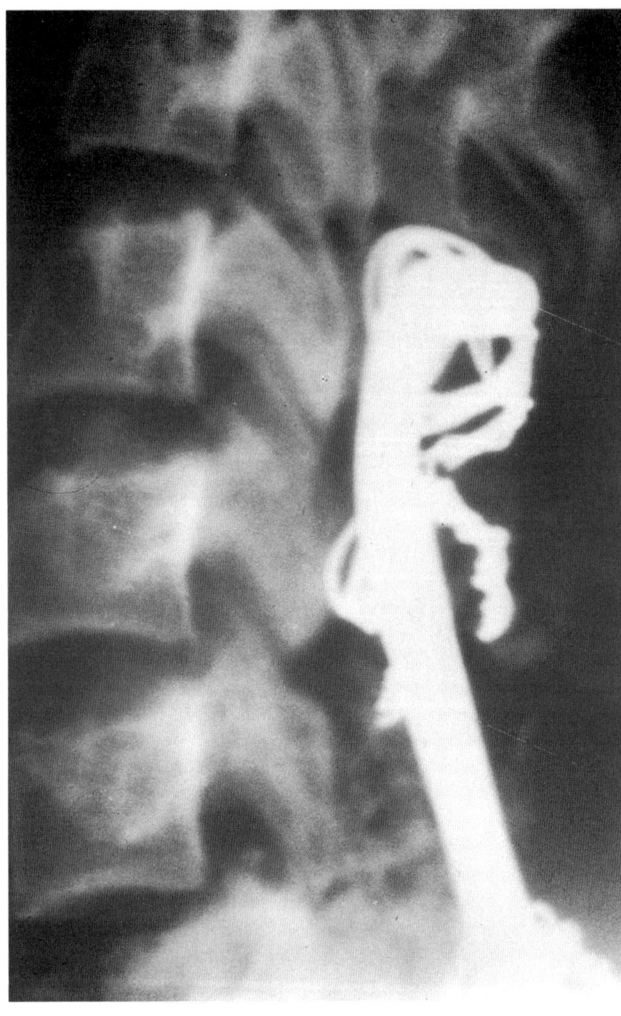
(b)

Fig. 18.47 (a) Old unstable bilateral dislocation with root pressure. (b) The symptoms were relieved and the position improved following laminectomy and fixation using the Hartshill system. (Courtesy of Dove.)

Immense diagnostic difficulties arise in medico-legal practice when the question of malingering is raised in chronic cases. In the author's opinion, the distinction can seldom be made with absolute confidence. The interested reader is referred to the standard works on hysteria (Roy 1982).

Rehabilitation

The aims of rehabilitation are the development and preservation of a high standard of physical fitness combined with a satisfactory mental adjustment. Incomplete lesions usually show a substantial recovery but this is sometimes offset by spasticity — an eminently treatable condition in the vast majority of patients. Complete tetraplegia is a catastrophic injury and it would be

disingenuous to suggest otherwise. The fact that people can readjust to such a high degree of disablement is a tribute to human nature and an indication of the individual's resources.

The principles involved are similar to those following other major injuries and need no detailed explanation here. Excellent accounts are available — Mooney *et al.* 1975; Danbrough & Kinrade, 1977; Bromley, 1985 and Ford & Duckworth, 1987.

After the immediate mental shock, which lasts for a few days, there follows a period of gradual recognition which varies with age, intelligence and pre-accident personality. This is the time to discuss the future prospects truthfully and sympathetically in the light of the clinical judgement. It will be but the first of many similar discussions, bearing in mind that the picture

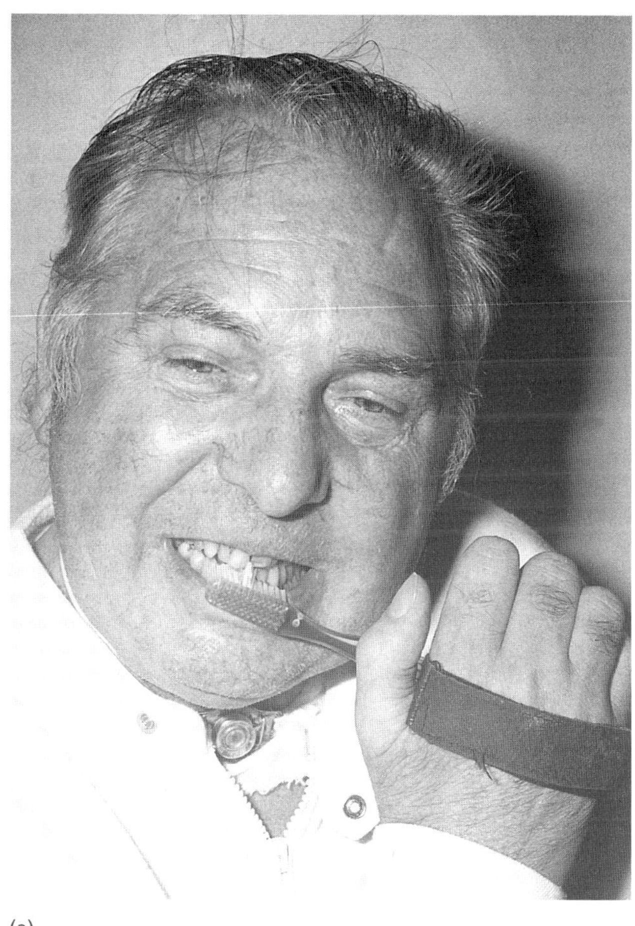

(a)

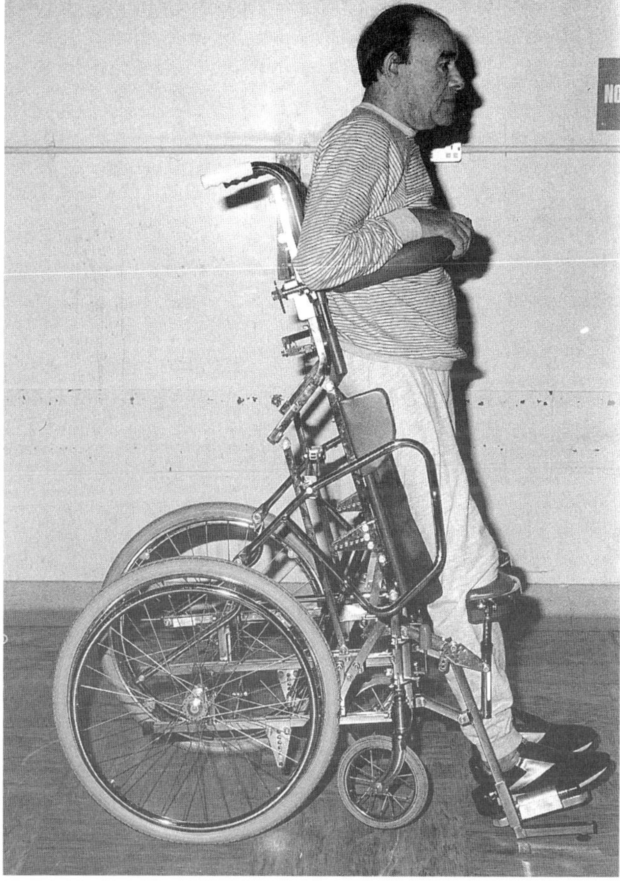

(b)

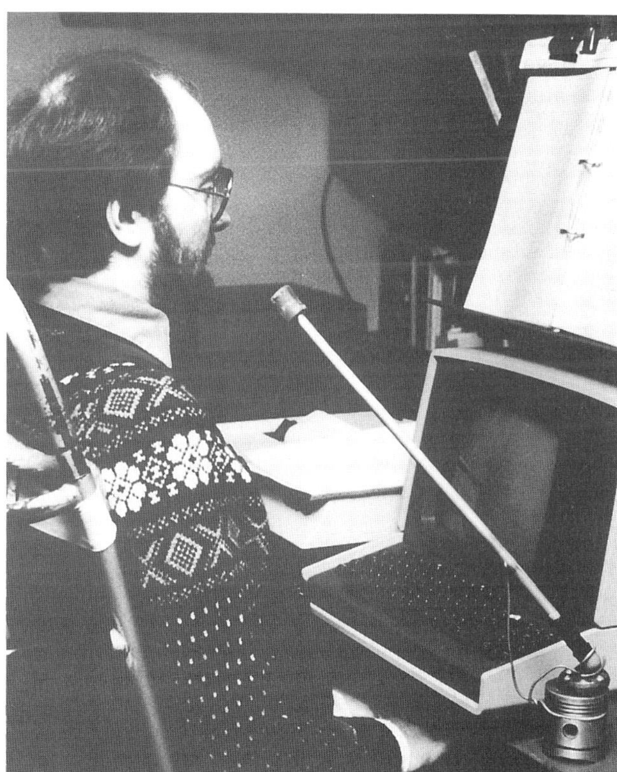

(c)

Fig. 18.48 (a) The traditional aids should not be forgotten, while at a later stage (b) stand-up chairs, and (c) home computers are available.

may alter considerably in the ensuing months. All para-medical staff should be aware of the content of the discussions, and their support and empathy is most important. Once the grief reaction has passed, a stage of active rebellion or latent aggression is often encountered. It is a testing period for all, but when properly directed it is a more favourable feature than the profound apathy which may affect some older patients. When the intermediate phase is reached the tempo is increased, more time is spent in the Rehabilitation department than on the ward (Fig. 18.48) and the necessary orthoses are made available. Later, home visits are arranged and regular case conferences with the social services and industrial and educational authorities are arranged. This policy of graduated discharge should be closely integrated with the family, general practitioner and community nursing service (McSweeney 1983).

Resettlement

This is the complementary process which enables the patient to live in the community with as much independence as the disability will allow (Jones & Jones 1975). While great progress has been made in enlightened countries, some vulgar misconceptions remain. There are three fundamental requirements for the severely disabled; namely, a caring relative or companion, appropriate housing and a reliable means of transportation. Entitlement to social security benefits varies and the advice of a well-informed professional is essential. The present system of compensation is not always satisfactory, and in civil cases the huge single payment award is open to serious criticism. An annuity payment with the early award of an appropriate capital of sum for housing and incidental expenses would seem more sensible. For non-compensatable accidents a no-fault system has many advocates.

Conclusion

The cord and nerve roots are unharmed in most spinal injuries. Localized fusion is advised for those injuries where consequential instability is anticipated. The controversy centres around the place for surgical decompression in the acute phase. It seems to the author that this is of doubtful value once alignment of the spinal column has been restored, but many experienced surgeons take a more hopeful view. The future may lie in a pharmacological agent which would control the early post-traumatic changes in the spinal cord and which would lessen the neurological reaction.

References

Allen, A.R. Surgery of experimental lesion of the spinal column. Preliminary report. *J Am Med Assoc* 1911; **57**: 878–880.

Anderson, L.D. & d'Alonzo, R.T. Fractures of the odontoid process of the axis. *J Bone Joint Surg* 1974; **56A**: 1663–1674.

Andrade, R.J. de & MacNab, I. Anterior occipito cervical fusion using an extra pharyngeal approach. *J Bone Joint Surg* 1969; **51A**: 1621–1626.

Bachs, A., Barraquer-Bordas, L., Barraquer-Ferre, L., Candell, J.M. & Modolell, A. Delayed myelopathy following atlanto-axial dislocation by separated odontoid process. *Brain* 1955; **78**: 537–553.

Bailey, D.K. The normal cervical spine in infants and children. *Radiology* 1952; **59**: 712–719.

Baker, L.H.E. The first aid management of spinal cord injury. In: Harkness, J.W., Hughes, S.P.F. & Schulitz, K.P. (eds) *Seminars in Orthopaedics*, Vol. 4.1. Grune & Stratton: Philadelphia, 1989.

Beatson, T.R. Fracture dislocations of the cervical spine. *J Bone Joint Surg* 1963; **45B**: 21–35.

Beighton, P. & Craig, J. Atlantoaxial subluxation in Morquio syndrome. *J Bone Joint Surg* 1973; **55B**: 478–481.

Bell, H.S. Cruciate paralysis. In: Vinken, P.J. & Bruyn, G.W. (eds) *Handbook of Clinical Neurology*, Vol. 25. North Holland Publishing Co: Amsterdam, 1976.

Blockey, N.J. & Purser, D.W. Fractures of the odontoid process of the axis. *J Bone Joint Surg* 1956; **38B**: 794–816.

Bohlman, H.H. Acute fractures and dislocations of the cervical spine: an analysis of three hundred hospitalized patients and review of the literature. *J Bone Joint Surg (Am)* 1979; **61A**: 1119–1142.

Bohlman, H.H. Late anterior decompression and fusion for spinal cord injuries. Review of 100 cases with long term results. *Orthop Trans* 1980; **4(1)**: 42.

Bonney, G. & Williams, J.P.R. Transoral approach to the upper cervical spine. *J Bone Joint Surg* 1985; **67B**: 691–698.

Braakman, R. & Vinken, P.J. Unilateral facet locking in the lower cervical spine. *J Bone Joint Surg* 1967; **49B**: 249–257.

Braakman, R. & Vinken, P.J. Old luxation of the lower cervical spine. *J Bone Joint Surg* 1968; **50B**: 52–60.

Bracken, M.B., Shepard, M.J., Collins, W.F., Holford, T.R., Young, W., Baskin, D.S., Eisenberg, H.M., Flamm, E.S., Leo, L.S., Maroon, J., Marshall, L.F., Perot, P.L., Piepmeir, J., Sonntag, V.K.H., Wagner, F.C., Wilbergen, J.E. & Winn, R.H. A randomised, controlled trial of methylprednisolone or naloxone in the treatment of acute spinal cord injury. Results of the Second National Acute Spinal Cord Injury Study. *N Engl J Med* 1990; **322**: 1405–1411.

Bracken, M.B., Shepard, M.J., Hellenbrand, K.G., Collins, W.F., Leo, L.S., Freeman, D.F., Wagner, F.C., Flamm, E.S., Eisenberg, H.M., Goodman, J.H., Perot, P.L., Green, B.A., Grossman, R.G., Meagher, J.N., Young, W., Fisher, B., Clifton, G.L., Hunt, W.E. & Rilkinson, N. Methylprednisolone and neurological function 1 year after spinal cord injury. Results of the National Acute Spinal Cord Injury Study. *J Neurosurg* 1985; **63**: 704–713.

Breig, A. *Biomechanics of the Central Nervous System*. Alamgyist & Wilksells: Uppsala, 1960.

Bromley, I. *Tetraplegia and Paraplegia*. Churchill Livingstone: Edinburgh, 1985.

Bucholz, R.W. & Burkhead, W.Z. The pathological anatomy of fatal atlanto occipital dislocations. *J Bone Joint Surg* 1979; **61A**: 248–250.

Burke, D.C. Hyperextension injuries of the spine. *J Bone Joint Surg* 1971; **53B**: 3–12.

Burke, S.W., French, H.G., Roberts, J.M., Johnston, C.E., Whitecloud, T.S. & Edmunds, J.O. Chronic atlanto axial instability in Down's syndrome. *J Bone Joint Surg* 1985; **67A**: 1356–1360.

Cattell, H.S. & Filtzer, D.L. Pseudo subluxation and other normal variations in the cervical spine in children. *J Bone Joint Surg* 1965; **47A**: 1295–1309.

Cheshire, D. The stability of the cervical spine following the conservative treatment of fracture and fracture dislocations. *Paraplegia* 1969; **7**: 193–203.

Clark, C.R. & White, A.A. Fractures of the dens. A multicenter study. *J Bone Joint Surg* 1985; **67A**: 1340–1348.

Cone, W. & Turner, W.G. The treatment of fracture dislocations of the cervical vertebrae by skeletal traction and fusion. *J Bone Joint Surg* 1937; **19**: 584–602.

Cornish, B.L. Traumatic spondylolisthesis of the axis. *J Bone Joint Surg* 1968; **50B**: 31–43.

Crockard, H.A. The transoral approach to the base of the brain and upper cervical cord. *Ann R Coll Surg Engl* 1988; **67**: 321–325.

Crutchfield, W.G. Skeletal traction in treatment of injuries to the cervical spine. *J Am Med Assoc* 1954; **155(1)**: 29–33.

Crutchfield, W.G. Redesigned Crutchfield skull tongs. *J Neurosurg* 1966; **25**: 656–657.

Danbrough, A. & Kinrade, D. *The Directory for the Disabled.* Woodhead-Faulkner: Cambridge, 1977.

Delargy, M.A., Peatfield, R.C. & Burt, A.A. Successful rehabilitation in conversion paralysis. *Br Med J* 1986; **292**: 1730–1731.

DeLorme, T.L. Axis pedicle fractures. *J Bone Joint Surg* 1967; **49A**: 1471–1472.

Denis, F. The three column spine and its significance in the classification of acute thoracolumbar spinal injuries. *Spine* 1983; **8(8)**: 817–831.

Dohrmann, G.J. Experimental spinal cord trauma. A historical review. *Arch Neurol* 1972; **27**: 468–473.

Ducker, T.B. Experimental injury of the spinal cord. In: Vinken, P.J. & Bruyn, G.W. (eds) *Handbook of Clinical Neurology*, Vol. 25. North Holland Publishing Co: Amsterdam, 1976.

Ducker, T.B., Kindt, G.W. & Kempt, L.G. Pathological findings in experimental spinal cord trauma. *J Neurosurg* 1971; **35**: 700–708.

du Toit, G. Lateral atlanto axial arthrodesis. A screw fixation technique. *S Afr J Surg* 1976; **14**: 9–12.

Eismont, F.J., Arena, M.J. & Green, B.A. Extrusion of an intervertebral disc associated with traumatic subluxation or dislocation of cervical facets. *J Bone Joint Surg (Am)* 1991; **73A**: 1555–1560.

Elliot, G.R. & Sachs, E. Observation on fracture of odontoid process of axis with intermittent pressure paralysis. *Ann Surg* 1912; **56**: 876–882.

Evans, D.K. Reduction of cervical dislocations. *J Bone Joint Surg* 1961; **43B**: 552–555.

Evans, D.K. Anterior cervical subluxation. *J Bone Joint Surg* 1976; **58B**: 318–321.

Evans, D.K. Dislocations at the cervico thoracic junction. *J Bone Joint Surg (Br)* 1983; **65B**: 124–127.

Fang, H.S.Y. & Ong, G.B. Direct anterior approach to the upper cervical spine. *J Bone Joint Surg* 1962; **44A**: 1588–1604.

Fielding, J.W. & Hawkins, R.J. Atlantoaxial rotary fixation. *J Bone Joint Surg* 1977; **59A**: 37–44.

Ford, J.R. & Duckworth, B. *Physical Management for the Quadriplegic Patient*. FA Davis; Philadelphia, 1987.

Forsyth, H.F. Extension injuries of the cervical spine. *J Bone Joint Surg* 1964; **64A**: 1792–1797.

Frankel, H.L., Mathias, C.J. & Spalding, J.M.K. Mechanism of reflex cardiac arrest in tetraplegic patients. *Lancet* 1975; **ii**: 1183–1185.

Gallie, W.E. Fractures and dislocations of the cervical spine. *Am J Surg* 1939; **46**: 495–499.

Gardner, B.P., Theocleous, F. & Watt, J.W.H. Ventilation or dignified death for patients with high tetraplegia? *Br Med J* 1985; **291**: 1620–1622.

Gardner, B.P., Watt, J.W.H. & Krishnan, K.R. The artificial ventilation of acute spinal cord damaged patients: a retrospective study of forty-four patients. *Paraplegia* 1986; **24**: 208–220.

Gardner, W.J. The principle of spring-loaded points for cervical traction. *J Neurosurg* 1973; **39**: 543–544.

Geisler, F.H., Dorsey, F.C. & Coleman, W.P. Recovery of motor function after spinal cord injury: a randomized placebo-controlled trial with GM-l ganglioside. *N Engl J Med* 1991; **324**: 1829–1838.

Giannestras, J.J., Mayfield, F.J., Provencio, F.P. & Maurer, J. Congenital absence of the odontoid process. *J Bone Joint Surg* 1964; **46A**: 839–843.

Glenn, W.W.L. & Phelps, M.L. Diaphragm pacing by electrical stimulation of the phrenic nerve. *Neurosurgery* 1985; **17**: 974–984.

Glenn, W.W.L., Hogan, J.F. & Phelps, M.L. Ventilatory support of the quadriplegic patient with respiratory paralysis by diaphragm pacing. *Surg Clin North Am* 1980; **60**: 1055–1078.

Grundy, D., McSweeney, T. & Jones, H.W.F. Cranial nerve palsies in cervical injuries. *Spine* 1984; **9(4)**: 339–343.

Guarantors of *Brain. Aids to the Examination of the Peripheral Nervous System*. Baillière Tindall: London, 1986.

Guttmann, L. Spinal shock. In: Vinken, P.J. & Bruyn, G.W. (eds) *Handbook of Clinical Neurology*, Vol. 26. North Holland Publishing Co: Amsterdam, 1976.

Guttmann, L. & Whitteridge, D. Effects of bladder distension on autonomous mechanisms after spinal cord injuries. *Brain* 1947; **70**: 361–404.

Hall, M. *On the Diseases and Derangement of the Nervous System*. Balliere: London, 1841.

Head, H. & Riddoch, G. The autonomic bladder, excessive sweating and some other reflex conditions in gross injuries of the spinal cord. *Brain* 1917; **40**: 188–263.

Hensinger, R.N., Lang, J.R. & MacEwan, G.D. The Klippel–Feil syndrome: a constellation of related anomalies. *J Bone Joint Surg* 1974; **56A**: 1246–1253.

Holdsworth, F. Fractures, dislocations and fracture dislocations of the spine. *J Bone Joint Surg* 1963; **45B**: 6–20.

Hutchinson, J. Case of fracture of the odontoid process with peculiar symptoms: notes of the case by Robert Debenham. *Clinical Lectures and Reports, The London Hospital*, vol 4, pp. 210–12. John Churchill: London, 1867–68.

Jefferson, G. Fractures of the atlas vertebra; report of four cases and a review of those previously recorded. *Br J Surg* 1920; **20**: 407–422.

Jefferson, G. Discussion on fractures and dislocations of the cervical spine. *Proc R Soc Med* 1940; **33**: 657–660.

Jefferson, G. *Selected Papers*. Pitman Medical: London, 1960.

Jeffreys, E. (ed.) *Disorders of the Cervical Spine*. Butterworth: London, 1980.

Johnson, D.P. & Fergusson, C.M. Early diagnosis of atlanto axial rotatory fixation. *J Bone Joint Surg* 1986; **68B**: 698–703.

Johnson, R.M., Owen, J.R, Hart, D.L. & Callahan, R.A. Cervical orthosis: a guide to their selection and use. *Clin Orthop* 1981; **154**: 34–42.

Jones, H.W.F. & Jones, G. The resettlement process. *Paraplegia* 1975; **12**: 251–253.

Kelly, D.L., Lassiter, K.R.L. & Calogero, J.A. Effects of local hypothermia and tissue oxygen studies in experimental paraplegia. *J Neurosurg* 1970; **33**: 554–563.

Khan, E.A. & Yglesias, L. Progressive atlanto axial dislocation. *J Am Med Assoc* 1935; 105: 348–352.

Ladd, A.L. & Scranton, P.E. Congenital cervical stenosis presenting as transient quadriplegia in athletes. *J Bone Joint Surg* 1986; **68A**: 1371–1374.

Lipschitz, R. Stab wounds of the spinal cord. In: Vinken, P.J. & Bruyn, G.W. (eds) *Handbook of Clinical Neurology*, Vol. 25. North Holland: Amsterdam, 1976.

Lipschitz, R. & Block, J. Stab wounds of the spinal cord. *Lancet* 1962; 169–172.

Louw, J.A., Mafoyane, N.A., Small, B. & Neser, C.P. Occlusion of the vertebral artery in cervical spine dislocations. *J Bone Joint Surg (Br)* 1990; **72B**: 679–681.

Magerl, F. *New Experimental Implants: Cervical Hook Plates*. Technical Bulletin No 61: Association for the Study of Internal Fixation, 1983.

McCall, I.W., Park, W.M. & McSweeney, T. The radiological demonstration of acute lower cervical injury. *Clin Radiol* 1973; **24**: 235–240.

McGraw, R.W. & Rusch, R.M. Atlantoaxial arthrodesis. *J Bone Joint Surg* 1973; **55B**: 482–489.

McMillan, B.S. & Silver, J. Extension injuries of the cervical spine resulting in tetraplegia. *Injury* 1987; **18**: 224–233.

McSweeney, T. Discussion on manipulation. International Medical Society of Paraplegia. *Paraplegia* 1975; **13**: 217–218.

McSweeney, T. Injuries of the Spine. In: London, P.S. (ed.) *Operative Surgery* 3rd edn. Butterworth: London, 1978.

McSweeney, T. Traumatic atlantoaxial dislocation in a child. *Paraplegia* 1979; **17**: 372–376.

McSweeney, T. Fractures, fracture dislocations and dislocations of the cervical spine. In: Jeffreys, E. (ed.) *Disorders of the Cervical Spine*. Butterworth: London, 1980.

McSweeney, T. Management of tetraplegia and paraplegia. In: Harris, N.H. (ed.) *Postgraduate Textbook of Clinical Orthopaedics*. Wright: Bristol, 1983.

McSweeney, T. Injuries to the upper cervical spine. In: Findlay, G. & Owen, R. (eds) *Surgery of the Spine*, Vol. 2. Blackwell Scientific Publications: Oxford, 1992.

Melzak, J. Spinal deformities in two sisters with Brailsford–Morquio syndrome. *Paraplegia* 1969; **6**: 246–258.

Merriam, W.F., Taylor, T.K.F. *et al.* A reappraisal of acute traumatic central cord syndrome. *J Bone Joint Surg* 1986; **68B**: 708–713.

Minns, R.J. & Sutton, R.A. The mechanics of skull traction calipers. *Injury* 1985; **16**: 464–468.

Mixter, S.J. & Osgood, R.B. Traumatic lesions of the atlas and axis. *Am J Orthop Surg* 1910; **7**: 348–355.

Mooney, T.O., Cose, T.M. & Chilgren, R.A. *Sexual Options for Paraplegics and Quadriplegics*. Little, Brown & Co: Boston, 1975.

Murphy, M.J. & Southwick, W.O. Modified Harrington instrumentation of the cervical spine. *Orthop Trans* 1983; **7**: 119–121.

Newman, P. & Sweetman, R. Occipitocervical fusion. *J Bone Joint Surg* 1969; **51B**: 423–431.

Nicoll, E.A. Fractures of the dorso-lumbar spine. *J Bone Joint Surg* 1949; **31B**: 376–394.

Norrell, H.A. The role of early vertebral body replacement in the treatment of certain cervical spine fractures. In: *Proceedings of the Eighteenth Spinal Cord Injury Conference* 1971; 35–39.

Osgood, R.B. & Lund, C.C. Fractures of the odontoid process. *N Engl J Med* 1928; **198**: 61–72.

Osterholm, J.L. & Matthews, Altered norepinephrine metabolism following experimental spinal cord injury. Parts I and II. *J Neurosurg* 1972; **36**: 386–401.

Osti, O.L., Fraser, R.D. & Griffiths, E.R. Reduction and stabilisation of cervical dislocations. *J Bone Joint Surg (Br)* 1989; **71B**: 275–282.

Parsons, K.F. Management of the neuropathic bladder. In: Findlay, G. & Owen, R. (eds) *Surgery of the Spine*, Vol. 2. Blackwell Scientific Publications: Oxford, 1992.

Pearman, J.W. & England, E.J. *The Urological Management of the Patient Following Spinal Cord Injury*. Charles C. Thomas: Springfield, 1973.

Penning, L. Prevertebral haematoma in cervical spine injury. *Am J Neuroradiol* 1980; **1**: 577–565.

Pierce, D.S. Spinal cord injury with anterior decompression, fusion and stabilization and early rehabilitation. *J Bone Joint Surg* 1969; **51A**: 1675–1683.

Pringle, R.G. Effects of injury on the spinal cord. In: Findlay, G. & Owen, R. (eds) *Surgery of the Spine*, Vol. 2. Blackwell Scientific Publications: Oxford, 1992.

Ramsay, A.H., Waxman, B.P. *et al.* A case of traumatic atlanto-occipital dislocation with survival. *Injury* 1986; **17**: 412–413.

Ransford, A.O., Crockard, H.A. *et al.* Craniocervical instability treated by contoured loop fixation. *J Bone Joint Surg* 1986; **68B**: 173–177.

Ransohoff, J. Cervical spinal cord injury medical and surgical therapy. In: Guttmann, L. (ed.) *Proceedings of the Nineteenth Veterans Administration Spinal Cord Injury Conference, Scottsdale, Ariz., 29–31 Oct. 1973*. U.S. Government Printing Office: Washington, D.C., 1977.

Ravichandran, G. & Silver, J. Missed injuries of the spinal cord. *Br Med J* 1982; **284**: 953–956.

Raynor, R.B. & Koplik, B. Cervical cord trauma. The relationship between clinical syndromes and force of injury. *Spine* 1985; **10(3)**: 193–197.

Roaf, R. A study of the mechanics of spinal injuries. *J Bone Joint Surg* 1960; **42B**: 810–823.

Robertson, P.A. & Ryan, M.D. Neurological deterioration after reduction of cervical subluxation. Mechanical compression by disc tissue. *J Bone Joint Surg (Br)* 1992; **74B**: 224–227.

Roy, A. *Hysteria*. John Wiley & Sons: Chichester, 1982.

Roy-Camille, R., Saillant, G. & Benazet, J.P. Treatment of lower cervical spine injuries C3 to C7. *Spine* 1992; **17**: 442–446.

Scher, A. & Vambeck, V. An approach to the cervico dorsal junction following injury. *Clin Radiol* 1977; **28**: 243.

Schiff, D.C.M. & Parke, W.W. The arterial supply of the odontoid process. *J Bone Joint Surg* 1973; **55A**: 1450−1456.

Schneider, R.C. A syndrome in acute cervical spine injuries in which early operation is indicated. *J Neurosurg* 1951; **8**: 360−367.

Schneider, R.C., Livingstone, K.A., Cave, A.J.E. & Hamilton, G. Hangman's fracture of the cervical spine. *J Neurosurg* 1965; **22**: 141−153.

Selecki, B.R. & Williams, H.B.L. *Injuries to the Cervical Spine and Cord in Man*. Australian Medical Publishing Co: Sydney, 1970.

Silberstein, M., Brown, D., Tress, B.M. & Hennessy, O. Suggested MRI criteria for surgical decompression in acute spinal cord injury. Preliminary observations. *Paraplegia* 1992; **30**: 704−710.

Spillane, J.D. Craniovertebral anomalies. In: Williams, D. (ed.) *Modern Trends in Neurology*. Butterworth: London 1957.

Steel, H.H. Anatomical and mechanical considerations of the atlanto axial articulations. *J Bone Joint Surg* 1968; **50A**: 1481−1482.

Stevens, J.M., Kendall, B.E., Crockard, H.A. & Ransford, A. The odontoid process in Morquio−Brailsford's disease. *J Bone Joint Surg (Br)* 1991; **73B**: 851−857.

Stringa, G. Traumatic lesions of the cervical spine. Statistics, mechanism, classification. In: *Neuviene Congres. Société International de Chiurgie Orthopaedique et de Traumatologie, Vienna 1963*. Imprimerie des Sciences: Brussels, 1964.

Taylor, A.S. Fracture dislocations of the neck. A method of treatment. *Arch Neurol Psychiatr* 1924; **12**: 625−639.

Taylor, R.G & Blackwood, W. Paraplegia in hyperextension cervical injuries with normal radiographic appearances. *J Bone Joint Surg* 1948; **30B**: 245−248.

Thorburn, W. Cases of injury to the cervical region of the spinal cord. *Brain* 1887; **9**: 510−514.

Torg, J.S., Pavlov, H. *et al.* Neuropraxia of the cervical spinal cord with transient quadriplegia. *J Bone Joint Surg* 1986; **68A**: 1354−1370.

Wadia, N.H. Myelopathy complicating congenital atlantoaxial dislocation (a study of 28 cases). *Brain* 1967; **90**: 449−463.

Walton, G.L. A new method of reducing dislocation of cervical vertebrae. *J Nerv Ment Dis* 1893; **20**: 609−611.

Watson-Jones, R. Spontaneous hyperaemic dislocation of the atlas. *Proc R Soc Med* 1932; **25**: 586.

Watson-Jones R. *Fractures and Joint Injuries*, Vol. 2. Churchill Livingstone: Edinburgh, 1955.

Watson, N. An outbreak of hysterical paraplegia. *Paraplegia* 1982; **20**: 154−157.

Webb, J.K., Broughton, R.B.K., McSweeney, T. & Park, W.M. Hidden flexion injury of the cervical spine. *J Bone Joint Surg* 1976; **58B**: 322−327.

Weir, D.C. Roentgenographic signs of cervical injury. *Clin Orthop* 1975; **109**: 9−15.

White, A.A. & Panjabi, M.M. *Clinical Biomechanics of the Spine*. Lippincott: Philadelphia, 1978.

White, A.A., Johnson, R.M. *et al.* Biomedical analysis of clinical stability in the cervical spine. *Clin Orthop* 1975; **109**: 85−95.

Whitesides, T.E. & Kelly, R.P. Lateral approach to the upper cervical spine for anterior fusion. *South Med J* 1966; **59**: 879−883.

Whitley, J.E. & Forsyth, H.F. The classification of cervical spine injuries. *Am J Roentgenol* 1960; **83**: 633−644.

Wood-Jones, F. The ideal lesion produced by judicial hanging. *Lancet* 1913; **i**: 53−56.

Thoracic and lumbar spine

D.K.EVANS

Clinical and radiological investigations

Clinical

Injuries to the dorsal and lumbar areas are quite often overlooked, although less frequently so than those in the cervical region. The two circumstances in which mistakes may occur because attention is not drawn to the spine are (i) when the patient has other multiple painful injuries and (ii) when the patient is unconscious. Failure to examine the spine in these circumstances leads to error. It is easy to forget to examine the part of the body which is hidden because the patient is lying on it. Examination of the spine must be routine in the multiply injured or unconscious patient. On the other hand, when an injured patient does complain of back pain it should be initially assumed that a spinal injury is present and that the injury is unstable. Turning the supine patient to examine the spine must therefore be done with the trunk in one plane with the shoulders and the pelvis, maintaining the same alignment at all times.

Inspection. An inspection of the dorso-lumbar region may reveal obvious deformity and loss of alignment of the spinous processes in the sagittal or coronal plane. Bruises or abrasions may suggest the mechanism of injury. For example, flexion−rotation injuries at the dorso-lumbar junction occur when force is applied to one scapula and the spine is twisted. Bruising or grazing on that scapula are not uncommon in such injuries.

Palpation. This confirms the spinal malalignment and may also reveal a tender defect between spinous processes, indicating rupture of the interspinous ligaments. Such a gap is certain evidence that the damaged spinal segment is unstable. In less severely injured spines localized tenderness often indicates the level on which radiological examination must be focused.

Lack of tenderness should not be taken as an indication that the spine is undamaged. In burst fractures of the vertebral body (see p. 604) damage to the posterior ligaments and the spinous processes may not occur even though the body is severely comminuted. Tenderness may then be absent.

Neurological assessment

A detailed neurological examination, repeated regularly in the first 2—3 days after injury and accurately recorded, is absolutely essential if rational treatment is to be offered and the treatment subsequently assessed. Sensation, motor power and reflex activity must all be carefully noted. The examiner must assess each modality of *sensation* in each lumbar and sacral dermatome below the level of cord injury in a regular and systematic way. It is best to start from the fifth sacral segment around the anus and work upwards. Dorsal column sensations of light touch, vibration and position sense, and spinothalamic tract pain and temperature sensation must be determined. The upper level of sensory disturbance should be accurately recorded. Significant changes, which may be temporary, often occur in the first week or two after injury.

Motor power. This is conventionally assessed by muscle groups rather than individual muscles and should be recorded on the Medical Research Council scale of 0—5. Hip flexors and extensors, and abductors and adductors should be noted. Knee flexion and extension and ankle dorsiflexion, plantar flexion, inversion and eversion and toe movements should all be recorded. Abdominal muscle action can be assessed roughly by palpation and by displacement of the umbilicus on raising the head and shoulders from the bed (Beevor's sign).

Reflex activity. Such activity must be looked for. It returns in the transected cord from below upwards and rises like a tide. The anal skin (S5) and glans-bulbar reflexes (S3/4), which have early prognostic significance, are usually the first to return and, indeed, may never be lost. The plantar responses (S1), at first flexor, appear in a day or two and after several days become extensor. The ankle jerks (L5/S1) may not be elicited for 2 weeks and the knee jerks not, perhaps, for 6 weeks (L3/4). In an apparently complete neurological lesion the presence of reflex activity at a level, or time, that is not expected should lead to a guarded prognosis and suggests that the cord damage is incomplete. Reflex activity is significant since spinal shock must have passed off in the cord segments through which the reflex arc passes (Fig. 18.49).

If the cooperative patient shows no signs of motor or sensory function, i.e. the cord lesion is a complete one, after 24 hours and *in the presence of expected reflex activity below the level of cord damage*, then further recovery is unlikely under any circumstances. A complete cord injury means that there is no voluntary motor

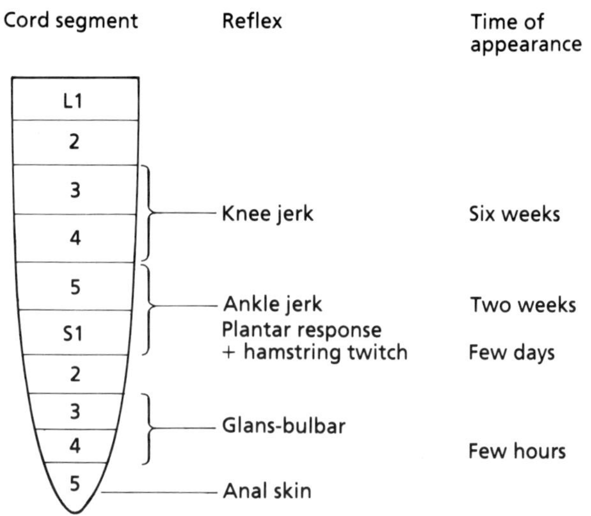

Fig. 18.49 The return of reflex activity after complete spinal cord transection.

activity in the muscles, nor the slightest sensory appreciation in the dermatomes, below the level of spinal cord damage. Should an incomplete lesion of the cord be present, however, some degree of functional recovery in the lower limbs is likely and this recovery may be very considerable, even when no attempt at reduction of the bony displacement has been made. The incomplete nature of the cord damage may be shown merely by a small area of sensory appreciation in the skin around the anus (S5 dermatome).

A neurological examination should be repeated at least daily in the first week or two after the injury.

Radiology

Physical examination can indicate a level of injury and suggest a mechanism, but the exact nature of the bony damage is revealed only by imaging techniques. Radiology in two planes centred on the injured segment is the first step. The posterior spinal elements should be seen as clearly as the vertebral bodies. A double-cassette technique using two films with an interposed filter allows both anterior and posterior elements to be seen with one exposure (Fig. 18.50). Oblique radiographs are occasionally helpful to show the middle column (see below) more clearly.

Tomography has been largely superceded by computerized axial tomography (CAT) scanning in spinal injuries. It is still useful, however, in the visualization of sagittal displacements in the upper dorsal spine (Fig. 18.51). Resolution is poor but this is usually of little consequence since most displaced injuries in this region

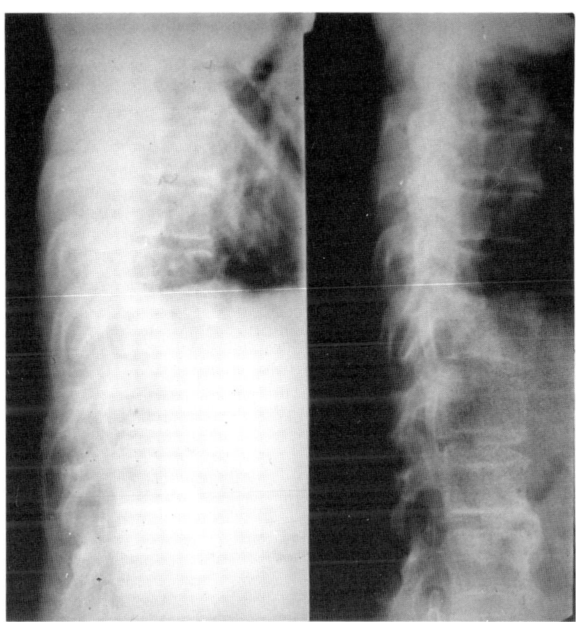

Fig. 18.50 Double-cassette exposure.

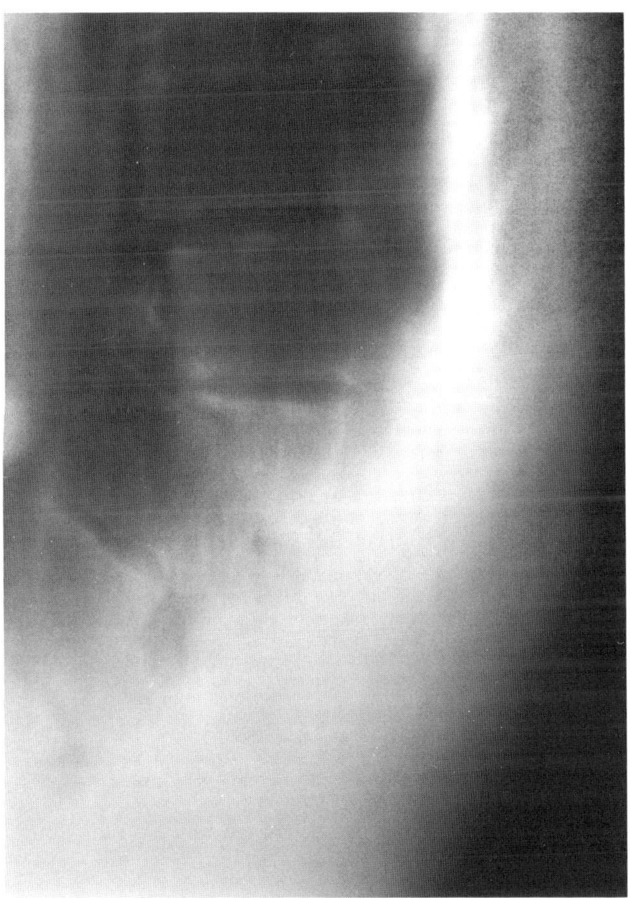

Fig. 18.51 Tomogram of the upper dorsal spine.

are associated with complete cord damage and the displacement is rarely physically disabling or a source of symptoms. There is therefore very little indication for exact reduction of the injured segments in such circumstances.

Encroachment on the spinal canal by bone fragments may be inferred by close examination of the lateral radiograph. Distortion of the posterior wall of the vertebral body (Fig. 18.52a) and shortening of the pedicles are pointers (Fig. 18.53a). CAT scanning, however, certainly reveals fractured fragments and their exact position relative to the spinal cord and nerve roots (Figs 18.52b and 18.53b). These fractures are not otherwise demonstrable (McAfee *et al.* 1983). How helpful such exact knowledge is in treatment is discussed later.

Nuclear magnetic resonance (NMR) imaging demonstrates ligamentous soft tissue damage and, especially, displacements of the intervertebral disc. It is more exact than myelography or simple manometry in the diagnosis of the injured spinal soft tissues. Manometric block of the flow of cerebrospinal fluid (csf) is not always the result of compression of the theca by disc or bone fragments. It is frequently due to oedema. Moreover, the result of manometric investigation has no prognostic significance. A complete block may be present in an incomplete neurological lesion even when recovery is occurring. Conversely, complete and irrecoverable cord lesions can be associated with an incomplete manometric block.

Pathology of spinal cord injury

Pathological changes in the injured spinal cord develop very rapidly. It has been shown experimentally that within 15 minutes red cell diapedesis produces small petechial haemorrhages in the central grey matter; these enlarge and may extend into the white matter within 2 hours. At 4 hours after injury most of the central grey matter has been destroyed by this advancing coagulation necrosis (Fig. 18.54). The changes spread longitudinally as well as radially and may affect several cord segments.

The white matter is also affected and within 4 hours of injury many of the myelinated fibres show swelling and disintegration of the axonal material and the myelin sheaths. These changes cause oedema of the cord, which becomes so tense that the subarachnoid and subdural spaces are obliterated. The extent of these changes varies considerably from transient interruption of function with rapid, complete recovery to total anatomical transection.

The haemorrhagic changes are associated with pro-

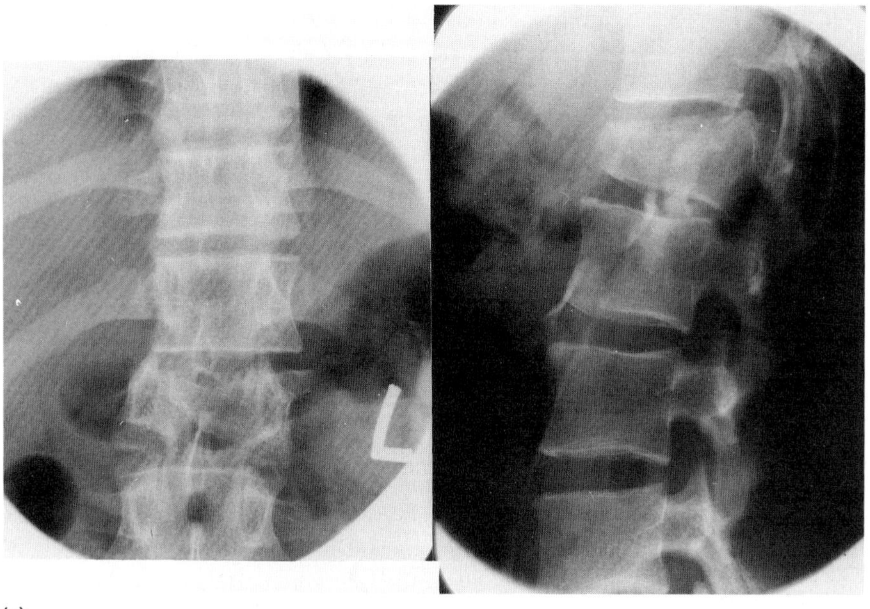

(a)

(b)

Fig. 18.52 (a) The displaced fragment of the posterior wall of the vertebral body can be seen here. (b) The bony fragment in the canal revealed by CAT scan.

found changes in the norepinephrine metabolism. The amount of this substance in the damaged cord increases remarkably and it is suggested that it causes intense vasospasm and ischaemia, thus increasing the necrosis of the cord substance. Efforts to halt or reverse these haemorrhagic and ischaemic changes have been made. The use of hypothermia to reduce the oxygen demand of the cord has been found to be beneficial, but only if cord damage is not severe and if the cooling is initiated within an 8-hour period. The method involves laminectomy which may compromise spinal stability. It has not proved very useful in practice (White 1973).

To reverse the dramatic decrease in oxygen tension in the injured tissue, hyperbaric oxygen has been used. Yeo *et al.* (1977) noted an improved neurological outcome in sheep but, so far, the technique has been little used in clinical practice.

It is difficult to deliver pharmacological agents to the

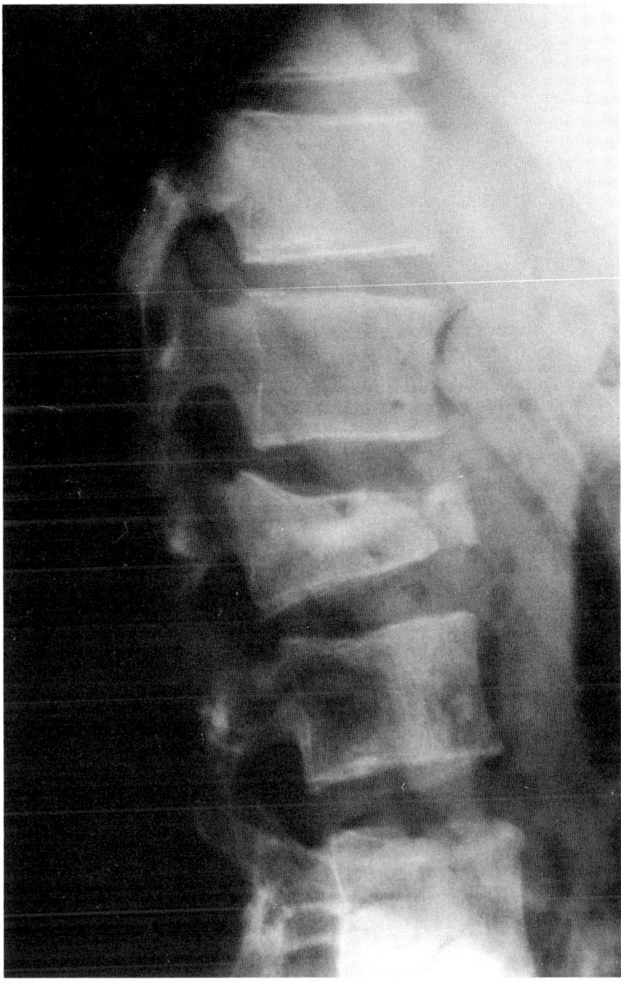

(a)

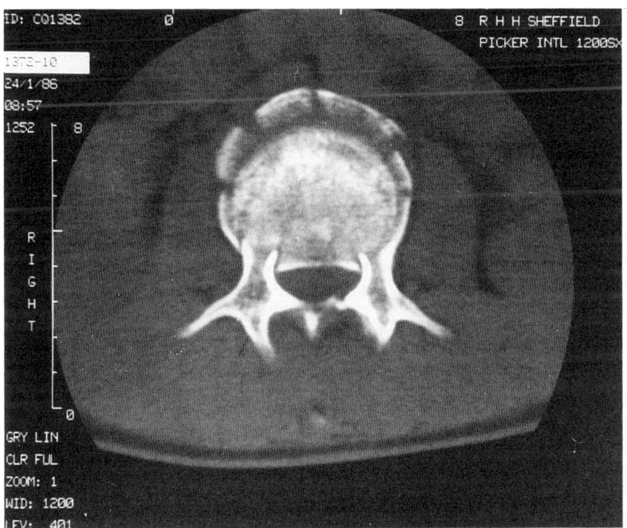

(b)

Fig. 18.53 (a) Apparent shortening of the pedicles suggesting spinal canal narrowing. (b) CAT scan of the fractured vertebral body shown in (a).

injured spinal cord, partly because of the ischaemia and partly because the exact local dosage is impossible to assess. Intravenous infusion of alpha methyl tyrosine might inhibit the changes caused by norepinephrine, since it inhibits tyrosine hydroxylase. This enzyme is essential for the conversion of tyrosine in norepinephrine synthesis. Steroids, which are known to have a dramatic effect in diminishing cerebral oedema, have been used in spinal cord injuries. Recently, favourable results have been reported in patients who received high-dose methylprednisolone for the treatment of spinal cord trauma, providing that the cord injury has been identified within 8 hours of injury (Bracken *et al.* 1990).

At the present time, therefore, it may be possible to influence the development of the pathological process in the injured spinal cord by non-surgical means. If the force has been sufficient to cause complete haemorrhagic necrosis of the whole cord however, then a complete paraplegia will inevitably result. The position is not so clear when the damage to the cord leads to partial disruption of the neural elements, particularly when bone or disc fragments occupy the spinal canal and can be shown to impinge on the cord and theca. If the tracts and cells in the cord remain distorted by the pressure of bone fragments, then the situation might be similar to that occurring in conditions such as tuberculosis, where the pressure on the cord by an abscess produces paraplegia slowly. Decompressing such a cord can lead to remarkable recovery, even when paralysis has persisted for many weeks. There are those that argue that the force of the injury has already been spent in these cases, and that at the time of impact the distortion of the cord was considerably greater. They argue that removal of small fragments cannot 'decompress' the cord since some degree of recoil and decompression after the immediate impact has already occurred. Although it has been said that the force applied to the cord is usually greater than the minimum necessary to produce the maximum damage, this cannot be so in the partially damaged cord.

The work of Bohlman (1982) and Riska *et al.* (1987) suggests that the partially damaged cord, still under some pressure, can recover when the pressure is removed and distortion corrected. Accurate assessments of the value of surgery are difficult to make as spontaneous improvement in partial lesions is the rule. There are no documented controlled results at present to prove that such 'decompression' procedures improve cord recovery.

Below the second lumbar vertebra, however, there is no doubt that relieving the nerve roots of the cauda

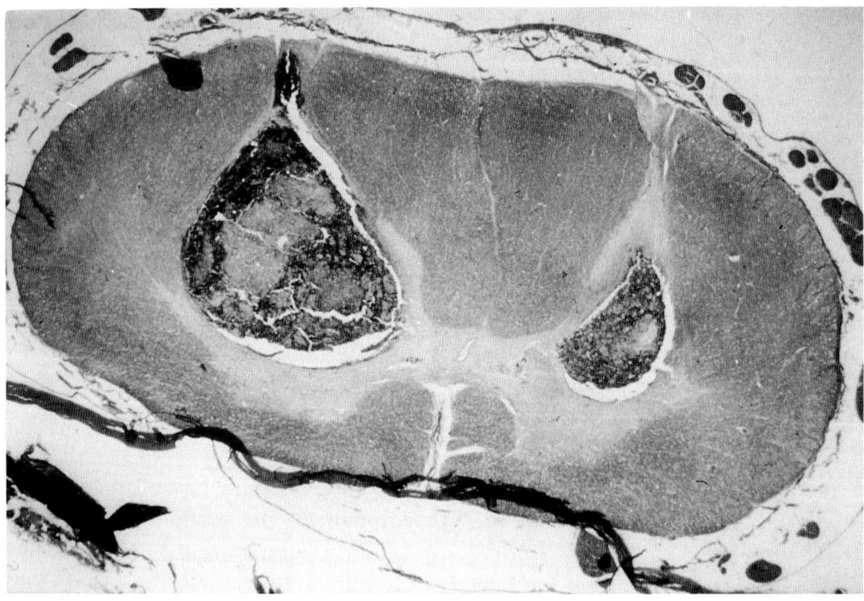

Fig. 18.54 Haemorrhagic necrosis of the central area of grey matter.

equina from pressure does frequently improve neurological recovery, as it does in other peripheral nerve entrapment syndromes.

Classification

Böhler recognized varieties of flexion fractures and dislocations of the spine but did not attempt a classification. He stated that most injuries of the dorsal and lumbar spines were produced by compression. Illustrations of burst fractures and fracture–dislocations, and even the Chance fracture, appear in his book (Böhler 1935). He described the palpable gap between the spinous processes in severe flexion injuries when the posterior ligaments were torn. Böhler recognized also that paralysis was likely to occur if the posterior wall of the vertebral body fractured or if displacement of the vertebral bodies occurred. Roaf (1960) came close to classifying the various spinal injuries in an experimental study of isolated spinal units subjected to forces of different magnitude and direction. He was able to produce the various compression, flexion and rotational injuries with ease and concluded that, in general, rotational forces produced dislocations, whereas compression forces produced fractures.

Sir Frank Holdsworth (1963) clarified treatment by classifying spinal injuries into stable and unstable injuries, and in defining stability divided the spinal column into two distinct pillars: anterior and posterior. The anterior pillar, or joint system, consisted of the intervertebral disc joint with its associated anterior and posterior longitudinal ligaments. The posterior system

was composed of the facet joints, their associated capsular ligaments and the accessory supraspinous, interspinous and interlaminar ligaments. If one joint system was disrupted he thought that the spine should be considered stable, and if both were damaged then instability was present (Fig. 18.55).

Such a pure 'black and white' concept, while excellent in serving the purpose of simplifying the understanding and rationalizing the treatment of most spinal injuries, did not embrace a large number of 'grey' injuries. Even the bursting fracture of the vertebral body, as he illustrated it, very seldom occurred without damage to the posterior elements.

The classification of White and Panjabi (1978) was based on a biomechanical analysis of the motion of spinal segments. It is complex and difficult to use.

An extended classification was proposed by Denis (1982). That posterior ligamentous division alone could not produce instability has long been recognized, especially by surgeons fusing scoliotic spines. Holdsworth's dictum, that rupture of these ligaments was certain evidence of instability, was stated in the context of injury and is still valid. Denis proposed a third spinal pillar or column: namely, the posterior wall of the vertebral body, the posterior annulus and the posterior longitudinal ligament (Fig. 18.56). This concept has drawn attention to the 'grey' injuries and, in particular, to the vertical compression or bursting fractures already mentioned. CAT scanning of such injuries of the vertebral body confirms that the posterior elements are seldom intact and, in most cases, the splaying of the posterior joints and the increase in interpedicular dis-

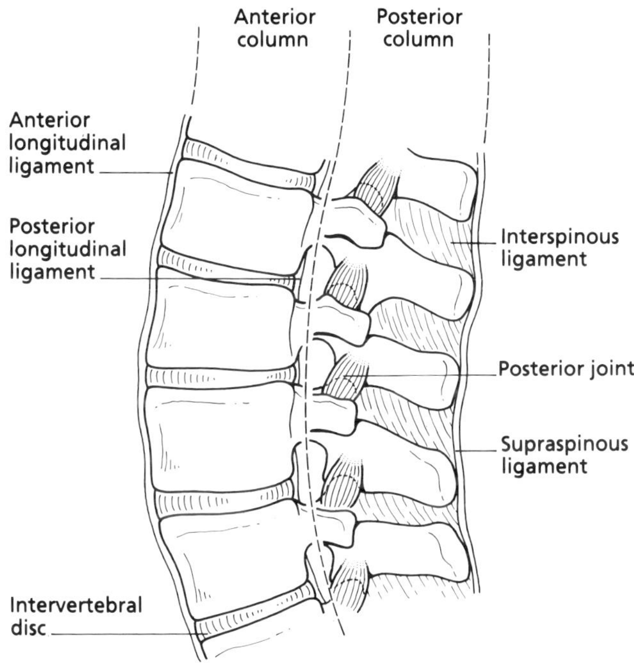

Fig. 18.55 The two-column spine.

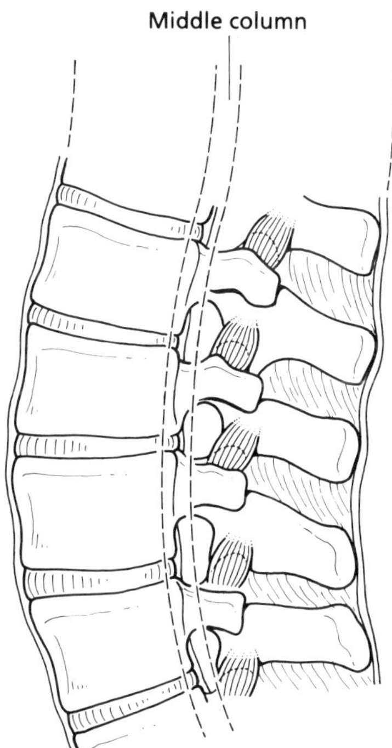

Fig. 18.56 The three-column spine.

tance is not just due to a greenstick fracture of the lamina, as described by Denis, but is rather the result of a much greater disruption of the laminae, pedicles, or the junction of pedicles and body. Although the posterior ligamentous complex may be largely intact in such cases, a considerable degree of abnormal movement — instability — is possible at the damaged segment. Denis complicated his classification by introducing the term 'neurological instability' to describe a lesser degree of instability for these burst fractures not showing neurological damage, although some of his cases later developed neurological deficits. It is safer to assume that all burst fractures are potentially unstable and capable of further displacement.

A more readily remembered and useful classification would be:

Stable

Flexion−compression fracture.

Unstable

Fractures and dislocations of the Chance variety.

Vertical compression (burst) fractures.

Rotational fracture−dislocations.

Shear fracture−dislocations.

There are obviously degrees of instability, as Denis describes, and therefore these unstable injuries might be further subdivided (Table 18.1). The term 'stable' should be defined since it means different things when different fractures are discussed. When referring to spinal injuries it may be considered that a spine is unstable if abnormal movement can be produced when the spine is gently flexed, rotated or axially loaded. The 'looser' the spine is, the greater the degree of instability. In the classification in Table 18.1 a first-degree injury is unstable only in the direction of the original force. In the second degree, instability is also present, to some extent, in directions other than the original, while in third-degree injuries the disruption is so great that abnormal movement is possible in all directions.

Injury patterns

Anatomical factors determine the pattern of injury when a force is applied to the spinal column. The thoracic spine has a smooth kyphotic curve which converts any vertical compression force into one of flexion. Typical vertical compression burst fractures are seldom seen, therefore, in the thoracic region. Similarly, because of its mobility, a direct horizontally applied force to the lumbar area is converted to a flexion, or flexion−rotation force, and the shearing fracture, produced so often by such a force in the thoracic region, is rare.

Flexion injuries

Flexion−compression

Flexion of the spine is resisted by the very strong

Table 18.1 Classification of unstable injuries

Injury	Mechanism
First degree	
Injuries of the Chance variety	Flexion–distraction
Horizontal displacement of the dorsal spine (the intact ribs confer stability)	Shear
Burst fractures with intact posterior column	Vertical compression
Second degree	
Burst fractures with damage to all three columns	Vertical compression
Third degree	
Rotational dislocations and fracture–dislocations	Flexion–rotation

posterior ligaments. These structures, designed to resist tension, withstand forces which are expended on the front of the vertebral body and produce a compression fracture (Fig. 18.57). The body is not comminuted, no ligaments are torn, and further displacement will not occur unless a force greater than the original flexion force is applied. The injury is a stable one, although some consider anterior wedging greater than 50% of bony height to be a sign of instability (Walters *et al.* 1986). Neurological damage is unusual. Symptomatic treatment only is required. There is no need to reduce the compressed bone and healing rapidly occurs. These injuries are seen in both the thoracic and upper lumbar regions. Although they heal rapidly, it is not unusual for some back pain, below the fracture, to persist.

Flexion–distraction

An unusual type of fracture occurs at the dorso-lumbar junction by a flexion and distraction force. Such injuries were first described by Chance in 1948. They are rare in the UK but are not uncommon in countries where road traffic accidents are frequent and where the car occupant is restrained only by a lap strap. Sudden deceleration throws the trunk upwards and forwards over the fulcrum of the lap strap. Several varieties of the injury are possible (Gumley *et al.* 1982). They are characterized by a relatively horizontal fracture line through the posterior elements and the posterior part of the vertebral body (Fig. 18.58). Rarely, the injury is entirely ligamentous and a flexion–dislocation results. As would be expected, there is a high incidence of associated intra-abdominal injuries, caused by the lap strap.

Vertical compression injuries

Vertical compression fractures occur in the lumbar spine if the vertical force is applied with the spine slightly flexed so that the lumbar lordosis is corrected. Such injuries occur by falling from a height and landing in a sitting position. The most commonly affected vertebrae are L1, L2 and L3. The longitudinal force squeezes the intervertebral disc through the vertebral endplate, burst-

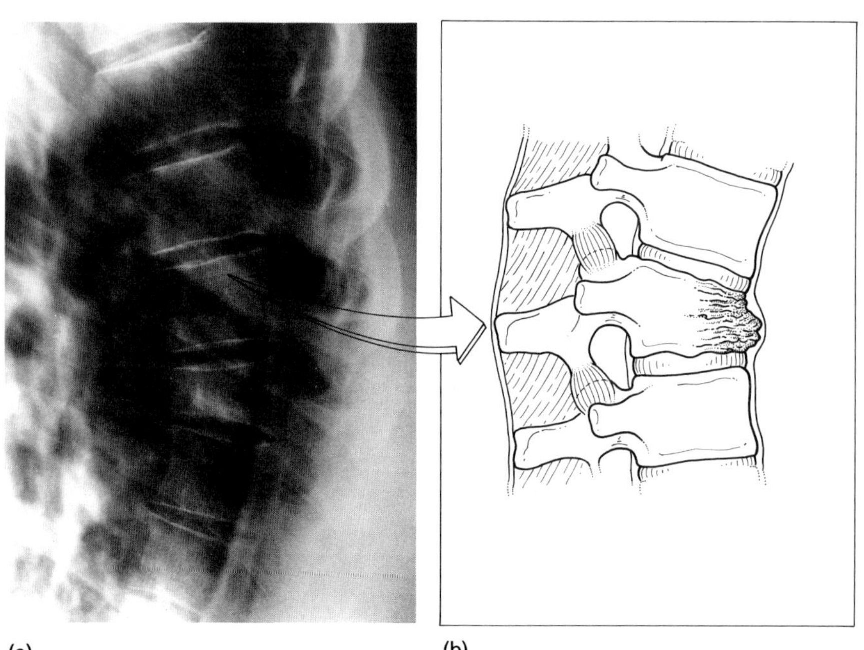

(a)   (b)

Fig. 18.57 (a) Flexion–compression fracture. (b) Flexion–wedge fracture.

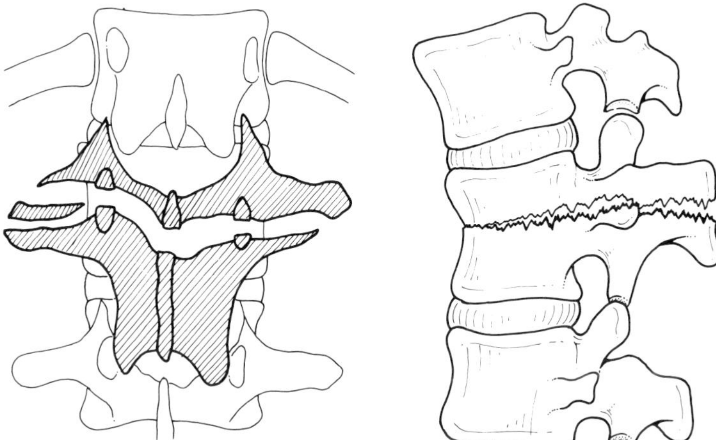

Fig. 18.58 Flexion–distraction 'Chance' fracture.

ing the cancellous vertebral body (Percy 1957, Roaf 1960). Fragments of the body may be displaced forwards or backwards and, in addition, variable damage is done to the posterior vertebral ring (Fig. 18.59). Retropulsion of fragments of the posterior vertebral wall frequently causes spinal cord or nerve root damage. Variable degrees of instability of the injured segment occurs depending upon the amount of comminution of the vertebral body and the amount of damage to the pedicles and laminae. These bursting fractures have been classified by Denis into five groups, depending on the manner of endplate disruption and whether there is associated rotatory or lateral flexion displacements.

The five types of burst fracture are:

1 Both endplates of the vertebra are fractured.

2 Fracture of the superior endplate.

3 Fracture of the inferior endplate.

4 Burst with rotation.

5 Burst with lateral flexion.

If decompression is performed, then the surgical exposure should be directed to the endplate fracture level(s).

Knowledge of the extent of these bursting injuries has increased with the use of CAT scanning. That the posterior wall of the vertebral body has been fractured can be deduced from the lateral radiographs but scanning shows by exactly how much the fragments of bone have encroached into the canal. The scan does not, however, indicate how much neurological damage has occurred, nor how mobile such displaced fragments are. There is no simple direct relationship between canal compromise and neurological deficit. NMR imaging will show distortion of the spinal cord and may prove invaluable in assessment and treatment.

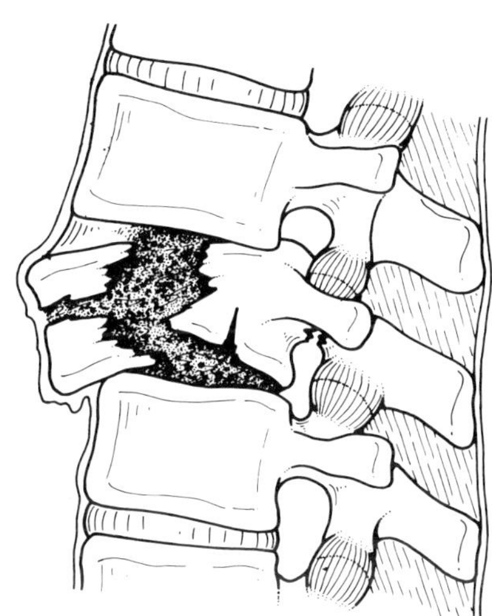

Fig. 18.59 Vertical compression burst fracture; note the fracture of the pedicle.

Flexion–rotation injuries

Flexion and rotational forces applied to the upper trunk are transmitted to the next mobile lower segment: namely, the dorso-lumbar junction. The flexion and twisting force ruptures the posterior ligaments and the weight of the trunk on the vertebral body shears off a slice of the body below the displacement. The facet joint on one side is frequently fractured or dislocated (Fig. 18.60). Such an injury disrupts all three spinal columns and gross displacement can result. The instability is so severe that the displacement may reduce completely when the rotational force is reversed and the patient placed supine. The bony movement usually causes considerable neurological damage and, frequently, complete paraplegia but, surprisingly, rupture of the theca is rare.

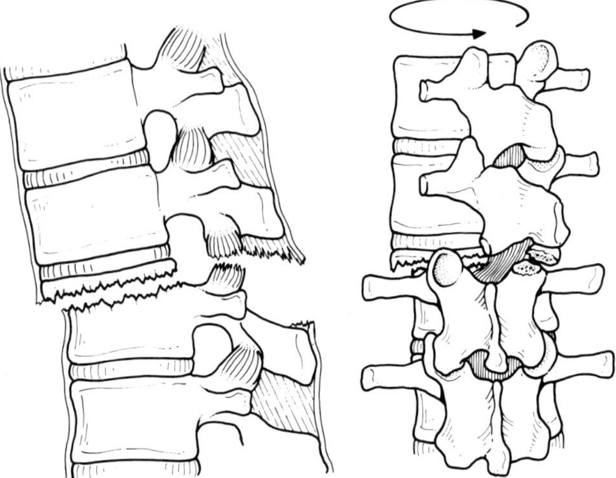

Fig. 18.60 Flexion–rotation fracture–dislocation.

Horizontal translation ('shearing') fracture–dislocations

Such injuries occur in the dorsal spine as a result of direct violence to the spine. The upper spinal segment usually displaces forwards and there is frequently an added flexion component to the force (Fig. 18.61). There are usually fractures of the pedicles, laminae, transverse processes and vertebral body, together with posterior rib fractures at the damaged level (Fig. 18.69). Although all the spinal columns are disrupted, considerable stability is conferred by the remainder of the intact rib cage. As would be expected from the displacement and the relatively poor vascular supply to the dorsal spinal cord between T3 and T9, (Domisse 1974) complete destruction of the cord and permanent paraplegia commonly results.

Management of paraplegia

Complete loss of voluntary muscle power and sensation in the spinal cord segments below the level of injury, which is immediate and which persists for more than 24 hours, is usually permanent. An important prognostic sign is the return of reflex activity in the cord segment below the injury. Such activity reveals that spinal shock in these segments has passed off. The absence of voluntary power and sensory appreciation in the myotomes and dermatomes served by those segments indicates interruption in the long spinal tracts. If the spinal paralysis and sensory loss is incomplete, then the prognosis should be guarded as considerable spontaneous improvement is possible.

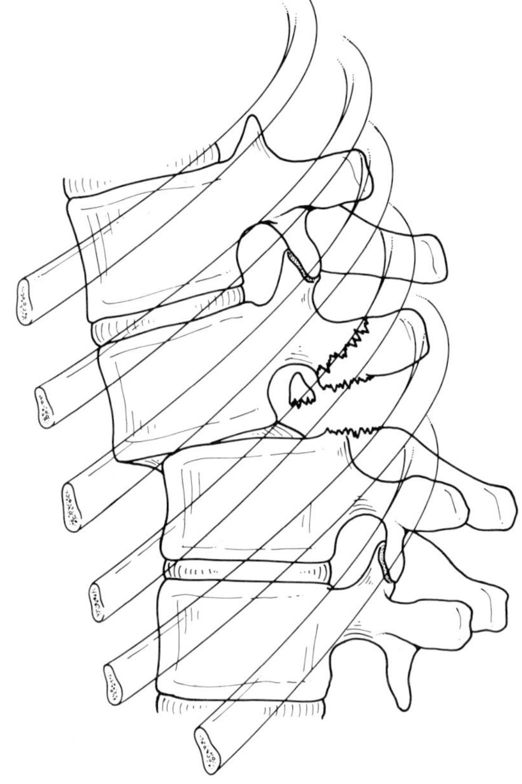

Fig. 18.61 The horizontal 'shearing' fracture–dislocation.

Muscles and joints

In the completely paraplegic patient the muscles having reflex activity will remain bulky, but those whose motor nerve, or its anterior horn cell, has been destroyed will remain flaccid and waste.

The joints of the paralysed limbs must be put through a full range of passive motion every day to prevent joint stiffness, to control spasticity and to prevent the development of contractures. Spasticity is improved if the muscles are stretched. A routine morning 'work-out' often controls spasticity for the rest of the day. The physiotherapist may need the help of drugs to control more severe spasticity. Diazepam, baclofen and dantrolene sodium are used singly or in combination. They are thought to act at cerebral, spinal and peripheral levels respectively. Such measures may not overcome very fierce spasm and muscle contractures may develop. The spasms, which may be painful in the incomplete cord lesion, and the contractures are an added burden for the paraplegic patient to bear. In the severest cases independence may be prevented, nursing becomes almost impossible and pressure sores inevitable. Spasticity can be relieved by breaking the reflex arc centrally, by destruction of the cord with intrathecal phenol or absolute alcohol, or peripherally, by various combinations of the routine orthopaedic procedures of myotomy, tenotomy and neurectomy. The latter measures are particularly indicated in those cases where satisfactory reflex bladder function is present and where sensation is preserved in the paralysed limb, since they do not interfere with existing bladder function nor with useful sensation.

The bladder

The paralysed bladder requires drainage to prevent overdistension, and guarding from infection until a pattern of bladder action is developed. The bladder may be drained by an indwelling urethral catheter which is changed once a week. It may be drained by one of the newer fine suprapubic catheters or, and this is the method now favoured by most Spinal Injury units, drainage may be by intermittent catheterization three or four times a day. The latter method has a lower incidence of infection and spontaneous bladder function occurs sooner. When reflex activity returns, care must be taken that the bladder empties satisfactorily and that there is no build-up of back pressure which could lead to upper tract distension and kidney damage. Monitoring of the residual bladder urine by catheterization after voiding is simple, but the urodynamic investigation and treatment of bladder dysinergia is a sophisticated and specialized discipline.

In lesions of the conus of the spinal cord the second, third and fourth sacral segments containing the detrusor motor centres may be completely destroyed. Such patients have flaccid, compressible bladders, are con-

tinuously incontinent, and require some form of permanent drainage appliance. During the period of catheterization an adequately high fluid intake should be maintained. After a period of catheterization a cystoscopy should always be performed to ensure that the bladder is free from stones and calcareous debris.

The bowel

Like the bladder, the lower bowel may be reflexly innervated or flaccid. A pattern of bowel emptying should be established at an early stage. The completely flaccid bowel requires digital evacuation by the patient or an attendant. If reflex activity is present, then spontaneous emptying may be precipitated by anal stimulation by a gloved finger, or better still, by the insertion of a mildly aperient liquid. Such bowel activity is established by training to occur daily or every other day.

Skin

Anaesthetic skin and subcutaneous fatty tissue is prone to damage by injury and, especially, by excessive and prolonged pressure. The relative immobility of the paralysed patient increases the risk of pressure necrosis of areas on which the patient sits or lies. The sacral, ischial and trochanteric areas are particularly vulnerable (Fig. 18.62). To prevent necrosis and ulceration these vulnerable areas must not suffer pressure for periods exceeding 2 hours. The position of the paralysed patient must therefore be changed at 2-hourly intervals and this routine must be continued day and night in the early weeks after injury. Later, the skin develops some resist-

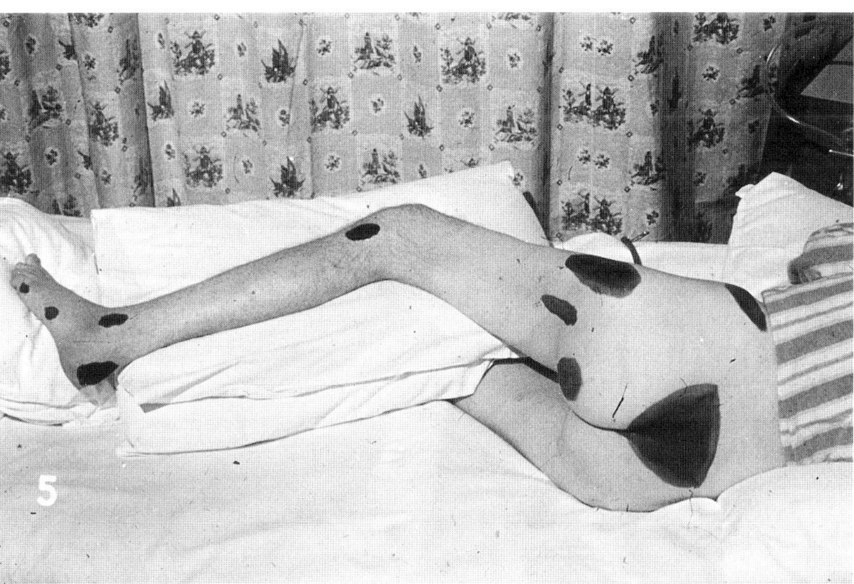

Fig. 18.62 Areas of skin vulnerable to pressure sores in the paraplegic patient.

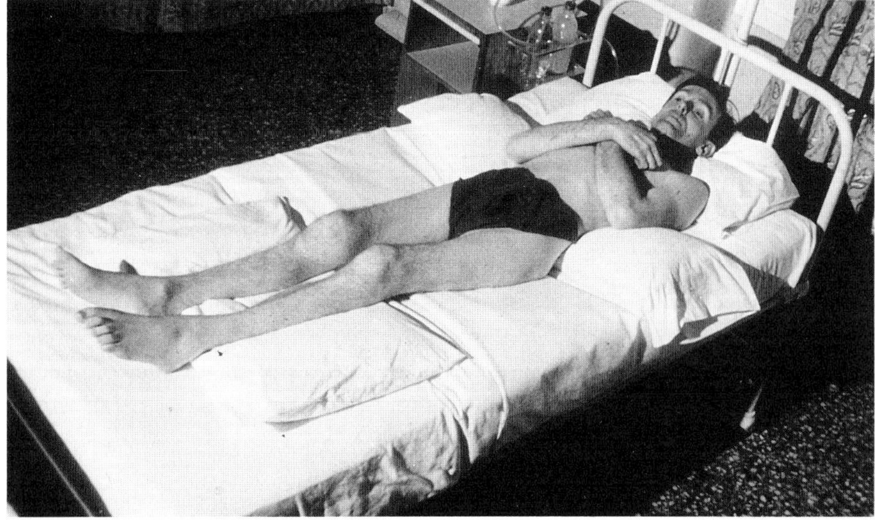

Fig. 18.63 Nursing the paraplegic patient — the long lumbar pillow.

ance and one position may be tolerated safely for 3–4 hours.

These nursing turns may be performed easily by two or three attendants with the aid of a long lumbar pillow. This pillow extends the width of the bed and its depth is tailored to the patient's lumbar lordosis, or to the posture dictated for maintenance of reduction of the spinal injury (Figs 18.63 & 18.64). Very heavy and obese patients are more easily managed in some form of electric bed, which performs the turns automatically and continuously. Such beds are also valuable if trained nurses are not freely available.

Rehabilitation

Rehabilitation of the patient with an injury to the spinal cord should commence very early. Care of the bladder, bowel and skin is started immediately, and as soon as pain allows, active exercises for the upper limbs are commenced (Fig. 18.65). A graduated exercise programme to develop the upper limbs is carried out, since strength in the arms will be essential to make easy wheelchair mobility and transfer from wheelchair to bed, toilet and car. Later, when calipers can be fitted to the paralysed lower limbs, standing and balancing between parallel bars and then walking with a plough and crutches are activities which increase well-being, control spasticity, prevent urinary stasis and minimize skeletal porosis.

Specific training is also necessary towards making the patient independent, as far as is possible, in the activities of daily living. Most paraplegics can be taught to attend to their own toilet, dress themselves and put on their calipers. They can be taught to transfer themselves

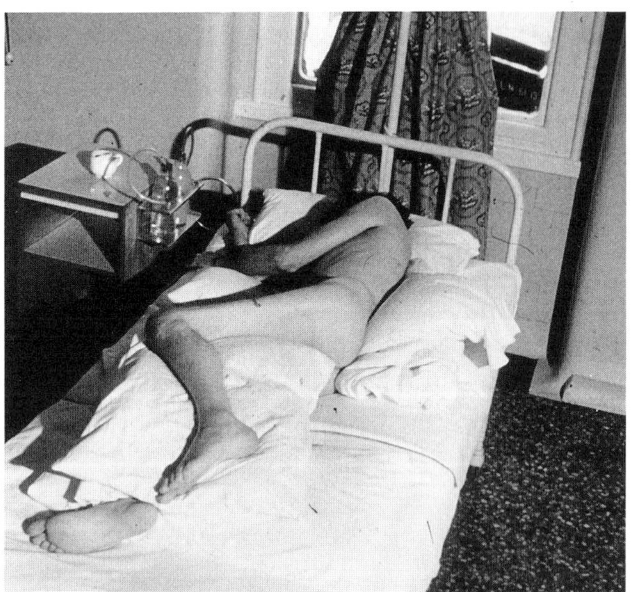

Fig. 18.64 The paraplegic patient turned to the lateral position.

from bed to chair; many drive modified cars and are usually employed. Their environment has, however, to be modified. Ramps have to be built alongside steps and some form of lift is necessary to negotiate stairs. Normal housing needs modification so that doorways are wide enough to take wheelchairs and suitable handles are adjacent to baths and toilets.

Treatment

The two aims of treatment of spinal injuries are:
1 To achieve a stable, painless spine, in a position that

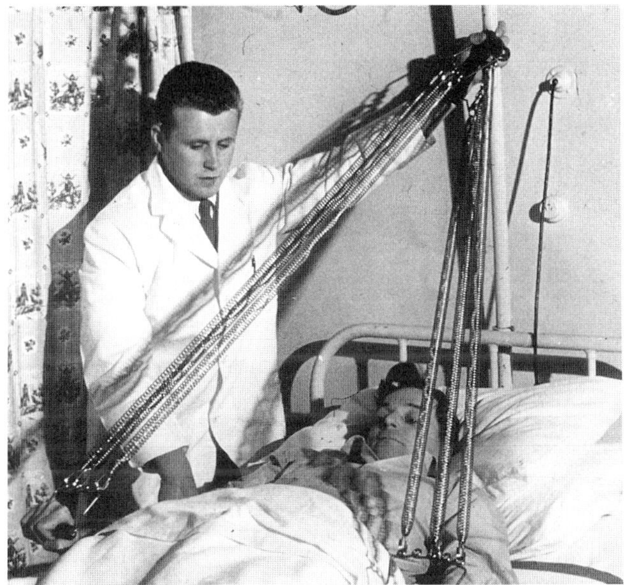

Fig. 18.65 Strengthening the upper limbs.

does not produce functional disability.

2 To preserve spinal cord and nerve root function and prevent further neurological deterioration.

It is important to remember that in the natural course of healing, an unstable spinal segment will, as a rule, gradually become stable. If the vertebral body has fractured, then such stability is often bony. In other injuries fibrous union is often sufficient to abolish abnormal movement and prevent compromise of the neural elements. However, this fibrous union, especially in the lumbar region, is sometimes a cause of pain. When a fibrous union has developed it is essential that the strength of the natural scar be assessed. Before mobilizing the patient gentle flexion and extension strain radiographs should be made. If, after a reasonable period of conservative treatment (6–8 weeks for the cervical spine, 10–12 weeks for the dorso-lumbar spine), stability is not present, a bone grafting and internal fixation procedure is appropriate, just as in a long bone fracture treated conservatively.

When the injury is purely ligamentous, for example, a cervical subluxation unaccompanied by fracture, spontaneous stability is less certain. Operative reduction, internal fixation and bone grafting are more likely to achieve stability in such cases. Such is also the case when gross spinal displacements are not corrected. It is thus sensible to reduce gross bony displacements, although reduction need not be anatomically accurate to achieve satisfactory spinal column function.

There is a view, however, that operative internal fixation and bone grafting should be performed on all unstable injuries so that the patient can be mobilized and rehabilitation accelerated. It is suggested that such a programme is justified because it leads to increased well-being and early discharge from hospital.

In most spinal cord injuries the extent and pattern of damage is determined at the time of injury. Neurological deterioration may occur by extension of the pathological haemorrhage and oedema inside the spinal medulla and may be beyond the control of the physician. Deterioration can also occur by injudicious handling of the patient and, occasionally, by surgical manoeuvres. The recognition of the degree of spinal instability is therefore essential. The reduction of gross spinal displacement and the promotion of stability then follows. The most the surgeon can do, as far as the cord is concerned, is to avoid further cord damage by reducing unstable bony displacements and preventing abnormal movement by skilled nursing or surgical fixation.

If the reduction of displacement can be achieved by closed manipulation or postural methods, and if skilled nursing care is available, then spontaneous stability without redisplacement can be expected in most cases. If, however, reduction requires an open operation, then it is usually a simple matter to add localized bone grafting to the procedure to ensure bony fusion. In addition, an internal fixation device ensures that redisplacement does not occur. When trained nursing care is not available, internal fixation is advisable in the unstable injury even when displacement is not great and reduction is not necessary.

The degree of neurological damage must also be taken into account. When the spinal cord injury is complete and irrecoverable, perfect anatomical reduction of bony displacements is not so important, and if conservative treatment achieves bony fusion then it is acceptable. Even in the completely paraplegic patient, however, some consider that the ability to mobilize the patient rapidly justifies a surgical stabilization operation, even if this can do nothing to improve neurological recovery.

Treatment of unstable lumbar injuries

Flexion–distraction (Chance fracture; Fig. 18.66)

Most of such injuries can be reduced to an acceptable position by postural extension over pillows with subsequent immobilization of the patient in a body jacket. Healing is usually rapid as the anterior part of the injury occurs through the cancellous bone of the vertebral body. Those fractures which have separated widely, and are therefore more unstable, are best treated by open reduction and fixation. A Harrington com-

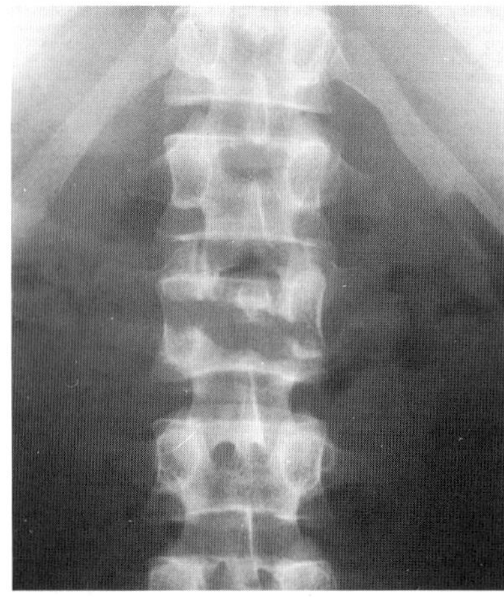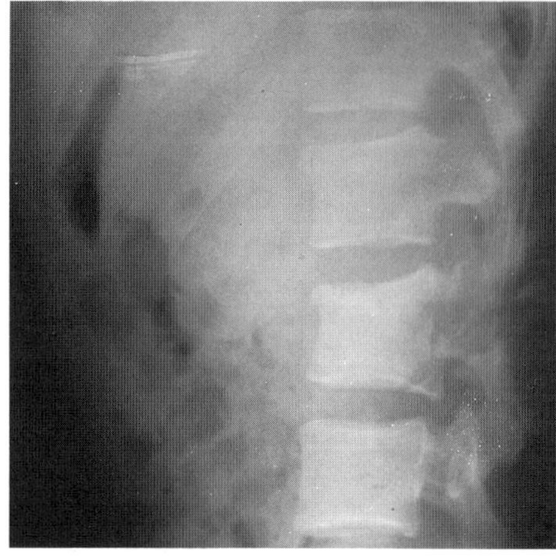

Fig. 18.66 Flexion−distraction fracture.

pression device or a simple Zadik clamp (Zadik 1959) may be used to keep the posterior elements together (Fig. 18.67).

Shearing fractures of the dorsal spine

The horizontal displacement of these fractures is often accompanied by lateral wedging or anterior angulation, depending upon the direction of the force applied to the upper part of the thoracic spine (Fig. 18.68). Displacement is accompanied by fracture of the laminae and pedicles, transverse processes and ribs (Fig. 18.69). The remaining intact rib cage stabilizes the damaged segment. Since deformity of the upper thoracic spine, at which level most of these injuries occur, rarely interferes with function, and complete high dorsal paraplegia is the rule, operative reduction and fixation is rarely indicated. In those rare cases where pain and gross displacement are marked, then the application of two contoured Harrington rods is an acceptable method of reduction and immobilization.

Bursting fractures

These comminuted fractures are painful and require immobilization. If displacement is slight and there is no neurological damage, bedrest for a few weeks, followed by mobilization in a body jacket, is safe and acceptable.

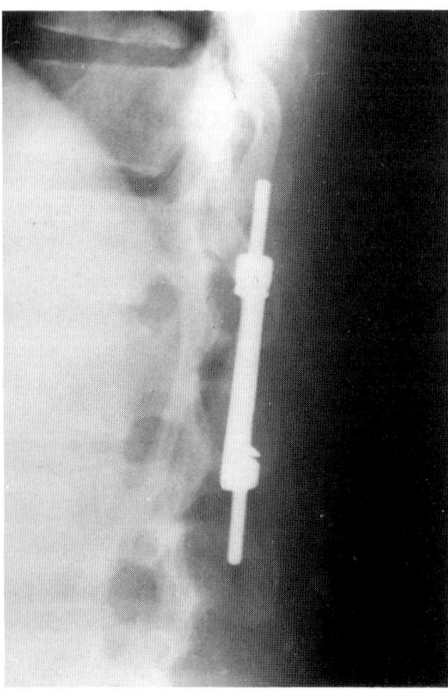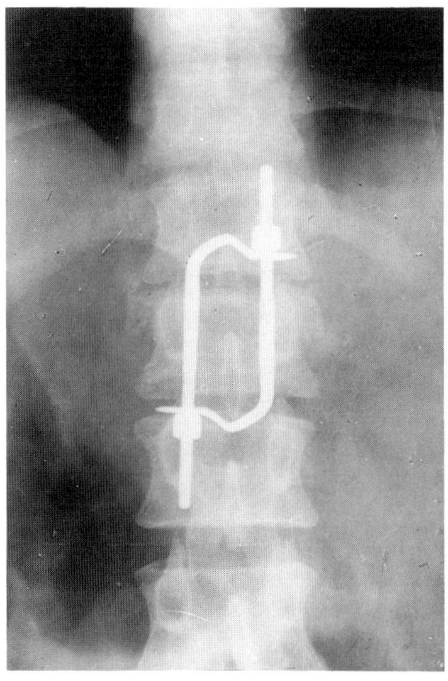

Fig. 18.67 Zadik clamp.

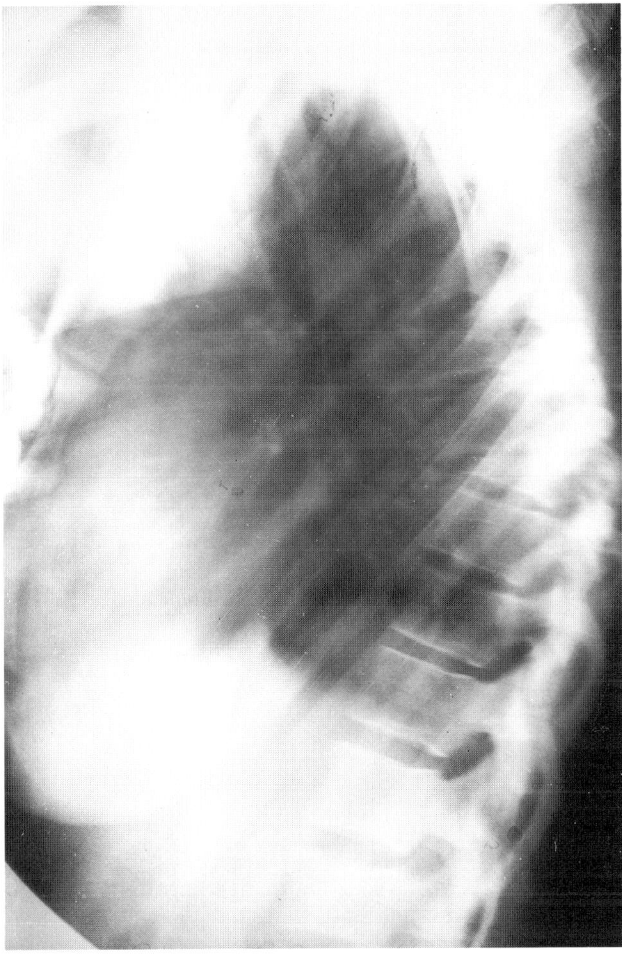

Fig. 18.68 Shearing fracture—dislocation of the dorsal spine; flexion is also marked.

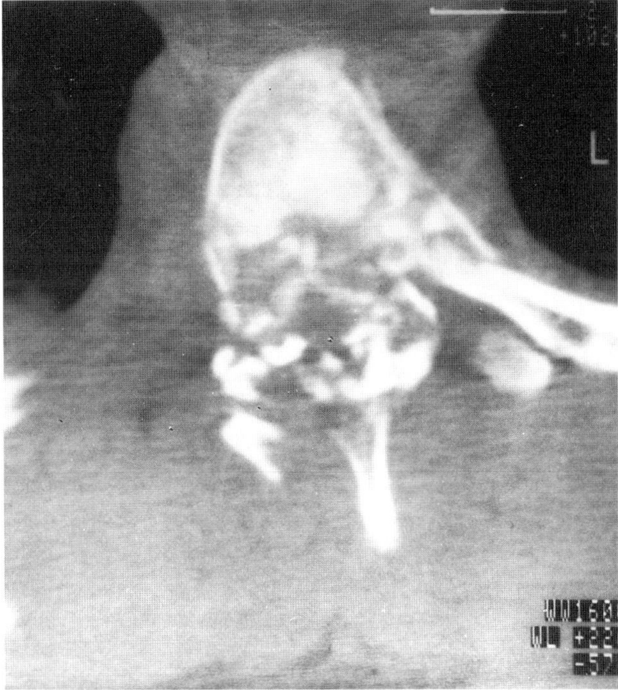

Fig. 18.69 CAT scan of dorsal shearing fracture—dislocation. Cord damage was complete.

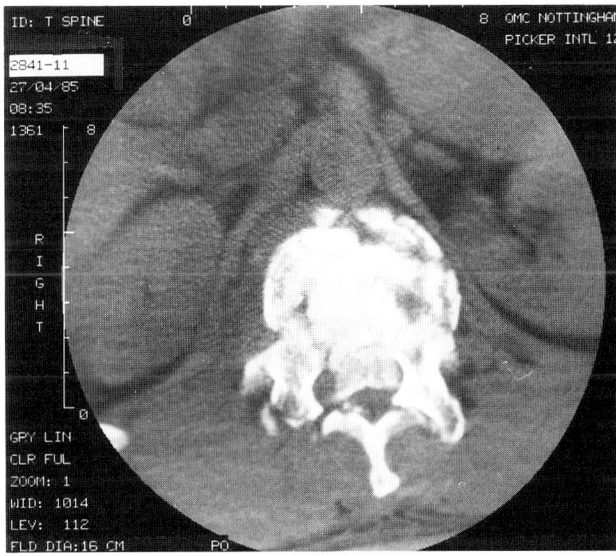

Fig. 18.70 CAT scan of bursting fracture showing extent of spinal canal compromise.

Bony union of the vertebral body fragments nearly always occurs.

If there is damage of the lumbar nerve roots by the posteriorly displaced fragments of the vertebral body, this may be reversible if the pressure on the roots is relieved. The exact state of affairs in the spinal canal is revealed by CAT scanning (Fig. 18.70). Distraction reduction by contoured Harrington instrumentation has been frequently employed and is superficially attractive in that it would tend to reverse the original compression force. However, because, in many cases, the anterior vertebral body is badly damaged, posterior distraction reduction, relying as it does on anterior column integrity, frequently fails (Gertzbein *et al.* 1982).

The addition of sublaminar wires to the rods, or to a frame, increases the fixation strength and avoids the need for an external cast or brace (Fig. 18.71). Bony union, however, is ultimately essential and to ensure that this occurs bone grafts are frequently applied pos-teriorly across the damaged segments. The need to span normal segments to obtain firm fixation has led to the technique being termed 'fuse short, rod long'.

The stability conferred on the injured spinal segments by Harrington rods is not sufficient to allow early weight-bearing. Without a stable anterior column the

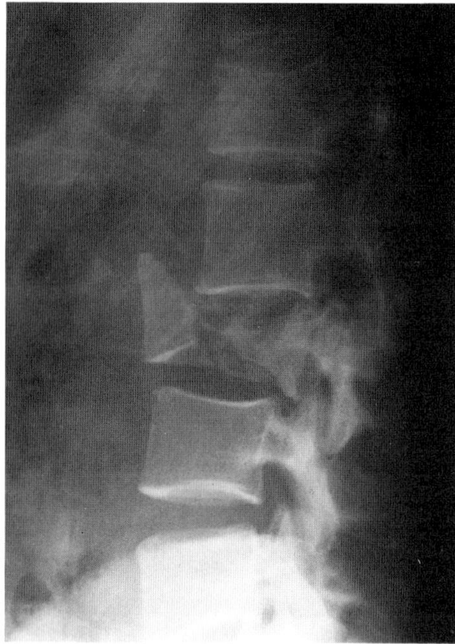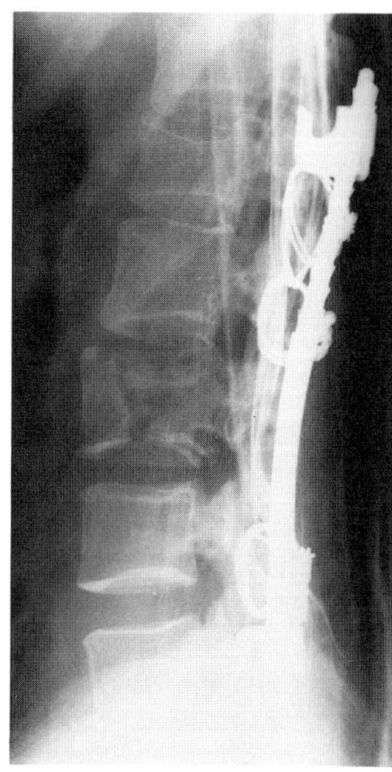

Fig. 18.71 Vertical compression burst
fracture treated by contoured
Harrington distraction rods and
sublaminar wires.

rods cannot resist flexion forces. An adequate period of
bedrest following the application of rods is essential. A
disadvantage of the Harrington system is the need to
span normal joints with the fixing rods. Even though
the rods are removed in 6—12 months (this second
operation is another disadvantage), there is evidence
that the normal distracted joints are permanently damaged and show the histological appearance of osteoarthritis (Jacobs & Casey 1984, Kahanovitz *et al*. 1984).

A more attractive method of fixation employs screws,
through the pedicles and into the vertebral bodies,
attached to an external or internal fixation device. Only
the damaged segments need be immobilized. The original external device of Magerl (1982) has been shown to
be more secure than rods or plates but has the disadvantages of screws protruding from the skin and a
cumbersome external frame. The development of an
internal metal block or plate attached to the pedicular
screws (Roy-Camille *et al*. 1976, Luque 1986, Steffee
et al. 1986) answers many of the criticisms of the 'fuse
short, rod long' concept (Figs 18.72 & 18.73).

These posterior devices are perfectly satisfactory if
their application results in reconstruction of the diam-
eters of the spinal canal. If, in comminuted fractures of
the vertebral body, some fragments are still thought to
be compressing the theca after posterior stabilization,
then these fragments must be removed by an anterior
approach. Both an anterior and a posterior operation
may thus be necessary. The development of more secure
anterior implant systems (Dunn 1984, Kostuik 1984)
allows decompression of the theca, reduction of the

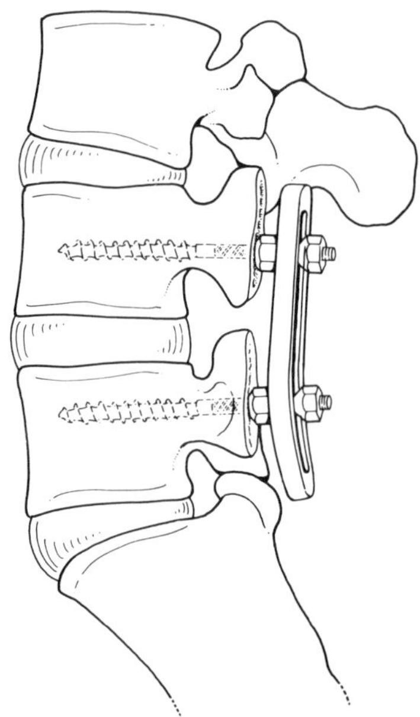

Fig. 18.72 Intrapedicular screws and plate.

spinal deformity and fixation of the damaged segments
together with bone grafting (Fig. 18.74) (Kostuik 1988,
Kaneda *et al*. 1984); the aims of surgery are thus achieved
by one operation.

Rotational fracture—dislocation

These grossly unstable injuries occur at, or on each side
of, the dorso-lumbar junction (Fig. 18.75). They deserve
special consideration owing to the neurological anatomy

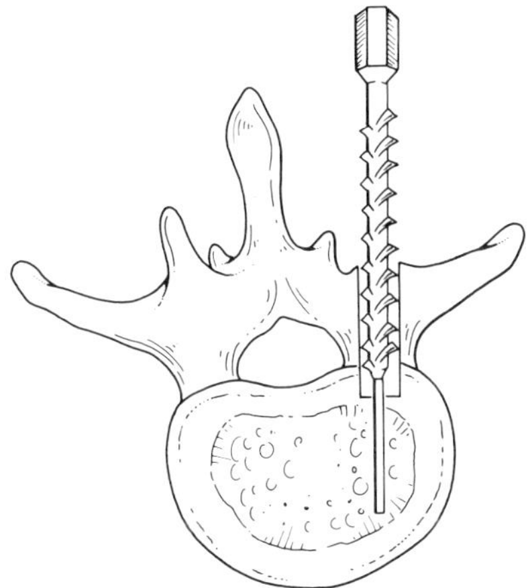

Fig. 18.73 Intrapedicular fixation: the direction of the screws.

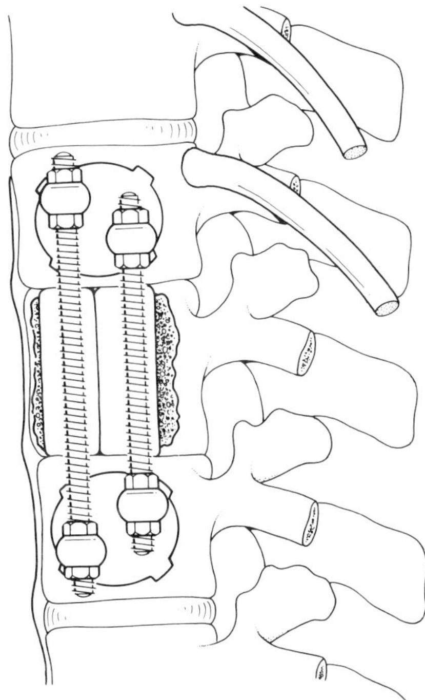

Fig. 18.74 The Kaneda anterior fixation device.

at that level. The conus of the spinal cord, containing all the sacral segments, lies behind the body of the first lumbar vertebra and all the lumbar nerve roots pass downwards alongside the conus (Fig. 18.76). A dislocation at the T12/L1 level will thus damage the tip of the very vulnerable spinal cord and the more resistant lumbar nerve roots. The cord damage is more serious and ascending haemorrhagic necrosis often extends to the lower lumbar cord segments. Anterior horn cells in these segments can therefore be destroyed, even though the corresponding nerve roots are intact. Complete paraplegia, often above the L1 spinal segment, is not unusual in such injuries. In these cases, if postural reduction can be achieved and skilled nursing is available, then conservative treatment can achieve satisfactory spinal function.

Operative reduction and fixation is preferred for the grossly displaced injuries, when the unfractured facets have dislocated and locked, and when the patient is irritable and restless and cannot be controlled. Re-

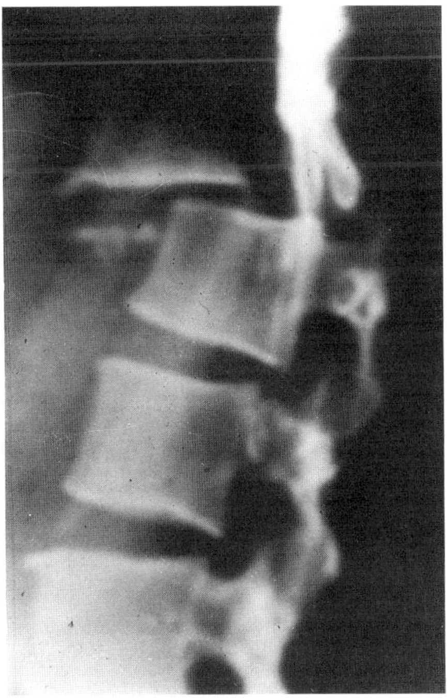

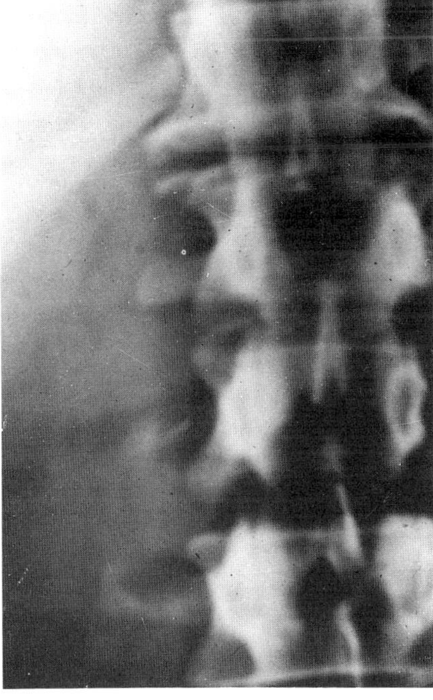

Fig. 18.75 Tl2/L1 flexion–rotation ('slice') fracture–dislocation. Note the wide separation of the spinous processes — the palpable gap.

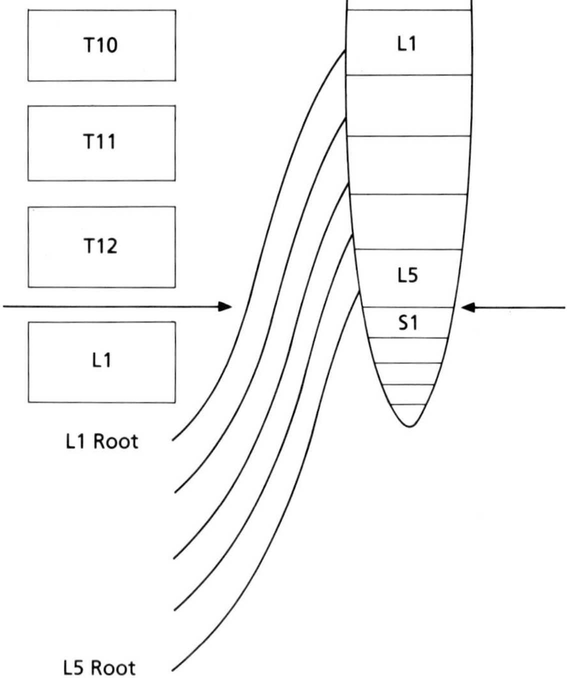

Fig. 18.76 Diagrammatic representation of the neurological anatomy at the dorso-lumbar junction.

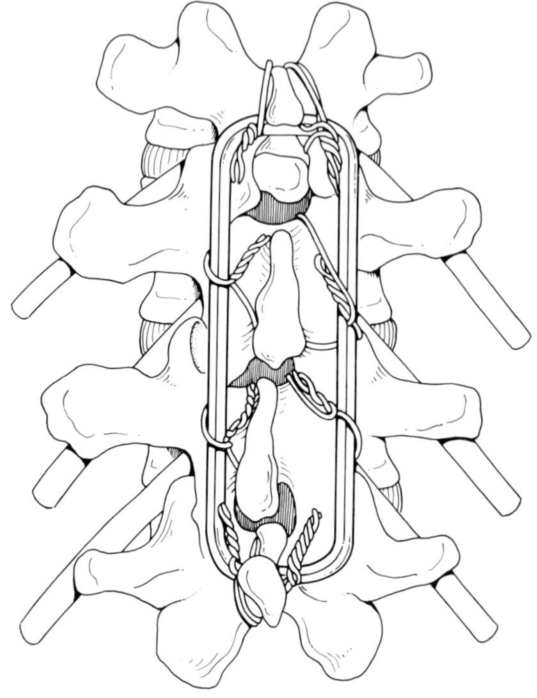

Fig. 18.77 The Hartshill rectangle.

duction is usually easy, and since the vertebral body is in two main pieces, reduction restores the normal configuration of the spinal canal and achieves satisfactory 'decompression'. Fixation by a Zadik clamp is sufficient to maintain reduction if the patient is kept in bed until body union is advanced. If more rapid mobilization of the patient is considered essential, then square-ended double Harrington rods, or a Hartshill rectangle (Fig. 18.77) with sublaminar wires may be used. The disadvantages of long Harrington rods have already been mentioned. Sublaminar wires in an acute spinal cord injury have hazards too, not only at the time of insertion but possibly also when they need to be removed. The more localized internal fixation devices, which have already been discussed, utilizing intact pedicles and vertebral bodies, are likely to prove simpler and safer and will avoid the need for a second procedure to remove the metalware.

These operative procedures reduce displacement and guard against further damage to the vulnerable spinal cord and nerve roots by movement of the spine. There is no evidence, however, that they improve existing cord damage. Hardy (1965) stated that the pattern of spinal cord damage was established at the time of the initial injury and was not substantially altered by (posterior) surgery. Similar conclusions have been reached by other workers (Dickson *et al.* 1978, Davies *et al.* 1980).

Whether anterior surgery betters these results remains to be proved.

References

Bohler, L *The Treatment of Fractures* 4th edn. Wright: Bristol, 1935.

Bohlman, H.H. Indications for late anterior decompression and fusion for cervical spinal cord injuries. In: Tator, C.H. (ed.) *Early Management of Acute Spinal Cord Injury.* Raven Press: New York, 1982.

Bohlman, H.H. & Anderson, P.A. Anterior decompression and arthrodesis of the cervical spine; long term motor improvement. Part I. *J Bone Joint Surg* 1992; **74A**: 671–682.

Bracken, M.B., Shephard, M.J., Collins, W.F., Holford, T.R., Young, W., Baskin, D.S., Eisenberg, H.M., Flamm, E.S., Leo, L.S., Maroon, J., Marshall, L.F., Perot, P.L., Piepmeir, J., Sonntag, V.K.H., Wagner, F.C., Wilbergen, J.E. & Winn, R.H. A randomised controlled trial of methylprednisolone or naloxone in the treatment of acute spinal cord injury. Results of the Second National Acute Spinal Cord Injury Study. *N Eng J Med* 1990; **322**: 1405–1411.

Chance, C.Q. Note on a type of flexion fracture of the spine. *Br J Radiol* 1948; **21**: 452–453.

Davies, W.E., Morris, J.H. & Hill, V. An analysis of conservative (nonsurgical) management of the thoraco lumbar fractures and fracture dislocations with neural damage. *J Bone Joint Surg* 1980; **62A**: 1324–1327.

Denis, F. Updated classification of thoraco lumbar fractures. *Orthop Trans* 1982; **6**: 8–9.

Dickson, J.H., Harrington, P.R. & Erwin, W.D. Results of reduction and stabilisation of the severely fractured thoracic and lumbar spine. *J Bone Joint Surg* 1978; **60A**; 799−805.

Domisse, G.F. The blood supply of the spinal cord. *J Bone Joint Surg* 1974; **56B**: 225−235.

Gertzbein, G.D., MacMichael, D. & Tile, M. Harrington instrumentation as a method of fixation in fractures of the spine (a critical analysis of deficiencies). *J Bone Joint Surg* 1982; **64B**: 526−529.

Gumley, G., Taylor, T.K.F. & Ryan, M.D. Distraction fractures of the lumbar spine. *J Bone Joint Surg* 1982; **64B**: 520−525.

Hardy, A.G. The treatment of paraplegia due to fracture dislocations of the dorso lumbar spine. *Int J Paraplegia* 1965; **3**: 112−123.

Holdsworth, F.W. Fractures, dislocations and fracture−dislocations of the spine. *J Bone Joint Surg* 1963; **45B**: 6−20.

Jacobs, R.R. & Casey, M.P. Surgical management of thoraco lumbar spinal injuries. *Clin Orthop* 1984; **189**: 22−35.

Kahanovitz, N., Bullough, P. & Jacobs, R.R. The effect of internal fixation without arthrodesis on human facet joint cartilage. *Clin Orthop* 1984; **189**: 204.

Kaneda, K., Abumi, K. & Fujiya, M. Burst fractures with neurological deficits of the thoraco-lumbar spine. *Spine* 1984; **9**: 788−795.

Kostuik, J.P. Anterior spinal cord decompression for lesions of the thoracic and lumbar spines; techniques, new methods of internal fixation, results. *Spine* 1988; **8**: 512−531.

Luque, E.R. Interpeduncular segmental fixation. *Clin Orthop* 1986; **203**: 54−57.

Magerl, F. External skeletal fixation of the lower thoracic and lumbar spine. In: Uhthoff, H.K. (ed.) *Current Concepts of External Fixation of Fractures*. Springer-Verlag: Berlin, 1982.

McAfee, P.C., Yuan, H.A., Frederickson, B.E. & Lubicky, J.P. The value of computed tomography in thoraco lumbar fractures. *J Bone Joint Surg* 1983; **65A**: 461−473.

Perey, O. Fracture of the vertebral end plate in the lumbar spine: an experimental study. *Acta Orthop Scand* 25, 1957.

Riska, E.B., Myllynen, P. & Bostman, O. Anterolateral decompression for neural involvement in thoraco-lumbar fractures. *J Bone Joint Surg* 1987; **69B**: 704−708.

Roaf, R. A study of the mechanisms of spinal injuries. *J Bone Joint Surg* 1960; **42B**: 810.

Roy-Camille, R., Guillant, G., Berteaux, D. & Salgado, V. Osteosynthesis of thoraco lumbar spine fractures with metal plates screwed through the pedicles. *Reconstr Surg Traumatol* 1976; **15**: 2.

Steffee, A.D., Biscup, R.S. & Sitkowski, D.J. *Clin Orthop* 1986; **203**: 45−53.

Walters, C.L., Schmidek, H.H., Krag, M.H. & Brier, L. The management of thoraco lumbar fractures. In: Dinsker, Schmidek, Frynoyer, & Kahn, (eds) *The Unstable Spine*. Grune & Stratton: New York, 1986.

White, A.J. Current status of spinal cord cooling. *Clin Neurosurg* 1973; **20**: 400.

White, A.W. & Panjabi, M.M. *Clinical Biomechanics of the Spine*. J.B. Lippincott, 1978.

Yeo, L.J.D., Stabback, S. & McKenzie, B. A study of the effects of hyperbaric oxygen on the experimental spinal cord injury. *Med J Aust* 1977; **2**: 145.

Zadik, F.R. Fracture-dislocation of thoraco lumbar spine. *J Bone Joint Surg* 1959; **41B**: 772−773.

19: The Pelvis and Acetabulum

P.H.WORLOCK AND M.TILE

Major injuries of the pelvis and acetabulum are becoming more common with the increasing incidence of high-energy trauma in the western world. However, the management of such injuries remains difficult because of the complexity of the fractures. The objective of this chapter is to outline the main problems and provide a logical approach to injury management.

Pelvic fractures

The forces required to disrupt the pelvic ring in an adult are major and therefore damage to structures within the pelvis is common; such damage may be life threatening. Mortality after major pelvic fracture remains at approximately 10%, despite therapeutic advances (McMurtry *et al.* 1980, Hesp *et al.* 1985, Goldstein *et al.* 1986).

As well as this high mortality, there is significant disability amongst the survivors. Holdsworth (1948) reported that 15 out of 27 patients with sacro-iliac dislocation were unable to return to work because of pain. Raf (1966) reported that after pelvic fracture 33% of patients had significant pain, but this figure rose to 52% after sacral fracture or sacro-iliac dislocation. Tile (1984) reviewed 218 patients with displaced ring fractures of the pelvis: 40% of patients complained of significant pain. This pain was usually posterior and often associated with sacro-iliac dislocation or non-union. When only patients with a vertically unstable injury were considered, 60% were left with pain. Non-union was seen in 3.5% of patients and malunion (with leg length discrepancy >2.5 cm) was observed in 4%. Tile felt that stable injuries gave few long-term problems.

Prognosis appears to be related to the type of injury and the instability that results. Classification should be based on stability, so that attention can be directed to those injuries that are liable to long-term problems, particularly the unstable vertical shear fracture with sacro-iliac joint dislocation.

Pelvic biomechanics

The pelvis is a ring. If the ring is broken in one place, with displacement of the fracture fragments, there must be a fracture or dislocation in another portion of the ring. Stability of the pelvic ring depends on the posterior sacro-iliac complex. The strong posterior sacro-iliac ligaments maintain the normal position of the sacrum in the ring. The sacrospinous ligaments join the sacrum to the ischial spine and resist external rotation of the hemipelvis. The sacrotuberous ligaments resist both rotational and vertical shearing forces.

The major force patterns resulting in pelvic fractures are external rotation, lateral compression (internal rotation) and vertical shear. External rotation usually results from forced external rotation/abduction of the legs and typically produces the open-book injury. The symphysis pubis is disrupted, together with the anterior sacro-iliac and sacrospinous ligaments. Usually, the injury stops when the posterior ilium impacts against the sacrum, but continued application of force may shear off the hemipelvis completely.

Lateral compression ('closed-book') forces result either directly from a blow to the lateral iliac crest or indirectly from forces transmitted via the femoral head. These forces typically produce compression fractures posteriorly with fractures of the pubic rami. The anterior and posterior fractures can be either on the same side of the pelvis (ipsilateral type) or on opposite sides (bucket-handle type). Major rotational deformity and malunion can result from bucket-handle injuries.

Vertical shear forces are usually massive, across the main trabecular pattern, causing marked displacement of bone and disruption of soft tissue. There may literally be no end point to such forces, resulting in traumatic hemipelvectomy (Tile 1984).

Fracture classification

Classification is based on the force applied to the pelvis and the stability of the resulting fracture (see Table 19.1). These groups will now be discussed in detail.

Type A

Avulsion fractures of the iliac spines or the ischial tuberosity and isolated fractures of the iliac wing are all examples of type A1 injuries. In type A2 injuries, although the pelvis ring is broken the fracture(s) is undisplaced and stable.

Type B

In type B1 injuries (open-book fractures) the hemipelvis is unstable in external rotation and stable in internal rotation. There are three stages: I — disruption of the symphysis pubis <2.5 cm with no posterior lesion; II — separation >2.5 cm with unilateral disruption of a sacro-iliac joint; and III — separation >2.5 cm with bilateral disruption of the sacro-iliac joints (see Fig. 19.1).

The common type of B2 lesion is seen where the pubic rami are fractured anteriorly together with a crush, impaction fracture posteriorly. Less commonly, the rami may remain intact, but the symphysis pubis is disrupted, overlapped and locked. Occasionally, the ramus fracture rotates around the disrupted symphysis,

Table 19.1 Classification of pelvic fractures

Type A	Stable
A1	Fractures not involving the ring
A2	Minimally displaced fractures of the ring
Type B	Rotationally unstable, vertically stable
B1	Open book
B2	Lateral compression (ipsilateral or bucket-handle)
B3	Bilateral type B injury
Type C	Rotationally and vertically unstable
C1	Unilateral
C2	Bilateral
C3	Associated with an acetabular fracture

causing a fragment of bone to protrude into the perineum — the tilt fracture (see Fig. 19.1).

Less commonly, the affected hemipelvis rotates anteriorly and superiorly, like the handle of a bucket. Even with a relatively intact posterior complex, leg length inequality may result. Reduction of such fractures requires derotation of the hemipelvis rather than traction in a vertical plane (see Fig. 19.1). Type B3 injuries are bilateral.

Type C

These major disruptions may be unilateral (C1) or bilateral (C2) (see Fig. 19.2). Radiological signs of instability include posterior displacement of the hemipelvis by more than 1 cm, avulsion of the transverse process of

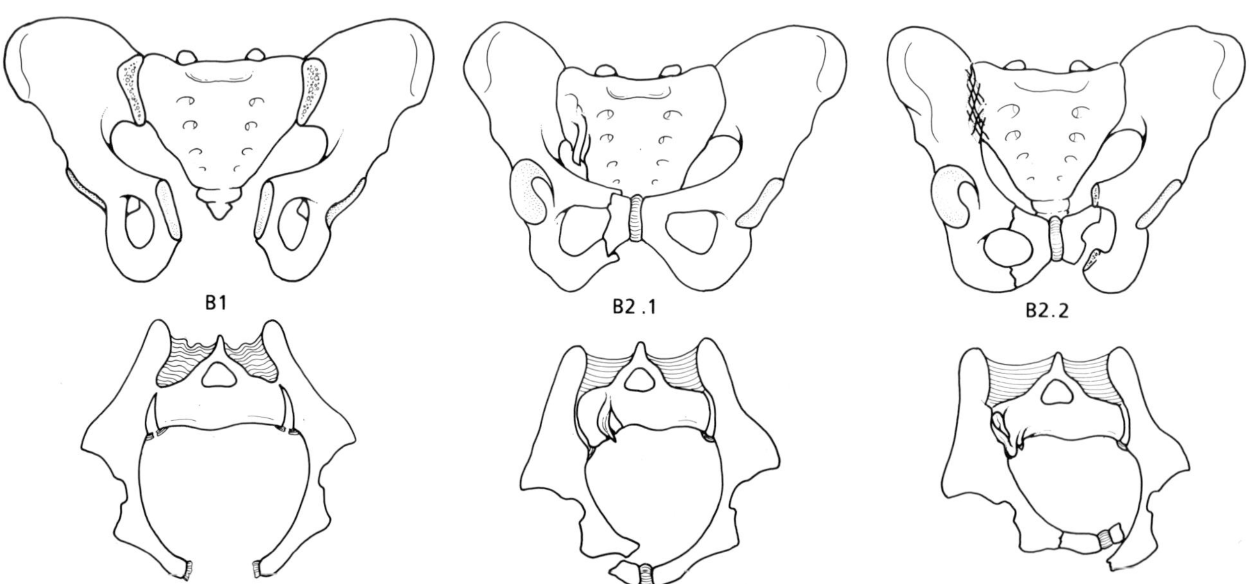

Fig. 19.1 Type B pelvic fractures. B1, Open-book injury; B2.1, lateral compression injury (ipsilateral); B2.2, lateral compression injury (bucket-handle).

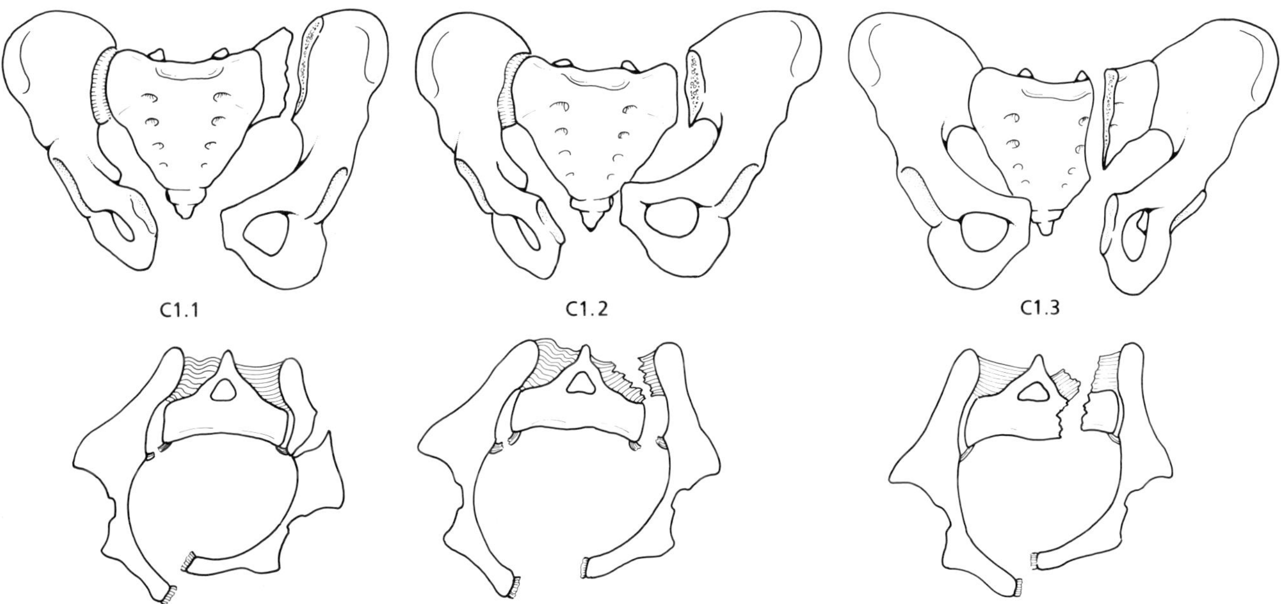

Fig. 19.2 Type C pelvic fractures. C1.1, Iliac wing fracture; C1.2, sacro-iliac joint dislocation; C1.3, sacral fracture.

the fifth lumbar vertebra, or detachment of the bony insertion of the sacrospinous ligament from the sacrum or ischial spine. Recognition of posterior disruption is best achieved with computerized tomography (CT) scanning. C3 lesions with associated acetabular fractures require careful assessment and management of both injuries.

Pelvic fracture management

Patients with major pelvic fractures are often critically ill and have associated major injuries. Assessment and resuscitation should be carried out simultaneously and systematically using trauma management protocols, such as those recommended by the American College of Surgeons (1988) and the Royal College of Surgeons of England in the Advanced Trauma Life Support (ATLS) course.

The stability of the pelvis is assessed clinically and radiologically. Rotational and vertical instability are assessed by manual rotation of the hemipelvis and traction/compression via the leg, respectively. Major displacement clinically, marked posterior bruising, associated vessel/nerve injury and open wounds all suggest major disruption and, therefore, instability.

Three initial radiographs of the pelvis should be obtained in the resuscitation room (Tile 1984): the anteroposterior view, the 45° inlet view (showing posterior displacement), and the 45° outlet view (showing vertical displacement and rotation). CT scan-

ning is essential to accurately define the posterior injury, but should be delayed until the patient is haemo-dynamically stable.

Resuscitation

This should proceed along conventional lines with securing and maintaining an airway, ensuring adequate oxygenation and ventilation, and massive fluid replacement via two large-bore peripheral intravenous (IV) lines. Other techniques, such as use of the pneumatic antishock garment, embolization of pelvic vessels and direct surgical intervention, have been advocated in the past to control major bleeding (McMurtry *et al.* 1980). However, there is now considerable clinical experience to suggest that application of an external fixator will reduce venous and bony bleeding, so that other intervention is rarely indicated (Tile 1988).

Those pelvic fractures which result in an increase in pelvic volume (namely the type B1 open-book lesion or the type C unstable vertical shear injury) may require early stabilization of the ring during the resuscitation phase. This can be safely and quickly carried out with an external fixator applied percutaneously to the iliac crests. This may need to be performed in the resuscitation room.

A simple configuration of the frame is desirable in these seriously ill patients. Two pins are placed percutaneously into each iliac wing (one at the anterior superior iliac spine and the other at the iliac tubercle) and joined in the form of an anterior rectangle. The more complex frames that have been described do not confer enough added stability to justify the extra operative procedure (Tile & McBroom 1982). The simple frame described will control pelvic volume and stabilize the pelvic ring enough to allow the patient to be nursed in an upright position.

Definitive management

Stable fractures (types A1 and A2) require only symptomatic treatment and early mobilization. For type B and C injuries consideration has to be given to reduction and fixation by operative means. Assessment of the fracture pattern by CT scanning is essential to define the pattern exactly *before* taking any decision to operate.

If operative treatment is indicated, it is generally agreed that a delay of 5–7 days from injury is beneficial to allow the patient's general condition to improve. Exceptions to this general rule are:

1 When early laparotomy gives access for plating the symphysis pubis.

2 When vascular repair of the femoral artery gives access to the superior pubic ramus.

3 When a posterior open fracture exposes the sacro-iliac complex (Tile 1988).

The role of immediate open reduction and internal fixation is currently under evaluation at some major trauma units, but cannot be recommended routinely at present.

TYPE B1 FRACTURES

When the symphysis is opened less than 2.5 cm, operative stabilization is not usually required. However, in some cases anterior pain may persist and necessitate surgery. If the symphysis is opened more than 2.5 cm, this should be closed and stabilized. If laparotomy is necessary (and there is no faecal/urinary contamination) a single four-hole superior plate is recommended. In other circumstances, an anterior external fixator should be used to 'close the book'.

TYPE B2/B3 FRACTURES

In most cases of ipsilateral lateral compression injuries the elastic recoil of the pelvis ensures that there is no significant displacement, and operative stabilization is rarely required.

With a bucket-handle type injury there is usually a compression fracture posteriorly, rendering the ring stable. It is preferable to accept a leg length discrepancy of up to 1.5 cm, together with some internal rotation of the hemipelvis, rather than disimpact the fracture to achieve reduction as this will then require stabilization by internal or external fixation.

If the leg length discrepancy is greater than 1.5 cm or if the displacement of the fracture is severe, reduction and stabilization is necessary. This is most easily achieved by insertion of the external fixator pins into the iliac crests, and the hemipelvis is reduced by external rotation via the pins. When reduced, the anterior external fixator is completed to stabilize the fracture. Rarely, a 'tilt' fracture may occur, with bone protruding into the perineum. In such cases open reduction and internal fixation is indicated.

TYPE C FRACTURES

Options for definitive care include external fixation, with or without added skeletal traction, or open reduction and internal fixation. Although complex external fixator frames have been recommended (Mears & Fu 1980), Tile and McBroom (1982) have shown that they confer only a slight biomechanical advantage over the simple anterior frame and *no* external fixator frame will restore enough stability in these injuries to allow walking.

The combination of anterior frame and skeletal traction (via a supracondylar pin) is a safe method of treatment and gives satisfactory results in certain cases. This method of treatment is particularly suitable when the posterior injury is a fracture of the ilium (rather than a fracture through the sacrum or a dislocation of the sacro-iliac joint) and this posterior fracture can be reduced. Traction entails bedrest for 8 to 12 weeks and involves all the attendant complications of prolonged immobilization.

Open reduction and internal fixation in type C injuries offers many advantages, but the risks are high. Malunion and non-union can be prevented and the restoration of stability to the pelvic ring allows early mobilization. However, major complications include bleeding, infection and nerve damage. The risk of major haemorrhage during reconstructive surgery has led some units to recommend preoperative arteriography and selective embolization (Goldstein *et al.* 1986).

Posterior skin wounds are at risk of breakdown. Kellam *et al.* (1987) reported skin necrosis in 25% of patients in whom crush injuries had been treated by posterior open reduction and internal fixation. High infection rates were also noted by Goldstein *et al.* (1986). Nerve damage can also occur: the lumbo-sacral trunk is at risk in the anterior approach to the sacro-iliac joint,

Table 19.2 Indications for open reduction and internal fixation of unstable pelvic fractures

Anterior
For disruption of the symphysis/rami fractures:
1 To improve pelvic stability
2 In association with laparotomy (non-contaminated)
3 Bone protrusion into perineum (tilt fracture)
4 In association with acetabular fracture, requiring open reduction and internal fixation

Posterior
1 Inadequate reduction (especially sacro-iliac dislocation)
2 Presence of open posterior wound (*never* open perineal wound)
3 In association with acetabular fracture, requiring open reduction and internal fixation

and when screws are introduced posteriorly cauda equina damage can occur (Tile 1984).

In some patients, the benefits of surgery may outweigh the risks. The main indications for anterior and posterior surgery of the unstable pelvis are given in Table 19.2.

If anterior surgery is undertaken in a type C fracture, two plates should be placed across the symphysis pubis at 90° to each other if no posterior fixation is planned (see Fig. 19.3). If posterior stabilization is carried out in addition, then a single anterior four-hole plate will suffice. The fixation of fractures of the pubic rami is technically more complex and may require an ilio-inguinal approach (Letournel 1980). In inexperienced hands the risks of this major dissection are usually greater than the benefits. It is therefore rarely indicated, except where an associated anterior column fracture of the acetabulum requires fixation. In other cases it may be more appropriate to stabilize the posterior injury by open reduction and internal fixation, and control the anterior injury with an external fixator.

Posterior stabilization is indicated for inadequate reduction of the posterior sacro-iliac complex, especially

an unreduced sacro-iliac dislocation or where there is a gap of more than 1 cm between the fragments. For posterior fractures, with a minimal gap, especially those through the ilium, external frames and skeletal traction will suffice.

The surgical approach to the posterior disruption may be either anterior or posterior. The anterior approach has the advantage of good soft tissue cover and is indicated if there is posterior skin injury.

For sacral fractures, two sacral bars from one posterior iliac spine to the other provide stability and compression of the sacral fracture with no risk of nerve damage. This technique is possible only when both posterior iliac spines are intact, and care most be taken to avoid overcompression (see Fig. 19.4).

For sacro-iliac dislocation, with or without an associated iliac fracture, an anterior approach to the sacro-iliac joint is recommended (Tile 1988); plates should be placed across the sacro-iliac joint and any iliac fracture. The lumbo-sacral trunk runs approximately 1.5 cm medial to the sacro-iliac joint; this should be identified and then protected throughout the procedure. The articular cartilage of the sacro-iliac joint is removed and bone graft may be added to promote fusion (see Fig. 19.5).

Using standard techniques iliac fractures should be fixed with plates to apply interfragmentary compression (see Fig. 19.6). The pelvic reconstruction plates are recommended for easier use. The anterior approach is preferred, but for posterior iliac fractures the posterior approach has to be used. The patient is normally placed supine for anterior approaches and prone for posterior approaches. However, for simultaneous access to both posterior and anterior structures, a lateral position may be used.

Summary

Pelvic ring disruption is a serious injury with significant mortality and morbidity. Early and adequate resuscitation of the patient using ATLS protocols is essential. Simple anterior external fixation has a major role in the acute phase in multiply injured patients with either type C (unstable vertical shear) or type B1 (open-book) injuries. The need for operative intervention is rare. In a series of 494 consecutive pelvic fractures only 19% required stabilization, which was achieved by open means in only 5% (Tile 1988).

These injuries often occur in multiply injured patients and the problems are complex. Assessment and management techniques are difficult and should only be carried out in centres with experience and expertise in this

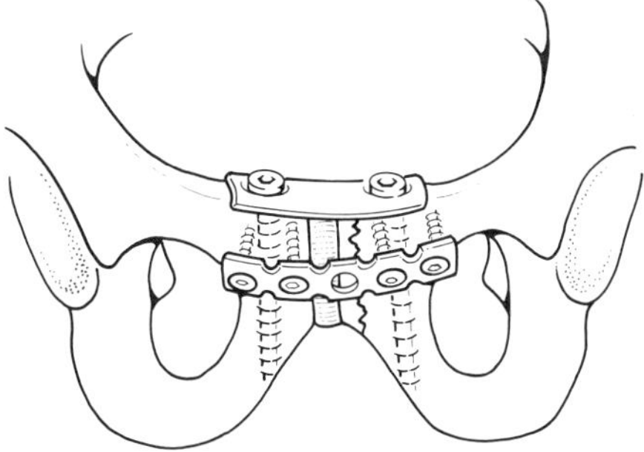

Fig. 19.3 Double plating of the symphysis pubis with two plates at 90° to each other.

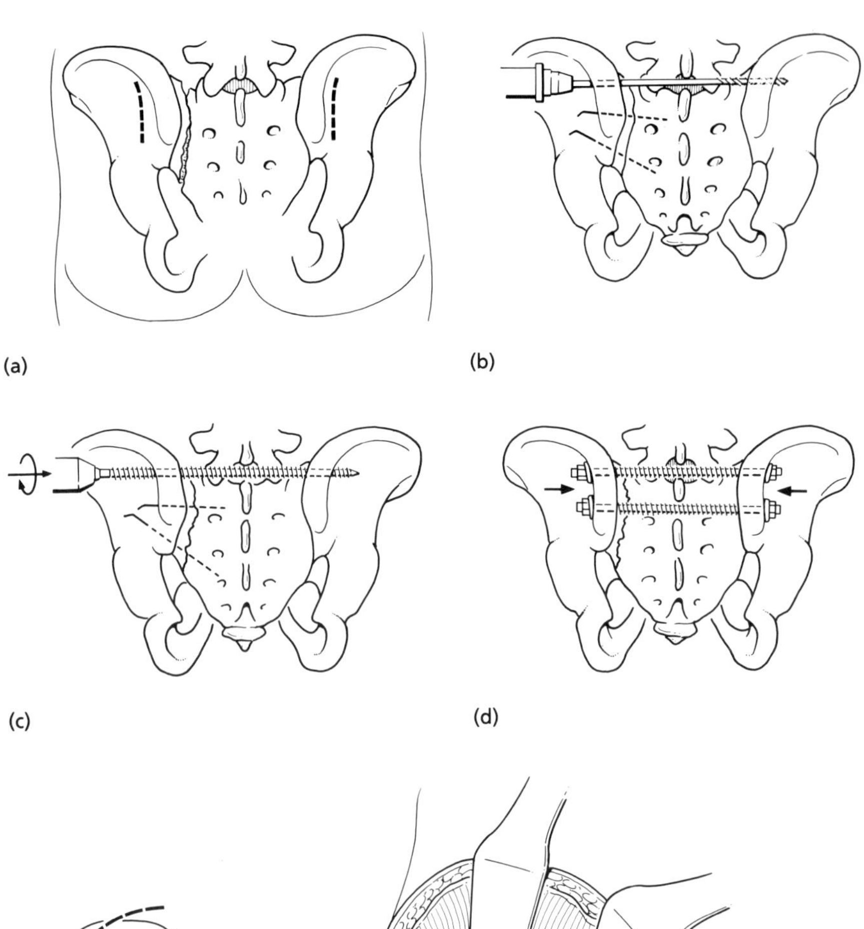

Fig. 19.4 Stabilization of a sacral fracture with posterior sacral bars. (a) Two posterior vertical skin incisions. (b) Drilling of the post-iliac crest to accept 6.4-mm Harrington sacral bars. (c) Insertion of posterior sacral bar, superficial to sacrum. (d) Two bars *in situ*, tightened to provide compression.

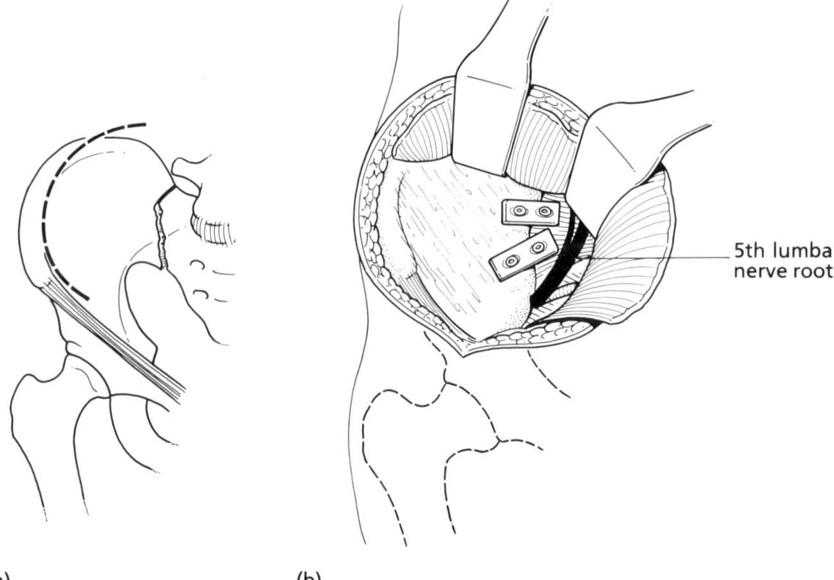

Fig. 19.5 Anterior approach to the sacro-iliac joint. (a) Skin incision. (b) Dislocation fixed with two short dynamic compression plates. Only one screw should be placed in the sacrum to protect the L5 nerve root.

field. Most pelvic fractures are stable and may be managed by simple techniques. However, the vertically unstable pelvic fracture does badly with traditional methods and consideration should be given to operative stabilization.

Acetabular fractures

It is now widely accepted that intra-articular fractures require anatomical reduction to ensure good long-term function. If anatomical reduction cannot be achieved by closed means, then open reduction, stable internal fixation and early movement are essential. These principles of management apply just as much to a displaced acetabular fracture as to a displaced ankle fracture. However, the technical problems of operating on the acetabulum have prevented many surgeons from adopting these logical principles.

A review of the published reports on treatment of acetabular fractures confirms the necessity for achiev-

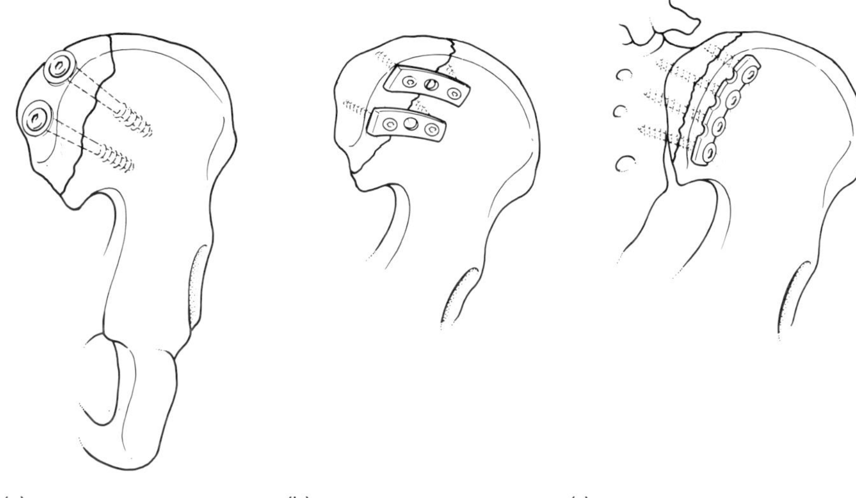

Fig. 19.6 Ilial wing fractures fixed with; (a) cancellous lag screws; (b) two dynamic compression plates; (c) 3.5 reconstruction plate.

(a)   (b)   (c)

ing an anatomical reduction if good results are to be obtained. The work of Rowe and Lowell (1961) is often quoted as an argument for non-operative treatment of acetabular fractures. Yet, a careful study of this paper reveals a different message. Of the 93 fractures reviewed by Rowe and Lowell, 50 were low-energy, undisplaced fractures or medial wall fractures in older patients. The results of non-operative treatment in this group were, unsurprisingly, satisfactory. However, the other 43 fractures were high-energy injuries that resulted in marked incongruity or instability of the hip joint. Results were uniformly poor when there was a failure to achieve anatomical reduction and/or stability of the hip joint. Operative treatment was more likely to achieve these goals, and in this high-energy group of fractures operative treatment gave better results than non-operative management.

Judet *et al.* (1964) reached the same conclusion. In their series, if anatomical reduction was achieved, 90% of such patients had a good long-term result. However, they were only able to achieve an anatomical reduction in 74% of patients. In the remaining 26%, incongruity of the hip joint led to the development of post-traumatic osteoarthritis. The necessity of obtaining an anatomical reduction of a displaced acetabular fracture to ensure good long-term hip function has also been confirmed by Larson (1973), Carnesale *et al.* (1975), Pennal *et al.* (1980) and Senegas *et al.* (1980).

Thus, it is clear that if closed reduction of a displaced fracture of the acetabulum fails, open reduction and stable internal fixation is needed. However, such treatment will improve results only if an anatomical reduction is obtained and complications are avoided.

Anatomy

From the lateral view, the acetabulum forms an inverted 'Y', with one limb forming the anterior column and the other limb the posterior column. The anterior column extends from the iliac crest to the symphysis pubis and includes the anterior wall of the acetabulum. The posterior column begins at the superior gluteal notch and descends through the acetabulum, the obturator foramen and the inferior pubic ramus (see Fig. 19.7). The superior weight-bearing area (including a portion of both the anterior and posterior columns) is the acetabular dome.

The type of acetabular fracture produced depends on the position of the femoral head at impact. Fractures of the posterior column occur when the femoral head is internally rotated, and fractures of the anterior column occur when the femur is externally rotated. If the femoral head is adducted the superior part of the dome will be involved, and if it is abducted the inferior part of the dome is damaged.

Diagnosis

Sensible decision-making depends on an accurate diagnosis, based on a careful history, thorough physical examination and standard radiographic protocol. The history will determine the so-called patient factor, to involve age, pre-existing medical conditions and treatment, and some estimate of the magnitude of the force resulting in the fracture.

The physical examination is directed at assessing the whole patient for other injuries (and treating these if

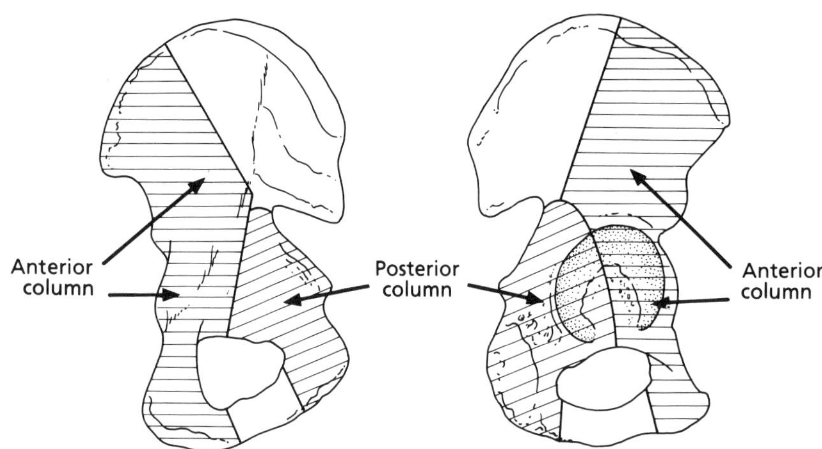

Fig. 19.7 The extent of the anterior and posterior columns of the acetabulum.

appropriate) and defining the neurovascular status of the injured side. Once life-threatening injuries have been diagnosed and managed, a standard set of radiographs of the acetabulum/pelvis is obtained to assess the acetabular fracture. These radiographs include standard views, special views and CT scans.

Standard views The anteroposterior, inlet and outlet views of the pelvis allow a basic assessment of the acetabulum and will reveal whether the pelvic ring is involved in the fracture.

Special views Three views of the affected hip joint are obtained. These are the anteroposterior view, the 45° internal rotation (obturator oblique) view and the 45° external rotation (iliac oblique) view. These latter two views are also known as the Judet views.

The anteroposterior film will allow the following to be defined: the iliopectineal line, showing the extent of the anterior column; the ilio-ischial line, showing the extent of the posterior column; the medial wall of the acetabulum and teardrop; and the anterior and posterior acetabular lips (see Fig. 19.8).

The obturator oblique view outlines clearly the iliopectineal line, throwing the whole anterior column into view. The posterior lip of the acetabulum is seen best on this view (see Fig. 19.9). The iliac oblique view throws the ilio-ischial line and posterior column into view. The greater sciatic notch and ischial spine are clearly seen, as is the anterior lip of the acetabulum (see Fig. 19.10).

CT scan The overall pattern of the fracture can be defined with the plain radiographs described above, but CT scanning is essential to show the fine detail of the acetabular fracture. It demonstrates with greater precision fragments of the anterior or posterior wall, marginal impaction, retained fragments in the joint, the degree of comminution and persistent hip dislocations, and allows an assessment of associated sacro-iliac pathology.

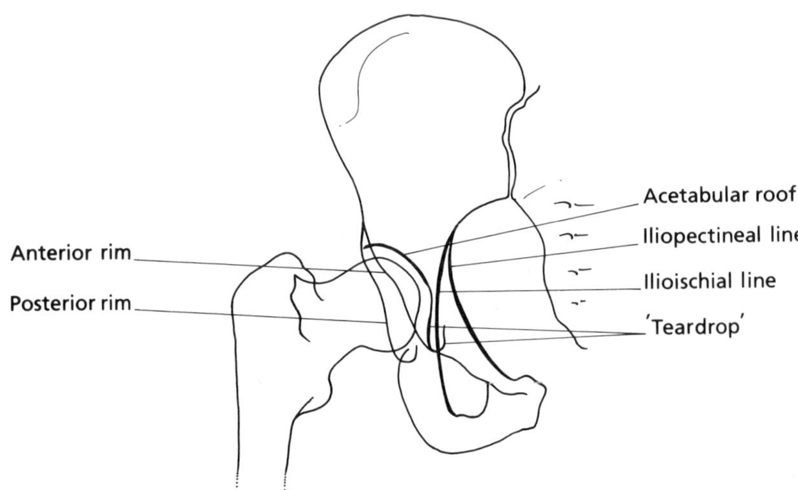

Fig. 19.8 Radiographic features of the anteroposterior view of the acetabulum.

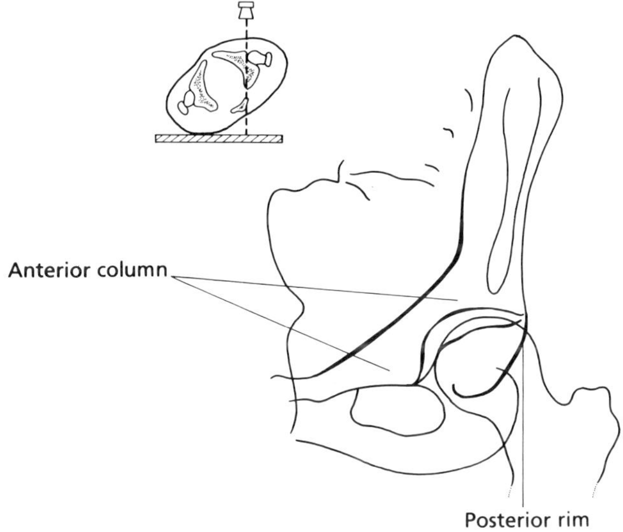

Fig. 19.9 Obturator oblique view of the acetabulum.

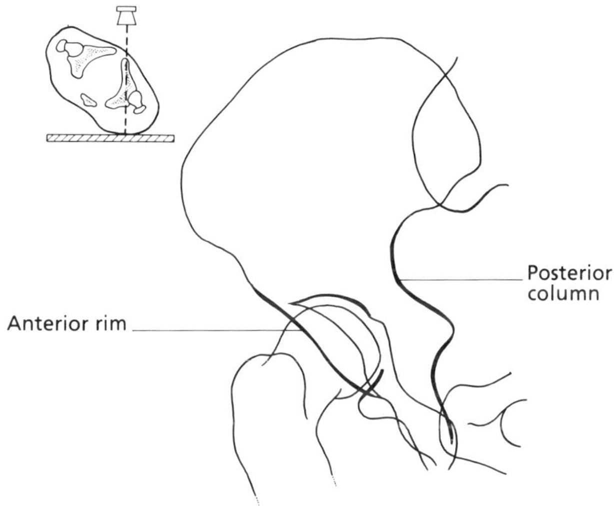

Fig. 19.10 Iliac oblique view of the acetabulum.

Classification

Classification is based on the anatomical character of the fracture, together with the direction of the force applied. It should allow grouping of fractures, so that treatment can be compared, and should give the surgeon some guidance on the optimum method of treatment. However, the surgeon must also consider other aspects of the 'fracture personality' namely: (i) displacement; (ii) comminution; (iii) integrity of the dome fragment; (iv) state of the bone; and (v) presence or absence of associated dislocation. The Association for Osteosynthesis (AO) classification is given in Table 19.3 and shown diagramatically in Fig. 19.11.

Table 19.3 AO classification of acetabular fractures

Type A	Only one column involved, the other column remains intact
A1	Posterior wall fracture and variations
A2	Posterior column fracture and variations
A3	Anterior wall/anterior column fractures
Type B	Transverse fracture component, where a portion of the dome remains attached to the intact ilium
B1	Transverse fracture/transverse plus posterior wall fracture
B2	T-fracture and variations
B3	Anterior wall/column with posterior hemitransverse fracture
Type C	Both-column fractures, with all articular surfaces (including dome) detached from intact ilium
C1	Anterior column fracture extending to ilial crest
C2	Anterior column fracture extending to anterior ilium
C3	Fracture lines enter sacro-iliac joint

Management

Major acetabular trauma is rarely a single event. In patients with multiple injuries, resuscitation should proceed according to recognized ATLS guidelines. Following this, the 'personality' of the fracture should be defined using the radiographic techniques described above. Decision-making then follows the algorithm given in Table 19.4.

If there is a dislocation of the hip joint — either anterior, posterior or central — this should be reduced, if possible, under general anaesthetic as soon as is practicable. Reconstructive acetabular surgery is usually delayed for 5–7 days from injury to allow it to be performed in optimal circumstances. Indications for urgent surgery include irreducible dislocation, increasing neurological deficit following closed reduction, associated vascular injury and open fracture.

After closed manipulation, the limb should be placed in skeletal traction. However, such traction should *never* be via a trochanteric pin as this may be over the site of a proposed incision. If, as often happens, the pin becomes septic, this will compromise the planned surgery (Tile 1984). Traction should be via a supracondylar femoral pin with 9–14 kg (20–30 lbs) weight.

If, after closed reduction, the hip joint is both congruous and stable, closed treatment on traction may be definitive. Traction is maintained for 8–12 weeks and a satisfactory reduction confirmed by serial radiographs. Non-operative management is indicated for: (i) dome displacement <2 mm; (ii) low anterior column fractures; (iii) low transverse fractures; and (iv) associated both-

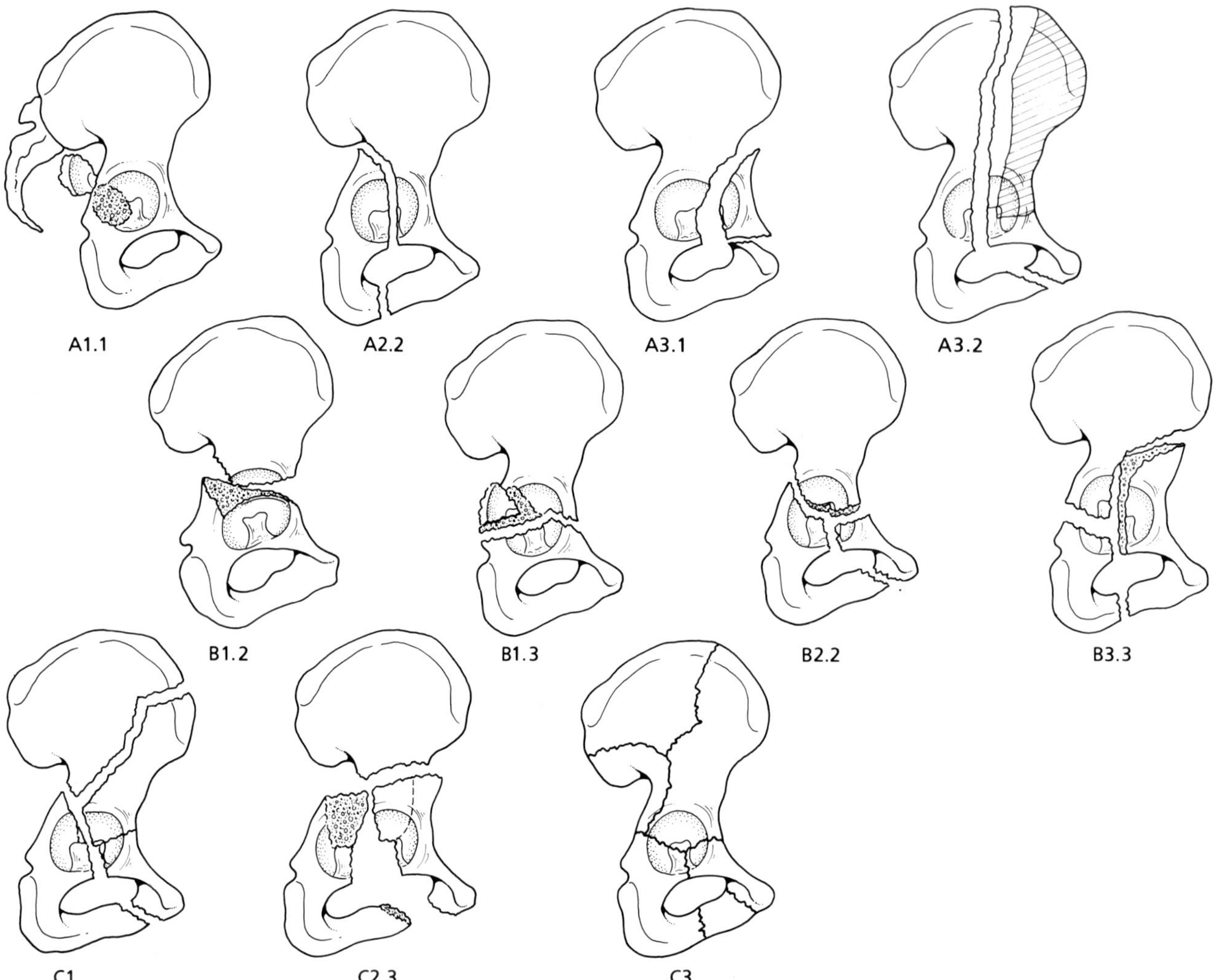

Fig. 19.11 AO classification of acetabular fractures. Type A: fractures involving only one column. Type B: transverse fracture component; dome fragment still attached to ilium. Type C: both-column fractures; no part of dome remains attached to ilium.

column fracture without major posterior column displacement.

If the reduction of the fracture is incongruous or the hip joint is unstable, the operability of the fracture must be assessed. Operability depends on: (i) the anatomical pattern of the fracture; (ii) the degree of comminution; (iii) the general state of the patient; (iv) the state of the bone; and (v) the skills of the surgeon and associated team. The questions that must be asked are: 'Can I fix this fracture?' and 'Can this fracture be fixed at all?' If there is any doubt, the patient should be transferred as soon as possible to a centre that is capable of assessing and managing these complex injuries.

As a general rule, the following fractures are likely to require surgery:

1 Any acetabular fracture with a large posterior wall fragment causing instability. If in doubt, the stability should be assessed under general anaesthetic.

2 Displaced dome fragments rarely reduce with closed manipulation, and thus surgery is essential to ensure joint congruity.

3 High transverse or T-fractures are shearing injuries. If they occur through the superior weight-bearing area, they are grossly unstable (and often associated with central dislocation). Even at operation, reduction can be difficult.

4 Displaced both-column fractures.

5 Retained bone fragments within the joint, causing incongruity and/or instability, are an absolute indication for surgery.

6 Fractures of the acetabulum associated with a fracture of the femoral head.

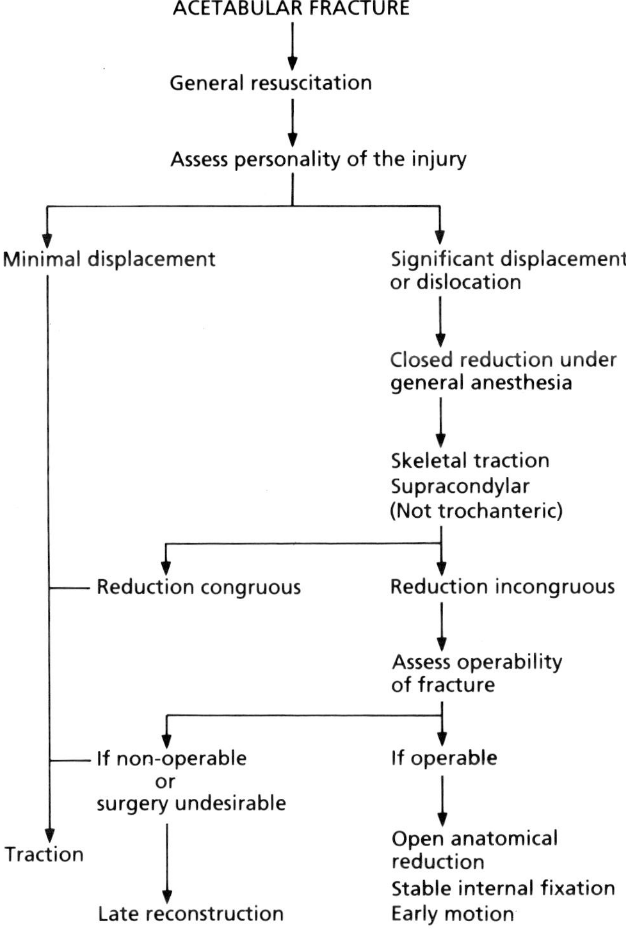

Fig. 19.12 Management algorithm for acetabular fracture.

If surgery restores joint congruity and stability, the long-term results will be improved. However, if surgery fails to achieve these objectives, the long-term outlook will not have improved *and* the patient will have been exposed to the possible risks and complications of surgery. Such surgery is demanding and complex — if in doubt, transfer the patient to a centre experienced in acetabular reconstruction.

Surgical technique

Reconstructive acetabular surgery is not usually an emergency procedure, but closed reduction of a dislocated hip is. Definitive surgery should be delayed until optimal conditions prevail, but should ideally be performed within 7 days. Prophylactic intravenous antibiotics should be given. There is a distinct possibility of major haemorrhage and 6—10 units of blood should be made available.

Surgical approaches

The approach is governed by the type of fracture and guidelines are given in Table 19.5. For a detailed description of the approaches, the reader is referred to the standard texts (Letournel & Judet 1981, Tile 1984). Nevertheless, there are important points to be made regarding each approach.

POSTERIOR KOCHER—LANGENBECK

This allows access to the posterior column and posterior wall only, but exposure is limited proximally by the superior gluteal vessels and the greater trochanter. The sciatic nerve is at risk in this approach, and the knee *must* be kept flexed at all times to protect the nerve. The muscle bellies of the short external rotators should be used to protect the sciatic nerve during retraction. It is also essential to avoid damage to the superior gluteal artery and nerve as they exit the pelvis via the greater sciatic notch. Arterial injury may cause massive bleeding, which can be difficult to control if the artery retracts within the pelvis. Embolization or direct surgical control may be necessary if packing does not control bleeding. The superior gluteal nerve supplies the abductor muscles of the hip and injury causes major disability.

TRANSTROCHANTERIC

For transverse or T-fractures the same posterior skin approach is used, but the greater trochanter can be detached, giving a better view of the dome. The detach-

Table 19.4 Choice of approach for acetabular fractures

Type of fracture	Approach
Posterior wall fractures	Posterior Kocher—Langenbeck
Posterior wall with associated posterior column or transverse fracture	Transtrochanteric
Transverse or 'T'-fracture	Transtrochanteric or ilio-inguinal
Anterior types (all)	Ilio-inguinal
Double-column fractures	Ilio-inguinal extended iliofemoral or combined anterior plus posterior approach

ment of the greater trochanter also removes tension from the superior gluteal neurovascular bundle. If the heads of rectus femoris are also detached and deflected, part of the anterior column can be visualized. However, it is only possible to use a retrograde interfragmentary lag screw to fix the anterior column through this approach.

It is difficult to gain anterior access with a transtrochanteric approach using a posterior skin approach only. If this access is a problem, for instance with a difficult double-column fracture with major displacement, the approach should be extended to the triradiate transtrochanteric approach. The additional skin incision runs from the greater trochanter to the anterior superior iliac spine and, after detaching the greater trochanter, a triangular musculofasciocutaneous flap is reflected superiorly, giving excellent access to the entire side wall of the pelvis as well as the whole of the posterior column.

ILIO-INGUINAL

This approach is ideal for difficult anterior column fractures with anterior displacement and when access to the whole of the anterior column is required. It also allows access to the symphysis pubis. Some double-column fractures can be dealt with by this anterior approach, but only if the posterior fragment is single and large. To allow intra-articular visualization of the hip, a 'T' extension of the incision is recommended; this is made just medial to the anterior superior iliac spine and runs axially down the anterior thigh to allow anterior exposure of the hip joint. This 'T' extension follows the plane of the iliofemoral approach between tensor fascia lata and sartorius. The dissection for the ilio-inguinal approach is complex and great care must be taken to protect the vital structures on the anterior aspect of the hip joint. It is advisable to practise this approach on a cadaver before trying it on a patient!

ILIOFEMORAL

This approach gives excellent visualization of the outer table of the ilium, the dome and the posterior column. It gives virtually the same exposure as the triradiate approach, but with better exposure of the anterior column down to the iliopectineal eminence. The danger of this approach is that the whole muscle mass of the gluteus medius and minimus depends on the superior gluteal neurovascular bundle exiting the greater sciatic notch. Any tension or other damage to this bundle can render the entire muscle mass ischaemic.

COMBINED

If visualization is not going to be adequate by use of one of the extensive lateral approaches, combined anterior and posterior approaches may be used. The patient is placed in the lateral position to stabilize the posterior column via a posterior approach and then, either during the same anaesthetic or at a later date, the anterior column is stabilized via an ilio-inguinal approach.

Surgical reduction and fixation

Anatomical reduction of an acetabular fracture may still be difficult to achieve despite adequate visualization. However, anatomical reduction is essential to ensure good long-term results. The operating surgeon therefore requires adequate human and technical resources. A minimum of two assistants is required — preferably with some experience or knowledge of acetabular reconstruction. Special pelvic reduction clamps are manufactured by the AO/ASIF group and are very useful, especially for posterior column and transverse fractures. There are also some other 'tricks' which help with reduction or fixation:

1 The articular surface of the hip joint must be seen adequately by wide capsulotomy.

2 A corkscrew inserted up the femoral neck will allow direct traction of the femoral head to visualize the hip joint.

3 A corkscrew inserted into the ischial tuberosity allows rotation or traction of the posterior column in transverse and posterior column fractures.

4 Provisional fixation with Kirschner wires allows the accuracy of the reduction to be checked before screw or plate fixation is carried out. The use of 2-mm Kirschner wires is recommended as a 4.0-mm cancellous screw can later be introduced via the Kirschner-wire hole.

Stable internal fixation is achieved by use of interfragmentary lag screws. In pelvic and acetabular fractures both 4.0- and 6.5-mm cancellous screws are used. Plates are used to neutralize the fracture once stable interfragmentary compression has been achieved. The 3.5-mm reconstruction plate is the implant of choice.

Before fixation, plates must be carefully contoured to provide an exact fit. Great care must be taken to ensure that no screws penetrate the joint, as this is a potent cause of chondrolysis.

Postoperative care

In general, the patient should be maintained on traction,

with continuous passive motion, for 7–10 days. If the bone stock was adequate and satisfactory stability was achieved at operation, the patient is then mobilized non-weight-bearing. Partial weight-bearing may commence at 6 weeks and should be gradually increased to full weight-bearing at 12 weeks (Tile 1984).

If there is concern regarding bone quality or if major comminution was present, traction should be maintained for 6 to 8 weeks. This is followed by walking non-weight-bearing for a further 6 weeks and then introducing progressive weight-bearing.

Complications

As well as the general complications that may arise following hip surgery, there are certain specific problems that may occur after acetabular fractures.

The sciatic nerve may be damaged at the time of injury or during surgery. Judet *et al.* (1964) reported that the risk to the sciatic nerve following posterior surgery was 17.4%. In the first 102 cases of acetabular fractures treated at Sunnybrook Medical Centre, there were 22 sciatic nerve lesions: 16 post-traumatic and six post-operation. All the postoperative cases recovered, but in the post-traumatic cases four recovered fully, eight partially and four showed no signs of recovery.

The femoral nerve is also at risk after anterior column fractures, either from the fracture itself or during surgery. The superior gluteal nerve is particularly vulnerable as it leaves the pelvis via the greater sciatic notch; great care must be taken at operation.

Heterotopic ossification remains a major problem. Among the first 102 patients at Sunnybrook Medical Centre there were 18 cases of significant heterotopic ossification, resulting in reduced hip movements. All these instances of heterotopic ossification followed surgical approaches with the reflection of muscles from the wall of the ilium (posterolateral, triradiate transtrochanteric or iliofemoral). The patient most at risk is the young male undergoing a posterolateral approach with muscle stripping. Diphosphonates have not been shown to be of value. Indomethacin has been shown to be of value in reducing the heterotopic ossification rate when given as a dose of 25 mg tds 3 weeks from surgery.

Avascular necrosis of the femoral head may be partial or complete, but is a serious complication. Judet *et al.* (1964) report an incidence of 6.6%, mainly occurring after high-energy injuries or after posterior fracture or dislocation. Avascular necrosis of the acetabulum has also been reported and resulted in collapse of the hip joint.

Summary

The critical decisions regarding acetabular fractures are the early ones. Factors determining the outcome are injury related, including the amount of damage to the femoral head/acetabulum and the development of avascular necrosis, or surgeon related, including the adequacy of reduction and iatrogenic complications.

Fractures with significant displacement, especially posterior types, transverse types or T-fractures involving the dome, require accurate open reduction and internal fixation, to allow early movement. If joint congruity and stability are restored (and complications avoided) good results can be expected. Nevertheless, much acetabular reconstructive surgery is both demanding and complex; such cases should be referred to centres with special experience and expertise.

Conclusions

Major fractures of the pelvis and acetabulum remain among the most major therapeutic challenges in modern orthopaedic trauma surgery. The first priority is to save the patient's life and this is particularly a problem after major pelvic fracture. Unstable pelvic ring injuries require stabilization, although the exact technique will vary depending on the circumstances. Displaced fractures of the acetabulum should be treated as any other displaced intra-articular fracture — via anatomical reduction and stabilization by internal fixation — to allow early movement.

The management of such complex injuries is difficult and demanding. In any situation where adequate resources are not available to manage the patient to the highest possible standard, the patient should be transferred as soon as possible to a centre that is experienced in the assessment and management of major pelvic and acetabular trauma.

References

American College of Surgeons *Advanced Trauma Life Support Course Manual*. American College of Surgeons: Chicago, 1988.

Carnesale, P.G., Stewart, M.J. & Barnes, S.N. Acetabular disruption and central fracture–dislocation of the hip. *J Bone Joint Surg* 1975; **57A**: 1054–1059.

Goldstein, A., Phillips, T., Sclafani, S.J.A. *et al.* Early open reduction and internal fixation of the disrupted pelvic ring. *J Trauma* 1986; **26**: 325–333.

Hesp, E.L., Van Der Werken, C., Keunen, R.W. *et al.* Unstable fractures and dislocation of the pelvic ring: results of treatment in relation to severity of injury. *Neth J Surg* 1985; **37**: 148–152.

Holdsworth, F.W. Dislocation and fracture–dislocation of the pelvis. *J Bone Joint Surg* 1948; **30B**: 461–466.

Judet, R., Judet, J. & Letournel, E. Fractures of the acetabulum: Classification and surgical approaches for open reduction. *J Bone Joint Surg* 1964; **46A**: 1615–1647.

Kellam, J.F., McMurtry, R.W., Paley, D. & Tile, M. The unstable pelvic fracture: Operative treatment. *Orthop Clin North Am* 1987; **18**: 25–41.

Larson, C.B. Fracture–dislocation of the hip. *Clin Orthop* 1973; **92**: 147–154.

Letournel, E. & Judet, R. *Fractures of the Acetabulum*. Springer-Verlag: Berlin, 1981.

Letournel, E. Acetabulum fractures: Classification and management. *Clin Orthop* 1980; **151**: 81–106.

McMurtry, R.W., Walton, D., Dickinson, D. *et al*. Pelvic disruption in the polytraumatised patient: A management protocol. *Clin Orthop* 1980; **151**: 22–30.

Mears, D.C. & Fu, F.H. Modern concepts of external skeletal fixation of the pelvis. *Clin Orthop* 1980; **151**: 65–72.

Pennal, G.F., Davidson, J., Garside, H. *et al*. Results of treatment of acetabular fractures. *Clin Orthop* 1980; **151**: 115–123.

Raf, L. Double vertical fractures of the pelvis. *Acta Chir Scand* 1966; **131**: 298–305.

Rowe, C.R. & Lowell, H.D. Prognosis of fractures of the acetabulum. *J Bone Joint Surg* 1961; **43**: 30–59.

Senegas, J., Liourzou, G. & Yates, M. Complex acetabular fractures, a transtrochanteric lateral surgical approach. *Clin Orthop* 1980; **151**: 107–114.

Tile, M. & McBroom, R. Disruption of the pelvic ring. *Orthop Trans* 1982; **6**: 493.

Tile, M. *Fractures of the Pelvis and Acetabulum*. Williams & Wilkins: Baltimore, 1984.

Tile, M. Pelvic ring fractures: Should they be fixed? *J Bone Joint Surg* 1988; **70B**: 1–12.

20: The Hip Joint

Introduction

Injuries about the hip joint may be conveniently classified as:

1 Acetabular fractures (see Chapter 19).
2 Dislocations of the hip
  (a) Anterior.
  (b) Posterior.
  (c) Central (see Chapter 19).
3 Femoral head fractures.
4 Proximal femoral fractures
  (a) Intracapsular.
  (b) Extracapsular.

Dislocations and fracture — dislocations

D.J.WOOD AND J.STEVENS

Traumatic dislocations of the hip are the result of major trauma; they require early diagnosis and prompt reduction. The three major types, posterior, anterior and central, are named according to the position of the femoral head in relation to the acetabulum. Central dislocation is essentially a 'stove-in' pelvis with a different aetiology, treatment and prognosis from the other two types (Proctor 1973) and is dealt with in the section on acetabular fractures. About 10% of traumatic hip dislocations are anterior, where the femoral head is forced through the anterior ligamentous structures. Conversely, posterior dislocations are frequently associated with acetabular rim fractures.

Classification

Posterior dislocations and fracture−dislocations have been classified in many ways, but the most widely accepted classification is that of Thompson and Epstein (1951); its prognostic value has been verified in a series of 559 dislocations of the hip reported by the latter author (Epstein 1973). There are five groups of injuries in this classification:

Type I — posterior dislocation with nothing more than a minor fracture (Fig. 20.1).

Type II — posterior dislocation with a large single fracture of the posterior acetabular rim.

Type III — posterior dislocation with a comminuted fracture of the acetabular rim.

Type IV — posterior dislocation with a fracture of the posterior acetabular rim and the floor of the acetabulum.

Type V — posterior dislocation with an associated fracture of the femoral head.

Anterior dislocations are classified according to the position of the femoral head and associated fractures (Epstein 1973):

1 Pubic (superior)
  (a) No fracture (simple).
  (b) With a fracture of the femoral head (Fig. 20.2).
  (c) With an acetabular fracture.
2 Obturator (inferior)
  (a) No fracture (Fig. 20.3).
  (b) With a fracture of the femoral head.
  (c) With an acetabular fracture.

Mechanism of injury

Most dislocations of the hip result from road traffic accidents, when the flexed knee strikes the dashboard forcing the femoral head out of the acetabulum posteriorly. This happens if the hip is flexed on impact and the femur held in internal rotation. The exact type of fracture acquired may be determined by the alignment of the femur in the sagittal plane. In other words, with the hip more adducted there will be less of an acetabular fragment than with the hip in a relatively abducted position (Thompson & Epstein 1951). A blow

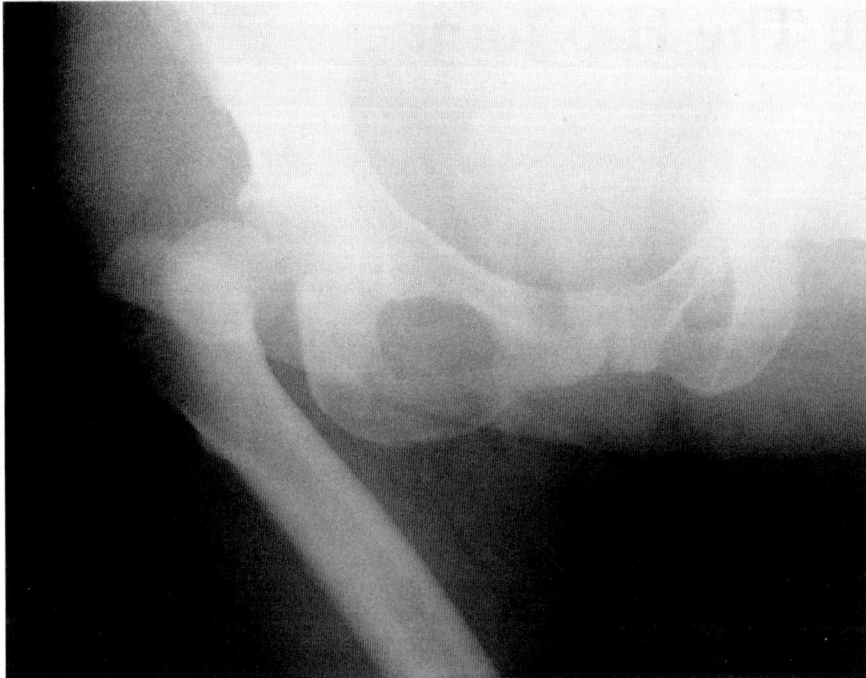

Fig. 20.1 Posterior dislocation of the femoral head.

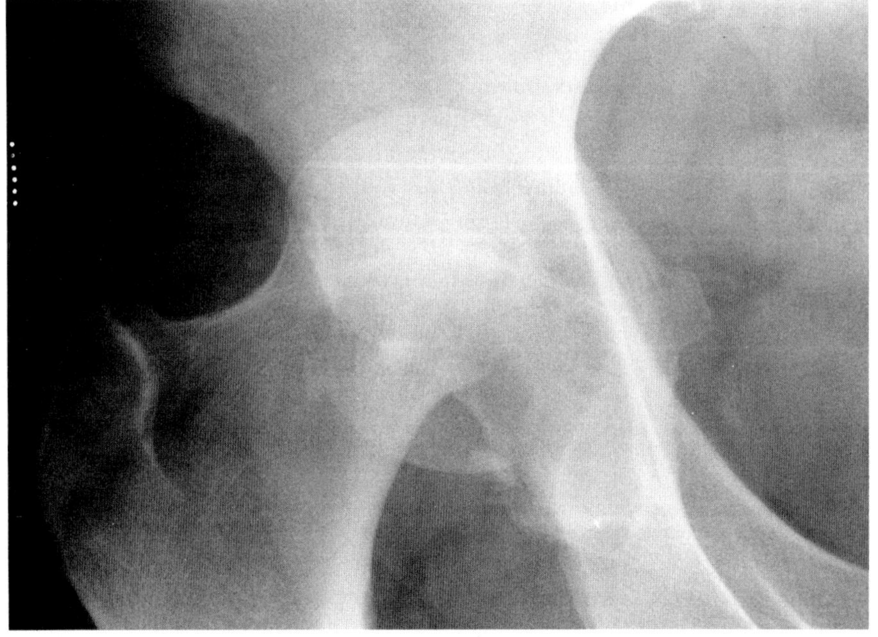

Fig. 20.2 Anterior (pubic) dislocation of the hip.

to the knee, when the hip is abducted and held in external rotation, would exaggerate this position and lead to anterior dislocation. The femoral neck or greater trochanter impinges on the posterior rim of the acetabulum and the femoral head is levered out through a tear in the anterior joint capsule. Both anterior and posterior dislocations may occur when a passenger is ejected from a vehicle or when a motor vehicle is overturned (Epstein 1973). Clearly, most of these injuries may be prevented by the proper use of seat belts.

In all categories of hip dislocation the inverted Y-shaped ligament of Bigelow remains intact. This very strong ligament is the major component in producing ultimate stability of the hip.

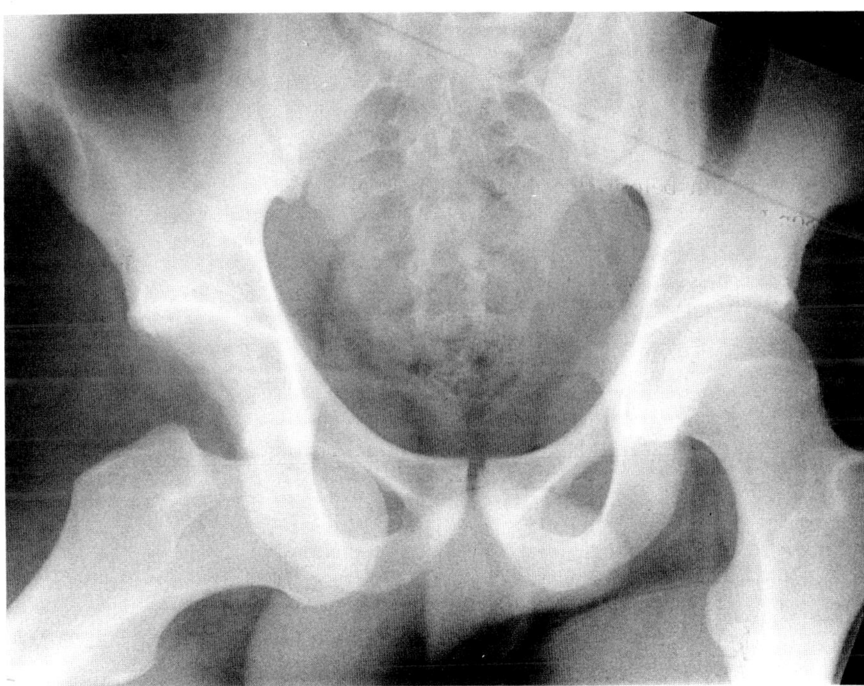

Fig. 20.3 Anterior (obturator) dislocation of the hip.

Clinical features

Traumatic dislocation of the hip is the result of major trauma and is often associated with multiple injuries. In posterior dislocations there is a typical attitude of shortening, adduction and internal rotation of the lower limb. In anterior dislocations the lower limb is shortened, abducted and externally rotated. These classical features may be confounded by an associated fracture of the ipsilateral femur or tibia. Dislocation of the hip is often overlooked with multiple injuries of the same leg. Delay in diagnosis increases the risk of avascular necrosis of the femoral head, secondary osteoarthritis and sciatic nerve palsy (Epstein 1973).

Standard anteroposterior and lateral radiographs should be accompanied by internal and external oblique views of the pelvis. These views, which are taken with the patient lying supine and alternately lifting the affected side of the pelvis 45° forward and then the non-affected side of the pelvis 45° forward, will then demonstrate anterior and posterior columns of the acetabulum (Judet *et al.* 1964). In any dislocation of the hip there is an almost mandatory requirement for transverse computerized axial tomography (CAT). This is to show (i) the presence or absence of small fragments of bone which are not regularly seen on a normal radiograph, (ii) the relationship of the femoral head to the acetabulum and (iii) the relationship of fracture fragments, which may be present in the joint, to one another.

Treatment of posterior dislocations

Type I

Most of these are manageable by closed reduction; this should be conducted without delay, after early diagnosis, with a fully relaxed anaesthetized patient. Several techniques of closed reduction have been described. The Bigelow technique involves the patient lying supine on the floor while the surgeon holds the leg, flexes it to 90° at the hip and knee, and then lifts the patient off the floor (the patient may have to be held down) with abduction, adduction and internal and external rotation movements until the reduction is achieved, usually with a distinct click. Epstein recommends traction in the line of deformity, restoration of alignment and apposition in the absence of muscle spasm (Allis 1896). Alternatively, the patient may be placed prone on the table with the affected lower extremity hanging over the edge; gentle pressure on the flexed knee with rotatory movement may achieve reduction, and may occasionally be used when general anaesthesia is contraindicated (Stimson 1889). It is the author's practice to reduce the dislocated hip by a modification of the Bigelow method, with the anaesthetized relaxed patient supine on an operating table. The surgeon sits on the table facing away from the patient and an assistant puts counter-traction on the pelvis. Hip and knee are both flexed to 90° and the lower leg is held over the surgeon's shoulder. Traction may then be efficiently applied either by straightening the surgeon's back or by pulling down on the lower leg, which is also used to control hip rotation.

Unstable long bone fractures should be stabilized by internal fixation before closed reduction is attempted (Watson-Jones 1943). Small fragments of bone or muscle can act as a block to reduction and a single failed attempt at closed reduction by an experienced orthopaedic surgeon is an indication for immediate open reduction.

In a series of 54 patients with dislocation of the hip and no fracture, nine required open reduction either because the original injury was irreducible or because, having been reduced, there was no concentricity of the hip joint. With use of a posterior approach for open reduction not a single case of avascular necrosis of the femoral head was recorded (Canale & Manugian 1979).

There is controversy about the timing of weight-bearing after closed reduction. The period of non-weight-bearing recommended in the literature varies from 2–4 weeks (Stewart *et al.* 1975) to up to 1 year (Stuck & Vaughan 1949). The authors' policy is to maintain non-weight-bearing for 12 weeks; this may reduce the overall complication rate, although the incidence of avascular necrosis remains unchanged (Brav 1962).

Type II

A dislocation should be reduced as soon as possible because a delay of more than 24 hours makes subsequent avascular necrosis of the femoral head much more likely. There is disagreement as to whether dislocations with significant acetabular fractures should be primarily reduced by open or closed means. Primary open reduction has been recommended so that loose fragments of bone and debris, present in 91% of patients at arthrotomy, may be removed from the joint (Epstein 1980). The joint may be anatomically reduced and fracture fragments stabilized by internal fixation. In reality, the ideal conditions to undertake technically demanding surgery with adequate preoperative radiographic information do not always prevail. In these circumstances it is safer to reduce the dislocated hip by closed means, but without delay. Once the femoral head has been accurately reduced within the intact part of the acetabulum, open reduction of the acetabular fragments can be delayed for up to 5–10 days. Having achieved a reduction and reduced the risk of avascular necrosis, CAT scanning can be performed and a detailed examination of the radiographs can be conducted. If, however, the reduction of a type II fracture–dislocation is con-

gruent, with no radiographic or clinical evidence of intra-articular fragments and stability in 90° of flexion, then no surgery at all is warranted.

Any operation undertaken is best performed with the anaesthetized intubated patient positioned prone and by making a posterolateral incision which extends from the posterior superior iliac spine to the greater trochanter (Griswold & Herd 1929). The gluteus maximus is split by blunt dissection to expose the areolar fatty tissue around the short external rotators of the hip. The exposure may be widened by lateral extension through the aponeurosis of the gluteus maximus and tensor fascia lata (King & Richards 1941). The sciatic nerve is identified and preserved, and then the short rotators are divided at the point of their attachment to the greater trochanter. If further exposure of the hip joint is needed, the gluteus medius may be divided at its point of attachment to the greater trochanter. This gives an excellent approach to the posterior rim of the acetabulum. When the joint has been found to be free from small fragments, the acetabular fragments can be replaced and accurately fixed with one or two screws.

The ilio-inguinal approach to the hip joint is contra-indicated in posterior dislocations of the hip. In 11 such procedures not a single good result was achieved (Epstein 1973). Posterior dislocation disrupts some of the blood supply to the proximal femur and, in addition, the lateral circumflex femoral artery is divided during the ilio-inguinal approach.

Postoperatively, skeletal traction of 4.5–6.8 kg (10–15 lb) is applied and gentle active and passive movements may be started after several days. The period of traction depends on the stability of internal fixation, fracture comminution and radiographic evidence of bony union, but usually lasts for between 6 weeks and 3 months.

Types III and IV

These are treated similarly, but are more likely to need open reduction. The argument as to whether primary reduction should be open or closed remains and is determined by local factors. Postoperatively, the patient can start active exercises at around 4 weeks and can start weight-bearing (partially) at 3 months or so. The actual timing will depend on the degree of security with which the small fragments have been fixed.

Type V

Type V fracture–dislocations were further subdivided according to the type of femoral head fracture (Pipkin

1957). Pipkin classified fractures of the femoral head as:

Type I — fracture of the femoral head caudal to the fovea centralis.

Type II — fracture cephalad to the fovea centralis.

Type III — fracture of the femoral head associated with fracture of the femoral neck.

Type IV — type I, II, or III femoral head fracture associated with a fracture of the acetabulum.

These injuries are quite unusual; there were only 15 cases reported in the literature by 1926 (Christopher 1926). It is most uncommon to get a fracture of the head of the femur, either superior or inferior, whether or not there is an associated fracture of the pelvic rim in a posterior dislocation of the hip. In this particular circumstance the value of CAT scanning is very well demonstrated. Of course, when the hip is reduced, the fragment of the head may 'wander' and block the reduction to the normal position. In so doing, it may well maintain the injury, damage the vessels to the femoral head and lead to avascular necrosis.

Pipkin type I injuries may be treated by excision of the femoral head fragment (Stewart 1974), but other authors have found that patients treated by excision of the fragment did not do as well as those treated by simple closed reduction (Kelly & Yarborough 1971). Excision of fragments has also been recommended in Pipkin type II fractures when they are less than one-third of the area of the articular surface (Epstein 1980). However, if the larger fragments cannot be reduced anatomically by closed means, they require open reduction and internal fixation with a screw or Smillie pins. To do this, of course, the hip must be dislocated which, in itself, carries some risk of avascular necrosis.

In Pipkin type III injuries the femoral neck fracture not infrequently occurs during manipulation of a type I or II fracture. In this situation the alternatives are open reduction and internal fixation, primary total hip replacement or primary hip fusion in the younger patient (Stewart 1974). For older patients the insertion of a primary endoprosthesis may be more appropriate (Roeder & DeLee 1980).

The management of Pipkin type IV injuries, where a femoral head fracture is associated with an acetabular fracture, is determined by the degree and geometry of damage to the acetabulum (Stewart 1974).

Treatment of anterior dislocations

As with posterior dislocations, early diagnosis and prompt closed reduction under general anaesthetic with full muscle relaxation is the treatment of choice. Similarly, a failed attempt at reduction by a competent orthopaedic surgeon is an indication for open reduction.

In the reverse Bigelow method of closed reduction, traction is applied to the abducted leg which is flexed at the hip. A firm lift with counter-traction on the pelvis is frequently sufficient to reduce the hip unless the dislocation is pubic (Bigelow 1870). If this manoeuvre fails, it is the author's practice to apply traction in the line of deformity followed by adduction and internal rotation. This should be done under fluoroscopic control, mindful that the femoral neck is at risk of fracture during internal rotation. Some direct anterior pressure may be applied to the femoral head, pushing it posteriorly and laterally. If reduction fails after one or two attempts, then open reduction is carried out through an anterior iliofemoral approach. Interposition of soft tissues is the commonest block to reduction.

Complications

Avascular necrosis

The reported incidences of avascular necrosis vary from 6% (Upadhyay & Moulton 1981) to more than 40% (Stewart & Milford 1954). In the latter series the use of an anterior approach for open reduction of posterior dislocations of the hip may have exaggerated the problem of avascular necrosis. In the largest series of traumatic hip dislocations, the avascular necrosis rate in 426 patients with adequate follow-up was 13% (Epstein 1973).

Avascular necrosis most probably results from damage to the ligamentum teres and the ligament of Weitbrecht. The incidence of avascular necrosis depends on the severity of the initial trauma (Proctor 1973), the time for which the hip remains dislocated, particularly if this is more than 12 hours (Brav 1962), and repeated reductions (Morton 1959).

There is a consensus of opinion that the timing of weight-bearing does not influence the incidence of avascular necrosis. However, collapse or fracture of necrotic bone during resorption and repair by creeping substitution may be prevented if weight-bearing is delayed. Various periods of non-weight-bearing, from 3 months (Ghormley & Sullivan 1953) to 12 months (Stuck & Vaughan 1949), have been recommended; this discrepancy is an expression of the inadequacy of methods previously used to assess proximal femoral blood supply. It is possible to assess proximal femoral vascularity more accurately nowadays, using either single photon emission CT of ^{99m}-technetium bone scans (Collier 1985) or magnetic resonance imaging (MRI) (Mitchell *et al.* 1986, Markisz *et al.* 1987), and the scene is set for a more detailed follow-up using these techniques. Unfortunately, forces equivalent to four times the body weight pass through the hip joint when the patient rolls over in bed, so protection from weight-bearing for prolonged periods may not be beneficial. Avascular necrosis may not become clinically evident for up to 3 years or more after the initial injury, and long-term follow-up is recommended for this reason.

Post-traumatic osteoarthritis

Although the clinical picture of post-traumatic osteoarthritis is sometimes difficult to distinguish from avascular necrosis, the incidence in 426 patients with adequate long-term follow-up has been estimated at 23% (Epstein 1973). Fracture−dislocations are more likely to produce secondary osteoarthritis than are simple dislocations and the incidence of osteoarthritis is proportional to the severity of the trauma (Brav 1962). It has been suggested that early primary open reduction by the posterior approach may reduce the incidence of avascular necrosis in posterior dislocations to 17% (Epstein 1973).

Nerve palsy

The incidence of nerve palsy in traumatic dislocation of the hip is about 10% and two-thirds of such cases return to normal within 3−30 months (Epstein 1973). The peroneal part of the sciatic nerve is the most susceptible to trauma, usually by direct contusion. Dislocated hips with associated nerve palsy should be reduced as a surgical emergency to prevent permanent damage to the nerve from pressure-induced ischaemia. Occasionally, nerve palsy is noted immediately after reduction and immediate exploration should be undertaken to ensure that the nerve has not been trapped in the joint. Late sciatic paresis has also been noted in association with either recurrent dislocation or myositis ossificans.

Myositis ossificans

Myositis ossificans can be a problem in some of these patients; the incidence of 2% may be reduced by early active movements (Epstein 1973).

References

Allis, O.H. *The Hip.* Dornan Printer: Philadelphia, 1895.

Bigelow, H.J. Luxationa of the hip joint. *Boston Med Surg J* 1870; **5**: 1−3.

Brav, E.A. Traumatic dislocation of the hip. *J Bone Joint Surg* 1962; **44A**: 1115−1134.

Canale, S.T. & Manugian, A.H. Irreducible dislocations of the hip joint. *J Bone Joint Surg* 1979; **61A**: 7−14.

Christopher, F. Fractures of the head of the femur. *Arch Surg* 1926; **12**: 1049−1061.

Collier, B.D., Carrera, G.F., Johnson, R.P., Isitman, A.T., Hellman, R.S., Knobel, J., Mager, M.A., Gonyo, J.E. & Manoy, S.J. Detection of femoral 'head' necrosis in adults by SPECT. *J Nuc Med* 1985, **26**: 979−987.

Epstein, H.C. Traumatic dislocations of the hip. *Clin Orthop* 1973; **92**: 116−142.

Epstein, H.C. *Traumatic Dislocation of the Hip.* Williams & Wilkins: Baltimore, 1980.

Ghormley, R.K. & Sullivan, R. Traumatic dislocation of the hip. *Am J Surg* 1953; **85**: 298−301.

Griswold, R.A. & Herd, C.R. Dislocation of the hip with fracture of the posterior lip of the acetabulum. *J Indiana State Med Assoc* 1929; **22**: 150−153.

Judet, R., Judet, J. & Letournel, E. Fractures of the acetabulum: classification and surgical approaches for open reduction. *J Bone Joint Surg* 1964; **46A**: 1615−1646.

Kelly, R.P. & Yarborough, S.H. Posterior fracture−dislocation of the femoral head with retained medial head fragment. *J Trauma* 1971; **11**: 97−108.

King, D. & Richards, V. Fracture−dislocation of the hip joint. *J Bone Joint Surg* 1941; **23**: 533−551.

Markisz, J.A., Knowles, R.J.R., Altchek, D.W., Shneider, R., Whalen, J.P. & Cahill, P.T. Segmental patterns of avascular necrosis of the femoral heads: early detection with MR imaging. *Radiology* 1987; **162**: 717−720.

Mitchell, M.D., Kundel, H.L., Steinberg, M.E., Kressel, H.Y., Alavi, A. & Axel, L. Avascular necrosis of the hip: comparison of MR, CT and scintigraphy. *Am J Roentgenol* 1986; **147**: 67−71.

Morton, K.S. Traumatic dislocation of the hip: a follow-up study. *Can J Surg* 1959; **3**: 67−74.

Pipkin, G. Treatment of grade IV fracture−dislocation of the hip. *J Bone Joint Surg* 1957; **39A**: 1027−1042.

Proctor, H. Dislocations of the hip joint (excluding 'central' dislocations) and their complications. *Injury* 1973; **5**: 1−12.

Roeder, L.F. & DeLee, J.C. Femoral head fractures associated with posterior hip dislocations. *Clin Orthop* 1980; **147**: 121−130.

Stewart, M.J. Management of fractures of the head of the femur complicated by dislocation of the hip. *Orthop Clin North Am* 1974; **5**: 793−798.

Stewart, M.J. & Milford, L.W. Fracture−dislocation of the hip. *J Bone Joint Surg* 1954; **36A**; 315−342.

Stewart, M.J., McCarroll, H.R. & Mulhollan, J.S. Fracture−dislocation of the hip. *Acta Orthop Scand* 1975; **46**: 507−525.

Stimson, L.A. Five cases of dislocation of the hip. *NY Med J* 1889; **50**: 118−121.

Stuck, W.G. & Vaughan, W.H. Prevention of disability after traumatic dislocation of the hip. *South Surg* 1949; **15**: 659−675.

Thompson, V.P. & Epstein, H.C. Traumatic dislocation of the hip. *J Bone Joint Surg* 1951; **33A**: 746−778.

Upadhyay, S.S. & Moulton, A. The long term results of traumatic posterior dislocation of the hip. *J Bone Joint Surg* 1981; **63B**: 548−551.

Watson-Jones, R. *Fractures and Other Bone and Joint Injuries* 2nd edn. Williams & Wilkins: Baltimore, 1943.

Proximal femoral fractures

D.J.WOOD AND J.STEVENS

Fractures of the proximal epiphysis and metaphysis of the femur are included in this category. The overwhelming majority of proximal femoral fractures are sustained by the elderly; some 90% of these fractures occur in the population over 65 years of age (Boyce & Vessey 1985). There is concern about a fracture epidemic as the incidence of proximal femoral fractures increases within an ageing population. The authors' local proximal femoral fracture incidence of 56 cases per 100 000 per year is equally divided between intracapsular and extracapsular fractures. The two predominant fracture types are intertrochanteric and subcapital femoral fractures. Fractures of the femoral head are rare and are usually associated with hip dislocation; subtrochanteric fractures constitute 5% of all extracapsular fractures and are often associated with secondary deposits.

Classification

Anatomical classification is crucial to the surgical management and prognosis of these fractures. Fractures contained wholly within the confines of the anatomical fibrous capsule may have their blood supply compromised and are more susceptible to non-union and avascular necrosis. Conversely, extracapsular fractures have at least part of the fracture line outside the capsular limits (Fig. 20.4) and rarely suffer non-union and avascular necrosis, although they are prone to malunion.

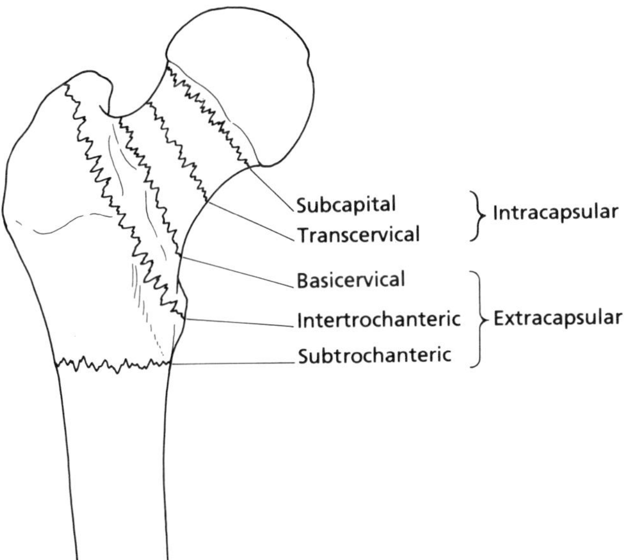

Fig. 20.4 The anatomical sites of proximal femoral fractures.

Intracapsular fractures

Historical review

Hip fractures were reported in the literature over 350 years ago (Pare 1634), but intracapsular fractures were first described as a separate entity by Sir Astley Cooper. He stated, 'In the examinations which I have made of fractures of the cervix femoris, entirely within the capsular ligament, I have only met one in which a bony union had taken place' (Cooper 1823). He concluded that non-union of subcapital femoral fractures was due to the loss of blood supply to the femoral head and that consequent fibrous union would result in 'permanent lameness'. Only if the 'reflected ligament' of the neck (Weitbrecht 1742) remained intact did Cooper believe that bony union was possible. His perceptive work, before the advent of radiographs, was based on clinical and post-mortem studies. The evolution of treatment for this fracture mirrors the development of orthopaedic surgery.

Treatment by traction developed in parallel with early attempts at internal fixation, as anaesthetic techniques improved. Both methods of treatment gave poor results. An inherently unstable fracture could not be satisfactorily held by traction and the metals used for internal fixation were impure and corrosive. The variety of ingenious methods of conservative treatment designed to achieve a stable reduction reflects the universally poor results. Against a background of inadequate conservative and surgical treatment, of non-union and avascular necrosis, this fracture was labelled the 'unsolved fracture' (Speed 1935).

An anterolateral approach to the hip joint was refined to facilitate open reduction and internal fixation with flanged nails (Smith-Petersen 1917, Smith-Petersen *et al.* 1931). The widespread acceptance of these techniques was due, in part, to the parallel development of inert and biocompatible metals (Venable *et al.* 1937). Introduction of a cannulated nail (Johansson 1932, Westcott 1934) enabled closed reduction of fractures on the fracture table under radiographic control. This technique was a significant advance but was not universally successful, as expressed by the plethora of implant designs that followed.

The problems of non-union and late segmental collapse persisted and surgeons, frustrated with the complications of subcapital femoral fractures, turned to primary prosthetic replacement. Austin Moore originally designed his hemiarthroplasty to replace a giant cell tumour of the proximal femur (Moore & Bohlman 1943). 'Thompson's' hemiarthroplasty was designed as a salvage prosthesis for a patient with non-union and collapse of a femoral neck fracture. Initial successes rapidly led to the use of these prostheses in the primary treatment of subcapital femoral fractures (Moore 1952, Thompson 1954).

Whether prosthetic replacement or internal fixation should be used for the primary treatment of displaced intracapsular fractures remains a matter of controversy, and the issue is further clouded by the variety of available implants and a paucity of controlled clinical trials. The fact that uncertainty still exists as to the best method of management was recently highlighted by a survey of all United Kingdom orthopaedic surgeons (Anderson *et al.* 1991). This showed that for patients under 70 (relatively young) almost one-third of surgeons perform primary femoral head replacement; the other two-thirds perform closed reduction and some form of internal fixation. Approximately one-third use cannulated screws, one-third use a dynamic compression screw/plate and the remaining one-third use a variety of other internal fixation devices which include Garden screws (15%). With regard to the choice of prosthesis for femoral head replacement, one-third of surgeons prefer a Thompson prosthesis, one-third an Austin Moore prosthesis and one-third some type of bipolar design. A significant number of surgeons use a Thompson prosthesis without cement.

Classification

Intracapsular fractures of the proximal femur may be classified according to their anatomical site and fracture morphology. Intracapsular fractures have been divided according to their location in the femoral neck (Fig. 20.4). The majority of intracapsular fractures are subcapital, but many of these have a distal spicule of bone. Even when the entire fracture line is transcervical, there is no difference in clinical behaviour. Basicervical fractures are like extracapsular fractures: usually stable with a good blood supply and protection from non-union and avascular necrosis.

The most widely accepted classification of subcapital femoral fractures is that of Garden (1961a), based on the degree of fracture displacement; he separated femoral neck fractures into stages I–IV. Stage I fractures are incomplete or impacted in abduction, but with a continuous cortical buttress on radiographs. When treated by internal fixation these fractures have a 95% union rate (Bentley 1968) and a 16% incidence of late segmental collapse. Stage II fractures are rarely encountered (Barnes *et al.* 1976), and their prognosis does not differ from stage I. Stage III and IV fractures are displaced, and ac-

counted for all of Garden's original cases of non-union and late segmental collapse (Garden 1961b) (Fig. 20.5).

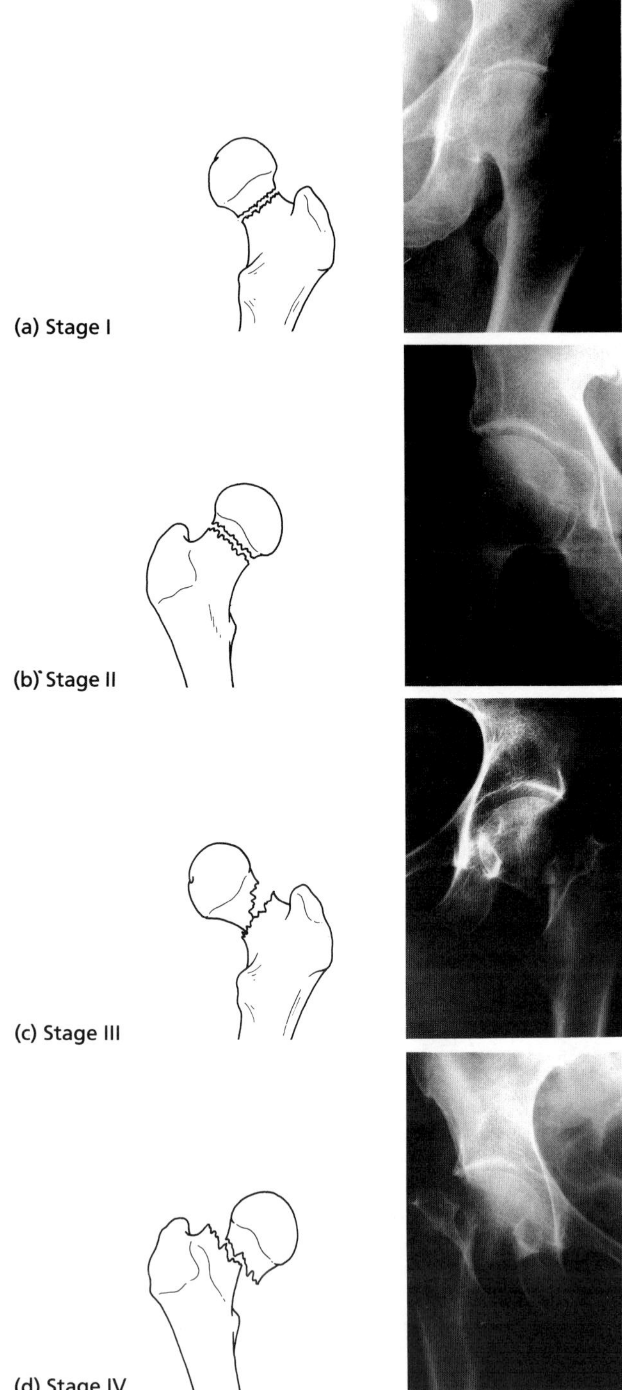

Fig. 20.5 Garden classification of subcapital femoral fractures. (a) Stage I — incomplete fractures and abduction-impacted fractures. (b) Stage II — complete fracture without displacement. (c) Stage III — complete, displaced fracture; the fracture ends are still in contact. (d) Stage IV — complete, displaced fracture; the fracture ends have lost contact.

Pauwels (1935) based his classification on the angle of inclination of the fracture line from the horizontal. Types I–III have a progressively more vertical fracture line. Pauwels' type I fracture has an angle of inclination 30° from the horizontal, type II is inclined 50° from the horizontal and type III 70° from the horizontal. Pauwels believed that non-union in his type III fractures was due to the increased shearing force. Other authors were unable to demonstrate a relationship between the angle of inclination of the fracture line and the complications of non-union and avascular necrosis (Cassebaum & Nugent 1963, Boyd & Salvatore 1964, Ohman *et al.* 1969). Garden (1971) stated that the radiographic projection of the fracture line in obliquity changed with the rotation of the distal fragment. Of fractures 85% have an angle of inclination between 45–80° (Linton 1944). In addition, the direction of the fracture line on the radiograph may be altered by changing the direction of the beam or the position of the limb (Linton 1944).

Classification of fractures into displaced and undisplaced is adequate for clinical purposes. Management may also be influenced by the age of the fracture, whether it is pathological and whether it is reducible. The patient's age, mental function, mobility, medication and intercurrent illnesses all have a bearing on the management of the fracture and are dealt with in more detail below.

Surgical anatomy

The head and neck of the femur lie within the hip joint. The head, unlike the head of prosthetic hemiarthroplasties, is not truly spherical (Cathcart 1972), and is only congruous with the acetabulum in the weight-bearing position (Walmsley 1928). It is directed upwards, medially and slightly forwards. A little below and behind its centre is a small pit, the fovea, for attachment of the ligamentum teres. The neck is a tube 3–4 cm long, which connects the head with the shaft at a mean angle of 127° (range 113–136°). The neck is anteverted by a mean of 10° but this angle varies from 20° of retroversion to 38° of anteversion. The neck is compressed in the anteroposterior direction, is almost cylindrical proximally, and becomes progressively elliptical distally where it joins the shaft at the intertrochanteric line. Posteriorly, the lateral half of the neck is extracapsular and joins the shaft at the intertrochanteric crest (Fig. 20.6).

The internal architecture of the proximal femur is dominated by the calcar femorale (Fig. 20.7), which represents the 'true' femoral neck (Bigelow 1900). This plate of bone lies deep to the lesser trochanter and fans out into the compression group of trabeculae. The lateral group of trabeculae consists of the primary tensile group, which passes from the fovea into the superior aspect of

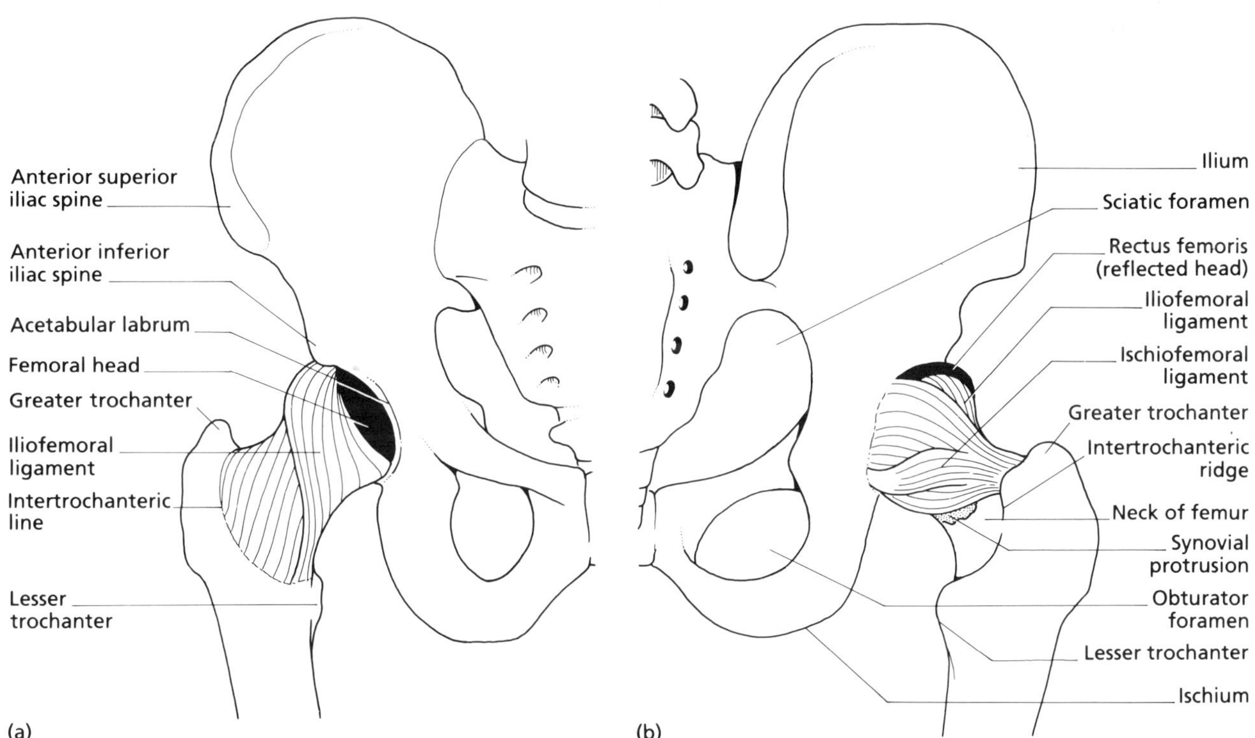

Fig. 20.6 (a) Anterior and (b) posterior views of the hip joint and proximal femur.

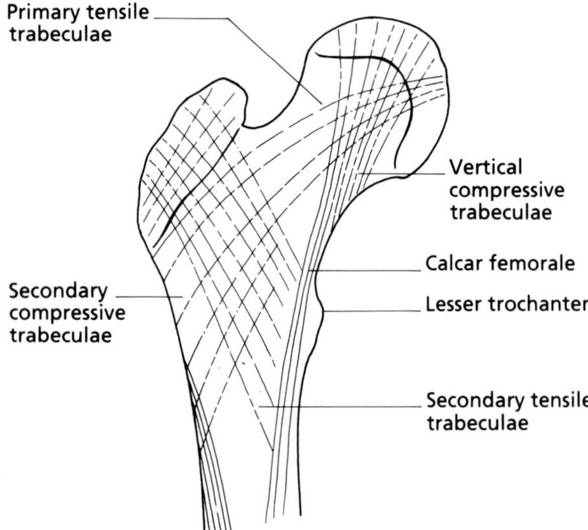

Fig. 20.7 The internal architecture of the proximal femur.

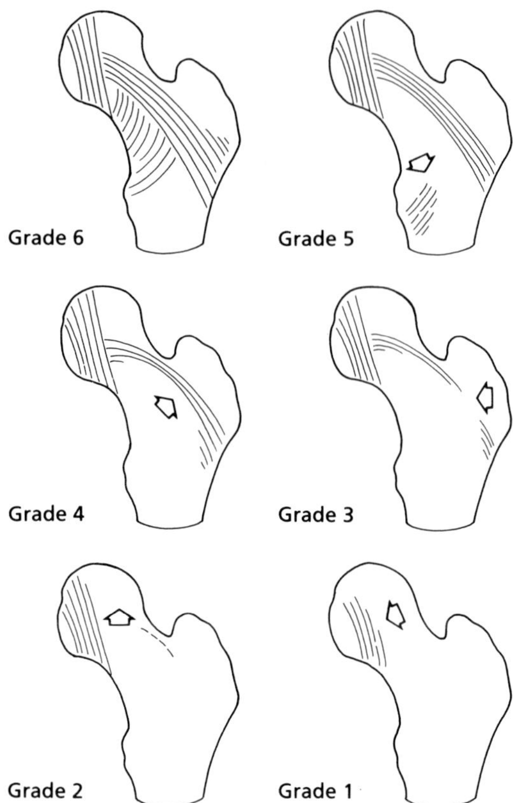

Fig. 20.8 Singh grading system for osteoporosis of the proximal femur based on the internal trabecular architecture. (After Singh *et al*. 1970.)

the femoral neck and to the lateral femoral cortex, where it is called the secondary tensile group. A secondary compressive group passes from the calcar to the greater trochanter where it abuts against the greater trochanteric group (Ward 1838) (Fig. 20.8). The lateral group of trabeculae was originally thought to be laid down in response to tensile forces, in accordance with Woolf's law (1870). However, it has been demonstrated that the whole of the femoral neck is in compression (Frankel 1960) and that the neutral axis (Koch 1917) does not exist. Tensile forces only pass across the femoral neck in unphysiological positions of increased abduction. With increasing age one or more of these trabecular groups may be absent, indicating age-related osteoporosis (Fig. 20.8) (Singh *et al*. 1970).

Blood supply

The femoral head receives its blood supply from three sources (Fig. 20.9):

1 Medial epiphyseal vessels (arteries of the ligamentum teres), derived from either the obturator artery or the acetabular branch of the medial circumflex femoral artery (Crock 1965).

2 Lateral epiphyseal vessels. Retinacular vessels arising from an extracapsular ring of arteries around the base of the femoral neck provide 90% of the blood supply to the femoral head. The retinacular vessels pierce the fibrous capsule and run subsynovially along the neck to penetrate the femoral head through nutrient foramina. Of these vessels 70% run posterosuperiorly on the femoral neck (Trueta & Harrison 1953, Sevitt & Thompson 1965). The extra-articular ring of vessels is derived from the

crucial anastomosis, with contributions from the medial and lateral circumflex femoral arteries and the superior and inferior gluteal arteries.

3 Metaphyseal vessels. Superior and inferior metaphyseal vessels are derived from the medial circumflex femoral artery. These run within the medullary cavity of the neck along with terminal ascending branches of the nutrient artery of the shaft.

Clearly, the metaphyseal and retinacular vessels may be disrupted by fracture, and the blood supply may be further compromised by the tamponade effect of raised intracapsular pressure (Harper *et al*. 1990). The medial epiphyseal blood supply is variable, and in a histological study of femoral heads obtained at various times after subcapital femoral fracture, a small medial vascular wedge of tissue was associated with more advanced avascular necrosis and late segmental collapse (Catto 1965a).

Venous drainage of the proximal femur has been demonstrated by injection of radiopaque dye into the marrow cavity of the inferomedial third of the femoral head (Phillips 1966). Dye was rapidly taken up by a group of tortuous medullary sinusoids: the lumino-

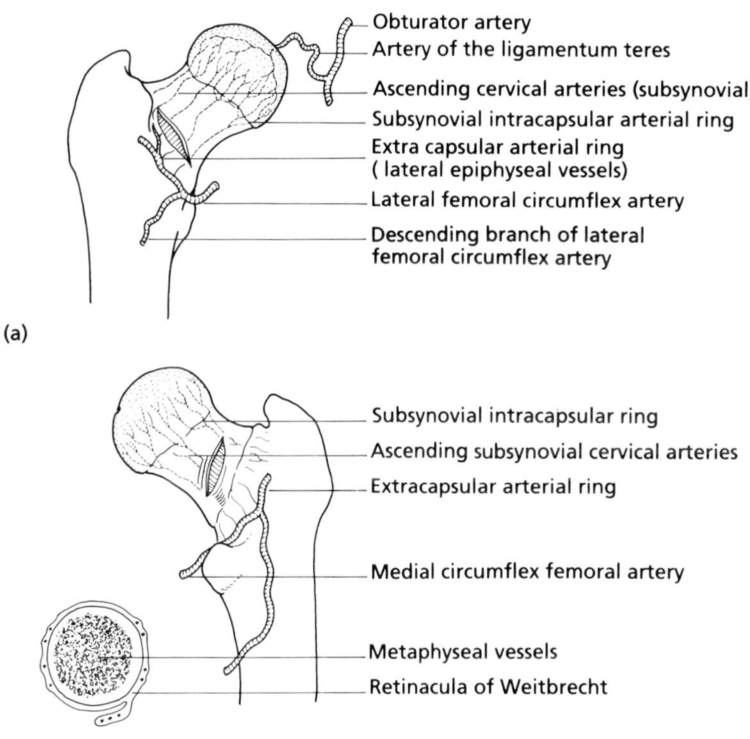

Fig. 20.9 Blood supply of the femoral neck and head. (a) Posterior view. (b) Anterior view.

capsular veins. A second group of well-defined channels drain the femur just proximal to the lesser trochanter and enter the common femoral veins. These vessels constitute the circumflex group (Meriel *et al.* 1955). A third group of veins arise in the digital notch of the greater trochanter, passing posteromedially towards the greater sciatic notch. A fourth group of veins arise on the posterior aspect of the femoral neck and drain towards the ischial tuberosity. A fifth group drains into the femoral shaft distal to the lesser trochanter. No drainage was seen through the ligamentum teres (Phillips 1966).

Mechanism of injury

The mechanism of production of proximal femoral fractures is a function of bone strength and a propensity to trauma. With increasing age, bone mass diminishes and there is an increase in the tendency to fall (Grimley Evans 1979, Grimley Evans *et al.* 1979b). Bone strength is directly proportional to density (Leichter *et al.* 1982); therefore fracture threshold is reduced by age-related osteoporosis (Frankel 1974). More than sufficient energy to fracture the proximal femur is produced by a simple fall. It has been calculated that 4000 kg cm^{-1} of potential energy would be produced by the fall of an average-sized woman. The energy-absorbing capacity of the

proximal femur is about 60 kg cm^{-1}. Under normal circumstances the energy is dissipated by active muscle contraction. Patients with dementia (Grimley Evans *et al.* 1979b), diabetes or rheumatoid arthritis (Alframm 1964) may be susceptible to proximal femoral fractures because they have a neuromuscular deficit and are unable to dissipate the energy produced by a fall.

Spontaneous fracture of the femoral neck is relatively rare (Alframm 1964), but is well recognized (Freeman *et al.* 1974). Severe trauma is more commonly associated with femoral neck fractures in younger patients, predominantly male (Alframm 1964), and may contribute to the higher incidence of avascular necrosis in this group of patients. The majority of proximal femoral fractures occur in elderly females and in these cases the injury is usually caused by mild or moderate trauma, such as a fall from a sitting or standing position (Alframm 1964).

The first proposed mechanism of injury described in the literature suggests an external rotation injury with a strong abductor force. The posterior acetabulum was said to act like an anvil on the posterior cortex of the femoral neck, producing an initial posterior fracture (Kocher 1896). This is consistent with observations that the anterior fracture line is a clean break, as if under tension, and that there is frequently posterior comminution (Meyers *et al.* 1973). However, in a recent study of CT scans of fresh subcapital femoral fractures, comminution of both anterior and posterior cortices was seen, indicating a lateral compressive component to the fracture force (Harper *et al.* 1990) (Fig. 20.10).

The role of the abductors in producing compression in the femoral neck, at both the superior and inferior aspects, was emphasized by Duhamell in 1947. By placing an axial load on the femoral neck, using a bolt through the head and neck, fractures similar to those seen clinically were produced in the laboratory (Hirsch & Frankel 1960). Without axial compression, atypical fractures were produced. It has been shown experimentally that an increase in the bending component of the force producing the fracture is more likely to lead to transcervical fractures (Frankel 1960). If the axial or compressive component of the resultant force is increased, a subcapital fracture is more likely.

Clinical features

Patients, usually elderly females, present, following a fall, with a painful hip and a short externally rotated leg. A small minority of patients sustain their fracture spontaneously or following a minor injury; this should alert the physician to the possibility of malignancy (Alframm 1964).

Critical clinical characteristics include the patient's age, general and mental health, the degree and type of trauma which produced the fracture and the presence of co-morbid conditions, including rheumatoid arthritis, Parkinson's disease, Paget's disease, renal failure, ipsi-

lateral stroke, immobility and metastatic malignant disease. The use of high-dose long-term steroids or local radiation therapy is also of some importance.

The most important prognostic indicator is mental function. A simple 10-question mental test score can be used to classify patients as demented, cognitively impaired or normal. In a study of more than 500 hip fracture patients, multivariate analysis demonstrated that mental function was a more reliable indicator of outcome than age, intercurrent infection, neoplasia, pressure sores or a wide variety of preoperative variables. Of demented patients over the age of 85 and with a subcapital femoral fracture, 75% were dead within 6 months; out of 31 surviving patients within this category only one was mobile a year after surgery. Many of these patients should probably be treated conservatively, provided that more time for nursing care is available.

Anteroposterior and lateral radiographs are usually sufficient to confirm the clinically suspected diagnosis. However, because bony impaction confers stability, a small proportion of patients will have minimal pain on weight-bearing, will not have a short externally rotated leg and may only experience discomfort at the extremes of motion. In the face of normal radiographs, and particularly in patients at risk of stress fractures (e.g. military recruits), sequential radiographs, a [99m]-technetium bone scan and tomograms of the affected hip are recommended (Prather *et al.* 1977). Tomograms may demonstrate extracortical or endosteal callus not visible on plain radiographs. An increased uptake on scintigraphy

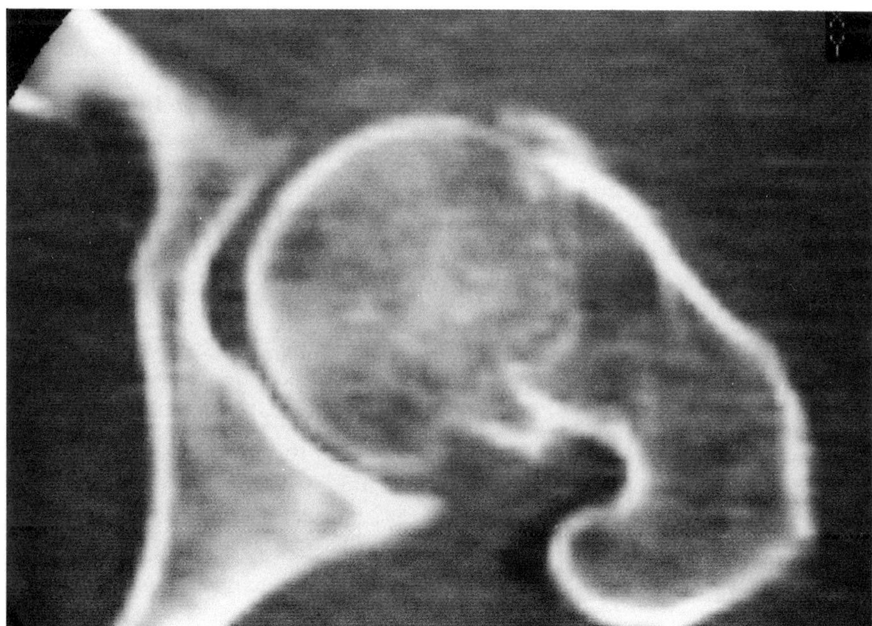

Fig. 20.10 CT scan of the femoral neck, following subcapital femoral fracture, showing comminution of both anterior and posterior cortices.

was reported in three out of four patients with a subcapital femoral fracture not seen on plain radiographs (Dorne & Lander 1985). A missed fracture may displace on weight-bearing with a consequent deterioration in prognosis; therefore a high index of suspicion of fracture is justified in elderly patients with hip pain.

Treatment

Undisplaced fractures

Undisplaced fractures, which include Garden grades I and II, account for 20% of all intracapsular fractures (Barnes *et al.* 1976) and mend well with internal fixation.

Conservative treatment of valgus impacted fractures has been repeatedly recommended (Crawford 1960, 1965, Anderson *et al.* 1964, Eklund & Eriksson 1964, Hilleboe *et al.* 1970). Crawford elaborated on this principle by carefully selecting patients with no shortening or external rotation deformity, minimal pain on active or passive movement, active internal rotation, and impaction on anteroposterior and lateral radiographs. These patients were treated by bedrest until pain-free and this was followed by a 4-month period of partial weight-bearing. Prolonged periods of partial weight-bearing, particularly in the elderly, represent an unrealistic goal and late displacement rates of 20% have been reported (Hansen & Solgaard 1978). In a comparison between conservative treatment and internal fixation of undisplaced fractures, 12% of fractures displaced on conservative treatment but none of the internally fixed fractures displaced (Bentley 1968). There was no difference between the groups in the incidence of late segmental collapse.

The authors would recommend early internal fixation using parallel cannulated screws. Large single screws may carry an additional risk of rotatory displacement (Wood 1990) and nails may disimpact the fracture. Great care should be taken to prevent displacement: the patient should be on light traction, no more than 22 kg (5 lb), until surgery. The surgeon should personally supervise transfer onto the fracture table with the patient's leg held extended at the hip in light traction and internal rotation. The anaesthetized relaxed patient is most vulnerable to fracture displacement, either by exuberant traction or by inappropriate manipulation.

With the patient supine on a fracture table, surgery is performed through a lateral approach, splitting the posterior part of the proximal vastus lateralis. The lower guide wire is introduced first, through a hole midway between the anterior and posterior femoral cortices and about 3 cm below the tubercle of vastus lateralis. The tip of the screw is advanced to within 0.5 cm of the joint line. Using a parallel barrel guide, two further suitable screw slots are selected, as far apart as possible — usually one posterior and one anterior (Figs 20.11 & 20.12). Cannulated screws are introduced over guide wires and are tightened to compress the fracture site. Postoperatively, patients are mobilized within 48 hours of surgery, following the removal of closed suction drains.

Stress fractures of the femoral neck in young adults are rare, associated with a sudden increase in activity and may be treated conservatively if the fracture is undisplaced. An initial 3-week period of balanced traction is followed by 6 weeks of non-weight-bearing on crutches. Progression to partial weight-bearing depends on plain radiograph and tomographic findings (Aro & Dahlstrom 1986).

Displaced fractures

There are contentious issues in the treatment of displaced subcapital femoral fractures. Should these fractures be treated by internal fixation or by prosthetic replacement? What type of fixation and which design of prosthesis should be used? The authors' algorithm for the management of displaced fractures is based on:
1 Mental function.
2 Age.
3 Intercurrent illness
  (a) Metastatic malignancy.

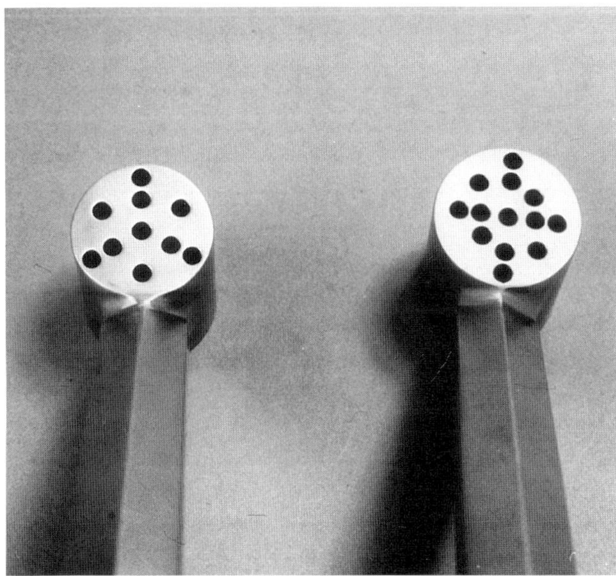

Fig. 20.11 The triangular (left) and parallelogram (right) barrel guides.

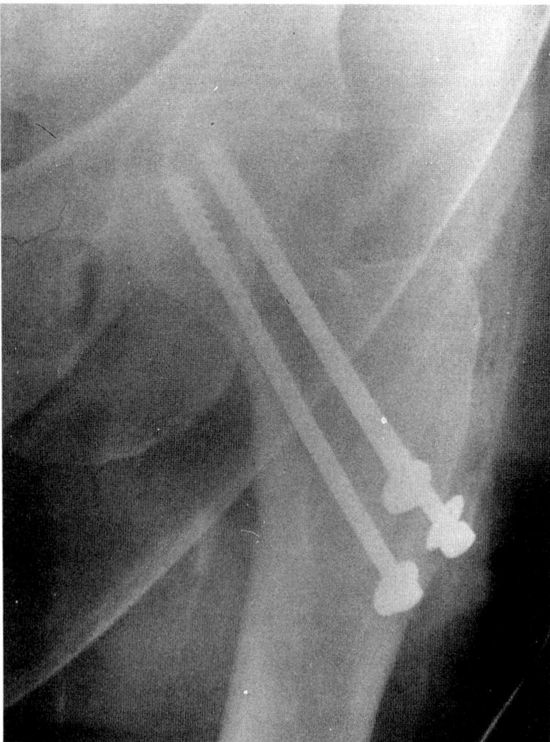

(a)

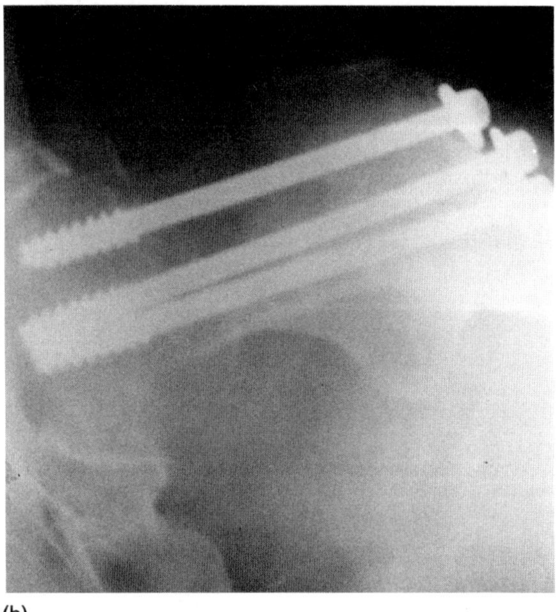

(b)

Fig. 20.12 (a) Anteroposterior and (b) lateral radiographs of a subcapital femoral fracture internally fixed with Asnis cannulated screws.

(b) Cerebrovascular accident.
(c) Parkinson's disease.
(d) Paget's disease of bone.
4 Mobility.

5 High-dose long-term steroids.
6 Inflammatory or degenerative arthritis of the affected hip.
7 Reducibility of the fracture.

The risk of death in hip fracture patients is greatly increased by dementia (Blessed *et al.* 1969, Ions & Stevens 1987). The authors treat demented patients over the age of 85 conservatively. Pain is controlled with a combination of analgesia and traction for 2–3 weeks, by which time the fracture surfaces are usually covered with fibrocartilage. This treatment results in a shortened limb with an unstable hip, but weight-bearing may be started as early as 3 weeks. These patients need more nursing care and may be better treated in a geriatric or rehabilitative unit rather than on a trauma ward where the more immediate requirements of perioperative patients place extra demands on the nursing staff. It must be emphasized that this conservative approach reflects the authors' opinion and is at odds with those who believe that hemiarthroplasty is an effective means of local pain control, which facilitates nursing care. A local prospective randomized trial of conservative treatment versus operative treatment in elderly demented patients with subcapital femoral fractures is underway, and is considered the most scientific way of resolving this difference of opinion.

Displaced fractures may be reduced and held by internal fixation. A 25–55% rate of non-union at 1 year, associated with mechanical failure, and a 28.5% rate of late segmental collapse (Barnes *et al.* 1976) (Tables 20.1–20.5), associated with revascularization of a previously avascular femoral head (Catto 1965a), have led many surgeons to abandon this method of treatment. The alternative — endoprosthetic replacement — has its own disadvantages. Hemiarthroplasty results in significant pain in 30% of patients at 3 years (Hunter 1969) and early work on total hip replacement suggests that the dislocation rate is higher than in the osteoarthritic population (Coates & Armour 1979, Sim & Stauffer 1980).

The authors prefer closed reduction and internal fixation in patients under 65 and in those patients between 65 and 80 years of age with good mental function. Patients over 80, and demented patients between 65 and 80 years of age who are physiologically older than their years, may be suitable for prosthetic replacement. Patients with severe osteoporosis from steroid therapy, immobility or paralysis are unsuitable for internal fixation and the motion of uncontrolled Parkinson's disease leads to non-union. Irreducible fractures (about 2% of displaced fractures in the authors' experience) and patients with ipsilateral inflammatory or degenerative arthritis are also unsuitable for internal fixation.

The authors' algorithm for the treatment of displaced fractures is summarized in Fig. 20.13 and individual methods of treatment are dealt with in more detail below.

As yet, no reliable preoperative method of recording femoral head vascularity in subcapital femoral fracture patients has been reported, although in non-traumatic avascular necrosis, single photon emission CT of ^{99m}-technetium bone scans has an 85% accuracy in predicting avascular necrosis in radiographically normal femoral heads (Collier *et al.* 1985). This technique has not yet been used as a prognostic indicator in intracapsular hip fractures and no reliable indicator of future complications has been developed.

Although damage to the blood supply to the femoral head at the time of fracture is an undoubted factor in the development of avascular necrosis, other possible aetiological factors have been suggested. The two most plausible hypotheses are delay between fracture and operation, and increased intracapsular pressure causing a tamponade effect on femoral head blood flow. Obviously, these two factors may be related.

It has been suggested by various authors (Soto-Hall *et al.* 1964, Crawfurd *et al.* 1988) that increased intracapsular pressure following femoral neck fractures may reach a sufficiently high level so as to obstruct the flow of blood to the femoral head. Experimental work with juvenile animals (Swiontkowski *et al.* 1986, Vegter 1987, Svalagosta 1989) has shown that sustained increases in intracapsular pressure, even with levels as low as 40 mmHg in the rabbit, can produce hypoxia and ischaemic changes in the femoral head. Levels of intracapsular pressure well above diastolic pressure have been reported in the literature (Crawfurd *et al.* 1988, Stromqvist 1988).

There is, therefore, good evidence that high intracapsular pressures may occur after proximal femoral fractures, more particularly in relatively undisplaced intracapsular fractures where capsular integrity is probably preserved. However, there is little direct evidence in man that these pressures can abolish or decrease blood flow to the femoral head. Two clinical studies have addressed this problem. Using radioisotope bone scanning techniques, femoral heads were shown to have increased isotopic uptake following aspiration (Stromqvist 1988). However, other factors may have influenced the results as hips were scanned 24 hours after operation and following osteosynthesis. Recent work has demonstrated changes in the intraosseous blood flow consistent with improved femoral head blood flow following aspiration of the hip (Harper *et al.* 1990).

The balance of opinion seems to be that increased

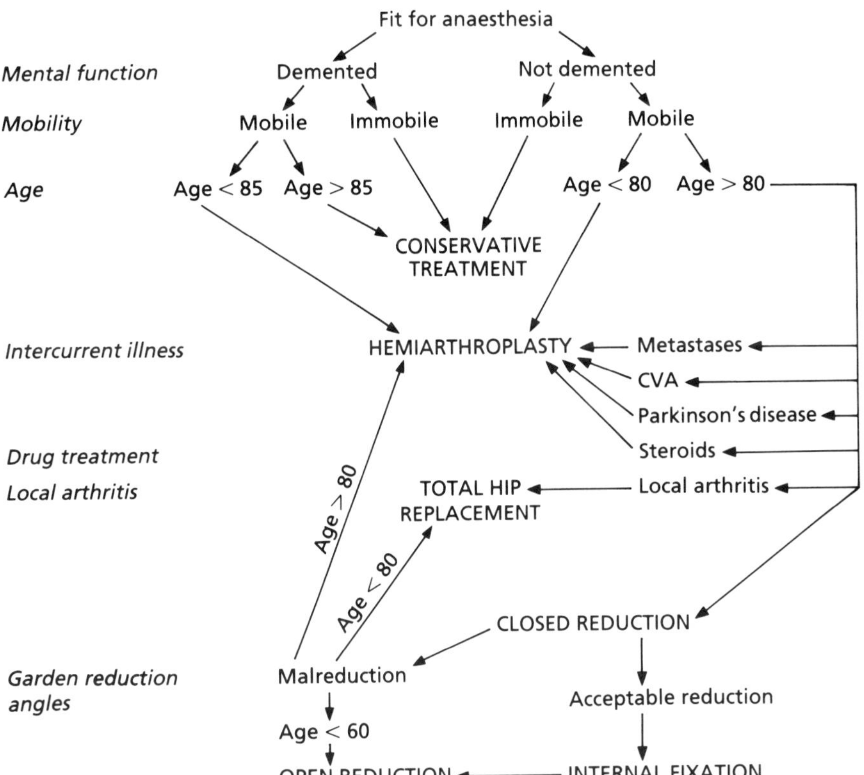

Fig. 20.13 Treatment algorithm for displaced subcapital femoral fractures. CVA = cerebrovascular accident.

intracapsular pressure can occur following fracture, and that this increased intracapsular pressure may have a deleterious effect on femoral head blood flow. The authors would therefore recommend that, until the results of randomized clinical trials are available, if fixation is contemplated, then consideration should be given to early aspiration of the hip joint.

Reduction

Closed reduction is usually performed on a fracture table with biplanar fluoroscopic control using an image intensifier. The proximal fracture fragment is comparable to a universal joint, except that the ligament of Weitbrecht confers some stability by acting as a soft tissue hinge (Smith 1953). Once reduction has been achieved, further stability may be achieved by internal rotation, increasing tension in the iliofemoral ligament, which is translated into compression across the fracture. This has been called the closed packed position (Flynn 1973) (Fig. 20.14).

Forced internal rotation, to stabilize the fracture, has been recommended (Massie 1964), but other authors have disagreed, arguing that gentle reduction minimizes further vascular damage and additional comminution of the fracture (Green 1960, Garden 1971). Reduction with both hips in extension, positioning the medial cortex of the distal femoral neck fragment beneath the corresponding medial cortex of the proximal fracture fragment, has been recommended (McElvenny 1945). Over-reduction of the fracture may be achieved by applying direct pressure to the greater trochanter as the

hip is internally rotated from an externally rotated position, with the hip held in extension (Deyerle 1959). The fracture may be disimpacted, with the hip in 90° of flexion and slight internal rotation. Subsequent extension and abduction of the fracture is performed to obtain a reduction (Leadbetter 1933). By disimpaction of the fracture and circumduction of the thigh, malrotation may occur and this is not readily detected radiographically.

Accurate evaluation of the reduction is imperative. A close correlation between the accuracy of reduction and the mechanical failure of internal fixation has been clearly demonstrated using Garden angles in over 1500 fractures (Barnes *et al.* 1976). The anteroposterior Garden angle is between the medial femoral shaft and the vertical trabecular buttress (Fig. 20.15). Failure rates were shown to increase significantly when Garden angles exceeded 180° or were less than 155° in the anteroposterior plane (Barnes *et al.* 1976). The lateral Garden angle is between a line along the centre of the femoral neck and a line from the centre of the femoral head to the mid-point of the distal fracture surface (Fig. 20.16). If the lateral Garden angle was more than 20° either side of 180°, the mechanical failure rate increased (Barnes *et al.* 1976).

The authors prefer to reduce the fracture on a fracture table with the hip in extension and slight external rotation. Gentle traction to correct shortening is applied under the control of image intensification. The leg is then internally rotated into the closed packed position. Biplanar fluoroscopy and formal plain radiographs are taken to ensure that the fracture is within the limits described above, and that the neck-shaft angle is as close to that of the contralateral hip as is possible before proceeding to internal fixation.

Internal fixation

The aim of internal fixation is to produce a load-sharing composite of bone and implant until fracture union occurs. The failure rate of internal fixation increases with age and approaches 50% 1 year postoperatively in patients over 84 years of age (Barnes *et al.* 1976). Bone density decreases with age and osteoporotic bone may be less able to share the load.

Following internal fixation, the incidence of postoperative complications is not increased by early weight-bearing (Abrami & Stevens 1964). About half the body weight is transferred across the hip joint when the patient is mobilized non-weight-bearing (Rydell 1966), and considerable stresses are transferred across the hip joint when moving in bed (Rydell 1973).

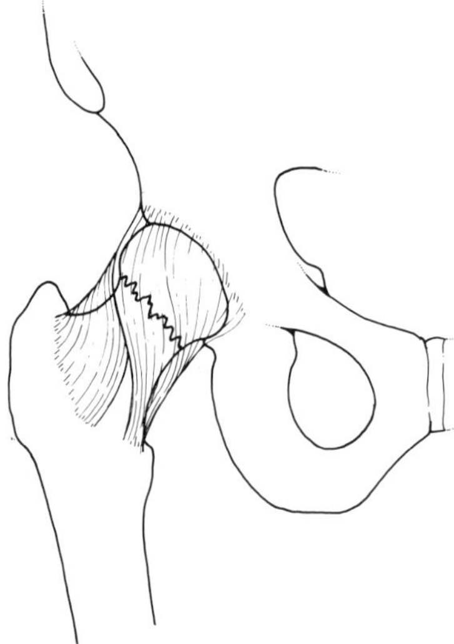

Fig. 20.14 Anterior view of the hip in the closed packed position with the iliofemoral ligament under tension. (After Flynn 1973.)

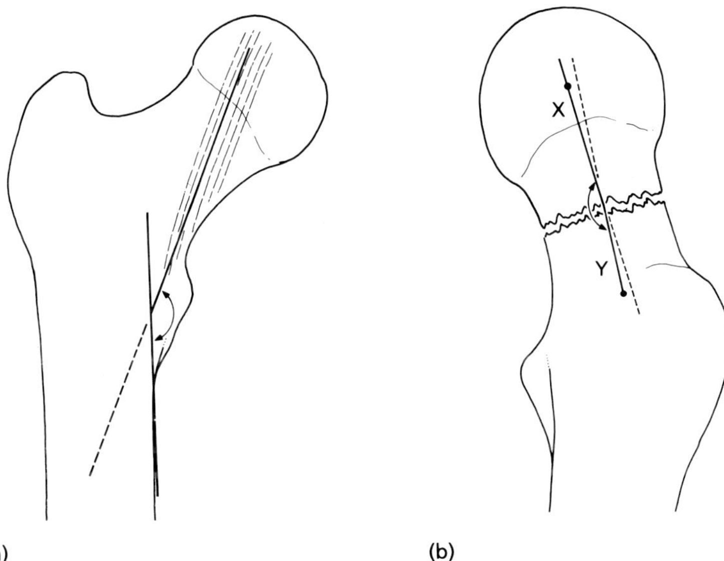

Fig. 20.15 Reduction angles of a subcapital femoral fracture before internal fixation with a dynamic compression screw. (a) Anteroposterior Garden angle between the medial femoral cortex and the vertical trabecular buttress. (b) Lateral Garden reduction angle between line (×) from the centre of the femoral head to the centre of the fracture and line (y) which lies along the central axis of the femoral neck.

MULTIPLE PINS OR SCREWS

With the advent of biologically compatible metals in the 1930s, relative success was achieved with multiple pin fixation (Moore 1934, Knowles 1936, Deyerle 1959). This success was enhanced with the introduction of accurate fluoroscopy. The methods mentioned are similar; the screws may be introduced either percutaneously, under local anaesthetic, or through a formal lateral incision, under general anaesthetic. The pins should be placed parallel, as convergence results in an increased incidence of non-union and, to prevent rotation, they should be placed peripherally in the femoral neck (Moore 1934). The pins should be placed in subchondral bone to give the best proximal fixation (Arnold *et al*. 1974).

Deyerle reported a 2% non-union rate and a 9% rate of avascular necrosis when up to 12 screws with a diameter of $\frac{1}{8}$ in. were used, and stabilized laterally by a side plate. He reduced the fracture into a slightly valgus position and placed the pins peripherally, tightening them to achieve compression at the fracture site (Deyerle 1959). Other authors have failed to reproduce such low complication rates using Deyerle pins (Chapman *et al*. 1975, Ryan *et al*. 1979).

Asnis has developed a cannulated cancellous screw system with a parallel barrel guide (Fig. 20.16h). The authors have used this method of internal fixation in 86 subcapital femoral fractures with a combined clinical and radiological failure rate of 17% at 1 year in displaced fractures (Wood 1990).

The results of various studies of multiple parallel screw internal fixation are summarized in Table 20.1.

FIXED-ANGLE NAIL PLATES

A four-flanged nail was originally introduced by Hey-Groves (1916). A similar triflanged nail was subsequently developed with the later addition of a side plate (Smith-Petersen *et al*. 1931). The Smith-Petersen side plate may be fixed at varying angles, unlike the Jewett nail (Fig. 20.16b & g) which is a one-piece flanged nail (Jewett 1941). The main disadvantages of this group of implants are penetration of the femoral head and disimpaction of the fracture during insertion. Failure rates with the fixed-angle nail plates are consistently 20% higher than with sliding nails (Barnes *et al*. 1976), which have now superceded this historically significant design. A summary of the results of fixed-angle nail plates is shown in Table 20.2.

SLIDING NAIL PLATES

These devices reduce the late incidence of femoral head penetration by accommodating collapse and impaction at the fracture site (Barr 1973). The barrel must not cross the fracture site and sufficient slide should be left in the system to allow for collapse.

A 135° angle nail was designed to rest on the calcar, with the tip placed low in the femoral head (Pugh 1955), thereby resisting downward displacement of the femoral

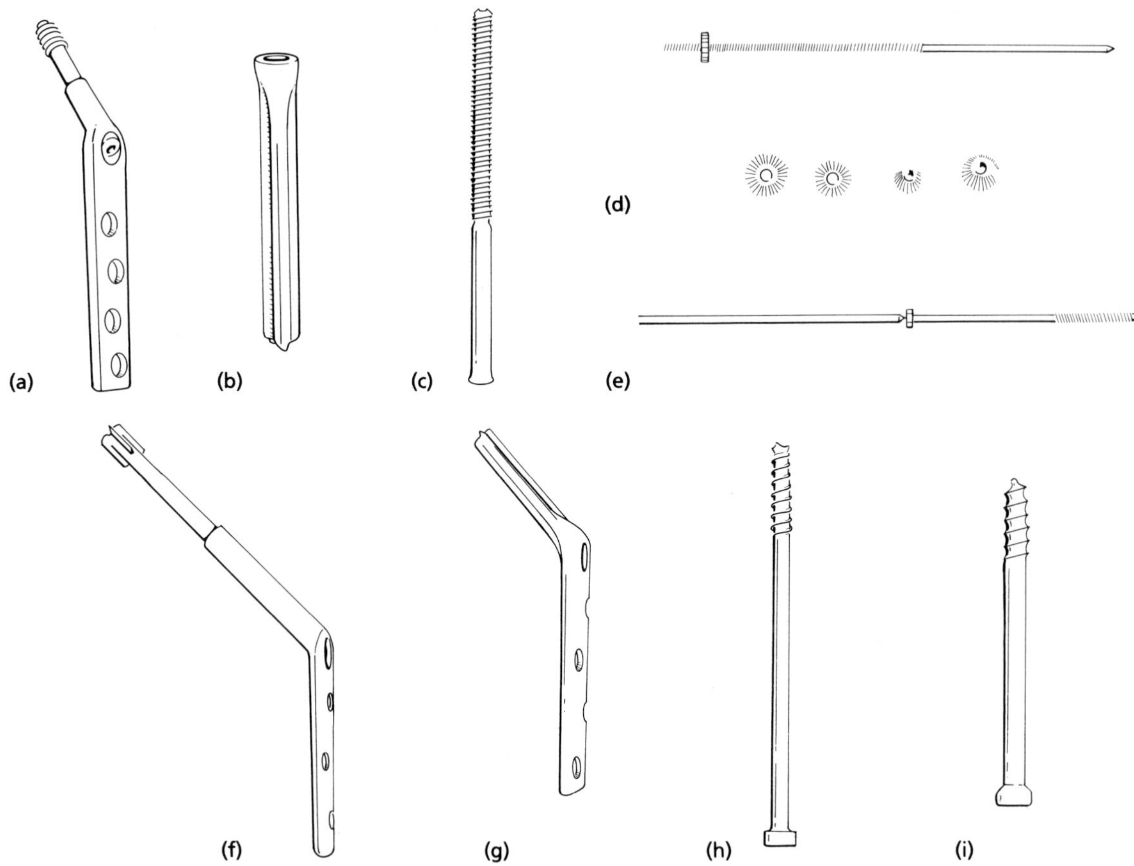

Fig. 20.16 A wide variety of implants used for internal fixation of subcapital femoral fractures. (a) Sliding compression screw. (b) Smith-Petersen Trifin nail. (c) Garden hip screw. (d) Moore adjustable pin. (e) Knowles pin. (f) Pugh sliding nail plate. (g) Jewett fixed-angle nail plate. (h) Asnis guided screw. (i) AO/ASIF cancellous screw.

Table 20.1 Results of internal fixation of displaced subcapital femoral fractures using multiple pins or screws

Reference	Implant	Number of patients	FU (months)	Patient age (years)	Non-union (%)	Avascular necrosis (%)
Arnold et al. (1974)	Knowles pins	505	6 (min.)	71	15	12
Bagby & Wallace (1971)	Knowles pins	35	12–54	All > 70	0	17
Deyerle (1965)	Deyerle pins & plate	29	12–60	70	0	1
Metz et al. (1970)	Deyerle pins & plate	63	24 (min.)	77	4.7	11.6
Jones (1966)	Moore pins	14	48 (mean)	67	4.3	7.1
Swiontkowski et al. (1984)	Cancellous bone graft	27	All > 48	32.4	0	20

Table 20.2 Results of internal fixation of displaced subcapital femoral fractures with fixed-angle nail plates

Reference	Implant	Number of patients	FU (months)	Patient age (years)	Non-union (%)	Avascular necrosis (%)
Boyd & George (1947)	Smith-Petersen nail	300	6–24	40–96	13.5	33.6
Boyd & Salvatore (1964)	Smith-Petersen nail	400	>12	68.7 males 72.9 females (all fractures)	11.2	36.8
Garcia et al. (1961)	Smith-Petersen nail	105				
Barnes et al. (1976)	Smith-Petersen nail	255	36	–	55.6	28.4
Hullinger (1966)	Smith-Petersen nail	43			26.6	
Hullinger (1967)	Smith-Petersen nail	64			11.0	
Svenningsen et al. (1984)	McLaughlin nail plate	68	36	All < 70	25	21

head by reducing the length of the lever arm between the femoral head and the lateral femoral cortex. A subsequent sliding nail with a 150° angle was designed so that the nail rested on the calcar and lay in the axis of weight-bearing (Massie 1964). However, the vertical trabecular buttress lies at an angle of about 165° to the shaft of the femur. A comparison of the two devices with different plate/nail angles demonstrated that there was no difference in the respective non-union and avascular necrosis rates (Brown & Court-Brown 1979). A summary of the results of studies using sliding nail plates is shown in Table 20.3.

SLIDING SCREW PLATE FIXATION

In 1955 a screw with a sliding barrel to accommodate impaction was introduced (Schumpelick & Jantzen 1955). Similar screws, but with blunt tips to reduce the risk of femoral head penetration, were produced by the Richards Company (Fig. 20.17). The flat surfaces of a screw provide a larger area per unit load, compared with a nail, when stressed, furnish firmer fixation and are less likely to cut through bone (Brodetti 1961).

An investigation of the sliding and jamming properties of four different designs of sliding screw concluded

Table 20.3 Results of internal fixation of displaced subcapital femoral fractures with sliding nail plates

Reference	Implant	Number of patients	FU (months)	Patient age (years)	Non-union (%)	Avascular necrosis (%)
Barnes et al. (1976)	Sliding nail plate	304	36	<65–>85	28	24
Brown & Court-Brown (1979)	Sliding nail plate	200	3	43–95	21	–
Massie (1964)	Sliding nail plate	57	12–72	<40–89	10.5	0.23
Jacobs et al. (1965)	Pugh nail	50	36	69	20	7

that high angle screw plates of 150° have better sliding characteristics than the lower 135° screw plates, and deep engagement of the screw in the barrel enhances sliding. Galling of adjacent metal surfaces, associated with jamming, was seen in stainless steel implants but not in chrome cobalt implants (Kyle *et al.* 1980).

A theoretical disadvantage of sliding compression screws is that they may rotate the femoral head during insertion, thereby altering the reduction and impairing the blood supply to the femoral head (Hayes & Groth 1967). To prevent this complication additional threaded screws have been inserted above the main screw (Calandruccio & Anderson 1980, Ort & Lamont 1984). The results of sliding screw fixation are summarized in Table 20.4.

CROSSED SCREWS

Crossed screws, used with an adjoining side plate, were introduced by Smyth *et al.* (1964). Garden (1964) pop-ularized the use of crossed screws without a side plate (Fig. 20.16c). These screws are cannulated and inserted over a guide wire and under fluoroscopic control. The screw threads cross the fracture line, holding the fracture out to length. There was no significant difference in the rates of non-union and avascular necrosis when the two devices were compared. Both designs of implant had a bony union rate which was consistently 20% higher than the fixed-angle nail plate (Barnes *et al.* 1976) (Table 20.5).

MUSCLE-PEDICLE BONE GRAFT

Local bone grafts have been elevated on muscle pedicles from the vastus lateralis (Stuck & Hinchey 1944), gluteus maximus (Hewson 1971) and the short external rotators of the hip (Judet *et al.* 1961, Judet 1962).

A vascularized bone graft, based on the quadratus femoris, has been used to improve the blood supply to the femoral head and across the fracture site in order to

Table 20.4 Results of internal fixation of displaced subcapital femoral fractures with sliding compression screws

Reference	Implant	Number of patients	FU (months)	Patient age (years)	Non-union (%)	Avascular necrosis (%)
Frandson *et al.* (1984)	Sliding screw plate	156	12	78 (original group)	26	22
Ort & Lamont (1984)	Sliding compression screw and two Knowles pins	21	6–42	61	0	24
Skinner & Powles (1986)	Compression screw	86	24	72.3	17.1	27.1
Svenningsen *et al.* (1984)	Compression screw	70	36	All < 70	11.4	21

Table 20.5 Results of internal fixation of displaced subcapital femoral fractures with crossed screws

Reference	Implant	Number of patients	FU (months)	Patient age (years)	Non-union (%)	Avascular necrosis (%)
Garden (1971)	Crossed Garden screws	406	Up to 180	–	25	21.3
Barnes *et al.* (1976)	Crossed screws	157	36	<65–>85	25	27.5
Sikorski & Barrington (1981)	Crossed Garden screws	74	24 (min.)	Over 70	2*	18

* 38.6% required revision for technical failure.

improve bony union and prevent late segmental collapse. A quadratus femoris muscle-pedicle bone graft procedure was carried out on 150 patients with fractures, which had been openly reduced and internally fixed with multiple pins (Meyers *et al.* 1973, Meyers *et al.* 1974, Meyers 1980). Only 11% of fractures failed to unite and 5% of patients suffered late segmental collapse of the femoral head. However, follow-up patient drop-out rate was high in patients attending the Los Angeles County Hospital and only a few patients were over 70 years of age and therefore the group was on the whole more likely to achieve bony union. The population was highly selected and therefore incomparable with other series. The current place of this technique remains uncertain in the authors' opinion.

Prosthetic replacement

HEMIARTHROPLASTY

The Austin Moore hemiarthroplasty (Fig. 20.17) was originally designed to replace a giant cell tumour of the proximal femur (Moore & Bohlman 1943). This prosthesis has a long fenestrated stem for insertion without cement, and the femoral neck is resected 12−19 mm proximal to the lesser trochanter (Anderson *et al.* 1964). The Thompson's hemiarthroplasty (Fig. 20.17) was introduced as a salvage prosthesis for non-union of intra-

capsular femoral fractures (Thompson 1952, Thompson 1954). Initial success led quickly to the use of these prostheses in the primary treatment of displaced intra-capsular fractures. The Thompson hemiarthroplasty is designed to be inserted into patients with femoral neck deficiency (Thompson 1954). In primary treatment, the femoral neck is resected so that the collar rests on the calcar at the superior surface of the lesser trochanter; this inevitably results in unnecessary shortening.

Hemiarthroplasty is contraindicated in younger patients because of progressive acetabular cartilage erosion and associated pain. After 3 years 30% of patients have disabling pain (Hunter 1980), and in some series up to 50% unsatisfactory results are reported (Coates 1975). However, the non-union rate in patients over 84 years of age, treated by internal fixation, approaches 50% (Barnes *et al.* 1976). Hemiarthroplasty is indicated in the chronologically and physiologically elderly patients who protect the prosthesis by their relative infirmity (Table 20.6).

Accurate sizing of the prosthesis is essential to ensure the maximum area of contact (Hinchey & Day 1964). If the prosthesis is too small, central stress concentration will lead to rapid articular cartilage erosion. Too large a prosthesis produces equatorial contact and a reduction in the range of movement.

The Thompson prosthesis has a collar and a banana-shaped stem which is much narrower than the medullary

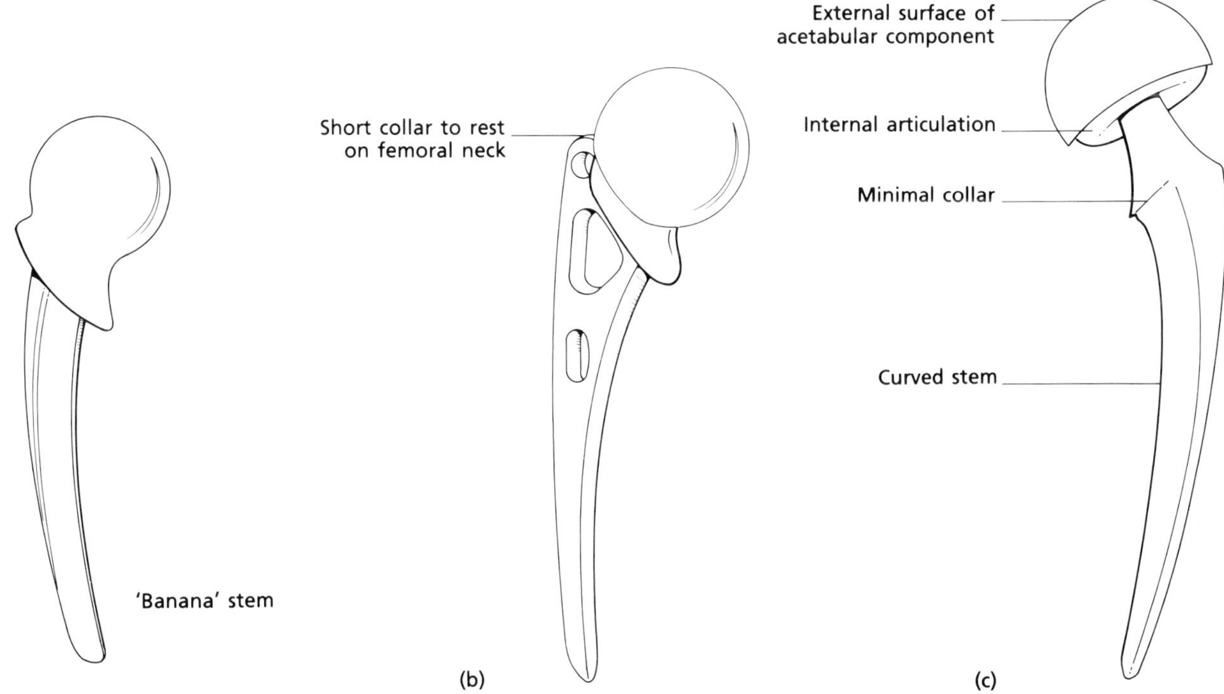

Fig. 20.17 (a) Thompson prosthesis. (b) Austin Moore prosthesis. (c) Hastings prosthesis.

cavity of the femur in the elderly. It was originally designed to be inserted without the use of acrylic cement, but femoral stem loosening may be reduced with application of cement (Wrighton & Woodyard 1971). The Thompson prosthesis should be placed in a neutral or slightly valgus position (Hinchey & Day 1964). Retroversion will predispose to dislocation in internal rotation and in external rotation to deformity of the foot. Anteversion will lead to an internally rotated foot and predisposes to dislocation in external rotation.

The posterolateral and posterior approaches are associated with an increased incidence of dislocation and sepsis (Chan & Hoskinson 1975). The anterolateral approach has been reported to have a lower dislocation rate than the posterior approach (D'Arcy & Devas 1976). However, some authors have been unable to demonstrate the superiority of either approach (Barr 1974).

Although the operation of hemiarthroplasty is a more extensive procedure than internal fixation (Boyd & Salvatore 1964), there is, contrary to popular thinking, no difference in the mortality rates for the two operative techniques in patients of similar age groups (Grimley Evans *et al.* 1979b).

BIPOLAR HEMIARTHROPLASTY

More recently, a variety of biarticular prostheses have been used in the treatment of displaced intracapsular fractures. These bipolar prostheses have an inner bearing to reduce the frictional forces at the prosthesis—articular cartilage interface (Bhuller 1982). In a comparative series between the Bateman bipolar prosthesis and a cemented Thompson prosthesis no difference could be demonstrated between the two groups of patients (Drinker & Murray 1979). These authors also found that the degree of motion at the inner bearing was unpredictable and decreased with time. Dislocations of bipolar prostheses are more troublesome, the two components may dissociate and, in one series, open reduction was required in five out of nine dislocations (Drinker & Murray 1979). More recent designs have been modified, with a more captive inner bearing, and this may have eliminated the problem of dissociation.

In a retrospective comparison between Austin Moore hemiarthroplasty and the Christiansen bipolar prosthesis, Harris scores for pain and range of movement were significantly better with the Christiansen prosthesis (Meyers 1980, Meyer 1981). Furthermore, 18.5% of the Austin Moore prostheses had to be revised, compared with 5% of the 40 patients treated with the Christiansen prosthesis.

A more recent report of a 5% acetabular erosion rate with the Monk hard-top prosthesis (Leyshon & Matthews 1984) casts some doubt on the theoretical advantages of the bipolar principle and, clearly, more carefully executed trials are required in this area.

TOTAL HIP REPLACEMENT

The consistently low percentage of satisfactory results obtained in patients treated by hemiarthroplasty has led to the use of total hip replacement in the primary treatment of displaced subcapital femoral fractures. An early report of excellent results in patients with Paget's disease, three of whom had pathological fractures (Stauffer & Sim 1976), preceded a more extensive series. Of 85 patients, 81% were pain free following total hip replacement. The dislocation rate was 13%, which was higher than the dislocation rate for elective total hip replacement in degenerative joint disease (Sim & Stauffer 1980). Dislocation rates of 8% (Coates & Armour 1979) and 14% (Cartlidge 1981) were also reported. The results of total hip replacement in intracapsular fractures differ from those in degenerative disease, probably because of the high proportion of patients with neuromuscular deficiency in the hip fracture group predisposing to dislocation. Furthermore, fracture patients were usually pain free before their injury and therefore had different expectations to patients who had been restricted by chronic pain for years.

Treatment of patients with special considerations

Young adults

Subcapital femoral fractures in young adults are rare (Protzman & Burkhalter 1976), have a male preponderance (Alframm 1964), are associated with high-velocity trauma and multiple injuries, and are more susceptible to non-union and avascular necrosis (Massie 1964, Protzman & Burkhalter 1976). In a series of 22 young adults, between the ages of 20 and 40 years with a mean age of 27, 33% of patients had non-union of their fracture and 86% had late segmental collapse (Protzman & Burkhalter 1976). A non-union rate of 25% and avascular necrosis rate of 45% was reported in young adults (Kuslich & Gustilo 1976). Anatomical reduction and internal fixation have naturally been advocated in this age group (Cave 1960) but, if closed reduction fails, there should be no hesitation in proceeding to open reduction. The primary use of a posterior muscle-pedicle

Table 20.6 Results of treatment of displaced subcapital femoral fractures by hemiarthroplasty

Reference	Prosthesis	Number of patients	FU (months)	Patient age (years)	Complications			
					Dislocation (%)	Femoral loosening (%)	Infection (%)	Erosion (%)
Hunter (1980)	Thompson & Austin Moore	100	18–36	79	7	—	8–44%	—
D'Arcy & Devas (1976)	Thompson	161	36	81	2	6	1.8	11
Gingras *et al.* (1980)	Thompson	27	17	73	—	18	0	8
Jensen & Holstein (1975)	Austin Moore	60	57	77	1	22	5	17
Lindholm *et al.* (1976)	Austin Moore	80	40	72	2	3	3	4
Whitaker *et al.* (1972)	Austin Moore	45	60	73	4.4	32	7	24
Hinchey & Day (1964)	Austin Moore	285	24	<60–>90	1	—	12	—
Montgomery & Lawson (1977)	Thompson (uncemented)	250	48	77.7 (mean)	1.4	—	24	—
Mandell (1972)	Austin Moore	35	42	74	0.3	—	12	9

bone graft in 23 patients under 40 years of age, with a 2% non-union rate and no cases of avascular necrosis, has been reported (Meyers 1980).

Stress fractures

Stress fractures occur in military recruits who are unaccustomed to strenuous physical exercise. If undisplaced, these fractures heal with conservative treatment (Kaltsas 1981).

Stress fractures also occur in elderly patients, and are frequently missed in the presence of a normal radiograph. Callus may be present on the radiograph 2 weeks after the onset of pain (Blickenstaff & Morris 1966) and bone scintigraphy may be positive before radiographs show a fracture (Prather *et al.* 1977). Treatment is by internal fixation.

Paget's disease

Non-union was reported in all the 11 fractures through Pagetic bone in one series (Grundy 1970). Five patients were treated conservatively and three were treated by subtrochanteric osteotomy without internal fixation. Of the three fractures that were internally fixed, two were with a Smith-Petersen nail, which is now considered obsolete, and one fracture was fixed with a Venable screw that fractured after 2 weeks. It is difficult to draw conclusions about the treatment of fractures through Pagetic bone from this series, because the treatment of nine of the fractures would be expected to result in non-union in non-pathological fractures.

Prosthetic replacement has been reported in a small number of cases. Three hemiarthroplasties — one Judet and two Austin Moore procedures — failed (Nicholas & Killoran 1965) in contrast to a report of three successful total hip joint replacements (Stauffer & Sim 1976).

A report of one procedure being abandoned because of haemorrhage (Grundy 1970) indicates that if Paget's disease is in an active vascular phase with a markedly raised alkaline phosphatase level, consideration should be given to treatment either with diphosphonates or with calcitonin given preoperatively to reduce perioperative bleeding.

Pathological fractures through neoplastic tissue

The majority of patients in this category suffer fractures

through the metastases and have a reduced life expectancy. Hemiarthroplasty has, therefore, been used to achieve rapid mobilization and pain relief (Parrish & Murray 1970). If insufficient bone remains, either at the calcar or at the lateral femoral cortex, then the prosthesis may become displaced. Long-stemmed cemented prostheses have been used to prevent this (Parrish & Murray 1970). Total hip replacement is the procedure of choice in patients with subcapital femoral fractures who also have metastatic disease of the acetabulum (Lane *et al.* 1980).

Opinion is divided as to whether prophylactic internal fixation with radiotherapy (Cameron *et al.* 1974) or prosthetic replacement (Lane *et al.* 1980) should be undertaken in impending pathological fractures of the femoral neck where more than 50% of the width of the femoral neck is occupied by a lytic lesion.

Parkinson's disease

Parkinson's disease is associated with osteoporosis, tremor, rigidity, impaired balance, soft tissue contractures and an increased mortality following femoral neck fractures (Rothermel & Garcia 1972). Endoprosthetic replacement is said to produce a higher mortality than internal fixation (Coughlin & Templeton 1980). In this series there were only three patients treated by internal fixation. The 12 patients treated by endoprosthetic replacement had a 6 month mortality of 75%. The authors' recommendation would be to treat displaced fractures by prosthetic replacement using a Thompson hemiarthroplasty, inserted by the lateral approach.

Complications

Mortality

Clearly, the most significant complication of intracapsular fractures is death. There are some patients in whom the fracture is simply part of an expression of multisystem failure. Recent reports indicate that dementia is the most reliable indicator of physiological ageing, and a simple measurement of cognitive function is essential in planning treatment (Grimley Evans *et al.* 1979b, Ions & Stevens 1987).

Standardized mortality rates 6 months after operation vary widely from 12 to 41% (Table 20.7). Consideration of the factors which influence mortality is essential in order to define this heterogenous population and so that valid comparisons may be made. Age (Alframm 1964) and dementia (Grimley Evans *et al.* 1979b) are associated with an increase in mortality in hip fracture patients. The relative importance of these factors has been recently defined in a multivariate analysis of preoperative predictors of survival (Ions & Stevens 1987). Demented patients over 75 years have a 6-month mortality rate of 50%. Their peers, with normal mental function, have a 6-month mortality rate of 11%; this is less than for demented patients under 75 years of age, who have a 6-month mortality rate of 17%. In the multivariate analysis, mental function was the most significant predictor of survival (Ions & Stevens 1987). Mortality rates at 6 months after operation are higher in patients who sustain an injury in their own home or in an institution than in patients who are injured in a public place (Grimley Evans *et al.* 1979b).

The grade of subcapital fracture (Alframm 1964) and type of proximal femoral fracture (Riska 1970−71) show no correlation to mortality.

There is a high incidence of chronic degenerative disease in the elderly hip fracture population. In particular, 70% of men and 58% of women have been shown to have arteriosclerosis (Niemann & Mankin 1968). Cerebrovascular disease and cancer carry a significant risk of death within 6 months of injury. Patients with more than four medical conditions, detected preoperatively, are at a greater risk of death (Kenzora *et al.* 1984).

Conservative management of subcapital femoral fractures has been associated with an increase in mortality (Riska 1970−71, Ions & Stevens 1987). In both reports, patients who were unfit for anaesthesia were treated conservatively; this preselection explains the increase.

A preoperative interval of up to 7 days is not associated with an increase in mortality, but patients operated on after this time had an increased risk of dying. This latter group included patients whose operation had been delayed for medical reasons and this accounts for the increased mortality rate (Grimley Evans *et al.* 1979b). In one series, 34% of patients operated on within 24 hours of admission were dead 1 year after injury; this mortality was significantly greater than for patients operated on during the following 4 days (Kenzora *et al.* 1984). This is an indication that patients should be adequately resuscitated, and that coexisting medical conditions should be treated, before surgery.

Although some reports show a higher death rate in patients treated by endoprosthetic replacement (Raine 1973), valid comparisons may only be made if populations are standardized for age and mental function. Epidemiological series have failed to demonstrate

Table 20.7 Mortality in subcapital femoral fracture patients

Reference	Number of patients	Patient age (years)	Treatment	Mortality	Time from operation (months)
Nystrom (1935)	29	67	Excludes surgically treated patients	6.9	3
King (1939)	50	<60−98	Excludes conservatively treated patients	14	>12
Boyd & George (1947)	300	40−96	Smith-Petersen nails (285) Knowles pins (15)	9.3	6
Cleveland & Fielding (1954)	100	72.1	Internal fixation and hemiarthroplasty	12	2
Addison (1959)	53	79	Austin Moore hemiarthroplasty	30	1.5
Garcia et al. (1961)	105		Smith-Petersen nails	18	6
Hinchey & Day (1964)	288	<60−>90	Austin Moore hemiarthroplasty	14	6
Frangakis (1966)	179	40−>80	Internal fixation	21	12
Burwell (1967)	131	73.8	Acrylic hemiarthroplasty	27	6
Davie (1968)	39	80.5	Austin Moore hemiarthroplasty	31	3
Hunter (1969)	94	79	Hemiarthroplasty	41	6
Riska (1970−71)	122	<45−94	Internal fixation (endoprosthesis and conservative groups included)	20	5
Wrighton & Woodyard (1971)	154	<70−>80	Austin Moore & Thompson hemiarthroplasty	39	6
Lucht (1971)	98	<70−>90	Thompson & Austin Moore hemiarthroplasty	31	6
Polyzoides (1971)	110	73 (59−93)	Austin Moore hemiarthroplasty	23	4
Raine (1973)	42 / 52	77	Internal fixation / Prosthesis	12 / 33	6 / 6
Kavlie & Sundal (1974)	269	60−>90	Christiansen prosthesis	23	6
Hunter (1980)	100	79	Mixture of uncemented Austin Moore, uncemented Thompson & cemented Thompson	20	6
Chan & Hoskinson (1975)	107 / 136	76.9 / 77.4	Overall / Anterior Thompson / Posterior Thompson	14.4 / 6.5 / 20.6	1.5

Continued on p. 656

Table 20.7 (*Continued*)

Reference	Number of patients	Patient age (years)	Treatment	Mortality	Time from operation (months)
Kavlie et al. (1975)	300	<60->90	Christiansen prosthesis	21	6
D'Arcy & Devas (1976)	361	81	Thompson hemiarthroplasty	23	6
Barnes et al. (1976)	1503	<65->85	Internal fixation	7.6 (females) 14.2 (males)	1
Tillberg (1976)	163	78 (66-95)	Arthroplasty	9	1.5
Sikorski & Barrington (1981)	57 57 74	Over 70	Anterior Thompson Posterior Thompson Internal fixation	20 38 35	6
Kreutzfeldt et al. (1984)	117	—	All groups	26	12

any difference in mortality between groups of patients undergoing different surgical procedures (Alframm 1964, Grimley Evans et al. 1979b).

A comparison of fatality rates between two main teaching hospitals in one city showed a significantly higher mortality in the hospital with lower non-medical staffing ratios serving the socio-economically deprived area of the city (Grimley Evans et al. 1980). This finding substantiated the 'inverse care law' (Hart 1971), which states that patients in socio-economically deprived areas have poorer healthcare facilities and suffer as a consequence.

Non-union

The tenuous blood supply to the femoral head may be completely obliterated by fracture. Furthermore, the absence of a cambium layer of periosteum on the intracapsular femoral neck further reduces the vascularity at the fracture site and results in a non-union rate of 26% of displaced fractures treated by closed reduction and internal fixation (Barnes et al. 1976). An increased incidence of non-union of intracapsular fractures is associated with avascular necrosis of the femoral head as a result of vascular insufficiency (Phemister 1939, Boyd 1957).

The incidence of non-union increases with increasing age and is greater in displaced fractures (Barnes et al. 1976). Most patients with non-union are elderly and many have associated avascular necrosis of the femoral head. Under these circumstances prosthetic replacement of the femoral head is necessary, and if the acetabular surface has been damaged a total hip replacement is appropriate (Salvati et al. 1974). If the patient is young and the femoral head is considered viable, treatment by bone grafting, valgus osteotomy, or a combination of these, may be considered. Either cortical (Bonfiglio 1969) or cancellous (Deyerle 1959) bone grafting may be used. If the fracture has displaced into a varus position, a valgus corrective osteotomy may be used.

Avascular necrosis and late segmental collapse

The tenuous blood supply to the femoral head renders it susceptible to avascular necrosis following fracture of the femoral neck. Collapse of the weight-bearing segment of the femoral head occurs months, or years, after surgery, probably because the bone is temporarily weakened during the repair process of trabecular bone by creeping substitution. Late segmental collapse is found in about 30% of displaced fractures treated by internal fixation, and one-third of these patients are symptomatic 3 years after surgery (Barnes et al. 1976).

Histologically, in about 80% of all patients with subcapital femoral fracture, at least partial avascular necrosis of the femoral head occurs. In femoral heads removed after fracture, this is distinguishable from physiological osteonecrosis at 2 days after injury by the agglomeration of blood-forming cells in the marrow, and by the loss of lipocyte nuclei and necrosis of small vessels from 4 days after injury (Catto 1965a).

Histology of femoral heads, removed between 16 days and 10 months after fracture, invariably show callus at the fracture site. When there is a large viable medial wedge of bone based on the arteries of the ligamentum teres, revascularization is more rapid and is sometimes complete as early as 4–8 weeks (Sevitt 1964). In patients treated conservatively, before the advent of the Smith-Petersen nail, non-union was four times more common with a necrotic capital fragment than with a live one (Phemister 1949). When necrosis of the femoral head is complete, and contributions from the medial epiphyseal artery are negligible, union may occur but late segmental collapse follows. The subchondral region of the femoral head is the last to be revascularized and is the most susceptible to late segmental collapse.

The radiographic appearance of areas of increased density surrounded by relatively lucent osteoporotic bone is suggestive of avascular necrosis (Bohr & Larsen 1965) and such areas may appear months after the original injury. As repair bone is laid down on necrotic trabeculae, by the process of creeping substitution, the increase in mineralized bone is evident as an absolute increase in the radiodensity of the femoral head.

A number of different techniques, used preoperatively, to predict non-union and late segmental collapse have been tried and found wanting. More recently, interest has been directed towards the use of radio-pharmaceutical imaging. Planar and collimator scintigraphy suffer from the disadvantage of photon emission from the posterior rim of the acetabulum. In a recent investigation of 20 patients with avascular necrosis of the femoral head, diagnosed clinically and with normal radiographs, single photon emission CT correctly identified 17 of the 20 affected hips (sensitivity 0.85) by the presence of focal photon-deficient areas (Collier *et al.* 1985). In the same series investigated by planar imaging, only 11 out of 20 avascular hips were detected. It would seem prudent to investigate patients with displaced intracapsular fractures preoperatively by simple photon emission CT. This technique avoids image interference from the posterior acetabulum and may provide vital information about the vascularity of the femoral head, particularly in the region supplied by the medial epiphyseal vessels. Clearly, MRI can demonstrate avascularity in the femoral head, but no reports of preoperative studies in subcapital femoral fracture patients have emerged.

Only 30% of patients suffering late segmental collapse have symptoms severe enough to warrant revision surgery (Barnes *et al.* 1976). However, most, if not all, hips with late segmental collapse will undergo arthritic change if they bear weight for long enough (Boyd & George 1947). The operative options for painful late segmental collapse are the same as those for secondary osteoarthritis of the hip, and include osteotomy with bone grafting in younger patients and prosthetic replacement in the elderly. Satisfactory results have been reported in 78% of patients treated by bone grafting. The results are better in those patients with avascular necrosis but without late segmental collapse (Bonfiglio 1969). When late segmental collapse is established in younger patients, osteotomy is indicated to preserve the femoral head (Calandruccio & Anderson 1980). In elderly patients the femoral head may be replaced either by hemiarthroplasty or by total hip replacement if acetabular cartilage is compromised (Salvati *et al.* 1974).

Infection

The incidence of wound infection is reduced by prophylactic perioperative antibiotics (Boyd *et al.* 1973) and their use is now widespread. In a randomized double-blind trial of cephalothin prophylaxis in 307 hip fracture patients, the cephalothin group had a significantly lower deep wound infection rate (0.7%) than did the controls (4.7%) (Burnett *et al.* 1980). Deep wound infection is more likely to require major reconstructive surgery in intracapsular fractures than in extracapsular fractures because the hip joint is directly affected in the former (Barr 1974).

Venous thromboembolism

In a report of routine ascending venography of sub-capital femoral fracture patients, deep venous thromboses (DVT) were identified in 40%, and it was estimated that one-third of these occurred before surgical intervention (Stevens *et al.* 1968). Fatal pulmonary emboli are said to occur in 4–7% of patients undergoing emergency hip surgery, compared with an incidence of up to 2% in those undergoing elective hip surgery (Hull & Raskob 1986).

DVT may occur in the calf and propagate into the femoral veins (Kakkar *et al.* 1969) or may arise *de novo* in the femoral veins (Mavor & Galloway 1969). Some thrombi lyse spontaneously during the first 72 hours (Kakkar *et al.* 1969); those that do not may obliterate the venous channel and irreversibly damage the valves. Recanalization of veins may occur, but incompetence leads to post phlebitic syndrome with varicose veins, ulceration and chronic oedema (Mudge & Hughes 1978).

The incidence of DVT and pulmonary embolism both increase with age (Nillius & Nylander 1979), obesity (Kakkar *et al.* 1970), immobility (Sevitt 1962), malignancy (Bauer 1946), varicose veins and a previous history of deep venous thrombosis (Kakkar *et al.* 1970). Clinical diagnosis is notoriously unreliable, giving false positive results of up to 49% (Milne *et al.* 1971) and false negative results of up to 73% in some series (Evans & Cockett 1969, Cranley *et al.* 1976).

Ascending phlebography is usually employed after clinical suspicion and is the yardstick by which other techniques are measured. False positive results may occur with inadequate mixing of blood and dye (Browse 1978) and may cause thrombosis of veins and skin necrosis locally (Berge *et al.* 1978). Venography cannot be used repeatedly in the same patient; this is a distinct disadvantage in hip surgery where 25% of thrombi occur after 1 week (Sikorski *et al.* 1985). The alternative method using ^{125}I-labelled fibrinogen is less invasive but cannot be used to detect thrombi proximal to the inguinal ligament (Sikorski *et al.* 1985). False positive results may occur at rates between 8 and 35% (Harris *et al.* 1976, Loudon 1976).

Pleuritic chest pain or the onset of dyspnoea should raise the suspicion of pulmonary embolism. Changes on chest radiographs and electrocardiographs are often inconclusive. The most accurate method of diagnosis is a ventilation perfusion scan. A positive diagnosis is made when an area of lung is ventilated but not perfused. However, to exclude preoperative defects, a baseline scan should be taken (Williams *et al.* 1974).

The main issue facing orthopaedic surgeons is whether to institute prophylaxis. Intermittent pneumatic calf compression is not a practical preoperative proposition in hip fracture patients. The anti-platelet action of aspirin has led to several studies. One randomized double-blind trial has shown aspirin to be effective in reducing the incidence of DVT in men (Harris *et al.* 1982); other studies have failed to show any beneficial effect (Saltzman 1983, Harris *et al.* 1985). Intravenous dextran is effective in reducing the incidence of postoperative venous thrombosis in both elective and emergency hip surgery (Evarts & Feil 1971, Harris *et al.* 1974). However, cardiac failure from volume overload is the main problem, and bleeding and rare allergic reactions, particularly with dextran 70, are also recognized complications. A randomized trial comparing a fixed low dose of heparin with heparin adjusted to maintain a normal partial thromboplastin time, showed the latter to be a more effective method of preventing DVT (Leyvraz *et al.* 1983).

On balance, the use of prophylaxis in the elderly patient undergoing emergency hip surgery offers effective protection against venous thromboembolism.

Epidemiology

Subcapital femoral fractures pose a significant public health problem in Great Britain. Of the 46 000 people in England and Wales who sustain a proximal femoral fracture each year about 25% die and less than one-third of the survivors consider themselves to be fully mobile (Grimley Evans 1979). The cost of acute hospital care alone has quadrupled over the last decade to about £160 million and these patients occupy 20% of all orthopaedic beds in the National Health Service.

The annual incidence of proximal femoral fractures in the elderly, arbitrarily described as those over 65 years of age, is about 5 cases per 1000 people (Rees 1982) and increases exponentially with age (Grimley Evans *et al.* 1979a). The authors' findings suggest that this pattern of increase is maintained in a fixed population for males and females, and for trochanteric and subcapital fractures. In contrast, reports from Scandinavia indicate an increase in the proportion of trochanteric fractures from 40% of all proximal femoral fractures in the 65–74 age group to about 70% in the over 85 age group (Falch *et al.* 1985). These trends may be related to cultural, climatic or other population differences (Alframm 1964).

Age-specific incidence rates are about twice as high in females as in males in Great Britain in the over 65 age group (Grimley Evans *et al.* 1979a). In those under 50 the trend is reversed with a 2:1 male to female ratio, but proximal femoral fractures in young adults are rare and are usually associated with more severe trauma (Alframm 1964, Baker 1980).

There are racial differences in proximal femoral fracture incidence. People of European origin are more susceptible to such fractures than are Israeli-born Jews, or Negroes (Solomon 1968, Levine *et al.* 1970). A striking racial difference was reported in South Africa where the incidence of proximal femoral fractures in the Bantu tribe was one-tenth of the incidence reported in western European populations, in spite of an appreciably lower calcium intake in the former group (Solomon 1968).

Several authors have noted that more fractures occur in the winter months (Grimley Evans *et al.* 1979a, Baker 1980); this may be linked to a reduction in plasma 25-hydroxyvitamin D (Beadle *et al.* 1980).

Increasing age, being of the female sex, dementia (Grimley Evans *et al.* 1979a), osteoporosis (Cooper *et al.* 1987), a tendency to fall (Grimley Evans *et al.* 1979a), low body mass, cigarette smoking, alcohol intake (Kelsey & Hoffmann 1987), physical inactivity and muscle weakness (Cooper *et al.* 1988) are all positive risk factors for proximal femoral fracture. It is clearly important to identify such aetiological factors if national campaigns are to be effective in preventing these common fractures which are associated with high mortality and morbidity (Grimley Evans *et al.* 1979a).

References

Abrami, G. & Stevens, J. Early weightbearing after internal fixation of transcervical fracture of the femur. *J Bone Joint Surg* 1964; **46B**: 204–205.

Addison, J. Prosthetic replacement in primary treatment of fractures of the femoral neck. *J R Soc Med* 1959; **52**: 908–910.

Alframm, P.A. An epidemiological study of cervical and trochanteric fractures of the femur in an urban population. *Acta Orthop Scand* 1964; **65** (Suppl.): 1–109.

Anderson, G.H., Harper, W.M. & Gregg, P.J. Management of intracapsular fractures of the proximal femur in 1990: a cause for concern? *J Bone Joint Surg* 1991; **73B** (Suppl.): 70.

Anderson, L.D., Hamsa, W.R. & Waring, T.L. Femoral head prostheses. *J Bone Joint Surg* 1964; **46A**: 1049–1065.

Arnold, W.D., Lyden, J.P. & Minkoff, J. Treatment of intracapsular fractures of the femoral neck. *J Bone Joint Surg* 1974; **56A**: 254–262.

Aro, H. & Dahlstrom, S. Conservative management of distraction-type stress fractures of femoral neck. *J Bone Joint Surg* 1986; **68B**: 65–67.

Bagby, G.W. & Wallace, G.T. Femoral neck fractures in the elderly treated by multiple pins (Knowles). *North West Med* 1971; **70**: 696–698.

Baker, M.R. *The Epidemiology and Aetiology of Femoral Neck Fracture*. MD thesis: University of Newcastle-Upon-Tyne, 1980.

Barnes, R., Brown, J.T., Garden, R.S. & Nicoll, E.A. Subcapital fractures of the femur. *J Bone Joint Surg* 1976; **58B**: 2–24.

Barr, J.S. Experiences with a sliding nail in femoral fractures. *Clin Orthop* 1973; **92**: 63–68.

Barr, J.S. Diagnosis and treatment of infections following internal fixation of hip fractures. *Orthop Clin North Am* 1974; **5(4)**: 847–864.

Bauer, G. Thrombosi; early diagnosis and abortive treatment with heparin. *Lancet* 1946; **i**: 447–454.

Beadle, P.C., Burton, J.L. & Leach, J.F. Correlation of seasonal variation of 25-hydroxycholecalciferol with UV indication dose. *Br J Dermatol* 1980; **103(3)**: 289–293.

Bentley, G. Impacted fractures of the neck of the femur. *J Bone Joint Surg* 1968; **50B**: 551–561.

Berge, T., Bergquist, D., Elsing H.O. & Hallböök, T. Local complications of ascending phlebography. *Clin Radiol* 1978; **29**: 691–696.

Bhuller, G.S. Use of the Giliberty bipolar endoprosthesis in femoral neck fractures. *Clin Orthop* 1982; **162**: 165–169.

Bigelow, H.J. *The Mechanism of Dislocation and Fracture of the Hip*. Little, Brown & Co: Boston, 1900.

Blessed, G., Tomlinson, B.E. & Roth, M. The association between quantitative measurements of dementia and of senile change in the cerebral grey matter of elderly subjects. *Br J Psychiatr* 1969; **114**: 368–374.

Blickenstaff, L.D. & Morris, J.M. Fatigue fractures of the femoral neck. *J Bone Joint Surg* 1966; **48A**: 1031–1047.

Bohr, H. & Larsen, E.H. On necrosis of the femoral head after fracture of the neck of the femur. A microradiographic and histological study. *J Bone Joint Surg* 1965; **47B**: 330–338.

Bonfiglio, M. Fracture of the femoral neck : early recognition and treatment of complications. *J Iowa Med Soc* 1969; **59**: 303–312.

Boyce, W.J. & Vessey, M.P. Rising incidence of fracture of the proximal femur. *Lancet* 1985; **1**: 150–151.

Boyd, H.B. Avascular necrosis of the head of the femur. *AAOS Instructional Course Lectures* 1957; **14**: 196–204.

Boyd, H.B. & George, L.L. Complications of fractures of the neck of the femur. *J Bone Joint Surg* 1947; **46A**: 1066–1068.

Boyd, H.B. & Salvatore, J.E. Acute fractures of the femoral neck: internal fixation or prosthesis. *J Bone Joint Surg* 1964; **46A**: 1066–1068.

Boyd, R.J., Burke, J.F. & Colton, T. A double blind clinical trial of prophylactic antibiotics in hip fractures. *J Bone Joint Surg* 1973; **55A**: 1251–1258.

Brodetti, A. An experimental study on the use of nails and bolt screws in the fixation of fractures of the femoral neck. *Acta Orthop Scand* 1961; **31**: 247–271.

Brown, T.I.S. & Court-Brown, C. Failure of sliding nail-plate fixation in subcapital fractures of the femoral neck. *J Bone Joint Surg* 1979; **61B**: 342–346.

Browse, N.L. Diagnosis of deep vein thrombosis. *Br Med Bull* 1978; **34**: 163–167.

Burnett, J.W., Gustilo, R.B., Williams, D.N. & Kind, A.C. Prophylactic antibiotics in hip fractures. *J Bone Joint Surg* 1980; **62A**: 457–461.

Burwell, H.N. Replacement of the femoral by a prosthesis in subcapital fractures. *Br J Surg* 1967; **54**: 741–749.

Calandruccio, R.A. & Anderson, W.E. Post-fracture avascular necrosis of the femoral head. Correlation of experimental and clinical studies. *Clin Orthop* 1980; **152**: 49–84.

Cameron, H.J., Fornasier, V.L. & McNab, I. Pathological fractures of the femoral neck. *Can Med Assoc J* 1974; **111**: 791–792.

Cartlidge, I.J. Primary total hip replacement for displaced subcapital femoral fractures. *Injury* 1981; **11**: 249–253.

Cassebaum, W.H. & Nugent, G. The predictability of bony union in displaced intracapsular fractures of the hip. *J Trauma* 1963; **3**: 421–424.

Cathcart, R.F. The shape of the normal femoral head and results from clinical use of more normally shaped non-spherical replacement prostheses. *J Bone Joint Surg* 1972; **54A**: 1559.

Catto, M. A histological study of avascular necrosis of the femoral head after transcervical fracture. *J Bone Joint Surg* 1965a; **47B**: 749–776.

Catto, M. The histological appearances of late segmental collapse of the femoral head after transcervical fracture. *J Bone Joint Surg* 1965b; **47B**: 777–791.

Cave, E.F. Fractures of the femoral neck. *AAOS Instructional Course Lectures* 1960; **17**: 79–93.

Chan, R.N.W. & Hoskinson, J. Thompson prosthesis for fractured neck of femur: a comparison of surgical approaches. *J Bone Joint Surg* 1975; **57B**: 439–443.

Chapman, M.W., Stehr, J.H., Eberle, C.F., Bloom, M.H. & Bovill, E.G. Treatment of intracapsular fractures by the

Deyerle method. *J Bone Joint Surg* 1975; **57A**: 735−744.

Clawson, D.K. Intracapsular fractures of the femur treated by the sliding screw plate fixation method. *J Trauma* 1964; **4**: 753−756.

Cleveland, M. & Fielding, J.W. A continuing end result study of intracapsular fractures of the neck of the femur. *J Bone Joint Surg* 1954; **36A**: 1020−1030.

Coates, R.L. A retrospective survey of eighty one patients with hemiarthroplasty for subcapital fracture of the femoral neck. *J Bone Joint Surg* 1975; **57B**: 256.

Coates, R.L. & Armour, P. Treatment of subcapital femoral fractures by total hip replacement. *Injury* 1979; **11**: 132−135.

Collier, B.D., Carrera, G.F. & Johnson, R.P. Detection of femoral head avascular necrosis by SPECT. *J Nuc Med* 1985; **26(9)**: 979−987.

Cooper, A.P. *A Treatise on Dislocations and on Fractures of the Joints* 2nd edn. Longman: London, 1823.

Cooper, C., Barker, D.J.P., Morris, J. & Briggs, R.S.J. Osteoporosis, falls and age in fracture of the proximal femur. *Br Med J* 1987; **295**: 13−15.

Cooper, C., Barker, D.J.P. & Wickham, C. Physical activity, muscle strength, and calcium intake in fracture of the proximal femur in Britain. *Br Med J* 1988; **297**: 1443−1446.

Coughlin, L. & Templeton, J. Hip fractures in patients with Parkinson's disease. *Clin Orthop* 1980; **148**: 192−195.

Cranley, J.J., Canos, A.J. & Sull, W.J. The diagnosis of deep venous thrombosis. Fallibility of symptoms and signs. *Arch Surg* 1976; **111**: 34−36.

Crawford, H.B. Conservative treatment of impacted fractures of the femoral neck. *J Bone Joint Surg* 1960; **42A**: 471−479.

Crawford, H.B. Experience with the non-operative treatment of impacted fractures of the neck of the femur. *J Bone Joint Surg* 1965; **47A**: 830−831.

Crawfurd, E.J.P., Emery, R.J.H., Hansell, D.M., Phelan, M. & Andrews, B.G. Capsular distension and intracapsular pressure in subcapital femoral fractures of the femur. *J Bone Joint Surg* 1988; **70B**: 195−198.

Crock, H.V. A revision of the anatomy of the arteries supplying the upper end of the human femur. *J Anat* 1965; **99**: 77−88.

Cummings, S.R. Are patients with hip fractures more osteoporotic? *Am J Med* 1985; **78**: 487−494.

DaCosta, J.C. Nailing of a fracture of the femoral neck. *Am J Orthop Surg* 1907−1908; **5**: 35.

D'Arcy, J. & Devas, M. Treatment of fractures of the femoral neck by replacement with the Thompson prosthesis. *J Bone Joint Surg* 1976; **58B**: 279−286.

Davie, B. Experience with the Austin Moore prosthesis with special reference to mortality from recent femoral neck fractures. *Med J Aust* 1968; **1**: 92−93.

Deyerle, W.M. Absolute fixation with contact compression in hip fractures. *Clin Orthop* 1959; **13**: 279−297.

Deyerle, W.M. Multiple pin peripheral fixation in the fractures of the neck of the femur: immediate weight-bearing. *Clin Orthop* 1965; **39**: 135−156.

Dickson, J.A. The high geometric osteotomy with rotation and bone graft for ununited fractures of the neck of the femur. *J Bone Joint Surg* 1947; **29**: 1005−1018.

Dorne, H.L. & Lander, P.H. Spontaneous stress fractures of the femoral neck. *Am J Roentgenol* 1985; **144(2)**: 343−347.

Drinker, H. & Murray, W.R. The universal proximal femoral endoprosthesis. A short term comparison with conventional hemiarthroplasty. *J Bone Joint Surg* 1979; **61A**: 1167−1174.

Duhamel, G. *Progress Med* 1947; **75**: 584−587.

Eklund, J. & Eriksson, F. Fractures of the femoral neck: with special regard to the treatment and prognosis of stable abduction fractures. *Acta Chir Scand* 1964; **127**: 315−337.

Evans, D.S. & Cockett, F.B. Diagnosis of deep vein thrombosis with an ultrasonic Doppler technique. *Br Med J* 1969; **2**: 802−804.

Evarts, C.M. & Feil, E.J. Prevention of thromboembolic disease after elective surgery of the hip. *J Bone Joint Surg* 1971; **53A**: 1271−1280.

Falch, J.A., Uebeck, A. & Slungaard, U. Epidemiology of hip fractures in Norway. *Acta Orthop Scand* 1985; **56**: 12−16.

Flynn, M. A new method of reduction of fractures of the neck of the femur based on anatomical studies of the hip joint. *Injury* 1973; **5**: 309−317.

Frandson, P.A., Anderson, P.E., Christofferson, H. & Thomsen, P.B. Osteosynthesis of the femoral neck fracture. The sliding screw plate with or without compression. *Acta Orthop Scand* 1984; **55**: 620−623.

Frangakis, E.K. Intracapsular fracture of the neck of the femur: factors influencing nonunion and ischaemic necrosis. *J Bone Joint Surg* 1966; **48B**: 17−30.

Frankel, V.H. Biomechanics of the hip. In: *Function, Fracture Mechanism and Internal Fixation*. Charles C. Thomas: Springfield, 1960.

Frankel, V.H. In: Tronzo, R.G. (ed.) *Surgery of the Hip Joint*. Lea & Febiger: Philadelphia, 1974.

Freeman, M.A.R., Todd, R.C. & Pirie, C.J. The role of fatigue in the pathogenesis of senile femoral neck fractures. *J Bone Joint Surg* 1974; **56B**: 698−702.

Garcia, A., Neer, C.S. & Ambrose, G.B. Displaced intracapsular fractures of the femur. *J Trauma* 1961; **1**: 128−132.

Garden, R.S. The structure and function of the proximal end of the femur. *J Bone Joint Surg* 1961a; **43B**: 576−589.

Garden, R.S. Low angle fixation in fractures of the femoral neck. *J Bone Joint Surg* 1961b; **43B**: 647−663.

Garden, R.S. Stability and union in subcapital fractures of the femur. *J Bone Joint Surg* 1964; **46B**: 630−647.

Garden, R.S. Malreduction and avascular necrosis in subcapital fractures of the femur. *J Bone Joint Surg* 1971; **53B**: 183−197.

Gingras, M.B., Clarke, J. & Evarts, C.M.C. Prosthetic replacement in femoral neck fractures. *Clin Orthop* 1980; **152**: 147−157.

Green, J.T. Management of fresh fractures of the neck of femur. *AAOS Instructional Course Lectures* 1960; **17**: 94−105.

Grimley Evans, J. Fracture of proximal femur in Newcastle-upon-Tyne. *Age Ageing* 1979; **8**: 16−24.

Grimley Evans, J., Prudham, D. & Wandless, I. A prospective study of fractured proximal femur: incidence and outcome. *Public Health London* 1979a; **93**: 235−241.

Grimley Evans, J., Prudham, D. & Wandless, I. A prospective study of fractured proximal femur: factors predisposing to survival. *Age Ageing* 1979b; **8**: 246−50.

Grimley Evans, J., Wandless, I. & Prudham, D. A prospective study of fractured proximal femur: hospital differences. *Public Health London* 1980; **94**: 149−154.

Grundy, M. Fractures of the femur in Paget's disease of bone. *J Bone Joint Surg* 1970; **52B**: 252−263.

Hansen, B.A. & Solgaard, S. Impacted fracture of the femoral treated by early mobilisation and weight-bearing. *Acta Orthop Scand* 1978; **49**: 180−185.

Harper, W.M., Barnes, M. & Gregg, P.J. Femoral head blood flow in proximal femoral fractures; an analysis using intraosseous pressure measurement. *J Bone Joint Surg* 1990; **72B**: 735−736.

Harris, W.H., Athanasoukis, C.A., Waltman, A.C. & Salzman, E.W. Cuff impedance phlebography and ^{125}I-fibrinogen scanning versus roentgenographic phlebography for diagnosis of thrombophlebitis following hip surgery. *J Bone Joint Surg* 1976; **58A**: 939−944.

Harris, W.H., Athanasoukis, C.A., Waltman, A.C. & Salzman, E.W. High and low dose aspirin prophylaxis against venous thromboembolic disease in total hip replacement. *J Bone Joint Surg* 1982; **64A**: 63−66.

Harris, W.H., Athanasoukis, C.A., Waltman, A.C., Salzman, E.W. Prophylaxis of deep vein thrombosis after total hip replacement. Dextran and external pneumatic compression compared with 1.2 or 0.3 gram of aspirin daily. *J Bone Joint Surg* 1985; **67A**: 57−62.

Harris, W.H., Salzman, E.W. & Athanasoukis, C.A. Comparison of warfarin, low molecular weight dextran, aspirin and subcutaneous heparin in the prevention of venous thromboembolism following total hip replacement. *J Bone Joint Surg* 1974; **56A**: 1552−1562.

Hart, J.T. The inverse care law. *Lancet* 1971; **i**: 405−412.

Hayes, A.G. & Groth, H.E. The influence of rotational malposition on intracapsular fracture of the femoral neck. *Surg Gynecol Obstet* 1967; **124**: 40−48.

Hewson, J.C. Treatment of intracapsular fracture of the hip with primary pedicle bone graft from the greater trochanter. *Clin Orthop* 1971; **76**: 100−101.

Hey-Groves, E.W. *On Modern Methods of Treating Fractures.* Wright: Bristol, 1916.

Hilleboe, J.W., Staple, T.W., Lansche, E.W. *et al.* The nonoperative treatment of impacted fractures of the femoral neck. *South Med J* 1970; **63**: 1103−1109.

Hinchey, J.J. & Day, P.L. Primary prosthetic replacement in fresh femoral neck fractures. *J Bone Joint Surg* 1964; **46A**: 223−240.

Hirsch, C. & Frankel, V.H. Analysis of forces producing fractures of the proximal end of the femur. *J Bone Joint Surg* 1960; **42B**: 633−640.

Hull, R.D. & Raskob, G.E. Prophylaxis of venous thromboembolic disease following hip and knee surgery. *J Bone Joint Surg* 1986; **68A**: 146−150.

Hullinger, C.W. Intracapsular fractures of the neck of femur. *Int Surg* 1967; **47(2)**: 166−171.

Hunter, G.A. A comparison of the use of internal fixation and prosthetic replacement for fresh fractures of the neck of femur. *Br J Surg* 1969; **56**: 229−232.

Hunter, G.A. Should we abandon primary prosthetic replacement for fresh fractures of the neck of the femur. *Clin Orthop* 1980; **152**: 158−161.

Ions, G.K. & Stevens, J. Prediction of survival in patients with femoral neck fractures. *J Bone Joint Surg* 1987; **69B**: 384−387.

Jacobs, B., Wade, P.A. & Match, R. Intracapsular fractures of the femoral neck treated by the Pugh nail. *J Trauma* 1965; **5**: 751−760.

Jensen, G.G. & Holstein, P. Long term follow-up of Moore arthroplasty in femoral neck fractures. *Acta Orthop Scand* 1975; **46**: 764−774.

Jewett, E.L. One piece angle nail for trochanteric fractures. *J Bone Joint Surg* 1941; **23**: 803−810.

Johansson, S. On the operative treatment of medial fractures of the femoral neck. *Acta Orthop Scand* 1932; **3**: 362−385.

Jones, K.G. Fractures of the femoral neck, fixation by multiple threaded wires. *South Med J* 1966; **59(5)**: 541−546.

Judet, R. Treatment of fractures of the femoral neck by pedicled graft. *Acta Orthop Scand* 1962; **32**: 421−427.

Judet, R., Judet, J., Lord, G., Roy-Camille, R. & LeTournel, E. Treatment of fractures of the femoral neck by pedicled graft. *Presse Med* 1961; **69**: 2452−2453.

Kaltsas, D.S. Stress fractures of the femoral neck in young adults: a report of seven cases. *J Bone Joint Surg* 1981; **63B**: 33−37.

Kakkar, V.V., Flanc, C. & Howe, C.T. Treatment of deep vein thrombosis. A trial of heparin, streptokinase and arvin. *Br Med J* 1969; **1**: 806−810.

Kakkar, V.V., Howe, C.T. & Nicolaides, A.N. Deep vein thrombosis of the leg: is there a 'high risk' group? *Am J Surg* 1970; **120**: 527−530.

Kavlie, H., Nordeval, Y. & Sundal, B. Femoral head replacement with the Christiansen endoprosthesis. *Acta Chir Scand* 1975: **141**: 96−103.

Kavlie, H. & Sundal, B. Primary arthroplasty on femoral neck fractures: a review of 269 consecutive cases treated with the Christiansen endoprosthesis. *Acta Orthop Scand* 1974; **45**: 590−597.

Kelsey, J.L. & Hoffmann, S. Risk factors for hip fracture. *N Engl J Med* 1987; **316**: 404−406.

Kenzora, J.E., McCarthy, R.E., Lowell, J.D. & Sledge, C.B. Hip fracture mortality: relation to age, treatment, preoperative illness, time of surgery. *Clin Orthop* 1984; **186**: 45−56.

King, T. The closed operation for intracapsular fractures of the femur. *Br J Surg* 1939; **26**: 721−748.

Knowles, F.L. Fractures of the neck of the femur. *Wis Med J* 1936; **35**: 106−109.

Koch, J.C. The laws of bone architecture. *Am J Anat* 1917; **XXI**: 177−298.

Kocher, T. *Beitrage zur Kentruss eineger praktisch wichtiger Fracturformen.* Carl Sallman: Basel and Leipzig, 1896.

Kreutzfeldt, J., Haim, M. & Bach, E. Hip fractures among the elderly in a mixed urban and rural population. *Age Ageing* 1984; **13(2)**: 111−119.

Kuslich, S.D. & Gustilo, R.B. Fractures of the femoral neck in young adults. Proceedings of AAOS. *J Bone Joint Surg* 1976; **58A**: 724.

Kyle, R.F., Wright, T.M. & Burstein, A.H. Biomechanical analysis of the sliding characteristics of compression hip screws. *J Bone Joint Surg* 1980; **62A**: 1308−1314.

Lane, J.M., Sculco, T.P. & Zolan, S. Treatment of pathological fractures of the hip by endoprosthetic replacement. *J Bone Joint Surg* 1980; **62A**: 954−959.

Leadbetter, G.W. A treatment for fracture of the femur. *J Bone Joint Surg* 1933; **15**: 931−940.

Leichter, I., Margulies, J.Y., Weinreb, A. Mizrahi, J., Robin, G.C., Conforty, B., Marin, M. & Bloch, B. The relationship between bone density, mineral content and mechanical strength in the femoral neck. *Clin Orthop* 1982; **162**: 272−281.

Levine, G., Makin, M., Menczel, J., Robin, G., Naor, E. & Steinberg, R. Incidence of fractures of the proximal end of the femur in Jerusalem. *J Bone Joint Surg* 1970; **52A**: 1193−1202.

Leyshon, R.L. & Matthews, J.P. Acetabular erosion and the Monk hard top prosthesis. *J Bone Joint Surg* 1984; **66B**: 172−174.

Leyvraz, P.E., Richard, J., Bachmann, F., van Melle, G., Treyvand, J.M., Livio, J.-J. & Candardjis, G. Adjusted versus fixed dose subcutaneous heparin in the prevention of deep vein thrombosis after total hip replacement. *N Engl J Med* 1983; **309**: 954−958.

Lindholm, R.V., Puranen, J. & Kinnuren, P. The Moore vitallium femoral neck prosthesis in fractures of the femoral neck. *Acta Orthop Scand* 1976; **47**: 70−78.

Linton, P. On different types of intracapsular fractures of the femoral neck. *Acta Chir Scand* 1944; **90**: 1−122.

Loudon, J.R. ^{125}I-Fibrinogen test. *Br Med J* 1976; **2**: 793.

Lucht, U. A prospective study of accidental falls and resulting injuries in the home among elderly people. *Acta Sociomed Scand* 1971; **2**: 105−120.

Mandell, R.M. Fracture of the femoral neck treated with Austin Moore prosthesis: clinical assessment and review of 60 cases. *J Am Orth Assoc* 1972; **71**: 953−967.

Massie, W.K. Fractures of the hip. *J Bone Joint Surg* 1964; **46A**: 658−690.

Mavor, G.E. & Galloway, J.M. Iliofemoral venous thrombosis: pathological considerations and surgical management. *Br J Surg* 1969; **56**: 45−59.

McElvenny, R.T. The roentgenographic interpretation of what constitutes adequate reduction of femur neck fractures. *Surg Gynecol Obstet* 1945; **80**: 97−106.

Meriel, P., Ruffie, R. & Fournie, A. La phlebographie de la hanche dans les coxarthroses. *Rev Rhum Mal Osteoartic* 1955; **22**: 238.

Metz, C.W., Seller, T.D., Feagin, J.A., Levine, M.I., Onkey, R.G., Dyer, J.W. & Eberhard, E.J. The displaced intracapsular fracture of the neck of the femur. *J Bone Joint Surg* 1970; **52A**: 113−127.

Meyer, S. Prosthetic replacement in hip fractures. A comparison between the Moore and Christiansen endoprostheses. *Clin Orthop* 1981; **160**: 57−72.

Meyers, M.H. The role of posterior bone grafts (muscle-pedicle) in femoral neck fractures. *Clin Orthop* 1980; **152**: 143−146.

Meyers, M.H., Harvey, J.P. & Moore, T.M. Treatment of displaced subcapital and transcervical fractures of the femoral neck by muscle-pedicle bone graft and internal fixation. *J Bone Joint Surg* 1973; **55A**: 257−264.

Meyers, M.H., Harvey, J.P. & Moore, T.M. Delayed treatment of subcapital and transcervical fractures of the neck of the femur with internal fixation and muscle-pedicle bone graft. *Orthop Clin North Am* 1974; **5**: 743−756.

Milne, R.M., Gunne, A.A. & Griffiths, J.M. Postoperative deep vein thrombosis; a comparison of diagnostic techniques. *Lancet* 1971; **ii**: 445−447.

Montgomery, S.P. & Lawson, L.R. Primary Thompson prosthesis for acute femoral neck fractures. *Clin Orthop* 1977; **137**: 62−68.

Moore, A.T. Fracture of the hip joint (intracapsular): a new method of treatment. *J South Carolina Med Assoc* 1934; **30**: 199−205.

Moore, A.T. Metal hip joint: a new self locking vitallium prosthesis. *South Med J* 1952; **45**: 1015−1019.

Moore, A.T. & Bohlman, H.R. Metal hip joint: a case report. *J Bone Joint Surg* 1943; **25**: 688−692.

Mudge, M. & Hughes, L.E. The long term sequelae of deep vein thrombosis. *Br J Surg* 1978; **65**: 692−694.

Nicholas, J.A. & Killoran, P. Fracture of the femur in patients with Paget's disease. *J Bone Joint Surg* 1965; **47A**: 450−461.

Niemann, K.M.W. & Mankin, H.J. Fractures about the hip in the elderly indigent population. *Geriatrics* 1960; **Oct**: 150−158.

Nillius, A.S. & Nylander, G. Deep vein thrombosis after total hip replacement: a clinical and phlebographic study. *Br J Surg* 1979; **66**: 324−326.

Nystrom, S. Some experiences with the treatment of fractura collifemoris medialis by the pegging method of Smith Petersen−Sven Johansson. *Acta Chir Scand* 1935; **76**: 1−24.

Ohman, U., Bjorkegren, N. & Fahlstrom, G. Fracture of the femoral neck. *Acta Chir Scand* 1969; **135**: 27−42.

Ort, P.J. & Lamont, J. Treatment of femoral neck fractures with a sliding compression screw and two Knowles pins. *Clin Orthop* 1984; **190**: 158−162.

Pare, A. *The Work of That Famous Chirugian Ambroise Pare*, Vol. XV. Johnson, T. (trans.). Cotes & Young: London, 1634.

Parrish, F.F. & Murray, J.A. Surgical treatment for secondary neoplastic fractures. *J Bone Joint Surg* 1970; **52A**: 665−686.

Pauwels, F. *Der Schenkenholsbruck, ein Mechanisches Problem. Grundlagen des Heilungsvorganges. Prognose und Kausale Therapie.* Ferdinand Enke: Stuttgart, 1935.

Phemister, D.B. The pathology of un-united fractures of the neck of the femur with special reference to the head. *J Bone Joint Surg* 1939; **21A**: 681−693.

Phemister, D.B. Treatment of the necrotic head of the femur in adults. *J Bone Joint Surg* 1949; **31A**: 55−66.

Phillips, R.S. Phlebography in osteoarthritis of the hip. *J Bone Joint Surg* 1966; **48B**: 280−288.

Polyzoides, A.J. Prosthetic replacement after femoral neck fractures. *Injury* 1971; **2**: 283−286.

Prather, J.L., Nusynowitz, M.L., Snowdy, H.A., Hughes, A.D., McCartney, W.H. & Bagg, R.J. Scintigraphic findings in femoral neck fractures. *J Bone Joint Surg* 1977; **59A**: 869−874.

Protzman, R.R. & Burkhalter, W.E. Femoral neck fractures in young adults. *J Bone Joint Surg* 1976; **58A**: 689−695.

Pugh, W.L. A self adjusting nail-plate for fractures about the hip joint. *J Bone Joint Surg* 1955; **37A**: 1085−1093.

Raine, G.E.T. A comparison of internal fixation and prosthetic replacement in recent displaced subcapital fractures of the neck of the femur. *Injury* 1973; **4(5)**: 25−30.

Rees, J.L. Secular changes in the incidence of proximal femoral fracture in Oxford. *Commun Med* 1982; **4**: 100−103.

Riska, E.B. Factors influencing the primary mortality in the treatment of hip fractures. *Injury* 1970−71; **2(2)**: 107−115.

Rothermel, J.E. & Garcia, A. Treatment of hip fractures in patients with Parkinson's disease on Levadopa therapy. *J Bone Joint Surg* 1972; **54A**: 1251−1254.

Ryan, J.R., Salciciolli, G.C. & Pederson, H.E. Deyerle fixation for intracapsular fractures of the femoral neck. *Clin Orthop* 1979; **144**: 178−182.

Rydell, N.W. Forces acting in the femoral head prosthesis. A study in strain gauge supplied prostheses in living persons. *Acta Orthop Scand* 1966; Suppl **88**: 1−132.

Rydell, N.W. Biomechanics of the hip joint. *Clin Orthop North Am* 1973; **92**: 6−15.

Saltzman, E.W. Progress in preventing venous thromboembolism. *N Engl J Med* 1983; **309**: 980−982.

Salvati, E.A., Artz, T., Aglietti, P. & Asnis, S.E. Endoprostheses in the treatment of femoral neck fractures. *Orthop Clin North Am* 1974; **5(4)**: 757−777.

Schumpelick, W. & Jantzen, P.M. A new principle in the operative treatment of trochanteric fractures of the femur. *J Bone Joint Surg* 1955; **37A**: 693−698.

Sevitt, S. Venous thrombosis and pulmonary embolism; their prevention by oral anticoagulants. *Am J Med* 1962; **33**: 703−716.

Sevitt, S. Avascular necrosis and revascularisation of the femoral head after intracapsular fractures. *J Bone Joint Surg* 1964; **46B**: 270−296.

Sevitt, S. & Thompson, R.G. The distribution and anastomoses of arteries supplying the head and neck of the femur. *J Bone Joint Surg* 1965; **47B**: 560−573.

Sikorski, J.M. & Barrington, R. Internal fixation versus hemiarthroplasty for the displaced subcapital fracture of the femur. *J Bone Joint Surg* 1981; **63B**: 357−361.

Sikorski, J.M., Davis, N.J. & Senior, J. Rapid transit system for patients with fractures of the proximal femur. *Br Med J* 1985; **290**: 439−443.

Sim, F.H. & Stauffer, R.N. Management of hip fractures by total hip arthroplasty. *Clin Orthop* 1980; **152**: 191−197.

Singh, M., Nagrath, A.R. & Maini, P.S. Changes in the trabecular pattern of the upper end of the femur as an index of osteoporosis. *J Bone Joint Surg* 1970; **52A**: 457−467.

Skinner, P.W. & Powles, D. Compression screw fixation for displaced subcapital fracture of the femur. Success or failure. *J Bone Joint Surg* 1986; **68B**: 78−82.

Smith, L.D. The role of muscle contraction or intrinsic forces on the causation of fractures of the femoral neck. *J Bone Joint Surg* 1953; **35A**: 367−383.

Smith-Petersen, M.N. A new supra-articular subperiosteal approach to the hip joint. *Am J Orthop Surg* 1917; **15**: 592−595.

Smith-Petersen, M.N., Cave, E.F. & Van Gorder, G.W. Intracapsular fractures of the neck of the femur. *Arch Surg* 1931; **23**: 715−759.

Smyth, E.H.J., Ellis, J., Mannifold, M.C., Dewey P.R. Triangular pinning for fracture of the femoral neck. A new method based on the internal architecture. *J Bone Joint Surg* 1964; **46B**: 664−673.

Solomon, L. Osteoporosis and fracture of the femoral neck in the South African Bantu. *J Bone Joint Surg* 1968; **50B**: 2−13.

Soto-Hall, R., Johnson, L.H. & Johnson, R.A. Variations in intra-articular pressure of the hip joint in injury and disease. A probable factor in avascular necrosis. *J Bone Joint Surg* 1964; **46A**: 509−516.

Speed, K. The unsolved fracture. *Surg Gynecol Obstet* 1935; **60**: 341−351.

Stauffer, R.N. & Sim, F.H. Total hip arthroplasty in Paget's disease of the hip. *J Bone Joint Surg* 1976; **58A**: 476−478.

Stevens, J., Fardin, R. & Freeark, R.J. Lower extremity thrombophlebitis in patients with femoral neck fractures: a venographic investigation and a review of the early and late significance of the findings. *J Trauma* 1968; **8**: 527−534.

Stromqvist, B., Nilsson, L.T., Egund, N., Thorngren, K.G., Wingstrand, H. Intracapsular pressures in underplaced fractures of the femoral neck. *J Bone Joint Surg* 1988; **70B**: 192−194.

Stuck, W.S. & Hinchey, J.J. Experimentally increased blood supply to the head and neck of the femur. *Surg Gynecol Obstet* 1944; **78**: 160−163.

Svalastoga, E., Kiaer, T., Jensen, P.E. The effect of intracapsular pressure and extension of the hip on oxygenation of the juvenile femoral epiphysis: a study in the goat. *J Bone Joint Surg* 1989; **71B**: 222−226.

Svenningsen, S., Benum, P., Nesse, O., Furset, O.I. Internal fixation of femoral neck fractures. A compression screw compared with nail plate fixation. *Acta Orthop Scand* 1984; **55**: 423−429.

Swiontkowski, M.F., Tepic, S., Perren, S.M., Moor, R., Ganz, R. & Rahn, B.A. Laser Doppler flowmetry for bone blood flow measurement: correlation with microsphere estimates and evaluation of the effect of intracapsular pressure on femoral head blood flow. *J Orthop Res* 1986; **4**: 362−371.

Swiontkowski. M.F., Winquist, R.A. & Hansen, S.T. Fractures of the femoral neck in patients between the ages of twelve and forty nine years. *J Bone Joint Surg* 1984; **66A**: 837−846.

Thompson, F.R. Vitallium intramedullary hip prosthesis; preliminary report. *NY Med J* 1952; **52**: 3011−3020.

Thompson, F.R. Two and a half years experience with a vitallium intramedullary hip prosthesis. *J Bone Joint Surg* 1954; **36A**: 489−500.

Tillberg, B. Treatment of fractures of the femoral neck by primary arthroplasty. *Acta Orthop Scand* 1976; **47**: 209−213.

Trueta, J. & Harrison, M.H.M. The normal vascular anatomy of the femoral head in adult man. *J Bone Joint Surg* 1953; **35B**: 442−461.

Vegter, J. & Cubsen, C.C. Fractional necrosis of the femoral head epiphysis after transient increase in joint pressure. An experimental study in juvenile rabbits. *J Bone Joint Surg* 1989; 69B: 530−535.

Venable, C.S., Stuck, W.G. & Beach, A. The effect on bone of the presence of metals; based on electrolysis. *Ann Surg* 1937; **105**: 917−938.

Walmsley, T. Articular mechanism of diarthroses. *J Bone Joint Surg* 1928; **10**: 40−45.

Ward, F.O. *Human Anatomy* Renshaw: London, 1838.

Weitbrecht, J. *Syndesmologia sive Historia Ligamentorum Corporis Humani Quain Seeundum. Observationes Anatomicas Concinnavit et Figuris ad Objecta Reentia Adumbratis Illustravit.* Typographia Academiae Scietiarum: Petropoli, 1742.

Westcott, H.H. A method for the internal fixation of transcervical fractures of the femur. *J Bone Joint Surg* 1934; **16**: 372−378.

Whitaker, R.P., Abeshaus, M.M., Scholl, H.W. & Chung, S.M.K. Fifteen years experience with metallic endoprosthetic replacement of the femoral head for femoral neck fractures. *J Trauma* 1972; **12**: 799−806.

Williams, O., Lyall, J., Vernon, M. & Croft, D.N. Ventilation perfusion lung scanning for pulmonary emboli. *Br Med J* 1974; **1**: 600−602.

Wood, D.J. *Hip Fractures in the Elderly*. MS thesis: London University, 1990.

Woolf, J. *Virchows Archiv Orth Anat* 1870; **50**: 389.

Wrighton, J.D. & Woodyard, J.E. Prosthetic replacement for subcapital fractures of the femur: a comparative study. *Injury* 1971; **2**: 287–293.

Extracapsular fractures (fractures in the trochanteric region)

R.HORNBY

Isolated fracture of the greater trochanter

In contrast to the clean apophyseal separation which occurs as an apparently pure traction-avulsion of the greater trochanter in children, the pattern of fracture in

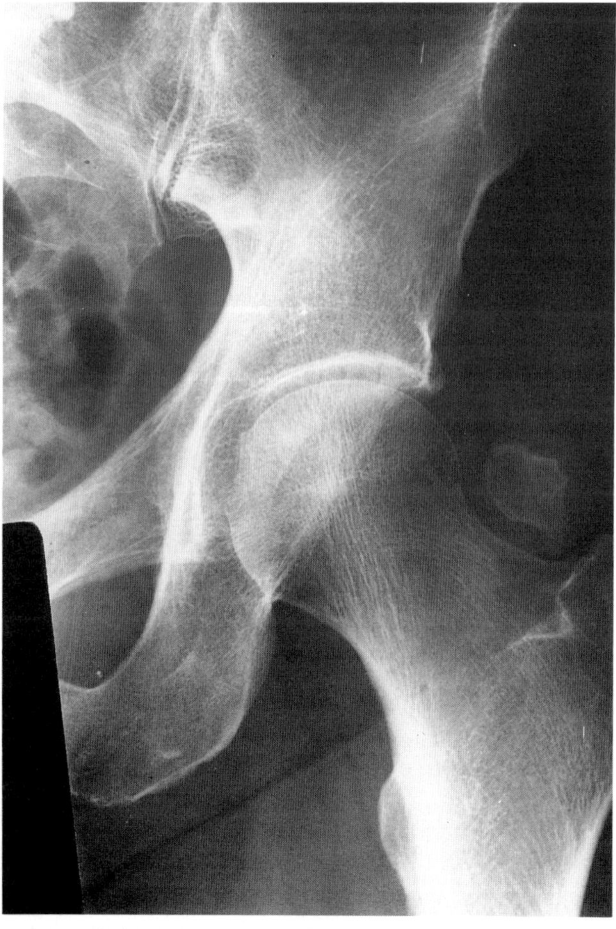

Fig. 20.18 This fracture of the greater trochanter was sustained by an athletic 54-year-old anaesthetist who fell whilst running, but within 2 months, was running once again.

adults is usually one of irregular comminution with minimal displacement, usually at the posterior part of the tip of the trochanter (Fig. 20.18). A history of a direct blow is usually present and the most obvious features on clinical examination are local tenderness and painful, inhibited active hip abduction.

In most cases, all that is required is recumbency with the hip abducted, until pain subsides, and then a gentle mobilization programme can be tailored to the patient's recovery. Operative reattachment of the greater trochanter is only indicated where there is a large fragment, minimal comminution and significant displacement in a young adult. A lag screw or tension-band wiring technique may be used, as appropriate.

It should be recalled that the insertion of the gluteus medius and minimus is over a wide area distal to the apex of the greater trochanter, so that unless the major part of the former apophysis is widely avulsed, the functional deficit from these fractures, even when associated with fibrous or non-union, is generally slight. In elderly patients, administration of analgesic drugs may be sufficient to allow walking in abduction, using a frame, after only 1 or 2 days (Watson-Jones 1955, Merlino & Nixon 1969).

Isolated fracture of the lesser trochanter

The lesser trochanter develops as a traction apophysis and is, therefore, susceptible to avulsion fracture before growth is complete, along the margin of the zone of calcification. Such injuries are fairly uncommon in children, even less common in adolescents and extremely rare in adults. The combined ilio-psoas tendon inserts not only into the lesser trochanter but also to a more extensive area of the femur surrounding it, and separation is therefore seldom very great. In most instances there is the history of resisted powerful contraction of the hip flexors, typically occurring in the course of athletic or contact sports.

The area over the lesser trochanter is tender and flexor power, tested at 90° of flexion is reduced. The relative infrequency of the injury prevents sound comparisons, but the apparently excellent late function in patients who have had widely avulsed fractures ignored suggests that surgical repositioning of such lesions is rarely necessary. In young, serious athletes, where anatomical perfection may be demanded, open reduction and fixation by a cortical lag screw has been recommended for separation greater than 2 cm. A medial approach to the upper femur, via a Ludloff (1908) incision, gives adequate access to this region.

Occasionally, the lesser trochanter base may be weakened by secondary tumour deposits, or by other pathological processes, and the trochanter may be spontaneously avulsed by the ilio-psoas muscle during quiet activity. Such episodes may be clinically silent and symptomatic treatment is all that is required. In most cases of fracture in non-athletic adults, a decision not to operate will be taken. The patient should be placed in a position of comfort, usually in some degree of hip flexion, and given pain-relieving drugs until the discomfort becomes tolerable. A rapid return to normal activity should then be encouraged and minimal attention directed to the radiographic appearances (Howard & Phia 1965, DeLee 1984).

Extracapsular (trochanteric) fractures proper

Nomenclature

In contrast to the relatively infrequent 'isolated' fractures of the individual trochanters, trochanteric fractures which traverse the diameter of the upper femur are now occurring in almost epidemic proportions in the enlarging elderly population of many western societies. These injuries occur in the zone bounded proximally by the base of the femoral neck along a line joining the most proximal limits of the greater trochanter and lesser trochanter, and distally by a line drawn across the upper femur at the lower limit of the lesser trochanter (Fig. 20.19).

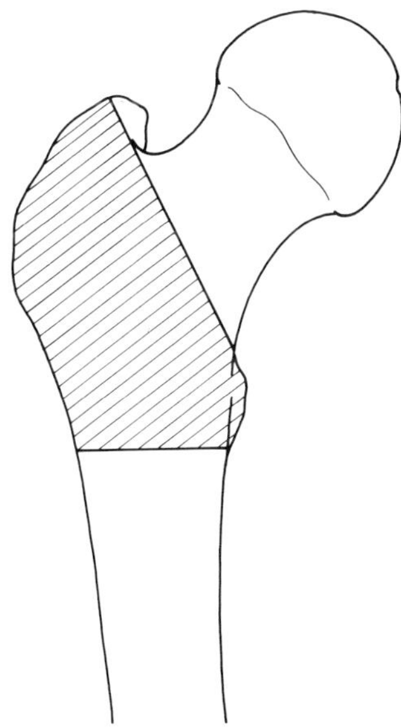

Fig. 20.19 Boundaries of the trochanteric zone of the femur.

In the majority of instances fractures which link the apices of the trochanters along an oblique line provide no difficulty in classification as 'trochanteric'. When the fracture lies more medially it may be difficult to decide from radiographs, obtained under emergency conditions, whether or not the femur has broken at a presumed 'intracapsular' level, and is therefore more correctly described as 'basicervical', or whether the fracture is 'extracapsular', and therefore falls more appropriately into the trochanteric group. The original purpose of such groupings was to distinguish more medial fractures, regarded as intracapsular and known to be prone to avascular necrosis, from more lateral trochanteric injuries, believed to be entirely extracapsular and carrying a minimal vascular risk.

Unfortunately, plain radiographs do not depict the hip capsule nor do they demonstrate blood vessels, neither of which conform to the arbitrary straight lines of conventional fracture classifications. Reports of paradoxical avascular necrosis in series of 'trochanteric' fractures are therefore difficult to evaluate unless the exact method of demarcation in this junctional 'basal' zone is explicit. In the same way, the proportion of basal fractures reported in case series of intracapsular injuries alters the significance of such complication rates (Mann 1973).

It is not unusual for comminution of trochanteric fractures to extend beyond the lesser trochanter limit. Traditionally, such fractures have been classified as 'trochanteric', as distinct from more distal injuries in which the femur is broken at a subtrochanteric level. In clinical practice, fractures are encountered which do not fit neatly into either category and which may well deserve special consideration. Subtrochanteric fractures are prone to non-union or delayed union and raise particular problems of mechanical fixation in highly stressed, cortical bone. Trochanteric fractures, on the other hand, occur in cancellous bone which has an excellent capacity for union and a different stress pattern. Non-uniformity in classification, again, may explain variations in complication rates reported after fractures in this more distal junctional area.

A further difficulty arises from different applications of the latin prefixes 'inter' and 'per' meaning 'between' and 'through', respectively. The term intertrochanteric has been applied by some authors to mean a fracture line which links the trochanters (Fig. 20.20a) and by other authors as one which separates them (Fig. 20.20b), or to mean running between the trochanters in the opposite obliquity (Fig. 20.20c). The term pertrochanteric has been used in the context of Fig. 20.20a and

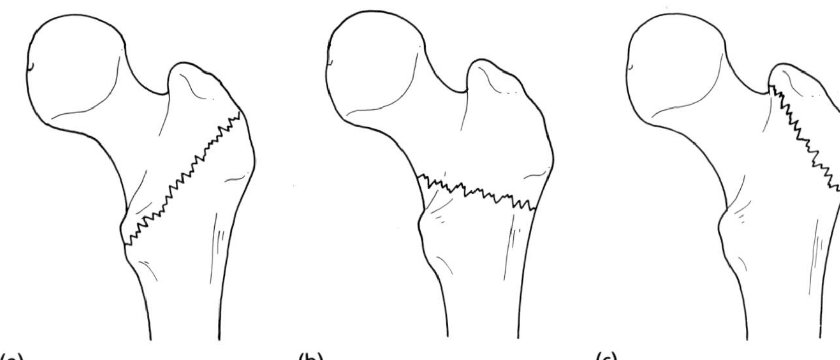

Fig. 20.20 Extracapsular (trochanteric) fracture lines. (a) Usual form of trochanteric fracture. (b) Reverse oblique pattern. (c) Isolated fracture of the greater trochanter.

Fig. 20.20c with similar ambiguity. The use of such confusing prefixes is best avoided in favour of a simple description of the actual fracture lines conveyed in plain language.

In fact, the vast majority of trochanteric fractures occur along a line joining the greater trochanter to the lesser trochanter with additional comminution in other directions, i.e. the pattern shown in Fig. 20.20a. These are usually known as 'typical' trochanteric injuries and are in contrast to the less common variety where the obliquity runs in the opposite direction, commencing proximally at the lower calcar femorale and passing distally to the lateral cortex. This latter group is sometimes known as the 'reverse oblique type' (Fig. 20.20b) (Evans 1949, Bremner & Graham 1958, Müller *et al.* 1970, Muckle 1977, James & Hunter 1983).

Clinical features

With the rare exception of undisplaced linear fractures, which are barely detectable on initial radiographs (Fig. 20.21), the majority of trochanteric fractures are attended by a complete inability to bear weight, a shortening of the thigh and an externally rotated attitude of the lower limb (Fig. 20.22). In comparison to intracapsular fractures, where the distal fragment is moored to the pelvis by the hip capsule, trochanteric fractures show a greater degree of deformity, with the femur being drawn upwards by the combined effects of adductors, the superficial abductors, the rectus femoris and the hamstrings. The additional effects of the short hip rotators, the gluteus medius and minimus and the ilio-psoas muscles depend on whether or not their attachments remain intact or are separated by additional comminution. Appreciation of the latter aspect is of some help in planning manipulative reduction (Horn & Wang 1964, May & Chacha 1968).

Pain and tenderness over the trochanteric area is usual, and bruising is often detected within the first few days after injury.

Epidemiology

In European orthopaedic practice, trochanteric fractures affect three more-or-less distinct sections of the adult population in increasing frequency (Boyce & Vessey 1985). These are:

1 Young adults who sustain the fracture in high-speed accidents. The incidence is low and generally reflects road safety and/or working practices. These patients are usually otherwise fit and have received a direct blow to the upper femur, which is of normal strength.

2 Middle-aged to elderly adults with impaired neuromuscular capacity and varying degrees of bone weakness. A history of alcoholism, anticonvulsant therapy, gastrectomy or drug addiction is often obtained. At present, this group appears to be increasing in size.

3 Frail, elderly (average 80 years), osteoporotic adults who are often mentally impaired and show a tendency to fall: there is a preponderance of females. Many patients in this category have already become socially dependent or are living in institutions.

The twentieth century has seen more people live to old age and an extension of the duration of survival; thus, the numbers of the very old have grown rapidly in developed countries. At the age of 60 years the incidence of proximal femoral fractures rises exponentially with age, doubling with every 5-year increment. In the United States the female population doubled in size between 1900 and 1960, whereas the incidence of hip fractures rose sixfold. In a British study, confined to the elderly, Evans (1979) noted an annual incidence rate of 5 per 1000 in those over the age of 65 years and observed that the percentage of trochanteric fractures rose from 40%

at the age of 70 years to 70% at the age of 85 years and above. Jensen (1981), studying a Scandinavian population, noted a reversal of the proportion of cervical to trochanteric fractures at approximately 80 years of age in females: at age 50 years, trochanteric fractures accounted for 20% of hip fractures, at 80 years the incidence was 50%, and at 90 years it rose to almost 65%. In males the percentage of trochanteric fractures remained constant and independent of age (Bauer 1960, Gallanaugh *et al.* 1976, Alffram 1964, Jensen 1980a, Editorial 1982, Frandsen & Kruse 1983, Zetterberg *et al.* 1984).

In populations of European origin, most trochanteric fractures occur in patients over the age of 75 years. A recent population-based study found that one-third of the patients were living alone, exhibiting varying degrees of mental impairment and needing support from their family or the community. The high incidence of hip fractures in psychiatric hospitals, and the associated high mortality and morbidity, have long been recognized, but the value of a quantitative assessment of dementia as a predictor of survival and the probability of rehabilitative success has only recently been appreciated (Evans 1979b).

Further details of the epidemiology of proximal femoral fractures as a whole are discussed in the section on intracapsular fractures. These aspects were recently summarized by Parker and Prior (1993).

Biomechanics

With the exception of that minority of young adults who sustain trochanteric fractures in high-energy trauma, most of these injuries in elderly patients are sustained in a simple indoor fall. In the majority, a direct blow to the greater trochanter appears to be the

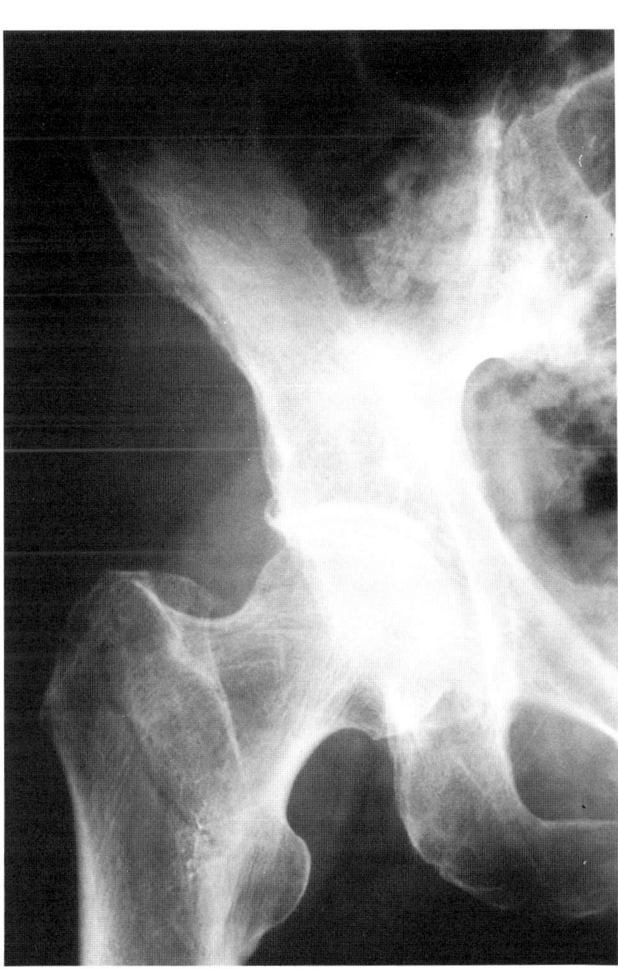

Fig. 20.21 Undisplaced trochanteric fracture.

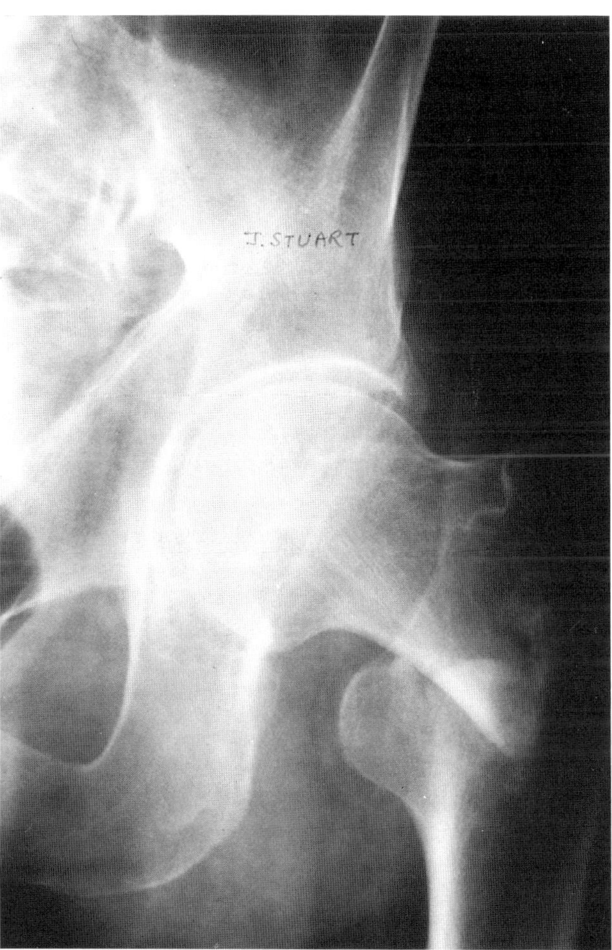

Fig. 20.22 Displaced trochanteric fracture. The distal fragment has moved proximally and is externally rotated.

initiating injury, but the precise external and internal force patterns which operate have not been clearly identified. In laboratory tests on post-mortem femora, fractures similar to those encountered clinically have been generated by combined axial compression with medially directed forces on the hip. Other mechanisms have been described, but the relevance of such cadaveric studies to the situation which occurs *in vivo* remains uncertain. A more accessible approach to the biomechanics of fracture is that of energy transfer, rather than the uncertainties of force distribution. When a person falls from a standing position, the potential energy available is equal to the product of the mass times the height of the centre of gravity (roughly at sacral level) above the floor. A 50-kg adult, of height 160 cm, with a centre of gravity approximately 70 cm above the floor, thus produces 3500 kg cm of energy, which is available for dissipation on the greater trochanter at impact. This is more than enough to fracture a normal femur, which will fail after absorbing only 60 kg cm (Hirsch & Frankel 1960, Gozna & Harrington 1982, Lawton *et al.* 1983, Aitken 1984).

The rarity of fracture in young persons who fall in this way is explicable not so much by their stronger bones, as by their greater efficiency in dissipating the energy in other ways, for example, elastic strain in other skeletal members and soft tissues, in particular by protective, energy-absorbing movements in the upper limbs. Whether or not a fracture occurs after a fall on to the hip is largely determined by the extent to which such protective mechanisms are efficiently retained: loss of this capacity leads to greater residual energy being transferred to the upper femur. The role of osteoporosis would seem to be in lowering the threshold at which absorbed strain energy results in fracture: the more violent the fall, and the more fragile the bone, the greater is the likelihood of fracture and of comminution (Aitken 1984).

These biomechanical concepts go some way to help with an understanding of the increased incidence of trochanteric fractures in relation to age and osteoporosis, and may explain Jensen's observation of an increase in the proportion of unstable, and generally more comminuted, fractures with age; however, until the variables can be quantified, interactions will remain obscure (Frankel & Burstein 1970, Jensen 1981).

Outcome of trochanteric injury: 'determinants' and the role of treatment

For a young adult, trochanteric fracture carries no material risk to life. Simple fractures may be managed by operation or by non-operative means with equal success. Even when fractures are comminuted, interfragmentary compression by supplementary lag screws may yet be achievable where the secondary fragments have a thick, strong cortex. The architecture may be preserved and a stable configuration be obtained, so that rapid mobilization is feasible. When such anatomical restoration is deemed likely to fail, a period of traction, either as a primary method of treatment or as a supplement to surgical reconstruction, provides a safe, albeit slow, alternative approach. Perhaps the most important index of the success of treatment in a young adult is the degree of any residual deformity, or loss of agility. In this context, varus malunion, with its reduction in abductor efficiency and shortening of the limb by, for example, 2 cm, would be a hindrance to an otherwise fit, athletic individual (Fig. 20.23).

The situation for the typical elderly victim of a trochanteric fracture is entirely different. The affected population, with an average age of 80 years, is already

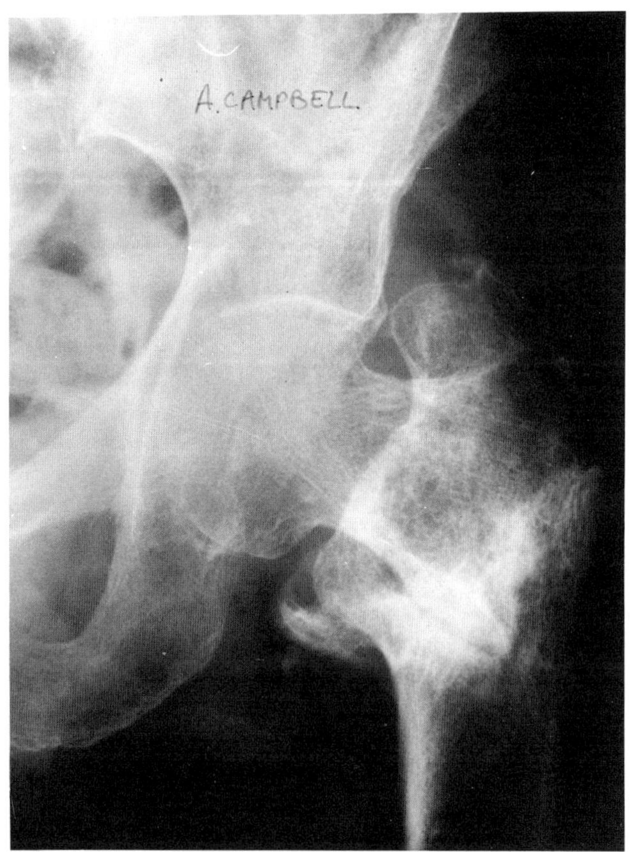

Fig. 20.23 Malunion in varus.

facing mortality, in a more urgent sense than the younger patient, even before fracture. Teetering on the brink of social independence, or already institutionalized, many of these patients display dementia of varying degrees and have very limited motivation or ability to move from place to place, or to carry out everyday tasks. For this overwhelmingly larger group of elderly patients, the preservation of life and retention of any residual intellectual or motor functions are the most important aims of treatment. The maintenance of upper femoral anatomy is only relevant to the extent that its loss interferes with these aims.

In all age groups the economics of treatment cannot be ignored — particularly by those individuals or bodies who bear the financial burden. In this respect, the duration of treatment which a method entails, particularly in the hospital inpatient phase, has received much direct and implicit attention. Because of this disparity in incidence, these social and economic aspects have achieved greater prominence in the elderly patient groups. The incidence and gravity of general complications of treatment, such as DVT, pulmonary embolism, pneumonia and pressure sores, plus the specific complications of individual methods, for example, nerve injury, implant breakage or detachment or surgical wound infection, must all be taken into consideration when the outcome is being evaluated (Ceder 1980a, Jensen & Tondevold 1980, Jensen *et al.* 1980b, Jensen 1984).

The outcome of care of trochanteric fractures has generally been viewed in terms of the perceived success or failure of various regimens. Thus, the rates for mortality and complications may be reported in an apparently unambiguous way, but the difficulty in measuring rehabilitative success and in estimating the total costs of treatment has often been given less precise, if not entirely subjective, evaluation. Mortality, surely the clearest of all end-points, has been reported at variable periods after fracture, and is sometimes not even stated, so that useful comparisons are scarce. The observation that the introduction of surgical treatment, refined by 30 years of 'development', had not improved the survival rate, when compared with non-operative care, led to a reappraisal, from the 1970s onwards, of the precise factors which determine the outcome (Hunter 1975).

Mortality

Few reports exist on the patterns of survival in defined populations after hip fractures. Evans (1979) reported

that approximately 50% of deaths occurred within 3 weeks of injury, with a secondary high risk period after 4–6 weeks, in a population-based study in the United Kingdom. Dahl examined the survival in a Norwegian population served by a single centre for the treatment of hip fractures (Dahl 1980). The death rate during the first month was found to be 15 times, and during the second month seven times, the expected death rate for an age-matched sample of the general population of the region; patients who had survived the first 2 months showed no significant excess mortality during the next 4 years, indicating the same survival as the general population. By means of life tables, several authors have shown excess mortality from these fractures to be essentially attributable to death in the first 6 months (Jensen & Tondevold 1979). Alffram (1964) identified the first 3 months as the time when survival curves matched those of the general population, i.e. the same phase which Gordon (1972) identified as producing the greatest mortality. If an arbitrary end-point is to be chosen for the comparison of series, then 6 months appears to be a reasonable time when mortality may be usefully measured. Jensen, who studied a hospital-based series of trochanteric fractures, has pointed out the secondary rise in mortality which occurs 3–4 months after discharge from hospital in the case of patients treated operatively and has criticized the limited value of reports of 'hospital' mortality (Acheson 1966, Kolind-Sorensen 1975, Jensen & Tondevold 1979).

Determinants

In 1979, Evans reported a prospective study of all cases of proximal femoral fracture in a defined population of persons aged 65 and over in northeast England (Evans 1979a, b). This area had an annual incidence rate of 6.5 per 1000 in females and 2.4 per 1000 in males. All patients were admitted to one of the two teaching hospitals in the city. A mental function test was carried out using a shortened form of a questionnaire first described by Blessed *et al.* (1969). This modified questionnaire had a score range of 0–13, standard errors for test–retest, and the between-observer variation was approximately 1.0. Patients were assessed within a few hours of admission until 6 months from injury. It was found that age, mental test score, type of residence, place of injury and hospital of admission were all significantly associated with the likelihood of survival to 6 months. When these factors were taken into account, no additional association was demonstrated between survival and social class, type of fracture, type of operation, grade of operator, associated disease or cigarette smoking. It was concluded that existing factors must be taken into account in comparisons of management.

Of the predictor factors identified by Evans, the magnitude of the effect of mental test score on survival was the most striking. This point has subsequently been reinforced by Ions and Stevens (1987), who used multivariate analysis in the context of intracapsular injuries. They identified mental test score as the most useful single predictor of the 6-month mortality risk.

The observation of better survival in those patients who sustained fractures outdoors, and were implicitly more mobile than the more infirm who were already confined to a home or institution, has been explored by Jensen (1984). The level of social dependence, pre-fracture, was measured according to a shortened four-point classification that was originally proposed by Thomas and Stevens (1974). Formal mental testing was not carried out in this Danish study. Life expectancy after hip fracture was found to be determined by the patient's social dependence prior to fracture and, secondarily, by the age of the patient. Neither type of fracture, method of treatment, technical failure, sex nor type of accommodation after hospital discharge were found to have any significant influence on the survival rate.

Trials of different forms of management in this field have usually been based on cases admitted to particular hospitals, but different hospitals, even in the same city, may receive cases that are different in important ways with respect to factors associated with the prognosis. In addition, the effective catchment area of a hospital may vary with time. Evans found that two British teaching hospitals, less than 1 mile apart, differed in the proportion of elderly hip fracture patients who survived for 6 months. The hospital with the worse results received a higher proportion of patients with a poorer prognosis in terms of mental function and residence in institutions, and this reflected differences in the catchment area and referral policy. Patients admitted to the hospital with the better results were also more likely to have been injured in public places rather than indoors (Evans *et al.* 1980). It is now clear that survival can be related to at least four 'determinants' or characteristics of the patient which are readily accessible at the time of injury. Though measurable, they are, unfortunately, beyond the control of the surgeon. These 'determinants' are:
1 Mental function.
2 Age.
3 Type of residence.
4 Place of injury.

In practice, residence or place of injury can be reduced further to a composite predictive variable:
1 Resident in an institution — fractured in an institution.
2 Living in a private household — fractured indoors.
3 Capable of going outside a residence — fractured outdoors.

An alternative approach, in societies with a well-organized, uniform provision for the needs of the elderly infirm, is to record the extent to which patients used such services prior to a fracture (Thomas & Stevens 1974, Ceder *et al.* 1980). When the factors in Table 20.8 were taken into account, Evans found no differences in mortality at 6 months between males and females with proximal femoral fractures, and Jensen found an apparently higher long-term mortality in males which could be accounted for by differences in social dependence after trochanteric fracture (Jensen 1984). An absence of information on these factors in the majority of orthopaedic surgical publications on trochanteric injury limits the extent to which conclusions can be drawn about the outcome of treatment. Most series have been hospital-based and patients have been defined only by age and sex.

A simple method of assessing pre-fracture mobility has been reported by Parker and Palmer (1993) as a useful predictor of mortality after hip fracture.

Influence of treatment on outcome

If the outcome of trochanteric fracture is, to a large extent, determined by factors in the patient's previous health, and therefore outside the surgeon's control, it

Table 20.8 Definition of different social function groups

Social function group	Definition
Independent	Manages everything; possibly working
Slightly dependent	Manages household and personal needs; receives 'meals on wheels' and/or home help <4 hours per week
Moderately dependent	Home help >5 hours per week; possibly visited by district nurse
Totally dependent	Living in a nursing home or receiving long-term nursing at home

Source: Jensen and Michaelsen (1975).

may well be asked what influence specific methods of treatment have on survival? Where differences have been shown between two hospitals using the same general plan of management, any residual differences in survival, which could not be accounted for by known determinants, were not attributable to the method of treatment or to the grade of operating surgeon. In one study the between-hospital differences were thought to be traceable to differences in the patient: nurse staffing ratio and/or to the levels of non-medical support services, such as physiotherapy. Subsequent improvements in these factors in the hospital with a poorer service almost, but not entirely, eliminated these residual differences, suggesting that the choice of method is less important than the hospital environment in which it is employed (Evans *et al.* 1980).

In 1951, Scott reported a prospective comparison of traction against internal fixation by nail plate, in the care of trochanteric fracture in a hospital-based series carried out in Oxford. No appreciable difference for the 3-month mortality rate was found between the two treatment groups. A further comparison of this type was carried out in Newcastle-upon-Tyne, in 1978, where the 6-month mortality was 25% for both methods of treatment, in a series defined by age and mental function. These results cast doubt on the validity of the proposal by E.M. Evans that the nail plate method was the treatment of choice on the grounds of reduced mortality, and on his report of a fall in mortality rate from 34 to 18% after the introduction of internal fixation (Evans 1949 & 1951, Hornby *et al.* 1986).

Many authors have reported comparable survival rates with operation and with non-operative care, but the lack of information on important determinants of outcome in the treated populations make useful comparisons difficult, if not impossible (Murray & Frew 1949, Horn & Wang 1964, Frew 1972, Bong *et al.* 1981, James & Hunter 1983). An epidemiologically based study, designed to overcome some of these limitations, was reported in 1985 (Hornby *et al.* 1986, 1989). All elderly patients, from a defined population, admitted to hospitals in the city of Newcastle-upon-Tyne in northeast England during a 12-month period, were studied and followed up to 6 months from injury. These arriving at one of the admitting hospitals were stratified according to mental test score, age and stability of the fracture, and were randomized to treatment by an AO (Association for Osteosynthesis) dynamic hip screw or by traction. Compared with traction, operation gave better anatomical results and a shorter hospital stay, but there were no significant differences between the treatments

in terms of survival, functional outcome or overall general complication rates. However, the operations in this series were nearly all the work of one surgeon who was working to a strict protocol using a well-rehearsed technique with a mean duration of less than 30 minutes and no technical or implant-related complications of clinical significance were encountered. Whether more complex, prolonged or traumatic procedures, such as intramedullary fixation, osteotomy or valgus displacement, would give similar survival rates and complication rates remains uncertain (Hornby *et al.* 1989).

The available evidence suggests that, at least for the relatively simple procedures such as nail plate and compression screw fixation, operative treatment gives the same survival rates as non-operative methods. Both methods are sensitive to the level of nursing care. Until a particular method of fracture management is shown to improve survival rate after trochanteric fracture, the decision as to whether to operate or not must be based on other measurements of outcome such as the overall cost and duration of treatment, the extent of any residual deformity, disability or discomfort and, not least, the seriousness and probability of specific and surgical implant-related complications which operative methods have introduced to an already rich field of morbidity. Horn and Wang (1964) have rightly warned that operations should not be used as a substitute for good nursing care.

Mobility and social dependence

The ability to walk before trochanteric fracture and survival afterwards are obvious prerequisites for long-term mobility. Thus, the success of management in this regard may be assessed by the sum of the rates for mortality and for loss of walking ability. Rates for independent walking, expressed as a percentage of survivors, are, perhaps, of some general interest, but gratifyingly high rates for walking postoperatively may be attributable to sample bias in favour of low-risk factors determining the outcome or to a 'weeding-out' of high-risk cases, via excess early mortality, rather than to any inherent advantage of the particular method; such information must be interpreted with caution (Shaftan *et al.* 1967). Miller (1978) reported 51% of patients regaining their original ability to walk. Horn and Wang (1964), reporting a series treated conservatively, claim that all patients who walked unaided before fracture were able to do so after their fracture had united. The average age in this series was 69.6 years and the mortality 'during treatment' was only 5.3%, but the follow-up was acknowledged to be under 50%. Scott (1951), in a comparative study, noted no great differences between treatments and observed that the results of conservative treatment were 'if anything slightly the better'. However, in a prospective study taking into account known risk factors, 16% of patients allocated to treatment with a dynamic hip screw had lost independence at 6 months after injury compared with 31% of those allocated to traction ($p < 0.05$) (Hornby 1989).

Interestingly, Ceder *et al.* (1980), in a Swedish investigation of rehabilitation after hip fracture in the elderly, found that postoperative mobility at 2 weeks, rather than prefracture mobility, proved to be a better indicator of the patient's chances of returning home. It was suggested that this could be used to plan aftercare. The author stated that the need to plan active rehabilitation was only relevant to those patients who lived at home at the time of injury. Institutionalized patients could hardly ever be rehabilitated to non-institutionalized living. Mobility grading, in which points are allocated according to the degree of independence in walking, was recommended.

In a British study of proximal femoral fractures in patients over 60 years of age, Thomas and Stevens (1974) noted that 25% of the survivors of operative treatment had become more dependent 1 year after injury. Great age, established dependence and 'a poor clinical result' were found to be principal contributory factors. They also noted that the presence of a spouse or companion appeared to be a powerful spur to physical recovery. Ceder (1980) noted that the main obstacles to rehabilitation were more often of a medical or social nature and pertained less often to 'mechanical aspects'. Jensen and Bagger (1982) found that the risk of social deterioration was related to the destination on discharge from hospital, as well as to age and the previous dependence level. They recommended discharge of patients to their own homes wherever possible.

Medical complications

It has been widely believed that conservative treatment is attended by an unacceptably high rate of general complications in comparison with operative methods, and that it carries a higher mortality rate. In centres where conservatism is reserved for the relatively unfit and surgery is offered only to the remainder, it is easy to see how such an impression has arisen. Retrospective studies are often seen to be skewed in this way by preselection. Even when treatments are being compared prospectively, it is important that any exclusions should

be made before patients are allocated to treatment groups in order to prevent sample bias. Thus, for example, the test of fitness for surgery, usually assessed by an anaesthetist preoperatively, must be applied to all cases before the stage of separation into treatment groups (Shaftan *et al.* 1967, Heyse-Moore *et al.* 1983, Sher *et al.* 1985, Esser *et al.* 1986).

Low rates of general complications have been consistently reported from centres routinely practising non-operative methods (Murray & Frew 1949, Lawson 1957, Horn & Wang 1964, Frew 1972).

In a study of patients matched for known risk factors no significant differences were found, between traction and operations using a dynamic hip screw, with respect to urinary and faecal incontinence, the need for tranquillizer prescriptions, the occurrence of pressure sores, DVT, pneumonia or pulmonary embolism during hospital stay. At 6 months after injury, there were no differences in frequency or severity of pain, the presence of leg swelling or persistence of unhealed pressure sores. Mental confusion was commonly observed but was not influenced by the choice of fracture treatment. Some patients recovered from the acute delirium of injury and showed an improvement in mental test scores, but no improvement in dementia occurred and, overall, there was no statistical difference between treatments (Hornby *et al.* 1989).

The reported incidence rates for pressure sores vary from 4 to 40% or more and appear to be most often initiated in the period between injury and admission into a hospital bed; during this interval patients may lie for several hours unattended and without moving position (Heyse-Moore 1983b, Versluysen 1985). Davis *et al.* (1988) were unable to detect any effect on the risk of this complication in patients whose operations were delayed for more than 3 days after admission. Whatever the method of treatment chosen, the incidence of such general complications will inevitably remain a problem in the elderly patients who make up the majority of the relevant population.

Prolonged operations may also initiate sacral pressure sores or aggravate pre-existing problems, particularly in very elderly subjects.

Duration and cost of treatment

Trochanteric fractures which are not internally splinted usually require 6–10 weeks of external splintage, or traction, for union to occur, and a further period of 3 months with protection from full weight-bearing may be necessary if late deformity is to be minimized. Once the period of acute discomfort is over, further extension of the period in traction is largely dependent on the surgeon's attitude to late deformity. Operation, on the other hand, allows the possibility of leaving the hospital bed long before fracture union could be expected. This potential to reduce the period spent in acute surgical wards appears to be the most definite single advantage of operation over traction. Scott has pointed out, however, that this advantage in saving hospital beds, by an average of 60 days in his series, may be illusory to some extent because the time spent in 'second line' hospital beds or other institutions is not taken into account (Scott 1951). In a similar prospective trial 20 years later the advantage of accelerated discharge conferred by operation was found to be highly dependent on fracture stability when fixed-length nail plates were compared with Hamilton Russell traction. Operations for stable fractures led to an average shortening of the hospital stay by 1 month, but no such benefit occurred in the case of unstable fractures, which were attended by an unacceptably high rate of local complication (Hornby *et al.* 1986). When a compression screw plate device was substituted for the McLaughlin nail, a subsequent trial, which took account of the known risk factors as well as of fracture stability, demonstrated that the advantage for operation was no longer dependent on fracture stability: patients treated by the AO dynamic hip screw left hospital on average 28 days earlier than 'control' patients managed in traction (Hornby *et al.* 1989). Unlike the patient-related determinants of age, mentality and mobility, on which the surgeon can have no influence, the choice of implant and the care taken in its insertion may have a profound effect on the rehabilitation time. This observation, that the potential benefit of an operation to accelerate the process of rehabilitation may be seriously offset by a mechanical failure, has long exercised orthopaedic minds: the search for ways of reducing such risk has been the theme of countless publications (Hunter 1975, Jensen *et al.* 1980b, James & Hunter 1983, Jensen 1984).

Fracture mechanics

The resultant hip joint force acts on the femur along a line medial to the mid-point of the trochanteric region. The effect is thus to produce a bending moment which tends to produce a varus deformity after trochanteric fracture (Gozna & Harrington 1982).

In a simple, undisplaced, linear fracture, linking the trochanters, residual soft tissue anchorage at the injured cortical margins plus the compressive action of the overlying lateral muscles will be sufficient to prevent material displacement. Fractures showing wider initial separation may yet be capable of accurate reduction by gentle traction, abduction and appropriate rotation of the distal fragment to align it with the capital element. Such two-part fractures are conventionally described as 'stable' because of their inherent capacity for staying reduced (Figs 20.21 & 20.22).

In fact, trochanteric injuries are often more complex and avulsion of the lesser trochanter is common. When this apophyseal structure is avulsed at its tip the integrity of the tubular structure of the upper femur is not greatly altered and, thus, even in these three-part fractures, if the larger two elements are accurately apposed, cortex-to-cortex, they may also be regarded as stable. However, if the lesser trochanteric fragment is large enough to include the medial cortex of the neck and shaft regions, a medial fulcrum for a stable reduction is no longer available. The larger the fragment the less is the capacity to resist varus deformation, unless the medial fragment can be soundly held in position by a lag screw. Most three-part fractures are therefore regarded as unstable. With increasing comminution there is a greater degree of instability and increased likelihood of varus collapse.

Coronal plane fractures, noted on a lateral radiograph, are another source of instability; in these cases a seemingly accurate reduction is likely to be lost unless the anterior and posterior elements can be secured one to the other by lag screws, a feat not always practicable in the osteoporotic bone of many elderly patients (Fig. 20.24). Under load, these posterior and anterior elements displace in front of and behind the distal fragment, producing shortening and adduction deformity.

The rarer form of trochanteric fracture, in which the fracture line occurs in the opposite obliquity to the intertrochanteric ridge, sometimes called the reverse trochanteric pattern, is subject to loading more or less parallel to the line of the fracture and this shearing is the dominant deforming mechanism (Fig. 20.25).

In the usual form of trochanteric fracture, shear forces are resisted by opposing fracture surfaces after impaction around implants but, until impaction occurs, such implants must be strong enough to withstand the shear forces. In fractures managed conservatively, shearing is often a recognizable element in the residual deformity, despite longitudinal traction on the distal femur (Fig. 20.26). Rotation of the femoral shaft, in relation to the capital fragment, is one of the cardinal signs for clinical diagnosis of a fracture of the proximal femur (Fig. 20.22). Regard must be paid to the muscle forces producing

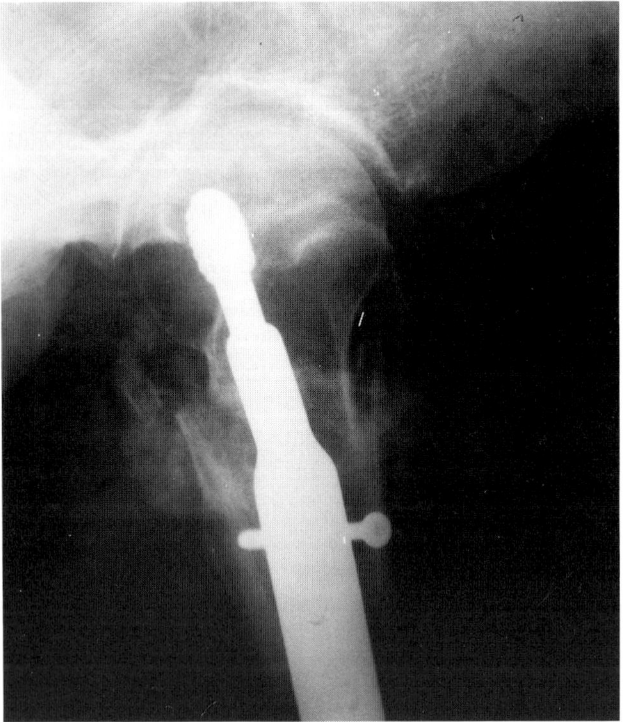

Fig. 20.24 Interfragmentary compression of a coronal plane fracture by a lag screw.

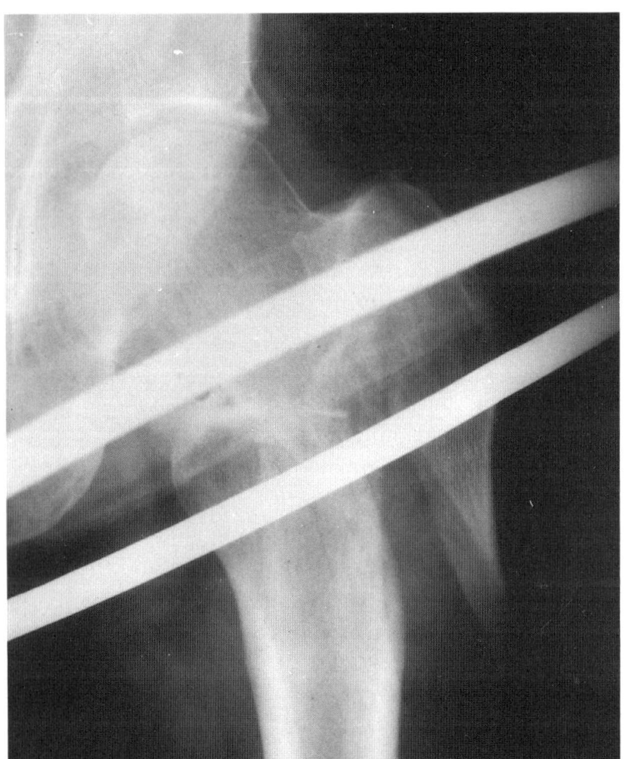

Fig. 20.25 Reverse oblique fracture.

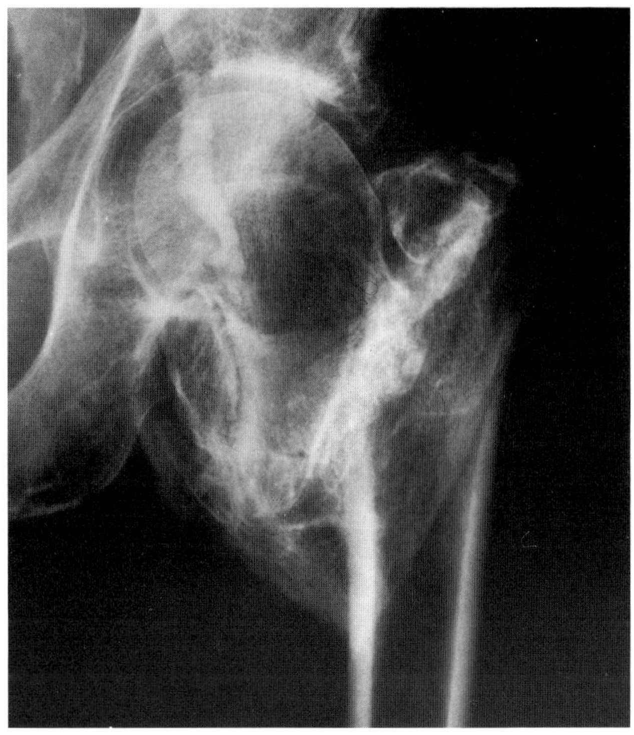

Fig. 20.26 End result of conservative management: shearing has occurred and there is plentiful callus in this region of cancellous bone.

this rotation, particularly during attempts at reduction, whether by closed or open technique (Horn & Wang 1964, May & Chacha 1968).

Classification of fracture patterns

Until World War II, non-operative management was the accepted practice: at that time the simple grouping into displaced and undisplaced fractures was helpful only in so far as it drew attention to the greater demands made by displaced fractures and the need for careful positioning of the limb so as to minimize deformity. The change of emphasis from external to internal splintage by fixed-length nail plates was followed by the emergence of mechanical complications not previously met after conservative treatment. Reduction of certain patterns of fracture was found to be difficult to achieve and to maintain, with a variable risk of secondary displacement of the bone fragments relative to each other and to the implant. However, generally simple patterns retained their stable reduction and allowed body weight and muscle forces to be shared between bone and implant without troublesome migration or mechanical failure of the nail plate.

Evans' system of classification (Fig. 20.27)

Evans classified trochanteric fractures according to whether or not stable reduction could be obtained (Evans 1949, 1951). He recognized two basic anatomical patterns: in type 1 the fracture line connected the greater and lesser trochanters; in the less common type 2 the fracture line was in the opposite diagonal, separating the two trochanters. In fact, type 2 fractures have more in common with subtrochanteric fractures, are nearly always displaced and are always unstable. A fundamental point in Evans' concept is that the term 'stability' should refer to the mechanical characteristics of the fragment assembly after attempted reduction and internal fixation by a nail plate. Thus, type 1 fractures, the undisplaced two-part fracture and the displaced two-part fracture, which has been reduced cortex-to-cortex, will usually remain stable after internal fixation. More comminuted type 1 fractures, where a separate third medial fragment is present, will buckle into varus under the normal compression load to which the proximal femur is subject. The only exception to this rule is the pattern in which the lesser trochanter is separated at its base from the adjacent medial femoral cortex, but which leaves the weight-transmitting tube of cortical bone intact. Most avulsions of the lesser trochanter involve significant amounts of surrounding posteromedial cortex, which leave a defect in the tubular compression-resisting structure and are therefore unstable. Posterior comminution, usually of the greater trochanter, allows the neck and shaft fragments to deform into extension, or, if the coronal fracture extends to the medial cortex, allows the neck fracture to shear into varus. Type 2 fractures are almost in the same line as the

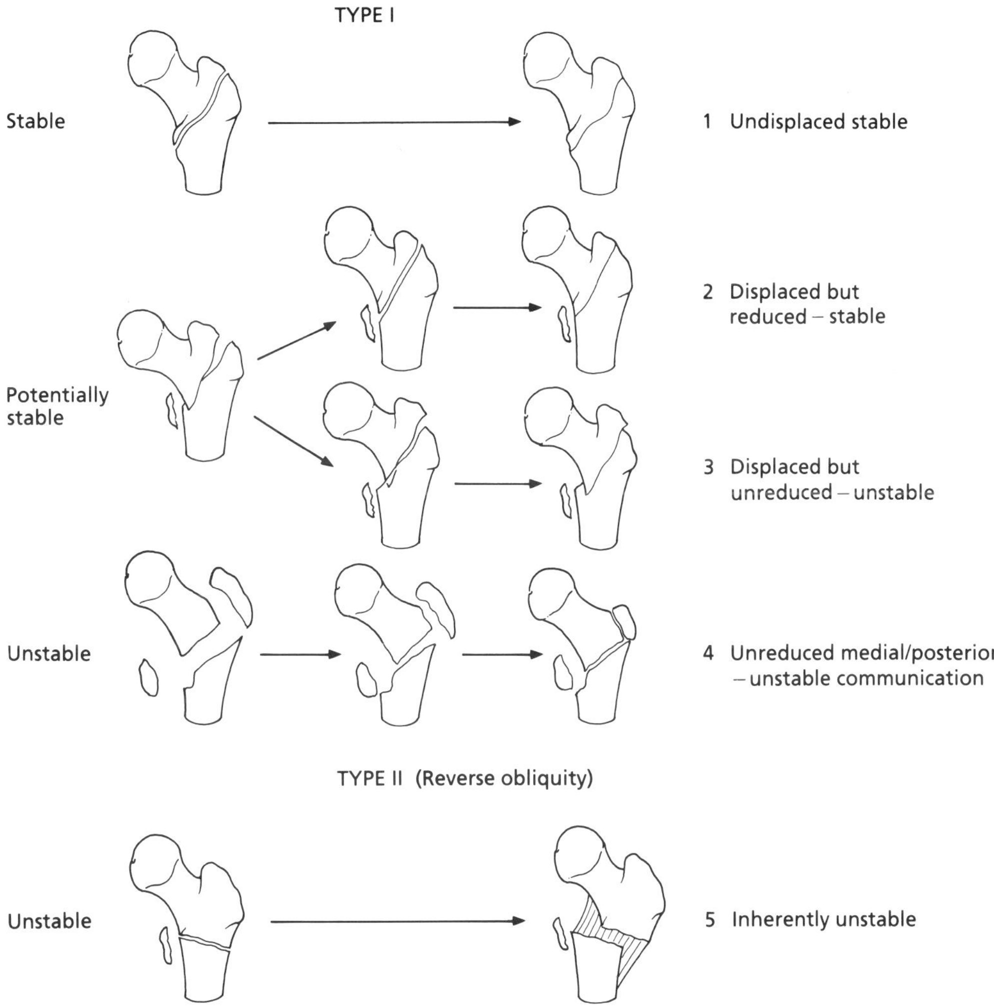

Fig. 20.27 Evans' classification of trochanteric fractures.

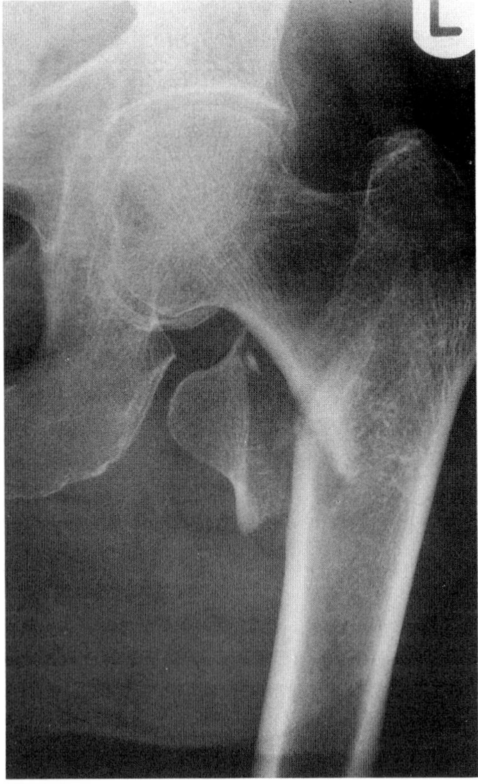 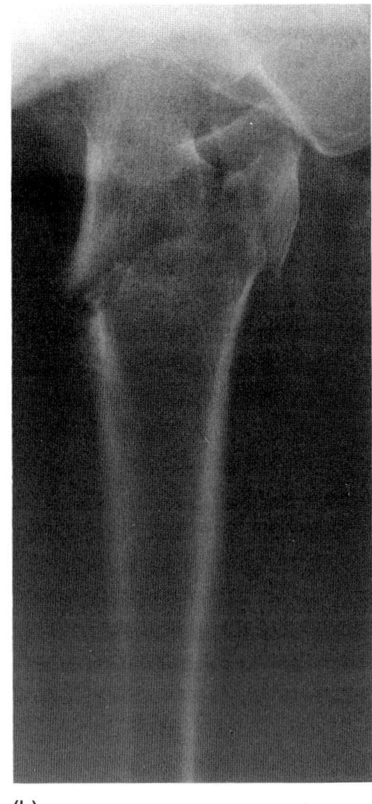

(a)   (b)

Fig. 20.28 (a) Posterolateral and (b) medial instability visible on these radiographs foretell secondary displacement.

trajectory of load and have no inherent resistance to shearing: thus, they are always unstable. Evans advised internal fixation of trochanteric fractures and recommended that classification be applied at the stage of attempted reduction on the basis of good anteroposterior and lateral radiographs (Fig. 20.28).

An ideal classification would allow the surgeon to predict, from scrutiny of the preoperative radiographs alone, the likelihood of a reduction being obtainable and the risk of subsequent displacement. Unfortunately, no such system has yet been revealed, although some are more effective than others. Another difficulty is that reduction and displacement are not independent of the type of operative treatment so that a universal classification is probably unattainable.

The Evans' system was slightly modified by Jensen and Michaelsen in 1975; they based the assessment on the primary radiographs after the accident and reduced the number of groups by including the reverse oblique fracture into group 3 (Table 20.9). In comparison with the systems of Ender, Tronzo and the AO method of classification, the Evans' grouping was found to be superior in its ability to predict the possibility of achieving anatomical fracture reduction and the risk of secondary displacement of trochanteric fractures treated by compression screws (Fig. 20.29). The degree of comminution thus determines the quality of reduction and the existence of residual fracture separation leads to secondary displacement. The Evans' classification, as modified by Jensen and Michaelsen, is therefore recommended (Müller *et al.* 1970, Tronzo 1973, Ender 1976, Jensen 1980b, 1981).

Table 20.9 Modification of the Evans' classification

Group	Anatomical reduction (%)*	Secondary displacement (%)
1	96	8
2	89	11
3	33	56
4	21	61
5	8	78

* Values are for anteroposterior/lateral.

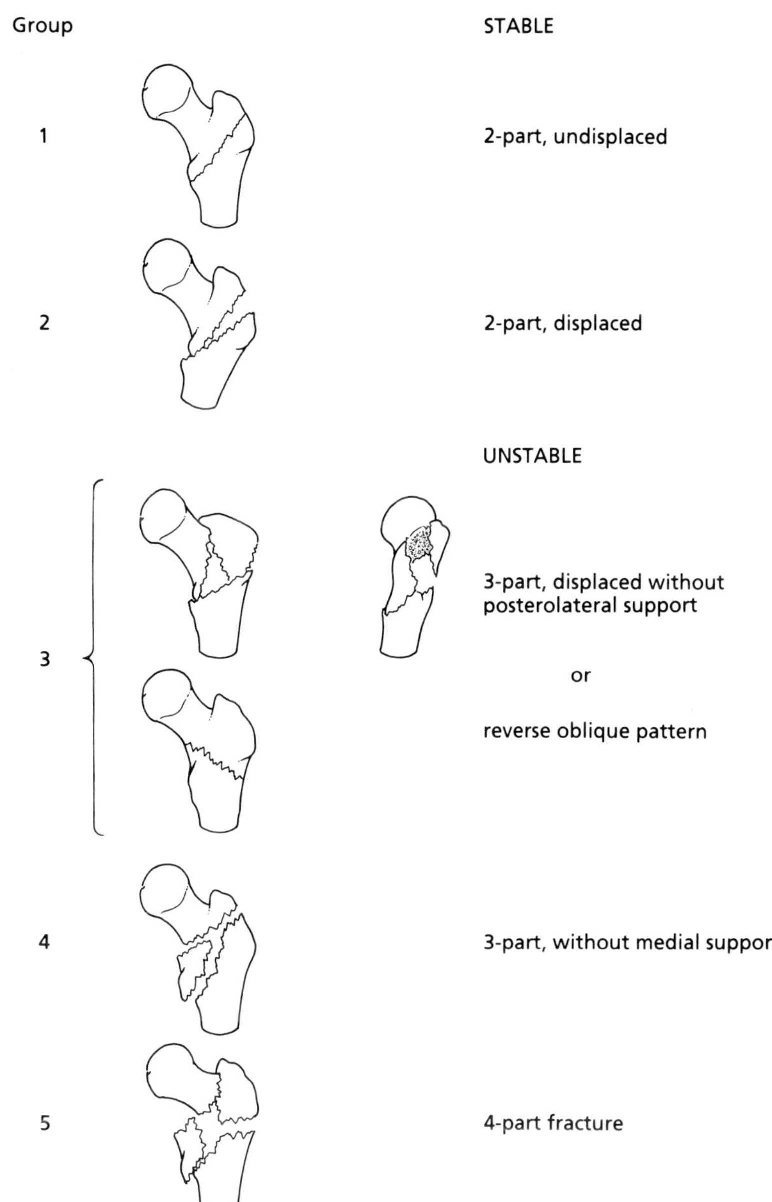

Fig. 20.29 Evans' classification as modified by Jensen and Michaelsen.

Biomechanics of internal fixation in trochanteric fractures

Stable fractures

Undisplaced fractures may heal without deformity when treated by 'benign neglect' — clearly the demands on implants inserted into such fractures must be minimal. Even when displaced, most two-part fractures can be held reduced by simple implants, either nail plate or intramedullary devices (Fig. 20.30) (James & Hunter 1983).

Implants that rely on a lateral plate screwed to the upper femoral shaft are further from the line of the hip joint force than intramedullary devices, and are therefore subjected to greater bending moments. In the case of a two-part fracture, reduced into a position of good overall alignment and without cortical overlap as judged on anteroposterior and lateral radiographs, but with a gap remaining between the two elements, the bending moments are resisted by the implant alone. The sequence of events after such operations depends on several mechanical factors. If the implant is strong, the bone is of good texture and the nail has a relatively blunt tip, then the fracture gap may be maintained and non-union may occur. Fatigue failure of the implant may eventually lead to varus collapse which may, in turn, lead to bony contact and fracture union. Where the implant is less rigid the nail may deform until the medial cortices abut, with slow union progressing from medial to lateral ends of the fracture line.

When the nail has a small cross-section, particularly if it has been sharpened to ease insertion by hammering or where the bone quality of the head fragment is poor, body weight and muscle forces may combine to drive the nail further into the head — even penetrating the hip joint, when a long nail has been inserted close to the subchondral bone plate, or emerging from the anterior cervical cortex. This relative motion of implant and capital fragment occurs in three dimensions, with the nail tip cutting forwards in the head and rotating laterally as well as migrating vertically. Fortunately, these movements are usually limited as the fracture surfaces impact and the excess forces on the nail are progressively reduced; the fracture thereby comes under compression.

Unstable fractures

In three- and four-part fractures there is no inherent stability in the fracture assembly, even when reduced. Medial comminution prevents the buttressing which resists varus bending moments in unstable injuries and/or there may be separate large posterior elements in relation to the greater trochanter (Fig. 20.31).

Recognizing that such fractures could not be safely or

reliably treated by fixed-length nail plates, because of the inevitable varus bending moments, rotational and shear forces which led either to mechanical failure or to cutting-out of the nail, Evans considered that varus deformity was the lesser evil and advised that unstable fractures should be fixed in a varus position. When such unstable fractures are nailed in anatomical alignment, the limitations of fixed-length devices are more obvious. A nail which is long enough to prevent rotation of the head fragment is more likely to protrude as impaction occurs: a shorter nail may not project into the hip joint, but may fail to stop rotation into varus and external rotation. Another complication of too short a nail is subcapital fracture at the tip of the nail, which acts as a stress-riser (Cleveland *et al.* 1947, Kauffer *et al.* 1974, 1980, Baker 1975, Jensen *et al.* 1980a).

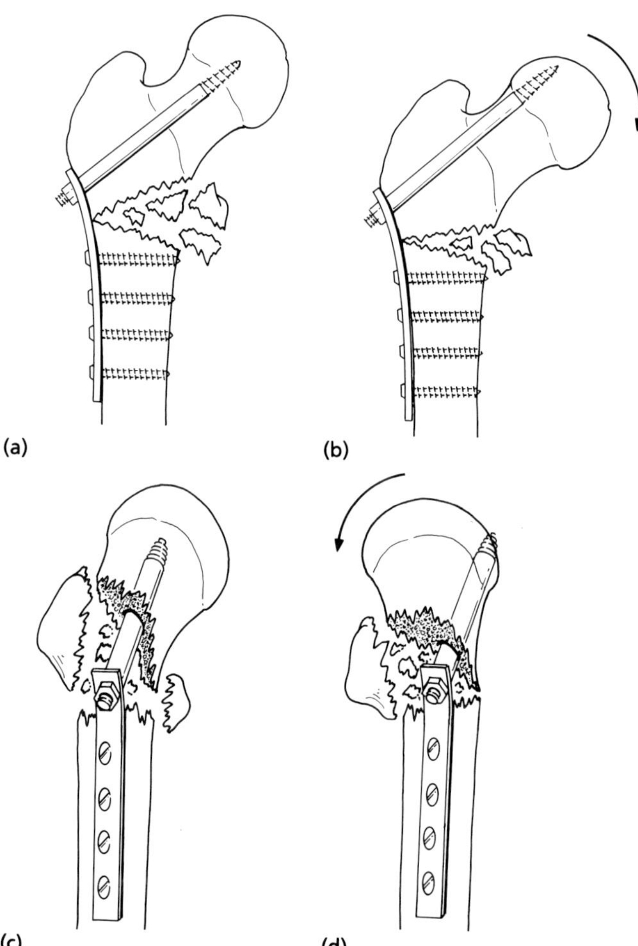

Fig. 20.31 Unstable fractures. (a) Lack of medial support. (b) Varus bends around the nail — the nail cuts upwards in the head and neck fragment. (c) Lack of posterior support. (d) Extension collapse of a capital fragment — the nail cuts out through the anterior cortex of the neck.

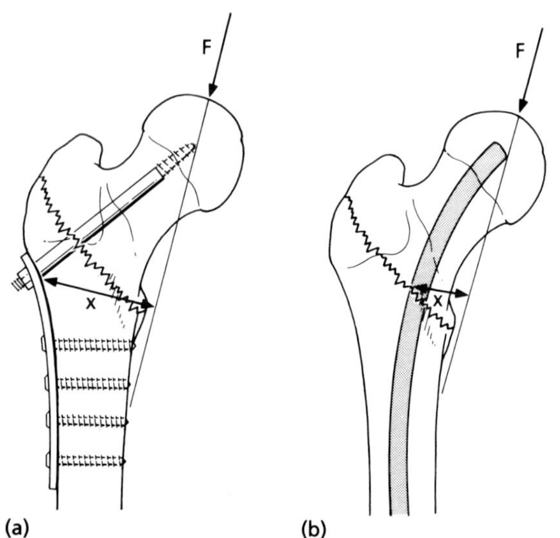

Fig. 20.30 Stable fractures. (a) Nail plates sustain bending stresses at the junctional region, which is at the maximum distance from the line of the hip joint resultant force. (b) Intramedullary implants lie nearer to the trajectory of hip joint force and are less prone to bending.

Surgeons who are unwilling to accept Evans' fatalistic approach have exercised considerable ingenuity in trying to combine internal fixation at the same time as avoiding adduction deformity. Sarmiento advocated trimming the fracture surfaces so that the capital fragment could be adducted into extreme valgus, placing the new 'fracture line' under almost pure compression. He inserted a short strong nail of an appropriately steep angle to fix this non-anatomical arrangement (Fig. 20.32) (Sarmiento 1967, 1970, 1973).

Dimon and Hughston (1967) advocated jamming the inferior calcar spike into the medullary canal of the medially displaced upper femoral shaft. A short nail was then driven up into the neck fragment through the open fracture site and the greater trochanter. From a biomechanical point of view both these methods aim to reduce the bending lever arm by moving the fracture site medially and closer to the line of hip joint force (Fig. 20.33).

Displacing unstable fractures into valgus has the virtue of tending to restore leg length. Fixing unstable fractures by sliding screw devices almost invariably produces a medializing effect on the shaft (Fig. 20.34).

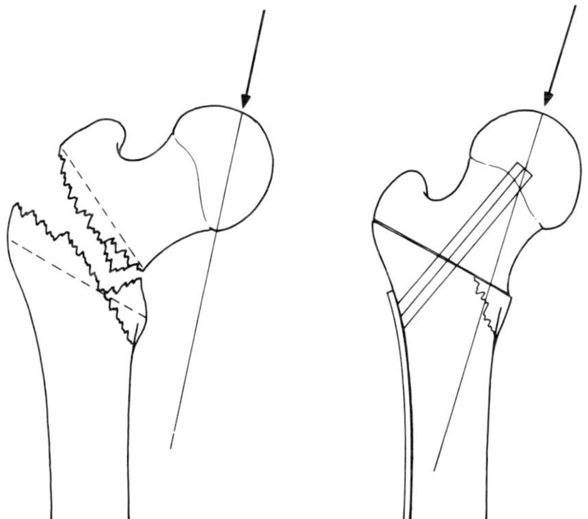

Fig. 20.32 Valgus reduction, after trimming of the fracture surfaces, brings the assembly under compression. A short, steeply angled nail is then required. (A compression screw/plate may be used as an alternative implant.)

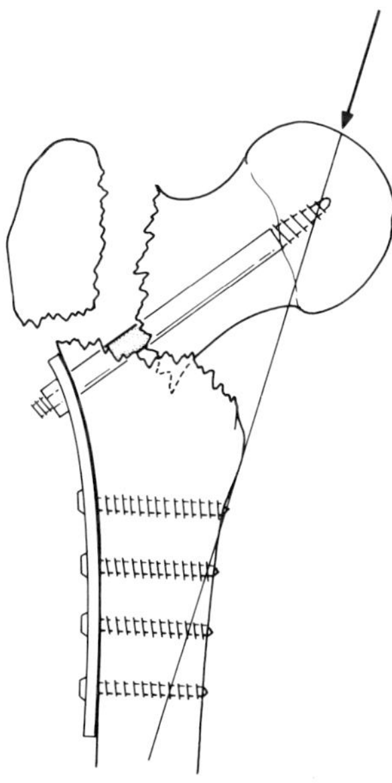

Fig. 20.33 Deliberate medial displacement: the inferior spike of the calcar femorale is jammed into the medullary canal of the shaft. The greater trochanteric fragment is ignored.

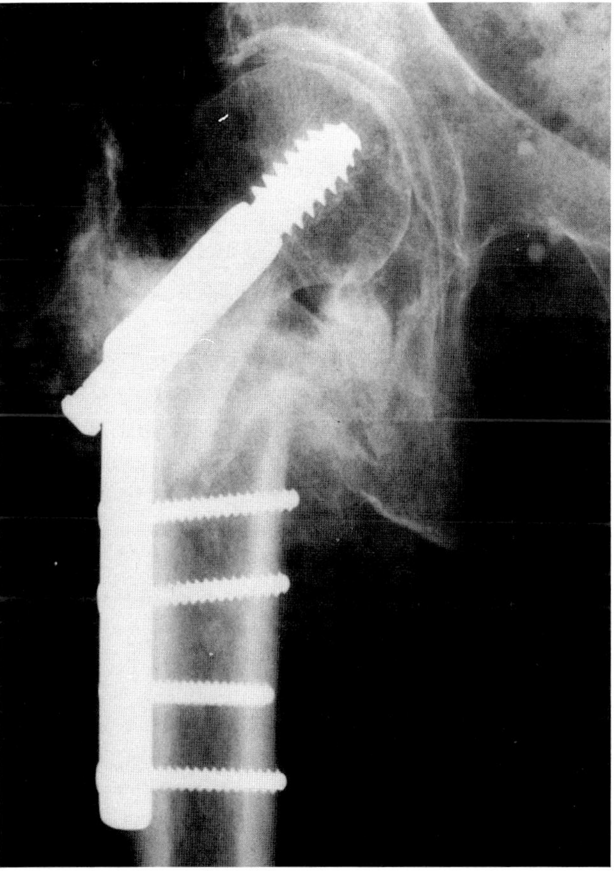

Fig. 20.34 Displacement of an unstable fracture treated with an AO dynamic hip screw.

Evolution of surgical treatment

Nail plates (Fig. 20.35)

Until 1945 conservative treatment was generally accepted as appropriate for the typical elderly patient with a trochanteric fracture. A mortality rate of, roughly, one in five was regarded as almost inevitable, as was the general morbidity associated with age, recumbency and fracture.

In 1948, Evans presented the results of a case series of 22 fractures treated by fixation with a nail plate at the Birmingham Accident Hospital. No 'fatalities' were observed, hospital stay was shortened by half and the patients were reported to be more comfortable and mobile than when treated by non-operative methods. Evans was careful to point out that internal fixation

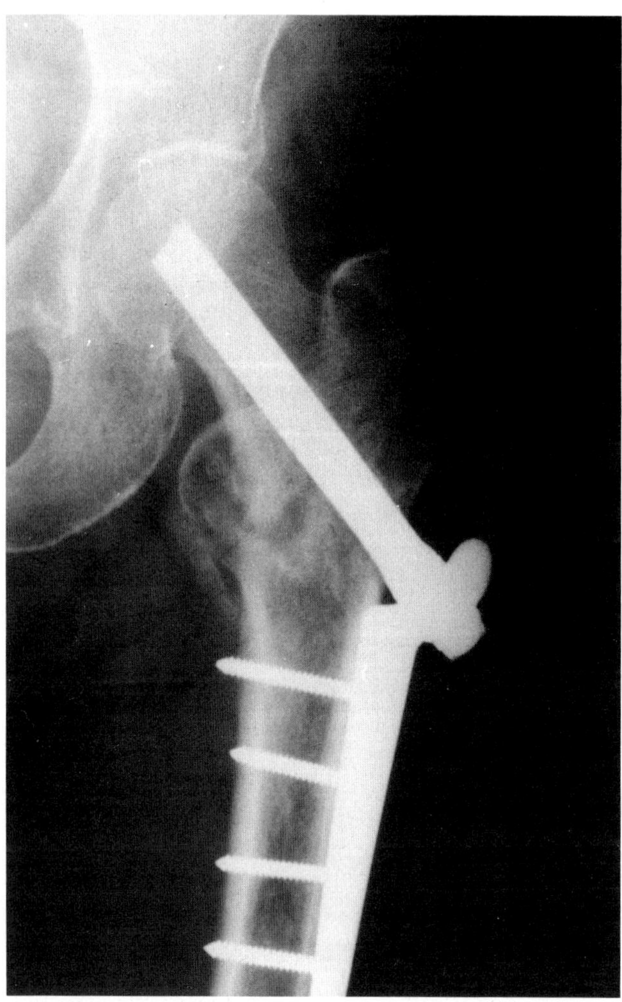

Fig. 20.35 Nail plate. The nail angle can be varied on the curved proximal end of the plate.

with the relatively weak nail plate then available could not be expected to maintain reduction of fractures in which there was a discontinuity in the medial cortical buttress. The nail would either bend into varus or break, usually at the nail–plate junction. He presented a carefully considered classification, which has subsequently been vindicated, and suggested that unstable fractures (29% in his series) should be nailed in a position of varus deformity. He argued that great age and great frailty, rather than being contraindications as had hitherto been thought, were, in fact, no bar to internal fixation which was presented as a life-saving measure.

It is an interesting comment on surgical behaviour that the least well-founded part of Evans' case — that operation improved mortality and morbidity — should have been accepted, almost without question, for the subsequent three decades, and that the risks of nailing unstable fractures in anatomical alignment rather than varus position was received with less enthusiasm (Foster 1958, Hunter 1975, Jensen 1981).

The hoped- for rapid mobilization after nail plating was observed most consistently in patients with simple linear fractures that could be rendered stable by bringing the medial cortices into accurate reduction. Such patients, particularly if they were relatively young, appreciated the early discharge from hospital. However, unstable fractures appeared to be more numerous than had been thought and other fractures, which were apparently 'stable' on admission radiographs, were all too often discovered to be difficult to reduce without cortical overlap and later displacement. The following 10 years saw the emergence of stronger and stiffer nails which were more resistant to bending and breakage and were used in an attempt to cope with the instability of often imperfect reductions (Tronzo 1974, James & Hunter 1983).

Blade plates (Fig. 20.36)

The blade plate, proposed by the Swiss AO group of surgeons, differed from the conventional nail plates by having the proximal segment directed horizontally; it was then better able to resist downward displacement of the capital fragment than were nails co-axial with the femoral neck. A high stress concentration at the junctional area, as occurs with nail plates, leads to fatigue fracture after a predictable number of load cycles if deformation is not prevented by medial bone buttressing. Complex interfragmentary fixation is often required if this complication is to be avoided in unstable injuries.

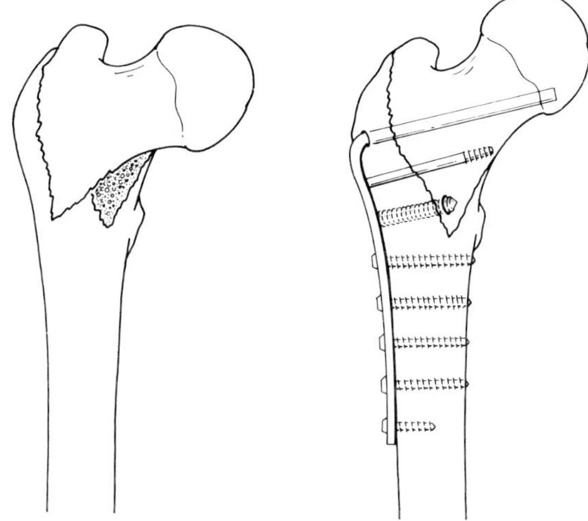

Fig. 20.36 Angled blade plate.

An additional limitation of these intramedullary implants is the need to create a cortical hole in the distal femur: the stress-riser effect may then result in fractures at the lower end of the femur, in addition to those already present at the proximal end! Because load is borne over a longer segment, intramedullary devices are theoretically less prone to bending and fatigue failure than are nail plates. Resistance to torsional loads is not an outstanding feature of the solitary intramedullary nail and the use of multiple pins inserted in a fan-like arrangement within the femoral head is a way of overcoming this defect (Ender 1976, 1978, Kuntscher 1977, Harris 1980, Chapman *et al.* 1981).

When bone grafting is used as an alternative, the uncertain outcome of the race between graft maturation and implant fracture is mechanically unattractive. In reality, sound mechanical stability may only be achieved at the expense of prolonged and technically difficult surgery, even in younger subjects with good quality bone, and in the typical osteoporotic, elderly patient stabilization may be unrealistic. In the English-speaking countries the method of angle blade plate fixation was never popular. Regazzoni has contrasted the biomechanical characteristics of this type of implant and its clinical outcome as unfavourable compared with the characteristics of the sliding screw (Müller *et al.* 1970, Ganz *et al.* 1979, Regazzoni *et al.* 1985).

Intramedullary devices (Fig. 20.37)

As has already been observed, implants which are enclosed within the medullary cavity of the femur lie nearer to the line of force across the hip joint and therefore sustain lower bending stresses than nail plates which are more laterally placed. However, unless intramedullary nails are free to slide, they are no less likely to perforate a hip than are conventional nails. The surgeon must gauge very accurately how much impaction is likely to occur and insert the nail so that the tip(s) is kept far enough from subchondral bone, to allow for this relative motion, but not left so short as to be ineffectual in resisting bending stresses. When nails are inserted more loosely, so as to allow for sliding in the event of impaction, there is usually a price to pay in soft tissue discomfort at the distal end of the femur as the nail backs out.

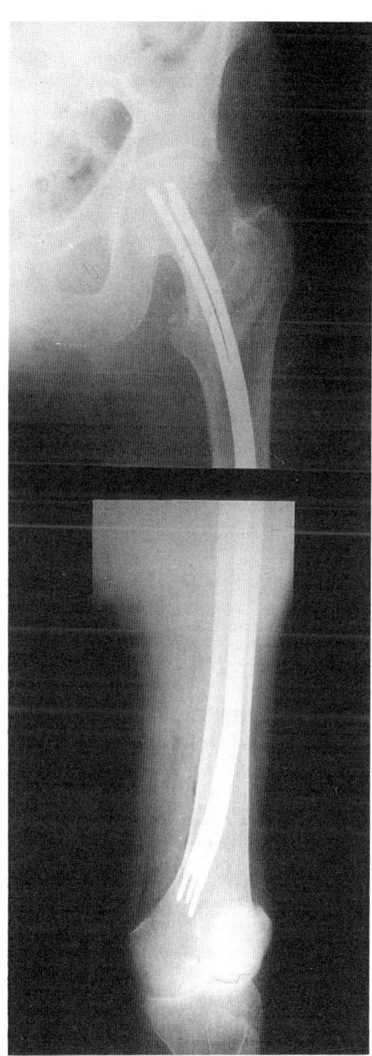

Fig. 20.37 Ender's flexible pins.

Sliding nail and screw plates (Figs 20.38 & 20.39)

One way of avoiding the risks of joint penetration and cutting-out, which are inherent in the fixed-length devices, is to make the part of the implant which crosses the fracture zone of variable length by using a separate 'capital' element which is allowed to slide within a tubular extension of the side plate. The chief benefit of this group of implants is that they allow controlled collapse of the fractured fragments into a stable configuration so that load is shared between bone and implant. The capital element is firmly held by the nail or screw, and track-bound collapse occurs along the axis of the screw, which descends within the barrel of the plate element. In unstable fractures, with a large separate medial fragment, collapse may bring the shaft fragment much closer to the hip force line, thus effectively reduce the bending moment — as occurs in medial displacement osteotomy. In the case of stable fractures, however, in osteoporotic bone a slow shearing in the plane of the fracture is commonly observed, indicating that migration of the head fragment is occurring in a downwards and medial direction and/or some resorption is occurring at the fracture surfaces (Heyse-Moore & MacEachern 1983). One benefit of the sliding screw over sliding nails is the ability to create compression of the impacted fracture surfaces at the time of operation by arranging for the tip of the capital screw shank to be drawn down, under tension, by a secondary screw inserted into the tip of the capital screw shank (Schumpelick & Jantzen 1955, Callender 1957, Clawson 1964, Ecker *et al.* 1975).

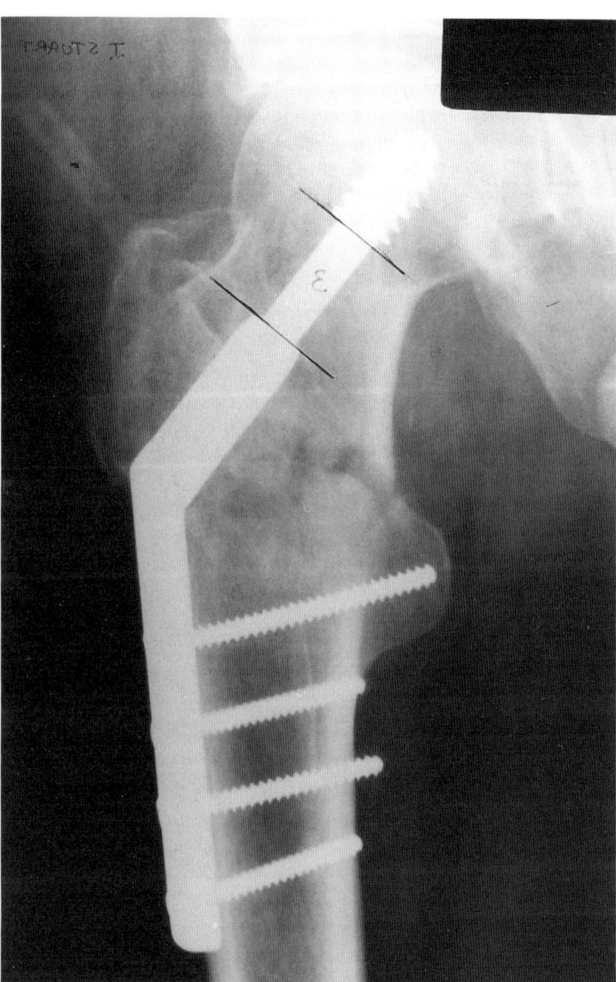

Fig. 20.38 Posterolateral instability has led to 2 cm displacement along the axis of the screw. Compare the postoperative film (this Fig.) with the radiograph 6 months later (Fig. 20.39).

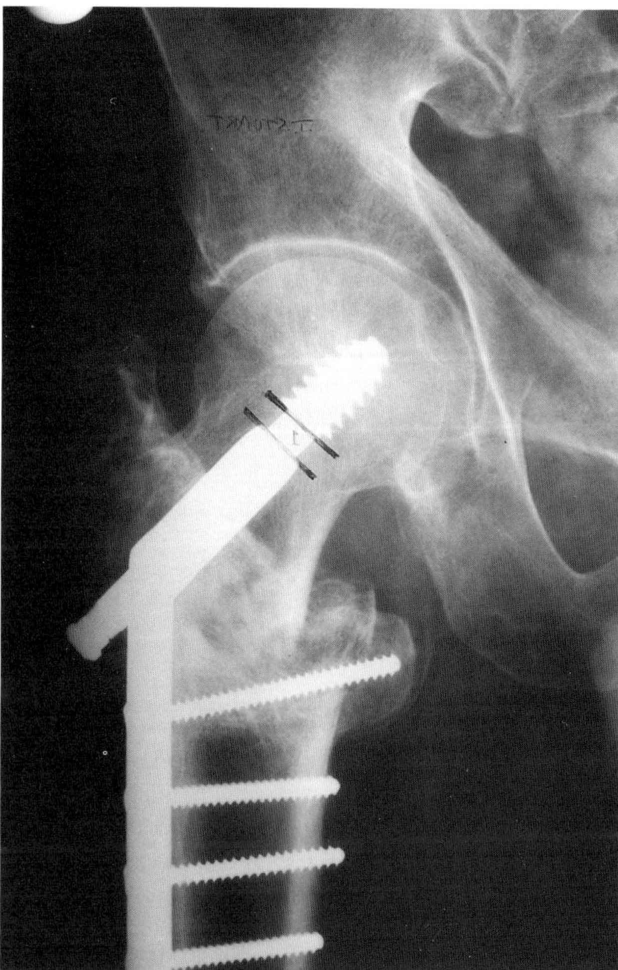

Fig. 20.39 The effect on the shaft is to produce a medializing effect.

The mechanical considerations relating to reduced bending and shearing and to increased compression forces obtained by valgus reduction, with or without medial displacement as described in relation to fixed-length nail plates, apply equally well to sliding devices (Friedenberg *et al.* 1972, Harrington & Johnston 1973, Regazzoni *et al.* 1985).

Two-component intramedullary nails

The Kuntscher 'Y' nail, which has a perforated capital element to allow passage of an intramedullary nail inserted via the greater trochanter, is clearly subjected to smaller bending moments than the nail plate. It allows the collapse of trochanteric fractures in a vertical direction only, and once this capacity has been used up any residual medial evidence of instability is liable to generate the same problems of penetration and cutting-out as occurs with nail plates (Cuthbert & Howat 1976).

The Zickel nail, in which the capital element passes through a hole in the shaft element, is, like the Kuntscher 'Y' nail, better suited to accommodate axial shortening in the subtrochanteric region (Fig. 20.40). A shorter variant is the 'Gamma nail'. The vertical element is wide at the proximal end, curving distally to match the femoral shaft, and tapers in the subtrochanteric part. The screw segment has a thick, heavy shank with a smaller threaded tip and is designed for insertion without prior tapping. Collapse along the axis of the

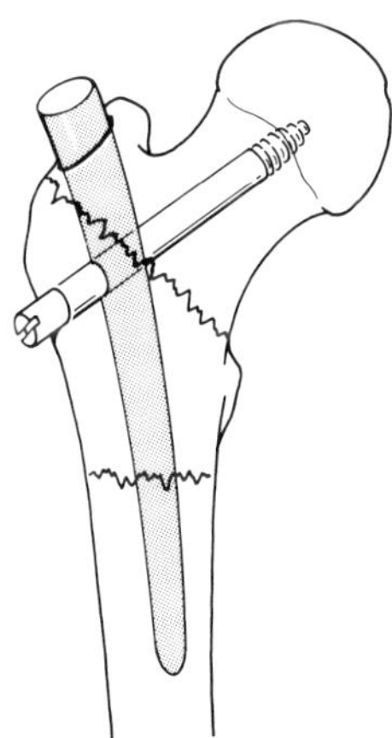

Fig. 20.40 The two-component intramedullary device accommodates subtrochanteric collapse around the shaft of the nail. Unless the capital element is capable of sliding, it is liable to problems of all fixed-length implants — cutting-out anteriorly and superiorly when instability is present.

femoral neck may be accommodated by leaving the capital screw loose in the shaft element (Halder & Gill 1988). Controlled trials have not supported the use of 'Gamma nails' in preference to *et al.* the AO dynamic hip screw (Bridle *et al.* 1991, Leung *et al.* 1992, Radford *et al.* 1993).

Two problems associated with conventional devices which employ side plates are loosening and pulling-out of the screws which secure the plate to the femoral shaft, and a more dramatic secondary fracture through the area weakened by the screw holes. Securing the capital screw by an intramedullary nail elegantly avoids these mechanical problems, as well as reducing the bending moments.

For a quantitative treatment of the biomechanical aspects of trochanteric fractures and their fixation, the review by Jensen (1981) and the earlier work of Kauffer (1974, 1980) are useful starting points. For the historically-interested reader Tronzo (1974) has catalogued the wide variety of implants which have been designed for trochanteric fractures.

Treatment

Typical elderly patients

Surgical treatment allows the possibility of earlier discharge from hospital and better preservation of leg length and social independence than does conservative treatment, but it introduces specific additional complications, such as infection and mechanical failure, which non-operative management avoids. As neither method confers any significant advantage in respect of general medical complications or ultimate survival, and as they are equally sensitive to the level of nursing care, a logical choice of treatment must take other factors into account.

Thus, nursing care, operating theatre environment and type of implant available, as well as patient factors, such as suitability for anaesthesia, intercurrent illness and injury, type of fracture and personal attitudes to surgical and other risks, must all be considered. Unless the operating theatre environment can be shown to have an overall infection risk close to zero, for example, $< 2\%$, it is difficult to justify what is, effectively, elective surgery in these patients. Such infection rates are commonly achieved in the context of total hip replacement, but significantly higher rates have been reported for trochanteric fractures without apparent embarrassment (Jacobs *et al.* 1976, James & Hunter 1983). In the writer's view, no less an exacting technique is appropriate and a 'clean air' operating enclosure is recommended. If nursing care is poor, operation will not improve the overall results. Some patients with stable fractures, well-preserved in mind and body, may escape early and enjoy a good outcome, but this fortunate minority will be offset by the larger group of very old, mentally impaired, osteoporotic patients with unstable fractures who will never recover from their injury.

The use of fixed-length implants, now less popular, can no longer be justified in the context of unstable fractures, although a reasonably satisfactory outcome is usually obtained in Jensen type I and type II injuries, if the nail is inserted correctly. Unfortunately, in the real world, the estimation of fracture stability from preoperative radiographs cannot always be achieved and few surgeons avoid the dismal discovery of unwelcome and unexpected secondary fracture lines at the time of operation. Stability is a function of the particular arrangement of bony fragments obtained at the end of the procedure and a lack of it can only be assessed in retrospect from serial postoperative films. In the event of miscalculation the patient may pay an unacceptably high price, unless the implant is designed to accommodate collapse. Not least for this reason, traditional nail plates cannot be recommended, even for stable fractures, if more forgiving implants, capable of shortening with fracture displacement, are available (Jensen & Michaelsen 1975, Jensen 1978, Jensen *et al.* 1980c).

The presence of infection, particularly in the affected limb and most often from pressure sores, is a contra-indication to operation. In many cases such lesions precede the injury which led to fracture. More often, they are generated in the period between the fall and arrival in a hospital bed. Long periods lying on stretchers are probably the most dangerous in this respect (Versluysen 1985). Clinical diagnosis of hip fracture is sufficient reason to institute preventive measures: sacral padding and sheepskin bootees for the heels are basic requirements before radiographic examination. Once admitted to hospital, and after anteroposterior and lateral radiographs have been obtained, the patient should have light balanced skin traction applied: 2.2–4.5 kg (5–10 lb), with the limb in slight abduction, is usually sufficient to achieve an immediate improvement in the level of discomfort. Heavy sedation and powerful analgesic drugs are seldom necessary, and in the typical case are often harmful.

Routine assessment of electrolyte and water balance not uncommonly reveals significant dehydration in elderly subjects. Failure to rectify this promptly is a frequent cause of worsening of the patient's general well-being and level of mentation. An assessment of mental function by one of the well-established numerical scales will give an accurate prediction of survival outcome (Blessed *et al.* 1969, Denham & Jeffreys 1972). When taken in conjunction with information about the previous social circumstances, this information allows a realistic plan to be formulated for long-term care and enables appropriate family and community support to be organized. A positive attitude to rehabilitation needs to be displayed by the whole nursing and surgical team from the earliest stage, but goals must be realistic. Maintenance of whatever mobility and independence remains is the best that can be expected and unrealistic plans to improve on the pre-injury status are best avoided by a careful appraisal of the background and circumstances of the patient. The typical patient presenting with a trochanteric fracture has evidence of some degree of impairment in at least three body systems other than the skeleton (Fitzgerald 1965). Preparation for anaesthesia may therefore take several hours or days for optimum improvement to be obtained. No absolutely reliable evidence is available regarding the effect of delay in operation and similar uncertainty applies to the choice between spinal and general anaesthesia (Davis *et al.* 1988). If the patient cannot be made fit for operation in a reasonable length of time or if, for whatever reason, surgery is not appropriate, further management in balanced traction may be confidently offered as carrying no increased risk to life. The view that 'the most frail patients have most to gain from surgery', and the conclusion that operations should seldom be withheld, was first propounded when operation carried serious risks. Even with safer modern procedures there is little or no evidence to support this view and its survival, during an era when nail plates were repeatedly demonstrated as having baneful complication rates of up to 40%, is difficult to explain on purely scientific grounds (James & Hunter 1983).

The load-sharing characteristics of the sliding screw implant, and its ability to produce track-bound impaction of fracture surfaces without material risk of penetration of the acetabulum or anterior cortex of the femoral neck, has reduced the former importance of preoperative radiographs in assessing fracture patterns and potential stability. Indeed, unless the surgeon plans to improve stability in type III, IV and V fractures by some embellishment of technique, such as medial displacement and osteotomy or valgus alignment of the capital fragment, the exercise of classification is little more than a predictor of the extent of ultimate displacement after reduction, and makes no material contribution to the management when these telescoping implants are used. The increased morbidity, arising from more prolonged operations, greater blood loss and soft tissue dissection with these complex techniques has not been shown to confer any advantage over conventional fixation and such procedures are not recommended (Laros & Moore 1974).

Practical details of operative treatment (AO dynamic hip screw)

The following technique has been found to be satisfactory. The patient is placed on an orthopaedic operating table with leg extensions. Longitudinal traction is applied to the affected leg and somewhat less powerful traction to the opposite limb, which is abducted as near to 45° as possible. The affected limb is held in very slight abduction. The opposite limb is not flexed at the hip as this leaves the pelvis free to move, usually throwing the iliac crest into the line of the horizontal X-ray beam and so obscuring the view. A mild internal rotation force may be of benefit in this regard. Surgical and nursing teams wear protective lead aprons and thyroid shields. A C-arm image intensifier, preferably with image retention facility, is then positioned over the upper femur to give a satisfactory anteroposterior image and its height is adjusted so that it can be rotated for a horizontal projection without the need for further repositioning. The fractured limb is then positioned so as to restore, as closely as possible, the normal relationships between the femoral neck and shaft. To some extent, the requisite manoeuvres can be predicted by the fracture pattern, but not all patients are equally obliging and trial of internal and external rotation, in combination with varying amounts of longitudinal traction, is the most dependable approach. Rarely, open reduction may be necessary, when the ilio-psoas tendon is caught between fragments or when stubborn impaction is present (Tronzo 1973).

When the best reduction has been obtained, the skin is prepared with alcoholic povidone—iodine solution applied from the knee to the iliac crest. A large sterile sheet of clear polythene is stuck to the proximal aspect of the thigh and suspended from a horizontal rail about 2 m in height and extending down to the floor level; this divides the clean air zone of the operating theatre into a sterile area for the surgical team and a dirty area for the radiological and anaesthetic teams.

A mid-lateral incision is made, extending 15 cm distally from the tip of the greater trochanter and continuing down through the deep fascia and fascia lata. The glistening fibrous layer of the vastus lateralis is then carefully incised in approximately the same line and the posterior edge is retained in three or four artery forceps. The underlying muscle fibres are then gently teased away from the deep surface of the fibrous layer, which is held out horizontally by an assistant. A rounded periosteal elevator of the Cobb or Dewar pattern is most suitable. When the periosteum comes into view, the perforating vessels are cauterized and divided and the muscle is then held anteriorly by a self-retaining retractor whose posterior jaws engage the posterior deep fascia, superficial to the muscle layer which is generally too friable for retraction purposes. A 135° angle guide is then placed firmly on the lateral cortex and an aiming wire is placed in front of it and the soft tissue in front of the femoral neck for preliminary anteroposterior screening. It is important that the operator appreciates that the ultimate target is the centre of the femoral head, not merely the centre of the neck; the commonest error is to place the guide too high (Mulholland & Gunn 1972). A pointed guide wire with a threaded tip is then passed through the guide, drilled through the cortex and inserted into the middle of the femoral head under X-ray screening (Fig. 20.41). The requisite angle, in relation to the coronal plane, can be estimated roughly from the alignment of the patella, allowing for femoral neck anteversion, but some realignment is usually necessary when the horizontal radiograph is obtained. The repositioning must be done with care and the C-arm should be held in the horizontal mode whilst it is being done. The pin is withdrawn, almost to the lateral cortex, and then, keeping the guide firmly pressed on to the femur, the pin is rotated in the guide anteriorly or posteriorly until it can be passed exactly through the centre line of the femoral head and until the threaded tip engages the subchondral bone 2 mm short of the apparent joint line. The C-arm is then replaced in the anteroposterior position to confirm satisfactory alignment. If difficulty is encountered in obtaining a good lateral alignment, then the most likely explanation is that the cortical hole has been made too far anteriorly or posteriorly to allow medullary drilling. This results in attempts to rotate the pin as desired merely causing jamming on the inner aspect of the cervical cortex. Drilling the pilot hole a few millimetres in the appropriate direction, forwards or backwards, at the same level on the femur is the remedy.

When a satisfactory pin placement has been obtained, as judged on anteroposterior and lateral views, the intraosseous length of the pin from the cortex to subchondral bone is measured to the nearest millimetre

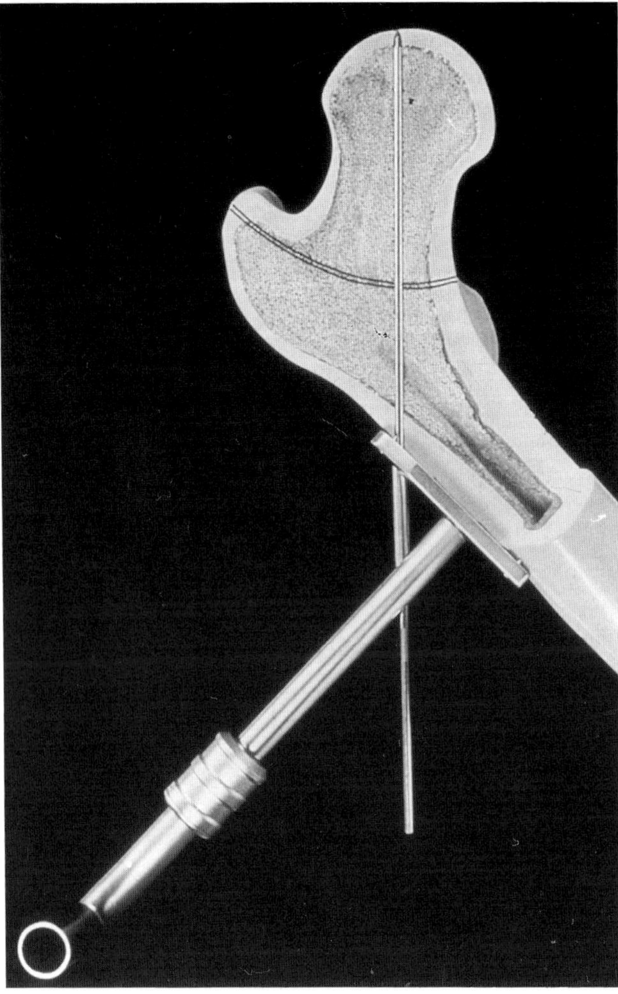

Fig. 20.41 A 135° guide is used to introduce a guide wire into the centre of the femoral head.

(Fig. 20.42). The reamer is then adjusted to a length 10 mm shorter and a screw, 20 mm shorter than the pin length, is selected. The outer cortex and femoral neck are then reamed and the screw is inserted on its guide wire until its tip comes to lie between 5 and 10 mm from the joint, as judged on anteroposterior and lateral views. Prior tapping of the reamed track is seldom required in elderly patients but in young patients it may be advantageous. A four-hole plate is then passed over the shank of the capital screw and secured with a small, fine-threaded screw inserted into the base of the shank (Figs 20.42, 20.43 & 20.44).

The plate is then aligned in the long axis of the femur. The distal end may need rotating slightly and it is then pressed firmly against the cortex as the distal screw is inserted. A reversible power drill for thread tapping and screw insertion shortens the operating time, and if two separate drills are available the procedure can be further accelerated. Finally, traction should be released and preliminary impaction encouraged by further tightening of the small compression screw to draw the capital and shaft elements closer together. The fibrous layer of the muscle and the deep fascial layer are then sutured and a suction drain applied to the subfascial space. The adhesive seal is then elevated at the skin edges which are wiped again with povidone−iodine and the skin is closed with interrupted sutures or staples. Systemic antibiotics are given with premedication and for 48 hours thereafter.

The above is a summary of the current technique as applied to typical elderly osteoporotic females with trochanteric fractures and to the group of middle-aged patients whose health is not uncommonly impaired by alcohol or other drugs and in whom osteopenia is usually less severe.

In younger adults, stable fractures may be treated in the same way. In contrast, unstable fractures usually reflect high-energy accidents and the risk of shortening after sliding screw fixation may be unacceptable. In such cases attempts at interfragmentary compression, to produce a stable configuration, may be feasible, but if this appears unattainable then judicious use of traction, either as an alternative or as a supplement to operation, is recommended.

The less common reverse oblique fracture has an inherent tendency to displace. Stability may be obtained by interfragmentary compression screws, which are passed in front of and behind the main implant, or by notching the apposing surfaces to provide interlocking (Tronzo 1973).

Postoperative care is centred on meticulous attention to skin pressure areas, adequate hydration and nutrition and a realistic programme of mobilization. For many senior victims of trochanteric injury, their normal life is predominantly sedentary and a return to the level of activity enjoyed prefracture should be the aim. A cheerful, optimistic environment, familiar clothing and kind encouragement all help to revive the will and ability to remain active. Once a patient's wound drains have been removed, he or she should be helped to stand and dress and to take a few steps. The process should be repeated several times a day and modest goals should be set for the mentally alert to achieve. For the infirm, demented inmates of psychogeriatric institutions, the ability to sit without support may be the best that can be achieved. The whole rehabilitation team should be aware of the overriding effects of mental impairment and age on the outcome. Between 10 and 14 days after operation it is generally clear whether a patient is going to return to somewhere near the pre-injury state and what form of accommodation, family support or social service help may be required. By 3 months most fractures will have united but unstable injuries may have produced some degree of shortening, for which a shoe raise may be appropriate if the patient is troubled by it.

In very osteoporotic or obese subjects, refracture through the screw hole in the femoral shaft may occur or the screws may pull out and the side plates separate

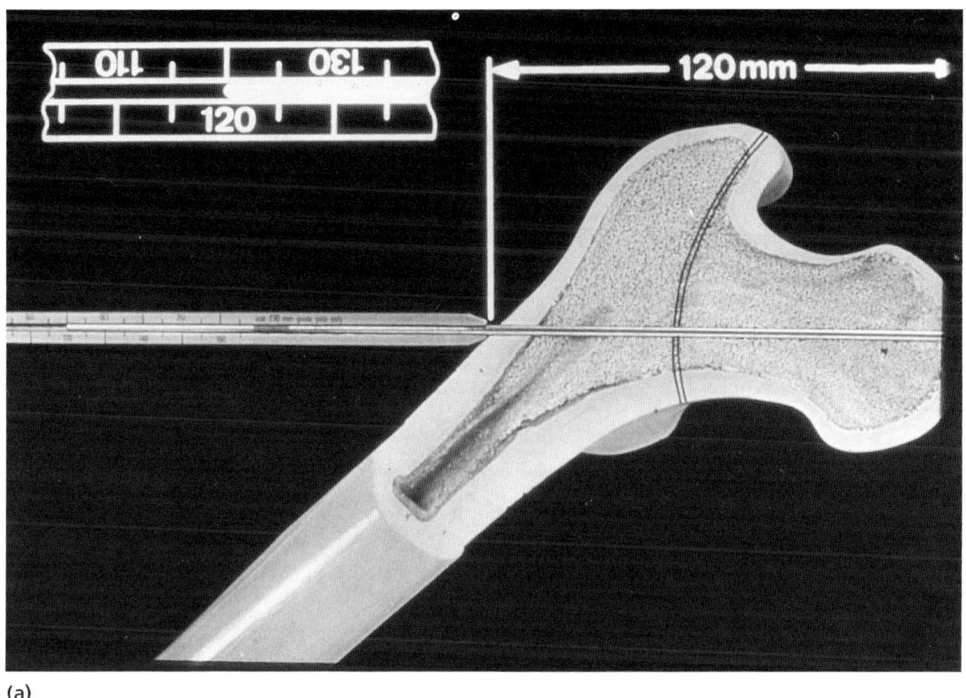

(a)

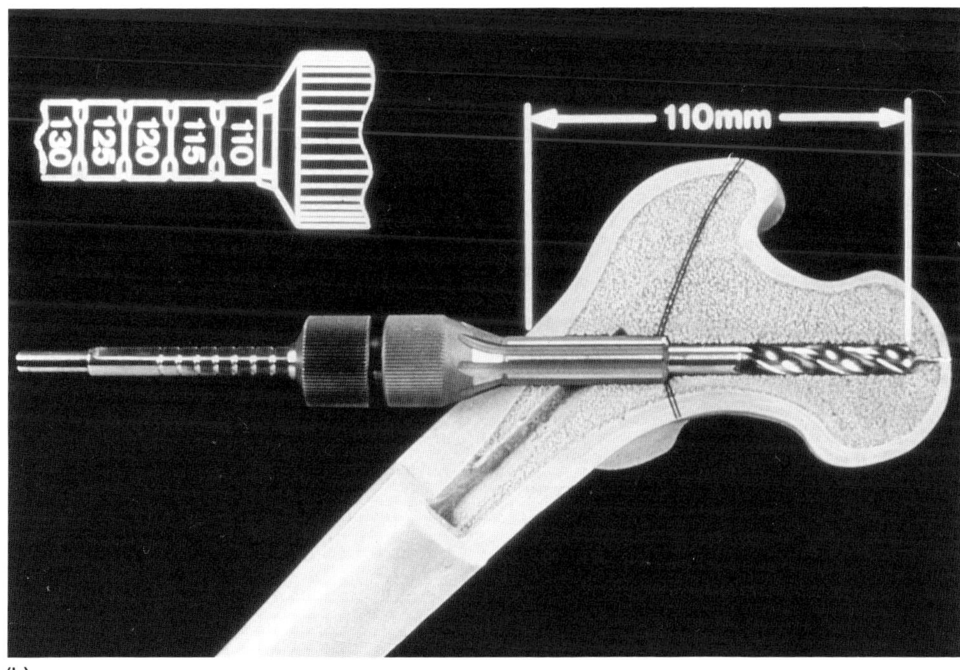

(b)

Fig. 20.42 (a) Measuring the length of the neck. (b) Reaming.

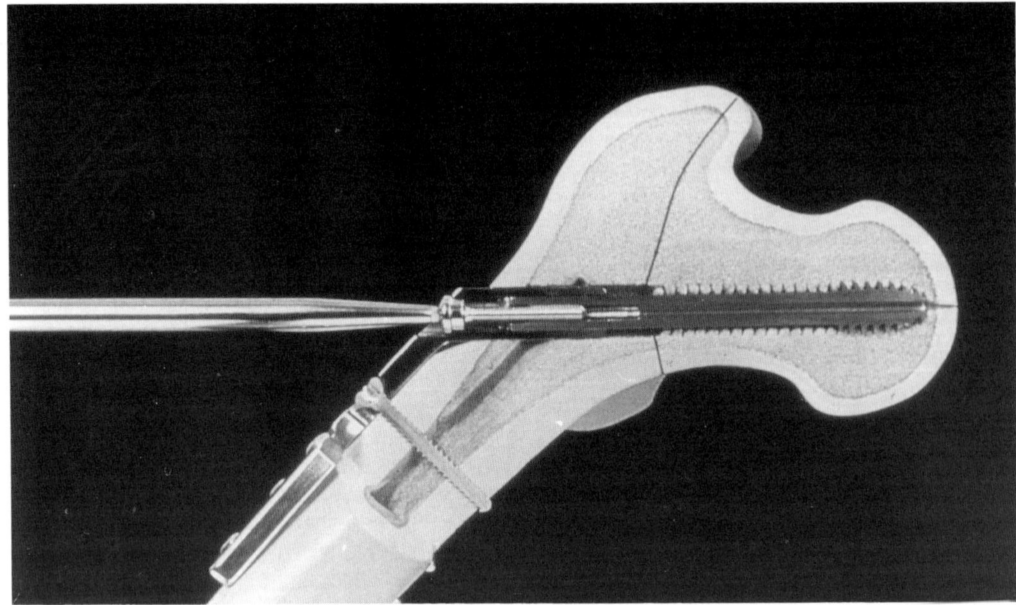

Fig. 20.43 Applying compression.

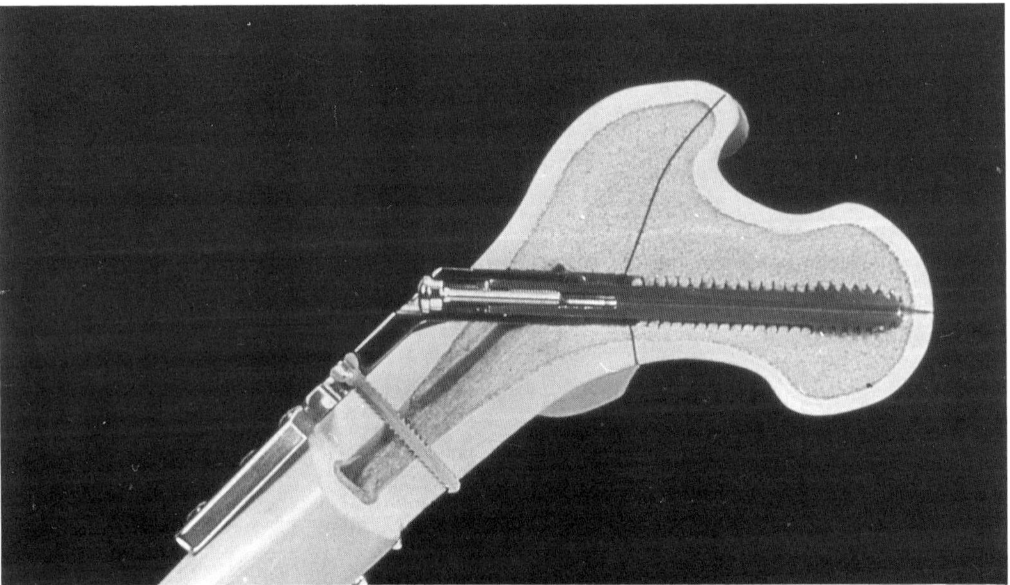

Fig. 20.44 Final position.

from the lateral cortex. According to the circumstances refracture may be managed by substituting a longer side plate or by traction in recumbency. Loosening of the side plate may be clinically undetectable and should only be treated if symptoms are progressive and disintegration of the internal splintage appears imminent. The plate may be reattached using longer screws with medially placed lock-nuts, or else a longer side plate may be substituted to spread the load.

Non-operative treatment

If predictably safe operation cannot be offered, then balanced traction is an alternative which requires more prolonged care and is less efficient in preventing shortening, but which has few serious complications and is no worse than surgical methods in respect of mortality and general morbidity (Fig. 20.45).

A heavy Steinmann pin is passed through the upper

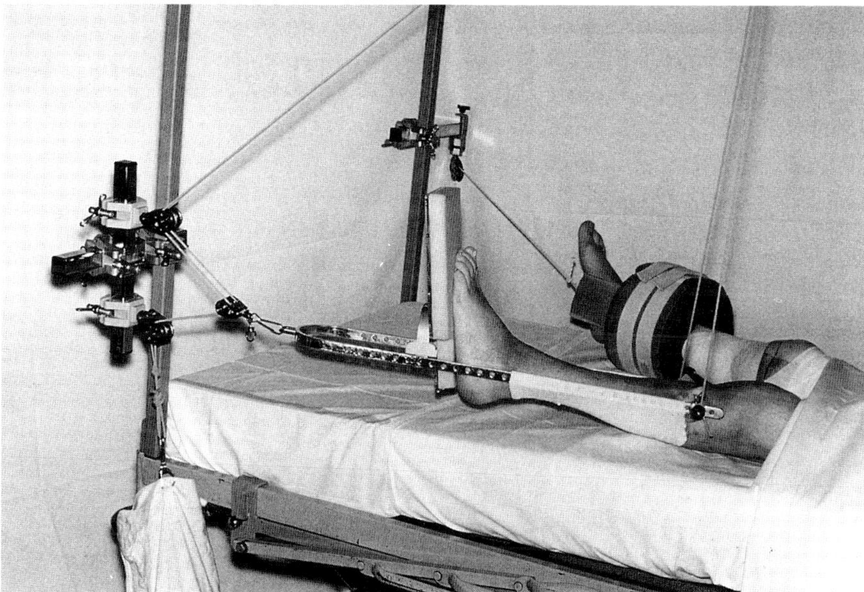

Fig. 20.45 Hamilton Russell traction via tibial Steinmann pin. Note the abducted contralateral limb and heel skin position.

tibia just distal to the tubercle under local anaesthesia. A Tulloch Brown aluminium 'U' loop is then fitted to the pin and secured with collars, to which traction cords may be connected. This U loop encloses the distal part of the limb and supports the calf by elasticated stockinet which is stretched between the side bars. A Hamilton Russell system of traction is then employed with the cords attached to the medial and lateral ends of the Steinmann pin. By increasing or decreasing the weight on the lateral cord system mediolateral rotation is produced. The total weight required is half the traction load in the femoral axis by virtue of the multiplier pulley system. The limb should be positioned in slight abduction and serial radiographs obtained as the traction is adjusted to give the best position of the fragment. Clinical union is often rapid and many patients can lift their limb in the air without pain in less than 6 weeks. Late adduction deformity will occur if traction is abandoned prematurely, and radiological union should be awaited in cases where varus is unacceptable (Figs 20.46 & 20.47). As with operative treatment, the same high level of nursing care is required but the absence of post-anaesthetic drowsiness is a notable benefit and most patients are able to move about in bed with little or no pain in a matter of days. The chief drawback to this method is that hospital care is prolonged by 1 month and rehabilitation is retarded (Hornby *et al.* 1989).

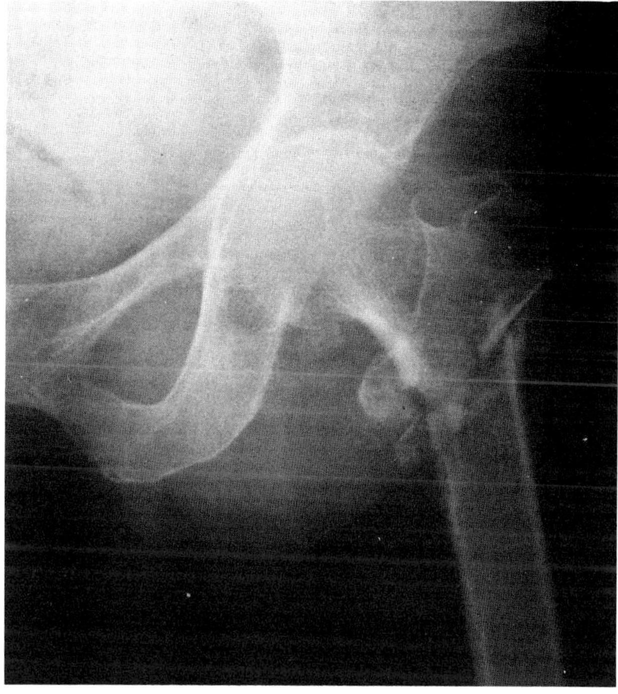

Fig. 20.46 Good overall alignment obtained on traction.

Pathological trochanteric fractures

Although the subtrochanteric zone of the femur is more often affected by secondary tumour, such lesions may occur proximal to the lesser trochanter. The addition

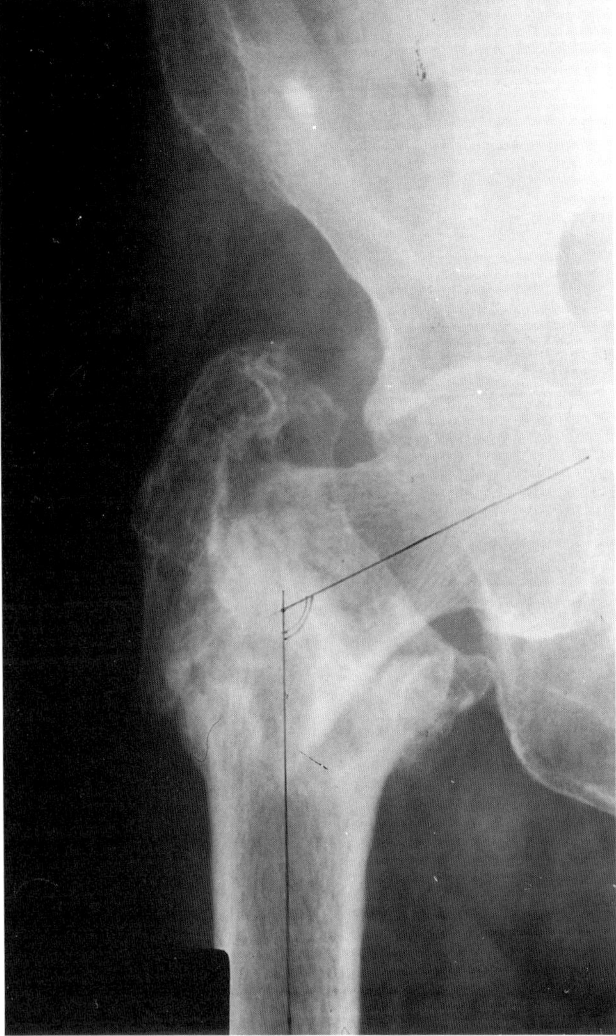

Fig. 20.47 Mild varus deformity of which the patient was unaware. Normal hip function.

of methylmethacrylate bone cement, to stabilize the fracture at the time of operative fixation, is often worthwhile.

References

Acheson, E.D. *Oxford Record Linkage Study*. 1966. Cited in Editorial (1982).

Aitken, J.M. Relevance of osteoporosis in women with fractures of the femoral neck. *Br Med J* 1984; **288**: 597–601.

Alffram, P.A. An epidemiologic study of cervical and trochanteric fractures of the femur in an urban population. *Acta Orthop Scand Suppl* 1964; 65.

Baker, D.M. Fractures of the femoral neck after healed intertrochanteric fracture. *J Trauma* 1975; **15**: 73–81.

Bauer, G.C.H. Epidemiology of fracture in aged persons. *Clin Orthop* 1960; **17**: 219–225.

Blessed, G., Tomlinson, B.E. & Roth, M. The association between quantitative measures of dementia and of degenerative changes in cerebral grey matter of elderly subjects. *Br J Psychiatr* 1969; **114**: 797–811.

Bong, S.C., Lau, H.K., Leong, J.C.Y. & Fang, D. The treatment of unstable intertrochanteric fractures of the hip: a prospective trial of 150 cases. *Injury* 1981; **13**: 139–146.

Boyce, W.J. & Vessey, M.P. Rising incidence of fracture of the proximal femur. *Lancet* 1985; **i**: 150–151.

Bremner, R.A. & Graham, W.D. Pertrochanteric fractures. *J Bone Joint Surg* 1958; **40B**: 694–700.

Bridle, S.H., Pale, A.D., Bircher, M. & Calvert, P.T. Fixation of intertrochanteric traction of the femur: a randomised prospective comparison of the gamma nail and dynamic hip screw. *J Bone Joint Surg* 1991; **73B**: 330–334.

Callender, R.G. The Callender hip assembly. *J Bone Joint Surg* 1957; **49A**: 1235.

Ceder, L. Differentiated care of hip fracture in the elderly. *Acta Orthop Scand* 1980; **51**: 157–162.

Ceder, L., Svensson, B.S. & Thorngren, K.-G. Statistical prediction of rehabilitation in elderly patients with hip fractures. *Clin Orthop* 1980; **152**: 185–190.

Chapman, M.W., Bowman, W.E. & Csongrad, I. The use of Ender's pins in extracapsular fractures of the hip. *J Bone Joint Surg* 1981; **63A**: 14.

Clawson, D.K. Trochanteric fractures treated by the sliding screw plate fixation method. *J Trauma* 1964; **4**: 737–751.

Cleveland, M., Bosworth, D.M. & Thompson, F.R.C. A ten-year analysis of intertrochanteric fractures of the femur. *J Bone Joint Surg* 1947; **29A**: 1399.

Cuthbert, H. & Howat, T.W. The use of the Kuntscher Y-nail in the treatment of intertrochanteric and subtrochanteric fractures of the femur. *Injury* 1976; **8**: 135–142.

Dahl, E. Mortality and life expectancy after hip fractures. *Acta Orthop Scand* 1980; **51**: 163–170.

Davis, T.R.C., Sher, J.L., Porter, B.B. & Checketts, R.G. The timing of surgery for intertrochanteric fractures. *Injury* 1988; **19**: 244–246.

DeLee, J.C. Fractures and dislocations of the hip. In: Rockwood, C.A. & Green D.P. (eds) *Fractures in Adults* 2nd edn. Lippincott: Philadelphia, 1984.

Denham, M.J. & Jeffreys, P.M. Routine mental testing in the elderly. *Mod Geriatr* 1972; **2**: 275–279.

Dimon, J.H. & Hughston, J.C. Unstable intertrochanteric fractures of the hip. *J Bone Joint Surg* 1967; **49A**: 440–450.

Ecker, M.L., Joyce, J.J. & Kohl, E.J. The treatment of trochanteric hip fractures using a compression screw. *J Bone Joint Surg* 1975; **57A**: 23–27.

Editorial. The old woman with a broken hip. *Lancet* 1982; **ii**: 419–20.

Ender, H.G. Richtlinien zur Behandlung per- und subtrochanter Brüche mit Federnägeln. *Aktuel Traumatol* 1976; **6**: 155.

Ender, H.G. The treatment of pertrochanteric and subtrochanteric fractures of the femur with Ender nailing. In: *Proceedings of the Hip Society*. CV Mosby: St Louis, 1978.

Esser, M.P., Kassab, J.Y. & Jones, D.H. A randomised prospective trial of Jewett nail vs dynamic hip screw in trochanteric fractures. *J Bone Joint Surg* 1986; **68B**: 557−560.

Evans, E.M. The treatment of trochanteric fractures of the femur. *J Bone Joint Surg* 1949; **31B**: 190−203.

Evans, E.M. Trochanter fractures. *J Bone Joint Surg* 1951; **33B**: 192.

Evans, J.G. Fractured proximal femur in Newcastle upon Tyne. *Age Ageing* 1979; **8**: 16−24.

Evans, J.G., Prudham, D. & Wandless, I. A prospective study of fractured proximal femur. Incidence and outcome. *Public Health London* 1979a; **93**: 235−241.

Evans, J.G., Prudham, D. & Wandless, I. A prospective study of fractured proximal femur: factors predisposing to survival. *Age Ageing* 1979b; **8**: 246.

Evans, J.G., Wandless, I. & Prudham, D. A prospective study of fractured proximal femur; hospital differences. *Public Health London* 1980; **94**: 149−154.

Fitzgerald, J.A. Fractures of the neck of the femur: factors affecting hospital stay. *NZ Med J* 1965; **64**: 637−640.

Foster, J.C. Trochanteric fractures treated with McLaughlin nail-plate. *J Bone Joint Surg* 1958; **40B**: 684.

Frandsen, P.A. & Kruse, T. Hip fractures in the county of Funen, Denmark. *Acta Orthop Scand* 1983; **54**: 681−686.

Frankel, V.H. & Burstein, A.H. *Orthopaedic Biomechanics*. Lea & Febiger: Philadelphia, 1970.

Frew, J.F.M. Conservative treatment of intertrochanteric fractures. *J Bone Joint Surg* 1972; **54B**: 748.

Friedenberg, Z.B., Gentchos, E. & Rutt, C. Fixation in intertrochanteric fractures of the hip. *Surg Gynecol Obstet* 1972; **135**: 225.

Gallanaugh, S.C., Martin, A. & Millard, P.H. Regional survey of femoral neck fractures. *Br Med J* 1976; **2**: 1496−1497.

Ganz, R., Thomas, R.J. & Hammerle, C.P. Trochanteric fractures of the femur: treatment and results. *Clin Orthop* 1979; **138**: 30.

Gordon, P.C. The probability of death following fracture of the hip. *Can Med Assoc J* 1972; **105**: 47−51.

Gozna, E.R. & Harrington, I.J. *Biomechanics of Muscoloskeletal Injury*. Williams & Wilkins: Baltimore, 1982.

Halder, S.C. & Gill, J.G. The Halifax nail (gamma). *Report to Spring Meeting of British Orthopaedic Association, March 1988, Plymouth*.

Harrington, K.D. & Johnston, J.O. The management of comminuted unstable intertrochanteric fractures. *J Bone Joint Surg* 1973; **55A**: 1367−1376.

Harris, L.J. Closed retrograde intramedullary nailing of pertrochanteric fracture of the femur with a new nail. *J Bone Joint Surg* 1980; **62A**: 1185.

Heyse-Moore, G.H. & MacEachern, A.G. Stable intertrochanteric fractures − a misnomer? *J Bone Joint Surg* 1983; **65B**: 582.

Heyse-Moore, G.H., MacEachern, A.G. & Jameson Evans, D.C. The treatment of intertrochanteric fractures of the femur. *J Bone Joint Surg* 1983; **65B**: 262−267.

Hirsch, C. & Frankel, V.H. Analysis of forces producing fractures of the proximal end of the femur. *J Bone Joint Surg* 1960; **42B**: 633−640.

Horn, J. & Wang, Y.C. The mechanism, traumatic anatomy and non-operative treatment of intertrochanteric fracture of the femur. *Br J Surg* 1964; **54**: 574−580.

Hornby, R., Evans, J.G. & Vardon, V. Trochanteric fractures in the elderly. *J Bone Joint Surg* 1986; **68B**: 157.

Hornby, R., Evans, J.G. & Vardon, V. Operative or conservative treatment for trochanteric fractures of the femur. A randomised epidemiological trial in elderly patients. *J Bone Joint Surg* 1989; **71B**: 619−623.

Howard, F.M. & Phia, R.J. Fractures of the apophyses in adolescent athletes. *J Am Med Assoc* 1965; **192**: 150−152.

Hunter, G.A. The results of operative treatment of trochanteric fractures of the femur. *Injury* 1975; **6**: 202−205.

Ions, G.K. & Stevens, J. Prediction of survival in patients with femoral neck fractures. *J Bone Joint Surg* 1987; **69B**: 384−387.

Jacobs, R.R., Armstrong, J.H. & Whitaker, J.H. Treatment of intertrochanteric hip fractures with a compression screw and a nail-plate. *J Trauma* 1976; **16**: 599.

James, E.T.R. & Hunter, G.A. The treatment of intertrochanteric fractures − a review. *Injury* 1983; **14**: 421−431.

Jensen, J.S. A photoelastic study of a model of the proximal femur. *Acta Orthop Scand* 1978; **49**: 54−59.

Jensen, J.S. Incidence of hip fractures. *Acta Orthop Scand* 1980a; **51**: 511−513.

Jensen, J.S. Classification of trochanteric fractures. *Acta Orthop Scand* 1980b; **51**: 803−810.

Jensen, J.S. Trochanteric fractures. *Acta Orthop Scand Suppl* 1981; **52(188)**.

Jensen, J.S. Determining factors for the mortality following hip fractures. *Injury* 1984; **15**: 411−414.

Jensen, J.S. & Bagger, J. Longterm social prognosis after hip fractures. *Acta Orthop Scand* 1982; **53**: 97.

Jensen, J.S. & Michaelsen, M. Trochanteric fractures treated by McLaughlin osteosynthesis. *Acta Orthop Scand* 1975; **46**: 795.

Jensen, J.S. & Tondevold, E. Mortality after hip fractures. *Acta Orthop Scand* 1979; **50**: 161−167.

Jensen, J.S. & Tondevold, E. A prognostic evaluation of the hospital resources required for the treatment of hip fractures. *Acta Orthop Scand* 1980; **51**: 515−522.

Jensen, J.S., Sonne-Holm, S. & Tondevold, E. Unstable trochanteric fractures − a comparative analysis of 4 methods of internal fixation. *Acta Orthop Scand* 1980a; **51**: 949−962.

Jensen, J.S., Tondevold, E. & Hove-Sorensen, P. Costs of treatment of hip fractures. *Acta Orthop Scand* 1980b; **51**: 289−296.

Jensen, J.S., Tondevold, E. & Sonne-Holm, S. Stable trochanteric fractures − a comparative analysis of 4 methods of internal fixation. *Acta Orthop Scand* 1980c; **51**: 811−816.

Kauffer, H., Matthews, L.S. & Sonstegard, D. Stable fixation of intertrochanteric fractures. *J Bone Joint Surg* 1974; **56A**: 899−907.

Kauffer, H. Mechanics of the treatment of hip injuries. *Clin Orthop* 1980; **146**: 53−61.

Kolind-Sorensen, V. Mortality in intertrochanteric fracture of the femoral neck. *Acta Orthop Scand* 1975; **46**: 654−656.

Kuntscher, G. A new method of treatment of pertrochanteric fractures. *Proc R Soc Med* 1977; **63**: 1120.

Laros, G.S. & Moore, J.F. Complications of fixation in intertrochanteric fractures. *Clin Orthop* 1974; **101**: 110−119.

Lawton, J.O., Baker, M.R. & Dickson, R.A. Femoral neck fractures − two populations. *Lancet* 1983; **ii**: 70−72.

Leung, R.S., Gruber, M.A. & Zimmerman, A.J. Gamma nails and dynamic hip screws for peritrochanteric fractures: a randomised prospective study in elderly patients. *J Bone Joint Surg* 1992; **74B**: 345−351.

Ludloff, K. Zurblutigen Einrenkung der angeborenen Huftlaxation. *Zentralbl Orthop Chir* 1908; **22**: 272.

Mann, R.J. Avascular necrosis after trochanteric fracture. *Clin Orthop* 1973; **92**: 108–115.

May, J.M.B. & Chacha, P.B. Displacements of trochanteric fractures and their influence on reduction. *J Bone Joint Surg* 1968; **50B**: 318–323.

Merlino, A.F. & Nixon, J.E. Isolated fractures of the greater trochanter. *Int Surg* 1969; **52**: 117–124.

Miller, C.W. Survival and ambulation following hip fracture. *J Bone Joint Surg* 1978; **60A**: 930.

Muckle, D.S. *Femoral Neck Fractures*. Chapman & Hall: London, 1977.

Mulholland, R.C. & Gunn, D.R. Sliding screwplate fixation of intertrochanteric fractures. *J Bone Joint Surg* 1972; **55A**: 1367–1376.

Müller, M.E., Allgower, M. & Willenegger, H. *Manual of Internal Fixation*. Springer-Verlag: New York, 1970.

Murray, R.C. & Frew, J.F.M. Trochanteric fractures of the femur. *J Bone Joint Surg* 1949; **31B**: 204.

Parker, M.J. & Palmer, C.R. A new mobility score for predicting mortality after hip fracture. *J Bone Joint Surg* 1993; **75B**: 797–798.

Parker, M.J. & Prior, G. *Hip Fracture Management*. Blackwell Scientific Publications: Oxford, 1993.

Radford, P.J., Needoff, M. & Webb, J.K. A prospective randomised comparison of the dynamic hip screw and the gamma locking nail. *J Bone Joint Surg* 1993; **75B**: 789–793.

Regazzoni, P., Ruedi, T., Winquist, R. & Allgower, M. *The Dynamic Hip Screw Implant System*. Springer-Verlag: Berlin, 1985.

Sarmiento, A. Avoidance of complications of internal fixation of trochanteric fractures. *Clin Orthop* 1967; **53**: 47–59.

Sarmiento, A. The unstable intertrochanteric fracture: treatment with valgus osteotomy and an I-beam nailplate. *J Bone Joint Surg* 1970; **52A**: 1309–1318.

Sarmiento, A. Unstable trochanteric fractures of the femur. *Clin Orthop* 1973; **92**: 77–85.

Schumpelick, W. & Jantzen, P.M. A new principle in the operative treatment of trochanteric fractures of the femur. *J Bone Joint Surg* 1955; **73A**: 693–698.

Scott, J.C. Treatment of trochanteric fractures. *J Bone Joint Surg* 1951; **33B**: 508–512.

Shaftan, G.W., Herbsman, H.H. & Pavlides, C. Selective conservatism in hip fractures. *Surgery* 1967; **61(4)**: 524–527.

Sher, J.L., Stevens, J., Porter, B.B. & Checketts, R.G. A comparison of operative and conservative treatment for unstable trochanteric fractures. *J Bone Joint Surg* 1985; **67B**: 495.

Thomas, J.G. & Stevens, R.S. Social effects of fractures of the neck of the femur. *Br Med J* 1974; **3**: 456–458.

Tronzo, R.G. *Surgery of the Hip Joint*. Lea & Febiger: Philadelphia, 1973.

Tronzo, R.G. Hip nails for all occasions. *Orthop Clin North Am* 1974; **5(3)**: 479–491.

Versluysen, M. Pressure sores in elderly patients: the epidemiology related to hip fractures. *J Bone Joint Surg* 1985; **67B**: 10–13.

Watson-Jones, R. *Fractures and Joint Injuries*, Vol. 2, 4th edn. Churchill Livingstone: Edinburgh, 1955.

Zetterberg, C., Elmerson, S. & Anderson, G.B.J. Epidemiology of hip fractures in Goteborg, Sweden 1940–1983. *Clin Orthop* 1984; **191**: 43–52.

21: The Thigh

A.T.CROSS AND B.F.MEGGITT

Introduction

The thigh is the segment between the hip and knee joints and functions mechanically in load transmission, length maintenance and muscle anchorage for weight-bearing and locomotion. In normal life the central femur, surrounded by the large muscle groups, is subjected to high axial, bending and torsional stresses that may approach 50% breaking force. Displaced femoral fractures with muscle spasm result in malalignment, length loss, muscle damage and failure of load-bearing. Thus, the main problems arising from femoral fractures are malunion, shortening, knee stiffness and functional impairment, but less commonly non-union, because of the good muscular blood supply to the bone.

The commonest mechanisms of injury causing femoral fractures in young adults and children are major external violence from road traffic accidents and falling from a height, and in the elderly are lower forces from falls. The high-energy thigh fractures are also often associated with extensive local soft tissue damage and other distant injuries which may be limb- and life-threatening. In the younger age group, subject to high-energy forces, femoral shaft fractures are more common. In the elderly group with age-related osteoporosis, the weaker metaphyseal areas are more often fractured by much lower energy trauma, which produces supracondylar, condylar and subtrochanteric fractures.

Historical review

Hippocrates (*c.* 400 BC) is attributed with the first description of femoral fractures in a scientific treatise on fractures (Hippocrates 1849). He stressed the importance of keeping adequate extension with femoral shaft fractures to prevent shortening after manual reduction. He also described wooden splints and wax-impregnated fabric bandages used in their treatment. Albucasis (*c.* AD 958), an Arabic physician, wrote in his *Third Book on Surgery* of fractured femur treatment with splinting of the flexed lower leg to the thigh using wooden splints and plaster casing of egg white and flour on fabric bandages (Spinks & Lewis 1973). Plaster of Paris, described originally by the ancient Egyptians, was reintroduced by Mathijsen (1852) as plaster bandages that then rationalized fracture treatment.

Continuous traction, to oppose muscle contraction and maintain leg length, was first used in femoral fractures. James (quoted by Rocyn-Jones 1953) described one of the earlier systems with traction strings that were attached to splints, bandaged to the calf, and taken over a pulley at the end of the bed to a suspended weight. The patient was fixed to the headboard by a harness as the concept of bed elevation had not been developed. Buck popularized straight-leg traction using adhesive plaster skin traction and coaptation splints to the thigh in 1860. The advent of radiographs in the 1890s visualized the problem of providing adequate reduction of femoral fractures using skin traction alone. Early skeletal traction was described by Kirschner (1909) who used transverse bone pins above and below the fracture with a distraction apparatus originally. Steinmann developed thicker pins, initially two short ones, that could be driven into the upper tibia or femur (Fig. 21.1) on each side and then, later, he developed a long pin, drilled through the bone, for the application of skeletal traction. He also identified the sites for this skeletal traction in the femoral condyle, tibial tubercle and calcaneum. One further development for stabilizing the acute fracture, and mobilizing the patient in the later healing phases, was the Thomas' splint (Thomas 1875, Peltier 1968) (Fig. 21.2). The introduction of the Thomas' splint during World War I had a dramatic effect in reducing the mortality of soldiers with fractured femurs from 80% in 1916 to 20% in 1918, when the splint was applied to injured soldiers on the battlefield and used during their transport (Jones 1925). Various modifications of the Thomas' splint and

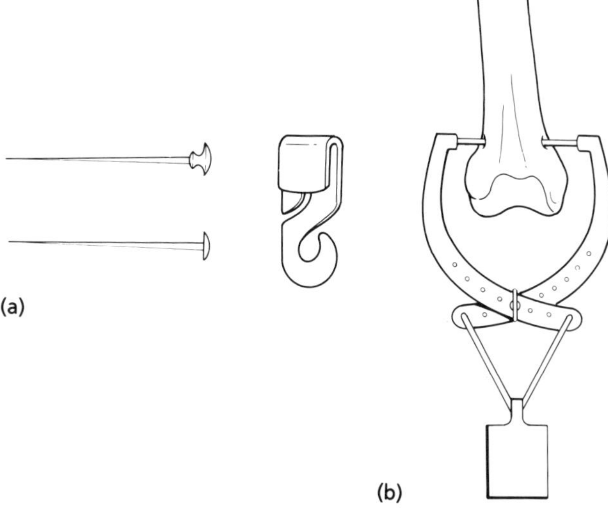

Fig. 21.1 Original skeletal traction apparatus of Steinmann.
(a) Two small bone pins and traction hook. (b) Single pin and
traction stirrup.

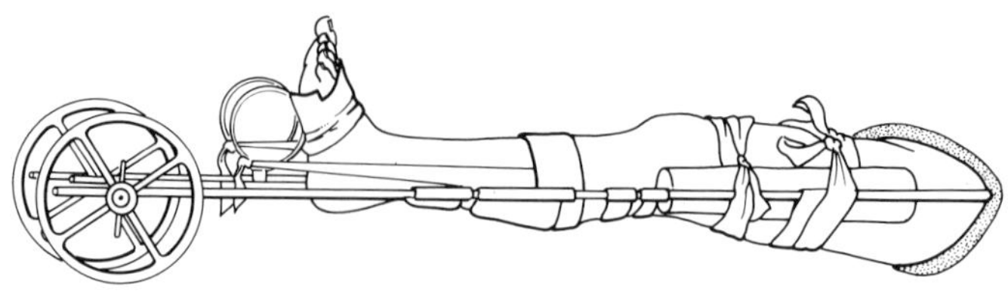

Fig. 21.2 The original Thomas' ring splint with adjustable
track secured to steel spring hoops (or to fixed end of splint)
with counter-traction through the proximal ring. (After
Thomas 1975).

alternative systems for traction have been described
over the years (Fig. 21.3), as discussed by Charnley
(1961). Practical additions involved an attachable knee
flexion piece (Pearson & Drummond 1919), the use of a
below-knee plaster cast traction unit (Charnley 1961)
and the major modification of a dynamic hinged lower
half to the splint (Fisk 1944). Alternative traction systems
evolved with various static, free-standing splints, such
as the Böhler–Braun frame, with direct skeletal traction
over a pillow and split bed (Perkins 1958) and with the
vertical '90–90' method. In the 1970s, further support to
conservative treatment was given by the development of
the functional femoral cast brace, which allowed early
mobilization of the patient and the knee with distal half
femoral fractures, by use of a knee-hinged long leg cast
(Mooney *et al.* 1970). Wider acceptability occurred with
the introduction of lighter multiple synthetic casting
materials.

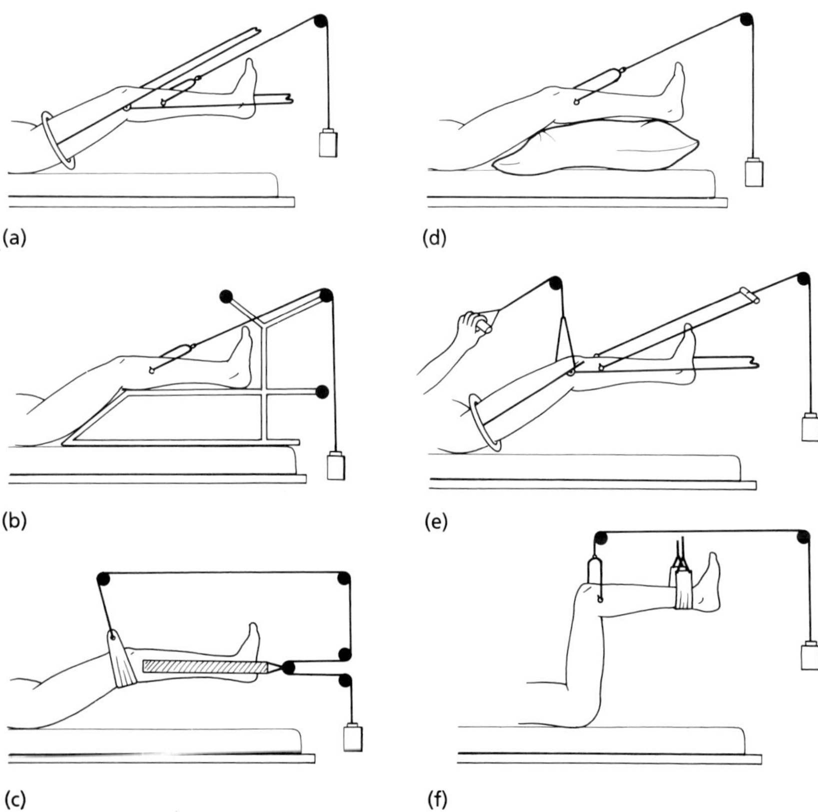

Fig. 21.3 Various forms of sliding
traction: (a) Thomas' splint and
Pearson knee flexion piece; (b) Braun
frame; (c) Russell traction; (d) Perkins
traction; (e) Fisk splint; (f) '90–90'
vertical traction.

Operative treatment of femoral fractures became a serious alternative to conservative treatment with the introduction of asepsis in surgery and radiographic imaging at the end of the nineteenth century. In England, Lane (1914) originated the 'no-touch technique' and developed plates with screws for internal fracture fixation. Hey Groves (1916) reported the first use of intramedullary fixation using solid and hollow steel rods, but metal rusting and infection were major problems. Lambotte (1913) developed the 'fixateur externe' for supporting fractures, usually after open reduction. The technique of intramedullary nail fixation was reintroduced by Küntscher (1958) using a V-shaped rod. This technique was further developed by him to include medullary reaming, the cloverleaf-shaped nail and proximal introduction under radiographic control (Küntscher 1957, 1967). In the 1960s, a group of Swiss surgeons and engineers (the 'AO group') further developed the concept, previously described by Danis (1947) and Charnley (1953), of 'primary bone healing' with rigid internal fixation, using newer interfragmentary compression screws and plates, of all fractures, including those of the femur (Müller *et al.* 1965). They also described a more elastic tubular intramedullary nail.

More recently, new internal fixation devices have been developed for treatment of femoral fractures. The locked intramedullary nail, with proximal and distal cross screws, has facilitated closed internal fixation of most femoral shaft fractures. Immediate stabilization of the thigh and mobilization of the knee and patient are possible and have been a major advance in treatment (Kempf *et al.* 1985). A reconstruction nail for combined femoral shaft and neck fractures is now an important addition to the management of complex fractures, as is the development of locked intramedullary devices for the treatment of subtrochanteric fractures. Improved fixation devices have also been developed very recently for the distal femoral fracture, with the dynamic condylar screw and plates and the heavy condylar plates being added to the previous condylar blade plate devices.

Classification

Selection of the optimum treatment and audit of the results of femoral fractures requires essentially four classifications of the injury to be defined. These involve the fracture site, pattern, comminution and the soft tissue damage.

Site

Anatomically, the shaft has been divided into thirds from the lesser trochanter to the supracondylar expansion. However, a more functional classification defines the mid-shaft section with the tubular medullary canal as being approximately three-fifths of the shaft and the proximal and distal sections, with the medulla flaring out, as approximately one-fifth each. The proximal shaft section is also termed the subtrochanteric region, the distal section is called the supracondylar region and the terminal articular area is the condylar segment (Fig. 21.4).

Fracture pattern

This classification gives the complexity of the fracture and is an index of the force producing it. Oblique and spiral fractures result from torsional stresses, usually applied at a distance from the fracture. Transverse fractures, with or without butterfly fragments at one or two levels, which give a segmental fracture, are all produced

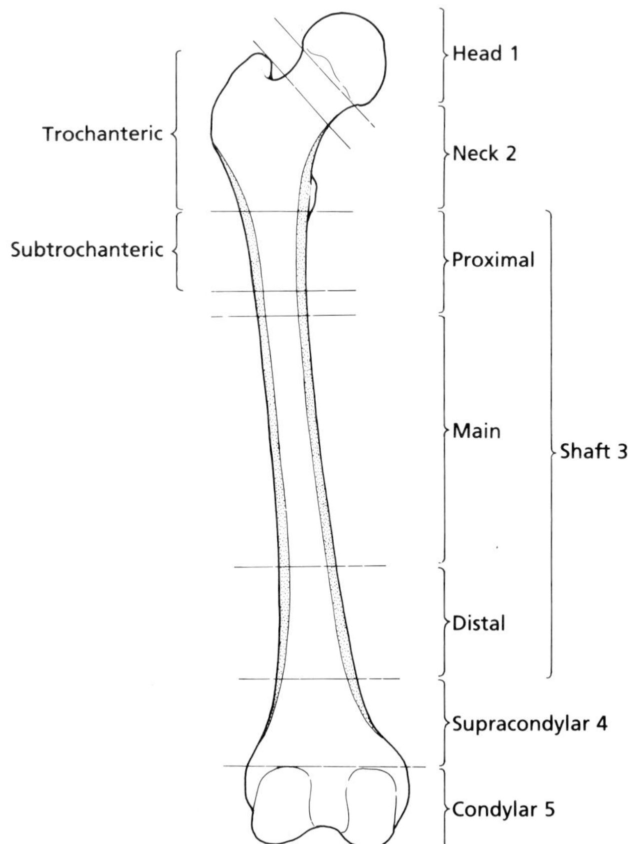

Fig. 21.4 Femoral bone segments.

by mainly bending forces. Comminuted fractures of increasing severity occur from impaction or crushing forces and bone loss may occur with soft tissue penetration and bone extrusion.

Comminution degree

This reflects the severity of fracture impaction and crushing forces and the stability of the fracture possible with treatment. Four grades are represented: type 1 has 75% of the cortex intact, type 2 has 50–75% intact, type 3 has 25–50% intact type 4 has no contact (Winquist & Hansen 1980).

Soft tissue injuries

Fractures may be classified simply as 'closed' or 'open', with the latter often consistent with greater damage to bone and soft tissues. Open fractures have received various grading criteria but two systems have been most widely used. Gustillo and Anderson (1976) classified open fractures into three types according to the main injuries. This was upgraded by Gustillo *et al.* (1984) to become more comprehensive:

Type 1 — Small wounds of 1cm or less from low-velocity trauma with minimal soft tissue damage.

Type 2 — Wounds extensive in length and width but with little foreign material.

Type 3 — Wounds of moderate or massive size with considerable devitalized soft tissue or foreign material, or both, or traumatic amputation.

Type 3a — Wounds with extensive soft tissue laceration or flaps, or wounds caused by high-energy trauma but with adequate soft tissue to cover the fractured bone.

Type 3b — Wounds with extensive soft tissue injury or loss with periosteal stripping and bone exposure.

Type 3c — Open fractures associated with arterial injuries requiring repair.

Lange *et al.* (1985) reported the use of a similar widely applicable classification in a series of open tibial fractures; this system can be used with all open fractures and is now becoming more widely accepted:

Grade 1 — In-out skin wound <1 cm with minimal contusion.

Grade 2 — Skin wound >1 cm with skin and soft tissue or extensive contusion.

Grade 3 — Large severe wound with extensive skin, soft tissue and muscle contusion and/or loss of soft tissue and with bone penetration with three subgrades:

3(a) Wound associated with severe bone and muscle loss, and nerve or tendon injury.

3(b) Open wounds with major arterial injury:

3(c) Traumatic amputation.

With the continuing advances in new treatment methods for this most serious of limb injuries, the open fractures, it is essential that different studies are comparable and this requires a comprehensive description of the injuries and standardization of the grading systems.

Biomechanics

In someone of average build the centre of gravity lies in the area of the sacral promontory. During normal gait, body weight has to be shifted laterally through the hip into the femoral shaft. Mechanically, it is not possible to bring the centre of gravity over the axis of weight-bearing through the hip, knee and ankle, and in order to prevent loss of equilibrium, the glutei must oppose the downward thrust of the body weight. This arrangement can be converted quite simply into balancing forces (Fig. 21.5). It will be seen that in order to maintain

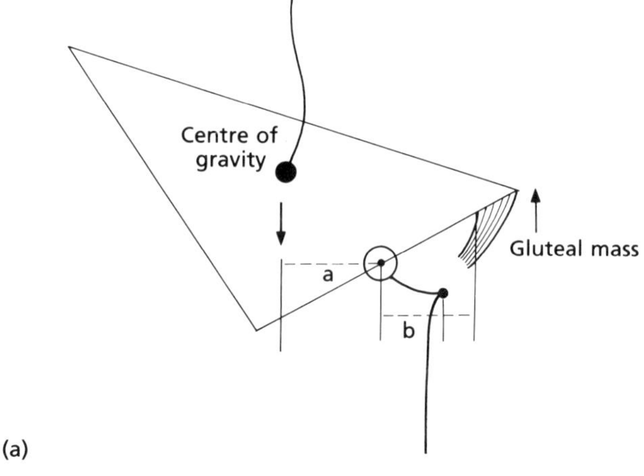

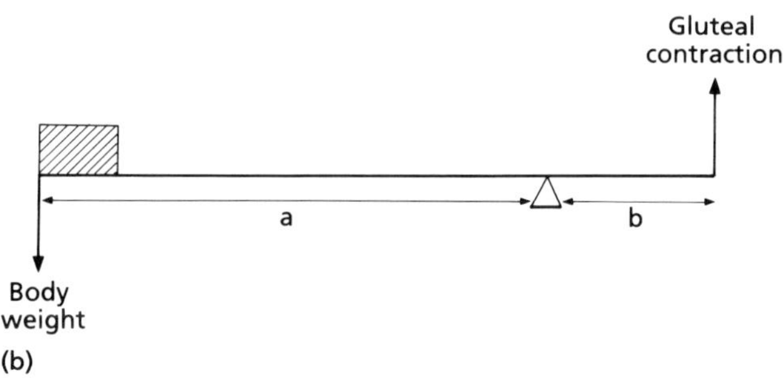

Fig. 21.5 (a) Can easily be translated into component forces as in (b). The distance a represents the horizontal distance between the centre of gravity and the fulcrum of the hip. Distance b is between the hip and the gluteal attachment to the pelvis. Body weight multiplied by a must equal gluteal contraction multiplied by b. Since a is greater than b, the force exerted by the gluteal contraction must be greater than the force exerted by the body weight.

equilibrium the force generated by gluteal contraction must be greater than the body weight. Thus, the force applied through the hip joint, the fulcrum, has been estimated as rising to between two and three times the body weight during normal gait.

The femur itself is part of a cantilever system (Fig. 21.6a). Compression forces occur in the medial femoral cortex and tension forces occur laterally. These forces are greater in the subtrochanteric region (Cochran *et al.* 1980) and the difference in tension and compression decreases along the length of the femur because the line of weight-bearing approaches the mid-line of the femur at the knee joint.

The unique shape of the shaft of the femur means that load transmission for the greater part of the proximal two-thirds is medial to the medial cortex, resulting in compression forces on the medial shaft and tension forces laterally. As long ago as 1917, Koch showed that forces acting across the medial femoral cortex in the

subtrochanteric region under a static load would be twice those passing through the head of the femur and, in addition, when the muscle forces of the abductors and adductors are taken into account, the dynamic load of over 14.0^6 Pa can be demonstrated. The action of the adductors will further tend to cause compression on the medial femoral cortex and, also, the gluteal mass attached to the greater trochanter will tend to increase the tension on the lateral cortex, thus causing medial compression. Although the tensor fascia lata acts as a neutralizing force, rather like a tension-band, surgical approaches often compromise its function. These mechanical factors have an important bearing on the stability of the femoral shaft following a fracture and on subsequent internal fixation.

Internal fixation of the fracture needs to balance these unequal forces. The effect of the tension/compression system is shown in Fig. 21.6. The force applied on the inner limb produces a compressive force on the medial

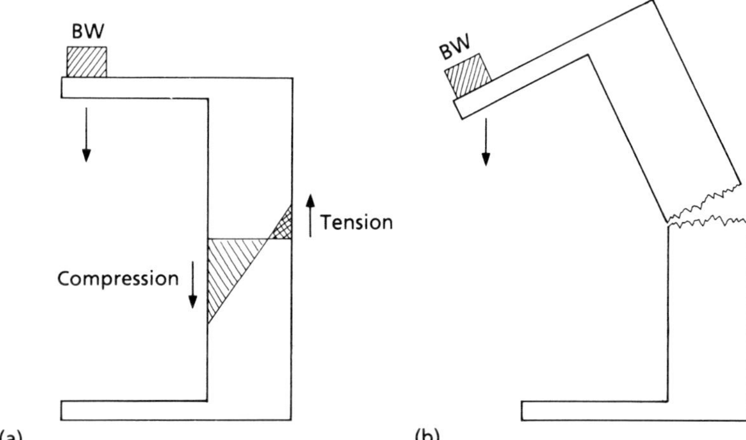

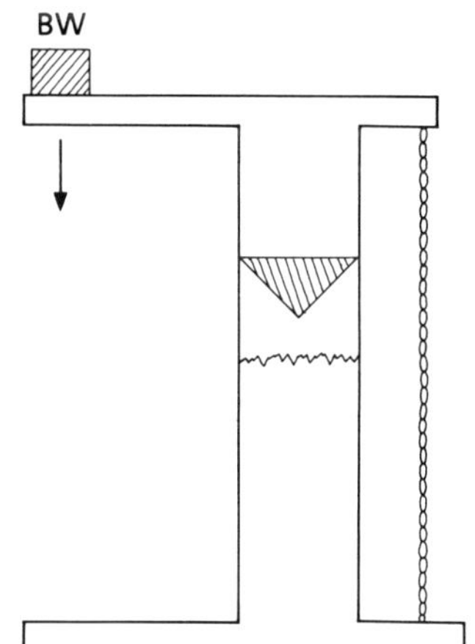

Fig. 21.6 (a) (b) (c) See text. (From Müller *et al.* 1979.) 1 pascal (Pa) is equal to a force of 1 newton/m^2, 10 newtons equal the gravitational force exerted by 1 kg.

side of the column. If the column is fractured (Fig. 21.6b) then there will be a loss of equilibrium. In order to counteract this loss, a tension-band (Fig. 21.6c) can be applied to restore the equilibrium. This is the rationale of plating techniques.

In summary, it is clear that the medial femoral cortex has to withstand an extremely high compressive load. If there is marked medial comminution, and fixation is considered, then it will be necessary for any implant to be able to withstand such loading forces. The belief that no loading occurs if the patient is confined to bed or is allowed to mobilize non-weight-bearing is naive since it is clearly impossible to abolish muscle tone.

The subtrochanteric area is of special interest. A fracture here is subject to the unequal forces of muscles which are attached to it, namely the glutei and the ilio-psoas. The action of these muscles results in flexion and external rotation (ilio-psoas) and abduction (gluteus). In addition, the femoral shaft will always lie adducted in relation to the proximal fragment because of the unopposed action of the adductor muscles. Shortening will occur through hamstring and rectus femoris spasm (Fig. 21.7). The relevance of this to the management of subtrochanteric fractures is discussed in the specific section.

There has been little reported work on the biomechanics of human fracture healing. The best criterion of fracture healing is probably the return of ultimate breaking strength. This can only be applied in experimental fracture models where four stages of fracture healing have been identified: unstable, plastic, rigid and clinical union. A biomechanical study has been reported (Meggitt *et al.* 1981) on monitoring the functional recovery of load-bearing strength in a series of human fractured femurs treated with cast bracing. Vertical loads taken through the fracture site were determined throughout fracture healing using a standard leg load test (10-second steady standing test) and subtracting the load through the brace with transducer hinges from the total leg load on a force plate, with both measured simultaneously. By taking the obtained fracture load as a percentage of the body load, a fracture strength index was obtained. The study showed that it was the fracture itself which controlled the loading and appeared to exhibit a biological feedback system on a mechanoreceptor basis, producing a protective mechanism against overload to the healing fracture. Four mechanical phases were described during fracture healing and were correlated with the clinical, histological and radiographic patterns (Fig. 21.8). A further simplified fracture union index was reported and this allowed regular monitoring of the mechanical recovery

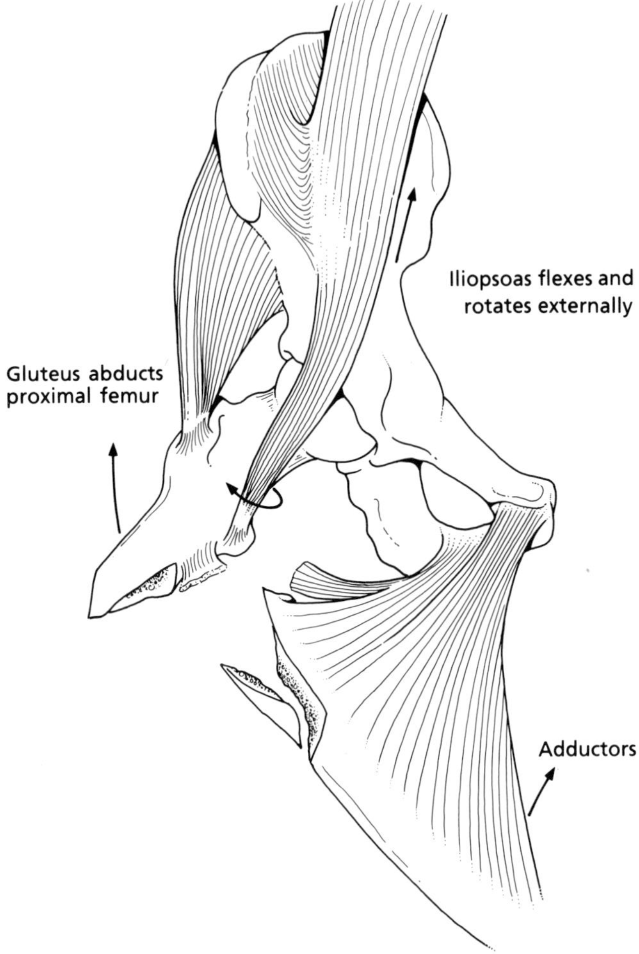

Fig. 21.7 Diagram of pathological anatomy of a subtrochanteric fracture. The proximal fragment is flexed, abducted and externally rotated while the femoral shaft is shortened and adducted. (From Froimson, A.I. *Surg Gynecol Obstet* 1970; **131**: 465. Reproduced with permission from *Surgery, Gynecology and Obstetrics*.)

of the fracture in and out of the cast brace until a full 100% loading was taken to confirm bone union. This biomechanical test is not applicable to fractures treated with fixation with a rigid plate, locking nails or stable external fixation.

Blood supply

The proximal thigh soft tissues receive their circulation from the four perforating branches of the profunda femoris artery which pass circumferentially behind the femur, penetrating the muscle attachments to the linea aspera. These arteries are at risk when damaged by fracture fragments or during posterolateral surgical exposure of the femur shaft. The metaphyses of the femur

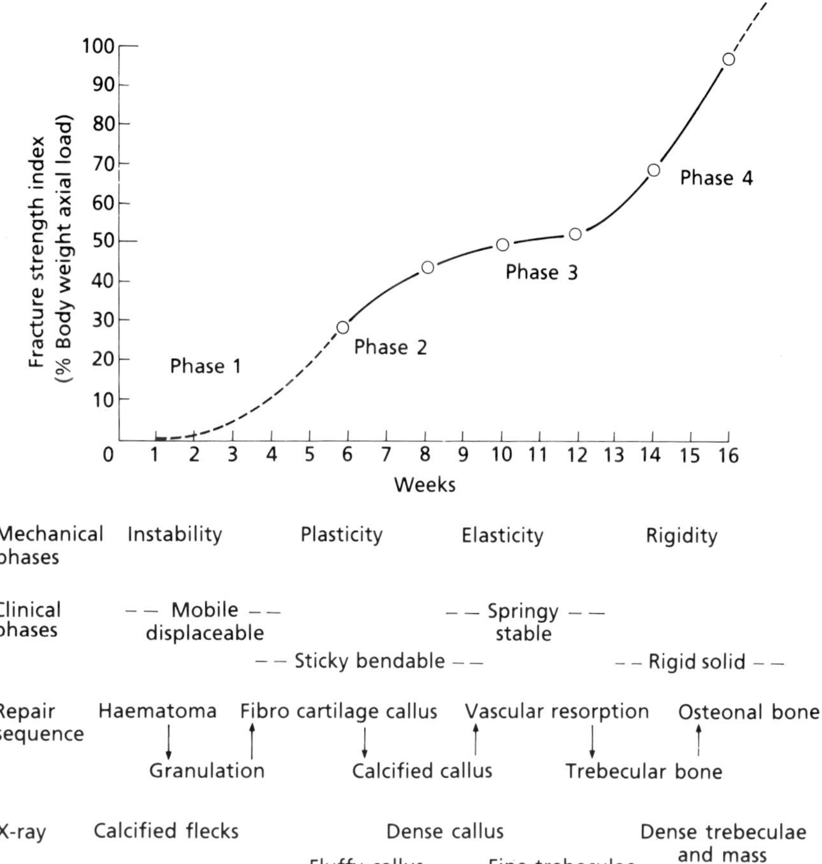

Fig. 21.8 Femur fracture: four phases of union expressed as 'fracture strength index' and correlated with mechanical, clinical and radiographic phases of recovery.

also have a rich anastomosis from the circumflex vessels proximally and from the genicular arteries distally in the vascular cancellous bone. It is uncommon for either shaft or metaphyseal fractures to experience significant avascular necrosis or non-union unless there are major, completely detached fragments.

The main arterial supply to the thigh (Fig. 21.9) is derived from branches arising from the femoral artery and the profunda femoris artery in the proximal and main thigh regions. Distally, genicular branches from the popliteal artery supply the supracondylar region. The blood supply to the femur follows that of all long bones, with the periosteal and endosteal circulation to the shaft and the circumferential anastomoses to the metaphyseal region. The nutrient arterial supply is derived from perforating branches of the profunda femoris artery penetrating, as one or two vessels, the femoral shaft along the linea aspera. The periosteal blood supply is derived from the muscle attachments to the shaft of the femur and thus provides an extensive surface network. Vessels enter the cortex from the periosteal and nutrient artery systems, showing complex patterns of distribution but essentially following the

Haversian systems. There are direct anastomoses between the endosteal and periosteal circulation at all levels, and this allows change in flow patterns with surface or medullary damage from fracture, plating or medullary nailing.

It has been shown that the endosteal circulation is a much more important component of blood supply. This gains access to the shaft of long bones through nutrient arteries. Under normal circumstances the blood flow is centrifugal and drainage occurs through both the endosteal circulation and the periosteal circulation. There is virtually no centripetal flow in the normal bone (Brookes 1988). Following fracture, the endosteal circulation will be disrupted but since there are both proximal and distal nutrient arteries, bone necrosis at the fracture ends is minimal. However, comminuted fragments may well lose all their endosteal blood supply and will be dependent on viability by virtue of their attachments to the periosteum. An understanding of what happens to these comminuted fragments has been advanced by the work of Brookes (1988) and Perren (1989) in experimental operations on animals using plates and intramedullary techniques.

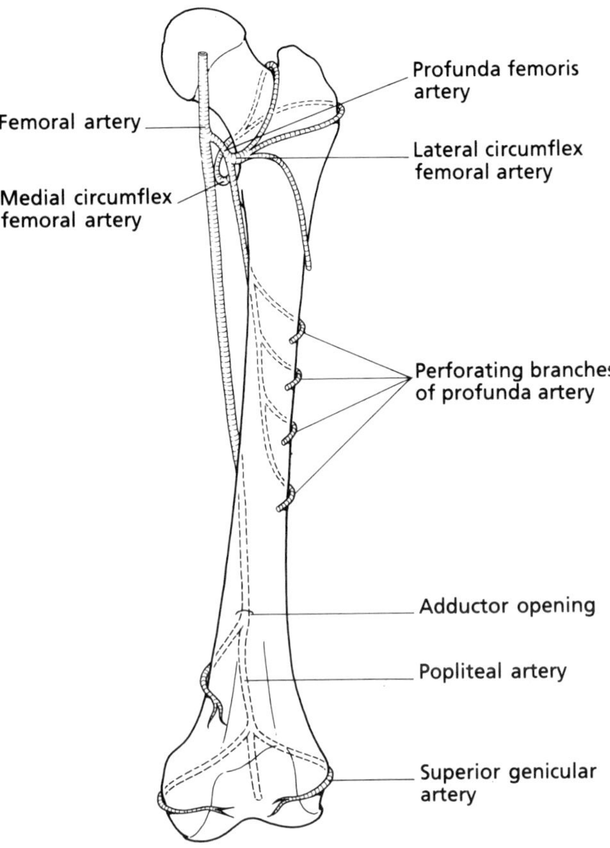

Fig. 21.9 Main arterial circulation of the thigh.

Rigid plating can result in a disturbance of the periosteal blood supply (Rhinelander & Wilson 1982). In addition, there is an element of stress protection which will result in an initial hyperaemia from the endosteal blood supply, and osteoporosis of the area of bone immediately adjacent to and below the plate. During fracture healing, stress protection becomes less and the circulation returns to normal.

Intramedullary reaming completely destroys the endosteal circulation and results in a temporary loss of blood supply to at least inner two-thirds of the cortical bone, regardless of whether or not an implant is used (Fig. 21.10). However, at an early stage there is a reversal of the centrifugal aspect of blood supply and the periosteal blood supply takes on a more important role. Over the next 2−3 weeks the endosteal circulation starts to recover (Brookes, personal communication). The use of unreamed nails in the canine tibia has been shown to produce much less disturbance of the cortical circulation, resulting in only 31% cortical area loss as opposed to 70% following reaming (Klein *et al.* 1989).

Treatment of femoral fractures

The object of fracture management is the restoration of optimum function of the limb and a return to normal for the patient in the shortest time by the safest and most reliable method. Early mobilization, with return to the home environment, provides a psychological stimulus to recovery. In the fractured femur, treatment requires stabilization of the main fragments in continuity with-

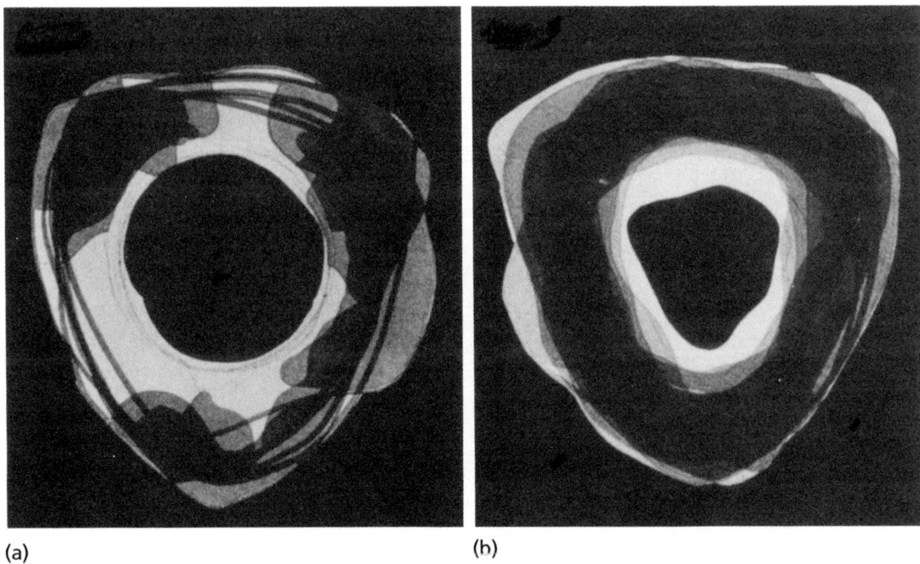

(a)   (b)

Fig. 21.10 Superimposition of the cross-sections of six (a) reamed and (b) unreamed tibiae. Normal circulation stains black. Absent circulation is white.

out malalignment, rotation or shortening. This should be followed by early muscle and knee recovery with safe mobilization from bed and hospital without jeopardizing the fracture union.

Treatment of the fractured femoral shaft is considered in five sections:

1 Diaphyseal fractures.
2 Subtrochanteric fractures.
3 Distal, supracondylar and condylar fractures.
4 Fractures in children.
5 Pathological fractures.

Diaphyseal fractures

Classification

Classification of femoral shaft fractures has to reflect the increasing complexity of the fracture pattern as an index of the force producing it, and the stability of the fracture possible with treatment. These patterns range from simple single fractures through butterfly fragments, two-level segmental fractures to comminuted fractures of increasing severity. Four grades of comminuted fracture have been described (Fig. 21.11) (Winquist & Hansen 1980):

Type I — with 75% of the cortex intact.
Type II — with 50–75% intact.
Type III — with 25–50% intact.
Type IV — with no contact.

Recently, a comprehensive classification of all long bones has been developed (Müller *et al.* 1988) with an alpha-numeric computer diagnostic code. The fracture is coded by bone and segment numbers, and type with subdivision for increasing severity; the main groups of this OA classification of fractures involving the femoral shaft are shown in Fig. 21.22.

Treatment options

Options for the treatment of femoral shaft fractures have evolved over a long period and now form three groups:

1 Closed manipulation with traction and casting.
2 External fixation with percutaneous pins and side bar(s).
3 Internal fixation with intramedullary nails or plates with screws.

Bed traction management was the standard method of treatment for most femoral shaft fractures in the first half of the twentieth century. Although the union rate was high, the average time in traction was 12 weeks (Watson-Jones 1960) and there was an expected knee recovery period of 12 months (Charnley 1961) with a high rate of knee stiffness occurring (Nichols 1963).

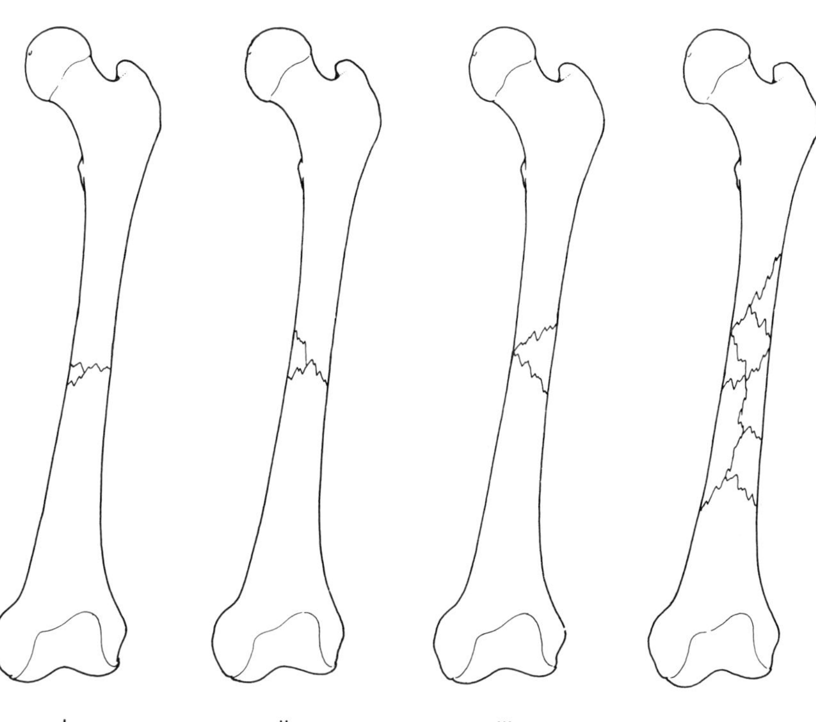

Fig. 21.11 Winquist and Hansen classification of comminution.

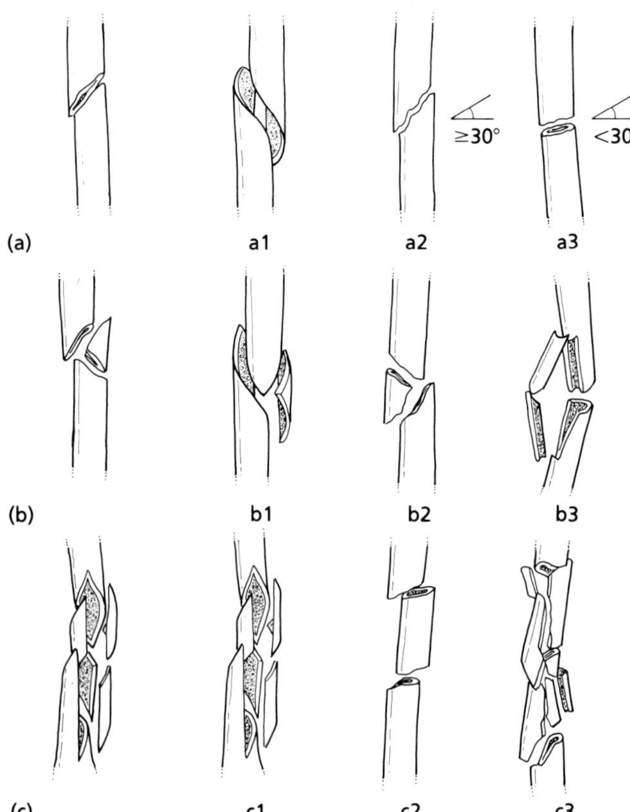

Fig. 21.12 AO classification of femoral shaft fractures.
(a) Femur diaphysis, simple fracture: 1, spiral; 2, oblique;
3, transverse. (b) Femur diaphysis, wedge fracture: 1, spiral
wedge; 2, bending wedge; 3, fragmented wedge. (c) Femur
diaphysis, complex fracture: 1, spiral; 2, segmental;
3, irregular.

Further developments in the non-operative care were
the use of functional fracture bracing systems for distal-
half femoral shaft fractures (Mooney *et al.* 1970,
Sarmiento 1972); these considerably reduced the traction
and hospital time to half that of the bed traction alone
(Thomas & Meggitt 1981).

The introduction of the intramedullary nail
(Küntscher 1967) provided treatment for the middle
and proximal-half femoral shaft fractures with the early
mobilization of patient and knee. This method was not
suitable for stabilizing distal shaft fractures at the point
of widening of the medullary canal or for the severe
comminuted type with shortening. The introduction,
by the Swiss AO group, of anatomical reduction and
rigid internal fixation with compression screws and
plates (Müller *et al.* 1965) extended the operative treatment with complex and exacting surgery for femoral
shaft fractures. Significant advances were made with
the development of the locking intramedullary nail
(Kempf *et al.* 1985) with proximal and distal cross screws

permitting stable fixation of all shaft fractures, even
with severe comminution beyond the scope of conventional intramedullary nails or plates. The closed
technique performed under image-intensifier control
has reduced the operation time and infection risk, and
allows almost immediate mobilization of the knee and
patient. This rapidly changing technology in the treatment of femoral shaft fractures is shown in a review of
the Cambridge experience from 1970 to 1990 (Fig. 21.13).

External fixation with percutaneous pins and bars has
only a limited acceptance in the treatment of femoral
shaft fractures. Severe fractures with open wounds,
which carry a high risk of infection with internal fixation, can be stabilized with the external fixator and this
allows easy access to the wounds for further treatment.
External fixation is usually considered a valuable temporary emergency measure for 'untreatable' fractures
(Dabezies *et al.* 1984), with very few reports existing on
its use in all femoral shaft fractures (De Bastiani *et al.*
1984).

Selection factors

Selection of the optimum method for treatment of each
patient with a femoral shaft fracture depends mainly
upon the following criteria:
1 *Fracture*: site, pattern, comminution and soft tissue
injury.

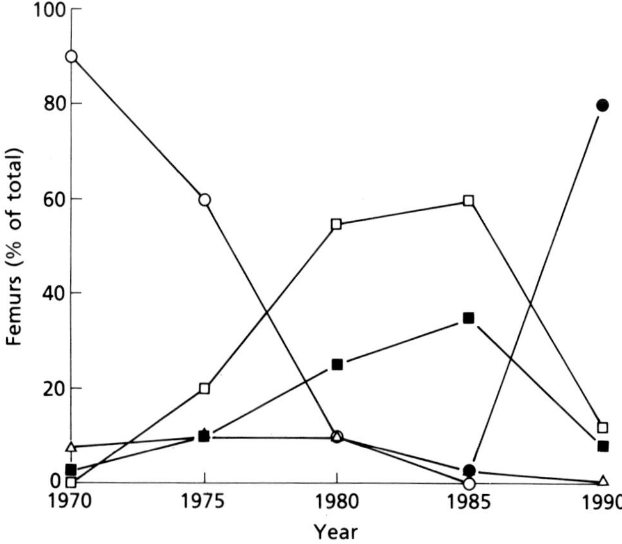

Fig. 21.13 Femoral shaft fractures: treatment profile
1970–1990 from Addenbrooke's Hospital, Cambridge.
○, Traction; ●, plate; □, cast brace; ■, intramedullary nail;
△, lock nail.

2 *Bone*: osteoporosis, infection, deformity and disease.
3 *Patient*: age, general condition and associated injuries.
4 *Expertise*: skill and experience of surgeon and team.
5 *Technology*: instrumentation and equipment available.

It is necessary for the surgeon to undertake a full evaluation of these factors before selecting and proceeding with treatment. The most recent advances, of closed locking intramedullary nails for femoral shaft fractures, require a high level of surgical expertise and modern technology (traction table, complex instrumentation, air tools and image-intensifier). However, in many situations this level of surgical expertise and technology is not available, requiring either transfer of the patient to a centre where they are, or utilization of a lower level of technology. In many parts of the developing world, treatment must be adapted with low technology levels of traction and casting or intermediate levels with external fixation. Also, there are occasional situations where surgical treatment is not indicated or possible in any unit and non-operative methods must be used. Thus, it is necessary for the surgeon dealing with fractures to have a working knowledge of all the options available and to select the optimum treatment for the patient in that particular situation.

Initial assessment

Fractures of the femoral shaft are not usually isolated injuries and the patient may have multiple injuries which may involve the head, chest and abdomen, and may include other extremity fractures. These injuries can result in severe shock and life-threatening complications which require emergency treatment, by various specialists in the trauma team. A full evaluation of the fractured limb is required to assess other injuries, open wounds and evidence of neurovascular damage. Treatment for the fractured femur itself requires immediate analgesia, immobilization with skin traction and blood replacement, as there is often extensive internal thigh bleeding with muscle damage; 2–4 units of whole blood may be required. Open wounds require clinical description and documentation with instantly developed photographs before they are sealed with sterile dressings, the leg is elevated and intravenous antibiotics are administered; debridement and surgical treatment follow later. A radiological assessment of the entire lower extremity, including the pelvis, may be required to exclude the not uncommon associated ipsilateral injuries of fractures or dislocations of the hip, fractures involving the distal femur, patella and tibia, and knee ligament or foot injuries. Contralateral lower limb injuries and spine fractures also require exclusion

with radiographs if suspected. If there are clinical signs of any vascular injury, then an urgent arteriogram is essential when the femoral or translumbar approach should be used.

Non-operative treatment methods

Early casting of femoral shaft fractures is only possible in small children because an unacceptable position is produced by the powerful limb muscles. Closed reduction and maintenance of alignment and length require traction to the femur. In the first half of the twentieth century, the bed traction suspension method was the standard treatment for union of most femoral shaft fractures. This was then followed by a plaster hip spica or a weight-bearing caliper until consolidation occurred. Development of femoral cast bracing in the 1970s reduced the use of skeletal traction to the early period only. Today, with the majority of femoral shaft fractures being treated operatively, bed traction is only used during the primary phase while the patient is awaiting definitive fixation. The development of modern Trauma centres and the immediate availability of operative fixation are reducing skeletal traction even further and this is to the benefit of patients.

TRACTION SYSTEMS

These involves the use either of 'fixed' traction on a Thomas' splint or of 'sliding' traction with or without a splint. These two traction methods differ in that isometric reduction is involved in fixed traction and isotonic reduction in sliding traction, where the splint then acts only for suspension. The fixed traction method of Thomas required manipulative reduction of the fracture and maintenance of the reduction by skeletal traction applied through a transverse pin, inserted behind the tibial tubercle and attached by cords to the distal splint cross bar. Counter-traction was provided by the Thomas' splint ring against the perineum and groin; any excessive pressure was relieved by a small additional weight attached to the distal end of the splint. Charnley (1961) reported good results with this fixed traction system, but problems with knee stiffness and patient discomfort resulted in the sliding traction system being widely used. The Thomas' splint then functions only as a leg suspension device, with the continuous traction being applied directly to the skeletal traction tibial pin. The Pearson knee-flexion piece is an additional attachment to the centre of the Thomas' splint, and allows the knee to be held comfortably flexed with the leg elevated. The Fisk splint was a hinged variety of the Thomas' splint, and allowed active mobilization of the knee by the patient at the appropriate time. These, and other variations of traction and splinting systems, have been described and discussed by Charnley (1961) (see Fig. 21.3).

BALANCED TRACTION TECHNIQUE

A suitable size of Thomas' splint is selected with a Pearson knee piece attached, both being approximately 10 cm longer than the normal limb and having a thick ring size 5 cm larger to allow for swelling. This is prepared by the addition of non-stretchable slings passed across the thigh and calf sections of the splint. Skeletal traction is applied following the insertion of a Denham or Steinmann pin just behind the tibial tubercle under local or general anaesthetic, as necessary. If the fracture requires manual reduction, this is undertaken with a short relaxant anaesthetic and the Thomas' splint is threaded over the leg. Skeletal traction is applied via a cord attached to a hoop applied to the skeletal pin; 8–10 kg weight is usual for an average adult. A large, firm wool pad is applied just distal to the fracture and the whole splint is suspended via cords, pulleys and weights from an overhead beam (Fig. 21.14). Elevation of the foot of the bed provides counter-traction to the skeletal traction. Biplanar radiographs are taken and appropriate adjustments made to the pads, sling or pulleys until correct alignment and reduction of the femoral fracture has been obtained. A tape measure is useful when comparing lengths with the uninjured limb, and attention to any posterior, varus or rotational deformities is undertaken and corrected as necessary. Distraction should be avoided, particularly with transverse fractures, as delayed union may result. Clinical and radiographic assessment of the fracture, with the necessary adjustments, is made to maintain the reduction until callus union stabilizes the fracture. Late problems of varus and posterior angulation, particularly around weeks 4–6 when callus union occurs, must be prevented. The optional use of a Charnley plaster traction unit with a below-knee cast incorporating the skeletal pin may give better control of the lower limb during the early unstable fracture period. Quadricep exercises are started as soon as possible and once the patient can lift the lower leg from the splint then knee flexion exercises are begun. Change of the Thomas' splint to a Fisk splint at this stage allows the physiotherapist to start active mobilization of the knee. Once the union is clinically stable and radiologically well advanced, non-weight-bearing mobilization with crutches is allowed. In adults, union varies on average from 8 weeks for a spiral fracture to 16 weeks for a transverse fracture, but clinical evaluation is always necessary. Intensive knee and quadriceps exercises are undertaken and weight-bearing is delayed until consolidation of the fracture has occurred; this may well take 12–24 weeks. Earlier mobilization is possible but requires stabilization of the fracture with a plaster hip spica or modified long-leg caliper brace.

FEMORAL CAST BRACING

Principles

The problem of long stays in bed and hospital with sliding traction suspension treatment of femoral fractures was reduced to 50% with the introduction of femoral functional cast bracing. This system involved the application of an above-knee thigh cast connected to a below-knee walking cast with lateral and medial polycentric hinges, giving essentially a long-leg knee-

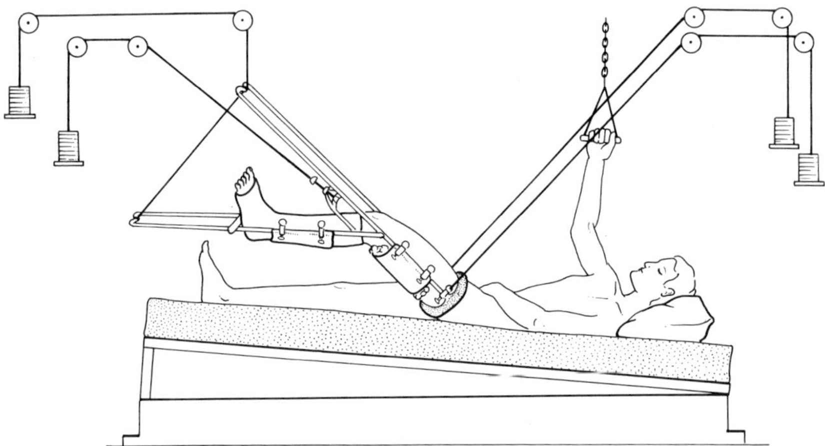

Fig. 21.14 Balanced sliding skeletal traction with Thomas' splint, Pearson knee piece and a Charnley plaster traction unit.

hinged weight-bearing cast. With early functional weight-bearing, mobilization of the patient and leg, knee stiffness and high wasting were greatly reduced. The original concept that the cast brace functioned as a weight-relieving caliper or as a soft tissue hydraulic compression cylinder of the thigh, required that high loads would be taken through the brace. Biomechanical studies (Meggitt *et al.* 1981) showed that the brace carried small loads throughout healing and that it was the fracture itself which controlled the increase in the loading of the leg. This was considered to function as an anti-buckling hinged tube and a steady increase in permissible load-bearing was determined by the fracture healing itself.

Indications

In the absence of other technology, cast bracing is indicated for all closed fractures of the distal half of the femoral shaft, provided that adequate reduction and fracture stability can be maintained.

Management

Functional femoral fracture bracing has three phases of treatment:
1 Reduction and maintenance with traction suspension until the fracture is stable.
2 Cast brace mobilization with maximal weight-bearing until union occurs.
3 Post-bracing period with intensive physiotherapy.
The application time for the femoral cast brace should ideally be when the fracture has reached the sticky, stable, plastic state and is bendable but not displaceable; this usually takes between 4 and 6 weeks (Fig. 21.15). Too early application can lead to malposition, and too late application to a waste of bed and hospital time. A cast brace application technique involves a full-length thigh and below-knee cast section of plaster of Paris or resin cast, with quadrilateral moulding of the proximal thigh. Paired hinges are plastered in at the correct knee axis, i.e. the mid-patella or adductor tubercle level and just behind the mid-axial lateral thigh line. The foot section is reinforced for weight-bearing with a walking cast shoe (Fig. 21.16). Radiographs are obtained immediately after brace application, to check the femoral fracture position, and again after full mobilization.

Variations of the most basic and economical plaster femoral cast brace involve laminated castings with elasticated plaster bandages, and resin or acrylic lightweight cast rolls. Stable metal hinges with locking screws or plastic types are available, but they should ideally be stable in the medial-lateral plain, especially for lower shaft fractures. A number of variations are available with the thigh section incorporating a pre-shaped or externally mouldable plastic brim, or with the two sections constructed from thermo-mouldable plastic sheets (Hall & Stenner 1985). For non-obese limbs, an even more functional 'cylinder' cast brace (Fig. 21.17) may be used with a total contact, well-moulded plastic cast being supported from a waist belt with suspension straps, and with elimination of the restricting foot section (Vaughan-Lane & Meggitt 1980). After cast bracing, the patient is allowed to mobilize, maximally weight-bearing with elbow crutches and undertaking knee exercises before discharge from hospital, usually at around 5−6 weeks after the fracture. Monitoring of the fracture healing progress can be followed using the 10-second steady standing test on bathroom scales (Meggitt *et al.* 1981). The average 10-second-maximum of weight-bearing in the cast brace is used as a percentage of the body weight to determine the fracture union index. A steady increase in this index to 100% at between 12 and 20 weeks indicates satisfactory bone healing (Fig. 21.18). A failure of steady recovery suggests that there are union problems which need to be investigated. Cast brace removal is undertaken when full weight-bearing in the braced limb is possible. An intensive course of mobilization and strengthening physiotheraphy then follows, with good functional limb recovery expected.

Operative treatment methods

There is little doubt that the locked intramedullary nail has overshadowed, and in some centres supplanted, most other surgical options in the management of this fracture. In 1967, Küntscher published what is generally regarded as the definitive treatise on intramedullary nailing and, in 1968, described the development of a locking technique. In parallel with this, the AO school was developing its own plating techniques for long bone fractures (Müller *et al.* 1979). Acceptance of an operative approach to femoral shaft fractures was slow in the English-speaking world, partly because of the strong influence of a powerful conservative school but also because of anxiety about the supposedly high incidence of infection, often amounting to 7−15% following. open surgical procedures of the femur.

Surgical options can be divided into three groups:
1 External fixation.
2 Tension-band techniques (i.e. plating).
3 Intramedullary devices.

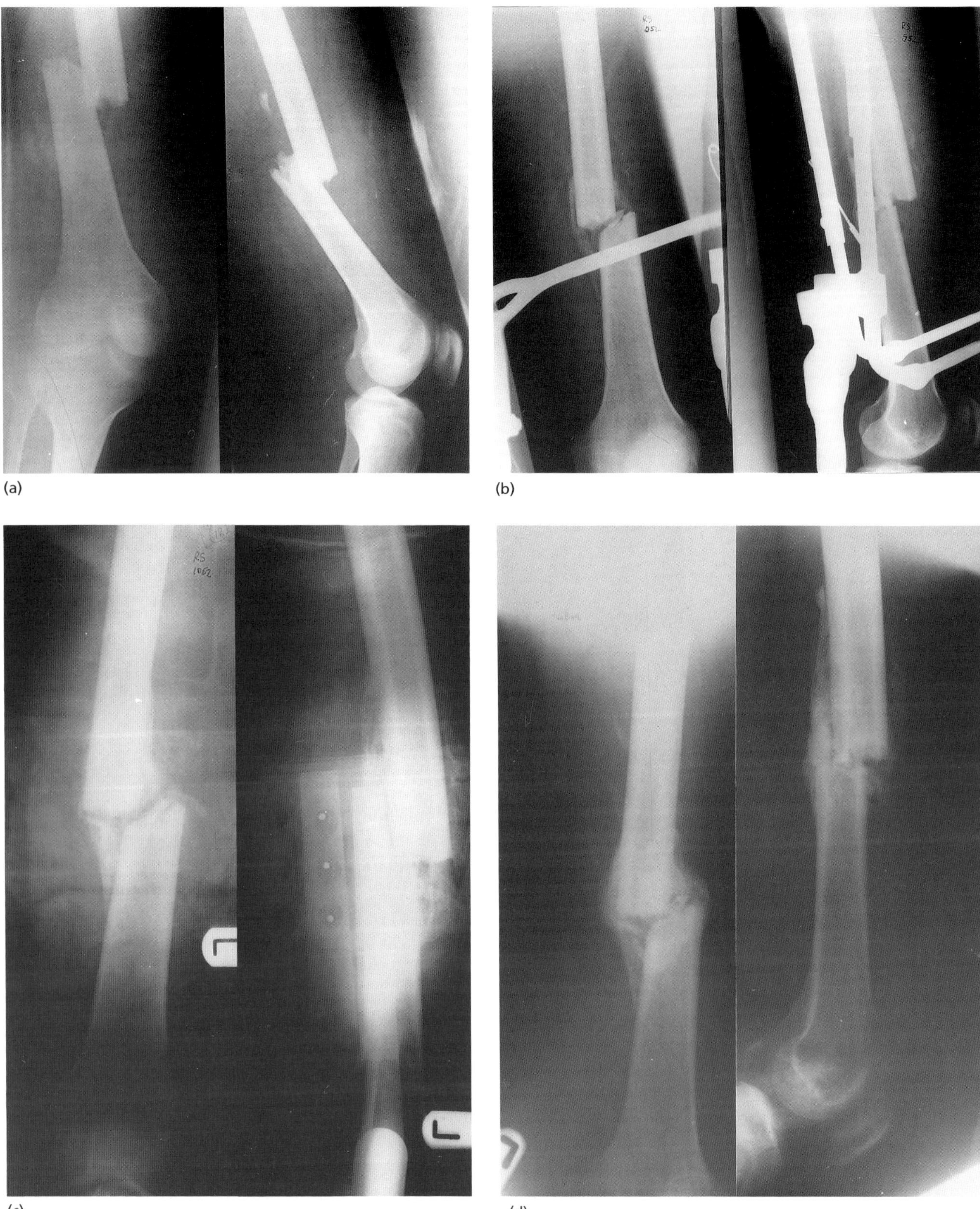

Fig. 21.15 Cast brace treatment stages: (a) acute fracture for skeletal traction treatment; (b) sticky callus phase for cast bracing at 6 weeks; (c) mobile in cast brace at 12 weeks; (d) fracture union with brace removal at 16 weeks.

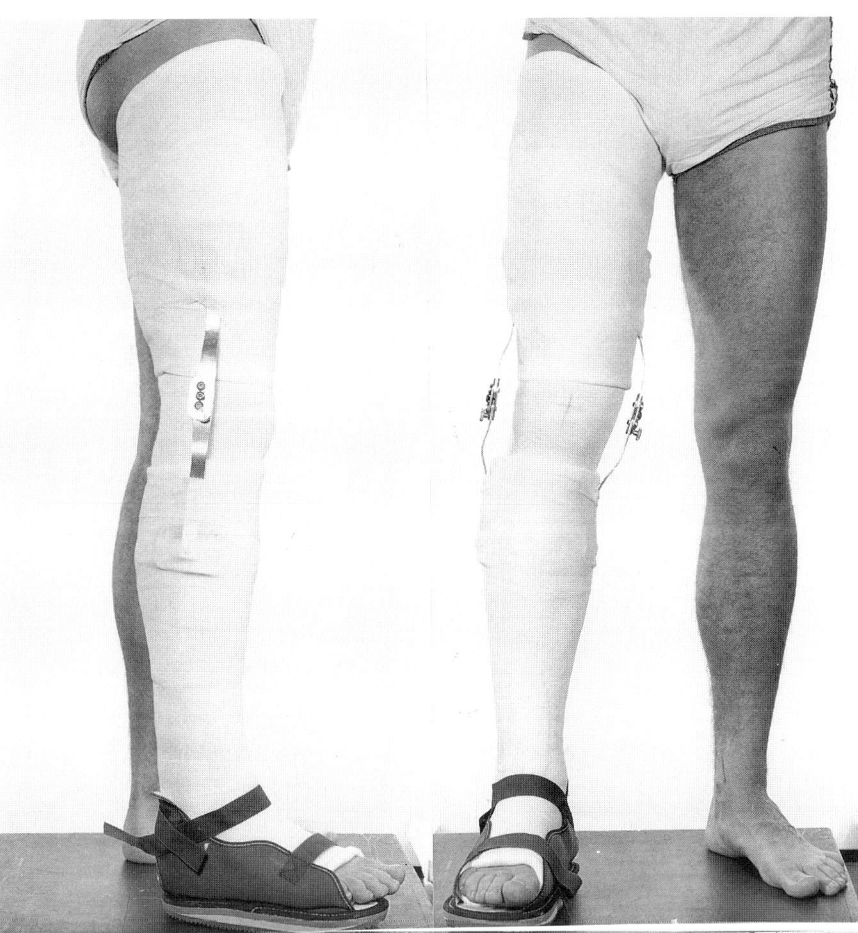

Fig. 21.16 Femoral cast brace with a composite plaster and plastic contoured casts, stable knee hinges with removable locking screws and a walking cast shoe.

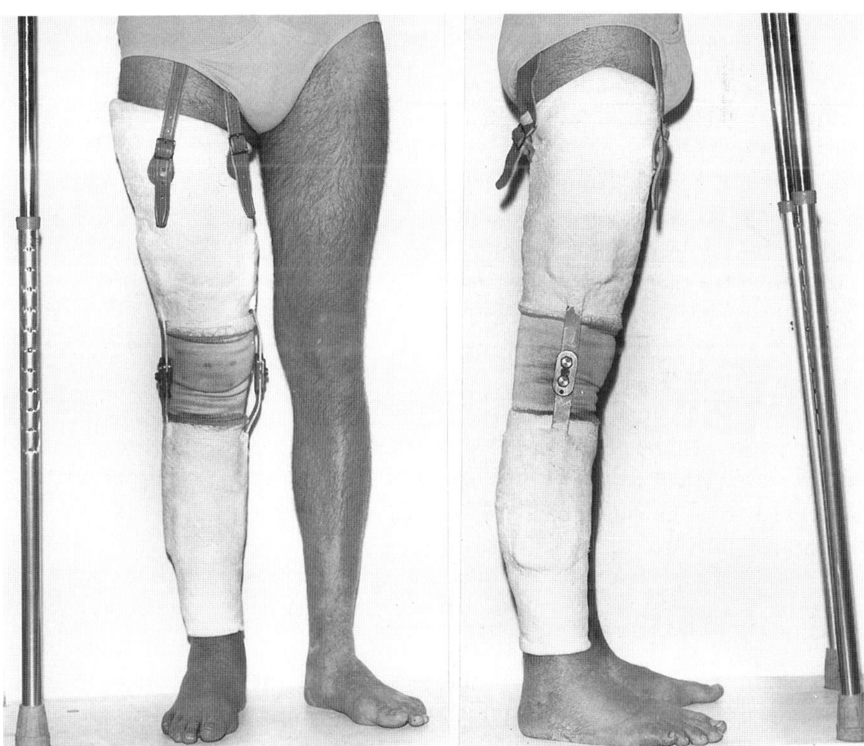

Fig. 21.17 Femoral cylinder cast brace with suspension straps from waist belt to cast buttons (elasticated posterior strap for sitting).

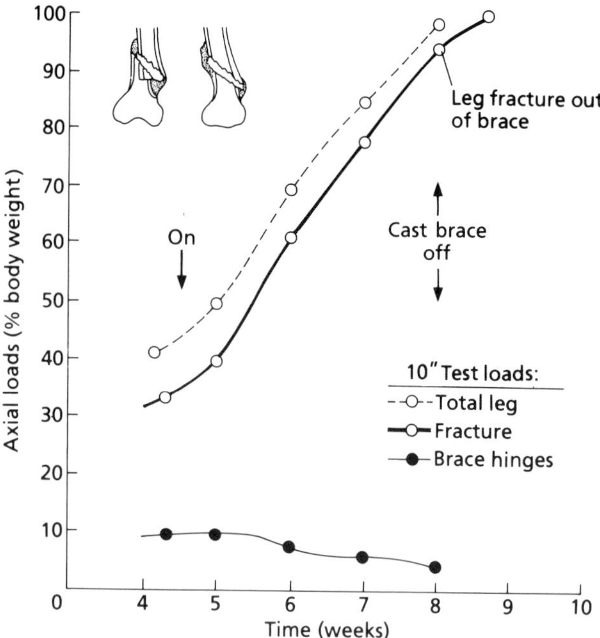

Fig. 21.18 Increase in load bearing through the femur as bony union proceeds.

EXTERNAL FIXATION

External fixation of femoral shaft fractures is usually reserved for open injuries where there is major soft tissue loss or damage. However, the work of De Bastiani *et al.* (1984) has promoted the concept of managing closed fractures with external fixators; they claim a 98% consolidation rate. This method of treatment has not gained popularity since, although it is relatively non-invasive, the bulk of muscle and soft tissue between the skin and the bone requires the fixator to be laterally placed; it also involves a moderate amount of local dissection in order to allow the muscles to slide around the pins. High mechanical forces have a much greater tendency to cause pin loosening. Alignment is also more difficult to control and varus deformity is not uncommon (Fig. 21.19). There is often difficulty both in achieving and maintaining full extension and flexion during bone healing. However, if the fracture is very comminuted, there is a 'floating knee' or the patient is otherwise too debilitated, then the use of an external fixator has much to commend it (Fig. 21.20).

PLATING TECHNIQUE

Prior to the wide availability of the locking nail for proximal, distal and comminuted fractures of the femur, plating techniques were the only forms of operative

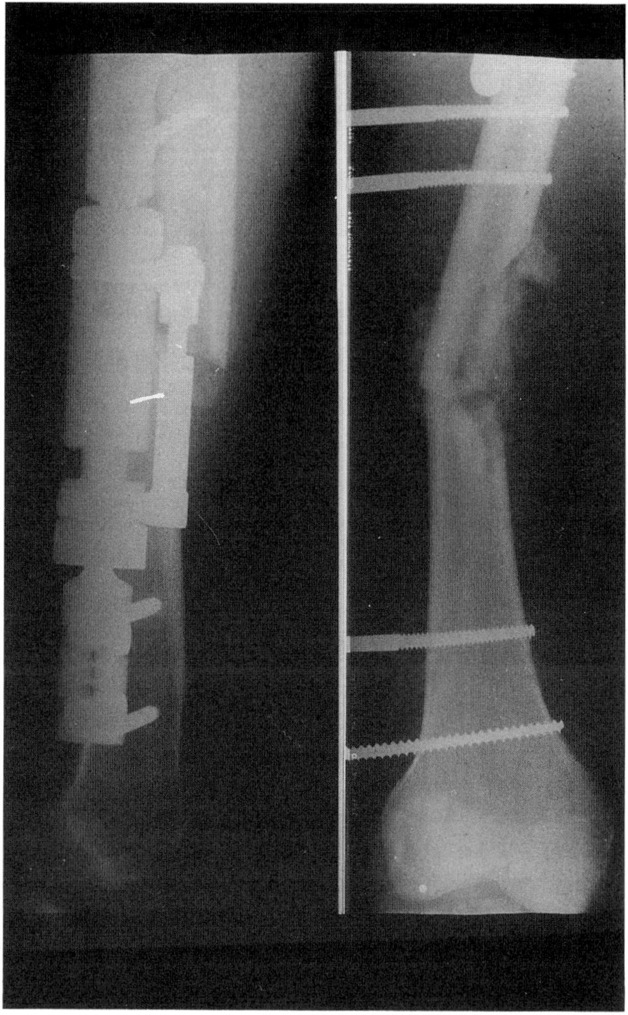

Fig. 21.19 Despite adequate fixation, this patient's sheer bulk was too great to allow full correction into axial alignment.

treatment available. Occasionally, plates were used in combination with an intramedullary nail as an anti-rotation device (Burwell 1971), although the resulting endosteal and periosteal circulatory destruction had the potential for major bone necrosis (Fig. 21.21). The role of plating remains controversial, but if a plate is to be used, then the AO system is the most versatile and reliable (Reudi & Luscher 1979).

Indications

As in all methods of surgical treatment, no one implant will cover all indications. Plating techniques are particularly useful in the following circumstances:
1 *Polytrauma*. In the polytraumatized patient with chest, abdominal or pelvic injuries, the use of a plate requires

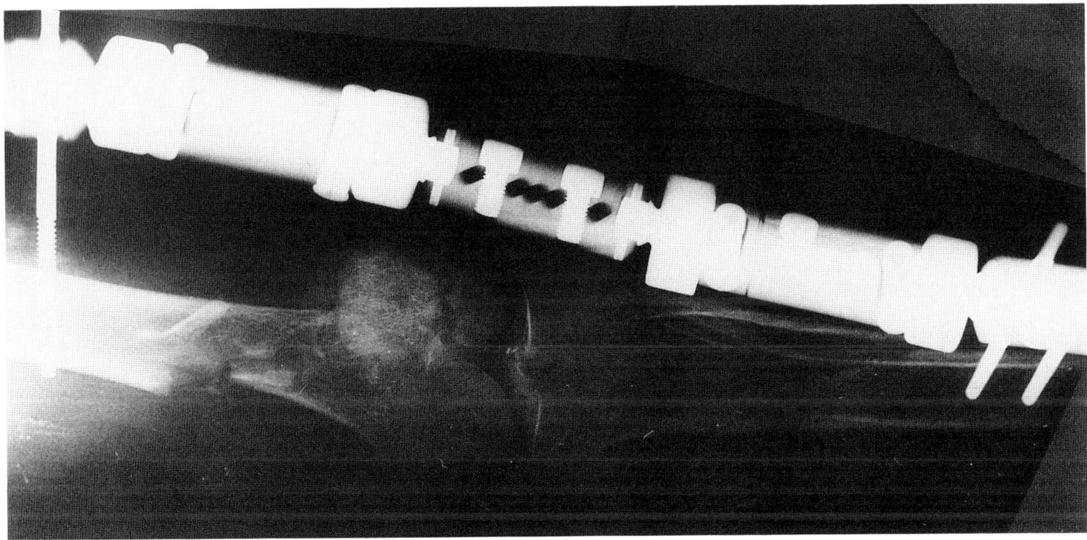

Fig. 21.20 This elderly female was too ill to tolerate major surgery and had extensive type III open injuries. Following consolidation of the fracture with an external fixator, she achieved a remarkably good range of knee movement.

only a standard operating table and is quicker and safer than the use of the locking nail. The slightly increased risk of deep infection is regarded as acceptable in association with the relative safety of the technique.

2 *Nerve or vascular injuries.* In an open femoral shaft fracture, vascular or nerve repair may need to be performed. Occasionally, it is necessary to shorten the femur in order to accomplish this. It is evident that plating under these circumstances is a logical and effective method of fixation, despite possible long-term risks of delayed or non-union.

3 *Pre-existing deformity* (in which the femur is too bent or sclerotic to allow passage of a locking nail). Refracture or fracture through a Pagetic bone with marked pre-existing deformity obviously precludes the use of a locking nail. Frequently, bone in this circumstance is pathological and the hold of external fixator pins would be poor. Careful contouring of a plate may well be necessary.

4 *Extension into the trochanteric or condylar regions.* The use of a blade plate or dynamic compression screw in the condylar and trochanteric regions in association with a femoral shaft fracture remains the best way of managing these fractures. At present, there is no satisfactory external fixator or locking nail which is able to cope totally with these injuries, particularly if there is an intracondylar extension.

5 *Unavailability of a locking nail system and associated expertise.* The use of the locking nail requires a large armamentarium of equipment, including a compatible operating table system and image intensifier. Absence of this will preclude satisfactory fixation. The technical tricks of locking nailing are much greater than those required for plating and for the occasional operator plating is probably safer.

6 *Fractures in children.* The inability to satisfactorily reduce a fracture in the older child with the epiphysis still open is an absolute indication for the use of a plate.

Technique

Careful preoperative assessment is particularly important when plating any femoral shaft fracture. Adequate anteroposterior and lateral radiographs must be available, to show the extent of the fracture, together with a radiograph of the opposite femur in its entirely so that a preoperative plan can be drawn up. In deciding the length and position of the plate, the basic AO principles of lag screwing must be considered, wherever possible, together with six cortical screw holds above and below the limits of the fracture. It is essential to use a broad dynamic compression plate.

The degree of comminution of the fracture will influence the plating technique used. If the fracture has only a minimal degree of comminution, as in Winquist and Hansen types I, II and III, then accurate reduction using lag screws will be necessary. However, if the comminution is greater than this, mobilization of the fragments will only cause devascularization and the aim should be to use a long plate bridging the comminuted area (biological fixation), in order to hold the femoral shaft out to length.

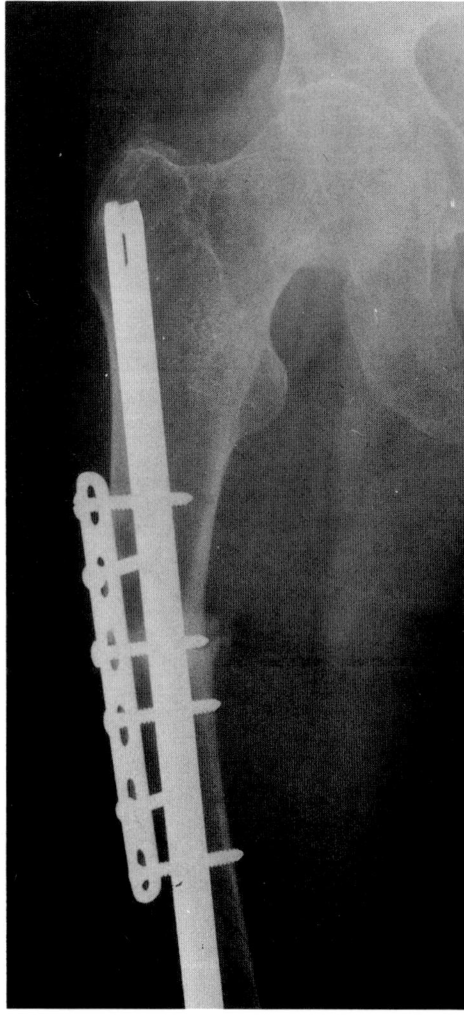

Fig. 21.21 The rotational instability of this fracture has been neutralized by the use of an anti-rotation plate, the screws of which are straddling the Küntscher nail. Even so, it has not been possible to maintain a perfect position.

A bone graft should always be placed on the medial side.

Surgical approach

The approach to the entire shaft of the femur is from a line joining the greater trochanter and the mid-part of the lateral femoral condyle. The fascia lata is divided along the same line to gain access to the vastus lateralis, which is dissected medially from the intermuscular septum and down to the linea aspera (Fig. 21.22). If the fracture extends down to the condylar area, it will be necessary to open the knee joint and extend the incision anteriorly to the tibial tubercle.

The linea aspera is invariably intact and is an excellent

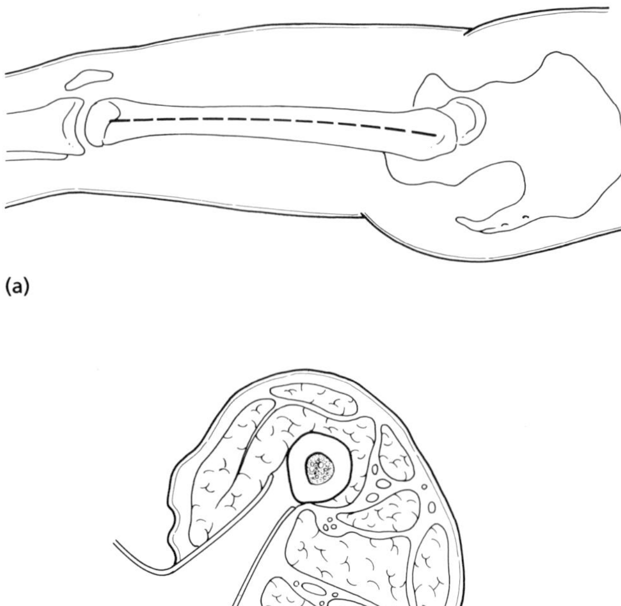

(a)

(b)

Fig. 21.22 (a) Exposure of the femoral shaft is along an imaginary line joining the trochanteric mass and the mid-part of the lateral femoral condyle. (b) The vastus lateralis is divided in the line of the skin and retracted anteriorly together with the vastus lateralis.

guide to alignment. It may need to be released for 1–2 cm at the ends of the bone in order to assist in the mobilization of other fragments and to achieve an accurate reduction. In the more simple fractures, where there is minimal comminution and interfragmentary compression will be achieved, it is sometimes helpful to provisionally reduce the fracture using cerclage wires, particularly if some of the interfragmentary screws have to pass through the plate. These cerclage wires can then be removed following the application of the plate. Reduction before plate fixation is necessary in order to adequately contour the plate for more distal fractures. It can then be applied according to the preoperative plan (see p. 726).

The addition of a cancellous bone graft to the medial wall of the fracture is mandatory.

In more comminuted fractures (Winquist and Hansen type IV), the plate will act as a buttress to hold the proximal and distal shafts in alignment with the comminuted fragments acting as bone graft between the two ends. In such circumstances, the linea aspera is particularly valuable as a guide to rotation of the bony fragments. The AO femoral distractor is of invaluable assistance in holding the bone ends out to length and once this has been applied, prior to plate fixation, a check of the shaft of the femur should be taken to ensure that there is no discrepancy between the planned and actual length. The contoured plate is then applied according to the plan, again ensuring that there are at least six, and preferably seven, cortical screw holds above and below the fracture ends (Fig. 21.23).

Again, bone graft should be used. Particularly in such circumstances, the old adage applies: one never regrets taking a bone graft but one often regrets not doing so.

The wounds are closed over suction drainage with meticulous closure of the fascia lata and skin.

Postoperative management

With the advent of the continuous passive motion (CPM) machine, passive knee flexion can start immediately. Some physiotherapists are unhappy about these machines because they feel that their use increases the extensor lag. Nevertheless, starting passive and active knee flexion in the early postoperative period is of vital importance since the potential for quadriceps tethering is extremely high. Once adequate quadriceps control is present, the patient can be mobilized non-weight-

bearing. It will depend very much on the configuration and stability of the fracture as to the timing of partial weight-bearing. It is important that in the first 8–12 weeks regular radiographs should be obtained in order to detect the presence of irritation callus, which would indicate weakening and possible fatigue of the plate (see p. 739). Only when there is good evidence of a satisfactory bony buttress medially should full weight-bearing be allowed.

INTRAMEDULLARY NAILS

The middle third of the femur is the domain of the intramedullary nail' (Müller *et al.* 1979). Simple short oblique or transverse fractures in this region, even in association with type I or II Winquist and Hansen comminution, are suitable for simple nailing alone. Locking nailing extends the indications to fractures which are comminuted, oblique or spiral and also into the subtrochanteric and supracondylar regions (Kempf *et al.* 1985) (Fig. 21.24). The decision of whether to perform a simple nailing or locking nailing would depend on the preoperative evaluation of the fracture and its axial rotational and angulatory stability. For

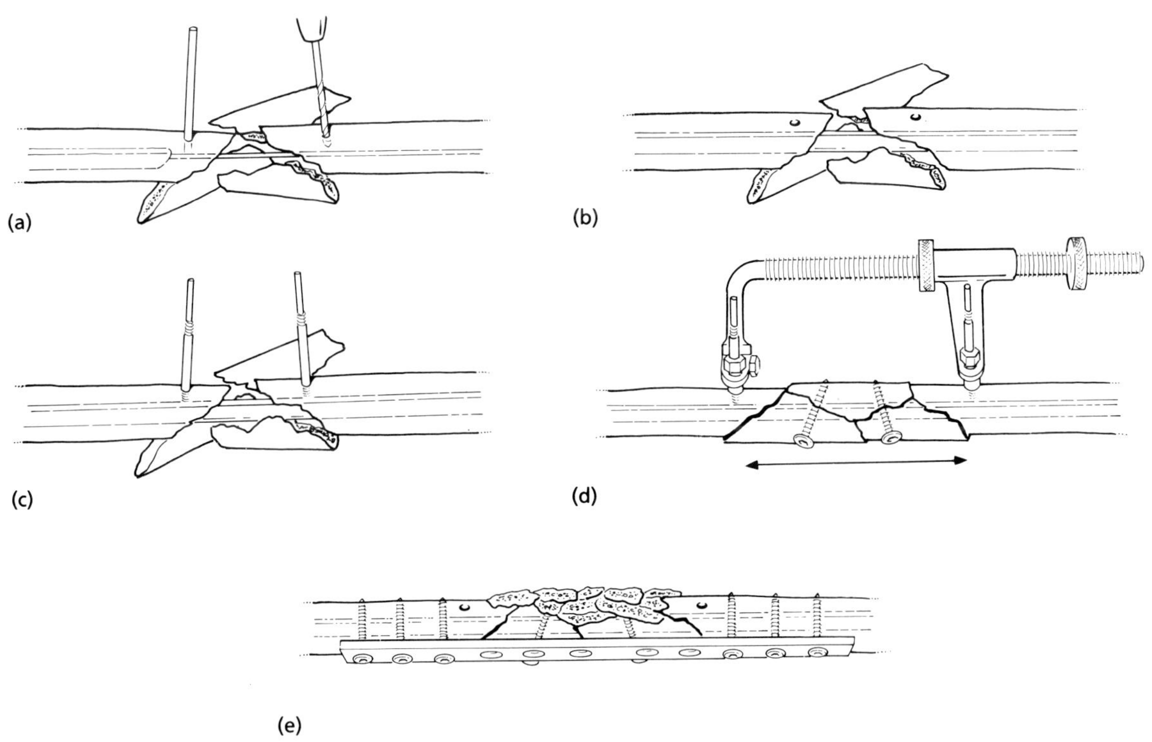

Fig. 21.23 (a) Temporary insertion of shantz screws in proximal and distal fragments. (b) Removal of pins to allow passage of IM nail. (c) Reinsertion of pins. (d) Application of distractor; advancement of distractor nut realigns femur and pulls it out to length. (e) Anti-rotation plate and bone graft.

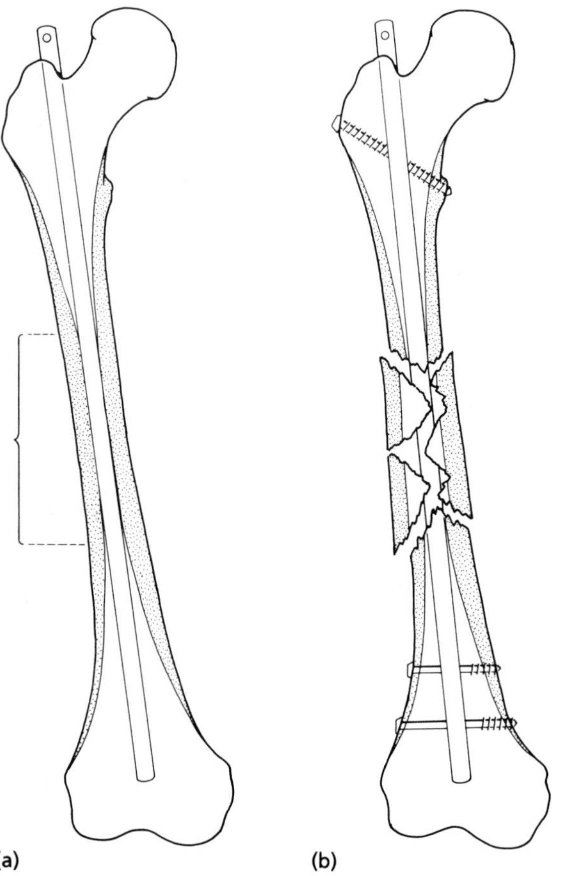

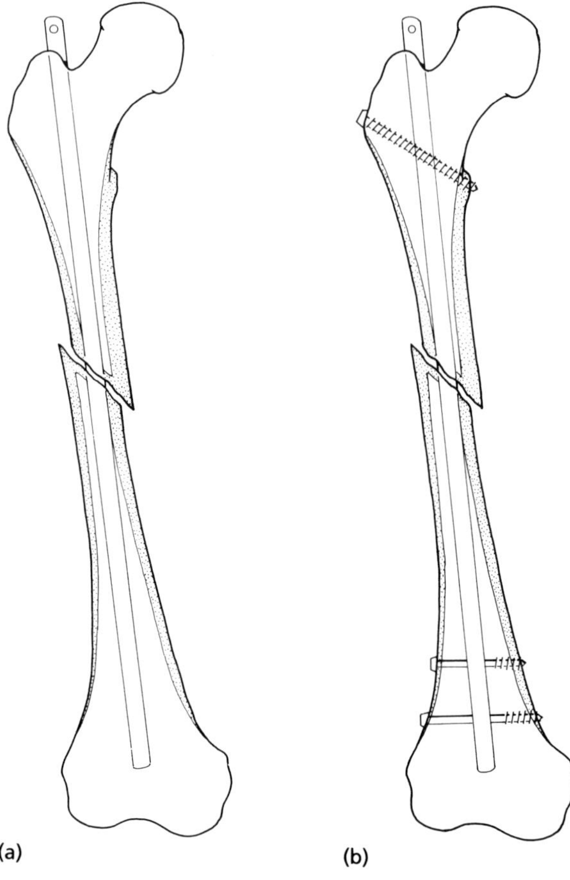

Fig. 21.24 (a) Fracture stability is achieved if the purchase of the nail on the cortex extends 3 cm distally and proximally. (b) But with the locking nail, cortical contact is not necessary at all provided that there is adequate purchase by the locking screws. A much greater spectrum of fracture configurations can therefore be treated.

Fig. 21.25 (a) A long spiral fracture will shorten by external or internal rotation along the line of the nail. Inevitably, the nail will tend to back out in the hip region and this will result in major complications. The only way to prevent this complication is by the use of adjunctive traction or, alternatively, cast bracing to prevent rotation of the distal fragment. (b) Static locking will prevent rotation of the proximal on the distal fragment and thus shortening.

instance, a long spiral fracture treated with a simple nail has the potential to shorten and rotate about the nail because there is no good proximal or distal hold of the bone on the nail (Fig. 21.25). Similarly, a distal-third fracture will have the potential for varus or valgus deformity because the nail has no good purchase in the soft cancellous bone in the supracondylar region (Fig. 21.26). In the first instance proximal and distal locking ('static' locking) is necessary and in the second instance only distal locking will be necessary, provided that there is an adequate purchase of the nail in the middle third of the femur ('dynamic' locking). In these more proximal and distal fractures, nailing can be used as an alignment method, although adjunctive fixation such as cerclage wires or anti-rotation plates should not be used because of the risk of devascularization of the periosteal supply. An alternative would be postoperative traction and cast bracing.

It goes without saying that although a formal pre-operative plan is not essential when using a nailing technique, since anatomical reduction of a comminuted fracture cannot be achieved, it is important to measure the opposite limb preoperatively in order to decide on the correct length of nail to be used.

Classically, three nailing techniques are available for consideration:

1 Open nailing using a retrograde technique. This method does not need a traction table. The lateral position is used and the fracture is exposed. The proximal and distal fragments are reamed up in 1-mm steps using a solid reamer. The nail is inserted through the fracture site in retrograde fashion, and at the point of its exit through the trochanteric region a stab skin incision is made and the nail advanced through the

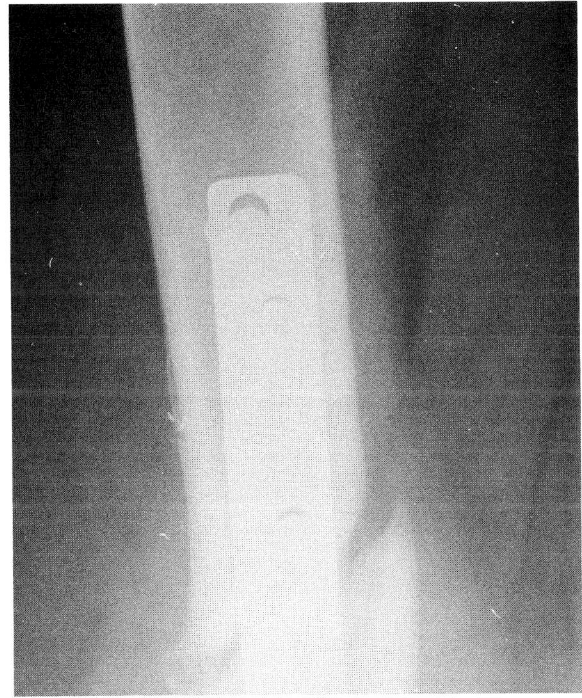

(a)

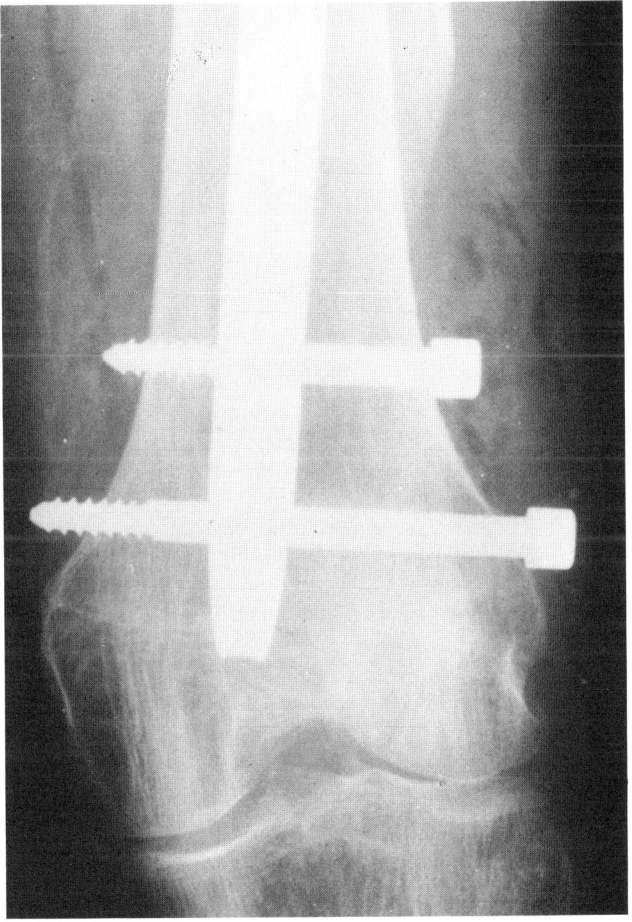

(b)

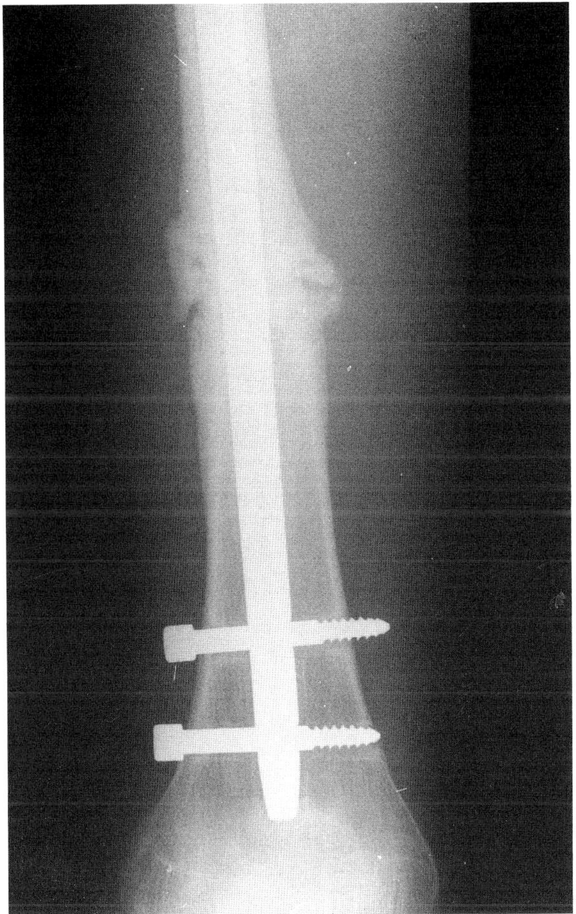

(c)

Fig. 21.26 (a) Although in this radiograph alignment was maintained by postoperative traction, there is a potential for varus or valgus, flexion or extension and flexion or extension deformities because of the large area of distal cancellous bone. (b) If the fracture is badly fixed with a locking nail then this deformity can persist. (c) Often these fractures are stable using distal locking screws only and this is known as dynamic locking.

skin. When the distal end of the nail is flush with the distal end of the proximal fragment the fracture is reduced and the nail is then advanced into the distal fragment, leaving approximately 2 cm of the nail proud of the trochanteric region in order to facilitate later removal (Fig. 21.27).

2 Open pro-grade nailing. This is a technique previously described by the AO group and it utilizes the traction table with the patient in the lateral or supine position. Image intensification is not strictly necessary. The fracture is approached through a small incision and reduced. Following reduction, an incision over the trochanteric region is made and the trochanter is opened through a point just medial and posterior to the tip; a guide wire is then passed through the fracture under direct vision. The femoral shaft is then reamed using 0.5-mm increments over the guide wire. After reaming is complete, the reaming wire is exchanged for a nailing rod and a nail is inserted over it (Fig. 21.28).

3 Closed technique. The development of closed nailing has been possible only with the advent of image intensification and digital memory. A traction table is necessary and, because of the need for image intensification, the draping procedure is much more complex. This method requires considerable manipulative skill. An accurate closed reduction of the fracture is essential before the knife touches the skin!

Open versus closed

The open retrograde nailing technique has little to commend it, although it is easy and quick. Considerable periosteal stripping is necessary for exposure and the incremental used of 1-mm solid reamers cannot now be

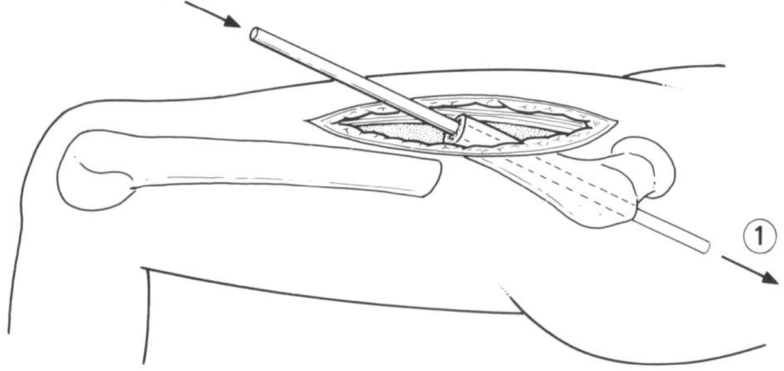

Fig. 21.27 The fracture is opened, proximal and distal reaming performed through the fracture ends and the nail hammered out through the greater trochanter through a stab incision in the skin. When the end of the nail is flush with the end of the proximal fragment, it is then hammered down into the distal fragment until the tip of the nail is just proud of the tip of the greater trochanter.

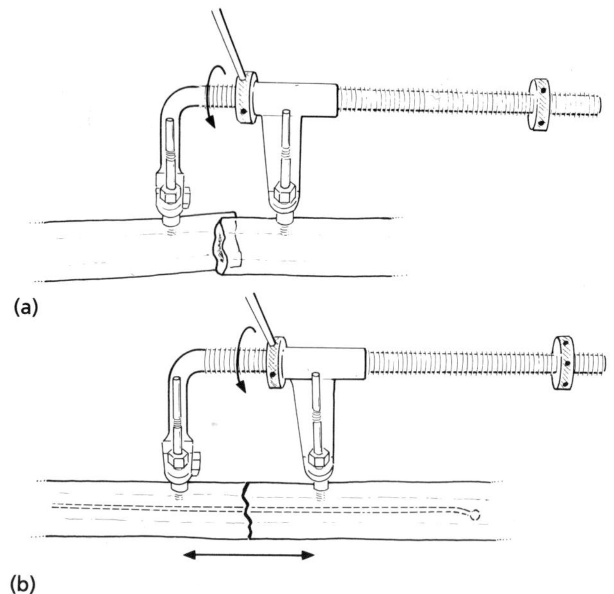

Fig. 21.28 The use of the AO femoral distractor; a traction table is not required for this. (a) The distractor is applied using a unicortical hold and opened out until the fragments fall into place. Note the prior insertion of a guide wire. (b) Following adequate reduction the guide wire can be passed along the shaft. In comminuted fractures, because the technique is open, bone grafting is mandatory. (From Müller *et al.* 1979.)

defended because of the potential for thermal destruction of the medullary canal during reaming. This method is associated with a high incidence of infection, varying between 7 and 15%, and has a significant incidence of delayed and non-union.

The pro-grade nailing technique described by the AO group has a less destructive exposure. The reaming technique is more sensitive and less liable to cause thermal destruction.

Providing the surgeon has the skill, there is little doubt that closed intramedullary nailing is now the treatment of choice. This is a technique which the authors recommend and is described in detail below. In published series the rate of infection in closed fractures is less than 1% (Winquist *et al.* 1984). In addition, closed intramedullary nailing can be combined with proximal or distal locking with a very small increase in operative time.

CLOSED LOCKING NAILING

The problem of radiation

Any closed manipulative reduction and internal fixation carries the risk of excessive radiation exposure to the surgeon and nursing staff. The radiation associated with reduction, reaming, nailing and locking techniques can be particularly great in inexperienced hands and it is important that this should be minimized. It has been estimated that the use of an image intensifier with an electronic memory reduces total radiation time by 60% and, for locking, the use of an image-intensifier-mounted distal target device further reduces the potential exposure to the surgeon (Fig. 21.29). The use of a lead apron is essential and provided that theatre staff keep more than 70 cm away from the radiation source, radiation exposure is negligible (Dupuis *et al.* 1984).

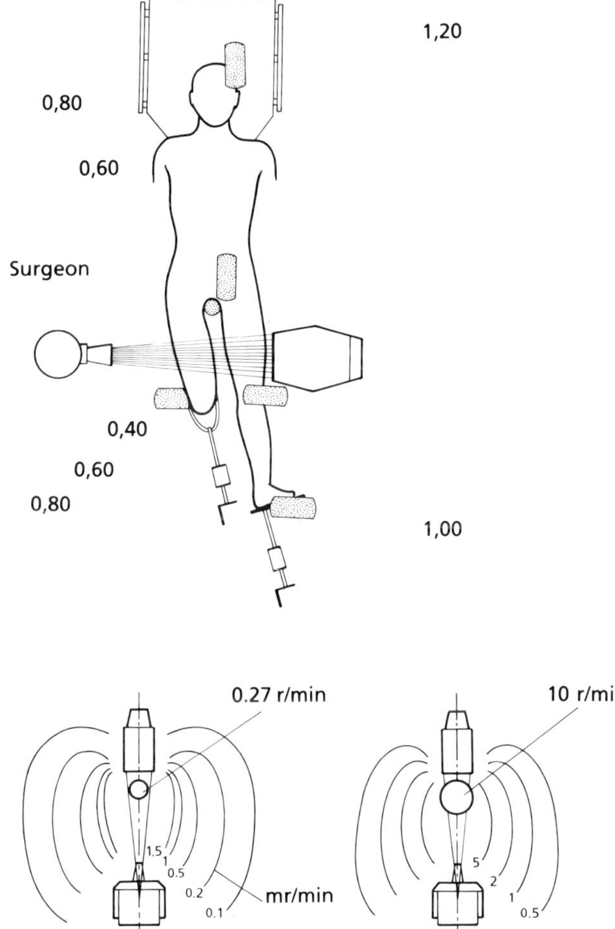

Fig. 21.29 X-ray dosage is measured in millirads per minute. Positioning of the tube should be such that minimal exposure is possible and this means that the tube should be invariably square with the limb to be imaged. Under these circumstances, with modern machines, scatter is minimal at 70 cm from the patient.

Technique

Timing. Closed nailing is a difficult technique and requires an experienced surgeon as well as properly trained theatre and radiological staff. Operations should usually be confined to daylight hours when a full complement of staff and back-up facilities are available. Nevertheless, it is important to avoid undue delay and if it is not possible to perform surgery within the first 12−24 hours, then the patient should be treated by skeletal traction of at least 10 kg through a tibial pin to maintain length. A delay of more than 7−10 days will make closed manipulation and reduction of the fracture extremely difficult and although delay in the fixation of femoral shaft fractures of up to 14 days has been suggested as increasing the rate of union, this may not be applicable in closed nailing (Lam 1964).

Open fractures require special consideration. Surgical debridement should be performed within the first 6 hours of admission; the wound should be sealed and nailing performed at the same time. Further discussion regarding open fractures follows later.

Setting up. Adequate reduction can only be achieved using a *transcondylar Steinmann pin*. This can be inserted either in the anaesthetic room or, alternatively, and particularly if the patient is obese, under image-intensifier control in the operating theatre. For distal-third fractures, the transcondylar pin should be placed anteriorly in the subchondral bone through the femoral condyles in order to extend the distal fragment (Fig. 21.30). A small traction loop is fixed rigidly to the traction extension of the table and the pin is trimmed. This allows access to the complete femoral shaft. The position of the patient on the operating table is in a 'banana' shape with the traction post resting squarely between the ischial tuberosities and with the shoulder of the affected side drawn towards the opposite side of the table. The fractured leg is placed in adduction relative to the operating table and the unaffected limb is flexed and stabilized on a support (Fig. 21.31).

The image intensifier is then positioned from the unfractured side and anteroposterior and lateral access to the whole femoral shaft, including the trochanteric region, is checked. The machine should not require constant adjustment during the course of the surgical procedure, and the unaffected leg must be positioned well out of the way of the intensifier. For distal locking it should be able to be positioned at a true right angle to the distal end of the femur in both anteroposterior and lateral planes.

Reduction can then be accomplished using a com-

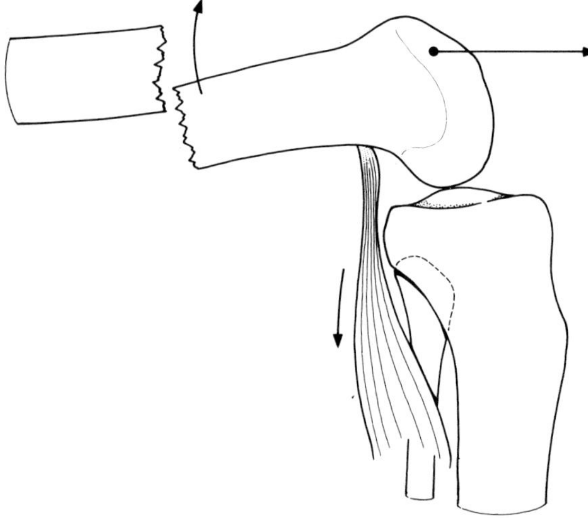

Fig. 21.30 In distal-third fractures positioning the patient with the leg in full extension will tighten the gastrocnemius muscle and cause difficulty in aligning the distal fragments. Extension of the distal fragment is achieved firstly by placing the transcondylar pin in the upper quadrant of the femoral condyles, and secondly by allowing the knee to flex and thus relax the gastrocnemius. Reduction of the distal fragment can then always be achieved.

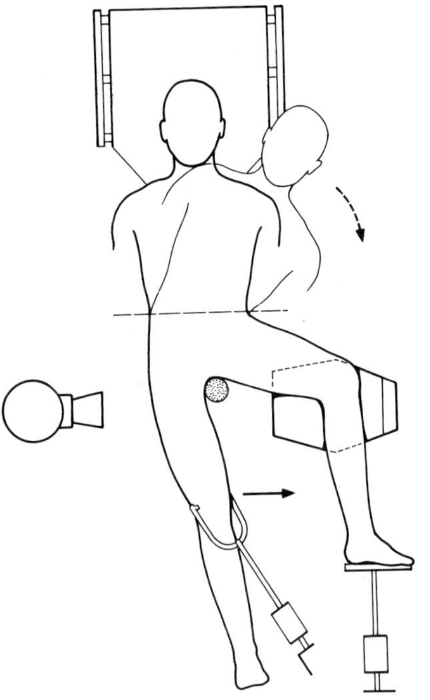

Fig. 21.31 Access to the trochanteric region is much easier with the leg abducted. However, if an excessive amount of traction is applied and the femur is then adducted, the net result is a tilting of the pelvis rather than femoral adduction. The patient needs to be draped for the whole length of the table and anaesthetic equipment, etc., should be on the opposite side.

bination of strong traction, adduction and rotation. The rotational deformity is usually corrected by allowing the lower leg to be dependent, although once satisfactory rotation has been established reduction is often aided by extension of the knee. In high fractures, reduction is usually difficult and it is sometimes necessary to accept that intraoperative manipulation will have to be performed.

Guide wire insertion and reaming The incision is centred over the greater trochanter and extended proximally for 7–10 cm, incising the tensor fascia lata in line with the incision. The gluteal muscle is split until the tip of the greater trochanter is palpated. The normal entry point for the guide wire is posterior and medial to the tip of the greater trochanter close to the piriform fossa. This area is broached with an awl. Because of the relatively compact cancellous bone in this region, it is sometimes necessary to ream up the proximal 12–15 cm using a solid reamer. The position of the entry point should be checked on the image intensifier to confirm that it is in direct line with the shaft of the femur. Too medial an insertion increases the risk of the nail acting as a stress riser with consequent potential fracture of the femoral neck (Fig. 21.32); too lateral a point of insertion carriers the risk of impingement of the nail on the medial cortex during insertion, causing the cortex to splinter.

The guide wire is advanced across the fracture. Bending the guide wire at its tip facilitates its passage across the fracture site if an anatomical reduction has not quite been obtained. It is important to ensure that the olive tip of the guide wire is situated in the middle of the condylar region both on anteroposterior and lateral films (Fig. 21.33). Failure to place the guide wire tip in the mid-part of the distal fragment is liable to result in a persistent varus or valgus deformity. In subtrochanteric fractures, where reduction is not possible, the proximal fragment is reamed to 10–11 mm. A Küntscher nail is inserted over the guide wire and used as a lever to aid reduction (Fig. 21.34). Reaming is accomplished in 0.5-mm steps, starting with an end-cutting reamer and continuing with side-cutting reamers. As the reamer passes through areas of comminution, the motor of the power reamer should be stopped to prevent it catching on the bony fragments and further devitalizing them. During reaming a considerable amount of bone debris comes out through the fracture fragments and acts as bone graft (Fig. 21.35). The shaft of the femur should not be washed out to clear bone debris. Except in exceptional cases reaming is continued until the femoral shaft is able to accept at least a 12-mm-diameter nail, and preferably a 13- or 14-mm nail.

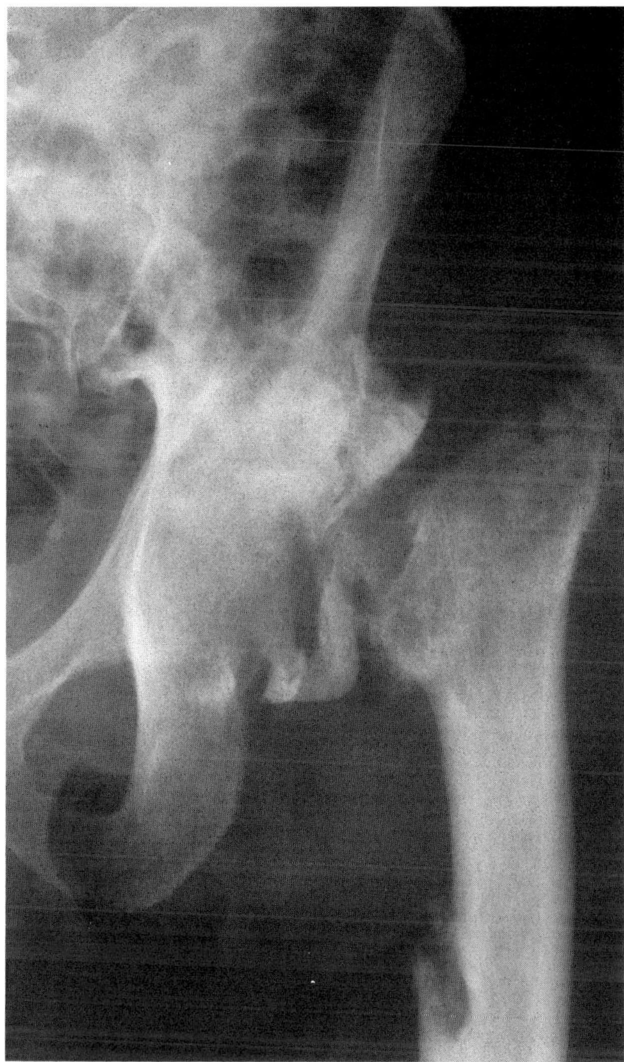

Fig. 21.32 This patient had a rather medial insertion point for the guide wire and had a delayed subcapital fracture of the femoral neck.

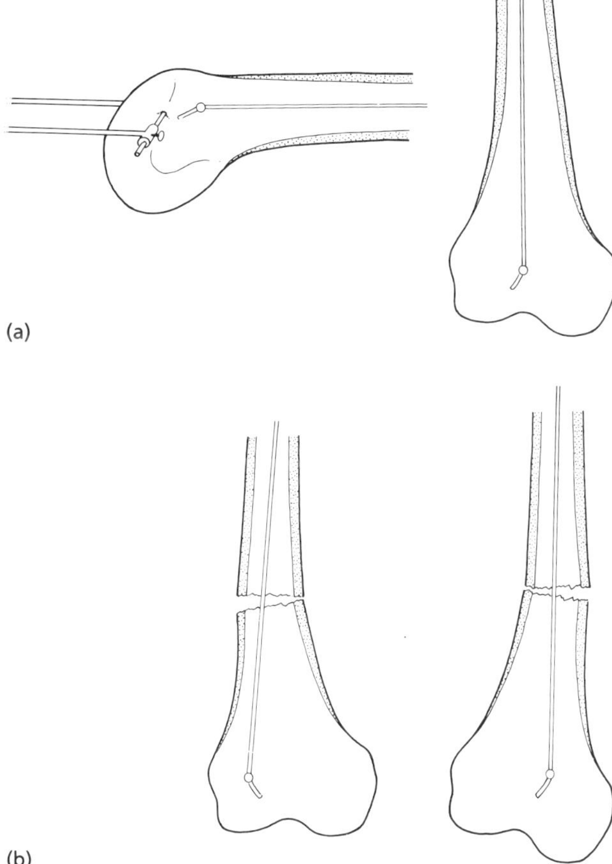

(a)

(b)

Fig. 21.33 (a) The end position of the guide wire determines the end position of the nail. In distal-third fractures positioning is particularly important and if, as in (b), the position of the guide wire is in a varus or valgus position, then the distal fragment will finish in the same configuration.

Insertion of nail The modern intramedullary nail should be inserted so that the tip is approximately 1–2 cm away from the intercondylar notch with the proximal end flush with the tip of the greater trochanter. A shorter nail, particularly in elderly patients with soft bone, has the potential for acting as a stress riser in the relatively soft supracondylar area. The nail is introduced and inserted under image-intensifier control with steady hammer blows. If the nail becomes stuck, it is sensible to withdraw it straightaway and ream up another 0.5– 1 mm. During insertion, regular checks are made to ensure that the distal locking holes remain in the horizontal plane. If an image-intensifier mounted target device is used for distal locking, rotation of the nail can

cause considerable difficulties (Fig. 21.36). If the fracture is a middle-third fracture and in a stable configuration, the proximal wound is then closed and the patient returned to the ward.

Targeting and the use of the locking nail Proximal locking is usually easy. Most devices are attached rigidly to the proximal end of the nail using a screw coupling, and targeting under image-intensifier control poses no problems. It is the procedure for distal locking that fills the average theatre nurse and surgeon with apprehension. Correct initial positioning of the patient together with ensuring that the nail does not rotate during insertion will considerably allay these fears. There are essentially three techniques in common usage:

1 *Freehand technique.* The distal locking holes are visualized under image-intensifier control and the beam is

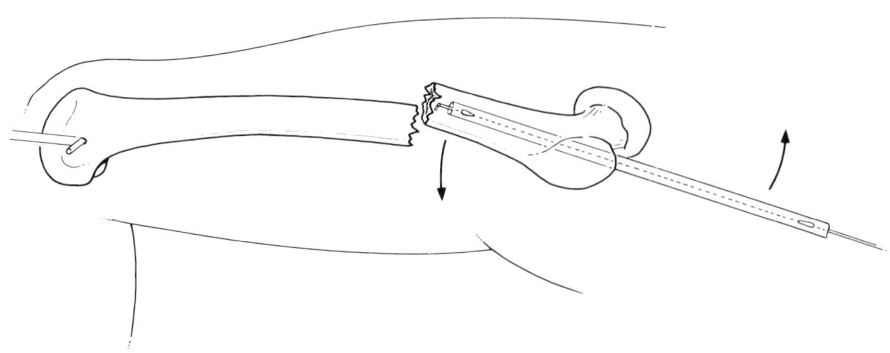

Fig. 21.34 In high fractures, where reduction cannot be accomplished prior to surgery, a guide wire is inserted down to the level of the fracture and the medullary canal is opened in the usual fashion. A Küntscher nail can be slipped over the guide wire and used as a lever to reduce the proximal fragment onto the distal fragment. Occasionally the use of a sling, fashioned out of swabs, can be helpful as a means of counter-traction.

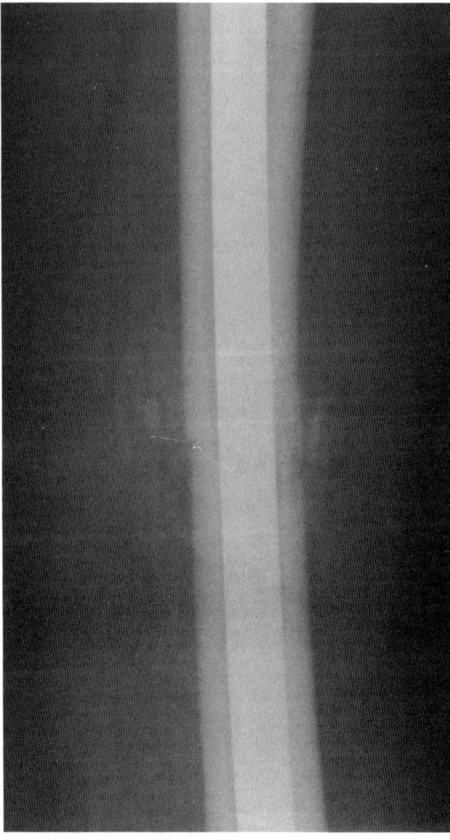

Fig. 21.35 This powdery appearance around the fracture site is not callus. The radiograph was taken immediately postoperatively and shows the copious reamings from around the fracture site. It is believed that this acts as a very effective bone graft.

adjusted so that it passes through the centre of one of them. On the screen the hole should appear round. A 4-cm incision is made in the distal femur under direct vision, and then a Steinmann pin or drill bit is centred under image-intensifier control in the middle of the hole. The pin or drill is swung in line with the beam and the outer cortex drilled. With some practice it is usually possible to get the drill or Steinmann pin straight through the distal locking holes, following which insertion of the screw or bolt is easy.

2 *Nail-mounted target device*. This system relies on a jig attached to the proximal nail and requires pre-setting on each individual nail before its insertion. It still relies on the image intensifier to check that the holes in the target device and nail are in line, because of the possibility of minor deformities occurring to the nail during insertion, and of the whip effect of the long extension.

3 *Remote target devices*. A large variety of remote target devices are available. All of them except the image-intensifier-mounted device of Grosse and Kempf are handheld but have the potential for reducing irradiation of the surgeon. The use of these target devices is strongly recommended since, particularly in inexperienced hands, irradiation of the surgeon's hand in the freehand technique can be extremely high.

Postoperative care

Immediate active mobilization of the knee, hip and ankle is encouraged. If the fracture is of a stable configuration with dynamic locking, then immediate weight-bearing can be started. Discharge is as appropriate for the patient, level of mobilization and social circumstances, and in the younger patient can usually

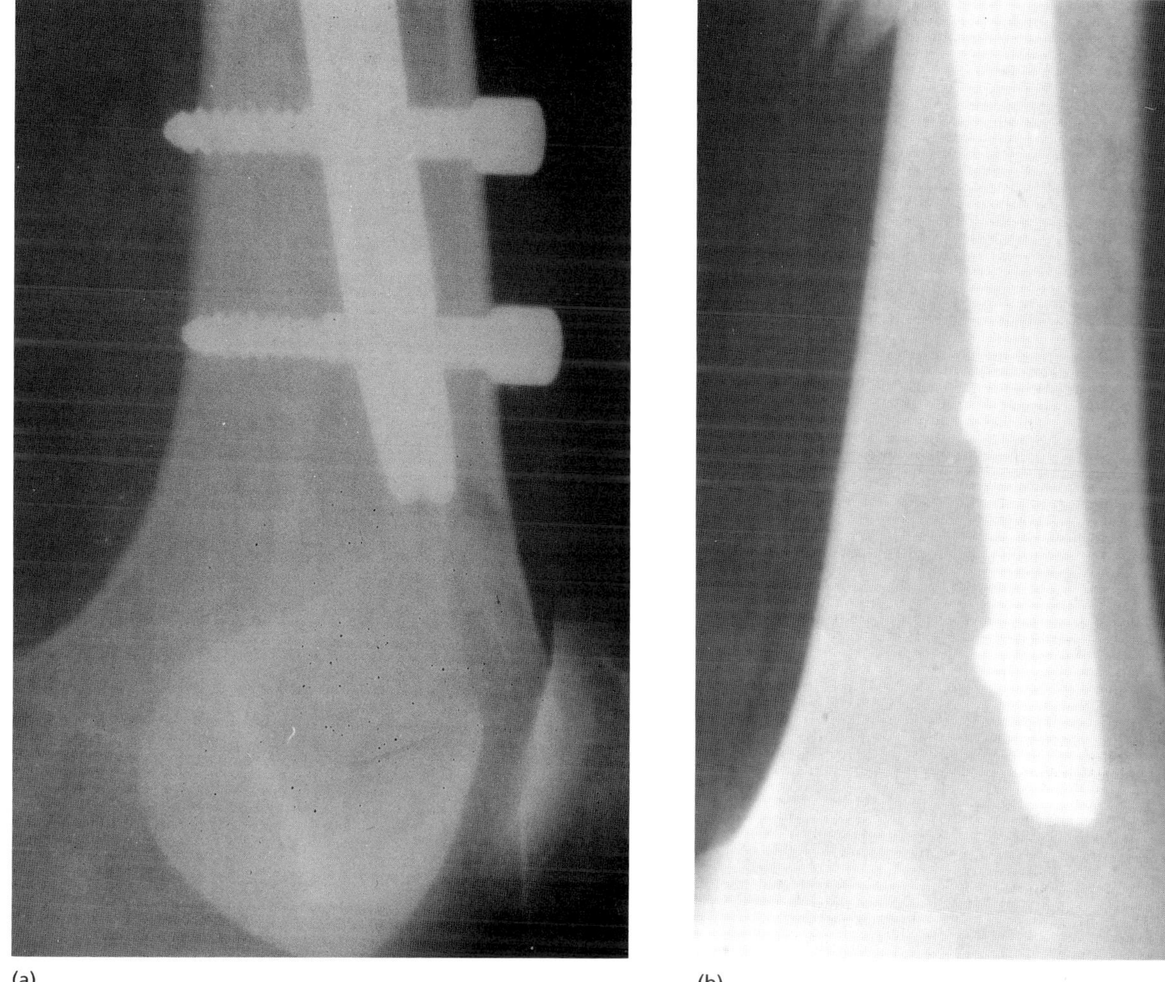

(a)   (b)

Fig. 21.36 Rotation of the nail is usually only a problem in slotted nails and occurs less frequently in unslotted nails. Rotation is usually due to an incorrect insertion point and is a feature particularly in distal-third fractures. (a) Note the anteroposterior position of the nail in the lateral view and (b) vice versa.

be achieved within 3–4 days. Those patients who have comminuted fractures with static locking (and thus have had a high-energy injury) may have associated soft tissue problems, and thus mobilize more slowly; in these cases partial or non-weight-bearing only is permitted. Early nailing seems to reduce the incidence of pulmonary dysfunction and fat embolus syndrome (Johnson *et al.* 1985) and systemic complications relating to nailing are rare.

The problem of 'dynamization' of statically locked nails is controversial. It would seem, however, that if the appearance of callus is slow, it is reasonable to remove the locking screw remote from the fracture site and to encourage active weight-bearing, accepting that there might be some settling of the fracture.

Variants on intramedullary nails

At present, the most widely used types of locking nail are those of Grosse and Kempf, the AO universal nail and the Russell—Taylor nail. All these systems employ proximal and distal locking screws and the techniques of insertion are similar. Variations in the design of all three nails account for minor advantages for certain types of fracture, but under most circumstances these nails are able to fix the majority of fractures of the femoral shaft reliably and safely.

The Huckstep nail (Huckstep 1986) is a variant of the locking nailing system (Fig. 21.37) and was one of the first locking nails available. The system relied upon an open approach to the fracture and thus had the disadvantages of destruction of the endosteal circulation as well as devitalization of the remaining periosteal circu-

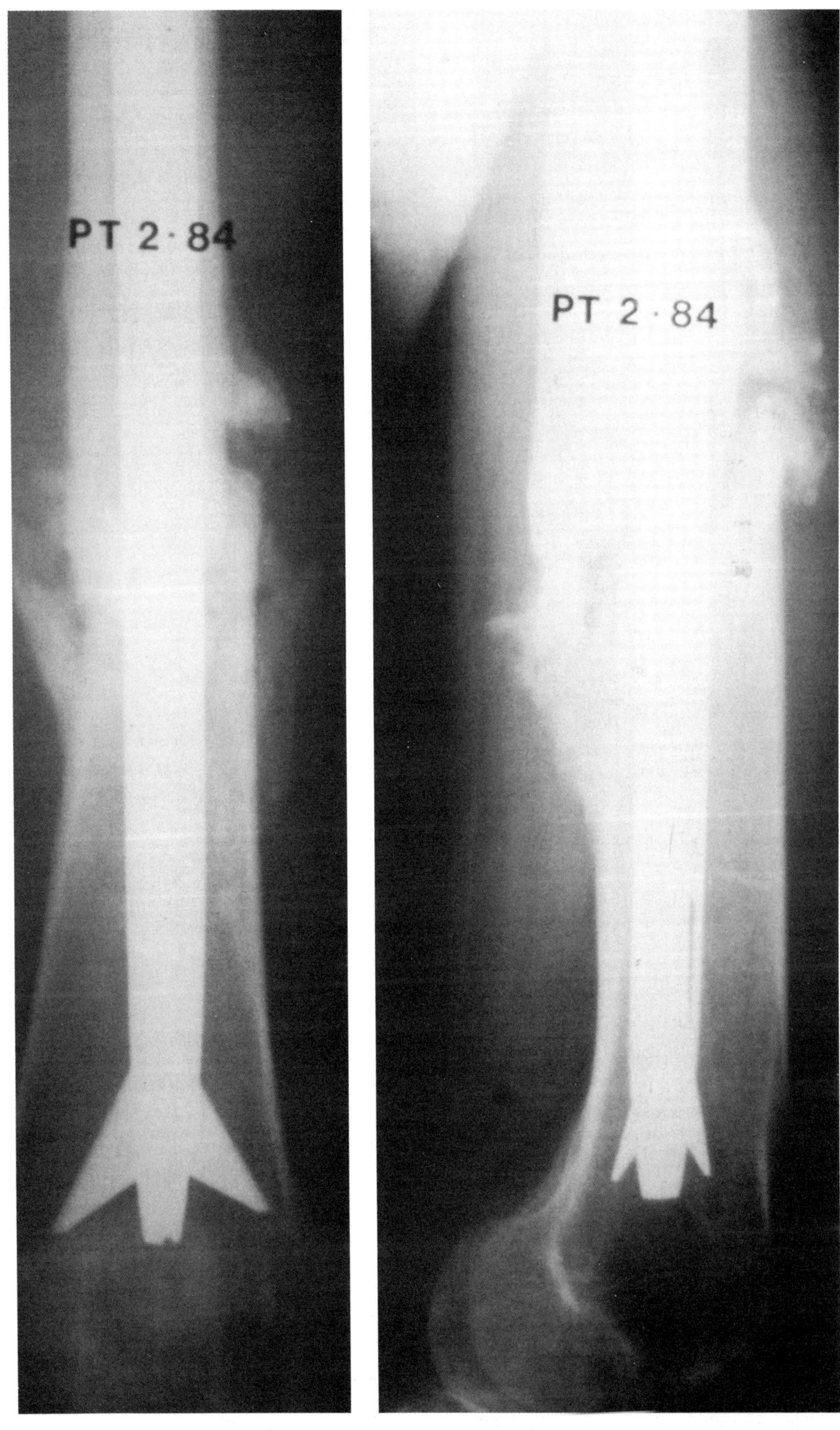

Fig. 21.37 The Brooker–Wills nail system.

lation. Locking was performed by the use of an external jig with multiple screw holes, and for fixation of complex fractures it is highly versatile. It has now largely been superseded by conventional closed techniques.

The Derby nail system (Papagianoupoulos & Clement 1987) and the Brooker–Wills system (White *et al.* 1986) with distal locking fins, as opposed to screws, were developed because of early difficulties in distal targeting. The distal fins are intramedullary (Fig. 21.38) and thus have no cortical grip — often the strongest part of the distal femur in an elderly patient. There is, therefore, less ability of the implant to prevent collapse of the fracture site and to resist torsion. However, the system performs well in good-quality bone with minimal comminution. More recent developments are the Variwall nail, which has the facility for being a truly 'universal' nail. This can be used for proximal locking screw insertion either into the neck of the femur or into the conventional subtrochanteric area, and is thus able to treat high subtrochanteric fractures or combined neck

and shaft fractures. The AO unreamed femoral nail, which is of modular design, further extends proximal locking possibilities.

Subtrochanteric fractures

Because of the difficulties in the management of subtrochanteric fractures, this fracture has always been neglected in the literature or lumped together with either shaft or trochanteric fractures. Nevertheless, the biomechanical forces acting across the subtrochanteric region are so different from those that influence the trochanteric or mid-shaft region of the femur that separate consideration for this fracture is justified.

The subtrochanteric area is not included in the muscle tube of the mid-shaft and distal shaft of the femur, and when fractured is subject to unequal muscle forces producing the classic flexion/external rotation/abduction deformity of the proximal fragment (see Fig. 21.7). This has major implications in terms of management.

Classification

Despite appreciating that subtrochanteric fractures pose separate problems from trochanteric or shaft fractures, the Fielding's or Seinsheimer's classifications are rarely used (Fig. 21.39). Between 6 and 15% of all proximal femoral fractures are in the subtrochanteric region, depending on the definition of the fracture and the population sample. The recently published AO classification defines three types of subtrochanteric fracture with trochanteric extension. Otherwise, true subtrochanteric shaft fractures are classified by adding the digit 1 to the alpha-numeric code of the general shaft classification (Fig. 21.40). As with all fractures, a distinction has to be made between the high-velocity injuries which occur mainly in younger patients and those of low velocity which occur chiefly in elderly patients. These latter injuries, which are frequently comminuted, may be pathological, and in themselves have particular surgical difficulties.

Treatment options

Options can be divided into two groups: those using conservative methods and those using operative methods. Because of the adverse biomechanical conditions described above, holding the position of the fracture is only rarely possible using conservative methods. Operation is invariably undertaken now.

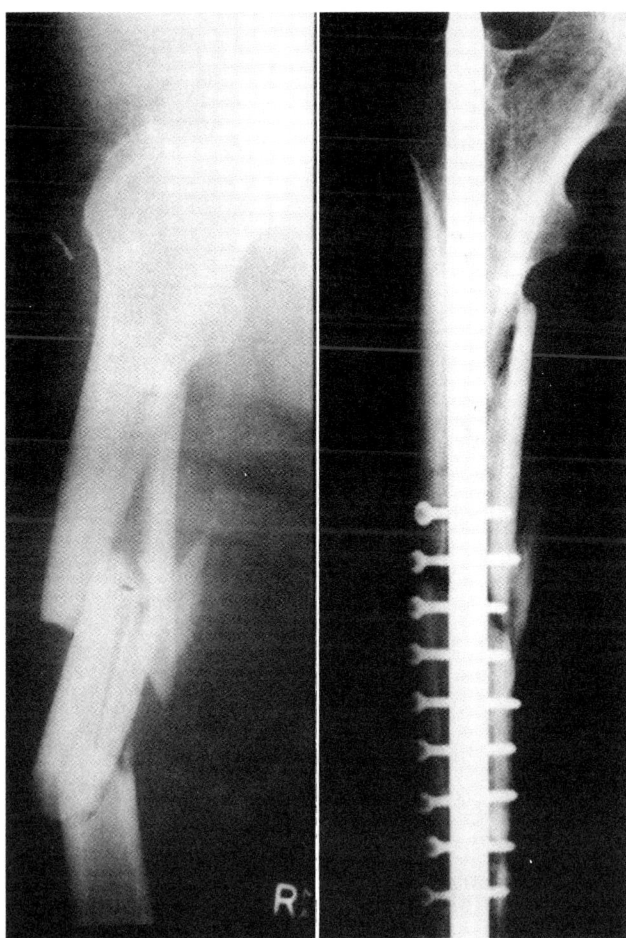

Fig. 21.38 The Huckstep nail.

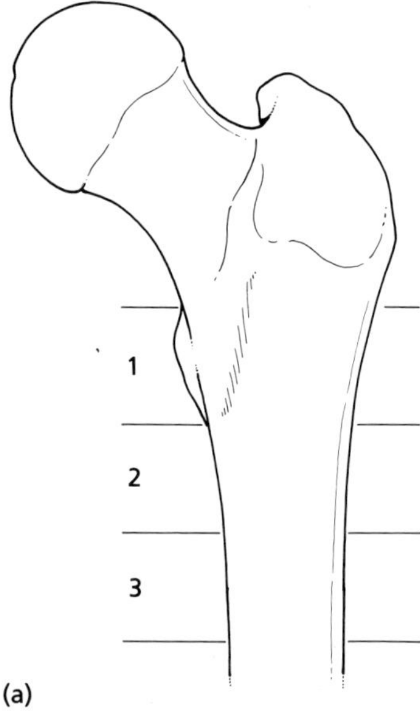

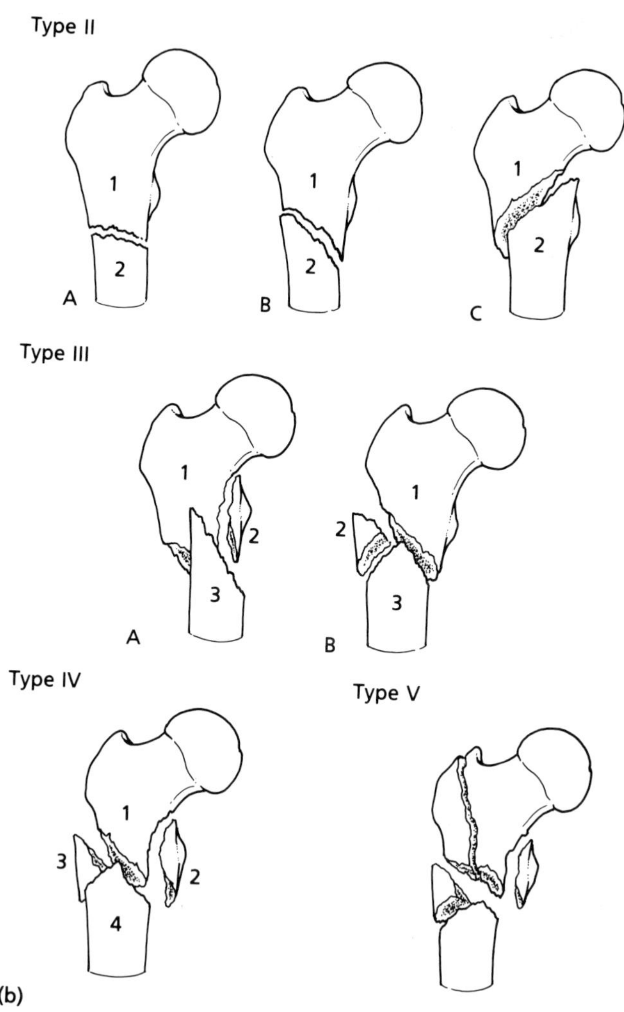

(a)

(b)

Fig. 21.39 (a) Fielding's classification of subtrochanteric fractures. Type I at level of lesser trochanter, type II between 2.5 and 5 cm below lesser trochanter and type III between 5 and 7.5 cm below lesser trochanter. (From Fielding, J.W. & Magliato, J.H. *Surg Gynecol Obstet* 1966; **122**: 555. Reproduced with permission from *Surgery, Gynecology and Obstetrics*.) (b) Seinsheimer's classification of subtrochanteric fractures of the femur based on the number of fragments and the location and configuration of fracture lines. Type I: any configuration of non-displaced fracture or those with less than 2 mm displacement. (Not illustrated.) Type II: two-part fractures; IIa, transverse; IIb, spiral configuration with lesser trochanter attached to proximal fragment; IIc, spiral configuration with lesser trochanter attached to distal fragment. Type III: three-part fractures; IIIa, three-part spiral configuration with lesser trochanter a part of the third fragment; IIIb, three-part spiral configuration with the third part a butterfly fragment. Type IV: comminuted with four or more fragments. Type V: subtrochanteric−intertrochanteric configuration. (From Seinsheimer, P. III *J Bone Joint Surg* 1978; **60A**: 300.)

Selection factors

As in femoral shaft fractures, selection of the patient for the particular procedure, whether conservative or operative, will depend on many conditions.

PATIENTS WITH DEBILITY

Generally speaking, younger patients with isolated injuries are more likely to tolerate conservative treatment better. However, of course, bone quality is better than in elderly patients and accurate surgical realignment and fixation is more reliable and successful than in the older patient. Nevertheless, younger patients have usually sustained high-velocity injuries and may well be polytraumatized and require considerable resuscitation before surgery is possible. In the presence of multiple injuries aggressive surgical treatment is the treatment of choice.

Elderly patients are less able to tolerate conservative treatment. Bony union is frequently poor and unsatisfactory alignment with shortening and deformity often occurs. Many patients are poor anaesthetic risks because of the frequency of secondary deposits in the subtrochanteric region, and because many are terminally ill. Internal fixation is difficult because of poor bone stock and, frequently, suboptimal fixation has to be accepted with some restriction in postoperative mobilization. Nevertheless, in view of the significant problems in managing elderly patients for a long period of time in bed and in their subsequent rehabilitation, operative stabilization of the fracture is still the best option.

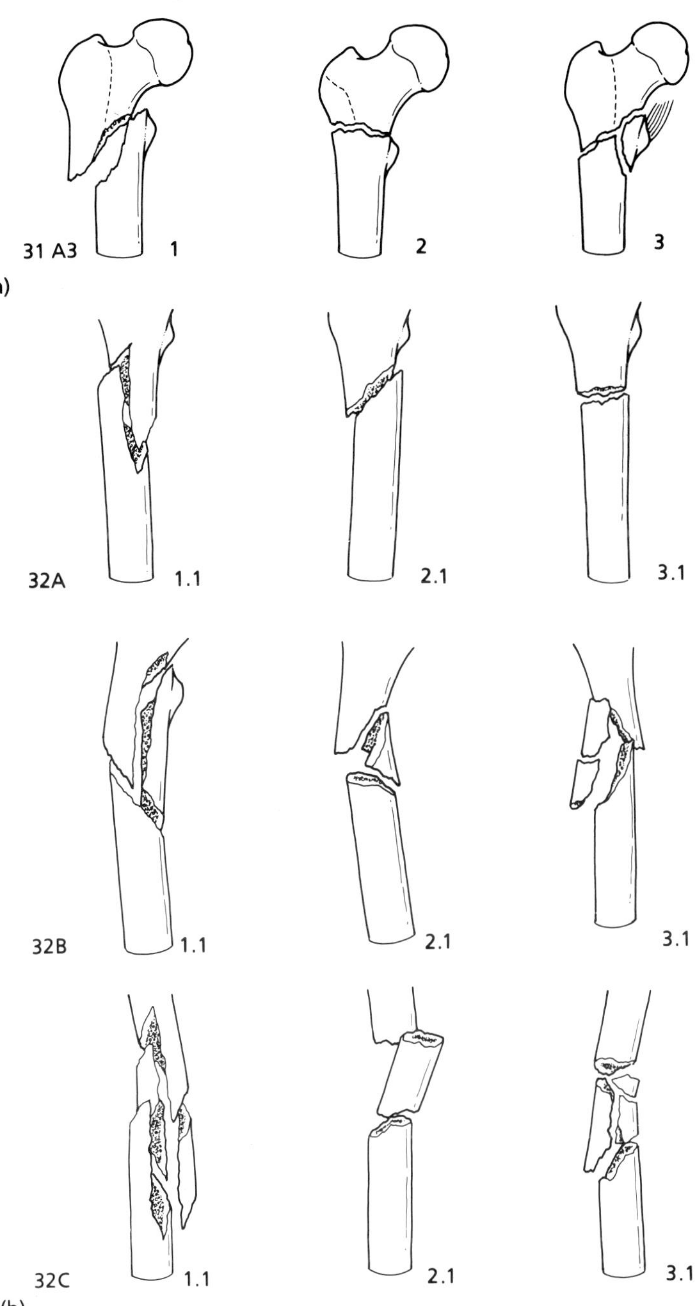

31 A3 — 1, 2, 3

32A — 1.1, 2.1, 3.1

32B — 1.1, 2.1, 3.1

32C — 1.1, 2.1, 3.1

(a)

(b)

Fig. 21.40 This group is classified with the proximal segment of the femur and often has a trochanteric extension: code 31C. (b) True subtrochanteric fractures are diaphyseal, and their proximal position in the diaphysis is designated by an additional digit (in this case 1) at the end of the code.

AVAILABILITY OF ADEQUATE FACILITIES

There is no one method of adequately treating subtrochanteric fractures. Poor quality or pathological bone may not be strong enough to hold screws and plates and intramedullary techniques may be better. Both methods of stabilization are difficult and the availability of adequate implants, nursing and radiological facilities are essential.

SURGICAL AND ANAESTHETIC STAFF

It is clear that, particularly for elderly patients and for polytraumatized patients, sophisticated anaesthetic skills are required. The management of both groups of patients should not be undertaken in the middle of the night in suboptimal conditions. In addition, it goes without saying that before surgery is performed, proper training needs to be given to the surgeon and assistants.

Non-operative treatment methods

The proximal fragment lies in flexion, abduction and external rotation. The fracture is not enclosed within the muscle tube of the thigh muscles and strong traction in a straight line will not realign the fragments fully. External rotation and flexion of the proximal fragment remains a problem and the patient is often left with a significant anterior bow at the fracture site with resulting shortening. Watson-Jones (1940) recommended, in the first edition of his book on fractures and dislocations, skin traction on a Thomas' splint. However, this was soon modified to a more rational method of treatment using Hamilton Russell traction with the limb in flexion and abduction. Alignment is easier to maintain using this method, although it is difficult for the patient to tolerate (Fig. 21.41).

If good control has been obtained using traction in fit patients, it is often possible to convert treatment to cast

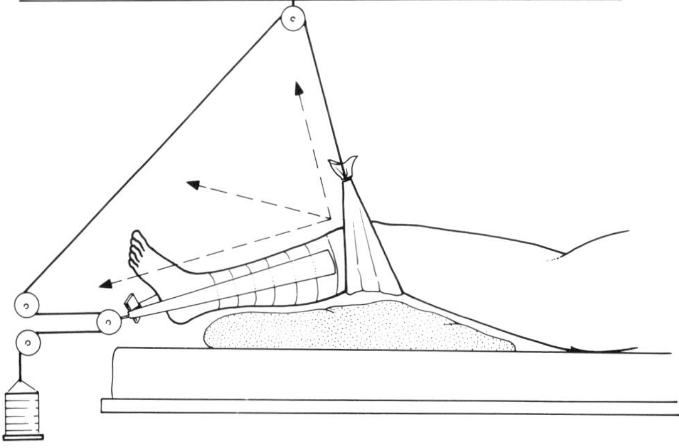

Fig. 21.41 The use of Hamilton Russell traction with the hip in flexion and abduction. The fact that the knee is flexed gives some control of rotation.

bracing. It is, however, necessary for the limb to be placed in abduction with a pelvic extension and a hip hinge.

Operative treatment methods

EXTERNAL FIXATION

In practice, external fixation is difficult to achieve in subtrochanteric fractures, although it is an attractive concept where the proximal third of the femur is markedly comminuted. It requires the use of a traction table and accurate reduction of the fracture before the external fixation pins can be inserted. There is little discussion of this method of treatment in the literature but De Bastiani has described it using a system with a proximal angled T-clamp (Fig. 21.42). He claimed good results for this, although when used in high-velocity injuries delayed union is common. In addition, because of the large mechanical forces transmitted through the pins (compounded by the lateral placement of the barrel), there is often failure to hold the position. Local movement at the pin tract sites, where they penetrate the vastus lateralis, can result in serious sepsis.

PLATES

Until the importance of the biomechanics of the proximal femur was appreciated, subtrochanteric fractures were treated as an extension of a trochanteric fracture and nail plate techniques for internal fixation were used. Methods of fixation commonly used were a Jewett fixed angle nail or a McLaughlin nail. Frequently, it was not possible to place any form of fixation in the proximal fragment other than the nail itself and in the presence of an inadequate medial buttress the system often failed (Fig. 21.43). In a review of 30 consecutive cases of subtrochanteric fracture, treated between 1965 and 1975, less than half the patients had satisfactory functional or radiological results (Cross & Murphy 1977).

The reasons for failure were invariably related to the following:

1 Inadequate medial buttress with failure to bone graft.
2 Failure to appreciate the strong biomechanical forces acting on the plate.
3 The use of weak materials with mechanically unsatisfactory blade plate welds or articulations.

Because of their high failure rate, there is no place for the use of fixed angle tri-fin nail plates of the McLaughlin system in the management of subtrochanteric fractures.

The present generation of sliding hip screws have been more successful when applied to subtrochanteric

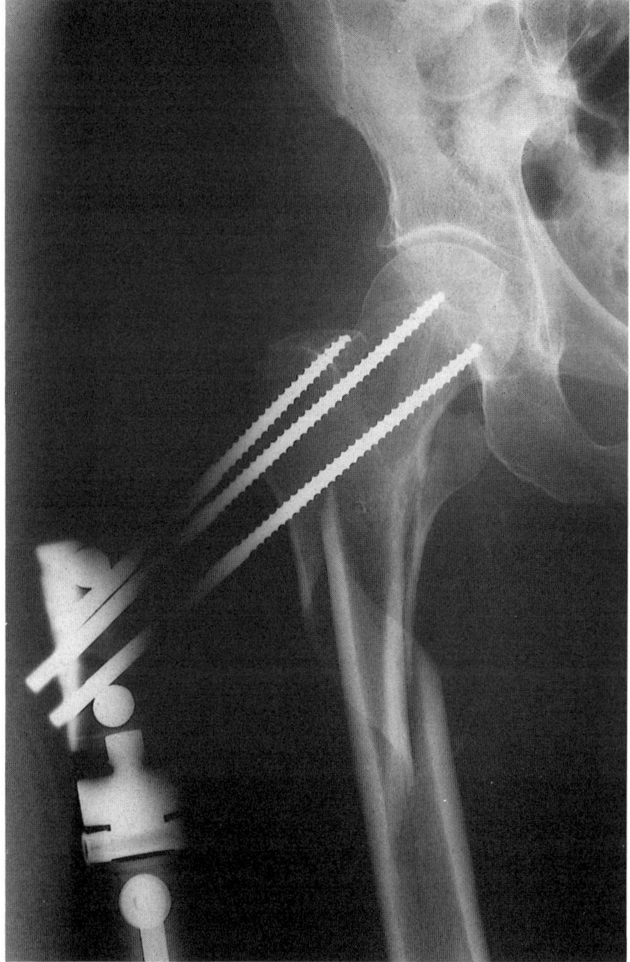

Fig. 21.42 This comminuted fracture has an angled clamp. Probably three cancellous pins are better because if the bone quality is poor fixation is improved.

fractures. This is due to better implant design, use of stronger materials and avoiding the presence of local stress risers. However, there is still the potential for plate failure to occur if there is any delay in healing.

The condylar screw systems, designed primarily for the condylar and supracondylar areas of the distal femur, can be used in place of the condylar blade plate, and many surgeons now prefer to use this as a method of internal fixation of the proximal femur rather than the blade plate which is more technically demanding.

The 95° AO blade plate system uses a pure tension-band principle. The advantage of this method over the sliding hip screw system is that the blade enters the trochanter and the neck of the femur at a much higher level than does the barrel of the hip screw system, and it is thus possible to place a proximal screw above the level of the lesser trochanter. Although originally it was

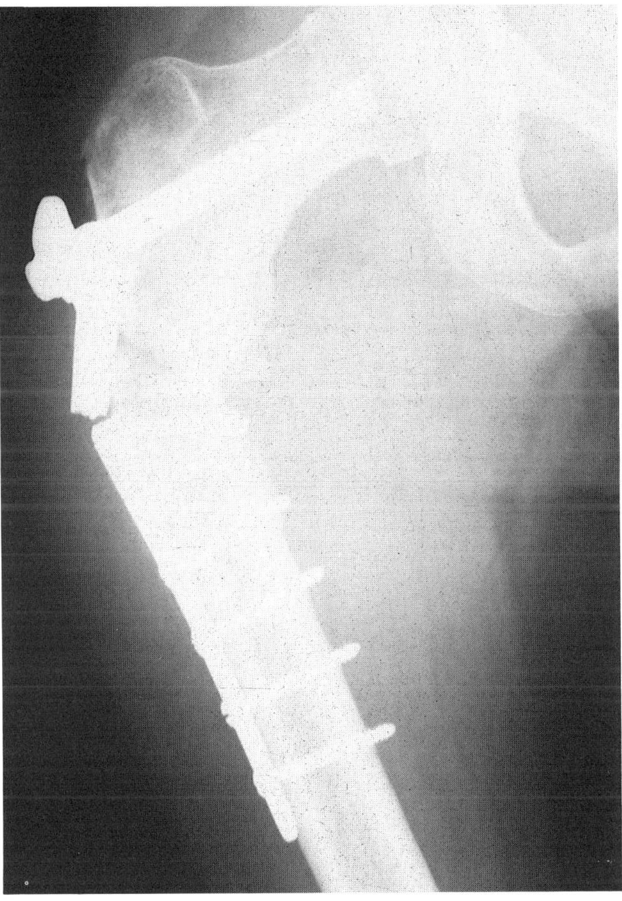

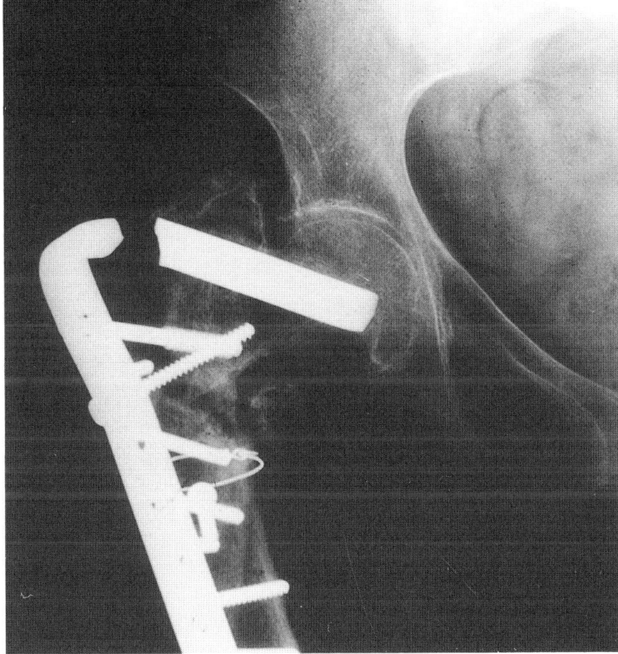

Fig. 21.44 This elderly patient with a comminuted subtrochanteric fracture was not bone grafted because of her age and general debility. The plate 'lost the race'.

Fig. 21.43 This film is a classical example of the surgeon's failure to appreciate the 'tension-band' concept of fixation of proximal-third fractures.

recommended that bony fragments should be accurately reduced and fixed using lag screws, simple alignment of the proximal and distal fragments in comminuted fractures appears to be adequate; however, copious bone grafting is necessary. The principle still depends on adequate bony healing within a reasonable period of time. The unholy race between bony union and plate fatigue' is never more evident in plate fixation than in the subtrochanteric region (Fig. 21.44).

Preoperative planning is mandatory in comminuted fractures in order to achieve satisfactory leg length equality and rotation. On admission of the patient the whole of the femoral shaft on the opposite side is radiographed and, using tracing paper, the bony fragments of the injured side are transposed onto the copy of the uninjured side. When this has been done, with use of templates supplied by the manufacturers it is possible to get an estimate of the size of blade plate that will be needed (Fig. 21.45). There is clearly nothing

more disastrous than setting out to do a surgical procedure and finding that the equipment available is inadequate for the procedure planned (Mast *et al.* 1989).

INTRAMEDULLARY DEVICES

Intramedullary fixation in subtrochanteric fractures is attractive because the medial position of the nail reduces the moment of the lever arm (Fig. 21.46), and thus the high stresses on the implant device. However, in practice, the use of a straight nail of the Küntscher type is limited because it relies on the soft bone of the trochanteric region to withstand the still considerable varus forces and, in addition, there can be no rotational control. Reliance on a straight intramedullary nail alone is akin to the insertion of a rod through the apex of a hollow cone (Fig. 21.47). In 1971 Burwell described the use of an anti-rotation plate (usually a small four- or five-hole plate) in conjunction with a nail, placing the screws through the lateral cortex only. However, any technique involving a combination of intramedullary and extramedullary fixation is likely to compromise bone vascularity for a considerable period of time (Brookes 1988). Before his death in 1972, Küntscher was developing a locking nailing system which was subsequently further developed by Grosse in Strasbourg

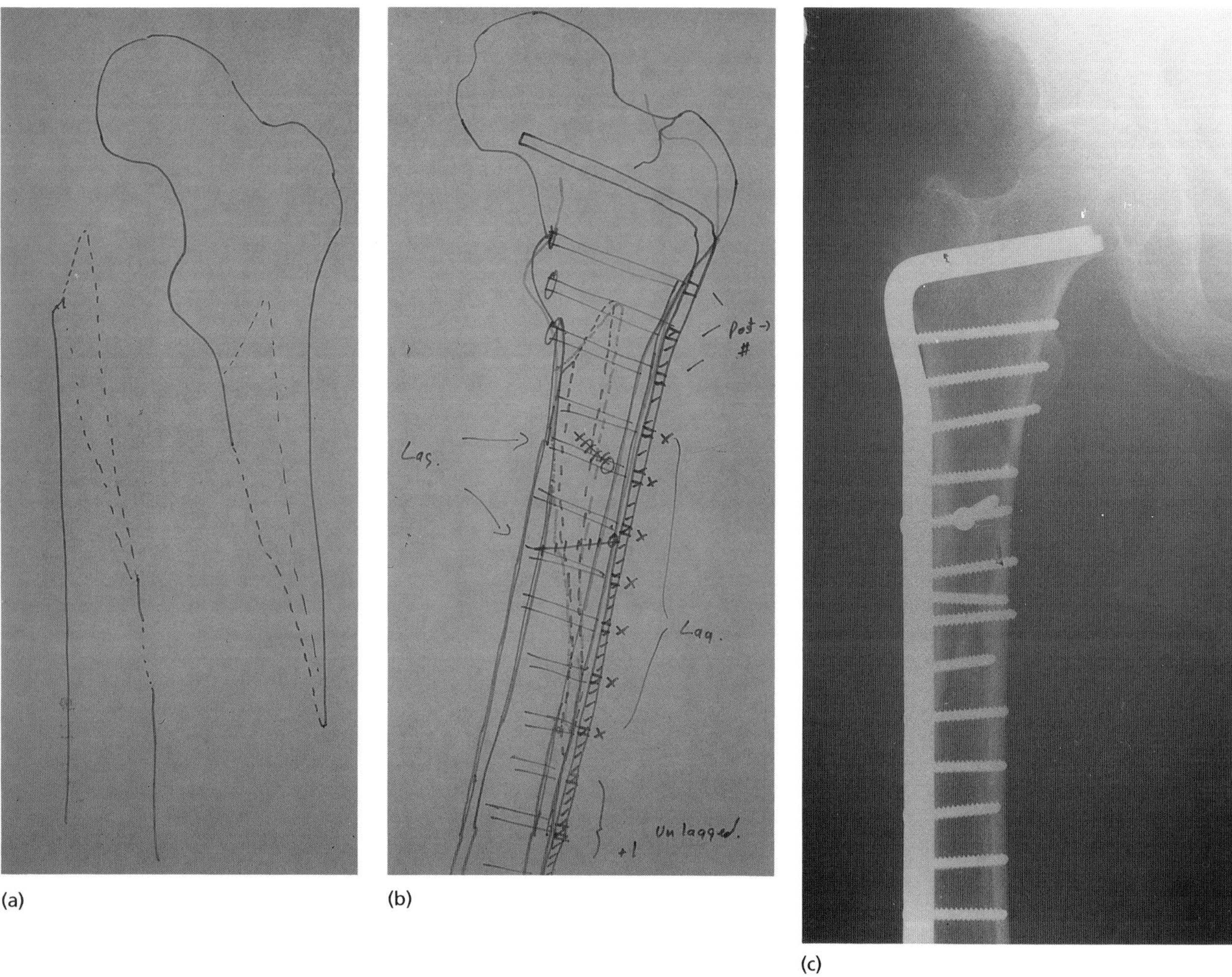

(a)

(b)

(c)

Fig. 21.45 (a) A tracing is made of the fracture fragment on an anteroposterior film. (b) These are superimposed on a tracing of the intact femur, using landmarks such as the flare in the subtrochanteric region and cortical thickness. Lag screws are planned and a suitable plate template is superimposed on the 'reduction'. (c) The completed tracing should match the postoperative film. Sometimes, it is useful to use this technique with lateral films but, in practice, it is extremely difficult to get adequate standard magnification radiographs of the injured femur.

and Klemm in Hanover. In the meantime, Zickel *et al.* (1977) in New York were developing a modification of the signal arm principle already proposed by Küntscher many years before.

The Zickel nail

The Zickel nail is an intramedullary signal arm device which is square in cross-section, solid and contoured to conform approximately to the average curvature of the femur. The proximal end of the Zickel nail has a fixed angled hole for the insertion of a tri-flanged hip nail which is locked into position by a screw inserted through a vertical channel at the top of the nail. The nail

itself is fashioned in chrome cobalt and is extremely strong. The square cross-sectional area gives a four-point grip in the medullary cavity and its resistance to rotation properties rely on this. The width of the nail varies from 11 to 17 mm and two lengths are available. Biomechanically, it is an extremely strong implant at the level of the medial femoral cortex.

Surgical technique The original technique describes open reduction and insertion of the nail in the supine position with image intensification. The technique has since been modified with insertion of the nail in the lateral position. An incision is centred over the greater trochanter, and if the fracture is very proximal the

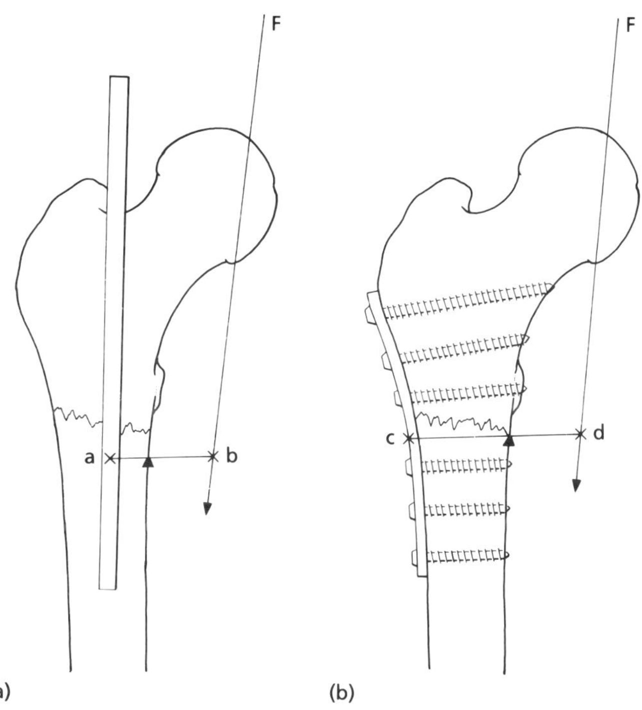

(a)   **(b)**

Fig. 21.46 The tension forces on the nail (a) will be much less than the tension forces on the plate (b) because the distance a−b is much greater than c−d.

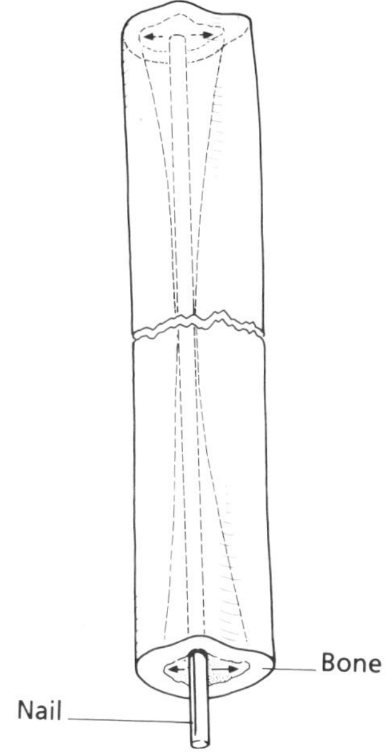

Fig. 21.47 In this example the only stable point of the cone can be around the centre of the configuration. Rotation, sideways angulation and forwards angulation can occur about this point.

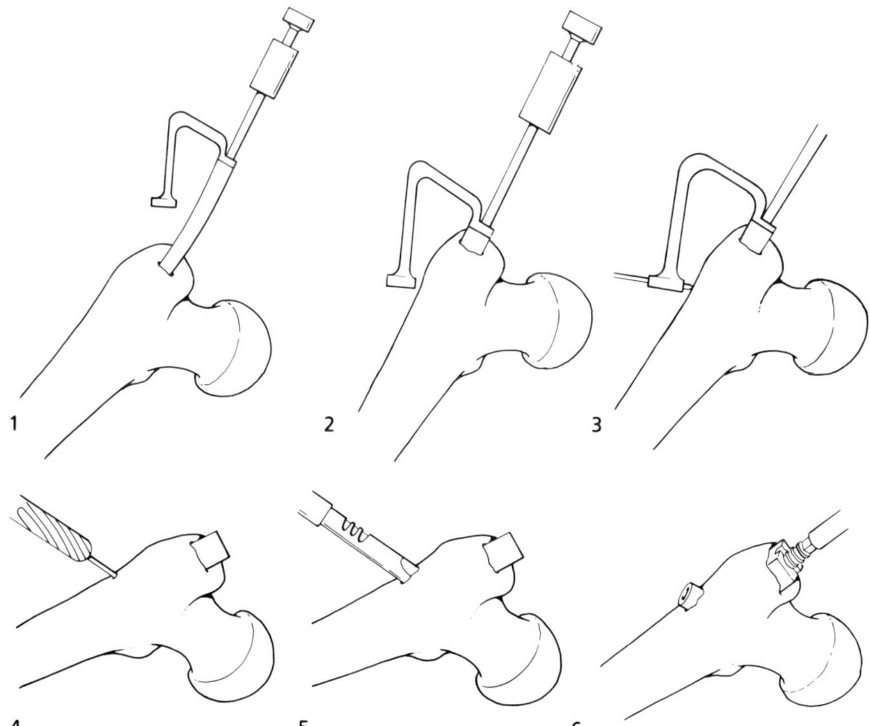

Fig. 21.48 Stages in the insertion of the Zickel nail. Disadvantages of this technique include that the guide pin is initially positioned in the head by trial and error. If the position of the reduction slips after the guide pin is removed, then there is potential for the hip nail to enter the slot in the intramedullary rod in the wrong position.

fracture site is exposed sufficiently in order to attain some control of the proximal and distal fragments. The proximal medullary canal is opened, a guide wire passed through the fracture fragments and reamed up to an appropriate size. The guide wire is removed and while maintaining control of the fragments, the nail assembly is inserted, using the hip nail guide as a handle. It is important to maintain correct rotation of the nail during its introduction. When the nail is fully home, a standard guide wire is put through the guide handle of the nail into the neck of the femur and this is checked on an image intensifier. Lateral films can be taken flexing the hip and obtaining a 'frog lateral'. The lateral cortex is opened with a special drill, the guide pin is removed and a suitable hip nail inserted and locked into position (Fig. 21.48).

For transverse fractures in good-quality bone the Zickel nail offers excellent stability. It is quick and relatively easy to insert. The main technical problems include malposition of the hip nail in the neck of the femur or in the prosthesis (Fig. 21.49). Late problems include shortening in long spiral fractures, although this can be avoided by use of cerclage (Fig. 21.50). Delayed union is common in patients with Paget's disease and this can be associated with rotational instability of the distal femur and eventually fatigue of the hip nail or the intramedullary nail (Fig. 21.51). Removal of the implant is not recommended since there is a significant incidence of stress fracture in young patients (Cross, personal observation). The use of the Zickel nail should now be restricted to elderly patients. It is an ideal method of fixation of simple fractures in pathological conditions such as metastasis and osteomalacia. The weakness of the Zickel nail is that it is not adequate to cope with the rotational or axial stability in comminuted or long spiral fractures and the concept of the antirotational lock of the 'square peg in a round hole' is dubious.

Other devices

A similar biomechanical concept of a signal arm system has been modified by Cuthbert and Howar (1976–77) (initially for trochanteric fractures) and refined by Straughan using various thicknesses of standard Küntscher nails. This system has never really gained wide acceptance.

The gamma nail has recently come on to the market and it is proposed that this nail has significant advantages over the nail plate configuration for trochanteric fractures. However, it has yet to prove itself and is technically difficult to use. The facility for distal locking

of the gamm nail suggests that it may have limited advantages for subtrochanteric fractures, particularly in elderly patients with wide medullary cavities, but this role has yet to be evaluated. Initial literature has concentrated on the use of this device in both trochanteric *and* subtrochanteric fractures: complications include external rotational deformities when distal locking is not performed, and fracture at the tip of the nail due to high stress rising properties. Further evaluation of this device in subtrochanteric fractures may improve its acceptability, and in the authors hands, it has certainly been valuable. A longer version of the gamma nail is now available and this will considerably increase its scope

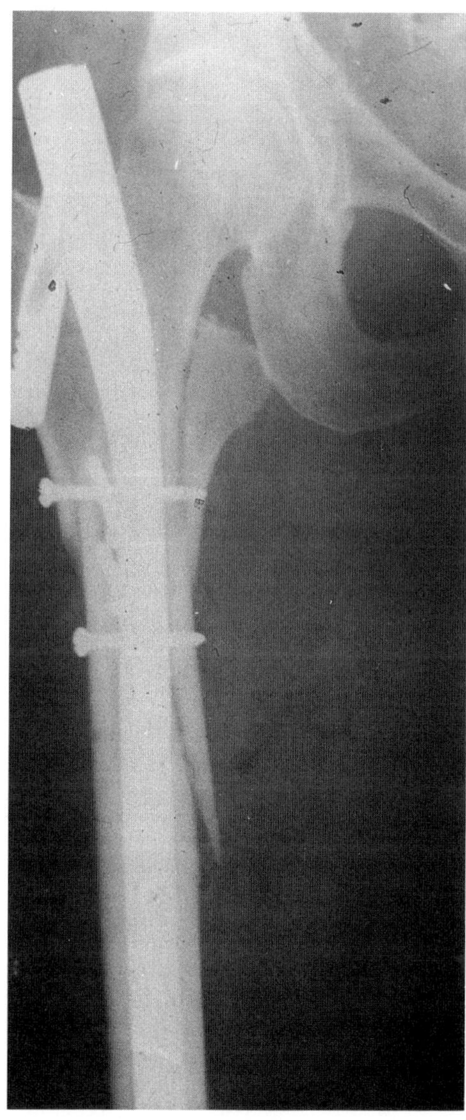

Fig. 21.49 In this example the surgeon wondered why the stability of the fracture was so poor after fixation! This is the reason for the adjunctive fixation.

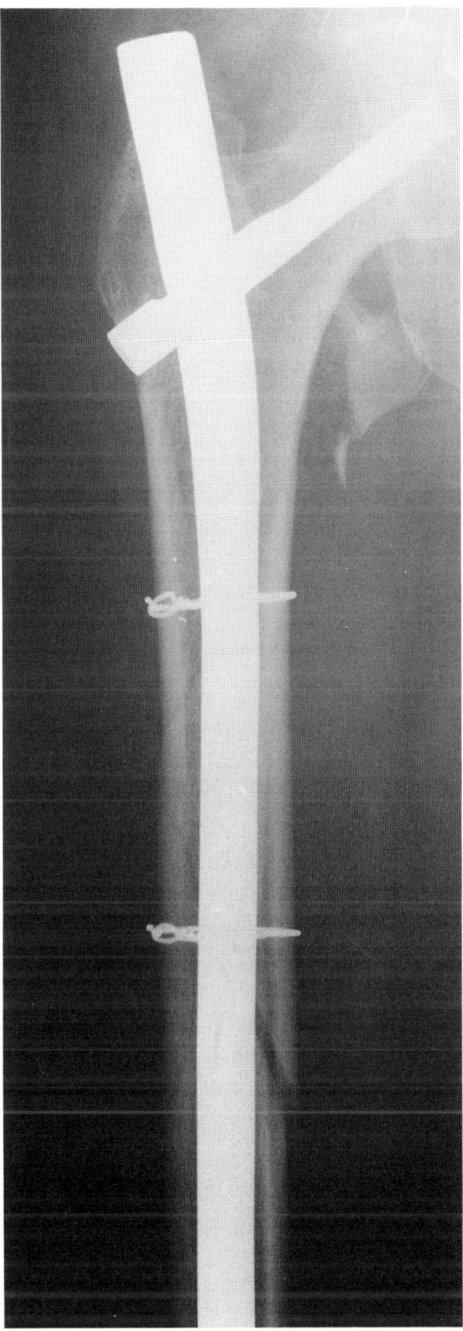

Fig. 21.50 Stabilization of long spiral fractures achieved by open reduction and cerclage.

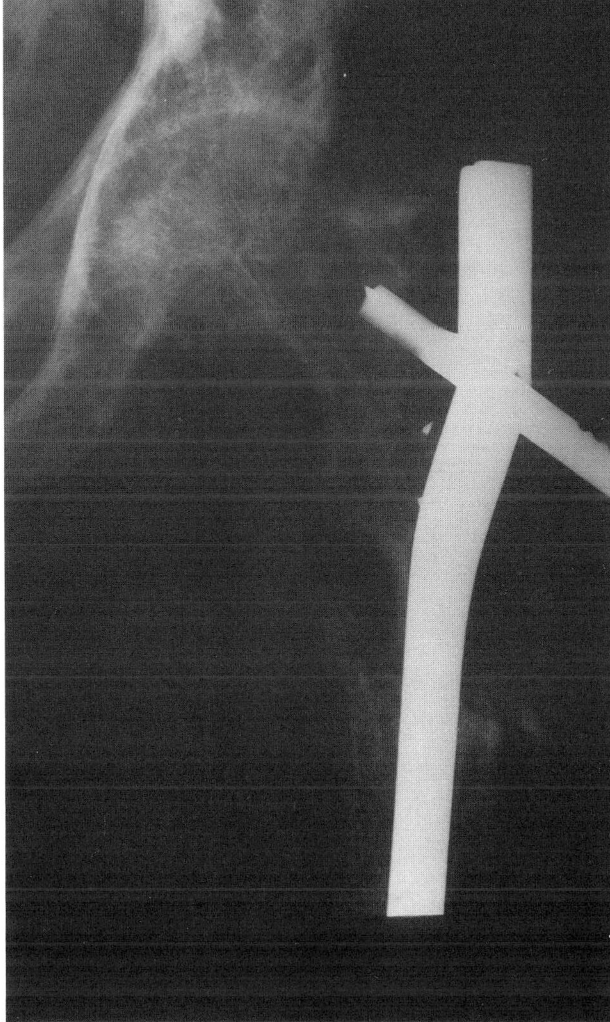

Fig. 21.51 Delayed union in Pagetic bone resulted in fatigue of the nail at its weakest point — the hip screw hole.

for highly comminuted subtrochanteric fractures with distal extension.

The locking nail

The locking nail has revolutionized current concepts in the management of femoral diaphyseal fractures, and this includes subtrochanteric fractures. The facility for both distal and proximal locking (static locking) allows comminuted fractures to be stabilized in correct axial and rotational alignment and, by comparison with the uninjured side, allows correct leg length to be maintained. Although open subtrochanteric fractures are rare, the minimal soft tissue dissection involved in the insertion of the locking nail makes it the treatment of choice for such fractures.

There are a number of specific technical difficulties associated with subtrochanteric fractures, namely:
1 Difficulty in achieving a preoperative reduction. The manoeuvre demonstrated in Fig. 21.34 may need to be used to achieve reduction and passage of the guide wire.

2 In soft bone the guide wire tends to lie against the posterior cortex (Fig. 21.52a). It is possible to ream away the whole of the posterior cortex with resultant catastrophic failure of the device when mobilization is started (Fig. 21.52b).

3 Because of the persistent flexion and external rotational deformity it is very easy for the initial insertion point to be too anterior and too lateral. In a high subtrochanteric fracture this can cause an extension of the fracture in the medial femoral diaphysis (see p. 742).

In Grosse and Kempf's original series of subtrochanteric fractures (Moncade 1984) they describe 30% of patients as having a varus deformity with 20% of secondary displacement and 16% of shortening. Subsequent series have revealed a marked improvement in the management of these fractures, but the lessons learned are clear: these fractures are extremely difficult to manage and are not for the inexperienced surgeon.

Femoral supracondylar and condylar fractures

Fractures of the distal end of the femur are very severe injuries and are usually the result of direct violence to the knee region. In the younger patient, high-velocity trauma is involved and often results in a more severe fracture with greater intra-articular damage or segmental comminution. Associated injuries may also occur in the same limb with ligamentous knee disruptions and patellar, tibial shaft or plateau fractures being more common. In the older patient, low-velocity trauma more often occurs with simple falls onto the knee but, with the ageing osteoporotic bone, severe comminution may still result.

The main problems in the treatment of distal femoral fractures result from fracture displacement and intra-articular disruption. With supracondylar fractures the distal fragment is often flexed, adducted and shortened by the contracture of the gastrocnemius, hamstring and quadriceps muscles. In a condylar fracture joint displacement depends upon the applied force direction with often vertical displacement of one or both condyles, with or without comminution, involving articular surfaces. Unless the fracture can be accurately reduced and the knee mobilized early, then malunion, shortening, angular deformities and knee stiffness will occur.

Classification

The AO classification is the most functional, defining the fracture type and its severity, and provides a guide to surgical treatment for optimum prognosis (Fig. 21.53).

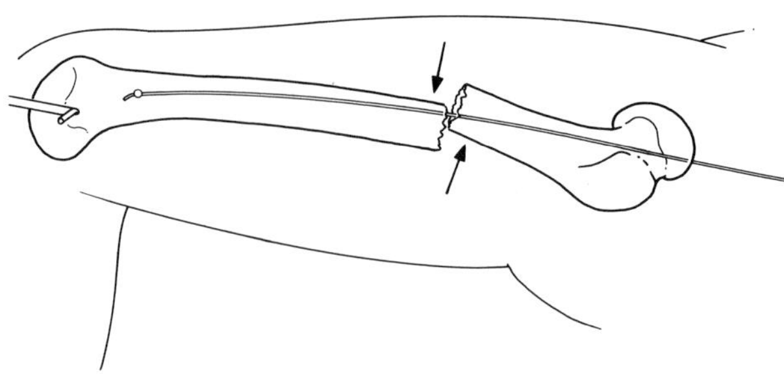

(a)

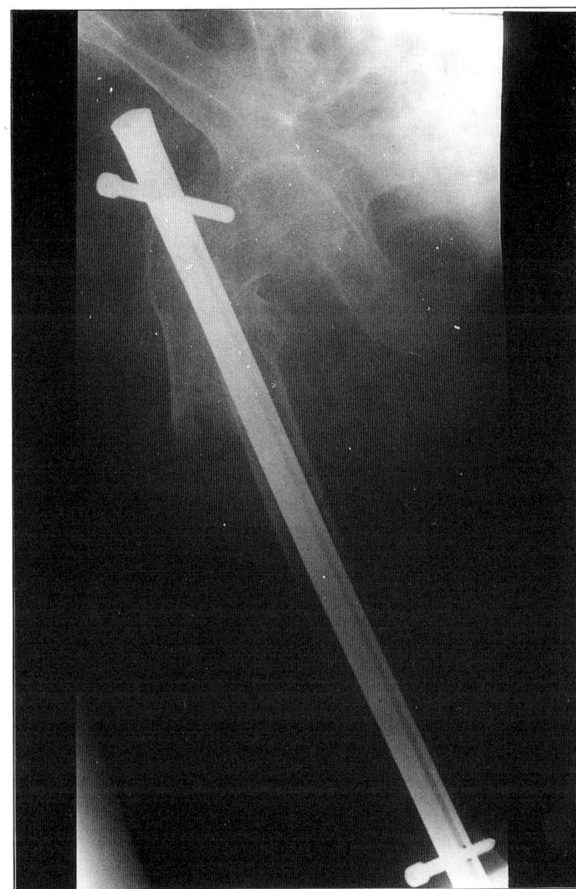

(b)

Fig. 21.52 (a) A combination of inaccurate reduction and soft bone may result in complete loss of the proximal posterior and distal anterior cortex; (b) shows resultant failure of the device.

Type A fractures are supracondylar extra-articular, type B fractures are intra-articular condylar and type C involve both. These main types are further divided into subgroups (1−3) with increasing complexity, stabilization difficulties and worsening prognosis.

Treatment options

Fractures of the distal femur may be very difficult to

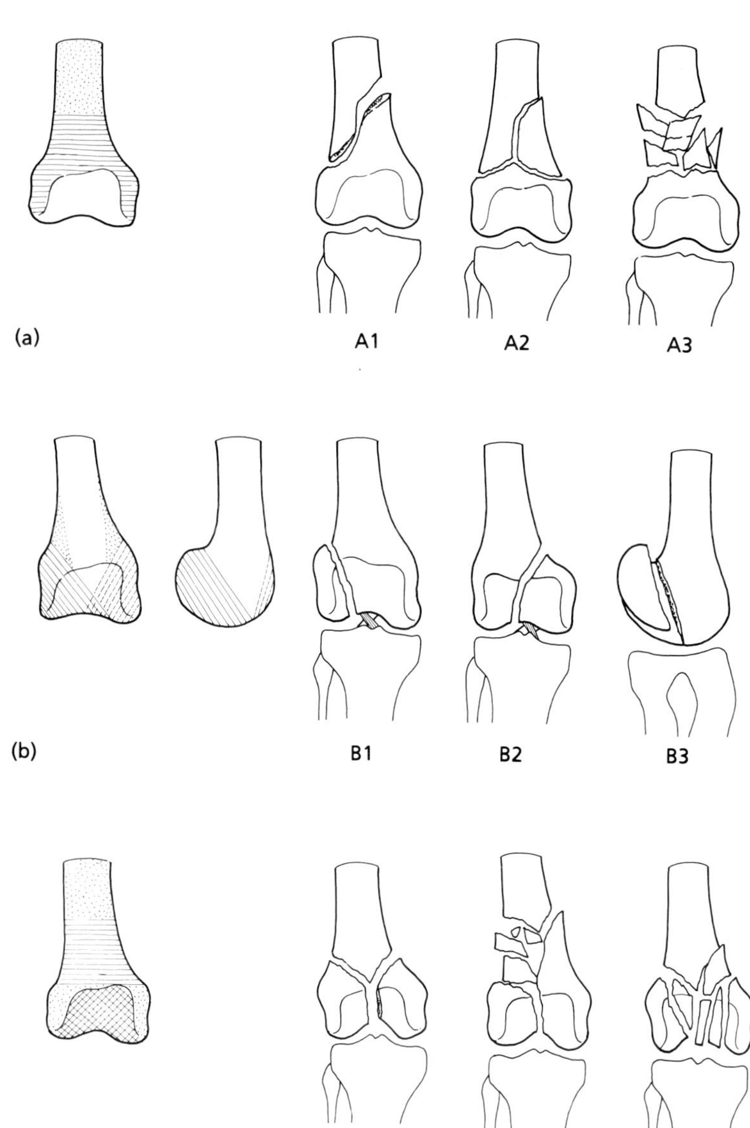

Fig. 21.53 AO classification of distal femoral fractures. (a) Extra-articular. A1, simple; A2, metaphyseal wedge; A3, metaphyseal complex. (b) Partial articular. B1, lateral condyle, sagittal; B2, medial condyle, sagittal; B3, in the frontal plane. (c) Complete articular. C1, articular simple, metaphyseal simple; C2, articular simple, metaphyseal multi-fragmentary; C3, multifragmentary.

treat, irrespective of the non-surgical or surgical method selected. They have, until recently, carried a poor prognosis with a high incidence of permanent disability. The options for treatment now form two groups: (i) closed reduction and traction with cast bracing; or (ii) open reduction and stable internal fixation. Until recently, the generally accepted treatment for the majority of distal femoral fractures was closed reduction, traction and splinting using one tibial tubercle pin or, sometimes, use of a second pin through the flexed supracondylar fragment for elevation. The knee was immobilized in a suitable splint, usually a Thomas type, with sliding traction to maintain optimum reduction until union. The problems included long hospital stays, an inability to control the displaced fragments, especially intra-articular ones, and residual knee contractures. Surgical treatment with open reduction and internal fixation, using various screws and plates, was reported at times but the results were generally very poor. This was due to the lack of surgical expertise and of suitable implants required for stable fracture fixation and necessary early knee mobilization. Complications included malunion and non-union of fractures, infection and knee stiffness. Comparisons between studies of large series of closed and open fixation of supracondylar fractures showed the general superiority of the conservative method. Thus, Stewart *et al.* (1966) reported 67% good or excellent closed fracture treatment results and 54% success for open fracture treatment. Neer *et al.* (1967) showed 90% success for closed treatment against 52% for open, although these success criteria are low in comparison with today's assessment.

The conservative method received furher support with the development of earlier mobilization 4 to 6 weeks after traction with functional fracture cast bracing (Mooney *et al.* 1970). At the same time, the advance in surgical treatment using the AO group principles with open anatomical reduction, rigid internal fixation with screws and condylar blade plates and early mobilization showed that high success could be obtained (Wenzl *et al.* 1970, Slatis *et al.* 1971, Olerud 1972). The reported comparative series from Toronto, 1961–1972 (Schatzker *et al.* 1974), showed closed treatment to give 32% and operative AO methods to give 75% good to excellent results. The application of the AO principles in these complex distal femoral fractures involves very demanding surgery, and if not achieved, then poor results are obtained (Schatzker & Lambert 1979). Another device, the Zickel double intra-medullary nail, was developed for supracondylar fracture reduction and fixation but with variable stability. Traction and cast bracing was often additionally required (Zickel *et al.* 1977). A more recent development, and of particular advantage in supracondylar fractures above knee replacements and below hip prostheses, is an intramedul-

lary device inserted proximally through the intercondylar notch. The locking principle is very similar to that of the Huckstep nail.

The most recent advance in the treatment of supracondylar fractures has been the development of the dynamic condylar screw (DCS) by the Swiss AO/ASIF group (Fig. 21.54). The DCS is replacing the condylar blade plate because it overcomes the difficulty of impacting the blade section by using a large compression screw which mounts into a cylinder on the side plate, allowing correction of any malalignment. The easier insertion technique of the DCS with avoidance of some of the complications of the condylar blade plate has been shown in practice and it is also usable in osteoporotic bone (Schatzker *et al.* 1989).

Selection factors

These are essentially the same as in femoral shaft fractures and involve the patient's condition, fracture characteristics, bone status, surgical expertise available and technology levels provided. The AO classification of distal femoral fractures gives a practical guide to the complexity of the fracture, the relative difficulty of treatment and the prognosis. The surgeon's expertise and the technology level available are significant factors in

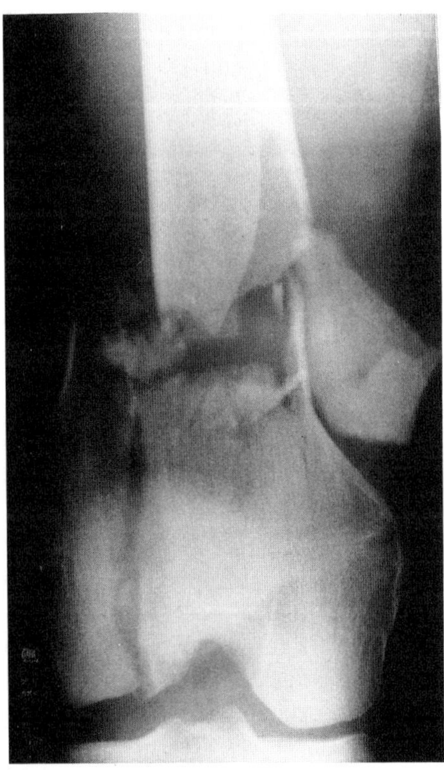

(a)

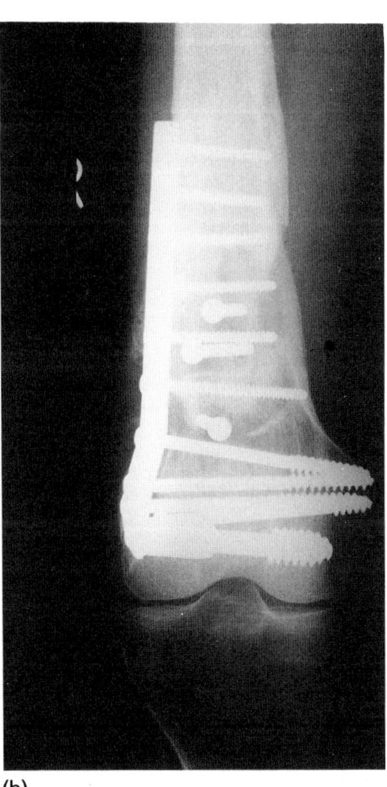

(b)

Fig. 21.54 (a) Multifragmentary supracondylar fracture (Type 33-C2). (b) Stable fixation with interfragmentary lag screws and a dynamic condylar screw.

closed or surgical treatment selection. Open reduction and stable internal fixation of these distal femoral fractures are often very difficult operations, requiring high skill and advanced instrumentation. If anatomical reduction and stable fixation are not obtained then the results may be worse than those from non-operative treatment (Schatzker & Lambert 1979).

Many supracondylar extra-articular fractures can be treated by closed reduction, skeletal traction and early mobilization with a cast brace. If reduction is not possible, or not maintained, then open reduction and fixation is necessary. Condylar intra-articular fractures with joint surface displacement cannot usually be reduced closed and require open fixation and early joint movement. Multiple lower-limb fractures give problems in traction and knee mobilization, with operative treatment being indicated. Thus, distal femoral fracture with ipsilateral tibial fracture or bilateral femoral fractures are best treated with internal fixation. Polytrauma patients with associated head, chest and abdominal injuries should have their fractures internally stabilized as soon as possible to reduce the respiratory distress complications and allow optimal nursing. Fixation following associated vascular damage requiring repair also benefits elderly patients who are at high risk with prolonged bedrest. Also, some patients with fixable fractures accept the option of surgical treatment to avoid long bedrest and traction periods. Finally, pathological fractures in patients with a limited life-span require open reduction and internal fixation, assisted by bone cement augmentation.

Controversy remains over the management of open fractures by immediate or delayed open reduction and internal fixation; both demand immediate thorough surgical debridement, intravenous administration of antibiotics and, also, local sterilization using depot gentamycin polymethylmethacrylate (PMMA) beads. Internal fixation would be contraindicated with severe open contaminated wounds and with pre-existing sepsis. Severe osteoporotic and comminuted fractures may not be fixable for technical reasons.

Non-operative treatment methods

Skeletal traction is applied through a Denham or Steinmann pin inserted behind the tibial tubercle transversely with a slight medial angulation to counter the external rotation of the proximal fracture. Balanced suspended traction is then set up using a Thomas' splint with a Pearson knee piece to allow knee flexion. With persistent posterior angulation from gastrocnemius contraction, a second transverse traction pin is

inserted through the femur at the level of the patellar superior pole in order to correct this defect. Many supracondylar fractures can be reduced with skeletal traction alone and held until callus forms. When a fracture has reached the sticky stable phase at 4 to 6 weeks, a well-moulded knee-hinged femoral cast brace is applied. The patient is then mobilized maximally weight-bearing and discharge from hospital is assessed using the union index and radiographs to monitor union as for femoral shaft fractures.

Operative treatment methods

In most cases the treatment preferred by the authors for complex distal femoral fractures is now by operative methods. Good functional results have been obtained in the majority of patients using open anatomical reduction of the fracture, stable internal fixation and very early knee mobilization with the CPM machine. The Swiss AO/ASIF instrumentation is used with the majority of cases having interfragmentary compression screws and with the DCS device replacing the previously used condylar plate technique. Preoperative planning is vital in order to determine the expected position of the device and screws; it is achieved by obtaining biplanar radiographs of the fractured distal femur and overlay templates of the implants. Surgical exposure of the distal femur is through a mid-lateral approach for supracondylar fractures (Fig. 21.55). With condylar fractures and where access is required medially, extended exposure is required, opening the knee to the tibial tubercle which can be osteotomized (Mize *et al*. 1982). The operative technique involves anatomical reduction of the fracture, compression screw fixation and then insertion of the DCS at the correct alignment using the triple reamer and tap. The large threaded condylar screw provides good fixation of the distal fragment and compression can be applied to the supracondylar fracture with the side plate screwed to the lower shaft (Fig. 21.54). With a medial cortical defect bone graft is required. For the stable fixation early mobilization with the CPM machine follows and the patient is then mobilized non-weight-bearing until union. With osteoporotic bone and less-than-rigid fixation a femoral cast brace is added for support.

Femoral fractures in children

Femoral shaft fractures

Children tolerate immobilization well for long periods. The femur heals quickly and only rarely are there joint

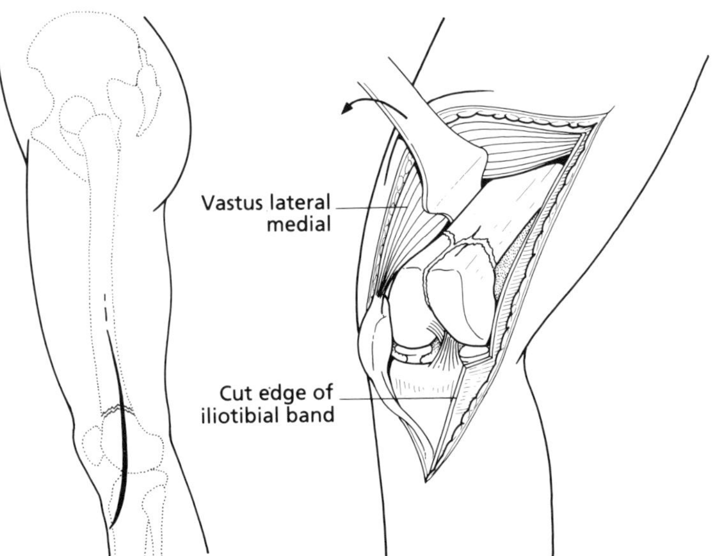

Fig. 21.55 Lateral approach to the distal femur and knee joint with optional tibial tubercle detachment for access to the medial side, and also for fixation and bone graft.

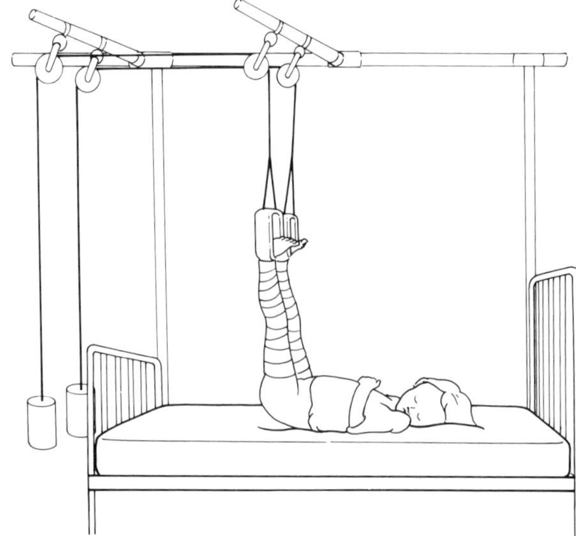

Fig. 21.56 Gallows traction for femoral fractures with skin traction and counterweight to hold buttocks clear of the bed.

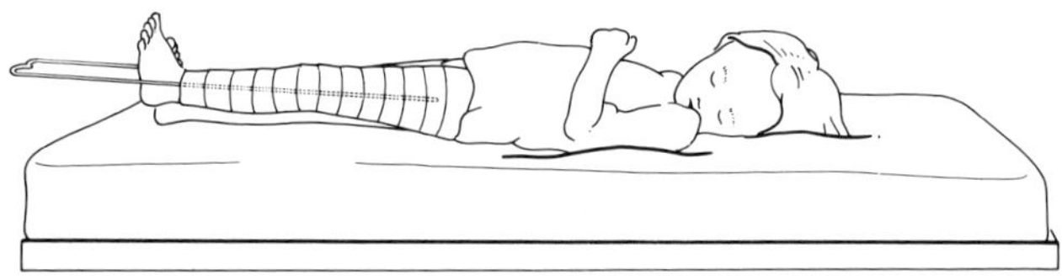

Fig. 21.57 Fixed skin traction on a simple splint is usually satisfactory for younger children.

stiffness problems. Thus, conservative treatment is indicated in most cases of femoral shaft fractures in children. The method of treatment depends upon the size of the child, the level of the fracture and the presence of any significant shortening.

For children who weigh under 13 kg (30 lb), usually up to the age of 18 months, skin traction is applied to both legs and the gallows vertical traction system is used. The infant's sacrum just rests on the bed with the buttocks clear (Fig. 21.56). With heavier children there is a risk of ischaemic damage to the limb if this method is used.

For children up to about 6 years of age, fixed traction with a Thomas' splint, using skin traction to the fractured limb, is usually satisfactory. The reduction can be maintained without difficulty. Initially, regular radiographs are necessary to allow for adjustment of the fracture (Fig. 21.57) if angulatory deformity and excessive shortening should occur. Overlap of the fracture ends by 1−2 cm is to be encouraged, as these limbs tend to overgrow for a period after fracture consolidation.

In children over 6 years, skin traction may not be sufficient to prevent excessive shortening because of stronger muscular contraction. Depending on the size and muscular build of the child, an early decision is required to use skeletal traction through the tibia rather than skin traction. An upper tibial pin is used for middle- and distal-third fractures together with a Thomas' splint suspension and Pearson knee piece.

Fractures of the proximal third tend to angulate from abductor/flexor muscle action and require treatment with vertical traction, with the hip and knee flexed in 90°, using a distal femoral pin. Alternatively, these cases may be suitable for an external fixator.

In any fracture in childhood, once a fracture has been stabilized with traction and early callus formation has been noted, it is possible for the child to be mobilized with the application of either a full leg cast or a hip spica. Once skeletal maturity is achieved, the treatment options are similar to those in the adult.

With unreducible fractures in children, or fractures in children who are uncooperative (following a severe head injury), external or internal stabilization of the fracture may be considered. The possibilities are a single bar external fixator on the lateral femur or, alternatively, a small intramedullary nail of the Rush pin type inserted below the greater trochanter. There are occasionally indications for open reduction and the use of a dynamic compression plate if the fracture remains unreducible by either of these two methods.

Distal femoral fractures

The thick growth plates of the distal femur are the weakest points in children, leaving them at risk from injury with any high stresses applied to the knee. The classification which has been generally accepted for injuries of the epiphyses (Salter & Harris 1963) is applicable to the distal femur; this classification is based on the mechanism of injury, relationship of the fracture line to the growing cells of the plate and to the prognosis in terms of potential angular deformity (Fig. 21.58). It includes the following types:

Type 1 — Simple epiphyseal plate fracture separation in which the plate remains intact and the germinal matrix remains on the epiphyseal side. These are more commonly seen as birth injuries, particularly breech presentations and also towards the end of the growth period. Closed reduction, if required, is usually stable but accurate replacement is not essential in the neonate with excellent remodelling potential; however, it is essential in the adolescent. Growth disturbances rarely occur.

Type 2 — This is the commonest variety with the epiphyseal plate intact and the fracture line passing through the metaphysis, leaving a peripheral fragment. Closed reduction and casting, often with the knee flexed, is usually satisfactory but if unstable, percutaneous K-wires are used also. The growth matrix is undamaged and disturbances are very unusual.

Type 3 — The fracture is intra-articular, extending from the articular surface through the epiphysis and along the plate to the periphery. This injury is uncommon and usually occurs towards the end of the growth period. Accurate reduction is essential both for restoration of the articular surface congruity and for realignment of the growth plate. This is best undertaken with open reduction and either a small transverse cancellous screw or two percutaneous wires. The prognosis is good providing the blood supply to the separated portion has been preserved.

Type 4 — This is an intra-articular fracture which extends from the articular surface through the growth plate and then through the metaphysis to the periphery, usually with vertical displacement. Accurate reduction of the epiphyseal plate is essential for restoration of the joint congruity. The best method of fixation is open reduction and use of either a small screw through the metaphyseal segment or percutaneous K-wires. With accurate reduction the prognosis is good but with any displacement a bone bridge will form and growth abnormalities develop.

Type 5 — These impact injuries produce crushing of the epiphyseal plate with loss of varying areas of the matrix. The seriousness of this injury is not always appreciated initially. Rest in a cast and non-weight-bearing is required for any epiphyseal recovery. The prognosis is poor with cessation of growth from a segment resulting in angular deformities. These may require open wedge lengthening osteotomies later when the deformity develops.

Type 6 — This results from exposure of the plate from damage to the periosteum as a result of local violent trauma, a penetrating injury or burns. A bony bridge bands the segment of the plate, producing local retardation of growth and angular deformities. Early treatment by excision of the bridge and replacement with a fat graft is necessary before angular deformities become significant.

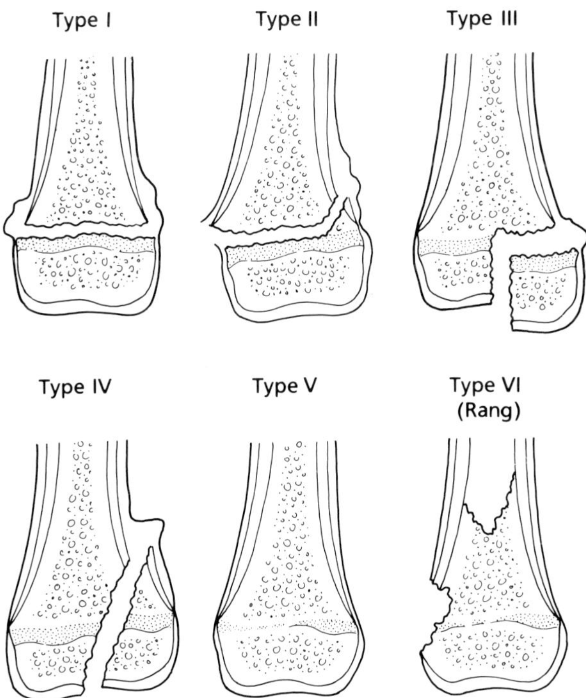

Fig. 21.58 Classification of growth plate injuries (Salter and Harris) into five types plus type 6 (Rang).

Pathological fractures

Pathological fractures usually occur through a mechanically weak segment of bone as the result of an abnormal condition. There are two main bone changes producing this state: one is a local lesion causing bone resorption and the other is a more generalized structural change in the bone resulting in brittleness. The commonest localized lesion in the femur is metastatic malignancy from, most commonly, carcinoma of the breast, lung, thyroid, prostate or colon. These lesions in the femur may produce pain before overt fracture evidence is present and they are readily localized with isotope bone scans. These fractures, most commonly in the shaft, are ideally treated with closed locked medullary nailing with the strongest available nail, although bone union often occurs with chemotherapy and radiotherapy. Other localized pathological lesions occasionally associated with fractures are osteogenic sarcomas, osteoclastomas, leukaemias and pyogenic abscesses.

The second form of pathological fractures occurs in mechanically generalized weakened bone of the femur secondary to metabolic bone disease such as osteoporosis, osteomalacia and osteitis deformans (Paget's disease). In osteomalacia the subtrochanteric area is the most frequent site of pathological fractures in the femur because of a high stress concentration. In osteoporosis fractures are most frequent in the neck region but can also occur in the subtrochanteric and supracondylar regions. The most stable treatment is with a short locking medullary nail or a Zickel nail proximally and a dynamic condylar screw plate distally. In patients with Paget's disease the femur is the most commonly fractured bone. The most frequent deformity of the femoral shaft is a lateral varus bowing with high-tension stress over the convexity, usually proximally; this means the subtrochanteric region and upper shaft are the commonest sites of fracture in Paget's disease. With the high fractures a short locking medullary nail may be feasible but lower down the large bone may prevent this so that treatment with a contoured femoral compression plate or conservative treatment is necessary. If held satisfactorily most of these fractures do unite eventually.

The third, and much less common, pathological fracture in the femur is the stress or fatigue fracture, which is probably the result of a mechanically induced local weakening condition of the bone. Repeated high stresses to the femur, far in excess of those usually experienced, result in local pain, periosteal new bone formation and a fatigue fracture, which usually starts on the convex side of the bone. The sort of sudden increase in physical activity which is liable to produce fatigue fractures occurs in the early intensive training period of athletes and military recruits. An early symptomatic warning often occurs in the thigh before complete fracture, and with restricted activity most cases proceed to full union.

Complications of femoral fractures

The prognosis for healing of femoral fractures is generally very good but, in spite of this, a considerable number of complications can occur. These may result from associated soft tissue injuries, may be associated with the acute femoral fracture or may arise from its method of treatment; specific complications may be connected with fractures of the proximal and distal ends of the femur. An appreciation of this wide variety of complications is necessary if they are to be minimized or if early treatment is to be instigated.

Associated soft tissue injuries

Open fractures

The management of open fractures is detailed elsewhere (see Chapter 9). Open fractures of the femoral shaft are less common than those of the tibia and are usually associated with high-velocity injuries and polytrauma. It is doubtful whether Gustillo and Anderson type I open fractures exist and most fractures will be type II or type III. Surprisingly, there remains controversy over the role of surgical stabilization in these fractures. There is, however, little doubt that surgical stabilization reduces long-term morbidity and mortality, and provided that the principles of wound care are followed meticulously, stabilization of type II and type IIIa fractures, using either a plate or (preferably) a nail, carries no significant increase in the risk of infection. Type IIIb and IIIc fractures are probably best treated using an external fixator, although problems with pin-tract sites can compromise any further surgery, particularly if there is delay in bone union.

Nerve and vascular injuries

Nerve injuries associated with acute femoral fractures are uncommon owing to the wide separation of the nerve from the bone by a thick muscle layer. High-stress fractures with extrusion or penetrating injuries posteriorly may involve the sciatic nerve directly or, with traction, indirectly. The commonest nerve complication that may occur during treatment of femoral fractures is damage to the common peroneal nerve as a result of either traction from excessive skin or skeletal pull, or from direct pressure at the fibular neck from external rotation against an incorrectly placed splint.

Vascular injuries are also uncommon in that femoral fractures may be associated with high-velocity injuries with the vessels becoming snagged or lacerated by the fracture fragments. This occurs more commonly in the distal thigh where the vessels are more fixed by their branches and fascial attachments. Intimal damage and secondary thrombosis are commoner in the main shaft area. Major arterial occlusion must be recognized early, with pain, parasthesia, paresis, pallor and pain on calf stretch giving the clinical picture. This may take some time to present but the early pulselessness, confirmed by a Doppler probe and followed by arteriography and, if indicated, by venography, will identify the site of the occlusion. Urgent exploration with compartment decompression and repair, and with a vein graft as indicated, is essential to restore the limb circulation and prevent distal necrosis which will occur within an 8-hour period. Stabilization of the fracture also provides splintage for the repaired artery; if necessary some degree of shortening is possible in order to relax the repair tissue. Vascular damage may also occur as a complication of internal fixation, most commonly while drilling a screw hole in the shaft of the femur. Partial laceration of the vessels, from the acute fracture or during internal fixation, may result in immediate haemorrhage or in a delayed arteriovenous fistula formation which may require separation and repair or grafting once diagnosed and confirmed by arteriography.

Finally, neurovascular injuries may occur in association with a compartment compression syndrome which is uncommon following femoral shaft fractures but occurs more frequently with Volkmann's contracture in children, usually following the selection of an inappropriate traction technique (Mubarak & Carroll 1979). The clinical signs are similar to arterial obstruction, with a tense, painful thigh, but the pulses are intact until very late. This thigh compartment syndrome may also develop after an ischaemic period following vascular damage and repair. Intramuscular pressure measurement, using the wick or split catheter with a pressure transducer and recorder, will give more accurate monitoring of the tissue pressures, However, if the signs are present clinically then urgent fasciotomy decompression of the thigh is necessary.

Polytrauma

The principles of management of polytraumatized patients are described elsewhere. A rapid initial assessment of such patients, the provision of adequate intravenous lines and airway control are all priorities.

Between 30 and 40% of polytraumatized patients will have a femoral shaft fracture. The risk of adult respiratory distress syndrome (ARDS) in polytraumatized patients is high and it has been shown that early stabilization of the femoral shaft fracture within 24 hours of the injury has the potential to reduce the incidence of ARDS by 500%. In addition, intensive care (Johnson *et al.* 1985) requirements are also reduced and Johnson *et al.* do not feel that there is any place for conservative management of femoral shaft fractures in such circumstances. The controversy as to whether to stabilize the fracture with a plate or nail continues. In closed fractures treated with plate fixation blood loss is significant and Pennig (personal communication) found that because of this it was possible to operate on only 44% of all femoral shaft fractures within the first 24 hours. Using the locking nail for closed fractures and the external fixator for open fractures, he was able to fix 80% of femoral shaft fractures within 24 hours of the injury with a related drop in mortality and ARDS. The use of the intramedullary nail does not appear to increase the risk of respiratory dysfunction.

Knee ligament injuries

In high-velocity trauma and in multiple injuries, associated knee ligament injuries must always be suspected with femoral shaft fractures. The incidence of injuries, particularly to the medial and anterior cruciate ligaments, in high-velocity trauma is high; estimates vary between 25 and 70%. Suspicion may be aroused by a knee effusion, particularly if the femoral shaft is in the mid or proximal diaphysis (Walling *et al.* 1982). Aspiration of the knee will reveal blood and it has been recommended that in order to confirm a knee ligament injury radiographically, prior to any form of surgery, a transcondylar or supracondylar pin should be inserted through the femur and the knee examined using counter-traction through this pin. Radiographic examination can be performed at the same time.

The suspicion of a knee ligament injury is now generally regarded as an absolute indication for internal fixation of the femoral shaft fracture, followed by knee ligament repair if this is indicated. The use of a lightweight cast brace with a flexion and extension block, following medial or lateral ligament repair, will control knee extension and flexion and yet allow satisfactory knee mobilization postoperatively.

If internal fixation is not performed then tibial traction is, of course, contraindicated. The hazards of long-term femoral traction include pin-tract sepsis and fracture through the pin site.

Associated with the fracture

Blood loss

Fractured femurs may cause high blood loss internally in the thigh with muscle damage, perforating vessel injury and bone fragment bleeding, which may vary from 1 to 3 l. Hypovolaemic shock is common unless replacement of the blood and fluid is undertaken. In the younger patient with a better ability to compensate, the bleeding may be very deceptive until sudden circulatory collapse occurs. This blood loss is greater in comminuted and open fractures, and in those associated with other fractures. However, before attributing the blood loss entirely to the fractured femur, it is essential that a full assessment is undertaken to exclude other causes of bleeding, particularly within the chest and abdomen. All fractured femurs should have an intravenous line established early with adequate fluid replacement.

ARDS and the fat embolism syndrome

This is an acute deterioration of pulmonary function that is characterized by progressive hypoxaemia with damaging systemic effects. Unless treated, the hypoxic cellular dysfunction can become life-threatening. The exact causes of ARDS are unknown but specific conditions are associated with its development, these being either sepsis or non-sepsis related. ARDS may develop following femoral fractures, particularly if associated with fat embolism, shock, other massive trauma, other fractures, chest trauma or burns. ARDS following fat embolism appears clinically with tachypnoea and dyspnoea, excessive bronchial secretions, irritability and confusion which may proceed to coma, pyrexia, tachycardia and a falling arterial blood oxygen level. Diffuse interstitial infiltrates appear on the chest radiograph, often with a 'snow storm' appearance. The diagnostic criteria are hypoxaemia ($Po_2 < 70$ mmHg on 40% oxygen), low platelet count ($<150\,000$ ml^{-1}) and fat detected in the sputum and urine. Petechial haemorrhages may occur in the skin over the anterior chest wall and in the conjunctiva. The fat in the lung produces both mechanical obstruction and chemical damage of the capillaries with fluid exudate, alveolar architecture damage and pulmonary arteriovenous shunting. The objectives of treatment are to minimize the fat embolization from the fracture and the hypoxaemia from the pulmonary damage. Specific treatment involves gentle handling and adequate splint immobilization of the fracture with careful transport, together with the pre-vention and early treatment of hypovolaemic shock. Early and regular blood gas monitoring and administration of 40% oxygen to all fracture patients is required. If this treatment is inadequate for the patient to maintain a reasonable blood gas level, assisted respiration with intubation is necessary. As ARDS occurs most commonly within the first 72 hours after significant skeletal trauma, immediate stabilization of all fractures with internal or external fixation has been advocated when adequate facilities are available; this results in a significant reduction in the morbidity and mortality from this potentially life-threatening complication.

Non-union

DEFINITION

There is no hard and fast definition of delayed or non-union in the femur, as there is in the tibia. However, failure of the femoral shaft fracture to unite within 18–20 weeks is generally regarded as indicating delayed union. Failure to unite after 1 year was regarded by Winquist and Hansen as a non-union, although Grosse and Kempf define non-union as being present at 6–8 months.

INCIDENCE

Because of the discrepancy in the definition of delayed and non-union, the incidence is difficult to assess. Conservative management using Pyrford traction in a consecutive series of 50 patients (Buxton 1981) revealed no patients with non-union, and delayed union over 18 weeks occurred in only three patients. In all patients the bone had united by 28 weeks.

Both Meggitt and Wardlaw, using traction and cast bracing, suggested that a non-union rate of less than 5–6% was the norm (Wardlaw 1977, Meggitt et al. 1981).

Using internal fixation, plating yields a non-union rate of approximately 5% (Reudi & Luchner 1979) and in 1980 Winquist and Hansen published a series of over 100 subtrochanteric fractures treated with various methods of fixation which resulted in an incidence of 5% non-union. The use of closed intramedullary nailing (Grosse 1988) resulted in a non-union rate of 1%. It is thus obvious that delayed and non-union are rarer in femoral shaft fractures than in tibial shaft fractures. Non-union, of course, is much more common if a fracture becomes infected.

AETIOLOGY

The factors associated with delayed or non-union are as follows:

1 Open fractures with bone loss.
2 Deep infection.
3 Failure to graft internally fixed fractures.
4 Open reduction and ineffective stabilization of the fracture (Fig. 21.59).

TREATMENT

Watson-Jones advocated prolonged immobilization of the fracture on a Thomas' splint and claimed a high rate of bony union. Sometimes the immobilization was continued for well over 6 months.

In considering the treatment of non-union it has been conventional to consider the difference between atrophic and hypertrophic non-union. This distinction is important, particularly in fractures of the upper limb and, to some extent, in the tibia. However, the distinction does not seem to be so important in femoral shaft fractures.

There are three main stimuli to healing ununited femoral shaft fractures. These are: (i) the use of autologous bone graft; (ii) restoration of the normal mechanical axis and forces; and (iii) electrical stimulation.

It has been regarded by some as essential to remove the fibrous bridge between the ununited fragments in order to achieve bony union. However, success of closed intramedullary nailing has proven this not to be the case. Removal of the fibrous bridge between the fragments is technically extremely difficult and often results in catastrophic haemorrhage.

Bone grafting alone requires a further period of immobilization, either on traction or in a cast brace, in an already wasted and compromised lower limb. Restoration of mechanical forces and alignment would seem to be a more potent factor in stimulating bony union. In this respect the intramedullary nail is an ideal solution as a load-sharing device. Grosse (1988), in a series of 27 patients with non-union, achieved a 93% success rate using a closed or semi-closed technique. The failures were treated by re-nailing with a larger nail. One patient became infected and required an external fixator.

It is not always possible to achieve a closed reduction in an established non-union. Particularly if there is significant deformity or overlap, it is often necessary to

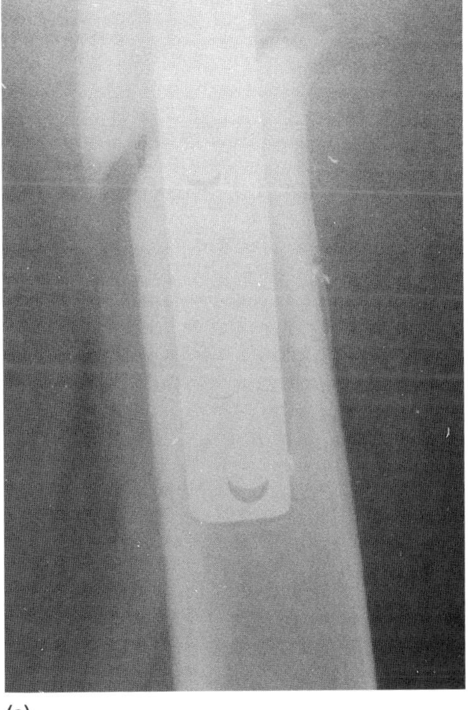
(a)

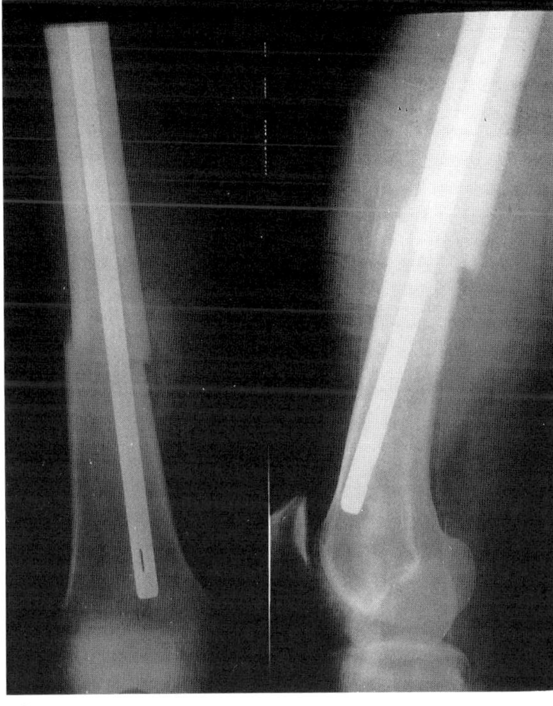
(b)

Fig. 21.59 (a) This fracture was inaccurately reduced and plated. Irritation callus can be seen, indicating delayed union. The patient went on to develop non-union and required bone grafting. (b) This nail is too small for the large conical medullary cavity. If the fracture unites, malunion is a strong possibility.

partially unpick the fracture site and, having achieved reduction, it is then usually possible to nail the fracture (Fig. 21.60). In cases where failure of union follows a previous implant, it is advisable to remove the implant, close the wound and then perform a closed nailing (Fig. 21.61).

The use of external fixators has been advocated but, as yet, their advantages are unproven; experience would tend to suggest that the rate of union is lower than after a closed nailing procedure. Pin sepsis is significant.

Malunion

Malunion of femoral fractures is almost entirely a problem of conservatively treated femoral fractures. The significance of a minor degree of malunion may well not be important, although if the malalignment is close to the knee joint, the development of late osteoarthritis may well be a problem (Fig. 21.62).

It is sometimes difficult to maintain adequate alignment, particularly in distal fractures, using conservative methods and, indeed, malposition of an intramedullary nail, particularly if it is not locked proximally or distally, can produce an unacceptable deformity. Because of the mechanical pull of the adductors a varus deformity is invariable. If this is in association with a surgical approach using either plates or nails, then technically the problem should be avoidable. Deformities following locking nailing are almost entirely due to the wrong entry point in the trochanteric region for proximal fractures and to incorrect reduction and placement of the guide wire for distal fractures (Fig. 21.63).

Malunion is often multidimensional, and if it is significant enough to require correction, then either closed or open osteotomy (Winquist *et al.* 1978) (Christie & Court Brown 1988) should be used in combination with an intramedullary nail.

De Bastiani has described the use of the external fixator in correcting multiplanar malunions following osteotomy and gradual distraction of the bone, and this may be particularly useful where there is significant shortening associated with the malunion.

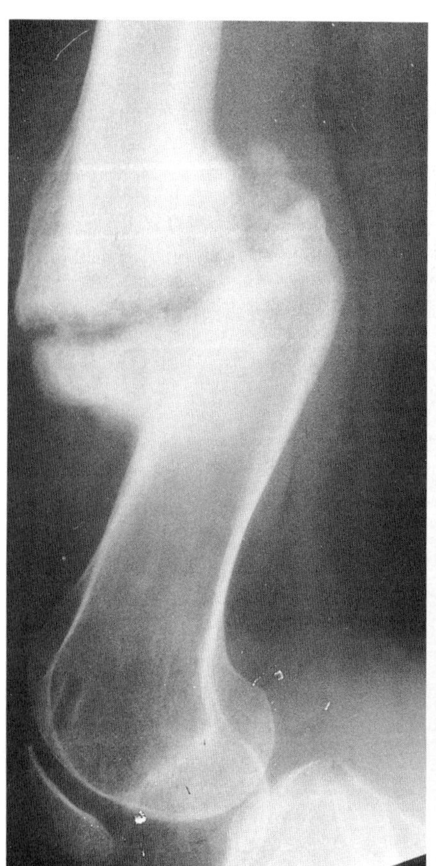
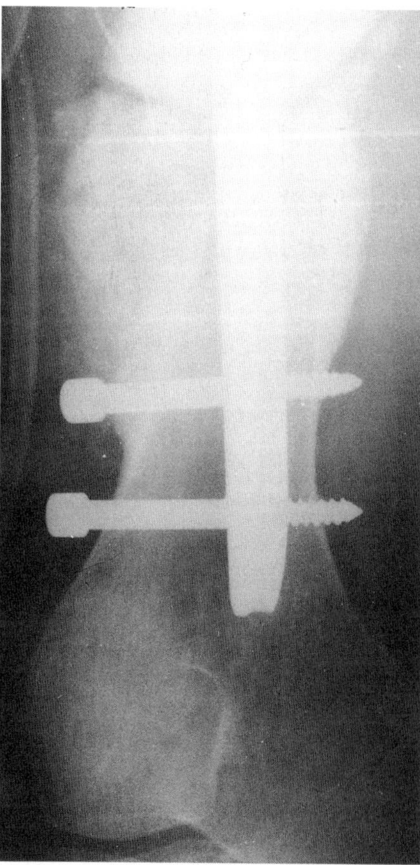

(a)   (b)

Fig. 21.60 This patient exhibited severe overlap. It was necessary to perform an open reduction, unpicking and osteotomizing the hypertrophic callus. In this case it was necessary to shorten the femur slightly, but having achieved reduction, it was possible to insert a dynamically locked nail.

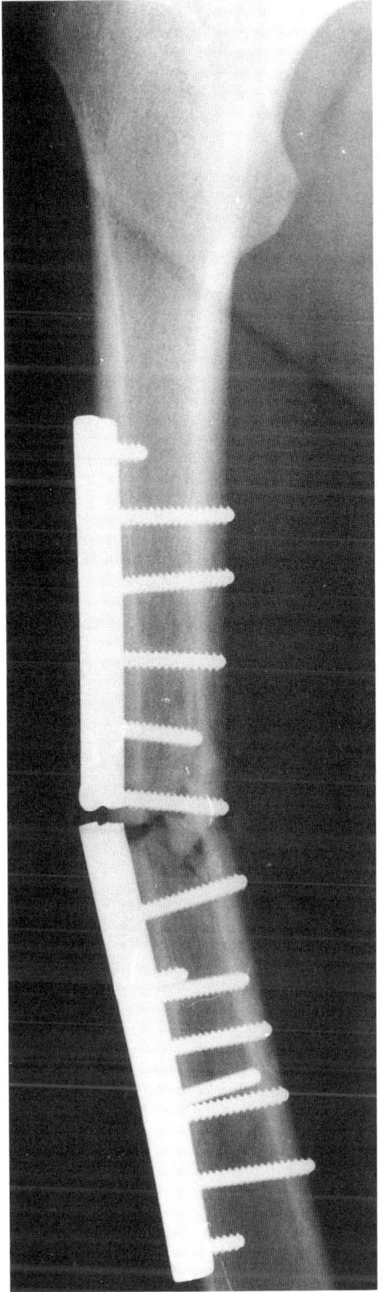

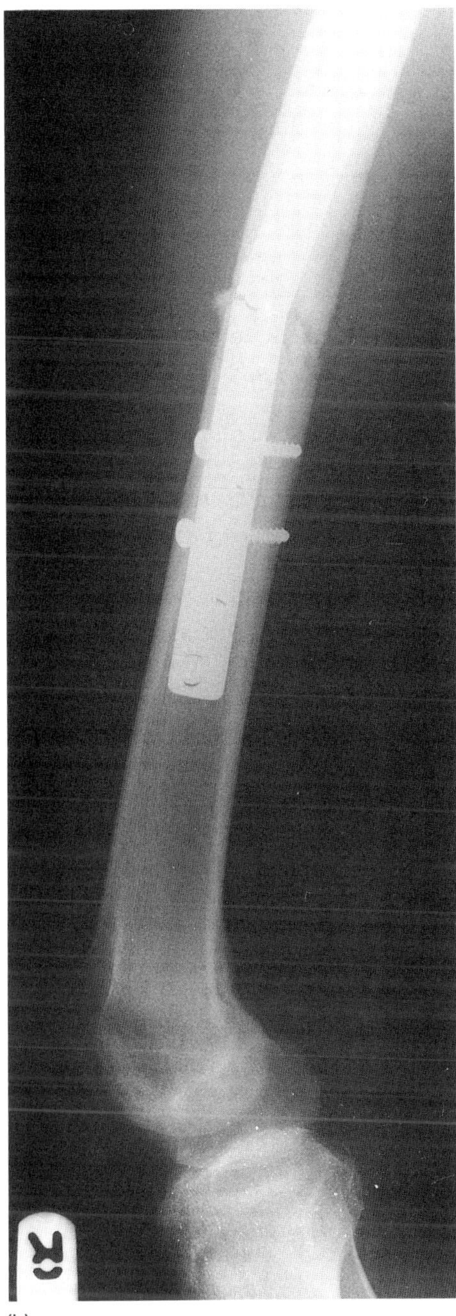

Fig. 21.61 This implant failed because the fracture was not bone grafted. Removal of the implant was straightforward and the fracture went on to satisfactory bony union following nailing.

Complications of supracondylar and condylar fractures

Complications arising from the fracture and its treatment in the distal femur are generally similar to those already discussed. There are, however, more specific complications associated with supracondylar and inter-condylar fractures. There is a higher incidence of vascular damage to the femoral or popliteal vessels because of their relative fixation and the posterior angulation; often with comminution of the distal fragment there may be tearing of the posterior tissues. Malunion is a common complication of conservatively treated fractures in this region because of the difficulty in reducing and maintaining alignment of the posterior, and often medially, angulated distal fragment. Intercondylar fractures involving the articular surface with displacement are also very difficult to reduce closed and may result in loss of articular congruity with resulting knee stiffness. Both articular incongruity and axial malalignment will produce high point loading stresses, with the develop-

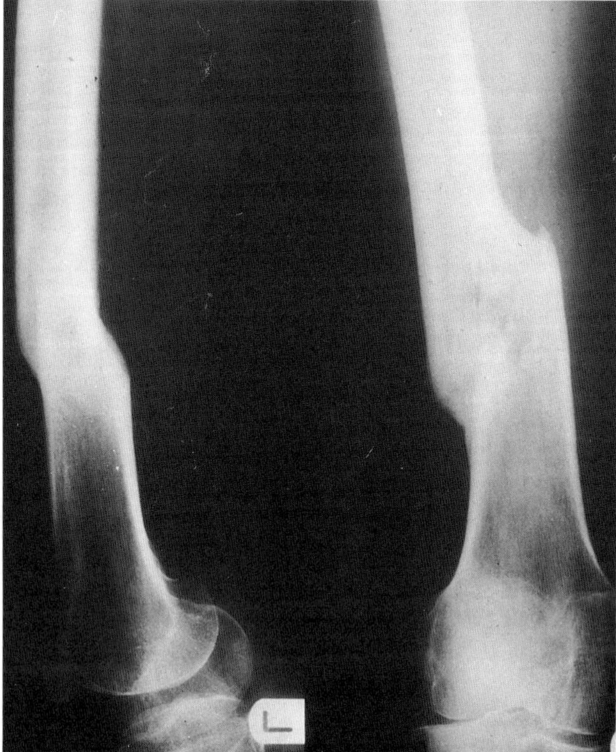

Fig. 21.62 This patient had a femoral shaft fracture treated with traction. This resulted in a significant varus deformity and late radiographs showed early development of osteoarthritis over the medial joint line.

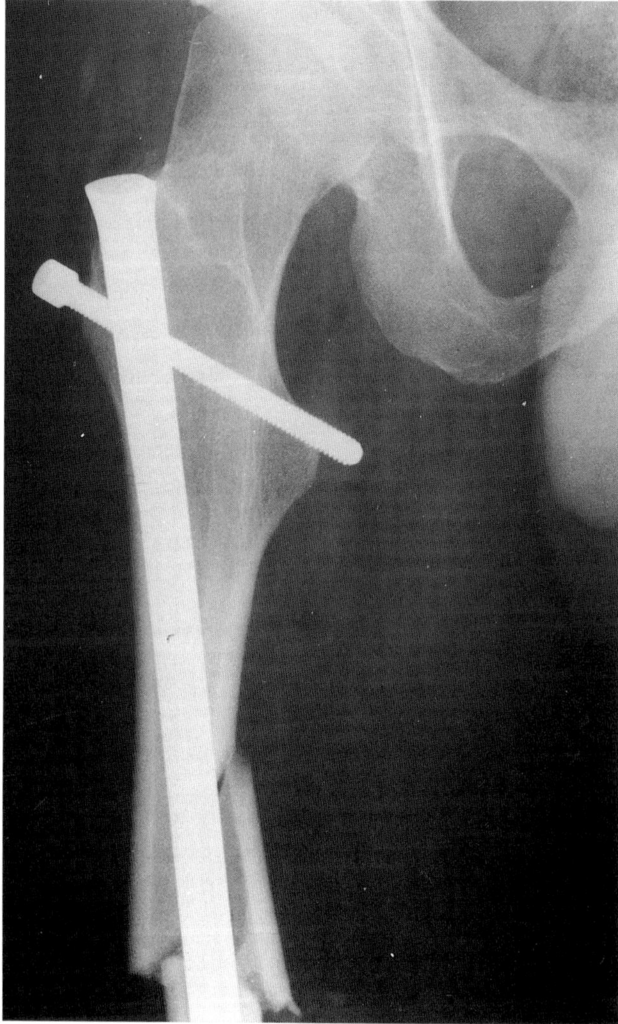

Fig. 21.63 Too lateral an entry point was used in this patient and the medial cortex was blown off. An unacceptable varus deformity results.

ment of early osteoarthritic changes. Delayed or non-union may also occur with traction treatment and can prevent early mobilization of the knee, which may then develop a contracture. This may also occur from damage to the distal quadriceps and knee joint from the proximal fracture shortening into these tissues. Significant angular malunion requires realignment with an osteotomy and plate or dynamic screw plate. An articular incongruity malunion may be very difficult to treat. Delayed or non-union, more common in the supracondylar section, requires similar internal fixation with compression after excision of the fibrous union and with the addition of a bone graft after cortical surface 'petalling'. It should be possible to correct knee contracture from intra-articular supracondylar adhesions to give a functional range of movement by surgical release and very early passive mobilization.

Many of these complications can be avoided by carefully preplanned open reduction and internal fixation with adequate devices, instrumentation and expertise. However, the surgical management of these distal femoral fractures is also fraught with a wide range of potential complications unless the principles of accurate

reduction and stable internal fixation are fully adhered to. Problems with delayed wound healing, infection, delayed or non-union, malunion, joint contracture, loosening or breakage of the fixation device, refracture and post-traumatic arthritis have all been recorded in the reported series of these injuries. Device failure, with the plate and screws cutting out and with the fracture displacing, is a significant problem in the osteoporotic, and often comminuted, fracture in the elderly.

Knee stiffness

Loss of knee movement with a flexion contracture has previously been a serious complication of femoral fractures and is most commonly caused by adhesions within the quadriceps muscle. With the conservatively treated traction methods, temporary knee stiffness was very commonly seen and the recovery in knee flexion was consistent with union of the fracture. However, with delayed union and more prolonged periods of traction, permanent knee contracture was not uncommon. Recently, however, the incidence of knee stiffness has decreased considerably with the advent of early mobilization following the use of stable internal fixation of the fracture. Very early fixation of femoral shaft fractures, using the locked intramedullary nail, and immediate post-operative use of a CPM machine has resulted in knee contractures being rarely seen, and a very good, often full, range of knee flexion movement is recovered, even in the severely comminuted closed fracture. With severe quadriceps muscle damage, and particularly with open contaminated fractures, treatment with traction or external fixation is necessary and the delayed soft tissue, and often also bone, healing is likely to lead to varying degrees of quadriceps fibrosis and contracture.

Treatment of the stiff knee, once the femoral fracture is soundly united, depends upon the site of the main adhesion. Although these are most likely to be within the quadriceps muscle, there can also be fibrotic contractures within the fascia lata and within the skin subcutaneous tissues. With associated injury to the knee joint, adhesions may be quite dense in the suprapatellar pouch and lateral recesses, or in the capsule and peri-articular tissue, presenting with a bound-down patella and a knee joint contracture. Treatment of a quadriceps fibrosis involves an examination under anaesthetic with gentle manipulation. If the fibrosis is mature, then little increased movement will be gained. If the disability is severe enough to the patient, then a quadricepsplasty procedure is undertaken (Thompson 1944, Nicoll 1963). In this procedure entry is through the anterior thigh, the rectus femoris is preserved, and the fascia are divided on each side, separating the lateralis and medialis muscles from the upper-third junction to the capsule of the knee joint. The vastus intermedius, which is commonly fibrotic and binds the rectus femoris and patella to the femoral surface, is excised completely. Any remaining adhesions are broken down with manipulation and the vastus medialis and lateralis are sutured back to the sides of the rectus down to the lower-third junction of the thigh. Modifications depend upon the area of scarring, with only one side of the vastus being released to expose the intermedius if the other side is undamaged, or with further excision extended to fibrosis within the vastus muscle. With extensive fibrosis an interpositional silastic sheet may be used in the lower femur to prevent fibrosis recurring. Prolonged vacuum drainage and early passive mobilization, with either auto-assisted exercises on a Fisk splint or a CPM machine, are necessary postoperatively. Any attempt at lengthening the contracture should be carefully balanced against the danger of producing an extension lag which may, in the long term, leave the knee unstable.

Complications relating to treatment

Skin traction

Skin traction of up to 4.5 kg can be applied safely in most adults and children. However, this is only enough to control fracture length in children up to the age of about six years. Heavier traction than this may result in slipping of the traction system, shearing of the skin, traction on the common peroneal nerve with foot drop and compression effects upon the calf muscles with potential compartment syndrome, deep vein thrombosis and arterial damage.

Skeletal traction

The main complications may involve necrosis of the skin at the percutaneous pin level, infection of the pin tract, loosening of the pin and, in osteoporotic bone, the pin may pull out. These complications may be prevented by the use of a central-threaded Denham pin or a full-threaded Steinmann pin, introduced by a hand drill and not by a power drill, (which may cause a thermal ring sequestrum). Release of the skin distally after insertion of the skeletal pin will prevent pressure necrosis and regular hygiene to the pin–skin interface reduces local infection. If deep sepsis does occur, the pin will require relocation with debridement and, occasionally, ring sequestrectomy and antibiotics.

Also, indirectly, varying degrees of malunion, particularly varus and posterior angulation and shortening, are complications of the traction method of femoral fracture treatment. These are not always due to treatment error as in many fractures, particularly the widely displaced and comminuted types, fragments become snagged on the muscle and fibrous elements, preventing accurate reduction and functional alignment. To avoid these potential malunion complications from an unacceptable closed reduction, operative treatment is required ideally with the locking intramedullary nail technique. Non-union related to skeletal traction is uncommon but can occur if distraction occurs, particularly with transverse and short oblique fractures. The early high traction weight required for reduction could be decreased after radiographic examination has shown that satisfactory alignment has been obtained, and thus, any associated complication should be avoided.

Cast bracing

This technique requires expertise in both the traction reduction method and in the application of the specialized long-leg hinged walking plaster cast. The main complications involve malunion and shortening, which are often present prior to the application of the brace but may also develop after its application if the brace is used too early, when the fracture is still unstable, or if the fracture is too high (in the upper third of the shaft) and receiving inadequate support. A well-fitting total contact cast for the thigh section is essential with immediate radiographic examination after brace application and with change of the thigh cast, or wedging, if required. Fractures in the upper third can be held, once callus union is advancing, using a uniaxial stable metal hip hinge with a rigid pelvic band and waist belt; the hip and fracture must be held in the abducted position during application. Cast brace application at the knee causes tissue swelling so that an elastic tubular knee support is required; restricted knee movement resulting from incorrectly placed knee hinges outside the knee joint axis requires reapplication of the brace.

External fixation

As indicated previously, external fixation is a system which is rarely indicated in fresh closed femoral shaft fractures except as a provisional stabilization in polytrauma and in major contaminated wounds. There are three major complications with the use of external fixation:

1 *Pin tract sepsis.* Because the pins pass through the quadriceps muscle, pin-tract sepsis is much more common than in the tibia where there is little skin movement over subcutaneous bone. Not only does pin-tract sepsis lead to bony infection and thus pin loosening, but it also compromises any secondary procedure such as intramedullary nailing or plating.

2 *Stability.* Because of the strong muscle forces and lateral placement of the pins, most external fixators are not strong enough to cope with the enormous varus forces. If the external fixator is used for any length of time in such circumstances, then varus deformity is common.

3 *Knee flexion.* It is inevitable that pins transfix the vastus lateralis in unilateral fixators. This usually restricts knee motion. Although this returns to normal following removal of the external fixator, intensive

physiotherapy is usually necessary. Although perhaps this cannot be called a complication, it is certainly a side-effect, and negates one of the requisites of operative treatment — that of early mobilization of adjacent joints.

Plating

EARLY COMPLICATIONS

Many complications associated with plating are related to the soft tissues. Particularly in open fractures, infection is a potential problem since exposure is extensive. Deep infection will lead to non-union. An infected non-union of a femoral shaft following plate or intramedullary nail fixation is a major surgical disaster. The risk of infection is increased by inadequate fixation, particularly in open fractures.

Secondary knee stiffness is an additional complication of femoral shaft fractures and if the surgeon is not confident of the adequacy of the fixation and further immobilizes the fracture, then the additional scarring of the retracted muscles will make subsequent knee mobilization even more difficult.

LATE COMPLICATIONS

Plate fatigue

The main problem following plate fixation of a femoral shaft fracture is delay in union of the fracture and plate fatigue — the race between non-union and plate failure. Reudi and Luchner (1979) quote an incidence of 6% in their series. Almost inevitably, plate failure is related to a failure to consider bone grafting at the time of the initial operation (see Figs 21.59 & 21.61).

Other problems

These include late failure of the screw—bone interface, again associated with delayed or non-union. In both circumstances salvage is relatively easy and involves removing the appropriate metalwork and inserting a locked intramedullary nail. The internal bone graft that occurs during reaming of the femur seems to stimulate bony union and Grosse (1988) quotes a union rate of 25 out of 27 femoral non-unions.

TECHNICAL PROBLEMS

Intramedullary nailing

Overall, intramedullary nailing is a safe and reliable

method of fixing most femoral shaft fractures. The main complications relate to technical inadequacies of the surgeon, of the patient's bone and of the implant material.

Incorrect insertion point

Too lateral a point of insertion will result in impingement of the nail on the medial femoral cortex, particularly in upper-third fractures, and this may well increase the comminution of the medial femoral cortex. The inevitable result of this is the development of a varus deformity and the necessity to statically lock the nail (Fig. 21.63).

Too medial a point of insertion through the neck of the femur is associated with the possibility of late avascular necrosis and subsequent neck fracture. Sometimes this configuration is inevitable, particularly in high femoral shaft fractures (see Fig. 21.32).

If the nail is inserted anteriorly, particularly in subtrochanteric fractures with associated osteoporosis, reaming may destroy the posterior cortex. This may result in a flexion deformity of the proximal fragment and, worse, (see Fig. 21.52) cutting out of the device.

Guide wire insertion

Placement of the guide wire poses no particular difficulty when the middle third of the femur is fractured. However, failure to align a guide wire in the centre of the knee joint in distal-third fractures will result in an inevitable varus or valgus deformity of the distal femur (Fig. 21.64). In soft bone it is possible for the guide wire, particularly the nailing wire, to enter the knee joint with the possibility of placement of the nail within the knee joint (Fig. 21.65).

Reaming and nailing

A statically locked nail does not require a tight fit in the medullary canal. It is only necessary to ream to a size that will allow the insertion of a strong enough nail for the patient. However, over-reaming to allow the easy insertion of the nail is better than reaming just enough to have a tight fit of the nail with consequent difficulties in insertion. It has been suggested that iatrogenic neck fractures (Christie & Court Brown 1988) are the result of too tight a nail insertion and excessive hammering to get the nail down (Fig. 21.66). In addition, too tight a fit of the nail can result in overdistraction of the fracture and this again will cause problems.

The reamer should be switched off and pushed

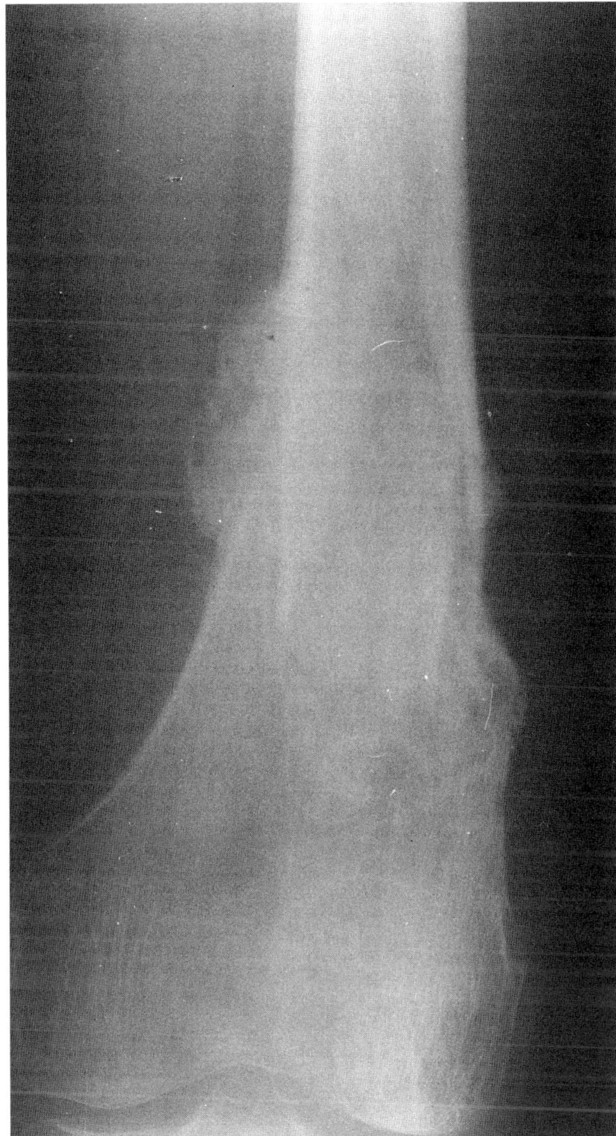

Fig. 21.64 Unsatisfactory guide wire placement resulted in a grossly unsatisfactory varus deformity in this elderly patient with a distal-third fracture.

through grossly comminuted areas of the femoral shaft because of the possibility of the reamer snagging on bony fragments and causing further devitalization of the femoral shaft fragments.

It is important that the correct length of nail is selected and the ideal position for the tip of the nail is 1–2 cm from the top of the intercondylar notch. The proximal end should be flush with the tip of the greater trochanter. Particularly in distal fractures, preoperative planning is essential to ensure that there is enough space for two screws to be able to get adequate purchase in the distal fragment.

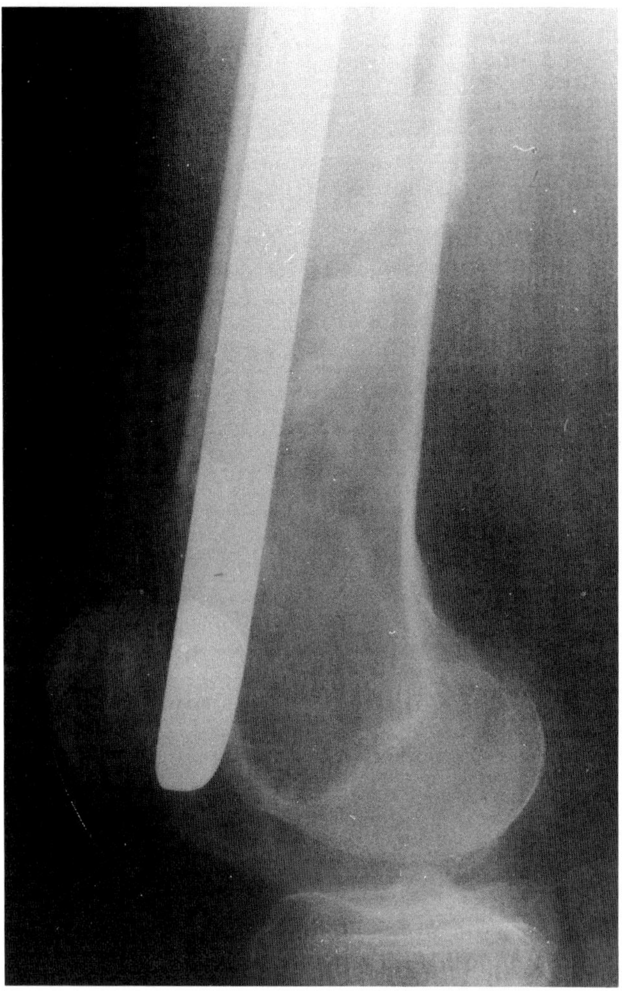

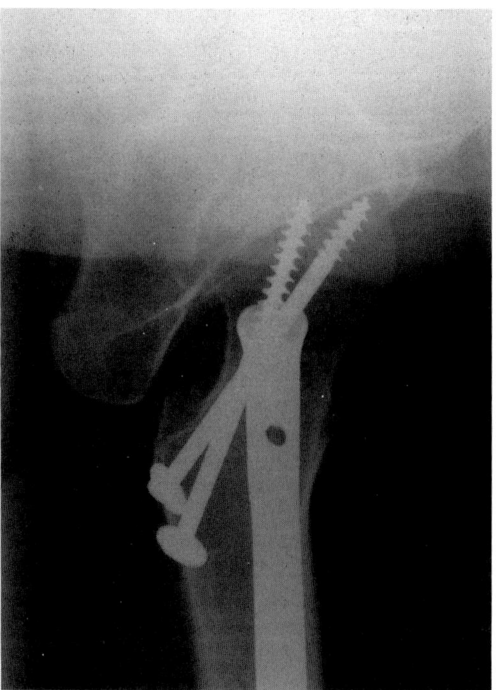

Fig. 21.66 This patient sustained a crack fracture of the femoral neck during nail insertion. The problem was salvaged satisfactorily with two screws placed behind the nail.

Fig. 21.65 The fracture in this patient was extremely distal and the nailing wire was not adequately controlled during its insertion. The nail penetrated the knee joint and required revision.

Particularly with distal targeting, it is possible to miss the distal holes. Failure of adequate transfixation can result in loss of stability of the fracture. If only one screw locks distally, then there may be excessive movement at the fracture site leading to delayed union or non-union. Alternatively, it can lead to an explosion of callus and very rapid union! Failure to achieve both proximal and distal locking can result in gross shortening of the fracture with backing out of the nail (Fig. 21.67).

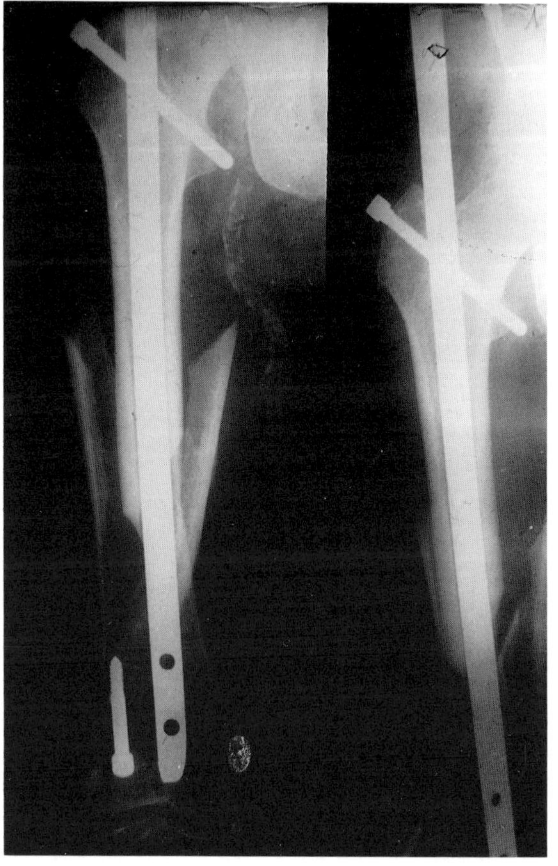

Fig. 21.67 (*Right.*) In this unfortunate patient, both proximal and distal holes were missed, causing predictable shortening.

Technical inadequacies

The use of too narrow a nail, associated with unrestricted weight-bearing or in the absence of any further protection, will inevitably result in nail fracture (Fig. 21.68). This is more the fault of the surgeon failing to appreciate the mechanical forces rather than a fault of the materials themselves.

Early versions of the Grosse–Kempf nail had a tendency to fail at the weld between the proximal tube and the forged cloverleaf section. This problem has now largely been overcome. Failure of locking nails at the more proximal of the two distal screws is associated with low fractures with inadequate distal insertion of the nail (Fig. 21.69). Occasionally, better purchase of the locking nail in the shaft of the femur can be enhanced by reduction of the distal tip by sawing off the distal centimetre of the nail peroperatively.

Removal of implant

Since the locking nail is a load-sharing device, removal is not strictly necessary. However, occasionally, the distal screws are too long and cause medial ligament irritation. Removal under these circumstances is indicated when the fracture has consolidated. Frequently, because it is not now the practice to wash all the reamings away from the fracture site, the nail is hidden in bony involucrum over the tip of the greater trochanter and it is sometimes extremely difficult to find the proximal end of the nail. This surgical procedure, when removal is contemplated, should never be underes-

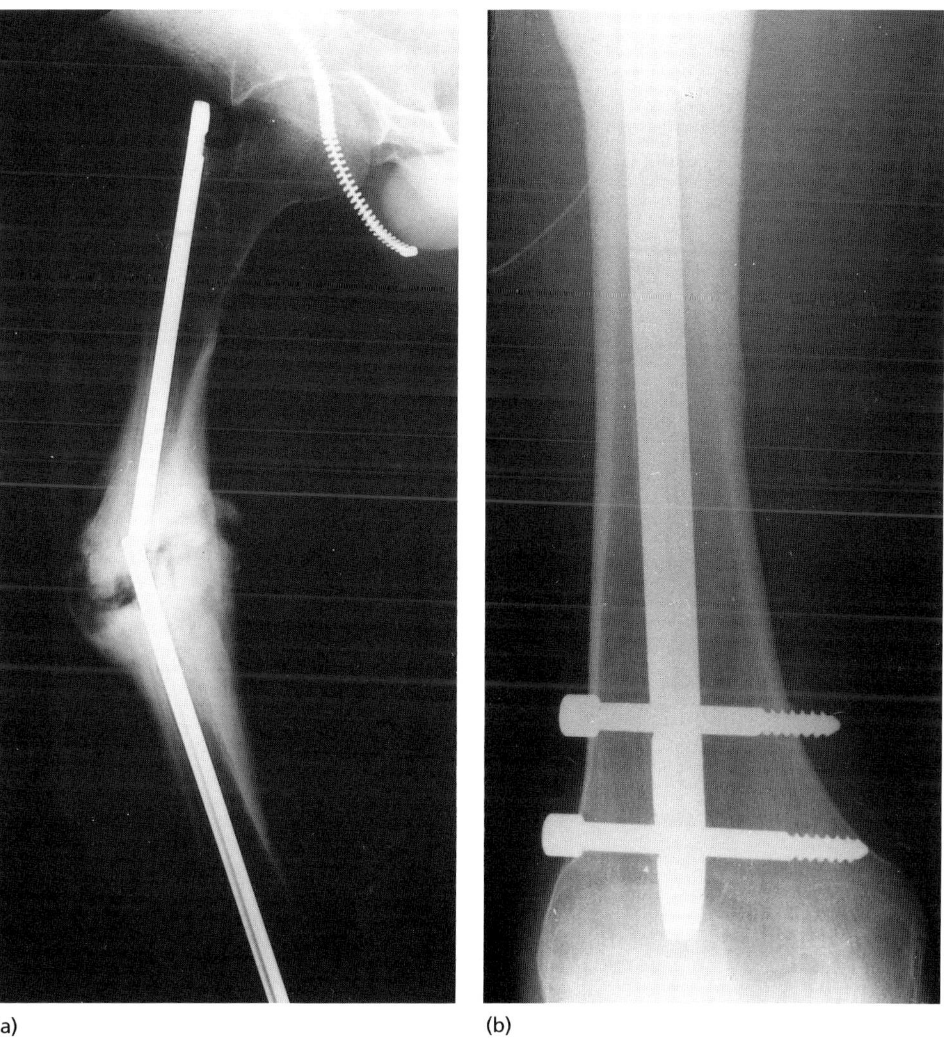

(a)   (b)

Fig. 21.68 This patient had a 9-mm nail inserted down a femoral shaft fracture. This was inadequate, the nail fractured and non-union resulted (a). It was salvaged by use of a stout intramedullary locking nail, leading to the development of strong and satisfactory callus (b).

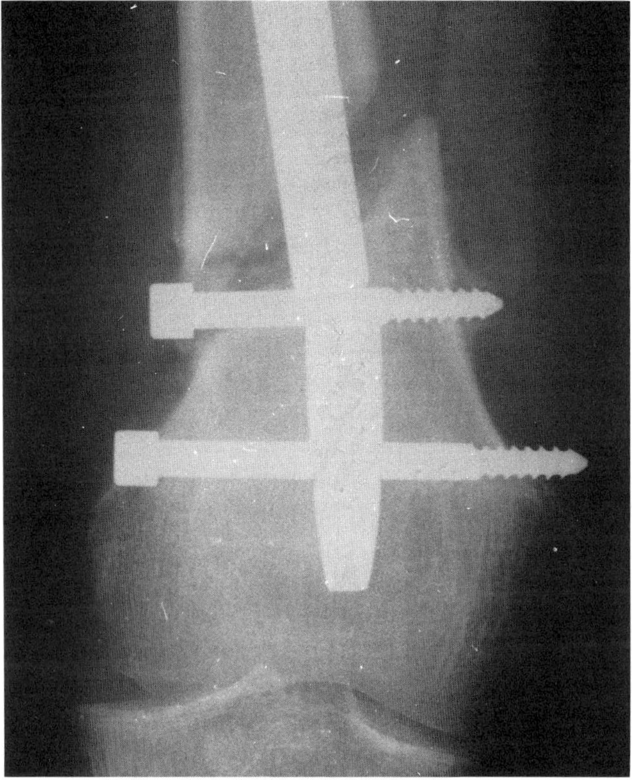

(a)

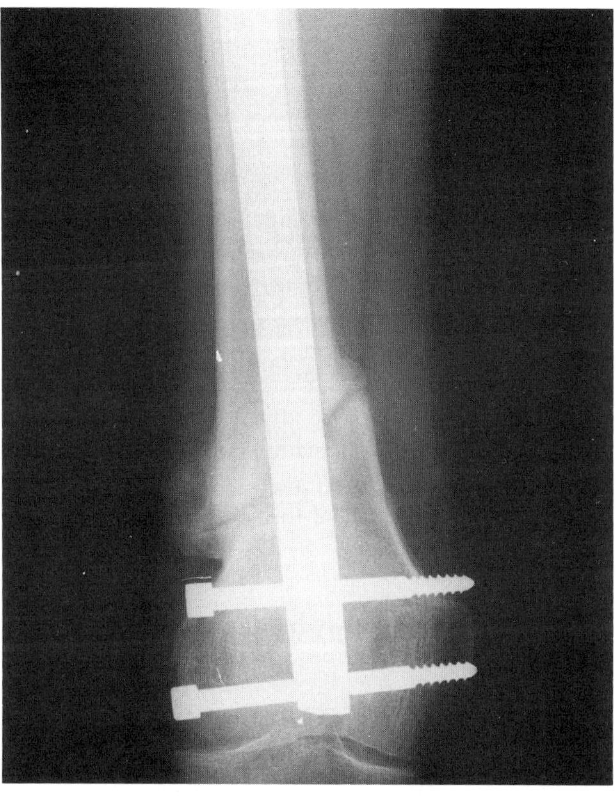

(b)

Fig. 21.69 In this distal fracture the more proximal of the two screws passed through the fracture site and the nail broke at its weakest point (a). This was overcome by cutting the tip off the nail and reinserting it more distally with good purchase of two distal screws through the distal fragment (b).

timated and complications relating to blood loss and wound haematoma are common. Failure to appreciate that distal locking screws are still present during extraction of the nail has been described with predictable and disastrous results!

Infection

Infection of pin tracts and plates in femoral shaft fractures is treated in the same way as in any other situation. It is essential that as soon as infection is suspected the wound is swabbed and appropriate antibiotics commenced. Failure to arrest infection within 48 hours should make the surgeon consider formally reopening the fracture site or pin-tract area, evacuating haematomas and dead tissue and treating the area locally with PMMA gentamycin beads.

The problem of the infected nail is, however, unique to the femur and in the past, particularly in an era when antibiotics were not so efficacious as they are at present, this led many surgeons to adopt a policy of avoiding intramedullary nailing altogether. The series by Weber,

in 1964, quoted a 29% above-knee amputation rate following infection after nailing procedures. Fortunately, with more sophisticated surgical techniques, including the closed nailing techniques described above, deep infection is now rare and prompt recognition of infection, together with appropriate antibiotic treatment, has reduced the morbidity of this major complication to a considerable extent. Nevertheless, infection following nailing is the more serious because of the easy passage of the infection along the whole length of the femoral shaft. It is therefore necessary to treat aggressively an established infection. It is now considered important that the stability of the fracture is maintained and if the fracture has not united at the time that the infection is diagnosed, then, provided that the intramedullary nail is still holding the fracture securely, it should be left in position. A suitable scheme for irrigating such fractures is shown in Fig. 21.70.

If the infection is established and the nail is loose, it is important that stability is obtained urgently. It has been suggested that the nail is removed, the infected membrane along the shaft of the femur is reamed out

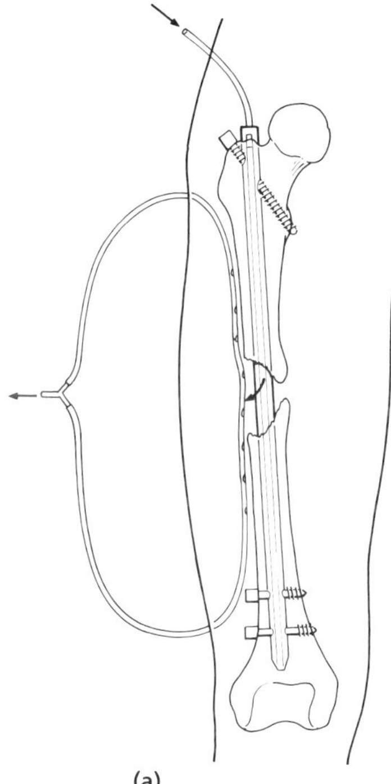 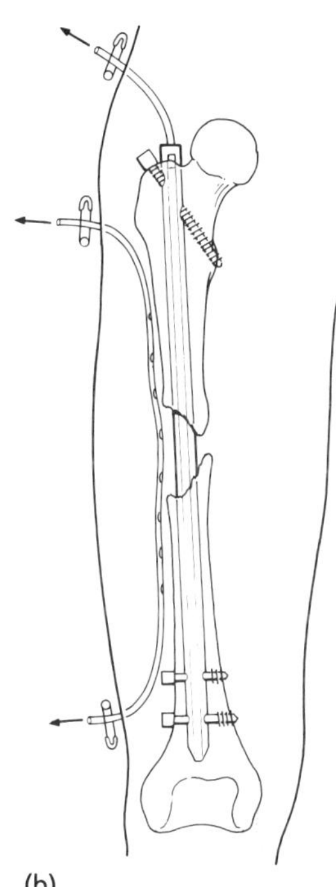

Fig. 21.70 (a) Insertion of drainage tubes for irrigation suction drainage in interlocking nailing of infected pseudarthrosis. (b) Permanent drainage until consolidation of the infected pseudarthrosis.

and a thicker nail is inserted and stabilized by static locking. Following this, the irrigation system outlined above can be used.

If the fracture is soundly united, then there is no difficulty in removing the nail itself, reaming out the infective pseudo-membrane, together with an additional millimetre of femoral shaft in order to remove infected bone, and using PMMA gentamycin beads along the shaft of the femur and at the site of the exit hole of the infective material along the shaft. Grosse reports a high percentage of clearance of infections and a minimal amputation rate.

Refracture after fixation

Following removal of a Zickel nail, which is a strong, curved and rigid implant, refracture appears to be a common feature, particularly in young adults (Fig. 21.71).

Fractures above and below implants in elderly patients pose difficult management problems, and are often associated with the poor condition of the patient rather than the initial method of fixation itself. Experience suggests that if such a fracture occurs it is frequently a terminal event, or at least one which is associated with a complete loss of walking ability, however complex and innovative the surgical solution (Fig. 21.72).

Difficult fracture configurations

Many femoral shaft fractures are produced by high-velocity injury which not only affects that limb but also the other leg and the rest of the body, as previously discussed. The high forces transmitted through the area of impact, usually distal, may result in almost any combination of structural damage from the foot to the pelvis. However, certain patterns of combined injuries are more common and present considerable difficulties in diagnosis and treatment.

Shaft fracture with dislocated hip

Clinically, it is difficult to diagnose a dislocation of the hip in the presence of a fractured femoral shaft but, with the standard mandatory radiographs of the pelvis and hips, this combined injury should not be missed. Urgent reduction of the dislocation is necessary to reduce the chance of aseptic femoral head necrosis. This may prove difficult if it is not possible to get sufficient purchase on the thigh but closed reduction can be effected by inserting a T-handle auger (the femoral head extractor 'cork-screw') through the greater trochanter into the base of the femoral neck, and using this for traction to lever the head back into the acetabulum. Internal fixation of the shaft fracture with a locking medullary nail and traction for 3 weeks with hip and

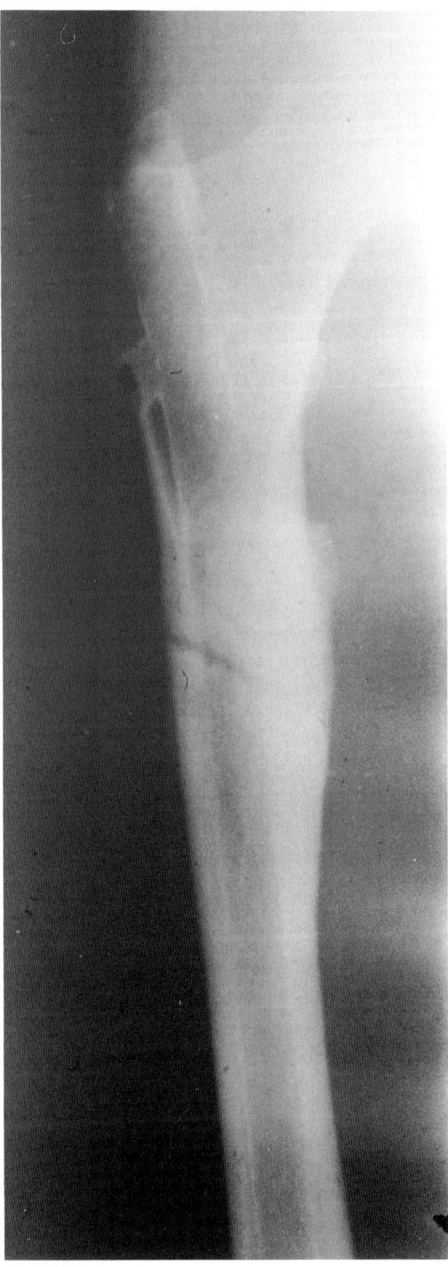

Fig. 21.71 This patient with a comminuted proximal-third fracture was treated with a Zickel nail and seemed to achieve adequate bony consolidation. However, shortly after removal of the implant, it was noted that there was a large crack in the medial femoral cortex.

knee movement then allows the patient to mobilize (Fig. 21.73).

If the dislocation was unrecognized, then after approximately 2 weeks closed reduction would not be possible and an open exposure, with extensive dissection, would be necessary to obtain a reduction. Stiffness and later aseptic necrosis with femoral head collapse would then be likely.

Shaft fracture with femoral neck fracture

Diagnosis may be difficult initially as the fracture may not be displaced. However, a standard anteroposterior radiograph of the pelvis and hips should reveal the fracture, if looked for. Also, a basal femoral neck fracture may be a complication of internal fixation using an intramedullary nail. This was seen with the older retrograde open fixation technique where the nail emerged at the base of the neck. More recently, the complication is occasionally seen in closed locking medullary nailing with the entry point being made too medial to the neck. The fracture occurs with impaction of the nail.

Treatment of combined femoral neck and shaft fractures are ideally treated closed by a reconstruction type nail, controlling the insertion of two proximal locking screws into the femoral neck with the image intersifier. Other methods available include use of a femoral intramedullary nail for the shaft and appropriate femoral neck pins being inserted along either side of the nail into the head, the use of the Zickel subtrochanteric medullary nail with locking cervical pin, the Huckstep nail or, finally, a hip screw and plate for the neck and either an extension of the plate for the proximal fracture or a second compression plate if the fracture is distal.

Ipsilateral tibial fracture

This is a very difficult combination of fractures to treat conservatively, as the centre 'floating knee segment' cannot be held reduced at both ends. Significant malunion, shortening and knee stiffness are inevitable. Early reduction and early fixation with intramedullary nails or compression plates allows early mobilization of the knee, limb and patient.

Ipsilateral patellar fracture

An associated fracture of the patella is invariably found in males and is associated with motorcycle accidents (Fig. 21.74). Fracture of the patella is invariably an absolute indication for internal fixation of a femoral shaft fracture in order to avoid knee stiffness. Similarly, in the displaced or comminuted fracture of the patella, internal fixation of the patella is again mandatory and under no circumstances should excision of the patella be considered as a primary procedure. It is frequently not possible in these injuries to reconstitute accurately the comminuted patellar surface but the cerclage technique, either holding all the bony fragments together or, alternatively, suturing the proximal pole around a screw placed across the tibial tubercle, will provide

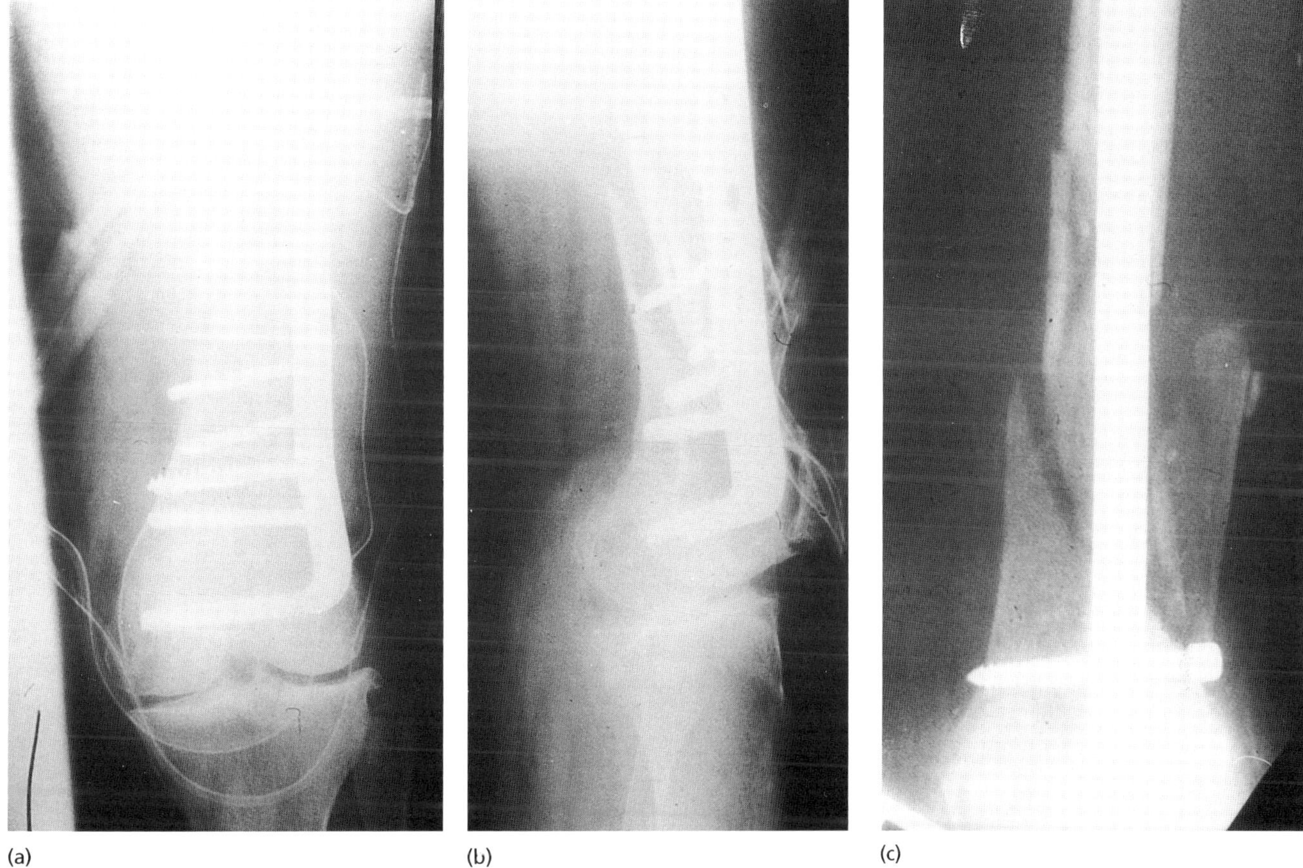

(a)   (b)   (c)

Fig. 21.72 (a) This patient sustained a supracondylar fracture which was treated with a blade plate. It may be argued that the plate was a little short. (b) A fracture was sustained at the top of the blade plate in the early period of mobilization; (c) this was treated by insertion of a locked intramedullary nail.

adequate stability to allow knee mobilization. If retro-patellar pain becomes a problem later, then the patella can be sacrificed.

Bilateral femoral fractures

Patients with bilateral femoral fractures frequently have other major injuries and the general principles for the management of polytraumatized patients, of course, apply. The method of treatment will depend upon the individual circumstances and particularly if the fractures are massively comminuted, it may be necessary to accept that the patient will not actually be able to weight-bear until such time as adequate consolidation is progressing. Nevertheless, it is important that the patient does not lie in the position of 'horizontal crucifixion' in two splints for 12 weeks. Rehabilitation after such conservative treatment wil be virtually impossible and during recovery the patient will be subject to all the problems of immobilization, both psychologically and physically.

Internal fixation of such fractures will allow the patient at least to sit out of the hospital bed at an early stage of convalescence and, of course, if the fractures are stable and weight-bearing is possible, will allow rapid rehabilitation as the fracture heals (Fig. 21.75).

Fractures in elderly patients

As in all fracture groups elderly patients have a specific pattern of injury. These are frequently low-velocity injuries and yet they have moderate comminution. The majority of femoral shaft fractures in these patients occur in females with osteoporotic bone and the presence of ipsilateral hip or knee arthritis (Moran *et al.* 1990). Post-operative mobilization in such patients is slow, partly because static locking is invariably performed, but also because of general debility and unsatisfactory social circumstances. No comparative literature on internal fixation of femoral shaft fractures is available but the conclusion of Moran *et al.* (1990) was that the

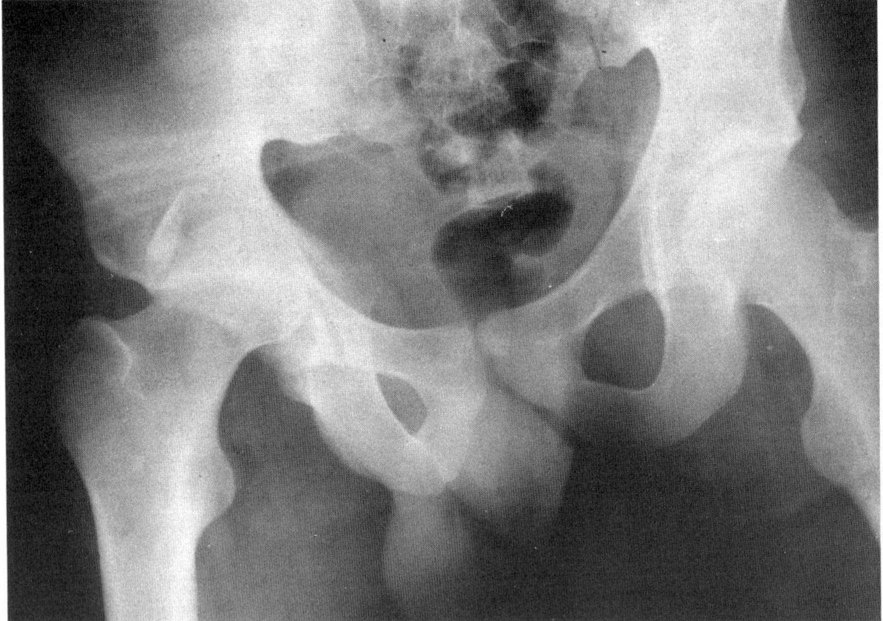

(a)

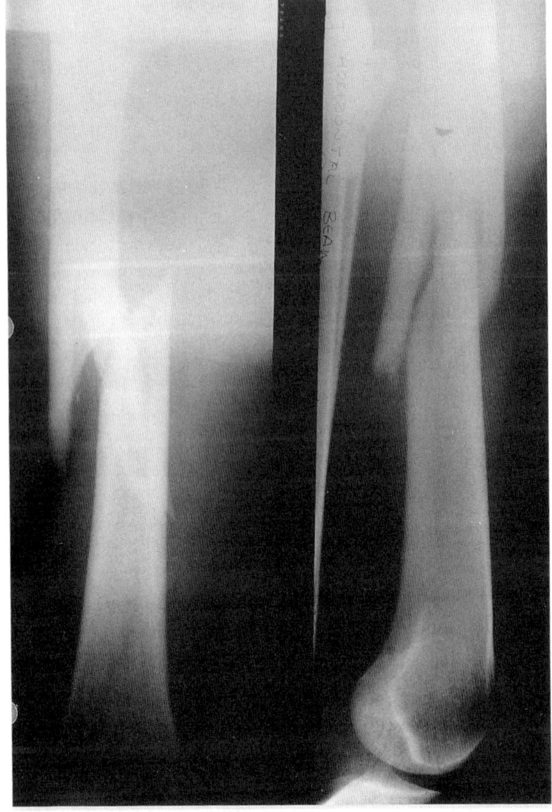

(b)

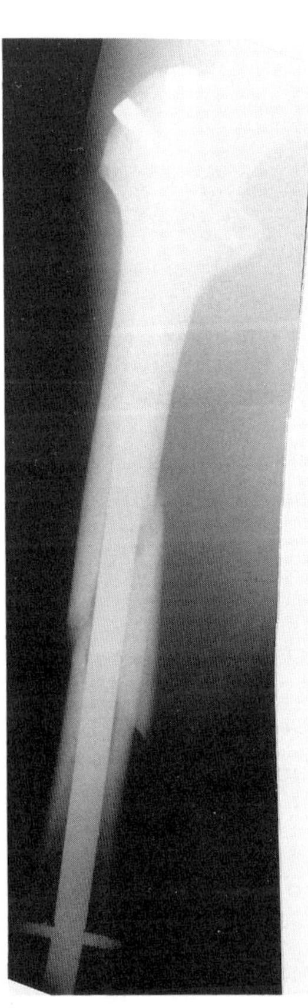

(c)

Fig. 21.73 Difficult combined injuries:
(a) posterior dislocation of the hip;
(b) comminuted fracture mid-shaft
ipsilateral femur; (c) closed hip
reduction and closed Russell-Taylor
locking nail fixation.

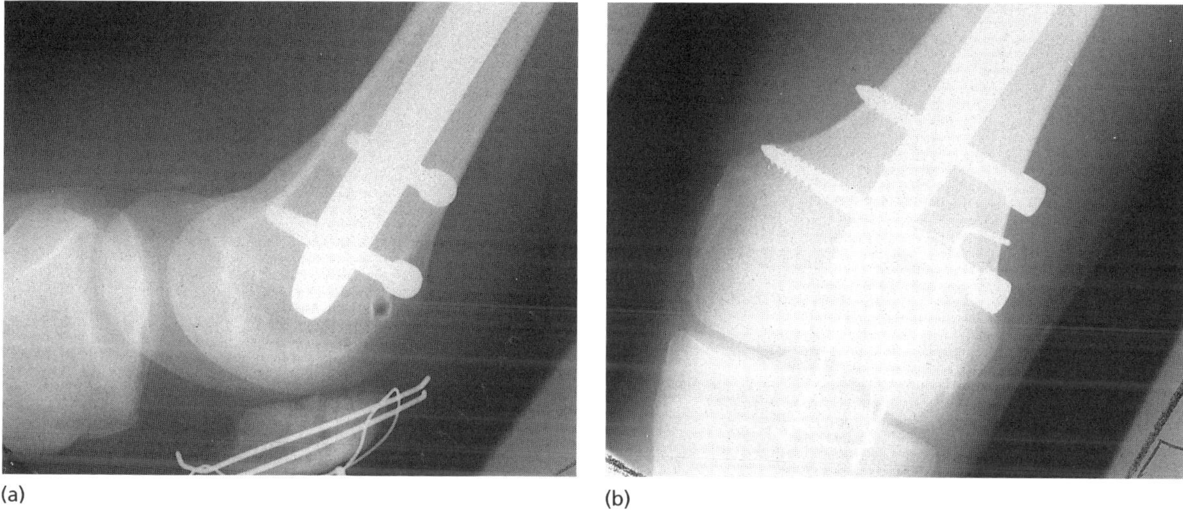

Fig. 21.74 Ipsilateral femoral and patellar fractures treated by locking nail and AO patellar wiring.

use of the locking nail in such patients was an effective means of stabilizing these fractures, despite a higher rate of general and local complications than occurs in the younger group of patients. The use of plates and external fixators for the management of these fractures is associated with a relatively high failure rate because the quality of bone for the screw holes is poor. Adjunctive cement can be used if a plate is applied to the shaft of the femur but it would seem likely that this has the potential for delaying, or even preventing, bony union. If the locking nail is used, then holding the distal fragment is frequently difficult because of the soft osteoporotic bone. Vecsei dowel bolts can provide a rigid fixation. Alternatively, following insertion of conventional bolts, a blob of bone cement can be inserted around the nail percutaneously through a stab incision in the front of the thigh (Fig. 21.76).

Associated joint replacement

Fracture around the prosthesis

This is a torsional injury and invariably occurs in elderly and debilitated patients. It commonly occurs in association with hemiarthroplasty rather than with total hip arthroplasty at the proximal end of the femur. Internal fixation following this injury is not recommended (Johansson *et al.* 1981) and in most cases the fracture heals satisfactorily using conservative management. However, subsequent loosening of the prosthesis is a problem and later revision is sometimes necessary (Fig. 21.77).

Fractures at or below the tip of the prosthesis

These fractures are difficult to control using conservative methods and are usually best treated by internal fixation. Providing it can be established that the hip prosthesis is not loose, then the use of broad dynamic compression plates allows for angulation of screws and stable fixation. If possible, bone graft should be used and protected weight-bearing postoperatively is mandatory. The use of Partridge straps has been advocated (Partridge & Evans 1982). This is normally combined with longitudinal support in the form of nylon plates (Fig. 21.78). The implant is bulky and is not applicable for very frail and thin patients, and the fixation is not rigid. There has been some anxiety as to the biological effect of cerclage; in most cases there appears to be a large amount of sclerotic bone associated with the procedure and it is difficult to be certain when bony union has actually occurred.

Supracondylar fractures associated with hip prostheses can usually be treated in a conventional manner, using either a blade plate or a compression screw system.

Fractures also occur in association with knee replacement arthroplasty. Results following fracture associated with knee arthroplasty are invariably bad. Frequently, the only method of salvage is immobilization of the patient, either on a splint or in a cast of plaster of Paris; there is consequent stiffness of the knee and often instability of the implanted prosthesis. Union of the bone in this situation is unreliable and any form of internal fixation is fraught with difficulties.

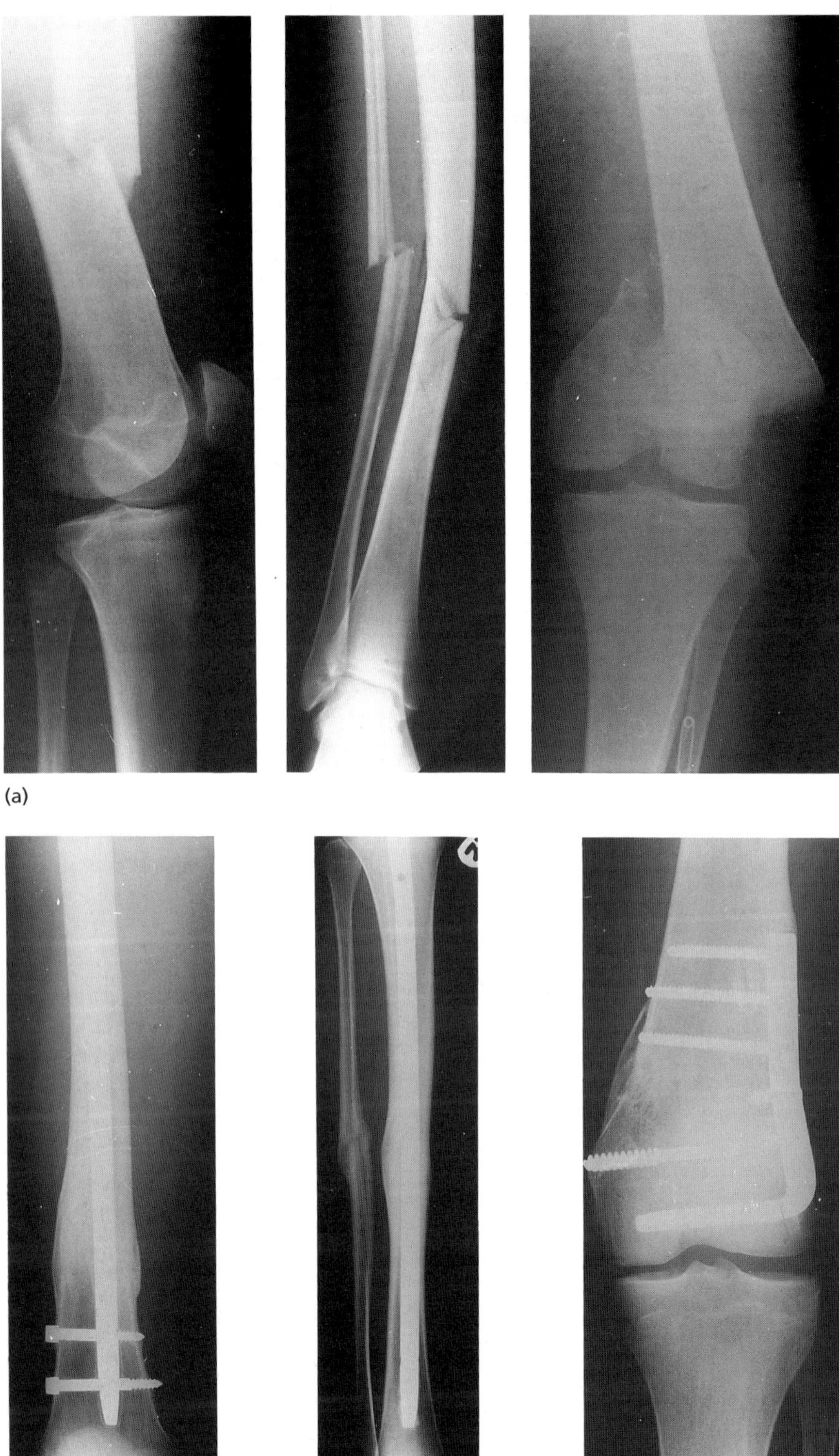

(a)

(b)

Fig. 21.75 This patient had mid-shaft femoral and tibial fractures together with supracondylar fracture on the left. Stable internal fixation (a) was possible and the patient was able to walk out of hospital 3 weeks after receiving the injuries (b).

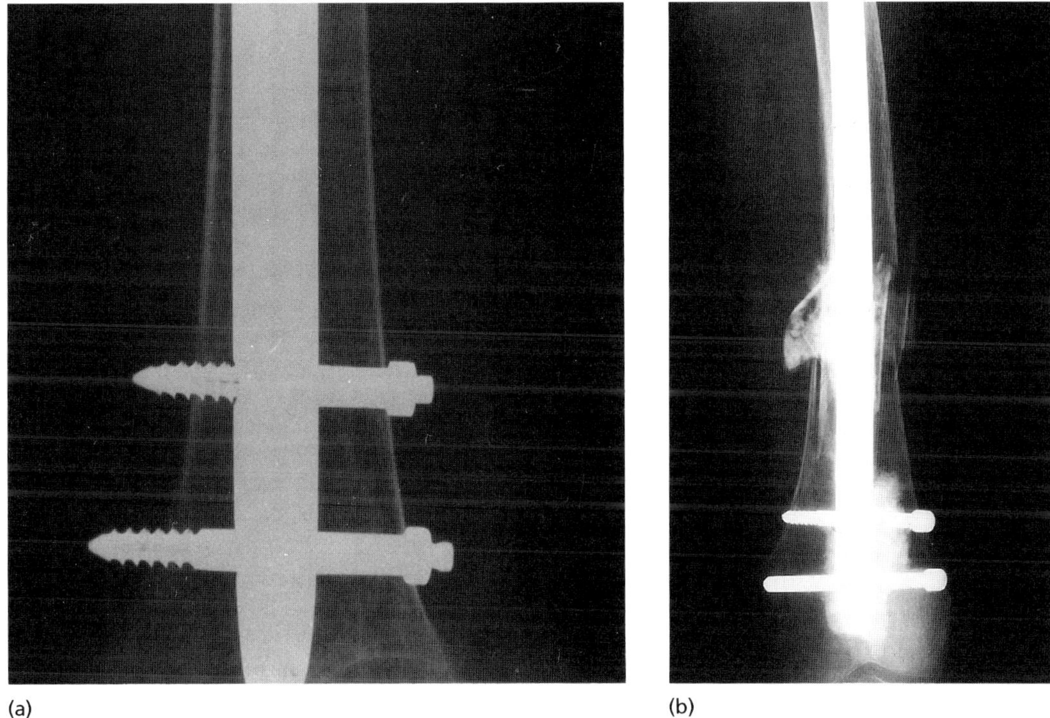

(a)

(b)

Fig. 21.76 (a) This example shows the use of dowel bolts in distal locking. The centre portion of the transverse screw expands, locking the screw to the nail (b). A blob of cement has been inserted percutaneously around the distal screws in this patient. Adequate stability was satisfactorily obtained.

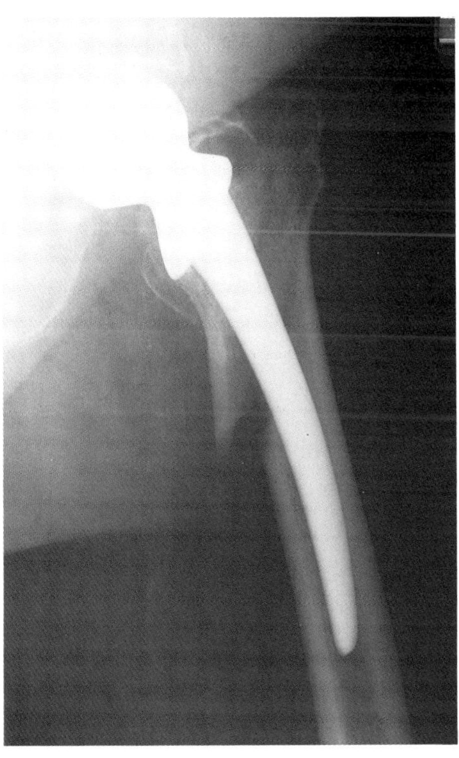

Fig. 21.77 This spiral fracture occurred around an existing prosthesis. It was treated on traction and satisfactory stabilization eventually occurred.

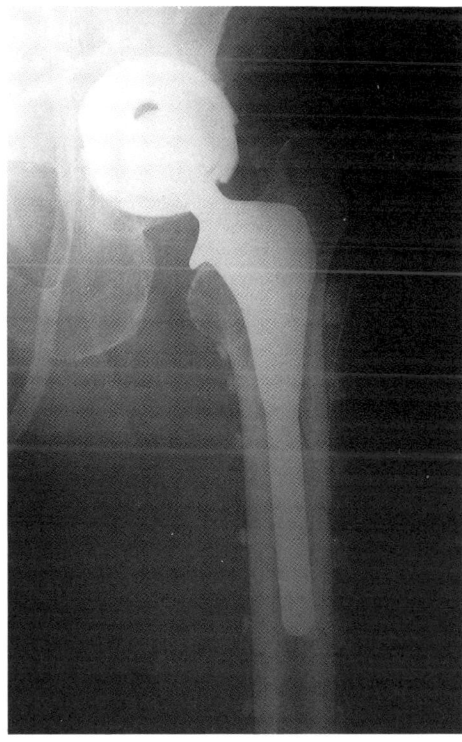

Fig. 21.78 The use of Partridge straps has always been controversial. Note that there is a considerable reaction in association with the Partridge straps and this causes some sclerosis. It is difficult to know when union has occurred.

References

Brookes, M. Blood flow in the diaphysis of long bones. In: *Proceedings of Advanced Course in IM Locking*. Courcheval, 1988.

Burwell, H.N. Internal fixation in the treatment of the fracture of the femoral shaft. *Injury* 1971; **2**: 235–244.

Buxton, R. Treatment of femoral shaft fractures using Perkins traction. *J Bone Joint Surg* 1981; **63B**: 362–366.

Charnley, J. *Compression Arthrodesis*. Livingstone: Edinburgh, 1953.

Charnley, J. Fractures of the shaft of the femur. *The Closed Treatment of Common Fractures* 3rd edn. Livingstone: Edinburgh, 1961.

Christie, J. & Court Brown, C. Femoral neck fractures during closed intramedullary nailing: a brief report. *J Bone Joint Surg* 1988; **70B**: 670.

Cochran, G.V.B., Zickel, R.E. & Fielding, J.W. Stress analysis of subtrochanteric fractures; effect of muscle forces and internal fixation devices. In: Uthof, H.K. (ed.) *Current Concepts of Internal Fixation of Fractures*. Springer-Verlag: Berlin, 1980.

Cross, A.T. & Murphy, W.M. Subtrochanteric fractures and the Zickel apparatus. *J Bone Joint Surg* 1977; **59B**: 498–499.

Cuthbert, H. & Howat, T.W. Use of the Küntscher Y nail in the treatment of intertrochanteric and subtrochanteric fractures of the femur. *Injury* 1976–77; **8**: 135–142.

Dabezies, F.J., Ambrosia, R. & Shoji, H. Fractures of the femoral shaft treated by external fixation with Wagner device. *J Bone Joint Surg* 1984; **66A**: 360–364.

Danis, R. 1947 Le traitemente operatoire des fractures. *J Internat Chir 7*: 311–314.

De Bastiani, G., Aldegheri, R. & Renzi Brivioz, The treatment of fractures with dynamic axial fixator. *J Bone Joint Surg* 1984; **66B**: 538–545.

Dupuis, M., Dosch, J.C. & Siedel, J.M. Distribution de l'irradiation lors de l'enclouage centro-medullaire, et radioprotection. In: *Dix Ans d'Enclouage Centro-Medullaire avec Verrouilage*. 1984.

Fisk, G.R. The fractured femoral shaft. New approach to the problem. *Lancet* 1944; **i**: 659–661.

Grosse, A. Aseptic pseudarthrosis. In: *Proceedings of Advanced Course in IM Locking*, Courcheval, 1988.

Gustillo, R.B. & Anderson, J.P. Prevention of infection in the treatment of 1,025 open fractures of long bones. *J Bone Joint Surg* 1976; **58A**: 453–458.

Gustillo, R.B., Mendoza, R.M. & Williams, D.N. Problems in the management of Type III fractures. *J Trauma* 1984; **24**: 742–746.

Hall, A.J. & Stenner, R.W. (eds) *Manual of Fracture Bracing*. Churchill Livingstone: Edinburgh, 1985.

Hey Groves, E.W. (ed.) *On Modern Methods of Treating Fractures*. Wright: Bristol, 1916.

Hippocrates. *Genuine Works of Hippocrates*. Adams, F. (trans.). New Sydenham Society: London, 1849.

Huckstep, R.L. The Huckstep IM compression nail. (Indications, technique, and results.) *Clin Orthop* 1986; **212**: 48–61.

James, J.H. (quoted by Rocyn-Jones, A.) *J Bone Joint Surg* 1953; **35B**: 651–666.

Johansson, J.E., McBroom, R.J., Barrington, T.W. & Hunter, G.A. Fractures of the ipsilateral femur, in patients with total hip replacements. *J Bone Joint Surg* 1981; **63A**: 1435–1442.

Johnson, K.D., Kadambi, A. & Seibert, G.B. Incidence of ARDS in patients with multiple musculo-skeletal injuries: effect of early operative stabilisation of fractures. *J Trauma* 1985; **25**: 375–383.

Jones, R. Thomas splint. *Br Med J* 1925; **1**: 909–913.

Kempf, I., Grosse, A. & Beck, G. Closed locked intramedullary nailing. *J Bone Joint Surg* 1985; **67A**: 709–720.

Kirschner, M. Ueber Nagelextension. *Beitr Klin Chir* 1909; **64**: 266–279.

Klein, M.P.M., Rahm, B.A. & Perren, S.M. Reaming versus non-reaming in the medullary cavity. *AO Dial* 1989.

Koch, J.C. The laws of bone architecture. *Am J Anat* 1917; **21**: 177–298.

Küntscher, G. Die Marknagelung von Knockenbruchen. *Arch Klin Chir* 1940; **200**: 443–455.

Küntscher, G. The Küntscher method of intramedullary fixation. *J Bone Joint Surg* 1958; **40A**: 17–24.

Küntscher, G. (ed.) *Practice of Intramedullary Nailing*. Charles C. Thomas: Springfield, 1967.

Lam, S.J.S. The place of delayed internal fixation of fractures of long bones. *J Bone Joint Surg* 1964; **46B**: 373–397.

Lambotte, A. (ed.) *Chirugie Operatoire des Fractures*. Masson: Paris, 1913.

Lane, W.A. (ed.) *Operative Treatment of Fractures*. Publishing Co: London, 1914.

Lange, R.H., Back, A.W., Hansen, S.T. Jr. & Johansen, R.H. Open tibial fractures with associated vascular injuries: prognosis for limb salvage. *J Trauma* 1985; **25**: 203.

Mast, R., Jacob, R. & Ganz, R. *Planning and Reduction Technique in Fracture Surgery*, 1st edn. 1989.

Mathijsen, A. *Een Mieuwe Wijzevan het Gipsverband bij Beenbrenken*. J.B. van Lochum: Haarlem, 1852.

Meggitt, B.F., Juett, D.A. & Smith, J.D. Cast-bracing for fractures of the femoral shaft: a biomechanical and clinical study. *J Bone Joint Surg* 1981; **63B**: 12–23.

Mize, R.D., Bucholz, R.W. & Grogan, D.P. Surgical treatment of displaced comminuted fractures of the distal end of the femur. *J Bone Joint Surg* 1982; **64A**: 871–879.

Moncade, N. Les fractures hautes du femur. In: *Dix Ans d'Enclouage Centro-Medullaire avec Verrouilage*. 1984.

Mooney, V., Nickel, V.L., Harvey, J.P. & Snelson, R. Cast-bracing treatment for fractures of the distal part of the femur. *J Bone Joint Surg* 1970; **52A**: 1563–1578.

Moran, C.J., Gibson, M.J. & Cross, A.T. Intramedullary locked nails for femoral shaft fractures in elderly patients. *J Bone Joint Surg* 1990; **72B**: 19–22.

Mubarak, S.J. & Carroll, N.C. Volkmann's contracture in children: aetiology and prevention. *J Bone Joint Surg* 1979; **61B**: 285–293.

Müller, M.E., Allgower, M., Schneider, R. & Willinegger, H. *Manual of Internal Fixation*. Springer-Verlag: Berlin, 1979.

Müller, M.E., Allgower, M. & Willenegger, H. *Technique of Internal Fixation of Fractures*. Springer-Verlag: New York, 1965.

Müller, M.E., Nazarian, S. & Koch, P. *The AO Classification of Fractures*. Springer-Verlag: Berlin, 1988.

Neer, C.S., Grantham, S. & Shelton, L. Supracondylar fractures of the adult femur. *J Bone Joint Surg* 1967; **49A**: 591–613.

Nichols, P.J.R. Rehabilitation after fractures of the shaft of the femur. *J Bone Joint Surg* 1963; **45B**: 96–102.

Nicoll, E.A. Quadriceps plasty. *J Bone Joint Surg* 1963; **45B**: 483–490.

Olerud, S. Operative treatment of supracondylar—condylar fractures of the femur. *J Bone Joint Surg* 1972; **54A**: 1015—1032.

Papagianoupoulos, G. & Clement, J.D. Treatment of fractures of the distal third of the femur. (Prospective trial of the Derby intramedullary nail.) *J Bone Joint Surg* 1987; **69B**: 67—70.

Partridge, A.J. & Evans, P.E.L. Treatment of fractures of the shaft of the femur, using nylon cerclage. *J Bone Joint Surg* 1982; **64B**: 210—214.

Pearson, M.C. & Drummond, J. *Fractured Femurs: Their Treatment by Caliper Extensions.* Oxford University Press: Oxford, 1919.

Peltier, L.F. A brief history of traction. *J Bone Joint Surg* 1968; **50**: 1603—1617.

Perkins, G. *Fractures and Dislocations.* Athlone Press: London, 1958.

Perren, S.M. *Basic Aspects and Scientific Background of Internal Fixation.* AO Group Publications, 1989.

Reudi, T.P. & Luscher, J.N. Results after internal fixation of comminuted fractures of the femoral shaft with dynamic compression plates. *Clin Orthop* 1979; **138**: 74—76.

Rhinelander, F.W. & Wilson, J.W. Blood supply in developing, mature and healing bone. In: Sumner-Smith, G. (ed.) *Bone in Clinical Orthopaedics.* WB Saunders: Philadelphia, 1982.

Salter, R.B. & Harris, W.R. Injuries involving the epiphyseal plate. *J Bone Joint Surg* 1963; **45A**: 587—622.

Sarmiento, A. Functional bracing of tibial and femoral shaft fractures. *Clin Orthop* 1972; **82**: 2—13.

Schatzker, J. & Lambert, D.C. Supracondylar fractures of the femur. *Clin Orthop* 1979; **138**: 77—83.

Schatzker, J., Horn, S. & Waddell, J. The Toronto experience with supracondylar fracture of the femur. *Injury* 1974; **6**: 113—128.

Schatzker, J., Mahomed, N., Schiffman, K. & Kellam, J. Dynamic condylar screw: a new device. *J Orthop Trauma* 1989; **3(2)**: 124—132.

Slatis, P., Ryoppy, S. & Huittinen, V. AOI osteosynthesis of fractures of the distal third of the femur. *Acta Orthop Scand* 1971 **42**: 162—172.

Spinks, M.S. & Lewis, G.L. *Albucasis on Surgery and Instruments,*

Vol. 3. Wellcome Institute of the History of Medicine: 1973.

Stewart, M.J., Sisk, T.D. & Wallace, S.H. Fractures of the distal third of the femur — a comparison of methods of treatment. *J Bone Joint Surg* 1966; **48A**: 784—807.

Thomas, H.O. (ed.) *Disease of the Hip, Knee and Ankle Joints.* Dobbs: Liverpool, 1875.

Thomas, T.L. & Meggitt, B.F. A comparative study of methods for treating fractures of the distal half of the femur. *J Bone Joint Surg* 1981; **63B(1)**: 3—6.

Thompson, T.C. Quadricepsplasty to improve knee function. *J Bone Joint Surg* 1944; **26**: 366—379.

Vaughan-Lane, T. & Meggitt, B.F. New casting material and improved function design for lower femoral fracture bracing. *Prosthet Orthot Int* 1980; **4**: 145—149.

Walling, A., Seradge, H. & Spiegel, P. Injuries to knee ligaments with fractures of the femur. *J Bone Joint Surg* 1982; **64A**: 1324—1327.

Wardlaw, D. Cast brace treatment of femoral fractures. *J Bone Joint Surg* 1977; **59B**: 411—416.

Watson-Jones, R. *Fractures and Other Bone and Joint Injuries,* 1st edn. Livingstone: Edinburgh, 1940.

Watson-Jones, R. (ed.) *Fractures and Joint Injuries,* Vol. 2. Williams & Wilkins: Baltimore, 1960.

Wenzl, H., Casey, P.A., Hebert, P. & Berlin, J. Die operative Behandlung der distalen Femurfraktur. *OA Bull* 1970.

White, G.M., Healy, W.L., Brumback, R.J., Burgess, A.R. & Booker, A.F. Treatment of femoral shaft fractures with the Brooker—Wills distal locking intramedullary nail. *J Bone Joint Surg* 1986; **68A**: 865—876.

Winquist, R.A. & Hansen, S.T. Comminuted fractures of the femoral shaft treated by intramedullary nailing. *Orthop Clin North Am* 1980; **11**: 633—648.

Winquist, R.A., Hansen, S.T. & Clawson, D.K. Closed intramedullary nailing of femoral fractures; a report of five hundred and twenty cases. *J Bone Joint Surg* 1984; **66A**: 529—539.

Winquist, R.A., Hansen, S.T. & Pearson, R.E. Closed intramedullary shortening of the femur. *Clin Orthop* 1978; **136**: 54—61.

Zickel, R.E., Fieti, V.S., Lawsing, J.F. & Cochran, G. van B. A new intramedullary fixation device for the distal third of the femur. *Clin Orthop* 1977; **125**: 185—191.

22: The Knee

M.L.HARDING

Soft tissue injuries

With the exception of joints of the hand, the knee joint is the most vulnerable in the body to soft tissue injury. All soft tissues may be injured, but most commonly ligaments and/or menisci are disrupted. All combinations can occur.

Ligaments

These may tear or disrupt when overstretched beyond strain limits. The precise pattern and degree of disruption may vary depending on a number of factors and certainly with velocity of strain applied (Kennedy *et al.* 1976). There are three degrees of severity of ligamentous injury. This designation refers to individual ligament damage and the classification that follows is largely reproduced, with permission, from *The Knee* (Müller 1983).

First degree ligamentous injury (mild sprain, 'stretch') — the continuity of the ligament is preserved, but it is lax *in situ* and allows abnormal displacement of the joint ends. At operation these segments appear glossy and swollen with traces of ecchymosis.

Second degree ligamentous injury (moderate sprain, partial rupture, interstitial tear) — gross continuity is maintained but torn fibre bundles hang loosely from the ligament. Some areas are overstretched and there are varying degrees of ecchymosis, again associated with marked oedema swelling. The ligament is elongated and can no longer ensure stable joint function.

Third degree ligamentous injury (severe sprain, rupture) — complete disruption of continuity by either a straight or multilevel tear. The torn ends can be reflected and lie loosely within the joint.

Müller distinguishes between the healing problems in the three degrees of ligament injury. In summary, first degree injuries can be treated conservatively and have the best prospect for optimum repair, provided that the ligament is not constantly stretched to its new length which leads to consequent healing in the elongated state. These knees require 2 weeks in plaster cast immobilization until the pain is relieved and then 'middle' range active knee joint movement with protected weight-bearing using crutches or a brace with a range of motion stop. Complete healing takes 4–8 weeks.

In second degree injuries gross ligament continuity is preserved; that is, the overall ligament 'form' is intact. Mechanical rest is required to allow the development of a stable scar. There is a conflict in allowing movement; this will maximize the early mechanical strength of the ligament but cause consequent instability problems. In clinical practice, this is often the dilemma with isolated anterior cruciate ligament (ACL) ruptures which fall into this category. With these injuries, it is impossible to protect the ligament in an optimal way and, hence, for young patients with athletic aspirations and with second degree or partial tears it is likely that surgical repair is required. Thus, the current debate is whether to treat second degree ACL injuries conservatively or offer primary repair. However, it is recognized that the prospects for primary repair are not promising. Feagin and Curl (1976) have demonstrated that 70% of patients who had had simple surgical repair of isolated ACL ruptures were athletically compromised at a 5-year follow-up. Hence the need to consider some form of tissue augmentation. Bracing is not used for these second degree injuries but it is recognized that there may be a useful place for this mode of treatment.

In third degree injuries there is no prospect of satisfactory tissue repair without some form of ligament end approximation and, therefore, surgical repositioning is required to provide the best prospect of a stable knee. Clancy *et al.* (1988) have shown that for ACL ruptures better results can be obtained for complete tears by early augmentation surgery using a free patellar tendon graft technique, than can for incomplete tears treated conservatively. The clear implication is, therefore, that all significant (second and third degree) ACL tears should be treated surgically with an efficient repair technique which recognizes that without tissue augmentation, adequate repair, in terms of mechanical strength and stability, will not ensue. This is discussed further on p. 767.

These three degrees of ligament injury may convert to a clinical laxity picture, which is conventionally expressed as follows, but only if the ligament injury is a pure one, i.e., all the ligaments have been injured to the same degree. The laxity measurement refers to the joint space difference between the stressed and unstressed lax compartments.

Grade I — laxity less than 5 mm.

Grade II — laxity 5—10 mm.

Grade III — laxity more than 10 mm (Committee of the Medical Aspects of Sport [CMAS], 1968)

However, ligament injuries are often multiple and complex. Thus, in reality, third degree tears (severe sprain or complete ruptures) are easy to diagnose, although it should be recognized that complete tears are often less painful than mild or moderate sprains (first and second degree tears). The problem lies in the distinction between these latter tears, and the mixed pattern of injury either in the same ligament or in two or more different ligaments. To complicate matters further, it appears that some ligaments are more important (or crucial) than others; for example, if the cruciate ligaments are intact in grade III medial collateral ligament (MCL) injuries, the latter can be treated conservatively (Indelicato 1983). Lateral ligament grade III injuries, by contrast, should always be offered early surgical repair even if the cruciate ligaments appear undamaged.

The exact pattern of injury will vary according to the magnitude, direction and complexity of the injury mechanism. Either one or nearly all of the ligaments may be injured. There are many classifications available in the literature. As Müller (1983) points out, Slocum and Larson (1968), Trillat *et al.* (1977), Hughston *et al.* (1976) and Kennedy *et al.* (1978) are often quoted as references for knee ligament injury classification. Nicholas (1973) added a new rotational concept to the discussion. Müller's account of rotatory instability classification, which is based on the work of Trillat *et al.* (1977), deserves close attention.

Most orthopaedic surgeons use a lesion-based classification and record which anatomical structures are damaged; they conduct their clinical examination with the questions 'What are the injured structures?' and,

consequently, 'What do I have to do to achieve a knee which has no instability problems?' Noyes and Grood (1988) report the most comprehensive approach to knee ligament injury and propose a classification utilizing four clinical concepts. These are:

1 The diagnosis of a ligament injury must be expressed as a specific anatomical defect.

2 The clinical ligament examination must be performed and interpreted using knowledge of the three-dimensional motion of the knee.

3 The so-called rotational instabilities can be characterized by the separate subluxations that occur to the medial and lateral tibial condyles.

4 The diagnosis of ligament and capsular defects requires the use of selected laxity tests for which the primary and secondary restraints have been experimentally determined.

This summarizes the means of examination and interpretation of the injured knee. A series of forces are applied to the knee; the knee, as a consequence, moves according to the six independent degrees of freedom. This movement profile is analysed according to a knowledge of the normal and abnormal three-dimensional motion of the knee, and further or coincident testing is performed in which individual ligaments are 'unmasked' by selective and precise positioning with the knowledge that in those positions the secondary restraints are slack. Thus, abnormal and maximal excursions will be revealed.

It is crucial to determine which cruciate ligaments are damaged. The tests for ACL rupture are well defined, although care must be taken to be aware of which, if any, tibial rotational movement is also being permitted when the anterior drawer tests are being performed. However, a practical difficulty seems to lie in assessing posterolateral instability and specifically concerns the integrity of the posterior cruciate ligament (PCL). This is discussed further on p. 772.

The broad list of ligament tissue groups to consider are:

1 MCL — superficial, deep, posterior oblique.

2 Lateral structures — lateral collateral ligament (LCL) or fibular collateral ligament (FCL), lateral complex structures which include the arcuate ligament and popliteus tendon, the 'popliteus corner' (Müller 1983).

3 ACL.

4 PCL.

5 Posterior capsule (PC).

6 Patellar dislocation with medial retinacular rupture with or without patellar avulsion fractures.

It should be remembered that avulsion fractures may be present, particularly in injuries in adolescents

(Fig. 22.1) and in lateral capsular disruptions at any age. Acute MCL bone fragment avulsions are uncommon.

Anatomy

The reader is referred to standard anatomy textbooks for a general description of ligament anatomy, and is also advised to undertake a revision dissection course to fully appreciate the form of these structures. For a helpful account of functional anatomy there is none better than that given by Jackson (1984). There are, however, some points to emphasize and these are summarized as follows.

MCL

This is a large fan-shaped structure passing from the medial femoral epicondyle to the medial aspect of the upper tibia. Noyes *et al.* (1980b) describe it as the prime static stabilizer controlling valgus laxity. Trickey (1984) emphasizes that division of the MCL results in anterior subluxation of the medial tibial condyle (external tibial rotation). Harding (1981), in a cadaveric study using the Goodfellow–O'Connor test rig, showed that the application of external rotation to the tibia after MCL division resulted in almost complete joint dislocation even with an intact ACL. However, such cadaveric ligament sectioning studies are notoriously misleading.

These three references serve to illustrate again the point that ligament function has to be seen in three dimensions. The MCL has a superficial and a deep component, the latter attaches to the rim of the medial edge of the tibial plateau and to the medial meniscus rim. It seems anatomically to be equivalent to the middle third of the medial capsule.

The superficial leaf attaches to the medial aspect of the proximal tibia 4–5 cm distal to the joint line and in a location deep to the pes anserinus tendon attachment. The latter has often to be reflected at surgery to find the avulsed superficial attachment of the MCL. Müller (1983) reminds us that the main MCL(s) does not attach to the medial meniscus and does require to remain free to glide to-and-fro in relation to the tibial plateau (and hence to the medial meniscus) in knee flexion and extension. However, the posterior oblique ligament (POL) does attach to the posterior third of the rim of the medial meniscus and it is this anatomical relationship which may result in the common association of a twisting injury and the peripheral tear of the posterior third of the medial meniscus; the Dandy type III concealed meniscus tear (Dandy 1981).

SEMIMEMBRANOUS TENDON

The semimembranosus tendon is an immensely impressive structure attaching like a 'sucker' (Müller 1983) to the posteromedial corner of the knee. There are five distinctive components to this insertion, namely:

1 Reflected portion which passes anterior below and parallel to the medial joint line passing deep to the medial collateral ligament (superficial leaf).

2 Direct insertion onto the posteromedial corner.

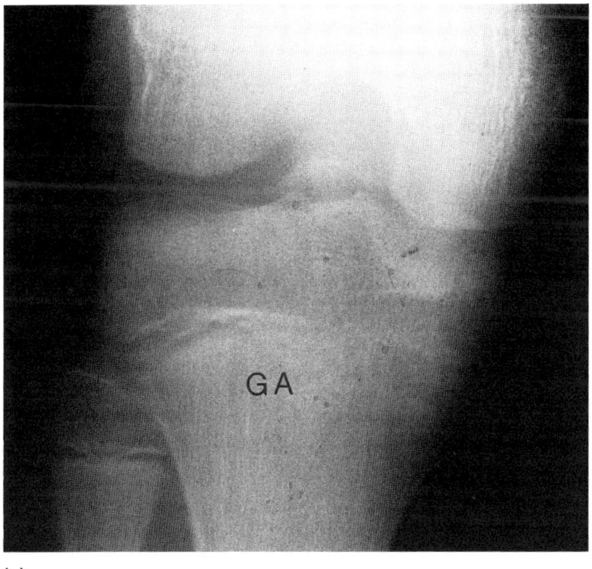

(a)

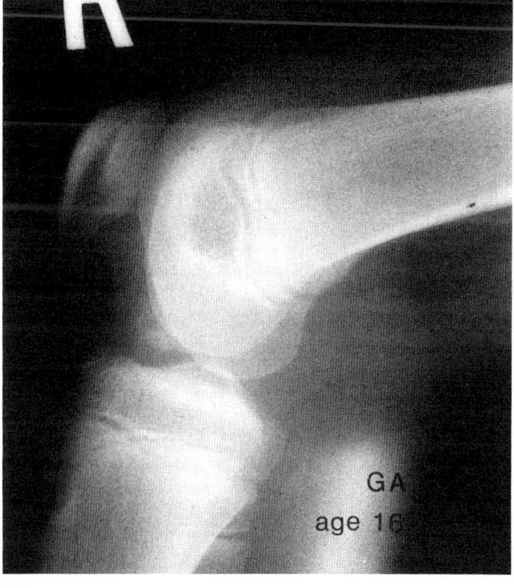

(b)

Fig. 22.1 (a) and (b) ACL avulsion fragment in an adolescent.

3 Oblique popliteal ligament which extends laterally and obliquely over the PC towards the fabella.
4 An expansion to the posterior fibres of the POL.
5 An expansion to the aponeurosis of the popliteus muscle.

CRUCIATE LIGAMENTS

A thorough knowledge of the anatomy of the cruciate ligaments is important. Essentially they are strong bands of dense connective tissue connecting the femur and tibia. Each ligament is approximately 3–4 cm in length. Tension yield studies show the posterior ligament to be the stronger (Kennedy *et al.* 1976).

Noyes and Grood (1976) report a maximum force, prior to failure, of 1730 ± 660 N at a strain rate of 100%/second in the ACL. It is important to be aware of the fibre orientation and its significance in different degrees of knee flexion, as clearly shown by Girgis *et al.* (1975), and of the attachment anatomy (Arnoczky 1983). Many authors, most recently Van Dijk (1983), have noted the two bands apparently present in the ACL. It appears that the anteromedial band is tight throughout flexion and extension. The posterolateral band is tight in extension and relaxes with flexion. Thus, the anteromedial band is the more isometric, but becomes even tighter as the knee is flexed. Arnoczky and Warren (1988) give an excellent account of all these features together with a description of the vascular anatomy and possible nerve supply and, hence, they allude to the function of these ligaments as proprioceptors.

Goodfellow and O'Connor (1978) have demonstrated the kinematics attributable to the cross four-bar linkage arrangement of the cruciate ligaments and attribute the first such description to Kapandji (1970). Harding (1981) has shown that there might be a variable 'axle' of knee flexion which centres at the cross-over point of the cruciates, in both the sagittal and coronal planes. This could afford flexibility in redistributing sudden twisting forces incurred during knee flexion and extension, which is lost when the cruciates are damaged.

LATERAL CAPSULAR LIGAMENTOUS COMPLEX

Andrews *et al.* (1988) consider that the lateral ligament/capsular structure can be divided into three parts: the anterior, middle and posterior thirds. The anterior third is essentially the patellar retinaculum. The middle third has the iliotibial band and tract: the former providing dynamic support and the latter static support. The middle third of the lateral capsular ligament attaches proximally to the lateral femoral epicondyle and distally

at the mid-coronal point onto the tibial joint margin. An avulsion injury at this latter site produces the Segond fragment (Segond 1879, Irvine *et al.* 1987) (Fig. 22.2). The posterior third capsular and non-capsular ligaments comprise the arcuate complex, the components of which are the FCL, the arcuate ligament and the aponeurotic sheath of the popliteus muscle. There is dynamic reinforcement from three muscles, namely the popliteus, biceps femoris and lateral head of gastrocnemius. The biceps femoris tendon and the FCL have conjoined insertion into the fibular head. The popliteus tendon and femoral end of FCL also have a combined or adjacent insertion: the latter into the epicondyle and the former into an area just anterior to this site. Figure 22.3 shows these ruptured structures in a typical lateral capsular injury.

General comments

One of the first important studies of knee ligament injury pattern was made by Palmer (1938). However,

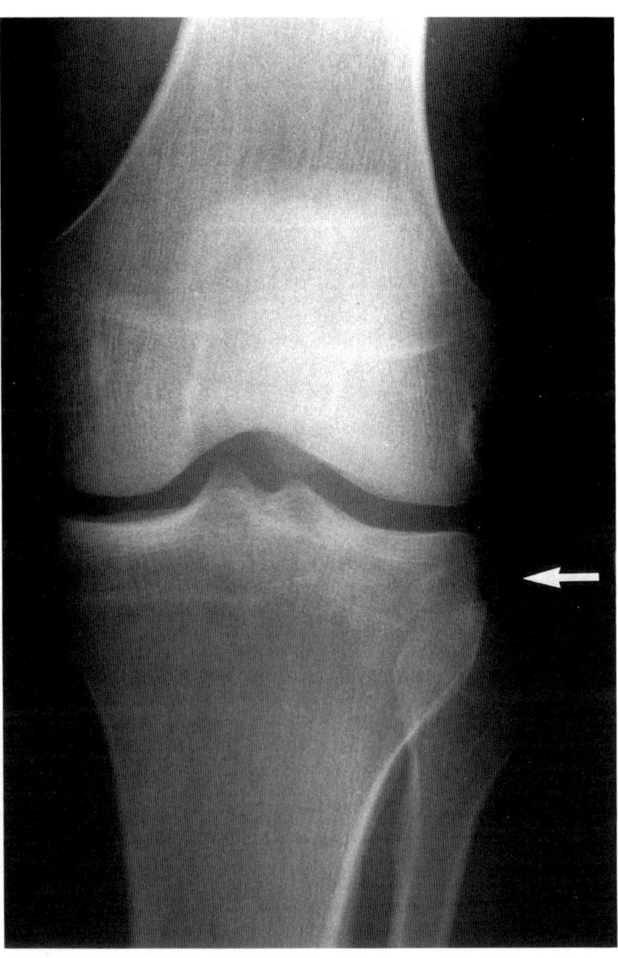

Fig. 22.2 A classical Segond fragment.

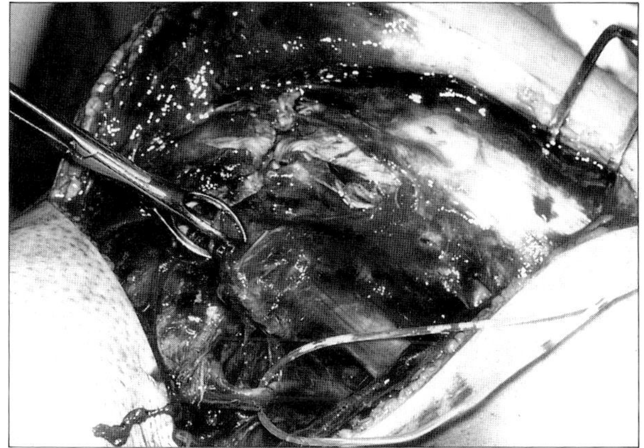

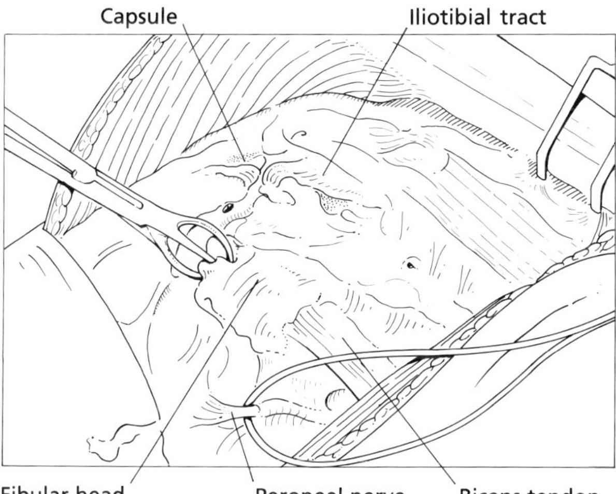

Fig. 22.3 (a) Photograph and (b) diagram of ruptured structures in a typical lateral capsular injury. ITT, iliotibial tract; CAPS, capsule; FH, fibular head; BT, biceps tendon; PN, peroneal nerve.

the message from this illuminating study was obscured by the intervention of World War II and for many years subsequently it was thought that the most common combination of ligament injury was the classical one described by O'Donoghue (1950), namely the triad of the disrupted ACL, MCL and medial meniscus. It is now believed that the most common single ligament rupture is to the ACL. Various studies have shown that 70% of knee joint injuries with significant haemarthroses have partial or complete ACL disruption (Noyes *et al.* 1980a, Jones & Allum 1989).

The history and clinical examination remain the mainstays of diagnosis together with a high index of suspicion. For example, certain sports like skiing and basketball are now associated with a high incidence of ACL ruptures by different mechanisms. Noyes *et al.* (1989) describe a non-contact injury in 81% of patients, of whom 62% had felt or heard a 'pop' at the time.

If the patient does not volunteer this information then it should be sought by appropriate questioning. It should be ascertained whether the patient was in collision with another person, the attitude of the leg at impact and whether the injured leg was weight-bearing at the time of injury. An immediate fall to the ground and inability to walk imply significant capsular and meniscal disruption whereas a patient with a cruciate injury can usually walk down a ski slope but cannot ski (Feagin 1988). Dashboard injuries were notorious for producing PCL ruptures but modification in car design with sloping shelves has lessened the incidence of these injuries. Particular difficulty in diagnosis will be had when there are associated femoral or tibial fractures. Sometimes the cruciate injury is impossible to diagnose until a femoral or tibial fracture has been stabilized, unless there are avulsion fragments. The insertion of a tibial pin for traction to treat a fracture of the femur may reveal joint laxity and a radiograph of the knee with skeletal traction applied in this way is a useful screening test.

Acute injuries

An acute ligament injury should be very carefully assessed by clinical examination and by radiographs, including stress films, which may yield important clues as to evidence of fracture fragments (Fig. 22.4). Oblique views can reveal undisplaced fractures in tibial plateaus which would explain a haemarthrosis and joint tenderness. Arthroscopic examination can be useful in limited circumstances. There are certain and important contraindications for the latter examination; namely, when capsular disruption is a major problem because fluid loss from the joint can cause compartment compression syndromes. MRI examination is now widely used.

Examination of the fresh knee injury

The examiner should ask direct questions of the patient, who should be relaxed and listened to carefully. Bruising patterns and the location of wounds should be observed.
1 Effusion — it needs to be determined whether a significant haemarthrosis is present. It is helpful to consider a simple algorithm (Fig. 22.5).

In a prospective study of 50 cases with haemarthrosis, Jones and Allum (1989) found 66% of knees with ACL tears. Of these 12% had completed previous partial ruptures, 26% had a fresh partial tear and 28% had a complete fresh tear of the ACL. There were a lot of associated meniscal injuries and other injuries. They concluded that a routine arthroscopic examination was

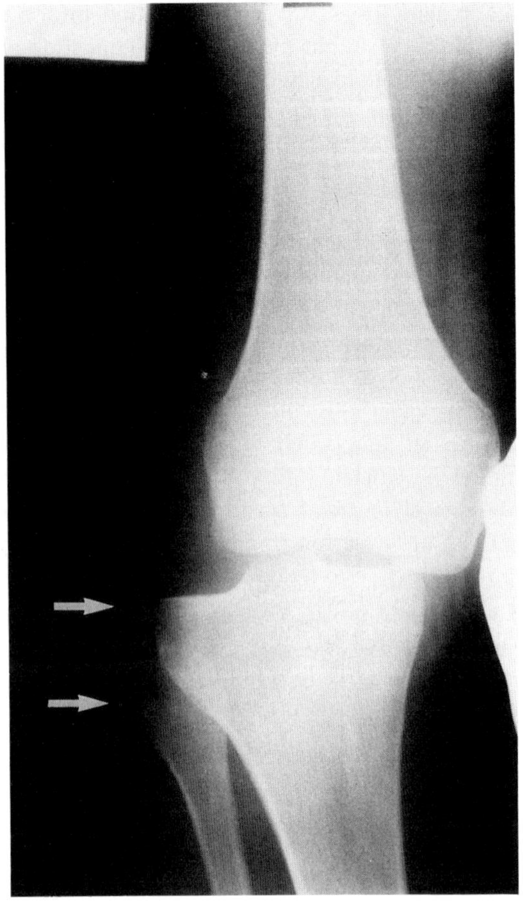

Fig. 22.4 Varus stress radiograph shows fibular head avulsion and a possible Segond fragment.

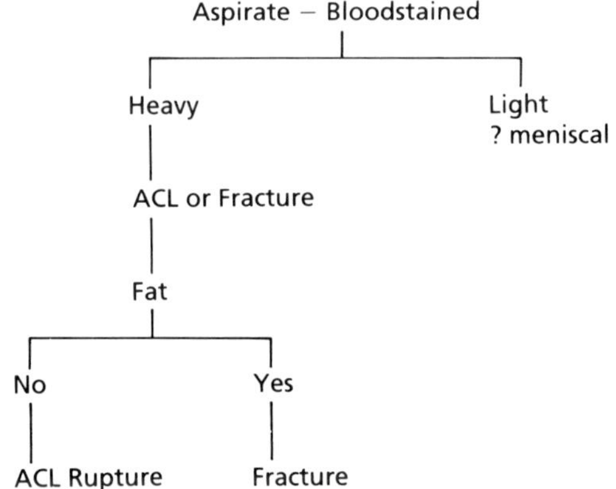

Fig. 22.5 Haemarthrosis algorithm.

justified in patients under the age of 35 years.

2 The extension position should be noted at the time of injury, i.e., whether this was normal, in flexion or hyperextended.

3 The range of movement should be recorded.

4 It should be noted whether there is a firm extension 'end-point' and whether this is painful.

5 Collateral ligament laxity and integrity should be assessed at 0° or in a hyperextended position and at 30° of flexion. This should be assessed in both a varus and valgus direction and recorded as I, II, or III grade of magnitude.

6 The Lachman test — the anterior drawer at 20° should be assessed. It should be noted whether there is a firm or a soft end-point. This is particularly important for the acute injury (Torg *et al.* 1976). With instrumented measurement using their KT1000 device, Daniel *et al.* (1985) reported that 96% of patients with unilateral ACL disruption show 2 mm or more anterior displacement than exists in the uninjured knee (mean 5.6 mm laxity). Forster *et al.* (1989) found, also using the KT1000 arthrometer, that 25% of normal subjects (9 out of 32) had right and left knee differences of more than 2 mm. Laxity measurements are therefore not generally used or relied on to assist diagnosis. Learmonth *et al.* (1991) has measured anterior knee stiffness in 139 patients with confirmed ACL ruptures, and found significant differences between injured and normal (uninjured) knees. The mean injured knee stiffness was 12 N mm^{-1} as compared to the mean normal knee stiffness of 37 N mm^{-1} ($p < 0.001$). This measurement, therefore, may yet prove to be a useful diagnostic aid in ACL rupture.

7 The anterior drawer at 90° should be noted.

8 Posterior drawer at 90° — this should be compared with the other knee and an observation made of the quadriceps active drawer test (Daniel *et al.* 1988). The test is performed by placing a hand behind the lower femur just above the popliteal fossa and supporting the weight of the knee with the latter flexed to about 40°, and with the heel resting lightly on the couch. The patient is asked to lift the heel and the movement of the tibial tubercle and posterior sag is assessed as the patellar tendon draws the tibia forward; this will happen in a posterior cruciate-deficient knee.

9 Pivot shift test — a variety of tests are available. The author's choice is that described by Galway *et al.* (1972) and is performed from a full resting extension position into flexion. Care should be taken to try and relax the patient completely. Most patients will be keen to watch the examination and they should be advised to rest their head back on the pillow of the examination couch. A brief description of the test is as follows for the examination of the right leg.

The knee is in extension and the heel is lifted off the couch by the right hand. The left hand is placed behind the fibular head, which is firmly rolled forwards, thus internally rotating the tibia. At the same time knee flexion will be occurring. Counterpressure is also applied between the two hands so that a strong valgus force is directed to close the lateral compartment so that the joint surfaces are firmly opposed. With continuing forward and internal rotation of the tibia, the latter will sublux forwards, initially into an abnormal position, and the patient will be aware that this is what occurs to the knee in clinical circumstances (positive for apprehension). As further knee flexion occurs, reduction follows as the fascia lata band passes behind the flexion axis. Three manoeuvres are therefore being performed by the examiner:

(a) Anterior tibial subluxation associated with internal tibial rotation.

(b) Knee flexion.

(c) A valgus strain.

The grade of positivity of the pivot shift test can be elicited (Noyes *et al.* 1983):

Grade I — normal (o).

Grade II — definite positive (1+), soft gliding movement, a slip.

Grade III — definite positive (2+), sharp movement with reduction of subluxation, a jerk.

Grade IV — grossly positive (3+), a jump.

This latter is also described as Finochietto's sign (Finochietto 1935); that is, it is impossible to proceed with knee flexion until the pressure producing anterior tibial subluxation is relaxed.

These grading categories help to select patients for surgery. Thus, patients with heavily positive pivot shift tests (III and IV) should be offered ACL reconstruction. Patients with a grade II test can be counselled and watched, after arthroscopy and meniscectomy. However, patients with a grade II instability who require a meniscal repair must have a supplementary ACL-stabilizing procedure, such as a Lamaire tenodesis, as the minimum requirement.

10 Local tenderness — direct palpation along the joint lines at the anterior, mid and posterior points on both the medial and lateral sides, and along the lines of the collateral ligaments, is effected to detect point tenderness at avulsion or sprain locations.

11 Patellar apprehension — this should be carefully assessed. Patellar dislocation may occur in association with medial capsular ligament rupture and may mimic a cruciate injury because medial patellar retinacular tears may give a positive Lachman test (ACL — false positive) and/or may produce some pronounced anterior and medial swelling so as to give the clinical impression of knee hyperextension (PCL — false posi-

tive). Patellar dislocation as an isolated problem is considered on p. 776.

ACUTE ACL TEARS

The ACL may be torn in isolation. It is difficult to envisage how this may occur with absolutely no further damage to secondary restraining structures, but experience shows that it may indeed be the only evident structure which is macroscopically disrupted in the acute injury. The acute ACL rupture may be incomplete. It is now conventional to accept that there are anteromedial and posterolateral band components of the ACL ligament. It may be possible to differentiate these partial tears by clinical examination, determining whether the anterior drawer laxity is present at 20° and 90°, and by the pivot shift test (Girgis *et al.* 1975, Furman *et al.* 1976, Van Dijk 1983). These authors describe that the anteromedial band is moderately tight in extension whereas the posterolateral band is very tight. With knee flexion, the anteromedial band tightens and the posterolateral band relaxes. Therefore, if the anteromedial band alone is torn the Lachman test could be equivocal but the anterior drawer test at 90° should be positive. The pivot shift test may well be equivocal or negative in these circumstances. With counselling, these knees may endure the partial tear without progression to full ACL insufficiency. In contrast, if the posterolateral band is torn whether or not the anteromedial band is intact, the prognosis is poor and full ACL insufficiency can be anticipated (Feagin 1988). In practice, the author has found this distinction difficult, and therefore inconsistently helpful.

Another approach has recently been described by Noyes *et al.* (1989) who list three predictive factors when partial ACL tears would be likely to progress to full insufficiency. These factors are:

1 The amount of estimated ACL tearing at the initial arthroscopy. (One-half of tears progressed to complete insufficiency in 50% of cases and three-quarters of tears progressed to a similar state in 86% of cases.)

2 An increase, even though subtle, in the initial anterior translation.

3 Subsequent occurrence of 'giving way' or re-injury.

Brand (1986), however, proposes that this surgical 'mechanistic' view is ill-founded and fails to explain many clinical contraindications: where an obviously unstable joint will cause no 'giving way' problems and yet, conversely, minimal laxity can yield significant ACL insufficiency symptoms. A neurosensorial concept of the function of the ligaments and capsules might be a better approach. Further evidence of the importance of joint proprioception has recently been provided by Barrett and MacKenny (1991).

Management

Jokl *et al.* (1984), in a small prospective but non-randomized study of MCL and ACL injuries, found no difference between a conservative group using early mobilization and a group using surgery. The detail of the latter was not described. The average follow-up was 3 years.

Ireland and Phen (1989) have shown that a selective approach may be adopted because 70% of patients can accept the consequences of ACL rupture if meniscal tears are dealt with. Bray and Dandy (1989) have confirmed that meniscal tears can be the consequence of ACL insufficiency. However, there is increasing evidence that complete tears should be treated with an efficient surgical technique (Clancy *et al.* 1988). The absence of any surgical treatment too often results in late instability sequelae (Fetto & Marshall 1980; Kannus & Jarvinen 1987).

There are few randomized prospective studies; three such studies are by Odensten *et al.* (1985), Sandberg *et al.* (1987) and Andersson *et al.* (1989). Odensten *et al.* pitched primary suture plus augmentation against conservative treatment and found no difference between the two groups at an average follow-up of 19 months except that stability was better in the operated knees. Sandberg *et al.* compared 200 consecutive patients with ACL and/or MCL tears by conservative versus operative treatment. Augmentation was not used. Injuries to the MCL did not benefit from surgery and those knees with ACL ruptures recovered more quickly with conservative treatment, but the final result differed significantly in only one respect: the pivot shift test was more often positive ($p < 0.001$) in the conservatively treated group. Andersson *et al.* compared surgical versus non-surgical treatment of acute rupture of the ACL and in the surgical repair group used either simple suture, if the tear was proximal, or augmentation. The term non-surgical referred to the ACL treatment. Thus, of the 59 patients in this group, the ACL was not repaired but the MCL was repaired in 15 out of 21 patients with a rupture of that ligament; the POL was repaired in 10 out of 12 patients with that injury; and curiously only one out of 11 patients with a rupture of the arcuate ligament complex had that structure repaired. There was also a very much higher incidence of arcuate ligament complex rupture in the conservatively treated group than in the surgically treated group. Notwithstanding, the knees treated with augmentation were significantly more stable and had fewer subsequent meniscal tears compared with the conservative ACL treatment. Augmentation was not shown to be clearly better than simple suture except with regard to activity-level scores. There was a high incidence of meniscal tear (64%) for which primary repair or excision was needed in more than one-half of those patients.

Conservative treatment

This may be considered for partial tears and the usual plan is for 6 weeks in plaster with the knee flexed to 40° and the tibia in neutral rotation because the ACL tenses with internal tibial rotation. The latter, of course, occurs coincidentally with knee flexion in the normal knee. In contrast, an ACL rupture associated with an MCL sprain or tear has been ruptured in external tibial rotation, and therefore the tibia should be internally rotated in the plaster. Thus, the position of the tibia in respect of rotation does require a distinction between these two patterns of injury.

Feagin (1988) advocates plaster treatment for the partial tear because of the potential benefit of the Wittek-type of healing phenomenon (Wittek 1927) where the ACL stump derives a useful blood supply from the intact PCL. Probably the worst results are obtained in patients who have no advice and no immobilization treatment. Noyes *et al.* (1989), however, found no benefit from plaster immobilization for partial tears compared with partial splinting with early movement.

Operative treatment

In the early stages operative treatment is only possible in the first 10 days after injury. The actual technique used depends upon whether there has been a bone fragment avulsion and upon the site of the rupture — whether the tear is near the end of the ligament or mid-substance in location.

1 The bone fragment should be reattached firmly, either with a screw and spiked washer or with a suture passed through the bone and fixed in some way onto the contralateral cortex. The avulsion area should be carefully defined and curetted prior to repositioning. Drill guides may be helpful. The author uses a simple wire pull-through method with parallel drill holes as advocated by O'Donoghue (1950).

2 Tears that have been avulsed from bone attachment can be satisfactorily reattached in the same way.

3 Proximal mid-substance tears occur in 80% of ACL ruptures (Steadman & Higgins 1988). Here the distal stump can be approximated to the lateral femoral condylar rupture site using three or four Dexon sutures.

4 True mid-substance or complex tears are the most difficult to repair. The author attempts a primary repair using three or four Dexon or Vicryl sutures in each stump. The sutures are then secured via parallel drill holes in the appropriate bone, taking care to secure the knot very tightly.

Feagin and Curl (1976) and Odensten *et al.* (1984) have reported that the prognosis for primary repairs of the type just described is not impressive. The current methods under trial in the author's unit are intra-articular augmentation either with semitendinosus or with an active biosynthetic composite (ABC) synthetic tow prosthesis. Steadman and Higgins describe an extra-articular lateral augmentation similar to that attributed to Andrews and Sanders (1983). Müller (1983) lists several evolving techniques and the indications for their current (1983) anterolateral femorotibial ligament (ALFTL) reconstruction alone or as a supplement to an ACL repair. Müller emphasizes the important association of the ALFTL disruption and ACL rupture. The ALFTL itself rarely ruptures in mid-substance. The ALFTL reconstruction is also indicated in adolescent ACL injury when the epiphyses are still open.

Attempts are being made to carry out arthroscopic repair in the acute injury and this is certainly possible using the ABC prosthetic cruciate ligament (Surgicraft), but the haemarthrosis makes the view difficult to maintain.

ACUTE MCL TEARS

First, second and even third degree tears may be treated conservatively provided that the ACL is intact (Indelicato 1983, Sandberg *et al.* 1987). For unstable third degree tears this means an above-knee plaster for 6 weeks with the knee flexed to 30° and the foot included. Optimum treatment is probably a shorter period in plaster followed by an efficient brace with a range of movement stop. First degree tears usually only require 1 week in plaster before commencing physiotherapy; and second degree tears seem more comfortable and ready to mobilize after 3−4 weeks. There are attractive concepts for early movement with regard to ligament healing. Experimental studies on rats by Hart and Dahners (1987) show that ligaments (MCL) that are *repaired* after transection are no stronger or less lax than those that are untreated. *Early motion* after transection gave stronger ligaments that were less lax (but not normal). There was an interaction effect *on laxity* of early motion and the status of the secondary stabilizing structures (ACL). Ligament stability was worse after early motion if the

ACL had been divided: however, when the ACL was intact early motion was beneficial and immobilization harmful. The *ligament strength* (as against the laxity) was better after early motion whether the ACL was intact or not. Thus, the critical feature that will determine whether the ligaments will be too long, and hence lax, after treatment will not depend on the treatment but on whether the ACL is intact or not.

If doubt exists about ACL integrity then an arthroscopic assessment is required but this has to be performed quickly and competently because of the danger of fluid leaking through the aperture in the torn capsule and causing compartment compression problems. Arthroscopy is required in any case, to assess possible meniscal tears.

Operative technique

Surgery for MCL rupture (third degree tears) will only usually be considered when there is, in addition, a rupture of one or both of the cruciate ligaments. The incision therefore, in addition to exposing the MCL, will need to provide exposure of the required sites for repair of those other ligaments. When the ACL is torn, this may mean the incision has to be long enough to allow retraction or dislocation of the patella to expose the lateral aspect of the lateral femoral condyle (LFC), or a separate lateral incision can be used. The incision is nearly straight and anteromedial. Care is required to avoid dividing the infrapatellar branches of the saphenous nerve (Müller 1983) but it is more difficult to define the fascial layers within 1−2 cm of the medial edge of the patellar tendon where they blend. Care should be taken because it is usually possible to finger dissect the tissues, thereby exposing and exploring the injured ligaments.

Once this has been done, the interior of the joint is inspected by extending the injury wounds by judicial incision as required. The anterior horns of the menisci can, on occasions, be divided to achieve access but it is preferable to avoid this and it is usually possible to do so by subcutaneous extension into the soft tissues peripheral to the menisci. Meniscal peripheral detachments are commonly found and should be repaired in a simple way. It is usually possible to distinguish between the rupture of the deep and superficial ligaments. If repairs are undertaken within a few days of injury, these can be accurately identified and repositioned in the anatomically correct locations. Care must be taken not to secure the superficial MCL to the proximal medial side of the tibia, thereby limiting subsequent flexion (Müller 1983). The author commonly uses cancellous AO screws with spiked washers for secure ligament fixation. Richards' staples are also useful. For interstitial tears or intersubstance stretching of ligaments, local 'box' type sutures are used to plicate and tighten as advocated by Müller (1983). Layered closure is performed after tourniquet release and an above-knee plaster is applied for 6 weeks.

POL TEARS

The same surgical approach described for MCL tears is used. The diagnosis is evident when the 20° valgus test produces external tibial rotation.

LCL TEARS

Isolated ruptures may occur with or without bone fragment avulsions. The diagnosis is usually obvious with varus testing at 20° of flexion and identification of local tenderness over the ligament.

Treatment

The LCL is the prime static stabilizer of the knee (Noyes *et al.* 1980b). Failure to effect surgical repair will result in varus laxity and troublesome instability. This will be more evident in a knee with an overall straight or varus alignment of the mechanical axis.

Technique

It is usually possible to reattach the avulsed ligament with a small cancellous AO screw and spiked washer (Müller 1983). Associated bone fragments are also amenable to this type of reattachment. Augmentation with composite ligaments or tows has been used when appropriate.

LATERAL COMPLEX (LCL, POPLITEUS TENDON AND LATERAL CAPSULE, FASCIA LATA, BICEPS FEMORIS, PC)

Two or more of these structures may be ruptured. These injuries give even more varus laxity at 20° and are often seen with bone flake avulsions (Figs 22.6 & 22.7). The surgical approach in the acute injury should be a curved lateral skin incision from Gerdy's tubercle distally, extending proximally along the line of the femoral epicondyle and shaft of the femur. Deep to the skin, the disrupted tissues should determine the route of access (Fig. 22.3). If it is intended to explore and repair cruciate ligaments, a long anterocentral skin incision is used.

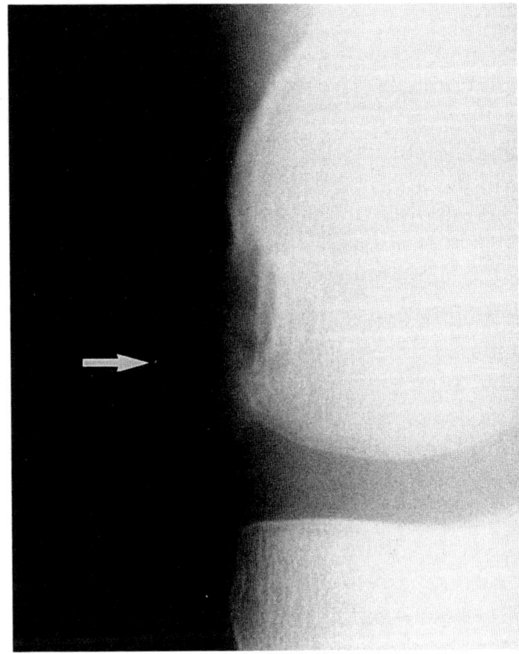

Fig. 22.6 A popliteus tendon femoral avulsion fragment.

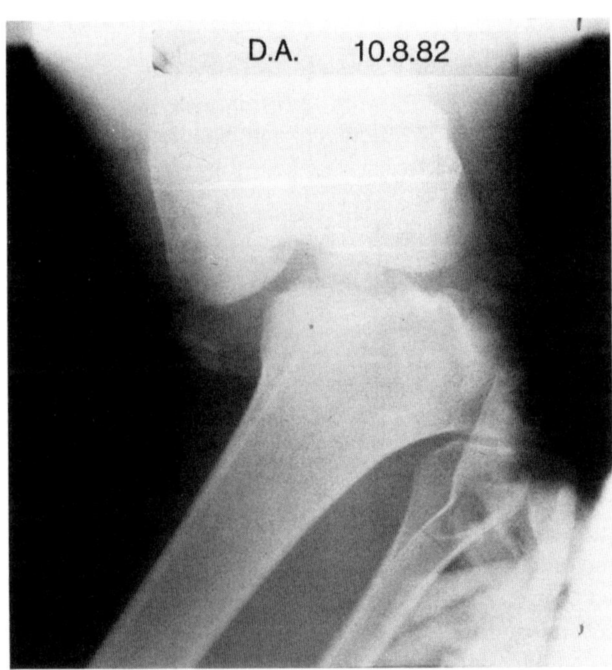

Fig. 22.7 There are lateral, medial and cruciate avulsion fragments in this gross varus dislocation injury.

Cruciate tears are repaired directly with 'pull-through' sutures (O'Donoghue 1950) and are optimally augmented with a patellar tendon or semitendinosus autograft and/or a Surgicraft ABC medium tow. Collateral ligament structures are directly sutured, and bone avulsions are secured with small fragment AO cancellous screws and spiked washers. The lateral popliteal nerve should always be sought in the surgical field. It should be noted that even with an intact PCL the varus laxity is evident at 0°. The question often arises as to whether a PCL rupture is present in these complex lateral ligament structure injuries. This has not been easy to determine clinically or at open operation. It has been the author's experience to proceed with surgery expecting to see a ruptured PCL, only to find that it is intact. Hughston's classification of rotatory instability (Hughston *et al.* 1976) assumes an intact PCL in posterolateral rotatory instability. This produces a clinical picture of posterior tibial drawer and sag, due to abnormal external rotational laxity.

ACUTE PCL TEARS

In association with other injuries, the torn PCL can be repaired by reattachment of the avulsed ends as previously described for ACL injuries, or by sutures for each stump-end for third degree mid-substance tears and augmentation with either an ABC Surgicraft tow or the semitendinosus tendon. In dislocated knees with patent vessels, meaning that ligament repair is appropriate, the torn PCL can usually be reached and, hence, repaired by a determined surgeon using the long, straight, anterior incision. Because one collateral ligament is intact in these circumstances, it will act as a soft tissue hinge. When the isolated PCL injury is diagnosed by virtue of an avulsed bone fragment, usually tibial, then the approach used by Trickey (1968) is required. When the isolated PCL rupture is mid-substance then diagnosis can be difficult and repair is equally so.

Ideally the tear should be confirmed arthroscopically. This should be safe to do if the PC is intact as shown by a normal extension position. A tear at or near the medial femoral condyle (MFC) can be reattached but with mid-point tears or those near the tibial attachment, then reconstruction is required. The author uses either a semitendinosus autograft or an ABC Surgicraft ligament for this purpose, and uses the technique and instrumentation described by Strover (personal communication). This has the invaluable advantage of allowing an anterior surgical approach for PCL reconstruction surgery.

Other associated injuries

PARALYSIS OF THE COMMON PERONEAL NERVE

This important injury occurs in severe lateral ligament disruption (Figs 22.4 & 22.7) or with dislocations of the knee. Assessment of function of this nerve should be a routine part of the examination. Inspection and protection of the nerve should be performed as a part of the operative procedure and preliminary identification of injured structures. The author's experience has been that the nerve sheath, although clearly bruised, appears to be in continuity. However, physiological neurotmesis is the usual outcome. Only one out of six cases recovered normal function; and even then subsequent application of a thigh tourniquet for a further surgical procedure resulted in a temporary neuropraxia.

For those patients who do not recover the function of strong ankle dorsiflexion, a tibialis posterior tendon transfer is performed in the standard manner. This is indicated if the ankle joint is reasonably normal and passive dorsiflexion can reach a neutral position; otherwise an ankle fusion may be required. It should be noted that ankle plantarflexion with an unstable hyperextended knee is a very adverse combination. With the latter therefore, plantarflexion must be avoided or corrected. A carefully observed period in a below-knee walking plaster must be proposed, in any event, before ankle fusion is undertaken.

DISLOCATION OF THE KNEE

Dislocation of the knee occurs with hyperextension injuries when the popliteal vessels are commonly compromised. Here the tibia is located anterior to the femur — an anterior dislocation. In severe flexion rotation injuries, as occur in American football and, less commonly now, with dashboard injuries, the tibia is posterior to the femur — a posterior dislocation (Kennedy 1963, Reckling & Peltier 1969). In Kennedy's series of 22 cases there were 14 anterior dislocations. The incidence of vascular disruption is about 30% (Green & Allen 1977). Sisto and Warren (1985) advocate an arteriogram for all cases of knee dislocation, whether or not there appears to be a vascular problem, to reveal any occult vascular damage, and hence potential ischaemia. Their caution is pertinent when tourniquets are to be used for ligament reconstruction. However, the vascular 'rescue' should not be delayed by an arteriogram (O'Donnell *et al.* 1977). It is helpful for the vascular surgeon to perform arteriography preoperatively (at the table) in all patients who have vascular occlusion and knee dislocation (Patel *et al.* 1988). An arteriogram should also be performed after reconstruction at this level, to ensure satisfactory patency.

When a dislocated knee has resulted in leg ischaemia due to popliteal artery injury, then it has not been the author's policy to attempt secure ligament reconstruction after the arterial repair has been achieved by the vascular surgeons. In such cases a simple plaster application secures the joint. However, the development of arterial shunt techniques now brings the combination of arterial *and* ligament repair within reach.

To-date, the author's management of knee dislocation, without vascular occlusion, has been to perform early surgery and repair adequately all injured ligaments, menisci and/or fractures. Adequate repair means careful and secure reattachment of ligament stumps by the O'Donoghue technique, box suturing of the stretched ligaments and the use of spiked washers and AO screws when appropriate. Simple suturing of the avulsed ligaments is not an adequate repair.

Levitsky *et al.* (1988) have described a case with bilateral open dislocation and fractures of the knee joints, each with arterial occlusion. One knee also had a transection of the popliteal vein. The conduct and timing of their surgery is very instructive and allowed a moderately secure ligament repair appropriate to the problem as a whole. The priorities were to secure vital limbs, with sound secondary closure of the compound joint injuries, and yet also to achieve pain-free joints in a mobile patient, albeit with some residual joint laxity.

Chronic ligament injuries

Residual chronic ACL laxity is the main problem. Controversy has existed over the natural history of the ACL-deficient knee but the clinical picture is clearing, as already discussed in the section dealing with acute injuries. McDaniel and Dameron (1983) have reported that at 14 years the 'giving way' symptoms were reduced compared with their incidence at 10 years, but at the expense of increasing radiological degenerative change (33%). Kannus and Jarvinen (1987) have shown that if the ACL is completely disrupted, 50% of patients will subsequently develop very significant meniscal tears and 'giving way' episodes over a 6-year period. Bray and Dandy (1989) confirm that meniscal lesions appear to be the result of instability and not the cause. In the prospective study by Jones and Allum (1989) of acute traumatic haemarthroses, 6 (12%) of the 50 knees were completed old partial tears. It is therefore necessary to address the logistics of avoiding chronic ACL problems and improving the early care of these important injuries. Each orthopaedic service should declare a policy giving due recognition to the considerable surgical requirements of early ligament repair.

For those patients with suspected chronic ACL problems, the author performs day-case arthroscopy after the usual thorough history, examination and plain radiographs have been taken. The patients may have already had arthrograms diagnosing meniscal tears. At arthroscopy the joint is generally assessed, particularly with regard to global joint laxity, the pivot shift test grading, the Lachman test, articular surface damage and presence or absence of ACL tissue. Meniscal tears are dealt with if excision is appropriate and a provisional opinion is given as to the advisability of ACL reconstruction. This is subsequently discussed with the patients when they return for review and suture removal. A patient under 35 years with a clearly positive pivot shift test (3+ or 4+) and with evidence of subluxation — induced surface changes, horizontal fissure tears/fibrillation and/or meniscal tears would be considered a clear candidate for further surgery. Account is also taken of the patient's intentions to play sport. However, the author usually advises that the patient should not return to contact sport activities, like soccer, even if the ligament repair is successful.

The Lemaire or MacIntosh I lateral substitution repairs are very safe, reliable techniques (Lemaire 1975, MacIntosh & Darby 1976), which confer considerable stability benefits (Ireland & Trickey 1980). These techniques are very similar. Both use a strip of fascia lata based distally on Gerdy's tubercle, which is then passed deep and secured to the FCL. In the Lemaire technique, the tube of tissue then passes back via a small bone tunnel from the lateral femoral condylar/shaft corner, *above* the FCL epicondylar attachment. The MacIntosh I technique secures the fascial strip through the lateral intermuscular septum (LIMS) with local sutures. However, some recent reports show some return of subluxation symptoms 6 years after this type of extra-articular tenodesis, even when combined with an intra-articular carbon tow (Bray *et al.* 1988).

The MacIntosh II repair takes a 15 cm long fascial strip wider (2 cm) proximally than distally (1 cm) and continues from the LIMS, over the top of the lateral femoral condyle (LFC), through the posterior capsule (PC) and the joint and exits the knee via a tibial bone tunnel sited at the ACL tibial attachment.

Review in the author's unit, with regard to measured anterior drawer laxity (Steingold *et al.* 1987), gave the MacIntosh II repair using the 'over the top' technique the best results, and this has been reported also by Bertoia *et al.* (1985); in 38 patients they achieved 91% good or excellent results at an average 3-year follow-up. Of the prosthetic ligaments, the Leeds–Keio Dacron implant without a lateral substitution repair gave reasonable results but a high early rupture rate was discouraging; this could certainly have been improved by a more adequate notch clearance, and by strict compliance with the recommended technique of insertion. There have been reports of very good results using this implant (Fujikawa *et al.* 1989). In the author's unit use has been made of the Surgicraft ABC synthetic ligament. O'Brien *et al.* (1989) have reported some promising early clinical results using this interesting composite scaffold ligament which does encourage fibrous tissue ingrowth, and is multifilament in design to allow this. It also has the merit of being implantable arthroscopically with only slight modification of the implant tools. However, the most recent review of this technique in the author's unit shows very disappointing results at a 2-year follow-up with a 12.5% neoligament rupture rate; laxity and stiffness measurements are barely better than in the chronic untreated ACL group.

The original Jones repair (Jones 1963, 1970), which directed attention to the patellar tendon as a donor graft site, appears to produce an unacceptable incidence of a significant extension block. The best current autologous repair available is probably the free one-third patellar tendon graft (Clancy *et al.* 1982, Trickey 1984); Rackemann *et al.* (1991) have reported 92% satisfactory results at a 6-year follow-up after using a combination of the intra-articular patellar tendon autograft and an extra-articular tenodesis. There is concern, however, at weakening the patellar tendon and risking a rupture of this structure; the surgical repair of this complication is not at all easy. There is also a definite risk of patellar fracture associated with the harvesting of patellar ligament autografts (Christen & Jakob 1992). For these reasons the author currently uses a semitendinosus autograft. Further reports on the use of allograft transplanted tendons are awaited with interest (Shino *et al.* 1988).

The safest technique for the orthopaedic surgeon who is not happy to embark on major, potentially troublesome intra-articular procedures is, therefore, the Lemaire, or the similar MacIntosh I, procedure which uses a distally based stump of fascia lata. An attractive modification of this is the Müller tenodesis which defines, but does not proximally divide, this strip of tissue and fixes it to the lateral femoral condyle at the distal end of the LIMS using a screw and spiked washer. This procedure can also be used as an augmentation technique with any intra-articular repair, such as an ABC ligament, or after an acute repair. In adolescents, where there are problems of open epiphyses, the lateral substitution tenodesis is virtually the only surgical procedure to consider.

CHRONIC MCL LAXITY

Pure MCL laxity rarely requires further surgery. The usual approach now, if there is a combination of ACL and MCL laxity, is to deal with the ACL laxity first and then consider an extra-articular augmentation with a carbon/Dacron composite ligament, if 'giving way' symptoms are still a persistent problem. If this is required, a double-strand MCL ligament procedure is advisable. Surgicraft now make a double-limbed medial collateral prosthetic ligament, of which the author has no practical experience.

It is important to remember that the superficial MCL slides posteriorly with knee flexion, and that the deep MCL tension does not change with knee flexion. Another feature which requires consideration is the natural varus or valgus stance of the knee (Trickey 1984). A knee with chronic MCL laxity with significant valgus will not benefit from MCL augmentation or plication unless the deformity is corrected by a supracondylar osteotomy. The Nicholas 'five-in-one' procedure (Nicholas 1973) is an option for chronic MCL laxity but it is harmful to sacrifice a normal medial meniscus which is a part of this operation. One might consider detaching the meniscus peripherally and re-attaching it after the medial capsular repositioning has been done.

Careful assessment of these patients is required to determine and deal with their ACL competence, and also to consider the mechanical axis alignment from long leg films. In addition, arthroscopic or arthrographic assessment of the location of ligament laxity may be required to determine whether a suprameniscal or inframeniscal laxity is the main problem because a distal advancement is logical with distal laxity and a proximal plication is logical with suprameniscal laxity. All these points need to be taken into account if the decision is made to proceed to MCL reconstruction for chronic MCL laxity.

CHRONIC LATERAL LAXITY (INCLUDING POSTEROLATERAL LAXITY)

It is helpful to palpate for an intact fibular (lateral) collateral ligament with the knee at 90° flexion and in varus strain, in the so-called figure-four or tailor position. Repair of pure lateral laxity can be effected using local tissue from the biceps tendon or fascia lata, or from a synthetic composite ligament such as a medium-duty Surgicraft ABC tow.

Posterolateral laxity is often, however, the main problem. Here there is varus laxity at 20° and recurvatum.

The external rotation recurvatum test is positive (Hughston & Norwood 1980), but the primary test for posterolateral ligament injury is the reverse pivot shift test (Jacobs 1981, Daniel & Stone 1988). Daniel and Stone describe the reverse pivot shift test as follows. 'Begin the test by supporting the limb with a hand under the heel. The knee joint is extended and in neutral rotation. The examiner's hand is applied to the lateral aspect of the calf and a mild valgus strain is applied as the knee is flexed. When the test is positive, at $20-30°$ flexion, the tibia will externally rotate and the lateral tibial plateau will sublux posteriorly and remain in this position during further flexion. When the knee is then extended, the tibia reduces. In the standard (anterior) pivot shift the tibia is anteriorly subluxed in early flexion and then reduces between $30-40°$ of flexion. In the reverse test, the tibia is initially reduced and then the lateral tibial plateau posteriorly subluxes at $20-30°$ of flexion'. They report that in a patient with combined ACL and posterolateral laxity, the tibia may go from an anterior subluxed position to reduction and then on to a posteriorly subluxed position. Tibial external rotation tests at $30°$ of flexion can also be helpful (Gollehon *et al.* 1985), by simply showing the available passive rotational laxity compared with the normal. This latter test is performed with the knees flexed to $90°$ and held lightly together. There should be no excessive internal tibial rotation at $30°$ unless there is concomitant anterolateral instability as well. The PCL at $30°$ is a secondary restraint structure, and even with an intact PCL these posterolateral laxity signs can be evident. Arthroscopic evaluation does not often seem to be conclusive in the author's experience, except when there is obviously no PCL tissue left. Attempts to advance the femoral insertion of the popliteus tendon and FCL as a bone block anterosuperiorly (Edmonson & Crenshaw 1980) has not been successful as an isolated procedure. Müller (1983) advocates separate tendon block advancements. It is likely that the central pivot must be restored (Trillat 1979), whether this be anterior or posterior. The current view is that both a central reconstruction *and* an extra-articular lateral bone block advancement should be performed if the poor results of surgery for this difficult type of instability are to be improved.

POSTERIOR LAXITY

Insall and Hood (1982) report the use of a PCL reconstruction using the medial head of gastrocnemius and describe the results as being moderately good. In a series of eight cases, there were three excellent, three good and two fair results. Significant patello-femoral pain was an important residual problem. Strover (personal communication) reconstructs the PCL using the Surgicraft ABC ligament and this is currently the author's choice of operation, although experience is limited to four cases only. The author has no personal experience of the Augustine (1956) procedure and experience of a semitendonosus graft is limited to two cases, neither of whom seemed to benefit. Clancy *et al.* (1983) give a comprehensive account of the repair of acute and chronic cases with PCL rupture using a free one-third patellar tendon graft. There were 48 patients in the series: 15 with acute and 33 with chronic tears.

To approach this problem the author carefully evaluates the clinical features, including the recurvatum and tibial rotational tests, and takes overall note of the leg alignment with regard to the mechanical axis and tibial rotational status of the normal leg. Routine radiographic examination is done to check on bone fragment clues, and an arthrogram is requested to determine the state of the posterior segments of the menisci. An examination under anaesthetic (EUA) and arthroscopic examination is done with careful probing of the posterior meniscal borders and the contents of the intercondylar notch. A decision is then made as to whether to proceed and attempt surgical reconstruction.

Bracing

The author uses bracing without conviction or enthusiasm. Perhaps because of this, except for 'range of motion' limitation, the results seem poor with unsatisfactory control of progressive laxity. Patients only seem to wear those braces which seem too flimsy to be of any conceivable value.

Menisci

The menisci are commonly injured and since their functions of load relieving (Walker & Erkmann 1975) and load distribution cannot be substituted, there has been an effort in recent years to preserve as much meniscal tissue as possible. Arthroscopic assessment and surgery have revolutionized treatment so that day-case meniscectomy is now routine in many centres.

Diagnosis

This is by the history of a relevant weight-bearing and coincident twisting injury in the younger patient. In the more mature individual meniscal posterior horns are easily trapped when squatting and twisting; the precipitating injury may go almost unnoticed in some cases but the resultant meniscal symptoms are both persistent and painful. A story of clear-cut locking and unlocking is almost diagnostic, together with the patient stating that 'something stretches like an elastic band and then has been relieved'. Plain radiographs will usually exclude the other common cause of locking: namely, a loose body. The third and least common cause is a chondral flap tear. Thus, a patient with a true negative arthrogram and normal radiographs may well have this latter problem.

ARTHROGRAPHY

This is a very useful technique for the diagnosis of meniscal tears. For a full description of the diagnostic possibilities and features the reader is referred to Butt and McIntyre (1969) and Stoker (1980). It might be argued that if arthroscopy is going to be performed in any case, then an arthrographic examination is a waste of time. However, as a screening procedure it is valuable. A negative result should not be taken as conclusive if the physical signs for a meniscal tear are strong. A clear, complete bucket-handle tear can readily be missed on arthrography if the rim is sharp because the attached segments are easily overlooked, being so small. The author's policy is to undertake an arthrographic examination of all patients with suggestions of meniscal tears, where the likelihood of a lesion is less than 50%. If the clinical signs are very suggestive then one can proceed straightaway to offer arthroscopic examination. Arthrography is proving to be particularly valuable with diagnosis of posterior horn tears of the medial meniscus where preservation and meniscal repair are appropriate; for example, when a positive posterior horn detachment is diagnosed arthrographically and it is shown at arthroscopy that the medial meniscus cannot be displaced even with firm probing beyond the summit of the femoral condyle. In these circumstances it is worthwhile proceeding to explore the posteromedial compartment of the knee and performing a meniscal suture. The author's current preference is to use a 2−0 Vicryl suture with an 8 mm strong needle (Ethicon). The patient is then advised to proceed with protected weight-bearing for 2 weeks but usually not with plaster immobilization. Limited experience suggests that this is a procedure well worth considering. Conventional advice is not to consider conserving the menisci when there is ligament instability, unless the latter is corrected. Arnoczky's research (Arnoczky et al. 1988) into meniscal and cartilage repair and conservation is setting new standards in meniscal and articular cartilage knee surgery.

ARTHROSCOPIC MENISCECTOMY

The reader is referred to the excellent textbooks on this technique (Dandy 1981). There is no doubt that in the argument of open versus arthroscopic meniscectomy, there is no contest: arthroscopic meniscectomy is more precise, more conservative and allows day-case surgery. In addition, the coincidental full joint and ligament examination is often very valuable. The mainstay techniques and instruments for arthroscopic meniscectomy are as follows.

1 Standard 30° arthroscope.
2 Meniscal hook (any make).
3 Strong grasping forceps (e.g. Wolf).
4 Straight hook scissors (any make).
5 Punch forceps (Acufex).
6 Small grasping forceps (e.g. Arthrex).
7 As an additional helpful extra: Dionics suction-type punches, both small and large.

The standard portals are the anterolateral and anteromedial. In addition, it is almost always necessary to use the supramedial (Patel 1982) entry and often the central transpatella route (Gillquist et al. 1979). The difficult tears are in the posterior third segment but the author rarely uses a posterior medial portal effectively, and instead relies on techniques which pull or push the hidden meniscal tears into view to allow access with punch forceps or, more frequently and recently, the power meniscotome or suction punches. Both these techniques suck the meniscal fragments into the jaws of the surgical tool and minimize articular surface damage.

Cystic menisci

These can be dealt with by closed arthroscopic techniques or by open arthrotomy. The author's preference, increasingly, is to arthroscope the knee joint and if there is a meniscal tear, then the meniscus is trimmed fairly radically in the abnormal segment where the tear is present. Meniscal pathology usually coincides with the cyst location and therefore meniscal excision, until the cyst is decompressed in this segment of the meniscus, is appropriate (Glasgow et al. 1991). Again, the power meniscotome is making this surgical exercise more feasible and practical. Open extra-articular excision of cysts, when the menisci are intact, has been advocated (Flynn & Kelly 1976), but the author's experience of this has been most disappointing. In particular, whilst cyst recurrence has not been a major problem, delayed healing and ugly scars are often a complication, no doubt due to the synovial fluid leakage into extra-articular tissue.

Hard tissue injuries

Osteochondral fractures

These can occur in association with direct impact or twisting injuries. Patellar dislocation is a frequent cause. Careful inspection of plain radiographs is required to diagnose and evaluate the problem (Fig. 22.8). If the fragments are small then these can be removed arthroscopically, if that is appropriate, or by open surgery, if that is being contemplated for other reasons, such as open ligament repair or patellar retinacular repair in patellar dislocation. Large fragments in important weight-bearing areas of the joint should be repositioned and secured. If necessary, AO small fragment screw fixation may be the best option (Fig. 22.9). The screw heads have to be recessed carefully and these can later be removed arthroscopically. Herbert screw fixation would also be a useful method if expense was no object. An alternative method of fixation is the use of carbon rods (Minns *et al.* 1982, 1987). Ultimately, no doubt, carbon screws will be an ideal compromise between the two techniques and will achieve the double objective of stable, non-obtrusive fixation with a biodegradable material which, in the case of carbon, has the additional benefit of encouraging fibrocartilage and fibroblastic tissue ingrowth. In the future, the use of osseo-cartilage autografts or allografts will become a routine additional technique, available for the solution of large defects in important weight-bearing joints (Meyers *et al.* 1989).

Rupture of extensor mechanism

With patellar fracture

If it is feasible to retain a major patellar fragment then this should be attempted. Thus, treatment should be directed towards excision of lower or upper pole fragments and suturing the relevant part of the extensor mechanism to the fragment to be retained. This should be done very securely with drill holes in the bone fragment. A period of plaster immobilization for a minimum 6-week period is inevitable.

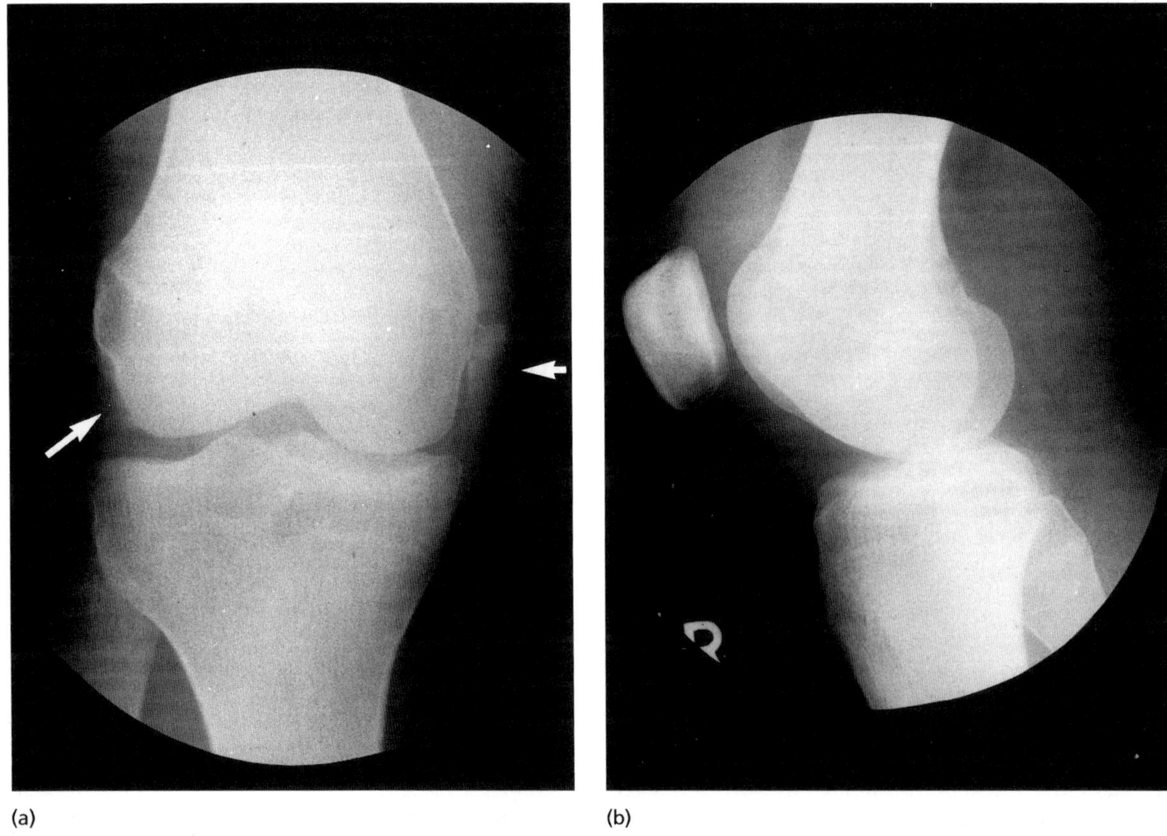

(a) (b)

Fig. 22.8 A lateral condylar chondral fracture. The fragment (left-pointing arrow) can be seen in the medial recess; the crater is more difficult to define (right-pointing arrow). Note the loss of cortical outline on the LFC in the lateral view and compare the appearance with Fig. 22.9.

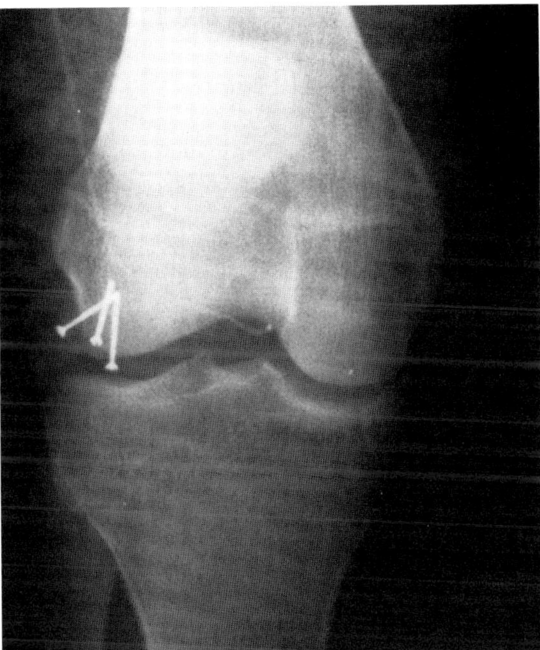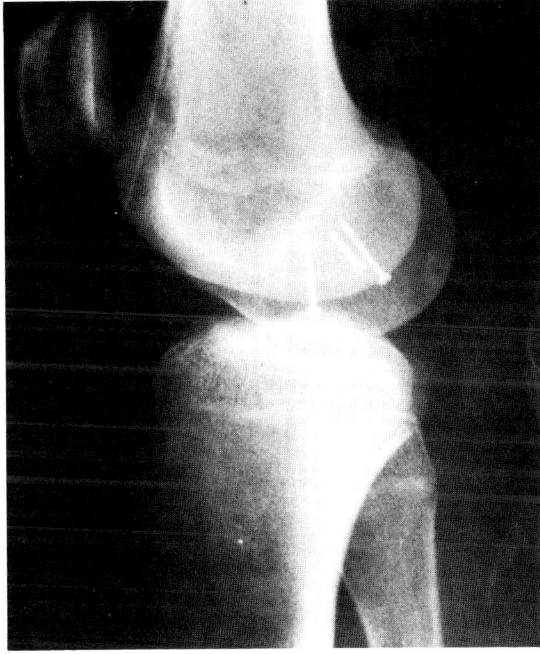

Fig. 22.9 The same knee as shown in Fig. 22.8, but after fixation of the chondral fracture fragment with mini AO screws.

Without patellar fracture

Injury usually follows a stumble or fall. The quadriceps muscles contract strongly, as a reflex, to maintain balance, presumably with a force/rate exceeding the ultimate tensile strength of the muscle or tendon fibres. Diagnosis is made by the history of such a mechanism and the clinical finding of a palpable tender gap in the injured segment of the extensor mechanism.

Rupture of the infrapatellar or suprapatellar tendons should be diagnosed early so that an early primary repair can be performed. Direct suture using a Bunnell-type of stitch with Vicryl is usually sufficient for primary repair, but local tissue augmentation with 'turn-down' or 'turn-up' flaps of the patellar retinaculum can be added if there is doubt about the security of the repair. Plaster immobilization follows for 6 weeks.

Late treatment of a missed rupture is very difficult. The problem relates to the low position (patella baja) of the patella with quadriceps tendon rupture and the high position (patella alta) with patellar tendon rupture. Surgicraft implants have not been an obvious success in the experience of the author, whose current practice for these injuries is to use a semitendonosus graft and, where appropriate, turn-down flaps of the superficial part of the patellar retinaculum and suprapatellar tendon.

Rupture of isolated parts of the quadriceps expansion are usually diagnosed late because early diagnosis is not particular easy. There is no evidence that early repair is effective, but it is evident that there is often a moderately significant morbidity from these injuries in the more mature patient. Late direct treatment is probably futile although the author has no personal experience to report.

Comminuted fractures of the patella

Undisplaced stellate fractures

These are caused by a direct blow. There is a haemarthrosis which requires relief by aspiration. Usually the patient can then show sufficient quadriceps control to achieve a near full extension lift, which is reassuring if conservative treatment is to be adopted. Plaster cylinder protection is advised for 6 weeks and this should be followed by physiotherapy.

Bipartite patellae

These are often found in the course of routine investigations for a possible fracture around the knee. The location is classically at the supralateral corner of the patella and it is this feature, together with the absence of local tenderness, which enables this to be excluded as a fracture. However, occasionally, a direct blow, such as on the corner of a goalpost, will dislodge the smaller patellar component and subsequent movement provokes local pain and tenderness. Treatment in these circumstances is either by excision of the small bipartite fragment or by screw fixation; the author has only used the former option.

Displaced comminuted patella fractures

The treatment of choice is operation, and where possible osteosynthesis is preferred to patellectomy (Marya *et al.* 1987). If the patella is hopelessly comminuted then patellar excision is the only option. An adequate transverse skin incision is used. The torn patellar retinacula should be repaired with due care. Where preservation of patellar fragments can be contemplated, then an 'S' incision can be employed. A straight, central, longitudinal incision gives the best exposure, and is better with regard to long-term planning for future surgery; however, it tends to heal poorly with a keloid scar. Osteosynthesis of the two major patellar fracture fragments is achieved after reduction by either tension-band with two longitudinal K-wires and a link figure-of-eight wire (Fig. 22.10a) or, more recently, by a single or double anterior tension circlage wire (Fig. 22.10b). Andrews and Hughston (1977) report the use of partial patellectomy for comminuted fractures and describe reliable results, providing at least three-fifths of the patella can be preserved: otherwise, with smaller retained fragments, the poorer results of patellectomy are approached. Böstman *et al.* (1981) confirm this latter observation with regard to the size of the retained patella. The authors analysed the results of 64 patients in three groups categorized by the measure of the initial displacement, in an attempt to clarify the effect on the results, of the magnitude of the original injury, using a numerical scoring system to assess their results. The Group IIa patients with the proximal pole intact and longitudinal displacement of more than 6 mm but with latitudinal displacement of less than 2 mm, scored as follows for the different treatment groups:

Tension band (3);−24.9
Partial patellectomy; proximal three-fifths intact (18)−23.6
Partial patellectomy; less than three-fifths intact (3)−21.5
There were no patellectomies in Group II patients.
In the worst group (III), the initial longitudinal displacement was more than 6 mm and latitudinal displacement more than 2 mm. There were 20 patients in Group III. Of these, four had been treated using the anterior circumferential tension-band technique and all four had unsatisfactory results. All Group III patients treated by

partial patellectomy (6) had less than three-fifths of the patella intact. The mean score for the 10 out of 20 Group III patients who had had total patellectomy was 20.1. Böstman *et al.* (1981) further point out that persistent steps of 1−2 mm in the articular surface seem to be of minor importance. Marya *et al.* (1987) compared the results of osteosynthesis and patellectomy in two identical groups of patients and found that patellectomy for fractures produces a negligible number of poor results, although excellent results will only be achieved in about half the cases compared with 80% excellent results after osteosynthesis. When functional disability is specifically analysed after patellectomy for fracture (Einola *et al.* 1976), a good subjective result is seen in only 16% of patients, with muscle power greater or equal to 75% of normal (other knee) in only 25% of cases.

Delay in patellar fixation causes treatment to be fraught with difficulties, because of quadriceps contraction and consequent fibrous shortening of the extensor mechanism. This delay is therefore to be avoided. However, if it is inevitable, preliminary attempts should be made at surgery to relengthen the quadriceps muscles, with skeletal traction if necessary, because it has been the author's experience that V-Y lengthening of the tendon together with prosthetic augmentation with Dacron can result in serious wound and tissue healing problems. Carbon fibre/Dacron tows (Surgicraft) have not been successful either for tissue augmentation and have failed to relieve pre-operative pain albeit in a different group of patients with a serious post-patellectomy quadriceps deficiency. A semitendinosus and gracilis autograft has been found to be a more efficient way of strengthening the deficient ventral extensor mechanism.

Dislocations of the patella

Classification (Aichroth 1984)

Dislocations can be:
1 Congenital (rare)*.
2 Acquired.
  (a) Recurrent — first episode usually associated with trauma.
  (b) Habitual*.
  (c) Persistent*.
  (d) Subluxation in extension*.
Recurrent dislocations usually occur in association

---

* Not considered further here.

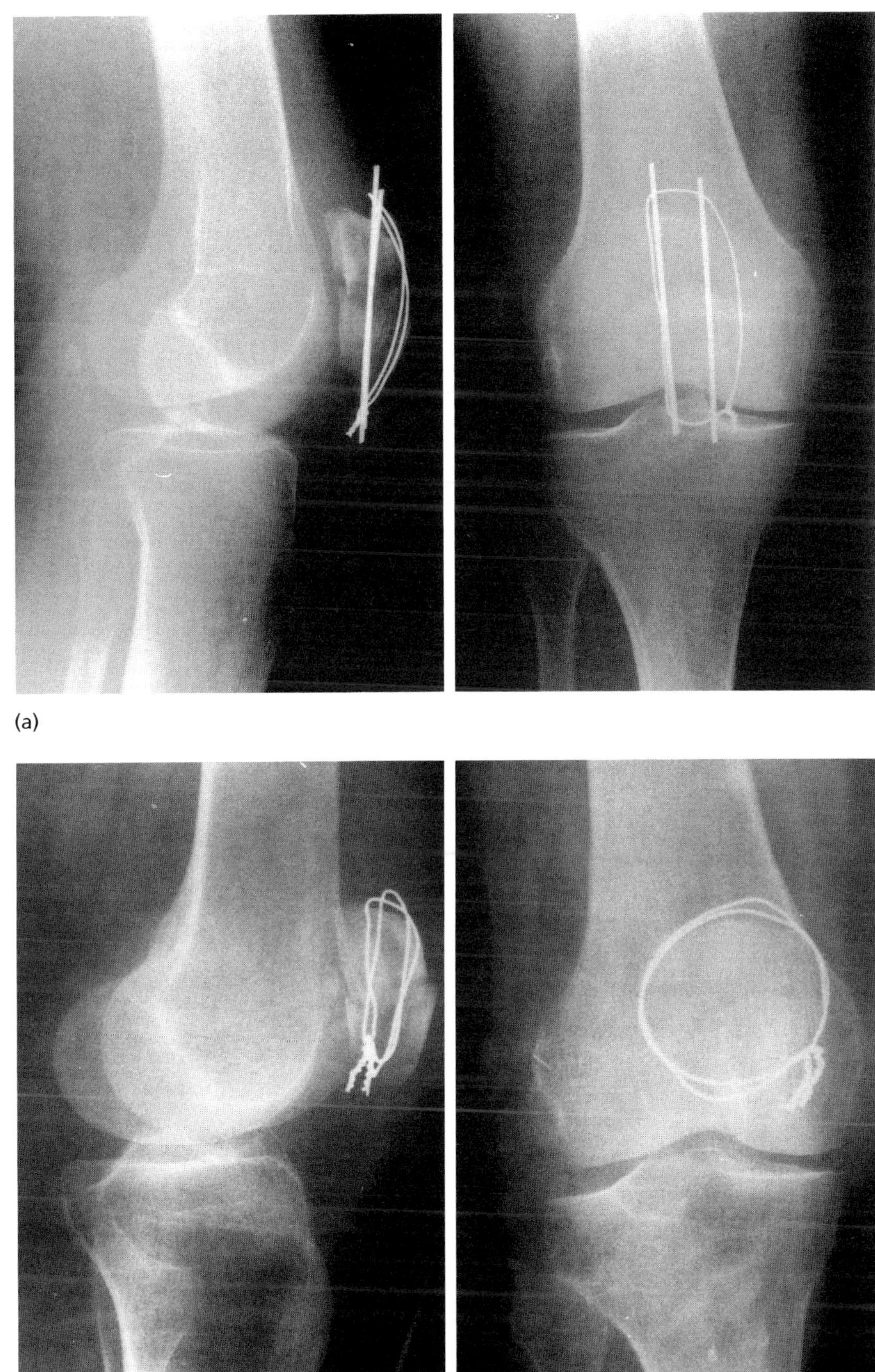

Fig. 22.10 (a) and (b) Fixation of patellar fractures with tension or double circlage wires.

with trauma and underlying malalignment problems, namely:

1 Lateral patellar subluxation.
2 Patella alta.
3 Lateral femoral condylar hypoplasia.
4 Shallow intercondylar groove.
5 Valgus deformity of the knee.
6 Internal distal femoral rotation.
7 External proximal tibial rotation.
8 Abnormal 'Q' angle (Insall 1984).
9 Vastus medialis origin dysplasia.

The mechanism is either a direct blow or a rotational

twisting injury. The latter may result in a clinical picture which can be confused with a MCL rupture.

Patients often describe that the patella shifted medially, and yet this happens very rarely and never in the author's experience. A prominent exposed medial condyle is responsible for the deception. Reduction is easily achieved by fully extending the knee. Aspiration is required to relieve the haemarthrosis. Fat globules may be observed in the aspirate because of associated avulsion or impaction fractures. These latter should, in any case, be looked for with skyline radiographs (Fig. 22.11) and may be a very helpful clue when the diagnosis is in doubt. The well-known classical patellar apprehension test should always be carefully elicited as a positive confirmation of the nature of the injury.

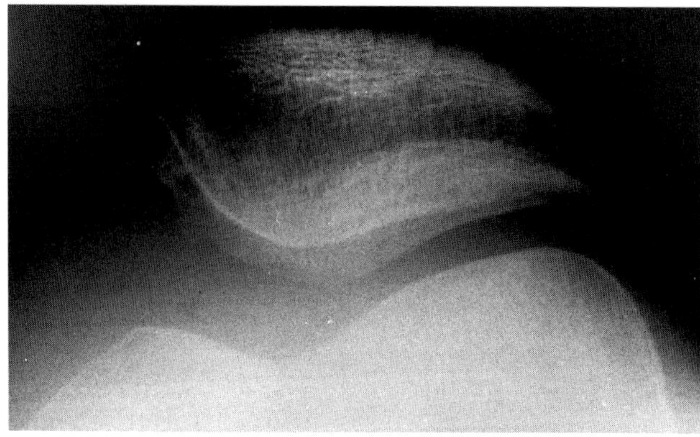

Fig. 22.11 Skyline patella radiograph showing typical post-dislocation features of medial facet avulsion and also calcification in the medial patellar retinaculum.

Treatment

There may be an argument for early repair of the ruptured medial patellar retinaculum but the logistics, with standard National Health Service (NHS) facilities and staffing, would rarely allow this luxury and there is no available evidence that it is beneficial in preventing further dislocation. Therefore, primary treatment is aspiration of the haemarthrosis, followed by 6 weeks immobilization in a plaster cylinder cast with the knee in full extension. Quadriceps activity should be encouraged in the plaster and subsequently when knee movement is regained. Particular attention should be directed towards vastus medialis strengthening. Patellar buttress bracing is often requested by patients to discourage redislocation when participating in sport and there would seem to be no harm in this.

When further dislocations occur surgery needs to be considered. In the skeletally mature patient, the author's preference is to perform an Elmslie–Trillat type of medial tibial tubercle displacement (Miller & LaRochelle 1986). It is often debated that such a procedure will recess the tubercle posteriorly and, hence, increase the patellofemoral pressure as the reverse to the benefit of a full Maquet procedure (Maquet 1976). However, this is probably not so in cases when the 'Q' angle is abnormally high (more than 15°). A pure lateral view of a knee before and after a tibial tubercle transfer usually shows the tubercle in clear profile postoperatively and yet invisible preoperatively. This implies elevation and, hence, patellofemoral load relief. In the author's series of tibial tubercle transfers for patellar dislocation, further subluxation/dislocation symptoms have occurred in only one patient. The vastus medialis plication after the style of Hughston *et al.* (1984) was performed to treat this resistant subluxation tendency, but has still failed to completely abolish patellar instability. Dandy and Griffiths (1989) have recently shown success with lateral release alone for patellar subluxation and dislocation. In patients requiring surgery before the epiphyses have closed this simple release would definitely be a reasonable proposal or, if more definitive patellar realignment is deemed necessary, a Goldthwait–Roux procedure might be offered (Roux 1888, Goldthwait 1904). However, the strong preference of this author is for a bony distal realignment, which maintains a strong bone–tendon junction, rather than this soft tissue procedure, which weakens the important bone–tendon junction; such surgery would be deferred until the epiphyses have closed.

References

Aichroth, P.M. Dislocation of the patella. In: Jackson, J.P. & Waugh, W. (eds) *Surgery of the Knee Joint*. Chapman & Hall: London, 1984.

Andersson, C., Odensten, M., Good, L. & Gillquist, J. Surgical or non-surgical treatment of acute rupture of the ACL. *J Bone Joint Surg* 1989; **71A**: 965–974.

Andrews, J.R. & Hughston, J.C. Treatment of patellar fractures by partial patellectomy. *South Med J* 1977; **70**: 809–813.

Andrews, J.R. & Sanders, R. A 'mini-reconstruction' technique in treating anterolateral rotatory instability (ALRI). *Clin Orthop* 1983; **172**: 93–96.

Andrews, J.R., Baker, C.L., Curl, W.W. & Gidumal, R. Surgical repair of the acute and chronic lesions of the lateral capsular ligamentous complex of the knee. In: Feagin, J.A. (ed.) *The Crucial Ligaments*. Churchill Livingstone: Edinburgh, 1988.

Arnoczky, S.P. Anatomy of the anterior cruciate ligament. *Clin Orthop* 1983; **172**: 19–25.

Arnoczky, S.P. & Warren, R.F. Anatomy of the cruciate ligaments. In: Feagin, J.A. (ed.) *The Crucial Ligaments*. Churchill Livingstone: Edinburgh, 1988.

Arnoczky, S.P., Warren, R.F. & Spivak, J.M. Meniscal repair

using an exogenous fibrin clot. *J Bone Joint Surg* 1988; **70**: 1209–1217.

Augustine, R.W. The unstable knee. *Am J Surg* 1956; **92**: 380–388.

Barrett, D.F. & MacKenney, R.P. Proprioception and stability in repairs of the anterior cruciate ligament. *J Bone Joint Surg* 1991; **73B**: (Suppl 1), 87.

Bertoia, J.T., Urovitz, E.P., Richards, R.R. & Gross, A.E. Anterior cruciate reconstruction using the MacIntosh lateral substitution over-the-top repair. *J Bone Joint Surg* 1985; **67A**: 1183–1188.

Böstman, O., Kiviluoto, O. & Nirhamo, J. Comminuted displaced fractures of the patella. *Injury* 1981; **13**: 196–202.

Brand, R.A. Knee ligaments: a new view. *J Biomech Eng* 1986; **108**: 106–110.

Bray, R.C. & Dandy, D.J. Meniscal lesions and chronic ACL deficiency. *J Bone Joint Surg* 1989; **71B**: 128–130.

Bray, R.C., Flanagan, J.P. & Dandy, D.J. Reconstruction for chronic anterior cruciate instability. A comparison of two methods after six years. *J Bone Joint Surg* 1988; **70B**: 100–105.

Butt, W.P. & McIntyre, J.L. Double contrast arthrography of the knee. *Radiology* 1969; **92**: 487–499.

Christen, C. & Jakob, R.P. Fractures associated with patellar ligament grafts in cruciate ligament surgery. *J Bone Joint Surg* 1992; **74B**: 4: 617–619.

Clancy, W.G., Nelson, D.A., Reider, B. & Narechania, R.G. Anterior cruciate ligament reconstruction using one-third of the patella ligament augmented by extra-articular tendon transfers. *J Bone Joint Surg* 1982; **64A**: 352–359.

Clancy, W.G., Shelbourne, K.D., Zoellner, G.B., Keene, J.S., Reider, B. & Rosenberg, T.D. Treatment of knee joint instability secondary to rupture of the posterior cruciate ligament. *J Bone Joint Surg* 1983; **65A**: 310–322.

Clancy, W.G. Jnr., Ray, R.M. & Zoltan, D.J. Acute tears of the ACL. Surgical versus conservative treatment. *J Bone Joint Surg* 1988; **70A**: 1483–1488.

Committee of the Medical Aspects of Sports (CMAS). Standard nomenclature of athletic injuries. *American Medical Association* 1968; pp. 99 & 101.

Dandy, D.J. *Arthroscopic Surgery of the Knee*. Churchill Livingstone: Edinburgh, 1981.

Dandy, D.J. & Griffiths, D. Lateral release for recurrent dislocation of the patella. *J Bone Joint Surg* 1989; **71B**: 121–125.

Daniel, D.M. & Stone, M.L. Diagnosis of knee ligament injury: tests and measurements of joint laxity. In: Feagin, J.A. (ed.) *The Crucial Ligaments*. Churchill Livingstone: Edinburgh, 1988.

Daniel, D.M., Malcolm, L.L., Losse, G., Stone, M.L., Sachs, R.S. & Burks, R. Instrumented measurement of anterior laxity of the knee. *J Bone Joint Surg* 1985; **67A**: 720–726.

Daniel, D.M., Stone, M.L., Barnett, P. & Sachs, R.S. Use of quadriceps active test to diagnose posterior cruciate ligament disruption and measure posterior laxity of the knee. *J Bone Joint Surg* 1988; **70A**: 386–391.

Edmonson, A.S. & Crenshaw, A.H. Knee injuries. In: *Campbell's Operative Orthopaedics* 6th edn. CV Mosby: St Louis, 1980.

Einola, S., Aho, A.J. & Kallio, P. Patellectomy after fracture. Long-term follow-up results with special reference to functional disability. *Acta Orthop Scand* 1976; **47**: 441–447.

Feagin, J.A. *The Crucial Ligaments*. Churchill Livingstone: Edinburgh, 1988.

Feagin, J.A. & Curl, W.W. Isolated tears of the anterior cruciate ligament: five-year follow-up study. *Am J Sports Med* 1976; **4**: 95–100.

Fetto, J.R. & Marshall, J.L. The natural history and diagnosis of anterior cruciate insufficiency. *Clin Orthop* 1980; **147**: 22–28.

Finochietto, R. Semilunar cartilages of the knee. The 'jump sign'. *J Bone Joint Surg* 1935; **17A**: 916–921.

Flynn, M. & Kelly, J.P. Local excision of cyst of lateral meniscus of the knee without recurrence. *J Bone Joint Surg* 1976; **58B**: 88–89.

Forster, I.W., Warren-Smith, C.D. & Tew, M. Is the KT1000 knee ligament arthrometer reliable? *J Bone Joint Surg* 1989; **71B**: 843–847.

Fujikawa, K., Iseki, F. & Seedhom, B.B. Arthroscopy after anterior cruciate reconstruction with the Leeds–Keio ligament. *J Bone Joint Surg* 1989; **71B**: 566–570.

Furman, W., Marshall, J.L. & Girgis, F.G. The anterior cruciate ligament. A functional analysis based on post-mortem studies. *J Bone Joint Surg* 1976; **58A**: 179–185.

Galway, R.D., Beaupre, A. & MacIntosh, D.L. Pivot shift: a clinical sign of symptomatic anterior cruciate insufficiency. *J Bone Joint Surg* 1972; **54B**: 763.

Gillquist, J., Hagberg, G. & Oretop, N. Arthroscopic visualization of the posteromedial compartment of the knee joint. *Orthop Clin North Am* 1979; **10(3)**: 545–547.

Girgis, F.G., Marshall, J.L. & Monajem, A.R.S. The cruciate ligaments of the knee joint. Anatomical, functional and experimental analysis. *Clin Orthop* 1975; **106**: 216–231.

Glasgow, M.M.S., Blakeway, C. & Allen, P.W. Arthroscopic management of the cystic lateral meniscus. *J Bone Joint Surg* 1991; **73B**: Suppl. I: 61.

Goldthwait, J.E. Slipping or recurrent dislocation of the patella with the report of eleven cases. *Boston Med Surg J* 1904; **150**: 169–174.

Gollehon, D.L., Torzilli, P.A. & Warren, R.F. The function of the posterolateral and cruciate ligaments in human knee stability (a biomechanical study). *Orthop Trans* 1985; **9**: 328.

Goodfellow, J.W. & O'Connor, J. The mechanics of the knee and prosthesis design. *J Bone Joint Surg* 1978; **60**: 358–369.

Green, N.E. & Allen, B.L. Vascular injuries associated with dislocation of the knee. *J Bone Joint Surg* 1977; **59A**: 236–239.

Harding, M.L. *Movement Under Load*. MS thesis: London, 1981.

Harding, M.L., Steingold, R.F., Howard, L. & Steven, R.O. Measurement of knee ligament laxity. *J Bone Joint Surg* 1987; **69A**: 159.

Hart, D.P. & Dahners, L.E. Health of the MCL in rats. The effects of repair, motion and secondary stabilizing ligaments. *J Bone Joint Surg* 1987; **69A**: 1195–1199.

Hughston, J.C. & Norwood, L.A. The posterolateral drawer test and external rotational recurvatum test for posterolateral rotatory instability of the knee. *Clin Orthop* 1980; **147**: 82–87.

Hughston, J.C., Andrews, J.R., Cross, M.J., & Moschi, A. Classification of knee ligament instabilities. Part I: the medical compartment and cruciate ligaments. Part II: the lateral compartment. *J Bone Joint Surg* 1976; **58A**: 159–179.

Hughston, J.C., Walsh, W.M. & Puddu, G. *Patellar Subluxation and Dislocation*. WB Saunders: Philadelphia, 1984.

Indelicato, P.A. Non-operative treatment of complete tears of the medial collateral ligament of the knee. *J Bone Joint Surg* 1983; **65A**: 323–329.

Insall, J.N. *Surgery of the Knee*. Churchill Livingstone: Edinburgh, 1984.

Insall, J.N. & Hood, R.W. Bone-block transfer of the medial

head of the gastrocnemius of posterior cruciate insufficiency. *J Bone Joint Surg* 1982; **64A**: 691–699.

Ireland, J. & Phen, H.T. Arthroscopy in knees with chronic anterior cruciate instability. *J Bone Joint Surg* 1991; **73B**: Suppl. I: 61.

Ireland, J. & Trickey, E.L. MacIntosh tenodesis for anterolateral instability of the knee. *J Bone Joint Surg* 1980; **62B**: 340–345.

Irvine, G.B., Dias, J.J. & Finlay, D.B.L. Segond fractures of the lateral tibial condyle: brief report. *J Bone Joint Surg* 1987; **69B**: 613–614.

Jackson, J.P. Surgical anatomy. In: Jackson, J.P. & Waugh, W. (eds) *Surgery of the Knee Joint.* Chapman & Hall: London, 1984.

Jacobs, R.P. Observations on rotatory instability of the lateral compartment of the knee. *Acta Orthop Scand* 1981; **52**: Suppl. 191.

Jokl, P., Kaplan, N., Stovell, P. & Kegg, K. Non-operative treatment of severe injuries to the medial and cruciate ligaments of the knee. *J Bone Joint Surg* 1984; **66A**: 741–743.

Jones, J.R. & Allum, R.L. Acute traumatic haemarthrosis of the knee: expectant treatment or arthroscopy? *Ann R Coll Surg Engl* 1989; **71**: 40–43.

Jones, K.G. Reconstruction of the anterior cruciate ligament using the central one-third of the patella ligament. *J Bone Joint Surg* 1963; **45A**: 925–932.

Jones, K.G. Reconstruction of the anterior cruciate ligament using the central one third of the patella ligament. A follow-up report. *J Bone Joint Surg* 1970; **52A**: 1302–1308.

Kannus, P. & Jarvinen, M. Conservatively treated tears of the anterior cruciate ligament. *J Bone Joint Surg* 1987; **69A**: 1007–1012.

Kapandji, I.A. *The Physiology of Joints*, Vol. II. Churchill Livingstone: Edinburgh, 1970.

Kennedy, J.C. Complete dislocation of the knee joint. *J Bone Joint Surg* 1963; **45A**: 889–904.

Kennedy, J.C., Hawkins, R.J., Willis, R.B. & Danylchuk, K.D. Tension studies of the human knee ligaments. Yield point, ultimate failure and disruption of the cruciate and tibial collateral ligaments. *J Bone Joint Surg* 1976; **58A**: 350–355.

Kennedy, J.C., Stewart, R. & Walker, D.M. Anterolateral rotatory instability of the knee joint. *J Bone Joint Surg* 1978; **60A**: 1031–1039.

Learmonth, D.J.A., Howard, L., Johnson, G.V. & Harding, M.L. Single measurement of anterior knee stiffness in patients with absent anterior cruciate ligaments. *J Bone Joint Surg* 1991; **73B**: Suppl. I: 61.

Lemaire, M. Instabilité chronique du genou. *J Chir* (Paris) 1975; **110**: 281–294.

Levitsky, K.A., Berger, A., Nicholas, G.G., Vernick, C.G., Wilber, J.H. & Scagliotti, C.J. Bilateral open dislocation of the knee joint. *J Bone Joint Surg* 1988; **70A**: 1407–1409.

McDaniel, W.J. & Dameron, T.B. The untreated ACL rupture. *Clin Orthop* 1983; **172**: 158–163.

MacIntosh, D.L. & Darby, T.A. Lateral substitution reconstruction. *J Bone Joint Surg* 1976; **59B**: 142.

Maquet, P.G.T. Advancement of the tibial tuberosity. *Clin Orthop* 1976; **115**: 225.

Marya, S.K.S., Bhan, S. & Dave, P.K. Comparative study of knee function after petellectomy and osteosynthesis with a tension band wire following patellar fractures. *Int Surg* 1987; **72**: 211–213.

Meyers, M.H., Akeson, W. & Convery R. Resurfacing of the knee with fresh osteochondral allograft. *J Bone Joint Surg* 1989; **71A**: 704–713.

Miller, B.J. & LaRochelle, P.J. The treatment of patellofemoral pain by combined rotation and elevation of the tibial tubercle. *J Bone Joint Surg* 1986; **68A**: 419–423.

Minns, R.J., Betts, J.A., Muckle, D.S., Frank, P.L., Walker, D.I., Strover, A. & Hardinge, K. Carbon fibre arthroplasty of the knee: preliminary clinical experience in a new concept of biological resurfacing. In: Noble, J. & Galasko, C.S.B. (eds) *Recent Developments in Orthopaedic Surgery.* Manchester University Press: Manchester, 1987.

Minns, R.J., Muckle, D.S. & Donkin, J.E. The repair of osteochondral defects in osteoarthritic rabbit knees by the use of carbon fibre. *Biomaterials* 1982; **3**: 81–86.

Müller, W. *The Knee. Form, Function and Ligament Reconstruction.* Springer-Verlag: Berlin, 1983.

Nicholas, J.A. The five-one reconstruction for anteromedial instability of the knee. *J Bone Joint Surg* 1973; **55A**: 899–922.

Noyes, F.R. & Grood, E.S. Strength of the anterior cruciate ligament in humans and rhesus monkeys. Age and species related changes. *J Bone Joint Surg* 1976; **58A**: 1074–1082.

Noyes, F.R. & Grood, E.S. Diagnosis of knee ligament injuries: clinical concepts. In: Feagin, J.A. (ed.) *The Crucial Ligaments.* Churchill Livingstone, Edinburgh, 1988.

Noyes, F.R., Bassett, R.W., Grood, E.S. & Butler, D.L. Arthroscopy in acute traumatic haemarthrosis of the knee. Incidence of anterior cruciate tears and other injuries. *J Bone Joint Surg* 1980a; **62A**: 687–695.

Noyes, F.R., Grood, E.S., Butler, D.L. & Malek, M. Clinical laxity tests and functional stability of the knee: biomechanical concepts. *Clin Orthop* 1980b; **146**: 84–89.

Noyes, F.R., Grood, E.S., Sunway, W.J. & Butler, D.L. The three-dimensional laxity of the anterior cruciate deficient knee as determined by clinical laxity tests. *Iowa Orthop* 1983; **3**: 32–34.

Noyes, F.R., Mooar, L.A., Moorman, III, C.T. & McGinniss, G.H. Partial tears of the anterior cruciate ligament. *J Bone Joint Surg* 1989; **71B**: 825–833.

O'Brien, T., Hughes, F., Strover, A. & Mowbray, M. Prosthetic ACL reconstruction — biomechanical and functional performance. In: Williams, K.R. & Lesser, T.H. (eds) *Proceedings of the First International Conference on Interfaces in Medicine and Mechanics.* Dotesios, Rowbridge T, Wilts, 1989.

Odensten, M., Hamberg, P., Nordin, M., Lysholm, J. & Gillquist, J. Surgical or conservative treatment of the acutely torn ACL. A randomised study with short-term follow-up observation. *Clin Orthop* 1985; **198**: 87–93.

Odensten, M., Lysholm, J. & Gillquist, J. Suture of fresh ruptures of the anterior cruciate ligament. A five-year follow-up. *Acta Orthop Scand* 1984; **55**: 270–272.

O'Donnell, T.F., Brewster, D.C., Darling, R.C., Veen, H. & Waltman, A.A. Arterial injuries associated with fractures and/or dislocations of the knee. *J Trauma* 1977; **17**: 775–784.

O'Donoghue, D.H. Surgical treatment of fresh injuries to the major ligaments of the knee. *J Bone Joint Surg* 1950; **32A**: 721–738.

Palmer, I. On the injuries to the ligaments of the knee joint: a clinical study. *Acta Chir Scand Suppl* 1938; **81**: 53.

Patel, D. Superolateral/medial approach to arthroscopic meniscectomy. *Orthop Clin North Am* 1982; **13(2)**: 299–305.

Patel, K.R., Semel, L. & Claus, R.H. Extended reconstruction rate for limb salvage with intraoperative pre-reconstruction angiography. *J Vasc Surg* 1988; **7**: 531–538.

Rackemann, S., Robinson, A. & Dandy, D.J. Reconstruction of the anterior cruciate ligament with an intra-articular patellar tendon graft and an extra-articular tenodesis. *J Bone Joint Surg* 1991; **73B**: 368–373.

Reckling, F.W. & Peltier, L.F. Acute knee dislocations and their complications. *J Trauma* 1969; **9**: 181–191.

Roux. Luxation habituelle de la rotule; traitment operatoire. *Rev Chir Paris* 1888; **8**: 682–689.

Sandberg, R., Balkfors, B., Nilsson, B.O. & Westlin, N. Operative versus non-operative treatment of recent injuries to the ligaments of the knee. A prospective randomised study. *J Bone Joint Surg* 1987; **69A**: 1120–1126.

Segond, P. Recherches cliniques et expérimentales sur epanchements sanguins du genou par entorse. *Progrès Méd* 1879; **7**: 379–381.

Shino, K., Inoue, M., Horibe, S., Nagano, J. & Ono, K. Maturation of allograft tendons transplanted into the knee. *J Bone Joint Surg* 1988; **70B**: 556–560.

Sisto, D.J. & Warren, R.F. Complete knee dislocation. A follow-up study of operative treatment. *Clin Orthop* 1985; **198**: 94–101.

Slocum, N.B. & Larson, R.L. Rotatory instability of the knee. *J Bone Joint Surg* 1968; **50A**: 211–255.

Steadman, J.R. & Higgins, R.W. ACL injuries in the elite skier. In: Feagin, J.A. (ed.) *The Crucial Ligaments*. Churchill Livingstone: Edinburgh, 1988.

Stoker, D.J. *Knee Arthrography*. Chapman & Hall: London, 1980.

Torg, J.S., Conrad, W. & Kalen, V. Clinical diagnosis of ACL ligament instability in the athlete. *Am J Sports Med* 1976; **4**: 84–93.

Trickey, E.L. Rupture of the posterior cruciate ligament of the knee. *J Bone Joint Surg* 1968; **50**: 334–341.

Trickey, E.L. Acute ligamentous injuries. Chronic ligamentous injuries. In: Jackson, J.P. & Waugh, W. (eds) *Surgery of the Knee Joint*. Chapman & Hall: London, 1984.

Trillat, A. Posterolateral instability. In: Schultz, K.P., Krahl, H. & Stein, W.H. (eds) *Late Reconstruction of the Injured Ligaments of the Knee*. Springer-Verlag: New York, 1979.

Trillat, A., Dejour, H. & Bousquet, G. *Chirurgie du Genou. Troisième Jornées Lyonnaises*. Simep, Villeurbanne, 1977.

Van Dijk, R. *The Behaviour of the Cruciate Ligaments in the Human Knee*. PhD thesis: University of Nijmegen, 1983.

Walker, P.S. & Erkmann, M.J. The role of the meniscus in force transmission across the knee. *Clin Orthop* 1975; **109**: 184–192.

Wittek, A. Zur Nacht Kreuzbandverletzung im Kniegelenk. *Zentralbl Chir* 1927; **54**: 1538–1541.

23: The Leg

J.R.W.HARDY AND J.K.WEBB

Introduction

This chapter is divided into two sections; the first considers fractures of the upper tibial metaphysis in the adult and the second fractures of the tibial and fibular diaphyses. Fractures of the fibular shaft are considered in the introduction to the second part. Distal tibial and fibular metaphyseal injuries are considered in Chapter 24.

Upper tibial metaphyseal fractures

J.R.W.HARDY

Introduction

For practical purposes, the upper metaphysis of the tibia is best described as the part, defined by a square, whose sides are the same length as the widest part of the epiphysis (Fig. 23.1). Fractures of the upper tibial metaphysis are uncommon. They occur mostly in the elderly, after high-energy trauma to the knee, as in bumper injuries, and only rarely as a result of sport (Hohl 1974). The fractures nearly always involve the joint, which makes management in the young different from that in the elderly, in whom late complications may be resolved by arthroplasty.

Fractures of the upper metaphysis commonly involve the lateral tibial condyle. The tibial condyles may not be involved at all or they may both be involved. Fracture of the lateral tibial condyle is caused by a valgus force at the knee with the foot well planted on the ground. In the young, a low-energy injury usually results in a medial collateral ligament injury, whereas a fall from a height results in a condylar fracture. Collateral ligament injury in association with condylar fracture is well recognized (Martin 1960). In the elderly, even a minor fall may result in the lateral condyle being broken or crushed. The medial tibial condyle, if involved, remains attached to the pes anserinus and mostly breaks with the tibial spines attached.

The pattern of fracture, which forms the basis of some classifications, is due not only to the force applied but also to the underlying condition of the bone. The tibial condyles are predominantly cancellous bone, which means fractures are comminuted and/or impacted. With fractures of this type, treatment that causes distraction prevents union (Charnley 1961).

Clinical features

Diagnosis

The history is usually that either of an elderly person being knocked down, or of a younger patient sustaining a bumper injury about the knee. Pain and the inability to weight-bear are the predominating symptoms.

Examination of the knee may show it to have a valgus deformity with a graze, swelling and bruising. Tenderness may be localized over the side of the fractured condyle and over a damaged ligament on the contralateral side.

Radiographs

Anteroposterior, lateral and oblique radiographs of the knee are enough to define the extent of injury in those to be treated conservatively (Moore & Harvey 1974). Following fracture, tomograms are difficult to obtain but computerized axial tomography (CAT) for tibial plateau fracture is less painful and useful in classifying the fracture (Dias *et al.* 1987). To make the diagnosis in patients with suspected tibial spine fractures, a tunnel view may be required when a haemarthrosis is discovered.

Classification

Many patterns of injury are found in the upper tibial metaphysis and these make it difficult to devise a classification that is a guide to treatment protocol. The Association for Osteosynthesis (AO) classification divides proximal tibial fractures into those not involving the condyles (non-articular), fractures of the lateral tibial condyle and fractures of both condyles.

Non-articular fractures include those of the tibial spines, tibial tubercle, intercondylar eminence, and the subcondylar fractures from the rare Segond fracture (Fig. 23.2) (Irvine *et al.* 1987) to the comminuted tibial metaphyseal injury. Tibial spine fractures have been classified by Meyers and McKeever, who found an association with other injuries, particularly medial collateral ligament injury (Meyers & McKeever 1959, 1970) (Fig. 23.3).

Fractures of the condyles can be classified according to type (Hohl & Luck 1956), degree of fracture displacement (Bick 1941, Roberts 1968, Apley 1979), alignment (Honkonen & Järvinen 1992) or anatomical type (Palmer 1951). Schatzker (1979) divided condylar fractures into those occurring in the medial condyle, those in the lateral condyle and those involving both condyles. The most commonly used classification of articular fractures is that devised by Hohl, following a review of 805 patients with this injury (Hohl 1967). He divided the fractures into those that had minimum fracture impaction or displacement (i.e. less than 3 mm), defined as undisplaced, and those with more than 3 mm impaction or displacement, divided according to the pattern of injury (Fig. 23.4). Hohl later revised his definition of the undisplaced fracture by describing minimal displacement as less than 4 mm of depression (Hohl 1984). A comprehensive classification that includes fracture—dislocations as well as the usual condylar injuries has been described by Moore (1981). Moore's classification of fracture—dislocations is divided into five types. These are split fracture, entire plateau fracture, rim avulsion, rim compression and four-part fracture. Finally, the newest classification is that of the AO/ASIF foundation (Müller *et al.* 1991). It is an amalgamation of nearly all the previous classifications, although it has missed out the Segond fracture.

Treatment

The treatment of tibial plateau fractures is either conservative or surgical and, as with most orthopaedic injuries, depends on the requirements of the patient, type of fracture, presence of significant displacement or

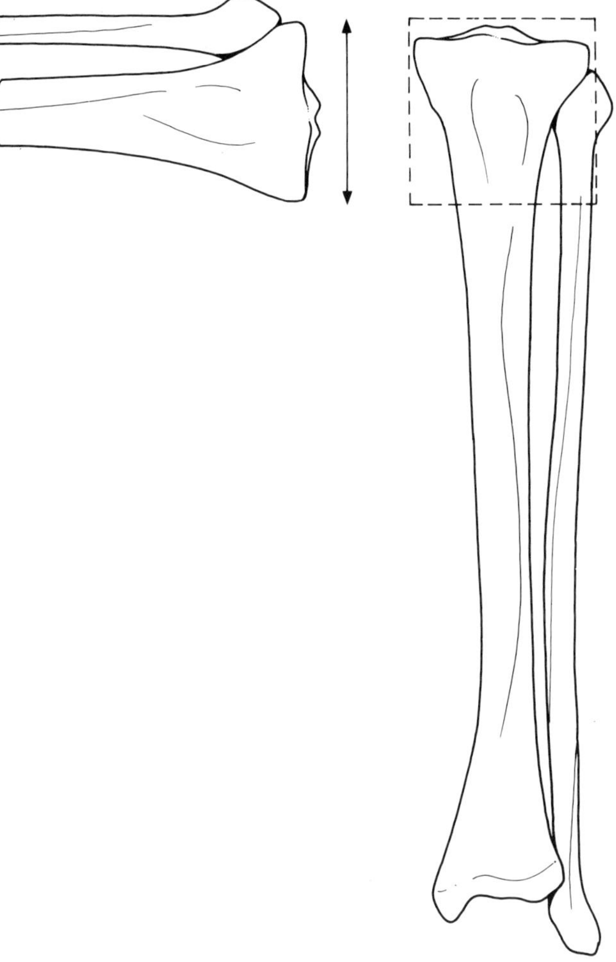

Fig. 23.1 The upper tibial metaphysis is defined by a square, whose sides are the same length as the widest part of the epiphysis.

complications, general condition of the patient, condition of the skin around the knee, age of the patient, aetiology of the underlying fracture and subsequent symptoms.

Depressed fractures of 5 mm or less treated conservatively may lead to instability and deformity, although the deformity is often minimal. Depressions of 5—10 mm lead to noticeable deformity and instability, and depression greater than 10 mm results in an unstable knee.

Conservative treatment

Conservative treatment is indicated in undisplaced fractures, minimally displaced fractures (i.e. those less than 4 mm), some moderately displaced fractures (i.e. those between 4 and 8 mm), fractures in patients over 65 years old with osteoporotic bone and in debilitated patients.

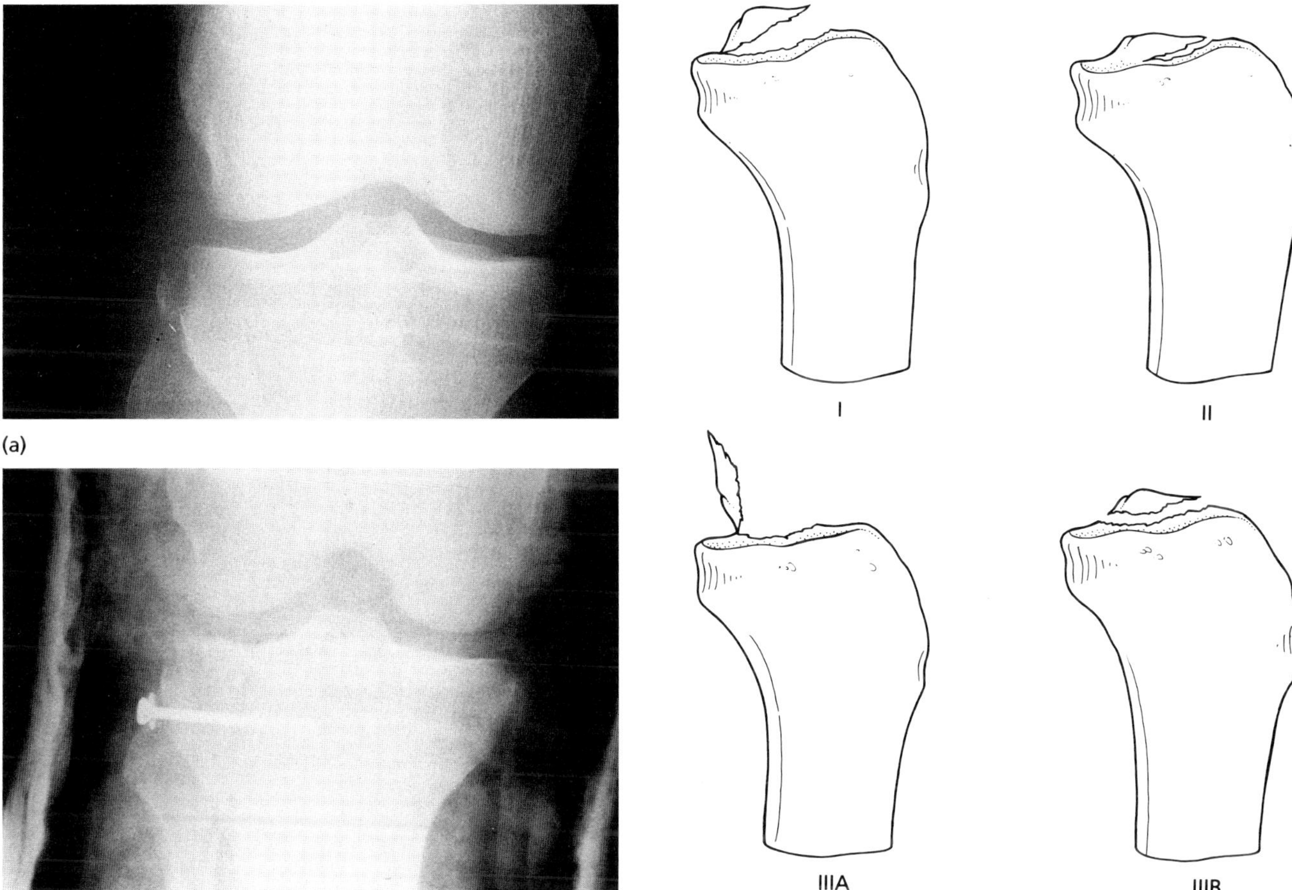

(a)

(b)

Fig. 23.2 Radiographs of a Segond fracture, not involving the joint, (a) before and (b) after fixation with a screw and washer.

Fig. 23.3 Classification of intercondylar eminence fractures. (Redrawn from Myers, M.H. & McKeever, F.M. Fractures of the intercondylar eminence of the tibia. *J Bone Joint Surg* 1970; **52A**: 1677–1684.)

The goal is to return knee function to a range of movement as near normal as possible. Extension is important, and may be almost guaranteed when the initial treatment maintains extension, as with immobilization in a plaster cylinder or traction. Most fractures should be examined for ligamentous injury with the patient under anaesthetic. A displaced, partial articular fracture of the pure split type may often be reduced by manipulation under anaesthetic with direct pressure on the lateral side, forcing it up and medially. Use of a large pair of reduction forceps or a few taps with a mallet over a bandaged knee sometimes helps. A haemarthrosis can be aspirated for comfort. Following reduction, the tendency to valgus displacement should be prevented with a full-length plaster or, preferably, a Thomas' splint (Charnley 1961) with graduation to knee flexion at 3–4 weeks using Perkins traction on a Hadfield split bed. The Denham pin for skeletal traction should not be placed within 2.5 cm of the lowest limit of the fracture

haematoma so that it cannot cause infection. The use of Simonis low friction swivel reduces pin site infections caused by pin–skin movement (Fig. 23.5). The cast is removed after 3–4 weeks, and thereafter treatment is by active exercise in a cast brace. Too early a return to weight-bearing can result in progressive deformity of the fracture, especially during the first few weeks after fracture. Thus, the patient should be re-examined frequently, clinically and with radiographs, in the first 3 months after fracture.

When a depressed fracture with fragmentation has occurred, it is near impossible to restore the articular surface with conservative management. Further displacement is unlikely as the forces induced by treatment are small compared with the force of fracture. If, because of the age and condition of the patient, the deformity is acceptable, then immobilization is avoided in favour of active and passive movement of the knee from as early as possible after fracture (Gausewitz & Hohl 1983). At

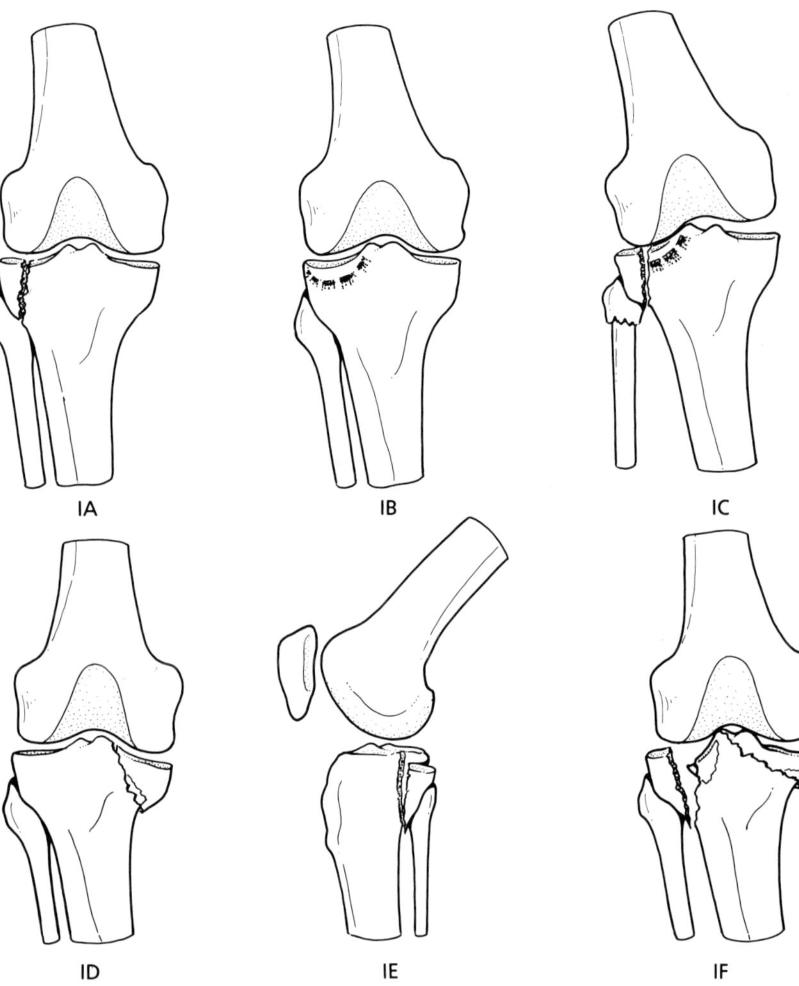

Fig. 23.4 Classification of tibial condylar fractures. (Redrawn from Hohl, M. Tibial condylar fractures. *J Bone Joint Surg* 1967; **49A**: 1455–1467.)

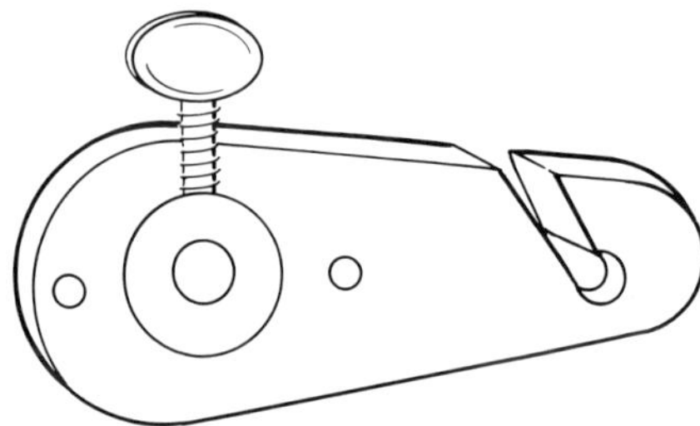

Fig. 23.5 The Simonis low-friction swivel.

night the limb may be rested in a back slab. If, following rehabilitation, the patient remains symptomatic, then arthroplasty may be considered. In those patients who are too debilitated for arthroplasty some symptoms may be controlled using walking aids and knee braces.

The prognosis for undisplaced tibial fractures is generally good, except in those with undiagnosed and unrepaired grade III ligament injury. Instability of a knee may result from either residual depression of a condyle or unrepaired ligament injury, or both, and repair of both is important in preventing late instability.

Surgical treatment

Surgical treatment is indicated in significantly displaced fractures (i.e. those with more than 8 mm depression) and moderately displaced fractures which, on examination with the patient under anaesthetic, demonstrate more than 5° of saggital laxity, even in extension. Surgery should also be considered in those under the age of 60 where the late complications of pain and instability are preferably not managed with arthroplasty. Hohl also recommends the repair of ruptured ligaments at the same time as open reduction and internal fixation (Hohl 1967).

Tibial spine fractures may benefit from arthroscopy, which helps classify the injury, allows accurate diagnosis of other intra-articular injuries, drains a haemarthrosis and removes loose fragments. Type I tibial spine fractures (Fig. 23.3) are effectively treated conservatively. Those classified as type II or III may be treated arthroscopically by reduction and immobilization with K-wires or small fragment cannulated screws. Open reduction is occasionally necessary, especially for avulsion of the posterior cruciate associated with a posterior capsule tear. Kendall *et al.* reviewed 31 patients of all ages treated variously and came to the conclusion that those injuries with associated intra-articular fractures or meniscal tears had the worse prognosis. They suggested that arthroscopy was useful for both diagnosis and treatment (Kendall *et al.* 1992). Avulsion of the tibial spine with the posterior or anterior cruciate ligament should be reduced and fixed with a screw when closed reduction has failed. The reduced fracture should

be protected in a plaster cast for 6 weeks in adults and 4 weeks in children, after which protected limited motion may be started.

Tibial condylar fractures should first be examined under anaesthesia and using image intensification to deduce the presence of a ligament tear. A grade III ligament rupture should be repaired if the condylar fracture is either displaced or undisplaced. Likewise, if a peripheral meniscal lesion is found associated with a condylar fracture it is recommended that it be repaired. A fracture depression of the central portion of a condyle can be elevated only by surgical means.

The approach for these injuries depends on the side of the major fragment. Lateral compression fractures should be approached through a lateral incision beginning from the femoral condylar attachment of the lateral

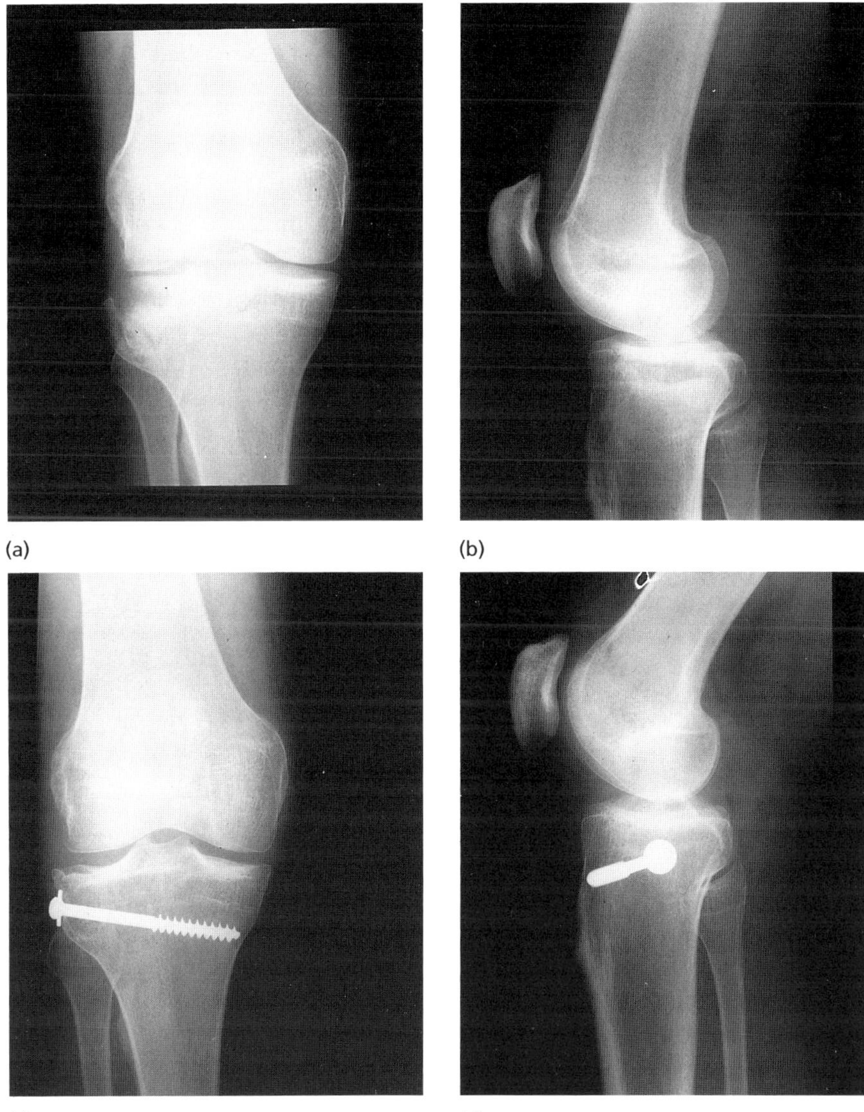

(a)

(b)

(c)

(d)

Fig. 23.6 (a)–(d) The split depressed fracture (1c from Hohl's classification) fixed by elevation grafting and a lag screw.

collateral ligament curving the incision to be just lateral to the patellar tendon. The incision should be deepened into the joint beneath the lateral meniscus, which can be elevated to reveal the lateral tibial condyle. Central-depressed fractures of the condyle are elevated through a cortical window cut with an osteotome in the flare of the metaphyseal part of the bone. A bone punch is used to separate the fragments and raise them level with the joint margins. The space that results is filled with corticocancellous graft from the ileum.

The split and depressed fracture fragments may be elevated by levering out the split fragment and elevating the depressed portions with a small osteotome. The split fragment is replaced and held with either a transverse lag screw into the opposite cortex or a plate and screws (Fig. 23.6a–d). Screws should not be used from anterior to posterior for fear of damaging the neurovascular structures behind the knee. Split fractures on their own that are not reducible manually are easily reduced by open operation and internal fixation. Occasionally, they may be reduced and held percutaneously using the new Richards cannulated screws (Smith & Nephew Richards, Memphis, USA) (Fig. 23.7a–c). As there is a tendency for depression of a raised tibial plateau fracture with weight-bearing, this should be avoided for at least 6 weeks after operation. After 3 weeks, rehabilitation of a range of movement may take place in a cast brace.

Comminuted and subcondylar fractures may be restored with a blade plate or a buttress plate and screws (Fig. 23.8a & b). Severely comminuted fractures tend to do best when treated by manipulation under anaesthetic, moulding and setting up in traction to prevent as much angular deformity as possible. The traction should be maintained for at least 6 weeks.

Prognosis

Poor prognosis following this injury is because of a loss of range of motion, persistent deformity, instability, loss of extension, pain from arthritis and weakness.

Hohl and Luck (1956) have suggested that the limitation of motion following fracture is because of the adhesions that develop between the fracture site and the retropatellar fat pad when a knee is immobilized. It has also been shown that prolonged immobilization increases the time for maximum recovery of motion and limits the degree of eventual recovery (Solonen 1963).

The paper by Honkonen and Järvinen (1992), which compared their combination of classifications with two others, found little difference between the conservatively treated and operated patients at a mean of 7 years

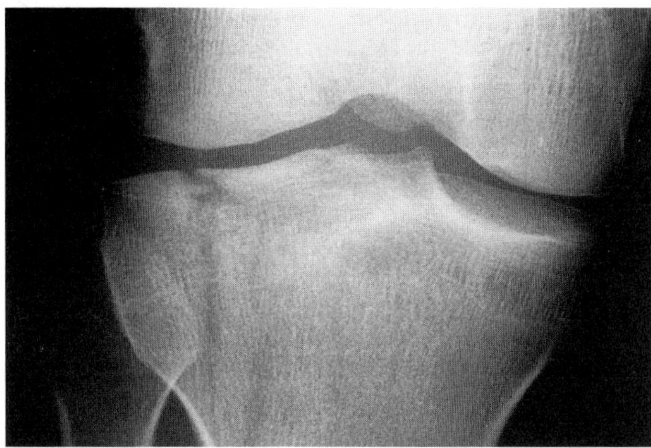

(a)

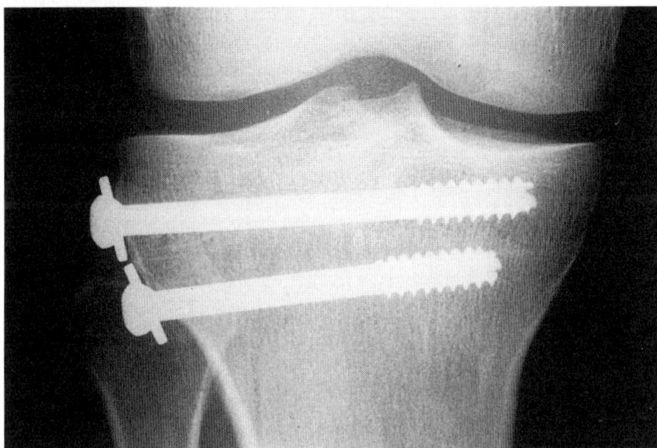

(b)

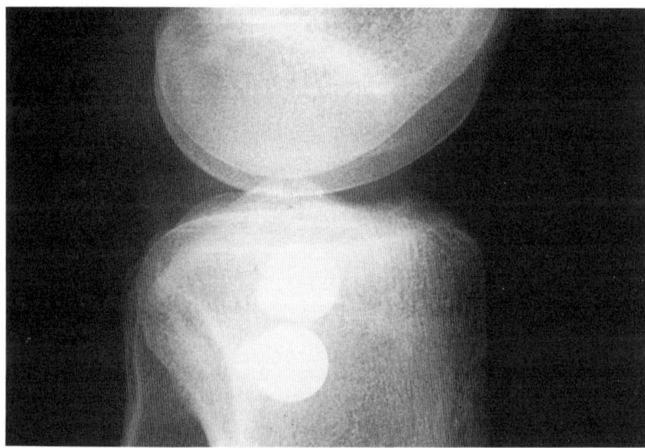

(c)

Fig. 23.7 (a)–(c) Split fracture of the lateral tibial condyle reduced and held by percutaneous screws over guide wire.

follow-up. They did show that a knee with a medial tilt fared worse than a knee with the same degree of lateral tilt on functional and subjective tests. The bigger the deformity the more significant the difference between the varus and valgus knees. On this basis an operative

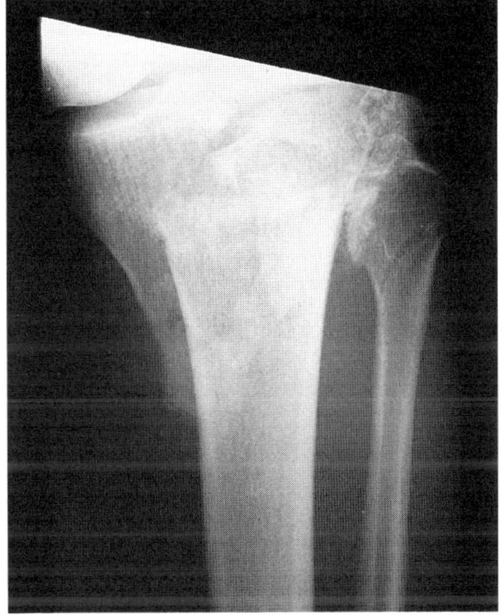
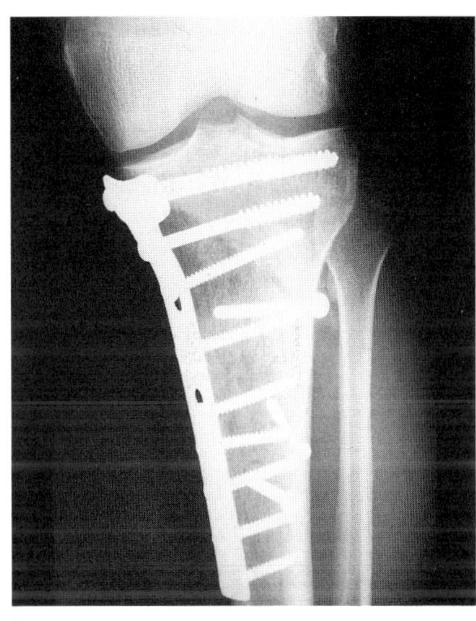

Fig. 23.8 (a) and (b) A comminuted bicondylar fracture (1f from Hohl's classification) fixed with a buttress plate and screws.

approach should be advised for those patients in whom operative reduction and immobilization will improve alignment. Correction of the angular deformity at the knee may also slow the inevitable progress towards osteoarthritis, although there is no evidence for this. It does, however, make late arthroplasty more easy.

Instability can be due to persistent depression of a condyle, loss of joint space owing to arthritic wear, ligamentous injury or all these factors. Operative open reduction and internal fixation and repair of grade III ligamentous injuries should prevent instability, except for that due to arthritic changes.

Loss of extension occurs with prolonged immobilization with the knee in a position of flexion. This may be due to adhesions or contracture of the posterior joint capsule. Muscle wasting as a result of immobilization rarely recovers fully.

Subcondylar fractures have a better prognosis. Late-onset osteoarthritis may be associated with injury to the condyles, but with restoration of good alignment the effects of the articular changes are not usually disabling.

References

Apley, A.G. Fractures of the tibial plateau. *Orthop Clin North Am* 1979; **10**: 61−74.

Bick, E.M. Fractures of the tibial condyles. *J Bone Joint Surg* 1941; **23**: 102−108.

Charnley, J. *The Closed Treatment of Common Fractures* 3rd edn. Churchill Livingstone: Edinburgh, 1961.

Dias, J.J., Stirling, A.J., Finlay, D.B.L. & Gregg, P.J. Computerised axial tomography for tibial plateau fractures. *J Bone Joint Surg* 1987; **69B**: 84−88.

Gausewitz, S.H. & Hohl, M. The significance of early motion in the treatment of tibial plateau fractures. *Orthop Trans* 1983; **7**: 68−69.

Hohl, M. Tibial condylar fractures. *J Bone Joint Surg* 1967; **49A**: 1455−1467.

Hohl, M. Tibial condylar fractures: Long-term followup. *Tex Med* 1974; **70**: 46−56.

Hohl, M. Fractures and dislocations of the knee. In: Rockwood, C.A. & Green, D.P. (eds) *Fractures in Adults* 2nd edn. Lippincott: Philadelphia, 1984.

Hohl, M. & Luck, J. Fractures of the tibial condyle: A clinical and experimental study. *J Bone Joint Surg* 1956; **38A**: 1001−1018.

Honkonen, S.E. & Järvinen, M.J. Classification of fractures of the tibial condyles. *J Bone Joint Surg* 1992; **74B**: 840−847.

Irvine, G.B., Dias, J.J. & Finlay, D.B.L. Segond fractures of the lateral tibial condyle: Brief report. *J Bone Joint Surg* 1987; **69B**: 613−614.

Kendall, N.S., Hsu, S.Y.C. & Chan, K.M. Fracture of the tibial spine in adults and children. *J Bone Joint Surg* 1992; **74B**: 848−852.

Martin, A.F. The pathomechanics of the knee joint. I The medial collateral ligament and lateral tibial plateau fractures. *J Bone Joint Surg* 1960; **42A**: 13−22.

Meyers, M.H. & McKeever, F.M. Fracture of the intercondylar eminence of the tibia. *J Bone Joint Surg* 1959; **41A**: 209−222.

Meyers, M.H. & McKeever, F.M. Fracture of the intercondylar eminence of the tibia: Follow-up note. *J Bone Joint Surg* 1970; **52A**: 1677−1684.

Moore, T.M. Fracture−dislocation of the knee. *Clin Orthop* 1981; **156**: 128−140.

Moore, T.M. & Harvey, J.P. Jr. Roentgenographic measurement of tibial-plateau depression due to fracture. *J Bone Joint Surg* 1974; **56A**: 155−160.

Müller, M.E., Allgöwer, M., Schneider, R. & Willenegger, H. *Manual of Internal Fixation* 3rd edn. Springer-Verlag: Berlin, 1991.

Palmer, I. Fractures of the upper end of the tibia. *J Bone Joint Surg* 1951; **33B**: 160−166.

Roberts, J.M. Fractures of the condyles of the tibia: An anatomical and clinical end-result study of one hundred cases. *J Bone Joint Surg* 1968; **50A**: 1505–1521.

Schatzker, J., McBroom, R. & Bruce, D. The tibial plateau fracture: The Toronto experience 1968–1975. *Clin Orthop* 1979; **138**: 94–104.

Solonen, K.A. Fractures of the tibial condyles. *Acta Orthop Scand* 1963; **63** (Suppl): 1–32.

Tibial and fibular diaphyseal fractures

J.K.WEBB AND J.R.W.HARDY

Introduction

The diaphyses of the tibia and fibula include only the shafts of these bones (Fig. 23.9). While fractures of the fibula only are relatively easy to manage, fractures of the tibia are accompanied by a high complication rate. This is in contrast to metaphyseal fractures, which mostly heal without complication. Most of this section will therefore deal with the management of tibial fractures but will include a foreword on fibular fractures.

Fibular diaphyseal fractures, without fracture of the tibia, usually arise from low-energy injury and occur either following a direct blow, as with the night stick injury of the ulna, or in association with a torsional injury to the ankle. The former are transverse or comminuted injuries. The latter are spiral fractures, the treatment of which depends on that of the ankle injury. Transverse fibular fractures occurring on their own can be managed conservatively with a crepe bandage and crutches, allowing the patient to increase weight-bearing as comfort allows. A fracture of the proximal third can be complicated by a common peroneal nerve injury. Fractures of the tibia without an associated fracture of the fibula are usually caused by low-energy injury and this is an indication that healing of the tibial fracture will usually be uncomplicated. Occasionally, an intact fibula may interfere with the healing of the tibial fracture, especially if an anatomical reduction of the tibia has not been achieved. This is probably because in this situation the fibula acts to hold the fracture apart. Some clinicians would advise the routine osteotomy of the fibula at the time of surgery for a severe tibial fracture, although no randomized trial has been performed to confirm the benefit of this extra procedure (Bone & Johnson 1986). One interesting observation to bear in mind is that fractures of the fibula at a different level to that of the tibia may be associated with a higher refracture rate (Böstman 1983). This has obvious medicolegal implications when considering the prognosis of a

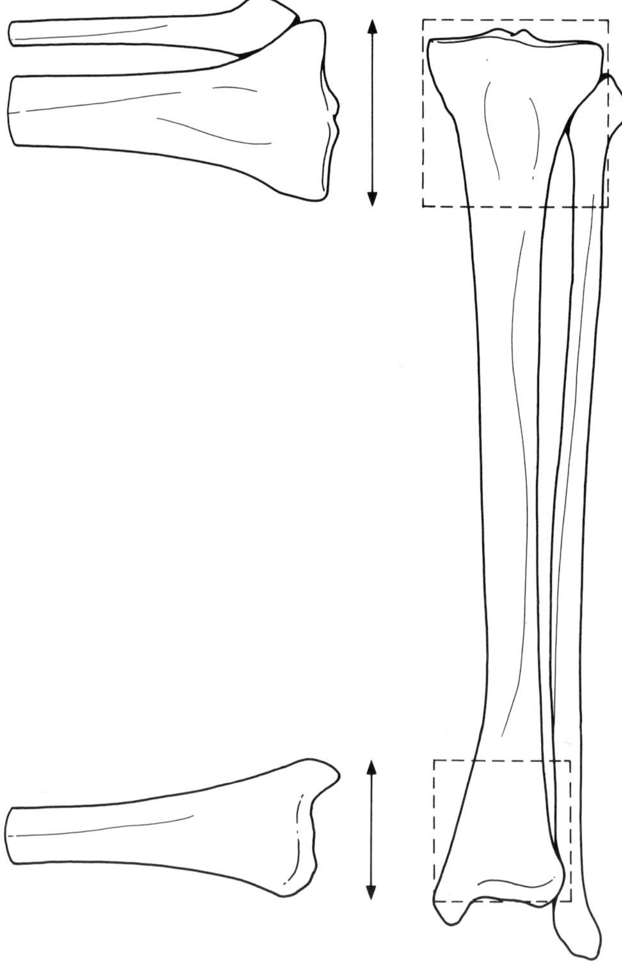

Fig. 23.9 The diaphysis is that part of the bone that excludes the upper and lower metaphysis.

patient with this injury. Delayed union of a fibular fracture in association with tibial fracture is rare as most have healed within 6–8 weeks of the injury (Böstman & Kyrö 1991). When both bones are fractured, the fibular fracture tends to be treated incidentally. Management of the tibial fracture becomes more important as it is the major weight-bearing bone.

Fractures of the tibial diaphysis are common. An accurate prospective survey in Leicester, England, showed 142 adult patients with tibial fractures admitted to one unit over 12 months. This was from a population of 918 549. The average age of the patient admitted with this injury was 37 years (range 16–94). The injury occurs most commonly in men. In Leicester, the commonest cause of injury was sport (38.6%), in particular football (33%) (Fig. 23.10). The national incidence for this injury is not available. These age and sex statistics are bound to vary geographically, as is the commonest aetiology of the condition.

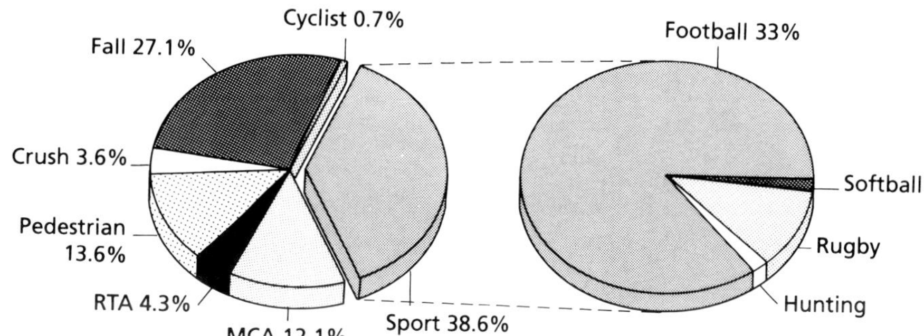

Fig. 23.10 A survey in Leicester showed that the commonest cause of tibial fractures was sport.

While trauma incurred on the football pitch and being knocked down by a vehicle are the commonest causes, other less common predisposing factors, such as tumour, infection, metabolic causes and stress fractures, seen in road runners and the military, must not be forgotten (Kuusela 1984, Micheli 1986).

Clinicians who attach as much importance to clinical examination as to looking at the initial radiographs will know that this injury involves damage to the soft tissues as well as to the bone. In most cases, the aim of management is to return the limb to its normal function by early restoration of weight-bearing, maintaining length and alignment while preventing the complications of malunion, delayed union, non-union or infection. Today's image-conscious patient is in the market for a return to normal with as little functional loss and deformity as possible. Unlike residual deformity of the femur, residual deformity of the tibia is much more noticeable. Shortening of more than 1 cm tends to be unacceptable, especially if the fractured limb was congenitally the shorter of the two limbs before fracture. An angulatory deformity of greater than 10° is noticeable clinically (Nicoll 1964). The effect on the line of weight-bearing through the ankle joint depends on the level of the deformity, as a high fracture has a greater effect than a low fracture. A radiographic assessment of angulation should take into account the effect of rotation, which is a much more noticeable and distressing deformity from the patient's viewpoint. For an accurate calculation from radiographs of the actual deformity, measure the angulation on each of the anteroposterior and lateral radiographs, then calculate the square root of the sum of the angles squared. The radiographs must be taken at 90° to each other. For small angles this gives an accurate estimate of the actual angulation at the fracture site.

Mechanisms of injury and fracture healing

The healing of a fracture in the tibial diaphysis depends firstly on the condition of the tissues, and therefore the mechanism of injury, and secondly on the method of immobilization of the fracture site. The pattern of injury seen in a fracture of the tibia depends on the magnitude of the injuring load, rate of loading, type of loading, structure of the tibia and surrounding soft tissues, and the material properties of the bone and soft tissues. The same energy injury may produce a different pattern of injury in an osteoporotic old person from that of an athletic young person.

The pattern of injury tells the surgeon something about the type of load that caused the fracture. A spiral fracture results from indirect injury and is caused by a torsional force. It is estimated that it requires 50% less force to break the bone in torsion than in bending (Oni 1988). A simple transverse fracture occurs with a bending load, and an oblique fracture occurs with bending while the bone is in compression. With a rapid rate or higher magnitude of loading comes comminution of the bone. Low-energy injuries of the tibia heal on average in 16 weeks when assessed by independent weight-bearing. High-energy injuries take much longer to heal (Ellis 1958a).

The best example of how a fracture heals is observed on the serial radiographs of a fracture sustained as a result of a low-energy bending injury. The patient is admitted with a transverse, displaced fracture with little swelling or bruising. With the patient under anaesthetic, the fracture is reduced by manipulation. The periosteal or soft tissue hinge is felt to be intact on at least two of the three surfaces of the tibia. If the fracture is stable to shortening it is treated in a plaster cast and the reduction maintained against the soft tissue hinge using the three-point fixation technique described by Sir John Charnley (Fig. 23.11). The patient with this pattern of injury may be encouraged to weight-bear early, as comfort allows. The fracture heals by passing through the three well-recognized phases of fracture healing: inflammation, reparation and, finally, remodelling (Fig. 23.12). The size of the callus is dependent on movement at the fracture site. Nature provides the callus to prevent the

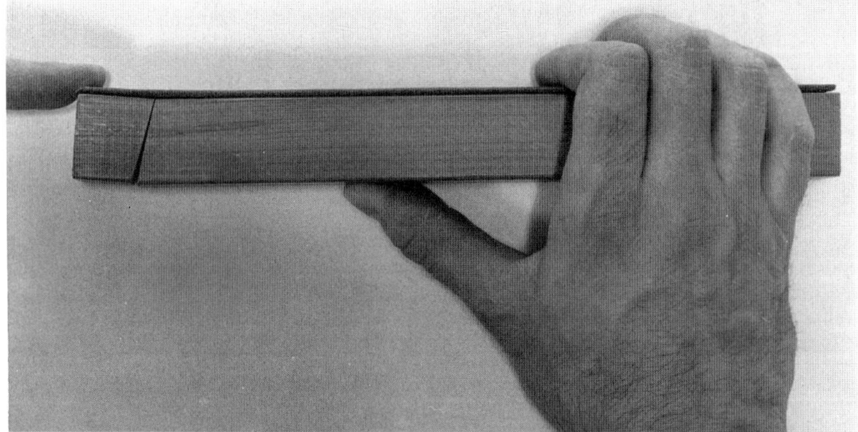

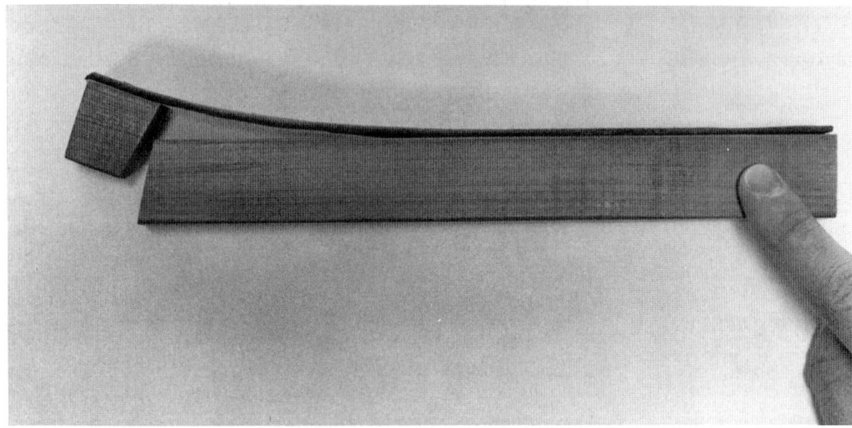

Fig. 23.11 The soft tissue hinge as described by Charnley to maintain the reduction of distal radial fractures can be used to maintain the reduction of a tibial fracture with three-point moulding of the plaster cast.

abnormal movement between the bone ends; in its usual efficient way it provides as much callus as is required to stop the abnormal movement and no more. Persistence of the abnormal movement in the presence of a healthy periosteum may cause a hypertrophic non-union (Fig. 23.13). The current hypothesis is that it is the size of the initial haematoma that determines the ultimate size of the callus (Hulth 1989). Clinical practice shows that when a patient with a transverse displaced fracture is treated by using rigid external fixation, or even more rigid internal fixation with a compression plate, then little callus forms and healing is by remodelling of the lamellar bone (Hutzschenreuter *et al.* 1969, Rahn *et al.* 1971, Perren 1979). The same patient treated in plaster, a less rigid unilateral external fixator or an intramedullary nail heals by the production of external callus.

All modern treatments carry complication risks peculiar to the particular treatment (Fig. 23.14), so any treatment can be justified so long as the surgeon has the necessary level of competence and expertise to reduce the risks of the procedure and the surgeon knows that the correct facilities are available for the procedure

proposed. It is the surgeon's duty to the patient to produce informed consent, discussing with the patient all the options and common complications. This means giving some estimate of the average time to removal of the support. As with all techniques, the best advice for surgeons is to use the method of reduction and immobilization with which they are most familiar and which, given the circumstances, is associated with the lowest risks of complication. However, if an unfamiliar immobilization technique is indicated, there is no excuse for not asking a colleague who is proficient in that method to help out.

Clinical features

The management of this injury requires an accurate diagnosis of the severity of injury and choice of the most appropriate treatment for the severity of injury.

Rarely will the orthopaedic trainee have the chance to manage the patient from the time of injury. Primary first aid will have been administered by the ambulance crew, paramedic or doctor from the flying squad. Each should have taken steps to reduce the fracture, if the

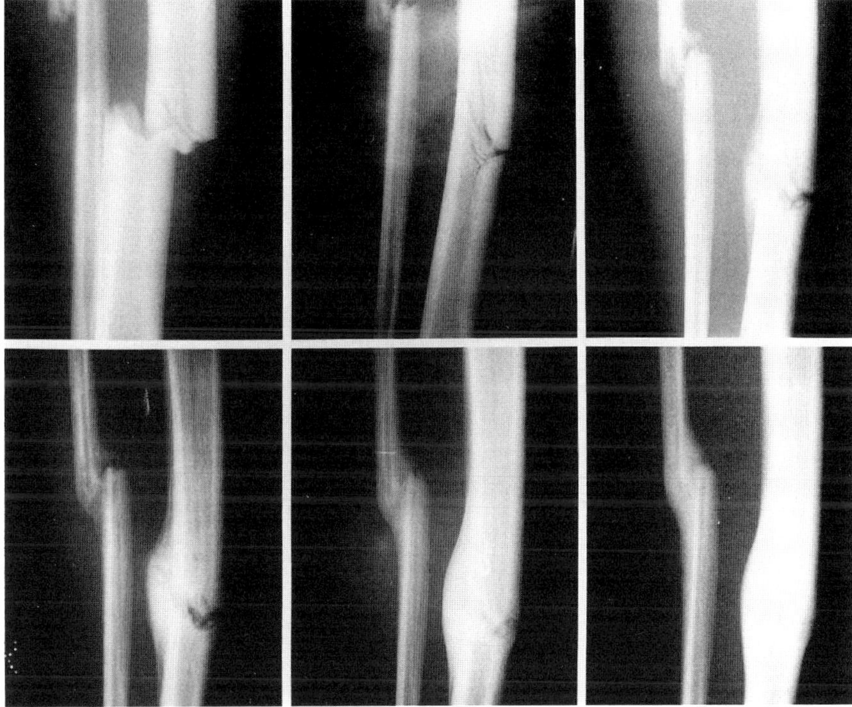

Fig. 23.12 Radiographs depicting the normal healing of a fracture. Top, left to right: displaced shortened fracture; same fracture following reduction; and callus at 8 weeks on the lateral surface. Bottom, left to right: the callus enlarges in response to weight bearing; the medial surface is bridged; and the remodelled fracture site at 1 year from injury.

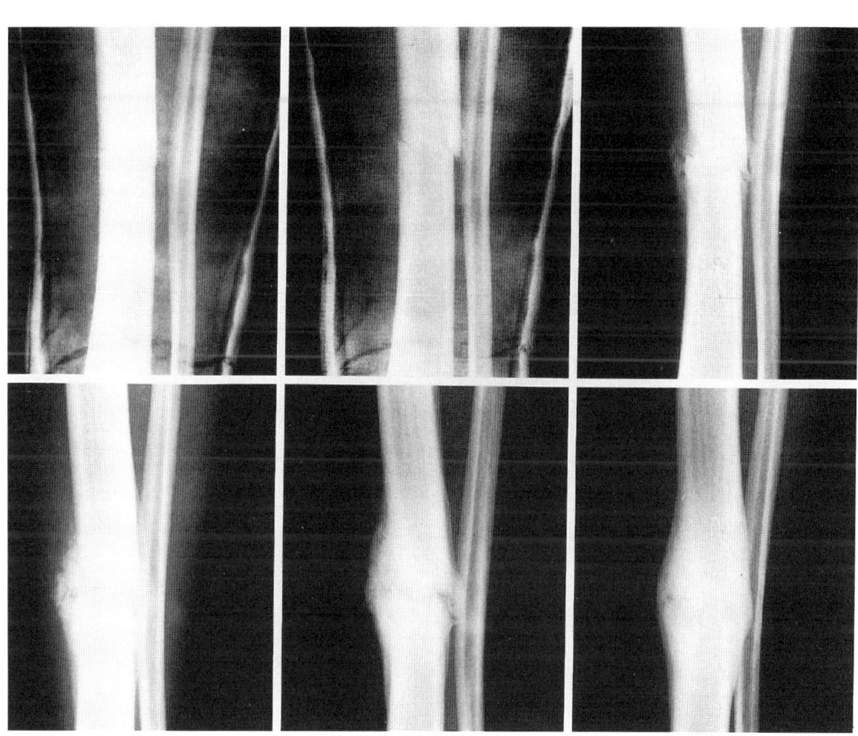

Fig. 23.13 Radiographs depicting hypertrophic delayed union. Top, left to right: an undisplaced fracture with intact fibula; endochondrial calcification seen at 6 weeks; further calcification but lack of bridge at 10 weeks. Bottom, left to right: abundant callus on both surfaces with fracture line running to periphery of callus bridges at 20 weeks; weight bearing reduced using crutches allows peripheral bridging; remodelling taking place 30 weeks after fracture.

skin integrity is threatened, cover a compound fracture with an iodophor-soaked dressing, and splint the fracture to prevent further soft tissue injury (Fig. 23.15).

Diagnosis

The resuscitation of a multiply injured patient takes priority over the management of the tibial fracture.

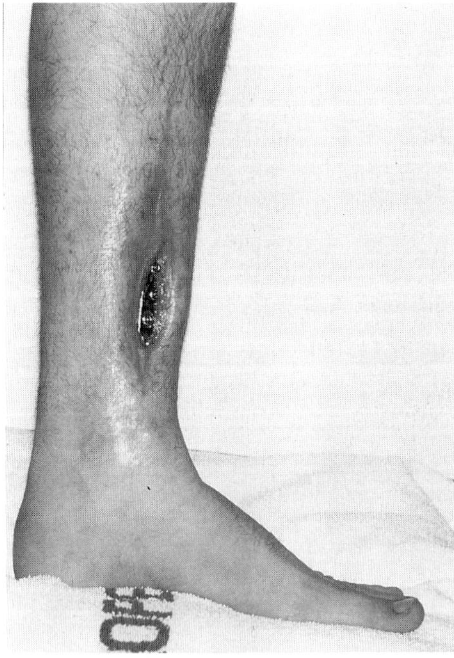

Fig. 23.14 Wound breakdown over a plate with underlying osteomyelitis following ORIF of a closed tibial fracture.

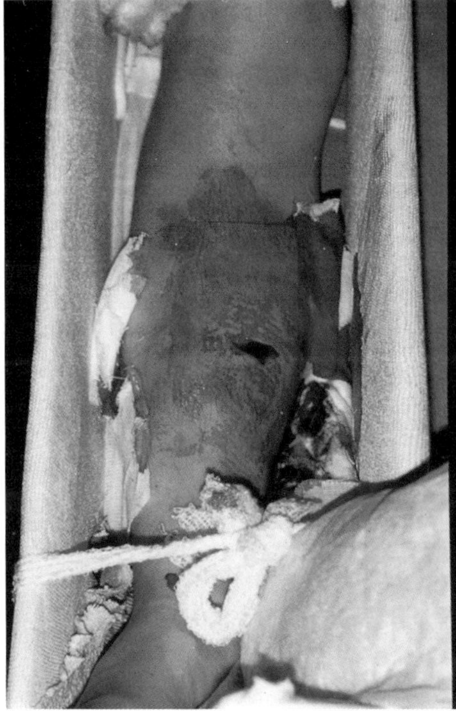

Fig. 23.15 Compound tibial fracture being undressed in the theatre for the first time since admission.

A full history should be taken. In particular, a history of the mechanism of injury should be sought from the patient or, if this is not possible, from eyewitness accounts of the accident. The patient's occupation and any coexisting illness should be ascertained as this will influence the method of treatment. Having established the level of energy involved in the accident one should compare this with the clinical examination findings.

Examination of the limb should include an assessment of the neurovascular status. The popliteal artery is anchored as it passes beneath the band that is the origin of the soleus muscle in the upper third of the tibia (Fig. 23.16). It is here that it may be damaged by the trauma of the accident or by the injudicious use of a drill or screw during open reduction and internal fixation. The posterior tibial, anterior tibial or peroneal arteries may be divided by the sharp edge of the fractured tibia on its way through the tissues in high-energy injuries. Likewise, the nerves of the leg may be damaged by the direct trauma or by the sharp edge of the broken tibia or a concomitant fibular fracture. Compartment syndrome should be suspected if the patient's pain is out of proportion to the injury, its splintage, and the amount of analgesia received. Clinical signs include a tense limb, inability of the patient to extend or flex the toes,

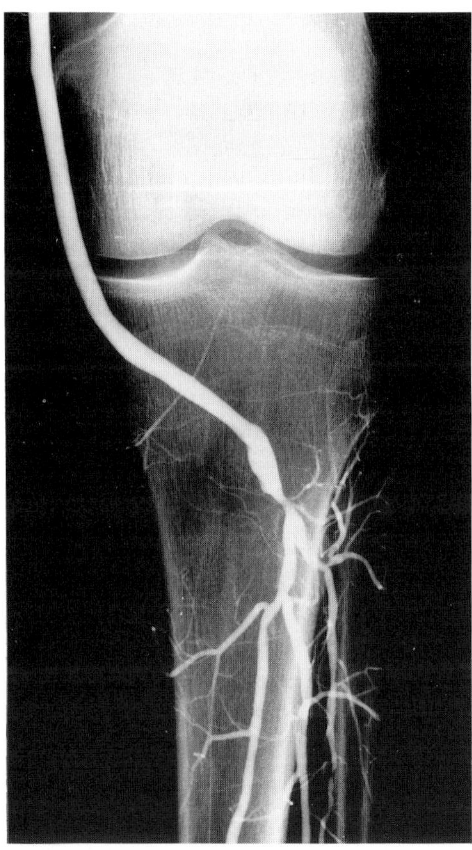

Fig. 23.16 Rare stricture of the popliteal artery at the soleal line demonstrating where the artery is anchored by the origin of soleus muscle.

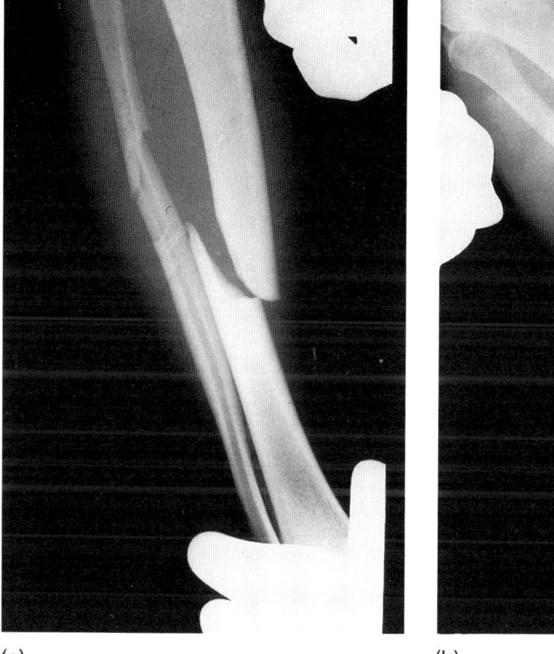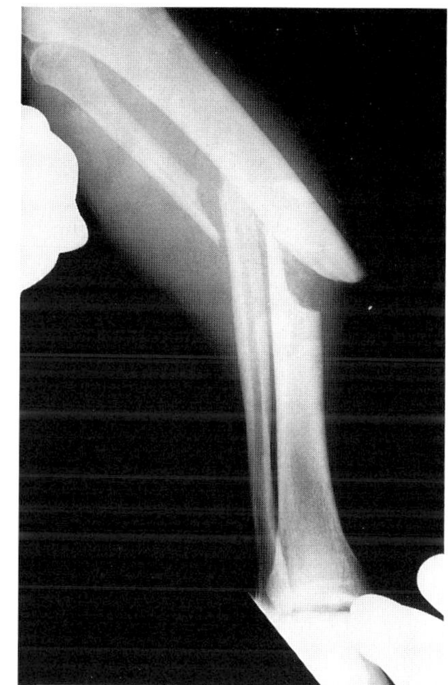

Fig. 23.17 Two radiographs of the same patient with a (a) varus and (b) valgus stress. The intact periosteal hinge is on the lateral surface.

excruciating pain on passive extension or flexion of the toes and signs of neurological compromise such as paraesthesia or numbness. Compartment syndrome may be present with a normal pulse, which is therefore an unreliable sign. Compartment syndrome must be excluded in unconscious patients with tibial fractures by the use of intracompartmental pressure measurements. The joints above and below a tibial fracture should be examined as associated injury to the knee or ankle is not uncommon.

Grazes, which may represent full-thickness burns, and the extent and degree of contamination of a compound wound should be noted. It is helpful to compare the site of the compound wound with the same area of the patient's clothing to see whether the clothing has been damaged, which increases the chance that clothing has been taken into the wound. The wound should be inspected once, a swab should be sent for culture and sensitivity reports; 70% of the organisms infecting a compound wound can be identified on the initial swab (Gustilo 1976). A Polaroid photograph of the wound prevents other clinicians from disturbing the dressing prior to definitive treatment. Compound wounds should be examined with sterile gloves to protect the patient and the examining surgeon.

Not all the assessment of the soft tissues is possible at the time of admission. Particularly for those patients who require a general anaesthetic, the examination of the degree of soft tissue injury may be continued prior

to definitive treatment. The presence or absence of a soft tissue hinge should be sought on reduction of the fracture. This is not only useful for deciding on the method of treatment, as outlined by Sir John Charnley (Fig. 23.17), but also the absence of the hinge alerts the clinician to the difficulty of treating the patient conservatively using three-point fixation. In high-energy injuries absence of the soft tissue hinge probably represents a badly damaged periosteum, which may predict delayed union or non-union. Evidence that it is the periosteum and supporting tissues rather than muscle or tendon that provides this hinge can be seen in the rare opportunities provided by examination of freshly dissected specimens from amputation following trauma (Fig. 23.18).

Imaging

Radiographs of the limb should include the whole of the tibia with the joints above and below the fracture on both the anteroposterior and lateral views. Oblique views rarely improve the management of a diaphyseal fracture.

Classification

A combination of classifications can help the clinician decide on the best treatment for the injury. A fracture of the tibia may be classified according to the usual

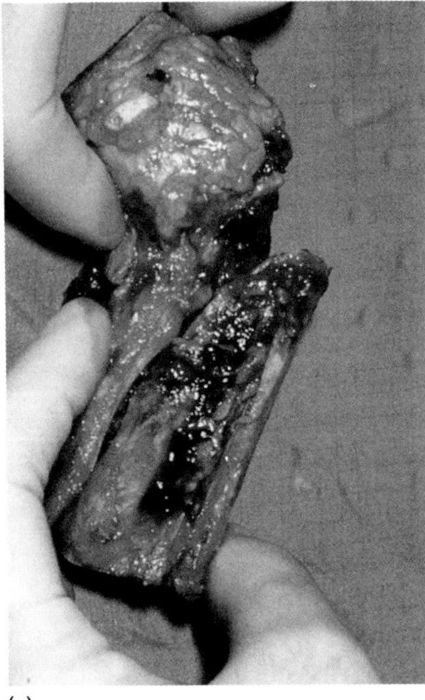
(a)

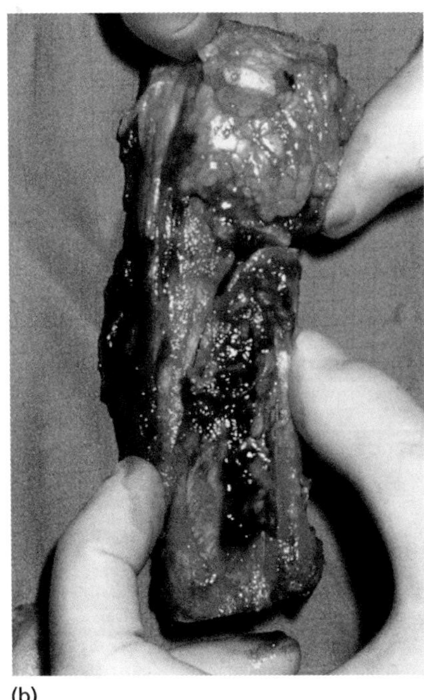
(b)

Fig. 23.18 (a) and (b) Freshly dissected tibia fracture from amputation following trauma showing the ability of the soft tissue hinge on the concave border to maintain a reduction.

descriptions of whether it is closed or open, simple or comminuted, the pattern of fracture, displacement and the level of fracture. The fracture may be pathological, traumatic or a stress fracture.

One of the newest classifications of closed injuries is the AO classification (Fig. 23.19), which is based on the pattern of tibial fracture, the degree of comminution and the level of fracture of the fibula. It is designed to allow an accurate description of the bony injury for the purposes of clinical comparisons of treatment. A complicated classification of soft tissue injuries has been developed by the same group to describe not only the bone injury but also injury to the skin, underlying muscle and tendon, and neurovascular system (Müller *et al.* 1991). It is too new a classification to be of use in guiding treatment, although with the advent of computer-aided audit it is proving very useful. The most commonly quoted classification for closed injuries is that of Tscherne, which also includes a classification of compound injuries (Table 23.1; Tscherne & Gotzen 1984). This classification is excellent at defining the soft tissue injury, and so is a good predictor of outcome, but it is not easily remembered. A memorable and most commonly quoted classification of compound fractures is a combination of the original types I—III of Gustilo and a modification of type III into types IIIa—IIIc (Table 23.2) (Gustilo 1976, Gustilo *et al.* 1984).

Depending on the local facilities and available technology it is worth standardizing the treatment of tibial fractures, using the available classifications, to create a treatment algorithm. This has the advantages of: (i) rationalizing the treatments available in one centre; (ii) ensuring similar fractures are treated in a similar fashion so that they may be compared for audit purposes or used in clinical trials; (iii) giving clear indications to junior staff of the minimum standards of care expected by a consultant; and (iv) ensuring that minor injuries are not at risk of the complications of overtreatment and major injuries are not at risk of undertreatment (Fig. 23.20).

Treatment

Treatment is best divided into treatment of the soft tissue injury and treatment of the bony injury. The bony injury can occur with little or no soft tissue damage and indeed these injuries, which are often a result of indirect trauma, usually heal as a model of normal fracture union (Fig. 23.21).

Treatment of the soft tissue injury

Compartment syndrome

Many patients treated in the past for 'uncomplicated' fractures of the tibia suffered from a minor degree of compartment syndrome. Pes cavus and clawing of the toes may be the only manifestation of an ischaemic contracture (Ellis 1958b).

The appreciation of compartment syndrome, as

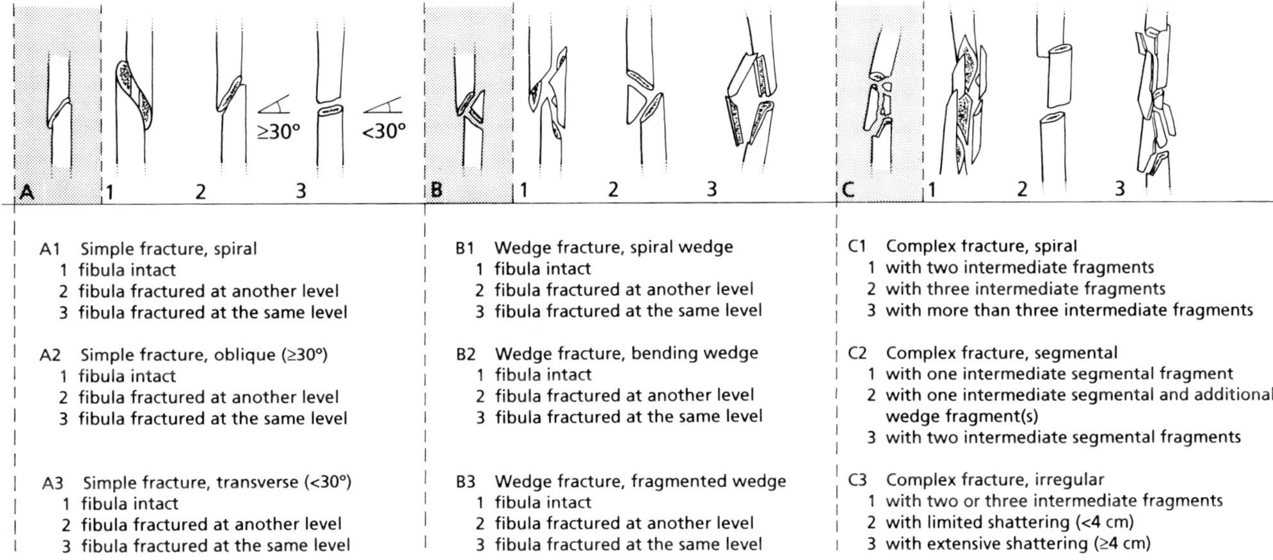

A1	Simple fracture, spiral	B1	Wedge fracture, spiral wedge	C1	Complex fracture, spiral
	1 fibula intact		1 fibula intact		1 with two intermediate fragments
	2 fibula fractured at another level		2 fibula fractured at another level		2 with three intermediate fragments
	3 fibula fractured at the same level		3 fibula fractured at the same level		3 with more than three intermediate fragments
A2	Simple fracture, oblique (≥30°)	B2	Wedge fracture, bending wedge	C2	Complex fracture, segmental
	1 fibula intact		1 fibula intact		1 with one intermediate segmental fragment
	2 fibula fractured at another level		2 fibula fractured at another level		2 with one intermediate segmental and additional wedge fragment(s)
	3 fibula fractured at the same level		3 fibula fractured at the same level		3 with two intermediate segmental fragments
A3	Simple fracture, transverse (<30°)	B3	Wedge fracture, fragmented wedge	C3	Complex fracture, irregular
	1 fibula intact		1 fibula intact		1 with two or three intermediate fragments
	2 fibula fractured at another level		2 fibula fractured at another level		2 with limited shattering (<4 cm)
	3 fibula fractured at the same level		3 fibula fractured at the same level		3 with extensive shattering (≥4 cm)

Fig. 23.19 Classification of tibia/fibula diaphysis. (Redrawn from Müller, M.E., Allgöwer, M., Schneider, R. & Willenegger, H. *Manual of Internal Fixation*, 3rd edn. Springer-Verlag: Berlin, 1991.)

Table 23.1 Classification of soft tissue injuries in closed and open fractures according to soft tissue damage, fracture severity and contamination. From Tscherne, H. & Gotzen, L. *Fractures with soft-tissue injuries*. Springer Verlag: Berlin, 1984.

Classification	Skin	Soft tissue damage	Fracture severity	Contamination
C o		−	+	−
C I	Closed	+	+ to ++	−
C II	Closed	++	+ to +++	−
C III		+++	+ to +++	−
O I		+	+ to ++	+
O II	Open	++	+ to +++	++
O III	Open	+++	+ to +++	+++
O IV		+++	+ to +++	+ to +++

C, closed; O, open; +, mild; ++, moderate; +++, severe.

Table 23.2 Number of malunions, bone grafts and time to union according to fracture grade

Fracture grade	Number	Malunions	Average union time (weeks)	Bone grafts
Closed + I	10	4	29.2	6
II	24	9	26.7	7
III	10	4	44.5	9

a major complication of tibial fracture, has become universal and failure to detect and correct such a condition is now considered unacceptable. It is important to appreciate that soft tissue injury alone, even without fracture, may give rise to compartment syndrome. Any one of the four anatomical compartments of the leg may be involved on its own and a compound fracture may be associated with compartment syndrome. Ischaemia of the soft tissues following trauma may be a result of direct trauma to the soft tissues or indirect trauma owing to arterial damage.

The pathology of compartment syndrome is not fully understood. It is recognized that as intracompartmental pressure increases, the tension in the deep fascia increases with expansion of the compartment. The increasing compartment pressure reduces the pressure gradient between the arterioles and the venules. Before the arteriovenous pressure gradient is reduced to zero,

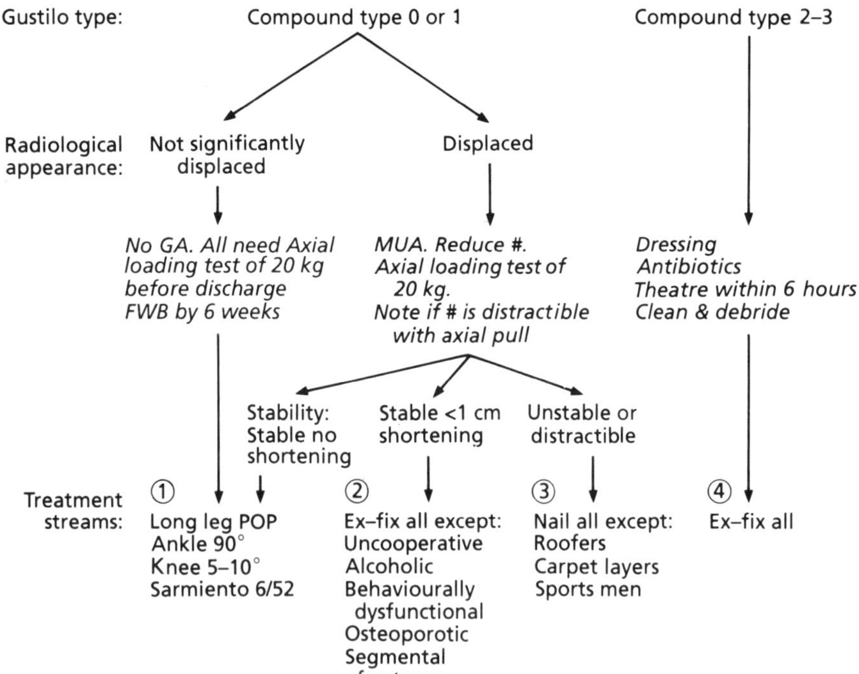

Fig. 23.20 Tibial diaphyseal fracture algorithm.

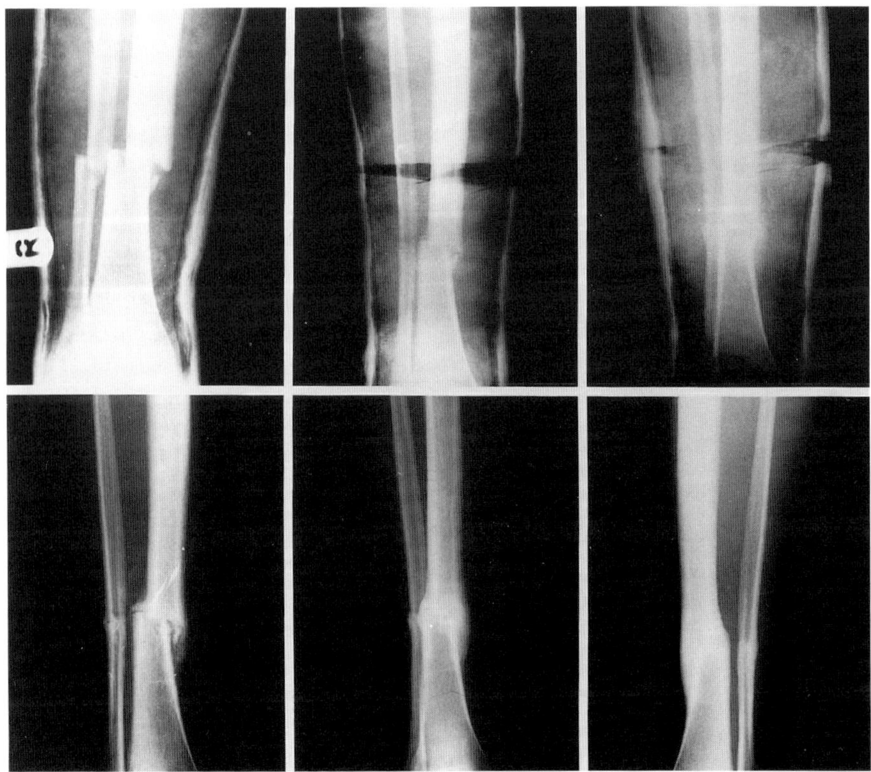

Fig. 23.21 Radiographs depicting how a stable but translated tibial fracture heals following a football injury. Note the wedging of the plaster to make use of the intact medial periosteal hinge.

the arteriolar circulation stops, owing to the intrinsic elasticity of the arteriolar walls, with a sudden cessation of blood flow (Button 1951, Ryder *et al.* 1953). At this stage, the tissues supplied by the vascular bed become ischaemic. Ischaemic muscle swells, particularly after the circulation is restored (Fuhrman & Crismon 1951). For this reason, a limited fasciotomy may prove inadequate.

DIAGNOSIS

Paraethesia, pain out of proportion to the degree of injury and level of analgesia, pain that persists when the plaster has been split down to the skin in an attempt to relieve swelling, and passive movement of the toes producing stretch pain are the clinical features of this condition. Distal pulses and capillary return are frequently normal. The use of wick, slit and needle catheters to measure compartment pressure has been well documented (Mubarek & Owen 1977) (Fig. 23.22). A conscious patient with the usual clinical signs and abnormal sensory or motor function in the territory of the peripheral nerve that traverses the affected compartment should not require compartment pressures before fasciotomy. If the same patient has normal motor or sensory function, then compartment pressure measurement is essential. Compartment pressure measurement in asymptomatic, conscious patients is of doubtful value (Triffitt *et al.* 1992). Using a slit catheter, a compartment pressure of greater than 30 mmHg is an indication for a fasciotomy (Bourne & Rorabeck 1989). The pressures should be measured in all four compartments. If no single compartment is above 30–35 mmHg, then the catheter is left in the compartment with the highest pressure until the patient is no longer felt to be at risk of a rise above 30 mmHg. Pressures lower than 30 mmHg can be detrimental in hypotensive patients.

TREATMENT

Early fasciotomy may be justified on clinical grounds where a high index of suspicion of compartment syndrome exists. This is especially true in the unconscious multiple-trauma victim, who should always be con-

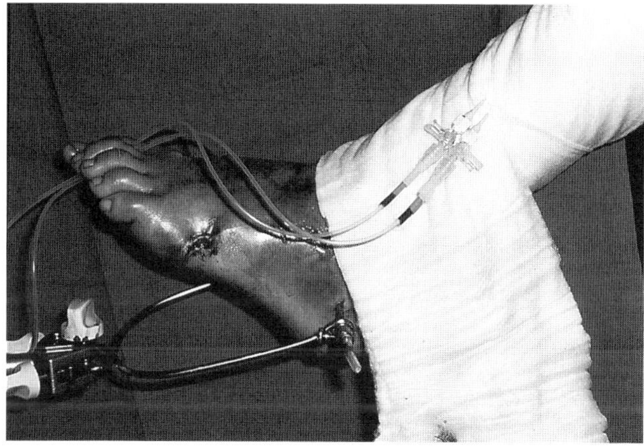

Fig. 23.22 The use of slit catheters to monitor compartment pressures after locked closed tibial nailing.

sidered for either fasciotomies or compartment pressure monitoring. The wise surgeon will proceed if clinical acumen indicates a compartment syndrome, even in the presence of low wick catheter measurements.

The medial and lateral double incision, advocated by Mubarek *et al.* (1978), is as good as excision of a segment of the fibula. Either an open wound or a degree of degloving makes hazardous the use of two incisions. In those cases where a single incision is used, it should be at least 5 cm from the wound or area of degloving to reduce the possibility of a necrotic skin bridge (Tscherne & Gotzen 1984). With extensive wounds, care must be exercised not to exceed a ratio of 3:1 between the length and the width of the skin bridge. It is important that all four compartments are decompressed widely at the time of surgery (Fig. 23.23). Fasciotomy should be performed without a tourniquet, as the quality of circulatory return must be witnessed, and a tourniquet

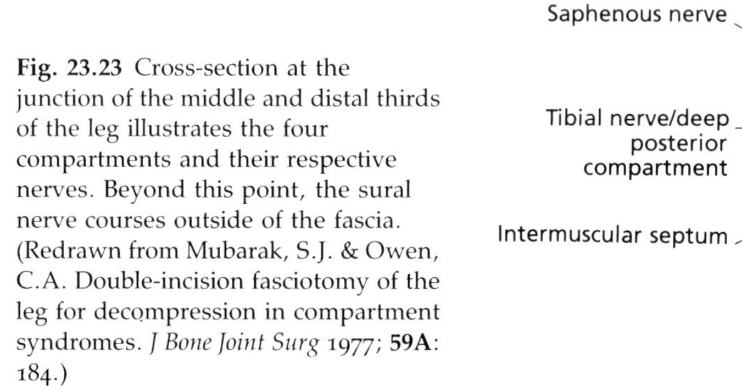

Fig. 23.23 Cross-section at the junction of the middle and distal thirds of the leg illustrates the four compartments and their respective nerves. Beyond this point, the sural nerve courses outside of the fascia. (Redrawn from Mubarak, S.J. & Owen, C.A. Double-incision fasciotomy of the leg for decompression in compartment syndromes. *J Bone Joint Surg* 1977; **59A**: 184.)

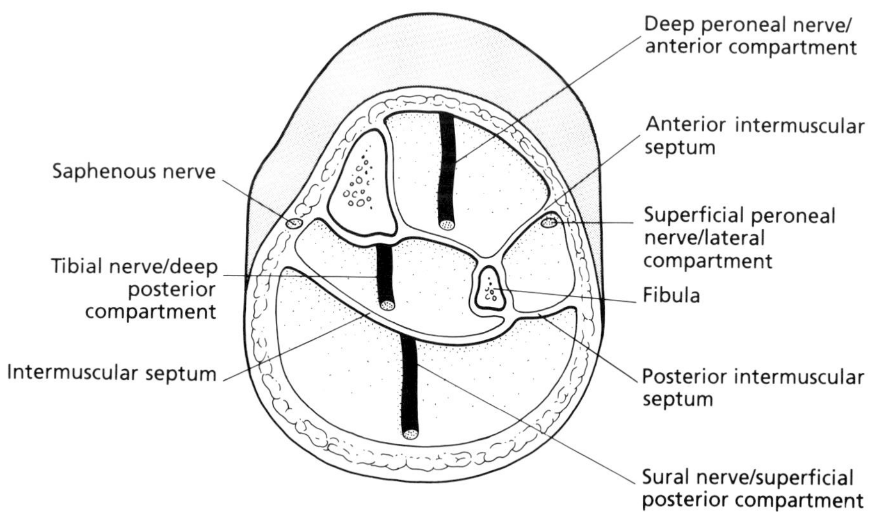

will compound the insult caused by the compartment syndrome (Fuhrman & Crismon 1951).

The use of diuretics has been shown to be effective in reducing compartment pressure but this must not be seen as a substitute for fasciotomy (Christenson & Wulff 1985).

Double-incision technique

The double-incision technique has been recommended as a simple and effective way of decompressing all compartments in the lower extremity. The anterior incision is centred over the anterior intermuscular septum between the anterior and lateral compartments, while the medial incision is located 1–2 cm behind the posteromedial border of the tibia (Mubarek & Owen 1977) (Fig. 23.24).

The anterior incision is made and the terminal branch of the deep peroneal nerve as well as the intermuscular septum are identified. Anterior and lateral compartment fasciotomies are made 1 cm in front of and 1 cm behind the intermuscular septum respectively. Through the posteromedial incision, the deep compartment is exposed by retracting the saphenous vein and nerve and releasing the fascia over the superficial posterior compartment. In order to expose adequately the deep posterior compartment, we have usually found it necessary to detach the soleal bridge to expose the fascia covering the flexor digitorum longus and tibialis posterior (Bourne & Rorabeck 1989). Fasciotomy converts a closed wound into an open one, which necessitates immobilizing the fracture with external fixation to allow easy inspection of the wounds and early closure of the fasciotomies. Long incisions are important as the skin envelope may contribute to an acute compartment syndrome (Cohen *et al.* 1991).

Crush injuries

When a limb has been crushed beneath a heavy object, the local and general complications of this injury must be considered. Local muscle necrosis may act as a nidus for sepsis. Myoglobin release from an extensive injury may cause the general complication of renal failure. Forced alkaline diuresis has been shown to be effective in preventing this renal failure (Reis & Michaelson, 1986).

Degloving injuries

The history of being run over by the wheel of a heavy vehicle, visible tyre marks and skin grazes should lead

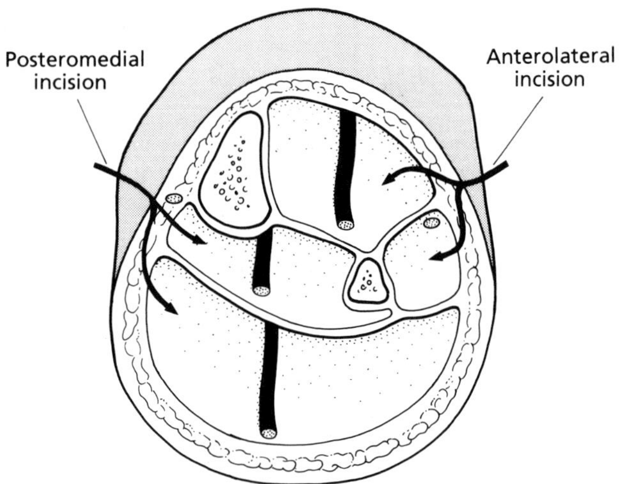

Fig. 23.24 Illustration of four-compartment decompression using a double-incision method. (Redrawn from Mubarak S.J. & Owen, C.A. Double-incision fasciotomy of the leg for decompression in compartment syndromes. *J Bone Joint Surg* 1977; **59A**: 184.)

to a high index of suspicion of a degloving injury (Hidaglo 1985, Letts 1985). The first step in management is to identify precisely the limits of skin viability. This is performed by repeated trimming of the wound edges until free bleeding occurs from the skin edges. Areas away from the main wound may be tested using a scalpel blade to make multiple perforations, which are less damaging than extensive excision. A fluorescine test may be employed to delineate the perfused tissues prior to excision. Split skin grafts can be harvested from a clean but ischaemic flap (Ziv *et al.* 1988). This regimen has the advantage that capillary bleeding from the donor bed indicates viability, whereas the absence of capillary bleeding identifies ischaemic flaps which may be removed after skin graft harvest.

Compound wounds

Initial treatment of the compound wound begins at the scene of the accident. The doctor or paramedic should ensure that extraneous matter, like torn clothing, is removed from the area of the wound. The tibial fracture should be reduced as well as possible to prevent further ischaemic insult to surrounding tissue under tension, and it should be dressed.

On arrival of the patient in the Accident department, and following necessary resuscitation, the wound should be swabbed to gauge the type of bacterial contamination, photographed to avoid repeated uncovering and then dressed with an iodophor dressing. The patient should be started on an appropriate intravenous antibiotic to cover the organisms likely to have been contaminants at the scene of injury, and the patient should be considered for revaccination for tetanus. Most surgeons continue giving antibiotics in a treatment regimen of 2–3 days (Gustilo 1976) but there is some evidence that 24 hours is sufficient (Dellinger *et al.* 1988). The patient with a compound wound should be operated on within 6 hours of injury as this has been shown to reduce the risk of late infection (Tscherne & Gotzen 1984).

Once the patient has been anaesthetized, the limb is cleaned with gloved hands using a chlorhexidine or cetrimide solution. A tourniquet may be applied but should not be used unless uncontrollable haemorrhage is expected. The dressings are removed, the skin of the limb disinfected with an aqueous solution of betadine and the limb towelled to exclude the unprepared skin and other surfaces. As copious amounts of irrigation fluids are to be used in an open bleeding wound, as many precautions as possible are taken to prevent soaking of the drapes and operating staff to avoid loss of the sterility of the operating surface and reduce the level of contact between the potentially hazardous body fluids of the patient and the operating staff.

The extent of the wound is now assessed for contamination, periosteal stripping and tissue ischaemia. All visible contaminants should be removed. The wound should be lavaged at this point with 2–5 l saline. Both bone ends need to be inspected and cleaned. Dirt engrained in the cortical bone should be nibbled free with bone nibblers, and bone chips devoid of periosteum should be removed. Unfortunately, even clean wounds with a nidus for infection can become secondarily infected from the haematogenous route (Elson 1977). Next, the skin edges should be excised and contaminated subcutaneous tissue debrided with it to leave healthy clean bleeding tissue behind. Clean periosteum should not be debrided with this first layer as the ideal is to preserve as much as possible. The wound should receive a final lavage with 2–5 l saline. Compound wounds should not be closed. The judicious repositioning of periosteum with a single tack of absorbable suture might help subsequent healing. Prior to the application of an immobilization device, the bone should be reduced by direct vision and the reduction held temporarily using bone reduction forceps. K-wires or drill holes should be avoided as the swarf is dead bone, which acts as a nidus for infection.

Early cover of the wound provides the best management for a compound fracture of the tibia. This should never be performed over tissue of doubtful viability as any dead tissue acts as a nidus for infection. In these circumstances delayed wound closure should be practised.

Other iatrogenic causes of deep infection include the formation of a haematoma by poor haemostasis at the time of surgery, insufficient drainage of a wound in the first 24 hours, and devascularization of previously viable tissue by rough handling, tight ligatures, prolonged retraction or skin closure under tension.

The assessment of tissue viability is never easy and comes with experience. Muscle viability is often the most difficult to assess (Heppenstall 1980) and presumably accounts for the students' mnemonic of looking for the four 'C's' of contractility, colour, consistency and capacity to bleed. When tissue viability is in doubt following initial debridement and cleaning, the wound is left open, dressed and reinspected 48–72 hours later, when further debridement of non-viable tissue is carried out. A period of more than 3 days between inspections is not acceptable as spreading infection will increase tissue damage. One should aim to cover a soft tissue defect between 3 and 5 days after injury.

A combined approach to achieving skin cover is often the best option, especially in busy units, where plastic and orthopaedic surgeons have the opportunity of working together (Glasson & Morrison 1988). Under these circumstances the plastic surgeon should be allowed to assess the wound from presentation and see it during the stages of debridement. Wounds left open lead to colonization by commensals which put at risk subsequent skin cover and add to the metabolic requirement of the patient.

The stability achieved by plaster casting techniques is not enough to rest the soft tissue to assist the body's defence against infection. The treatment of wounds of greater severity than Gustilo type I by plaster is problematical from the nursing point of view. The majority of surgeons will use an external fixator to avoid the potential risk of deep infection in association with implanted metal (Bach & Hansen 1989).

Secondary suture is most often employed once the traumatic oedema has subsided. It is best undertaken in stages if the oedema is slow to resolve and can be achieved using loose mattress sutures or steristrips to draw the wound edges further together after each inspection in theatre. Secondary suture is the method of choice for fasciotomy incisions for compartment syndrome.

Skin grafting needs to be employed where skin loss has occurred over soft tissue that will form a base of granulation tissue to support the graft with a blood supply. The easiest and most commonly used method of wound cover is split-thickness skin grafting. The split-thickness skin graft can be expanded to cover large areas using a purpose-built mill that makes cuts on the graft to turn it into an expandable mesh (Fig. 23.25).

Bone void of periosteum and tendon uncovered by tendon sheath will not granulate to support a split-thickness skin graft. When areas of exposed bone, tendon or metal fixation need to be covered, then pedicled skin flaps, myocutaneous flaps or free myocutaneous flaps should be employed, preferably by a surgeon with extensive experience in this area (see Chapter 9).

Vascular injuries

The severely injured lower limb with a vascular injury requires early assessment by experienced surgeons (Glasson & Morrison 1988, McAndrew & Lantz 1989). The early recognition of vascular impairment is imperative if secondary amputations and poor results due to ischaemic contracture are to be avoided. Arterial damage should be suspected in rapid-onset compartment syndrome in children (Friedman & Jupiter 1984) or adults.

In approximately 50% of cases a vascular lesion will occur with a neurological deficit and will be associated with a poor prognosis (Weaver et al. 1984). Amputation rates for limbs with vascular injury vary from 15% in blunt trauma (Meek & Robbs 1984) to 25% in gunshot wounds (Armstrong et al. 1988).

Angiography is the definitive investigation for vascular injury and may be performed quickly and easily with the minimum of equipment. It should be considered both pre- and postoperatively where a vascular injury is suspected or where the effectiveness of repair is in question (Allen et al. 1984). There is little doubt that an increasing proportion of severely injured legs are being preserved with modern treatment methods. Gustilo type IIIc injuries, however, continue to lead to high amputation rates (Caudle & Stern 1987). Where skin, muscle, nerve, bone and vascularity have been severely damaged, there is great potential advantage in performing a provisional amputation with delayed closure and fashioning of a stump (Heatley 1988). The quality of properly produced modern modular endoskeletal prostheses is such that a patient with a patellar tendon bearing suction prosthesis may have a near normal gait (Seiler & Richardson 1986). Added to this the cost in life from life-threatening infections (Herve et al. 1987) and resources (Bondurant et al. 1988) of inappropriate attempts at limb salvage makes less difficult the unpalatable decision to perform a primary amputation. The decision is best made at an early stage,

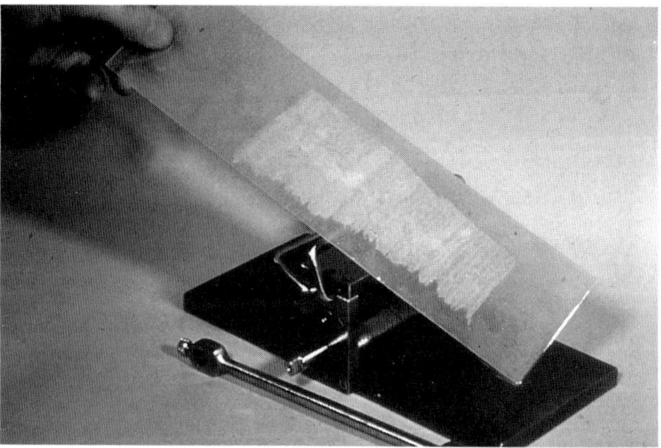

Fig. 23.25 Tibial split skin graft ready to be meshed.

and may be helped by the use of a severity grading system (Gregory et al. 1985, Bondurant et al. 1988), although these have not yet been validated (Lange 1989). A second opinion from an experienced and trusted colleague often helps to reassure the surgeon and patient of the benefits of amputation rather than protracted salvage.

Damage to the veins of the limb may occur directly as a result of trauma or internal fixation or indirectly as a result of superficial and deep venous thrombosis. Late venous insufficiency does not seem to be a common problem following tibial fracture.

Tradition teaches that a fracture should be stabilized before a vascular repair is carried out in order to protect the repair from damage due to manipulation of the fracture site. We recommend that this tradition is abandoned in favour of a combined management approach. Delay in the restoration of tissue perfusion is a greater threat to the patient than the fracture. It has been suggested that a delay of more than 6 hours results in a significantly increased rate of amputation (Howard & Makin 1990). A sensible approach would be to allow the vascular surgeon to establish the vascular supply to the limb first with the assistance of the orthopaedic surgeon. The advantage of this approach is minimization of the ischaemic insult to the soft tissues while allowing the orthopaedic surgeon to see the extent and site of the vascular repair required, so that it might be protected during subsequent immobilization of the reduced fracture. Whenever a loss in length of a vessel is being replaced, the length of the reduced fracture should be brought to the attention of the vascular surgeon by the assisting orthopaedic surgeon.

Treatment of the bony injury

In this section, treatment options for the fracture are discussed along with the potential local complications of each treatment. The trainee is reminded to inform the patient of the immediate, early, and late general complications of these procedures when seeking informed consent from the patient.

Treatment of the bony injury may be conservative or surgical. The advantages to be gained from non-operative methods of treatment are the lack of an incision resulting in a scar, the low risk of early superficial or deep infection, chronic osteomyelitis, and the low risk of late osteomyelitis due to haematogenous spread of bacteria.

In the absence of overlying metalware, the classical signs of fracture healing are visible on plain radiographs and can be used to gauge the state of progress towards union, although a healed fracture is difficult to diagnose from radiographs (Nicholls *et al.* 1979).

The indications for closed treatment generally include closed and type I open fractures with minimal fragmentation, shortening of <1 cm following attempts at reduction and assessment of stability, and minimal soft tissue injury. The contraindications for closed treatment include severe soft tissue injuries of types II and III, segmental fractures, fractures with a potential to shorten more than 1 cm (e.g. multifragmentary fractures) and fractures with an associated articular fracture.

If treatment by means of manipulation and plaster is to be undertaken, reduction is best performed as soon as possible. The injured leg tends to become swollen over the first 24 hours, and the distended soft tissue tends to cause shortening that is difficult to overcome.

Fractures suited to conservative treatment

THE UNDISPLACED FRACTURE

The undisplaced transverse diaphyseal fracture is stable to axial loading. This fracture may be treated initially by application of an above-knee plaster cast over a wool bandage, performed using a strong analgesic and constant reassurance. The patient should always be admitted for elevation and observation. As prevention of disuse osteoporosis depends on weight-bearing, this should be instituted as soon as possible. Most patients, when encouraged to weight-bear, will be fully weight-bearing by 6 weeks. Under these circumstances the patient may be given a below-knee Sarmiento type of plaster, plaster cast brace or one of the newer plastic braces, where the best results are seen in those able to weight-bear early (Digby *et al.* 1983, Sarmiento 1974).

Displacement of the truly undisplaced fracture treated in plaster is rare; however, the patient should be followed up on a regular basis to detect early radiographic evidence of displacement or delayed union due to an atrophic or hypertrophic callus. The plaster cast may be removed for assessment of clinical healing when the patient is fully weight-bearing and there are radiographic signs of bridging callus on at least three sides. Clinical healing is judged to have taken place when there is no movement detected between the fragments, stressing the fracture is pain free, there is no tenderness over the fracture site, and the patient is able to weight-bear comfortably without support. On removal of the cast or brace, the patient is shown the fracture line on the radiograph and advised not to return to contact sports for at least 12 months to reduce the incidence of refracture. The patient is further advised to continue to use crutches, in case of fatigue. This is noticed as aching at the fracture site after walking long distances. Patients should be reviewed 2 weeks after removal of the plaster cast, when most crutches are returned.

THE MINIMALLY DISPLACED FRACTURE

A minimally displaced fracture may be defined as one which is not shortened, one which is translated less than 50% of the diameter of the shaft at the level of the fracture, and one which is not angulated more than 10° (Fig. 23.21). The minimally displaced but axially stable fracture may be treated in an above-knee plaster cast until a callus response is seen. The patient may be allowed to weight-bear as comfort allows, but as the cast has been made without resort to a general anaesthetic, the position of the soft tissue hinge has not been diagnosed. This means that the patient must be warned that the plaster cast may need to be wedged to correct angulation.

Wedging of the cast is undertaken by marking the level of the fracture circumferentially on the cast with a pen. The anteroposterior radiograph laid over the cast acts as a guide. The point at which the plaster must hinge to correct the angulatory deformity is worked out from the anteroposterior and lateral radiographs. For example, a fracture with a valgus and anterior angulation must hinge posteromedially (Fig. 23.26). The cast is cut around its circumference, leaving one-quarter of the circumference where the proposed hinge should be. The divided plaster is gently opened for 1–2 cm using a three-point force with the hinge as the central fulcrum. The size of the wedge can be calculated more accurately (Gregson 1994). This reduces the patient's exposure to

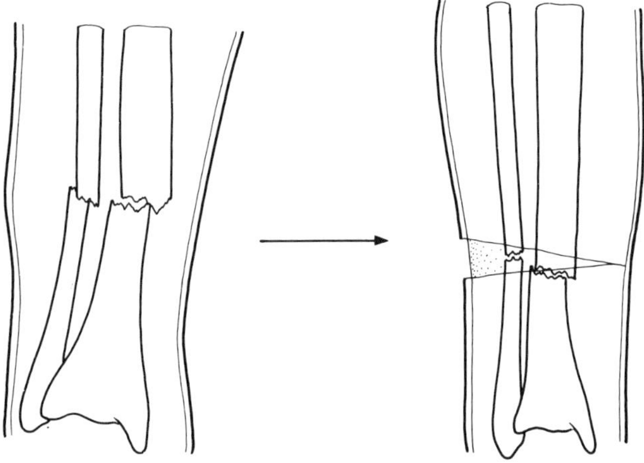

Fig. 23.26 Drawing of radiograph before and after a plaster is hinged posteromedially for a valgus and anterior angulatory deformity.

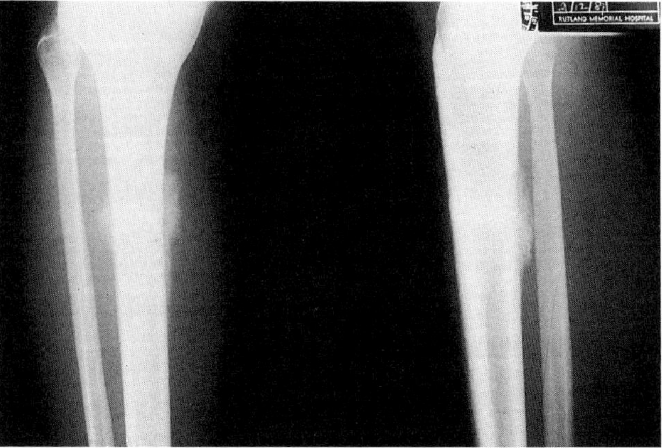

Fig. 23.27 Radiograph of a typical stress fracture of the tibia.

the excessive radiation of a trial-and-error approach. The wedge is maintained with a 1–2 cm half-cut cork and the limb radiographed to assess the correction achieved. When a satisfactory reduction has been obtained, wool is packed into the gap and the plaster strengthened with a plaster bandage. Follow-up of the patient should be regular to prevent further angulatory deformity.

Once a callus response is seen, a below-knee plaster may then be used until clinical healing is detected.

STRESS FRACTURES

Stress fracture of the tibia is common in road runners and new army recruits who undergo drilling and marching (Fig. 23.27). Most injuries are managed by rest and plaster casting or cast bracing.

COMPLICATIONS OF CONSERVATIVE TREATMENT

Refracture

This complication is seen mainly in patients who return to contact sport before 12 months after injury. The strength of healing callus has been studied in rats and shown to have a bimodal peak in the ultimate strength of the callus. The first peak occurs when the callus has reached its largest diameter, and the second peak occurs with remodelling of the fracture gap itself (Lindsay & Howes 1931). In adults, Böstman found the incidence of refracture to be 2.4%. Refracture occurred most commonly in patients with spiral fractures, those with a fracture of the fibula at a different level from that of

the fibula and those with marked initial displacement (Böstman 1983).

Delayed union and non-union

In a review on the natural history of union of 100 tibial fractures with closed treatment, Oni *et al.* (1988) showed 19% delayed union at 20 weeks. Four per cent were subsequently operated on as no progress was expected. All but four of the remaining 15% healed by 30 weeks.

Pressure sores

Patients should experience little or no discomfort in a well-moulded plaster cast. Localized pain should be investigated by windowing a plaster. Generalized pain should be investigated by either splitting the plaster to the skin and spreading the edges apart or bivalving the plaster.

Malunion and shortening

In the natural history of union study by Oni *et al.*, 65% of the patients were reviewed at 6 months. Of those reviewed, 78.9% had 0–5° residual angulation, 18.4% had residual angulation of 6–10° and only 2.6% had residual angulation of more than 10°. These were the maximum deformity as measured from either the antero-posterior or lateral radiographs. In a more recent study performed in Leicester, using the protocol described earlier in the chapter, 83% had 0–5° residual angulation, only 2% had residual angulation of 6–10° and 5% had residual angulation of more than 10°. This was a similar population in terms of age and sex but the more recent study also included patients with unstable and compound injuries.

In the study by Oni *et al.* of the 65% of patients reviewed at 6 months, 94.7% had less than 10 mm shortening and none had more than 20 mm shortening. In the more recent study performed in Leicester, 95% had less than 10 mm shortening and one had more than 20 mm shortening. During the more recent study we aimed at a stable fixation which would produce less than an acceptable 1 cm shortening; this was the consensus view of consultants in Leicester. Interestingly, only the patient with shortening of 2.5 cm complained of deformity. It would therefore seem reasonable to try to prevent more than 1 cm shortening.

Deep venous thrombosis (DVT)

Only two patients developed a clinical DVT in the most recent study of 100 tibial fractures from Leicester, and one of these patients developed thrombosis in the contralateral limb following external fixation and a prolonged period of bedrest for a soft tissue wound. The majority of patients with closed and Gustilo type I fractures were mobilized and discharged within 5 days of injury.

Sudeks atrophy

In the most recent study of 100 tibial fractures from Leicester, only two patients developed a Sudeks type atrophy of the foot. Both these patients were women, both showed an initial reluctance to weight-bear, and both showed a marked disuse osteoporosis of the tibia prior to the onset of the typical symptoms of Sudeks atrophy.

Fractures suited to operative treatment

THE DISPLACED SHORTENED FRACTURE

General anaesthesia is usually required if a satisfactory result is to be achieved in cases where there is shortening or more than 10° angulatory correction is necessary. Several practical points should be considered if good results are to be obtained. A fracture that is short with an intact soft tissue hinge is difficult to reduce and needs two strong operators to achieve a reduction. One should reduce the tibia as Charnley has demonstrated previously (Charnley 1961) and Rang has demonstrated for fractures of the forearm bones in children (Rang 1984). Transverse, shortened fractures with an intact soft tissue hinge are the most difficult to reduce.

The assistant is required to hold the patient's thigh during the manipulation. The soft tissue hinge is usually deduced to be on the concave border of the fracture when the tibia is manually angulated in the plane of least resistance. With the tibia in this position, the adjacent fracture ends are slid to meet each other as nearly as possible. The meeting of adjacent cortices acts as a fulcrum with which to guide the reduction of the fracture (Fig. 23.28). A check on rotation, by checking the alignment of the tibial tuberosity with that of the second toe, should be made before casting. It is helpful to drop both legs over the end of the operating table and compare foot progression angle in both feet. With the fracture ends reduced, the soft tissue hinge can be used to maintain the reduction in a plaster cast using the three-point moulding technique of Charnley (Fig. 23.11). This reduction is alarming to perform in the presence of the uninitiated, but is effective in producing a perfect reduction without causing more damage than that already caused by the original injury.

Once the fracture has been reduced, a diagnosis of the axial stability of the fracture may be made by producing an axial load of about 20 kg from the distal end of the bone. If the bone does not shorten, or shortens less than 1 cm, conservative treatment is acceptable. If the fracture shortens more than 1 cm, then it is likely to be similarly axially unstable in a plaster cast, as a cast will not prevent shortening. These unstable fractures used to be treated conservatively using skeletal traction followed by casting and yielded good results (Ellis 1958a). However, with increasingly good fixation techniques, either external fixation, intramedullary nailing or dynamic compression plating should be considered for the axially unstable fracture. If the fracture is easily reduced but distractible and unstable to angulation in all directions, because of a circumferential periosteal tear, then the limb should be hung dependent over the end of the operating table during plastering. If angulation persists, it can be corrected by wedging, as described above, when the plaster has dried. Angulatory and rotatory malunion, if corrected at an early stage, should not be a problem. For plastering the axially stable and reduced limb the patient should lie supine with the leg supported by a block behind the supracondylar region of the thigh, avoiding pressure on the popliteal fossa.

If an adequate reduction cannot be achieved, then open reduction and either external fixation, intramedullary nailing or dynamic compression plating should be performed. The plaster and two pins treatment, in anywhere but the poorest of countries, is mentioned only to be condemned because it combines fracture distraction with the risk of pin tract infection (Bassey 1989).

Sarmiento reported on the use of a functional cast for

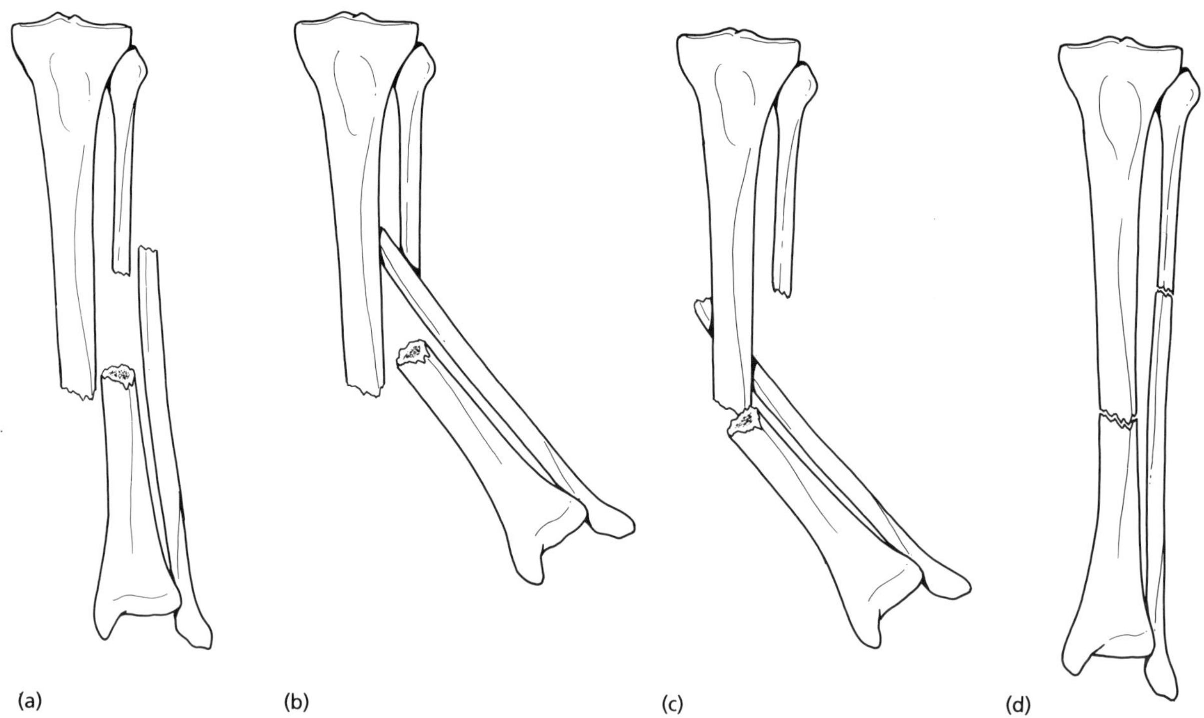

(a)   (b)   (c)   (d)

Fig. 23.28 A straight pull will not reduce a transverse fracture with an intact soft tissue hinge (a). The angulatory deformity should be reproduced (b) and the distal fragment slid distally until adjacent cortices match (c). The angulation is then corrected (d).

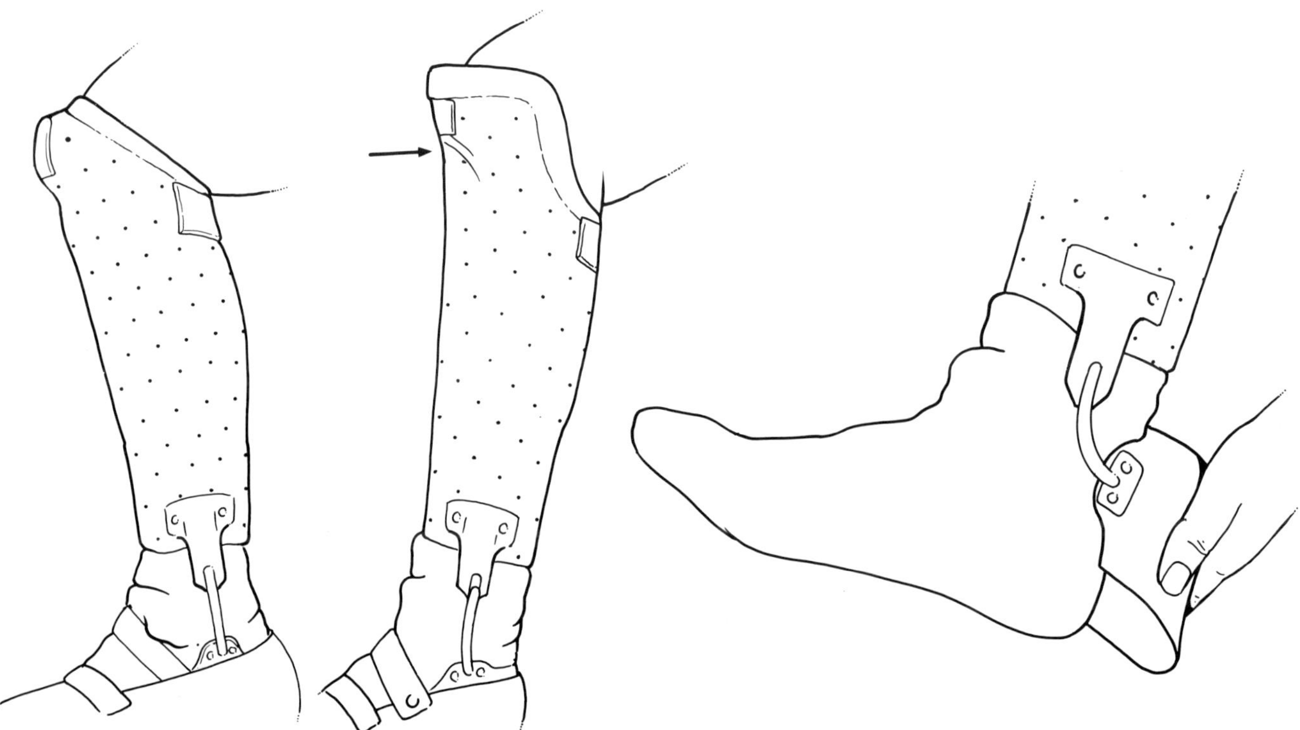

Fig. 23.29 Drawing of the original Orthoplast brace as published by Sarmiento, A. Functional bracing of tibial fractures. *Clin Orthop* 1974; **105**: 202–219. Note the patellar bar arrow.

the leg; this allowed motion at the knee whilst controlling rotation (Sarmiento 1967). The brace worked by means of the hydrostatic pressure generated within the tight-fitting plaster controlling axial alignment, whilst the patellar bar took minimal weight directly and the moulding at the tibial flares controlled rotation (Fig. 23.29). This method has less control over the rotational alignment of the fracture than does the conventional long leg cast. Tibial fractures managed in a long leg cast for 3–6 weeks post fracture are then placed in a functional cast. Early weight-bearing is essential to encourage bone healing and maintain the function of the soft tissues.

In a series of 185 patients, Sarmiento found that this method of treatment resulted in an average time to union of 14.5 weeks. There were no apparent cases of non-union but it must be emphasized that this is a series of treatments rather than a series of injuries. Segmental fractures healed in 17 weeks. Other series have not managed to emulate the low levels of non-union, delayed union and malunion seen in Sarmiento's series (Puno *et al.* 1986). Sarmiento has recently been using prefabricated tibial braces with good results (Sarmiento *et al.* 1989).

MULTIFRAGMENTARY FRACTURE

Multifragmentary fractures have a predictable tendency for shortening. Early operative techniques to manage these injuries avoid the shortening that inevitably occurs at 3–6 weeks when weight-bearing is encouraged. Multifragmentary complex fractures, which are the result of high-energy injuries, tend to produce atrophic non-union. For closed injuries of this sort, external fixation with delayed grafting, intramedullary nailing or dynamic compression plating with early grafting may be able to avoid atrophic non-union. In our opinion compound type II–III injuries should be treated by external fixation with delayed bone grafting, if necessary, once adequate skin cover has been achieved.

SEGMENTAL FRACTURES

Segmental fractures of the tibia have a tendency to produce one solid union and one non-union. Though it is the distal fracture which tends to unite more slowly, one patient, treated by external fixation, among a series of 220 tibial fractures had the proximal fracture unite last. It is not known whether this phenomenon was due to the central segment being ischaemic or the two fracture sites being involved in a race to stability, won by

only one of the fractures which then goes on to unite with a sleeve of controlling callus, whilst the other fracture accepts either no motion or all the unfavourable motions including shear. Research into this phenomenon would be interesting. As healing by callus is sought at both fracture sites, intramedullary nailing is an ideal treatment because it is biomechanically geared to the control of both fractures equally. Also, the process of reaming autografts both sites at the same time. During reaming of a segmental fracture the central fragment should be held to prevent devascularization by spinning the fragment.

MULTIPLE INJURIES

Injuries to the ipsilateral femur when combined with tibial fractures present a difficult problem for conservative management. The flexibility of the intervening joint defeats attempts to provide adequate mechanical control of either fracture. Operative treatment should be performed for all long bone fractures associated with ipsilateral or contralateral fractures as it eases nursing care and reduces the incidence of pulmonary problems from adult respiratory distress syndrome (ARDS) (Riska *et al.* 1976, Seibel *et al.* 1985, Broos *et al.* 1987, Svenningsen *et al.* 1987).

Operative treatments

External fixation

The external fixator allows stable fixation of the bone while preventing further damage to the bone and soft tissues involved in the injury. It allows ready access to the soft tissues. If bone loss has been encountered, then provision can be made with a fixator for shortening the limb at the fracture site to achieve healing, with subsequent calotasis at a more proximal site to restore length.

The indications for external fixation include axially unstable fractures, Gustilo type II–III open fractures and fractures with bone loss. Relative contraindications in the first category include patients who are either unco-operative, osteoporotic or have other implanted devices such as a total hip or knee replacement, where direct or haematogenous spread of infection from a pin site would result in a serious infection.

The application of an external fixator prior to plastic procedures allows ready access to the soft tissue. It will allow soft tissue cover by means of plastic flaps, almost regardless of the site of the defect. The external fixator may be used for rapid bone splintage to enable a vascular repair in the acute situation (Dreyfuss *et al.* 1987). Where fractures and injuries are combined with burns, the external fixator also allows suspension of the limb postoperatively.

The stability of the external fixator provides effective treatment of multifragmentary fractures, as mentioned above, with easy access for bone grafting, if necessary, after 12 weeks and evidence of delayed union. The unilateral and dynamizing frames are being used increasingly in favour of the very rigid frames which promote a slower union without callus (Sandberg *et al.* 1993).

The advantage of the external fixator in multiple injuries is:

1 A large number of injuries can be dealt with expeditiously.

2 The risk of fat embolus is theoretically less.

3 The correct application is relatively easy to learn.

The external fixator, when properly applied and supervised, is not associated with delayed or non-union. Callus growth enables the fixator to be removed. Callus builds up in response to movement at the fracture site, so it is important that this movement is encouraged through early weight-bearing. The poor reputation of external fixation probably stems from its predominant use in the more severe high-energy injuries, and the design of rigid external fixation which was the desire of many before De Bastiani showed the benefits of the unilateral telescoping frame. High-energy injuries and rigid external fixation are more likely to progress to delayed union (Clancey & Hansen 1978). Its use in closed stable fractures should not be undertaken lightly as pin tract infection is common and may lead to localized osteomyelitis. The use of interfragmentary compression using lag screws and an external fixator is to be deplored as the combination prevents fracture site movement, and therefore the callus response. This inhibition of callus also occurs with fixators like the 'A' frame, designed to be as rigid as a compression plate, and explains the recent trend towards using less rigid fixators (De Bastiani *et al.* 1984, Melendez & Colon 1989) (Fig. 23.30).

Some external fixators are better designed than others at allowing reduction of a fracture after pin insertion. An external fixator, like any immobilization device, is best applied to a well-reduced fracture. In compound injuries this is easily performed under direct vision. With closed injuries, the fracture should first be reduced, and the reduction maintained either by an assistant or by using skin or skeletal traction.

An aseptic technique and prophylactic antibiotics are essential. As far as possible, the pins should be placed

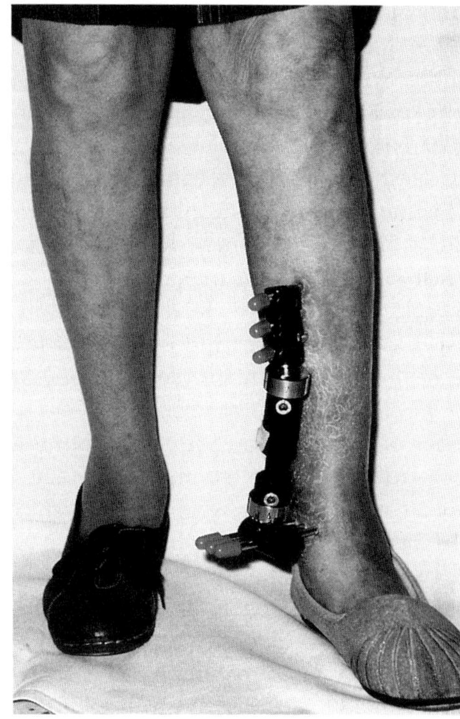

Fig. 23.30 A shortened spiral fracture of the distal tibia in a 77-year-old patient who was mobile from the 3rd postoperative day using a unilateral frame. The fracture healed by 14 weeks.

in the thick cortical bone of the diaphysis. The pins should be placed either side of the fracture and as far from the palpable fracture haematoma as possible. The pins are placed in the middle of the medial surface at an angle of about 30° medial to the anterior border of the tibia to avoid transfixing the anterior tibial nerve and vessels.

Longitudinal skin incisions are made and deepened to the periosteum with scissors. The pin tracts are made with a sharp slow-speed drill, well irrigated to reduce thermal injury (Matthews & Hirsch 1972). The swarf is removed from the drill bit before each subsequent hole is made, so as not to leave dead bone in the soft tissue tracts. The pins are inserted by hand, and if conical pins are used they should be guided with image intensification because a conical pin cannot be backed out without loosening. The use of six pins, instead of four, leads to a 30% increase in stiffness and this allows early weight-bearing and callus generation. When four uniaxial pins are used, the pins should be separated as widely as possible. Any skin left on the stretch after pin insertion and fracture reduction should be released or subsequent necrosis will promote infection.

After application of the fixator frame and reduction of the fracture, the pin sites are dressed and the limb is placed with the ankle at 90° into a back slab or orthosis for rest prior to mobilization. Rehabilitation begins immediately with quadriceps exercises during elevation. After about 5−7 days of elevation, when most skin wounds have healed, the patient is mobilized weight-bearing as comfort allows.

One of the advantages of external fixation is that rigidity may be altered with ease during the period of immobilization. A fixator's rigidity may be influenced by the size of the fracture gap, the distance between the pin−bone interface and the fixator, the number of pins, the spacing between the pins and the type of fixator used. Most of the newer designs of fixator allow dynamization; this term means many things to many people. It is probably best thought of in terms of the unlocking of the mechanism that controls stiffness, usually axial stiffness. Dynamization should not be confused with the physical state 'dynamic'. Dynamization of a fixator, especially where the fixator is biomechanically more rigid, should be performed early, probably between 1 and 2 weeks. A delay beyond 8 weeks, with no fracture site movement, probably causes a poor callus response (Green 1983).

McKibbin suggests that the callus response stops at between 6 and 8 weeks (McKibbin 1978). Where the soft tissue injury precludes early weight-bearing, cancellous bone grafting should be considered, to prevent the anticipated delay in bone union.

COMPLICATIONS

Pin tract infection

This is the commonest complication of external fixation. It may be due to preoperative conditions like peripheral oedema owing to right heart failure or to a lack of the ability to fight infection, as found in the immunocompromised. It can be due to poor operative technique or postoperative conditions such as swelling, dependency of the limb, pin site care and the proximity of the pins to a joint. Advice on routine pin care is very much a personal matter for the surgeon, but any antiseptic used should be of a non-occlusive nature. The mechanical effect of clearing encrustations from the pin-tract−skin junction is probably the principal measure required. Pin tract sepsis should be differentiated into minor and major. Minor pin tract sepsis can usually be managed by oral antibiotics, perhaps releasing tented skin, and paying attention to pin tract toilet. Rest and elevation are beneficial.

Major pin tract infection, producing pus, redness and discomfort, should be managed initially by a short trial of the appropriate antibiotics, rest and elevation. If the discharge continues, the pin should be removed and reinserted. This sort of infection probably forms because the granulation tissue sleeve, which forms along the pin tract, inevitably becomes contaminated. Encrustations of serum around the junction of pin and skin may cause a build-up of serum, which becomes heavily contaminated, leading to localized cellulitis. Motion of the pins relative to the skin, and tenting of the skin across the pins also predisposes to the development of pin tract sepsis and should be avoided. Underlying localized osteomyelitis may be seen as a ring sequestrum which should be removed by curettage following removal of the screw (Fig. 23.31).

If it is necessary to remove the fixator prematurely, then in most circumstances a functional brace is the best method for further management.

Aseptic loosening

Though this is a rare complication, it may occur in particularly comminuted fractures where few pins have a good cortical grip and the pin−bone interface

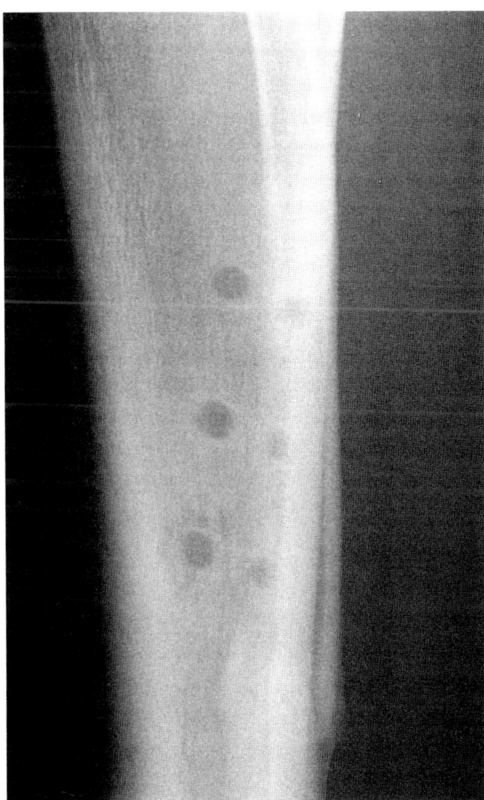

Fig. 23.31 Radiograph showing a localized osteomyelitis due to the presence of a ring sequestrum in the third pinsite from the top.

is undergoing repeated stressing by early heavy weight-bearing.

Refracture

Refracture, following premature removal of an external fixator, is a common complication of external fixation. It may occur in up to 3% of cases following external fixation (Rommens *et al.* 1986) and is twice as common when supplementary lag screws are used (Krettek *et al.* 1991). New methods of determining fracture healing by the serial measurement of fracture stiffness are helping to reduce this complication (Richardson *et al.* 1992), which probably occurs by fatigue failure of an immature callus.

Delayed union

Preoperative factors leading to delayed union are likely to be the severity of injury (Urist *et al.* 1954, Ellis 1958a) and initial displacement, which is probably a reflection of the severity of injury (Weissman *et al.* 1966). Where early weight-bearing is encouraged in a patient with a fracture considered to be low energy, delayed union is unlikely. In high-energy injuries, with periosteal stripping and soft tissue ischaemia, delayed union is inevitable and occurs even in the presence of fracture site micromovement. The operative skill with which the fixator is applied and choice of fixator are likely to influence healing to a lesser extent. A delay in union was seen with the attempts to emulate the rigidity of dynamic compression plating with early fixators. The combination of external fixation and lag screws has been shown to lead to a doubling of the incidence of refracture because the healing depended on cortical remodelling in this biomechanically rigid environment (Krettek *et al.* 1991). External fixation is difficult to maintain for the 12–18 months necessary for primary bone union. The worst scenario for healing may be where sufficient micromovement occurs to prevent primary bone healing, but insufficient movement exists to promote callus formation, although this has not been proven. The optimal amount of callus, and therefore micromovement, has yet to be determined. It probably depends on the micromovement that is set up by the patient weight-bearing, and the stability of the fracture configuration being moved. A stable configuration probably requires little callus to prevent micromovement and an unstable configuration needs a large callus. Fracture healing can be measured in terms of the micromovement taking place at a fracture gap (Cunningham *et al.* 1990). As fracture stabilization for independent

weight-bearing is more rapid via callus bridging, stimulation of callus through induced micromovement may be associated with more rapid healing (Goodship & Kenwright 1985). Fracture stiffness may provide the accurate end-point with which to compare the effects of different regimens of micromovement in externally fixed patients (Richardson *et al.* 1992).

There is some evidence that postoperative osteomyelitis or pin site infection may delay healing (Urist *et al.* 1954, Edwards & Nilsson 1965). Cancellous bone grafting should be undertaken in those known to have high-energy injuries, where radiographs show no evidence of a callus response, as soon as it is felt that the benefits will outweigh the risks for the patient. Possible operative causes of a delay in union are the distraction of a fracture gap where a periosteal injury has occurred.

Loss of reduction

This may be a complication following a fall, as most fixators are built to withstand the patient's weight but not the forces involved in a fall.

Malunion and shortening

In a paper describing the use of the Hughes external fixator, designed to provide rigidity, Court-Brown reported that 17 and the 44 fractures in this series healed in a malunited position (38.6%) (Table 23.2). No effect of pin angle, pin location, pin length or position of the fixator was found to affect the number of malunions or the average time to union.

In this paper, malunion was defined as being present if there were more than 5° of angular or rotational deformity or more than 1 cm of shortening. These criteria are identical to those used by Edge and Denham in discussing the results of their external fixator. This should be viewed in light of the variable degree of pathology present.

Malunion has been seen to occur in up to 38.6% of cases when an external fixator was used prospectively for severe injuries (Edge & Denham 1981, Court-Brown *et al.* 1985).

Neurovascular damage

External fixation of the tibia rarely leads to anterior tibial nerve palsy. However, if the pins are placed transversely in the upper portion of the distal third of the tibia it becomes more likely (Green 1983). An anteriorly sited pin in the distal third of the tibia is at risk of transfixing the tibialis anterior tendon. Where the anterior tibial compartment is penetrated, there exists a risk that the anterior tibial vessels could be penetrated, leading to a compartment syndrome.

When intramedullary nailing is to be undertaken following external fixation, there is a significant risk of osteomyelitis. Infected pin tracks are a contraindication to alternative methods of fixation, although the risk is lowered after a period of 6 weeks following removal of the pins (Gad 1991).

Internal fixation

Internal fixation by means of lag screws and a neutralization plate is a method of fracture care requiring a unique approach to the mechanical requirements of the fracture. Perren has shown that fractures fixed in the fashion described originally by Danis (1949) will unite by primary bony union only if the degree of movement is less than 10 μm (Perren 1979).

Dynamic compression plating is designed to withstand only a limited amount of cyclic loading. If the bone is not placed in compression (by the implant in tension), failure due to metal fatigue results; compression is a way of increasing the stability of fixation and does not in itself enhance bony union.

Plating is as technically demanding as any other technique of immobilization. As the technique relies on primary bone healing, the state of union cannot be judged radiographically. One normally therefore relies on the recommendations of the AO group for implant removal. The possibility of refracture after internal fixation is averted only if a generous allowance is made for the interval preceding implant removal; in the majority of cases, provided that the plate causes no discomfort, it does not require removal.

Implant removal itself inflicts a further operation on the patient, with the possibility of iatrogenic nerve and vessel injury, other general and local complications of surgery and a period of protected weight-bearing while the bone adapts to the new stresses imposed by the absence of an implant.

Stable fixation and early movement of adjacent joints underlie this form of management and the technique must be performed under the strictest of aseptic precautions with prophylactic antibiotics. Incisions should be placed 1 cm lateral to the anterior tibial crest, extending distally to follow the line of tibialis anterior tendon towards the medial maleollus (Fig. 23.32). The incision should pass directly to the deep fascia without undermining the skin edges. Minimal periosteal dissection should be undertaken to protect the vascular supply of soft tissue and bone.

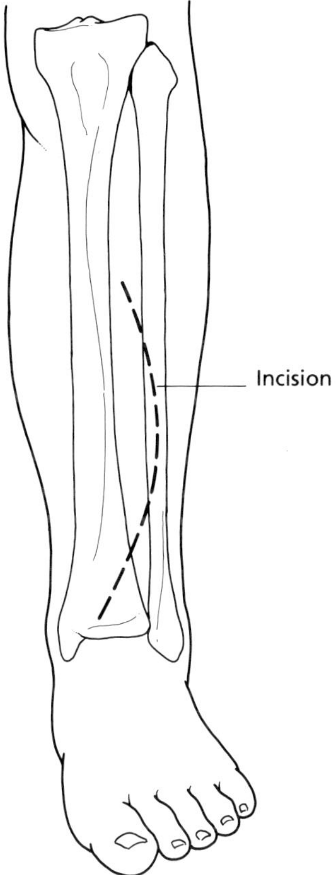

Fig. 23.32 Incision for ORIF of distal tibial fractures.

The fracture is immobilized using lag screws, with or without a neutralization plate if the fracture line is oblique or spiral. A dynamic compression plate is used if the fracture is transverse. The plate is normally placed on the medial (subcutaneous) surface of the tibia (Fig. 23.33), unless better purchase to the main fragments can be gained from the lateral surface. Contraindications to using the medial surface are: (i) skin damage on the medial side; (ii) correction of a varus deformity where the plate should be on the tension side; (iii) a posteromedial butterfly fragment; and (iv) multiple fragments medially. Complex multifragmentary fractures should not be reassembled anatomically as this will certainly devascularize fragments, leading to delayed union and a susceptibility to infection. The concept of 'biological fixation', fixation over an intact periosteum, is recommended. The diaphysis may require the use of a fracture distractor which tensions the soft tissues and realigns the fragments without stripping the periosteum (Fig. 23.34). A neutralization plate is placed across the fragmented area, the screws being placed to hold six cortices either side of the fracture (Fig. 23.35). Bone grafting provides a margin of safety in difficult cases,

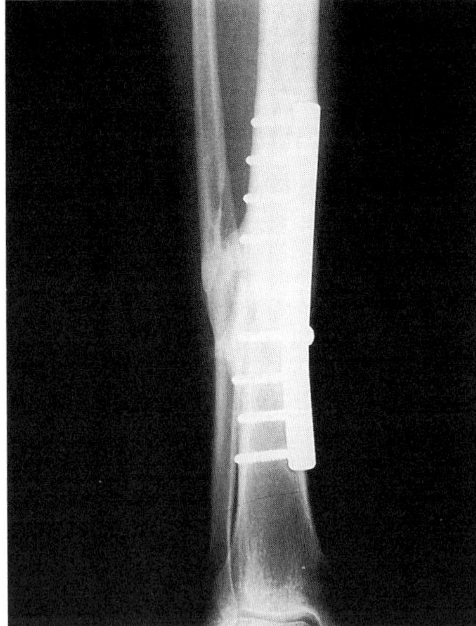

Fig. 23.33 Radiograph showing position of a DCP on the medial surface of the tibia.

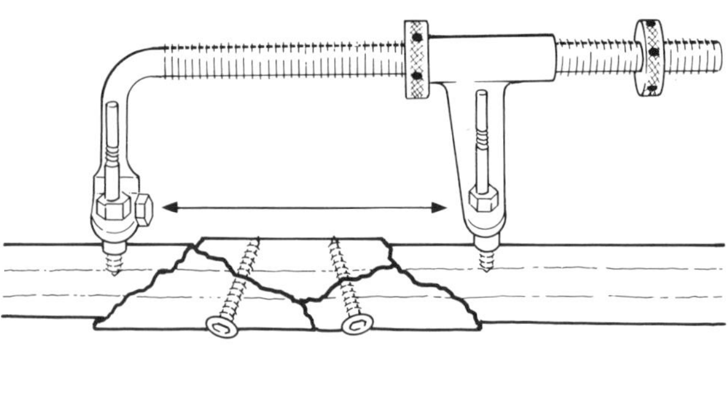

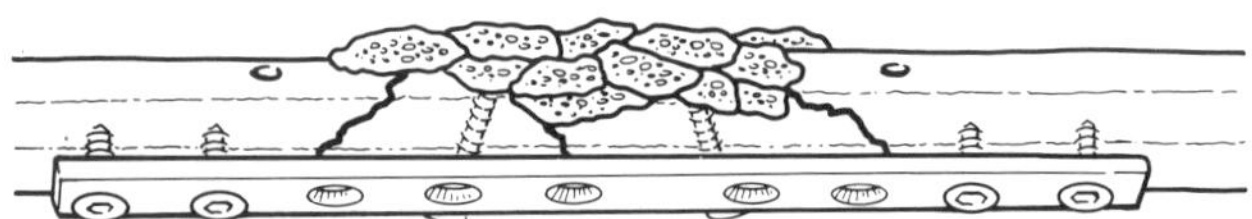

Fig. 23.34 Use of a femoral fracture distractor, a neutralization plate and bone grafting for a comminuted tibial fracture.

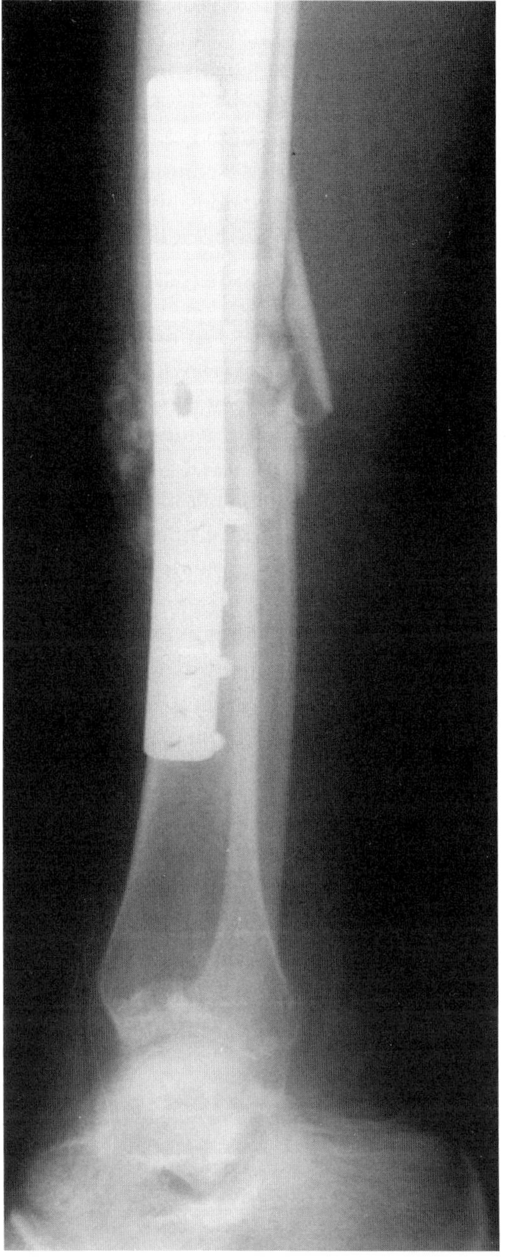

Fig. 23.35 Lateral radiograph of Fig. 23.33 showing the bone graft and plate with at least six cortices crossed by screws above and below the fracture.

especially where the compression side of the bone is comminuted.

Internal fixation is best utilized in fractures of the diaphysis that extend into the metaphysis, or even those associated with articular fractures of the knee or ankle joint which are difficult to immobilize using a locked nail or external fixator. They may be used in situations of compound type I and II fractures at the junction of the metaphysis and diaphysis so long as delayed closure is feasible. Gustilo type III fractures fare badly with internal plate fixation. Another situation where this technique is best avoided is with questionably viable skin that lies within 5 cm of the proposed site of the incision or plate.

If swelling prevents closure of the skin, then no attempt should be made to draw the skin edges together with tension sutures. Sutures should only be used on skin where the tension is not high. If the whole wound cannot be closed, the ends of the incision can often be closed, leaving the middle for a delayed secondary suture. This complication is the best reason for siting the incision over muscle and not bone. In these situations, relaxing incisions should not be used as there is a risk of producing skin necrosis of the bridge with exposure of the implant.

Attempts to piece together a complex fracture using multiple interfragmentary screws should not be made as this destroys the blood supply. These are the fractures that should be reduced by traction and held by a neutralization plate.

Type II open fractures of the diaphysis can be plated, although a risk of infection prevails. When delay occurs between injury and fixation, infection rates become unacceptably high, even in type I and II injuries. Infections that do occur can be managed conservatively by leaving the plate in place for bone healing to occur. However, this is a long drawn-out and expensive process with few alternatives for better treatment. In a series of 97 patients with compound fractures, who were all plated, the early sepsis rate was 5.4% for type I injuries, 7.8% for type II injuries and 44% for type III injuries (Clifford *et al.* 1988). At final review, which varied between 6 months and 2 years, all but one of the wounds had healed. An incidence of 10% significant joint stiffness, 7% implant failure and three cases of malunion were seen. This is good evidence that grade III injuries should not be treated by internal fixation. While type II−III open fractures are probably best treated by external fixation, lesser injuries may be either plated or externally fixed (Bach & Hansen 1989).

COMPLICATIONS

Wound infection

The complication with the most morbidity for this technique is infection, eradication of which cannot be achieved without removal of the metalware. The aetiology may be due to preoperative compounding of the wound, an immunocompromised patient prone to infection, or a patient with pre-existing infection which spreads into a fracture haematoma. Operative causes include poor prevention of endogenous or exogenous sources of infection, poor tissue handling and a long operating time. Postoperative causes may be dehiscence of the wound or haematogenous spread of infection. The safest treatment of this complication is to remove the plate, treat the infection by debriding the infected bone and using the antibiotics indicated by culture and sensitivity reports, and finally immobilizing the fracture in a removable cast brace, if it is stable to shortening, or by external fixation if it is not. If the fracture is not

amenable to immobilization by other techniques, then it can be successfully treated by drainage, dressings, antibiotics on occasion, and waiting for the fracture to heal enough to support the patient's weight when it is safe to remove the plate and debride the wound. This 'last resort' option works but may take 2−3 years of treatment (Fig. 23.14).

Failure of fixation

Fixation failure may occur because too much is expected of the quality of bone that has been fixed. Osteoporotic or osteomalacic bone is notorious for causing implant failure. The implant itself may fail if a plate or screws of adequate strength have not been used in a heavy patient who is fully weight-bearing too early. Poor operative technique when cutting and tapping screw holes may lead to early failure, as may siting the plate on the compression side of a fracture and leaving the tension side unprotected. Some of the signs of failure of fixation include callus formation, resorption of bone around screws, and an increase in the fracture gap, which usually means inadequate fracture site reduction and compression. If any of these signs are recognized then either the limb should be protected in a functional brace or the fixation should be revised and bone graft added.

Non-union

One of the difficulties with internal fixation by compression plating is that it is difficult to tell radiographically exactly when fracture healing has occurred. Most surgeons would not remove a plate before 18−24 months expecting to see any remaining fracture gap to have gone with remodelling. As the standard definition of non-union is an ununited fracture after 6 months, this complication is difficult to diagnose.

Refracture

Refracture is common after compression plating. Fracture may occur at the original site or through one of the screw holes. Contact sports should be avoided until at least 12 months after removal of a plate. In a prospective study of 278 closed fractures of the tibia, Pinder showed that this complication was more common following conservative treatment, 4% against 2.8% following compression plating. All refractures occurred during sport (Pinder 1973).

Intramedullary internal fixation

The best indications for this fixation technique are the axially unstable fracture, both simple and comminuted, and segmental fractures. This includes closed injuries and compound types I–II. Some large centres would accept the inevitable incidence of up to 11.1% intramedullary osteomyelitis that accompanies intramedullary nailing of type III fractures (Court-Brown *et al.* 1990). Nailing an infected pseudoarthrosis after a failed plating is absolutely contraindicated because nailing tends to devascularize the inner third of a cortex that has been devascularized by the application of a compression plate. The advantages of intramedullary fixation are that postoperative supervision, malunion and shortening are less than for other methods of immobilization. The disadvantages are that a second operation is necessary for removal of the device, there is a risk of osteomyelitis, even in closed injuries, and the high incidence of knee pain precludes its use in patients with occupations that require kneeling.

Current debate on intramedullary nailing concerns the advantages of nails that can be placed in unreamed tibias against placing nails in reamed tibias. Histological studies have shown that an unreamed nail causes less vascular damage to the endosteal circulation than does an interference nail placed following reaming to ensure a good fit. Apart from the thermal necrosis that reaming causes, it may also cause embolization of the inner two-thirds of Haversian vessels supplied by the endosteal circulation. There is some evidence to show that the use of unreamed nails reduces the incidence of infection in compound fractures (DeLong *et al.* 1989). However, the use of Ender's nails, as in the study by Delong *et al.*, is associated with an unacceptable incidence of late angulation and a lack of rotational control (Henley 1989). To some extent, the debate has been answered by the introduction of a nail engineered to be slim enough to be used unreamed yet strong enough not to fail under full weight-bearing. These unreamed tibial nails can be locked with screws either end to prevent shortening, but unless a reduced fracture is going to take the patient's weight it would be best to restrict the patient from full weight-bearing. Full weight-bearing with a fracture gap and a locked nail usually results in shearing of the proximal or distal screws.

The original Küntscher nails, which were so useful for femoral fractures, were difficult to introduce into the tibial canal as they were straight and not flexible. Furthermore, with the original interference fit nails only the fractures in the middle third of the diaphysis could be immobilized. The advent of the Herzog bend on the nail and proximal and distal locking extended the use of such devices to within a handsbreadth of either joint surface.

The modern intramedullary nail is inserted under the strictest of aseptic conditions using prophylactic antibiotics, an alcohol-based skin antiseptic, adhesive plastic drapes, and with the operation performed under laminar flow conditions, where possible (Lidwell *et al.* 1982), to avoid osteomyelitis. The operation may be performed on a radiolucent table with the limb dependent over the side. For more difficult reductions, or where the fracture is unstable, it is performed on a traction table with skeletal traction using an os calcis pin placed 2 cm below and 2 cm behind the lateral malleolus. A Denham pin is best placed from the lateral side with the operator's free hand palpating the posterior tibial neurovascular bundle on the medial side to prevent impaling it and to control insertion to ensure that the pin is horizontal with the long axis of the tibia. A Böhler stirrup is used to secure the traction pin to the traction device.

The patient is placed supine on the operating table with the hip and knee flexed to right angles. Before skin preparation and draping are undertaken it is important to ensure that reduction has been achieved and the radiographer using the image intensifier has good views of the tibia from the knee to the ankle in both the anteroposterior and lateral planes. It is the responsibility of the most senior surgeon to minimize the radiation exposure to the patient and theatre staff during what can be a radiographic-intensive procedure. When the patient has been draped, an incision is made in the mid-line of the patellar tendon from the middle of the patella to the tibial tubercle. The incision is deepened to the patellar tendon and either a tendon-splitting approach or a medial parapatellar approach is used to gain access to the extracapsular area between the tibial condyles, occupied by the retropatellar fat pad. A starter hole is made with an awl as far back as possible, using the tibial tubercle as a guide to entering the medullary canal in the mid-line of the tibia. Next, the proximal metaphysis is reamed with hand reamers of increasing diameter to allow the olive-tipped guide wire to be passed into the distal fragment. Check radiographically that the wire is in the medullary canal of the distal fragment in two planes. For a reamed nail a powered intramedullary reamer is used to expand the canal into a uniform diameter. Reaming is usually continued until the endosteal surface of the cortex is felt to provide some resistance to the reamer. A nail that is 1–1.5 mm smaller in diameter than the largest reamer passed is chosen. For the unreamed nail a series of olive-tipped sounds are passed and the appropriate nail diameter is chosen. The length of the nail is measured using a radio-opaque ruler and image intensifier. The length may be checked by measuring the length of the guide wire protruding from the proximal tibia and subtracting this from the total length of the guide wire. The olive-tipped guide wire is changed for the untipped guide and the nail of correct length is passed. It is often easier to remove the guide wire once the tip of the nail has passed into the distal fragment and before the nail has been hammered home.

Distal locking is easily performed freehand using a Steinman's pin and the image intensifier. If one knows how much distraction at the fracture site exists, how far the nail is from the distal ankle joint and how far into the proximal hole the nail is, one can decide on locking proximally or distally first. The advantages of distal locking first are that the fracture gap can be closed, the first screw hole, if too distal or too proximal to the nail hole, can be matched to the hole by tapping the nail further in or further out, and the more difficult task is undertaken while the surgeon is still relatively fresh. The distal locking screws should be proud of the distal cortex by about 5 mm. This is because if the screws should break, before dynamization or removal of the nail, the lateral half of the screw may be easily found and removed through a lateral incision.

Proximal locking is performed using the nail's own locking guides. Always check the position of the screws with the image intensifer. We apply a plaster backslab with the foot in the neutral position and elevate the limb for up to 5 days to reduce the risk of infection from leaking wounds at the sites of the screw and Denham pin. After this, the patient is mobilized partial weight-bearing, progressing to full weight-bearing depending on the axial stability of the fracture.

Like the external fixator, a locked tibial nail may be dynamized if this is thought necessary because a wide fracture gap is being maintained. The locked nail is dynamized by removing either proximal or distal locking screws. The proximal screws are removed if the distal end of the nail is down to the distal epiphyseal scar. The distal screws are removed if the proximal end of the nail is proud of the tibia. In general, the screws should be removed from the larger fracture fragment.

Removal of a nail when fracture healing and remodelling have taken place may or may not be necessary (Fig. 23.36a−f). We make this decision with patients, advising them on complications, their general condition, age, aetiology of the condition and symptoms.

Infection

In 1986, Bone and Johnson showed that in a series of closed nailings for fractures with grade II and III wounds there was 10 times the risk of infection compared with the closed or grade I wounds. Infection was successfully treated in all but one case. The average time to full weight-bearing was 4 weeks. Radiological union was estimated to have occurred at an average of 17.8 weeks with segmental fractures presenting little problem.

In a series of 401 complex tibial fractures that were nailed, Klemm reported an infection rate of 2.2% in a study containing 25% grade I compound wounds. The presence of a puncture wound led to a sevenfold increase in the risk of infection. As in the previous series, the delayed union rate was low at 0.7% (Klemm & Borner 1986).

The treatment of sepsis following intramedullary nailing is contentious. The colonizing organism must be sought prior to antibiotic therapy. One method of treatment advocates debridement of the infected tissue followed by closed continuous irrigation of the nail with antibiotic solution. If this is unsuccessful, then the nail is removed, the infected membrane reamed from the medullary canal and the canal lavaged, followed by a replacement nail along with polymethylmethacrylate (PMMA) gentamicin beads. Such treatment requires careful supervision and close co-ordination with the bacteriologists.

Malunion and shortening

The incidence of malunion is low, occurring in 2.4% in a series of closed, and 29% in a series of all injuries treated by nailing (Alho *et al.* 1990, Court-Brown *et al.* 1990). Attempts to nail very low fractures will result in angulation of the fracture. Rotational malalignment must and can be avoided by repeated checking of rotation using the greater trochanter, the patella and the big toe of both limbs as guides.

An unacceptable amount of shortening may occur on dynamization of a locked nail in a comminuted fracture. It is therefore wise to consider carefully the likelihood of this complication prior to removal of the locking screws.

If shortening has occurred once the fracture has consolidated, correction may be performed. Where the nail is not radiologically loose, then a step diaphyseal osteotomy is performed. Laminar spreaders are then employed to elongate the osteotomy to the required

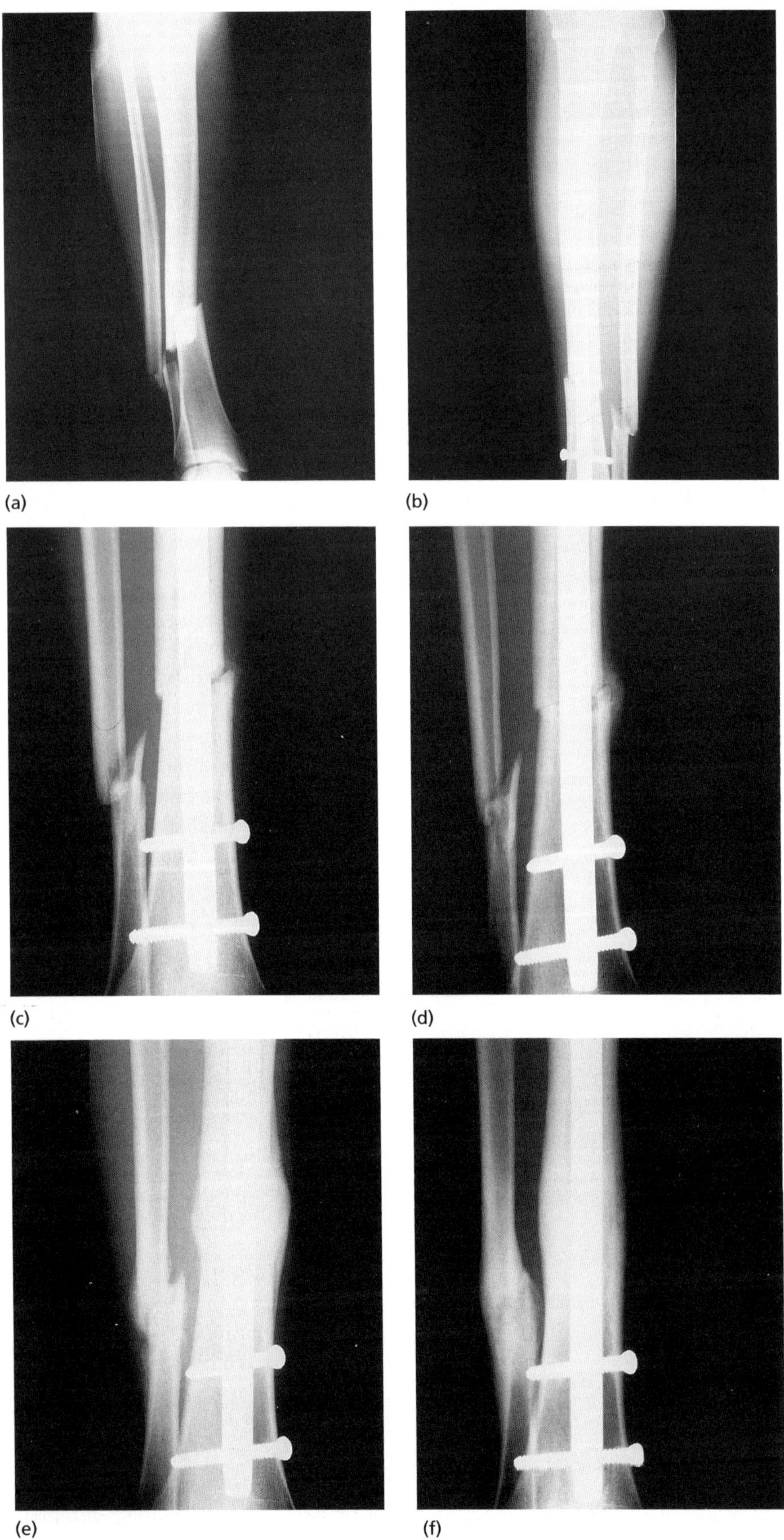

Fig. 23.36 (a)–(f) Radiographs of a fracture, treated by locked intramedullary nailing and the series of close-up radiographs showing healing by callus bridging in a full weight-bearing patient. The last radiograph shows the remodelled fracture site.

length and the gaps at the ends of the step osteotomy are grafted with autologous bone graft. The nail is fully interlocked at the new length and the patient mobilized in a light plastic gaiter, partially weight-bearing. If the nail is loose, then the medulla is reamed first and a tighter fitting nail inserted.

Knee pain

Failure to site the entry point of the nail sufficiently proximal or use of too long a nail may lead to difficulty with patellar tendon abrasion and pain on kneeling; this will necessitate nail removal. Knee pain and tenderness is a common complication, occurring in 40.8% of patients in one series (Court-Brown *et al.* 1990). It seems to occur regardless of the degree to which the top of the nail has been buried in the proximal tibia and even if the nail is removed. It does not seem to be altered by performing the operation through a low transverse incision rather than a longitudinal incision. For this reason, patients whose job requires kneeling should be informed of this complication at the time of consent.

Fracture of the tibial plateau may occur with nailing and is probably related to poor technique rather than the nail type (Court-Brown *et al.* 1990) (Fig. 23.37). Comminution of the bone can also occur.

Implant failure

Nail fatigue and failure can occur with any nail type. The screws are also prone to fatigue fracture.

Delayed union

As with all methods of fixation, this complication is most likely to be due to the severity of the original injury. This is a difficult diagnosis to make in the presence of a nail. Though delayed union occurs as in other methods of fixation (Court-Brown *et al.* 1990), it does not seem to be as great a problem, in terms of patient morbidity, as with other methods of fixation (Alho *et al.* 1990).

The problem fracture
Non-union

Aseptic fractures that fail to unite following conservative treatment are generally the ones which leave the surgeon with the greatest freedom with regard to possible operative treatment types.

The hypertrophic delay in union may be recognized by the extension of the fracture line out into the newly formed callus. Provided that undue motion can be eliminated at the fracture site, union will follow in the majority of cases. This motion may be eliminated conservatively by supplying a better fitting plaster cast and reducing weight-bearing. It is helpful to educate the patient by showing radiographs of the fracture that has occurred in the new callus as a result of continued motion through weight-bearing too much and for too long periods. If prolonged use of these methods results in a large callus or delayed union, then union will occur using surgical methods of reducing movement at the

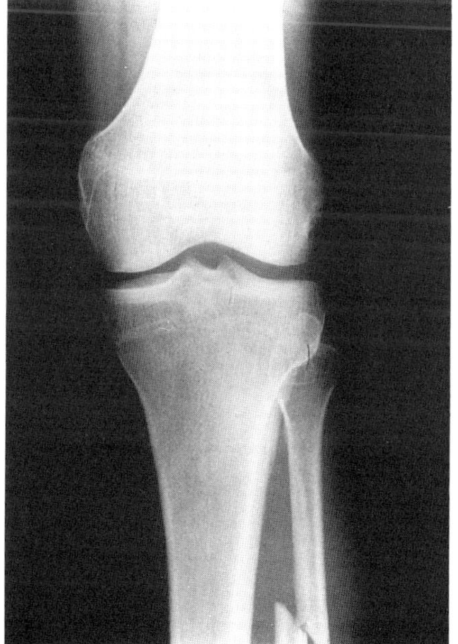

(a)

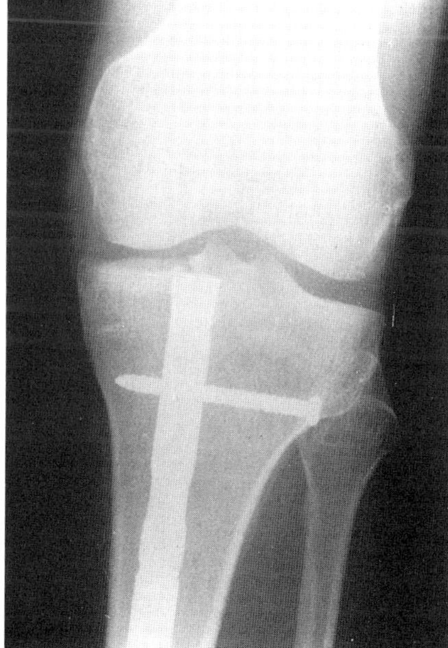

(b)

Fig. 23.37 (a) Radiograph showing a normal tibial plateau prior to nailing. (b) After nailing the tibial plateau has split. The patient made an uneventful recovery.

fracture site, without recourse to the use of bone graft and its attendant problems of donor site pain. Plating and reamed intramedullary nailing (Sledge *et al.* 1989) are both useful methods for this complication. Intramedullary nailing should be performed by an experienced surgeon using endcutting reamers to cross the endosteal callus at the fracture site.

The atrophic delay in union, and those that have progressed to non-union are difficult to predict. Most healing fractures have evidence of calcification of that callus between 6 and 8 weeks after injury (Hardy *et al.* 1993). Fracture stiffness measurements in patients with external fixators may be a useful early predictor of patients developing atrophic non-union because the lack of progress in stiffness, which is normally exponential with time, can be seen early (Richardson *et al.* 1992). The majority of cases of atrophic non-union arise from periosteal and soft tissue damage at the time of injury but a few may be associated with infection at the fracture site. Rarely, an apparent atrophic non-union may be due to failure of a callus to calcify. This occurs in patients with osteomalacia from various causes. Provided that infection has been excluded, plating or intramedullary nailing is appropriate when augmented by means of an autologous cancellous bone graft. The same bone-grafting technique may be used in the fracture immobilized with external fixation. If nailing is to be considered following external fixation, a period of 6 weeks in plaster following the removal of the fixator pins is recommended before nailing is performed. Pin site infections should first be treated with a course of antibiotics. Nailing following removal of a plate carries the theoretical risk of the devascularization of the endosteal bone supply that survived the original injury and in most cases should be avoided.

Osteomyelitis

The overriding principle in the management of this complication is the removal of those parts that can act as a nidus for infection. This necessitates the removal of metalware, dead bone sequestra and avascular scar tissue. Only viable tissue must be left and this is recognized either by bleeding from lacunae on using a sharp osteotome or with the occasional use of vital dyes. Radioisotope scans are not particularly reliable with respect to assessing bone viability. A stable locomotor environment is essential for the healthy recovery of the infected environment and this is best obtained by external fixation of the healthy bone away from the infected area. When bone graft is used to replace an infected segmental defect, the Papineau technique is improved by an irrigation system, using Hartmann's solution, to prevent desiccation of the graft fragments (Malkawi *et al.* 1984).

Bone loss

Where bone loss has become a problem, the Papineau technique of open on-lay grafting with fresh autologous cancellous graft to fill the defect is recommended (Papineau *et al.* 1979). The cancellous chips are slowly vascularized and, ultimately, granulation takes place over the surface, allowing split-skin grafting of the defect. Though the process takes months it is a safe and well-tested technique. Those experienced in the techniques of turning vascular flaps may, at the time of applying the cancellous graft, use a soft tissue flap to augment the blood supply to the area. Another technique is to use PMMA spacers to allow soft tissue healing, whilst preventing obliteration of the soft tissue tube, followed by cancellous grafting (Christian *et al.* 1989).

More substantial defects can be bridged with free fibular grafts (Nusbickel *et al.* 1989), although incorporation and functional hypertrophy may take a long time. Non-union at one end of the strut is not uncommon. Massive vascularized autologous bone grafting helps promote union when performed by experienced surgeons (Weiland 1981).

Bone transport, using a technique first proposed by Ilizarov, has aroused considerable recent interest with the introduction of unilateral external fixation frames that allow this technique to be performed more easily (Ilizarov 1976). Technical difficulties are considerable and experience is required in the use and manipulation of external fixators for this purpose. Much has been written in the context of tibial fractures as they are most prone to the complications seen in any bone. The management is complex and requires not only experience but a combined approach for the various techniques employed.

References

Alho, A., Ekeland, A., Stromsoe, K., Follerås, G. & Bjørn, O.T. Locked intramedullary nailing for displaced tibial shaft fractures. *J Bone Joint Surg* 1990; **72B**: 805–809.

Allen, M.J., Nash, J.R., Ioannidies, T.T. & Bell, P.R. Major vascular injuries associated with orthopaedic injuries to the lower limb. *Ann R Coll Surg Engl* 1984; **66(2)**: 101–104.

Armstrong, K., Sfeir, R., Rice, J. & Kerstein, M. Popliteal vascular injuries and war: Are Beirut and New Orleans similar? *J Trauma* 1988; **28(6)**: 836–839.

Bach, A.W. & Hansen, J.T. Jr. Plates versus external fixation in severe open tibial fractures. *Clin Orthop* 1989; **241**: 89–94.

Bassey, L.O. The use of POP integration transfixion pins as an improvisation on the Hoffmann's apparatus: Contribution to open fracture management in the tropics. *J Trauma* 1989; **29(1)**: 59−64.

Bondurant, F.J., Cotler, H.J., Buckle, R., Miller Crotchett, P. & Browner, B.D. The medical and economic impact of severely injured lower extremities. *J Trauma* 1988; **28**: 1270−1273.

Bone, L.B. & Johnson, K.D. The treatment of tibial fractures by reaming and intramedullary nailing. *J Bone Joint Surg* 1986; **68A**: 877−887.

Böstman, O.M. Rotational refracture of the shaft of the adult tibia. *Injury* 1983; **15(2)**: 93−98.

Böstman, O. & Kyrö, A. Delayed union of fibular fractures accompanying fractures of the tibial shaft. *J Trauma* 1991; **31(1)**: 99−102.

Bourne, R.B. & Rorabeck, C.H. Compartment syndromes of the lower leg. *Clin Orthop* 1989; **240**: 97−104.

Broos, P.L.O., Stappaerts, K.H., Luiten, E.J.T. & Gruwez, J.A. The importance of early fixation in multiply injured patients to prevent late death from sepsis. *Injury* 1987; **18**: 235−237.

Button, A.C. On the physical equilibrium of small blood vessels. *Physiol Rev* 1951; **34**: 619.

Caudle, R.J. & Stern, P.J. Severe open fractures of the tibia. *J Bone Joint Surg* 1987; **69A**: 801−807.

Charnley, J. *The Closed Treatment of Common Fractures* 3rd edn. Churchill Livingstone, Edinburgh, 1961.

Christenson, J.T. & Wulff, K. Compartment pressure following leg injury: The effect of diuretic treatment. *Injury* 1985; **16(9)**: 591−594.

Christian, E.P., Bosse, M.J. & Robb, G. Reconstruction of large diaphyseal defects, without free fibular transfer, in grade-IIIB tibial fractures. *J Bone Joint Surg* 1989; **71**: 994−1004.

Clancey, G.J. & Hansen, S.T. Open fractures of the tibia. *J Bone Joint Surg* 1978; **60A**: 118−122.

Clifford, R.P., Beauchamp, C.G., Kellam, J.F., Webb, J.K. & Tile, M. Plate fixation of open fractures of the tibia. *J Bone Joint Surg* 1988; **70B**: 644−648.

Cohen, M.S., Garfin, S.R., Hargens, A.R. & Mubarak, S.J. Acute compartment syndrome. Effect of dermotomy on fascial decompression in the leg. *J Bone Joint Surg* 1991; **73B**: 287−290.

Court-Brown, C.M., Christie, J. & McQueen, M.M. Closed intramedullary tibial nailing. *J Bone Joint Surg* 1990; **72B**: 605−611.

Court-Brown, C.M., McQueen, M.M., Quaba, A.A. & Christie, J. Hughes external fixator in treatment of tibial fractures. *J R Soc Med* 1985; **78**: 830−837.

Cunningham, J.L., Kenwright, J. & Kershaw, C.J. Biomechanical measurement of fracture healing. *J Med Eng Technol* 1990; **14(3)**: 92−101.

Danis, R. *Theorie et Pratique de l'Osteosynthese*. Masson: Paris, 1949.

De Bastiani, G., Aldegheri, R. & Brivio, L.R. The treatment of fractures with a dynamic axial fixator. *J Bone Joint Surg* 1984; **66B**: 538−545.

Dellinger, E.P., Caplan, E.S., Weaver, L.D., Wertz, M.J., Droppert, B.M., Hoyt, N., Brumback, R., Burgess, A., Poka, A., Benirschke, S.K., Lennard, E.S. & Lou, M.A. Duration of preventive antibiotic administration for open extremity fractures. *Arch Surg* 1988; **123**: 333−339.

DeLong, W.G. Jr, Born, C.T., Marcelli, E., Shaikh, K.A., Iannocone, W.M. & Schwab, C.W. Enders nail fixation in long bone fractures, experience in a level I trauma center. *J Trauma* 1989; **29(5)**: 571−576.

Digby, J.M., Holloway, G.M.N. & Webb, J.K. A study of function after tibial cast bracing. *Injury* 1983; **14**: 432−439.

Dreyfuss, D.C., Kaufman, J.L., Flancbaum, L., Stark, K.R. & Dinerstein, C.R. Improved operative exposure of infrapopliteal vessels in combined vascular and orthopaedic injuries. *J Vasc Surg* 1987; **6(4)**: 422−423.

Edge, A.J. & Denham, R.A. External fixation for complicated tibial fractures. *J Bone Joint Surg* 1981; **63B**: 92−97.

Edwards, P. & Nilsson, B.E.R. Graphic representation of healing time in fractures of the shaft of the tibia. *Acta Orthop Scand* 1965; **36**: 104−111.

Ellis, H. The speed of healing after fracture of the tibial shaft. *J Bone Joint Surg* 1958a; **40B**: 42−46.

Ellis, H. Disabilities after tibial shaft fractures. *J Bone Joint Surg* 1958b; **40B**: 190−197.

Elson, R.A., Jephcott, A.E., McGechie, D.B. & Verettas, D. Bacterial infection and acrylic cement in the rat. *J Bone Joint Surg* 1977; **59B**: 452−457.

Friedman, R.J. & Jupiter, J.B. Vascular injuries and closed extremity fractures in children. *Clin Orthop* 1984; **188**: 112−119.

Fuhrman, F.A. & Crismon, J.M. Early changes in distribution of sodium, potassium and water in rabbit muscles following release of tourniquets. *Am J Physiol* 1951; **166**: 424−432.

Gad, H.F. Treatment of open tibial shaft fractures by delayed closed intramedullary nailing. *J R Coll Surg Edinb* 1991; **36**: 417−420.

Glasson, D.W. & Morrison, W.A. Complex limb trauma requiring revascularization: Early multidisciplinary management. *Aust NZ J Surg* 1988; **58(7)**: 543−548.

Goodship, A.E. & Kenwright, J. The influence of induced micromovement upon the healing of experimental tibial fractures. *J Bone Joint Surg* 1985; **67B(4)**: 650−655.

Green, S.A. Complications of external skeletal fixation. *Clin Orthop* 1983; **180**: 109−116.

Gregory, R.T., Gould, R.J., Peclet, M., Wagner, J.S.M., Gilert, D.A., Wheeler, J.R., Snyder, S.O., Gayle, R.G. & Schwab, C.W. The mangled extremity syndrome (M.E.S.): A severity grading system for multisystem injury of the extremity. *J Trauma* 1985; **25**: 1147−1150.

Gregson, P.A. Tibial cast wedging: a simple and effective technique. *J Bone Joint Surg* 1994; **76B**: 496−497.

Gustilo, R.B. Prevention of infection in the treatment of one thousand and twenty five open fractures of long bones. *J Bone Joint Surg* 1976; **58A**: 453−458.

Gustilo, R.B., Mendoza, R.M. & Williams, D.N. Problems in the management of Type III (severe) open fractures: a new classification of type III open fractures. *J Trauma* 1984; **24**: 742−746.

Hardy, J.R.W., Conlan, D., Hay, S. & Gregg, P.J. Serum ionised calcium and its relationship to parathyroid hormone after tibial fracture. *J Bone Joint Surg* 1993; **75B**: 645−649.

Heatley, F.W. Severe open tibial fractures − the courage to amputate. *Br Med J* 1988; **229**: 296.

Henley, M.B. Intramedullary devices for tibial fracture stabilisation. *Clin Orthop* 1989; **240**: 87−96.

Heppenstall, R.B. *Fracture Treatment and Healing*. WB Saunders: Philadelphia, 1980.

Herve, C., Gaillard, M., Andrivet, P., Roujas, F., Kauer, C. & Huguenard, P. Treatment in serious lower limb injuries:

Amputation versus preservation. *Injury* 1987; **18**: 21–23.

Hidaglo, D.A. Lower extremity avulsion injuries. *Clin Plast Surg* 1985; **13(4)**: 701–710.

Howard, P.W. & Makin, G.S. Lower limb fractures with associated vascular injury. *J Bone Joint Surg* 1990; **72B**: 116–120.

Hulth, A. Current concepts of fracture healing. *Clin Orthop* 1989; **249**: 265–284.

Hutzschenreuter, P., Perren, S.M., Steinemann, S., Geret, V. & Klebl, M. Some effects of rigidity of external fixation on the healing pattern of osteotomies. *Injury* 1969; **1**: 77–81.

Ilizarov, G.A. Basic principles of trausosseous compression and distraction osteosynthesis. *Ortop Traumatol Protez* 1971; **32**: 7–11.

Klemm, K.W. & Borner, M. Interlocking nailing of complex fractures of the femur and tibia. *Clin Orthop* 1986; **212**: 89–100.

Krettek, C., Haas, N. & Tscherne, H. The role of supplemental lag-screw fixation for open fractures of the tibial shaft treated with external fixation. *J Bone Joint Surg* 1991; **73A**: 893–897.

Kuusela, T.V. Incidence of bone lesions in the lower extremities during endurance training. *Ann Clin Res* 1984; **16**: 17–19.

Lange, R.H. Limb reconstruction versus amputation: Decision making in massive lower extremity trauma. *Clin Orthop* 1989; **243**: 92–99.

Letts, R.M. Degloving injuries in children. *J Pediatr Orthop* 1985; **6(2)**: 193–197.

Lidwell, O.M., Lowbury, E.H.L., Whyte, W., Blowers, R., Stanley, S.J. & Lowe, D. Effect of ultraclean air in operating rooms on deep sepsis in the joint after total hip or knee replacement, a randomised study. *Br Med J* 1982; **285**: 10–14.

Lindsay, M.K. & Howes, E.L. The breaking strength of healing fractures. *J Bone Joint Surg* 1931; **13**: 491–501.

McAndrew, M.P. & Lantz, B.A. Initial care of massively traumatized lower extremities. *Clin Orthop* 1989; **243**: 20–29.

McKibbin, B. The biology of fracture healing in long bones. *J Bone Joint Surg* 1978; **60B**: 150–162.

Malkawi, H., Shannak, A. & Sunna, P. Active treatment of segmental defects of long bones with established infection. A prospective study. *Clin Orthop* 1984; **184**: 241–248.

Matthews, L.S. & Hirsch, C. Temperatures measured in human cortical bone when drilling. *J Bone Joint Surg* 1972; **54A**: 297–308.

Meek, A.C. & Robbs, J.V. Vascular injury with associated bone and joint trauma. *Br J Surg* 1984; **71(5)**: 341–344.

Melendez, E.M. & Colon, C. Treatment of open tibial fractures with the Orthofix fixator. *Clin Orthop* 1989; **241**: 224–230.

Micheli, L.J. Lower extremity overuse injuries. *Acta Med Scand* 1986; **711**: Suppl 171–177.

Mubarek, S.J. & Owen, C.A. Double incision fasciotomy of the leg for decompression of compartment syndromes. *J Bone Joint Surg* 1977; **59A**: 184–187.

Mubarek, S.J., Owen, C.A., Hargens, A.R., Garetto, L.P. & Akeson, W.H. Acute compartment syndromes: diagnosis of treatment with the aid of the wick catheter. *J Bone Joint Surg* 1978; **60A**: 1091–1095.

Müller, M.E., Allgöwer, M., Schneider, R. & Willenegger, H. *Manual of Internal Fixation* 3rd edn. Springer-Verlag: Berlin, 1991.

Nicoll, E.A. Fractures of the tibial shaft — a survey of 705 cases. *J Bone Joint Surg* 1964; **46B**: 373–387.

Nicholls, P.J., Berg, E., Bliven, F.E. & Kling, J.M. X-Ray diagnosis of healing fractures in rabbits. *Clin Orthop* 1979; **142**: 234–236.

Nusbickel, F.R., Dell, P.C., McAndrew, M.P. & Moore, M.M. Vascularized autografts for reconstruction of skeletal defects following lower extremity trauma. A review. *Clin Orthop* 1989; **243**: 65–70.

Oni, O.O.A., Gregg, P.J., Morrison, C. & Ponter, A.R.S. An investigation of the fracture characteristics of the tibia of mature rabbits. *Injury* 1988; **19**: 172–176.

Papineau, L.J., Alfageme, A., Dalcourt, J.P. & Pilon, L. Ostéomyélite chronique: Excision et greffe de spongieux a l'air libre après mises à plat extensives. *Int Orthop* 1979; **3**: 165–176.

Perren, S.M. Physical and biological aspects of fracture healing with special reference to internal fixation. *Clin Orthop* 1979; **138**: 175–196.

Pinder, I.M. Refracture of the shaft of the adult tibia. *J Bone Joint Surg* 1973; **55B**: 878.

Puno, R.M., Teynor, J.T., Nagano, J. & Gustilo, R.B. Critical analysis of results of treatment of 201 tibial shaft fractures at Hennepin County Medical Centre. *Clin Orthop* 1986; **212**: 113–121.

Rahn, B.A., Gallinaro, P., Baltensperger, A. & Perren, S.M. Primary bone healing — An experimental study in the rabbit. *J Bone Joint Surg* 1971; **53A**: 783–786.

Rang, M. *Children's Fractures* 2nd edn. Lippincott: Philadelphia, 1984.

Reis, N.D. & Michaelson, M. Crush injury to the lower limbs. Treatment of the local injury. *J Bone Joint Surg* 1986; **68A**: 414–418.

Richardson, J.B., Kenwright, J. & Cunningham, J.L. Fracture stiffness measurement in the assessment and management of tibial fracture. *J Biomech* 1992; **7**: 75–79.

Riska, E.B., von Bonsdorff, H., Hakkinen, S., Jaroma, H., Kiviluoto, O. & Paavilainen, T. Prevention of fat embolism by early internal fixation of fractures in patients. *Injury* 1976; **8**: 110–116.

Rommens, P., Broos, P. & Gruwez, J. External fixation of the tibial shaft fractures with severe soft tissue injuries by Hoffmann–Vidal–Audrey osteotaxis. *Arch Orthop Trauma Surg* 1986; **105(3)**: 170–174.

Ryder, H.W., Molle, W.E. & Ferris, E.B. The influence of collapsibility of veins on venous pressure, including a new procedure for measuring tissue pressure. *J Clin Invest* 1953; **23**: 334.

Sarmiento, A. A functional below the knee cast for tibial fractures. *J Bone Joint Surg* 1967; **49A**: 855–875.

Sarmiento, A. Functional bracing of tibial fractures. *Clin Orthop* 1974; **105**: 202–219.

Sarmiento, A., Gersten, L.M., Sobol, P.A., Shankwiler, J.A. & Vangsness, C.T. Tibial shaft fractures treated with functional braces: experiences with 780 fractures. *J Bone Joint Surg* 1989; **71A**: 602–609.

Seibel, R., Laduca, J., Hassett, J.M., Babikian, G., Mills, B., Border, D.O. & Border, J.R. Blunt multiple trauma (ISS 36), femur traction, and the pulmonary failure-septic state. *Ann Surg* 1985; **202**: 283–295.

Seiler, J.G. III & Richardson, J.D. Amputation after extremity injury. *Am J Surg* 1986; **152**: 260–264.

Sledge, S.L., Johnson, K.D., Henley, M.B. & Watson, J.T. Intramedullary nailing with reaming to treat non-union of the tibia. *J Bone Joint Surg* 1989; **71**: 1004–1019.

Svenningsen, S., Nesse, O., Finsen, V., Hole, A. & Penum, P. Prevention of fat embolism syndrome in patients with femoral fractures — immediate or delayed operative fixation?

Ann Chir Gynaecol 1987; **86**: 163—166.

Triffit, P.D., Konig, D., Harper, W.M., Barnes, M.R., Allen, M.J. & Gregg, P.J. Compartment pressures after closed tibial shaft fracture. Their relation to functional outcome. *J Bone Joint Surg* 1992; **74B**: 195—198.

Tscherne, H. & Gotzen, L. *Fractures with Soft Tissue Injuries.* Springer-Verlag: Berlin, 1984.

Urist, M.R., Mazet, R. & Mclean, F.C. The pathogenesis and treatment of delayed union and non-union. *J Bone Joint Surg* 1954; **36A**: 931—968.

Weaver, F.A., Rosenthal, R.E., Waterhouse, G. & Adkins, R.B. Combined skeletal and vascular injuries of the lower extremities. *Am J Surg* 1984; **50(4)**: 189—197.

Weiland, A.J. Current concepts review. Vascularized free bone transplants. *J Bone Joint Surg* 1981; **63A**: 166—169.

Weissman, S.L., Herold, H.Z. & Engleberg, M. Fractures of the middle two-thirds of the tibial shaft. *J Bone Joint Surg* 1966; **48A**: 257—267.

Ziv, I., Zeligowski, A., Mosheiff, R., Lowe, J., Wexler, M.R. & Segal, D. Split thickness skin excision in severe open fractures. *J Bone Joint Surg* 1988; **70B**: 23—26.

24: The Ankle

A.H.R.W.SIMPSON AND P.H.WORLOCK

Anatomical considerations

Both experimental and clinical studies have shown that even small displacements of the articular surfaces of the ankle joint from the anatomical position predispose to arthritis. Ramsey and Hamilton (1976) studied cadaver ankle joints using a carbon-black transference technique to investigate the tibio-talar contact area as the talus was shifted laterally. They found a dramatic drop (42%) with the first millimetre of lateral displacement and then a continuing reduction (Fig. 24.1).

Willeneger and Breitenfelder (1965) reported the effect of tilt of the talus on the contact area. A tilt of 2–4° had the effect of shifting the talus 2 mm laterally, and 2–3 mm of posterior shift of the lateral malleolus caused a rotation of 10° of the talus with a significant reduction in tibio-talar contact area.

Although reservations have been expressed as to how much these static cadaver studies can be used to predict the dynamic contact area, they do clearly show that minor displacements of the articular surfaces have a profound effect on joint congruity.

Physiological considerations

Determining the stability

Lauge-Hansen (1948, 1950) studied the way the ligamentous/bony structures failed in the ankles of cadavers. He then developed a classification (Fig. 24.2) which is useful for determining the type of force that has produced the injury and also for indicating the associated ligament damage and the degree of instability of the ankle. The former is useful in predicting which manoeuvre is needed for reduction, and the latter for determining whether internal fixation is likely to be needed; the more unstable a fracture the harder it is to hold the anatomical reduction by closed means.

Lauge-Hansen realized that the pattern of injury depends on the position of the foot and the type of

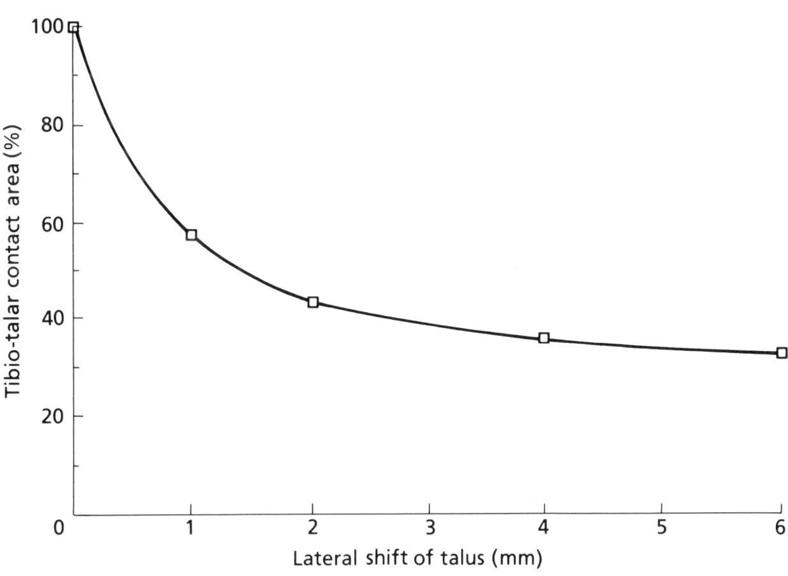

Fig. 24.1 Effect of lateral displacement of the talus on the contact area at the ankle joint.

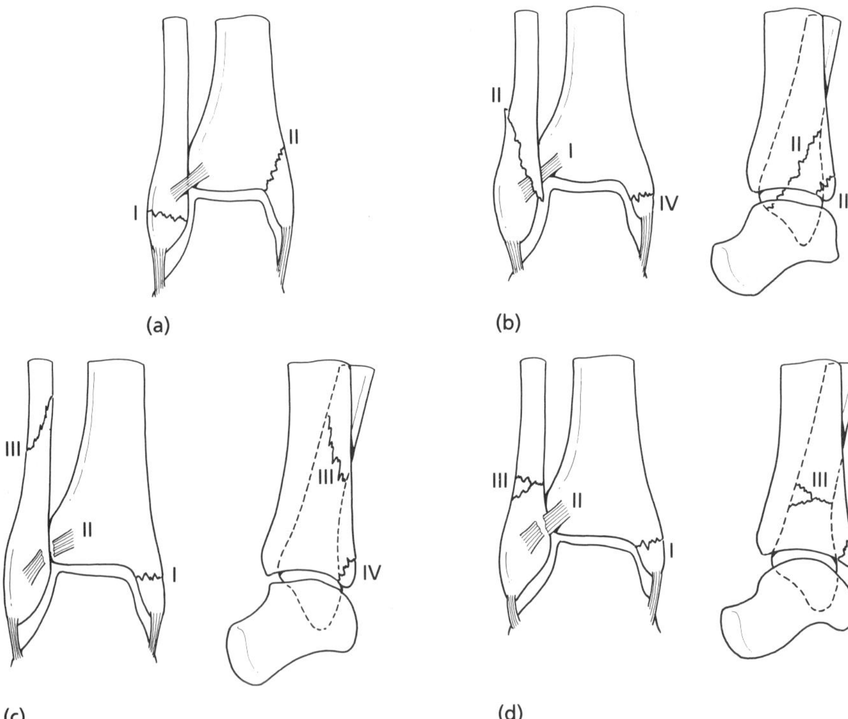

Fig. 24.2 (a) Supination–adduction (SA); (b) supination–external rotation (SE); (c) pronation–external rotation (PE); and (d) pronation–adduction (PA).

pathological force acting on the ankle. Therefore, in his classification, the first term refers to the position of the foot at the time of injury and the second term to the direction of the force applied to the talus.

Despite the many possible combinations of these two variables, which are also compounded by the amount of vertical compression and the amount of dorsiflexion and/or plantarflexion, the majority of patients can be placed into certain common groups.

For each type the injury is divided into stages and these refer to the sequence in which the structures failed.

1 *Supination–adduction (SA).*

Stage I — Transverse avulsion fracture of the fibula at, or inferior to, the tibial plafond or rupture of the collateral ligaments.

Stage II — Oblique or vertical fracture of the medial malleolus.

This mechanism of injury may also injure the talar dome by tilting the talus into varus and producing a crushing of the articular surface on the medial side or an osteochondral shear fracture on the lateral side.

2 *Supination–external rotation (SE).*

Stage I — Rupture of the anteroinferior tibio-fibular ligament within its substance or at the ligamento-osseous interface.

Stage II — Spiral fracture of the fibula at, or superior to, the level of the tibial plafond.

Stage III — Rupture of the posteroinferior tibio-fibular ligament or an avulsion fracture of the posterior malleolus.

Stage IV — Avulsion fracture of the medial malleolus or rupture of the deltoid ligament.

3 *Pronation–abduction (PA).*

Stage I — Transverse avulsion fracture of the medial malleolus or rupture of the deltoid ligament.

Stage II — Rupture of the syndesmosis, antero- and posteroinferior tibio-fibular ligaments within their substance or at the ligamento-osseous junction.

Stage III — Short oblique fracture of the fibula with the fracture line beginning immediately proximal to the ankle joint (occasionally, a butterfly fragment is present). Fractures of the talar dome are also associated with this injury mechanism.

4 *Pronation–external rotation (PE).*

Stage I — Transverse avulsion fracture of the medial malleolus or rupture of the deltoid ligament.

Stage II — Rupture of the anteroinferior tibio-fibular ligament and interosseous membrane.

Stage III — High spiral fracture of the fibula (the interosseous membrane is rupture to the level of the fibular fracture). This is also known as a Maisonneuve fracture.

Stage IV — Rupture of the posteroinferior tibio-fibular ligament or avulsion fracture of the posterior malleolus.

An avulsion fracture has the same effect on stability as rupture of the attached ligament. Therefore, in his analysis, Lauge-Hansen considered these fractures and ligament injuries as interchangeable. There are several eponyms for the fragments of these avulsion fractures: Tillaux fracture is an avulsion of the anterolateral part of the distal tibia by the anterior tibio-fibular ligament; Wagstaffe fracture is an avulsion of the anterior portion of the fibula by the anterior tibio-fibular ligament; and Volkmann fracture is an avulsion of the posterior lip of the lateral tibial plafond by the posterior tibio-fibular ligament.

Model for stability

The ankle joint can be considered to consist of two rings of stabilizing structures (Fig. 24.3). One ring lies in the coronal plane and is formed by the lateral and medial malleoli/collateral ligaments, the tibial plafond and the calcaneus; the other ring lies in the transverse plane and is composed of the anterior and posterior tibio-fibular ligaments, the malleoli and tibial margins with the interosseous ligament acting as a transverse tying cord. If either of the rings is unstable the ankle joint is unstable. The coronal ring is unstable if disrupted in two places on its circumference. The transverse ring is unstable if two of the three struts are disrupted.

The term stable is used here to indicate whether the fragments will displace when subjected to ordinary physiological forces.

Classification

To be of use a classification must address a question. For the question 'which patients are going to have a poor result?', the main factor determining the result is the adequacy of reduction of the articular surface, and a classification based on this is most appropriate, i.e. one based on the state of the reduction at fracture union. Phillips *et al.* (1985), in a follow-up of 71 patients for a mean of 3.5 years, found that a classification based on the talocrural angle (Fig. 24.4) had the best correlation with the patient outcome score. Similar results were found by Tile *et al.* (1977).

For the more common question 'what is the best way to treat this patient's fracture?', a classification based on the stability of the fracture complex is more useful. The more proximal fibular fractures have more extensive damage to the ligamentous structures that tie the fibula and tibia together; therefore, it is more likely that these fracture complexes are unstable. The Association for Osteosynthesis (AO) classification is an easy-to-apply

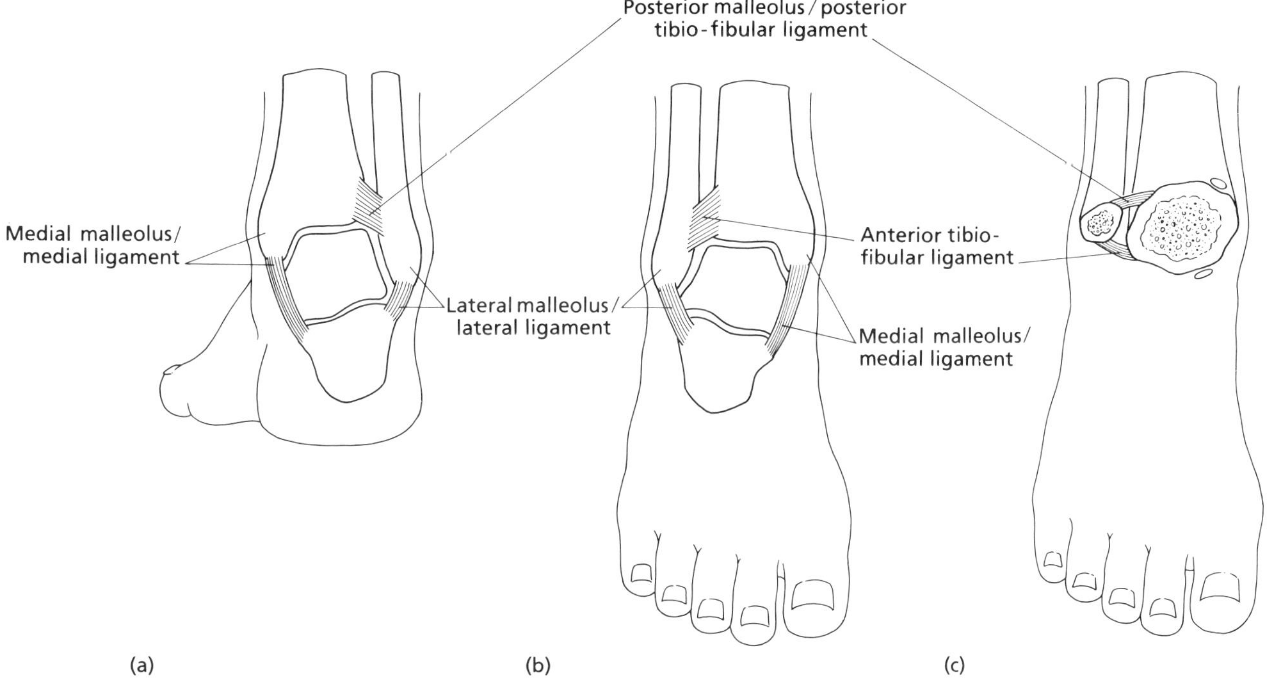

Fig. 24.3 (a)–(c) Ankle stability is dependent on the following structures: 1, the lateral malleolus/lateral ligament; 2, the medial malleolus/medial ligament; 3, the anterior tibio-fibular ligament; and 4, the posterior malleolus/posterior tibio-fibular ligament. As each successive group is lost, the ankle becomes more unstable. When all four groups have been lost, the ankle is completely unstable.

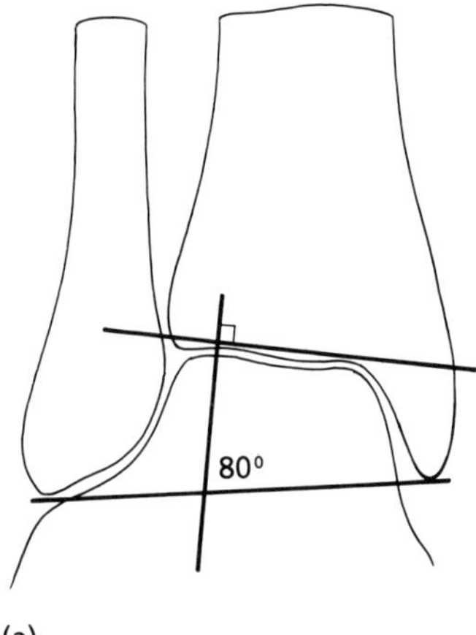

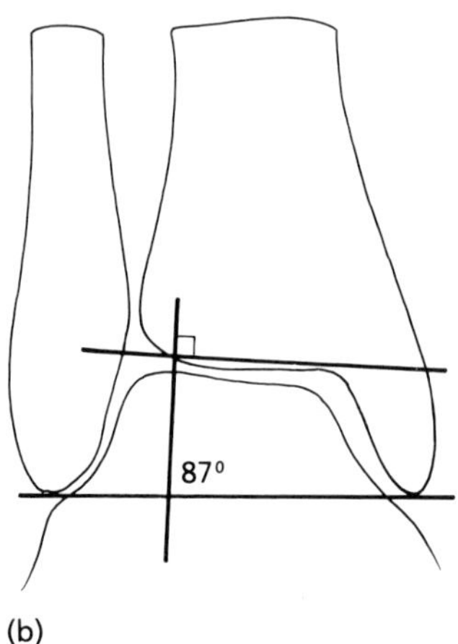

Fig. 24.4 The talocrural angle is the angle formed by the intersection of a line joining the tips of both malleoli and a line perpendicular to the articular surface. (a) The normal talocrural angle of 80°. (b) An abnormal angle secondary to shortening of the lateral malleolus.

system based on this. There are three patterns of injury determined by the level of the fibular fracture (Fig. 24.5) in relation to the syndesmosis.

Aims of treatment

The aims of treatment are: (i) to provide a pain-free joint with normal function; and (ii) to minimize the risk of post-traumatic arthritis.

Obtaining a pain-free functioning joint

There is general agreement that the best way to obtain a pain-free joint is to achieve union of the fracture in an anatomical position (Burwell & Charnley 1965, Hughes *et al.* 1979). However, there is still dispute over which method of treatment results in the fastest return of function.

The risk of post-traumatic arthritis

There is a correlation between poor reduction and early post-traumatic arthritis: Hughes *et al.* (1979) found arthritis in only one of 61 patients who had an anatomical reduction of their ankle fracture, but there was an incidence of 61 of 65 for those who had a poor reduction. Other workers have confirmed this (Burwell & Charnley 1965).

To obtain the maximum function and the minimum risk of post-traumatic arthritis, *union of the fracture should be obtained in an anatomical position.*

Operative versus non-operative management

To achieve an anatomical result it is necessary first to obtain the reduction and second to hold it until union.

Obtaining the reduction

For the majority of ankle fractures, reduction can be achieved by closed methods, reversing the forces that have produced the injury (see Lauge-Hansen 1948, 1950). There are some instances where closed reduction is impossible and open reduction is necessary:
1 Interposition of the deltoid ligament between the medial malleolus and the talus.
2 Interposition of the tibialis posterior tendon between the medial malleolus and talus (when the tendon sheath and deltoid ligament are torn).
3 Interposition of the lateral tendons may occur when the syndesmosis snaps open and traps them in the interosseous space.
4 Fracture dislocation with the fibula trapped posteriorly behind the tibia. With one such case it was possible to obtain a closed reduction. This required recognition on the preoperative radiographs and immediate manipulation under anaesthetic (Molinari *et al.* 1990). However, the majority of cases of this type of ankle fracture require open reduction.

An operative approach is also necessary in the following instances:
1 Displaced fractures of the medial malleolus that compromise the blood supply to the overlying skin of this area.
2 Fractures of the medial malleolus with small bone fragments within the joint.

Holding the reduction

For other fractures closed reduction is usually possible and the question is whether it is then possible to hold the reduction with closed means until union. The likelihood of this depends primarily on the degree of

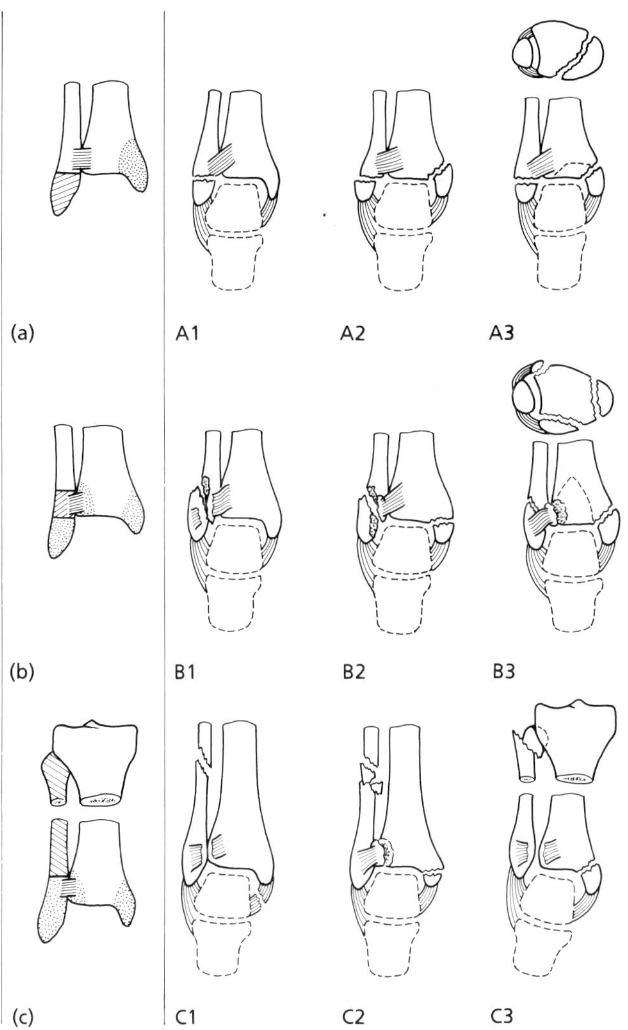

Fig. 24.5 AO classification of ankle injuries (a) A1, infrasyndesotic lesion, isolated; A2, infrasyndesmotic lesion, with fracture of medial malleolus; A3, infrasyndesmotic lesion, with posteromedial fracture. (b) B1, trans-syndesmotic fibular fracture, isolated; B2, trans-syndesmotic fibular fracture, with medial lesion; B3, trans-syndesmotic fibular fracture, with medial lesion and posterolateral fracture. (c) C1, suprasyndesmotic lesion, simple diaphyseasl fracture of fibula; C2, suprasyndesmotic lesion, diaphyseal fracture of the fibula, multifragmentary; C3, suprasyndesmotic lesion, proximal fibular lesion.

instability of the ankle, but also on the shape of the patient's leg, the degree of swelling and the compliance of the patient with any instructions.

Rowley *et al.* (1986), in a small trial with a short follow-up, did not find a significant difference in return to mobility between operative and non-operative treatment for unstable fractures. However, Hughes *et al.* (1979) reviewed the results of three series and concluded that for type B and C fractures the operative group had a better outcome.

In summary, if the joint is considered to be stable, the fragments will not shift and the fracture can be treated with a plaster cast or by early mobilization/analgesia only (Zeegers *et al.* 1989). If the joint is unstable, although it may be possible to hold the fracture to union by non-operative means, the most reliable method of ensuring a good result is internal fixation.

Operative principles

Originally, attention centred on the medial malleolus as being the most important bone to have correctly aligned. Now it is recognized that the fibula can take up to 20% of the body weight and it is essential to have the lateral malleolus as well as the medial malleolus correctly restored both in length and rotation.

Non-operative techniques

Sedation or regional or general anaesthesia can be used as long as the affected leg is completely relaxed. The direction of the injuring force is determined from the radiograph using Lauge-Hansen's classification. The force is reversed and the ankle reduced and then held in an above-knee padded cast using three-point moulding. If the swelling is severe, the cast may initially need to be changed each week to maintain reduction. As many as 50% of patients treated non-operatively may need a second manipulation as the swelling subsides. The rehabilitation regime depends on the stability of the ankle. If the fracture complex is stable, the patient can start to mobilize weight-bearing in a below-knee walking cast or an alternative orthosis as soon as the swelling has subsided. If the injury is unstable, then a long-leg non-weight-bearing cast is needed for 3–4 weeks, followed by a below-knee walking cast for 3–4 weeks.

Open technique

A single dose of intravenous antibiotic is given and then a thigh tourniquet is inflated. The skin incisions (Fig. 24.6) should not be directly over the subcutaneous border but adjacent to them. On both medial and lateral sides, the incisions can be curved in either direction. They should be designed to avoid any damaged areas of skin and to leave a large bridge between the two incisions. If the medial incision lies anterior and curves posteriorly, the saphenous nerve and vein are at risk. If the dissection is kept in front of the tibialis posterior

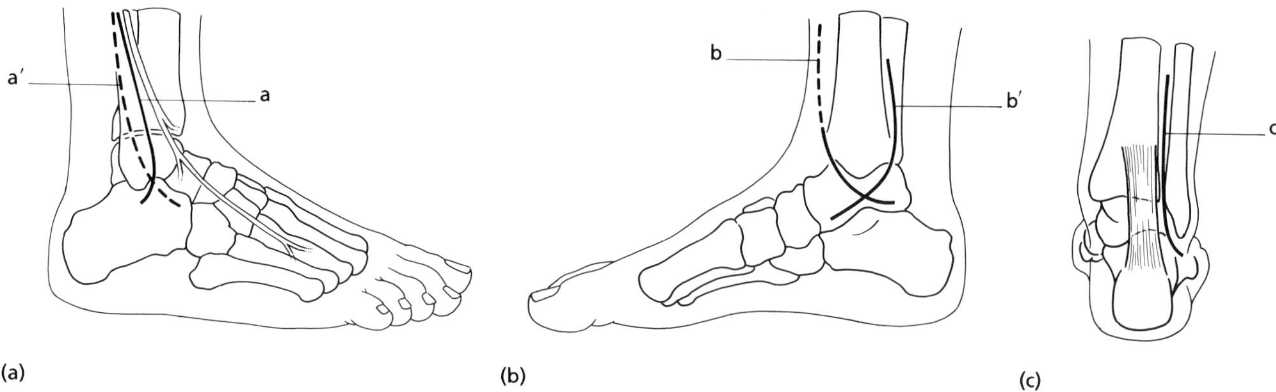

Fig. 24.6 Surgical approaches for malleolar fractures. (a) The anterolateral approach (a) is preferred to the posterolateral approach (a'). *Note*: Avoid superficial branch of the peroneal nerve. (b) Either an anteromedial incision (b) or a posteromedial incision (b') is used for the medial malleous. The posteromedial approach is used when there is a large posteromedial fragment. (c) The posterolateral approach (c) can be used for fixation of a fibular fracture, with an associated large posterolateral fracture.

tendon the neurovascular bundle is protected. On the lateral side, the superficial peroneal nerve lies in the proximal part of the wound and is at risk during incision.

ARTICULAR CARTILAGE DAMAGE

The talar dome should always be inspected for damage: Small loose fragments of the articular surface should be removed. Larger fragments should be reduced and fixed using a device such as the Herbert screw. The most common site for osteochondral fractures is the dome of the talus.

FRACTURES OF THE LOWER TWO-THIRDS OF THE FIBULA

The fibular fracture is fixed first to restore correct length and rotational alignment. Fractures of the lower two-thirds of the fibula should be plated. The lateral malleolus should be fixed with interfragmentary compression screws and either a 3.5-mm reconstruction plate or a one-third tubular plate used as a neutralization plate.

PROXIMAL FIBULAR FRACTURES

Type C ankle fractures involving the proximal third of the fibula should be reduced and held either by conventional plating or with a diastasis screw. Great care should be taken to ensure that the correct length and rotation of the fibula is obtained. If the fibula is plated in an anatomical position and if the medial injury is a fracture, also anatomically reduced and stably fixed, there is no need for a diastasis positioning screw.

MEDIAL MALLEOLUS

The medial malleolus should be fixed with two 4.0 cancellous screws perpendicular to the fracture line. These should not exceed 50 mm in length. Longer screws have a weaker grip because their thread lies proximal to the cancellous bone of the metaphysis. If the fracture is very comminuted a tension-band wire technique can be used for type B and C fractures. However, this is not suitable for type A fractures because they are caused by a compression force.

POSTERIOR MALLEOLUS

The posterior malleolus is best approached via a posterolateral incision, although it can be reached through a separate posterior incision. The fracture is reduced and K-wires inserted. If radiographs show an anatomical reduction, then screws can be inserted from the anterior surface across the fracture into the posterior malleolar fragment.

WOUND CLOSURE

Radiographs are obtained in the theatre; if talar shift is still present, the reduction of the lateral fragment is checked and if necessary corrected. It may be necessary to open the medial side to extract the deltoid ligament from the joint space. Suction drainage is used for all wounds. After closure of the wounds, it is essential to use a plaster back slab to prevent the foot dropping into equinus. The drains are removed after 24 hours, because after this period there is an increased risk of the drain tube acting as a portal of entry for infection. Mobilization is commenced at 24 hours.

Specific problems

The syndesmosis

The syndesmosis is the fibrous joint at the lower end of tibia and fibula. It is a variable structure both in size and strength. Monk (1969) found that its proximal extent varied from 2 to 6 cm superior to the joint line. If the syndesmosis has been disrupted, it is essential to hold the fibula in correct apposition with the tibia while this fibrous structure heals.

If there is a complete tear of the deltoid ligament and the fibular fracture is over 4.5 cm proximal to the joint line, there is a high probability that the distal tibio-fibular joint will be unstable (Boden *et al.* 1989). This should be checked by seeing whether it is possible to produce a diastasis using a bone hook to apply a lateral force to the fibula. If the syndesmosis opens, then a diastasis screw should be inserted. It should not pass through the syndesmosis as this may predispose to a bony synostosis. The screw may be a 4.5-mm or 3.5-mm cortical screw; all its cortices should be tapped and it should not be a lag screw. The fibula should be held firmly against the tibia with the ankle dorsiflexed. If the ankle is plantarflexed or a lag screw used, the mortice can be narrowed, which will restrict the range of movement. In cadaver studies, Needleman *et al.* (1989) have shown that the diastasis screw contributes to abnormal motion at the ankle joint. For this reason and the possibility that the screw may break at the tibio-fibular interface, removal of the screw at 6 weeks is recommended.

Posterior malleolus

Views differ on the necessity for internal fixation of the posterior fragment. Heim (1989) advised fixation of all articular posterior malleolar fragments. Other workers fix only fragments that remain displaced after fixation of the other malleoli and are larger than a third of the articular surface on the lateral radiograph.

There is little direct information on the question, but cadaver studies by Ramsey and Hamilton (1976) show where the main contact area between the talus and tibial plafond is on weight-bearing. When the talus is in its normal position, the weight-bearing area lies towards the anterior and lateral sides of the plafond. The posterior malleolar fractures mainly involve the postero-lateral corner of the plafond. Therefore, fractures of less than a quarter of the articular surface on the lateral radiograph should result in only a small decrease in the weight-bearing area.

However, these cadaver studies were performed with a static vertical load. The way the contact area varied with plantarflexion and dorsiflexion of the ankle was not studied, and this part of the plafond may have greater weight-bearing function than that suggested by these cadaver studies. Heim (1989) found that any sub-luxation of the talus was associated with a poorer prognosis, but slightly displaced fragments without any suspicion of talar subluxation had a good prognosis. In his study of 45 patients, the fragment was considered to be small in 20 and large in 25 cases. Four of the 45 patients went on to develop severe arthrosis and this was attributed to technical error.

To date, neither the cadaver nor the clinical studies provide good evidence for fixing all posterior malleolar fractures, so it seems reasonable to fix only those posterior malleolar fractures associated with subluxation of the talus or associated with a step in the articular surface, or fragments that contain more than a quarter of the articular surface as seen on the lateral radiograph.

Conditions for internal fixation

For internal fixation, it is essential that the right equipment and necessary expertise are available.

Two patient factors particularly increase the hazards of operative treatment: first, any endogenous source of infection (such as breaks in the skin resulting from chronic ulceration or psoriasis); and second, weak osteo-porotic bone. In a study of patients over 50 years of age Beauchamp *et al.* (1983) found a high incidence of failure. The complication rate was more marked in female patients (61% versus 27%), with a high rate of infection, thromboembolism and failure of fixation. The authors concluded that internal fixation should be avoided in female patients over 50 years. In contrast, Phillips *et al.* (1985) found that the outcome of all fractures in the elderly was worse than that in a younger group, but elderly patients treated by internal fixation fared better than those treated by closed means.

It is our practice to try and use closed methods for elderly patients, but if this fails we then proceed to internal fixation.

Removal of metalwork

It is our practice to remove diastasis screws at 6–8 weeks (see above). The remaining metal is removed only if the patient has symptoms attributable to the plate and screws. This is often the case with immediately subcutaneous implants.

Some surgeons have been using biodegradeable

implants in an attempt to avoid the problem of further surgery. Hirvensalo (1989) used polyglycolide rods in 41 patients, five of whom had some loss of position and two required re-operation. In a study of 102 patients, Bostman *et al.* (1989) found that six had transient sinus formation and discharge of the biodegradeable material between 2 and 4 months after surgery. Both series reported good functional outcomes at 1-year follow-up. At present, we continue to use metallic fixation devices until the problems of loss of fixation and sinus formation with the biodegradeable implants have been solved.

Rehabilitation

Postoperatively, the ankle is rested in the back slab for 24 hours. Providing stable fixation has been achieved, early mobilization should be commenced to regain ankle movement and muscle function. If the patient is sensible, partial weight-bearing (9−18 kg; 20−40 lb) with crutches is commenced.

In unreliable patients, a removable lightweight below-knee cast can be used to protect the ankle and yet allow mobilization under physiotherapy supervision. Ahl *et al.* (1988) have described the use of a plastic orthosis to allow weight-bearing and active movement; this facilitated rehabilitation after ankle fracture. Konradsen and Raun (1990) studied peroneal reaction time after ankle ligament injuries. They found that patients with chronic instability had prolonged peroneal reaction times, which can be improved by proprioceptive retraining; this form of therapy should be included in any rehabilitation regime.

Complications

Systemic

Any of the systemic complications of surgery can occur after open reduction and internal fixation. Thromboembolism appears to be more common after internal fixation, but deep-vein thrombosis and pulmonary emboli also occur with closed forms of treatment.

Local

Skin

Superficial wound infection can occur. If the wound is sutured under tension, sloughing of the wound edges may result. Pressure sores may occur as a result of the plaster, particularly if the patient has a concommitant head injury or reduced sensation from any other cause.

Nerve

The distal part of the superficial peroneal nerve may lie in the line of the lateral incision and is then at risk of division; this results in numbness on the dorsum of the patient's foot.

Bone

Deep infection is rare (less than 1% in most reports) and usually settles with appropriate management.

Malunion can occur with operative or non-operative treatments, but is obviously more common with the latter. Loss of fixation occurs mainly in patients who have osteoporotic bone.

Non-union can occur. It is particularly common (up to 10%) with medial malleolar fractures treated non-operatively. A flap of periosteum is described as being inverted and lying in the fracture gap. Non-union of the medial malleolus can result in pain, instability and tibialis posterior tendonitis (Burwell & Charnley 1965).

Joint

Reduced movement of the subtalar joint has been reported and appears to be slightly worse if a cast has been used. It normally recovers by 2 years. The rehabilitation regime should address this joint as well as the ankle joint.

Post-traumatic arthritis depends on the quality of the reduction and the degree of articular cartilage damage at the time of the original injury. The presence of a posterior lip fracture has also been reported as predisposing to post-traumatic arthritis.

Reflex sympathetic dystrophy

This complication can occur with any fracture or soft tissue injury. After ankle injuries, patients may develop a painful, hyperaesthetic swollen foot. The areas of maximum tenderness are often distant from the fracture sites. Vasomotor instability and hypersensitivity to cold may also be present. This condition should be treated by anti-inflammatory agents, physiotherapy and, if necessary, guanethidine.

Summary of management

History

The description by the patient of the actual direction of force of injury may be unreliable. However, the circumstances of the injury, in particular the energy of the impact, are very useful. The ability to weight-bear is also important, because someone with a normal perception of pain and who can weight-bear is unlikely to have an unstable ankle injury.

Examination

The ankle should be inspected for any wounds and the sites of swelling should be noted. Any sites of tenderness should be related to the underlying bony and ligamentous structures.

Radiographs

The positions of fracture lines are observed and the likely ligament damage is deduced. The talus is inspected for any shift or rotation. The articular surfaces are scrutinized for any osteochondral fractures. Occasionally, oblique views or a computerized tomography (CT) scan can be of use in further delineating the fracture complex.

Treatment

From the foregoing discussion, choose the best and safest means of obtaining and holding the reduction. Union in an anatomical position is the best way to achieve a good outcome.

Rehabilitation

Following surgery, ankle mobilization is commenced after 24 hours. Stable fractures and internally fixed fractures are mobilized partial weight-bearing in a removable below-knee walking cast. Non-operated fractures are mobilized when the fracture has clinically united. Physiotherapy includes gait education, strengthening of the leg muscles, passive mobilization of the ankle and subtalar joints and proprioceptive retraining.

References

Ahl, T., Dalen, N. & Selvik, G. Mobilisation after operation of ankle fractures. *Acta Orthop Scand* 1988; **59**: 302−306.

Beauchamp, C.G., Clay, N.R. & Thexton, P.W. Displaced ankle fractures in patients over 50 years of age. *J Bone Joint Surg* 1983; **65B**: 329−332.

Boden, S.D., Labbropoulos, P.A., McCowin, P., Lestini, W.F. & Hurwitz, S.R. Mechanical considerations of the syndesmosis screw. *J Bone Joint Surg* 1989; **71A**: 1548−1555.

Bostman, O., Hirvensalo, E., Vainionpan, S., Makila, A., Vihtonen, K., Rokkannen, P. & Tormala, P. Ankle fractures treated using biodegradeable internal fixation. *Clin Orthop* 1989; **238**: 195−203.

Burwell, H.N. & Charnley, A.D. The treatment of displaced fractures of the ankle by rigid internal fixation and early joint movement. *J Bone Joint Surg* 1965; **47B**: 634−660.

Heim, U.F. Trimalleolar fractures: late results after fixation of the posterior fragment. *Orthopaedics* 1989; **12(8)**: 1053−1059.

Hirvensalo, E. Fracture fixation with biodegradeable rods. Forty one cases of severe ankle fractures. *Acta Orthop Scand* 1989; **60**: 601−606.

Hughes, J.L., Weber, H., Willeneger, H. & Kuner, E.H. Evaluation of ankle fractures: non-operative and operative treatment. *Clin Orthop* 1979; **138**: 111−119.

Konradsen, L. & Raun, J.B. Ankle instability caused by prolonged peroneal reaction time. *Acta Orthop Scand* 1990; **61(5)**: 388−390.

Lauge-Hansen, N. Fractures of the ankle. Analytic historical survey as a basis of new experimental roentgenologic and clinical investigations. *Arch Surg* 1948; **56**: 259−317.

Lauge-Hansen, H. Fractures of the ankle. II. Combined experimental surgical and experimental roentgenologic investigations. *Arch Surg* 1950; **60**: 957−985.

Molinari, M., Bertoldi, L. & De March, L. Fracture dislocation of the ankle with the fibula trapped behind the tibia. *Acta Orthop Scand* 1990; **61**: 471−472.

Monk, C.J. Injuries of the tibiofibular ligaments. *J Bone Joint Surg* 1969; **51B**: 330.

Needleman, R.L., Skrade, D.A. & Stiehl, J.B. Effect of syndesmotic screw on ankle motion. *Foot Ankle* 1989; **10**: 17−24.

Phillips, W.A., Schwartz, H.S., Keller, C.S., Woodward, R., Rudd, W.S., Spiegel, P.G. & Laros, G.S. A prospective randomised study of the management of severe ankle fractures. *J Bone Joint Surg* 1985; **67A**: 67−78.

Ramsay, P.L. & Hamilton, W. Changes in tibiotalar area of contact caused by lateral talar shift. *J Bone Joint Surg* 1976; **58A**: 356−357.

Rowley, D.I., Norris, S.H. & Duckworth, T. A prospective trial comparing operative and manipulative treatment of ankle. *J Bone Joint Surg* 1986; **68B**: 610−613.

Tile, M., Steele-Scott, C., Gollish, J.D. & Begg, R. Fractures of the ankle − clinical and biomechanical considerations. *J Bone Joint Surg* 1977; **59B**: 510.

Willeneger, H. & Breitenfelder, H. *Principles of Internal Fixation.* Springer-Verlag: Berlin, 1965.

Zeegers, A.V., Van Raay, J.J. & van-der-Werken, C. Ankle fracture treated with a stabilising shoe. *Acta Orthop Scand* 1989; **60**: 597−599.

25: The Foot

Os calcis

P.D.TRIFFITT AND P.J.GREGG

Introduction

While the often poor outcome from fractures of the os calcis has long been recognized (Cotton & Wilson 1908), the treatment of these injuries remains controversial. Their comparative rarity, and their variability in form, have made controlled prospective studies difficult.

Clinical anatomy

The bone comprises four principal parts, all of which may be fractured (Fig. 25.1).

The *tuberosity* carries no articulation, but receives the insertion of the tendo Achillis. It has medial and lateral processes on its plantar aspect.

The *body* supports the posterior articular facet which, with its counterpart on the inferior aspect of the talus, forms the main articulation of the subtalar joint. The facet is angled at 40–50° to the long axis of the bone, and is convex both from front to back, and from side to side.

The *sustentaculum tali* carries the middle and anterior articular facets, which are separated from the posterior facet by the sulcus calcanei. This sulcus forms the floor of the sinus tarsi, and contains the insertion of the interosseous talocalcaneal ligament.

The *anterior process* articulates with the cuboid, and gives origin to the bifurcate ligament which inserts into the cuboid and the navicular.

Böhler's angle is that subtended by lines joining the superior points of both the anterior process and the posterior calcaneal border to the highest point of the posterior facet (Böhler 1931) (Fig. 25.2). In one series of subjects who had sustained a unilateral os calcis fracture, in 90% of cases the angle on the opposite uninjured side was between 30 and 45° (Aaron & Howat 1976).

The thin cortical shell of the bone is readily comminuted. The best purchase for screw fixation is provided by the dense subchondral bone of the articular facets.

Classification

Many forms of classification have been proposed, the principal ones being those of Böhler (1931), Essex-Lopresti (1952), Warrick and Bremner (1953) and Soeur and Remy (1975). Most variation in classification has concerned the description of intra-articular fractures, and that given here is considered to cover the distinctions that have appeared to be of clinical usefulness.

Extra-articular fractures may be classified as:

1 Fractures of the tuberosity
   (a) Avulsion of the insertion of the tendo Achillis.
   (b) Fracture of the medial process.
2 Fractures of the sustentaculum tali.
3 Fractures of the anterior process
   (a) Avulsion fractures.
   (b) Compression fractures of the calcaneo-cuboid joint.
4 Extra-articular fractures of the body. These comprise fractures passing behind the posterior subtalar facet.

Intra-articular fractures may be classified as:

1 Undisplaced.
2 Displaced
   (a) Tongue type.
   (b) Central depressed type.
   (c) Comminuted.

Extra-articular fractures

This group includes any fracture that does not involve the posterior subtalar joint, although fractures lying at the posterior margin of the posterior facet are sometimes considered to be intra-articular. Extra-articular fractures account for approximately 25% of all os calcis fractures and, in general, have a favourable prognosis.

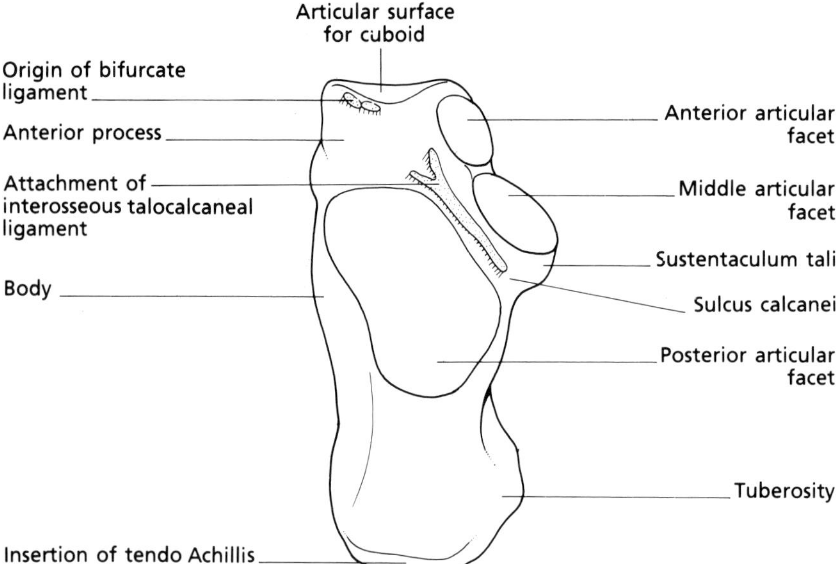

Fig. 25.1 The os calcis, superior aspect.

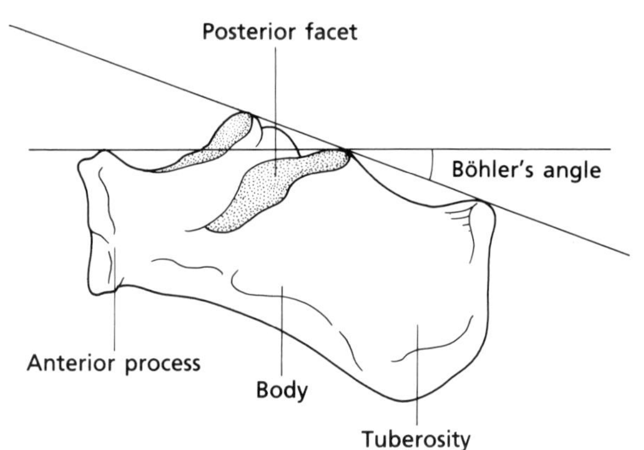

Fig. 25.2 The os calcis, lateral aspect.

Intra-articular fractures

These are fractures of the body that involve the posterior facet. They comprise some 75% of os calcis fractures (Essex-Lopresti 1952, Warrick & Bremner 1953, Allan 1955, Lindsay & Dewar 1958, Lance *et al.* 1963, Soeur & Remy 1975), and a higher proportion still of those fractures with a poor outcome.

Displacement of these fractures takes the form of depression of part or all of the posterior facet into the body of the bone, or occasionally of separation of the facet fragments, and is discussed below.

Mechanisms of injury

The great majority of intra-articular fractures are caused by a fall from a height, while the much less common extra-articular fractures often result from twisting injuries.

Fractures of the body

A fall onto the heel results in shear between the body weight, acting downwards through the subtalar joint, and the opposing reaction force, directed upwards through the tuberosity (Palmer 1948, Essex-Lopresti 1952, Burdeaux 1983) (Fig. 25.3). The primary fracture so formed splits the bone into two main fragments: a posteroinferior lateral part and an anterosuperior medial part. The medial part remains firmly attached to the talus by the interosseous ligament, and moves with it, while the lateral fragment includes the tuberosity. The fracture line may pass in front of, through or behind the posterior facet (Burdeaux 1983).

On displacement of the main fragments, the lateral fragment is forced upwards and outwards, resulting in shortening and widening of the bone. Further, it is the lateral fragment that is compressed between the talus and the ground. Any part of the facet that is carried by the lateral fragment may therefore be secondarily depressed into the cancellous body of the bone, the facet usually being tilted forwards, and often also to one side or the other (Fig. 25.4). Depression may occur when the primary fracture passes through, or anterior to, the facet, as all or part of the facet then lies on the lateral fragment. With the primary fracture behind the facet, the whole of the facet lies with the medial fragment and the underlying cancellous bone is not compressed, although the upward displacement of the lateral fragment may give rise to the appearance of depression.

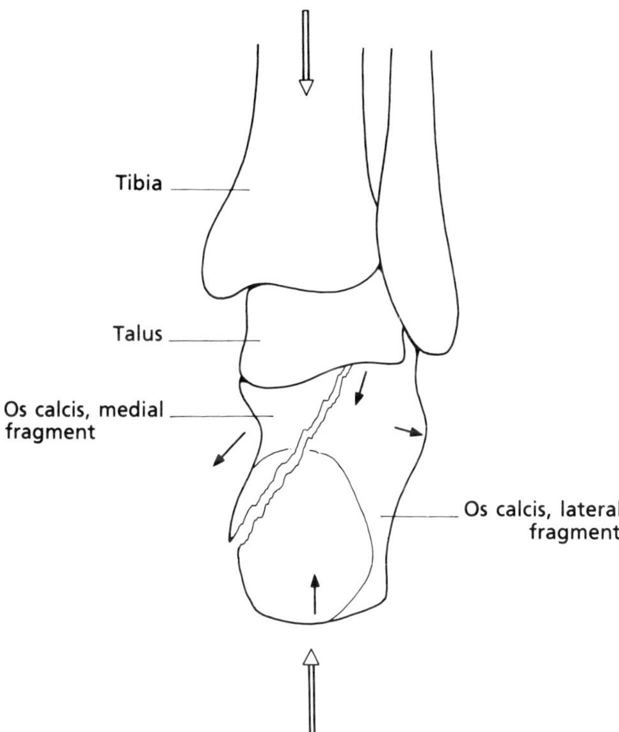

Fig. 25.3 Posterior aspect of the right hindfoot, showing the production of a primary fracture by shear forces. Large arrows indicate principal forces at impact and small arrows show the resulting displacements of different parts of the bone.

Secondary fractures of the lateral fragment result in two forms of depressed fracture, named by Essex-Lopresti (1952). In the *tongue* type, a secondary fracture divides the lateral fragment in the transverse plane, the upper part carrying the facet. Facet depression causes the posterior end to tilt upwards. In the *central depressed* type the secondary fracture lies along the posterior border of the facet (Fig. 25.5). With either type, lateral fragment compression results in secondary comminution of the lateral wall, which buckles underneath the lateral malleolus causing further widening of the bone. In severe fractures, the fragment is extensively comminuted.

Bone height is lost both by posterior facet depression and by the upward movement of the tuberosity with the lateral fragment. This has the effect of reducing, or even reversing, Böhler's angle. The talus assumes a more horizontal position and the talocalcaneal angle is reduced.

Secondary fractures may involve the anterior process, entering the calcaneo-cuboid joint.

Fractures of the tuberosity

The majority of these fractures are avulsions of the insertion of the tendo Achillis, although some may result from a direct blow. The superior extent of the tendon insertion is variable, and may reach almost to the upper limit of the posterior surface (Lowy 1969). The avulsed fragment takes one of two forms: triangular ('beak' fracture) or oval (Fig. 25.6). Overall, these avulsion injuries account for only 1–2% of os calcis fractures (Wilson 1933, Carey *et al.* 1965).

Pathological fractures of this type have been described in diabetic patients, in whom it is proposed that peripheral neuropathy is the main aetiological factor (Kathol *et al.* 1991). Concomitant conditions such as renal osteodystrophy and steroid treatment after renal transplantation may also be important in these patients.

Isolated *medial process* fractures are caused by the direct trauma of a fall, or possibly by avulsion of the origin of the plantar fascia (Böhler 1931).

The tuberosity is frequently involved secondarily in fractures of the body.

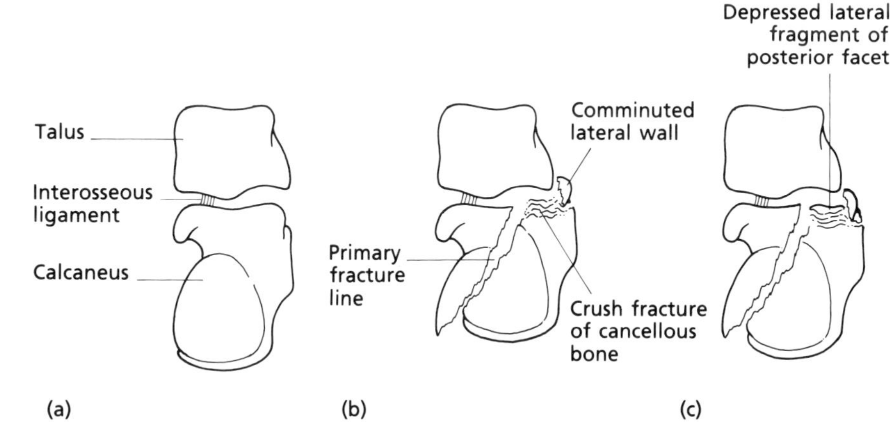

Fig. 25.4 Depression of the lateral facet fragment. (After Palmer 1948.)
(a) Before impact. (b) During impact.
(c) After impact.

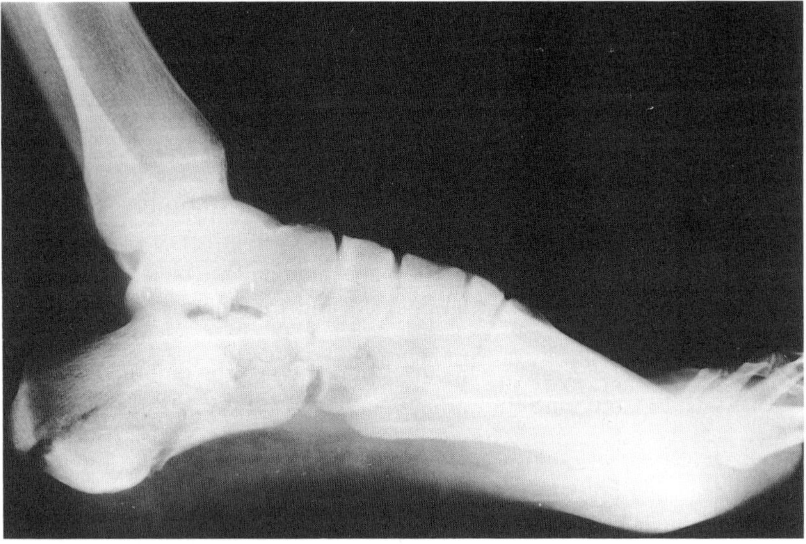 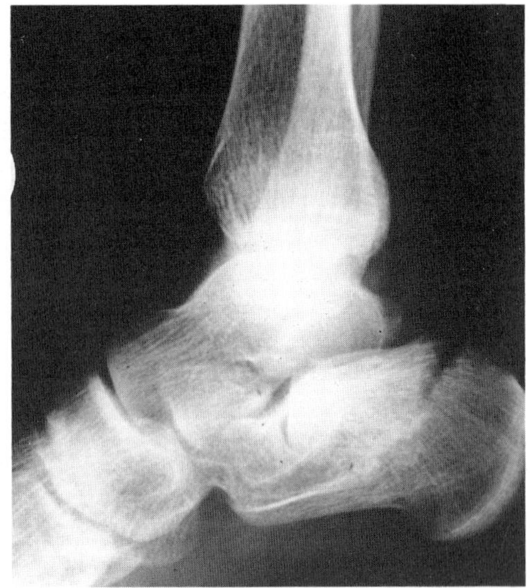

(a)   (b)

Fig. 25.5 Fractures of the body. (a) Tongue type. (b) Central depressed type.

Fractures of the sustentaculum tali

Isolated fractures of this structure are rare, accounting for 0.3–3% of calcaneal fractures, and little is known about the mechanism involved (Essex-Lopresti 1952, Warrick & Bremner 1953, Carey *et al.* 1965, Soeur & Remy 1975). It has been stated as most commonly resulting from a twisting injury (Carey *et al.* 1965).

Fractures of the anterior process

These injuries usually result from forced inversion with adduction, resulting in avulsion of the origin of the bifurcate ligament (Carey *et al.* 1965). Forced abduction of the forefoot, or eversion in dorsiflexion, may cause a compression fracture of the process which is usually intra-articular (Hunt 1970, Degan *et al.* 1982) (Fig. 25.7).

The anterior process is frequently involved secondarily in fractures of the body, with an incidence of up to 96% in displaced fractures of the posterior subtalar joint (Thompson 1973).

Epidemiology

INCIDENCE

The os calcis is the most commonly fractured tarsal bone, but accounts for only 1–2% of all fractures. It is fractured bilaterally in approximately 8% of cases (Wilson 1933), the highest incidence amongst bones of the extremities.

AGE AND SEX

As most injuries are sustained in a fall from a height, injury is commonest amongst males of working age. The average age in most series lies in the fifth decade, and men account for 80–90% (Wilson 1927, O'Connell *et al.* 1972). However, fractures resulting from other mechanisms are often sustained by women, who comprise between one- and two-thirds of those with fractures of the anterior process, tuberosity and sustentaculum tali (Carey *et al.* 1965). The role of osteoporosis in fractures of the elderly is not well defined.

SUBTALAR JOINT INVOLVEMENT

The posterior subtalar joint is involved in 75% of fractures, although approximately 20% of these appear by conventional radiography to be undisplaced (Essex-Lopresti 1952, Warrick & Bremner 1953, Allan 1955, Soeur & Remy 1975). The central depressed type is commoner than the tongue type by a ratio of 3:2 (Essex-Lopresti 1952, Warrick & Bremner 1953). Approximately 4% are too comminuted for classification (Essex-Lopresti 1952).

SOFT TISSUE INJURY

Only 1–2% of fractures are compound (Wilson 1933), although this proportion is higher in military practice, where the injury is often caused by explosions below deck or by landmines under vehicles (Böhler 1931, Harris 1946).

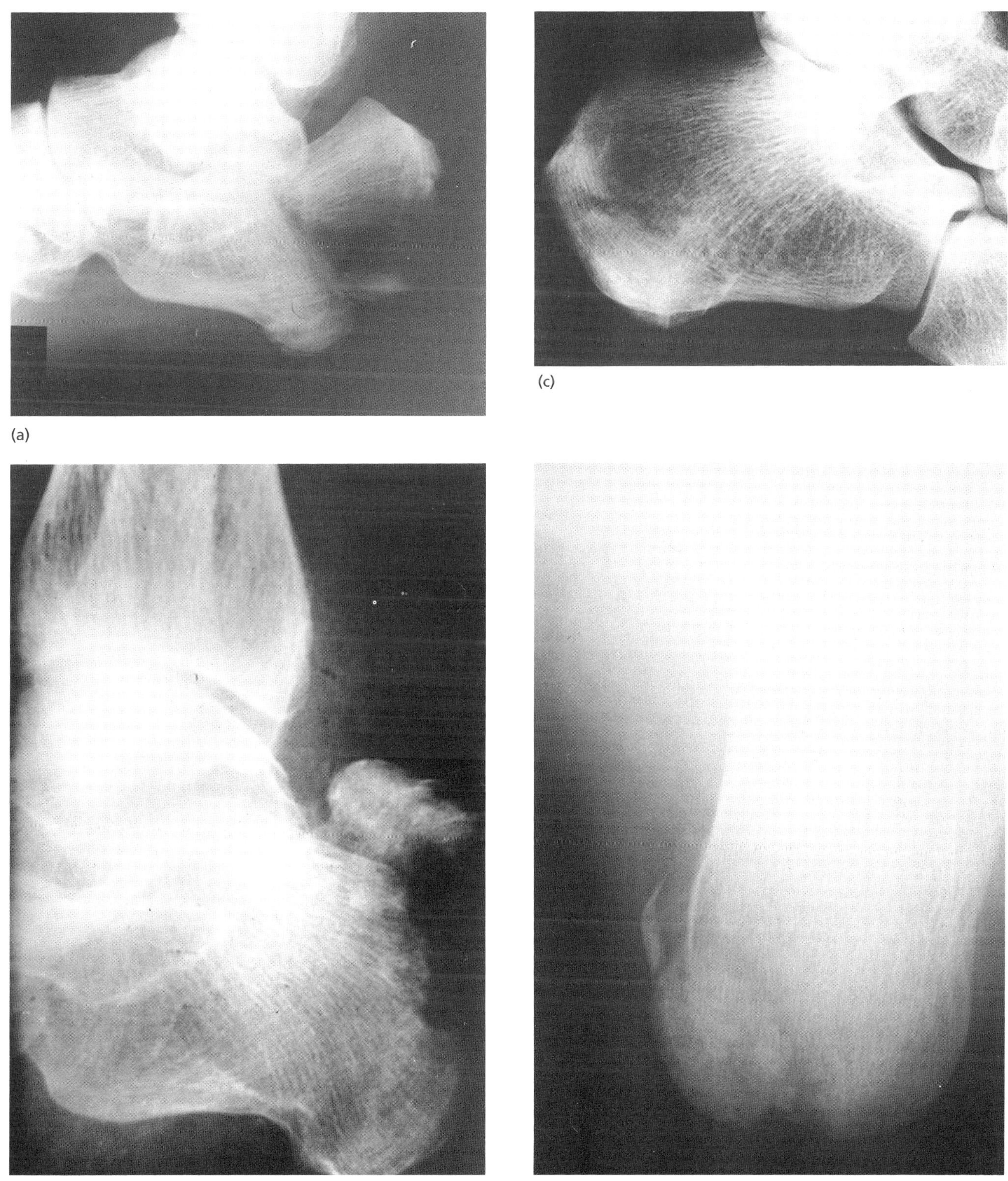

Fig. 25.6 Fractures of the tuberosity. (a) Beak type. (b) Oval type. (c) Medial process.

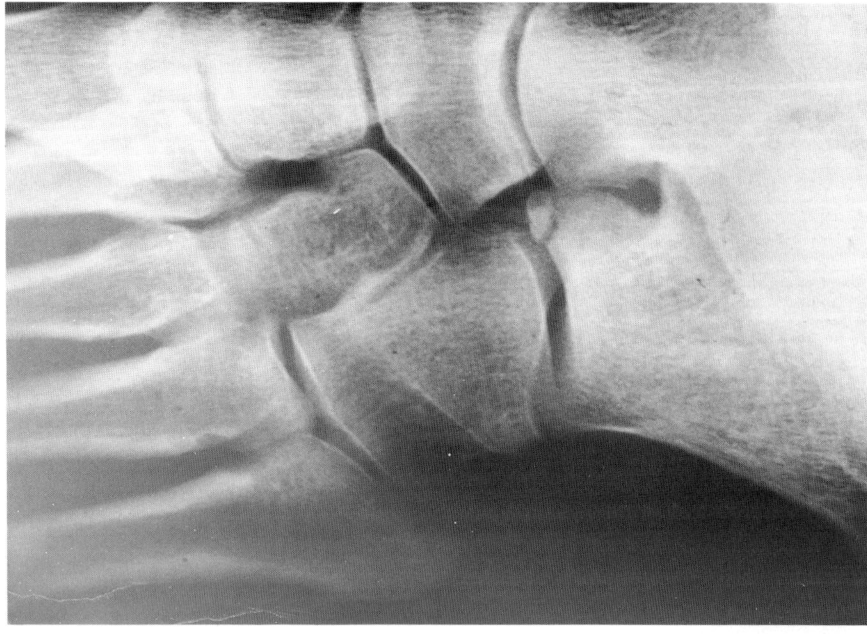

(a)

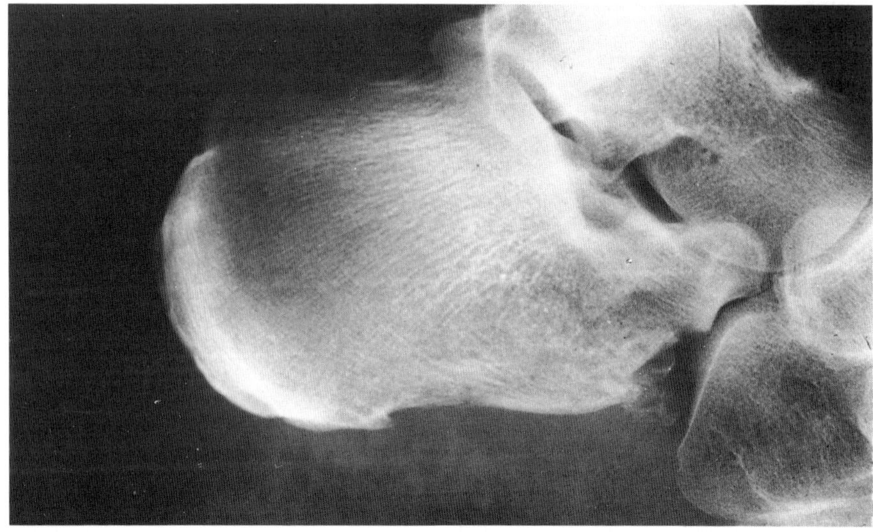

(b)

Fig. 25.7 Fractures of the anterior process. (a) Avulsion type. (b) Crush type.

ASSOCIATED INJURIES

The commonest associated injury is a compression fracture of one or more vertebrae; this has been found to occur in up to 10% of patients when radiographs of the spine were routinely taken (Hermann 1937). The incidence of concurrent ankle and talar fractures is under 5% (Wilson 1933, Soeur & Remy 1975). The navicular is fractured in over a third of patients with isolated fractures of the anterior process (Carey *et al.* 1965) (Fig. 25.8).

Clinical features

Diagnosis of fractures of the body of the os calcis is usually straightforward, although they may be missed in the multiply injured patient. A fracture should be suspected after any fall from a height, even if this is only 1–1.5 m (Wilson 1933).

Apart from local tenderness, swelling is often severe, and may be accompanied by fracture blistering (Fig. 25.9). Bruising that tracks around either side of the plantar fascia into the sole or sides of the heel is pathognomonic, but may take 24 hours to develop. The spine should always be examined, even in the absence of symptoms, as associated crush fractures may not be immediately symptomatic.

Avulsion fractures of the tuberosity are generally

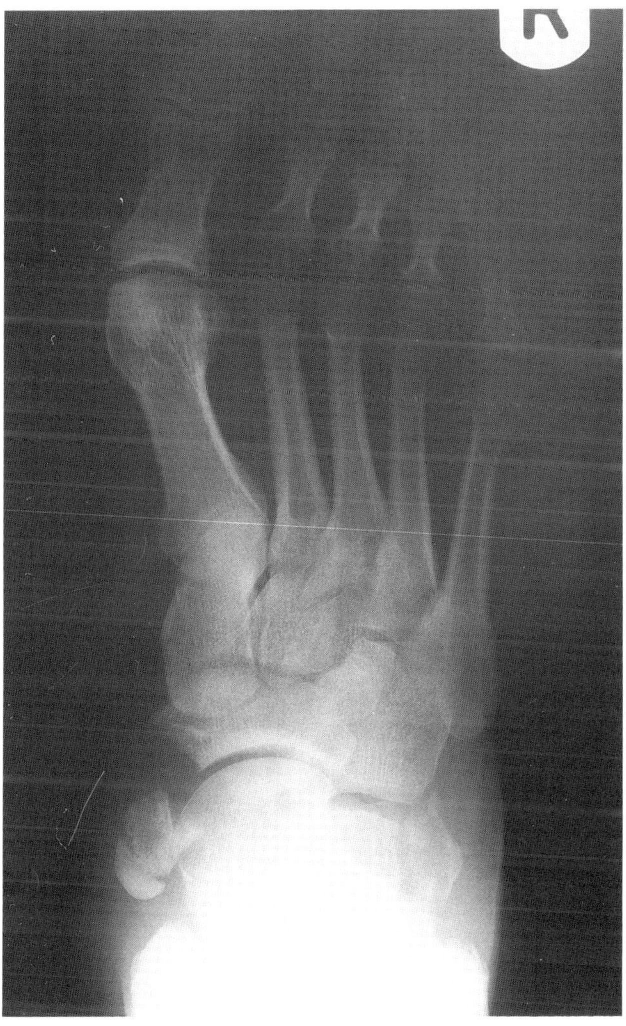

Fig. 25.8 Fracture of the navicular associated with an anterior process fracture.

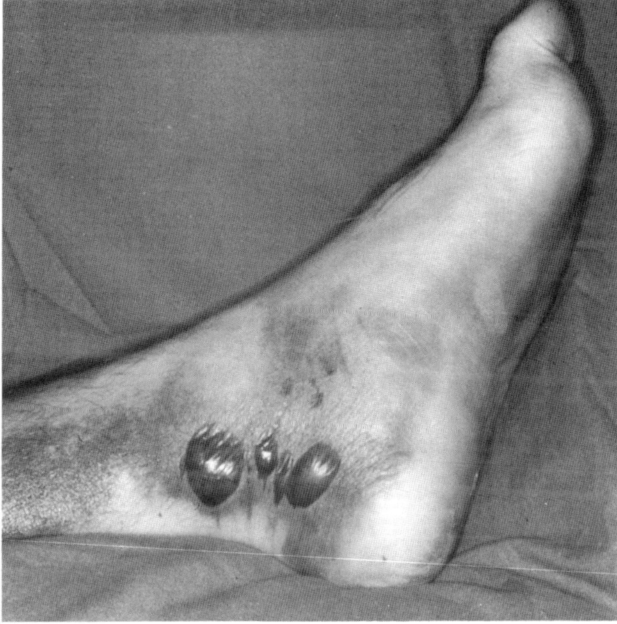

Fig. 25.9 Fracture blisters after an os calcis fracture.

isolated injuries, giving rise to localized pain and tenderness and characteristic radiographs.

In contrast, fractures of the anterior process are easily overlooked, the diagnosis being one of a sprain of the dorsal calcaneo-cuboid ligament or of the anterolateral ligament of the ankle.

Imaging

Diagnostic radiographic examination in suspected cases comprises lateral and axial views of the os calcis, together with anteroposterior views of the ankle and foot to show any associated injuries. Oblique projections and computerized tomography (CT) are of use in the characterization of fractures of the body, particularly if operative management is contemplated.

Consideration should be given to routine radiography of the spine, as crush fractures may otherwise be missed.

Plain radiographs

Lateral view

Depression and forward tilting of posterior facet fragments is usually well shown on a lateral view (see Fig. 25.5), but articular involvement of an undisplaced fracture is often not visible. The loss of height after a fracture can be assessed by measurement of Böhler's angle, preferably with comparison with the opposite side, if unfractured.

This view usually shows fractures of the anterior process.

Axial view

The axial view is, in effect, an oblique anteroposterior projection, avoiding the overlying forefoot. It is taken from the plantar aspect, with the beam angled 45–55° posteriorly. Adequate visualization of the subtalar joint in profile and of the sustentaculum tali requires the foot to be dorsiflexed, which is uncomfortable after a fracture, and the joint and tuberosity require different exposures for optimal demonstration of each. Within these limitations, the axial view will usually show both primary fractures of the body and fractures of the medial process of the tuberosity (Figs 25.6c and 25.10).

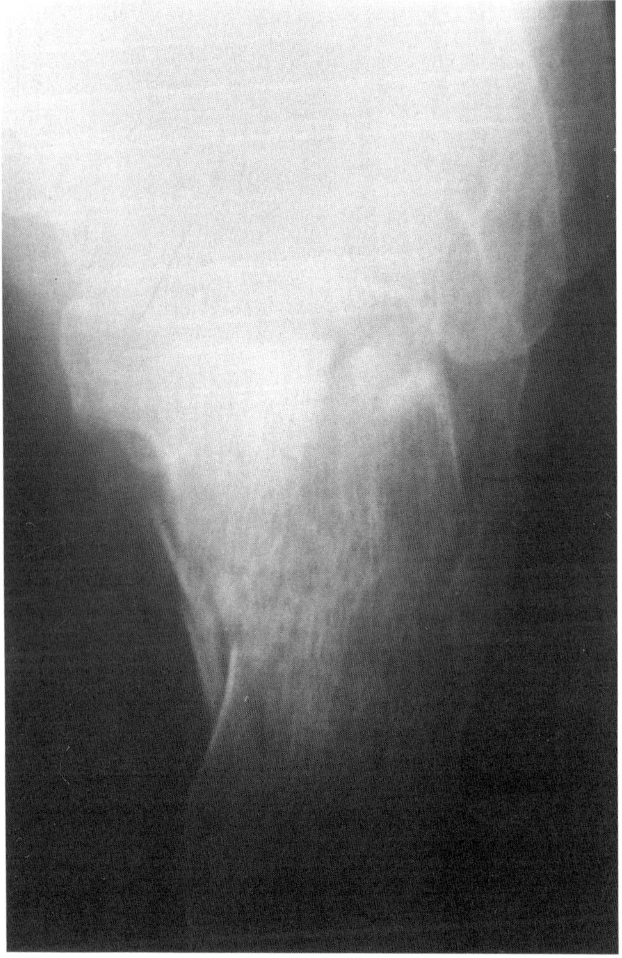

Fig. 25.10 Axial view of a primary fracture of the body.

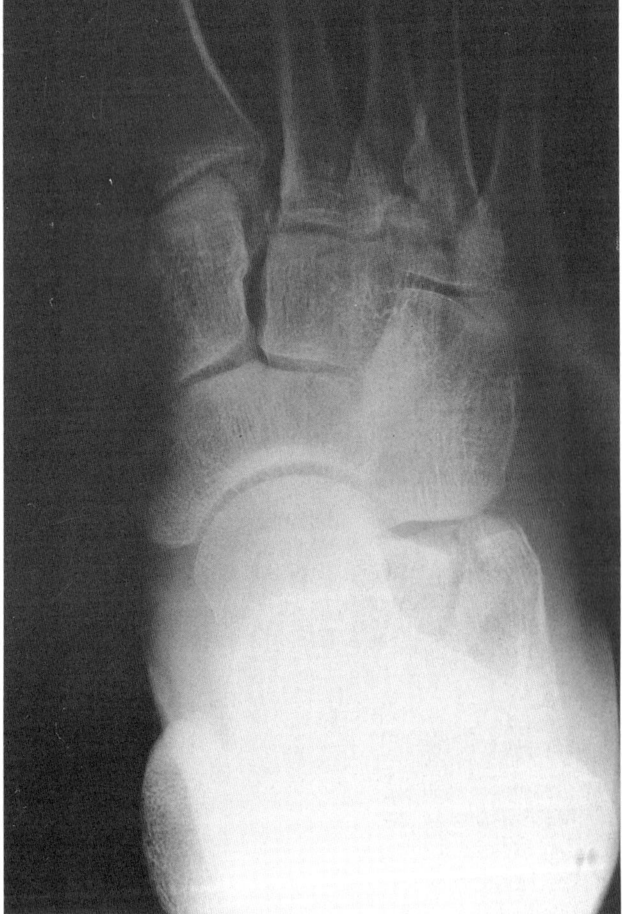

Fig. 25.11 Anteroposterior view of the foot demonstrating the involvement of the calcaneo-cuboid joint.

Anteroposterior views

The os calcis is obscured by the forefoot in standard anteroposterior views of the hindfoot, and their main utility is in the indication of an associated injury of the ankle. A dorsoplantar projection of the foot will show talo-navicular subluxation and associated navicular fractures, common after twisting injuries, and involvement of the calcaneo-cuboid joint by a fracture arising secondarily to a fracture of the body (Fig. 25.11).

Oblique views

Various oblique views have been used in an effort to demonstrate better the posterior subtalar joint. Of these, the most commonly used have been those of Anthonsen (1943) and Brodén (1949).

Anthonsen's view is taken along the axis of the sinus tarsi, with the beam directed from 25° above and 30° behind the medial malleolus. This shows the posterior and middle facets in profile (Fig. 25.12).

Brodén's views are taken along the longitudinal axis of the posterior facet, with the beam directed from the lateral side and angled at 45° to the parasagittal plane. Radiographs taken at intervals from 0 to 40° cranial inclination show most of the facet in profile, from back to front (Fig. 25.13).

Apart from gains in visualization of the subtalar joint, fractures of the anterior process may best be shown by oblique projections (Degan *et al.* 1982).

Tomography

Conventional tomography has not been extensively used in the assessment of fractures of the os calcis, and has now been largely superseded by CT scanning.

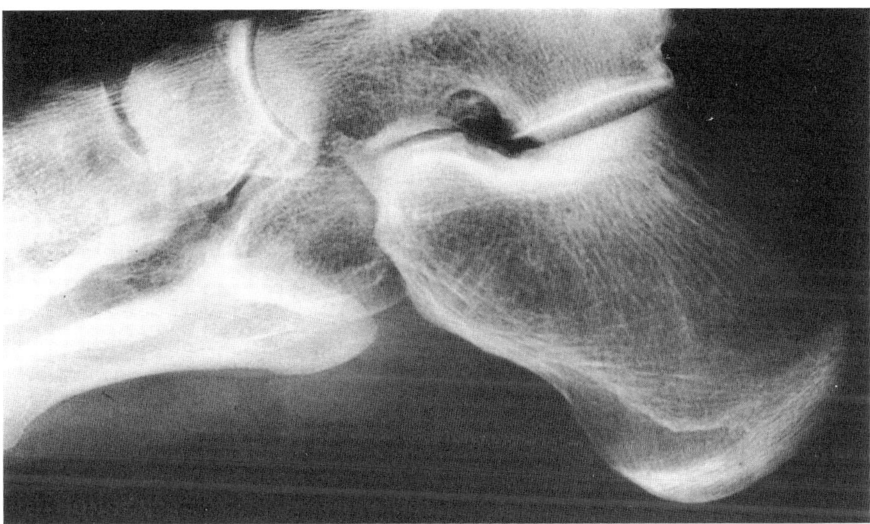

Fig. 25.12 Anthonsen's view.

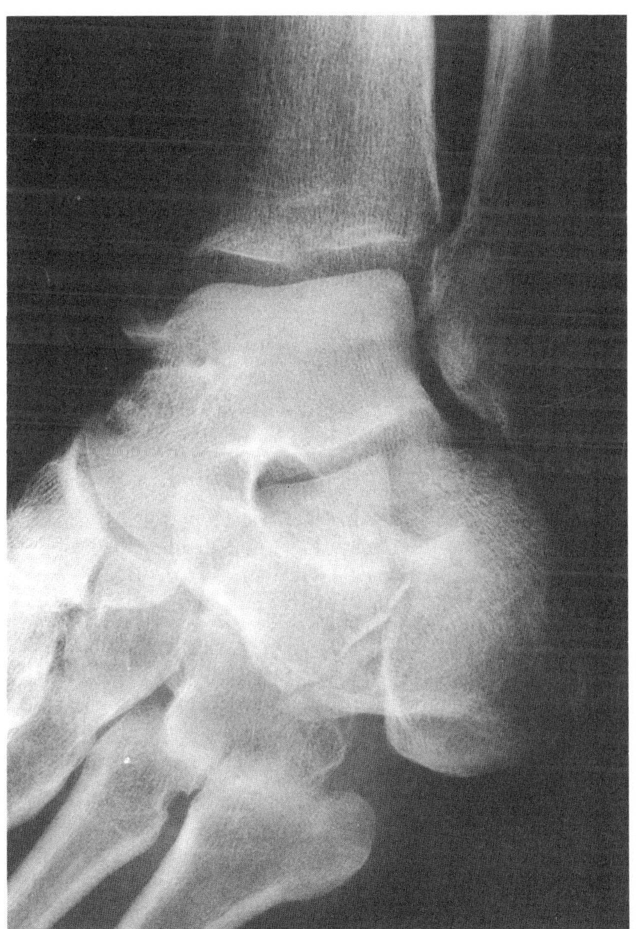

Fig. 25.13 A Brodén's view, demonstrating an intra-articular fracture.

CT scanning

This has been investigated with a view to assisting in the preoperative planning of open reductions. It may be performed with the foot comfortably plantarflexed or immobilized in plaster (Segal *et al*. 1985). Coronal scans are used for examination of the posterior subtalar joint, while the calcaneo-cuboid joint may best be demonstrated by transverse cuts. The radiation dosage administered is much lower than that given during conventional coronal tomography (Guyer *et al*. 1985).

Coronal or near-coronal scans, angled so as to be approximately perpendicular to the posterior facet surface, give an axial view of the joint which is far superior to plain axial radiographs in demonstrating the presence and nature of articular involvement and in showing the deformity of the lateral wall (Lowrie *et al*. 1988). In the great majority of intra-articular fractures the facet is seen to be in two main fragments, with the medial fragment undisplaced or minimally tilted in relation to the talus, and the lateral fragment rotated with or without depression (Fig. 25.14). However, the degree of displacement of the lateral fragment tends to be underestimated, and a plain lateral view or scans in other planes are important in order to assess parasagittal rotational and translational displacement of this fragment. Measurement of displacements from CT scans is unreliable without large numbers of narrow cuts, because the planes of scanning vary between patients and between repeated scans in the same patient.

The characterization of intra-articular fractures given by this technique is essential for the matching of study groups in comparative trials of treatment (Giachino & Uhthoff 1989).

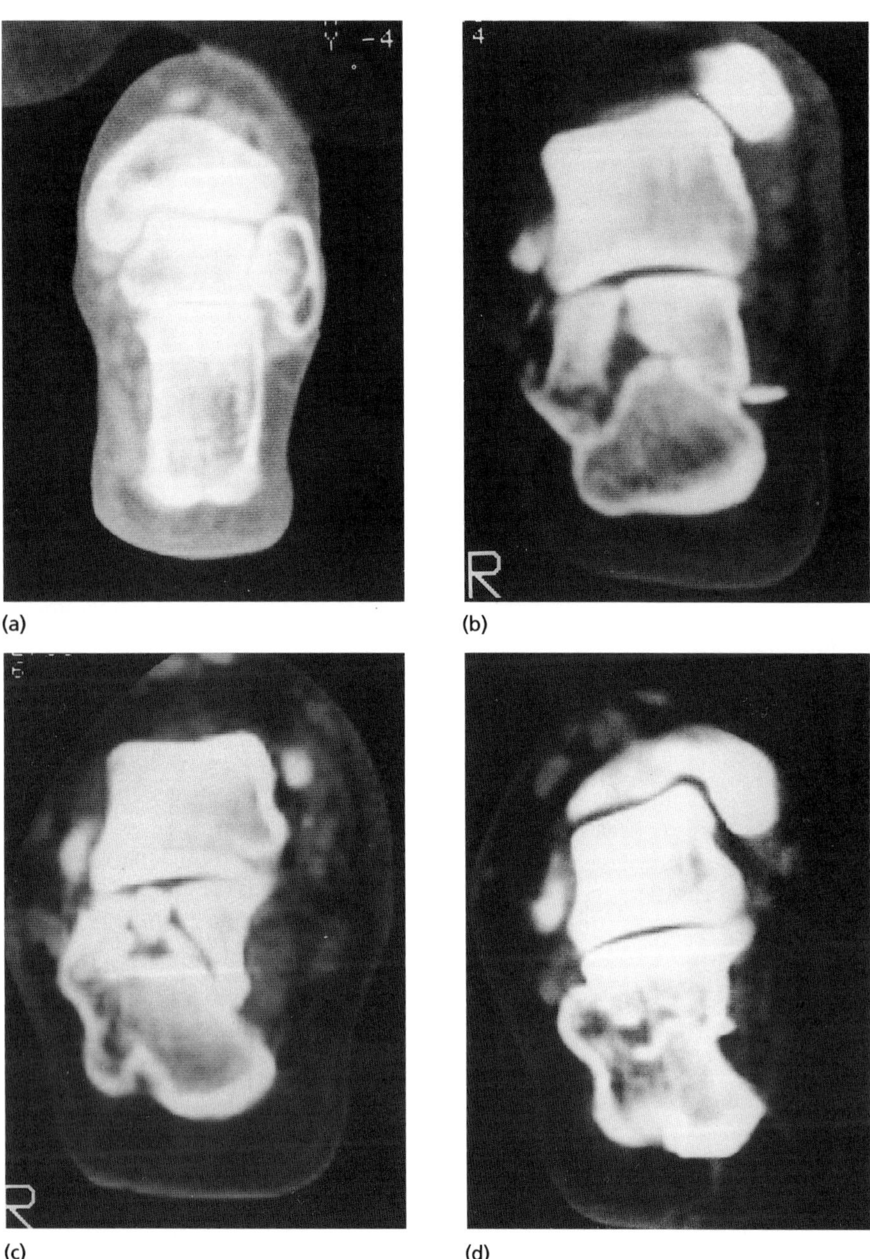

Fig. 25.14 Fractures of the body as seen on CT scanning. (a) Normal scan. (b) Intra-articular fracture, with two main facet fragments. (c) Comminuted facet fracture. (d) Extra-articular fracture.

Treatment

General principles

Fractures of the os calcis may result in considerable deformity of the bone, with consequent loss of leverage of the calf muscles, and almost invariably subtalar movement is reduced. However, these features are not usually the cause of significant long-term disability unless accompanied by pain. Treatment is thus aimed at those aspects of the injury perceived to be responsible for this symptom.

The assessment of pain is notoriously difficult, and the principal measure of recovery has been the time taken to the resumption of work. This measure is in itself subject to influences such as the nature of the work and the level of motivation of the patient.

General measures after injury start with elevation, usually as an inpatient unless the fracture is minor and extra-articular. Ice packs and compression bandaging may be used to reduce oedema, and mobilization of the subtalar and ankle joints may be started as soon as swelling permits. Whether treated by open or closed methods, the patient may be kept non-weight-bearing for up to 8 weeks, there being little likelihood of further displacement at that stage (Lance *et al.* 1963, 1964).

The occurrence of compartment syndromes in the foot from oedema or haemorrhage after fracture prompts vigilance in the first few days, as it may result in contractures (Mittlmeier *et al.* 1991, Myerson & Manoli 1993). The deep posterior compartment of the leg may also be involved (Matsen & Clawson 1975). The foot may be decompressed through the medial approach of Henry or through a plantar incision; alternatively, it has been suggested that a haematoma may be successfully evacuated through a large bore needle (Mittlmeier *et al.* 1991)..

Extra-articular fractures

In general, this type of fracture responds well to conservative methods, with the exception of displaced avulsion fractures of the tuberosity.

Avulsion fractures of the tuberosity

Displaced fractures in which the continuity of the flexor mechanism is lost, as determined by examination under anaesthesia, are best treated by open reduction and internal fixation (Lowy 1969), using a cancellous screw or a tension-band wire. The fixation is usually protected for 6 weeks in a below-knee cast with the foot in 5−10° of plantarflexion. Minimally displaced fractures may be treated by cast immobilization alone. Pathological fractures in diabetic patients with neuropathy may be prone to complications if treated operatively, and therefore closed treatment even of displaced fractures should be considered (Biehl *et al.* 1993).

Medial process fractures of the tuberosity

These fractures are usually minimally displaced, and respond well to conservative methods of treatment.

Fractures of the anterior process

The usual avulsion type of this injury responds well to conservative treatment. More than 95% of patients recover with minimal residual symptoms, with or without the use of a plaster cast (Carey *et al.* 1965), although they may take more than 12 months to do so (Degan *et al.* 1982). There is also evidence that delay in diagnosis adversely affects the outcome (Degan *et al.* 1982).

Displaced compression fractures may possibly respond better to operative elevation with internal fixation and bone grafting (Hunt 1970).

Isolated fractures of the sustentaculum tali

These rare fractures are generally treated closed. Displaced fragments may be manipulated into position before the application of a plaster cast.

Displaced intra-articular fractures of the posterior subtalar joint

It is the treatment of intra-articular fractures that has given rise to controversy. Many methods of therapy have been devised, but none has been positively demonstrated to be beneficial by prospective randomized controlled trials. This, and the supposed inevitability of a poor outcome (Cotton & Wilson 1908, Bankart 1942), has led many surgeons to adopt conservative measures whatever the fracture type.

Most techniques are based on the premise that subsequent symptoms arise predominantly from the deranged subtalar joint. Approximately 80% of fractures involving the subtalar joint are displaced (Essex-Lopresti 1952, Warrick & Bremner 1953), and while undisplaced fractures will usually be treated by closed methods, displacement may not be apparent on simple lateral and axial radiographs; these should therefore be supplemented by oblique views or CT scanning if open treatment is contemplated.

The methods available are simple mobilization of the foot, closed or percutaneous manipulation, open reduction with internal fixation, bone grafting or both, external fixation with or without internal fixation, and primary fusion.

Mobilization

Simple mobilization of the foot and a period of non-weight-bearing, with or without plaster, has been advocated by some (Barnard 1963, Parkes 1973) and practised by many. Complications of treatment are virtually non-existent, and better results after more interventionist management have yet to be proven. In view of the risk of severe swelling, patients should be admitted for this treatment rather than sent home in a cast.

A prospective study of this method indicates that with follow-up of at least 1 year and averaging 21 months, approximately half of patients have more than mininal pain, limitation in walking distance and difficulty in walking on uneven ground. However, three-quarters of men previously employed had returned to work, almost all to their original occupation (Parmar *et al.* 1993).

Closed manipulation

While operative intervention was fraught with hazard in the pre-antibiotic era, the outcome of this fracture has, in general, been thought so bad that attempts have been made to correct the many deformities by closed manipulation (Cotton & Wilson 1908, Böhler 1931, Harris 1946).

Reduction may be attempted by hand or by traction exerted on pins inserted through the tuberosity and distal tibia, the method popularized by Böhler (1931). This is supplemented by lateral pressure to reduce the bulging lateral wall. *Immobilization* of the fracture in the reduced position has been undertaken by re-impaction using a mallet (Cotton & Wilson 1908) or by incorporating the traction pins in plaster. However, when continuing poor results prompted some surgeons to fuse the joint primarily, it was seen at operation that these manoeuvres had no effect on the displacement of the facet fragments (Conn 1935), or even exaggerated it (Palmer 1948). A retrospective review suggested that results were little different to those obtained without manipulation (Lindsay & Dewar 1958).

Percutaneous manipulation

The depressed posterior facet fragments may be levered up onto the undersurface of the talus, a method particularly applicable to tongue fractures (Essex-Lopresti 1952, King 1973). The pin is then incorporated into a plaster, which is extended to the knee to avoid problems with re-displacement (King 1973). Overall results are not improved over those obtained with simple mobilization, and while subtalar joint movement is increased markedly in severe fractures, pain relief and improvement in function are much less so (Aaron & Howat 1976).

Open reduction

While practised sporadically since the turn of the century, open reduction became a major method of treatment after the work of Palmer (1948), who elevated the depressed lateral facet fragment from the lateral side and inserted bone graft into the cavity left beneath (Maxfield & McDermott 1955, Hazlett 1969). Open reduction is now routinely combined with internal fixation of the lateral facet fragment, with or without the lateral wall and tuberosity, to the stable anteromedial fragment. Kirschner wires or screws may be used for the facet fragment, while a plate is generally required to hold the comminuted lateral wall and tuberosity. Bone grafting is unnecessary if the fracture is stabilized (Soeur & Remy 1975, Stephenson 1983, 1987) (Fig. 25.15). Displaced fragments of the anterior process may require reduction in order to avoid impingement on the talus, causing a block to eversion (Langdon *et al.* 1994).

A longitudinal incision anterior to the tip of the fibula suffices for simple reduction of the lateral facet fragment, but reduction of the lateral wall and tuberosity requires a much larger approach. To limit problems with skin edge necrosis, this is probably best achieved by a curved incision near the posterior and inferior borders of the bone with subperiosteal elevation of the sural nerve and peroneal tendons (Benirschke & Sangeorzan 1993, Zwipp *et al.* 1993). The calcaneo-fibular ligament may be divided to improve exposure.

The medial wall will generally be subject to the primary fracture alone, with minor degrees of comminution, making alignment of the tuberosity more straightforward. With the reduction from the medial side introduced by McReynolds (1972, 1982), the interlocking of the cancellous fragments provides its own stability, which may be supplemented by a staple or axial pin (Hazlett 1969, Burdeaux 1983). Reduction of the depressed lateral facet fragment can be carried out by levering from the medial side, or by adding a lateral incision (Ross & Sowerby 1985).

Almost every study of this kind of management is based on an uncontrolled series, often retrospective, assessed with its own schemes of fracture classification and outcome grading. Further, in general the results are not independently reviewed. Thus, while improved results in comparison with closed methods are claimed, they have yet to be fully substantiated (Järvholm *et al.* 1984). In recent series good or very good results have been reported in 56–85% of cases (Bèzes *et al.* 1993, Fernandez & Koella 1993, Letournel 1993, Stephenson 1993). Complications have included deep infection rates of up to 6%, occasionally resulting in amputation, and skin edge necrosis in up to 10%, these complications arising most often in the first 100 or so cases treated (Benirschke & Sangeorzan 1993, Bèzes *et al.* 1993, Sanders *et al.* 1993, Zwipp, *et al.* 1993). Subtalar range of movement is not consistently restored, and a good reduction has not been found to ensure a good result (Benirschke & Sangeorzan 1993, Letournel 1993, Sanders *et al.* 1993). The only randomized controlled trial of which we are aware studied reduction of the lateral facet alone, and found no benefit over simple mobilization of the foot after follow-up of at least a year (Parmar *et al.* 1993). While it might be argued that reduction of the remainder of the bone might improve results, independent combined clinical and radiological

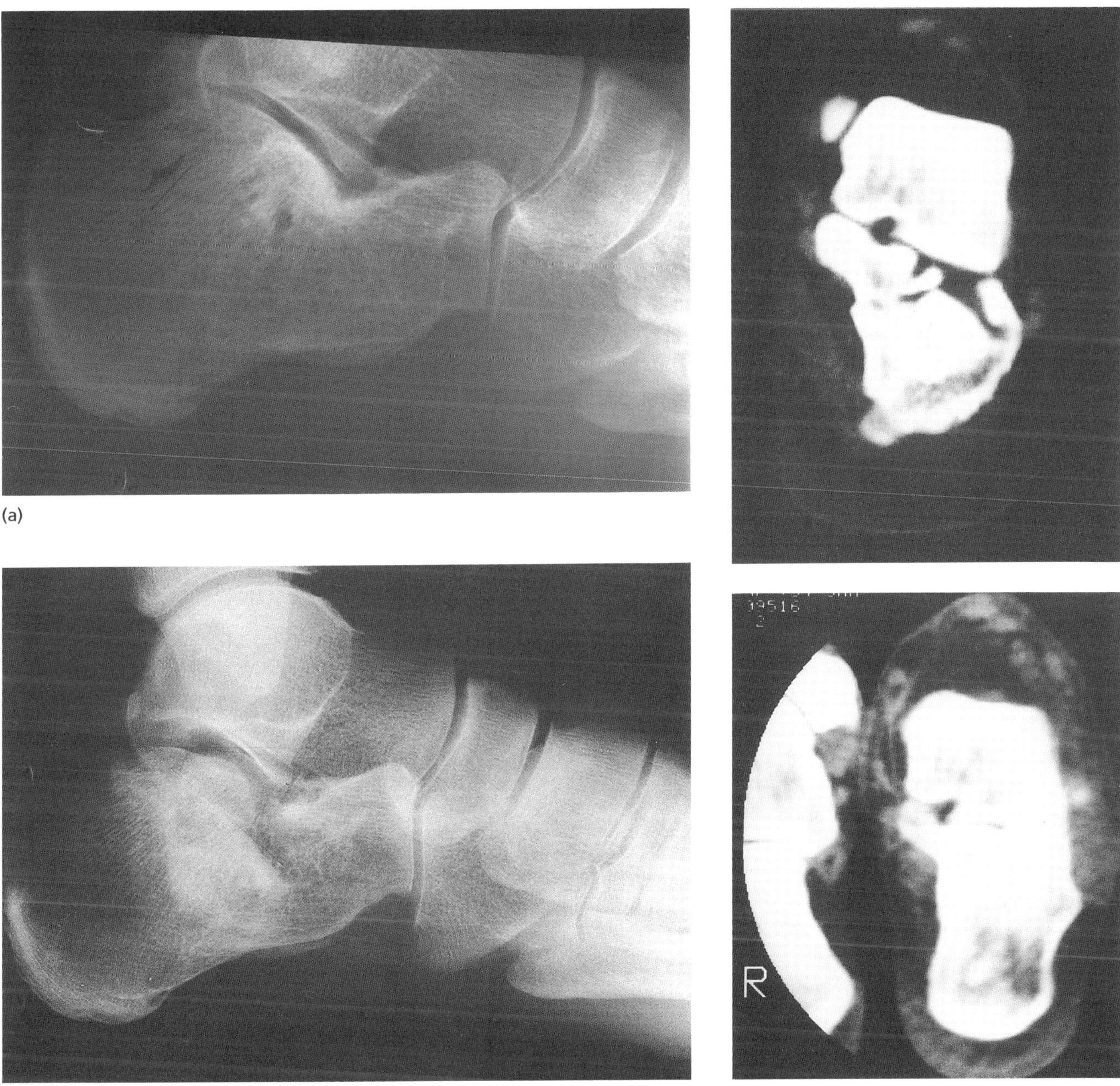

Fig. 25.15 Lateral radiographs and CT scans of a displaced intra-articular fracture. (a) On admission. (b) After open reduction. The pins were removed before the CT scan was obtained.

review of surgically and conservatively treated cases does not support this (Bradley & Davies 1990, Janzen *et al*. 1992).

Failure of open reduction to prevent subsequent symptoms may result from peroneal tendon damage or displacement (Bradley & Davies 1990), heel-pad injury (Paley & Hall 1993), irreparable articular cartilage damage (Dick 1953), or avascular necrosis of separated fragments of the posterior subtalar joint (Harris 1946).

Vascular derangement may also be involved, as there is early evidence that supplementation of treatment with impulse compression of the venous foot pump may improve results, although the mechanism is unclear (Erdmann *et al*. 1992). Paley and Hall (1993) have reviewed their results with fixation together with radiographs of the contralateral uninjured foot, and have described those patient characteristics presumed to be present before fracture and which were associated with a worse outcome. On comparison with the averages of the patients as a whole, these were greater body weight, shorter height, a flatter longitudinal arch, a reduced talocalcaneal angle and an increased fat pad height.

External fixation

Minimal internal fixation may be supplemented with external fixation in order to allow early weightbearing, in the hope of alleviating later heel-pad pain (Paley & Fischgrund 1993). Attempts to limit soft tissue problems after internal fixation by prior temporary reduction of the tuberosity with an external fixator have been associated with high rates of infection (Baumgaertel & Gotzen 1993). Experience with this approach is limited at present.

Primary subtalar fusion

While secondary fusion has long been used in the treatment of pain after intra-articular fractures, primary fusion was introduced by Wilson (1927) in an effort to prevent symptoms and to shorten the period of treatment (Harris 1946, Dick 1953, Hall & Pennal 1960). While fusion necessarily abolishes subtalar movement, this joint is almost invariably restricted after a displaced fracture, and a fused joint does not prevent heavy work or work involving ladders (Wilson 1933, Dick 1953).

Fusion may be carried out as soon as the reduction of swelling permits, either as the method of choice, or as second-line treatment if manipulation or open reduction is deemed to have failed (Wilson 1933, Harris 1946).

This procedure does not appear to result in a higher proportion of patients with mild symptoms or none (Hall & Pennal 1960, Noble & McQuillan 1979), although controlled series are lacking.

Primary triple fusion

The lack of universal success with primary subtalar fusion has been ascribed to associated injury to the mid-tarsal joints, both calcaneo-cuboid joint fracture and talo-navicular subluxation. Excellent results after triple fusion have been claimed but not substantiated (Conn 1935, Bankart 1942, Thompson & Friesen 1959). Long-term follow-up suggests that the calcaneo-cuboid joint is responsible for pain in less than 5% of unfused cases (Lindsay & Dewar 1958).

Local complications of open treatment

INFECTION

The use of percutaneous fixation is associated with a significant risk of bony infection, which may reach 11% (Pennal & Yadov 1973). As almost all fractures of the os calcis in civilian practice are closed injuries, any operative intervention will create a risk of infection. Deep infection after primary fusion occurs in 0–14% (Dick 1953, Thompson & Friesen 1959, Hall & Pennal 1960, Noble & McQuillan 1979), and in up to 6% after open fixation (see above).

NEUROVASCULAR DAMAGE

The sural nerve is at risk during any lateral approach to the fracture.

NON-UNION

Healing of the cancellous bone of the os calcis is reliable, and non-union of the fracture site is virtually unknown. The rate of non-union in primary fusions ranges from 0 to 10% (Dick 1953, Thompson & Friesen 1959, Hall & Pennal 1960, Thompson 1973, Noble & McQuillan 1979), although not all are symptomatic (Thompson 1973).

The role of plaster casts

Operative fixation of cancellous bone is not always reliable in the presence of comminution and therefore prompts the use of supplementary plaster cast support. While open treatment without external splintage is entirely feasible (Dick 1953, Hazlett 1969, Noble & McQuillan 1979, Burdeaux 1983, Ross & Sowerby 1985, Stephenson 1987), there is no indication that it results in better subtalar movement, and casts have not been found adversely to affect hindfoot movement after operative treatment of ankle fractures (Finsen *et al.* 1989).

Salvage

Treatment of chronic pain after a fracture of the os calcis is complicated by difficulties in defining the origin of the pain. The most obvious sites are a deranged posterior subtalar joint and structures compressed between a bulging lateral wall and the lateral malleolus. However, the mid-tarsal and ankle joints may also be to blame (Lance *et al.* 1964). Failures of secondary surgery may thus arise from misdiagnosis. A further complicating factor is that many of these are industrial injuries and are the subjects of compensation claims.

Symptoms may improve over a period of 12–18 months after injury (Essex-Lopresti 1952), and thus there is reason to delay further surgery until this period has elapsed. However, this may result in prolonged disability in a manual worker who has difficulties in obtaining a lighter job.

Secondary subtalar fusion

This procedure is the mainstay of secondary treatment of intra-articular fractures and may be combined with lateral decompression and correction of valgus deformity. Both the Gallie and the Grice fusions have the theoretical advantage of maintaining hindfoot height, further loss of which may exacerbate lateral abutment (Isbister 1974). Distraction fusion may assist with decompression of the peroneal tendons, and by restoring the normal talocalcaneal angle may reduce any anterior tibio-talar impingement arising from the horizontal position of the talus (Carr *et al.* 1988).

The Gallie fusion (1943) was developed specifically for this problem and is suitable in cases where the heel is in neutral alignment or only slight valgus. Through a posterolateral incision, a tunnel is cut through the posterior subtalar joint, its upper half lying in the talus and its lower half in the os calcis (Fig. 25.16). Corticocancellous bone graft, taken originally from the tibia but now more usually from the iliac crest, is punched into the defect. With a distraction fusion a bone graft is used to separate the bones, or alternatively the heel height may be restored by an osteotomy of the os calcis through the site of the original primary fracture (Romash 1993).

Patient selection is the problem, and variation in this probably accounts for much of the variation in published results. Methods of establishing that pain is arising from the subtalar joint include a trial period in a below-knee plaster cast, on the premise that it abolishes subtalar movement, and the injection of local anaesthetic into the subtalar joint. Successful relief of pain after operation is achieved in 45–100% of cases (Lindsay & Dewar 1958, Pennal & Yadov 1973, Kalamchi & Evans 1977, Johansson *et al.* 1982).

Secondary triple fusion

Adding the fusion of the mid-tarsal joints might offer the hope of more reliable pain relief, particularly with calcaneo-cuboid involvement, although there is no evidence for this (Gaul & Greenberg 1966).

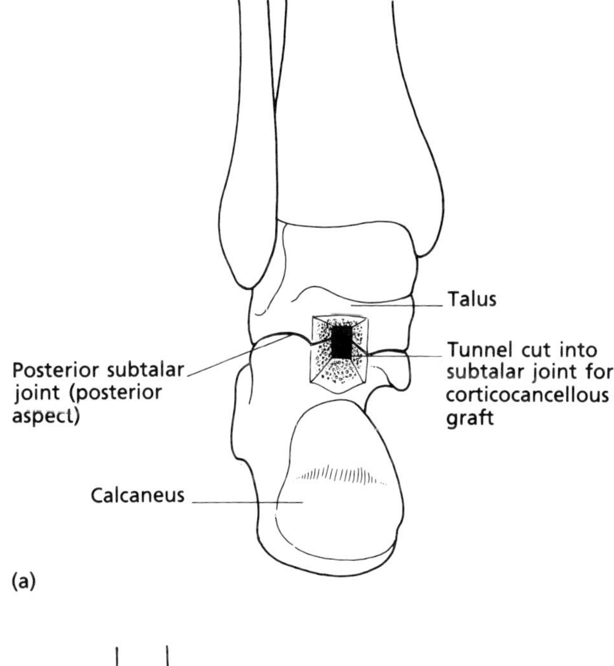

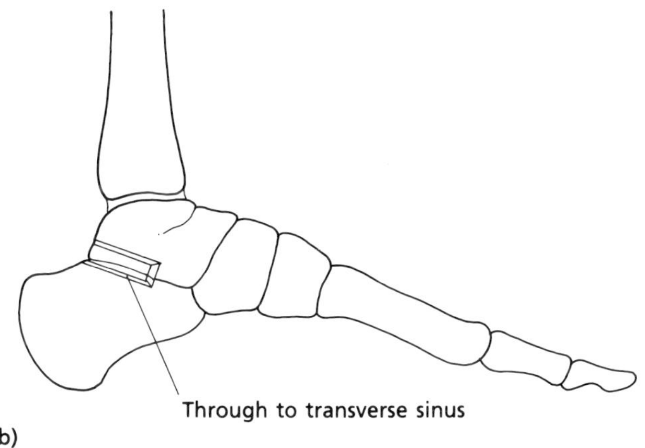

Fig. 25.16 The Gallie subtalar fusion. (After Gallie 1943.)

Lateral decompression

Lateral entrapment is suggested by lateral pain that is made worse by ankle movement rather than by subtalar movement (Braly *et al.* 1985), and CT scanning may show compromise of the peroneal tendons (Guyer *et al.* 1985). Combined clinical and radiological review suggests that tendon abnormality, such as rupture or stenosis of the sheath, is more important than subluxation or dislocation in those patients who are symptomatic (Bradley & Davies 1990).

While bony bosses may be excised alone, results appear to be improved if a subtalar fusion is included (Myerson & Quill 1993). Extra-articular excision of the distal end of the fibula appears reliable where pain arises from bone-to-bone contact (Isbister 1974).

Sural nerve damage after previous surgery may also be responsible for lateral pain. This may be managed by neurectomy and transfer of the stump into the peroneus brevis (Myerson & Quill 1993).

Minor procedures

EXCISION OF EXOSTOSES

Displaced fracture fragments may produce sufficient symptoms to warrant excision, particularly if they cause pressure points in the sole.

PERONEAL TENDON RELOCATION OR DECOMPRESSION

Tendon displacement may result from lateral calcaneal wall deformity. However, less than a quarter of cases are associated with symptoms (Lindsay & Dewar 1958). Stenosing tenosynovitis as demonstrated on CT scanning is associated with a poorer outcome after fracture (Bradley & Davies 1990) and decompression may be considered.

EXCISION OF ANTERIOR PROCESS FRAGMENTS

Symptomatic ununited avulsion fractures of the anterior process respond well to simple excision of the fragments if carried out within 2 years of the injury (Levine *et al*. 1959, Degan *et al*. 1982).

TARSAL TUNNEL DECOMPRESSION

Tarsal tunnel syndrome after fracture is not well recognized but is said to occur in up to 10% of cases, of which a quarter require operative release (Guillen Garcia *et al*. 1979). The results of surgery are, however, unpredictable (Myerson & Quill 1993).

Amputation

The ultimate salvage procedure is most commonly required as a tertiary measure to deal with infection, skin problems and continuing pain after fusion (James & Hunter 1983). For pain relief it has been found unreliable, prompting the suggestion of a 'regional pain syndrome' in these cases.

The future

The treatment of displaced intra-articular fractures of the os calcis is controversial, and will remain so until large prospective randomized trials of the treatment options are published. While it is likely that the efficacies of the treatments available will vary with the fracture configuration, much remains to be established concerning the soft tissue element of this injury.

References

Aaron, D.A.R. & Howat, T.W. Intra-articular fractures of the calcaneum. *Injury* 1976; **7**: 205–211.

Allan, J.H. The open reduction of fractures of the os calcis. *Ann Surg* 1955; **141**: 890–900.

Anthonsen, W. An oblique projection for roentgen examination of the talo-calcanean joint, particularly regarding intra-articular fracture of the calcaneus. *Acta Radiol* 1943; **24**: 306–310.

Bankart, A.S.B. Fractures of the os calcis. *Lancet* 1942; **ii**: 175.

Barnard, L. Non-operative treatment of fractures of the calcaneus. *J Bone Joint Surg* 1963; **45A**: 865–867.

Baumgaertel, F.R. & Gotzen, L. Two-stage operative treatment of comminuted os calcis fractures. Primary indirect reduction with medial external fixation and delayed lateral plate fixation. *Clin Orthop* 1993; **290**: 132–141.

Benirschke, S.K. & Sangeorzan, B.J. Extensive intraarticular fractures of the foot. Surgical management of calcaneal fractures. *Clin Orthop* 1993; **292**: 128–134.

Bèzes, H., Massart, P., Delvaux, D., Fourquet, J.P. & Tazi, F. The operative treatment of intraarticular calcaneal fractures. Indications, technique, and results in 257 cases. *Clin Orthop* 1993; **290**: 55–59.

Biehl, W.C., III, Morgan, J.M., Wagner, F.W. & Gabriel, R. Neuropathic calcaneal tuberosity avulsion fractures. *Clin Orthop* 1993; **296**: 8–13.

Böhler, L. Diagnosis, pathology, and treatment of fractures of the os calcis. *J Bone Joint Surg* 1931; **13**: 74–89.

Bradley, S.A., Davies, A.M. Computed tomographic assessment of old calcaneal fractures. *Br J Radiol* 1990; **63**: 926–933.

Bradley, S.A., Davies, A.M. Computed tomographic assessment of soft tissue abnormalities following calcaneal fractures. *Br J Radiol* 1992; **65**: 105–111.

Braly, W.G., Bishop, J.O. & Tullos, H.S. Lateral decompression for malunited os calcis fractures. *Foot Ankle* 1985; **4**: 90–96.

Brodén, B. Roentgen examination of the subtaloid joint in fractures of the calcaneus. *Acta Radiol* 1949; **31**: 85–91.

Burdeaux, B.D. Reduction of calcaneal fractures by the McReynolds medial approach technique and its experimental basis. *Clin Orthop* 1983; **177**: 87–103.

Carey, E.J., Lance, E.M. & Wade, P.A. Extra-articular fractures of the os calcis. *J Trauma* 1965; **5**: 362–372.

Carr, J.B., Hansen, S.T. & Benirschke, S.K. Subtalar distraction bone block fusion for late complications of os calcis fractures. *Foot and Ankle* 1988; **9**: 81–86.

Conn, H.R. The treatment of fractures of the os calcis. *J Bone Joint Surg* 1935; **17**: 392–405.

Cotton, F.J. & Wilson, L.T. Fractures of the os calcis. *Boston Med Surg J* 1908; **159**: 559–565.

Degan, T.J., Morrey, B.F. & Braun, D.P. Surgical excision for anterior-process fractures of the calcaneus. *J Bone Joint Surg* 1982; **64A**: 519–524.

Dick, I.L. Primary fusion of the posterior subtalar joint in the treatment of fractures of the calcaneum. *J Bone Joint Surg* 1953; **35B**: 375−380.

Erdmann, M.W.H., Richardson, J. & Templeton, J. Os calcis fractures: a randomized trial comparing conservative treatment with impulse compression of the foot. *Injury* 1992; **23**: 305−307.

Essex-Lopresti, P. The mechanism, reduction technique, and results in fractures of the os calcis. *Br J Surg* 1952; **39**: 395−419.

Fernandez, D.L. & Koella, C. Combined percutaneous and 'minimal' internal fixation for displaced articular fractures of the calcaneus. *Clin Orthop* 1993; **290**: 108−116.

Finsen, V., Saetermo, R., Kibsgaard, L., Farran, K., Engebretsen, L., Bolz, K.D. & Benum, P. Early postoperative weight-bearing and muscle activity in patients who have a fracture of the ankle. *J Bone Joint Surg* 1989; **71A**: 23−27.

Gallie, W.E. Subastragular arthrodesis in fractures of the os calcis. *J Bone Joint Surg* 1943; **25**: 731−736.

Gaul, J.S. Jr. & Greenberg, B.G. Calcaneus fractures involving the subtalar joint: a clinical and statistical survey of 98 cases. *South Med J* 1966; **59**: 605−613.

Giachino, A.A. & Uhthoff, H.K. Intra-articular fractures of the calcaneus. *J Bone Joint Surg* 1989; **71A**: 784−787.

Guillen Garcia, P., Garcia-Rubio, M., Concejero Lopez, V., Cachero Bernardez, D. Tarsal tunnel syndrome: a report of fifty-six cases. *J Bone Joint Surg* 1979; **61B**: 123.

Guyer, B.H., Levinsohn, E.M., Frederickson, B.E., Bailey, G.L. & Formikell, M. Computed tomography of calcaneal fractures: anatomy, pathology, dosimetry, and clinical relevance. *Am J Roentgenol* 1985; **145**: 911−919.

Hall, M.C. & Pennal, G.F. Primary subtalar arthrodesis in the treatment of severe fractures of the calcaneum. *J Bone Joint Surg* 1960; **42B**: 336−343.

Harris, R.I. Fractures of the os calcis. Their treatment by tri-radiate traction and subastragular fusion. *Ann Surg* 1946; **124**: 1082−1100.

Hazlett, J.W. Open reduction of fractures of the calcaneum. *Can J Surg* 1969; **12**: 310−317.

Hermann, O.J. Conservative therapy for fracture of the os calcis. *J Bone Joint Surg* 1937; **19**: 709−718.

Hunt, D.D. Compression fracture of the anterior articular surface of the calcaneus. *J Bone Joint Surg* 1970; **52A**: 1637−1642.

Isbister, J.F.St.C. Calcaneo-fibular abutment following crush fracture of the calcaneus. *J Bone Joint Surg* 1974; **56B**: 274−278.

Järvholm, U., Körner, L., Thorén, O. & Wiklund, L.-M. Fractures of the calcaneus. A comparison of open and closed treatment. *Acta Orthop Scand* 1984; **55**: 652−656.

James, E.T.R. & Hunter, G.A. The dilemma of painful old os calcis fractures. *Clin Orthop* 1983; **177**: 112−115.

Janzen, D.L., Connell, D.G., Munk, P.L., Buckley, R.E., Meek, R.N. & Schechter, M.T. Intraarticular fractures of the calcaneus: value of CT findings in determining prognosis. *Am J Roentgen* 1992; **158**: 1271−1274.

Johansson, J.E., Harrison, J. & Greenwood, F.A.H. Subtalar arthrodesis for adult traumatic arthritis. *Foot Ankle* 1982; **2**: 294−298.

Kalamchi, A. & Evans, J.G. Posterior subtalar fusion. A preliminary report on a modified Gallie's procedure. *J Bone Joint Surg* 1977; **59B**: 287−289.

Kathol, M.H., El-Khoury, G.Y., Moore, T.E. & Marsh, J.L. Calcaneal insufficiency avulsion fractures in patients with diabetes mellitus. *Radiology* 1991; **180**: 725−729.

King, R.E. Axial pin fixation of fractures of the os calcis (method of Essex-Lopresti). *Orthop Clin North Am* 1973; **4**: 185−188.

Lance, E.M., Carey, E.J. & Wade, P.A. Fractures of the os calcis: treatment by early mobilization. *Clin Orthop* 1963; **30**: 76−90.

Lance, E.M., Carey, E.J. & Wade, P.A. Fractures of the os calcis: a follow-up study. *J Trauma* 1964; **4**: 15−56.

Langdon, I.J., Kerr, P.S. & Atkins, R.M. Fractures of the calcaneum: the anterolateral fragment. *J Bone Joint Surg* 1994; **76B**: 303−305.

Letournel, E. Open treatment of acute calcaneal fractures. *Clin Orthop* 1993; **290**: 60−67.

Levine, J., Kenin, A. & Spinner, M. Non-union of a fracture of the anterior superior process of the calcaneus. *J Bone Joint Surg* 1959; **41A**: 178−180.

Lindsay, W.R.N. & Dewar, F.P. Fractures of the os calcis. *Clin Orthop* 1963; **30**: 76−90.

Lance, E.M., Carey, E.J. & Wade, P.A. Fractures of the os calcis: a follow-up study. *J Trauma* 1964; **4**: 15−56.

Langdon, I.J., Kerr, P.S. & Atkins, R.M. Fractures of the calcaneum: the anterolateral fragment. *J Bone Joint Surg* 1994; **70B**: 247−250.

Lowy, M. Avulsion fractures of the calcaneus. *J Bone Joint Surg* 1969; **51B**: 494−497.

McReynolds, I.S. Open reduction and internal fixation of calcaneal fractures. *J Bone Joint Surg* 1972; **54B**: 176−177.

McReynolds, I.S. The case for operative treatment of fractures of the os calcis. In: Leach, R.E., Hoagland, F.T. & Riseborough, E.J. (eds) *Controversies in Orthopaedic Surgery.* WB Saunders: Philadelphia, 1982.

Matsen, F.A. & Clawson, D.K. The deep posterior compartmental syndrome of the leg. *J Bone Joint Surg* 1975; **57A**: 34−39.

Maxfield, J.E. & McDermott, F.J. Experiences with the Palmer open reduction of fractures of the calcaneus. *J Bone Joint Surg* 1955; **37A**: 99−106.

Mittlmeier, T., Mächler, G., Lob, G., Mutschler, W., Bauer, G. & Vogl, T. Compartment syndrome of the foot after intra-articular calcaneal fracture. *Clin Orthop* 1991; **269**: 241−248.

Myerson, M. & Manoli, A. Compartment syndromes of the foot after calcaneal fractures. *Clin Orthop* 1993; **290**: 142−150.

Myerson, M. & Quill, G.E. Late complications of fractures of the calcaneus. *J Bone Joint Surg* 1993; **75A**: 331−341.

Noble, J. & McQuillan, W.M. Early posterior subtalar fusion in the treatment of fractures of the os calcis. *J Bone Joint Surg* 1979; **61B**: 90−93.

O'Connell, F., Mital, M.A. & Rowe, C.R. Evaluation of modern management of fractures of the os calcis. *Clin Orthop* 1972; **83**: 214−223.

Paley, D. & Fischgrund, J. Open reduction and circular external fixation of intraarticular calcaneal fractures. *Clin Orthop* 1993; **290**: 125−131.

Paley, D. & Hall, H. Intra-articular fractures of the calcaneus. A critical analysis of results and prognostic factors. *J Bone Joint Surg* 1993; **75A**: 342−354.

Palmer, I. The mechanism and treatment of fractures of the calcaneus. *J Bone Joint Surg* 1948; **30A**: 2−8.

Parkes, J.C. The nonreductive treatment for fractures of the os calcis. *Orthop Clin North Am* 1973; **4**: 193−195.

Parmar, H.V., Triffitt, P.D. & Gregg, P.J. Intra-articular fractures of the calcaneum treated operatively or conservatively. A prospective study. *J Bone Joint Surg* 1993; **75B**: 932–937.

Pennal, G.F. & Yadov, M.P. Operative treatment of comminuted fractures of the os calcis. *Orthop Clin North Am* 1973; **4**: 197–211.

Romash, M.M. Reconstructive osteotomy of the calcaneus with subtalar arthrodesis for malunited calcaneal fractures. *Clin Orthop* 1993; **290**: 157–167.

Ross, S.D.K. & Sowerby, M.R.R. The operative treatment of fractures of the os calcis. *Clin Orthop* 1985; **199**: 132–143.

Sanders, R., Fortin, P., DiPasquale, T. & Walling, A. Operative treatment in 120 displaced intraarticular calcaneal fractures. Results using a prognostic computed tomography scan classification. *Clin Orthop* 1993; **290**: 87–95.

Segal, D., Marsh, J.L. & Leiter, B. Clinical application of computerized axial tomography (CAT) scanning of calcaneus fractures. *Clin Orthop* 1985; **199**: 114–123.

Soeur, R. & Remy, R. Fractures of the calcaneum with displacement of the thalamic portion. *J Bone Joint Surg* 1975; **57B**: 413–421.

Stephenson, J.R. Displaced fractures of the os calcis involving the subtalar joint: the key role of the superomedial fragment. *Foot Ankle* 1983; **4**: 91–101.

Stephenson, J.R. Treatment of displaced intra-articular fractures of the calcaneus using medial and lateral approaches, internal fixation, and early motion. *J Bone Joint Surg* 1987; **69A**: 115–130.

Stephenson, J.R. Surgical treatment of displaced intraarticular fractures of the calcaneus. A combined lateral and medial approach. *Clin Orthop* 1993; **290**: 68–75.

Thompson, K.R. Treatment of comminuted fractures of the calcaneus by triple arthrodesis. *Orthop Clin North Am* 1973; **4**: 189–191.

Thompson, K.R. & Friesen, C.M. Treatment of comminuted fractures of the calcaneus by primary triple arthrodesis. *J Bone Joint Surg* 1959; **41A**: 1423–1436.

Warrick, C.K. & Bremner, A.E. Fractures of the calcaneum. With an atlas illustrating the various types of fracture. *J Bone Joint Surg* 1953; **35B**: 33–45.

Wilson, P.D. Treatment of fractures of the os calcis by arthrodesis of the subastragular joint. *J Am Med Assoc* 1927; **89**: 1676–1683.

Wilson, P.D. Fractures and dislocations of the tarsal bones. *South Med J* 1933; **26**: 833–845.

Zwipp, H., Tscherne, H., Thermann, H. & Weber, T. Osteosynthesis of displaced intraarticular fractures of the calcaneus. Results in 123 cases. *Clin Orthop* 1993; **290**: 76–86.

Talus, navicular, metatarsals and phalanges

H.P.J.WALSH AND L.KLENERMAN

The talus

The talus is unique in that it has no tendinous attachments and therefore no added blood supply to the extrinsic source it receives, unlike other bones. It is also the largest tarsal bone and as 60% of its surface is articular, intra-articular fractures are common (Hansen 1989). The body of the talus articulates superiorly with the tibia and medially and laterally with the malleoli of the ankle joint. Inferiorly, it articulates with the posterior facet of the calcaneum. The neck of the talus is somewhat slimmer than the body, and although supported by ligamentous and capsular attachments it is prone to fracture. The head articulates with the concave surface of the navicular and is supported inferiorly by the spring ligament and the sustentaculum tali.

There are two separate processes on the talus, both prone to fracture on occasions: the lateral and posterior bony processes. The former articulates with the fibula superiorly and the lateral part of the posterior calcaneal facet inferiorly. The posterior process is separated into medial and lateral tubercles by the tendon of flexor hallucis longus. These receive the insertion of the deltoid and posterior talo-fibular ligaments respectively.

Classification of talar fractures

Talar fractures may be classified as follows:
1 Fractures of the neck.
2 Fractures of the head.
3 Fractures of the body, including fractures of the lateral and posterior processes and talar dome.

Talar neck fractures

Talar neck fractures are uncommon injuries but carry a high complication rate. They make up the majority (50–60%) of all talar fractures.

Before discussing these fractures it is important to understand the blood supply to the body of the talus (Mulfinger & Trueta 1970). There are four major feeding arteries. The artery of the tarsal canal arises from the posterior tibial artery and anastomoses with the artery of the tarsal sinus (Fig. 25.17), which usually comes from the dorsalis pedis artery (Fig. 25.18). The posterior tibial artery also forms a deltoid branch, which supplies the body of the talus through a branch that runs within the deep part of the deltoid ligament (Fig. 25.19). Finally, also through the posterior tibial artery, the posterior tubercle branches form a posterior upper axis to supply the posterior aspect of the talus (Fig. 25.17).

CLASSIFICATION

Hawkins' (1970) classification is the most frequently used (Fig. 25.20).

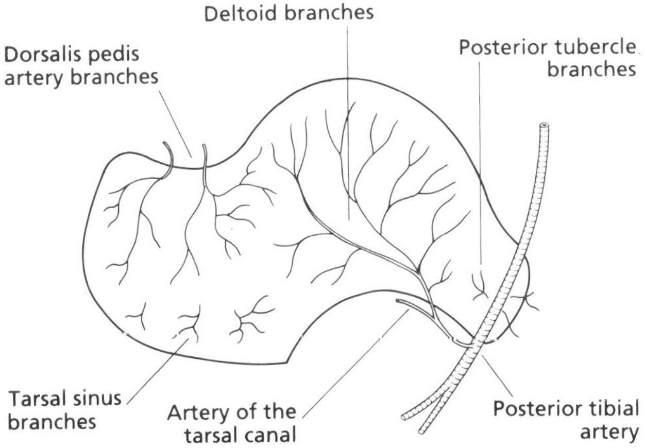

Fig. 25.17 The artery of the tarsal canal formed from the tibialis posterior artery and the interosseus anastomoses. Also note the posterior tubercle (calcaneal) branches.

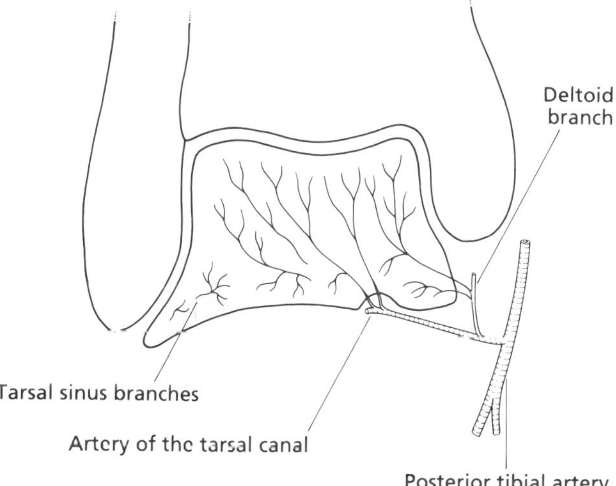

Fig. 25.19 The deltoid branch to the talar body is formed from the posterior tibial artery.

Type I — Undisplaced fracture through the neck of the talus with no disruption of either the ankle or subtalar joint (Fig. 25.21).

Type II — Some displacement of the body of the talus, owing to the fracture, with some subluxation or complete dislocation of the subtalar joint; the ankle joint remains intact (Fig. 25.22).

Type III — The body of the talus is so significantly displaced that there is dislocation at both the subtalar and ankle joints (Fig. 25.23).

Type IV — In this injury, which was not in Hawkins' original description, there is complete dislocation of the body of the talus and ankle and subtalar joint; in addition, there is a dislocation of the head of the talus from the talo-navicular joint (Fig. 25.20).

MECHANISM OF INJURY

Most of these injuries are caused by hyper-dorsiflexion of the foot in relationship to the tibia. Very occasionally, such an injury can occur due to a direct blow to the dorsal aspect of the foot. The hyper-dorsiflexion injury was most commonly seen in flying accidents when the foot was forced into dorsiflexion while resting on the rudder bar on impact (Coltart 1952). More commonly now, however, the injury is seen following road traffic accidents or following a fall from a height, landing on the foot in the neutral position. The forced dorsiflexion, which causes impaction of the talar neck on the under-surface of the anterior aspect of the tibia, gives rise to the injury.

CLINICAL PRESENTATION

Patients give a history of a high-velocity injury which, in most cases, has given rise to a hyper-dorsiflexion injury to the ankle. Patients are usually in great pain and, on clinical examination, swelling is the most obvious finding; this can be seen even when the fragments are not significantly displaced. However, in types II, III and IV distortion of the hindfoot and ankle may be obvious and as the degree of displacement increases so

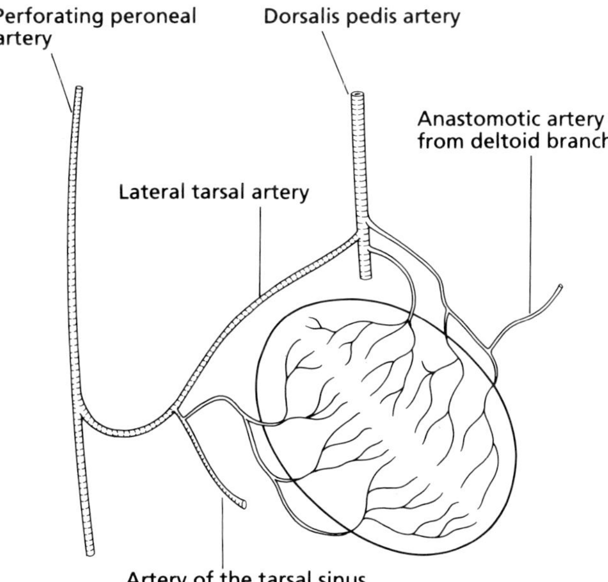

Fig. 25.18 The artery of the tarsal sinus is a branch of the anterior tibial dorsalis pedis artery. Also shown are the anastomoses within the head of the talus at this level.

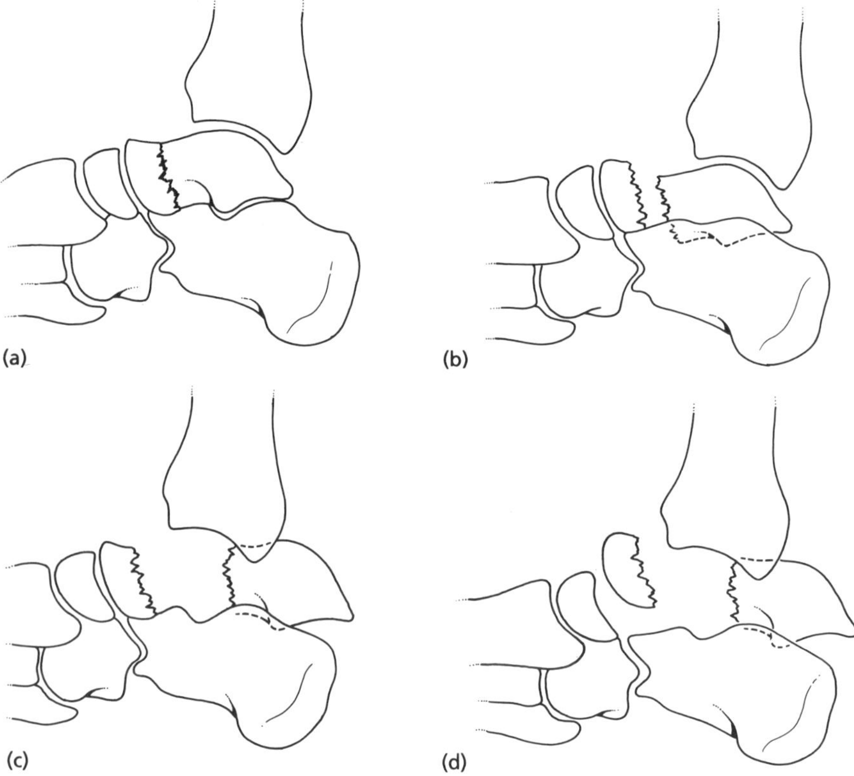

Fig. 25.20 Hawkins' gradings with Canale's addition.

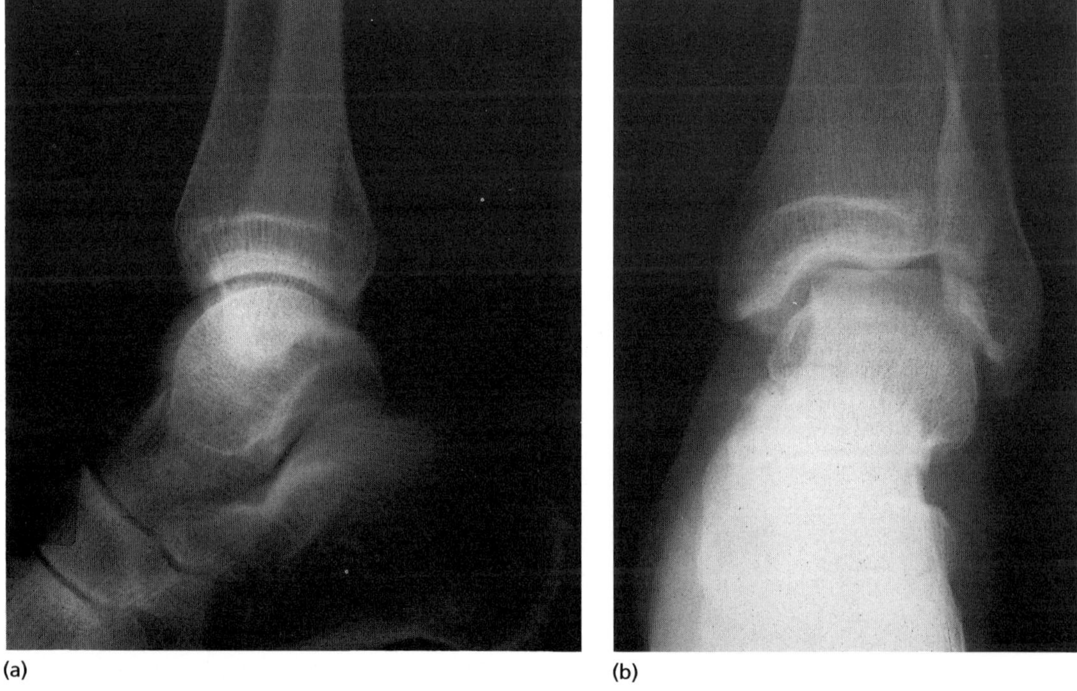

Fig. 25.21 Type I talar neck fracture.

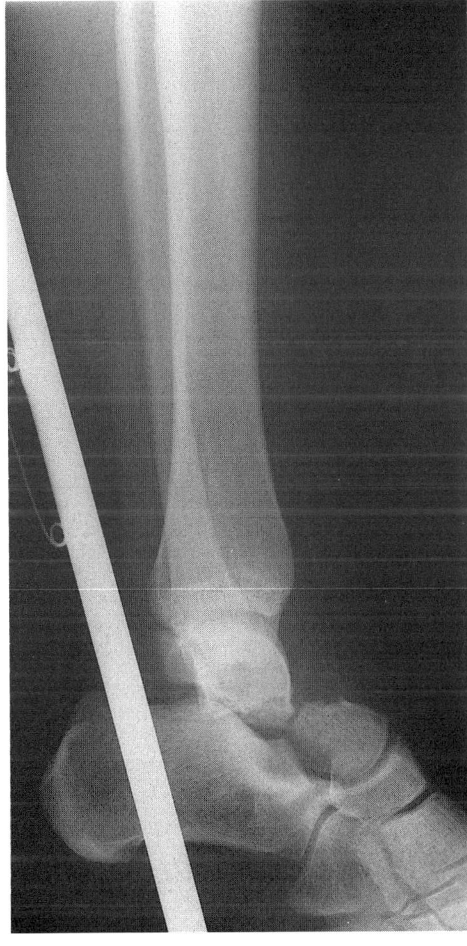

Fig. 25.22 Type II fracture of the talus with subtalar disruption.

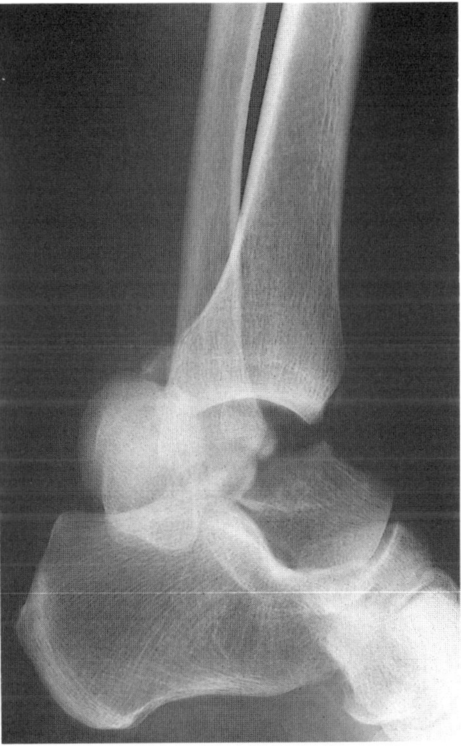

Fig. 25.23 Type III fracture of the talar neck with subtalar and crural disruption. Note also the fracture of the medial malleolus.

locally and distally, require careful clinical and radiological assessment.

TREATMENT

The risk of avascular necrosis following talar neck fractures increases from type I, where the risks are low (0%), to type III, where the risk is as high as 91% (Hawkins 1970). Displaced injuries represent a true orthopaedic emergency. Rapid reduction is essential to prevent skin necrosis, as discussed earlier, and compound injuries in particular require early assessment of the soft tissues and appropriate repair.

Once the diagnosis has been made, the authors agree with many others (Hansen 1989) that early open reduction and rigid internal fixation is indicated. This applies even to undisplaced type I fractures because it is thought that early mobilization of the foot and ankle is essential. The formerly accepted treatment of reduction of type II injuries, by application of a below-knee cast with the ankle in full equinus to hold the reduction, is both uncomfortable for the patient and also slows down rehabilitation.

When performing open reduction and internal fixation the surgeon must take care not to further com-

the risk of a compound injury arises (Canale & Kelly 1978). The skin should be carefully monitored because with displaced injuries pressure from the bony fragments on the soft tissues can give rise to skin necrosis and breakdown.

It is essential that the distal circulation is monitored carefully, particularly with the more severe injuries. It has also been noted in the past that there is a high incidence of medial malleolar fractures (Canale & Kelly 1978) as well as injuries to more remote structures (Hawkins 1970).

RADIOLOGY

It is important to get good-quality anteroposterior and lateral views of the ankle and hindfoot as well as a good mortice view of the ankle joint itself. One must always be aware that these injuries quite often are associated with other injuries and so the relevant parts, both

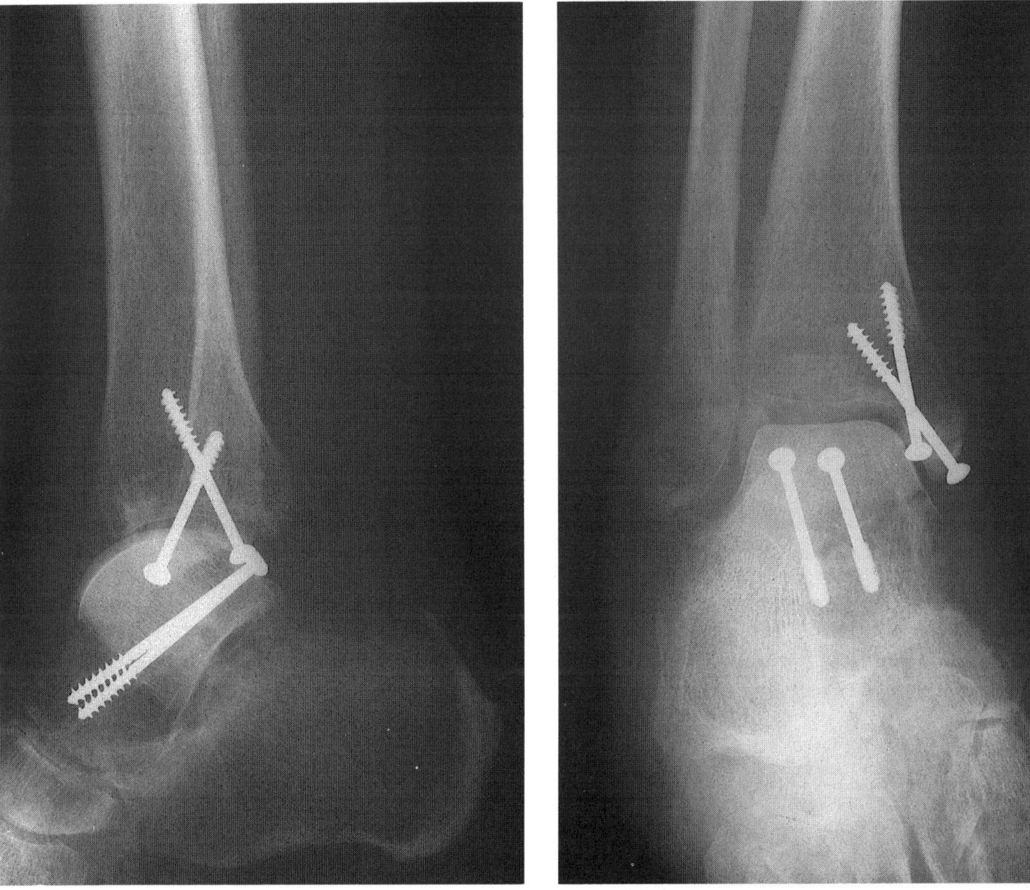

Fig. 25.24 Case as shown in Fig. 23. Despite open reduction and internal fixation the talar body is dense 6 weeks after injury.

promise the blood supply to the talus. An anteromedial incision is the one most commonly used or, alternatively, a lateral Ollier approach. Access to the talus through the medial site can be enhanced by turning down the medial malleolus, either through a fracture site, if present, or by osteotomy of the bone and subsequent fixation with Association for Osteosynthesis (AO) cancellous screws or tension-band wiring. Once the talar fracture has been reduced it can be held with Kirschner wires; intraoperative radiographs are required to decide whether anatomical reduction has been achieved. The fracture can then be fixed with 4- or 6.5-mm AO cancellous screws, depending on the size of the fragments. Early mobilization can be permitted, provided that fixation is rigid. The patient should remain non-weight-bearing for approximately 3 months.

Follow-up should include regular radiographs to make sure the reduction is maintained and to watch for signs of avascular necrosis (Fig. 25.24). A bone scan may be helpful and in the occasional case where internal fixation has not been used, magnetic resonance imaging (MRI) of the area can reveal evidence of avascular necrosis within the talus; however, the presence of metalwork may preclude this investigation (Adelaar 1989).

Should avascular necrosis develop, it may not mean that collapse of the talus will occur. This is thought to be due to the fact that the avascularity may be patchy and there are areas of good bone stock. Hawkins (1970) described a radiological sign apparent on the anteroposterior radiograph at 2 weeks after a talar neck fracture: a crescent of osteolysis below the articular surface (Fig. 25.25). This radiological sign suggests that the vascularity within the body of the talus is relatively normal because the radiolucency represents an area of osteoporotic bone, which is secondary to the disuse around the area of injury and can only occur if blood is reaching this particular subchondral area. In contrast, subchondral collapse or marked density are poor radiological signs and suggest there is avascularity in this region. Should avascular necrosis be evident or suspected, then a patellar tendon-bearing orthosis, (Fig. 25.26) which allows free ankle movement, is

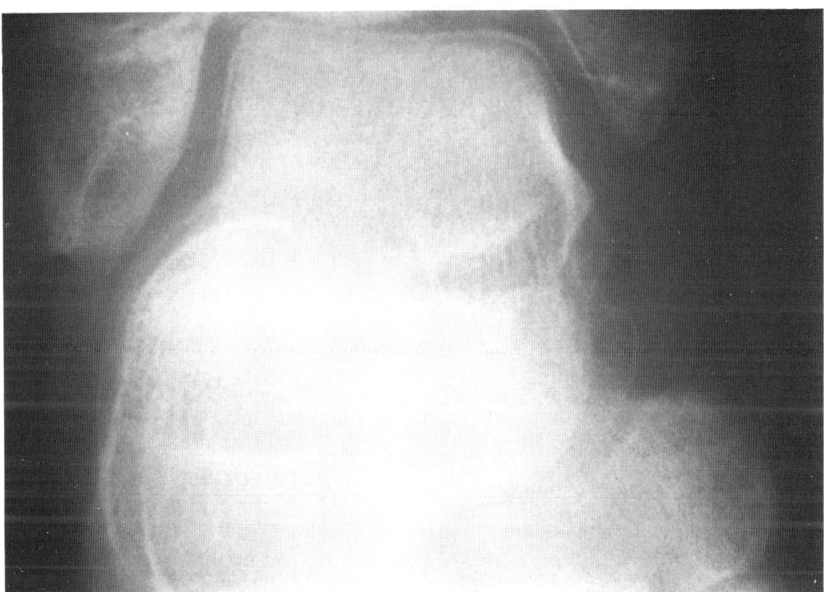

Fig. 25.25 Subchondral radiolucency on the anterior posterior radiograph in a patient 7 weeks after a talar neck fracture.

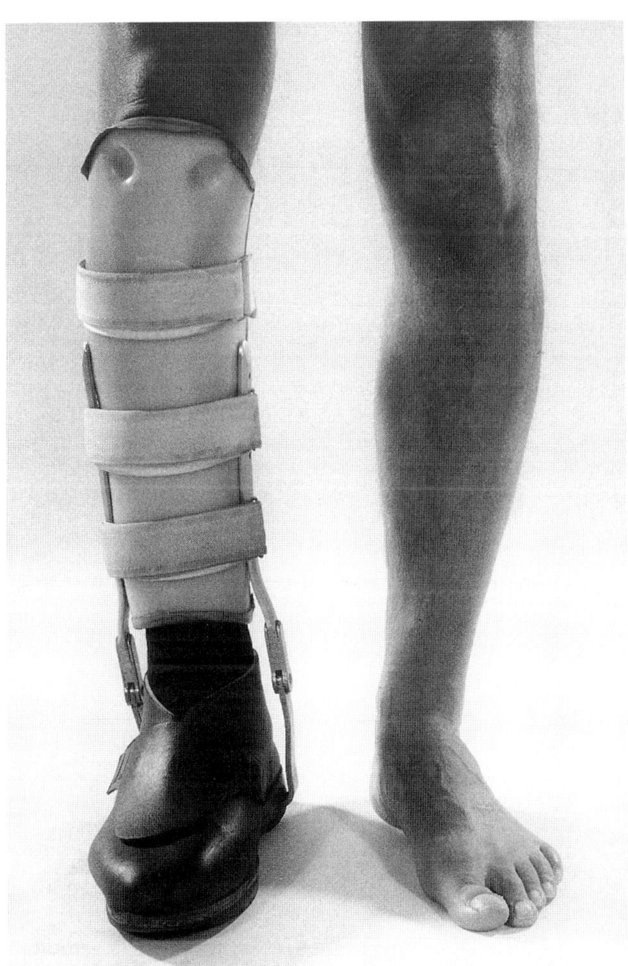

Fig. 25.26 A patellar tendon weight-bearing orthosis in a patient with avascular necrosis of the talus following a type III injury.

thought by the authors to prevent collapse but allow relative mobility of the joints.

If the joints become painful, stiff and degenerate (Fig. 25.27) as a result of the fracture then there are several salvage procedures available. These include talectomy with or without tibiocalcaneal fusion, sub-

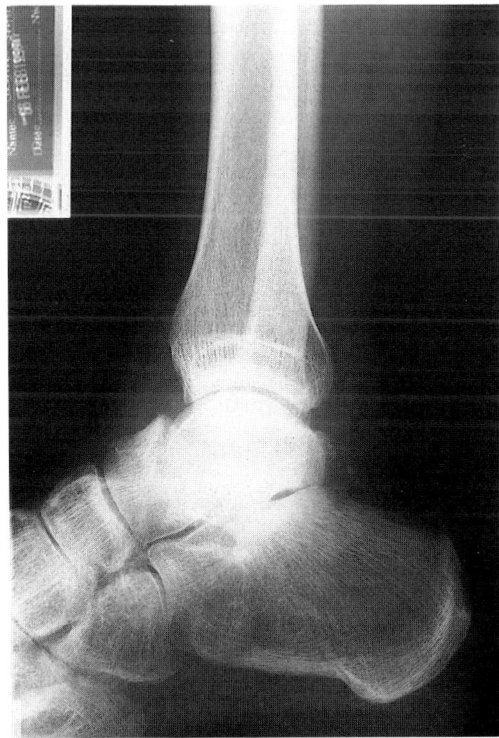

Fig. 25.27 A missed type II injury presented 2 years later with malunion and a stiff subtalar joint.

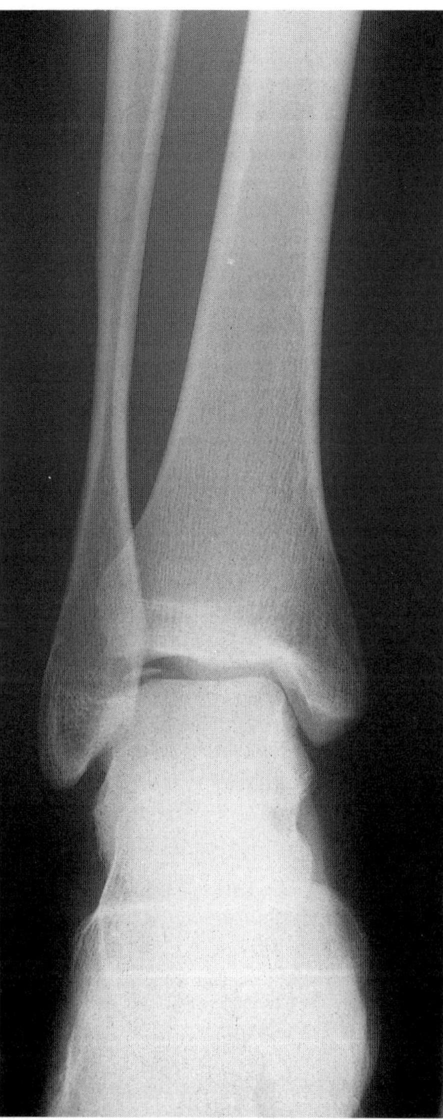

Fig. 25.28 Fracture of the lateral dome of the talus, which was treated by excision.

talar fusion if the ankle joint is satisfactory, a Blair fusion (Blair 1943), which is a fusion of the distal tibia to the residual viable head of the talus after removal of the avascular body, or pantalar fusion. If the injury has been treated conservatively and delayed union develops, then open reduction and internal fixation with compression is indicated. Occasionally, malunion occurs and symptoms can develop from bony prominences which hinder movement and require excision or local fusion.

Talar head fractures

These injuries frequently accompany Chopart's dislocation but can occur in isolation. The mechanism of injury is thought to be a longitudinal impaction of the talar head as a result of a high-velocity trauma when the force is transmitted along the first ray while the foot is in a relatively plantigrade position. This is similar to the impaction seen with rudder bar injuries (Coltart 1952). The injuries can be either displaced or undisplaced and the fragments, when displaced, can be either small or large. Clinically, the patient presents with pain and tenderness over the region of the talo-navicular joint and as there is so often little swelling the injury can be easily overlooked (Heckman 1991). However, if adequate anteroposterior, lateral and oblique views of the foot are taken, then the talar head fracture becomes apparent. The remainder of the foot should be scrutinized for other bony injuries.

Treatment depends on whether the fracture is undisplaced or not. The authors feel that undisplaced injuries can be managed by use of a well-moulded below-knee cast, with the patient remaining non-weight-bearing for 3 weeks. In the case of displaced injuries, if the fragment is small then excision is indicated because incongruity of the joint may develop once the fracture has healed. In instances where the fragments are larger, then internal fixation is more appropriate and this could be achieved by the use of K-wires (Heckman 1991) or a more rigid internal fixation device similar to those described for talar dome fractures, for example the Herbert screw (Lange *et al.* 1986).

This fracture in isolation may be associated with degenerative change later within the talo-navicular joint and the authors feel that an isolated talo-navicular fusion to maintain a longitudinal arch may suffice. However, if the joint changes are long standing, then disorganization of the subtalar and calcaneo-cuboid joints may be present and a triple arthrodesis will be more effective.

Talar dome fractures

Talar dome fractures can be looked upon as osteochondral fractures and constitute 0.8% of all ankle fractures (Mukerjee & Young 1973). They can be either medial or lateral (Figs 25.28 & 25.29); the latter are often missed. The mechanism of injury for the medial fracture is a compression injury to this area while the ankle is inverted and plantarflexed. The more common lateral injury is not infrequently encountered amongst sportsmen, especially soccer players, and occurs when

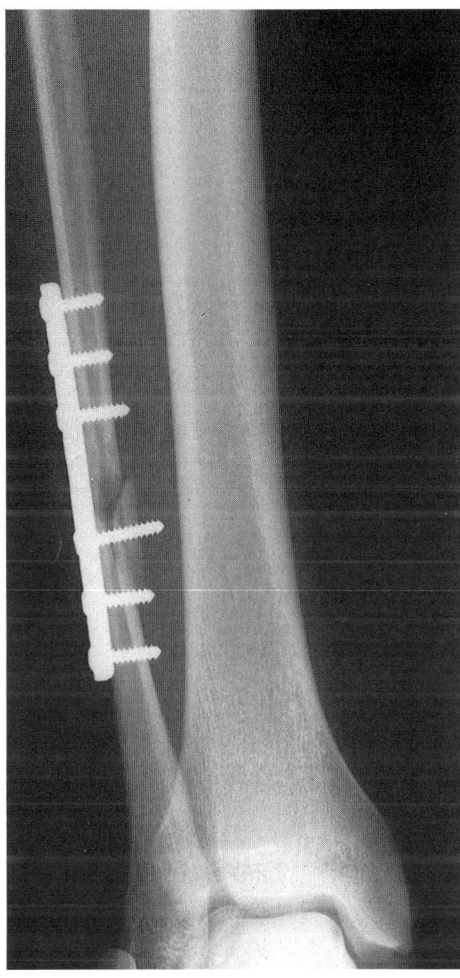

Fig. 25.29 Missed fracture of the lateral dome with major ankle disruption; this was treated by internal fixation of the fibula and deltoid ligament repair.

the ankle is in the dorsiflexed and inverted position (Wilson 1991). Patients often feel that they have had just a severe sprain of the ankle and may not seek medical advice.

However, the clinician should be aware of the possibility of the diagnosis and should look for tenderness and swelling over the appropriate areas; this is usually associated with a decreased range of motion. Diagnosis can be confirmed on anteroposterior and lateral views of the ankle with the medial lesion identified by a view taken with the ankle in maximum plantarflexion. The lateral lesion can be seen on a mortice view of the ankle. Medial lesions are usually posterior and their extent can be confirmed on the lateral radiograph. Lateral injuries tend to be a little more anterior but if there is any doubt computerized axial tomography (CAT) or magnetic resonance scan (Fig. 25.30) can confirm the diagnosis. There is sometimes a medial malleolar fracture associated with the medial injury.

Treatment depends upon the size of the lesion. Conservative treatment has no role. If the fragment is very small it should be excised and the subchondral bone drilled. If the lesion is large, then open reduction and internal fixation using a screw with a buried head, e.g. the Herbert screw (Lange *et al.* 1986), and early movement is good treatment. As medial lesions tend to be a little posterior a medial malleolar osteotomy may be necessary to aid the exposure. Lateral lesions are usually accessible via an anterolateral incision over the ankle joint.

Osteochondritis dissecans is thought by many experts

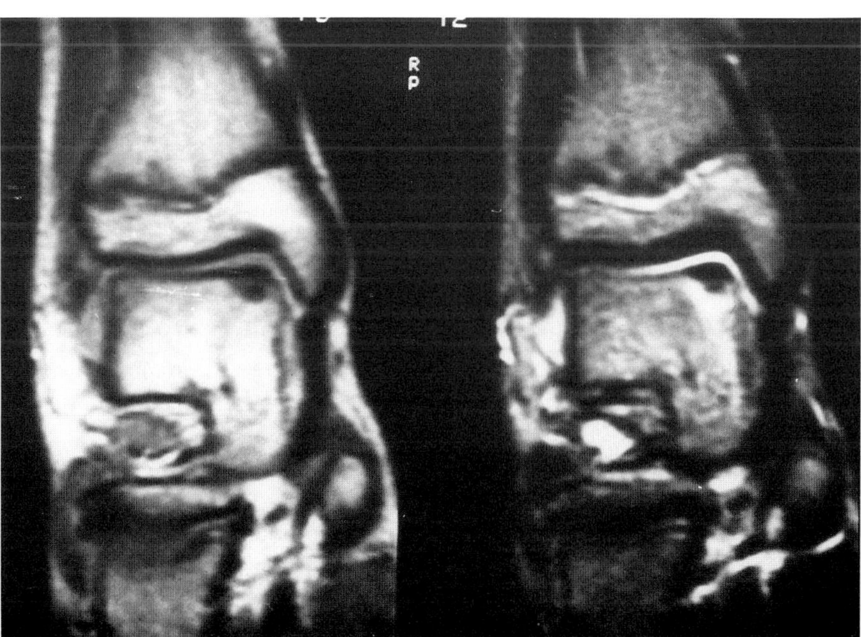

Fig. 25.30 A magnetic resonance image to show an osteochondral fracture of the talus medially.

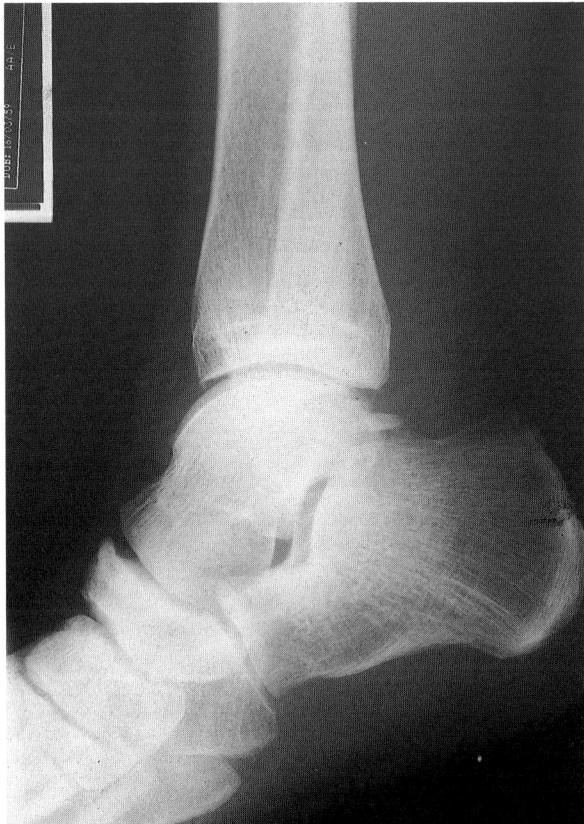

Fig. 25.31 The os trigonum is seen posterior to the body of the talus and above the os calcis.

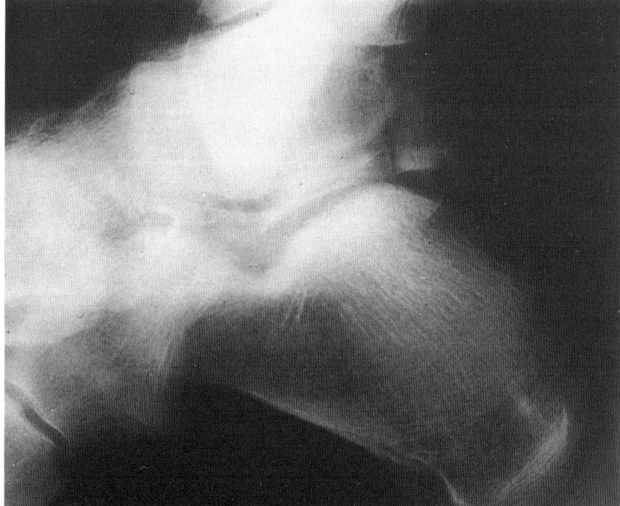

Fig. 25.32 Fracture of the posterior process of the talus.

to be one of the long-term effects of the above injuries (Berndt & Harty 1959). Therefore, recognition and appropriate treatment of these acute fractures is necessary to prevent the possible long-term sequelae seen once the fragment has become avascular and separated, causing locking of the ankle joint and later osteoarthrosis.

Fractures of the posterior process of the talus

The posterior process of the talus is made up of two tubercles, the lateral and medial, separated by the tendon of the flexor hallucis longus. The lateral tubercle is larger and is the site of insertion of the posterior talo-fibular ligament; the medial tubercle accepts the posterior fibres of the deltoid ligament. Injuries in this area include fractures of either tubercle, separately or together (Heckman 1991). The os trigonum (Fig. 25.31) is a smoothly delineated accessory ossicle found behind the posterior process of the talus in 4–6% of feet and bilaterally in 60% (Heckman 1991). In the acutely injured ankle it can cause confusion to the unwary because it is clearly seen on a lateral radiograph.

Pennal (1963) believed the mechanism of posterior process fractures to be due to compression of the process between the os calcis and the posterior aspect of the tibia while the ankle is in marked plantarflexion. Separate fractures of the tubercles making up the posterior process are thought to occur due to avulsion of either the posterior aspect of the deltoid ligaments, for the medial tubercle, or the posterior talo-fibular ligament, for the lateral tubercle. Diagnosis can be made if, on movement, there is tenderness and pain over the region of the process. The pain is exacerbated by passive movement of the great toe owing to the proximity of the tendon of flexor hallucis longus to the bony process. True lateral radiographs should show a separate fragment of bone with an irregular edge separating from the main body of the talus (Fig. 25.32), and a technetium bone scan may be useful if there is any doubt (Heckman 1991).

Because it is a rare fracture we have little experience of management, but would immobilize an undisplaced fracture in a below-knee cast for 4–6 weeks until union had occurred. If it does not heal, then excision of the fragment is indicated if the patient has symptoms. Excision of a widely displaced fragment would be the treatment of choice if there was significant disability (Wilson 1991). Malunion can cause subtalar degeneration (Fig. 25.33).

Fractures of the lateral process of the talus

The lateral process makes up approximately one-third of the posterior talocalcaneal joint on the inferior surface and articulates superiorly with the distal end of the

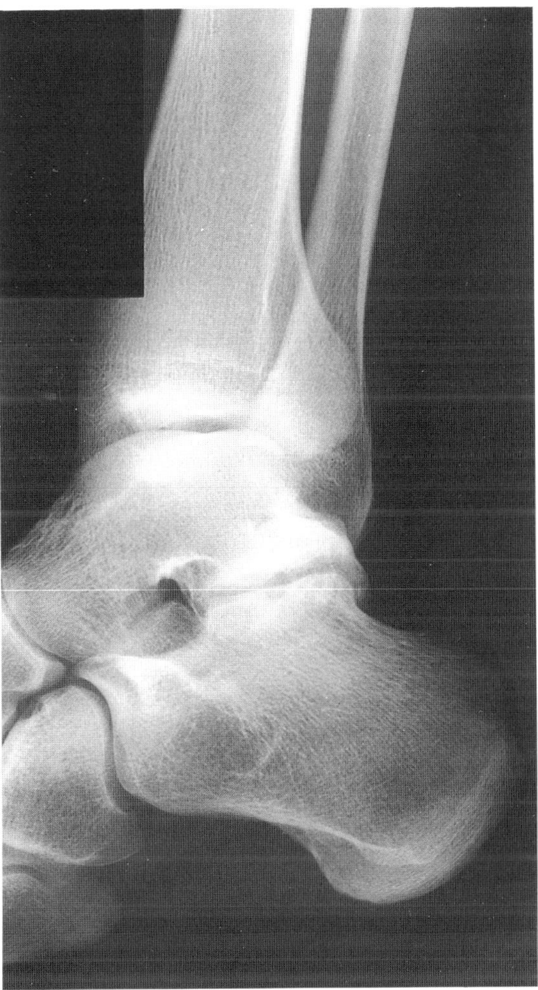

Fig. 25.33 Malunion of a fracture of the posterior process of the talus with a subtalar extension which years later has produced degeneration of the posterior subtalar joint.

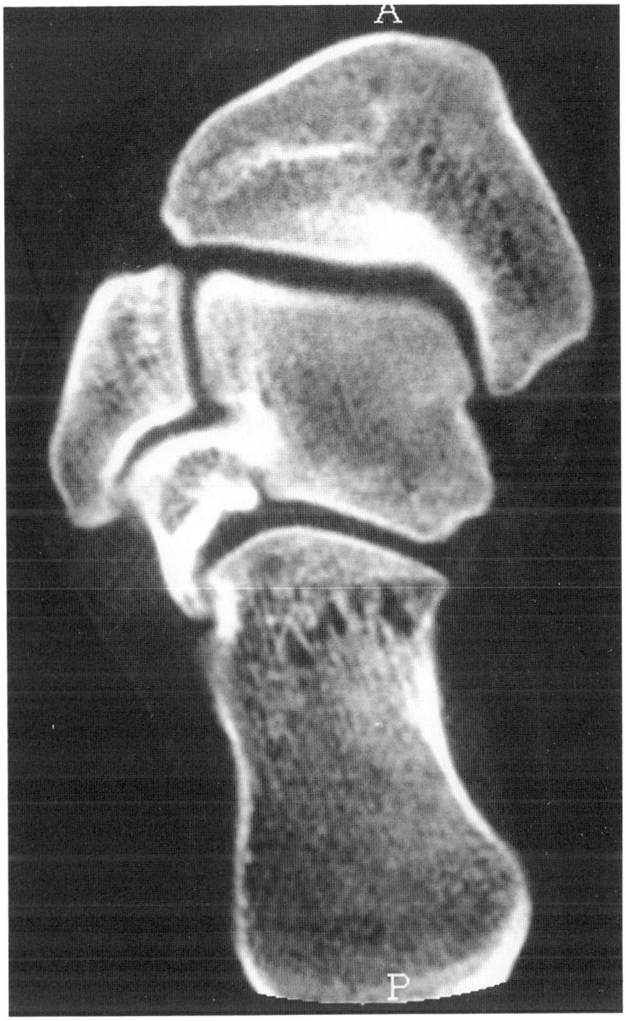

Fig. 25.34 A type II lateral process fracture of the talus clearly seen on a computerized tomogram.

fibula. The lateral ligament complex of the ankle has some attachment to the tip of this process. Hawkins (1965) classified this injury into three types: First, a fracture involving the articulation of the talocalcaneal joint only: type II is an injury in which there is involvement not only of the talocalcaneal joint but also of the talo-fibular articulation; and finally, more severe injury would be suggested by a fracture of the lateral process of the talus with marked comminution.

It has been postulated (Hawkins 1965, Mukerjee *et al*. 1974) that this injury is caused by forced dorsiflexion of the inverted heel, so that the superior aspect of the lateral part of the calcaneum shears off or compresses the lateral process. Patients usually present with a history of a violent inversion injury to the heel with pain and tenderness just beneath the fibula. Radiologically,

the fracture may be difficult to see, particularly on the lateral view, but is usually apparent on the antero-posterior veiw. It is recommended, however, that perhaps a special internal rotation view of 45° with 10° plantarflexion (Wilson 1991) would show the fracture more clearly, although this may be impractical in an acutely injured patient. Computerized tomography is also of use (Fig. 25.34).

Conservative treatment is advised only for undisplaced fractures and involves immobilization in a below-knee cast for 6 weeks with no weight-bearing for 4 weeks (Heckman 1991). For displaced injuries internal fixation is required and the earlier this is performed the better the results (Mukerjee *et al*. 1974). The fragment is approached through an incision over the sinus tarsi and fixed back with a suitable screw. If the fracture is very

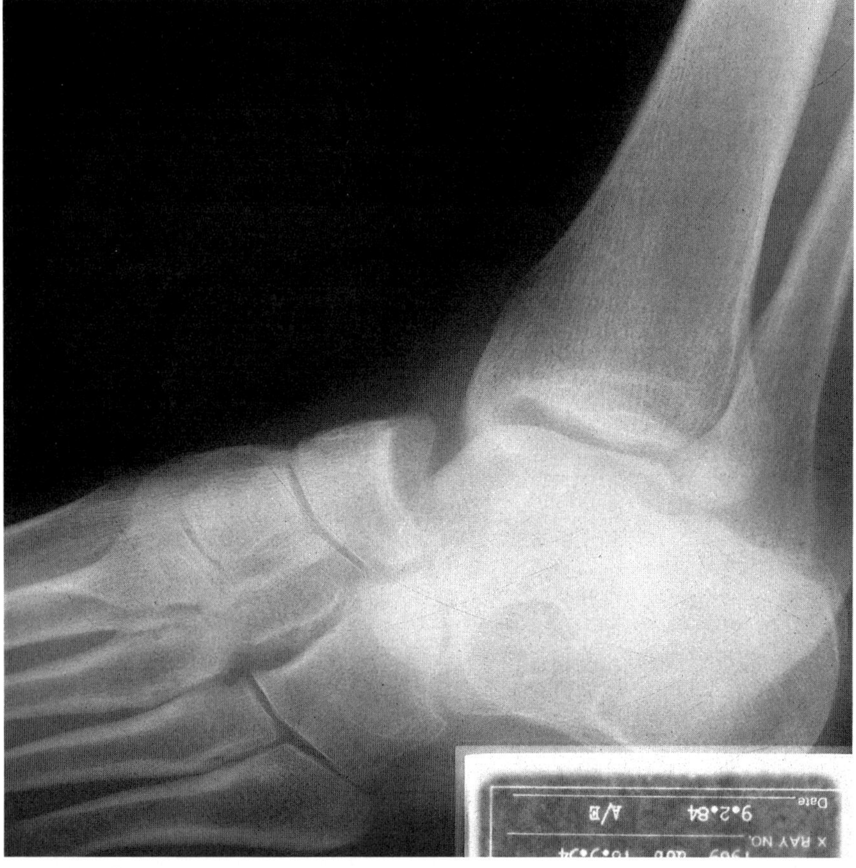

Fig. 25.35 A subtalar dislocation.

comminuted, then excision of loose fragments is more effective to prevent degenerative changes.

In the long term, the fracture may not unite, leading to resultant irregularity of the subtalar joint and arthrosis; when there are small fragments these may produce local irritation, causing pain and stiffness. As this is an intra-articular injury, the larger the fragment the more important it is to realign the articular surface accurately to avoid long-term sequelae (Hawkins 1965, Mukerjee *et al.* 1974). If late problems develop then subtalar fusion is the only option, provided that the patient's symptoms warrant a surgical solution (Heckman 1991).

Dislocations around the talus

These can be classified as: (i) talo-crural, i.e. dislocations of the ankle (see Chapter 24); or (ii) subtalar dislocations (De Lee 1986) (Fig. 25.35).

Subtalar dislocations

These are classified according to the displacement of the calcaneum and the foot in relationship to the talus. The talus stays within the ankle mortice while the calcaneum and the remainder of the foot move relative to it. Medial subtalar dislocations (Fig. 25.36) account for 85% of these injuries (De Lee & Curtis 1982). Here, the calcaneum and the navicular come to lie medial to the talus and the talar head is felt to be prominent on the dorsum of the foot. Conversely, the lateral dislocation, which carries a more serious prognosis (Heckman 1991), is typically found with displacement of the calcaneum and the remainder of the foot lateral to the talus which is felt medially on the dorsum of the foot. Rarer types of dislocation of the subtalar joint have been described but the majority contain a significant component of medial or lateral displacement.

The mechanism of injury of subtalar dislocation is an excessive inversion injury, resulting in subtalar displacement, or an excessive eversion injury, leading to a lateral subtalar displacement. The reason the whole foot and navicular displace with the calcaneum during the dislocation but the talus remains *in situ* is that the calcaneo-navicular ligaments are relatively stronger than the talocalcaneal or talo-navicular ligaments. In consequence, the latter two ligaments tear while the former remains intact. Frequently, there are associated injuries

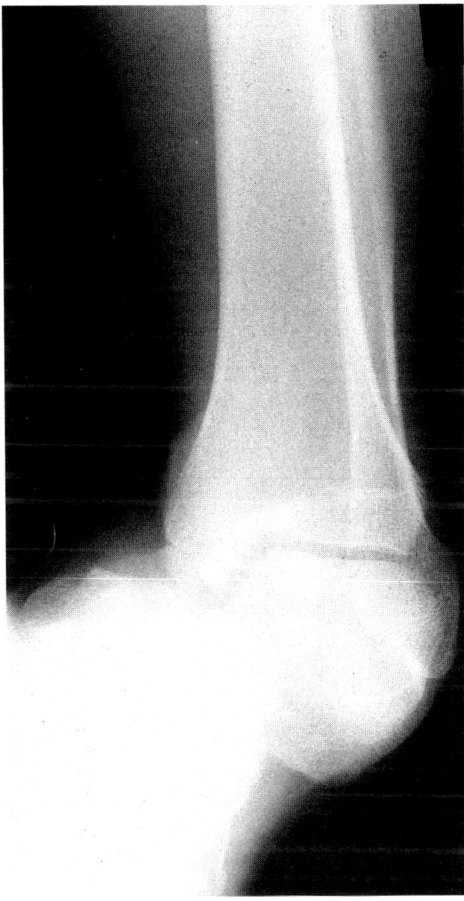

Fig. 25.36 Medial subtalar dislocation.

and De Lee and Curtis (1982) described associated intra-articular fractures in 45% of cases. The fact that medial dislocations are more common than lateral dislocations may suggest that increased forces are required (Heckman 1991). The usual history is of a violent incid-

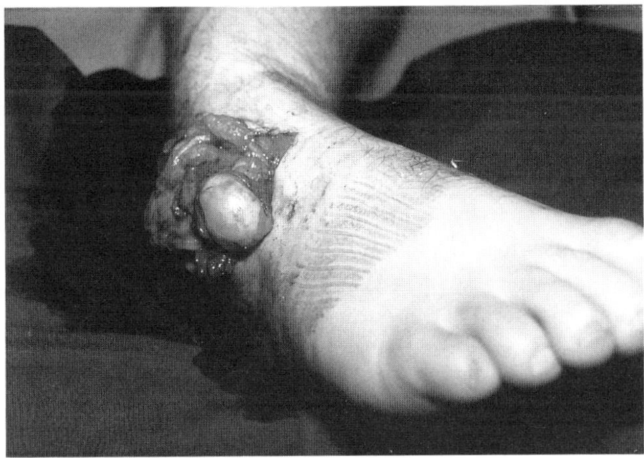

Fig. 25.37 Compound subtalar dislocation. Note that the head of the talus is exposed.

ent, such as a road traffic accident, but may alternatively involve sport (Grantham 1964).

The clinical appearance is typical and radiographs are hardly necessary before reduction. However, antero-posterior, lateral and oblique radiographs of the ankle and hindfoot are mandatory to confirm the diagnosis and eliminate other injuries around the tarsus.

Because of tenting of the skin, necrosis of the soft tissues may follow prolonged displacement if the dislocation is left unreduced. Approximately 10–15% of cases are open injuries (Fig. 25.37). A distal neuro-vascular injury is uncommon but one should be aware of the possibility (Heckman 1991).

Reduction of these dislocations is an orthopaedic emergency. An attempt can be made with the patient under sedation in the Accident room should there be any cause for delay in obtaining theatre time. Reduction is achieved with the knee flexed to relax the gastro-cnemius and gentle traction on the heel to relocate the calcaneum (De Lee 1986). However, if this is unsuccessful general or spinal anaesthesia will be necessary to achieve full muscle relaxation. The knee is kept in the flexed position to relax the gastrocsoleus complex and to allow the calcaneum to be moved (Heckman 1991). The deformity is then accentuated and, by traction on the calcaneum with counter-traction on the lower leg provided by an assistant, the calcaneum can usually be reduced by reversing the deforming force. Occasionally, pressure over the distal talus will also aid relocation (Heckman 1991). Further radiographs must then be taken to confirm the reduction and also to check for other bony injuries, particularly intra-articular fractures (De Lee & Curtis 1982). These injuries will require internal fixation, if they are of a significant size, or excision, if they are small. Failure to reduce the closed injury indicates that an open reduction is required through a dorsal approach. The incision should be based over the talar head. Any loose fragments of bone should be removed. The extensor retinaculum quite commonly prevents closed reduction of medially displaced injuries and this may have to be excised. For lateral injuries the tibialis posterior tendon may be a factor in preventing relocation and may have to be retracted to complete the procedure (Heckman 1991). In either case, removal of small bony fragments is necessary and internal fixation of any larger ones with K-wires or screws is indicated.

Once reduced, the injury is inherently stable because of the bony configuration. In open injuries full debridement of the wound is essential; the wound should be left open and secondary closure performed at 3–5 days (Heckman 1991).

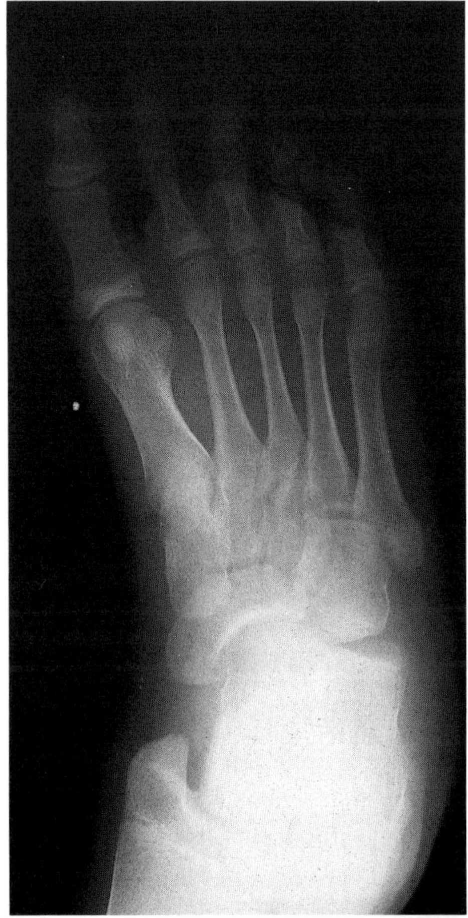

(a)

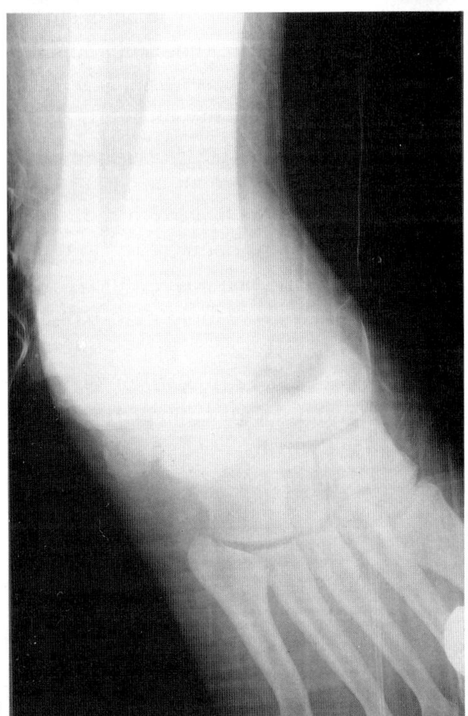

(b)

Fig. 25.38 (a) Subluxation of Chopart's joint. (b) Complete dislocation of Chopart's joint.

Whatever means is used to reduce the dislocation, the leg is immobilized for 4 weeks in a below-knee cast, non-weight-bearing; following this, the patient requires an aggressive rehabilitation programme to try and mobilize the joints and prevent long-term stiffness. If the patient has had a rapid reduction performed and it has been a closed injury with no associated skin necrosis, local infection or intra-articular fracture, then the prognosis is good (Heckman 1991). However, if there is a delay in reduction, an open injury, associated fractures, or more violent injuries, such as a road traffic accident, then the prognosis is worse (De Lee & Curtis 1982, Heckman 1991). Infection can occur, particularly following compound fractures or in association with soft tissue necrosis, but is unusual. As lateral injuries are associated with a more violent mechanism of injury these too carry a worse prognosis (Heckman 1991). Intra-articular fractures are certainly associated with an increased risk of degenerative changes (Monson & Ryan 1981) but avascular necrosis of the talus is rare (De Lee & Curtis 1982). Recurrent dislocations have been described but are uncommon (Janssen & Kopta 1985) and are thought to be due to either increased joint laxity (Larson 1957) or inadequate immobilization (less than 4 weeks) (Zimmer & Johnson 1989). Very occasionally, a patient will require further surgery to relieve symptoms of pain and stiffness associated with secondary degenerative changes, i.e. either a subtalar or triple arthrodesis.

Total talar dislocations

Total talar dislocation is an exceptionally rare injury and is thought to be the extreme continuum of subtalar dislocation. In other words, as a severe inversion/supination force, which causes medial subtalar dislocation, continues the talus itself is extruded laterally as the forefoot recoils (Pennal 1963). Conversely, in a violent pronation/eversion injury to the subtalar joint, lateral dislocation of the subtalar joint can occur and the talus can be extruded medially to come to lie in front of the medial malleolus. Not surprisingly, there is high incidence of vascular compromise following these injuries and the vast majority are compound. If the injury is closed, skin necrosis is a common problem because there is increased tension on the soft tissues. More frequently, this injury does not occur in isolation and there can be fractures of the medial or lateral malleoli.

Reduction should be immediate. For closed injuries Steinman's pins should be inserted into the calcaneum and into the distal tibia; while two assistants pull, to recreate the space for the talus, an attempt is made to push it back into place (De Lee 1986). If the reduction is unstable, then it can be held with K-wires and the leg incorporated into a well-moulded below-knee cast. The wires should be removed at 3 weeks to allow soft tissue healing. If a closed reduction should fail, then an open reduction has to be performed through either a lateral or medial incision corresponding to the displacement of the talus. Once it has been reduced, the same treatment is needed but the authors recommend that the wounds be left open and inspected after 48–72 hours. Similar treatment is recommended for compound injuries, with thorough debridement of the soft tissues to minimize infection.

This injury can be complicated by significant soft tissue infection, osteomyelitis or avascular necrosis of the talus. In the long term, if there is either infection or avascular necrosis of the talus degenerative arthritis can develop in the ankle or subtalar joint or in both.

It is recommended that a radiograph is obtained 6–8 weeks after injury to look for Hawkins' crescent sign (Fig. 25.25). If present, then it is suggested that avascularity may not become a problem. However, if the sign is absent then a patellar tendon-bearing ankle foot orthosis (Fig. 25.38) is worn to allow free ankle motion; this is similar to the treatment recommended after talar neck fractures. This may have to be kept on for up to 2 years. If osteomyelitis develops and is not controllable, then talectomy is recommended. If degenerative arthritis should develop, for whatever reason, then the authors recommend fusion of the appropriate joints, i.e. an ankle, subtalar or a pantalar arthrodesis.

Mid-tarsal (Chopart's) dislocation

Chopart's dislocation is usually associated with a fracture in the region of the talo-navicular and calcaneocuboid joints (mid-tarsal joints). Pure dislocations are uncommon (Wilson 1991) and a spectrum of injury from sprain to complete disruption is seen (Main & Jowett 1975) (Fig. 25.38). Careful scrutiny of the radiographs showing navicular, talar head, calcaneal or cuboid articular fractures is essential to exclude associated joint disruption. The injuries are classified according to the direction of the deforming force and the resultant displacement (Main & Jowett 1975), i.e. medial, longitudinal, lateral or plantar. Finally, a complete disruption with no distinct pattern is known as a 'crush' injury. Although most injuries are due to the indirect trauma (abduction or adduction injuries, etc.), the crush fracture–dislocations are usually secondary to direct violence.

Not surprisingly, the foot is very swollen and

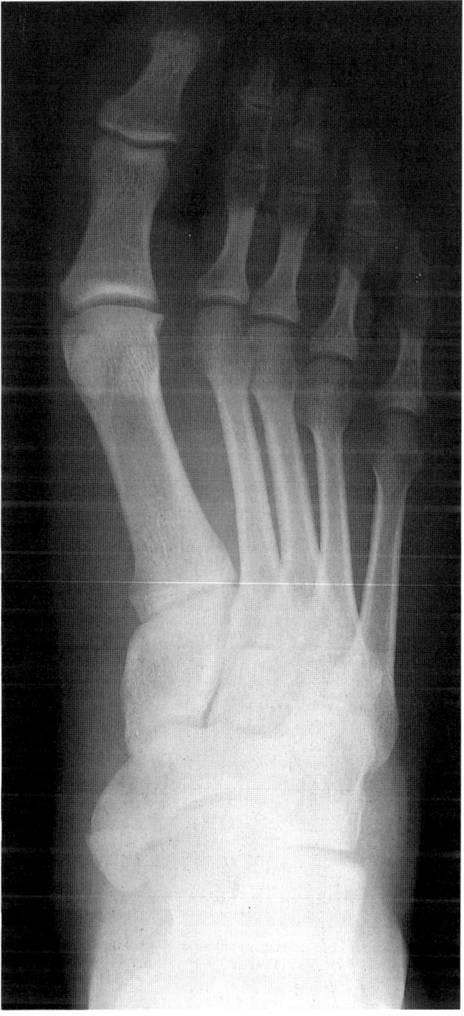

Fig. 25.39 Avulsion fracture of the navicular.

occasionally open injuries are seen. Circulatory damage must not be overlooked. Standard anteroposterior, oblique and lateral views are required for a full evaluation of the injury. Stress radiographs are occasionally helpful. Preliminary elevation to reduce swelling is invaluable. Treatment depends on the degree of displacement (De Lee 1986). Undisplaced medial, lateral, longitudinal or plantar 'sprains' simply require non-weight-bearing casts for 4 to 6 weeks. Displacement must be reduced either open or closed and then held with Kirschner wires, supplemented with plaster, for 6 weeks. Longitudinal displaced injuries may best be held with an AO lag screw across the commonly seen navicular fracture before application of the cast. Badly crushed mid-tarsal fracture–dislocations can be expected to produce stiff joints but, nevertheless, it is best to hold as anatomical a reduction as possible with multiple Kirschner wires.

Long-term sequelae are common. Recurrent dislocations can be minimized if Kirschner wires are used to hold the reduction. As with talar dislocations, intra-articular fractures or articular damage invariably leads to degenerative change if left unreduced, and long-term stiffness results (Pennal 1963). Arthrodesis of the damaged joints is the only possible salvage procedure (Main & Jowett 1975). Avascular necrosis of the navicular following these injuries has been documented (Kenwright & Taylor 1970).

Navicular fractures

Isolated navicular fractures are unusual (Heckman 1991). The navicular is a horseshoe-shaped bone with a concave proximal surface and a less convex distal surface. The navicular is at the maximum height of the longitudinal arch and is the keystone. It has a ligamentous attachment dorsally (the talo-navicular ligament) which is linked to the anterior fibres of the deltoid ligament. The tuberosity of the navicular receives attachment from the spring ligament on the plantar surface; the tibialis posterior has a wide insertion in this area and also to adjacent areas of the tarsus. The navicular receives its blood supply not only from dorsal and plantar vessels but also through the tuberosity itself. While the medial and lateral thirds of the navicular have good vascularity the central portion has a relatively poor blood supply (Torg *et al.* 1982). The vascularity of this bone diminishes with age.

Classification

The classification of navicular fractures has been well documented by De Lee (1986). There are four types:
1 Fractures of the tuberosity (Fig. 25.39).
2 Chip fractures of the dorsal surface (Fig. 25.40).
3 Fractures of the body — with or without displacement (Fig. 25.41).
4 Stress fractures.

The diagnosis of navicular fractures may be difficult but if a careful history has been taken and the patient has pain and tenderness of the appropriate area the level of suspicion should be raised. Good-quality anteroposterior, lateral and oblique radiographs of the injured area are essential. One must, however, be aware of the normal appearance of the accessory navicular, which is also known as the os tibiale externum (Fig. 25.42). This is a smooth sesamoid bone within the tendon of the tibialis posterior and is differentiated from the avulsion fracture which can occur in this area by its clearcut regular separation from the navicular with a smooth margin. It is found bilaterally in 90% of patients.

Fractures of the tuberosity

These are avulsion injuries caused by powerful contraction of the tibialis posterior during acute forced eversion of the foot. Because of the extensive insertion of this tendon around the tarsus these fractures are usually only minimally displaced. The diagnosis is readily made in the patient with the above history and with tender-

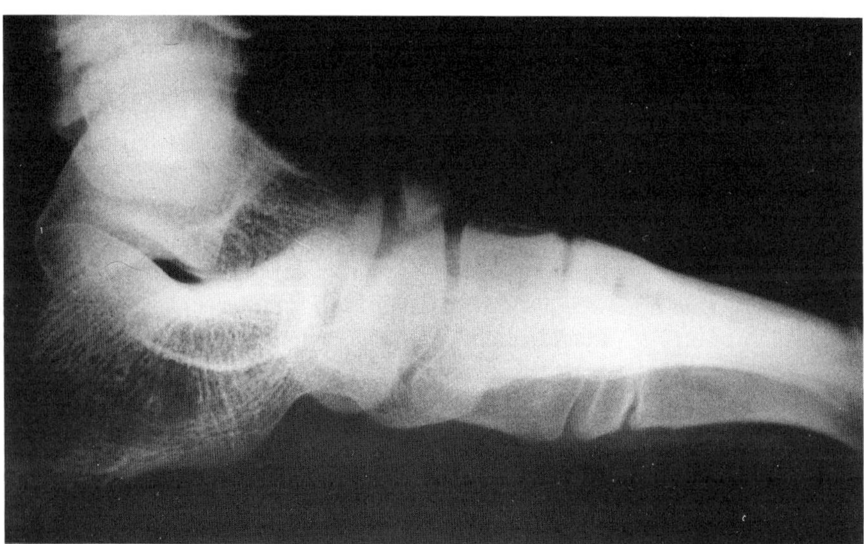

Fig. 25.40 Chip fracture off the dorsal surface of the navicular (old).

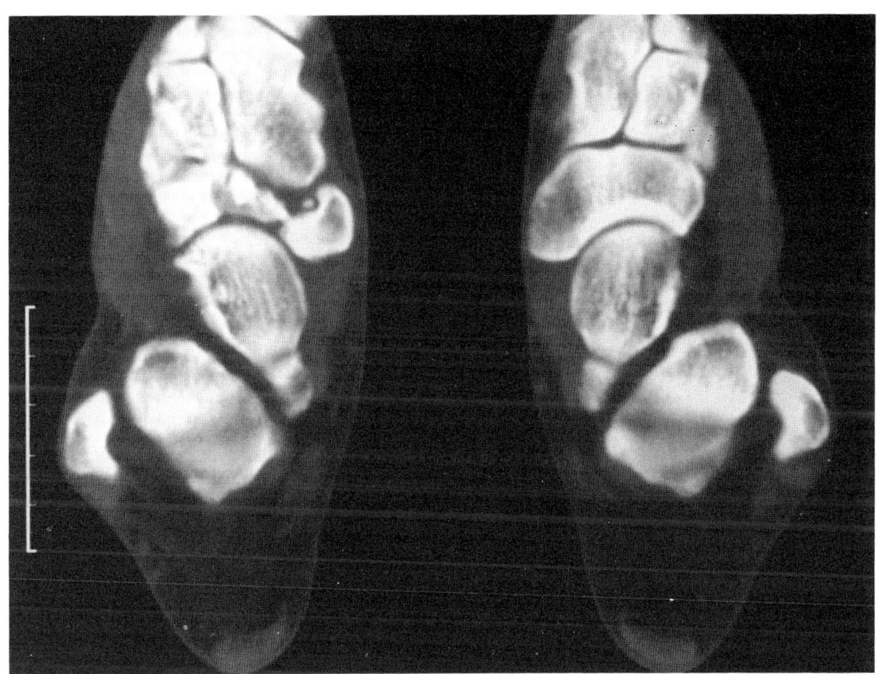

Fig. 25.41 Comminuted fracture of the navicular identified by computerized tomography.

ness over the navicular tuberosity and pain on weight-bearing. The diagnosis can then be confirmed with radiographs (Fig. 25.39). Treatment is by immobilization of the foot in a well-moulded below-knee cast for 4 weeks. Even if bony union fails to occur, long-term symptoms are unusual. If, however, the patient does have persistent pain, excision of the bony fragment is indicated and the tendon should be reinserted into the freshened bone. The leg should be placed in a below-knee cast for a further 4 to 6 weeks to allow the tendon to heal at the site of new attachment (De Lee 1986).

Fractures of the dorsal lip of the navicular

A fracture of the dorsal lip indicates that the patient has sustained an acute plantarflexion injury to the midfoot; this can be seen in association with ankle sprains (Heckman 1991). Once the diagnosis is suspected confirmation can be obtained from lateral radiographs (Fig. 25.40). One should be wary of missing a possible midtarsal disruption (Watson-Jones 1982). Four weeks in a below-knee walking plaster is adequate treatment. Occasionally, a persistent bony prominence requires secondary excision but long-term problems from this injury are exceptional.

Navicular body fractures

The minimally displaced fracture is often caused by an object dropped onto the foot. It will heal in 6 weeks in a

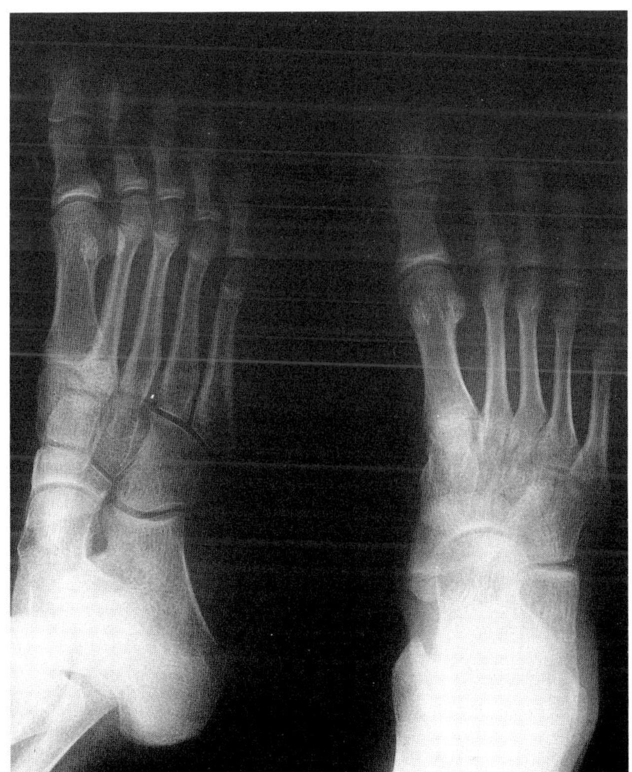

Fig. 25.42 Os tibialae externum.

quently there is wide displacement and extrusion of the navicular fragments (Fig. 25.43). In this case, open reduction and internal fixation is indicated, using either Kirschner wires or small AO cancellous screws to restore the contour of the bone (Fig. 25.44) (Nyska *et al.* 1989, Sangeorzan *et al.* 1989). This procedure can be carried out through an incision based over the medial aspect of the talo-navicular joint. If the fracture is very comminuted, an attempt can be made to reconstruct the articular surface of the bone and to hold this with multiple K-wires; the foot is then placed in a well-moulded cast for 6 weeks. In the long term, if articular degeneration supervenes local fusions are indicated, either of the talo-navicular or of the talo-navicular cuneiform joints. Persistent prominences, due to small fragments of bone, can be excised if they become troublesome.

Stress fractures of the navicular

Athletes may complain of pain in the medial arches of their feet during activity. Tenderness over the navicular and the above history differentiates stress fractures of the navicular from other over-use injuries of the foot (Hunter 1981). The diagnosis may be difficult because the radiographs may appear normal at first. A bone scan or repeat radiograph at 2 months will confirm the diagnosis (Hunter 1981, Torg *et al.* 1982). CT scans may also prove helpful (Fig. 25.45). A coned anteroposterior view of the navicular will usually show the fracture in the central portion of bone, but one must be aware of the normal variant, the bipartite navicular.

With a short history early treatment is essential. A below-knee cast for 4 to 6 weeks may suffice to allow healing in early cases. If, however, the patient's symptoms persist and the navicular develops an established non-union, then bone grafting and internal fixation, and immobilization, are required.

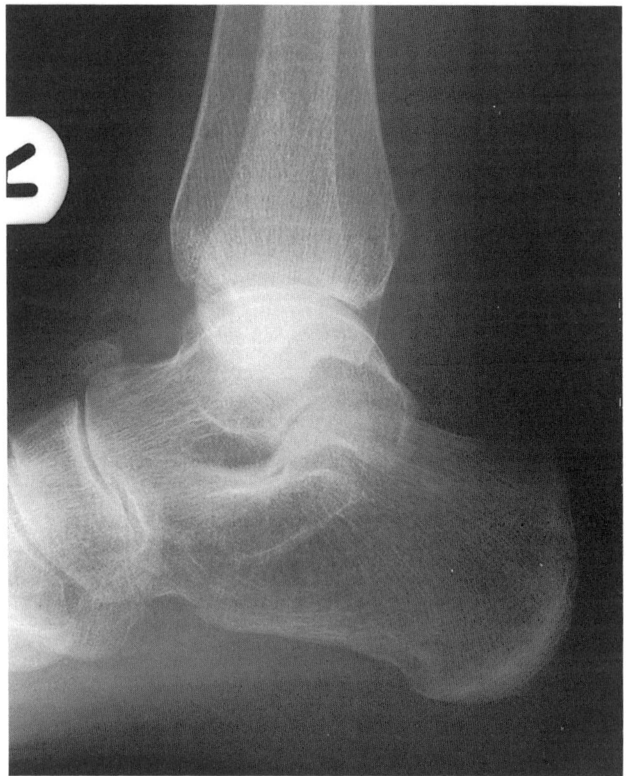

Fig. 25.43 Old avulsion injury of dorsal aspect of the navicular causing a persistent swelling that required excision.

below-knee cast. However, indirect injuries, such as a fall from a height with the foot in the plantarflexed position and the mid-tarsus adducted, can give rise to not only a fracture but also disruption of the navicular cuneiform ligaments; this can then lead to marked displacement and extrusion of the navicular. The navicular can be split by the head of the talus impacting it against the cuneiform bones. There is a definite risk of avascular necrosis of the navicular bone from this injury. If there is little displacement then non-operative treatment, as for direct injuries, is the treatment of choice, but fre-

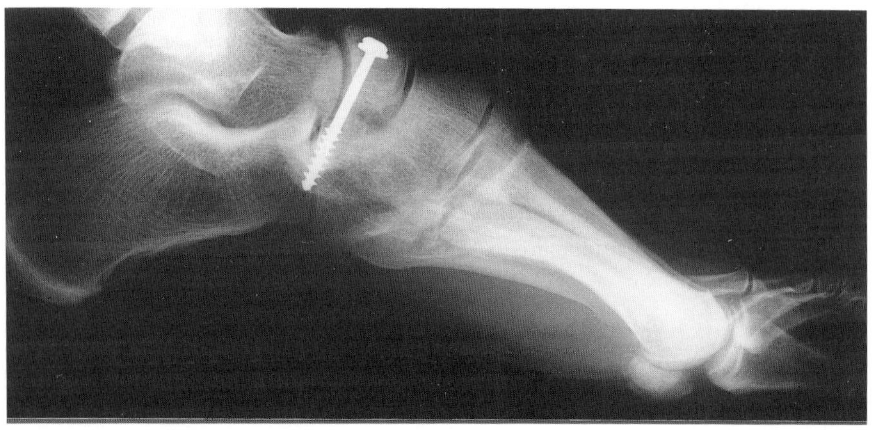

Fig. 25.44 Internal fixation and bone grafting of a comminuted navicular body fracture.

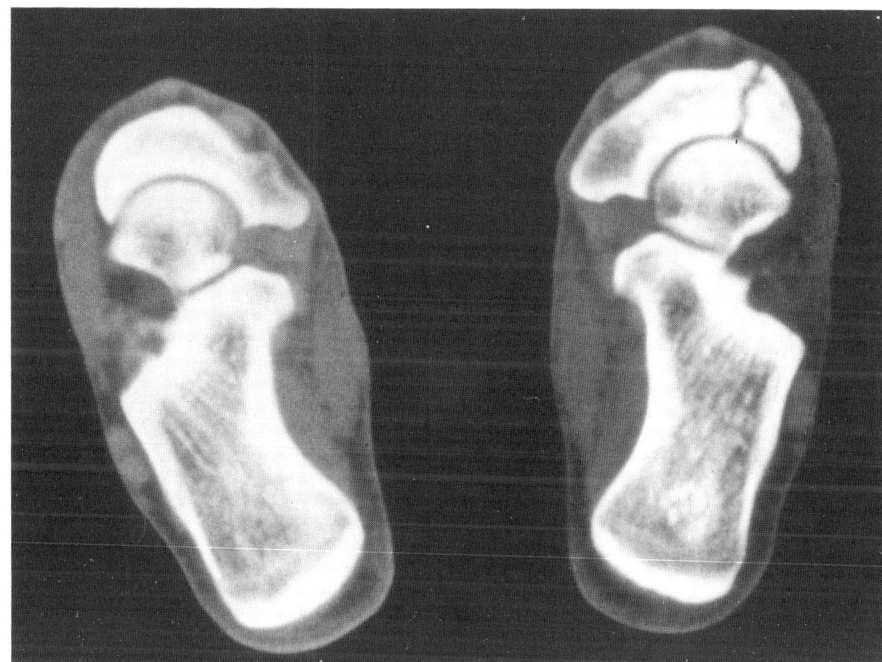

Fig. 25.45 Computerized tomogram of a stress fracture of the talar navicular in a soldier.

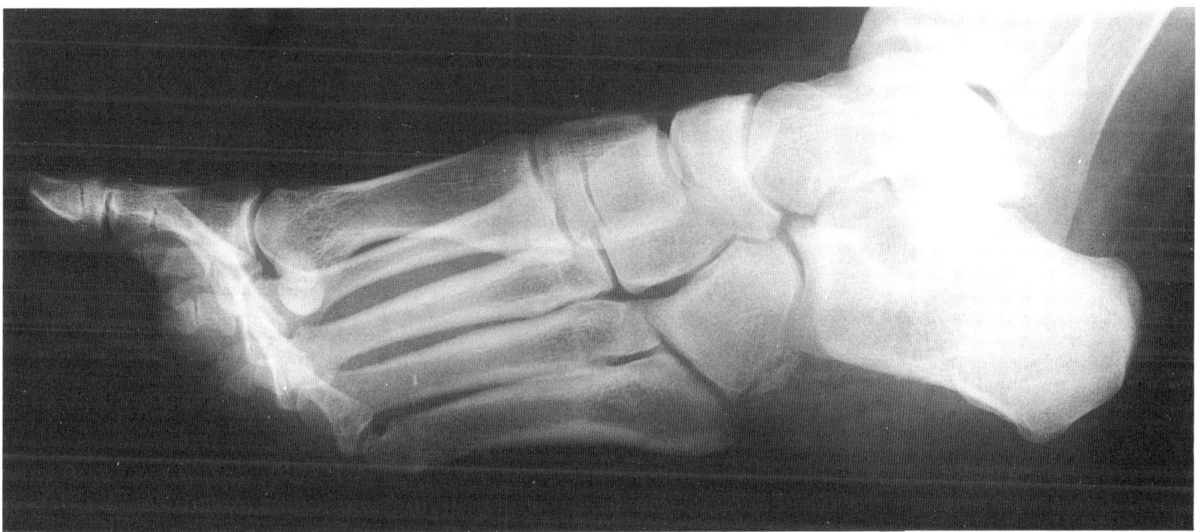

Fig. 25.46 Avulsion fracture of the cuboid.

Cuboid fractures

As is the case with navicular fractures, isolated cuboid fractures are rare because the cuboid is well protected and buttressed (McKeever 1950). However, isolated avulsion injuries can occur (Fig. 25.46), as can crush fractures (Fig. 25.47), fractures of the entire body or the nutcracker fracture (Hermal & Gershon-Cohen 1953). This last type occurs when there is an abduction of the mid-tarsus and the cuboid bone is crushed between the distal part of the calcaneum and the bases of the lateral two metatarsals. If a fracture is seen, the whole foot should be assessed for major damage as there may have been a tarsal disruption. Suspicion is raised if it is noted on radiographs that there is a concomitant navicular fracture. Avulsion injuries and minor fractures of the cuboid joint can be treated in a below-knee moulded cast for 4 to 6 weeks. Severely comminuted injuries with associated displacement are best treated by bone grafting and internal fixation prior to plaster immobilization to restore the length of the lateral border of the foot.

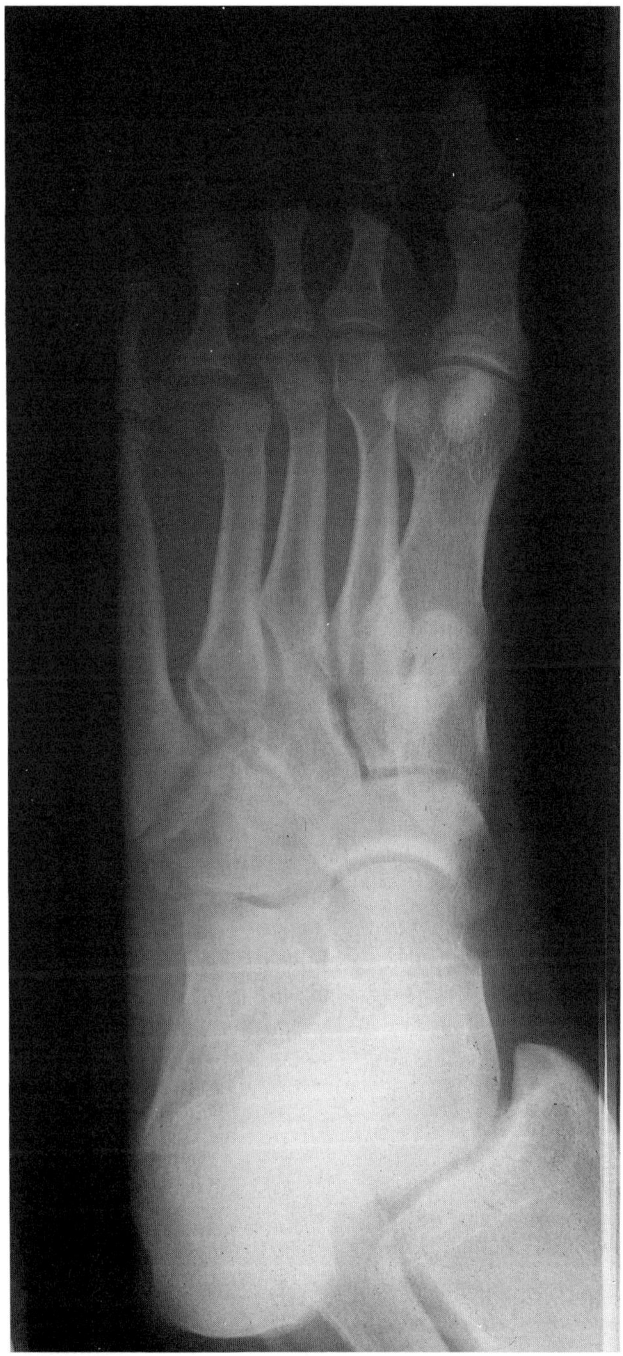

Fig. 25.47 Crush fracture of the cuboid joint in association with fractures of the bases of the metatarsals.

Cuneiform fractures

A direct blow to the foot is the usual cause for this quite rare isolated injury (Heckman 1991). The injuries are usually undisplaced and best treated in a cast for 4 to 6 weeks. If, however, radiographs show displacement then one should be aware of the possibility of severe tarsal disruption.

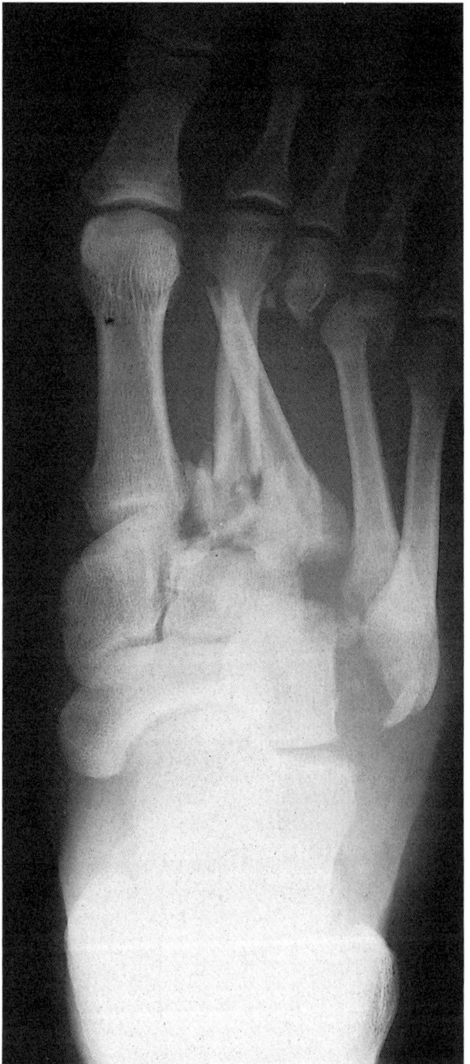

Fig. 25.48 Gross disruption of the tarsometatarsal joint with accompanying multiple metatarsal fractures.

Tarsometatarsal fracture–dislocations

Although Jacques Lisfranc's name has been permanently associated with dislocations and fracture–dislocations in the joints dividing the metatarsals from the cuneiform bones and cuboid (Hardcastle *et al.* 1982), his only association with this injury is that he was a Napoleonic surgeon who described an amputation through these joints for various forefoot war injuries. The injury itself is quite rare and decreasing in incidence (King 1987) since horseback riding has declined as a common means of transport. It frequently occurs following a fall from a horse where the foot is held firmly in the stirrup as the rider is dismounted, thus disrupting the foot at the tarsometatarsal level.

These injuries are often missed (20% in some series [Myerson 1989]), and very often they occur with other injuries (81%) and are given scant attention (Myerson *et al.* 1986). Clinical suspicion should be high if there is marked swelling and bruising around the midfoot (Arntz & Hansen 1987). Good-quality anteroposterior, lateral and oblique radiographs are essential. The diagnosis may be obvious (Fig. 25.48) but in doubtful cases one should look for incongruity in the line coming from the medial wall of the second metatarsal and the second cuneiform; this should be in continuity (Fig. 25.49) but is disrupted by this injury. In addition, increased gaping between the metatarsals is suspicious. Some authors advocate obtaining stress views with the patient under anaesthesia, while others have pointed out the 'fleck sign' (Fig. 25.50), which is positive if there is a flake of bone avulsed from the base of the second metatarsal while attached by strong interosseous ligaments to the medial cuneiform (Myerson *et al.* 1986). Ipsilateral ankle and other foot fractures are seen in 32% of cases (King 1987).

To understand the details of these injuries one has to remember some salient anatomical features (King 1987). First, the dorsal interosseous ligaments between the

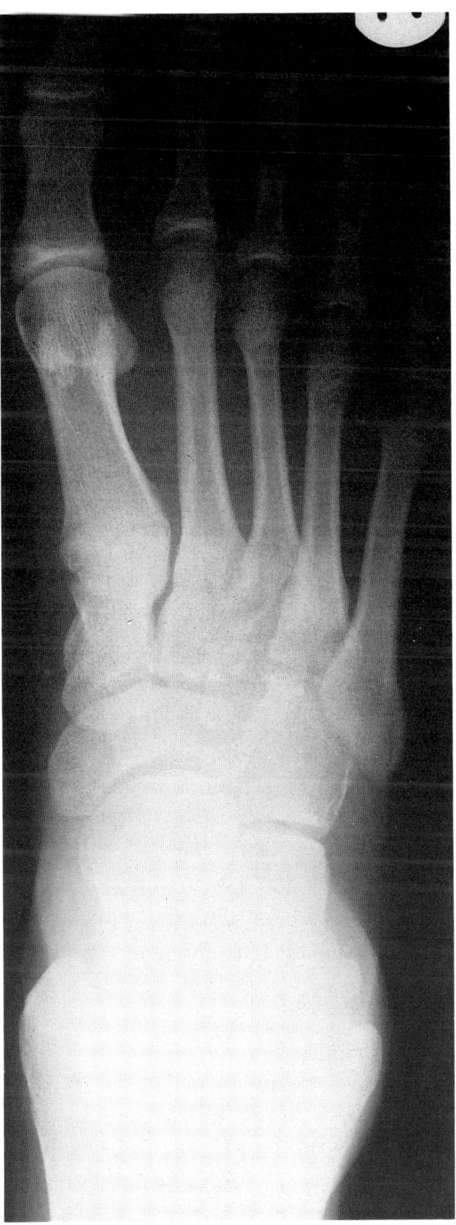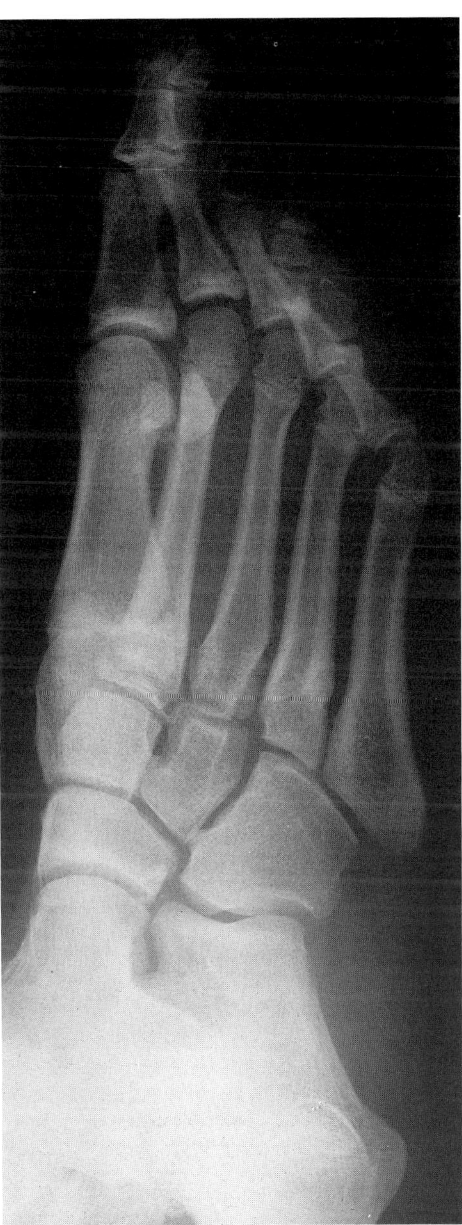

Fig. 25.49 Normal radiograph of the foot to show the clear continuity of the medial side of the second metatarsal on the middle cuneiform; this is lost subtly in Fig. 25.50 but obviously in Fig. 25.48.

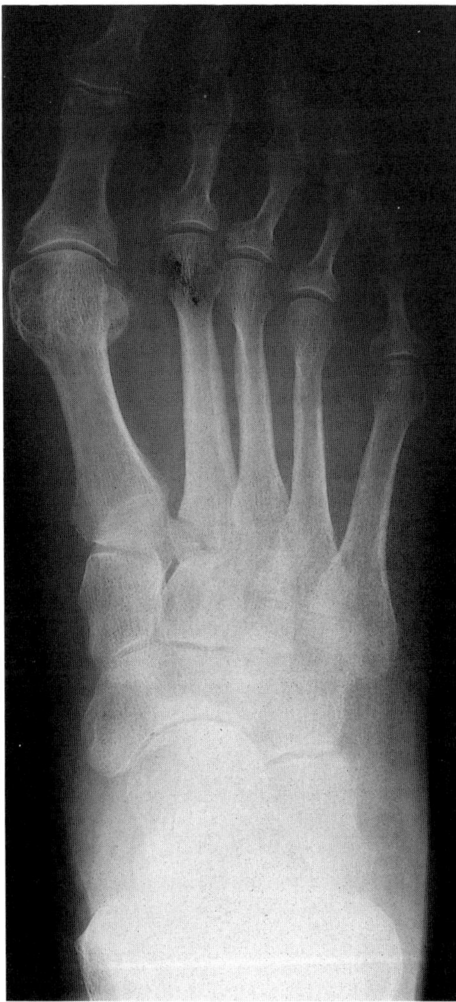

Fig. 25.50 The fleck sign or Lisfranc's fragment. Note the loss of continuity between the medial walls of the second metatarsal and the middle cuneiform.

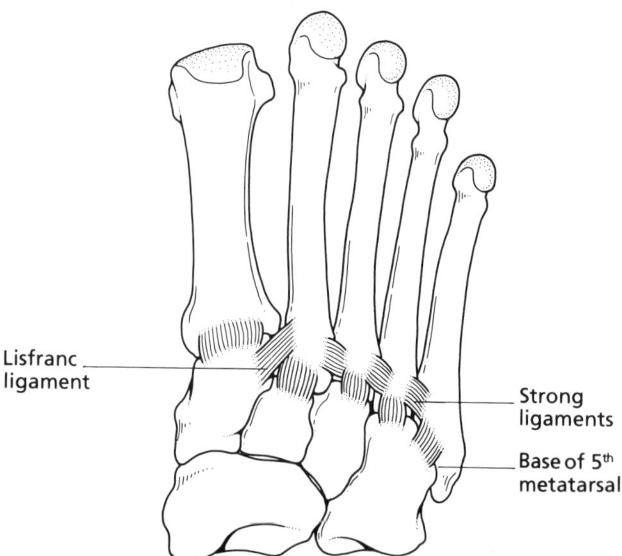

Fig. 25.51 Plantar view of right foot to show not only the strong ligaments at the base of the fifth metatarsal but also Lisfranc's ligament.

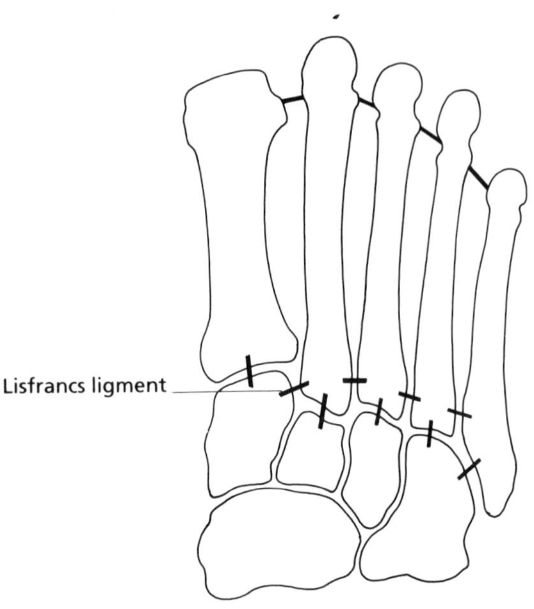

Fig. 25.52 Schematic drawing of the plantar ligaments to show the relationship of the metatarsal bases to these ligaments.

metatarsals are weak, while the plantar ligaments are strong. Each metatarsal base has a ligament linking it to its neighbour as well as the proximal bones, except the second which has an oblique strong plantar ligament (instead of the intermetatarsal ligament to the first metatarsal) attaching it to the medial cuneiform (Figs 25.51 & 25.52); known as Lisfranc's ligament this frequently remains intact during disruption and is responsible for the fleck sign. In general, the medial or first ray is more stable than the lateral rays (Myerson *et al.* 1986).

Second, the second ray is wedged in the apex of a 'Roman arch' as seen in the coronal plane with the other bones sloping away medially and laterally, giving an inherent stability to either side of the second ray (Fig. 25.53). Third, the base of the second metatarsal is like

a keystone in the groove between the medial and lateral cuneiforms and is the 'locking mechanism' of the tarsometatarsal joints (Fig. 25.51). Finally, there are secondary stabilizers, including the plantar fascia, the intrinsic muscles and the tendon attachments of the tibialis anterior and posterior, which have wide insertions in this region.

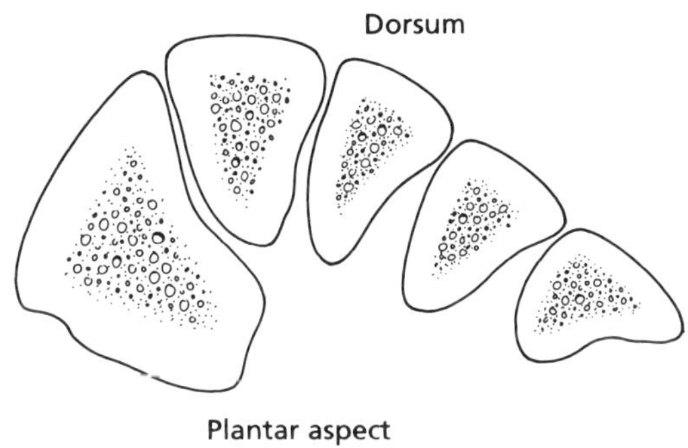

Fig. 25.53 The Roman arch arrangement of the metatarsal bases.

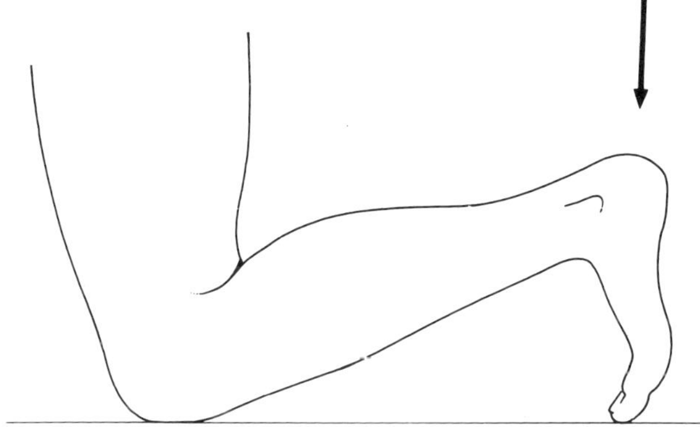

Mechanism of injury

Two basic mechanisms of injury are described. First, blows to the foot, such as a weight falling onto the heel, while the knee is flexed and the foot dorsiflexed (Fig. 25.54) cause acute plantarflexion of the joint and usually occur in industry (King 1987). The soft tissue damage may not be extensive and these injuries are rarely compound.

Second, direct blows, which occur in road traffic accidents when the foot strikes the floorboard during a head-on collision (Fig. 25.55) or a fall from a height when the patient lands in the ballerina position (Fig. 25.56), cause a compound injury with major soft tissue damage. The metatarsals are said to displace plantarwards in 57% of cases and dorsally in 43% (Myerson 1989).

Compartment syndromes may arise and should be looked for (Myerson 1987). There are four compartments in the foot: medial, lateral, central and the interossei (Fig. 25.57). The first contains the abductor hallucis and flexor hallucis brevis muscles as well as the tendons of flexor hallucis longus, peroneus longus and the tibialis posterior tendon. The central compartment contains the

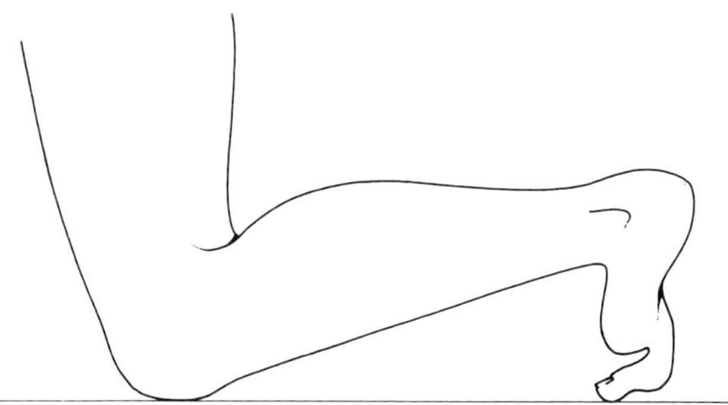

Fig. 25.54 'Industrial' mechanism for tarsometatarsal disruption. A heavy weight falls on the heel while the subject is in the kneeling position.

flexor digitorum brevis muscle, the flexor digitorum longus tendons and the lumbrical muscles as well as the quadratus plantar muscle, the adductor hallucis muscle and for part of their course the peroneus longus and the tibialis posterior tendons. The three intrinsic muscles of the small toe are bound down in the lateral compartment. The interossei form their own compartment between the metatarsals and can be considered a separate entity.

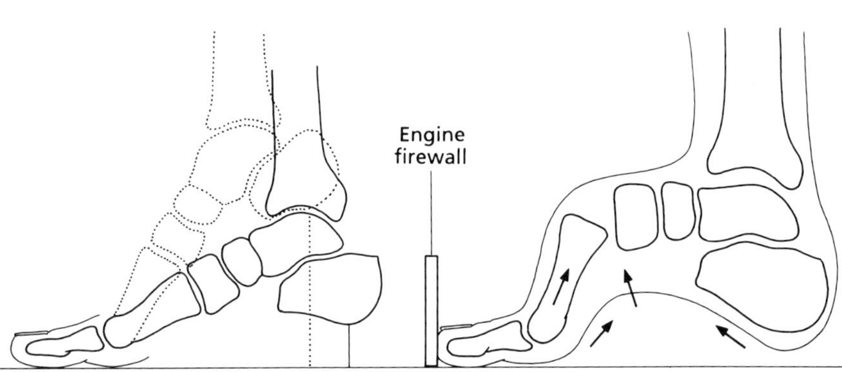

Fig. 25.55 Common mechanism of injury in road traffic accidents.

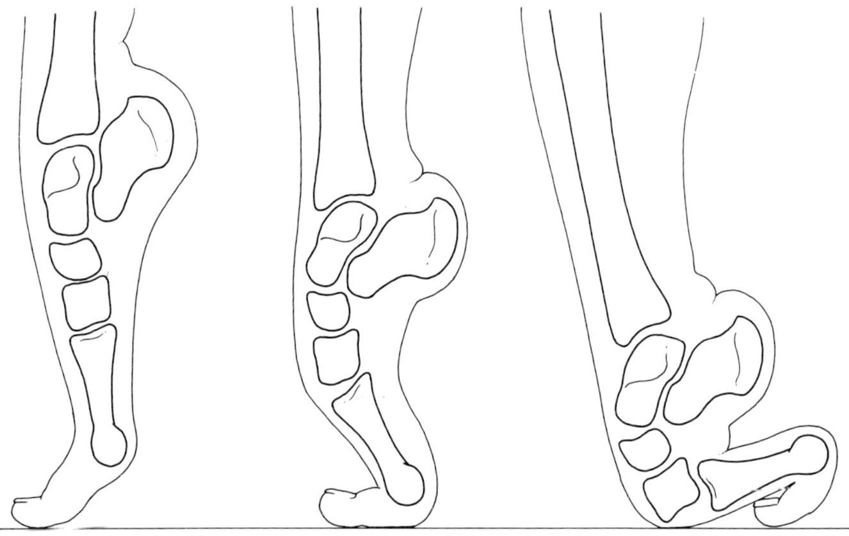

Fig. 25.56 Mechanism of injury when the patient falls from a height and lands on the ball of the foot.

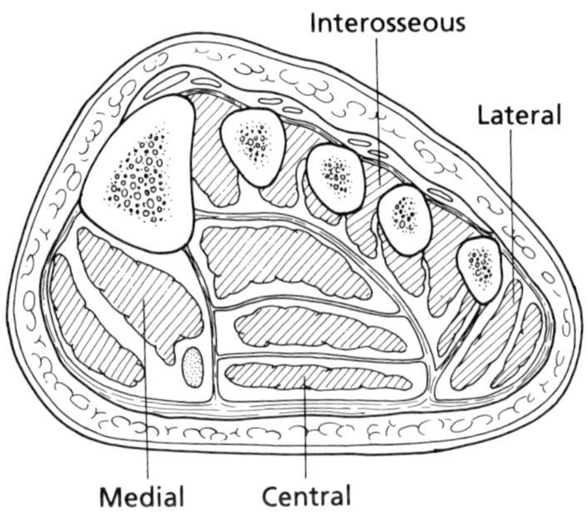

Fig. 25.57 Compartments of the foot.

With injuries to the midfoot, in particular those associated with crushing phenomena, the pressures within these compartments may be raised, just as occurs in the lower leg and forearm. The pressure can be measured with a slit catheter and a measuring device such as the quick pressure monitoring set (Stryker). For those who do not have this type of equipment, diagnosis must be suspected if the patient has a disproportionate amount of pain, complains of hypoaesthesia in the toes or, more suspiciously, has severe pain on passive extension of the toes, similar to the excruciating pain experienced by patients on this manoeuvre when testing for compartment syndromes in the lower leg or forearm (Myerson 1988).

Once the diagnosis is suspected, all four compartments need to be decompressed as an emergency. If

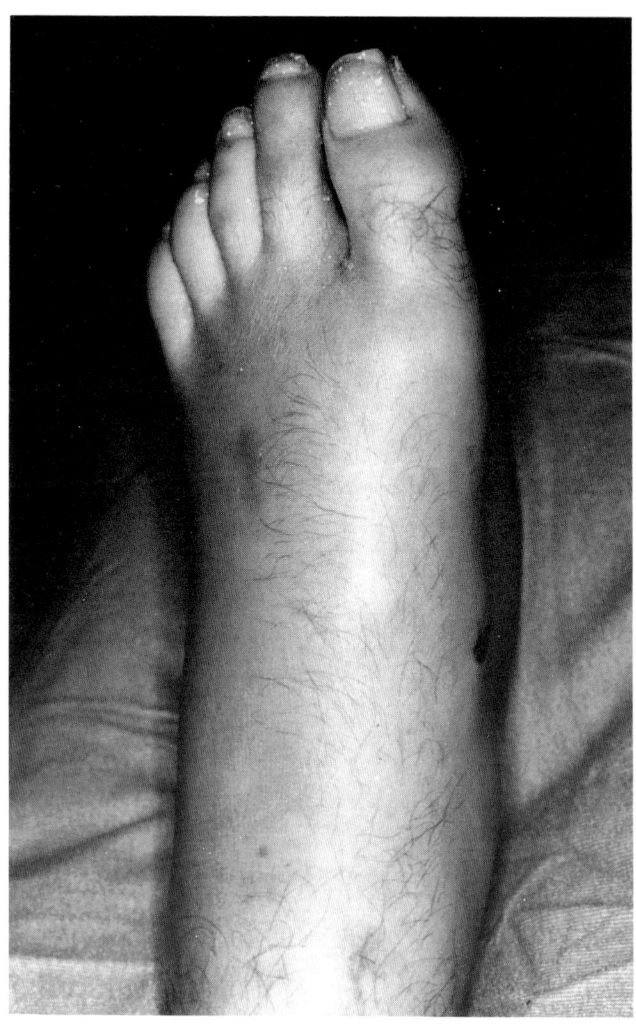

Fig. 25.58 Pallor of the toes in a patient with compartment syndrome secondary to a Lisfranc fracture dislocation.

this is not carried out then the muscles will become ischaemic, fibrosis will develop and a Volkmann-like contracture with clawing of the toes will subsequently arise. Worse still, venous obstruction can occur or arterial flow can be interrupted, leading to severe compromise of the distal circulation (Fig. 25.58). Myerson (1988) advocates two possible approaches. One involves a decompression carried through a medial plantar incision. This would allow full decompression of all four compartments but is really reserved for those surgeons familiar with the anatomy. More simply, decompression of all four compartments can be made through two separate incisions, one based over the shaft of the second metatarsal and the other over the shaft of the fourth metatarsal. Through these incisions dissection is continued through the interosseous spaces, thereby decompressing these compartments; then the medial and central compartments can be easily decompressed, as can the lateral compartment, by extending the dissection in the plantar direction. The other

added advantage of the dorsal approach is that if there is a Lisfranc's dislocation and/or multiple metatarsal fractures these can be fixed through the same incisions. Having performed the decompression and removed any non-viable tissue, the wounds should be left open for subsequent inspection at 24–48 hours and skin grafting as necessary.

Classification

Many classifications have been documented but that by Myerson *et al*. (1986), by expanding the best features of other descriptions, gives a worthwhile contribution as one can plan treatment accordingly.

Type A — Total incongruity. The whole of the metatarsal-tarsal joint is disrupted and is displaced in either the lateral (Fig. 25.48), dorsal or plantar direction.

Type B — Partial incongruity (Fig. 25.59). The joint is 'split' with shift of either the medial column (first ray) or lateral rays using the base of the second metatarsal as the reference point.

Type C — Divergent. Both columns are disrupted and displaced medially and laterally to a greater or lesser extent.

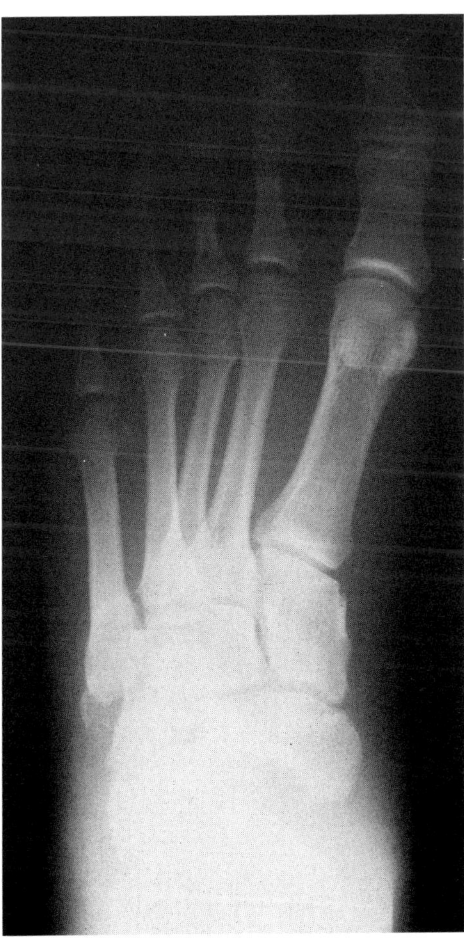

Fig. 25.59 Disruption of Lisfranc's joint with partial incongruity and lateral shift.

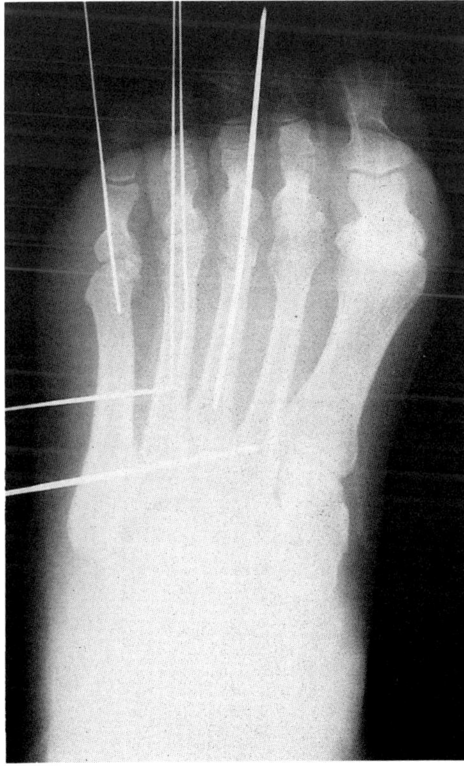

Fig. 25.60 Case as shown in Fig. 25.59 after open reduction and fixation with multiple Kirschner wires. Note also the fixation of the metatarsal neck fractures by the 'Sisk' technique.

Conservative treatment has only a small role in management (Myerson 1989). If reduction cannot be achieved by closed means with the aid of Chinese finger straps pulling down on the toes with the patient in the prone position (King 1987), then open reduction and internal fixation is necessary (Arntz & Hansen 1987, Myerson 1988). The aim is to achieve a stable anatomical reduction. Fixing the first and fifth metatarsals is inadequate as the central column also needs stabilization (Fig. 25.60). Small fragments of loose bone which cannot be reduced and fixed should be removed. Fixation of all rays may be necessary, depending on the degree of stability (Myerson 1989). Dorsal incisions are advocated and should be centred over the second and fourth rays; this also allows full decompression of the compartments of the foot.

Once reduction and fixation has been achieved,

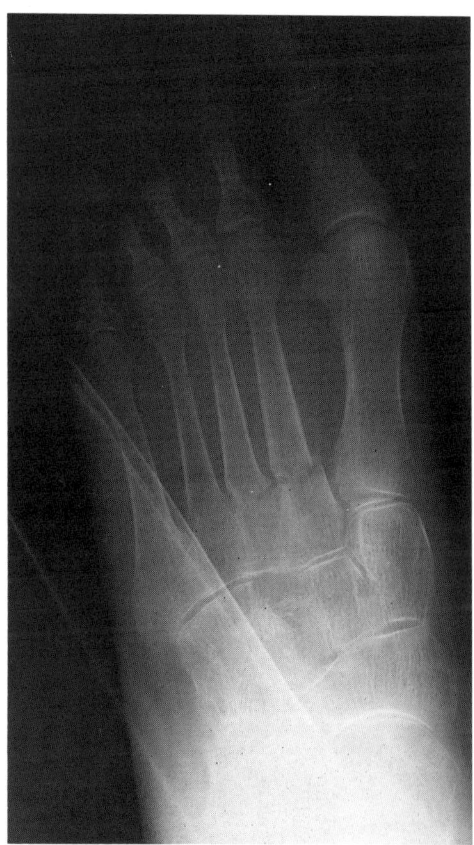

Fig. 25.62 Fracture of the second, third and fourth metatarsals as the result of a heavy object falling on the foot.

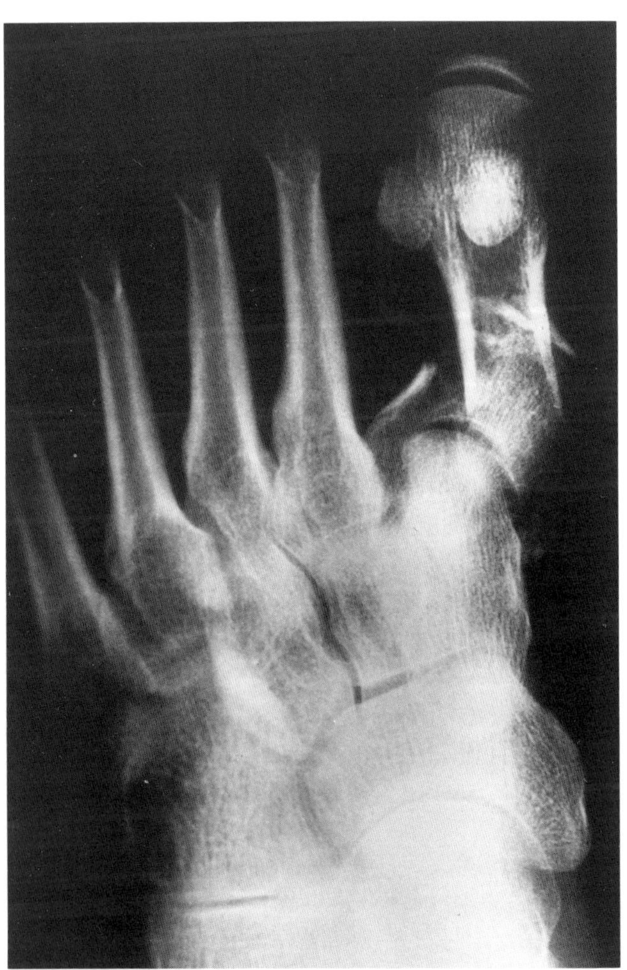

Fig. 25.61 Comminuted fracture of the base of the first metatarsal involving Lisfrancs joint carrying a potentially worse prognosis.

immobilization in a below-knee cast is necessary for 6 weeks but the wound should be inspected regularly as the percutaneous wires can cause local skin problems. Some authors advocate the use of AO screws to fix such a fracture because they feel that K-wires give inadequate hold on the fragments (Arntz & Hansen 1987). Redislocation has been described (Hardcastle *et al.* 1982) and the use of AO techniques prevents redisplacement or recurrent subluxation (Arntz & Hansen 1987); despite a short follow-up there is early evidence that post-traumatic arthritis is less frequent.

Vascular injuries are said to be rare (King 1987) but secondary degeneration is seen, especially if small fragments are retained or a poor reduction is accepted (Myerson *et al.* 1986). Closed reduction may be prevented by a displaced tibialis anterior tendon. The incidence of Sudek's atrophy can be high (25%) (Gossens & DeStoop 1983) and non-union of the metatarsals has been described. The incidence of problems due to secondary osteoarthritis is a cause for debate. Some authors (Arntz & Hansen 1987) feel that significant symptoms can be prevented if the patient is left with the plantar-grade stable foot that has been fixed by rigid internal fixation after an anatomical reduction has been achieved. Others suggest that the problems associated with post-traumatic osteoarthrosis in this area are exaggerated and problems arise only when the first ray is significantly involved (Brunet & Wiley 1987). Symptoms often decrease for some months after the operation and then tend to stabilize at about 12 months. Poor radiological results do not always match the clinical symptoms. However, if there is severe pain then mid-tarsal arthro-deses are the only salvage procedure.

Metatarsal fractures

Both single and multiple fractures of the metatarsal bone are commonly seen. The fifth metatarsal is most frequently injured. The metatarsals are bound both distally and proximally by strong interosseous ligaments, in addition to strong muscles attached around the interosseous spaces. Fractures are therefore usually undisplaced, unless there has been severe trauma and major soft tissue disruption. Fractures can occur at the neck, where the strong pull of the long flexors tends to displace the head plantarwards (Lindholm 1961) and proximally. Shaft fractures and basal fractures can also occur.

Fractures of the second, third and fourth metatarsals are usually the result of a direct blow (Fig. 25.62), whereas isolated fifth metatarsal fractures can occur following twisting injuries. Metatarsal head fractures are usually the result of crush injuries. The injuries are frequently seen in multiply injured patients and once suspected clinically are diagnosed by obtaining appropriate anteroposterior, lateral and oblique radiographs. Special attention should be paid to the soft tissues. The dorsalis pedis artery is disrupted only rarely.

Classification

Metatarsal fractures may be classified as follows:
1 Metatarsal neck fractures.
2 Metatarsal base fractures.
3 Metatarsal shaft fractures.
4 Fracture of the fifth metatarsal base.

Metatarsal neck fractures

Special sesamoid views (Fig. 25.63) are useful for checking the degree of plantar displacement of these fractures. If this is marked, then reduction under general anaesthesia with Chinese finger straps on the toes fol-

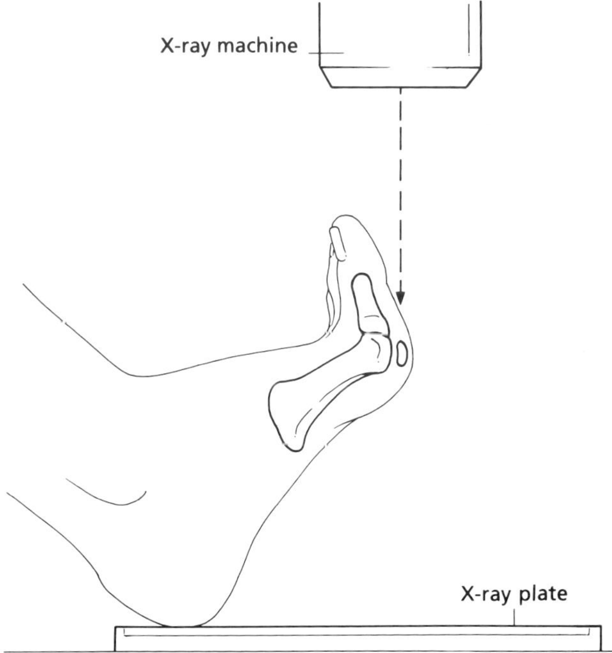

Fig. 25.63 Technique for performing sesamoid views to look not only at these ossicles but also metatarsal neck fractures.

lowed by Kirschner wire fixation may be attempted but usually open reduction is necessary (Sisk 1987) (Figs 25.64 & 25.65). The wires are taken out after 3 weeks and treatment completed in a cast for another 3 weeks.

Metatarsal base fractures

Metatarsal base fractures may result in dorso-plantar malalignment and malunion with subsequent callosity formation or incongruity of the metatarso-tarsal joint (De Lee 1986) (Fig. 25.66). To prevent this, reduction and wire fixation, as for metatarsal neck fractures, is indicated if significant displacement is present.

Metatarsal shaft fractures

It has been stressed in the literature that early weight-bearing with these injuries is essential to achieve union and a good functional result (De Lee 1986). Undisplaced fractures of the shafts of the lateral four metatarsals are best treated in compression bandages or below-knee walking casts for 4 to 6 weeks (Figs 25.67 & 25.68). Patients with isolated fractures of the first metatarsal may require a period of weight relief before being permitted to walk in the plaster for 4 to 6 weeks.

Displaced injuries may require internal fixation (Figs 25.69 & 25.70). This applies to the first metatarsal

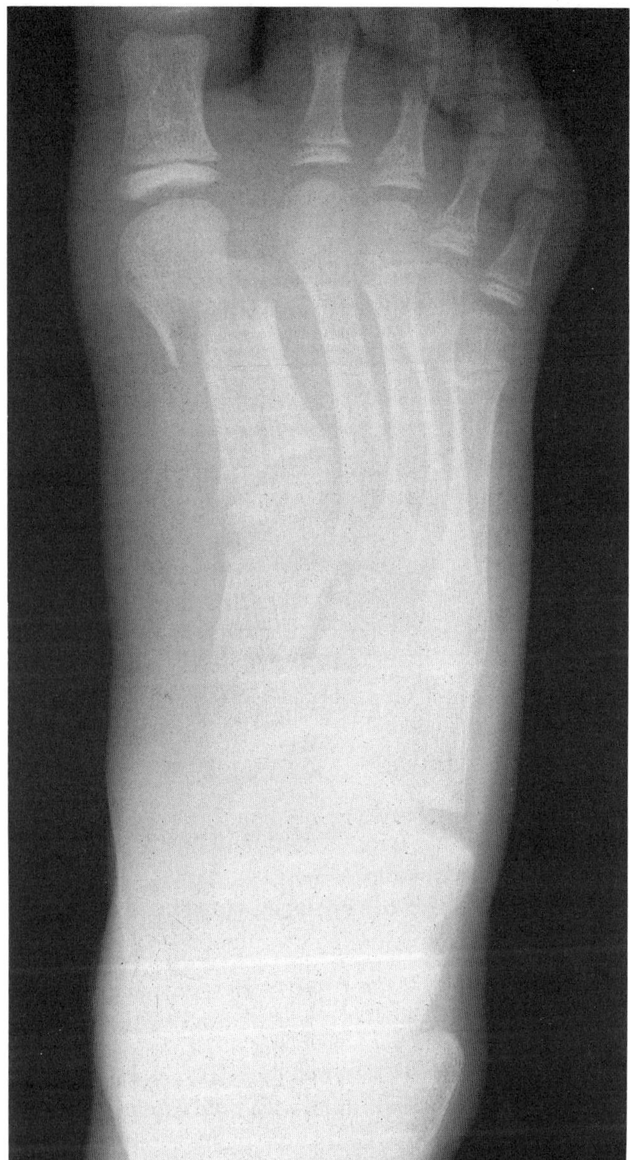

Fig. 25.64 Fracture of the neck of the first metatarsal in a child.

Fig. 25.65 Adequate reduction and fixation with Kirschner wire.

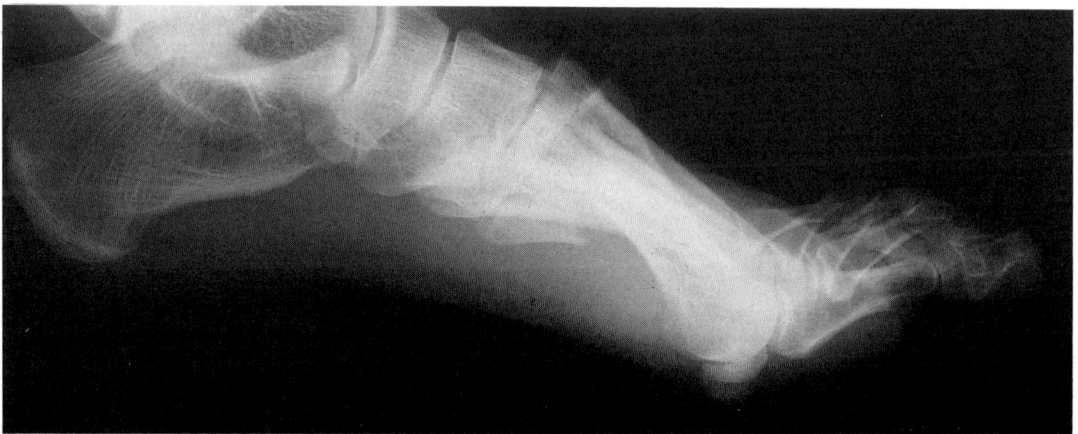

Fig. 25.66 Intra-articular fracture of the base of the first metatarsal with significant displacement.

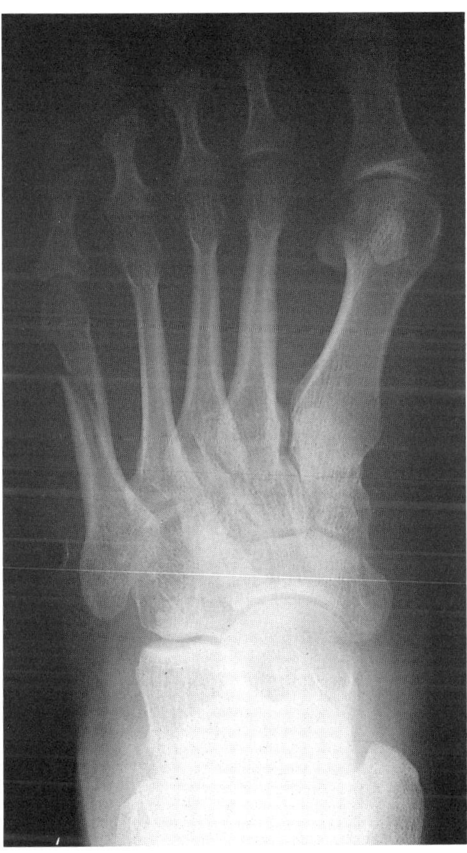

Fig. 25.67 Displaced fracture shaft of the fifth metatarsal displaced.

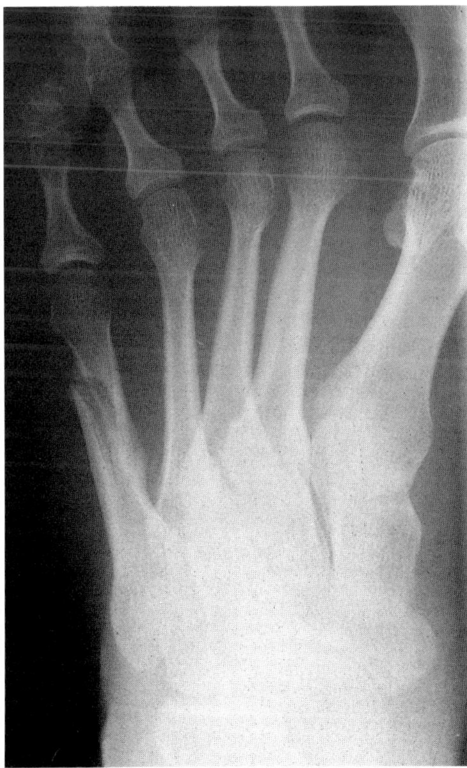

Fig. 25.68 Fracture as in Fig. 25.67 with union after conservative treatment.

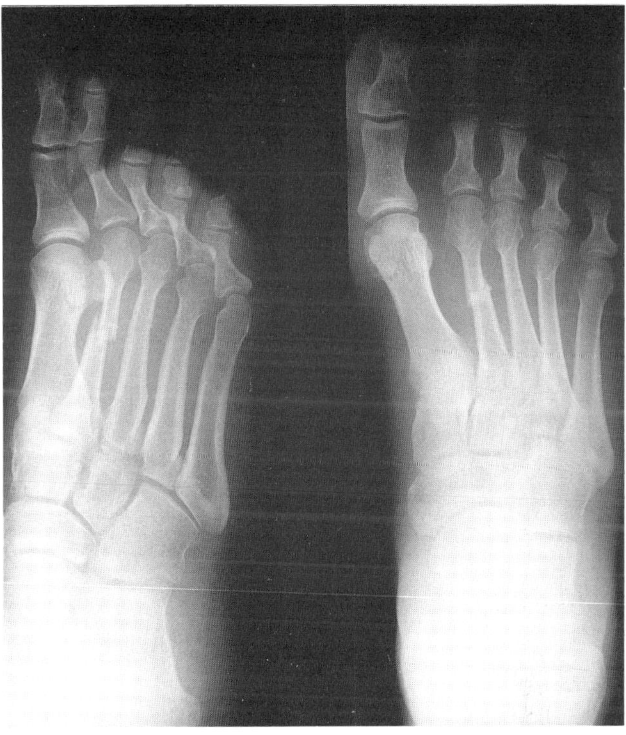

Fig. 25.69 Displaced fracture of the shaft of the 2nd metatarsal with an undisplaced fracture of the 3rd metatarsal.

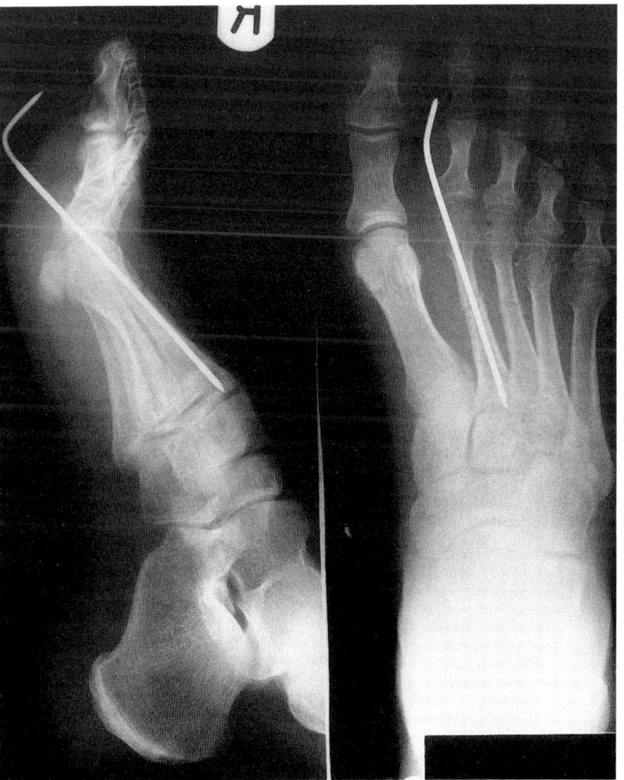

Fig. 25.70 Same case as Fig. 25.69 showing open reduction and internal fixation of the 2nd metatarsal fracture.

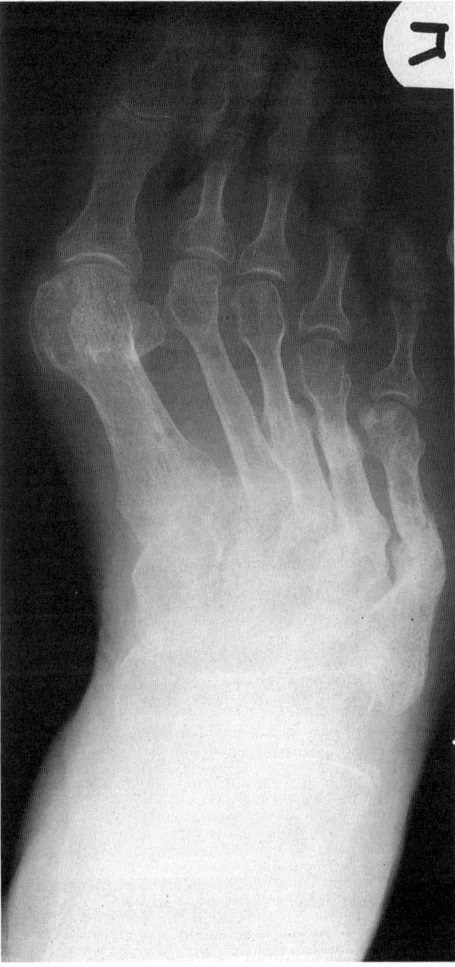

Fig. 25.71 Multiple metatarsal fractures which were neglected and led to malunion and foot adduction deformity.

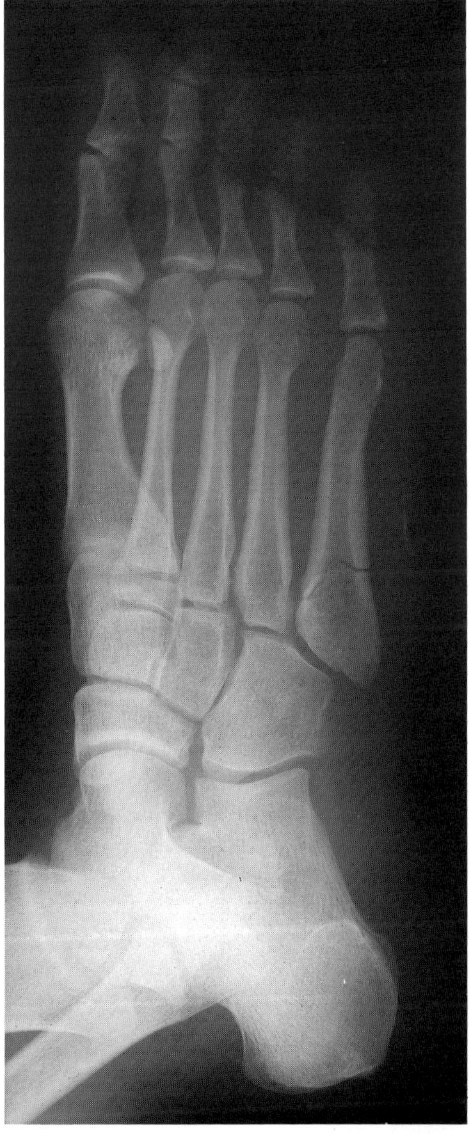

Fig. 25.72 Undisplaced fracture of the base of the fifth metatarsal at the metaphyseal—diaphyseal junction.

in particular. Prevention of relative 'lengthening' of the second metatarsal shaft is important to avoid subsequent metatarsalgia. The fixation is less critical in the other metatarsals unless the fractures are multiple (Fig. 25.71). Elevation for a few days before operation will reduce any swelling. The wires are usually removed after 2 weeks and then a weight-bearing cast is applied for 4 more weeks.

Fractures of the base of the fifth metatarsal

This is the commonest metatarsal fracture and ever since Robert Jones's article in the early part of the twentieth century (Jones 1902), confusion as to the classification has existed. He described a transverse fracture and not an avulsion fracture. De Lee's (1986) classification is the simplest and most appropriate.

Type I — Acute metaphyseal—diaphyseal fracture (traumatic), either undisplaced (Fig. 25.72) or displaced (Fig. 25.73)

Type II — Fracture at the metaphyseal—diaphyseal junction with clinical or radiological evidence of previous injury (Fig. 25.74).

Type III — Fracture of the styloid process of the fifth metatarsal, either extra-articular (Fig. 25.75) or intra-articular (Fig. 25.76).

Type II injuries are a form of stress fracture and are often seen in athletes; they may go on to non-union. They have been frequently recorded in basketball players (Kavanaugh *et al.* 1978). The base of the fifth metatarsal not only has an articulation with the cuboid

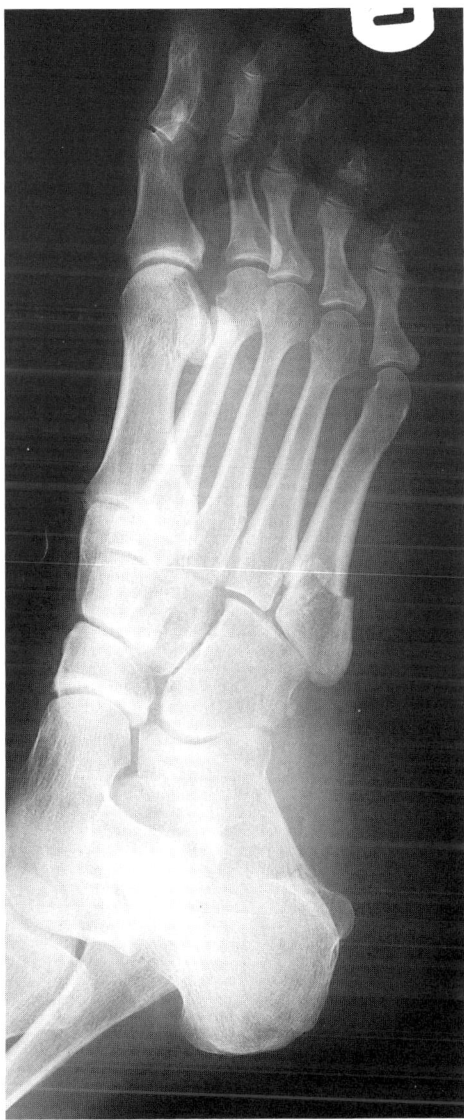

Fig. 25.73 Acute displaced fracture at the base of the fifth metatarsal at the diaphyseal–metaphyseal junction.

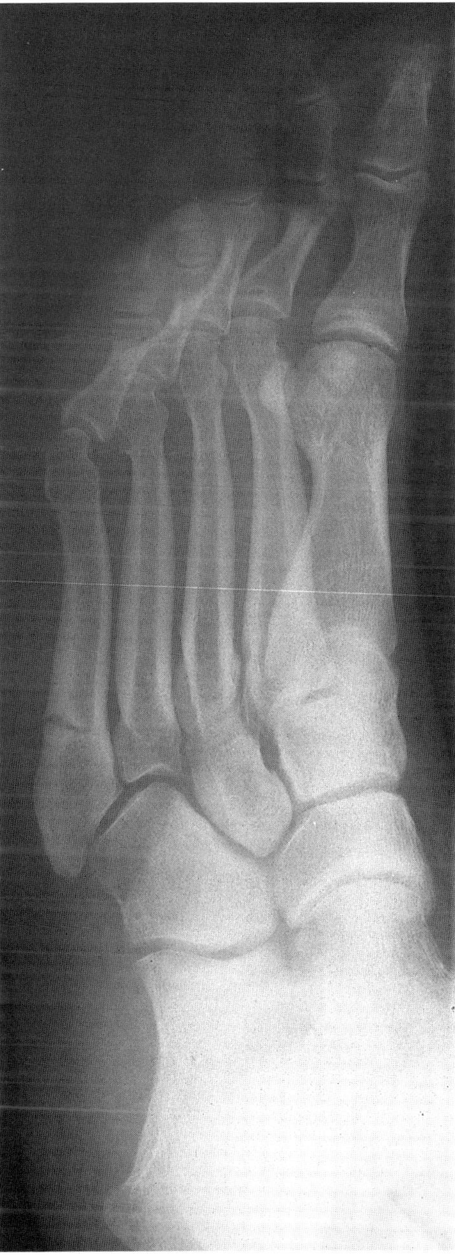

Fig. 25.74 Middle-aged patient presenting with pain on the lateral border of the foot with a sudden increase in severity. Type II metatarsal base fracture.

but also medially with the base of the fourth metatarsal. The peroneus brevis tendon can cause a simple avulsion fracture of the tip of the styloid process (Fig. 25.77) but because of strong intra-articular ligaments (Fig. 25.51) the force can be transmitted to the metaphyseal–diaphyseal junction and a transverse avulsion fracture may occur. Forced inversion during stance can cause these avulsion injuries (Heckman 1991). Some individuals have a more prominent styloid process (Dameron 1975) and as a result are more vulnerable to fracture of the base of the fifth metatarsal by direct trauma.

Standard anteroposterior and oblique radiographs will confirm the diagnosis. One must be aware of the anatomy of the apophysis at the proximal end of the fifth metatarsal. This centre of ossification appears after the age of 8 in about 20% of children and fuses at 12 years in girls and 15 years in boys (Dameron 1975). Characteristically, separation can occur but is parallel to the shaft of the bone and is extra-articular throughout, thereby distinguishing it from fractures. In addition, two accessory ossicles in this area can mislead the unwary (Dameron 1975). One is the os peroneum (Fig. 25.78), which is a sesamoid bone within peroneus longus

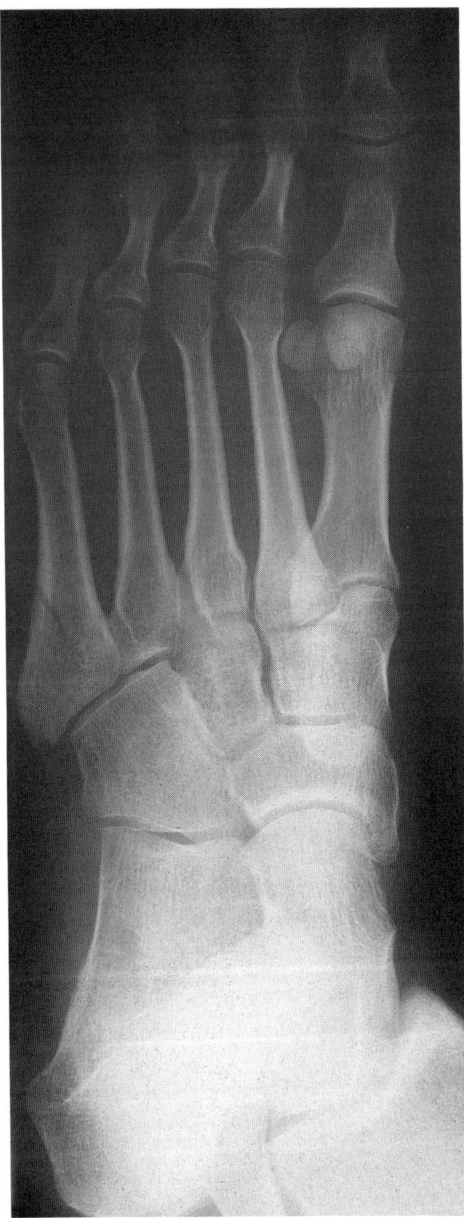

Fig. 25.75 Extra-articular fracture of the styloid process of the fifth metatarsal.

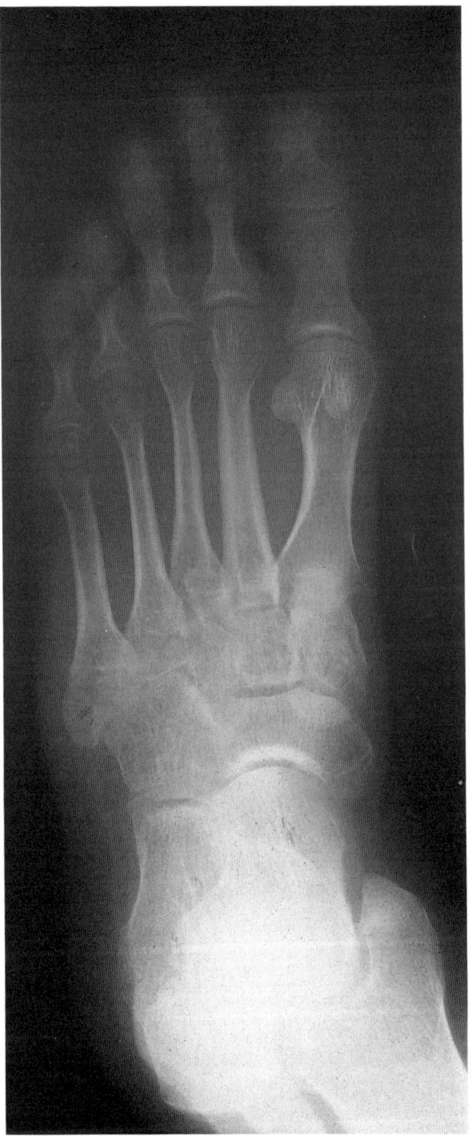

Fig. 25.76 Intra-articular avulsion fracture of the base of the fifth metatarsal.

found in 15% of people. The other, much less frequently seen, is the os vesalianum within peroneus brevis in one in 1000 people. It is smaller than the former and found more distally and usually bilaterally.

TREATMENT OF ACUTE FRACTURES IN THE BASE OF THE FIFTH METATARSAL

It is imperative to check by history and radiological examination that the injury is acute and not a stress fracture (De Lee 1986). Undisplaced type I fractures simply require 6 weeks weight-bearing in a below-knee cast. However, union may sometimes be delayed. Displaced type I injuries in very active patients should be fixed internally with an AO screw. Type III injuries are treated along similar lines, except that the period of immobilization is usually only 4 weeks and in active individuals the intra-articular type may require internal fixation. Non-union is rare and if it does occur excision of the fragment and reinsertion of peroneus brevis will suffice. Recognized stress fractures of the fifth metatarsal in athletes require open reduction and grafting and compression using an AO screw (Kavanaugh *et al.* 1978).

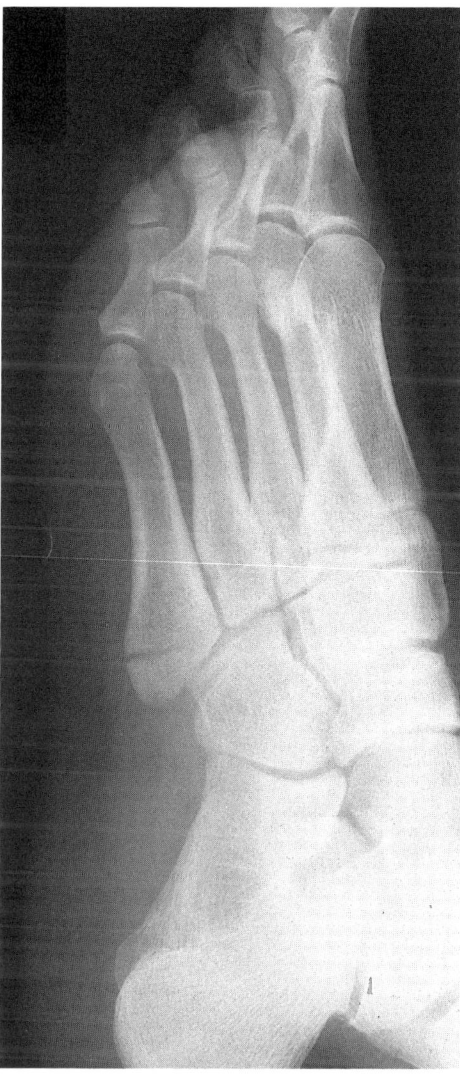

Fig. 25.77 Avulsion of the styloid process of the fifth metatarsal due to 'over pull' of the peroneum brevis.

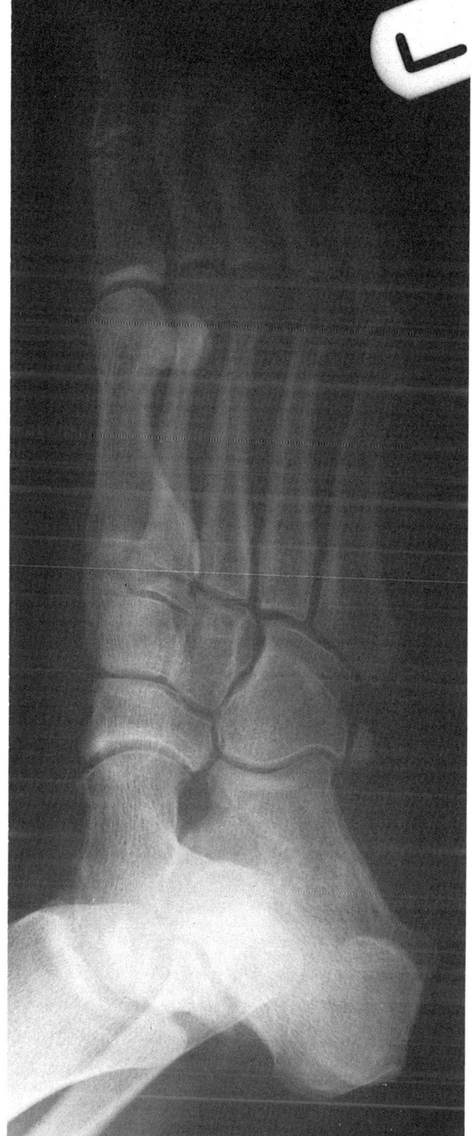

Fig. 25.78 Os peroneum.

Stress fractures of the metatarsals

All fatigue fractures are caused by abnormal stress in healthy bone; this leads to micro-fractures which, if allowed to rest, will heal. However, if activity continues a complete fracture will develop. The metatarsals are the commonest site for stress fractures and the second meta-tarsal is most frequently affected (Figs 25.79 & 25.80). Certain features are said to predispose patients to these problems. These include an excessively short first metatarsal (Wilson & Katz 1969), previous Keller's arthroplasty of the first metatarso-phalangeal joint and unaccustomed exercise, as experienced by new military recruits (Bernstern & Stone 1944). Certainly, the increase in athletic activities of the general population has led to a rise in the incidence.

The clinical diagnosis is easy. There is increasing pain on walking; this forces the patient to do less and less as a limp develops. The foot is swollen and tender over the fracture site. The pain can be reproduced by pressure on the affected metatarsal. At first the radio-graphs are normal but after a 2-week period there may be a faint line or periosteal reaction, followed by the obvious lesion at 21 days. Bone scans are positive from a very early stage.

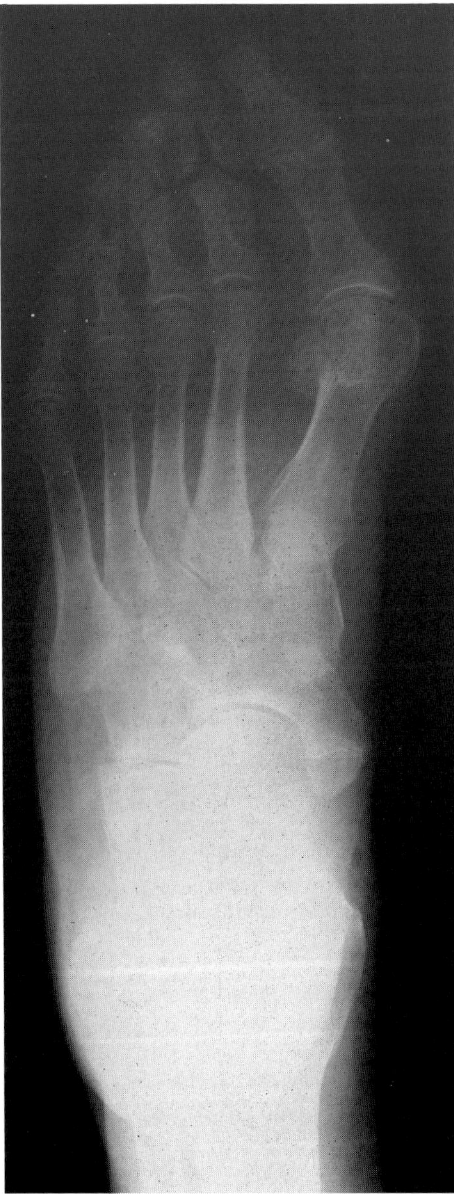 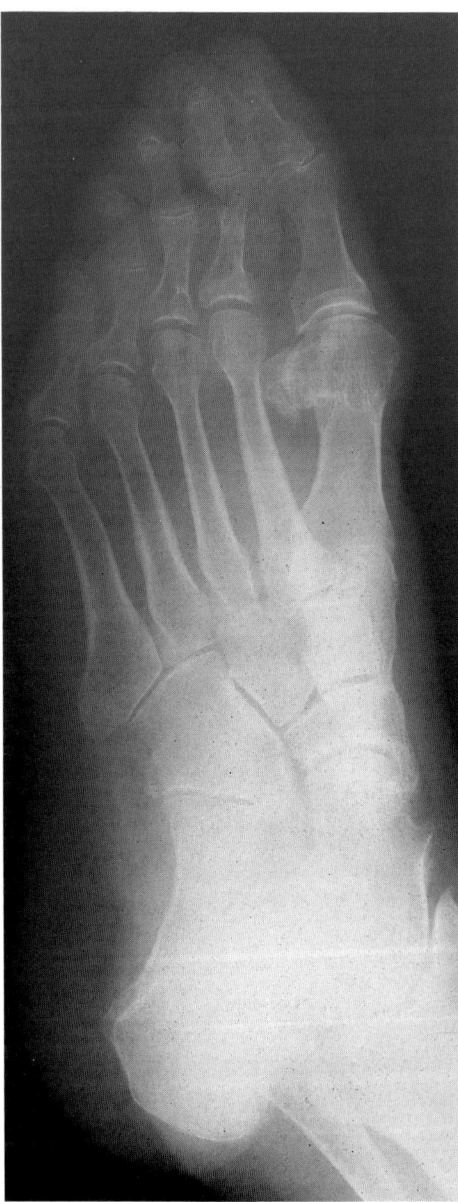

Fig. 25.79 This middle-aged patient presented with pain in the forefoot but a normal radiograph at first.

Treatment may need to be protracted, although there is often pressure from the patient to return to full sporting activity as soon as possible. If the symptoms are not severe and the fracture is recent, then rest with supportive strapping is all that is required. If, however, the symptoms are more severe a cast may be necessary. Recurrent fractures suggest that the metabolic status of the patient may require investigation as the patient may have diabetic neuropathy.

Metatarsal-phalangeal joint dislocations and toe dislocations

Dislocation of the first metatarsal-phalangeal joint

Of all the dislocations of the metatarsal-phalangeal joints, dislocation of the first is the most common (De Lee 1986). It is not unlike the equivalent injury in the hand in that it may not be reducible by closed means. Such dislocations usually result from hyperextension injuries in road traffic accidents or during sport (Clanton et al. 1986). They are usually dorsal dislocations with the

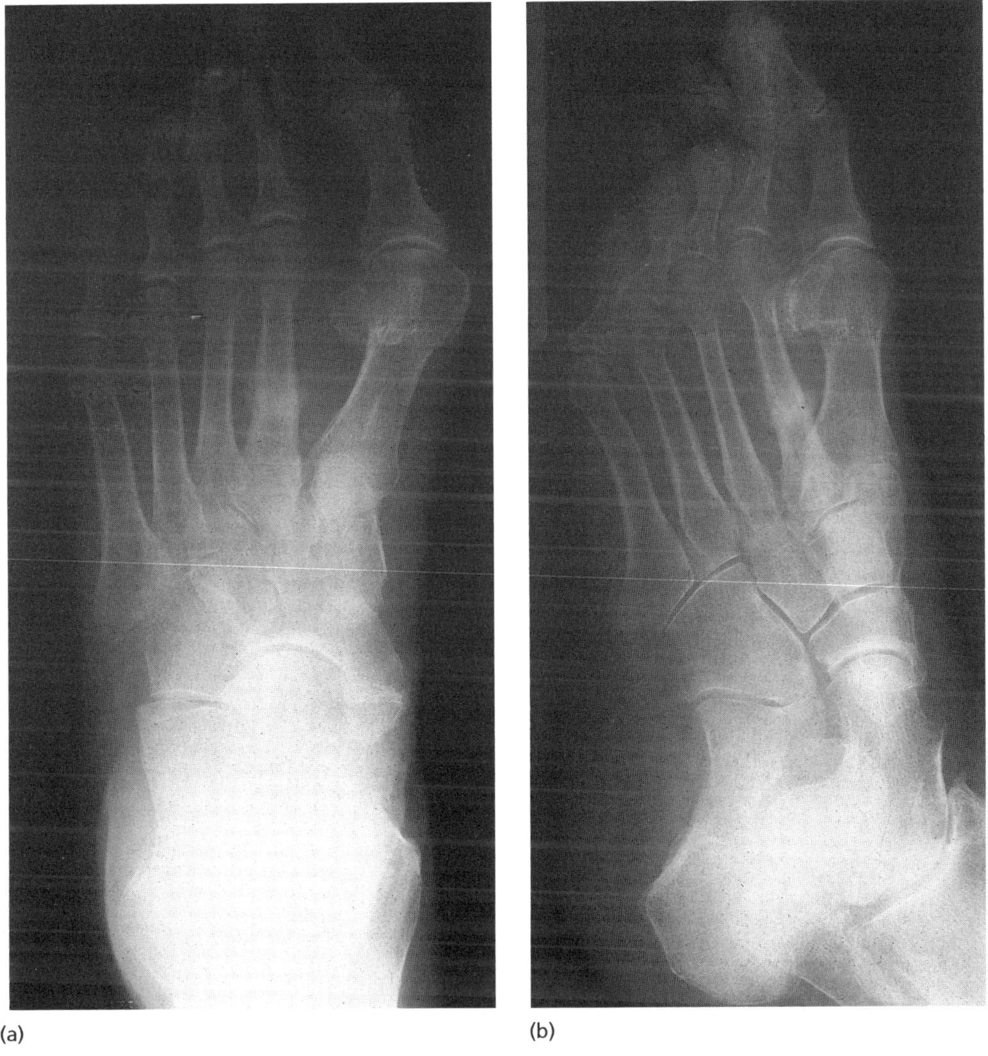

(a)   (b)

Fig. 25.80 One month later there is obvious callus formation in the proximal second metatarsal.

proximal phalanx coming to lie over the dorsal aspect of the head of the first metatarsal shaft with the two sesamoid bones and the plantar ligament which joins them. This is a type I injury (Fig. 25.81). With a type II injury there is a concomitant longitudinal fracture of a sesamoid bone or a rupture of the intersesamoid ligament, which causes wide separation of the sesamoid bones (Fig. 25.82). In the type I injury the intersesamoid ligament acts as a band preventing closed reduction, and open exploration is necessary. In the type II injury this obstruction to reduction is not present and closed reduction may be possible.

Patients present with a hyperextended great toe with a medial dimple and a prominent metatarsal head on the plantar surface. Radiographs confirm the diagnosis but should be scrutinized carefully for either a fracture of the sesamoid or separation of the sesamoids, which

indicates a type II injury. One attempt at reduction under local anaesthetic should be made and repeated under general anaesthetic if not successful (De Lee 1986). If reduced closed, a below-knee cast is applied with the toe held in slight plantarflexion. If open reduction is necessary this should be carried out using a tourniquet through a dorsal longitudinal incision centred over the first interspace. This approach is preferred because the distorted plantar neurovascular bundle can be avoided (Heckman 1991). The joint is opened longitudinally and with the aid of McDonald's dissector the phalanx can be levered into its correct position. However, occasionally, release of the adductor hallucis and the transverse metatarsal ligament may be necessary to allow a full reduction. The joint should be washed out and any loose fragments removed.

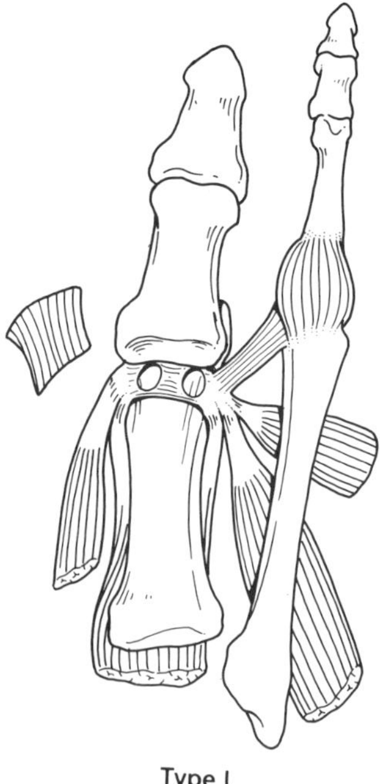

Type I

Fig. 25.81 Type I (irreducible) dorsal dislocation of the first metatarso-phalangeal joint.

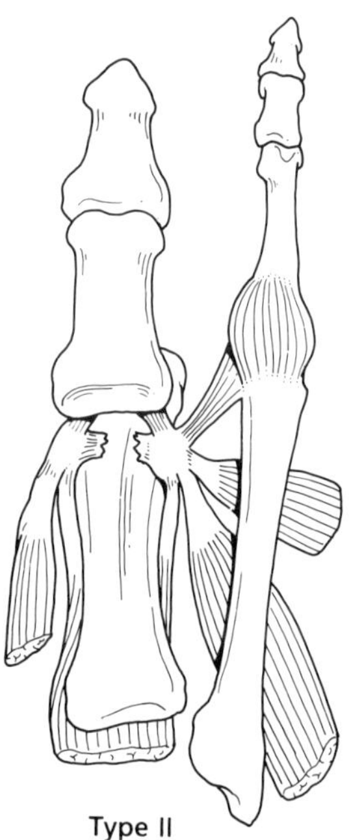

Type II

Fig. 25.82 An example of a type II dislocation of the first metatarso-phalangeal joint.

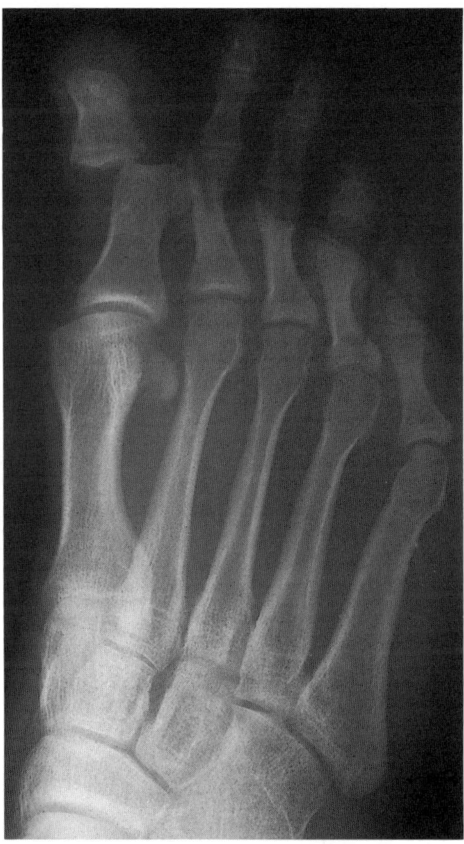

Fig. 25.83 Dislocation of the interphalangeal joint of the great toe.

Dislocations of the metatarsal-phalangeal joints of the lesser toes

These dislocations are similar to those of the great toe but are less common. The mechanism of injury is similar. Reduction can be difficult to achieve if the plantar metatarsal-phalangeal plate remains intact and the head of the metatarsal buttonholes between the lumbrical and flexor tendons. Radiographs are difficult to interpret and the injury can be associated with metatarsal neck fractures. Recurrent dislocation of the fifth toe has been described (Jahss 1981a). Treatment of these injuries is similar to that for dislocation of the metatarsal-phalangeal joint of the hallux. Occasionally, persistent or missed dislocations occur and if the patient presents late and with callosities in the plantar aspects of the foot, excision of the metatarsal head is indicated (Heckman 1991).

Dislocations of the interphalangeal joints of the toes

These are even more uncommon than metatarso-phalangeal dislocations (Heckman 1991). The great toe is again most commonly involved and dislocation is always dorsal (Fig. 25.83). The injury is of a hyperextension type and reduction is usually achieved by closed means. Great toe injuries require rest in a plaster for 3 weeks but lesser toe injuries can be splinted with 'neighbour strapping' or, if unstable, Kirschner wire fixation. It is rare for small bony fragments in the joints to require removal. If any long-term problems develop, such as stiffness or pain in the joint, particularly if the patient develops problems with footwear, then an interphalangeal joint arthrodesis is indicated (De Lee 1986).

Phalangeal fractures

Phalangeal fractures are the commonest fractures of the forefoot and the stubbed toe or 'night walking' fracture of the proximal phalanx is the most frequently seen (De Lee 1986, Heckman 1991) (Fig. 25.84). They rarely cause problems unless malunion occurs and produces local pressure problems. These injuries are always the result of direct trauma. The diagnosis is obvious clinically. It is important to obtain specific radiographs of the toes and not of the whole foot as a radiograph centred on the

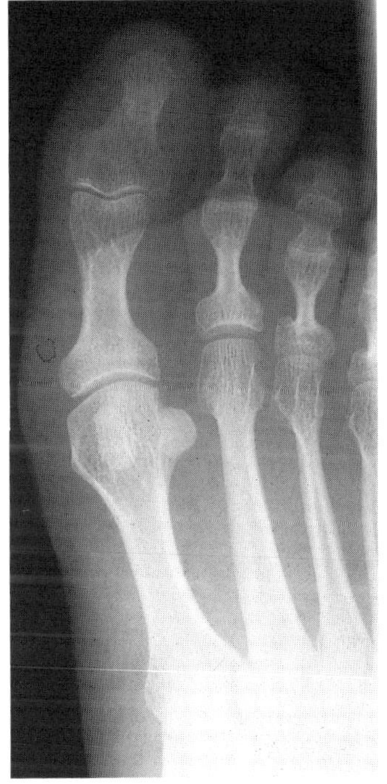
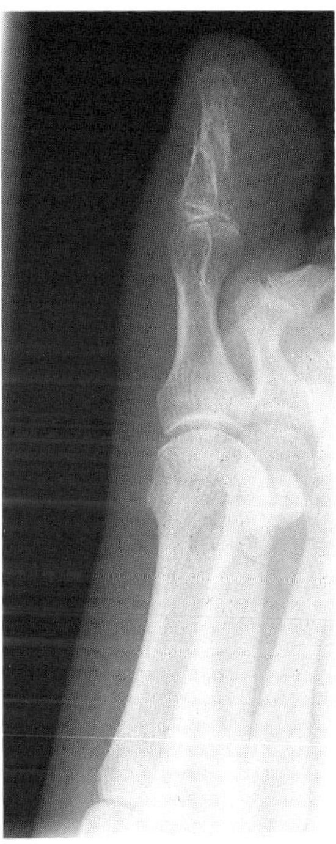

Fig. 25.85 Typical crush type fracture of the distal phalanx of the great toe. Note the marked soft tissue swelling.

area of injury allows a better assessment of the nature of the fracture. In addition, an attempt at obtaining a lateral radiograph of the toes should be made as it is necessary to exclude an associated dislocation.

The injuries may be compound and debridement followed by Kirschner wire fixation is necessary to stabilize the soft tissues (De Lee 1986). Hallux fractures may be undisplaced or displaced (Jahss 1981b). If they are undisplaced and involve the terminal phalanx, then trephining of the toe may be necessary to release the subungual haematoma which sometimes develops (Fig. 25.85). If phalangeal fractures of the hallux are displaced they may involve the interphalangeal joint (Fig. 25.86) or the metatarsal-phalangeal joint. Closed reduction may be necessary (in Chinese finger straps) and K-wire fixation performed. Immobilization with a toe platform for 4–6 weeks is necessary. Very rarely, the injury may be an avulsion type fracture (Fig. 25.87) and particularly if the fracture has intra-articular displacement, open reduction and fixation with a K-wire may be necessary (Fig. 25.88). Fractures of the lesser toes involving the middle and proximal phalanges only require treatment with neighbour strapping. Injuries of the distal phalanges are usually crush injuries and a supportive dressing is all that is necessary.

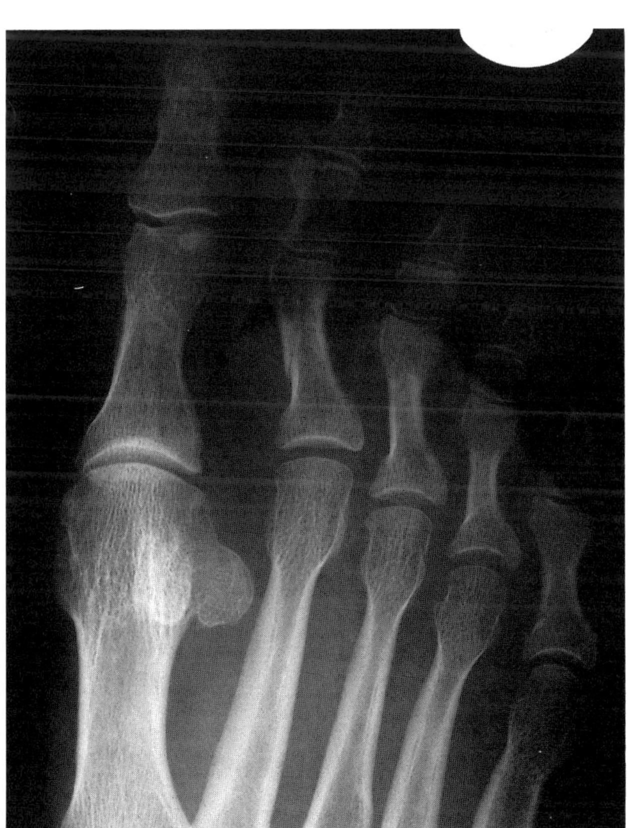

Fig. 25.84 'Night walking' fracture of the proximal phalanx of the second toe.

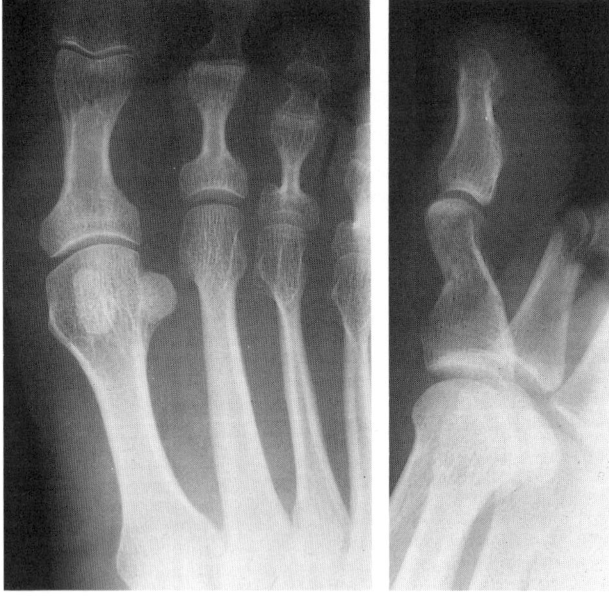

Fig. 25.86 Displaced intra-articular fracture of the great toe proximal phalanx.

Sesamoid fractures

Although rare injuries (Powers 1934), sesamoid fractures can cause problems of diagnosis and treatment. The great toe has two sesamoid bones. The tibial (medial) one is larger than its fibular (lateral) counterpart and, as it is under the weight-bearing area of the metatarsal head, is more frequently fractured, usually as the result of a fall from a height with the patient landing on the ball of the foot (Powers 1934). Occasionally, they are

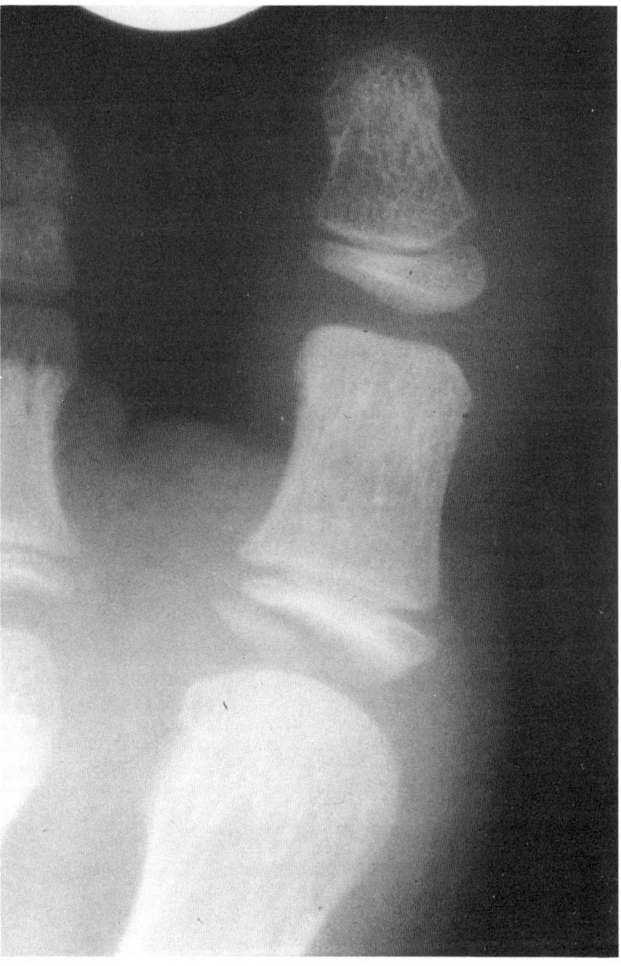

Fig. 25.87 A Salter–Harris type II fracture of the lateral aspect of the base of the proximal phalanx of the great toe.

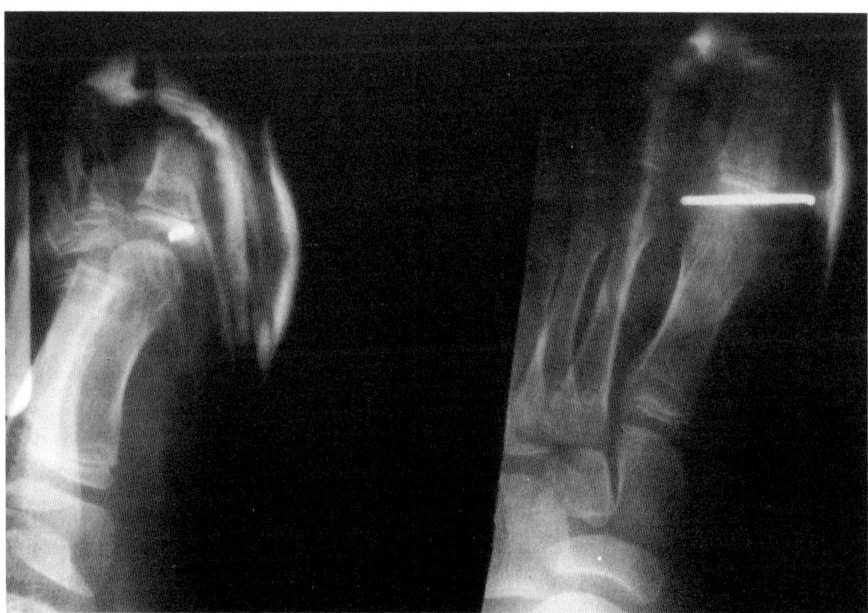

Fig. 25.88 Same case as Fig. 25.87 after open reduction and fixation with a Kirschner wire.

injured by forced dorsiflexion and abduction of the great toe, as seen in football injuries. The role of the sesamoids is to elevate the big toe so that it is level with the other metatarsal heads.

Suspicion of a fracture should be aroused by the history, as detailed above, and pain on weight-bearing, especially on toe off. Radiographs can be difficult to interpret, especially as about 15% of people have bipartite or multipartite sesamoids that are not always bilateral (Powers 1934). Anteroposterior views of the forefoot, and lateral and tangential views of the metatarsal heads should be requested (Fig. 25.63). The fractures are usually transverse or comminuted. Bipartite sesamoids have a smooth separation and are larger than their counterparts. Separation of these variants may occur following injury. Treatment of these fractures can be protracted as symptoms can persist for several months. A cast worn for 2 to 3 weeks in the acute phase will usually suffice. Excision may be indicated for recalcitrant cases.

Stress fractures of the sesamoids have been described in athletes (Van Hal *et al.* 1982).

References

Adelaar, R.S. The treatment of complex fractures of the talus. *Orthop Clin North Am* 1989; **20(4)**: oo−oo.

Arntz, C.T. & Hansen, S.T. Dislocations and fracture dislocations of the tarso-metatarsal joints. *Orthop Clin North Am* 1987; **18**: 105−114.

Berndt, A.L. & Harty, M. Transchondral fractures (osteochondritis dissecans of the talus). *J Bone Joint Surg* 1959; **41A(6)**: 1020.

Bernstern, A. & Stone, J.R. March fracture: a report of 307 cases and a new method of treatment. *J Bone Joint Surg* 1944; **26**: 743−750.

Blair, H.C. Comminuted fractures and fracture dislocations of the astragalus. *Am J Surg* 1943; **59(1)**: 37−43.

Brunet, J.A. & Wiley, J.J. The late results of tarso-metatarsal joint injuries. *J Bone Joint Surg* 1987; **69B**: 437−440.

Canale, S.T. & Kelly, F.B. Fractures of the neck of the talus. Long term evaluation of 71 cases. *J Bone Joint Surg* 1978; **60A**: 143−156.

Clanton, T.O., Butler, J.E. & Eggert, A. Injuries to the metatarsal phalangeal joints in athletes. *Foot Ankle* 1986; **7(3)**: 162−176.

Coltart, W.D. "Aviator's astragalas". *J Bone Joint Surg* 1952; **34B(4)**: 545−566.

Dameron, T.B. Fractures and the anatomical variations of the proximal portion of the fifth metatarsal. *J Bone Joint Surg* 1975; **57A**: 788−792.

De Lee, J.C. Fractures and dislocations of the foot. In: Mann, R.A. (ed.) *Surgery of the Foot* 5th edn. CV Mosby: St Louis, 1986.

De Lee, J.C. & Curtis, R. Subtalar dislocations of the foot. *J Bone Joint Surg* 1982; **64A**: 433−437.

Gossens, M. & DeStoop, N. Lisfrancs fracture dislocations: etiology, radiology and results of treatment. *Clin Orthop* 1983; **176**: 154−162.

Grantham, S.A. Medial subtalar dislocations: five cases with a common aetiology. *J Trauma* 1964; **4**: 845−849.

Hansen, S.T. Fractures of the talus and osteochondral fractures of the talus. *Comprehensive AAOS Foot and Ankle Course, California Nov. 8−11.* 1989.

Hardcastle, P.H., Reschauer, R., Kutscha-Lissberg, E. & Schoffman, W. Injuries to the tarsometatarsal joint. Incidence, classification and treatment. *J Bone Joint Surg* 1982; **64B**: 349−356.

Hawkins, L.G. Fractures of the lateral process of the talus. *J Bone Joint Surg* 1965; **47A**: 1170−1175.

Hawkins, L.G. Fractures of the neck of the talus. *J Bone Joint Surg* 1970; **52A**: 991−1002.

Heckman, J.D. Fractures and dislocations of the foot. In: Rockwood, C.A. Jr. & Green, D.P. (eds) *Fractures and Dislocations in the Foot*, Vol. II, 3rd edn. J.B. Lippincott: Philadelphia, 1991.

Hermal, M.B. & Gershon-Cohen, J. The nutcracker fracture of the cuboid by indirect violence. *Radiology* 1953; **60**: 850−854.

Hunter, L.Y. Stress fractures of the tarsal navicular. *Am J Sports Med* 1981; **9**: 217−219.

Jahss, M.H. Chronic and recurrent dislocations of the fifth toe. *Foot Ankle* 1981a; **I5**: 275−278.

Jahss, M.H. Stubbing injuries of the hallux. *Foot Ankle* 1981b; **I6**: 327−332.

Janssen, T. & Kopta, T. Bilateral recurrent subtalar dislocation. *J Bone Joint Surg* 1985; **67A**: 1432−1433.

Jones, R. Fracture of the base of the fifth metatarsal bone by indirect violence. *Ann Surg* 1902; **35**: 697−700.

Kavanaugh, J.H., Brower, T.D. & Mann, R.V. The Jones fracture revisited. *J Bone Joint Surg* 1978; **60A**: 776−782.

Kenwright, J. & Taylor, R.G. Major injuries of the talus. *J Bone Joint Surg* 1970; **52B**: 36−48.

King, R.E. Dislocation of the tarsometatarsal joints. *Bull Hosp J Dis* 1987; **47(2)**: 190−202.

Lange, R.H., Engber, W.D. & Tearse, D.S. Expanding Applications of the Herbert Screw. *AAOS Poster Exhibit.* 1986.

Larson, H.W. Subastragalar dislocation (luxatio pedis subtalo) — a follow up report of 8 cases. *Acta Clin Scand* 1957; **113**: 380−392.

Lindholm, R. Operative treatment of dislocated simple fractures of the neck of the metatarsal bone. *Ann Chir Gynaecol Fenn* 1961; **50**: 328−331.

Main, B.J. & Jowett, R.L. Injuries of the midtarsal joint. *J Bone Joint Surg* 1975; **57B**: 89−97.

McKeever, F.M. Fractures of the tarsal and metatarsal bones. *Surg Gynecol Obstet* 1950; **90**: 735−745.

Monson, S.T. & Ryan, J.R. Subtalar dislocation. *J Bone Joint Surg* 1981; **63**: 1156−1158.

Mukerjee, S.K. & Young, A.B. Dome fractures of the talus. *J Bone Joint Surg* 1973; **55B**: 319−326.

Mukerjee, S.K., Pringle, R.M. & Baxter, A.D. Fractures of the lateral process of the talus. *J Bone Joint Surg* 1974; **56B**: 263−273.

Mulfinger, G.L. & Trueta, J. The blood supply of the talus. *J Bone Joint Surg* 1970; **52B**: 160−167.

Myerson, M.S. Acute compartment syndromes of the foot. *Bull Hosp J Dis Orthop Inst* 1987; **47(2)**: 251−261.

Myerson, M.S. Experimental decompression of the fascial compartments of the foot — the basis of fasciotomy in acute compartment syndromes. *Foot Ankle* 1988; **8(6)**: 308–314.

Myerson, M.S. Fractures of the tarsometatarsal joint. *Second Annual Comprehensive Foot and Ankle Course, California.* 1989.

Myerson, M.S., Fisher, R.T., Burgess, A.R. & Kenzora, J.E. Fracture dislocations of the tarsometatarsal joints. End results correlated with pathology and treatment. *Foot Ankle* 1986; **6**: 225–242.

Nyska, M., Marguilies, J.Y., Barbarawi, M., Mutchlet, W., Dekel, S. & Segal, D. Fractures of the body of the tarsal navicular bone: case reports and literature review. *J Trauma* 1989; **29(10)**: 1448–1451.

Pennal, G.F. Fractures of the talus. *Clin Orthop* 1963; **30**: 53–63.

Powers, J.H. Traumatic and developmental abnormalities of the sesamoid bones of the great toe. *Am J Surg* 1934; **23**: 315–321.

Sangeorzan, B.J., Benirschke, S.K., Mosca, V., Mayo, K.A. & Hansen, S.T. Jr. Displaced intra-articular fractures of the talo-navicular joint. *J Bone Joint Surg* 1989; **71A**: 1504–1510.

Sisk, T.D. In: *Campbell's Operative Orthopaedics*, Vol. 3, 7th edn. 1987.

Torg, J.S., Pavlov, H., Cooley, L.H., Bryant, M.H., Arnoczky, S.P., Bergfield, J. & Hunter, L.Y. Stress fractures of the tarsal navicular. *J Bone Joint Surg* 1982; **64A**: 700–712.

Van Hal, E., Keene, J.S., Lange, T.A. & Clancy, W.G. Stress fractures of the sesamoids. *Am J Sports Med* 1982; **10**: 122–128.

Watson-Jones, R. *Fractures and Joint Injuries*, Vol. II, 6th edn. Churchill Livingstone: Edinburgh, 1982.

Wilson, D.W. Fractures of the foot. In: Klenerman, L. (ed.). *The Foot and Its Disorders*, 3rd edn. Blackwell Scientific Publications: Oxford, 1991.

Wilson, E.S. Jr. & Katz, F.N. Stress fractures: an analysis of 250 conservative cases. *Radiology* 1969; **92**: 481–486.

Zimmer, T.L. & Johnson, K.A. Subtalar dislocations. *Clin Orthop* 1989; **238**: 190–194.

26: Pathological Fractures

C.S.B.GALASKO

Introduction

There are basically three types of fracture:

1 Traumatic fractures: here the strength of the bone is normal, but the violence of the trauma to which the patient has been exposed is greater and the bone fractures.

2 Stress fractures: the strength of the bone is normal, but it is subjected to repeated stress. The bone gives way under the repeated stress, and it is the repeated nature of the stress that causes the fracture, e.g. 'march' fracture of a metatarsal.

3 Pathological fractures: by definition a pathological fracture develops under physiological stress in a bone that has been weakened by a disease process.

Causes of pathological fracture

1 Metabolic bone disease.

(a) Osteoporosis: this includes senile osteoporosis, and osteoporosis secondary to Cushing's syndrome. Disuse osteoporosis is not a metabolic disorder, but the osteoporosis is secondary to disuse. It is a local, rather than a generalized, condition but the bone is weakened and is subject to fracture under physiological stress (Fig. 26.1).

(b) Osteomalacia and rickets.

(c) Paget's disease.

(d) Hyperparathyroidism.

(e) Gaucher's disease.

2 Tumour.

(a) Metastatic: this may affect the spine, long bones and occasionally the small bones of the hand or feet.

(b) Primary malignant tumours.

(c) Primary benign tumours.

(d) Tumour-like conditions, e.g. fibrous dysplasia and unicameral bone cyst.

3 Infection.

4 Developmental disorders: for example, a fracture of the femoral neck in a patient with a marked coxa vara, irrespective of the cause of the deformity of the proximal femur. The fracture is probably due to repeated stress on a bone that has been weakened because of its changed architecture.

5 Neuropathic fractures: for example, Duchenne muscular dystrophy, spina bifida and cerebral palsy.

6 Dysplasias: for example, osteogenesis imperfecta and osteopetrosis. In the former condition the collagen is abnormal. The disease is classified depending on the collagen abnormality but, as a result of the abnormality, the bones are fragile and tend to fracture with minimal stress. The frequency of fracture depends on the type and severity of the osteogenesis imperfecta. The radiographic appearance also depends on the type of osteogenesis imperfecta. The bone may be expanded or abnormally thin, but is osteoporotic.

In osteopetrosis the bones are denser than normal and thickened, but they are brittle and tend to fracture with minimal trauma.

7 Miscellaneous.

(a) Rheumatoid arthritis.

(b) Haemophilia.

(c) Following irradiation.

(d) Sickle cell disease.

Diagnosis

In patients with pathological fractures, not only must the fracture be diagnosed but also the underlying abnormality. This may be due to:

1 A generalized metabolic or endocrine disorder.

2 A localized problem in a patient with generalized disease.

3 A localized disorder (e.g. a unicameral bone cyst).

4 Disuse (Fig. 26.1).

5 A surgical defect; e.g. following biopsy (Fig. 26.2).

As with traumatic fractures, the diagnosis of a fracture is made from the history and examination and is con-

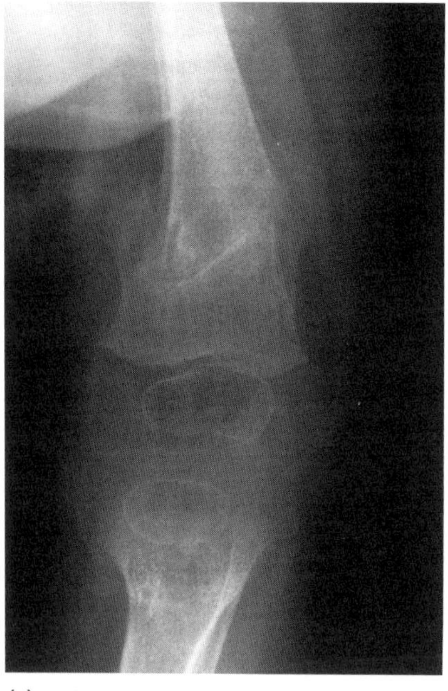

(a)

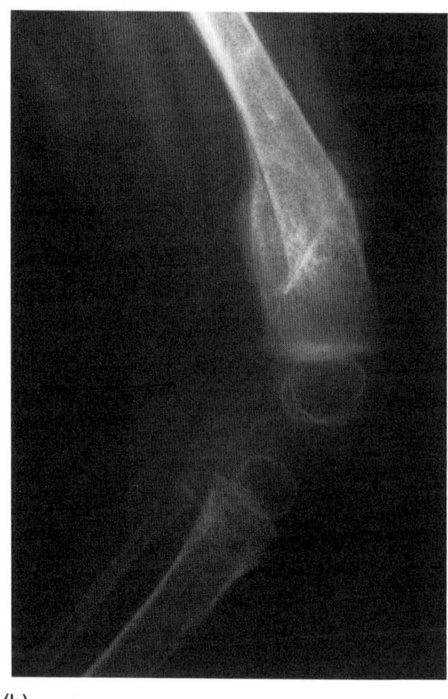

(b)

Fig. 26.1 Disuse osteoporosis. This child was born with irreducible dislocated hips which required open reduction and femoral osteotomy at the age of 7 months. Postoperatively immobilization in a double hip spica followed for 12 weeks. (a) and (b) The patient developed a supracondylar fracture 3 days after coming out of plaster; the fracture was immobilized in a plaster cast for a further 2 weeks.

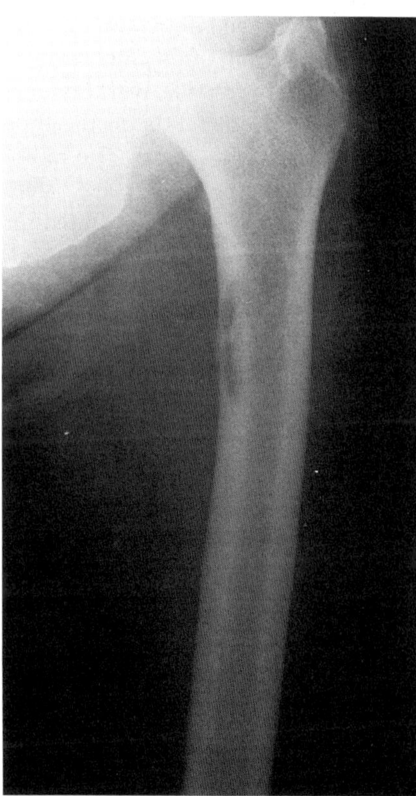

(a)

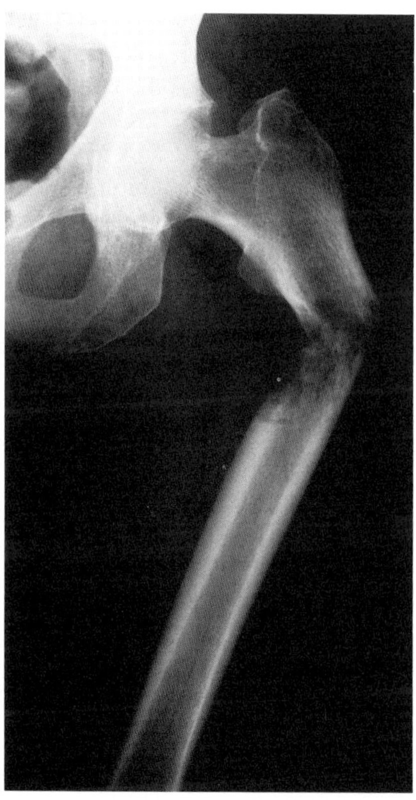

(b)

Fig. 26.2 (a) This female patient presented with pain in her left proximal thigh. A lytic lesion was seen on the X-ray. It was biopsied and found to be a metastasis from mammary carcinoma. (b) The patient developed a pathological fracture through the site of biopsy.

firmed on radiographs. A pathological fracture should be suspected if the patient suffers from a condition which predisposes to such fractures, the fracture occurs following minor trauma, the patient is elderly, there is a history of repeated fractures or there is a previous malignancy. The radiographs should be carefully inspected for any associated pathological abnormality such as a metastasis or osteopenia. Because the stress producing the fracture is usually much less than that required to produce a traumatic fracture, it is extremely rare for the patient to have associated vascular, nerve or visceral damage. Compound pathological fractures almost never occur. The diagnosis of the underlying condition can often be made from the history, examination and plain radiographs, for example a fracture occurring in a patient known to have Cushing's syndrome, metastatic mammary carcinoma, Duchenne dystrophy, etc., and with the typical radiographic features of that specific pathological condition. In many instances the diagnosis cannot be made without further investigation, including biopsy when indicated, and further tests may be required to reveal the extent of the disorder, e.g. skeletal scintigraphy in a patient with skeletal metastases. A full discussion on the methods of investigating each underlying disorder is beyond the scope of this chapter.

Complications

Complications occur more frequently than with traumatic fractures. The complications depend on the site and type of fracture and the underlying primary disorder.

Non-union

For example, pathological fractures of the femoral neck, secondary to metastatic disease, do not unite irrespective of the method of treatment and, therefore, some form of replacement arthroplasty is indicated, irrespective of the age of the patient or the degree of displacement.

Delayed union

This often occurs, and internal fixation is frequently indicated to obviate the prolonged immobilization required for healing of the fracture to occur.

Malunion

This occurs quite commonly in patients with osteogenesis imperfecta after multiple fractures.

Exuberant callus formation (Fig. 26.3)

Some pathological fractures heal very rapidly and with large amounts of callus, which occasionally may be mistaken for a primary malignant tumour. It may be difficult to differentiate immature callus from an osteo-

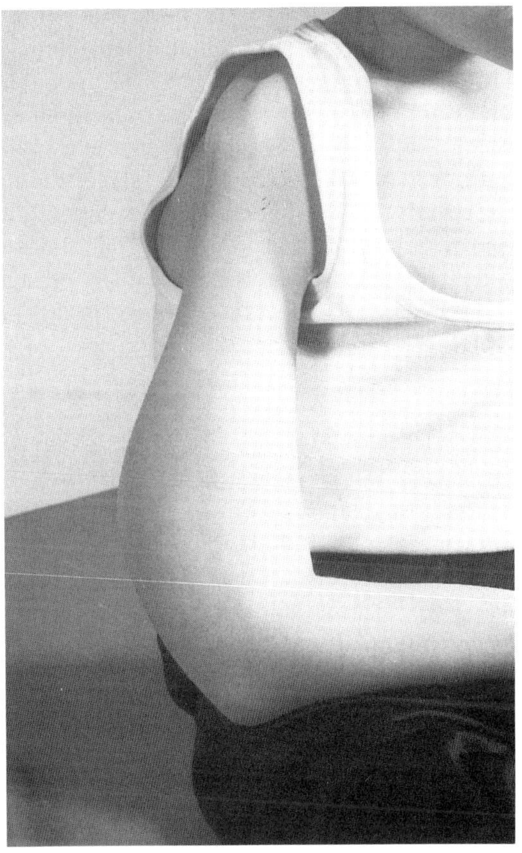

Fig. 26.3 Patient with osteogenesis imperfecta who has suffered recurrent fractures. The fracture of the right humerus has united with exuberant callus, responsible for the marked swelling of the upper arm.

sarcoma on histological examination but serial radiographs, taken over a period of a few weeks, show rapid maturation of the callus. This tends to occur with osteogenesis imperfecta and spina bifida.

Infection

Infection may complicate internal fixation of a pathological fracture but the risk should be no greater than with internal fixation of any other closed fracture.

Avascular necrosis

This depends on the site of the fracture; for example, pathological fractures of the femoral neck carry a high risk of avascular necrosis of the femoral head, as with traumatic fractures.

Metabolic disturbance

The fracture does not produce a significant metabolic

disturbance but may be associated with one. For example, patients with disseminated carcinoma may suffer from hypercalcaemia: this may be humoral, the tumour secreting osteolytic factors which stimulate osteoclast resorption of bone, as well as urinary calcium retention; or may be secondary to the skeletal metastases, the severity of the hypercalcaemia depending on the rapidity of bone destruction rather than the extent. The patient may be hypercalcaemic when presenting with the fracture. This must be excluded, or diagnosed and treated prior to internal fixation of a fracture.

General effects

The development of general complications, such as the adult respiratory distress syndrome, following a pathological fracture is rare, but many of these patients have generalized illnesses that may limit the treatment options. These illnesses include conditions such as cardiomyopathy with cor pulmonale in patients with neuromuscular disorders, respiratory failure due to chronic bronchitis and emphysema in the elderly, or respiratory insufficiency associated with distortion of the rib cage and gross kyphoscoliosis in children with osteogenesis imperfecta.

Treatment

The treatment depends on the fracture, as well as on the underlying pathological disorder. It is beyond the scope of this chapter to deal with every individual fracture in each pathological condition, but a few examples deserve special mention.

Fractures of the proximal femur in the elderly patient, secondary to osteoporosis and/or osteomalacia

This group of patients is probably more costly to the National Health Service than any other group, and these patients probably occupy more acute bed days than any other group. There are several reasons for this. These fractures occur commonly in the older age group and not only is there an increase in the numbers and proportion of older patients, but there also is an increase in the incidence of these fractures. Frequently these patients are unwell and are suffering from hypertension, cardiac failure, chronic bronchitis, emphysema, etc.; often these patients were barely able to cope at home prior to the fracture. Following the fracture they can no longer cope and have to spend weeks in hospital waiting for suitable aftercare. In England and Wales alone about 37 500 hip fractures occur annually at a cost of £165

million (Wallace 1987). It is estimated that by the age of 80 years 33% of women have sustained a fracture of their proximal femur, 24% a Colles fracture and 15% a vertebral compression fracture. By the age of 85 years 93% of elderly women have sustained at least one fracture (Woolf & Dixon 1988).

There is still much debate about the optimum method of treatment of these patients, but several principles emerge. Early surgery is recommended, providing the patient is generally fit; if not, their underlying medical condition must be treated before embarking upon surgery. These fractures are associated with a high mortality and morbidity, mainly associated with the patient's chronic respiratory disease and the most common cause of death is bronchopneumonia. It is possible to assess preoperatively the patient's prospects. Galasko *et al.* (1985) showed that mortality (within 3 months of sustaining a fracture) was related to the peak expiratory flow rate (PEFR) measured on admission to hospital. The mean PEFR in surviving patients was 185.5 ± 6.8 l min^{-1}, compared with 109.7 ± 7.7 l min^{-1} in those who died ($p < 0.001$). Similar significant differences were found for each age group. In patients whose PEFR was less than 100 l min^{-1} mortality was 69.6% but it was only 6.7% in patients whose peak flow was greater than 250 l min^{-1} (Tables 26.1 & 26.2). We now utilize the PEFR as one of our main criteria in assessing the suitability of an elderly patient for early surgery. If the PEFR is greater than 100 l min^{-1} and if the patient is otherwise fit, early internal fixation or replacement arthroplasty is indicated. However, if the PEFR is less than 100 l min^{-1} or if there are other contraindications to early surgery, operation is delayed for a few days in order to allow patients to receive intensive medical treatment and physiotherapy in an attempt to improve their general condition. Other factors that may affect the outcome include under-nutrition (Bastow *et al.* 1983), anaemia and mental test scores (Greatorex & Gibbs 1988).

Table 26.1 Fracture of the proximal femur: comparison of preoperative PEFR with mortality (From Galasko *et al.* 1985)

PEFR (l min^{-1})	Total number of patients	Surviving patients	Deceased patients	Mortality (%)
<101	46	14	32	69.6
101–150	50	39	11	22.0
151–200	45	40	5	11.1
201–250	26	23	3	11.5
251–300	15	14	1	6.7
>301	8	8	0	0

Table 26.2 Effect of age on mortality and PEFR in 190 patients who sustained a fracture of the proximal femur. In each age group the PEFR was less in those patients who died within 3 months of fracture

| | | | PEFR (l min^{-1}): mean ± SE | | |
Age (years)	Surviving patients	Deceased patients	Surviving patients	Deceased patients	Significance
<60	12	0	246.7 ± 36.9	–	–
60–69	22	2	200.7 ± 20.3	125.0 ± 75.2	NS
70–79	49	16	196.8 ± 10.1	125.0 ± 11.8	$p < 0.001$
80–89	49	25	161.6 ± 7.5	110.0 ± 12.4	$p < 0.001$
90+	6	9	113.3 ± 12.0	76.7 ± 7.5	$p < 0.02$

NS, not significant.

Early mobilization of these patients is indicated. The development of decubitus ulcers occurs more commonly in those patients whose injuries make regular turning difficult if not impossible. The development of these ulcers may prevent subsequent surgery and early stabilization of the fracture is often indicated to allow turning, even if patients cannot be mobilized because of their general condition. Prolonged immobilization in these patients is also frequently associated with respiratory infection, urinary infection, urinary incontinence, mental confusion and subsequent prolonged rehabilitation. These fractures are associated with a high incidence of deep vein thrombosis, but pulmonary embolism does not seem to be a major cause of death. The onset of the deep vein thrombosis may predate surgery and early surgery may not significantly diminish the incidence. If internal fixation of the fracture does not stabilize the fracture sufficiently to allow early mobilization, then the operation has failed to achieve its main purpose (Fig. 26.4).

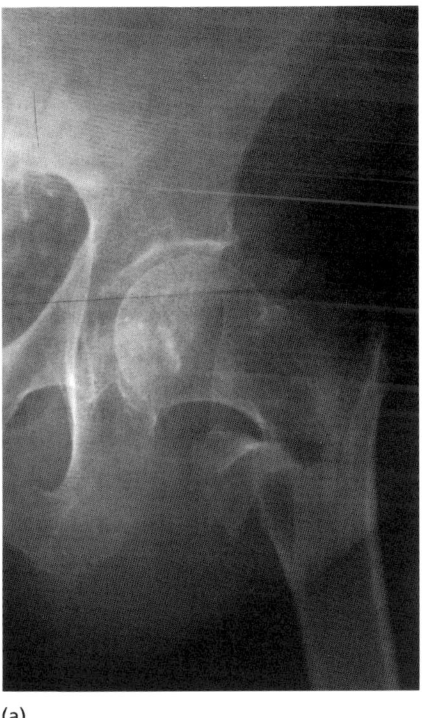

(a)

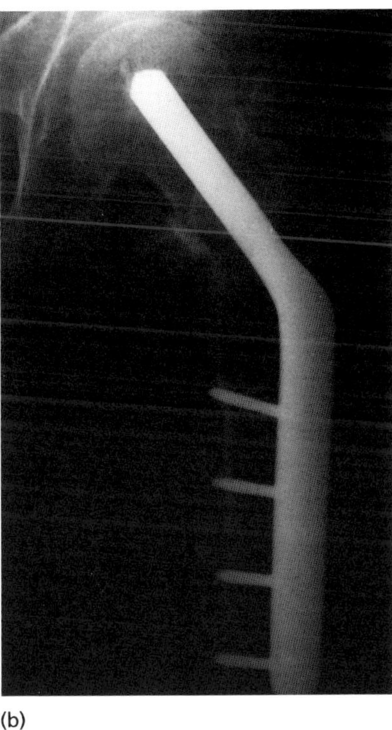

(b)

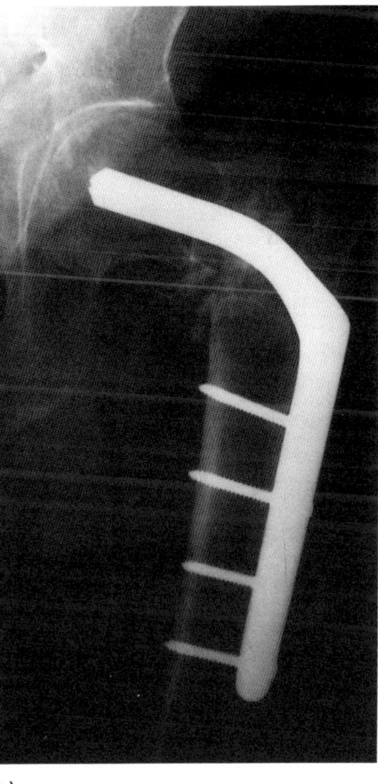

(c)

Fig. 26.4 (a) Elderly female patient with an unstable comminuted trochanteric fracture of the left femur. (b) Fixed with a nail plate; stabilization is inadequate. (c) Collapse at the fracture site and bending of the nail with weight-bearing. These patients require rigid stabilization which is sufficiently strong to allow them to weight-bear postoperatively. Therefore, this type of implant is no longer used.

Undisplaced or minimally displaced subcapital and transcervical fractures are probably best treated by a dynamic hip screw, although other alternatives are available. The choice of device is probably of secondary importance compared with the reduction of the fracture and stability of the fixation (Garden 1964).

Trochanteric fractures are probably best treated with a dynamic hip screw/plate. The basic principle of management of the latter is adequate stabilization to allow weight-bearing. It is not possible to mobilize those elderly patients who are unable to weight-bear or are only capable of very partial weight-bearing. The techniques of achieving stable fixation are described elsewhere in this book, but include the use of a sliding hip screw (Wyman 1982), abduction osteotomy (Sarmiento & Williams 1970) and medial displacement of the femoral shaft (Dimon & Hughston 1967).

There is some debate as to the optimum treatment for displaced (Garden 3 or 4) transcervical fractures. In Scandinavia these fractures are usually treated by closed reduction and internal fixation, whereas in the United Kingdom replacement arthroplasty is most frequently employed. The Scandinavians claim a lower mortality rate and a low complication rate, whereas in the United Kingdom replacement arthroplasty is carried out because of the high incidence of avascular necrosis and non-union. There are no controlled trials and the differences may lie in the general condition of the patients and the associated pathological abnormality of their bones.

Although fractures of the proximal femur are the most important fractures in this group of patients, other fractures occur and the principles of treatment are the same. Supracondylar femoral fractures require internal fixation to allow early mobilization of the patient. Fixation is sometimes extremely difficult to achieve because of the porosity of the bone and techniques include the use of a supracondylar angled blade plate supplemented by cerclage wires, and interlocking nails. The latter are particularly useful for subtrochanteric fractures.

Probably the most common fractures in this group of patients are compression vertebral fractures (Fig. 26.5) and fractures of the distal radius. The former may require bedrest for a few days until the acute pain has settled, but the emphasis of treatment is on mobilization. Fractures of the distal radius are treated by manipulation under anaesthesia to reduce the fracture (if it is displaced), followed by a short period of plaster immobilization and rehabilitation to maintain function in the joints of the upper limb.

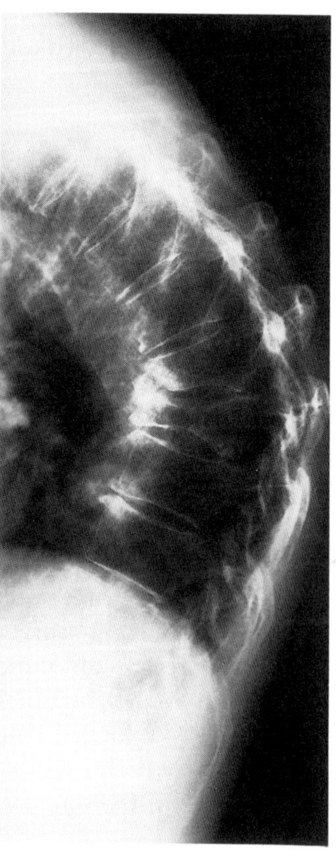

Fig. 26.5 Wedge compression fractures due to osteoporosis in an 83-year-old female.

Other fractures secondary to metabolic and endocrine disorders

These include fractures secondary to hyperparathyroidism, vitamin D deficiency and vitamin A excess, nutritional rickets, renal osteodystrophy, scurvy, Cushing's syndrome, liver disease which may cause osteoporosis, hyperthyroidism and hypogonadism. The underlying metabolic or endocrine disorder must be diagnosed and corrected (if possible), and the fracture is treated on its merits. Prolonged immobilization should be avoided to prevent disuse osteoporosis which may lead to an additional pathological fracture. Surgical stabilization is frequently required.

Patients with Paget's disease of bone have an increased tendency to fracture and pathological fractures of long bones are probably the commonest complication of Paget's disease. Such fractures are usually situated at right angles to the long axis of the bone. As with metastatic cancer, they may develop spontaneously or occur after minor trauma. They are more likely to develop during the osteolytic phase and may be the presenting manifestation of Paget's disease (Hamdy 1981).

The most common sites are the femur, tibia, humerus, spine and pelvis and multiple fractures may occur within the same bone. In the femur the most common site is in the subtrochanteric region and many fractures are heralded by localized pain, tenderness and, sometimes, the presence of local inflammation. These symptoms are probably due to the development of transverse stress fractures which may precede the development of a complete fracture by some weeks. The natural history of these transverse stress fractures is not well known. They may develop into complete fractures, may be painful and tender or may even be asymptomatic and remain so for some time. They are similar to Looser zones. As the risk of sarcoma is substantial in pathological fractures complicating Paget's disease, some authors recommend that a biopsy be taken for histological examination whenever a fracture develops (Nicholas & Killoran 1965, Milgram 1977). There is a high rate of non-union, particularly when these fractures are treated without internal fixation; Dove (1980) reported an overall incidence of 40%.

Management may be difficult because of the associated deformities, particularly bowing and widening of the medullary canal. In some cases the deformities are so severe that internal fixation is not possible but, in most cases, it is possible to correct the deformity at the time of surgery. Increased vascularity may produce serious bleeding problems during surgery; this should be controlled by a preoperative course of calcitonin or APD (3 amino-1-hydroxy-propylidene-1,1-biphosphonate).

Fractures of the femoral neck are probably best treated by replacement arthroplasty using a long-stemmed femoral component. For other fractures rigid internal fixation is usually the treatment of choice. Immobilization in traction may be associated with the development of hypercalcaemia or hypercalcuria with a high risk of nephropathy and renal stones (Hamdy 1981).

Fractures secondary to skeletal metastases or myeloma

These patients have a limited life expectancy and the aims of treatment are to relieve pain, provide early mobilization and early discharge from hospital. There are three aspects to the treatment: (i) adequate stabilization of the fracture to allow the patient early use of the affected limb; (ii) postoperative radiotherapy to control the metastasis responsible for the fracture; and (iii) chemotherapy or endocrine therapy to control the underlying disseminated cancer (Galasko 1986).

In the lower limb (excluding femoral neck) internal fixation provides the optimum form of stabilization. Treated conservatively, the majority of these fractures unite in patients who survive for more than 4 months, but union is delayed and prolonged immobilization is required. Internal stabilization provides better pain relief, easier nursing of the patient, more rapid mobilization and earlier discharge from hospital. The internal fixation must provide sufficient stability to allow the patient to weight-bear. Failure to achieve this implies that the aim of treatment has not been accomplished. Wherever necessary the internal fixation must be supplemented by methylmethacrylate to provide such stability.

The advantages of internal fixation over external immobilization are not as marked in the upper limb, but internal stabilization usually allows the patient earlier use of the affected limb. The internal fixation must provide sufficient stability to allow use of the limb (Fig. 26.6).

Fractures of the femoral neck fail to unite (Galasko 1974) and should be treated by replacement arthroplasty. If the acetabulum is involved a total hip arthroplasty is required, the tumour being curetted out of the acetabulum and the cavity filled with methylmethacrylate. If there is substantial involvement of the acetabulum some form of acetabular replacement is also required.

Prior to surgery a skeletal scintigram should be obtained and if there are other lesions in the affected bone, the entire bone should be stabilized in order to prevent a pathological fracture occurring at the edge of the implant at a later date. This may require the use of long-stemmed replacement arthroplasty, interlocking nails extending the entire length of the bone, or two separate implants (Figs 26.7 & 26.8).

Postoperative radiotherapy is essential to control the metastasis. Continual growth of the metastasis, with destruction of more bone, is likely to result in loosening of the implant and failure of the stabilization (Fig. 26.9).

Spinal instability

This is the equivalent of a pathological fracture in the spine. Back pain is a frequent symptom in patients with disseminated carcinoma. In about 10% of patients it is due to spinal instability (Galasko & Sylvester 1978). These patients present with severe back pain which is mechanical in nature. In its most severe form the patient is only comfortable when lying absolutely still and any movement, including log-rolling by two or three trained nurses, is associated with excruciating pain; although there may be no associated neurological abnormality, the patient may be unable to sit, stand or walk because

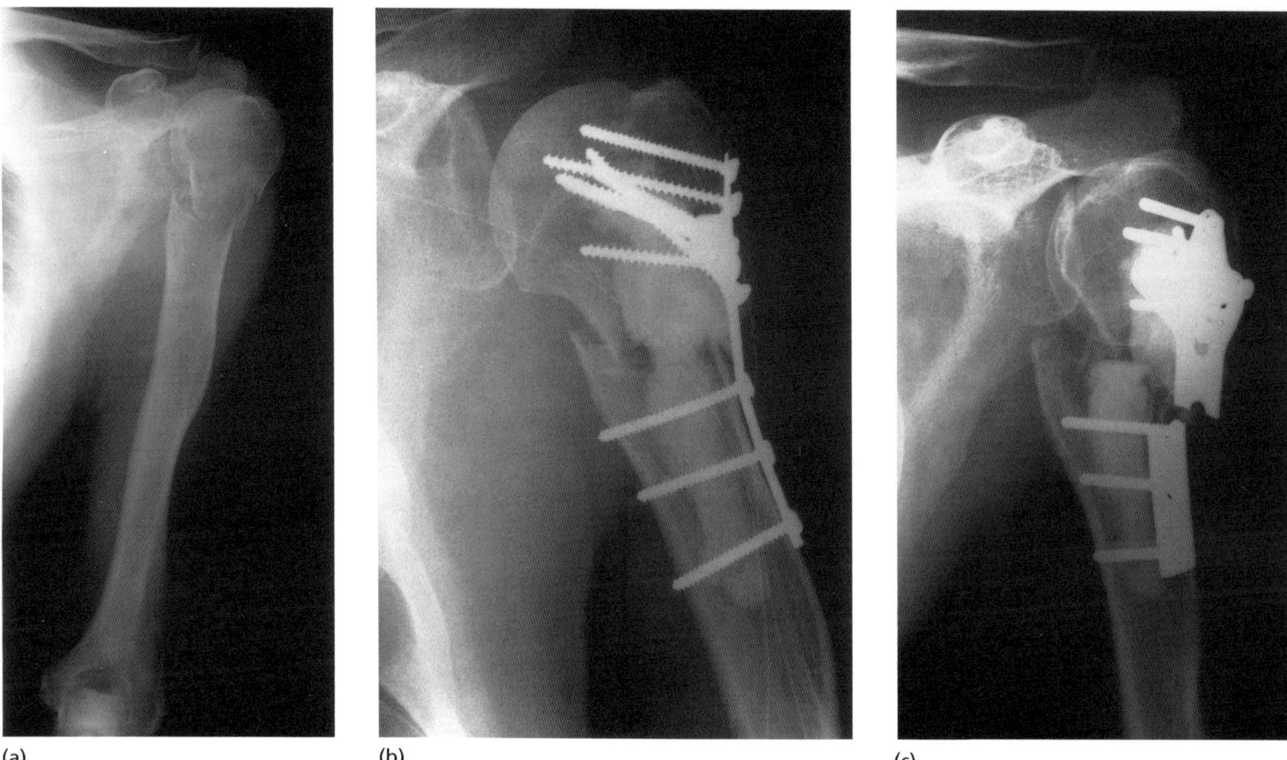

(a)   (b)   (c)

Fig. 26.6 (a) Pathological fracture through the left proximal humerus, secondary to a metastasis from bronchial carcinoma. (b) The fracture has been stabilized with a plate and cement. The plate is too thin and inadequate cement has been used; the fixation is inadequate. (c) The plate has broken and the fixation has failed. The aim of the operation is to provide sufficient stability to allow the patient unencumbered use of the limb; surgery is of little value if it does not provide such stability.

of the pain. In the milder form the patient may be relatively free from pain when wearing a rigid spinal orthosis but movement of the back, for example turning in bed, sitting or standing, is impossible without this support and in the more severe cases, the orthosis does not alleviate the pain sufficiently to allow the patient to mobilize. Radiographs show destruction of bone with vertebral collapse to a greater or lesser degree. No discrete fracture can be seen but, nevertheless, spinal instability should be considered as the equivalent of a pathological fracture in a long bone, as the pain is due to the instability and not to the metastasis. Radiotherapy or chemotherapy will not alleviate this mechanical pain although, as for pathological fractures, postoperative radiotherapy and chemotherapy, or endocrine therapy, is indicated. As with pathological fractures the commonest primary tumour is carcinoma of the breast followed by myeloma.

The principles of treatment are similar to those for pathological fractures, namely surgical stabilization to allow the patient use of the back for moving, sitting, standing and walking. Occasionally it is not possible to

give any further irradiation postoperatively because the patient has already received the maximum tolerable dose to the spinal cord but, where possible, post-operative radiotherapy should be given. Chemotherapy or endocrine therapy may also be indicated, depending on the primary tumour.

The pre-operative investigations should include a magnetic resonance (MR) scan to show whether there is any spinal cord or cauda equina compression, as well as a skeletal scintigram to indicate the degree of skeletal involvement. Where facilities are not available for MR imaging, computerized tomographic (CT) scanning with myelography should be used. If the spinal cord or cauda equina is compressed, it should be decompressed at the time of surgery, irrespective of whether there are any clinical signs of neurological involvement. There is some debate about the optimal treatment of these lesions. The spine can be adequately stabilized from behind using some form of segmental fixation such as a Hartshill rectangle with sublaminar wiring, or an implant fixed with intrapedicular screws. If there is any cord com-pression, the laminae should be removed at the level of

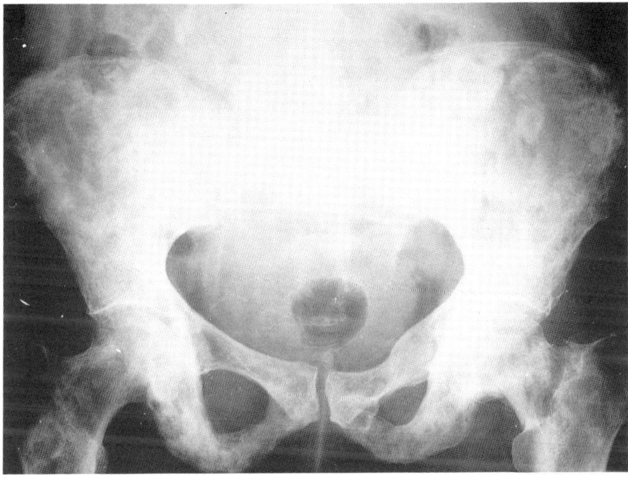

(a)

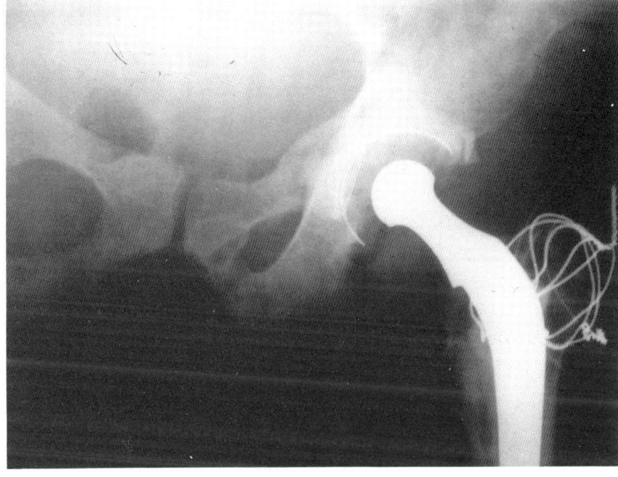

(b)

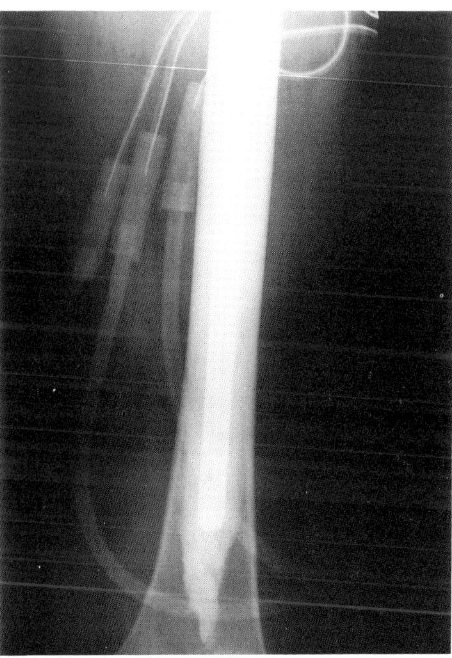

(c)

Fig. 26.17(a) Patient with mammary carcinoma who sustained an undisplaced fracture through the left femoral neck. X-rays and scintigrams indicate widespread metastatic disease involving the pelvis and femur. (b) The patient was treated by replacement arthroplasty using a long-stemmed Charnley prosthesis; (c) the stem of the prosthesis stabilizes the other lesions in the femoral shaft.

compression, the implant giving sufficient stability. The Hartshill rectangle should be fixed to at least two, and preferably three, vertebrae above and three vertebrae below the lesion. If pedicular screws are used it may be sufficient to fix the implant to only one vertebra above and one vertebra below the lesion. If the scintigram or MRI shows involvement of adjacent vertebrae, the fixation should be extended to support these vertebrae. If the instability affects the lower lumbar spine, posterior fixation should be supplemented by anterior fixation. Some surgeons prefer anterior stabilization using, for example, the Kaneda implant. There are now many suitable implants available for posterior and/or anterior stabilization of metastatic spinal instability.

We have treated 72 patients with instability of the thoracic or lumbar spine (Table 26.3). Four patients with destruction of L4 or L5 required a combined anterior and posterior approach (Fig. 26.10), as did a patient with a very acute kyphus, but in the other 67 patients posterior stabilization by means of a variety of implants was used (Figs 26.11, 26.12 & 26.13). The results are shown in Table 26.4. Thirty-four patients had associated neurological symptoms and the results are shown in Table 26.5.

Instability can also occur in the cervical spine. The principles of treatment are the same, namely, spinal stabilization and decompression, if there is any cord compression (Fidler 1987), followed by radiotherapy.

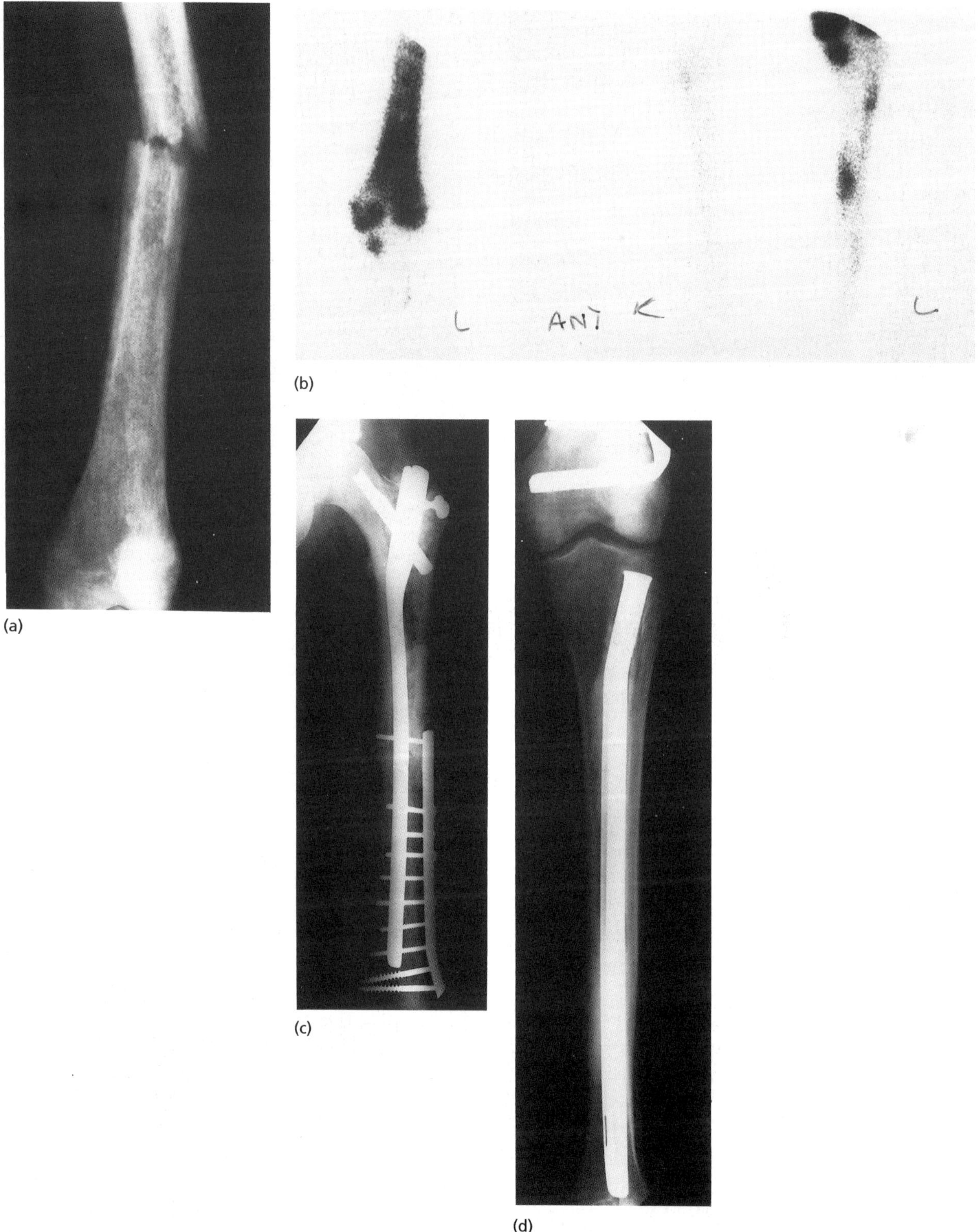

Fig. 26.8 Patient with rectal carcinoma who developed a pathological fracture. (a) Multiple permeative metastases affecting the left femur. These lesions are only a few millimetres in diameter and there is no large lytic lesion. Nevertheless, the bone has been weakened and is liable to fracture under physiological stress. (b) ^{99m}Tc-MDP scintigram shows involvement of the entire left femur, with metastases in the ipsilateral tibia. (c) and (d) The pathological fracture was stabilized with a Zickel nail, the distal femur being stabilized by a blade plate and the tibia with an AO nail. The stabilization was supplemented with methylmethacrylate.

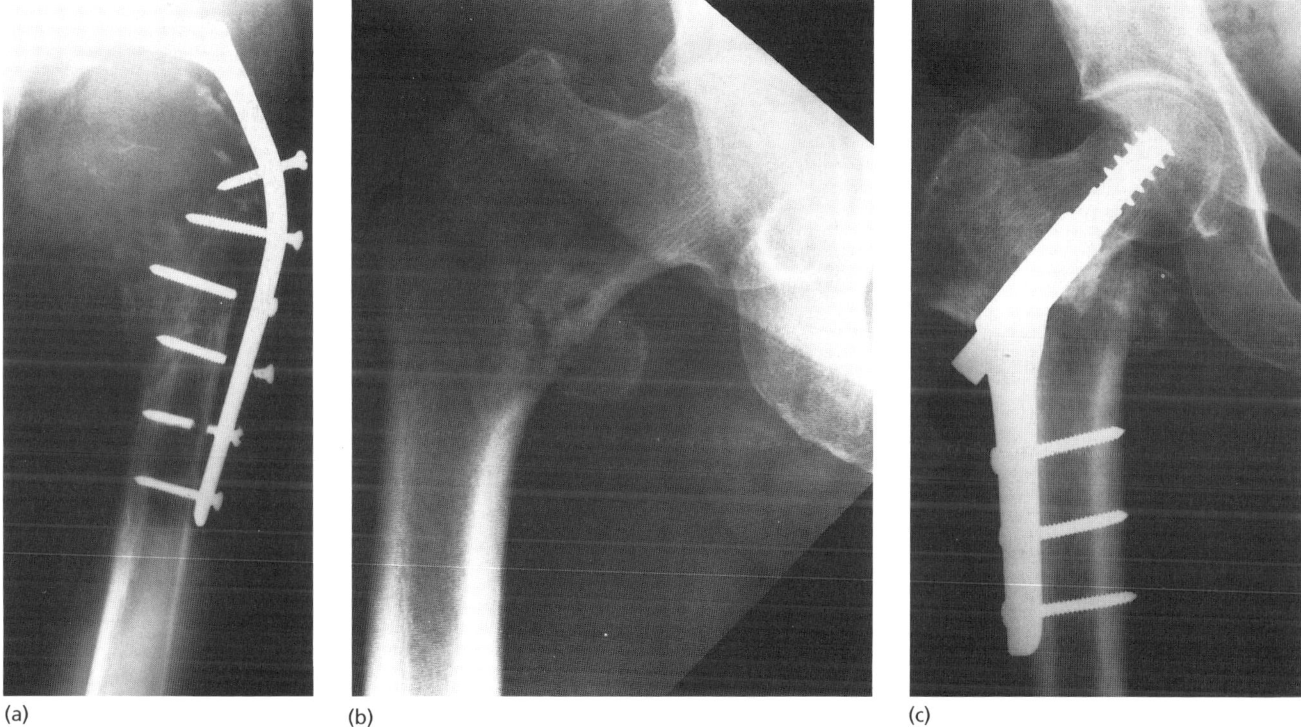

Fig. 26.9 (a) Patient with renal carcinoma who developed a trochanteric fracture stabilized elsewhere with a nail plate. Postoperative radiotherapy was not given. The tumour has continued to grow and destroy bone, resulting in failure of the implant. (b) Patient with mammary carcinoma who sustained a pathological trochanteric fracture of the right femur. (c) A stable fixation was obtained without the addition of methylmethacrylate. The patient received postoperative radiotherapy and endocrine therapy, and the fracture went on to unite with callus.

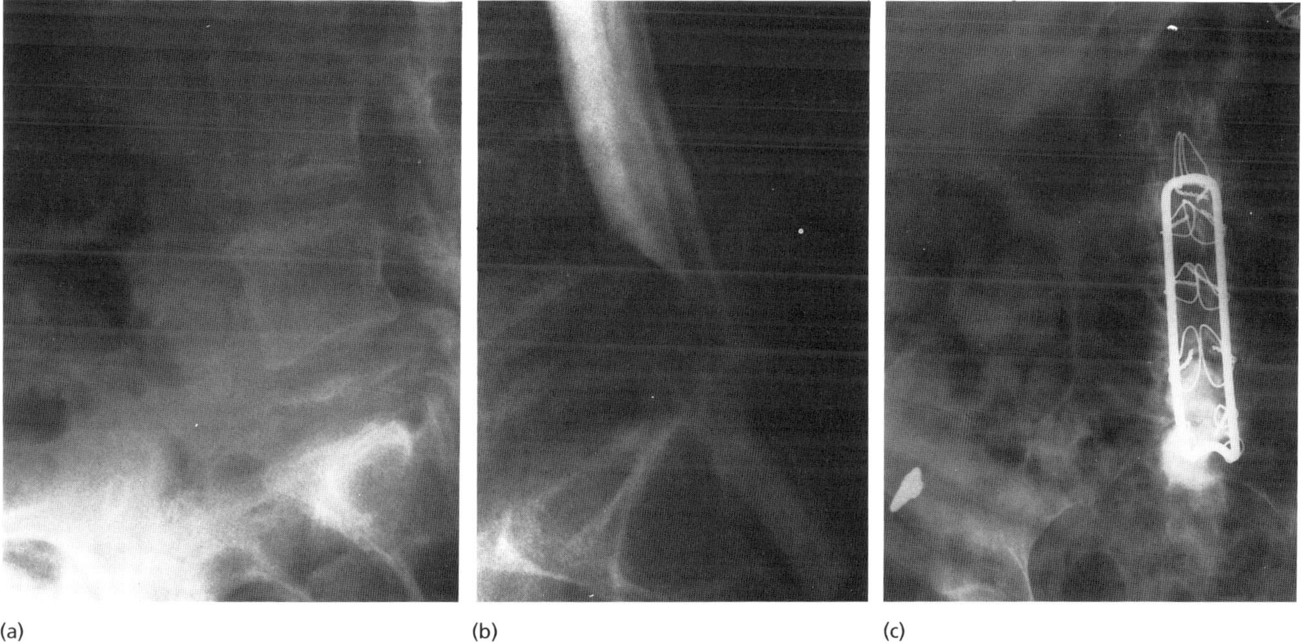

Fig. 26.10 (a) Patient with mammary carcinoma who developed spinal instability subsequent to destruction of the body of the L5 vertebra. (b) There were no neurological signs, although the radiculogram shows compression of the dural sheath at L5. (c) The patient was treated by anterior decompression and stabilization with methylmethacrylate, followed by posterior stabilization with a Hartshill rectangle.

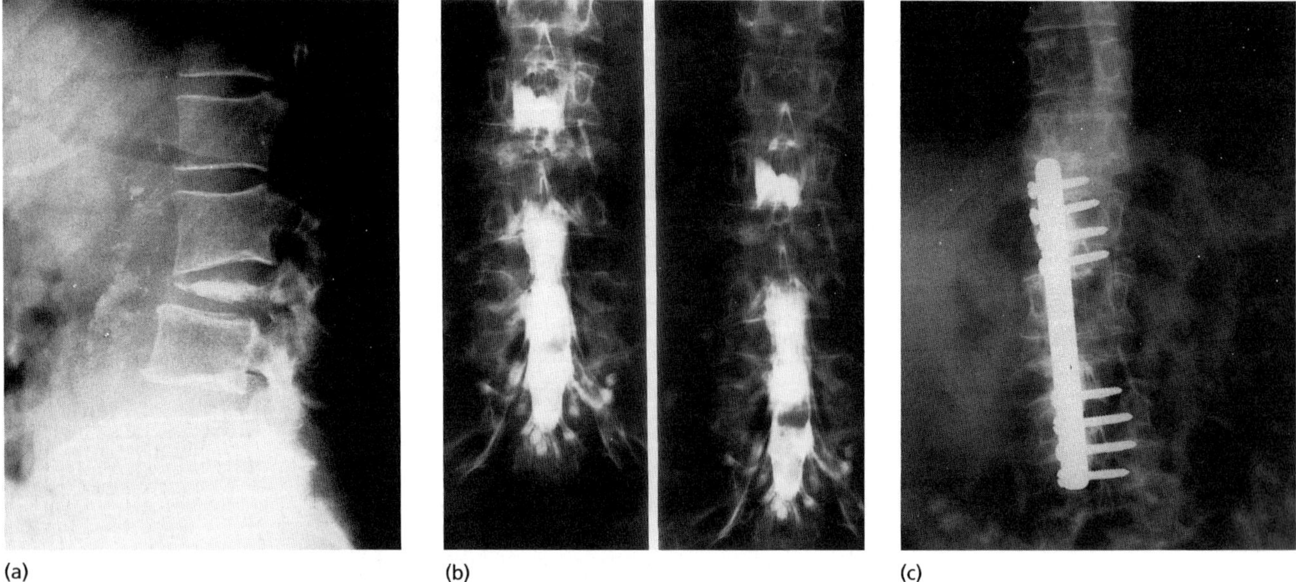

(a)   (b)   (c)

Fig. 26.11 (a) Patient with carcinoma of the cervix who presented with spinal instability due to destruction of the L3 vertebra. (b) This was associated with paraparesis and a complete block on the myelogram. (c) The patient was treated with posterior decompression, the laminae and spinous process of L3 being removed and stabilized with a Banks–Dervin rod. The patient made a full recovery, regaining bladder control and full motor power, and had complete relief of pain.

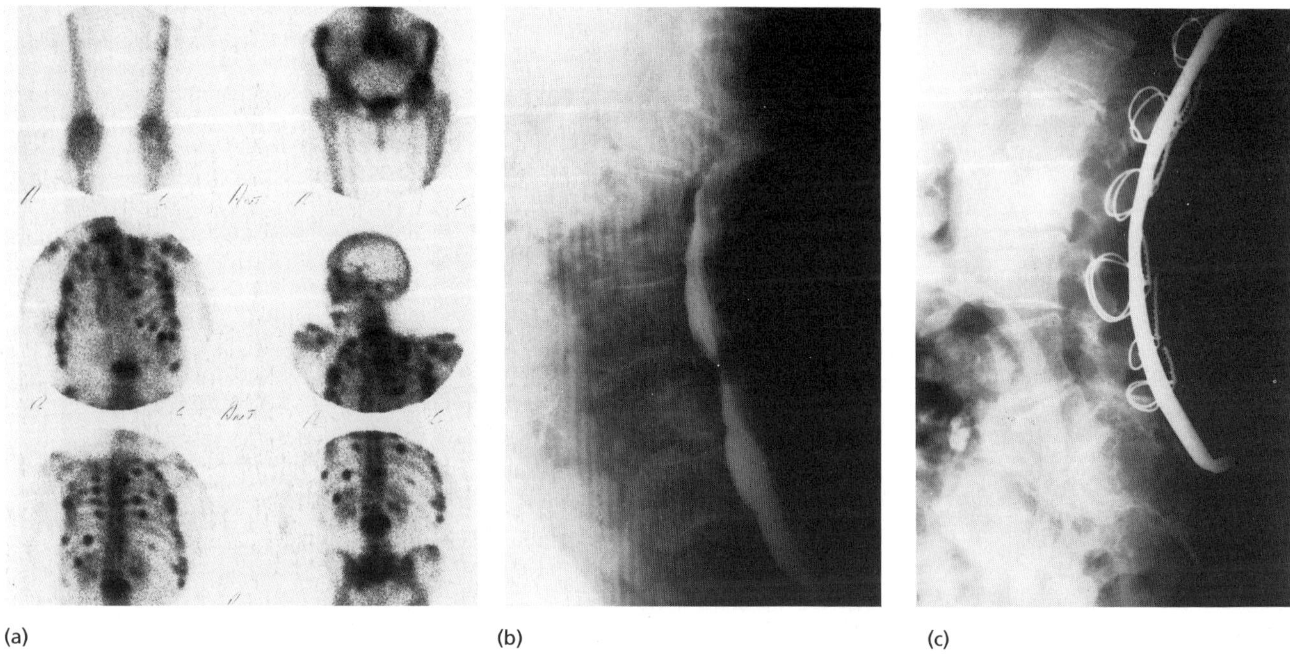

(a)   (b)   (c)

Fig. 26.12 Patient with mammary carcinoma who presented with severe back pain secondary to spinal instability, and profound weakness affecting the left lower limb. (a) The skeletal scintigram shows multiple skeletal involvement. (b) The plain radiographs show destruction of the body of L3, and the radiculogram shows marked compression of the dural sheath at that level. (c) The patient was treated by posterior decompression and stabilization using a Hartshill rectangle. The rectangle has been moulded to maintain a lumbar lordosis and the fixation has been extended to the sacrum. Postoperatively the patient received localized radiotherapy and endocrine therapy. This patient made a full recovery and was alive and well 5 years later, although still receiving endocrine therapy.

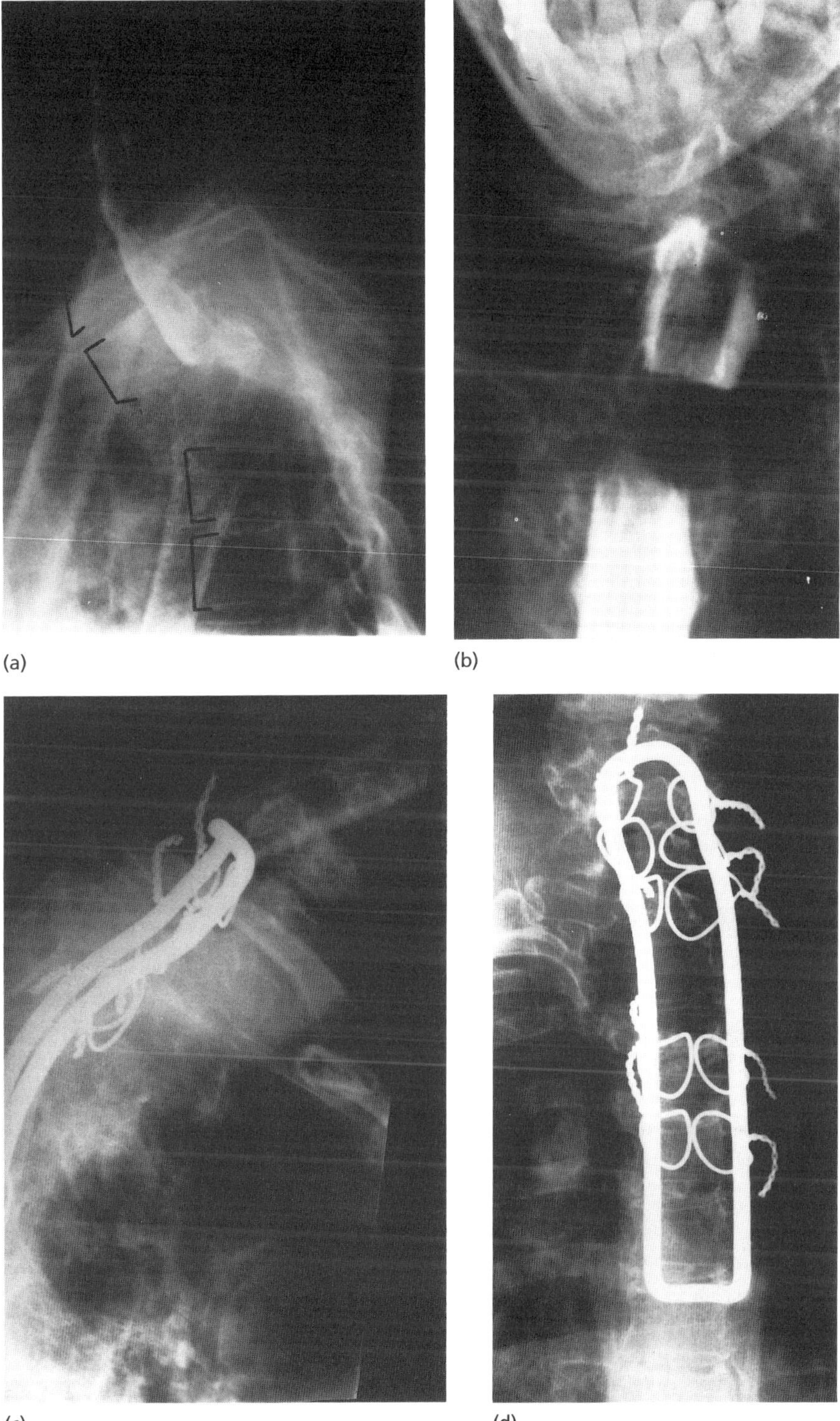

Fig. 26.13 Patient with disseminated mammary carcinoma. (a) Gross destruction of D3 with subluxation of D2 upon D4. (b) The myelogram shows a complete block at that level. The patient had been paraplegic for 12 hours and had urinary retention of 18-hours duration. (c) (d) After treatment by posterior decompression and stabilization with a Hartshill rectangle to correct the subluxation, the patient regained full bladder control and was able to walk independently when discharged from hospital 6 weeks later.

Minor degrees can sometimes be controlled by a collar, but if this does not relieve the pain surgical stabilization is indicated. Pathological fractures of the odontoid process may occur and can be easily overlooked (Lally *et al.* 1977). This lesion is particularly important if the patient is undergoing general anaesthesia. If the tumour is radiosensitive it can be treated by posterior stabilization and radiotherapy given anteriorly to the region of the odontoid. If the tumour is radioresistant the odontoid can be excised, via either a transoral or a lateral approach, and the spine stabilized posteriorly.

Lesions of the body of C2 also pose technical prob-

Table 26.3 Methods of spinal stabilization in cases of spinal instability

Method	Patients treated
Harrington rod	5
Harrington rod + sublaminal wiring	1
Banks–Dervin rod	26
Segmental sublaminal stabilization	
Double 'L' rod	1
Hartshill rectangle	31*
Isola	3
Combined anterior and posterior stabilization	5

* One patient had a lumbar stabilization 22 months after a successful dorsal stabilization.

Table 26.4 Results of spinal stabilization for instability secondary to metastatic cancer

Result	Number of patients
Infection resulting in removal of implant	1
Loosening	2
Extradural bleed in patient on anticoagulants for pulmonary embolus	1
Septicaemia	1
Relief of pain	
Complete	64
Partial	3
Complications in 67 patients with pain relief	
Infection, successfully treated	1
Wound breakdown requiring secondary suture/flap	2
Fracture of 'L' rod, requiring anterior graft	1
Fracture of Hartshill rectangle at 5 years	1

Table 26.5 Associated neurological complications in patients with spinal instability secondary to metastatic cancer

Number of patients	34
Number with complete/major* recovery following posterior decompression and stabilization	23
Late compression (8 months after stabilization)	1
Recurrence of compression	2
Extradural haematoma	1

* Major recovery indicates return of bladder function (if deficient) and sufficient power to allow independent ambulation.

(Harrington 1981). The proponents for anterior stabilization claim that they obtain a better spinal decompression, as the metastasis usually arises within the vertebral body. However, by the time spinal instability is complicated by dural sheath compression, the tumour has completely surrounded the dura and either anterior or posterior decompression will suffice, providing pressure is taken off the dural sheath and the decompression is combined with spinal stabilization.

Impending fracture

Patients with skeletal metastases may present with pain associated with a lesion which is liable to fracture. This occurs most commonly with a large lytic metastasis and the risk of fracture is related to the size of the lesion (Fidler 1981). However, bones riddled with permeative metastases are just as liable to fracture, even though a large discrete lytic deposit cannot be seen (Fig. 26.8).

Internal stabilization followed by postoperative irradiation after the wound has healed and chemotherapy or endocrine therapy is the treatment of choice. It is easier to stabilize a bone whilst it is intact. The limb must be carefully protected whilst the operation site is being prepared, otherwise a fracture may occur at this stage. As with pathological fractures it is essential that the internal stabilization of the lesion provides sufficient strength to allow unsupported use of the limb, including weight-bearing in the lower limbs. If the implant is not likely to provide this the stabilization should be supplemented with methylmethacrylate. The tumour is removed, the cavity filled with methylmethacrylate whilst still soft, and the implant fixed across the methylmethacrylate to normal bone above and below the lesion. Filling a large defect with methylmethacrylate was associated with a significant increase in both axial load and torque strength (Ryan & Begeman 1984).

lems. They are probably best treated by posterior stabilization using some form of occipito-cervical plate, such as the Ransford loop. Lesions of the lower cervical spine can be treated either by posterior stabilization using a Hartshill rectangle or by anterior resection and stabilization with a composite implant of methylmethacrylate and metal (Dunn 1977). The alternative treatment is anterior stabilization. The affected vertebral body is resected, the dural sheath is decompressed from in front and the spine is stabilized using methylmethacrylate

Internal fixation carries a theoretical risk of disseminating tumour cells both locally and into the circulation. However, this has never been proven providing the lesion is irradiated.

As with pathological fractures it is important that, prior to surgery, scintigrams and radiographs are obtained of the entire length of the affected bone, so that any other metastases, which may subsequently develop into a pathological fracture, can be stabilized and included in the radiotherapy field. A pathological fracture at the edge of a plate or intramedullary nail, particularly if the implant has been fixed with methylmethacrylate, is more difficult to treat than if there was no implant in the bone, and it is extremely difficult to irradiate a metastasis if part of the lesion has been included in a previous field.

Fracture through a benign tumour

There are two aspects to treatment; first, the treatment of the fracture, and secondly, the treatment of the underlying lesion.

The diagnosis of a unicameral bone cyst can usually be made from the radiographs but if there is any doubt, biopsy is indicated. The fracture is usually stable and can be treated by immobilization in a lightweight cast. The fracture may initiate healing of the cyst. If this does not occur, then excision, curettage and grafting of the cyst, or injection of steroids (Oppenheim & Galleno 1984), is indicated. Oppenheim and Galleno (1984) suggested that steroid injection resulted in a lower morbidity and lower recurrence rate.

Other benign tumours that fracture, for example, enchondroma, should be treated by curettage and bone grafting.

Giant cell tumours are benign in that they very rarely metastasize, but they tend to recur locally. They affect the epiphyseal and metaphyseal region of a long bone, most frequently at the knee, after the epiphysis has fused. When extensive they are usually associated with a fracture through the cortex, but occasionally may fracture through the subchondral bone into the joint. The treatment depends on their grade, size and location. They are usually treated by curettage and bone grafting, frequently combined with cryosurgery; excision with bone grafting; or prosthetic replacement.

Fracture through a malignant tumour

The fracture should be immobilized until the diagnosis is made. This may require radiographs, skeletal scintigrams, CT scans, magnetic resonance images and biopsy. The treatment depends on the tumour, the site of fracture and the general condition of the patient, but several principles apply. The development of a fracture usually implies that the tumour is too advanced for localized resection and prosthetic replacement; an amputation is generally indicated.

If the patient has disseminated disease and only palliative treatment is indicated, internal fixation of the fracture combined with radiotherapy and chemotherapy may provide the patient with useful function of the limb during the remaining months. A terminally ill patient should be made comfortable, usually with some form of external immobilization, for the remaining days.

Infection

A fracture through an osteomyelitic bone is a pathological fracture, whereas osteomyelitis complicating a compound fracture, or internal fixation of a traumatic fracture, is a complication of the fracture and is not pathological in the sense that the bone was normal prior to fracture.

Osteomyelitis still occurs commonly in the developing world, although the incidence has diminished in the Western world. Most cases are diagnosed early but neglected cases are still occasionally seen, by which time there may be much bone resorption. In most cases this is associated with new bone (involucrum) enveloping the necrotic bone (sequestrum) and this maintains the strength of the bone, but occasionally this is not the case and a pathological fracture occurs (Fig. 26.14). The aim of treatment is to eradicate the infection and then graft the defect. All pus must be drained and several operations may be required before all infected and necrotic material has been excised. The fracture should be stabilized and usually some form of external fixation is required. A modified external fixator may have to be made for a young child. Once the cavity is clean it should be bone grafted. In the young child bone grafting and immobilization will usually suffice, but in the older patient a more formal Papineau technique may be required (Vidal *et al.* 1976).

Figure 26.14 shows the radiograph of an adolescent female who, 10 years previously, had developed a pathological fracture through an osteomyelitic femur. Several attempts at bone grafting, including a vascularized fibular bone graft, had failed. When the patient was referred to this author's unit, the limb was 20 cm short and an amputation had been advised. The patient was wearing an orthosis to control the limb. This patient was treated by combined external fixation, bone grafting, electrical stimulation of the bone graft and immobil-

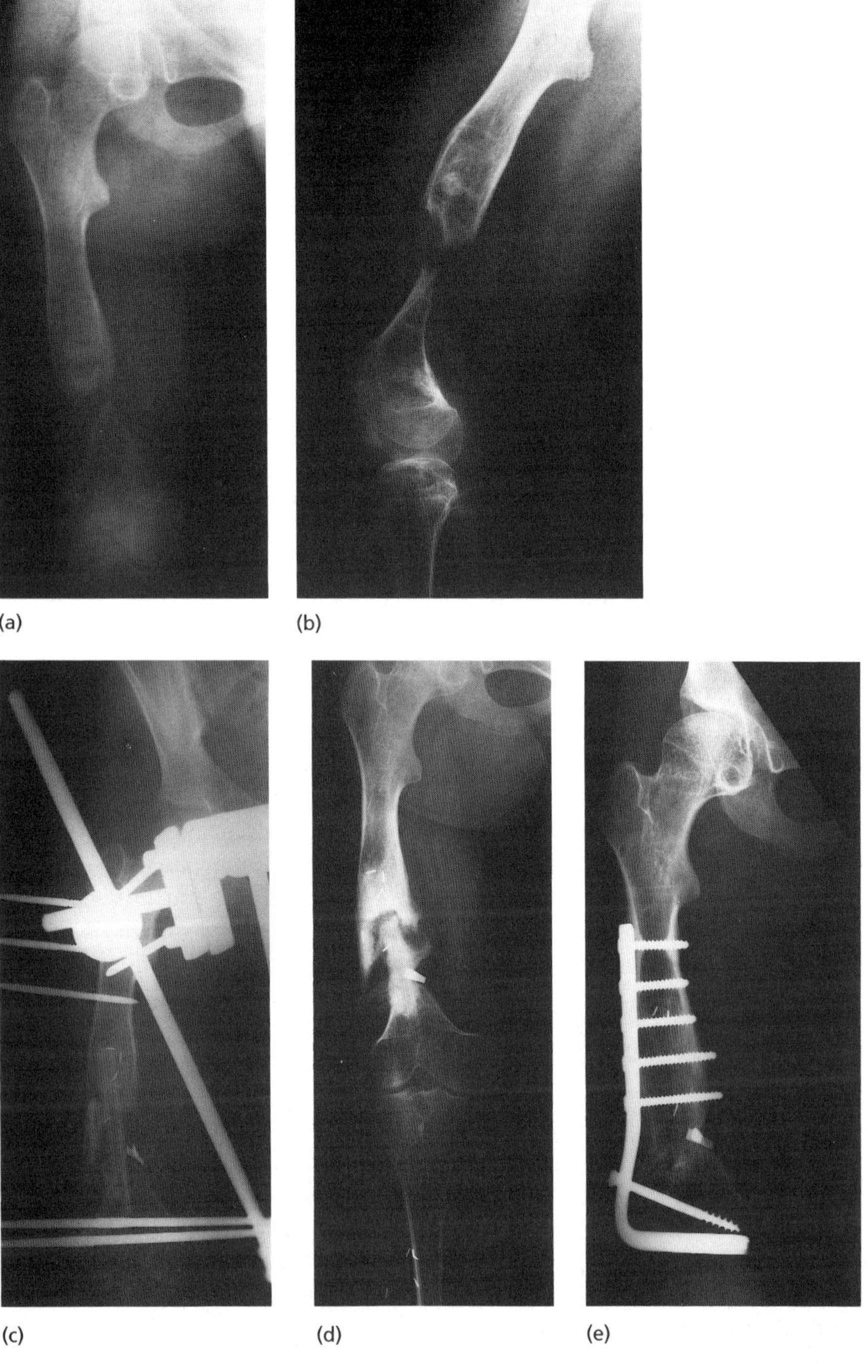

Fig. 26.14 This adolescent female had developed osteomyelitis of the right femur 10 years previously. Although the infection was treated, a pathological fracture developed and failed to unite. The patient wore an orthosis to control the limb. (a) and (b) Plain radiographs showing the shortened femur, pathological fracture and markedly thinned distal femoral metaphysis. (c) An attempt was made to treat the patient with a vascularized fibular graft. (d) The graft united distally but failed to unite proximally. (e) The patient was then treated by internal stabilization with a blade plate, bone grafting, electrical stimulation and external immobilization in a hip spica. The fracture went on to union and the patient has subsequently undergone femoral lengthening.

izization in a hip spica. The fracture united and the patient subsequently underwent a distal femoral and tibial lengthening procedure.

The development of the Ilizarov and similar frames has led to improvement in the treatment of infected non-unions. The frame is fixed and all infected and necrotic bone is excised. Subsequently, the defect is closed by transporting bone from a proximal or distal osteotomy site (the osteotomy site depending on the site of the infected non-union), using callus distraction at the osteotomy site. The timing of the osteotomy, callus distraction, and transport of healthy bone to close the defect, depends on the eradication of the infection.

Fractures in neuromuscular disease

Several factors predispose to pathological fracture in neuromuscular disease. The bones are osteoporotic, presumably secondary to disuse as a result of the underlying weakness. In many of these neurological conditions the bones grow normally in length but this is not always the case in spina bifida. However, appositional growth is sometimes inadequate and the shafts are much smaller in diameter than normal. If there is an associated sensory deficiency, for example, in myelomeningocoele, or congenital sensory neuropathy the patient is unable to protect against trauma and does not always realize that a fracture has been sustained because of the lack of pain. The osteoporosis is made worse by immobilization and the highest incidence of fractures occurs after surgery when the cast is removed.

Myelomeningocoele

Because of the risk of fracture following surgery (Fig. 26.15) these patients must be carefully mobilized when they come out of plaster. Their joints are frequently stiff and hydrotherapy is very useful: this not only helps to mobilize the joints but also encourages weight-bearing in the water before patients proceed to weight-bearing on land.

These fractures are often associated with exuberant callus and the limb may be red and swollen, but because of the sensory deficiency tenderness is usually absent. The fracture should be immobilized for as short a time as possible.

Muscular dystrophy

Fractures occur commonly (Fig. 26.16) (Hsu & Garcia-Aviz 1981). Mobile patients tend to fall frequently as a result of their muscle weakness and it is not uncommon for a patient to fall out of a wheelchair. The fracture should be treated by immobilization in a lightweight cast and the patient should be immediately mobilized. This is particularly important in a child who is still mobile. Immobilization in bed for 3–4 days can result in rapid muscle wasting, following which the child may no longer be able to walk. The aim of treatment is to maintain the mobility of the child and minimize the period of immobilization, even if this results in some shortening at the fracture site.

Cerebral palsy

Pathological fractures occur less frequently in patients with cerebral palsy than in patients with myelomeningocoele or muscular dystrophy, but they do occur.

There are two distinct varieties. Like all patients with neuromuscular disease, patients with cerebral palsy de-

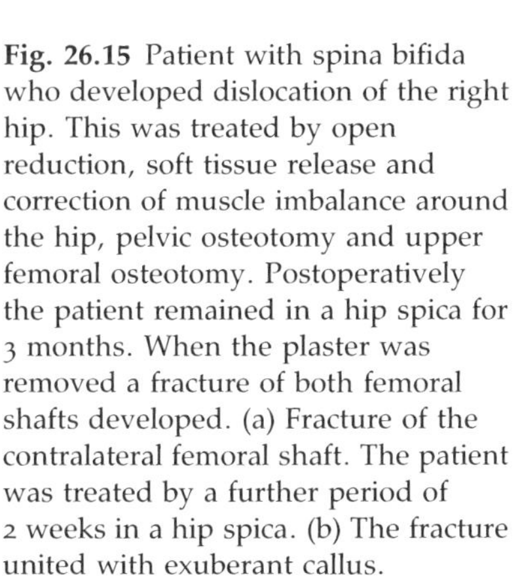

Fig. 26.15 Patient with spina bifida who developed dislocation of the right hip. This was treated by open reduction, soft tissue release and correction of muscle imbalance around the hip, pelvic osteotomy and upper femoral osteotomy. Postoperatively the patient remained in a hip spica for 3 months. When the plaster was removed a fracture of both femoral shafts developed. (a) Fracture of the contralateral femoral shaft. The patient was treated by a further period of 2 weeks in a hip spica. (b) The fracture united with exuberant callus.

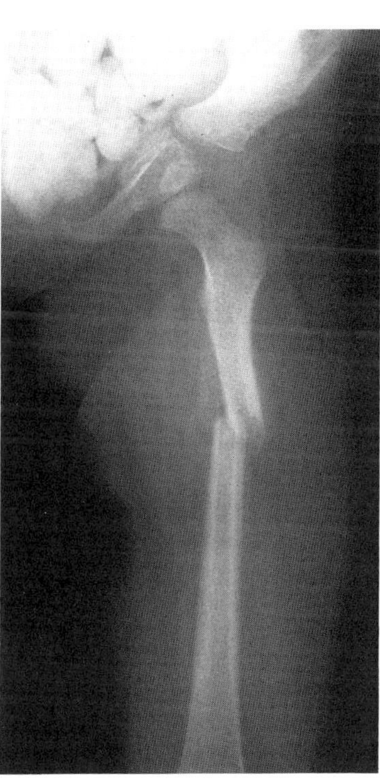

(a)

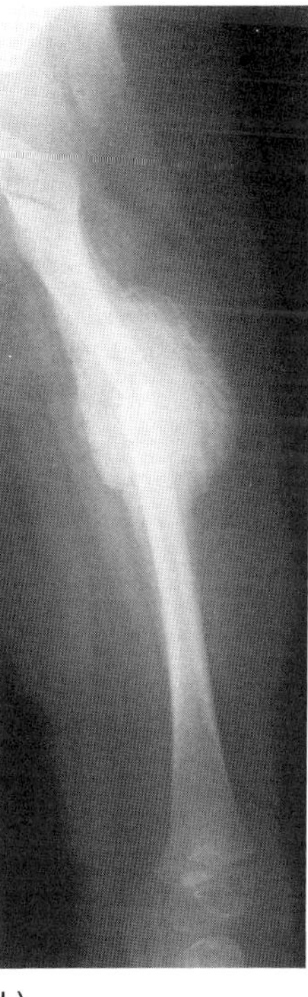

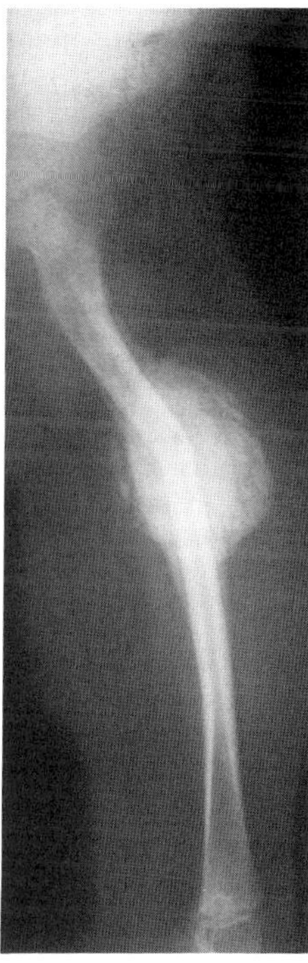

(b)

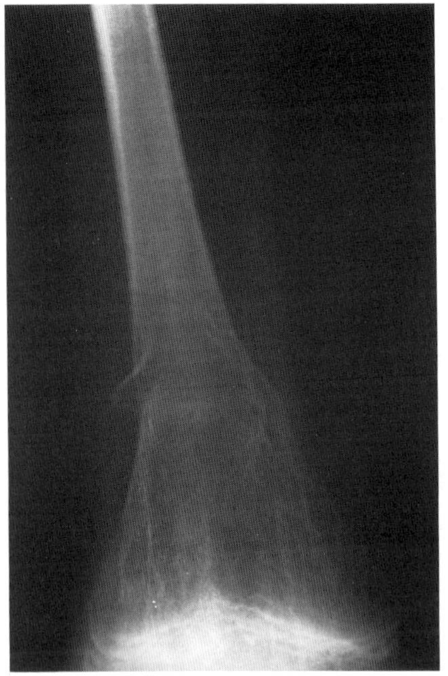

(a)

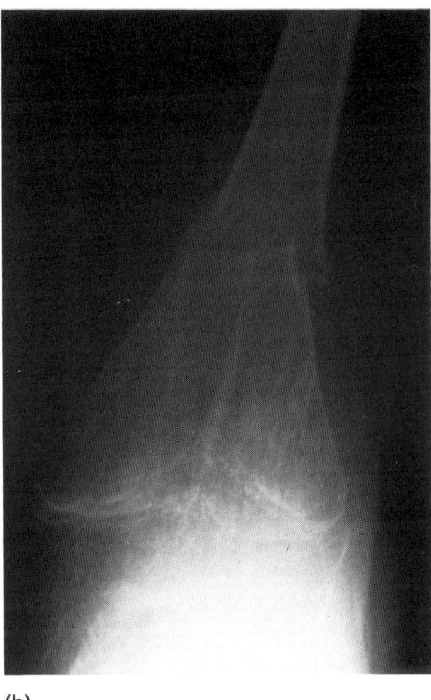

(b)

Fig. 26.26 (a) and (b) Patient with Duchenne muscular dystrophy who developed bilateral supracondylar femoral fractures.

velop marked disuse osteoporosis following surgery and immobilization in a plaster cast. Following removal of the cast there is a risk of fracture through the osteoporotic bone, although this risk is less than in spina bifida. Nevertheless, the same precautions must be taken in mobilizing the child. This is sometimes aggravated by spasm. Many patients with cerebral palsy develop increased spasm when they come out of plaster and suitable medication should be commenced prior to removal of the cast.

The second type of fracture is a stress fracture, secondary to the spasm. The most common site is at the patella. This is usually associated with a patella alta and tight hamstrings causing a fixed flexion deformity of the knee.

Dysplasias

Patients with osteogenesis imperfecta tend to have repeated and multiple fractures (Fig. 26.3). The aim of treatment is to immobilize the child as little as possible and early weight-bearing is to be encouraged. This is usually achieved by immobilization in a lightweight cast and in the smaller child a cotton wool compression bandage may suffice. Intramedullary rod fixation is indicated where patients suffer repeated fracture. At the time of surgery the previous deformity of the bone (usually secondary to previously healed fractures) can be corrected by osteotomy. Because of continuing growth of

the femur and tibia the rods rapidly become too short and fractures may occur at the extremities of the bone. Therefore, the rods need to be replaced at regular intervals. In an attempt to reduce the frequency of replacement expanding rods have been developed but these are more difficult to insert and have a high complication rate.

The Morel pneumatic orthosis (Morel 1971) can be used to rehabilitate a child who has become demoralized and chairbound by repeated fractures. This device is based on a pilot's 'G' suit, provides all-round support for the lower limbs and allows weight to be borne partially through the legs and partially through the inflated tubes of the suit. Corrective osteotomies may be required to straighten the limbs before the suit can be fitted. However, the suit is cumbersome and expensive and many children discard it. The author has no personal experience with the use of this device. Letts *et al.* (1988) recently described the use of 'vacuum pants' to prevent recurrent fractures of the lower limbs. The 'trousers' are filled with styrofoam beads that coalesce into a rigid system when air is evacuated and this allows the child to stand comfortably.

In osteopetrosis the fractures are transverse and slow to heal. They may require internal fixation, or external support for many months. Intramedullary rods can be difficult to insert because of the dense marrow cavity and hard dense bone.

Rheumatoid arthritis

The combination of osteoporosis (partly due to the disease process and partly due to the use of steroids) and stiff joints predisposes patients to fractures from trivial injuries. This applies both to the adult with rheumatoid arthritis and to the child with juvenile chronic arthritis. The most common site of fracture is the supracondylar region of the femur. Satisfactory internal fixation is often impossible to achieve because of the extreme porosity of the bone and the presence of adjacent total knee and/or hip arthroplasties. In the child, plaster immobilization is usually indicated, although the fracture should be immobilized for as short a time as possible. In the adult, external fixation with bone grafting may be of value to immobilize the fracture but allow movement of the adjacent joints and to minimize the period of bedrest.

Fractures in haemophilia

Boardman and English (1980) found that one-third of these fractures occurred at the elbow or knee and that a significant number were caused by trivial or minor trauma in severely affected patients. Bleeding must be controlled by factor VIII and the fracture must be rigidly immobilized. If surgery is required, either because the fracture cannot be controlled by splintage or because there is an associated compartment syndrome, a factor VIII level of 60% was found to be necessary for a period of 2 weeks (Boardman & English 1980). The majority of fractures can be adequately immobilized in a well-padded plaster, which must be split. Once the bleeding is controlled and the swelling has settled the plaster can be completed. If a fracture of the femur is being treated on a Thomas's splint, the ring must be split. Patients with auto-inhibitors pose a problem. Human factor VIII should be avoided, and in one case described by Boardman and English excessive bleeding was managed successfully by a simple blood transfusion.

Fractures secondary to irradiation

Fractures may occur in bones which previously have been irradiated; for example, fractures of the proximal femur may occur in patients treated by external irradiation for a carcinoma of the cervix. Union is usually delayed. Transcervical fractures should be treated by replacement arthroplasty, most frequently a total hip replacement, whereas other fractures require internal fixation and bone grafting.

Sickle cell disease

Ebong (1986) reported that pathological fracture of a long bone occurred in 26 out of 129 (20.2%) consecutive patients with sickle cell disease. In these patients the sickle cell disease was complicated by osteomyelitis, but the role of osteomyelitis in its causation is not defined (Bohrer 1970). In most instances the fractures occur in osteoporotic bones, the osteoporosis being secondary to the chronic anaemia and hyperplastic marrow, but occasionally pathological fractures occur at the site of acute infarcts.

Summary

There are two aspects to treating a pathological fracture. First, the underlying disease process must be diagnosed and, under certain circumstances, treatment must be instituted prior to the second aspect, that of definitive management of the fracture. Such treatment is necessary for patients with chronic bronchitis, etc., in the elderly patient with an osteoporotic fracture.

There are several phases to the management of the fracture. Temporary immobilization is required whilst the patient is being investigated for the cause of the underlying pathological process and treatment (where indicated) is started. Because many of the causative pathological processes are associated with osteoporosis, further osteoporosis secondary to disuse must be minimized by early mobilization.

In patients with a limited life expectancy (e.g. those with pathological fractures secondary to metastatic cancer) rigid internal fixation and early mobilization are indicated to provide maximum palliation for the patient. Where necessary, the implant must be supplemented by methylmethacrylate to allow the patient unsupported use of the limb (including weight-bearing in the lower limb).

Many fractures fail to unite unless they are rigidly immobilized, e.g. in Paget's disease or irradiated bone and primary bone grafting is sometimes indicated.

In some circumstances the treatment of the primary lesion takes precedence over the treatment of the fracture. For example, a fracture in an osteosarcoma with no evidence of distant dissemination is probably best treated by amputation and adjuvant chemotherapy, whereas a fracture through a giant cell tumour may be best treated by localized resection of the tumour and prosthetic replacement.

References

Bastow, M.D., Rawlings, J. & Allison, S.P. Under-nutrition, hypothermia and injury in elderly women with fractured femur: an injury response to altered metabolism? *Lancet* 1983; **1**: 143−146.

Boardman, K.P. & English, P. Fractures and dislocations in haemophilia. *Clin Orthop* 1980; **148**: 221.

Bohrer, S.P. Acute long bone diaphyseal infarcts in sickle cell disease. *Br J Radiol* 1970; **43**: 685−697.

Dimon, J.H. & Hughston, J.C. Unstable intertrochanteric fractures of the hip. *J Bone Joint Surg* 1967; **49A**: 440−450.

Dove, J. Complete fractures of the femur in Paget's disease of bone. *J Bone Joint Surg* 1980; **62B**: 12−17.

Dunn, E.J. The role of methylmethacrylate in the stabilisation and replacement of tumours of the cervical spine. *Spine* 1977; **2**: 15−24.

Ebong, W.W. Pathological fracture complicating long bone osteomyelitis in patients with sickle cell disease. *J Pediatr Orthop* 1986; **6**: 177−181.

Fidler, M. Incidence of fracture through metastases in long bones. *Acta Orthop Scand* 1981; **52**: 623−627.

Fidler, M.W. Pathological fractures of the spine including those causing anterior spinal compression: surgical management. In: Noble, J. & Galasko, C.S.B. (eds) *Recent Developments in Orthopaedic Surgery: Festschrift to Sir Harry Platt*. Manchester University Press: Manchester, 1987.

Galasko, C.S.B. Pathological fractures secondary to metastatic cancer. *J R Coll Surg Edinb* 1974; **19**: 351−362.

Galasko, C.S.B. *Skeletal Metastases*. Butterworth: London, 1986.

Galasko, C.S.B. & Sylvester, B.S. Back pain in patients treated for malignant tumours. *Clin Oncol* 1978; **4**: 273−283.

Galasko, C.S.B., Rushton, J., Sylvester, B.S., Steingold, R.F., Noble, J. & Boston, D.A. The significance of peak expiratory flow rate in assessing prognosis of elderly patients undergoing operations on the hip. *Injury* 1985; **16**: 398−401.

Garden, R.S. Stability and union in subcapital fractures of the femur. *J Bone Joint Surg* 1964; **46B**: 630−647.

Greatorex, I.F. & Gibbs, A.C.C. Proximal femoral fractures: some determinants of outcome. *J Epidemiol Community Health* 1988; **42**: 365−369.

Hamdy, R.C. *Paget's Disease of Bone*. Praeger: Eastbourne, 1981.

Harrington, K.D. The use of methylmethacrylate for vertebral-body replacement and anterior stabilization of pathological fracture−dislocations of the spine due to metastatic malignant disease. *J Bone Joint Surg* 1981; **63A**: 36−46.

Hsu, J.D. & Garcia-Aviz, M. Fractures of the femur in the Duchenne muscular dystrophy patient. *J Pediatr Orthop* 1981; **1**: 203−207.

Lally, J.F., Cossrow, J.I. & Dalinka, M.K. Odontoid fractures in metastatic breast carcinoma. *Am J Roentgenol* 1977; **128**: 817−820.

Letts, M., Monson, R. & Weber, K. The prevention of recurrent fractures of the lower extremities in severe osteogenesis imperfecta using vacuum pants: a preliminary report in four patients. *J Pediatr Orthop* 1988; **8**: 454−457.

Milgram, J.W. Orthopaedic management of Paget's disease of bone. *Clin Orthop* 1977; **127**: 63−69.

Morel, G. Revue de chérurgie orthopedique et reparatrice. *De L'Appareil Moteur* 1971; **54**: 409.

Nicholas, J.A. & Killoran, P. Fracture of the femur in patients with Paget's disease. Results of treatment in 23 cases. *J Bone Joint Surg* 1965; **47A**: 450−461.

Oppenheim, W.L. & Galleno, H. Operative treatment versus steroid injection in the management of unicameral bone cysts. *J Pediatr Orthop* 1984; **4**: 1.

Ryan, J.R. & Begeman, P.C. The effects of filling experimental large cortical defects with methylmethacrylate. *Clin Orthop* 1984; **185**: 306−310.

Sarmiento, A. & Williams, E.M. The unstable intertrochanteric fracture: treatment with a valgus osteotomy and I-beam nail plate. A preliminary report of 100 cases. *J Bone Joint Surg* 1970; **52A**: 1309−1318.

Vidal, J., Buscayret, C. & Paran, M. Utilisation de la technique de Papineau dans le traitement des fractures ouvertes. *Acta Orthop Belg* 1976; **42**: 42−49.

Wallace, W.A. The scale and financial implications of osteoporosis. *Int Med Suppl* 1987; **12**: 3−4.

Woolf, A.D. & Dixon, A. StJ. *Osteoporosis: A Clinical Guide*. Martin Dunitz: London, 1988.

Wyman, E.T. Jr. Fixation of intertrochanteric fractures. In: Leach, R.E., Hoaglund, F.T. & Riseborough, E.J. (eds) *Controversies in Orthopaedic Surgery*. WB Saunders: Philadelphia, 1982.

Index

Note: Page numbers in *italic* refer to figures and/or tables

Aa oxygen gradient 144
AARF 351
abbreviated injury score 112
abdominal trauma 114–26
abductor digiti minimi flap 231
abductor hallucis 871
 flap 231
abductor pollicis brevis 435
abductor pollicis longus 435
abrasion arthroplasty 83
accessory collateral ligament
 MP joint 529
 PIP joint 524
accessory ossicles 62, 858, 864, *865*, 879–80, *881*
acetabulum
 anatomy 623, *624*
 fracture 622–3, 629
  classification 625, *626*
  complications 629
  diagnosis 623–4, *625*
  and hip dislocation 631
  management 625–7
  postoperative care 628–9
  surgery 628
 radiography 53
Achilles tendon 833
 avulsion of inversion 835, *837*
 MRI 67, *68*
ACL *see* anterior cruciate ligament
acromio-clavicular joint
 anatomy 353
 dislocation 331, 353, 358–9
  age distribution 331
  classification 354, *355*
  early management 354–7
  late management 357
  outcome 357–8, *359*, *360*
  pathology 353–4
  postoperative care 356–7
  radiography 53, 354, 358, *359*, *360*
  surgical stabilization 355–6
  symptoms and signs 331, 354
 post-traumatic arthritis 348–9
 sprain 354, *355*
 subluxation 354, *355*
acromion 332
 fracture *398*, 399
acromionectomy 397
acute cardiocirculatory failure *see* shock

acute dislocation 35
adductor hallucis 871
ADH-vasopressin secretion in shock 93
adrenaline, systemic reactions to 201
adult respiratory distress syndrome (ARDS) 283, 298–9
 in femoral fracture 738
 following pathological fracture 892
 in long bone fracture 807
 pathophysiology 299
 in polytrauma 737
 and shock 96, 110
 treatment 299–300
age
 and chest injury 141
 and fracture healing 78
 and vascular damage 251
AIS 112
albumin
 in adult respiratory distress syndrome 300
 in septicaemic shock 101
alcohol, in fat embolism syndrome 285
aldosterone secretion in shock 93
algodystrophy 318
algoneurodystrophy 318
alpha-adrenergic blocking agents in haemorrhagic shock 99
alpha methyl tyrosine 601
aminoglycoside 209
amnesia in head injury 136
amputation
 in os calcis fracture 848
 in tibial shaft fracture 802
anabolic steroids in fracture healing 71, 78
anaesthesia 188
 assessment of risks 191–2
 awareness during 195
 and bleeding disorders 194
 choice of technique 193–202
 and concomitant medical disease 193
 and concurrent medication 188–9, 194
 and duration of surgery 194
 and fracture site 194
 and full stomach 190, 192, 194
 general 193, 194–5
  indications and contraindications 193–4
 in hand injury 496–7, *498*
 in head injury 137, 190–1, 192–3
 history of 188
 and hypovolaemia 194
 and incidence of DVT 290
 and infection 193–4
 preoperative assessment 188–91

 regional/local 193
  indications and contraindications 193–4
  techniques 195–202
 and sickle cell disease 194
 special investigations 189
 and timing of surgery 192–3
 in vascular injury 253
 volaemic status assessment 189–90
anal skin reflex 561, 598
analgesia in controlled ventilation 145
angiogenic growth factors 71
angiography 66
 abdominal trauma 116
 renal 151–2
 tibial shaft fracture 802
angulation 33
angulation fracture 32
anisotropic materials 4
ankle
 injury
  anatomical considerations 823
  associated with os calcis fracture 838
  classification 825–6, *827*
  complications 830
  management summary 830–1
  physiological considerations 823–5
  pronation–abduction 824
  pronation–external rotation 824
  radiography 54–5, *56–7*
  rehabilitation 830
  stability determination 823–5
  stability model 825
  supination–adduction 824
  supination–external rotation 824
  in talar neck fracture 851, *853*
  treatment
   aims 826
   non-operative 827
   operative 827–30
   reduction 826–7
 stress radiography 66
 tenography 66
ankle jerk 598
ankylosing spondylitis 588, *590*, 591
annular ligament 435
anosmia 137–8
anoxia 127–8
ANP, effect of shock on secretion 93
antegrade pyelography 154
anterior cord syndrome 555
anterior cruciate ligament (ACL)
 anatomy 762
 anteromedial band 765

anterior cruciate ligament (*cont.*)
injury 759–60, 763
acute tear 765–7
avulsion fracture 760–1
in femoral fracture 737
residual chronic laxity 770–1
tests 760, 763–5
MRI 67
posterolateral band 765
anterior drawer test
knee 764
shoulder 376
anterior longitudinal ligament 553
anterior sternoclavicular ligament 361
anterior tibial artery injury 794
anterior tibial nerve injury 810
anterior tibio-fibular ligament *825*
anteroinferior tibio-fibular ligament injury 824
anterolateral femorotibial ligament 767
Anthonsen's view 840, *841*
antibiotic therapy
adult respiratory distress syndrome 300
colonic trauma 126
following vascular injury repair 258
gas gangrene 298
head injury 134, 135
infected non-union 313–14
kidney injury 152
open fracture 209
proximal femoral fracture 657
septicaemic shock 103
tetanus 294, 296
tibial shaft fracture 801
vascular injury 254
anticoagulants
in anaesthesia 189
and compartment syndromes 272
in fat embolism syndrome 285, 286
following cervical spinal injury 562
prophylactic 289–90, 296, 658
therapeutic in DVT 289
in vascular injury 254
anus, trauma to 126
AO fixator 13, *212*
AO/ASIF group 18, 177, 695
aorta, injury 40, 258
aortic arch rupture 145–6
aortovelography in haemorrhagic shock 97
APD 895
appositional new bone 74
apprehension test 376–7
aprotinin in fat embolism syndrome 286
arcuate complex 762
arcuate ligament 760, 762
ARDS *see* adult respiratory distress syndrome
arm *see* forearm; upper arm
arterial injury *see* vascular injury
arteriography
following vascular repair 256–7
in vascular injury 253–4
arteriovenous fistula 252, 253
artery of the ligamentum teres 640, *641*
artery of the tarsal canal 850, *851*
artery of the tarsal sinus 850, *851*
arthrodesis
in scaphoid non-union 476
scaphoid-trapezium-trapezoid articulation 469, 478
triquetro-hamate articulation 469

arthrography 66
gleno-humeral joint instability 378
meniscal injury 773
wrist injury 451
arthroscopic surgery
anterior cruciate ligament injury 767
gleno-humeral joint instability 380–2
meniscal injury 773
arthroscopy
chronic anterior cruciate ligament laxity 770
gleno-humeral joint instability 378
in tibial spine fracture 786–7
articular cartilage
healing 79–80, 84–5
blunt impact 83–4
deep penetrating injury 81–3, Plate 5.1
superficial lacerative injury 80–1
necrosis 80
ASA physical status scale 191, *192*
ascending phlebography 658
aspiration pneumonitis 190
aspirin 258, 289, 658
Association for Osteosynthesis/Association for the Study of Problems of Internal Fixation group 18, 177, 695
atelectasis 139, 141
atherosclerosis 251–2
atlanto-axial joint
fusion
anterior 571, *578*
lateral 571
posterior 571, 578–9
instability 575, 577–9, *583*
in congenital abnormalities 575
rotatory injury 351, 572, *579*
subluxation with clavicle fracture 351
atlanto-occipital dislocation 566–7, *573*
atlas
congenital anomalies *567, 574*
fracture *567–8, 574, 575*
atracurium 295
atrial natriuretic peptide, effect of shock on secretion 93
Austin Moore hemiarthroplasty prosthesis 651, *653*
autonomic nervous system, effects of spinal cord lesions 554–5
avascular necrosis 322–3
and acetabular fracture 629
capitate 481
computerized tomography 326
and fracture healing 77
and hip dislocation 633, 635–6
humeral head 395
isotope bone scanning *323*, 324–6
lunate 477–8, *483*
magnetic resonance imaging 326, *327*
management 326
navicular 864, *866*
and non-union 326
in pathological fracture 891
in proximal femoral fracture 645, 656–7, 665
in radial neck fracture 428
radiography 323–4
in scaphoid fracture non-union 476, *477*
talus 853, 854–5, 862
avulsion fracture 32, 46
axial pattern flaps 227, 228, *229*
axillary artery injury 258, *259*, 387, *388*

axillary brachial plexus block 199–200, *201*
axillary nerve injury 369
axillary vein injury 387, *388*
axis, traumatic spondylolisthesis 572, 574, *580*
axonotmesis 41, 264, *265*
radial nerve 408

baclofen 606
bands of Büngner 266
Bankart lesion 368, 374–5, 378
Bankart operation 379–80, *381, 382*
baroreceptor system 91–2
Barton fracture 460, *461, 462*
Bateman bipolar hemiarthroplasty prosthesis 652
bend of bone 238–9
bending stress 5–6
Bennett's fracture 541–3
Bentzon procedure 476
benzodiazepines 196
biceps brachii 401
in cervical spinal injury 562
and displacement of humeral shaft fracture 402
biceps brachii tendon rupture 331, 397
biceps femoris 762
biceps femoris tendon 762
Bier's block 197–8, 497
bifurcate ligament 833
avulsion of insertion 836, *838*
Bigelow technique 633–4
biocompression 17
biodegradable implants 829–30
biological fixation 215, *216*, 811
biomechanics 3–6
clavicle fracture 334–5
femoral fracture 667–8, 673–4, 677–9, 696–8, *699*
of fracture healing 7–11, 698, *699*
of fracture production 6–7
pelvic fracture 617
sternoclavicular joint 361, 362
and treatment 11–24, 212–13
birth fracture 34, 350–1
bladder
injury 40, 155–6
clinical diagnosis 158–60
complications 162–3
management 158–61, *162*
mode of 156
in paraplegia 607
tear drop 160
Blair fusion 856
bleeding disorders and anaesthesia 194
blisters, fracture 249–50, 838, *839*
blood
assessment of loss 189–90
autotransfusion 97, 110
clotting 79
features in fat embolism syndrome 284–5
gas analysis 140, 189
letting 109
packed cells 110
plasma-reduced 110
preoperative sugar estimation 189
replacement
in haemorrhagic shock 97, *98*, 109–10
in septicaemic shock 101
substitutes 97, *98*, 101, 110–11

transfusion 109–10
warming devices 110
blood pressure 91
Boari technique 155, *156*
Böhler–Braun frame 694
Böhler stirrup 173, *174*
Böhler's angle 55, 833, *834*, 839
bone
cancellous, fracture healing 76
cortical, modulus of elasticity 4
cysts 63, 903
excision in open fracture 210
grafts
cancellous 310
in femoral shaft non-union 739
forearm fractures 442
in infected non-union 314, 315–16
inlay *310*
muscle-pedicle in proximal femoral
fracture 650–1
in non-union 309–10
onlay 310
in proximal humeral fracture 392, 394
in scaphoid fracture non-union 474
sliding 310
in tibial shaft fracture 818
primary healing 8, 74, 177, 215, 695
secondary healing 8, 314
structure and behaviour under stress in
childhood 237–8
bone morphogenic protein 71
bone transport 818
boutonnière deformity 49, 526–8
bowel, in paraplegia 607
bowing 29, 59
boxing glove bandage 503, 558, *559*
brachial artery 401, 407
angiography 66
injury 251, 259, 426
brachial plexus 332
anaesthesia 198–200, 497
injury 331
in birth fracture 34
in cervical spine injury 555
in clavicle fracture 345
neonatal 350–1
in proximal humeral fracture 387, *388*
in shoulder dislocation 369
with subclavian artery injury 258
brachial vein 401
thrombosis 337
brachialis 401
brachioradialis 401
bracing
functional
femur 694, 702, 704–5, *706–8*, 732, 744
forearm 435
humerus 404
in knee injury 772, 778
in tibial shaft fracture 805, *806*, 807
bradykinin and septic shock 100
brain swelling 133
Braun frame 175, *176*, *694*
breech delivery, clavicle fracture in 350
Bristow operation 379, 380
brittle materials, stress-strain curve 6
Broca lesion 378
Brodén's view 840, *841*
bronchial injury 142
bronchopleural fistula in chest drainage 148
bronchopneumonia 141

bronchospasm in fat embolism syndrome
284
Brown–Séquard syndrome 555, 584
bruising 38–9
buckle fracture 29, 238, *239*
distal radius 488
radiography 59, *60*
buddy taping 511
bulbocavernosus reflex 561, 598
bupivacaine 196, *197*, 497
burns and compartment syndromes 272
burrhole exploration in head injury 132–3
butterfly fragment 7, 31, 46, 824

calcaneo-cuboid joint
injury associated with os calcis fracture
840
in triple fusion 846, 847
calcaneofibular ligament rupture 66
calcaneo-navicular ligament 860
calcar femorale 639–40
calcitonin 71, 78, 895
calcium chloride
in blood transfusion 110
in septicaemic shock 102
callus 71, 791–2, *793*
asymmetrical formation 8, *9*
bridging 8, *9*, 62, 73–4
cartilaginous 73–4
external 73–4
formation 8
internal 74
in pathological fracture 891
provisional 71
radiography 61–2
capillary leak syndrome 101
capitate 448–9, *450*
avascular necrosis 481
dislocation 486
fracture 480–1
childhood 490
capitohamate ligament 448
carbon fibre, epoxy-reinforced 17
carbon rods 774
cardiac output determinants 91
cardiocirculatory failure *see* shock
cardiocirculatory monitoring in
haemorrhagic shock 96–7
cardiomyopathy 892
cardiovascular disease and anaesthesia 193
carotid artery injury 258, 345
carpal tunnel syndrome 270
following Colles' fracture 458
in lunate dislocation 483
in trans-scaphoid perilunate fracture–
dislocation 484
carpectomy, proximal row 475
carpometacarpal joint
injury 496, *497*, 538–9, *540*
thumb, dislocation 543–4
carpometacarpal ligament *448*
carpus 448–9
carpal arch injury 486–7
childhood injury 490
dislocations 481–7, 490
dorsal chip fracture 476, *477*
dorsal intercalated segment instability
466, 468
following Colles' fracture 459
fracture–dislocations 481–2, 484, 485, 490

fractures 469–81, 490
instability 465
childhood 490
classification 465–8
diagnosis 468–9
dynamic 466
static 465–6
treatment 469
osteoarthritis 469
volar intercalated segment instability 466,
467
Z-collapse *449*, 466
cartilaginous union 307
cast bracing *see* bracing, functional
casts 169–70
ankle injury 830
anterior cruciate ligament injury 766
biomechanical principles 11–12
in childhood 246
Colles' fracture 454, 456
and compartment syndromes 272
complications of use 170–1, *172*
following tourniquet use 204
hanging 168, 175, *177*, 403
humeral shaft fracture 168, 175, *177*, 403–4
in non-union 311
open fractures 211
os calcis fracture 846
pins through 211
scaphoid fracture 472
Smith fracture 461
sugar-tong/U-slab 403–4
thoraco-brachial spica 404
tibial shaft fracture 803–4
traction by 175–6, *177*
traction pin incorporation 173, *174*
wedging 171, *172*, 803–4
causalgia 318–21
cellulitis, anaerobic 297–8
central cord syndrome 552, 555
central venous pressure (CVP)
in compartment syndromes 276
in haemorrhagic shock 96
cephalic vein 407
cephalosporin 209, 298
cephalothin 657
CEPOD study 191
cerclage wire 177, 182, *183*
patellar fracture fixation 776, *777*
cerebral compression in head injury 128–34
cerebral contusion 130, *131*
cerebral palsy and pathological fracture 889,
905–6
cerebrospinal fluid, rhinorrhoea/otorrohoea
127, 135
cervical spine
injury 551
anterior subluxations 584–5, *586*, *587*
assessment and early management
556–64, *565–9*
associated injuries 559–60
atlanto-axial instability 575, 577–9, *583*
atlanto-axial rotatory injury 351, 572,
579
atlanto-occipital dislocation 566–7, *573*
atlas fracture 567–8, *574*, *575*
axial loading 588–9, *590*
bilateral facet dislocation 580–4
bursting fracture 553
childhood 574–5, *581*, 591
circulatory support 558

cervical spine (*cont.*)
    classification 551–2
    clinical features 556
    compression 551, 552, 553, 565
    distraction 551–2
    DVT prevention 562
    flexion 551–2, 553
    flexion–rotation 580–5, *586, 587*
    fracture–dislocation 553, *554*
    hyperextension 551–2, 553, 565, 585–8, *589, 590*
    and malformations 575, *582*
    mechanism 551
    mid and lower 580–92
    nerve injury in 555
    neurological examination 561–2
    odontoid process fracture 570–2, *576–8*
    operative procedures 589–90, *591*
    pharmacology 560–1
    pseudosubluxation in childhood 574
    psychological effects 555–6
    radiology 57, *58, 59*, 562–4, *565–9*
    rehabilitation 592–4
    respiratory care 556–7, *558*
    skin and joint care 558–9, *560*
    spinal cord injury in 553–5
    sprains 565
    stab and gunshot wounds 591
    stability 552–3
    subluxation 574–5, *581*
    suspected 39
    transverse ligament rupture 568, 570, *575*
    traumatic spondylolisthesis of axis 572, 574, *580*
    treatment 564–6, *570–2*
    unilateral facet dislocation 584
    upper 566–80, *581–3*
    urological care 559, *560*
    whiplash 565
  instability 897, 901–2
  MRI 68
  posterior ligamentous complex 552
  surgical approaches 580
  vertebral fusion
    anterior 590
    posterior 589–90, *592*
cervico-thoracic junction 551
Chance fracture 604, *605*, 609–10
Charnley traction unit 173, *174*
chemotherapy
  and fracture healing 78
  in spinal instability 896
chest drainage 147
  complications 147–8
  removal of drain 148
  subphrenic insertion 148
chest injury
  and age 141
  blood gas analysis in 140
  cardiocirculatory resuscitation 139
  co-existing injury 141–2
  gas exchange problems 139–40
  initial management 139–40
  occult 145–8
  pain relief 139, 143
  paradoxical ventilation 139–40
  penetrating 140
  pre-existing health status 141
  pulmonary contusions 140
  radiography 140–1
    severity
      assessment *142*
      classification 140–2
    treatment 142–5
      surgical 148
chest therapy in cervical spinal injury 557, *558*
childhood
  cervical spine
    hypermobility 563, *565*, 574
    injury 591
    pseudosubluxation 574
    subluxation 574–5, *581*
  chest injury 141
  clavicle fracture 349–52
  distal phalanx epiphyseal separation 507–9
  fractures
    classification 238–43
    complications 247
    diagnosis 245
    femur
      distal 735
      shaft 733–4
    healing 244–5
    indications for open reduction 246–7
    management principles 245–6
    radiography 57, 59, *60, 61*, 245
  head injury 136
  odontoid process fracture 572, *578*
  reflex sympathetic dystrophy in 320
  splenectomy in 119
  structure and behaviour of growing bone under stress 237–8
  urethral injury 164–5
  wrist injury 487–90
chlorpromazine
  adverse reactions to 293
  in haemorrhagic shock 99
chondral fracture 47
Chopart's dislocation 856, *862*, 863–4
Christiansen bipolar hemiarthroplasty prosthesis 652
chromotolysis 265
chronic obstructive airways disease 141
circulatory impairment due to plaster casts 170–1
classification
  dislocations 34–6
  fractures 29–34, 46–7
  see also under specific fractures
clavicle
  excision of lateral end 343, 357
  excision of medial end 344, 365
  fracture 148, 332
    age distribution 331
    biomechanics 334–5
    childhood 349–52
    classification 332–3, *334*
    clinical features 335
    complications 344–9
    distal with displacement 340–4
    malunion 348, *349*, 351
    mechanism of injury 334–5
    medial end 344
    neonatal 350–1
    non-union 345–8, 351
    post-traumatic arthritis 348–9
    radiology 335, 340–1, *342, 343*, 346, *347*, 351
    refracture 347, 352
    treatment
      conservative 335–7, 341–2
      incisions *337*, 339
      surgical 337–40, 343–4
    growth and development 349–50
    surgical anatomy 332
clavipectoral fascia 332
cleidocranial dysostoses 351
clindamycin 298
clinical union 302
clofibrate 286
closed dislocation 36
closed fracture 32–3
Clostridium histolyticum 297
Clostridium oedematiens 297
Clostridium perfringens 297
Clostridium septicum 297
Clostridium tetani 292
coagulation tests, preoperative 189
cock robin appearance 572
collagen
  in ligaments 87
  in tendons 86
collar 565
collateral ligament
  MP joint 529–30, 544
  PIP joint 524
Colles' fracture 270, 450, 452
  carpal tunnel syndrome following 458
  classification 452–3
  complications 458–9
  displaced 452–3, 455–8
  impacted, reduction *169*
  intercarpal collapse following 459
  long-term disability following 459
  malunion 458
  nature of injury 452
  and osteoporosis 452
  prevention of deformity 456, *457*
  radiography 454
  recovery of function 456
  reduction 455–6, 457
  reflex sympathetic dystrophy following 319, 458
  resolution of swelling 456
  reversed 459
  shoulder stiffness following 458–9
  signs and symptoms 453–4
  treatment 454–8
  undisplaced 452, *453*, 455
  wrist stiffness following 458
colonic injury 125–6
colostomy 125
coma 112, *113*, 133–4, 191
combination fracture 32
comminuted fracture 7, 31, 46
  radiography 45
common femoral artery injury 251
common femoral vein 641
common peroneal nerve injury 270, 736, 769, 790
compartment pressure measurement 799
compartment syndromes 40, 271, 737
  aetiology 272
  anatomical locations 271
  anterior thigh 275
  avoidance in open fracture management 210
  clinical signs and symptoms 273–6
  in combined vascular and orthopaedic injuries 281

definition 271
diagnosis 279
differential diagnosis 281
extensor 276
in external fracture fixation 186
following tourniquet use 204
foot 843, 871–3
forearm 271, *272*, 275–6, 280
leg 271, 275, 737, 794–5
  management 280, 796–800
  muscle abnormalities in *275*
  sensory changes in *275*
management 279–80
missed 280–1
and nerve injury 263, 267
pathophysiology 272–3
posterior thigh 275
pressure measurement in 276–9
volar *274*, 276
complete fracture 29, 46, 239, *240*
distal radius 489
complicated dislocation 34
complications
classification 249–50
detection 40–2
of dislocations 250
of fractures 249–50
immediate 40–2
see also specific complications and fractures
compression fracture 32, 46–7
distal radius 488
vertebral bodies 63
compression-band wiring 182
computerized tomography (CT) 63–4, *65*
abdominal trauma 116
acetabular fracture 624
ankle injury 831
avascular necrosis 326
bladder and posterior urethral injury 160
cervical spinal injury 564, *569*
clavicle fracture 335
head injury 130, *131*, 132
hip dislocation 633
intra-abdominal haematoma 108
kidney injury 152
liver trauma 121
os calcis fracture 841, *842*
pelvic fracture 619
spinal instability 896
sternoclavicular joint dislocation 363
thoracic and lumbar spinal injury 599, *600*,
  601
wrist injury 451
Cone calipers 566, *571*
Confidential Enquiry into Perioperative
  Deaths 191
confusion 140
consciousness, altered 112, *113*, 127, 133–4,
  141
consolidation 302
contamination 41
continuous passive motion (CPM)
effect on healing of articular cartilage 83
in femoral fracture healing 711
in phalangeal fracture healing 518
contracture following vascular injury repair
  258
contrast venography in DVT 287
cor pulmonale 892
coracoacromial ligament *353*
division 397

coracobrachialis 401, 402
coracoclavicular ligament 333, 340, 353
  ossification 358, *359*
  repair 344, 355, 356
coracoid fracture *398*, 399
cortex
  dying back 72, *73*
  in fracture healing 74–5
corticosteroids
  in fat embolism syndrome 286
  and fracture healing 78
corticotrophin releasing factor 92
cortisol secretion in shock 93
costoclavicular ligament 333, 361
cough in fat embolism syndrome 284
coxa vara 889
CPK 33
CPM *see* continuous passive motion
crack fracture 29
craniectomy, creeping 133
craniotomy 133
creatinine phosphokinase 33
creeping apposition 322
creeping substitution 322
CRF 92
cross leg flap 228, *229*, 315
Crutchfield calipers 565–6, *571*
csf, rhinorrhoea/otorrohoea 127, 135
CT *see* computerized tomography
cuboid 833
  fracture 867, *868*
cuneiform fracture 868
Cushing's syndrome and pathological
  fracture 889, 894
CVP *see* central venous pressure
cystourethrography in bladder and posterior
  urethral injury 159–60

D-dimer 288
Da Nang wet lung *see* adult respiratory
  distress syndrome
dantrolene sodium 606
DCS 732, 733
De Quervain's stenosing tenovaginitis 459
debridement 209, 210–11, 221–2
  in infected non-union 313
deep venous thrombosis (DVT) 189, 296
  in ankle injury 830
  clinical presentation 287
  diagnosis 287–8
  differential diagnosis 281
  incidence 287
  pathogenesis 286
  in pathological fracture 893
  prophylaxis 289–90, 562
  in proximal femoral fracture 657–8
  in tibial shaft fracture 805
  treatment 288–9
degloving injury 40, 222–3, 800
dehydration in proximal femoral fracture
  684
delayed primary closure in infected non-
  union 314
delayed union 75
  aetiology 305
  definition 303
  distal femoral fracture 742
  in external fixation 186, 214
  in internal fixation 183
  pathological fracture 891

talar neck fracture 856
tibial shaft fracture 804, 810, 817
delirium tremens 250
deltoid 332, 401
  in cervical spinal injury 562
  and displacement of humeral shaft
   fracture 402
deltoid ligament 858, 864
  injury 824, 829
delto-pectoral flap 315
dementia and proximal femoral fracture 642,
  644, 654, 666, 667, 669
denervation and fracture healing 77
Denham fixator 183
dermatomes 224, *226*, 562
developmental disorders and pathologcal
  fracture 889
dextran
  in fat embolism syndrome 286
  in hip surgery 658
  prophylactic 289
  in shock 97, *98*, 110–11
diabetes mellitus
  and anaesthesia 193
  fracture healing in 78
  pathological fracture in 835
  and vascular damage 251–2
diagnosis 37–42
  provisional 39
diaphragmatic injury 118–19
  and chest injury 141–2
diaphyseal fracture 30
diaphysis, structure and behaviour under
  stress in childhood 237
diastasis 47, *48*
diazepam
  in local/regional anaesthesia 196
  in paraplegia 606
  in tetanus 294
DIC
  and fat embolism syndrome 285
  in haemorrhagic shock 94, 95
digital nerve block 197, 496–7
digoxin 102
dihydroergotamine 289
DIP joint *see* distal interphalangeal joint
direct cutaneous vessel 227
direct flaps 227–8
DISI 466, 468
  following Colles' fracture 459
dislocation
  classification 34–6
  complications 250
  definition 34, 47
  radiography 44–5
displaced fracture 33
  clavicle 340–4
  Colles' fracture 452–3, 455–8
  femur
   intracapsular 643–53
   trochanteric 666
  humerus
   proximal 390–4
   shaft 401–2
  os calcis 843–6
  patella 776, *777*
  phalanges
   middle 510, *511*
   proximal 510, *511*, 519, *520*
  subtalar joint 843–6
  tibial shaft 805–7

disseminated intravascular coagulation
    and fat embolism syndrome 285
    in haemorrhagic shock 94, 95
distal interphalangeal (DIP) joint
    articular fracture 522
    in distal phalangeal fracture 503
    fracture–dislocation 507, *508*
distal phalanx
    epiphyseal separation 507–9
    fracture 503–4
        base 504–9
        tendon avulsion 505–7
distal radioulnar joint 447
    dislocation 464–5
        childhood 490
    fracture 463
    subluxation 464–5
distant flaps 227–8
distraction 33
distraction histogenesis 315
diuretics in haemorrhagic shock 99
dobutamine 98
dopamine
    in adult respiratory distress syndrome 300
    in haemorrhagic shock 98
    in septicaemic shock 102
Doppler ultrasound in DVT 288
dorsal intercarpal ligament *448*
dorsal interosseous ligaments 869–70
dorsal ligament *448*
dorsal radiocarpal ligament 447, *448*
dorsalis pedis artery 850, *851*
    injury 875
Down's syndrome 575, 577, *583*
dressings
    and compartment syndromes 272
    skin graft donor site 225
    skin graft recipient site 226
drilling, cooling during 19
drug reactions 188
    differentiation from tetanus 293
Duchenne muscular dystrophy and patho-
        logical fracture 889, 905, *906*
ductile materials, stress-strain curve 6
duodenal injury 124
duplex scanning in DVT 288
Dupuytren's disease 459
DVT *see* deep venous thrombosis
Dynabrace 13, 16
dynamics 3
dysphagia in tetanus 294
dysplasias and pathological fracture 889,
        891, 906
dyspnoea
    in diaphragmatic rupture 142
    in fat embolism syndrome 284

early management 105–65
ECG, preoperative 189
ECMO in adult respiratory distress
        syndrome 300
EGF
    in cartilage healing 84
    in fracture healing 71
elastin in ligaments 87
elbow
    anatomy 413–14
    dislocation 423
        anterior 425
        divergent 425

lateral 425
    neurovascular injury following 426
    posterior 423–5
    recurrent 425–6
    trapped medial epicondyle in 425
fracture
    coronoid process of ulna 428
    distal humerus 415–23
    olecranon 428–32
    radial head and neck 426–8
heterotopic calcification 426
hyperextension 373
radiography 51–2, *414*
types of injury 414
elderly
    femoral shaft fracture 751, 753, *755*
    proximal femoral fracture 666–7, 668–9
electrical stimulation
    and fracture healing 71, 77
    in non-union 311–12
electrocardiography, preoperative 189
electrolytes, preoperative assessment 189
Elmslie–Trillat procedure 778
emphysema, surgical 106
emprosthotonus 293
enchondroma 903
end-to-side anastomosis 235
endoneural tube 266
endoscopy
    in bladder and posterior urethral injury
        160
    in ureteric injury 154
endotenon 86
endotoxin 100, 101
endotracheal intubation 105
    in cervical spinal injury 557
    in chest injury 143–4
enteral feeding in tetanus 296
epidermal growth factor
    in cartilage healing 84
    in fracture healing 71
epidural anaesthesia 195–6
epidural analgesia 143
epiphyseal fracture 30–1, 239–43, 735
    avulsion by ligament 240
    compression 240
    osteochondral 240
    radiography 59, *60*
epiphysis *238*
    radiography 59, *61*
    structure and behaviour under stress in
        childhood 237
erythromycin 294
Escherichia coli 100, 103
Esmarch bandage
    in exsanguination 203
    as tourniquet 202
Essex–Lopresti fracture 464
examination under anaesthetic (EUA), in
        gleno-humeral joint instability 378
excretory urography
    in bladder and posterior urethral injury
        159
    in kidney injury 151, *152*
    in ureteric injury 153, *154*
exercise and fracture healing 77
exsanguination 202–3, *204*
extensor carpi ulnaris tendon 447, *448*
extensor digitorum brevis flap 231
extensor digitorum longus flap 231
extensor hallucis longus

flap 231
    weakness 274
extensor pollicis longus 435
extensor pollicis longus tendon rupture 458
extensor tendon avulsion 47, 49
external fixation 183, 211
    biomechanics 12–17, 212–13
    clavicle fracture 339–40, 348
    Colles' fracture 457–8
    complications 185–6, 214, 744
    devices
        application 184–5
        failure 13
        mechanical characteristics 13–17
        types 12–13, 183–4, *185*, 211–12, *213*
    dynamization 16–17, 214, 809
    femur
        shaft fracture 702, 708, *709*, 740, 744
        subtrochanteric fracture 724
    fixator rigidity 212, *213*
    forearm fractures 436, 440, *441*
    hand injury 499
    history 695
    humerus
        proximal fracture 391
        shaft fracture 407
    indications 214
    in infected non-union 314
    lumbar and thoracic spinal injuries 612
    metacarpal fracture 536
    middle and proximal phalangeal fracture
        513
    os calcis fracture 846
    outcomes 214
    pathological fracture 895, 903–4
    pelvic fracture 620
        initial management 619–20
    pin-bone interface stability 212–13
    pin-bone stress 212
    pin geometry and thread design 212
    and soft tissue cover 223
    supplementary internal fixation 15, *16*,
        214
    tibial shaft fracture 807–11
extra-articular fracture 30
extracorporeal membrane oxygenation in
        adult respiratory distress syndrome
        300
extradural anaesthesia 195–6
eye-shadow sign 135

FABER test 39
faciomaxillary injury with chest injury 141
failure of materials 6
false aneurysm 252–3
fasciocutaneous flaps 227, 232–3, 315
fasciotomy
    in compartment syndromes 279–80,
        799–800
    prophylactic 210–11, 223, 257
fat, excision in open fracture 210
fat cysts 72, *73*
fat embolism 140, 141, 283
    prevention 286
    sources 283
fat embolism syndrome 283
    clinical course 285
    clinical features 283–4
    definition 283
    in femoral fracture 738

pathophysiology 284–5
prognosis 285
treatment 285–6
fatigue failure 6
fatigue fracture *see* stress fracture
FCL *see* fibular collateral ligament
femoral artery 699, *700*
  angiography 66
  injury 259, 260
femoral nerve injury 629
femur 693
  anatomy 695
    surgical 639–41
  avascular necrosis 629
  blood supply 698–700
    effects of intramedullary reaming on
        700
    proximal 640–1
      assessment 635
      effect of fracture on 645–6
  condylar fracture 693, 730
    classification 730, *731*
    complications 741–2
    delayed union 742
    malunion 741–2
    non-union 742
    radiography 54, *56*
    refracture 749
    treatment
      non-operative 733
      operative 733, *734*
      options 730–2
      selection 732–3
  distal epiphyseal fracture in childhood
      735
  extracapsular/trochanteric fracture
    avascular necrosis following 665
    biomechanics 667–8, 673–4
    classification 674–6, *677*
    clinical features 666
    complications 672–3
    coronal plane 673, *674*
    displaced 666, *667*
    epidemiology 666–7
    isolated greater trochanter 664, *666*
    isolated lesser trochanter 664–5
    malunion 668
    mobility and social dependence
        following 671–2
    mortality 669
    nomenclature 665–6
    outcome 668–71
    pathological 689–90
    reverse oblique 666, 673, *674*, 686
    stable 675–6, 677–8
    treatment
      biomechanics 677–9
      duration and cost 672–3
      economics 669
      evolution of 680–2
      influence on outcome 670–1
      non-operative 688–9, *690*
      operative 683–6
    undisplaced 666, *667*
    unstable 675–6, *677*, 678–9
  fracture 693
    associated soft tissue injury 736–7
    biomechanics 696–8, *699*
    classification 637, 695–6
    degree of comminution 696
    fracture strength index 698, *699*

fracture union index 698
    historical review 693–5
    open 696
    pattern 695–6
    site 695
    soft tissue injuries 696
  intertrochanteric fracture 665–6
  intracapsular fracture 637–8
    avascular necrosis following 645, 656–7
    blood supply 645–6
    classification *45*, 53, 638–9
    clinical features 642–3
    complications 654–8
    displaced 639, 643–53
    DVT 657–8
    epidemiology 658–9
    with femoral shaft fracture 750
    Garden angles 646, *647*
    infection 657
    internal fixation 644, 646–51
    late segmental collapse 657
    mechanism of injury 641–2
    mortality 654–6
    non-union 656
    in Paget's disease 563, 652
    in Parkinson's disease 654
    pathological 653–4
    prosthetic replacement 644, 651–2, 653
    reduction 646, *647*
    spontaneous 641
    stress 643, 653
    treatment 643–53
    undisplaced 639, 643, *644*
    in young adults 652–3
  pathological fracture 653–4, 689–90, 735–6,
      892–4, 895, 897, 898, 899
  pertrochanteric fracture 665–6
  proximal fracture 637
    classification 637
    with hip dislocation 634–5
    incidence of DVT following 287
    radiography *45*, 53
  shaft 695
  shaft fracture 693
    associated with prostheses 753, *756*
    bilateral 751, *754*
    childhood 733–4
    classification 701, *702*
    complications 736–49, *750, 751*
    elderly patients 751, 753, *755*
    with femoral neck fracture 750
    with hip dislocation 749–50, *752*
    initial assessment 703
    with ipsilateral patellar fracture 750–1,
        753
    with ipsilateral tibial fracture 750
    malunion 740, *742*
    non-union 738–40, *741*
    open 736
    radiography 53–4
    refracture 749, *750*
    treatment
      non-operative 703–5
      operative 705, 708–21
      options 701–2
      selection 702–3
  stress fracture 736
  subtrochanteric fracture 665, 693, 721
    biomechanics 698
    classification 721, 722, 723
    treatment

    non-operative 723–4
    operative *216*, 724–30
    options 721
    selection 722–3
  supracondylar fracture 693, 730
    associated with prostheses 753
    classification 730, *731*
    complications 741–2
    delayed union 742
    malunion 741–2
    non-union 742
    refracture 749, *751*
    treatment
      non-operative 733
      operative 733, *734*
      options 730–2
      selection 732–3
FGF, and cartilage healing 84
fibreglass casts 170
fibrinogen uptake studies in DVT 288
fibroblast growth factor, and cartilage
      healing 84
fibrous dysplasia 77
fibrous union 307
fibula
  fracture
    distal 824, 828
    proximal in ankle injury 828
    shaft 790, *797*
  osteotomy 790
  radiography 54–5, *56–7*
fibula-protibia operation 316
fibular collateral ligament (FCL) 760, 762
  chronic laxity 771–2
  injury 768–69
fibular osteoseptocutaneous flap 315, 316
fibulectomy in non-union 310
figure-of-eight bandage 336–7, 352
fingers
  little
    fracture of base of proximal phalanx
        43
    proximal interphalangeal joint
        dislocation 45
  nerve blocks 197, 496–7
  tourniquet 205
  see also thumb
Finochietto's sign 765
flaps 227–35, 315
fleck sign 869, *870*
flexor carpi radialis 562
flexor digitorum brevis 871
  flap 231
flexor digitorum longus flap 231
flexor digitorum longus tendon 871
flexor digitorum profundus avulsion 47, 49
flexor digitorum superficialis avulsion *46*, 47
flexor hallucis brevis 871
flexor hallucis longus flap 231
flexor hallucis longus tendon 858, 871
flexor tendons, healing 87–9
flucloxacillin 298
fluid replacement
  in haemorrhagic shock 97, *98*, 109–10
  in head injury 137
  in septicaemic shock 101
foot
  compartment syndromes 843, 871–3
  radiography 55, 57, *58*
  see also specific bones
forearm

forearm (*cont.*)
    compartment syndrome 271, *272*, 275–6, 280
    fracture 435
        bone grafting 442
        classification 436, *439*
        complications 445
        indications for surgery 436–40, *441*
        management options 435–6, *437*, *438*
        open 440, 441
        plate application 438, 442, *445*
        plate removal 445–6
        postoperative care 444
        surgery
            approaches 440–2, *443–4*
            technique 440
            timing 440
        wound closure 442, 444
    radiography 51
four quadrant needle tap 108, 116
fracture
    childhood, classification 238–43
    choosing treatment method 186–7
    classification 29–34, 46–7, 238–43
    closed treatment 168–76, *177*
        see also casts; splint; traction
    and compartment syndromes 272
    complications 249–50
    definition 29
    external fixation *see* external fixation
    immobilization 169–76, *177*, 186–7
    internal fixation *see* internal fixation
    loading 10–11
    mechanics 6–7
    objectives of management 167
    reduction 18, 167
        closed 168–9, 186–7, 246
        open 187, 246–7
    stabilization 167, 211
    timing of surgery 192–3
    toughness 6
fracture blisters 249–50, 838, *839*
fracture–dislocation 47, 416
    carpus 481–2, 484, 485, 490
    cervical spine 553, *554*
    distal interphalangeal joint 507, *508*
    hip joint 631–5
    Lisfranc's/tarsometatarsal 55, 57, *58*, 868–75
    lumbar spine 606, 610, *611*, 612–14
    proximal interphalangeal joint 528–9, *530*
    thoracic spine 606, 610, *611*, 612–14
fracture gap 75
fracture healing 7, 71–2, 305, *306*
    and age 78
    and avascular necrosis 77
    biological process 7–8
    biomechanics 7–11, 698, *699*
    childhood 244–5
    cortical reaction 74–5
    and degree of trauma 76
    and denervation 77
    in diabetes mellitus 78
    and drugs 78
    effects of hormones on 78
    and electrical stimulation 71, 77, 311–12
    and exercise 77
    factors affecting 76–8
    fracture gap 75
    in hyperparathyroidism 77
    and immobilization 76

and infection 77
    inflammatory phase 72–3
    intra-articular fracture 77
    mechanical influences on 9–11
    mechanical properties 8–9
    medullary reaction 74, *75*
    in neurofibromatosis 77
    and nutrition 78
    in osteogenesis imperfecta 77
    in osteomalacia 77
    pathological fracture 77
    periosteal reaction 73–4
    radiography 61–2
    remodelling 75–6
    reparative phase 73–5
    in rickets 77
    and stress 77
    and type of bone involved 76
fracture line *43*, 44
fracture strength index 698, *699*
fracture union index 698
frames 12–13
    application 184–5
    bilateral 184
    biplanar 184
    configuration 184
    failure 13
    indications 184
    mechanical characteristics 13–17
    types 183, *184*
    unilateral 184
    uniplanar 184
    see also external fixation
free flaps 228–9, *230*, 233–5, 315
frusemide
    in adult respiratory distress syndrome 300
    in chest injury 142
    in fat embolism syndrome 285
    in haemorrhagic shock 99

G suit 99
Galeazzi fracture 51, 437, *439*, 464
Gallie subtalar fusion 847
gamekeeper's thumb 66
gangrene, gas 297–8
gap-healing 8
Garden angles 646, *647*
Gardner–Wells calipers 566, *571*
gas embolism 116
gas gangrene 297–8
gastrectomy 124
gastrocnemius 762
    flap 231, 232, 315
gastroenterostomy 124
Gaucher's disease and pathological fracture 889
gelatine-based infusion fluids 97, *98*, 111
Gelofusin 111
genitourinary tract injury 149–65
gentamicin
    in gas gangrene 298
    in infected non-union 314
    in polymethyl-methacrylate beads 314
giant cell tumours 903
Glasgow coma scale 112, *113*, 133–4, 191
gleno humeral joint
    dislocation 331, 367
        anterior 368, 369, 370–2
        diagnosis 369, *370*
        inferior 369, *370*

management 370–3
        mechanism of injury 368
        posterior 368, 369, *370*, 372–3
        radiography *369*, 370, *371*
        recurrent 373–86
    instability 373, *374*, 385–6
        AMBRI 374
        anterior 373
            pathogenesis 374–5
            treatment 379–82
        anterior and posterior drawer tests 376
        apprehension test 376–7
        assessment 376–8
        classification 379
        examination under anaesthetic 378
        expected outcome from surgery 373–4
        inferior 373
        multidirectional 373, 384–5
            treatment 384–5
        posterior 373
            treatment 382–4
        posterior stress test 377–8
        radiography 378
        sulcus sign 377
        symptoms 375–6
        treatment 379–85
        TUBS 374
        unidirectional 373
        voluntary 383, 385
    subluxation 367
        recurrent 373–86
    surgical anatomy 367–8
gleno-humeral ligaments 367, *368*
glenoid
    fracture 398–9
    posterior osteotomy 382–3, *384*
glenoid labrum, MRI 67
glucagon secretion, effect of shock on 93
gluteal muscles 696–7, 698
gluteus maximus, muscle-pedicle bone graft 650
GM-1 560–1
Goldman index of cardiac risk 191, *192*
Goldthwait–Roux procedure 778
gravity
    in closed fracture reduction 168
    in fracture immobilization 169
great occipital nerve injury 567
greenstick fracture 29, 46, 239
    distal radius 452, 488–9
    radiography 57, 59
groin flap 227, *228*, 315
growth arrest 243, 245
growth hormone
    effect of shock on secretion 93
    in fracture healing 71, 78
growth plate
    fractures 240, 241–3
    structure and behaviour under stress in childhood 237–8

Haemacel 111
haemarthrosis 309
haematoma
    extradural 129, 130, *131*, 135, *137*
    in fracture healing 7–8, 73
    intra-abdominal 108
    intracerebral 130, *131*, 132
    intracranial 129–32
        and altered consciousness 133–4

clinical diagnosis 132–3
intradural 129
perirenal 149, *150*, 151
pre-vertebral *564*
subdural 129–34
  acute 129, 130, *131*
  chronic 129–30
subungual 503
haematuria
  in fat embolism syndrome 284
  in genitourinary tract injury 149, 150, 151
haemobilia 122
haemodialysis
  in adult respiratory distress syndrome 300
  in chest injury 143
haemofiltration in adult respiratory distress
      syndrome 300
haemoglobin
  preoperative assessment 189
  stroma-free 111
haemopericardium 107
haemoperitoneum 117
haemophilia and pathological fracture 889,
      907
haemoptysis in fat embolism syndrome 284
haemorrhage 40
  control of 106–8
  in femoral fracture 738
  following vascular injury repair 258
haemostasis, in vascular injury 254
haemothorax 105, 107, 140, 144, 146–7
hairline fracture 29
hallux, phalangeal fracture 885, *886*
halo traction 566, *572*, 589
hamate 447, 448, 449
  dislocation 486
  fracture 480
hand injury 495
  anaesthesia 197, 496–7, *498*
  assessment 495
  carpometacarpal joint 538–9, *540*
  combined 499
  examination 495–6
  fracture
    articular 522, *523*
    distal phalangeal 503–9
    extra-articular phalangeal 519–20, *521–2*
    malunion 501
    management principles 501–3
    metacarpal 532–8
    middle and proximal phalangeal
        509–19
  isolated 499
  loss of motion following 501
  open 497–501
  phalangeal epiphyseal 524
  PIP joint 524–9, *530*
  position of safe splintage 501–3, 512
  radiography 47, 49, *50*, 496, *497*
  swelling in 501–3
  thumb 539–46, *547*
  wound cleansing 498
  see also fingers
hanging, judicial 572, 574
hanging arm method 370
hanging cast 168, 175, *177*, 403
hangman's fracture 574
Harrington rods 611–12, 614
Hartshill rectangle 614, 896–7
Hastings hemiarthroplasty prosthesis *651*
Hawkin's crescent sign 854, *855*, 863

head injury 126–7, 140
  admission criteria 136
  altered consciousness 133–4
  amnesia 136
  anaesthesia 190–1, 192–3
  anoxia 127–8
  blunt acceleration–deceleration 127
  cerebral compression 128–34
  clinical diagnosis 132–3
  closed 127
  compression 127
  consultation with neurosurgeon 136–7
  early management 135–7
  and infection 134–5
  minor/moderate 137–8
  open 127
  penetrating 127
  post-traumatic syndrome 138
  primary 127–35
  radiography 136
  severe 134
  skull base compound fracture 135
  skull vault compound fracture 134–5
healing time 302, *303*
heart, in haemorrhagic shock 94
hemiarthroplasty
  bipolar prosthesis 652
  femoral fracture associated 753, *756*
  history 637–8
  in proximal femoral fracture 644, *645*,
      651–2, 653
heparin
  in anaesthesia 189
  in fat embolism syndrome 285, 286
  in hip surgery 658
  prophylactic 289, 290, 296
  in vascular injury 254
HES 97, *98*, 111
heterotopic ossification following spinal cord
      injury 554
Hill–Sachs lesion 378
hip joint
  closed packed position 646
  CT scan 64, *65*
  dislocation 631
    anterior 631, *632*, *633*, 635
    central 631
    classification 631
    clinical features 633
    complications 635–6
    with femoral shaft fracture 749–50, *752*
    mechanism of injury 631–2
    posterior 631, *632*, 633–4
    treatment 633–5
  fracture–dislocation 631
    classification 634–5
    clinical features 633
    mechanism of injury 631–2
    treatment 634–5
  see also acetabulum
Hippocratic method of shoulder dislocation
      reduction 370, *371*
histamine and septic shock 100
history-taking
  in abdominal trauma 115
  in fracture 37–8
  in wrist injury 450–1
HIV infection 188
Hoffman fixator 13, 183, 184, 339
Holstein fracture *268*
Hooke's Law 4

humerus
  distal fracture
    capitellar 415–16
    epicondylar 415
    intercondylar 418–21, *422*
    lateral condylar 416, *417*
    medial condylar 416, *417*
    practical aspects 422–3
    supracondylar 52, 416–18
    transcondylar 52, 416–18
  functional bracing 404
  greater tuberosity fracture 395–6
  head replacement 393–4
  proximal fracture 386–7
    age distribution 331, 386, *387*
    associated injuries 387, *388*
    classification 387, *388*
    clinical symptoms 331
    complications of treatment 394–5
    displaced two-segment 390–2
    displaced three-segment 392
    displaced four-segment 392–4
    malunion 394–5
    management principles 387–9
    non-union 394–5
    radiography 387, *388*
    surgical approaches 389–90
    undisplaced 390
  shaft fracture 401
    anatomical aspects 401–2
    classification *402*
    complications 407–10
    diagnosis 402
    displacement 401–2
    management 168, 175, *177*, 403–7
    non-union 409–10
    pathological 410
hydronephrosis 150, 154
hydroureter 154
hydroxyethyl starch 97, *98*, 111
hyperacusis in tetanus 294
hypercalcaemia 892, 895
hypercalcuria 895
hypercapnia 140
hyperglycaemia 93
hyperlipidaemia 93
hyperparathyroidism
  fracture healing in 77
  and pathological fracture 889, 894
hyperpathia 586
hypertension
  and chest injury 141
  following kidney injury 152
  pulmonary 285
hyperthyroidism and pathological fracture
      894
hypoalbuminaemia 300
hypocalcaemia 284
hypogonadism and pathological fracture
      894
hypotension
  in general anaesthesia 194
  in head injury 128
  in regional anaesthesia 202
hypovolaemia
  and anaesthesia 194
  preoperative assessment 189–90
hypoxia
  in chest injury 140
  in fat embolism syndrome 284, 285
  in head injury 128

ICP, raised 133, 191
IGF 84
IL-1 *see* interleukin-1
ileostomy 125
iliac osteocutaneous flap 315, 316
iliofemoral ligament 646
iliopsoas 698
iliotibial band 762
iliotibial tract 87, 762
Ilizarov fixator 13, 14, 183
Ilizarov technique 315
immobilization and fracture healing 76
impedance plethysmography in DVT 288
impingement syndrome, MRI 67
impotence following bladder and posterior
        urethral injury 163, 165
incomplete fracture 29, 46
incontinence following bladder and
        posterior urethral injury 163
indirect bone healing 8, 314
indirect flaps 227, 228
indomethacin 629
infection 41
    and anaesthesia 193–4
    ankle injury 830
    bladder and posterior urethral injury 162
    in external fixation 13, 185–6, 214, 744, 809
    femoral shaft fracture 748–9
    forearm fractures 445
    and fracture healing 77
    and head injury 134–5
    implant-associated 24
    in internal fixation 182, 215, 217–18, 744,
        748–9
    kidney injury 152
    in non-union 307–8, 313–16
    open fractures 207, 208–9
    os calcis fracture 846
    in pathological fracture 891
    pathological fracture in 889, 903–4
    in proximal femoral fracture 657, 684
    tibial shaft fracture *794, 801, 809, 813, 815*
    in traction 743
    vascular injury repair 258
inferior acromio-clavicular ligament 353
inferior gluteal artery 640
inferior metaphyseal vessels 640, *641*
infertility following bladder and posterior
        urethral injury 163, 165
inflammatory response 79
    in fracture healing 72–3
infrapatellar tendon rupture 775
injury
    systemic response to 91–103
    tissue response to 79–80
injury severity score 112
insulin
    and anaesthesia 189
    and cartilage healing 84
    effect of shock on secretion 93
    in fracture healing 78
insulin-like growth factors 84
intercostal blockade 143
intercostal drainage 106, 107
interfragmentary compression 18
interleukin-1 (IL-1)
    and articular degradation 84
    and septic shock 100
intermetatarsal ligaments 870
internal fixation 176–82, *183*, 214–18
    acetabular fracture 628

ankle injury 827–8, 829
    biomechanical principles 17–23
    in childhood 246–7
    clavicle fracture 337–9, 343–4, 347, 348
    complications 182–3, 744–8
    femur
        distal fracture 731–2, 733
        extracapsular/trochanteric fracture
            677–88
        intracapsular fracture 643, 644, 646–51
        shaft fracture 702, 708–21, 744–8
        subtrochanteric fracture 724–30
    forearm fractures 435–6, *438*, 442, *445*
    fracture stability 18
    hand injury 499
    history 695
    humerus
        proximal fracture 391–2, 394
        shaft fracture 405–7, 410
    implants
        application of biomechanics to 18–23
        material characteristics 17–18
        removal 23–4
    indications 187
    lumbar and thoracic spinal injuries 612,
        613, 614
    materials 17–18
    metacarpal fracture 536, 537–8
    middle and proximal phalangeal fractures
        514–19
    objectives 17
    os calcis fracture 844–6
    pathological fracture 895, 903
    pelvic fracture 620–1
    reverse Barton fracture 463
    scaphoid fracture non-union 474, *475*
    Smith fracture 461
    supplementary 15, *16*, 214
    talus
        lateral process fracture 859–60
        neck fracture 853–4
    tibia
        metaphyseal fracture 787–8, *789*
        shaft fracture 811–17
internal iliac artery ligation 259
interosseous ligament 435, *448*
interosseous membrane injury 824
interosseous talocalcaneal ligament 833
interosseous wiring 516
interphalangeal (IP) joints
    fingers
        dislocations 49
        immobilization in hand injury 501,
            502–3
        see also distal interphalangeal joint;
            proximal interphalangeal joint
    toes, dislocations 894–5
interscalene block 199, *200*
intersesamoid ligament 883
interspinous ligament 552
    ossification 563, *566*
intra-abdominal haemorrhage 107–8
intra-abdominal injury with chest injury
        141, 145
intra-articular fracture 30, 47
    healing 77
intracranial pressure, raised 133, 191
intramedullary nail 177, 179–81, *182*
    AO 180–1, 719
        unreamed femoral 721
    biological response to 23

Brooker–Wills 721
    cross-section 22–3
    Derby 721
    Ender's 181, *681*, 814
        humeral 406
    flexible 181
    gamma 683, 728–9
    Grosse–Kempf 719, 747
    Hansen–Street 181
    history 695
    Huckstep 181, 719, *720*, 721
    implant failure 817
    Küntscher 180–1, 683, 814
    locking 23, 181, *182*, 406, 695, 711–12,
        714–19, 729–30
        dynamic 712, *713*
    Lottes *181*
    mechanical characteristics 21–3
    optimal insertion 23
    removal 24
    rigid 179–81
    Russell–Taylor *180*, 719
    Sampson *181*
    Schneider *181*
    solid 181
    techniques
        clavicle fracture 338, 348
        closed 714–19
        complications 744–8
        dynamization 719
        femur
            extracapsular/trochanteric fracture
                677–8, 681, 683–5
            shaft fracture 702, 711–21, 744–8
            subtrochanteric fracture 725–30
        forearm fractures 436, *438*
        humeral shaft fracture 406–7, 410
        indications 217–18
        in non-union 310, *311*
        open pro-grade 714
        open retrograde 712, 714
        phalangeal fractures 518–19
        stacked nailing 406
        tibial shaft fracture 814–17
    Variwall 721
    working length 180
    Zickel 683, 726, *727, 728, 729, 732, 749, 750*
intravenous regional anaesthesia 197–8, 497
inverse care law 656
IP joints *see* interphalangeal joints
irreducible dislocation 34
isoprenaline 98
isotope bone scanning 64–5
    avascular necrosis *323*, 324–6
    in non-union 303–4
    proximal femoral fracture 642–3
    in reflex sympathetic dystrophy 320
    wrist injury 451–2
isotropic materials 4
ISS 112
IVRA 197–8, 497

jaundice 188
Jefferson fracture 568, *575*
Jewett fixed angle nail plate 647, *648, 649*
joints
    care in cervical spinal injury 558–9, *560*
    instability 35, 373
    laxity 373

mobility restriction in external fracture
    fixation 186
  in paraplegia 606–7
  radiography of fractures around 45–6
  stiffness and non-union 309
  see also specific joints
Jones repair 771

K wire *see* Kirschner (K) wire
Kaneda device 612, *613*, 897
keloid 337, 344
kidney
  in haemorrhagic shock 94–5
  injury 149
    associated pathology 150
    clinical presentation 150–1
    closed 149–50, *151*
    management 151–2
    post-traumatic complications 152, *153*
  spontaneous rupture 149, 150
Kienböck disease 477–8
Kirschner (K) wire 177, 182
  fixation
    clavicle fracture 343–4
    hand injury 499, 513–14, *515*, 516
    interosseous 516
    patellar fracture 776, *777*
    proximal humeral fracture 391, 392, 394
  in traction 173, 175
Klebsiella 103
Klippel–Feil syndrome 575, 577, 588
knee
  CT scan 64
  dislocation 769–70
    anterior 769
    posterior 769
  extensor mechanism rupture 774–5
  fat fluid level 54, *55*
  gas in joint 54, *55*
  hard tissue injury 774–8
  hyperextension 373
  ligaments
    anatomy 761–3
    in femoral fracture 737
    injury 759–61
      acute 763, *764*
      associated injury 769–70
      chronic 770–2
      classification 760
      examination 763–5
      first degree 759
      haemarthrosis 763, *764*
      and laxity 760
      management 765–69
      second degree 759
      third degree 759–60
  menisci
    cystic 773
    injury 67, 772–3
    suture 773
  MRI 67–8
  osteochondral fracture 774, *775*
  pain following tibial shaft fracture fixation
    817
  replacement arthroplasty, femoral fracture
    associated 753
  soft tissue injury 759–73
  stiffness following femoral fracture 742–3,
    744
  stress radiography 66, 763

  see also patella
knee jerk 598
knives, skin graft 225, *226*
Kocher manoeuvre 370
KT1000 arthrometer 764

labetalol 296
Lachman test 764
laparoscopy in abdominal trauma 116
laparotomy 117–18
lateral circumflex femoral artery 640, *641*,
    699, *700*
lateral collateral ligament (LCL) 760, 762
    chronic laxity 771–2
    injury 768–69
lateral ligament *825*
lateral malleolus *825*
    radiography 54
latissimus dorsi 401
    and displacement of humeral shaft
      fracture 402
    flap *230*, 231, 234–5, 315
LCL *see* lateral collateral ligament
LD$_{50}$ 112
lead-pipe fracture 59
Leeds–Keio Dacron implant 770–1
Lemaire technique 770, 771
ligament of Bigelow 632
ligament of Weitbrecht 635, 646
ligamenta flava 552
ligaments
    accessory 87
    capsular 87
    healing 89–90
    injury to 41–2
    sprain/rupture 34
    structure and function 87
    synthetic 767, 769, 771
    vertebral 87
ligamentum teres 635, 639
lignocaine 196, *197*
limb ischaemia in skin traction 173
linea aspera 698, 699, 710
linear fracture 31
Lisfranc's fracture–dislocation 868–70, *871*
    classification 873
    mechanism of injury 871–3
    radiography 55, 57, *58*
    treatment *873*, 874–5
Lisfranc's fragment 869, *870*
Lisfranc's ligament 870
liver
    control of haemorrhage 121–2, *123*
    disease and pathological fracture 894
    function tests 189
    in haemorrhagic shock 95
    injury 40
    regeneration 122
    trauma to 121–2
load–extension curve 3
local anaesthetic agents 196, *197*
    allergic reactions to 201
    cardiovascular toxicity 201
    CNS toxicity 201
    dosage 196–7
local flaps 227
lock jaw 292
Looser zones 895
lumbar spine
    CT scan 64

injury
    classification 602–3, *604*
    clinical investigation 597–8
    cord decompression 601–2
    flexion–compression 603–4
    flexion–distraction 604, *605*, 609–10
    flexion–rotation 605, *606*
    horizontal translation (shearing) frac-
      ture–dislocation 606, 610, *611*
    pathology 599–602
    patterns 603
    radiology 57, *60*, 598–9, *600*, *601*
    rotational fracture–dislocation 612–14
    stable 603
    treatment 608–14
    unstable 603, *604*, 609–14
    vertical compression/burst fracture
      604–5, 610–12, *613*
  instability 895–7, *899*, *900*, *902*
lumbrical muscles 871
luminocapsular veins 640–1
lunate 447, 448–9, 450
    avascular necrosis 483
    dislocation 482–3
    fracture 476–8
    fracture–dislocation *50*
lunatomalacia 477–8
lunotriquetral ligament *448*
luxatio erecta 369, *370*

Mach effect 62, *63*
MacIntosh I technique 770, 771
MacIntosh II technique 770
magnetic resonance imaging (MRI) 67–8
    avascular necrosis 326, *327*
    cervical spinal injury 562, 564
    gleno-humeral joint instability 378
    kidney injury 152
    knee injury 763
    spinal instability 896
    thoracic and lumbar spinal injury 599
    wrist injury 452
Maisonneuve fracture 55, *56–7*, 824
Major Trauma Outcome Study 113–14
malalignment and non-union 309
malingering 591–2
mallet finger 49, *50*, 505
malunion 250
    ankle injury 830
    childhood fractures 247
    clavicle fracture 348, *349*, 351
    Colles' fracture 458
    in external fixation 214
    femur
      distal fracture 741–2
      proximal fracture 668
      shaft fracture 740, *742*
    humeral fractures 394–5, 401
    pathological fracture 891
    talar neck fracture 856
    tibial shaft fracture 797, 804–5, 810, 815,
      817
mammillary processes 237
manipulation 168–9
mannitol
    in haemorrhagic shock 99
    in raised intracranial pressure 191
Maquet procedure 778
march fracture *48*
marginal fracture 30

MAST suit 99, 272
MCL *see* medial collateral ligament
mechanics 3
medial circumflex femoral artery 640, *641,*
699, 700
medial collateral ligament (MCL)
anatomy 761
chronic laxity 771
injury 760, 783
acute tear 767–8
avulsion fracture *56,* 761
in femoral fracture 737
medial ligament *825*
medial malleolus *825*
fracture 824, 828
non-union 830
radiography 54
median nerve 401, 407
block 497, *498*
injury
in Colles' fracture 270, 458
in distal radial fracture 452
in elbow dislocation 426
in forearm fracture management 445
and numbness 38
medical anti shock trousers suit 99, 272
medullary canal, and fracture healing 74, *75*
medullary vasomotor centre 92
meningitis 135
meniscectomy, arthroscopic 773
mesenteric injury 124–5
mesotenon 86
metacarpal block 496–7
metacarpal fracture
head 532–3
neck 49, 533–4
shaft 496, *497,* 534–8
thumb 539–43
metacarpophalangeal (MP) joint 529–30
articular fracture 522
dislocation 530–1, 546, *547*
hyperextension 373
immobilization in hand injury 501–3, 512
locking 531–2
thumb, injury 544–6, *547*
metaphyseal fracture 30
radiography 59, *61*
metaphysis *238*
structure and behaviour under stress in
childhood 237
metastatic carcinoma and pathological
fracture 63, 889, 895–903
femur 47, 653–4, 736
humeral shaft 410
metatarsal fractures *874, 875*
base 875, *876*
base of the fifth 878–80, *881*
classification 875
neck 875, *876*
shaft 875, *877, 878*
stress 881–2, *883*
metatarsal-phalangeal joint dislocations
882–4
methylprednisolone 560, 601
metoclopramide 293
metronidazole 103, 209
micromovement 214
microscope, operating *229*
microstrain 4
microvascular free flaps 228–9, *230,* 233–5,
315

middle meningeal artery 129
middle meningeal vein 129
middle phalangeal fracture 509–10
angulation 510
articular 510, 522
classification 510–11
closed reduction
with external splintage 511–12, *513*
with percutaneous pin fixation 513–14,
515
epiphyseal 524
external fixation 513
extra-articular 510
open reduction and internal fixation
514–19
protected active motion 511
rotational displacement in 510, *511*
traction 512–13
minihep 289
see also heparin
minute volume 144
missile fracture 32
Mitek anchor 379
modulus of elasticity 4
Monk hard-top hemiarthroplasty prosthesis
652
monoamine oxidase inhibitors 189
monosialotetrahexosyl-ganglioside 560–1
Monteggia fracture 51, 247, 423, 438–9, *440*
Morel pneumatic orthosis 906
morphine 295
morphology of fractures 31
Morquio–Brailsford syndrome 577
motor power
assessment 267, 598
in compartment syndromes 274
MP joint *see* metacarpophalangeal joint
MRI *see* magnetic resonance imaging
MTOS 113–14
mucopolysaccharidoses 577
Müller tenodesis 771
multiple injuries 105–6, 737
muscle
grading scale 267
injury to 42
in paraplegia 606–7
viability assessment 210, 801
muscle flaps 221, 227, 229
free 234–5
in infected non-union 315
local 229, *230,* 231
muscle-pedicle bone graft in proximal
femoral fracture 650–1
muscle relaxants 145
muscular dystrophy and pathological
fracture 889, 905, *906*
musculocutaneous nerve 401, 407
myeloma 63, 895–903
myelomeningocoele 905
myocardial contusion 146
myocardial ischaemia 141
myocutaneous flaps 227, 229, *230,* 232
myoglobinuria 94
myositis ossificans
and elbow injury 413, 421, 426
and hip dislocation 636
myotomy in paraplegia 607

nail-bed injury 503–4, 507, *508*
naloxone 140, 560

nasotracheal intubation 143–4
navicular 833
avascular necrosis 864, 866
fracture 864
associated with os calcis fracture 838,
839
body 864, 865–6
classification 864
dorsal lip 864, 865
stress 864, 866, *867*
tuberosity *863,* 864–5
navicular cuneiform ligaments 866
necrosis 79
Neer humeral head prosthesis 393–4
neonate
brachial plexus injury 34, 350–1
clavicle fracture 350–1
nerve grafts 269–70
nerve injury 41, 263–4
in ankle injury 830
in cervical spinal cord injury 555
in childhood fractures 247
classification 264, *265*
in clavicle fracture 344–5, 351
degeneration
distal 265–6
retrograde 265
transneuronal 265
traumatic 264–5
diagnosis 267
due to tourniquet use 204
in elbow dislocation 426
in external fixation 186
in femoral fracture 736–7
in forearm fractures 445
in hip dislocation 636
in knee injury 769
late exploration 269
in os calcis fracture 846
postreduction compression lesions 270
in proximal humeral fracture 387, *388*
regeneration 266–7
in regional anaesthesia 202
in shoulder injury 331
in skin traction 173
stretch lesions 41
tibial shaft fracture 794, 810–11
treatment 267–71
neurectomy 607
neurofibromatosis 77
neurological disease and anaesthesia 193
neuropraxia 41, 264, *265*
differential diagnosis 281
radial nerve 408
neurotmesis 41, *263,* 264, *265*
radial nerve 408
Nicholas five-in-one procedure 771
night walking fracture 885
nightstick fracture 439
nitric oxide 100
non-accidental injury 38, 63
radiography 59, *61*
non-steroidal anti-inflammatory drugs
(NSAIDs)
in adult respiratory distress syndrome 300
and fracture healing 78
non-union 75
aetiology 305
ankle injury 830
associated pathological conditions 308–9
atrophic 62, 307

avascular 307
and avascular necrosis 326
blood supply 307
cartilaginous union 307
characteristics 303–5
classification 305–8
clavicle fracture 345–8, 351
definition 303
in external fixation 214
femur
  distal fracture 742
  proximal fracture 656
  shaft fracture 738–40, *741*
fibrous union 307
histology 307, *308*
humerus
  proximal fracture 394–5
  shaft fracture 409–10
hypertrophic 62, 306–7
infection 307–8, 313–16
in internal fixation 183
and joint stiffness 309
and malalignment 309
os calcis fracture 846
pathological fracture 891
radiography 62, 306–7
and Sudek's syndrome 309
tibial shaft fracture 792, *793*, 804, 813,
    817–18
and tissue defects 308
treatment 309–13
vascular 307
NSAIDs *see* non-steroidal anti-inflammatory
    drugs

obesity
  and anaesthesia 193
  and chest injury 141
oblique fracture 31, 46
observation 38–9
obturator artery 640, *641*
obturator internus 53
occipito-cervical fusion 567, *573*, 579–80
odontoid process
  congenital anomalies 575, *582*
  fracture 570–2, *576–8*
old unreduced dislocation 35
olecranon fracture 428–9
  classification 429–32
  comminuted *431*, 432
  oblique 430
  pseudarthrosis 432
  transverse 429–30
olive wires 15
open dislocation 36
open fracture 32, 207
  in childhood 247
  classification 32–3, 207–8, 221
  fasciotomy 210–11, 223
  infection 207, 208–9
  management
    initial 208–11, 221–3
    see also external fixation; internal fixation
  plaster casts 211
  wound excision 209–10, 221–3
  wound phases *223*
  wound surgery 209–11
operating microscope *229*
opisthotonus 293
optic nerve injury 137

oral contraceptives 189
oropharyngeal intubation 105
Orthofix fixator 13, 16, *213*
Orthoplast brace 805, *806*, 807
os calcis
  clinical anatomy 833, *834*
  fracture
    age and sex distribution 836
    anterior process 836, *838*, 843
    anterior process fragment excision 848
    associated bony injury 838, *839*
    associated soft tissue injury 836
    of the body 834–5, *836*
    classification 833–4
    clinical features 838–9
    epidemiology 836, 838, *839*
    excision of exostoses 848
    extra-articular 833
    imaging 839–41, *842*
    incidence 836
    infection 846
    intra-articular 833, 834
    mechanisms of injury 834–6
    non-union 846
    pathological 835
    subtalar joint involvement 826
    sustentaculum tali 836, 843
    treatment
      complications 846
      displaced intra-articular fractures
          843–6
      extra-articular fractures 843
      minor procedures 848
      principles 842–3
      salvage 846–8
    tuberosity 835, *837*, 843
os naviculare *62*
os odontoideum *582*
os peroneum 879–80, *881*
os tibiale externum 864, *865*
os trigonum 858
os vesalianum 880
osteoarthritis
  carpus 469
  following ankle injury 826, 830
  following Bennett's fracture 541–2
  following hip dislocation/
      fracture–dislocation 633, 636
  intercarpal 481
  secondary degenerative 323, 326
osteoarthrosis 309
osteoblasts 8
  in fracture healing 71, 74
osteochondral fracture 30, 47, *48*
osteochondritis dissecans 857–8
osteoclast-activating factors 71
osteoclasts 8
  in fracture healing 71, 74
osteogenesis imperfecta 34, 63
  fracture healing in 77
  and pathological fracture 889, *891*, 906
osteomalacia 63
  fracture healing in 77
  and pathological fracture 736, 889, 892–4
osteomyelitis *794*, 811, 818
  pathological fracture in 903–4
  pin hole 185
osteonal bone healing 8, 74, 177, 215, 695
osteons, secondary 8
osteopetrosis and pathological fracture 889,
    906

osteophony and non-union 304
osteoporosis
  and Colles' fracture 452
  disuse 889, *890*
  following spinal cord injury 554
  implant-induced 23, 446
  and non-union 409–10
  and os calcis fracture 836
  and pathological fracture 726, 889, 892–4
  proximal femur 640, 666, 668
  secondary to Cushing's syndrome 889
  senile 889
osteoprogenitor cells 8
osteotaxis 183
otorrhoea, cerebrospinal fluid 127, 135
overgrowth 245
overtransfusion 96
oxygen, hyperbaric 298

$P\text{AO}_2$ 144
$P\text{aCO}_2$ 144
Paget's disease
  and fracture healing 77
  and pathological fracture 736, 889, 894–5
  proximal femoral fracture in 652, 653, 728,
      729
pain
  in compartment syndromes 273, 274
  following tibial shaft fracture fixation 817
  referral 37
  relief in chest injury 139, 143
  in vascular injury 253
painful arc syndrome of shoulder instability
    373, *374*
pallor 253
palmar ligament 541
palpation 39
pancreatic injury 122–3
Papineau technique 314, 315, 818, 903
paprika sign 313
paradoxical ventilation 139–40
paraesthesiae
  following peripheral nerve block 497
  in vascular injury 253
paralysis
  regimen in tetanus 295
  in vascular injury 253
paralytic ileus 125
paraplegia 601
  management 606–8, *609*
  rehabilitation 592–4, 608, *609*
  simulated 591–2
paratenon 86, *87*
parenteral feeding 141, 296
Parkinson's disease, proximal femoral
    fracture in 654
Partridge straps 753, *756*
parturition, clavicle fracture during 350–1
passive stimulation 15–16
patella
  bipartite 775–6
  buttress bracing 778
  dislocation 240, 760
    apprehension test 765, 778
    classification 776–8
    treatment 778
  fracture
    comminuted 775–6
    displaced 776, *777*

patella (*cont.*)
    with ipsilateral femoral shaft fracture 750–1, *753*
    with knee extensor mechanism rupture 774
    undisplaced stellate 775
  retinaculum 762
  shaving in chondromalacia 79
  skyline radiography 778
patella alta 775
patella baja 775
patellar tendon
  graft 771
  weight-bearing orthosis 854–5, 863
patellectomy 776
  partial 776
pathological dislocation 36
pathological fracture 34, *36*, 47, 889, 907
  avascular necrosis 891
  causes 889, *890*
  childhood 243
  complications 891–2
  delayed union 891
  diagnosis 889–91
  in dysplasias 889, *891*, 906
  exuberant callus formation 891
  femur 653–4, 689–90, 735–6, 892–4, 895, *897–9*
  following radiotherapy 889, 907
  fracture healing 77
  in haemophilia 889, 907
  history taking 38
  humeral shaft 410
  in infection 903–4
  infection in 891
  malunion 891
  metabolic disturbance in 891–2
  in metabolic and endocrine disorders 894–5
  in neuromuscular disease 905–6
  non-union 891
  os calcis 835
  radiography 62–3
  in rheumatoid arthritis 889, 907
  and sickle cell disease 889, 907
  spinal instability 895–7, *900*, 901–2
  treatment 892–907
  and tumours 889, 895–903
PCL *see* posterior cruciate ligament
peak expiratory flow rate and mortality in proximal femoral fracture 892, *893*
Pearson knee flexion piece *175*, *176*, *694*, 703, 704, 733
pectoralis 332, 401, 402
PEFR and mortality in proximal femoral fracture 332, 401
pelvic fracture 158, 617
  assessment 619
  associated vascular injury 259
  biomechanics 617
  and bladder injury 156
  bucket-handle 617, 618, 620
  with chest injury 141
  classification 618–19
  CT scan 64, *65*
  incidence of DVT following 287
  management 620–2, *623*
  open-book 617, 618, 620
  radiography 53
  resuscitation 619–20
  tilt 618

and urethral injury 156–7
pelvic reduction clamps 628
pendelluft 139
penetrating fracture 32
penicillin
  in gas gangrene 298
  in head injury 134, 135
  in tetanus 294
penile injury 163–4
peptic ulceration, stress 95–6, 296
  and fat embolism syndrome 284
percussion–auscultation 304
perfluorochemicals 111
pericardial tamponade 146
perichondrial ring 238
perineum, and urethral injury 158
periosteal hinge 168, *169*, 791, *792*, 795, *798*
periosteum
  in fracture healing 73–4
  structure and behaviour under stress in childhood 238
peripheral regional nerve blocks
  complications 200–2
  facilities 196
  hand 496–7, *498*
  inadequate 200
  local anaesthetic agents 196–7
  patient preparation 196
  in reflex sympathetic dystrophy 321
  techniques 197–200, *201*
peritoneal lavage 108, 116–17
peroneal artery
  injury 794
  pin damage to 220
peroneal tendon, relocation/decompression 794
peroneus brevis tendon 879, *881*
peroneus longus tendon 871
PFC 111
phalanges
  fingers *see* distal phalanx; middle phalangeal fracture; proximal phalangeal fracture
  toes, fractures 885, *886*
pharyngeal obstruction 105
phenindione 289, 290
phenothiazines 293
phenoxybenzamine 99
physical examination
  in abdominal trauma 115
  fracture 38–9
Physiogel 111
physiotherapy in reflex sympathetic dystrophy 321
physis *see* growth plate
pin external fixator 13, 183, *184*, 211, 212, *213*
pins
  Denham 173, *174*, 743, 785
  Deyerle 647
  external fixation 183
    geometry and thread design 212
    half pin 407
    iatrogenic injury 220
    insertion techniques 213
    mechanics of bone-pin interface 14–15, 212
    principles of application 15
  internal fixation
    intracapsular femoral fracture 647, *648*
    migration 338
    see also screws

Knowles 338
Moore adjustable *648*
percutaneous fixation
  Bennett's fracture 542
  metacarpal 535–6
  phalangeal 513–14, *515*
proximal femoral fracture fixation 647, *648*
Rush 181, 391–2
Schanz 391
Smith-Petersen Trifin nail 647, *648*
Steinmann 173, *174*, 518–19, 688–9, 693, *694*, 743
through plaster 176, 211
traction 173, *174*, 688–9, 693, *694*, 743, 785
Pio$_2$ 144
PIP joint *see* proximal interphalangeal joint
pisiform
  dislocation 486
  fracture 478
pivot shift test 764–5, 772
plantar ligaments 87, 870
plantar responses 598
plasma expanders 97, *98*, 101, 110–11
plasma protein fraction 97, *98*, 101, 111
plaster of Paris bandage 169–70
  see also casts
plaster sores 171, 804, 830
platelet-derived growth factor
  in cartilage healing 84
  in fracture healing 71
plates 177, 178, *179*
  biological response to 20
  blade 680–1, 724
  buttress 20, *21*, 178, 461
  condylar 522, *523*, 724
  dynamic compression 178–9, *180*, 811, *812*
  Eggers' 178
  fatigue/failure *739*, *741*, 744
  fixed angle nail 647, *648*, *649*
  mechanical characteristics 20
  neutralization 20, 178
  non-rigid 178
  optimal fixation 20–1, *22*, *23*
  pelvic reconstruction 338
  rigid 178
  sliding nail 647, *648*, *649*, 682
  sliding screw *648*, 649–50, 724
plating
  acetabular fracture 628
  clavicle fracture 338–9, 348
  complications 744
  compression 178–9, *180*, 811, *812*
  femur
    extracapsular/trochanteric fracture 677–9, 680–1
    shaft fracture 708–11, 744
    subtrochanteric fracture 724–5, *726*
  forearm fractures 435–6, *438*, 442, 445–6
  humerus
    proximal fracture 391, *392*, 394
    shaft fracture 405–6, 410
  indications 215, *216*
  metacarpal fracture *536*, 537–8
  in non-union 310, *311*
  pelvic fracture 621, *622*, *623*
  phalangeal fractures 517–18
  proximal femoral fracture 647–50
  reverse Barton fracture 463
  Smith fracture 461
  tibia

metaphyseal fracture 788, *789*
  shaft fracture 811–13
pleural space, haemorrhage into 106–7
pneumoperitoneum 116
pneumothorax
  in chest injury 140, 144, 146–7
  in IPPV 195
  tension 105–6, 147, 195, 556
POL *see* posterior oblique ligament
polyglycolide rods 830
polymethylmethacrylate cement 17
polytrauma 105–6, 737
popliteal artery 699, *700*
  angiography 66
  injury 251, 260, *261*, 769–70, 794
popliteus 762
popliteus tendon 760, 762
  injury 768–69
porta hepatis injury 122
posterior capsule 760
posterior cord syndrome 555
posterior cruciate ligament (PCL)
  anatomy 762
  chronic laxity 772
  injury 760, 769
  MRI 67
posterior drawer test
  knee 764
  shoulder 376
posterior interosseous nerve injury 445
posterior longitudinal ligament 553
posterior malleolus *825*
  fracture 824, 828, 829
posterior oblique ligament (POL) 761
  injury 768
posterior sacro-iliac ligaments 617
posterior sternoclavicular ligament 361
posterior stress test 377–8
posterior talo-fibular ligament 858
posterior tibial artery 850, *851*
  injury 794
posterior tibio-fibular ligament *825*
posteroinferior tibio fibular ligament injury
  824
postphlebitic syndrome 287, 289
post-traumatic dystrophy 318
postural vertigo in head injury 138
posture in compartment syndromes 274
PPF 97, *98*, 101, 111
pregnancy and anaesthesia 188
Preiser disease 476, *477*
premedication in peripheral regional nerve
  blocks 196
pressure index 202
pressure sores
  prevention in cervical spinal injury 558,
  559
  in proximal femoral fracture 672, 684
  in skin traction 173
  under figure-of-eight bandage 336
  under plaster casts 171, 804, 830
prilocaine 196, *197*, 497
primary bone healing 8, 74, 177, 215, 695
prochlorperazine 293
profunda artery 401
profunda femoris artery 698, 699, *700*
  injury 251
profundus tendon avulsion 506–7
pronator quadratus 435, *436*, 562
pronator teres 435, *436*, 562
propanolol 296

propofol 295
prostaglandin inhibitors 300
prostaglandins
  in adult respiratory distress syndrome 300
  in fracture healing 71
  and septic shock 100
proteinases 100
proximal interphalangeal (PIP) joint 524–5
  articular fracture 522
  dislocation 45
    dorsal 525, *526*
    lateral 528
    palmar 525–8
  in distal phalangeal fracture 503
  dorsal fracture–dislocation 528–9, *530*
  immobilization in hand injury 502–3, 512
  lateral strains 528
proximal phalangeal fracture 509–10
  angulation 509, *510*
  articular 510, 522, *523*
  base *43*, 546
  classification 510–11
  closed reduction
    with external splintage 511–12, *513*
    with percutaneous pin fixation 513–14,
    515
  epiphyseal 524
  external fixation 513
  extra-articular 510, 519–20, *521–2*
  open reduction and internal fixation
    514–19
  protected active motion 511
  rotational displacement in 510, *511*, 519,
    520
  traction 512–13
pseudoarthrosis 75, 303, *304*, 307, *308*
  congenital 351
  following olecranon fracture 432
Pseudomonas aeruginosa
  and septic shock 100
  in skin grafting 226
Pugh sliding nail plate 647, *648*, 649
pulmonary contusions 140
pulmonary embolism
  in abdominal and pelvic injuries 141
  in ankle injury 830
  clinical presentation 287
  in pathological fracture 893
  in proximal femoral fracture 657
  in spinal injury 562
pulmonary function tests, preoperative 189
pulmonary hypertension in fat embolism
  syndrome 285
pulmonary oedema
  in fat embolism syndrome 284, 285
  interstitial *see* adult respiratory distress
    syndrome
pulmonary wedge pressure measurement in
  haemorrhagic shock 96–7
pulses
  absence of 273
  in vascular injury 253
Putti–Platt operation 379
pyrexia 293

quadratus femoris, muscle-pedicle bone
  graft 650–1
quadratus plantar 871
quadriceps injury in femoral fracture 742–3
quadricepsplasty 743

racoon sign 135
radial collateral ligament 447, *448*
  rupture 546
radial forearm flap *232*, 233
radial nerve 401, 407
  block 497, *498*
  injury
    in Colles' fracture 458
    in distal radial fracture 452
    in humeral fracture *268, 269*, 408
    management 408–9
    in shoulder dislocation 369
    and wrist drop 270
radiocarpal joint 447
  fracture of radial styloid process 463
  fracture–subluxation 461–3
radiography 43–6
  in abdominal trauma 116
  acetabular fracture 624, *625*
  acromio-clavicular joint injury 53, 354,
    358, *359, 360*
  ankle 54–5, *56–7*
    injury 831
  avascular necrosis 323–4
  before manipulative reduction 168
  Bennett's fracture 541
  carpal instability 468–9
  cervical spinal injury 562–4, *565–9*
  chest, preoperative 189
  chest injury 140–1
  childhood fractures 57, 59, *60, 61*, 245
  and classification of fractures 46–7
  clavicle fracture 335, 340–1, *342, 343*, 346,
    347, 351
  Colles' fracture 454
  defensive 37
  diaphragmatic rupture *118*, 119
  dislocations 44–5
  elbow 51–2, *414*
    dislocation 423, *424*
  in fat embolism syndrome 284
  femur
    neck *45*, 53
    shaft 53–4
  finger injury 47, 49, *50*
  foot 55, 57, *58*
  forearm 51
  fracture healing 61–2
  gleno-humeral joint
    dislocation *369, 370, 371*
    instability 378
  hand injury 47, 49, *50*, 496, *497*
  head injury 136
  hip, dislocation 633
  humerus, proximal fracture 387, *388*
  knee 54, *55, 56*, 66
    injury 763, *764*
  Lisfranc's fracture–dislocation *868*, 869,
    870
  in liver trauma 121
  non-union 62, 306–7
  normal structures mimicking fractures 62,
    63
  os calcis fracture 839–40, *841*
  patella 778
  pathological fracture 62–3
  pelvis 53
    fracture 619
  and radiation exposure 714–15
  in reflex sympathetic dystrophy 320
  reports on 39

radiography (*cont.*)
  scaphoid fracture 470–1
  sesamoid *875, 887*
  shoulder *47,* 52–3, 332
  Smith fracture *460,* 461
  spine 57, *58, 59, 60*
  sternoclavicular joint dislocation 363, *364*
  stress 66
  talus neck fracture 853
  thoracic and lumbar spinal injury 598–9,
      600, 601
  tibia
      proximal metaphyseal fracture 783
      shaft fracture 795
  wrist 49–51
      injury 451
radiological union 302
radiolunate ligament 447, *448*
radiolunocapitate angle 459
radioscaphocapitate ligament 447, *448,* 450
radioscaphoid ligament *448*
radioscapholunate ligament 447, *448*
radiotherapy
  and fracture healing 77, 78
  pathological fracture following 889, 907
  in spinal instability 896
radiotriquetral ligament *448*
radioulnar ligaments 435
radio-ulnar synostosis 445
radius
  deviation 450
  distal epiphyseal injury 487–8
  distal fracture
      childhood 452, 487–9
      with dorsal displacement *see* Colles'
          fracture
      with volar displacement *see* Smith
          fracture
  head
      dislocation *51*
      prosthesis 427
  proximal fracture *44,* 426–8
  radiography 51
  shaft fracture 435
      bone grafting 442
      classification 436, *439*
      complications 445
      Galeazzi 51, 437, *439,* 464
      malunion *437*
      management options 435–6, *437, 438*
      open 440, *441*
      plate application *438,* 442, *445*
      plate removal 445–6
      postoperative care 444
      surgery
          approach 440–2, *443–4*
          indications 436–40, *441*
          technique 440
          timing 440
      wound closure 442, 444
  styloid process fracture 463
  styloidectomy 475
raised intracranial pressure 133, 191
random pattern flaps 227
ranitidine 296
rectal injury 126
rectus abdominis flap 231, 234–5
recurrent dislocation 35–6
red cells, frozen 111
reducible dislocation 34
reflex sympathetic dystrophy, post-

  traumatic 309, 318–21, 458, 830
reflexes in spinal injury 561, 598
refracture following implant removal 24
remodelling 8, 71, 75–6
  in childhood 244–5
  and implants 24
  osteonal 8
renal artery thrombosis 150
renal failure
  in haemorrhagic shock 95
  in limb crush injury 800
renal osteodystrophy 835, 894
respiratory disease and anaesthesia 193
respiratory failure in septicaemic shock *102*
restlessness in head injury 137
resuscitation 105–6
retrograde pyelography 151
reverse Barton fracture 460, 461, *462,* 463
reverse Bennett's fracture 538, *540*
reverse Bigelow technique 635
reverse pivot shift test 772
revised trauma score 112, 113, *114*
rheumatoid arthritis
  and chest injury 141
  and pathological fracture 889, 907
rhinorrhoea, cerebrospinal fluid 127, 135
Rhys-Davies exsanguinator 203, *204*
rib fracture 106
  strapping 143
  see also chest injury
rickets
  fracture healing in 77
  and pathological fracture 889, 894
ring fixator 13, 183, *184,* 211
  full 184
  half 184
  stiffness 14
  wire insertion 15
Ringer's lactate 110
Roger Anderson fixator 183, 184
rotation 33
rotational fracture 32
rotator cuff
  degeneration 331
  and displacement of humeral shaft
      fracture 401
  injury 67, 396–7
  strengthening exercises 379
RTS 112, 113, *114*

sacral bars 621, *622*
sacro-iliac joint
  CT scan 64
  dislocation 617
sacrospinous ligaments 617
sacrotuberous ligaments 617
Salter and Harris classification of epiphyseal
      injuries 30–1, 59, *60, 240,* 735
Saturday night palsy 272
scaphocapitate diastasis 466
scaphocapitate syndrome 485
scaphoid 447, *448,* 449
  bone scans 65
  dislocation 485
  fracture 49–51, 469–71
      childhood 490
      classification 471–2
      non-union 469, 472, *473–6*
      with perilunate dislocation 484, *485*

  treatment 472, *473*
  prosthesis 476
scaphoid fat pad 50–1, 471
scaphoid-trapezium-trapezoid (STT)
      articulation 449
  arthrodesis 469, 478
  dislocation 486
  instability 466
scapho-lunate advanced collapse wrist 469
scapholunate angle 459
scapholunate dissociation 450, 466, *467,* 469,
      483
scapholunate ligament *448*
  injury 454, 457
scaphotrapezial ligament *448*
scapular injury 331, 332, 397–9
Schwann cell 265–6
Schwann tube 266
sciatic nerve injury 629, 633, 636, 736
scintigraphy *see* isotope bone scanning
screws
  AO dynamic hip 685–8
  Asnis guided *647, 648*
  cancellous 177, *178, 648*
  cannulated 643, 788
  carbon 774
  coracoclavicular 343, 344
  cortical 177, *178*
  crossed 650
  dynamic condylar 732, 733
  external fixation
      mechanics of interface with bone 14–15
      principles of application 15
  Garden *648,* 650
  Herbert
      in knee injury 774
      in scaphoid fracture 484
      in scaphoid non-union 474, *475*
      in talar dome fracture 857
  internal fixation 177, *178,* 215, *216*
      biological response to 19
      femoral intracapsular fracture 643, *644,*
          647, *648*
      intrafragmentary 177–8, *179*
      mechanical characteristics 18–19
      optimal insertion 19–20
      phalangeal fractures 517–18
  intrapedicular 612, *613*
  machine 177
  malleolar 177, *178,* 344
  sliding compression *648,* 649–50
  wood 177
scurvy 894
seat belts, injuries associated 114
secondary bone healing 8
  in infected non-union 314
secondary centres of ossification 237
sedation
  in controlled ventilation 145
  in head injury 137
  in tetanus 294, 295
segmental fracture 31, 46
Segond fragment/fracture 762, 784, *785*
seizures and shoulder dislocation 368
semimembranosus tendon 761–2
sensory deficit in compartment syndromes
      274
sepsis and trauma 99–100
septicaemia *see* shock, septicaemic
septocutaneous flaps 227, 228, 232–3
serotonin 100

serum glutamic oxaloacetic transaminase 121
serum glutamic pyruvic transaminase 121
sesamoid 883
  bipartite/multipartite 887
  fracture 886–7
  radiography *875*, 887
sexual dysfunction following bladder and posterior urethral injury 163, 165
SFH 111
SGOT 121
SGPT 121
shear stress 5
Shearer fixator 183
shift 33
shock 40, 91, 108–9
  cardiogenic 91
  cold 101
  endotoxic 100
  haemorrhagic 91–3, *94*
    effect on heart 94
    effect on kidneys 94–5
    effect on liver 95
    in femoral fracture 738
    monitoring 96–7
    and peptic ulceration 95–6
    treatment 97–9
    vasomotor response 94
  in head injury 128
  septicaemic 91
    factors in development *102*
    mediators 100
    presentation 100–1
    re-exploration in 102–3
    respiratory failure in *102*
    treatment 101–3
  spinal 558, 561, 606
  warm 100, 101
shock lung *see* adult respiratory distress syndrome
shortening 33
shoulder
  dystocia 350
  frozen 318
  injury
    age distribution 331
    patterns 331
    radiography *47*, 52–3, 332
    signs and symptoms 331–2
  MRI 67
  stiffness
    following Colles' fracture 458–9
    following proximal humeral fracture fixation 394
  see also gleno-humeral joint
shoulder–hand syndrome 318
sickle cell disease
  and anaesthesia 194
  and pathological fracture 889, 907
  and use of tourniquet 205
sickle cell status, preoperative assessment 189
silicone implants, synovitis due to 478
Simonis swivel 173, *174*, 785, *786*
simple dislocation 34
simple fracture 31
single photon emission CT in proximal femoral fracture 657
sinus tarsi 833
skin
  care

in cervical spinal injury 558, *559*
  in paraplegia 607–8
damage in skin traction 173
excision in open fracture 210
in fat embolism syndrome 284
grafts 224–7
  in hand injury 499
  in infected non-union 314–15
  in tibial shaft fracture 801–2
injury 40–1, 222–3, 800
meshed 224, *225*
skin flaps 227
SLAC wrist 469
sling
  broad arm
    in acromio-clavicular dislocation 355
    in clavicle fracture 336, 352
    in gleno-humeral dislocation 371, *372*
  collar-and-cuff 168, 169
  Gilchrist 371, *372*
slit catheter 276, *277*
small bowel injury 124–5
Smith fracture 450, 459–61
soft tissue cover
  flaps 227–35
  general principles 220–4
  in hand injury 499
  in infected non-union 314–15
  reconstructive methods 224–35
  skin grafts 224–7, 314–15, 499, 801–2
  in tibial shaft fracture 801–2, 818
soft tissue injury and compartment syndromes 272
soleus flap 231, 315
space blanket in haemorrhagic shock 99
space of Poirier *448*
SPECT in proximal femoral fracture 657
spina bifida 39, 889, 905
spinal anaesthesia 195–6
spinal cord injury
  incomplete 554–5
  pathology 553, *554*
  physiological effects 554–5
  psychological effects 555–6
  stability 553
spinal instability 895–7, *899*, *900*, 901–2
spine
  injury
    associated with os calcis fracture 838
    DVT following 287
    posterior ligamentous complex 552, 553
    three-column theory 552–3
    see also cervical spine; lumbar spine; thoracic spine
spiral fracture 7, 31, 46
  radiography 59
spleen
  autotransplantation 120
  conservation 119–20
  function 119
  rupture 40
  trauma to 119–20
splenectomy 120
  in childhood 119
  complications 120
  sepsis following 119
splint 169, 175
  in Colles' fracture 455
  and compartment syndrome 272
  during examination 39
  extension block 529

Fisk 175, *176*, *694*, 703–4
  in hand injury 501–3, 505, 512, *513*
  in mallet finger 505
  in middle and proximal phalangeal fracture 512, *513*
  Stack 505
  Thomas' 175, *176*, 693–4, 703, 704, 731, 733, 734, 785
  Tulloch Brown 175, 689
  ulnar gutter 512, *513*
spring ligament 864
stab wounds 106, 114, 117
Staphylococcus albus 103
Staphylococcus aureus
  contamination of open fracture 209
  and septic shock 100, 103
Starling diagram 93, *94*
statics 3
sternoclavicular joint
  biomechanics 361, *362*
  dislocation 360–1
    acute traumatic anterior 362–3, 365
    acute traumatic posterior 362, *363*, 363–5
    classification 362–3
    mechanism of injury 361–2
    radiology 363, *364*
    treatment 363–5
  post-traumatic arthritis 348
  subluxation 360, 362
    treatment of chronic recurrent 365–7
  surgical anatomy 361
sternocleidomastoid 332
sternum 332
stiffness 3
  frame–fracture configuration in external fixation 13–14
  return during fracture healing 8–9, 305
stomach
  injury 124
  regurgitation of contents during anaesthesia 190, 195
stopwires 15
strain 4
  definition 3
  level at fracture site 10
  normal 4
  relationship to size of fracture gap 10
streptococcus Lancefield group A 226
Streptococcus pneumoniae 100
stress
  analysis 3
  average normal 4
  compressive 4
  concentrations 4
  definition 3
  and fracture healing 77
  normal 3
  at point of screw insertion 14
  raisers 4
  response 92–3
  tensile 3–4
stress fracture 7, 34, *35*, 889
  bone scans 65
  femur 736
  history taking 38
  metatarsals 881–2, *883*
  navicular 864, 866, *867*
  proximal femur 643, 653
  radiography 47, *48*, *49*
  tibial shaft 804

stress fracture (*cont.*)
    transverse 895
stress shielding 23
stress–strain curve 4
strychnine poisoning 293
STT articulation *see* scaphoid-trapezium-
        trapezoid articulation
stupor 133
subarachnoid anaesthesia 195–6
subclavian artery
    angiography 66
    injury 251, 258, 345, 351
subclavian vein injury 345, 351
subclavius 332
subluxation
    classification 34–5
    definition 34, 47
subtalar joint 830, 833
    dislocation 860–2
    displaced fracture 843–6
    fusion 855–6, 860
        primary 846
        secondary 847
    in os calcis fracture 826
    in talar neck fracture 851, *853*
subtotal syndrome 554–5
Sudek's syndrome/atrophy 318
    in Lisfranc's fracture-dislocation 874
    and non-union 309
    in tibial fracture 805
sulcus calcanei 833, *834*
sulcus sign 377
sulphadimidine 134, 135
Sunderland's classification of nerve injuries
        263, 264, *265*
super flap 232
superficial femoral artery injury 251
superficial peroneal nerve injury 830
superficialis finger 506
superior acromio-clavicular ligament 353
superior genicular artery 699, *700*
superior gluteal artery 640
superior gluteal nerve injury 629
superior interclavicular ligament 361
superior metaphyseal vessels 640, *641*
supinator 435, *436*
supraclavicular block 198–9
suprapatellar tendon rupture 775
suprapubic cystotomy 160, 161
supraspinatus, lesions 396
supraspinatus tendon injury
    age distribution 331
    signs and symptoms 331
supraspinous ligament 552
sural nerve
    injury 846, 848
    in nerve grafting 269–70
Surgicraft ABC synthetic ligament 767, 769,
        771
sustentaculum tali 833, *834*
    fracture 836, 843
swan-neck deformity 505–6, 525, *526*
swelling 38, 46
    in Colles' fracture 456
    in compartment syndromes 273, 275
    following vascular injury repair 258
    in hand injury 501–3
    tourniquet-induced 203–4
sympathectomy in reflex sympathetic
        dystrophy 321
synovial fluid and fracture healing 77

T-fracture 30
tachypnoea in fat embolism syndrome 284
talectomy 855
talocalcaneal joint 858–9
talocalcaneal ligament 860
talocrural angle 825, *826*
talofibular joint 55
talo-navicular cuneiform joint, fusion 866
talo-navicular joint
    fusion 856, 866
    in talar neck fracture 851
    in triple fusion 846
talo-navicular ligament 860, 864
talus 833, 850
    blood supply 850, *851*
    dislocations
        mid-tarsal/Chopart's 856, *862*, 863
        subtalar 860–2
        total talar 862–3
    effect of displacement on contact area in
        ankle joint 823
    fracture
        dome 824, 828, 856–8
        head 856
        lateral process 858–60
        neck 850
            classification 850, 850–1, *852–3*
            clinical presentation 851, 853
            malunion 856
            mechanism of injury 851
            radiology 853
            treatment 853–6
        posterior process 858, *859*
    injury, associated with os calcis fracture
        838
tapping fracture 32
tarsal tunnel syndrome 848
tarsometatarsal fracture–dislocation *see*
        Lisfranc's fracture–dislocation
teardrop fracture 588, *590*
temazepam 196
tendon transfer 270–1
    in Colles' fracture 458
    Jones 409
    in knee injury 769
    in radial nerve injury 409
tendons
    chondroapophysial attachment 86
    diaphysoperiosteal attachment 86
    healing 87–9
    injury to 41–2
    structure and function 86, *87*
    synovial sheaths 86, *87*
tenoblasts 86
tenocytes 86
tenography 66
tenotomy 607
tension-band wiring 182
    in clavicle fracture 344
    in patellar fracture 776, *777*
    in phalangeal fractures 516
    in proximal humeral fracture 391–2, 394
tension pneumothorax 40
tensor fascia lata 697
teres major 401
    and displacement of humeral shaft
        fracture 402
terminology 29–36
Terry-Thomas sign 466, *467*
tetanolysin 292
tetanospasmin 292

tetanus 292
    antisera 295
    cephalic 294
    classification 293–4
    clinical presentation 292–3
    diagnosis 293
    dysautonomic/hypothalamic 295–6
    immunization 297
    incubation period 293–4
    investigations 294
    nutritional problems 296
    onset period 293, 294
    outcome 296–7
    pathogenesis 292, *297*
    treatment 294–6
tetraplegia
    rehabilitation 592–4
    simulated 591
thermography in reflex sympathetic
        dystrophy 320
Thompson hemiarthroplasty prosthesis
        651–2, *653*
thoracic outlet syndrome 345
thoracic spine
    CT scan 64
    injury
        classification 602–3, *604*
        clinical investigation 597–8
        cord decompression 601–2
        flexion–compression 603–4
        flexion–distraction 604, *605*, 609–10
        flexion–rotation 605, *606*
        horizontal translation (shearing) frac-
            ture–dislocation 606, 610, *611*
        pathological fracture *63*
        pathology 599–602
        patterns 603
        radiology 57, *60*, 598–9, *600*, *601*
        rotational fracture–dislocation 612–14
        stable 603
        treatment 608–14
        unstable 603, *604*
        vertical compression/burst fracture
            604–5, 610–12, *613*
    instability 895–7, *901*, *902*
three-point fixation 170
thrombocytopenia in fat embolism syndrome
        284–5
thromboembolism 830
thrombosis
    after vascular reconstruction 258
    brachial vein 337
    renal artery 150
    in vascular injury *252*, 253
    see also deep venous thrombosis
thromboxane 100
thumb
    avulsion fracture at proximal phalangeal
        base 546
    CMC joint dislocation 543–4
    hypermobility 373
    metacarpal fractures 539–43
    MP joint injury 544–6, *547*
    radial collateral ligament tear 546
    stress radiography 66
    ulnar collateral ligament rupture 544–6
thyroid hormones
    effect of shock on secretion 93
    in fracture healing 71, 78
tibia
    condylar fracture 783, 784, *786*, 787–8, *789*

distal *see* ankle
external rotation test 772
fracture
  incidence of DVT following 287
  soft tissue cover 231
  vascular injury associated 260–2
proximal metaphyseal fracture 783, *784*
  classification 784, *785, 786*
  clinical features 783
  diagnosis 783
  prognosis 788–9
  radiography 54, *55*, 783
  treatment 784–8, *789*
shaft fracture 790–1
  bone loss 818
  classification 795–6, *797*
  clinical features 792–5, *796*
  complications 792, *794*
  compound wounds 800–2
  crush injury 800
  degloving injury 800
  delayed union 804, 810, 817
  diagnosis 793–5, *796*
  displaced shortened 805–7
  healing 791–2, *793, 794*
  with ipsilateral femoral shaft fracture
    750
  malunion *797*, 804–5, 810, 815, 817
  mechanism of injury 791–2
  minimally displaced *798*, 803–4
  multifragmentary 807
  in multiple injuries 807
  neurovascular injury 810–11
  non-union 792, *793*, 804, 813, 817–18
  osteomyelitis following *794*, 811, 818
  reduction 805, *806*, 807
  refracture 804, 810, 813
  segmental 807
  and shortening 804–5, 810, 815, 817
  stress 804
  and Sudek's atrophy 805
  treatment
    algorithm 796, *798*
    bony injury 803–18
    complications 804–5, 809–11, 813, 815,
     817
    operative 805–18
    soft tissue injury 796–802
  undisplaced 803
  vascular injury 802
tibial tubercle transfer 778
tibialis anterior, flap 231
tibialis anterior tendon 870
  injury 810–11
tibialis posterior tendon 861, 870, 871
  in navicular fracture 864–5
  transfer 769
tibiocalcaneal fusion 855
tibio-fibular syndesmosis
  injury 824, 829
  radiography 54–5, *56*
Tillaux fracture 825
tissue repair 79–80
Tivaloy 12 17
Tivanium 17
TNF *see* tumour necrosis factor
toddler's fracture 59
tomography 64
  clavicle fracture 335
  os calcis fracture 840
  proximal femoral fracture 642

thoracic and lumbar spinal injury 598–9
torticollis 351
torus fracture *see* buckle fracture
total hip replacement
  femoral fracture associated 753, *756*
  in proximal femoral fracture 644, *645*, 652,
    653, 895
tourniquet 106, 202
  complications of use 203–5
  cuff width 203
  digital 205
  double-cuff 198
  in initial management of open fracture
    210, 222
  pneumatic 202–3
  time limit 203
  in vascular injury 254
trachea
  injury 142
  obstruction 105
tracheostomy
  in cervical spinal injury 557
  in chest injury 143–4
  emergency 105
  in tetanus 295
traction 171–2
  acetabular fracture 625
  application of force 175–6, *177*
  Bennett's fracture 543
  biomechanical principles 12
  Bryant's 175, *176*, 246, 734
  Buck's 175, *176*
  by casts 175–6, *177*
  in childhood 246
  in closed reduction 169
  and compartment syndromes 272
  counter- 175
  Dunlop system 175, *176*, 246
  femoral fracture 688–9, 693–4, 701, 703–4,
    723, 731–2, 733
    childhood 734
    complications 743–4
  fixed 175, 703
  gallows 175, *176*, 246, 734
  halo 566, *572*, 589
  Hamilton Russell 175, *176*, 689, 723
  history of 693–4
  humeral shaft fracture 404–5
  middle and proximal phalangeal fracture
    512–13
  90–90 175, *176*, 694
  pelvic fracture 620
  Perkins 175, *176*, *694*
  Russell *694*
  skeletal 173, *174*
    complications 173, 175, 743–4
  skin 172, *173* 246
    complications 173, 743
  skull 565–6, *570–2, 581–2*, 589
  sliding 169, 175, *176, 694*, 703
    balanced 704
  tibial metaphyseal fracture 785
traction fracture 32, 46
traction unit 173, *174*
transcutaneous electrical nerve stimulation
    in reflex sympathetic dystrophy
    321
transuretero-ureterostomy 155
transverse fracture 7, 31, 46
transverse ligament rupture 568, 570, *575*
trapeziocapitate ligament 448

trapeziometacarpal joint 541
trapeziotrapezoid ligament 448
trapezium 448, 449
  dislocation 486
  fracture 478–9
trapezius 332, 340
trapezoid 448, 449
  dislocation 486
  fracture 480
trauma
  abdominal 114–26
  direct/indirect 31
  and sepsis 99–100
trauma scoring 112–14
traumatic fracture 889
triangular cartilage 447
triangular ligament 435
triceps 401
  in cervical spinal injury 562
trigger finger 459
triple fusion 856
  primary 846
  secondary 847
triquetro-hamate articulation 449
  arthrodesis 469
triquetro-hamate dissociation 466–7, *468*,
    469
triquetro-lunate dissociation 466, 469
triquetrum 447, 449
  dislocation 486
  fracture 476, 478
trismus 292
TRISS 113–14
tumour necrosis factor (TNF)
  in fracture healing 71
  and septic shock 100
tyrosine hydroxylase 601

ulna
  coronoid process fracture 428
  deviation 450
  dislocation of head of 464–5
  distal fracture in childhood 452, 487–9
  radiography 51
  shaft fracture 435
    bone grafting 442
    classification 436, *439*
    complications 445
    isolated 439–40
    malunion *437*
    management 435–6
    Monteggia 51, 247, 423, 438–9, *440*
    open 440, *441*
    plate application *438*, 442, *445*
    plate removal 445–6
    postoperative care 444
    surgery
     approach 440, *442*
     indications 436–40, *441*
     technique 440
     timing 440
    wound closure 442, 444
  styloid process fracture 463–4
  see also olecranon
ulnar collateral ligament 447
  rupture 544–6
ulnar nerve 401, 407
  block 497, *498*
  injury
    in Colles' fracture 458

ulnar nerve (*cont.*)
    in distal humeral fracture 415, 416
    in distal radial fracture 452
    in elbow dislocation 426
    in hamate fracture 480
    and numbness 38
ulnocarpal complex 447–8, 463
ulnocarpal meniscus 447, *448*
ulnolunate ligament 447, *448*
ultrasound
  abdominal trauma 116
  bladder and posterior urethral injury 160
  DVT 288
  kidney injury 152
  liver injury 121
  non-union 304
  ureteric injury 154
undisplaced fracture 33
upper arm
  anatomy 401–2
  compartments 401
urea, preoperative assessment 189
ureteric injury 152–5, *156*
uretero-ureterostomy 155
urethra
  injury 40
    anterior 163–4
    in children and females 164–5
    posterior 155–63
  stricture 162–3, 164
urinalysis 189
urinary catheterization
  in cervical spinal injury 559, *560*
  diagnostic 159
  in paraplegia 607
urinoma 153, 154

V ligament *see* volar intercarpal ligament
vascular foramina 62
vascular injury 40, 250–1
  and age 251
  and arterial insufficiency 251
  arteriovenous fistula *252*, 253
  and atherosclerosis 251–2
  in cervical spinal injury 591
  in childhood fractures 247
  in clavicle fracture 344–5, 351
  closed 252
  and compartment syndromes 272
  compression *252*, 253, 254–5
  and diabetes mellitus 251–2
  diagnosis 253–4
  differential diagnosis 281
  division 252
  emergency resuscitation 254
  in external fixation 186, 220
  false aneurysm 252–3
  in femoral fracture 736–7
  following elbow dislocation 426
  in hand injury 499
  in humeral shaft fracture 407
  intimal tears *252*, 253, 255–6
  in knee dislocation 769–70
  laceration 255, *256*

local factors in 251
management 254–7
  algorithm *261*, 262
  complications 258
  results *261*, 262
open 252–3
outcome 251–2
postoperative care 257–8
in proximal humeral fracture 387, *388*
surgery 254–6
symptoms and signs 253
thrombosis *252*, 253
in tibial shaft fracture 794, 802, 810–11
timing of repair 257
tourniquet-associated 204–5
types 252–3
venous 40, 257
see also specific vessels
vascular unit and haemorrhagic shock 93, *94*
vasodepressor material and septic shock 100
vastus intermedius 74
vastus lateralis muscle-pedicle bone graft
    650
vastus medialis plication 778
VDM and septic shock 100
*V*E 144
vein
  grafts 255, 256
  injury 40, 257
    see also vascular injury
  patch 255–6
venography 658
venous thromboembolism *see* deep venous
    thrombosis
ventilation
  controlled
    in adult respiratory distress syndrome
      299
    in cervical spinal injury 556
    in chest injury 144–5
    discontinuation 145
    in fat embolism syndrome 285
    pharmacological aids to 145
    in raised ICP 191
    risk of pneumothorax 195
    in septicaemic shock 102
    in tetanus 295
  intermittent mandatory 145
  paradoxical 139–40
ventilation perfusion scan 658
ventilator lung *see* adult respiratory distress
    syndrome
vertebral artery injury 258, 591
vertebral bodies
  compression fracture 63
  congenital fusion 588
vertex delivery, clavicle fracture in 350
vertical fracture 46
viscoelasticity 5
VISI 466, *467*
Vitallium 17
vitamin A
  excess and pathological fracture 894
  in fracture healing 71
vitamin D

deficiency and pathological fracture 894
  in fracture healing 71
VMC 92
volar intercarpal (V) ligament *448*
  rupture 466–7, *468*, 469
volar ligament *448*
volar plate
  MP joint 529–30, 544
  PIP joint 524, *525*
    arthroplasty 529, *530*
    chronic laxity 525, *526*
volar radiocarpal ligaments 447, *448*, 465
Volkmann fracture 825
Volkmann's ischaemic contracture
  in childhood 247
  in elbow dislocation 426
  following compartment syndromes 271,
    280, 737
  following tourniquet use 204
  in proximal humeral fracture 259, 417
vomiting during anaesthesia 190, 195

Wagstaffe fracture 825
warfarin 289
Weaver–Dunn procedure 343
whiplash injury 565
Whipple's operation 123
wick catheter 276
Wolff's law 76
wrist
  anatomy 447–9
  dinner fork deformity 451, 454
  dislocations *50*, 51
  dorsiflexion 450
  drop 270, 408
  injury
    carpal 465–87
    childhood 487–90
    classification 450
    diagnosis 450–2
    distal radioulnar joint 463–5
    dorsal radial fracture 452–61
    examination 451
    history 450–1
    radiocarpal 461–3
    radiology 49–51, 451–2
  laxity 451
  ligaments *448*
  movements 449–50
  pain following radial neck and head
    fracture 428
  palmar flexion 450
  scapho-lunate advanced collapse 469
  stiffness following Colles' fracture 458

Y-fracture 30
Young's modulus 4

Zadik clamp 610, 614
Zimaloy 17
Ziter view 50